Clinical Nephrotoxins

Renal Injury from Drugs and Chemicals

Third Edition

Clinical Nephrotoxins

Renal Injury from Drugs and Chemicals

Third Edition

Editors
Marc E. **DE BROE**
University of Antwerp, Belgium

George A. **PORTER**
Department of Medicine, The Oregon Health Sciences University
Portland, Oregon, USA

Associate Editors
William M. **BENNETT**
Northwest Renal Clinic, Legacy Good Samaritan Hospital
Portland, Oregon, USA

Gilbert **DERAY**
Groupe Hôspitalier Pitié Salpétrière, Service De Néphrologie
Paris, France

Springer

Editors
Marc E. De Broe
University of Antwerp
Belgium

George A. Porter
Oregon Health Sciences University
Portland, Oregon, USA

William M. Bennett
Oregon Health Sciences University
Portland, Oregon, USA

Gilbert Deray
Hopital Pitie-Salpetriere
Paris, France

ISBN-13: 978-0-387-84842-6 e-ISBN-13: 978-0-387-84843-3
DOI: 10.1007/978-0-387-84843-3

Library of Congress Control Number: 2008931970

Editorial support: Dirk De Weerdt: text processing, correspondence, lay-out, figure design, index, cover design, cover illustration. Contact: ddwdesign@telenet.be

Printed on acid-free paper

springer.com

Clinical Nephrotoxins

Renal Injury from Drugs and Chemicals

Third Edition

TABLE OF CONTENTS

Preface

As with our two previous editions we remained true to our concept of a multi-nationally author book. Our belief remains strong that scientific information is an international commodity whose interpretation and application are significantly influenced by both the cultural and ethnic background of the observer. The opportunity to share in the rich diversity of the international scientific community continues as a fundamental goal of this endeavor. The sharing of intellectual resources fostered by this effort continues to facilitate the advancement of sound science.

As the profession develops new and improved methods for treating disease, there has occurred a parallel increase in the recognition of adverse drug reactions. Also, as more of the world industrializes the occurrence of unexpected injury to organisms because of exposure to environmental/industrial toxins gains prominence. Nephrotoxicity is truly a worldwide problem and we recognize this with the addition of several new chapters. As with the two prior editions, drugs/substances were selected for inclusion based on both the frequency of use and current knowledge, thus new additions include: bisphosphonates, proton pump inhibitors, phosphate containing laxatives, oxalate, smoking and the use of star fruit. Similar criteria were used for including environmental/industrial exposure with the addition of trace metals in chronic kidney disease patients. We have also included chapters dedicated to specific circumstances, drugs associated with acute kidney injury in the intensive care unit, plus the use of dialytic therapies for poisoning.

The nature of scientific inquiry has remained unchanged through all editions. As stated previously, one approach is the application of Koch's postulates, aided and abetted by various experimental animal models. Another involves population based epidemiologic associations to identify potentially causal relationships. Each has its advocates and disciples, and each provides valuable information that can be used by the clinician in better managing his/her patient. However, each technique yields data that must be interpreted with an understanding of the drawbacks and pitfalls inherent in each approach. By enlisting multiple authors for each chapter, plus rigorous editing we hope the final product is a balanced, rationale statement of the field, as it exists today. The statement remains a guiding principle for developing the content of this third edition.

As with previous editions we strive to provide a text which is useful, not only to the clinician, but of equal interest to the investigator. The addition of nine new chapters is in response to topics of current interest and we are looking forward to suggestions by the reader (marc.debroe@ua.ac.be). We continue to stress the contribution of cell biology and pathophysiology, believing they provide both a better understanding of toxic injury when known, and a rational direction for therapy and prevention. Since the last edition the application of known risk factors as a means of stratifying acute kidney injury patient outcomes has made a significant contribution to management. With the validation of risk factor stratification the use of preventative techniques is becoming a reality. We continue to include risk factors as a prominent feature with the expectation of a reduction in the incidence of nephrotoxic injury.

On a more personal note we confess that without the diligent and tireless polyvalent contribution of Dirk De Weerdt, there would have been no preface for there would have been no book. We also applaud the timely contributions of our authors and their willingness to negotiate compromise when asked. Finally, to our wives Myriam and Marthel, two individuals whose gift of time made this labor possible, we are forever in your debt.

Marc E. DE BROE
George A. PORTER
Summer 2008

Clinical Nephrotoxins

Renal Injury from Drugs and Chemicals

Third Edition

Editors

Marc E. **DE BROE**
Department of Nephrology and Hypertension, University of Antwerp, Belgium

George A. **PORTER**
Department of Medicine, The Oregon Health Sciences University, Portland, Oregon, USA

Associate Editors

William M. **BENNETT**
Northwest Renal Clinic, Legacy Good Samaritan Hospital, Portland, Oregon, USA

Gilbert **DERAY**
Groupe Hôspitalier Pitié Salpétrière, Service De Néphrologie, Paris, France

LIST OF CONTRIBUTORS

ABDELRAHEEM Mohamed B.
University of Khartoum, Soba University Hospital
Pediatric Nephrology Unit
PO Box 8081 Amarat
Khartoum
Sudan

ABRAMOWICZ Daniel
Erasme Hospital
Nephrology Department
Route de Lennik, 808
1070 Brussels
Belgium

AGGARWAL Nidhi
Columbia University College of Physicians and Surgeons
Department of Medicine, Division of Nephrology
622 West 168th Street
PH 4124, New York, New York 10032
USA.

APPEL Gerald B.
Columbia University College of Physicians and Surgeons
Department of Medicine, Division of Nephrology
622 West 168th Street
PH 4124, New York, NY 10032
USA.

ARANY Istvan
Central Arkansas Veterans Health Care System
4300 West 7th Street 111/LR
Little Rock, AR 72205
USA

BATLLE Daniel C.
Northwestern University, Feinberg School of Medicine
Division of Nephrology/Hypertension
303 E. Chicago Avenue
Chicago, IL 60611
USA

BENGHANEM Gharbi M.
Centre Hospitalier Universitaire Ibn Rochd
Service de Néphrologie
Quartier Des Hôpitaux
Casablanca
Morocco

BENNETT William M.
Legacy Good Samaritan Hospital
1015 NW 22nd Avenue, W004
Portland, OR 97210
USA

BERNS Jeffrey S.
University of Pennsylvania School of Medicine
Renal-Electrolyte and Hypertension Division
3400 Spruce Street, 1 Founders
Philadelphia, PA 19104
USA

BLOCKMAN Marc
Groote Schuur Hospital
Division of Pharmacology
Cape Town, 7925 Western Cape
South Africa

BRANCH Robert A.
Center for Clinical Pharmacology
Thermo Fisher Scientific Building, Suite 450
100 Technology Drive
Pittsburgh, PA 15219
USA

BREWSTER Ursula C.
Yale University School of Medicine
Section of Nephrology
FMP 107, 330 Cedar Street (PO Box 208029)
New Haven, CT 06520-8029
USA

BURDMANN Emmanuel A.
São José do Rio Preto Medical School (Nephrol Div)
Faculdade de Medicina de São José do Rio Preto
Av. Brigadeiro Faria Lima 5416
150090-000 São José do Rio Preto SP
Brazil

CAPITANO Blair
5934 Elwood Street
Pittsburgh, PA 15232
USA

CAROLINO Ruither O.
University of Sao Paulo
Department of Biochemistry and Immunology
Campus Monte Alegre 14048-900
Ribeirao Preto, Sao Paulo
Brazil

CARVALHO Decio
University of Miami, Miller School of Medicine
Division of Nephrology
1600 N.W. 10th Street Room 7168 (R126)
Miami, FL 33136
USA

CHAFFER Sheldon C.
The Department of Medicine
Division of Nephrology and Hypertension
The Texas A&M College of Medicine/Scott & White Clinic
Temple, TX 76508
USA

COJOCEL Constantin
Kuwait University
Kuwait
† 2007

CONTRERAS Gabriel N.
University of Miami, Miller School of Medicine
Division of Nephrology
1600 N.W. 10th Street Room 7168 (R126)
Miami, FL 33136
USA

COVINGTON Marisa D.
Medical University of South Carolina
280 Calhoun Street
MSC 140
Charleston, SC 29425-1400
USA

DEBELLE Frédéric
Erasme Hospital, Université Libre de Bruxelles
Nephrology Department
Route de Lennik 808
1070 Brussels
Belgium

DE BROE Marc E.
University of Antwerp
Laboratory of Pathophysiology
Universiteitsplein 1
B-2610 Wilrijk
Belgium

DECKER Brian
Indiana University School of Medicine,
Division of Nephrology
1001 West 10th Street, OPW 526
Indianapolis, IN 46202-5115
USA

DE JONG Paul E.
Groningen University Medical Center
Hanzeplein 1
NL-9713 Groningen
Netherlands

DERAY Gilbert
Groupe Hôspitalier Pitié Salpétrière
Service De Néphrologie
83, Boulevard de l'Hôpital
F- 75013 Paris
France

DE WEERDT Dirk L.
University of Antwerp
Laboratory of Pathophysiology
Universiteitsplein 1
B-2610 Wilrijk
Belgium

D'HAESE Patrick C.
University of Antwerp
Laboratory of Pathophysiology
Universiteitsplein 1
B-2610 Wilrijk
Belgium

DIEGO Jorge M.
University of Miami, Miller School of Medicine
Division of Nephrology
1600 N.W. 10th Street Room 7168 (R126)
Miami, FL 33136
USA

DJUKANOVIC Ljubica
Clinical Centre of Serbia
Institute of Urology and Nephrology
Pasterova 2
11000 Beograd
Serbia

DOYLE Alden
University of Pennsylvania School of Medicine
Renal-Electrolyte and Hypertension Division
3400 Spruce Street, 1 Founders
Philadelphia, PA 19104
USA

EDELSTEIN Charles L.
University of Colorado
Health Sciences Center
Renal Box C281, 4200 East 9th Avenue
Denver
USA 80262 CO

EGBERTS Toine C.
Department of Pharmacoepidemiology
Utrecht Institute for Pharmaceutical Sciences
PO Box 90107
Nl-3508 TB Utrecht
The Netherlands

ELINDER Carl Gustaf
Department of Renal Medicine
Karolinska University Hospital
Huddinge & Solna
S-141 86 Stockholm
Sweden

ELSEVIERS Monique M.
University of Antwerp
Faculty of Medicine
Universiteitsplein 1
B-2610 Wilrijk
Belgium

ENDRE Zoltan H.
Christchurch School of Medicine, University of Otago
Department of Medicine
Po Box 4345
Christchurch, 8001 Canterbury
New Zealand

ERLEY Christiane M.
St. Joseph-Krankenhaus Berlin
Bäumerplan 24
D-12101 Berlin
Germany

ESPINAL Isabel
University of Miami, Miller School of Medicine
Division of Nephrology
1600 N.W. 10th Street Room 7168 (R126)
Miami, FL 33136
USA

FEINFELD Donald A.
Beth Israel Medical Center, Division of Nephrology & Hypertension, Baird Hall, 18BH26
350 East 17th Street
New York, NY 10003
USA

FINN William F.
University of North Carolina
UNC Kidney Center
7030 Burnett-Womack Bldg CB #7155
Chapel Hill, NC 27599
USA

FLORQUIN Sandrine
Academic Medical Center, University of Amsterdam
Department of Pathology
Meibergdreef 9
NL-1105 AZ Amsterdam
The Netherlands

FOURNIÉ Gilbert J.
INSERM U563, Centre de Physiopathologie Toulouse Purpan,
31024 -Toulouse cedex 3
France

FOWLER Bruce A.
Agency for Toxic Substances and Disease Registry
4770 Buford Hwy NE
Atlanta, GA 30341
USA

GARCIA-CAIRASCO Norberto
University of Sao Paulo, Department of Physiology
Faculty of Medicine of Ribeirao Preto,
Campus Monte Alegre 14048-900
Ribeirao Preto, Sao Paulo
Brazil

GREEN Jonathan R.
Musculoskeletal Diseases
Novartis Institutes for BioMedical Research
CH-4002 Basel
Switzerland

HAKKAPAKKI Santosh
Northwestern University, Feinberg School of Medicine
Division of Nephrology/Hypertension
303 E. Chicago Avenue
Chicago, IL 60611
USA

HAMDOUK Mohamed I.
Bahry Renal Centre
PO Box 1544
Kartoum North
Sudan

HARBORD Nikolas
Beth Israel Medical Center, Division of Nephrology & Hypertension, Baird Hall, 18BH26
350 East 17th Street
New York, NY 10003
USA

ISNARD-BAGNIS Corinne
Groupe Hôspitalier Pitié Salpétrière
Service De Néphrologie
83, Boulevard de l'Hôpital
F- 75013 Paris
France

JARNBERG Per O.
Department of Anesthesiology and Peri-Operative Medicine
3181 S.W. Sam Jackson Pk. Rd., UHS-2
Portland, OR 97239-3098
USA

JENNINGS Paul
Innsbruck Medical University, Department of Physiology and Medical Physics, Division of Physiology
Fritz-Pregl Strasse 3
A-6020 Innsbruck
Austria

KARIE Svetlana
Groupe Hôspitalier Pitié Salpétrière
Service De Néphrologie
83, Boulevard de l'Hôpital
F- 75013 Paris
France

KASBEKAR Nishaminy
PENN Presbyterian Medical Center, University of Pennsylvania Health System, Department of Pharmacy
51 North 39th Street
Philadelphia, PA 19104
USA

KAUSHAL Gur P.
Central Arkansas Veterans Health Care System
4300 West 7th Street 111/LR
Little Rock, AR 72205
USA

KIDO Teruhiko
Kanazawa University, Faculty of Medicine
School of Health Sciences
5-11-80 Kodatsuno
Kanazawa 920-0942
Japan

KOPPELSTÄTTER Christian
Innsbruck Medical University, Department of Internal Medicine, Division of Nephrology
Anichstrasse 35
A-6020 Innsbruck
Austria

KUNIS Cheryl L.
Columbia University College of Physicians and Surgeons
Department of Medicine, Division of Nephrology
622 West 168th Street
PH 4124, New York, NY 10032
USA.

LAUNAY-VAUCHER Vincent
Groupe Hôspitalier Pitié Salpétrière
Service De Néphrologie
83, Boulevard de l'Hôpital
F- 75013 Paris
France

LECHNER Judith
Innsbruck Medical University, Department of Physiology and Medical Physics, Division of Physiology
Fritz-Pregl Strasse 3
A-6020 Innsbruck
Austria

LERMA Edgar V.
University of Illinois at Chicago College of Medicine/ Associates in Nephrology, S.C.
Department of Medicine, Section of Nephrology
Chicago, IL 60612
USA

LEUFKENS Hubert G.
Utrecht University, Institute for Pharmaceutical Sciences
Division of Pharmacoepidemiology & Pharmacotherapy
PO Box 80 082
NL-3508 TB Utrecht
The Netherlands

LOPES Norberto P.
University of Sao Paulo
Department of Physics and Chemistry
Campus Monte Alegre 14048-900
Ribeirao Preto, Sao Paulo
Brazil

MARKOWITZ Glen
Columbia University, College of Physicians and Surgeons, Department of Pathology
630 West 168th Street, VC14-224
New York, NY 10032
USA

MEGYESI Judit
Central Arkansas Veterans Health Care System
4300 West 7th Street 111/LR
Little Rock, AR 72205
USA

MOCELIN CARVALHO Cristiane
University of Miami, Miller School of Medicine
Division of Nephrology
1600 N.W. 10th Street Room 7168 (R126)
Miami, FL 33136
USA

MOLITORIS Bruce A.
Indiana University School of Medicine
Division of Nephrology, FH 115 E
1120 South Drive
Indianapolis, IN 46202-5115
USA

MUNIZ-MARTINEZ Marie-Carmen
Erasme Hospital, Université Libre de Bruxelles
Nephrology Department
Route de Lennik 808
1070 Brussels
Belgium

NAAZ Parveen
Northwestern University, Feinberg School of Medicine
Division of Nephrology/Hypertension
303 E. Chicago Avenue
Chicago, IL 60611
USA

NETO Miguel M.
University of Sao Paulo, Division of Nephrology
Faculty of Medicine of Ribeirao Preto
Campus Monte Alegre 14048-900
Ribeirao Preto, Sao Paulo
Brazil

NORDBERG Gunnar
Umea University
Environmental Medicine
Department of Public Health and Clinical Medicine
S-90187 Umea
Sweden

NORTIER Joëlle
Erasme Hospital, Université Libre de Bruxelles
Nephrology Department
Route de Lennik 808
1070 Brussels
Belgium

OKUSA Mark D.
University of Virginia Health System
Division of Nephrology
Box 133
Charlottesville, VA 22908
USA

OLYAEI Ali J.
Oregon Health Sciences University, Division of
Nephrology, Hypertension and Clinical Pharmacology
3181 SW Sam Jackson Park Road
Portland, OR 97201
USA

PELLETIER Lucette
INSER U563, Centre de Physiopathologie Toulouse
Purpan,
31024 -Toulouse cedex 3
France

PERAZELLA Mark A.
Yale University School of Medicine
Section of Nephrology, Dept. of Internal Medicine
330 Cedar Street
New Haven, CT 06520-8029
USA

PFALLER Walter
Innsbruck Medical University, Department of Physiology
and Medical Physics, Division of Physiology
Fritz-Pregl Strasse 3
A-6020 Innsbruck
Austria

PORTER George A.
Oregon Health Sciences University, Division of
Nephrology, Hypertension and Clinical Pharmacology
3181 SW Sam Jackson Park Road
Portland, OR 97201
USA

PORTILLA Didier
Central Arkansas Veterans Health Care System
4300 West 7th Street 111/LR
Little Rock, AR 72205
USA

PRICE Peter M.
Central Arkansas Veterans Health Care System
4300 West 7th Street 111/LR
Little Rock, AR 72205
USA

PUSCHETT Jules B.
Texas A & M Health Science Center College of Medicine/
Scott & White, Central Texas Veterans Healthcare System
Medical Education Building 407 L, 2401 S. 31st St.
Temple, TX 76508
USA

RADOVANOVIĆ Zoran
Kuwait University, Faculty of Medicine, Department of
Community Medicine and Behavioural Sciences
POB 24923
13110 Safat
Kuwait

RITZ Eberhard
Medizinische Universitatsklinik Heidelberg
Department of Internal Medicine, Division Nephrology
Im Neuenheimer Feld 162
D-69120 Heidelberg
Germany

ROCH-RAMEL Françoise († 2001)
Université de Lausanne
Switzerland

ROELOFS Joris J.
Academic Medical Center, University of Amsterdam
Department of Pathology
Meibergdreef 9
NL-1105 AZ Amsterdam
The Netherlands

ROELS Harry A.
Industrial Toxicology and Occupational Medicine Unit
Université catholique de Louvain
Avenue E. Mounier, 53/02
B-1200 Brussels
Belgium

ROSNER Mitchell H.
University of Virginia Health System
Division of Nephrology
Charlottesville, VA 22908
USA

SAFIRSTEIN Robert L.
Central Arkansas Veterans Health Care System
4300 West 7th Street 111/LR
Little Rock, AR 72205
USA

SAOUDI Abdelhadi
INSERM U563, Centre de Physiopathologie Toulouse-Purpan
Hôpital Purpan
BP 3028
31024 Toulouse Cedex
France

SCHNELLMANN Rick G.
Medical University of South Carolina
280 Calhoun Street
MSC 140
Charleston, SC 29425-1400
USA

STURMER Til
German Centre for Research on Aging
Bergheimer Strasse 20
D-69115 Heidelberg
Germany

SWANEPOEL Charles
Groote Schuur Hospital
Renal Unit (E 13) Observatory
Cape Town, 7925 Western Cape
South Africa

TAHA Ahbab
Bahry Renal Centre
Po Box 1544
Khartoum North
Sudan

TALMUD Joe
Groote Schuur Hospital
Division of Pharmacology
Cape Town, 7925 Western Cape
South Africa

UEDA Shiro
Chiba University, Department of Drug Information and Communication, Graduate School of Pharmaceutical Sciences
1-8-1 Inohana, Chiba City 260-8675
Japan

VANHERWEGHEM Jean-Louis
Erasme Hospital, Université Libre de Bruxelles
Nephrology Department
Route de Lennik 808
1070 Brussels
Belgium

VERHULST Anja
University of Antwerp
Laboratory of Pathophysiology
Universiteitsplein 1
B-2610 Wilrijk
Belgium

WAHBA Ihab
Oregon Health Sciences University, Division of Nephrology, Hypertension and Clinical Pharmacology
3181 SW Sam Jackson Park Road
Portland, OR 97201
USA

WEDEEN Richard P.
Department of Veterans Affairs New Jersey Health Care System
385 Tremont Ave
East Orange, NJ 07018-1095
USA

WHELTON Andrew
Universal Clinical Research Center
Johns Hopkins University
615 North Wolfe Street
Baltimore, MD 21205
USA

WHITTAKER Margaret
Toxservices
1326 18th Street N.W.
Washington, DC 20036
USA

WINCHESTER James
Beth Israel Medical Center, Division of Nephrology &
Hypertension, Baird Hall, 18BH26
350 East 17th Street
New York, NY 10003
USA

YACOOB Muhammed
The Royal London Hospital
Department of Renal Medicine and Transplantation
Whitechapel
London E1 1BB
UK

ZGHEIB Nathalie K.
Pharmacology and Therapeutics
American University of Beirut
PO Box 11-0236
Riad El-Solh / Beirut 1107 2020
Lebanon

A

GENERAL

01

Clinical relevance

George A. PORTER

Oregon Health Sciences University, Portland, Oregon, USA

General incidence and outcome

Drugs are a frequent cause of both in-hospital and community-acquired acute kidney injury (AKI). Nephrotoxic drugs share the spotlight with renal hypoxia as primary etiologic factors for hospital acquired AKI [1,2,3]. With the increasing capacity of the medical community to treat the most serious life-threatening conditions, the in-hospital exposure to nephrotoxic drugs has increased as has the risk of drug-induced AKI, while the expanded drug treatments available for outpatient use is contributing to the rise in community acquired AKI.

Definition

Acute kidney injury (AKI) is easily defined as a syndrome characterized by a sudden decrease in GFR accompanied by azotemia [4]. However; the reported incidence of AKI varies depending on a number of independent variables. For example, was the patient population surveyed derived from a community wide database or was it restricted to hospitalized patients? What definition was adopted to designate acute kidney injury (AKI)? The lack of a universally agreed upon definition of acute kidney injury (AKI), makes it difficult to compare clinical reports as to the incidence, severity and outcome. Recently, the Acute Dialysis Quality Initiative [5] has attempted to address this issue involving both nephrologists and critical care physicians in the discussion. Success of this project is critical for it will allow the sharing of information regarding interventions which, in turn, will improve the dismal outcomes that currently exist for patients with acute kidney injury. This dismal outcome is especially true if the patient suffers from the constellation of multiple organ failure which is becoming common place in ICUs. Encouragement comes from the success of the KDOQI classification of Chronic Kidney Disease (CKD) [6] that is being adopted world wide and allows consistent stratification based on glomerular filtration rate (GFR) [7].

Additional variables exist, for example, in-hospital surveys enroll both post-surgical and medical patients, and it is important to isolate the contribution from ICU patients with multi-organ failure! With what precision was the AKI diagnoses established? Were multiple centers involved in providing the information? These are the often unanswered questions that complicate meaningful estimates of the incidence of AKI. In addition, as detailed by Turney et al. [8] and Nash and co-workers [3], significant changes have occurred in both the age of the AKI patients and also the etiologies, with older and sicker patients being admitted for treatment.

Incidence

The incidence of in-hospital AKI attributed to drug nephrotoxicity is estimated at between 18 and 40% of cases [9-16], while earlier reports, derived from community-based statistics set the incidence from 0 to 7% of cases [10, 11]; however, more recent series report incidence from 17 to 29% [17,18] which is still lower than the 37% reported by Baraldi et al. [14]. In both series that included hospital acquired AKI [17,18], the contribution of nephrotoxic drugs was slightly higher, 22 and 35%. The recently reported increase in the contribution of nephrotoxic drugs to community acquired AKI is particularly important since the total number of all cause cases of AKI, as derived from community based studies, is 2 to 3.5 times greater that reported from in-hospital statistics [17,19]. This suggested that patients who are hospitalized are either exposed to more nephrotoxic agents and/or they are more vulnerable to the drugs inducing an adverse renal effect. Community acquired AKI is associated with a significantly reduced mortality as compared to hospital acquired AKI [21], (41% vs. 59%, $p<0.001$ [18])and for elderly patients this equated to a risk of mortality that was 2.2 times greater for the hospital acquired AKI group. Irrespective of which aspect of the drug interaction is more important, it has been observed that hospital-acquired AKI is usually associated with one of three renal insults, either a pre-renal event, exposure to nephrotoxins, or sepsis [1], and that nephrotoxins, alone or in combination, contribute to at least 25% of all cases of hospital acquired AKI [2] and have an in-hospital mortality rate similar to ATN [20]

A one-year survey of 2,175 cases of AKI, 398 (18.3%) were considered to be drug-induced [11]. Antibiotics were the most frequently cited drug followed by analgesics, NSAIDs and contrast media and this relationship persists [3]. More than half of the patients had non-oliguric AKI. The mortality rate of 12.6% is much lower than for patients who develop AKI following surgery or trauma [22]. At 6-month post-AKI, 47.7% were fully recovered, 15.3% had regained previous renal function, and 23.1% had some degree of residual renal impairment. Chronic hemodialysis was required in only 2 patients (0.5%). This is a better outcome than reported for a group of patients post-AKI due to multiple causes [20,23]. Of the 39% who survived AKI, 41% had residual renal insufficiency and 10% required chronic dialysis. Residual renal impairment was more frequent in both older and oliguric patients, in those with previous chronic renal insufficiency, those who received antibiotics, and those whose duration of AKI was prolonged. The percentage of residual renal impairment is higher than that reported in the series of Davidman et al. [24] or Pru et al. [25], but is in accordance with that found 5 years later in the same country [26] and is supported by an earlier report from the European Dialysis and Transplant Association [27].

Table 1 summarizes the incidence of drug-induced AKI reported for the last two decades. As can be seen, the incidence of AKI due to contrast media and antibiotics is variable depending on the population included. If the population is drawn from hospital acquired AKI, then contrast media and antibiotics are prominent; however, if the population is mixed hospital and community acquired, as in the case of Sesso et al [18], the NSAID's are major contributors. Since the 1990's two

Table 1. Incidence of drug-induced AKI reported for the last two decades.

Author	Year	N	% acute renal failure due to					
			Antibiotic	Contrast	Analgesic	NSAIDs	ACEI	Total
Rasmussen & Ibels [9]	1982	143	11%	11%				**22%**
Hou et al [10]	1983	129	7%	12%				**20%**
Frankel et al [29]	1984	64	8%	5%				**19%**
Kleinknecht et al [11]	1986	2175	6%	2%	4%	3%	0.5%	**18%**
Fleury et al [26]	1990	700	5%	2%	3%	3%	3%	**21%**
Kaufman et al [12]	1991	100	3%			1%	6%	**19%**
Baraldi et al [14]	1998	109	5%	2%		22%	7%	**36%**
Nash et al [3]	2002	332	11%	13%	1%	4%	1%	**30%**
Wang et al [15]	2002	209						**39%**
Sesso et al [18]	2004	325	8%	3%		12%		**23%**

new categories of offending agents have appeared, e.g. NSAIDs and ACE inhibitors. This trend has been confirmed in the survey conducted by Ronco et al. [28]. Recently, Nash et al have repeated a survey of hospital acquired renal insufficiency 17 years after the first published report from this group of investigators [3]. Due to the more wide-spread use of antibiotics and contrast media, while the percentage contribution has fallen, the total number has increased. The class of antibiotic has changed dramatically. In the original report aminoglycosides nephrotoxicity accounted for nearly 80% of the drug induced renal insufficiency, while in the more recent analysis aminoglycoside accounted for less than 30% of the cases with significant contributions from amphotericin and pentamidine. In the series reported by Sesso et al [18], antibiotics(aminoglycosides, vancomycin, cephalosporines, quinolones), and NSAID's (diclofenac, ibuprofen, ketoprofen and indomethacin) were the two dominate classes of drugs leading to AKI for all patients irrespective of whether community or hospital acquired, while in the hospital acquired AKI group, 6.5% of the patients had contrast nephropathy [18].

The estimated incidence of 18-33% drug-induced AKI in hospitalized patients contrasts with the extremely low incidence of drug-induced renal disease in outpatients as reported by Beard et al. [30], i.e., 1:300,000 person/year. This low incidence is in part due to the author's exclusion of chronic renal disease. On the other hand, acute iatrogenic renal disease developed in 1% of all patients admitted to a Canadian hospital and in as many as 5.6% of those admitted directly to the nephrology unit of the same institution [25]; the AKI was due to multiple etiologies in 50% of these patients.

Outcome

Despite improved dialysis techniques and more aggressive supportive treatment, conventional wisdom is that mortality from AKI has not improved in the last decade. Support for this belief comes from a systematic review of mortality rates in nearly 16,000 patients with AKI, reported in 80 clinical studies, which concluded that mortality rates were unchanged over the 3+ decades covered by the review [31] However, 2 recent retrospective studies using nation wide databases have reported on the secular trends regarding both the incidence and mortality rates for AKI over the 10 years from 1992 to 2001 [32] or the 15 years between 1988 and 2002 [33] Both studies are unique for they are the first to use multi-year data to determine trends both in incidence and mortality for AKI. Xue et al [32] used a Medicare 5% sample beneficiary standard analytical file and collected data both for community-acquired AKI, eg AKI as the primary diagnosis at time of admission, and hospital-acquired AKI, eg AKI as a secondary diagnosis occurring during hospitalization. During the 10year period 2.4% of hospitalization involved AKI, 24% were community-acquired and 75% were hospital-acquired which is a reversal of the findings reported in 1997 [19]. Importantly, the over all incidence of AKI more than doubled over the 10 year period, with an annual increase of 11% ($p<0.0001$). Paralleling this increase in incidence was an increase in sepsis, ICU stay, and multiple organ failure [32]. Patients with AKI were older, more often male, and African -American. In hospital death rates declined as did death rates within 90 days of hospital discharge. However, using logistic regression analysis in cases of multi-organ failure, AKI was still a significant cause of death. While this represents a retrospective study which is complicated by coding changes which occurred during the study interval, there is reason to believe that the frequency of AKI is underreported in Medicare claims. The recent report by Ali et al [32a] would support this concept of underreporting. They reported, based on a comprehensive population-based study, an AKI prevalence of 1811 per million population. This estimate exceeds that of Waikar et al [33] by six fold. The second report by Waikar et al [33] uses the Nationwide Inpatient Sample which is the largest all-payer administrative database of hospitalizations in the United States. ICD-9 codes were used to identify AKI subjects from 1988 thru 2002. The incidence of annual discharges with AKI rose from 0.4% in 1988 to 2.1% in 2002, while in-hospital mortality declined from 40.4% in 1988 to 20.3% in 2002 ($p<0.001$). This decline was observed across groups stratified for age, gender, race/ethnicity, co morbidity index and a broad array of concomitant conditions. Interestingly, in hospital mortality was lower from AKI with CKD than AKI without CKD although rates declined in both groups over time. A significant decline in length of stay was also documented, decreasing from 10.3 days to 7.0 days. So both studies confirm an increased incidence in AKI with a predominance of in hospital acquired AKI , but a significant decline in annual mortality indicating that newer dialysis techniques coupled with aggressive supportive treatment are improving overall survival of AKI patients.

One of the significant changes in management strategies for patients with AKI is the introduction of severity score systems to address issues of treatment effectiveness, quality of care, and allocation of limited resources. Two classification used in ICU patients that have gained wide acceptance are APACHE-II [34] and the system introduced by Liano [35]. However, neither system is useful for non-dialyzed AKI patients. The Stuivenberg Hospital Acute Renal Failure (SHARF) score, has proven to be a predictive model for in-hospital mortality in cases of AKI [36] More recently, this same scoring system has be evaluated as a predictor of mortality over the first post-AKI year [37]. The 11% additional mortality 1 year after the episode of AKI occurred in patients who had significantly higher SHAKI scores as compared to either APACHE II or Liano scores. At the time of hospital discharge 32% of patients were CKD I-II, 58% CKD III-IV, and 10% CKD V. Interestingly, the degree of renal impairment had an inverse correlation with the 1 year death rate being 33%, 18% and 14%, respectively.

Although the search for an ideal definition of AKI continues, Chertow et al [38], recently evaluated the effect of AKI on mortality, hospital stay and cost using changes in serum creatinine as the marker of renal injury. The surprising result was that changes in serum creatinine of ≥ 0.3 mg/dl occurred in 31% of the study population and was associated with a 4.1 multivariable odds ratio of mortality (3,1-5,5), and the OD rose to 6.5 at serum creatinines ≥ 0.5 mg/dl, 9.7 at serum creatinines ≥ 1.0 mg/dl, and 16.4 at serum creatinines ≥ 2.0mg/dl. Patients with de novo AKI and serum creatinine ≥0.5 mg/dl had a significantly higher risk of death than patients with AKI superimposed in CKD. Even small increases in serum creatinine (0.3-0.4 mg/dl) had a multivariable OR of 1.7 [1.2-2.6]. In addition to the increased mortality risk, both hospital length of stay and cost had a direct linear correlation with the increase in serum creatinine. This association between serum creatinine and hospitalization outcomes occurred over a wide spectrum of clinical conditions. Similar conclusion regarding utilization of hospital resources for individuals with acute kidney injury was reported by Fischer et al [39].

Mechanisms of drug induced acute kidney injury

Because of the rich blood flow to the kidney (25% of the resting cardiac output), plus the enormous oxygen supply required to support active ion and solute transport, the kidneys are vulnerable to any change in blood flow and/or oxygen deprivation. In particular, acute tubular necrosis involving thick ascending limb (TAL) is a prominent manifestation of a sudden reduction in renal blood flow with accompanying hypoxia. This anatomic site is especially vulnerable to oxygen deprivation due to the marginal oxygen balance that results from high oxygen consumption related to the active NaCl reabsorption and the limited blood supply due to the anatomic structure of the vasa recti [40]. A second important contributor to AKI occurs when the tubulo-glomerular feedback system fails. Tubuloglomerular feedback is an auto regulatory mechanism that reduces glomerular filtration rate (GFR) and decreases the sodium load that is delivered to the TAL. The net result of the diminished sodium load is to minimize the oxygen required for active NaCl reabsorption [40,41].

When considering the mechanism by which drug causes nephrotoxicity, two components of renal function are decisive. The first are the renal transport processes which are critical to recovering essential minerals and nutrients from the glomerular filtrate and the second are the renal enzyme systems which are essential to both detoxification of xenobiotics and maintaining the body's acid/base homeostasis [41,42]. Recently, these two components have been merged into a single scheme of vectorial drug transport in both liver and kidney cells [43]. As can be appreciated, in addition to the traditional phase 1 and 2 metabolism steps, three new phases have been added (figure 1). The new phases are: phase 0 (entry via transporter), transcellular translocation (phase 3) and phase 4 (cell elimination via transporter). Solute carriers (SLC) are responsible for cellular entry of the xenobiotic, while ATP-dependent carriers (ABC) are responsible for cellular elimination or recycling. This concept allows for both intracellular metabolism and recycling or transcellular transport to eliminate xenobiotics.

The principle renal transport systems, which contribute to drug nephrotoxicities, reside in the proximal tubule. These transporters are involved in both secretion and reabsorption and share properties with hepatic drug transporters. Five different drug transport families have been identified in human kidneys [44]. Organic anion transporters (OATs) are present in both the brush border and basolateral membrane of the proximal tubule. Among the drugs transported by OATs are PAH, methotrexate, NSAIDs and antiviral nucleoside analogues. This is the transporter with affinity for ochratoxin A. P-glycoprotein (P-gp), better knows as multi-drug resistant transporter (MDR) , is located on the brush border of the proximal tubule and acts as an efflux transporter of drugs. Substrates for P-gp include anticancer drugs such as vincristine, vinblastine and doxorubicin, cyclosporine, verapamil, digoxin and steroids including aldosterone. Peptide transporters (PEPT1, PEPT2)) are localized to the brush border of the proximal tubule where they facilitate the uptake of β-lactams, ACE inhibitors, and valacyclovir. Organic Cation Transporters (OCTs)) are localized in the basolateral membrane of the proximal tubule and are primarily involved in tubular secretion. In addition to tetraethyl ammonium (TEA), other substrates for the OCTs include cimetidine, choline, dopamine, acyclovir and zidovudine. OCTN is a novel organic cation transporter which is located in the brush border of the proximal tubule. While OCTN1 accepts a variety of drugs, cephaloridine, verapamil, quinidine and TEA, its exact role in either reabsorption or secretion remains to be define. PEPT1 is an example is the organic ion transport system, which is instrumental in the intracellular accumulation of nephrotoxic cephalosporin's due to the lower transport capacity of the luminal membrane when compared to the basolateral membrane [45]. Another way in which proximal tubular transport is implicated in nephrotoxicity involves glutathione S-conjugates of xenobiotics, a phase 2 reaction. Once transported into the cell, these xenobiotic conjugates undergo biotransformation to electrophils, which then bind to macrophilic sites of intracellular macromolecules such as DNA. An example is tris (2, 3 dibromopropyl) phosphate, which undergoes metabolic activation and eventually covalently binds to DNA [46]. Other examples are cadmium-metallothionein complexes which are formed in the liver but eventually are filtered by the kidneys where they are reabsorbed in the proximal tubule by the same proc-

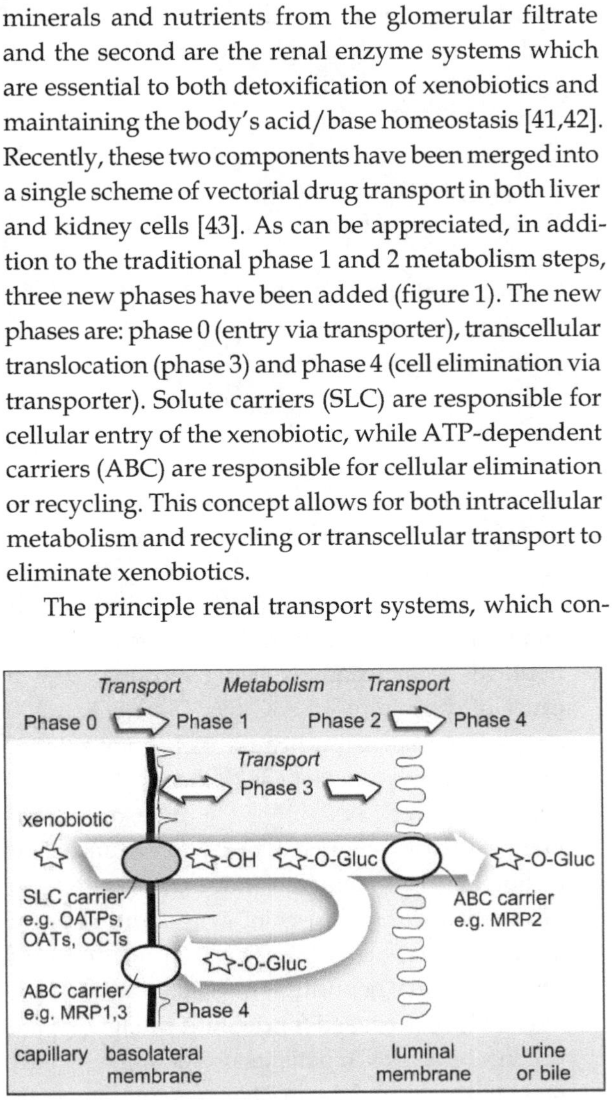

Figure 1. *Schematic principle of vectorial drug evasion in liver and kidney. Phase 0 = drug uptake out of blood, Phases 1 and 2 = biotransformation exemplified by hydroxylation and glucuronidation, Phase 3 = transport of xenobiotics/metabolites towards excretion, Phase 4 = efflux into excreted fluids and/or backward into blood. Adapted with permission from [43].*

ess as other low molecular weight proteins. Following lysosomal uptake, metallothionein production is stimulated, but once saturated; the inorganic cadmium is released within the renal cell causing cell death [47]. In a similar manner, aminoglycoside antibiotics, due to their cationic charge, attach to the proximal tubular membrane where they undergo pinocytotic uptake and accumulate within the cell inducing phospholipidosis, which leads to mitochondrial damage and cell death [48]. For more distal portions of the nephron, passive concentration of xenobiotics can occur due to the physiologic concentrating mechanism that provides a favorable gradient for the xenobiotic to undergo back-diffusion into the papillary region of the kidneys [42].

Another aspect of renal function, which contributes to drug nephrotoxicity, involves the renal enzyme systems that play key roles in maintaining body homeostasis. The flame retardant tris, which enters the proximal tubular cell conjugated with glutathione, undergoes bioactivation by glutathione-S-transferase resulting in reactive episulfonium ions that can cause cell death [46]. While the P-450 system of the liver is more abundant, substantial sex-linked renal P-450 activity causing bioactivation of xenobiotics has been documented in animals [42]. A similar role in human nephrotoxicity has yet to be established. However, medullary prostaglandin synthetase has been assigned a prominent role in analgesic nephropathy where it is hypothesized to co-oxidize acetaminophen to N-acetyl-p-benzoquinoneimine that then arylates cellular macromolecules to cause cell death [49]. Thus, the unique role of the kidneys in regulating body solute and water content, also make them targets for nephrotoxic drugs.

It is worth emphasizing that the same drug is capable of inducing several types of renal injury, e.g. NSAIDs may lead to intrarenal hemodynamic disturbances as well as to acute tubular necrosis, acute interstitial nephritis with or without nephrotic syndrome, and sometimes to various glomerular and arteriolar diseases [50,51].

Traditionally, when searching for the etiology of AKI, the clinician's will subdivides the potential causes of a sudden decline of GFR into one of three general pathophysiologic processes: pre renal failure, intrarenal failure or post renal failure [1]. Recently, Miet et al [52] in discussing drug-induce acute kidney injury detailed two additional mechanisms that need to be considered in addition to those outlined in Table 2. The 8 mechanisms recognized as causing drug induced AKI include:

1. **Vasoconstriction**: Two of the most common drugs which induce AKI are calcineurin inhibitors and contrast agents, both involve significant renal vasoconstriction. In addition, amphotericin also share this mechanism.
2. **Altered intraglomerular hemodynamics**: This mechanism is also responsible for two of the most common drugs which induce AKI, inhibitors of Renin-Angiotensin System and Non-steroidal Anti-inflammatory drugs. Recently, Huerta et al [53] reported a nested case-control study involving almost 400,000 patients. Their analysis indicated that NSAID users had a 3-fold greater risk of developing AKI compared to non-users. Risk factors that were important included hypertension and heart failure.
3. **Tubular cell toxicity**: This involves the cellular transport systems mentioned previously and is thus dose dependent to a degree. Examples of tubular cell toxins include: aminoglycosides, calcineurin inhibitors, amphotericin, antiviral agents, cisplatin, methotrexate, contrast agents and cocaine.
4. **Interstitial nephritis**: This is immunologically mediated event involving the activation of cytokines and is non-dose dependent. Examples include several antibiotics, NSAIDs, diuretics, anticonvulsants and a variety of other drugs [54]. Acute interstitial nephritis is increasingly being recognized as a cause of drug-induced AKI [56, 58-61]. Over 100 drugs have been implicated in kidney-related hypersensitivity reactions [62], the most common being listed on Table 3. For the other drugs, the number of cases reported is low and often anecdotal. In humans, cell-mediated immunity is probably involved with most cases of drug-induced acute interstitial nephritis [62].The true incidence of acute interstitial nephritis is difficult to assess since renal biopsy is needed for definitive diagnosis [56, 62]. In a series of 976 patients presenting with AKI, renal biopsy was done in 218 cases for diagnostic purposes; drug-induced interstitial nephritis was found in only 8 patients, i.e. 0.8% of all cases of AKI [58]. A similar frequency was found in the French collaborative study [11]. The proportion of patients with interstitial nephritis is higher in biopsied AKI patients, ranging from 2.5% [60] to 8.3% [55] to 54%

Table 2. Classification of various drugs based on pathophysiologic categories of acute kidney injury.

1.	*Vasoconstriction/altered intraglomerular hemodynamics (prerenal failure)* NSAIDs, ACE-inhibitors, cyclosporine, norepinephrine, angiotensin receptor blockers, diuretics, interleukins, cocaine, mitomycin C, Tacrolimus, Estrogen, quinine.
2.	*Tubular cell toxicity (acute tubular necrosis)* Antibiotics: aminoglycosides, cephaloridine, cephalothin, amphotericin B, rifampicin, vancomycin, foscarnet, pentamidine. NSAIDs, glafenin, contrast media, acetaminophen, cyclosporine, cisplatin, mannitol, heavy metals.
3.	*Acute interstitial nephritis* Antibiotics: ciprofloxacin, methicillin, penicillin G, ampicillin, cephalothin, oxacillin, rifampicin. NSAIDs, glafenin, ASA, fenoprofen, naproxen, phenylbutazone, piroxacam, tolemetin, zomepirac, contrast media, sulfonamides, thiazides, phenytoin, furosemide, allopurinol, cimetidine, omeprazole, phenindione.
4.	*Tubular obstruction* Sulfonamides, methotrexate, methoxyflurane, glafenin, triamterene, ticrynafen, acyclovir, ethylene glycol, protease inhibitors, cidoforvir, adeforvia.
5.	*Hypersensitivity angiitis* Penicillin G, ampicillin, sulfonamides, methamphetamine.
6.	*Thrombotic microangiopathy* Mitomycin C, cyclosporine, oral contraceptives, ticidipine, clopidogrd, cocaine.
7.	*Osmotic Nephrosis* Immunoglobulins, dextrans, starches, maltose and sucrose
8.	*Rhabdomyolysis* Statins, cocaine, methamphetamines, heroin.

Adapted from ref. [1] and ref [32]

Table 3. Outcome of drug-induced acute interstitial nephritis with and without granulomas (modified from ref. [61]).

	Granulomas	No granulomas
Number of cases	12	31
Drugs involved		
NSAIDs	8%	29%
Analgesics	50%	19%*
Beta-lactams	17%	26%
Other	25%	29%
Oliguria	50%	29%
Permanent renal damage	50%	13%**

*$p<0.05$; **$p<0.01$*

[15]. In the combined biopsy series [11,29] a diagnosis of interstitial nephritis was recorded in 16.8% of patients with drug-induced AKI. Schwarz et al. [56] reviewed over 1000 diagnostic renal biopsies of which 6.5% were judged to be acute interstitial nephritis. Eighty-five percent of the cases of acute interstitial nephritis were drug-induced, with the majority being due to analgesics and NSAIDs. While recovery of renal function following acute interstitial nephritis can be anticipated when the responsible drug is promptly withdrawn, certain drugs have a higher rate of permanent renal insufficiency [56]. When Schwarz et al. analyzed the outcome of drug-induced acute interstitial nephritis, 60% of NSAID induced acute interstitial nephritis were left with chronic renal insufficiency [56]. Naturally, persistent renal failure or even death is observed when the offending agent is continued or discontinued too late. Rossert [62] analysis of seven small, non-randomized, retrospective studies which compared patients who received corticosteroids and others who did not concluded that corticosteroids do not decrease the risk of chronic renal failure. While the pathologic similarities with acute transplant rejection support such a treatment approach, no controlled randomized studies have been reported. The best prognostic factors for recovery may be the duration of renal failure, with recovery being more frequent in non-oliguric than in oliguric patients [57]. Interestingly, a higher incidence of persistent renal impairment is found in cases with renal interstitial granulomas than in those without granulomas [61] (Table 3).

5. **Crystal deposition**: Particularly important with acyclovir and indinavir, but also noted with sulfonamides, methotrexate and triamterene. This mechanism is becoming more recognized due to the rise in the incidence of tumor-lysis syndrome with AKI. Acute kidney injury caused by tubular obstruction can also occur with a number of drugs (Table 2), due to intratubular precipitation of the

drug itself or of its metabolites. Of particular note have been the reports of obstruction associated with high-dose intravenous acyclovir used to treat systemic and genital herpes infections [63]. More recently, cidofivir and adeforvir have been added to the list of antiviral nucleotide analogues associated with tubular obstruction [64].

6. **Drug-induced thrombotic microangiopathy**: Only a few cases of angiitis due to drugs have been reported, the most prominent being secondary to methamphetamine [65]. In adults, drug-induced thrombotic microangiopathy leading to hemolytic uremic syndrome has been associated with both the use of oral contraceptives [66], and cyclosporine [67]. However, this complication has been reported with a wide range of immunosuppressive drugs plus mitomycin, ticlopidine, clopidogrel and cocaine [68]
7. **Osmotic nephrosis**: When the proximal tubules are exposed to hyper osmotic, non-reabsorbable solutes such as mannitol, osmotic nephrosis can lead to AKI. [69]. More recently the use of hydroxyethylstarch for resuscitation of hypotensive patients has been associated with increased incidence of AKI [70] The addition of sugar excipients to Intravenous immunoglobulin's, while reducing the constitutional symptoms associated with their administration have increased in the risk of acute kidney injury [71].
8. **Rhabdomyolysis**: While most frequently reported associated with high dose statin treatment in patients with compromised renal function [72] , it has also occurred with other drugs [73]. In addition to impaired renal function, other factors which contribute to the development of statin-induced rhabdomyolysis include: hepatic insufficiency, hypothyroidism, and diabetes [74]. A common presentation for drugs of abuse is Rhadomyolysis, with approximately one out of 3 patients developing severe renal failure [75] often requiring dialysis and extending hospital stay. Interestingly, the particular abuse drug varies depending on which side of the coast one practices. For the east coast of the United States, heroin and cocaine seem to be the preferred drugs [75] while for the west coast methamphetamine is the more prevalent [76] Far less common causes of rhabdomyolysis leading to acute kidney injury are "magic mushroom" abuse [77] and laxative abuse leading to hypokalemic induced rhabdomyolysis [78].

Pre-renal failure occurred 14.5% of one study [11] and 37.6% in another study of patients with drug induced AKI [24]. In the latter series, NSAIDs and ACE inhibitors were responsible for three fourth of the cases, presumably by blocking the normal adaptive responses to renal hypoperfusion. Bridoux et al. [55] demonstrated that, in sodium depleted patients, azotemia could occur in response to ACE inhibitors therapy, without stenosis of the renal arteries. Usually, ACEI-induced renal failure is rapidly reversed by discontinuing the drug. In an analysis of 131 biopsies of drug-induced AKI [11, 26], acute tubular necrosis occurred in 61.1% of the cases while acute interstitial nephritis was the diagnosis in 16.8%. Most cases were due to aminoglycoside antibiotics, NSAIDs and analgesics. Interestingly, acute tubular necrosis may occur in a significant proportion of patients developed AKI due to ACE inhibitors. In a recent report, 5 of 10 biopsied patients with AKI related to ACE inhibitors had acute tubular necrosis [57]. Moreover, in a series of the Société de Néphrologie, a diagnosis of acute tubular necrosis was made in 30 of 50 cases following the use of various contrast agents. Most patients were oliguric, and in one-third of them serum creatinine values did not return to baseline level [57].

Zhang et al [79] recently reported the results of renal biopsies in 104 cases of acute kidney injury complicating CKD. Drug related acute tubulointerstitial neprhritis accounted for 31% of all cases, while an additional 5% had evidence of drug-related acute tubular necrosis by biopsy. NSAIDs were the most common drug responsible for the AKI.

Particular features due to specific drugs

Antibiotics, in combination with NSAIDs, ACE inhibitor and contrast media, are responsible for the majority of cases with drug-induced AKI. The antibiotic class most often implicated is the aminoglycosides [9, 10, 13]. Acute kidney injury complicating treatment with aminoglycosides occurs in about 10% of therapeutic courses [12]; most of these patients have received inappropriate dosing regimens of the drug [80]. Because of aminoglycosides' narrow therapeutic range, once daily dosing has been popularized as a method of optimizing maximum drug concentration and minimizing toxicity due to the prolonged period of low or no drug concentration. Olsen et al have reported over a 50% reduction in the incidence of tobramycin nephrotoxicity using this approach [81] which confirms earlier reports of reduced aminoglycoside nephrotoxicity using single day dosing [82]. More recently Rougier et al [84] have reported a deterministic model which they claim describes the pharmacokinetic behavior of aminoglycosides, the kinetics of renal cortical accumulation, including the effect on renal cells, factoring in the effect on glomerulotubular feedback and determining the effect on serum creatinine. Interestingly according to their model the best time for single day dosing of aminoglycosides is 1:30PM. The value of careful monitoring of aminoglycoside dosing was confirmed by a recent report of the audit of aminoglycoside dosing by Zahar and colleagues [85].

Over 30 billion analgesic tablets were dispensed in the United States in 2000; approximately 16% represent prescriptions for NSAIDs [86]. These compounds enjoy a remarkable benefit/risk ratio when used in the treatment of acute self-limited pain syndromes. However, when taken chronically by the elderly or individuals with certain co-morbid conditions, the frequency of adverse reactions rises dramatically. Unfortunately, the real incidence of nephrotoxicity due to NSAIDs is unknown due to a lack of an accurate method of detection. The overall incidence could be very low, considering that up to 40 million people in the United States take NSAIDs on a regular basis [87]. In the 10 year-period 1972-1982, 8 million prescriptions for mefenamic acid were given in the United Kingdom, and only 23 cases of mefenamic acid nephropathy were observed [88]. This is in contrast to the higher incidence of nephrotoxicity in selected and prospective studies. Corwin and Bonventre [89] found that renal insufficiency secondary to NSAIDs accounted for approximately 6% of cases of AKI seen during a two-year period. In a prospective collaborative study, NSAIDs represented 15.6% of total patients with AKI [90]; half of prescriptions for NSAIDs could be considered as therapeutic errors, e.g. excessive or prolonged doses given in older and high-risk patients. While nephrotoxicity remains a risk with NSAIDs [91], much more attention has been focused on their cardiovascular risk [92]. In particular their effect on increasing blood pressure may account for the increased frequency of serious cardiovascular events in the recently reported polyp prevention trails [93].

Acute kidney injury has been associated with the use of ACE inhibitors in patients with heart failure, renal artery stenosis and acute volume depletion [14,24,55,94,95]. While these drugs are routinely recommended for renoprotective treatment of patients with proteinuria with or with diabetes [96] questions as to the risk of progressive renal failure and hyperkalemia exist. In fact ACE inhibition followed by AKI may sometimes result in severe irreversible renal damage [55,95] and even death [55] To address this question of renal risk, Bakris and Weir [97] reported a systematic review evaluating the effect of ACE inhibition in patients with pre-existing renal insufficiency on progression of renal disease. They found a strong association between acute increases of serum creatinine up to 30% that stabilized in 2 months and long term preservation of renal function. If serum creatinine rise exceeded 30% or serum potassium was ≥ 5.6 mmol/L then ACE inhibition should be abandon. These recommendation were adopted by the American Heart Association in 2001 [98]. However, the renal safety of long term inhibition of the RAAS has been called in to question by a recent report by Suisse and co-workers [99]. This was a retrospective population based cohort study of patients. While the rate ratio for the occurrence of ESRD during the first three years of ACEI therapy was comparable to other anti-hypertensive agents, at 10 years the rate ratio was 2.5 and significantly greater than thiazide diuretics. While the study is provocative, several questions arise regarding interpretation. Patients were enrolled in the early 1980's so the issue of ACEI dosing in important, also, there is no information as to the degree of reduction of proteinuria achieved which is central to the renoprotective effect of inhibiting the RAA system. Continuing evidence supporting the beneficial effects of inhibiting the RAA system continue to be published [100]

The frequency of contrast-media induced AKI is variable, but is judged to represent between 2 to 10% of all AKI patients. The incidence clusters in high-risk patients (see below) and cases of AKI that develop while hospitalized [10,101,102], with contrast-induced nephropathy being the third leading cause of hospital-acquired renal failure [3]. At present, the majority of CIN reports involve its frequency after percutaneous coronary interventions where it may be present in nearly 15% of patients [103]. While the majority of patients with contrast-associated nephropathy present as non-oliguric renal failure, in diabetic patients this presentation may be one of oliguric renal failure [104]. The majority of cases result from parenteral administration of triiodinated agents, but oral contrast agents used for cholecystography has been implicated. In the French collaborative survey, acute tubular necrosis was diagnosed in 60% of contrast-associated cases, and mortality was double that in AKI due to other drugs [11].

As with other cases of AKI, AKI due to drugs is most often the consequence of multiple simultaneous insults. For example, Rasmussen and Ibels [9] found that 62% of 143 patients had more than one acute insult, including excessive aminoglycoside exposure and radiocontrast material administration. In the series of Davidman et al. [24], multiple causes of AKI were also present in 50% of 38 patients with drug-related renal disease. Clearly, CIN is associated with prolonged hospitalizations, increased need for dialysis support and increased mortality [105]. In a recent review of guidelines to prevent the development of CIN, Thomsen and Morcos [106] found inconsistency regarding advise on prophylactic use of drugs and isoosmolar dimer to reduce CIN; however, they did find consistency in the importance of pre-administration hydration, stopping nephrotoxic drugs and administering the lowest effective dose of contrast medium.

Monitoring of renal function

The use of potentially nephrotoxic drugs requires close monitoring of renal function. The serum creatinine concentration is the most common method utilized to assess renal function but suffers from its lack of sensitivity. In patients with normal baseline renal function substantial renal injury can occur before there is a demonstrable rise in the serum creatinine concentration. A rise in the serum creatinine concentration that just exceeds the normal range may reflect as much as a 50% decline in the GFR. The failure of the serum creatinine to accurately reflect the degree of renal injury is particularly evident in patients with decreased muscle mass or those with chronic liver failure. Creatinine is produced from the metabolism of creatine in skeletal muscle. In turn, creatine is derived from the liver. In the setting of chronic liver disease or malnourished patients with decreased muscle mass creatinine synthesis becomes impaired. As a result more profound decreases in the GFR may occur before the serum creatinine concentration begins to rise above normal values [107]. By contrast, the serum creatinine concentration is a sensitive indicator of changing renal function in patients with chronic renal failure. In these patients a small decline in the GFR is associated with a large increase in the serum creatinine concentration.

Measurement of the creatinine clearance with a 24-hour urine collection is a more sensitive way to detect early impairment in renal function , although a 25% variation has been reported with this method [108]. At normal levels of renal function only a small percentage of creatinine appears in the urine by tubular secretion while the bulk of creatinine is filtered by the glomerulus. As a result, creatinine clearance is an accurate measurement of the GFR. However, the accuracy of creatinine clearance declines with advancing renal insufficiency. With a progressive decline in creatinine clearance, the proportion of creatinine which reaches the final urine by tubular secretion increases. As a result the creatinine clearance tends to overestimate the GFR in patients with renal insufficiency [109].

The most accurate way of assessing changes in the GFR is to measure the clearance of a compound that is freely filtered by the glomerulus but is neither secreted nor reabsorbed by the tubule. Radiolabeled sodium iothalamate and diethylenetriaminepenta-acetic acid (DTPA) are substances commercially available for this purpose. GFR calculation is based on computer programs that use either double pool or single pool data, with the single pool requiring less plasma samples. However, because the terminal elimination phase is prolonged in patients with impaired renal function, samples may be required up to 24 hours after injection [110]. The use of radiocontrast agents has gained popularity, especially for clinical investigation, since they offer the advantage of radioisotopes without the radiation risk. Iohexol may be the agent of choice due to it efficacy and ease of administration [111].

Because of the problems with changes in creatinine production and secretion, other endogenous compounds have been evaluated in an effort to provide a more accurate estimation of GFR. Perhaps the most promising is cystatin C, a low molecular weight protein that is a member of the cystatin super family of cysteine protease inhibitors [112]. Cystatin C is produced by all nucleated cells and its rate of production is relatively constant, being unaltered by inflammatory conditions or changes in diet. When compared to the GFR as determined by the clearance of radioactive iothalamate, serum cystatin C levels began increasing when the GFR was 88 ml/min while the serum creatinine concentration only increased when the GFR was 75 ml/min [113].

There is growing popularity of the formulae used to predict eGFR. While Cockcroft/Gault is the oldest, the MDRD formulae has gained greater use since it is most useful at GFR < 60 ml/min/1.73m^2 [111]. How reliable these values are with rapidly changing serum creatinine values is problematic.

In summary, monitoring changes in the creatinine clearance or directly measuring the GFR using markers that are not acted upon by the tubule are the best tools to detect early drug-induced renal toxicity in patients with a normal baseline creatinine concentration. Serial monitoring of the serum creatinine concentration is usually adequate in those chronic renal failure patients whose creatinine is already increased. The role of other endogenous compounds such as cystatin C as a way to monitor renal function is evolving.

Populations at risk

The changes in renal function of patients experiencing nephrotoxicity can be as dramatic as a sudden, acute deterioration requiring immediate dialysis to an insidious asymptomatic decline. This difference in presentation probably represents the level of exposure, i.e., dose and duration, to a drug or environmental toxin plus a component of genetic susceptibility. This formulation is supported experimentally since it has been shown that the rapidity with which renal failure occurs is dependent on the rate at which a known nephrotoxin is administered [114]. Similar observations regarding the influence of time-dosage effects have come from our laboratory using an experimental model of aminoglycoside nephrotoxicity [115]. The human counterpart is a study reported by Nicolau et al. [116] involving once daily aminoglycoside dosing in over 2000 patients. They found that in addition to dosing schedule, age and duration of treatment were factors in precipitating aminoglycoside-induced AKI. While this postulated dependency on time and *in vivo* drug concentration remains speculative for human renal disease, it provides a convenient approach to explaining many of the observations related to suspected environmental toxicants. The clinical course of renal failure has been defined to a great extent by observing the natural history of AKI [117]. Recently, Molitoris [118] has redefined the phases of AKI in hopes of improving therapeutic interventions such that intervention in the initiation phase would be for prevention, while interventions later in the course would be to limit either the extension phase or the maintenance phase (figure 2). It follows that much of our information regarding risk factors for the development of renal failure have also come from analysis of patients with AKI [1,2,8-10, 13]. However, with the advent of ESRD registers, i.e., EDTA and USRDS, data regarding risks factors for progressive renal failure are being accumulated [119,120].

Population characteristics which are candidates to correlate with increased susceptibility to toxin induced renal injury include: 1) genetic susceptibility, 2) occupational or environmental exposure, 3) gender, 4) age, 5) race, 6) nutritional status, 7) socio-economic status, 8) addictive personality, and 9) co-existing chronic disease. By defining populations at increased risk it is hoped that greater care will be exercised in either drug prescribing or removal of subjects from offending environments.

Sharing importance with individual susceptibility is the previously mentioned concept of critical body burden of toxicant as a prerequisite for inducing renal cell injury. It is this concept of body burden that helps explain why the various clinical manifestations

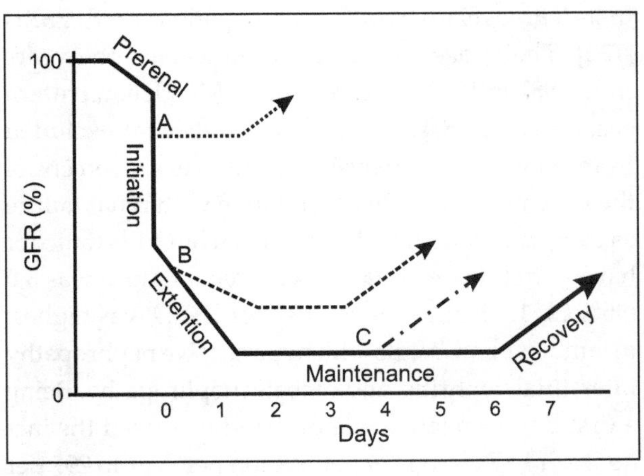

Figure 2. *Phases of ischemic acute renal failure. A, B, and C refer to therapies aimed at preventing (A); limiting the extension phase (B); and treating established AKI (C). Adapted with permission from [118].*

of toxin induced renal disease run the gamut from sudden deterioration of renal function to the insidious loss of function.

Genetic/hereditary susceptibility

Inherited renal disease is an infrequent cause of ESRD, cystic kidney disease being the most prevalent accounting for about 3% of all cases [119]. However, experimentally inbred strains of rats are selected because of their known susceptibility to toxic injury, an example of which is the Fischer 344 rat [121]. This selective animal susceptibility has led to speculation that a similar situation might exist for humans. A possible relationship between occupational exposure and genetic susceptibility comes from a study conducted by the Michigan Renal Registry [122]. The study design was a case-control involving 325 men with ESRD in which an occupational exposure was sought. The results found that the strongest association for ESRD patients was a family history of renal disease (odds ratio = 9.30). Patients with ESRD that were excluded from consideration included; diabetic nephropathy, polycystic kidney disease, heroin nephropathy, lupus nephropathy, nephropathy due to malignancy, Alport's syndrome, unspecified chronic renal failure, obstructive nephropathy and uncommon nephropathies, leaving only patients with diagnoses compatible with toxin-induced renal injury, i.e., glomerulonephritis, nephrosclerosis and interstitial nephritis, for evaluation.

O'Dea et al. reported a higher risk of renal failure in first-degree relatives of Canadian patients with ESRD [123]. Their case-control study bracketed the years from 1987 to 1993. Diseases with a Mendelian pattern accounted for 8.4% of all cases and were excluded from relative risk analysis. Twenty-seven percent of the probands had at least 1 relative with renal failure as compared to 15% of the controls. The Odds Ratio for have a first degree relative with renal failure was 3.0 (95% CL 1.7-5.2), while the risk for ESRD was highest in families of probands with hypertensive nephropathy, interstitial nephritis, and diabetic nephropathy. Being a first-degree relative of a proband increased the incidence of ESRD from 79 per million per year to 297 per million per year, nearly a four fold increase. Freedman et al. [124] using a case-control format investigated the incidence of familial clustering of ESRD in African-Americans suffering from HIV-associated nephropathy. After controlling for age, family size, and sex, they found a 5.4 fold increase in the incidence of ESRD in close relatives of HIV-associated nephropathy patients compared to HIV patients without evidence of nephropathy. Although they could not completely eliminate environmental factors as contributing to the significant difference ($p=0.004$), they raised the possibility of an inherited susceptibility in the families studied.

Genetic polymorphism has also been identified as possibly contributing to progression of renal disease. Chew and associates [125] were the first to report an association between apolipoprotein E allele group and the post-operative response of serum creatinine. Because of the key role that inflammation plays in sepsis and its association with AKI, interest in human polymorphism as it influences cytokine balance is receiving increasing interest and study. While much is speculative concerning the role of genetically determined cytokine response in patients with AKI, clear progress is being made. This has recently been summarized by Jaber and coworkers [126]. Based on the pathobiology of AKI, these authors suggest that produces of many genes act concomitantly, culminating in a beneficial or deleterious balance of pre- and anti-inflammatory molecules, which in turn, determine the extent of tissue injury. In addition a relationship that has been identified between endothelial nitric oxide synthase (ecNOS) polymorphism and abnormal hemodynamics, Wang and associated [127] investigated the frequency of gene polymorphism of ecNOS intron 4 in patients with ESRD as compared to health controls. These authors found that the frequency of the allele of endothelial nitric oxide synthase (ecNOS) was significantly higher in cases of non-diabetic ESRD when compared to healthy controls. Using similar reasoning, that ESRD is a complex phenotype that combines preexisting renal disease with environment and genetic factors, Gumprecht et al. [128] evaluated the role of gene polymorphism in the renin-angiotensin system as it occurs either during the development or progression of chronic renal failure. Two hundred and forty-seven CRF patients and their parents were enrolled in the study. The angiotensin 235 T allele was transmitted significantly more frequently to CRF patients than would be expected if no association existed. However, the significant transmission was limited to patients with interstitial nephritis. Fabris et al [129] have recently reported on three gene polymorphisms related to nephropathic risk to hypertensive patients. The D allele, T235 allele of AGT M235T polymorphisim and CYP11B2 gene polymorphism were all consistently associated with hypertensive nephropathy. Nobilis et al. [130] examined the association between very low birth weight newborns and AKI. They reasoned that since the neonate requires high RAS activity to maintain GFR, genetic polymorphism could impair either ACE activity or angiotensin II-type I receptor functions in very low birth weight newborns. Neither the frequency of the ACEI allele and/or ATIR CII66 variant differed between the AKI group (n=42) and these with normal renal function (n=68). Thus, no correlation was evident between genetic polymorphism and the development of neonatal AKI. However, in a study of heat shock proteins in neonates, Fekete et al [131] found that very low birth weight neonates that carried HSP 72 were at increased risk of AKI.

Occupational/environmental exposure

While there are well-recognized instances of drugs and toxins inducing AKI, the evidence supporting their causality in CRF / ESRD is circumstantial and thus less compelling. This is to be expected given the insidious nature of progressive renal failure, an observation that suggests a long latency between exposure and onset of disease. This problem is compounded by the superimposition of associated chronic conditions which can lead to renal failure independently of toxin exposure. Additionally, the lack of a uniform system of classifying renal disease (mixture of clinical and pathologic terms) and the distinct possibility of multifactorial causes for renal failure because of the many potential nephrotoxins, which exist in our environment [132]. At the Workshop on Chronic Disease in the Workplace, conducted by the Workplace Health Fund in 1983, it was estimated that nearly 4 million workers were exposed to known or suspected nephrotoxins during the 1971-72 interval [133]. Of interest was the list of nephrotoxins cited which are identical to those we currently believe to be candidates to produce chronic renal failure and eventually lead to ESRD. They included: I) heavy metals, i.e., lead, mercury, uranium and cadmium; 2) solvents, especially light hydrocarbons; 3) silica; 4) beryllium; 5) pesticides; 6) arsenic.

The effects of lead exposure on renal function continue to occupy investigators interest. While the association between exposure to lead and disease has been recognized since the time of Socrates, its involvement in kidney failure has been a more recent observation. Data from the Normative Aging Study provided a positive and significant association between blood lead levels and progressive elevations of serum creatinine values [134]. Much of the controversy regarding the role that lead plays in inducing renal failure is due to the fact that with progressive loss of renal function, the body lead burden rises since renal elimination of lead is restricted [135]. In an attempt to resolve this quandary, Lin et al [136] followed a group of patients with chronic renal failure over 2 years to determine the rate of deterioration. They then identified 64 patients from the group with a high body lead burden, and treated 32 with chelation therapy. The result was a significant improvement in the renal function of the chelated patient compared to the high lead burden controls supporting their hypothesis that it is the lead burden rather than the chronic renal failure that comes first. Additional support for the association between high lead body burden and progressive loss of renal function has been provided by the study of Yu and associates [137]. Linking race with environmental lead exposure, Vupputuri el al [138] reported a significant correlation between blood lead levels in both African American men and women and suggested that this might be one factor which contributes to the higher incidence of ESRD in that population.

Exposure to solvents have been implicated as inducers of glomerulonephritis [139], while the association between chronic interstitial nephritis and analgesic abuse is acknowledged [140] and the association between hypertensive renal disease (nephrosclerosis) and lead nephropathy continues to be explored [141,142]. According to data provided by USRDS for 2000 through 2004, glomerulonephritis accounted for 16.1% of ESRD, hypertensive renal disease was present in 24.4%, secondary glomerulonephritis and vasculitis involved 3.3%, 4.1% were unknown etiology and interstitial nephritis/pyelonephritis accounted for 4.6% of all cases of ESRD being treated in USA [119,]. From EDTA [120], 24.1% of new ESRD patients in 1987 were due to glomerulonephritis, 16.6% due to pyelonephritis/interstitial nephritis, 2.8% due to analgesic and other nephrotoxic agents, 9.9% due to renal vascular disease and 14.4% due to chronic renal failure of unknown etiology for a total of almost

68%. Thus, there exist a substantial number of ESRD patients whose etiology could involve a component of long-term, low level exposure to either environmental or occupational toxicants.

In addition to workplace exposures, there are acknowledged geographic regions of environmental contamination that expose the general population and can increase their risk of chronic renal damage. An example of such an environmental contamination is methyl mercury poisoning by industrial effluents in Minimata Bay region of Japan, which lead to both neurological and renal impairment in several hundred adults who ingested tainted fish [143]. In evaluating the occurrence of lead nephropathy in the general public, Staessen et al. concluded that while such exposure could impair renal function they were unable to demonstrate a cause/effect relationship [144].

Reports linking Chinese herb remediesto fatal renal failure have appeared [145, 146]. The remedies have been taken for weight loss or the treatment of eczema. The offending compound is thought to be aristolochic acid which is the acknowledged nephrotoxin that was identified as contributing to the progressive interstitial nephritis that lead to renal failure and death in the Belgian experience [145]. In an editorial, De Broe [146] speculates that combining a potentially nephrotoxic agent, such a Chinese herbs with a renal vasoconstrictive agent, may account for the observation that not all patients who use the herbal product develop AKI. In the UK it is estimated that over 3000 clinics were prescribing Chinese herbs in 1999 [147].

Gender

Experimentally gender predilection for various nephrotoxins is well recognized. Examples include the male rat's sensitivity to the nephrotoxic effects of both carbon tetrachloride and aminoglycosides [115]. Recently, Moore et al. [148] demonstrated an increased susceptibility of women to the nephrotoxic effects of aminoglycosides using multi variant analysis. These observations make two important points, first is that the extrapolation of animal results to predict human response must be done with caution since the experimental data predicted a male susceptibility. Secondly, gender can impart either susceptibility or resistance depending upon your point of view.

In searching for an explanation of the slower rate of progression to ESRD for female patients, Miller et al. [149] have identified a gender dependent difference in the renal hemodynamic effect of angiotensin II. The infusion of angiotensin II in women was associated with a parallel decline in GFR and effective renal plasma flow (ERPF), while in men GFR was maintained despite the angiotensin II-induced fall in ERPF. Thus, for women, the decline in filtration fraction (FF) paralleled the fall in GFR, while in men FF remained unchanged. The authors speculate that the gender difference in progression to ESRD is due to the angiotensin II associated sustained FF in men which is absent in women. It has been recognized for some time that glomerular hypertension, which would be required to sustain FF in the face of a fall in ERPF, is a known contributor to the progression of renal failure [150]. In the logistic model used to predict risk of AKI after cardiac surgery, female gender proved to be a significant risk factor along with the co morbidities of congestive heart failure, diabetes and COPD [151]. However, female gender as a post CABG risk was not confirmed in the report of Athanasiou et al [152]. In the analysis of incidence and mortality of AKI in Medicare beneficiaries, Xue et al [32] found that male gender, along with older age and being African American were all significantly associated with AKI ($P<0.0001$). Thus, the data is conflicting as to the contribution of gender as a risk factor for AKI.

Race

Although being African American was significantly associated with AKI [32], direct evidence linking a patients' race with the risk of toxin induced renal injury is lacking; however, an indirect association is suggested based on the clinical course of hypertensive renal disease (nephrosclerosis) in black versus white males. From incidence data provided by USRDS, ESRD occurs 8 times more frequently in black males with hypertensive renal disease than white males with a similar diagnosis [119]. This relationship has been defined in greater detail by the case-control study conducted by Freedman et al. [153]. Based on their results, the presence of a first-degree relative with ESRD increased the risk for developing ESRD nine fold, with OR of 9.13 (95% CL 2.6 to 31.8). Hypertensive nephrosclerosis and Diabetes, type II was more prevalent than chronic glomerulonephritis. In a recent retrospective survey of the incidence of AKI in African-Americans, Obialo et al.[17,154] found that while patients > 64 year of age had a high incidence of AKI, this was shared by the age group < 40 years of age. However, they noted that patients > 64 years of age were less likely to receive dialysis. If one were to pursue the concept of multi-toxin injury as contributing to nephrotoxic chronic renal failure, then the hypertensive kidney would be receptive substrate upon which a toxic insult could be superimposed. There is evidence from clinical studies involving in-hospital cases of AKI that hypertension is a risk factor [1, 2, 8-10]. This might explain the findings of the higher lead body burden correlating with blood pressure elevations in African Americans sited above [17].

Nutrition

Glomerular hyperfiltration regularly follows the ingestion of a protein rich diet. Furthermore, experimentally induced hyperfiltration induces glomerulosclerosis and chronic renal failure in animals deprived of their renal reserve [155]. In addition, pathologic variations in the body's mineral content has been linked with chronic renal injury in the case of severe hypokalemia induced by eating disorders [156], and shown to augment toxin induced injury in the case of calcium depletion and lead nephropathy [157], or salt depletion and analgesic nephropathy [158].

The assessment of the nutritional state of renal patients has come under scrutiny in recent years. While serum albumin has served as the common index of nutritional status, evidence is mounting that interpretation of this parameter is influence by other factors. Recently, Ikizler et al. [159] provided evidence of an interaction between depleted nutritional status and active inflammatory disease as providing markers for increased risk of hospitalization for chronic hemodialysis patients. This awareness of the impact of inflammation on nutrition status requires further evaluation in order to properly assess the contribution of each to the progressive atherosclerotic disease, which characterized ESRD patients [160].

Alcohol consumption has been reported to potentate the nephrotoxicity of lead [161] and anti-inflammatory drugs [162]. However, in a recent case-controlled study reported by Perneger et al. [163], these authors found the OR for developing ESRD was 4.0 (95% CL 1.2-13.0) among persons who self-reported consuming an average of >2 drinks/day. This was after adjusting for age, race, sex, income, and history of hypertension, history of diabetes mellitus, acetaminophen intake, cigarette smoking and opiate use. Fortunately, alcohol intakes of 2 drinks/day or less did not increase the risk of renal failure. However patients with a BMI>40 have almost triple the rate of AKI following cardiac surgery [164]. Increasing the energy intake in patients with AKI from 30 kcal/kg/day to 40 kcal/kg/day did not improve estimated nitrogen balance and was associated with more artificial nutrition-related side-effects [165]. In a 15 year survey of outcomes associated with AKI, Radovic et al [166] reported an improvement in the outcome of patients with AKI despite an increase both disease severity and average age. During this interval catabolism intensity did not change which may correlate with more aggressive and efficient dialysis treatment.

Socio-economic status

The exposure to lead based paints and subsequent lead nephropathy and encephalopathy, in the USA, is concentrated in substandard housing [162]. Individuals at the lower end of our economic ladder often are denied access to preventative health care thus putting them at additional risk for toxin exposure. Another example is the consumption of "moonshine" whiskey that has been associated with the development of lead nephropathy [167].

Age

Age, along with pre-existing renal disease and volume depletion, are well-recognized risk factors for in-hospital AKI [1, 9, 10, 13-14,18-19]The high risk of nephrotoxicity associated with age can be traced to normal age-related changes in renal function [168]. Aging is associated with a progressive decline in the GFR and renal blood flow, which correlate with an increase in renal vascular resistance (Table 4). Importantly, the renal vasculature is less responsive to vasodilators, while the response to vasoconstrictors remains unchanged. In addition to age-related changes in renal function, changes in the rate and manner that drugs are metabolized by elderly patients also increase their susceptible to renal toxicity [169]. Elderly pa-

Table 4. Risk factors for drug-induced nephrotoxicity in the elderly.

Age-related changes in renal function
↓ in glomerular filtration rate
↓ in renal blood flow
↑ in renal vascular resistance
Age-related changes in pharmacokinetics
↑ free drug concentration
• hypoalbuminemia
• retained metabolites
↓ total body water
↓ hepatic metabolism with longer drug half-life

tients, particular those with chronic illness, often have lower albumin levels, which reduces protein binding of drugs resulting in higher free drug concentrations. Protein binding is further interfered with by retained metabolites, which accumulate as a result of the normal age-related impairment in renal function. Increased drug levels also occur as a result of the age-related decrease in total body water. Finally, decreased hepatic metabolism, which is often present in the elderly, contributes to a longer half-life of drugs potentially resulting in unexpectedly high drug levels (Table 4). An additional mechanism for the progressive decline in GRF noted with aging can be correlated with the levels of inflammatory and prothrombic markers. Fried et al [170] found that the decline in GFR was greater in the group of elderly patients whose inflammatory and prothrombotic markers were above the median. This is true after adjusting for race, gender, baseline creatinine, systolic and diastolic blood pressure, lipid levels, weight and smoking history. For all of these reasons a given dose of a potentially nephrotoxic agent might be well tolerated in a young person but result in marked renal injury in an older person. In the community based study reported by Feest et al. [21], the annual rate of severe AKI rose from 83 per million populations (pmp) in the six decade of life to 949 pmp in the ninth decade of life, a nearly tenfold increase. In the hospital based study of Khan et al. [19], the annual incidence of AKI increased from 606 pmp for the age range of 50 to 69, to 4266 pmp for individuals older than 80 years. On the other hand, Kohli and co-workers prospectively examined the incidence of treatment-related AKI in elderly hospitalized patients [171]. During a one-year interval, these authors identified treatment-related AKI occurring in 1.2% of patient's > 60 years of age. Multiple insults were identified in most cases of AKI; however, drugs contributed 66% of the time, sepsis and hypotension 46% of the time, contrast media 17% of the time, and the post-operative state 25% of the time. The development of treatment-related AKI doubled the death rate (25.4% vs. 12.7%).

Since toxin induced chronic renal failure is theorized to occur after years of low-level toxin exposure, it stands to reason that the incidence would be clustered in elderly patients. The study of Chester et al. [172] provides indirect support that elderly patients may be at greater risk. Of the 79 patients with chronic renal failure who met age criteria of 70 year or more, 29% were classified as having chronic interstitial nephritis, a clinical diagnosis quite compatible with toxin induced renal failure and an incidence substantially higher than the 10.4% in accumulated series in which patients 50 year and older were included [173]. Furthermore, in the 2006 USRDS survey of causes of ESRD, the average age for patients with a diagnosis of interstitial nephropathy was 56 year compared to 58 years for the entire population reported [119]. In the recent analysis of the PICARD database, advanced age was associated with increased mortality in AKI patients both at time of consultation and after initiation of dialysis treatment [38].

Co-existing chronic diseases

Conventional wisdom dictates that pre-existing renal insufficiency is a well-established significant risk factor in the AKI of contrast-associated nephropathy [174]. However, a study by Levy et al. [175] questions this wisdom. These authors performed a cohort analytical study involving over 16,000 patients undergoing radiocontrast procedures. One hundred and seventy-four patients diagnosed with contrast-associated nephropathy were paired to a like number of nephropathy-free patients matched for age, baseline creatinine and similar radiocontrast procedures. Mortality in contrast-associated nephropathy patients was 34% compared to 7% in match control group. When the authors considered the contribution of co-morbid conditions, the mortality rate in the AKI group was consistently higher for patients with: diabetes, hypertension, cancer, lymphoma, liver disease, heart failure, acute myocardial infarction, sepsis and gastrointestinal bleeding. The authors concluded that the high mortality rate in AKI is not explained by co-morbid conditions; rather AKI increases the risk of fatal, non-renal complications. A similar misconception may exist for NSAID given to patients with chronic renal failure [176]. Evans et al. [176] conducted a case-control study involving a population base of 420, 600 individuals. These authors found that for patients hospitalized with AKI, the risk was doubled for patients who ingested NSAIDs during the 90 days prior to admission. Interestingly, they could not identify any interaction between NSAID use in patients with chronic renal failure and subsequent hospitalization for AKI. However, for patients requiring intensive care treatment, evidence continues to mount correlating increased mortality in AKI with the number of failed internal organs [176-180].

For chronic renal failure the information is again circumstantial. Patients with sickle cell disease have a high frequency of papillary necrosis which is assumed to be the result of the slugging effect of the abnormal red cells as they course through the vasa recti and are exposed to the high osmolarity of the renal papillae [181]. However, these same patients have significant pain associated with' 'sickle crisis', for which they often take analgesics that are also associated with papillary necrosis [182]. This may represent a case of multiple insults superimposed to give an additive pathologic effect. Another example is the supposed increased risk of contrast associated nephropathy in patients with myeloma kidney due to a physical interaction between Tamm-Horsfall protein and the radiocontrast media leading to intraluminal obstruction and AKI [183]. Diabetic nephropathy is a documented risk factor for acute contrast induced nephropathy; however, the review of Mudge suggests that in up to 25% of such cases serum creatinine does not return to pretreatment levels and these patients end up with further deterioration of their renal function as a result of the acute insult induced by the contrast media [174]. The role of hypertension as a risk factor has already been described in the section entitled Race. Recently, Rihal et al. [184] reviewed the incidence of AKI post-percutaneous coronary intervention. Stratifying pre-percutaneous serum creatinine provided ample evidence that once serum creatinine exceeded 2 mg/dl that AKI risk was high irrespective of co-existing diabetes. This was confirmed by the report of Yehia et al [185]. However, the presence of a normal serum creatinine does not eliminate the risk of adverse drug reactions in the elderly. Corsonelle et al [186] found an increased incidence of adverse drug reactions in elderly patient exposed to hydrosoluble drugs as part of a polypharmacy prescribing.

Addictive behavior

With drug abuse being an increasingly common behavior for the younger generation, it is not surprising that it has been linked to renal injury. Heroin nephropathy is a well-described cause of focal sclerosing glomerulonephritis with associated nephrotic syndrome [187,188]. This particular pathologic entity often progresses to ESRD and may account for up to 10% of such patients in cities with large addictive populations [189]. Although cardiac and/or cerebral ischemia is the more common acute presentations of cocaine inhalation, renal ischemia also occurs [190,191]. The most frequent cause of cocaine associated AKI occurs in the setting of rhabdomyolysis [192]; however, a more recent association between habitual cocaine abuse and accelerated or malignant hypertension leading to deterioration of renal function have been identified [193]. Intravenous amphetamine or "speed" can induce polyarteritis nodosa with progressive renal failure and severe hypertension [194]. Recently, Bingham and coworkers have reported a case of chronic renal failure due to habitual intake of oral methamphetamine and 'ecstasy' [195]. More disturbing is a report by Richards et al. [76] in which 43% of rhabdomyolysis patients entering an emergency room had a positive toxicologic screen for methamphetamines.

Summary

While much of the data concerning nephrotoxic chronic renal failure is circumstantial and based on epidemiologic surveys involving ESRD patients [119], for certain xenobiotics the evidence is substantial. The two most obvious groups at risk are individuals that receive nephrotoxic drugs for treatment of a life-threatening illness in the hospital and individuals exposed to known or suspected nephrotoxins in the workplace. A similar conclusion is valid for people living in geographic regions of contamination. The possible link between a family history of renal disease and development of renal failure may represent an inherited susceptibility or could result from a common geographic exposure. Altered nutrition and certain co-existing diseases including addictive behavior are additional parameters by which relative risk to nephrotoxin, can be ascertained. While gender, race and socio-economic status provide tantalizing clues that these factors could contribute to risk stratification, solid confirmation is needed. Thus, targeting populations at risk for future evaluation and follow-up is the most efficient strategy for the identification of patients early in the course of their toxic renal injury plus introducing protective measures to impede the progression of patients into ESRD programs.

Individual risk factors

Individuals may be at increased risk for developing nephrotoxicity from various drugs based on unique circumstances. For example, several antibiotics are well recognized as having nephrotoxic potential [195] but it must be appreciated that they are often administered under clinical circumstances in which acute renal insults co-exist, i.e., hypotension, reduced cardiac output, depressed liver function, etc. Rasmussen & Ibels [9] used multivariant analysis to determine the role of acute insults such as hypotension, dehydration, pigmenturia, liver disease, sepsis, aminoglycoside administration and contrast media for patients developing AKI without a prior history of renal disease. In 41 of 121 patients a single insult was considered to be responsible for AKI, 80% of the time this was hypotension. The remaining 80 patients were exposed to 140 insults or 1.75/patient giving support to the concept of the multifactorial basis for inducing nephrotoxic renal injury. This same pattern of multiple insults causing AKI is evident from the report of Kohli et al. [171]. Contrast-associated nephropathy has been evaluated extensively for possible clinical conditions in which patients are at additional risk for the induction of AKI [196]. Swartz et al. [197] using a retrospective analysis of factors related to renal failure following major angiography, reported that in addition to renal insufficiency, abnormal liver function tests, hypoalbuminemia, diabetes mellitus and proteinuria all were significantly correlated with the patient group which developed renal failure. They also noted a prevalence of 2.5-risk factors/case of contrast-associated nephropathy. Cochran et al. [198] used an odds-ratio analysis of 28 clinical factors that might correlate with increased risk for the development of contrast-associated nephropathy. In addition to underlying renal disease and elevated serum creatinine, their data confirmed proteinuria as a risk factor but failed to substantiate diabetes mellitus or abnormal liver function. They did demonstrate that male gender, hypertension, and vascular disease all were associated with significant additional risk as well as the amount and type of contrast administered. In a review of 6 publications which analyzed risk factors for contrast-associated nephropathy in 1416 patients, renal insufficiency was the only uniformly consistent factor for all studies [183], however, in 3 of 5 studies in which it was tested, the amount of contrast was found to have a positive correlation. Cigarroa et al. [199] have used a modified contrast media dosing scheme for patients at high risk for contrast-associated nephropathy and reported that virtually every case of post procedure contrast-associated nephropathy occurred when the recommended limits of the calculated dose of contrast were exceeded. In a recent consensus report [200], it was concluded that "1) adequate intravenous volume expansion with isotonic crystalloid for 3-12 hours before the procedure and continued for 6-24 hours afterward can lessen the probability of CIN in patients at risk; and 2) no adjunctive medical or mechanical treatment has been proven to be efficacious in reducing the risk of CIN."

In a similar vein, Leehey et al. [201] have reported on the frequency of aminoglycoside-induced nephrotoxicity using three different dosing schemes, including two that were based on pharmacokinetic principles. It is noteworthy that despite careful calculation of the dosing scheme, this did not alter the incidence of nephrotoxicity. However, the duration of dosing correlated positively with nephrotoxicity incidence, as did treatment with furosemide, old age, and liver disease.

While cyclosporine is an intrinsically nephrotoxic drug due to a direct action on the kidney, under other circumstances it can become nephrotoxic in the presence of a second drug, exhibiting a so-called drug-drug interaction. For example, drugs that inhibit the hepatic P-450 drug-metabolizing enzymes can cause a significant change in cyclosporine pharmacokinetics and, thus, render an otherwise stable dose nephrotoxic [202]. Drugs that induce such changes in cyclosporine levels include: erythromycin, fluconazole, ketoconazole, and cimetidine.

Another example of drug-drug interaction occurs when non-steroidal anti-inflammatory drugs are given to patients receiving anti-hypertensive drugs [203]. Due to the action of the NSAID to inhibit prostaglandin synthesis, the loss of endogenous induced vasodilatation causes the blood pressure to become uncontrolled often necessitating increasing the current anti-hypertensive drug dosage or prescribing additional anti-hypertensive drugs [204]. Recently, Mehta et al. [205] have called attention to the increased mortality and permanent residual renal impairment in AKI patients who are treated with diuretics. Once again we are reminded that empirical treatment, for which pathophysiologic rationale can be developed, must be evaluated in a controlled clinical trial before being universally accepted as standard therapy. So not only is it important to understand the patient's diseases, but also a complete list of all medications that the patient takes on a regular basis including those purchased over the counter.

References

1. Nolan CR, Anderson RJ. Hospital–acquired acute renal failure. JASN 1998; 9: 710-718.
2. Vijayan A, Miller SB. Acute renal failure: prevention and non-dialytic therapy. Sem. Nephrol 1998; 18: 523-532.
3. Nash K, Hafeez A, Hou S. Hospital-acquired renal insufficiency. Am J Kid Dis 2002;39:930-936
4. Starr R Treatment of acute renal failure Kid Internat 1998;54:1817-1831
5. Kellum JA, Mehta RL, Ronco C: Acute dialysis quality initiative. Contrib Nephrol. 2001;132:258-265
6. K/DOQI clinical practice guidelines for chronic kidney disease: Evaluation, classification, and stratification. Am J Kid Dis 2002;39: S1-S266.
7. Warnock DG Toward a definition and classification of acute kidney injury. J Am Soc Nephrol 2005;16:3149-3150
8. Turney JH, Marshall DH, Brownjohn AM, Ellis CM and Parsons FM. The evolution of acute renal failure 1956-1988. Q J Med 1990; 73: 83-104.
9. Rasmussen HH, Ibels LS. Acute renal failure: multi variant analysis of causes and risk factors. Am J Med 1982; 73: 211-218.
10. Hou SH, Bushunsky DA. Wish BB, Cohen JJ, Harrington IT. Hospital-acquired renal insufficiency: a prospective study. Am J Med 1983; 74: 243-248.
11. Kleinknecht D. Landais P. Goldfarb B. Les insuffisances renales aigues associees 11 des medicaments OU 11 des produits de contraste iodes. Resultats d'une enquete cooperative multicentrique de la société de Néphrologie. Néphrologie 1986; 7: 41-46.
12. Kaufman J, Dhakal M, Patel B, Hamburger R. Community-acquired acute renal failure. Am J Kidney Dis 1991; 17: 191-198.
13. Bennett WM. Porter GA. Overview of clinical nephrotoxicity. In: Toxicology of the kidney. Hook IB, Goldstein RS (editors). Raven Press, New York 1993; p. 61-97.
14. Baraldi A, Ballestri M, Rapana R, Lucchi L, Borella P, Leonelli M, Furci L and Lusvarghi E. Acute renal failure of medical type in an elderly population. Nephol Dial Transpl 1998; 13(supp7): 25-29.
15. Wang Y, Cui Z, Fan M. Retrspective analysis on Chinese patients diagnosed with acute renal failure hospitalized during the last decade (1994-2003) Am. J Nephrol. 2005;25:514-519.
16. Jayakumar M, Prabahar MR,Fernando EM, Manorajan R, Venkatraman R, Balaraman V. Epidemiologic trend changes in acute renal failure- a tertiary center experience from South India. Renal Failure 2006;28:405-410
17. Obialo CI, Okonofua EC, Tayade AS, Riley LJ. Epidemiology of de novo acute renal failure in hospitalized African Americans. Arch Intern Med 2000;160:1309-1313,
18. Sesso R, Roque A, Vicioso B, Stella S. Prognosis of AKI in Hospitalized elderly patients. Am J Kid Dis. 2004;44:410-419
19. Khan IH, Catto GRD, Edward N, Macleod AM. Acute renal failure: factors influencing nephrology referral and outcome. Q J Med 1997; 90: 781-785.
20. Mehta R, Pascual MT, Soroko S. Savage BR, Himmelfarb J, Ikizler TA, Paganini EP, Chertow GM. Spectrum of acute renal failure in the intensive care unit: The PICARD experience. Kid Internat 2004;66:1613-1621
21. Feest TG, Round A, Hamad S. Incidence of severe acute renal failure in adults: results of a community based study. Br Med J 1993; 306: 481-483.
22. Pruchnicki MD, Dasta JF. Acute renal failure in hospitalized patients: part I. Ann Pharmacother 2002; 36: 1261-1267.
23. Margrra S, Kraft AK, Siebert G, Luft FC, Neumayer HH. Long-term outcomes in acute renal failure patients treated with continuous replacement therapies. Am J Kidney Dis 2002; 40: 275-279.
24. Davidman M, Olsen P, Kohen J, Leither T, Kjellstrand C. Iatrogenic renal disease. Arch Intern Med 1991; 151: 1809-1812.
25. Pru C, Ebben J, Kjellstrand C. Chronic renal failure after acute tubular necrosis. Kidney Int 1982; 21: 176.

26. Fleury D, Vanhille P, Pallot IL, Kleinknecht D. Drug induced acute renal failure: a preventable disease linked to drug misuse. Kidney Int 1990; 38: 1238.
27. Wing AJ, Broyer M, Brunner FP, Brynger H. Challah S. Challah S, Donckerwolcke RA, Gretz N, Jacobs C, Kramer P, Selwood NH. Combined report on regular dialysis and transplantation in Europe XIII Acute (reversible) renal failure. Proc Eur Dial Transpl Assoc 1983; 20: 64-71.
28. Ronco C, Zanella M, Brendolan A, Milan M, Canato G, Zamperetti N, Bellomo R. Management of severe acute renal failure in critically ill patients: an international survey in 345 centres. Nephrol Dial Transplant 2001; 16(2): 230-237.
29. Frankel MC, Weinstein AM, Stenzel KH. Prognostic patterns in acute renal failure: the New York Hospital, 1981-1982. Clin Exp Dialysis Apheresis 1983; 7: 1457.
30. Beard K, Perera DR, lick H. Drug induced parenchymal renal disease in outpatients. J Clin Pharmacol 1988; 28: 431-435.
31. Ympa YP, Sakr Y, Reinhart K, Vincent J.L. Has mortality from acute renal failure decreased? A systematic review of the literature. Am J Med 2005;118: 827-832).
32. Xue JL, Daniels F, Starr RA, Kimmel PL, Eggers PW, Molitoris BA, Hmmelfarb J, Collins AJ. Incidence and mortality of acute renal failure in Medicare beneficiaries, 1992 to 2001. J Am Soc Nephrol 2006;17:1135-42
32a. Ali T, Khan I, Simpson W, Puscatt G, Townsend J, Smith W and MacLeod A. Incidence and outcome in acute kidney injury: a comprehensive population-based study. J Am Soc Nephrol 2007;18:1292-1298.
33. Waikar SS, Curhan GC, Wald R, McCarthy EP, Chertow GM. Declining mortality in patients with acute renal failure, 1988 to 2002
34. Knauss WA Apache II: a ;severity of disease classification system, Crit Care Med 1985;13:818-829],
35. Liano F, Pascual J, Garcia-Martin F et al Prognosis of acute tubular necrosis: an extended prospectively contrasted study. Nephron 1993;63:21-31
36. Lins, R, Elseviers M, Daelemans R et al. Prognositic value of a new scoring system for hospital mortality in acute renal failure. Clin Nephrol. 2000;53:10-17L.
37. Lins RL, Elseviers MM, Daelemans R. Severisty scoring and mortality 1 year after acute renal failure. Nephrol Dial Transpl 2006;21:1066-1068
38. Chertow GM, Burdick E, Honour M, Bonventre JV, Bates DW; Acute Kidney Injury, Mortality, Length of Stay and Costs in Hospitalized Patients. J Am Soc Nephrol 2005;16:3365-70
39. Fischer MJ, Brimhall BB, Dezotte, DC, Glazner JE, Parikh CR. Uncomplicated Acute Renal Failure and Hospital Resource Utilization: A Retrospective Multi-center Analysis. Am J Kid Dis. 2005;46:1049-57
40. Heyman SN, Brezis M, Epstein FH, Spokes K, Silva P, Rosen S: Early renal medullary hypoxic injury from radiocontrast and indomethacin. Kidney Int 1991; 40: 632-642.
41. Dishart M, Kellum JA. An evaluation of pharmacological strategies fro the prevention and treatment of acute renal failure. Drugs 2000; 59: 79-91.
42. Dekant W, Vamvakas S. Biotransformation and membrane transport in nephrotoxicity. Crit Rev Toxicol 1996; 26: 309-334.
43. Petzinger E and Geyer J. Drug transporters in pharmacokinetics. Naunyn Schmiedeberg's Arch Pharmacol 2006;372:465-475
44. Shitara Y, Sato H, Sugiyama Y. Evaluation of drug-drug interaction in the hepatobiliary and renal transport of drugs. Annu Rev Pharmacol. Toxicol 2005;45:689-723
45. Tune B. The nephrotoxicity of cephalosporin antibiotics. Sturcture-activity relationship. Commun Toxicol 1993; 1: 145-157.
46. Pearson PG, Omichinski JG, Holme JA, McClanahan RH, Brunborg G, Soderlund EJ, Dybing E, Nelson SD: Metabolic activation of tris (2, 3, dibromopropyl) phosphate to reactive intermediates: Covalent binding, reactive metabolite formation and differential metabolite-specific DNA damage, *in vivo*. Toxicol Appl Pharmacol 1993; 118: 186-196.
47. Goyer RA. Mechanisms of lead and cadmium nephrotoxicity. Toxicol Lett 1989; 46: 153-176.
48. Kaloyanides GJ. Aminoglycoside-induced functional and biochemical defects in the renal cortex. Fundam Appl Toxicol 1984; 4: 930-942.
49. Albano E, Rundgren M, Harvison PJ, Nelson SD, Moldeus P. Mechanisms of N-acetyl-p-benzoquinone imine cytotoxicity. Mol Pharmacol 1985; 28: 306-315.
50. Whelton A. Nephrotoxicity of nonsteroidal anti-inflammatory drugs: physiological foundations and clinical implications. Am J Med 1999; 106: 13S-24S.
51. Kleinknecht D. Diseases of the kidney caused by nonsteroidal anti-inflammatory drugs. In. Stewart JH (editor). Oxford University Press, Oxford 1993; p. 160-173.
52. Miet S, Dasta J, Goldstein S, Golper T. Drug-induced acute kidney injury. Current Opinion in Critical Care 2005;11:555-565
53. Huerta C, Castellsague J, Varas-Lorenzo C, Gracia Rodriguez LA. Nonsteroidal anti-inflammatory drugs and risk of AKI in the general population. Am J Kid Dis 2005;45:531-539
54. Markowitz GS, Perazella MA. Drug induced renal failure: a focus on tubulointerstitial disease. Clin Chim Acta 2005;351:31-47

55. Bridoux F, Hazzan M, Pallot JL, Fleury D, Lemaitre V, Kleinknecht D, Vanhille Ph. Acute renal failure after the use of angiotensin-converting enzyme inhibitors in patients without renal artery stenosis. Nephrol Dial Transplant 1992; 7: 100-104.
56. Schwarz A, Krause PH, Kunzendorf U, Keller F, Distler A. The outcome of acute interstitial nephritis: Risk factors for the transition from acute to chronic interstitial nephritis. Clin Nephrol 2000; 54:179-190.
57. Kleinknecht D, Landais P, Goldfarb B. Pathophysiology and clinical aspects of drug-induced tubular necrosis in man. Contr Nephrol 1987; 55: 145-158.
58. Richet G, Sraer JD, Kourilsky O. La ponction-biopsic rénale dans l'insuffisance rénale aigue. Ann Med Interne 1978; 129: 335-337.
59. Linton AL, Clark W, Driedger AA, Turnbull DJ. Lindsey RM. Acute interstitial nephritis due to drug. Review of the literature with a report of nine cases. Ann Intern Med 1980; 93: 735-741.
60. Buysen JGM, Houthoff HJ, Kredict RT, Arisz L. Acute interstitial nephritis, a clinical and morphological study in 27 patients. Nephrol Dial Transpl 1990; 5: 94-99.
61. Grunfeld JP. Kleinknecht D. Droz D. Acute interstitial nephritis. In: Diseases of the kidney. Schrier RW, Gottschalk CW (editors). Little Brown, Boston 1993; p. 1331-1353.
62. Rossert J. Drug-induced acute interstitial nephritis. Kidney Int 2001; 60: 804-817.
63. Henrich WL Nephrotoxicity of several new agents. Kid Internat 2005;67(supp94):S107-S109
64. Choudhury D, Ahmed Z. Drug-induced nephrotoxicity. Med Clin N Am 1997; 81: 705-717.
65. Richards JR, Johnson EB, Stark RW, Derlet RW. Methamphetamine abuse and rhabdomyolysis in the ED: A 5-year study. Am J Emerg Med 1999; 17: 681-685.
66. Lieberthal W, Levinsky NG. Acute renal failure. In: The kidney: physiology and pathophysiology. Seldin W, Giebish G (editors). Raven Press, New York 1992; p 3181-3225.
67. Wolfe JA, McCann RL, Sanfillipo F. Cyclosporine-associated microangiopathy in renal transplantation: a severe but potentially - reversible form of early graft injury. Transplantation 1986; 41: 541.
68. Dioti J.S, Danielson CF, Blue-Hindy DE, McCarthy LJ: Drug-induced thrombotic thrombocytopenic purpura/hemolytic uremic syndrome. A concise review. Ther. Apher.2004;8:102-111
69. VIsweswaran P, Massin EK, Dubose TD Jr. Mannitol-induced acute renal failure. J Am Soc Nephrol. 1997;154:1985-1987
70. Schortgen F, Lacherade JC, Bruneel F. Effects of hydroxyethylstarch and gelatin on renal function in severe sepsis. A multi-centre randomized study Lancet 2001;357:911-916
71. Itkin YM and Trujillo TC. Intravenous immunoglobulin-associated acute renal failure: case series and literature review. Phamacotherapy 2005;25:886-892
72. McKenney JM, Davidson MH, Jacobson TA, Guyton JR. Final conclusions and recommendations of the national lipid association statin safety assessment task force. Am J Cardiol 2006;97(suppC):89C-94C
73. Coco TJ, Klasner AE: Drug-induced rhabdomyolysis. Curr. Opinion Pediatr. 2004;16:206-210
74. Thompson PD, Clarkson P, Karas RH. Statin-Associated Myopathy. JAMA 2003;289:1681-1690
75. Fine DM, Gelber AC, Melamed MI, Lin JC, Zhan L, Eustace JA. Risk factors for renal failure among 72 consecutive patients with rhabdomyolysis related to illicit drug use. Am J Med 2004;117:607-610
76. Richards Jr, Johnson EB, Stark RW, Derlet RW. Methamphetamine abuse and rhabdomyolsis in the ED: A 5-year study. Am J Emerg Med 1999;17:681-685
77. Bicket M, Ditting T, Watz H, Roesler A, Weidauer S, Volkmar J, Gueller S, Betz C, Fichtischerfer S, Stein J. Severe rhabdomyolysis, acute renal failure and posterior encephalopathy after "magic mushroom" abuse. Euro J Emerg Med 2005;12:306-308
78. Menahem SA, Perry GJ, Dowling J, Thomson NM. Hypokalaemia-induced acute renal failure. Nephrol Dial Transpl 1999;14:2216-2218
79. Zhang L, Wang M, Wang H. Acute renal failure in chronic kidney disease – clinical and pathological analysis of 104 cases. Clin Nephrol 2005;63:346-350
80. Bailey TC, Little JR, Littenberg B. A meta analysis of extended-interval dosing vs multiple dosing of aminoglycosides. Clin Invect Dis 1997;24:786-795
81. Olsen KM, Rudis MI, Rebuck JA, Hara J, Gelmont D, Mehdian R, Nelson, C and Rupp ME. Effect of once-daily dosing vs. multiple daily dosing of tobramycin on enzyme markers of nephrotoxicity. Crit Care Med 2004;32:1678-1682
82. Murry KR, McKinnon PS, Mitrayk B. Pharmacodynamic characterization of nephrotoxicity associated with once-daily aminoglycoside. Pharmacotherapy 1999; 19:1252-1260.
83. Nicolau DP, Freeman CD Belliveau PP. Experience with once-daily aminoglycoside program administered to 2184 adult patients. Antimicrob Agents Chemother 1995;39:650-655
84. Rougier F, Claude D, Maurin M, Sedoglavic A, Ducher M, Corvaisier S, Jelliffe R and Maire P. Aminoglycoside Nephrotoxicity: Modeling, simulation and control. Antimicrobial Agents Chemother. 2003;47:1010-1016

85. Zahar JR, Rioux C, Girou E, Hulin A, Sauve C, Bernier-Combes A, Brun-Buisson C, and Lesprit P. Inappropriate prescribing of aminoglycosides: risk factors and impact an antibiotic control team. J Antimicrob Chemother 2006;58:651-656
86. Personal communication, Evans, T, McNeil Consumer Health Care, 2000.
87. Henrich WL. Nephrotoxicity of non-steroidal anti-inflammatory agents. In: Diseases of the kidney. Schrier RW, Gottschalk CW (editors). Little Brown, Boston 1993; p 1203-1217.
88. Nicholls AJ. Shortland JR. Brown CB. Mefenamic acid nephropathy - A spectrum of renal lesions. Proc Eur Dial Transpl Assoc 1985; 22:991-996.
89. Corwin HL Bonventre JV. Renal insufficiency associated with non-steroidal anti-inflammatory agents. Am J Kidney Dis 1984; 4: 147-152.
90. Kleinknecht D, Landais P, Goldfarb B. Analgesic and nonsteroidal anti-inflammatory drug-associated acute renal failure. A prospective study. Clin Nephrol 1986; 25. 275-281.
91. Gambaro G and Perazella MA. Adverse renal effects of anti-inflammatory agents: evaluation of selective and nonselective cyclooxygenase inhibitiors. J Intern Med 2003;253:643-652
92. White WB. Cardiovasculr Effects of Cyclooxygenase Inhibitors. Hypertension 2007;49:408-418
93. Solomon SD, Pfeffer MA, McMurray JJV, Fowler R, Finn P, Levin B, Eagle C, Hawk E, Lechuga M, Zauber AG. Bertagnolli MM, Arber N, Wittes J, ACP and PreSAP Trial Investigators. Effect of Celecoxib on Cardiovascular Events and Blood Pressure in Two Trials for the Prevention of Colorectal Adenomas. Circulation 2006;114:1028-1035
94. Makdassi R, Andrejak M, Westeel PF, Schmit JL, Renaud H, Houhou S, Fournier A. Aetiology and prognosis of iatrogenic renal failure on the basis of a 6-year experience. Nephrol Dial Transplant 1990; 5: 660-661.
95. Boiskin M, Marcussen N, Kjellstrand C. ACE inhibitors are now the second most common cause of acute, iatrogenic renal failure. J Am Soc Nephrol 1992; 3: 720.
96. Karalliedde J and Viberti G. Evidence for reno-protection by blockade of the rennin-angiotensin-aldosterone system in hypertension and diabetes. J Human Hyperten 2006;20:239-253
97. Bakris GL and Weir MR. Angotensin-converting enzyme inhibitor- associated elevations in serum creatinine. Arch Intern Med 2000;160:685-693
98. Schoolwerth AC, Sica DA, Ballermann BJ and Wilcox CS. Renal considerations in angiotensin convering enzyme inhibitor therapy. Circulation 2001;104:1985-1991
99. Suissa S, Hutchinson T, Brophy JM, Kezouh A. ACE-inhibitor use and the long-term risk of renal failure in diabetes. Kid Internat 2006;69:913-919
100. Hou FF, Zhang X, Zhang GH, Xie D, Chen PY, Zhang WR, Jiang JP, Liang M, Want GB, Liu ZR, and Geng RW. Efficacy and safety of benazepril for advanced chronic renal insufficiency. N Eng J Med 2006;354:131-140
101. Schusterman N, Strom BL, Murray TG, Morrison G, West SL, Maislin G. Risk factors and outcome of hospital-acquired acute renal failure. Am J Med 1987; 83: 65-71.
102. Rudnick M, Berns JS, Cohen RM, Goldfarb S. Contrast media-associated nephrotoxicity. Curr Opin Nephrol Hyperten 1996; 5: 127-133.
103. McCullough PA, Wolyn R, Rocher LL. Acute renal failure after coronary intervention: incidence risk factors and relationship to mortality Am J Med 1997;103:368-375
104. Weisberg LS, Kurnik PB, Kurnik BR. Risk of radiocontrast nephropathy in patients with and without diabetes mellitus. Kid Internat 1994; 45: 259-265.
105. Rihal CS, Textor SC, Grill DE . Incidence and prognostic importance of acute renal failure after percutaneous coronary intervention. Circulation 2002;105:2259-2264
106. Thomsen HS and Morcos SK. Contrast-medium-induced nephropathy: is there a new consensus? A review of published guidelines. Eur Radiol 2006;16:1835-1840
107. Levey AS. Measurement of renal function in chronic renal disease. Kidney Int 1990; 38: 167-184.
108. Keevil BG, Kilpatrick ES, Nichols SP, Maylor PW. Biological variation of cystatin C: implications for the assessment of glomerular filtration rate. Clin Chem. 1998;44:1535-1539
109. Shemesh 0, Golbetz H, Kriss JP, Myers BD. Limitations of creatinine as a filtration marker in glomerulopathic patients. Kidney Int 1985; 28: 830-838.
110. Bouchner-Mortensen J. Current status on assessment and measurement of glomerular filtration rate. Clin Physiol 1985;5:1-17
111. Traynor J, Mactier R, Geddes CC, Fox JG. How to measure renal function in clinical practice. BMJ 2006;333:733-737
112. Newman DJ, Thakkar H, Edwards RG, Wilkie M, White T, Grubb AO, Price CP. Serum cystatin C measured by automated immunoassay: a more sensitive marker of changes in GFR than serum creatinine. Kidney Int 1995; 47: 312-318.
113. Coll E, Botey A, Alvarez L, Poch E, Quinto L, Saurina A, Vera M, Piera C, Darnell A: Serum cystatin C as a new marker for noninvasive estimation of glomerular filtration rate and as a marker for early renal impairment. Am J Kidney Dis 2000; 36: 29-34.

114. Aviv A. John E. Bernstein J, Goldsmith DI, Spitzer A. Lead intoxication during development. Its late effects on renal function and blood pressure. Kidney Int 1980; 17: 430-443.
115. Parker RA, Bennett WM. Porter GA. Animal models in the study of aminoglycoside nephrotoxicity. In: The aminoglycosides: microbiology, clinical use and toxicology. Whelton A, Neu HC (editors). Marcel Dekker Inc, New York, Basel, 1982; 235-268.
116. Nicolau DP, Freeman CD, Belliveau PP. Experience with once-daily aminoglycoside program administrated to 2184 adult patients. Antimicrob. Agent Chemother 1995; 39: 650-655.
117. Swan RC. Merrill JP. The clinical course of acute renal failure. Medicine 1953; 32: 215-292.
118. Molitoris B. Transitioning to therapy in ischemic acute renal failure. J Am Soc. Nephrol. 2003;14:265-267
119. US Renal Data System, USRDS 2006 Annual Data Report: Atlas of end-stage renal disease in the United States. National Institutes of Health, National Institute of Diabetes and Digestive and Kidney Diseases, Bethesda MD, 2006.
120. Combined report on regular dialysis and transplantation in Europe, XIX, 1988. Nephrol Dial Transplant 1989; 4(Suppl4): 5-29.
121. Porter GA. Bennett WM, Gilbert DN. Unraveling aminoglycoside nephrotoxicity using animal models. J Clin Pharmacol 1983; 23: 445-452.
122. Steenland NK, Thun MJ, Ferguson CW, Port FK Occupational and other exposures associated with male end-stage renal disease: a case/control study. Am J Pub Health 1990; 80: 153-159.
123. O'Dea DF, Murphy SW, Hefferton D, Parfrey PS. Higher risk for renal failure in first-degree relatives of white patients with end-stage renal disease: A population based study. Am J Kidney Dis 1998; 32: 794-801.
124. Freedman BI, Soucie M, Stone SM, Pegram S. Familial clustering of end-stage renal disease in blacks with HIV-associated nephropathy. Am J Kid Dis 1999; 34: 254-258.
125. Chew ST, Newman MF, White WD, Conlon PJ, Saunders AM, Strittmatter WJ, Landolfo K, Grocott HP, Stafford-Smith M. Preliminary report on the association of apolipoprotein E polymorphisms, with postoperative peak serum creatinine concentrations in cardiac surgical patients. Anesthesiology 2000; 93:325-331
126. Jaber BI, Pereira JG, Bonventre JV, Balakrishnan VS. Polymorphism of host response genes: Implications in the pathogenesis and treatment of acute renal failure. Kid Internat. 2005;67:14-33
127. Wang Y, Kikuchi S, Suzuki H, Nagase S, Koyama A. Endothelial nitric oxide synthase gene polymorphism in intron 4 affects the progression of renal failure in non-diabetic renal disease. Nephrol Dial Transplant 1999; 14(12): 2898-2902.
128. Gumprecht J, Zychma J, Grzeszczak W, Zukowska-Szczechowska E, and ESRD study group. Angiotension I converting enzyme gene insertion/deletion and angiotensiongen M235T polymorphism. Kidney Int 2000; 58: 513-519.
129. Fabris B, Bortoletto M, Candido R, Barbone F, Cattin MR, Calci M, Scanferla F, Tizzoni L, Giacca M, Carretta R. Genetic polymorphisms of the rennin-angiotensin-aldosterone system and renal insufficiency in essential hypertension. J Hyperten 2005;23:309-316
130. Nobilis A, Kocsis I, Toth-Heyn P, Treszl A, Schuler A, Tulassay T, Vasarhelyi B. Variance of ACE and AT1 receptor gene does not influence the risk of neonatal acute renal failure. Pediatr Nephrol 2001; 16(12): 1063-1066.
131. Fekete A, Treszi A, Toth-Hey P, Vannay A, Tordai A, Tulassay T, Basarhelyi B. Association between heat shock protein 72 gene polymorphism and acute renal failure in premature neonates
132. Sandler DP, Smith JC. Chronic renal disease risk associated with employment in industries with potential solvent exposure. In: Nephrotoxicity mechanisms: early diagnosis and therapeutic management. Bach PH, Gregg NJ, Wiks MF, Delacruz L (editors). Marcel Dekker Inc, New York 1991: p 261-266.
133. Landrigan PJ, Goyer RA, Clarkson TW, Sandler DP, Smith JH, Thun MJ, Wedeen RP. The work-relatedness of renal disease. Arch Environ Health 1984; 39: 225-230.
134. Kim R, Rotnitsky A, Sparrow D, Weiss S, Wager C and Hu H. A longitudinal study of low-level lead exposure and impairment of renal function. The Normative Aging Study. JAMA 1996;275:
135. Marsden PA Increased body lead burden – cause or consequence of chronic renal insufficiency? N Eng J Med 2003;348:345-347
136. Lin JL, Lin-Tan DT Hsu Kh and Yu CC. Environmental lead exposure and progression of chronic renal disease in patients without diabetes. NEngJMed 2003;348:277-286
137. Yu CC, Lin JL, Lin-Tan DT. Environmental exposure to lead and progression of chronic renal diseases: A four-year prospective longitudinal study. J Am Soc Nephrol 2004;15:1016-1022
138. Vupputuri S, He J, Muntner P, Bazzano LA, Whelton PK, Batuman V. Blood lead levels is associated with elevated blood pressure in blacks. Hypertension 2003;41:463-468
139. Bennett WM, Elzinga LW, Porter GA. Tubulointerstitial disease and toxic nephropathy. In: The kidney. Brenner BM, Rector FC Jr (editors). WB Saunders, Philadelphia 1991; p 1430-1496.
140. Gregg NJ, Elseviers MM, De Broe ME, Bach PH. Epidemiology and mechanistic basis of analgesic nephropathy Toxicol Lett 1989; 46: 141-151.

141. Sandler DP. Epidemiology in the assessment of nephrotoxicity. In: Nephrotoxicily in the experimental and clinical situation. Bach PH, Locke EA (editors). Martinus Nijhoff, Dordrecht 1987; 847-883.
142. Staessen J, Yeoman WB, Fletcher AE, Markowe HLJ, Marmot MG, Rose G, Semmence A, Shipley MJ, Bulpitt CJ. Blood lead concentration, renal function and blood pressure in London civil servants. Brit J Ind Med 1990; 47: 441-447.
143. Iesato K, Wakastin M, Wakastin Y. Renal tubular dysfunction in Minimata disease. Ann Intern Med 1977; 86: 731-733.
144. Staessen JA, Lauwerys RR, Buchet JP, Bulpitt CJ, Rondia D, Vanrenterghem Y, Amery A, Cadmibel Study Group. Impairment of renal function with increasing blood lead concentrations in the general population. N Engl J Med 1992; 327. 151-156.
145. Vanherweghem JL. Misuse of herbal remedies: the case of an outbreak of terminal renal failure in Belgium (Chinese herbs nephropathy). J Altern Complement Med 1998; 4: 9-13.
146. De Broe ME. On a nephrotoxic and carcinogenic slimming regime. Am J Kidney Dis 1999; 33: 1171-1173.
147. Lord G, Tagore R, Cook T, Gower P, Pusey CD. Nephropathy caused by Chinese herbs in the UK. Lancet 1999; 354: 481-482.
148. Moore RD, Smith CR, Lipsky JJ, Mellitus ED, Lietman PS. Risk factors for nephrotoxicity in patients treated with aminoglycosides. Ann Intern Med 1984; 100: 352-373.
149. Miller JA, Anacta LA, Cattran DC. Impact of gender on the renal response to angiotensin II. Kidney Int 1999; 55: 278-285.
150. Thakar CV, Arrigain S, Worley S, Yared JP, Paganini EP: A clinical score to predict acute renal failure after cardiac surgery. J Am Soc Nephrol. 2005;16:162-168
151. Athanasiou T, Al-Ruzzeh S, Stanbridge RD, Casula RP, Glenville BE, Amrani M. Is the female gender an independent predictor of adverse outcome after off-pump coronary artery bypass grafging? Ann Thorac Surg 2003;75:1153-1160
152. Anderson S, Rennke H, Brenner B. Therapeutic advantage of converting enzyme inhibitors in arresting progressive renal disease associated with systemic hypertension in the rat. J Clin Invest 1986; 77: 1993-2000.
153. Freedman BI, Spray BJ, Tuttle AB, Buckalew VM. The familial risk of end-stage renal disease in African Americans. Am J Kidney Dis 1993; 21: 387-393.
154. Obialo CI, Crowell AK, Okonofua EC. Acute renal failure mortality in hospitalized African Americans: age and gender considerations. J Natl Med Assoc 2002; 94(3): 127-134.
155. Porter GA. Risk factors for toxic nephropathies. Toxicol Lett 1989; 46: 269- 279.
156. Cremer W, Bock KD. Symptoms and causes of chronic hypokalemic nephropathy in man. Clin Nephrol 1977; 7: 112-123.
157. Wedeen RP. Poison in the pot. The legacy of lead. So Illinois Univ Press, Carbondale 1984.
158. Mudge GH. Analgesic nephropathy: renal drug distribution and metabolism. In: Nephrotoxic mechanisms of drugs and environmental toxins. Porter GA (editor). Plenum Med Book Co, New York, London 1982; p 209-225.
159. Itizler TA, Wingard RL, Harvell J, Shyr Y, Hakim RM. Association of morbidity with markers of nutrition and inflammation in chronic hemodialysis patients: A prospective study. Kidney Int 1999; 55: 1945-1951.
160. Stenvinkel P, Heimburger O, Paultre F, Diczfulusy U, Wang T, Berglund L, Jogestrand T. Strong association between malnutrition, inflammation, and atherosclerosis in chronic renal failure. Kidney Int 1999; 55: 1899-1911.
161. Morgan JM, Hartley MW. Etiologic factors in lead nephropathy. South Med J 1976; 69: 1445-1449.
162. Wen SF, Parthasarathy R, Iliopoulos O, Oberley TD. Acute renal failure following binge drinking and nonsteroidal anti-inflammatory drugs. Am J Kidney Dis 1992; 20: 281-285.
163. Perneger TV, Whelton PK, Puddey IB, Klag MJ. Risk of end-stage renal disease associated with alcohol consumption. Am J Epidemol 1999; 150: 1275-1281.
164. Wigfield CH, Lindsey JD, Munoz A, Chopra PS, Edwards NM, Love RB. Is extreme obesity a risk factor for cardiac surgery? An analysis of patients with BMI≥40. Eur J Cardio-Thoracic Surg 2006;29:434-440
165. Fiaccadori E, Maggiore U, Rotelli C, Giascosa R, Picetti E, Parenti E, Meschi T, Borghi L, Tagliavini D, Cabassi A. Effects of different energy intakes on nitrogen balance in patients with acute renal failure: a pilot study. Nephrol Dial Transpl. 2005;20:1976-1980
166. Radovic M, Tomovic M, Simic-Ogrizovic S, Stosovic M, Lezaic V, Ostric V, Djukanovic L. An improvement in the outcome of acute renal failure. Renal Failure.2004;26:647-653
167. Emmerson BT. Chronic lead nephropathy. Kidney Int 1973; 4: 1-5.
168. Rodriguez-Puyol D. The aging kidney. Kidney Int 1998; 54: 2247-2265
169. Bennett WM. Geriatric pharmacokinetics and the kidney. Am J Kidney Dis 1990; 16: 283-288.
170. Fried L, Solomon C, Shlipak M, Seliger S, Stehman-Breen C, Bleyer AJ, Chaves P, Furberg C, Kuller L, Newman A. Inflammatory and prothrombic markers and the progression of renal disease in elderly individuals. J Am Soc Nephrol. 2004;15:3184-3191
171. Kohli HS, Bhaskaran MC, Muthukumar T, Thennarasu K, Sud K, Jha V, Gupta KL, Sakhuja V. Treatment-related acute renal failure in the elderly: a hospital-based prospective study. Nephrol Dial Transpl 2000; 15: 212-217.
172. Chester AC, Rakowski TI. Argy WP, Giacalone A, Schreiner GE. Hemodialysis in the eighth and ninth decade of lite. Arch Intern Med 1979; 139: 1001-5.

173. Marcias-Nunez IE, Cameron IS. Renal function and disease in the elderly. London, Boston, Durban, Singapore, Sydney, Toronto, Wellington: Butterworth 1987: p 503.
174. Mudge GH. Nephrotoxicity of urographic radiocontrast drugs. Kidney Int 1980; 18: 540-552.
175. Levy EM, Viscoli CM, Horwitz RI. The effect of acute renal failure on mortality: a cohort analysis. J Am Med Assoc 1996; 275: 1489-1494.
176. Evans JMM, McGregor E, McMahon AD, McGilchrist MM, Jones MC, White G, McDevitt DG, MacDonald TM: Non-steroidal drugs anti-inflammatory drugs and hospitalization for acute renal failure. Q J Med 1995; 88: 551-557.
177. Brivet FG, Kleinknecht DJ, Loirat P, Landais PJM, the French Study Group on Acute Renal Failure. Acute renal failure in intensive care units: causes, outcome, and prognostic factors of hospital mortality; a prospective, multicenter study. Crit Care Med 1996; 24: 192-198.
178. Liano F, Junco E, Pascual J, Madero R, Verde E, and the Madrid Acute Renal Failure Study Group. The spectrum of acute renal failure in the intensive care unit compared with that seen in other settings. Kidney Int 1998; 66: S16-S24.
179. Cole L, Bellomo R, Silvester W, Reeves JH. A prospective, multicenter study of the epidemiology, management, and outcome of severe acute renal failure in a "closed" ICU system. Am J Respir Crit Care Med 2000; 162: 191-196
180. deMendonca A, Vincent JL, Suter PM, Moreno R, Dearden NM, Antonelli M, Takala J, Sprung C, Cantraine FP. Acute renal failure in the ICU: risk factors and outcome evaluated by the SOFA score. Intensive Care Med 2000; 26: 915-921.
181. De long PE, Statius van Eps LW. Sickle cell nephropathy: new insights into its pathophysiology. Kidney Int 1985; 27: 711-719.
182. Allen M, Lawson L, Eckman IR, Delaney V, Bourke E. Effects of nonsteroidal anti-inflammatory drugs on renal function in sickle cell anemia. Kidney Int 1988; 34: 500-506.
183. Porter GA. Contrast associated nephropathy. Am J Cardiol 1989; 64: 22E-26E.
184. Rihal CS, Textor SC, Grill DE, Berger PB, Ting HH, Best PJ, Singh M, Bell MR, Barsness GW, Mathew V, Garratt KN, Holmes DR Jr. Incidence and prognostic importance of acute renal failure after percutaneous coronary intervention. Circulation 2002; 105(19): 2259-2264.
185. Fried L, Solomon C, Shlipak M, Seliger S, Stehman-Breen C, Bleyer AJ, Chaves P, Furberg C, Kuller L, Newman A. Inflammatory and prothrombic markers and the progression of renal disease in elderly individuals. J Am Soc Nephrol. 2004;15:3184-3191
186. Corsonello A, Pedone C, Corica F, Mussi C, Carbonin P, Incalzi RA. Concealed renal insufficiency and adverse drug reactions in elderly hospitalized patients. Arch Intern Med 2005;165:790-795
187. Rao TK, Nicastri AD, Friedman EA. Natural history of heroin-associated nephropathy. N Engl J Med 1974; 290: 19-25.
188. Dubrow A, Mittman N, Ghali V, Flamenbaum W. The changing spectrum of heroin associated nephropathy. Am J Kidney Dis 1985; 5: 36-43.
189. Cunningham EE, Zielezny MA, Venuto RC. Heroin-associated nephropathy - a nationwide problem. JAMA 1983; 250: 2935-2938.
190. Warner E. Cocaine abuse. Ann Intern Med 1993; 119: 226-235.
191. Glauser J and Queen JR. An overview of non-cardiac cocaine toxicity. J Emer Med. 2007;32:181-186
192. Roth D, Alarcon FJ, Fernandez JA, Preston RA, Bougoignie JJ. Acute rhabdomyolysis associated with cocaine intoxication. N Engl J Med 1988; 319: 673-677.
193. van der Woude FJ. Cocaine use and kidney damage. Nephrol Dial Transplant 2000; 15: 299-301.
194. Citron BP, Halpern M, McCarron M. Lundberg GD, McCormick R, Pincus IJ, Tatter D, Haverback BJ. Necrotizing angitis associated with drug abuse. N Engl J Med 1970; 283: 1003-1007.
195. Bingham C, Beaman M, Nicholls AJ, Anthony PP. Necrotizing renal vasculopathy resulting in chronic renal failure after ingestion of methamphetamine and 3, 4-methylenedioxymethamphetamine ('ecstacy'). Nephrol Dial Transplant 1998; 13: 2654-2655.
196. Porter GA. Antimicrobial nephrotoxicity. In: Textbook of nephrology. Massry SG, Glassock JR (editors). Baltimore, Williams & Wilkins 1989; p 812-818.
197. Swartz RD, Rubin JE, Leeming BW, Silva P. Renal failure following major angiography. Am J Med 1978; 65: 31-37.
198. Cochran ST, Wong WS. Roe DJ. Predicting angiographic-induced acute renal impairment: clinical risk model. Am J Radiol 1983; 141: 1027-1033.
199. Cigarroa RG, Lange RA, Williams RH, Hillis LD. Dosing of contrast material to prevent contrast nephropathy in patients with renal disease. Am J Med 1989; 86: 649-652.
200. Stacul F, Adam A, Becker CR, Davidson C. Lameire N, McCullough PA, Tumlin J. Strategies to reduce the risk of contrast-induced nephropathy. Am J Cardiol. 2006, 98(6A):59K-77K
201. Leehey DJ, Braun DA. Tholl LS, Chung CA, Gross JA, Lentino JR. Can pharmacokinetic dosing decrease nephrotoxicity associated with aminoglycoside therapy? J Am Soc Nephrol 1993; 4: 81 -90.
202. Swann SK, Bennett WM. Nephrotoxic acute renal failure. In: Acute renal failure. Lazarus JM, Brenner BM (editors). Churchill Livingston, New York, 1993; p 357-392.

203. Levenson DJ, Simmons CE, Brenner BM. Arachidonic acid metabolism, prostaglandins and the kidney. Am J Med 1982; 72: 354-374.

204. Whelton A. Renal and related cardiovascular effects of conventional and COX-2 specific NSAIDs and non-NSAID analgesics. Am J Ther 2000; 7: 63-74.

205. Mehta RL, Pascual MT, Soroko S, Chertow GM. Diuretics, mortality, and nonrecovery of renal function in acute renal failure. JAMA. 2002; 288(20): 2547-2553.

02

Drug-associated acute kidney injury in the intensive care unit

Mitchell H. ROSNER and Mark D. OKUSA

Division of Nephrology, University of Virginia Health System, Charlottesville, VA, USA

Epidemiology of acute kidney injury in the intensive care unit

In critically ill patients the development of acute kidney injury (AKI) is frequent and occurs in 15-64% of ICU patients [1-4]. Uchino et al reported from 29,269 critically ill patients in the ICU from 54 study centers that 30% of patients had renal dysfunction upon entering in the ICU and the prevalence of AKI defined by the need for dialysis to be 6% [3]. Mehta reporting on the PICARD experience (Program to Improve Care in Acute Renal Disease) found 64% of patients in the ICU required renal replacement therapy. Most recently a new classification scheme for AKI was established by the Acute Dialysis Quality Initiative Mortality that defines grades of increasing severity of AKI - risk (class R), injury (class I) and failure (class F)-and two outcomes class (loss and end-stage kidney disease) [5]. Using this classification scheme, Hoste et al found that AKI occurred in 67% of ICU admissions with maximum R, I, F class of 12%, 27% and 28%, respectively [6]. Mortality rates in those requiring dialysis renal replacement therapy ranges between 20-70% [2, 3, 7].

Nephrotoxicity due to drugs contributes to between 8-60% of AKI cases in hospitalized patients [8-12]. However in the ICU, patients are more complex and thus the etiology of AKI is less certain and more multifactorial in nature. Thus, in the ICU the incidence of AKI from drug nephrotoxicity is likely less prevalent than that due to sepsis or hemodynamic alterations. In the ICU setting the incidence of AKI from drug nephrotoxicity ranges between 1-23% [2, 4, 7, 13]. Elderly patients are likely more susceptible to AKI from nephrotoxic agents related to the age related decline in glomerular filtration rate or renal blood leading to reduced clearance of the drug, decline in hepatic clearance, altered free drug concentration [14].

In general, drug-induced nephrotoxicity is reversible but given the high morbidity and mortality associated with AKI and the frequent and necessary use of drugs in critically ill patients clinicians should be aware of the potential nephrotoxicities and mechanisms. Thus this review will discuss mechanisms of drug-induced AKI and preventive strategies. We will discuss broadly different categories by which drugs cause toxic injury to the kidney with selected examples of each. Detailed discussions of various agents can be found in specific chapters elsewhere in the text.

Mechanisms of drug-induced acute kidney injury

There are several mechanisms by which drugs can lead to nephrotoxicity. Table 1 lists these mechanisms along with prototypical drugs that may induce nephrotoxicity. Understanding their mechanism of action will permit the optimal preventative measures.

Hemodynamically mediated nephrotoxicity

Complex factors maintain constancy of renal blood flow and glomerular filtration despite widely varying arterial pressures. Such factors such as the renal nervous system, prostaglandins, angiotensin II, adenosine, tubuloglomerular feedback as well as other factors participate in regulating glomerular filtration rate. Normally drugs that affect renal hemodynamics are unlikely to precipitate AKI alone unless patients have underlying concomitant predisposing factors.

Nonsteroidal anti-inflammatory drugs

Volume contraction from any cause or other forms of prerenal AKI (cirrhosis, congestive heart failure) will increase the incidence of and severity of nephrotoxicity due to nonsteroidal anti-inflammatory drugs (NSAIDs). Conditions such as congestive heart failure, hypotension, volume depletion, 3rd spacing, decrease effective arterial volume are conditions that predispose to NSAID-induced nephrotoxicity. Prostaglandins under these conditions have an important effect to maintain renal blood flow and glomerular filtration rate [15]. Similarly compensatory vasconstriction due to synthesis of angiotensin II, norepinephrine, vasopressin, and endothelin are balanced by vasodilatory prostaglandins. The use of other drugs that increase renin such as diuretics, angiotensin converting enzyme

Table 1. Common drugs associated with nephrotoxicity in the ICU.

Mechanisms	Drugs	Clinical Findings
Hemodynamic	Radiocontrast agents, calcineurin inhibitors, angiotensin inhibitors, angiotensin receptor blockers, NSAIDs, interleukin 2	Benign urine sediment, FENa <1%, UOsm >500
Acute tubular necrosis (exogenous toxins)	Aminoglycosides, amphotericin, cisplatin, radiocontrast agents, methoxyflurane, outdated tetracyclines, cephalosporins, mithramycin, calcineurin inhibitors, pentamidine, IVIG, ifosfamide, zoledronate, cidofovir, adefovir, tenofovir	FENa>2%, UOsm <350, urinary sediment contains granular casts, renal epithelial cells
Acute tubular necrosis (endogenous toxins-rhabodmyolysis)	Lovastatin (statins), ethanol, barbiturates, diazepam	Elevated CPK, granular casts
Acute tubular necrosis (hemoglobin)	Quinine, quinidine, sulfonamides, hydralazine, triamterene, nitrofurantoin	Elevated LDH, decrease haptoglobin
Allergic interstitial nephritis	Penicillins, rifampin, sulfonamides, thiazides, cimetidine,phenytoin, allopurinol, furosemide, NSAIDS, ciprofloxacin, pantoprazole, omeprazole, atazanavir, bevacizumab	Rash, fever, eosinophilia, eosinophiluria, pyuria
Osmotic nephrosis	Mannitol, immune globulin, dextrans, hetastarch	Urine sediment shows vacuole containing cells
Papillary necrosis	NSAIDs	Hematuria, renal tissue
Obstruction (intratubular precipitation)	Acyclovir, methotrexate, sulfonamides, triamterene, indinavir, foscarnet, gancyclovir	Sediment might be benign despite obstruction
Obstruction (post renal)	Methylsergide, ergotamine, methyl dopa, hydalazine	Benign sediment, hydronephrosis
Thrombotic microangiopathy	Mitomycin, cyclosporin, bevacizumab, gemcitabine	Decreased hemoglobin, haptoglobin, elevated LDH, schistocytes

inhibitors (ACEI) or angiotensin receptor blockers (ARBs) when used concomitantly with NSAIDs leads to a reduced prostaglandin synthesis, renal vasoconstriction and AKI [16]. Because the kidney medulla is relatively hypoxic [17], a decrease in medullary blood flow may exacerbate the already hypoxic medulla leading to AKI. Radiocontrast agents in addition to being a direct tubule toxin induces vasoconstriction [18] and when administered in patients using NSAIDS may lead to AKI[19]. Vasopressors, often used in the ICU's, as well as amphotericin can precipitate AKI when NSAIDs are concomitantly used. Similarly, acute nephrotoxicity due to calcineurin inhibitors, and vasopressors contributes to toxicity especially when used with NSAIDs. The renal effects of NSAIDS are dose, drug and duration related. Aspirin is the least likely to cause AKI but nonselective and selective NSAIDS were associated with AKI [20]. In a nested case-controlled study, new NSAID users were followed for hospitalization with a diagnosis of AKI. Within 30 days of therapy the relative risk for AKI was similar for rofecoxib (RR = 2.31, 95% CI: 1.73, 3.08), naproxen (RR = 2.42, 95% CI: 1.52, 3.85), and nonselective, non-naproxen NSAIDs (RR = 2.30, 95% CI: 1.60, 3.32) and celecoxib (RR =1.54, 95% CI: 1.14, 2.09 were similar [20]. Thus despite the selectivity of Cox-2 inhibitors they do not seem to have renal sparing effects and the nephrotoxic potential is similar to COX-1 inhibitors [20, 21, 22].

ACEI/ARBs

ACEI and ARBs are commonly prescribed drugs used for hypertension, congestive heart failure and in chronic kidney disease. These drugs affect renal hemodynamics through an decrease in efferent arteriolar tone and intraglomerular capillary pressure [23]. The use of these drugs under normal circumstances when renal perfusion is adequate poses very little problem. However when these drugs are used in states of prerenal azotemia, renal artery stenosis or concomitantly with other drugs such as NSAIDs, renal failure may ensue. In general AKI under these circumstances is reversible following their discontinuation.

Other drugs that cause altered glomerular hemodynamics

Drugs such as cyclosporine and tacrolimus, belong to a class of commonly used immunsuppressants for organ transplantation referred to as calcineurin inhibitors. Calcineurin inhibitors are associated with early prerenal azotemia and oliguria (<50 mL/h urine output) due to vasoconstriction [24]. Calcineurin inhibitor-induced vasoconstriction is thought to be due to: 1) effects on the endothelium, 2) an increase in sympathetic activity, 3) an increase in adenosine 4) a relative decrease of nitric oxide and transforming growth factor-beta 1, and 4) an increase in endothelin-1, reactive oxygen and nitrogen species [25-27]. Other factors that may lead to renal vasoconstriction are drugs such as NSAIDs and ACEI/ARBs. In addition, drugs that may increase blood levels of calcineurin inhibitors such as ketoconazole are likely to lead to an increase in nephrotoxicity. Cyclosporine metabolism occurs in the liver via hepatic cytochrome P-450 microsomal enzymes [28]. Ketoconazole, an imidazole derivative, inhibits the cytochrome P-450 enzyme system leading to an increase in cyclosporine levels and potential toxicity. The early AKI from calcineurin inhibitors associated with prerenal indices is rapidly reversible upon discontinuation of the drug.

Intrinsic acute kidney injury

Acute kidney injury may be due to tissue parenchymal injury as manifested by direct tubule toxicity, acute interstitial nephritis, osmotic nephrosis and thrombotic microangiopathy.

Acute tubular necrosis

Direct tubule injury occurs with different classes of drugs and is commonly associated with antibiotics, chemotherapeutic agents, bisophosphonates, immunosuppressive agents and contrast agents (Table 1).

Cidofovir or tenovir, antiviral nucleotide analogues with activity against DNA viruses are associated with dose dependent AKI in 12-24% of patients [29] with urinary abnormalities that resemble Fanconi's syndrome (proteinuria, glucosuria, and bicarbonate wasting [30, 31]. The predilection for proximal tubule injury is due to its uptake in this segment across the basolateral membrane by the human organic anion transporter (hOAT) [32]. Probenecid blocks this transporter and reduces the cytotoxicity by reducing intracellular accumulation of these drugs [32]. Renal function usually improves upon discontinuing antiviral nucleotide analogues however they can lead to end stage renal disease [33].

Aminoglycosides including gentamicin, tobramycin, amikacin, streptomycin, neomycin, kanamycin, paromomycin, netilmicin, and spectinomycin are approved by the Food and Drug Administration (FDA) for clinical use in the United States. Gentamicin, tobramycin, and amikacin are the most frequently prescribed for use intravenously although tobramycin has been prescribed for inhaled use especially in patients with cystic fibrosis. All forms have been associated with AKI (7-9%) [34-36] including inhaled tobramycin [37, 38]. The renal toxicity was reported to be 3.9%, 30%, 30% in the first week, during the second week and after 2 weeks of therapy, respectively [39]. Aminoglycosides are organic bases that are freely filtered and taken up by megalin located on the apical membrane of the S_1/S_2 segments of the proximal tubule and collecting duct. Aminoglycosides rapidly traffick retrogradely through the Golgi complex and to the ER and are finally released into the cytosol [40]. Renal toxicity is frequently reversible. Risk factors for aminoglycoside-induced nephrotoxicity include sepsis, preexisting renal disease, age, diabetes, liver disease, hypovolemia, concurrent use of other drugs or exposure to contrast and the use of diuretics [29].

Allergic interstitial nephritis (AIN)

Drugs may produce an idiosyncratic or allergic reaction leading to inflammation and infiltration of immune cells such as lymphocytes, monocytes, plasma cells and eosinophils leading to injury to the renal tubules and interstitium. Renal dysfunction in drug-induced AIN is believed to be the cause of AKI in 3-15% of all cases [41, 42] and 27% of undiagnosed cases with normal size kidneys by ultrasound [43]. Most cases of AIN in the ICU stem from antibiotics due to the frequency of sepsis encountered requiring multiple antibiotics. A number of drugs have been associated with AIN including beta-lactams, quinolones, rifampin, macrolides, sulfonamides, NSAIDS, diuretics, cimetidine, randitine and proton-pump inhibitors (Table 1). Recently bevacizumab, a recombinant humanized monoclonal immunoglobulin G antibody to vascular endothelial growth factor (VEGF) used in clinical trials to treat cancer, has been reported to cause interstitial nephritis [44]. In addition there are other causes of interstitial nephritis including infections, immune mediated diseases, glomerular diseases and other idiopathic causes [41, 42, 45]. The onset may range from 3 days to 20 days [22] and maybe accelerated following rechallenge [46]. In general the clinical presentation includes, fever, rash and eosinophilia. However this triad only occurs in one third of the patient who actually have the disease. In addition AIN is often accompanied by low grade proteinuria and biopsy findings consistent with interstitial infiltration of immune cells.

Nephrotic syndrome

Bisphoshonates are used for treatment of hypercalcemia, fracture prevention and in patients with metastatic cancer. This class of drugs reduce morbidity from hypercalcemia is increasingly recognized to cause nephrotoxicity [14]. Both pamidronate and zoledronate have been associated with nephrotoxicity that features nephrotic syndrome with a collapsing glomerular sclerosis [47]. The mechanism is unkown and the return of renal function is slow.

Crystal deposition

Drug crystallization and deposition in kidneys cause AKI [48]. The main cause of injury is due to the relative insolubility of drugs in urine leading to precipitation within the tubule lumen that in most instances are pH dependent [49]. Drugs such as acyclovir, sulfonamides, methotrexate, indinavir, and triamterene may lead to crystal deposition [21, 48]. Tumor lysis syndrome leading to uric acid and calcium phosphate crystals may occur in the setting of malignancies. Acyclovir commonly used to treat VZV and HSV infections is associated with AKI particularly in those receiving high doses (500 mg/m^2) over a relatively short period of time. The incidence is thought to be 12-48% [50] [51-54] and in approximately 50% of the cases, the renal insufficiency is reversible. Indinivar, a protease inhibitor used in the treatment of HIV induces crystal formation [55] and deposition in the kidney [56] due to its relative insolubility in urine.

Drug-induced thrombotic microangiopathy (TMA)

A number of drugs have been reported to be associated with TMA. Although a direct casual relation has not been established, cumulative evidence exist for some drugs. Generally they fall into several categories including antineoplastics, immunotherapeutics and anti-platelet agents [57] Chemotherapeutic agents often encountered in the ICU are associated with drug-induced TMA. Such drugs include: mitomycin, cyclosporine, tacrolimus, quinine, ticlodipine, clopidogrel and others (Table 1) [56, 58, 59]. Recently bevacizumab has been added to the list of drugs causing TMA [60].

Osmotic nephrosis

Osmotically active agents such as intravenous immunoglobulin (IVIG), mannitol and dextran induce tubule damage through swelling and vacuolization [29, 61]. Drugs that may induce high osmotic pressures include mannitol and IVIG. The latter case, hyperosmotic damage or the stabilizing agent, sucrose, may lead to AKI. Hetastarch, used in the ICU as a volume expander is known to be a risk factor for AKI, especially in septic patients [62].

Risks associated with acute kidney injury

Despite the significant progress made in understanding the biology and mechanisms of acute kidney injury (AKI) in animal models, translation of this knowledge into improved management and outcomes for patients has been limited. In fact, with few exceptions pharmacological therapies to prevent AKI have not been successful. Thus, prevention of AKI must be a priority to avoid the morbidity and mortality associated with this event.

Preventive strategies rely on knowledge of the risk factors that are commonly associated with diverse causes of AKI, here specifically focusing on acute tubular necrosis (ATN). Three major categories of insults can lead to ATN: renal ischemia, nephrotoxins and pigmenturia (hemoglobinuria or myoglobinuria). It is clear from multiple human and animal studies that several insults are usually present to result in AKI [12, 13, 63-65]. For example, patients may experience bacteremia, sepsis, hypotension, exposure to aminoglycoside antibiotics that individually may not lead to AKI, but collectively lead to severe ATN. This is especially true in critically ill patients. Rasmussen and Ibels examined the risk factors for the development of ATN in 143 carefully selected patients [66]. The following were considered possible acute and causative insults: hypotension (74%), sepsis (31%), contrast media (25%), aminoglycoside exposure (25%), pigmenturia (22%) and volume depletion (35%). Nearly two-thirds of the patients had suffered more than one insult before the clinical appearance of AKI. Other studies [67-69] have showed similar results with sepsis, volume depletion, impaired cardiac output and exposure to nephrotoxins being the most common exposures in those patients developing ATN.

Specific clinical settings are particularly prone to the appearance of AKI. One of the most common and lethal is AKI in the context of multi-organ failure. Liano and colleagues studied more than 200 cases of intensive-care unit (ICU)-associated AKI and demonstrated that 11% had none, 24% had one, 40% had two and 26% had concomitant failure of three or more organ systems [7]. Groeneveld et al found that 90% of ICU patients with AKI had multi-organ failure [70]. Most often, other organ systems failed before AKI was apparent. What these studies make evident is that AKI (especially in the ICU) usually occurs in the context of additional organ system dysfunction and multiple insults (hemodynamic instability leading to renal ischemia, impaired cardiac output, intravascular volume depletion, sepsis and exposure to nephrotoxins). Attention to these risks is paramount to any effort to protect the kidney.

Advanced age is one of the most important risk factors for AKI. Feest and colleagues performed a prospective 2-year study of 450,000 patients and found that more than 70% of AKI cases occurred in patients age > 70 years [70]. In those patients aged 80-89 years, the risk of AKI was 56-fold higher than the reference population of those aged < 50 years. Certainly, much of this risk is attributable to co-morbidities seen in the elderly (impaired renal reserve due to chronic kidney disease, impaired left ventricular dysfunction, diabetes mellitus, concomitant medicine use such as non-steroidal anti-inflammatory agents (NSAIDS), etc).

Other clinical settings that are at particularly high-risk for the development of AKI include: sepsis/infection [4], HIV infection [71], post-operative states [72], trauma and burns [73], non-renal solid organ transplantation [74], heart failure [75], cardiac surgery [76], liver disease [77], bone marrow transplantation [78], and rhabdomyolysis [79]. Within each of these clinical settings, studies have demonstrated several associated factors that significantly increase the risk for AKI (Table 2). Not surprisingly, these factors are remarkably consistent across these clinical settings. For example, in a study of patients with sepsis, AKI was associated with older age, higher baseline serum creatinine values, and hepatic failure [80]. In patients undergoing cardiac surgery, risk factors associated with the development of AKI in multiple studies have

Table 2. Common risk factors associated with the development of AKI.

Clinical settings	
	ICU/multiple-organ failure
	Sepsis/infection
	Post-operative (especially cardiac and vascular surgery)
	Trauma
	Burns
	HIV
	Non-renal solid organ transplantation
	Bone marrow transplantation
	Liver disease
Patient-specific factors	
	Advanced age
	Diabetes mellitus
	Impaired renal function
	Impaired cardiac function
	Volume depletion
	Multiple nephrotoxic medications
	Radiocontrast agent exposure
Medication use	
	NSAIDS/Cox-2 inhibitors
	Aminoglycoside antibiotics
	Amphotericin B
	ACE-inhibitors/angiotensin-receptor antagonists
	Calcineurin inhibitors
	Chemotherapeutic agents (cisplatin, ifosfamide)
	Illicit drug use (cocaine)
	Deliberate or accidental ingestion of toxins (ethylene glycol)
	Occupational toxins (heavy metals, organic solvents)
	Herbal remedies (aristolochic acid)

Table 3. An example of a risk-scoring scheme and its application in predicting the risk for contrast-induced nephropathy.

Risk factor	Score
Hypotension	5
Intra-aortic balloon pump	5
Congestive heart failure	5
Age > 75 years	4
Anemia	3
Diabetes	3
Contrast media volume	1 for each 100 ml
Serum creatinine > 1.5 mg/dL	4
or eGFR 40-60 ml/min	2
eGFR 20-40 ml/min	4
eGFR < 20 ml/min	6

Risk score	Risk of contrast-induced nephropathy	Risk of dialysis
≤ 5	7.5%	0.04%
6-10	14.0%	0.12%
11-16	26.1%	1.09%
≥ 16	57.3%	12.6%

Adapted from: Mehran R, et al. A simple risk score for prediction of contrast-induced nephropathy after percutaneous coronary intervention: development and initial validation. J Am Coll Cardiol 2004; 44: 1393-1399.

been: severe left ventricular dysfunction (especially that requiring use of an intra-aortic balloon pump), prolonged cardiopulmonary bypass, older age, diabetes mellitus, and pre-existing renal impairment [81-83]. This last factor is perhaps the most important with the risk of AKI requiring dialysis approaching 10-20% in those patients undergoing cardiac surgery with a baseline serum creatinine between 2.0 and 4.0 mg/dL [84]. In patients exposed to radiocontrast agents, the key risk determinants for AKI include: chronic kidney disease stage III or greater (estimated GFR < 60 ml/min), diabetes mellitus, volume depletion, nephrotoxic drug use, preprocedural hemodynamic instability, anemia, congestive heart failure and hypoalbuminemia [85]. The importance of baseline renal function in this setting is exemplified by one registry study that demonstrated an incidence of AKI of 2.5% in patients with mild renal impairment (serum creatinine 1.2 to 1.9 mg/dL), which rose to 30.6% in those patients with more severe renal impairment (serum creatinine ≥ 3.0 mg/dL) [86].

Identification of risk factors has been used to produce clinical AKI predictive scoring systems that attempt to better quantify cumulative risk. These scoring systems are most useful *in situ*ations where a possible nephrotoxic exposure is to occur at a defined time (such as cardiac surgery or radiographic contrast exposure). They provide a very useful framework to identify patients who are at risk and thus may benefit from renal protective strategies. For example, a scoring system developed at the Cleveland Clinic utilizes 13 pre-operative variables to predict a risk for post-cardiac surgery AKI [87]. Similar scoring systems have been developed by others for cardiac surgery and for other settings such as radiocontrast media exposure [88-90]. An example of one such risk-scoring scheme for contrast-induced nephropathy is shown in Table 3 [90]. These scoring systems attempt to identify a small number of high-risk patients and thus will have good negative predictive power but will often lack positive predictive power. Many of these predictive scoring systems have not been validated across different population groups and thus are limited in their utility.

One important factor that limits the determination of risk for AKI is the poor sensitivity of serum

Table 4. General approaches for the prevention of AKI.

1.	Avoidance of nephrotoxins Recognition of potential nephrotoxic agents Recognition of high risk patients and clinical settings Avoidance of concomitant use of multiple nephrotoxins Use of lowest dose and for shortest time possible If applicable, monitoring of drug dose Frequent monitoring of renal function Maintain euvolemia
2.	Minimization of nosocomial infection
3.	Extracellular fluid expansion (maintain good urine output, stable hemodynamics)
4.	Avoid agents that impair renal blood flow autoregulation (NSAIDS, ACE inhibitors, ARBs)
5.	Pharmacological Interventions – if applicable (Table 5)
6.	Use of computer surveillance systems

Table 5. Examples of specific renal protective strategies.

Exposure	Strategy
Radiocontrast agents	IV hydration (normal saline) [95] IV sodium bicarbonate [96] N-acetylcysteine [108, 109] Vitamin C [123] Iso-osmolar contrast [124]
Aminoglycoside antibiotics	Once-daily dosing [125] Monitoring of drug levels
Tumor lysis (uric acid)	Allopurinol/rasburicase [126] IV hydration/urine alkalinization
Ethylene glycol ingestion	Ethanol/fomepizole [127] Hemodialysis
Rhabdomyolysis	IV hydration/urine alkalinization [128] ± mannitol [129]
Methotrexate	IV hydration/urine alkalinization [48]
Acyclovir	IV hydration [54]
Calcineurin inhibitors	Monitor drug levels [130] ± calcium-channel blockers [131]
Amphotericin B	Use of lipid formulation [132]

creatinine values for detection of mild degrees of renal injury. In fact, there is no practical, "real-time" method to provide accurate determination for mild degrees of kidney injury. Oliguria certainly heralds the presence of significant kidney dysfunction, but most causes of AKI are non-oliguric [91]. Thus, a relatively large decrease in glomerular filtration rate (GFR) may be associated with only small changes in the serum creatinine (especially true in those patients with normal baseline renal function). Furthermore, the serum creatinine is influenced by variables such as production rate, muscle mass and the volume of distribution. Thus, a cirrhotic patient who may be malnourished and volume expanded may appear to have a "normal" serum creatinine value when, in fact, there is significant kidney impairment [92]. All of this makes heightened awareness of the clinical setting and risks associated with AKI more important in the early detection of AKI. Careful attention to even small increases in serum creatinine as well as attention to urine abnormalities (presence of granular casts) is critical for the early detection of AKI. It is hoped that sensitive biomarkers of kidney injury may ultimately allow identification of patients at the earliest signs of AKI.

Renal protective strategies

Strategies used to prevent AKI can be broadly separated into generalized approaches and those approaches which are more specifically targeted to a particular risk factor (Tables 4 and 5). Certainly improvements in overall ICU care that focus on the risk factors identified above should reduce the incidence of AKI. In fact, early and aggressive therapy of hemodynamically unstable patients in the emergency department using a combination of IV hydration and pressor agents led to an impressive 88.5% reduction in the incidence of AKI [93]. Thus careful attention to volume status and maximization of cardiac output along with minimization of exposure to nephrotoxic agents should be employed in all at risk patients. Agents that impair the critical autoregulation of renal blood flow such as NSAIDs, ACE inhibitors, angiotensin-receptor antagonists (ARBs) should be avoided. Plasma concentrations of selected nephrotoxic drugs (aminoglycosides, calcineurin inhibitors) should be monitored closely and cumulative dose should be limited. Despite these clear recommendations, Weisbord and co-workers found that 16% of patients who were at clear risk for the development of contrast-induced nephropathy never received pre-procedural IV fluids and 8% of these patients were prescribed NSAIDS or COX-2 inhibitors [19].

One strategy to reduce the incidence of AKI has adopted a computer surveillance system that notifies physicians via e-mail messages whenever a small rise in serum creatinine occurs in their patients who are receiving potential nephrotoxic medications [94]. This notification system led to earlier cessation of offending drugs and a decrease in the incidence of severe AKI from 7.5 to 3.4%.

Specific strategies to reduce the incidence of acute kidney injury

Intravenous fluids clearly reduce the risk of AKI across a spectrum of etiologies. For example, in the prevention of contrast-induced nephropathy, one study compared IV hydration with 0.9% saline at 1 ml/kg/hour beginning 12 hours prior to the study with unrestricted oral fluids. The incidence of AKI (as defined by a 0.5 mg/dL or greater rise in serum creatinine) was 3.7% in the IV hydration group and 34.6% in the oral fluid group [95]. Saline-based therapies may not be as effective as a bicarbonate-based solution in this setting [96], however confirmation will be necessary from other centers.

In the setting of sepsis, while IV fluid resuscitation is clearly critical, the optimal form of volume support is not known. Three meta-analyses have compared crystalloid versus colloid solutions with at least no difference or perhaps a slight increase in mortality associated with colloid solutions [97-99]. In a multicenter randomized controlled trial of resuscitation fluids (saline versus albumin), there was no difference between the fluids in 28-day mortality, organ failure, days on renal replacement therapy, days on mechanical ventilation, or hospital days [100]. The Cochrane group concluded that albumin administration in severely ill patients was associated with increased mortality as compared with other IV fluids [101]. Other colloid solutions such as hydroxyethylstarch and gelatin have also been studied and do not seem to have an advantage over crystalloids [102]. In fact, hydroxyethylstarch was associated with a higher risk of AKI than gelatin [62]. In the preoperative setting, the use of IV fluids to "optimize" cardiac performance (as guided by pulmonary artery catheter measurements) has been shown to be beneficial with a reduction in the incidence of AKI from 4.8% to 1.5% in patients undergoing vascular surgery [103]. However, volume expansion to supranormal cardiac indices along with normal mixed venous oxygen saturation had no effect on the incidence of AKI and can not be routinely recommended [104].

In some patients, vasopressor agents are required to maintain hemodynamic stability. Few direct comparisons exist to support one vasopressor over another [105]. However, accumulating evidence supports the use of norepinephrine in patients with septic shock with a retrospective study demonstrating reduced mortality with norepinephrine over other vasopressors [106]. Furthermore, animal data demonstrates that reversal of septic hypotension with norepinephrine leads to increases in renal blood flow [107]. There are no studies that compare the renal outcomes between catecholamine therapy and vasopressin.

One renal protective strategy that is often overlooked is the intensive control of blood glucose levels in critically ill patients [107]. Insulin therapy reduced the risk of AKI that required dialysis by 41% in one trial [107]. While the mechanism of this effect is not known, this easily implemented strategy should be considered in all at risk patients.

N-acetylcysteine has been widely advocated as a renoprotective agent especially in the setting of radiocontrast media exposure. Several meta-analyses have shown that N-acetylcysteine can reduce the incidence of contrast-induced nephropathy by nearly 50% [108, 109]. However, in other settings such as post-cardiac surgery, N-acetylcysteine has not proved to be of benefit [110]. Furthermore, N-acetylcysteine may be of less benefit in those patients with moderate or severe chronic kidney disease [111].

Many other renal protective strategies have been attempted with poor results. Dopamine at doses between 0.5 to 5.0 ug/kg/minute has been promoted as a therapy to increase renal blood flow, induce natriuresis and diuresis and perhaps increase GFR. However, in multiple settings ranging from sepsis, contrast exposure, and cardiac surgery dopamine has not been shown to be beneficial in preventing AKI (reviewed in 56)[112]. Fenoldopam is a more selective dopamine A-1 agonist that increases renal blood flow to the cortex and outer medulla. A recent meta-analysis of 16 small trials has suggested that there may be a small benefit in reducing the risk of AKI [113]. However, most of the studies in this meta-analysis were underpowered and a larger, randomized clinical trial is required before this therapy can be recommended. Other agents that have been used and have shown no or at best marginal benefits include: atrial natriuretic peptide [114], clonidine [115], calcium channel blockers [116], furosemide [117], inotropic agents [118], growth factors [119, 120], and theophylline [121], as well as numerous others. These failures highlight the critical importance of nonpharmacological therapies.

One controversial strategy is the use of prophylactic dialysis to prevent AKI. This has been evaluated in the setting of high-risk patients undergoing coronary angioplasty [122]. In this study, patients with baseline serum creatinine values > 2 mg/dL were randomized to either IV fluids or IV fluids with hemofiltration that was commenced 4-6 hours prior to the procedure and continued for 18-24 hours after contrast administration. The group receiving extracorporeal therapy had a lower incidence of AKI requiring dialysis, a lower hospital mortality rate. However, the invasiveness and cost of this therapy as well as inherent flaws in the study (difference in total IV hydration, lack of N-acetyl cysteine use, difference in loop diuretic use between groups) prevents this strategy from being used more widely.

There are several preventative strategies that are specific to either clinical states (rhabdomyolysis) or nephrotoxic exposures. These are listed in Table 4 and discussed elsewhere in more detail. In these specific instances, these steps, in addition to the general strategies discussed above, may be employed to reduce the risk of AKI. However, it is critical to realize that these strategies are useful only when applied prophylactically to at-risk patients or are applied very soon after a renal insult.

Currently, the best evidence supports the use of non-pharmacological strategies in reducing the risk of AKI. Maintenance of blood pressure, avoidance of nephrotoxins, attention to risk factors and small changes in serum creatinine afford the greatest benefit. In certain specific instances, use of pharmacological agents such as N-acetylcysteine may be of use but more generalized pharmacological approaches to the prevention of AKI have not yet come to fruition. Thus, vigilance and rapid response with conservative measures are warranted in all patients.

References

1. Ronco C, and Bellomo R. 2003. Prevention of acute renal failure in the critically ill. *Nephron Clin Pract* 93:C13-20.
2. Mehta RL, Pascual MT, Soroko S, Savage BR, Himmelfarb J, Ikizler TA, Paganini EP, and Chertow GM. 2004. Spectrum of acute renal failure in the intensive care unit: the PICARD experience. *Kidney Int* 66:1613-1621.
3. Uchino S, Kellum JA, Bellomo R, et al. 2005. Acute renal failure in critically ill patients: a multinational, multicenter study. *Jama* 294:813-818.
4. Silvester W, Bellomo R, and Cole L. 2001. Epidemiology, management, and outcome of severe acute renal failure of critical illness in Australia. *Crit Care Med* 29:1910-1915.
5. Bellomo R, Ronco C, Kellum JA, Mehta RL, and Palevsky, P. 2004. Acute renal failure - definition, outcome measures, animal models, fluid therapy and information technology needs: the Second International Consensus Conference of the Acute Dialysis Quality Initiative (ADQI) Group. *Crit Care* 8:R204-212.
6. Hoste EA, Clermont G, Kersten A, Venkataraman R, Angus DC, De Bacquer D, and Kellum J.. 2006. RIFLE criteria for acute kidney injury are associated with hospital mortality in critically ill patients: a cohort analysis. *Crit Care* 10:R73.
7. Liano F, Junco E, Pascual J, Madero R, and Verde E. 1998. The spectrum of acute renal failure in the intensive care unit compared with that seen in other settings. The Madrid Acute Renal Failure Study Group. *Kidney Int Suppl* 66:S16-24.
8. Schetz M, Dasta J, Goldstein S, and Golper T. 2005. Drug-induced acute kidney injury. *Curr Opin Crit Care* 11:555-565.
9. Evenepoel P. 2004. Acute toxic renal failure. *Best Pract Res Clin Anaesthesiol* 18:37-52.
10. Choudhury D, and Ahmed Z. 2006. Drug-associated renal dysfunction and injury. *Nat Clin Pract Nephrol* 2:80-91.
11. Nash K, Hafeez A, and Hou S. 2002. Hospital-acquired renal insufficiency. *Am J Kidney Dis* 39:930-936.
12. Hou SH, Bushinsky DA, Wish JB, Cohen JJ, and Harrington JT. 1983. Hospital-acquired renal insufficiency: a prospective study. *Am J Med* 74:243-248.
13. Brivet FG, Kleinknecht DJ, Loirat P, and Landais PJ. 1996. Acute renal failure in intensive care units--causes, outcome, and prognostic factors of hospital mortality; a prospective, multicenter study. French Study Group on Acute Renal Failure. *Crit Care Med* 24:192-198.
14. Henrich WL. 2005. Nephrotoxicity of several newer agents. *Kidney Int Suppl*:S107-109.
15. Schlondorff D. 1993. Renal complications of nonsteroidal anti-inflammatory drugs. *Kidney Int* 44:643-653.
16. Dzeka TN, Townley R, and Arnold JM. 2003. Effects of enalaprilat on venoconstriction to norepinephrine: role of prostaglandins. *Cardiovasc Res* 59:250-256.
17. Brezis M, and Rosen S. 1995. Hypoxia of the renal medulla--its implications for disease. *N Engl J Med* 332:647-655.

18. Bakris GL, Lass N, Gaber AO, Jones JD, and Burnett JC. 1990 Jan. Radiocontrast medium-induced declines in renal function: a role for oxygen free radicals. *American Journal of Physiology* 258:F115-120.
19. Weisbord SD, Bruns FJ, Saul MI, and Palevsk, PM. 2004. Provider use of preventive strategies for radiocontrast nephropathy in high-risk patients. *Nephron Clin Pract* 96:c56-62.
20. Schneider V, Levesque LE, Zhang B, Hutchinson T, and Brophy JM. 2006. Association of selective and conventional nonsteroidal antiinflammatory drugs with acute renal failure: A population-based, nested case-control analysis. *Am J Epidemiol* 164:881-889.
21. Perazella MA. 2003. Drug-induced renal failure: update on new medications and unique mechanisms of nephrotoxicity. *Am J Med Sci* 325:349-362.
22. Taber SS, and Mueller BA. 2006. Drug-associated renal dysfunction. *Crit Care Clin* 22:357-374, viii.
23. Zatz R, Dunn BR, Meyer TW, Anderson S, Rennke HG, and Brenner BM. 1986. Prevention of diabetic glomerulosclerosis by pharmacological amelioration of glomeular capillary hypertension. *J. Clin Invest* 77:1925-1930.
24. Scott LJ, McKeage K, Keam SJ, and Plosker GL. 2003. Tacrolimus: a further update of its use in the management of organ transplantation. *Drugs* 63:1247-1297.
25. Lamas S. 2005. Cellular mechanisms of vascular injury mediated by calcineurin inhibitors. *Kidney Int* 68:898-907.
26. Guieu R, Dussol B, Devaux C, Sampol J, Brunet P, Rochat H, Bechis G, and Berland, Y.F. 1998. Interactions between cyclosporine A and adenosine in kidney transplant recipients. *Kidney Int* 53:200-204.
27. Buchler M, Leibenguth P, Le Guellec C, Carayon A, Watier H, Odoul F, Autret-Lec, E, Lebranchu Y, and Paintaud G. 2004. Relationship between calcineurin inhibition and plasma endothelin concentrations in cyclosporine-A-treated kidney transplant patients. *Eur J Clin Pharmacol* 60:703-708.
28. First MR, Schroeder TJ, Alexander JW, Stephens GW, Weiskittel P, Myre SA, and Pesce AJ. 1991. Cyclosporine dose reduction by ketoconazole administration in renal transplant recipients. *Transplantation* 51:365-370.
29. Joannidis M. 2004. Drug-induced renal failure in the ICU. *Int J Artif Organs* 27:1034-1042.
30. Vittecoq D, Dumitrescu L, Beaufils H, and Deray G. 1997. Fanconi syndrome associated with cidofovir therapy. *Antimicrob Agents Chemother* 41:1846.
31. Verhelst D, Monge M, Meynard JL, Fouqueray B, Mougenot B, Girard PM, Ronco P, and Rossert J. 2002. Fanconi syndrome and renal failure induced by tenofovir: a first case report. *Am J Kidney Dis* 40:1331-1333.
32. Ho ES, Lin DC, Mendel DB, and Cihlar T. 2000. Cytotoxicity of antiviral nucleotides adefovir and cidofovir is induced by the expression of human renal organic anion transporter 1. *J Am Soc Nephrol* 11:383-393.
33. Meier P, Dautheville-Guibal S, Ronco PM, and Rossert J. 2002. Cidofovir-induced end-stage renal failure. *Nephrol Dial Transplant* 17:148-149.
34. Bertino JS Jr, Booker LA, Franck PA, Jenkins PL, Franck KR, and Nafziger A. 1993. Incidence of and significant risk factors for aminoglycoside-associated nephrotoxicity in patients dosed by using individualized pharmacokinetic monitoring. *J Infect Dis* 167:173-179.
35. Eisenberg JM, Koffer H, Glick HA, Connell ML, Loss, LE, Talbot, GH, Shusterman NH, and Strom BL. 1987. What is the cost of nephrotoxicity associated with aminoglycosides? *Ann Intern Med* 107:900-909.
36. Baciewicz AM, Sokos DR, and Cowan RI. 2003. Aminoglycoside-associated nephrotoxicity in the elderly. *Ann Pharmacother* 37:182-186.
37. Cannella CA, and Wilkinson ST. 2006. Acute renal failure associated with inhaled tobramycin. *Am J Health Syst Pharm* 63:1858-1861.
38. Izquierdo MJ, Gomez-Alamillo C, Ortiz F, Calabia ER, Ruiz JC, de Francisco AL, and Arias M. 2006. Acute renal failure associated with use of inhaled tobramycin for treatment of chronic airway colonization with Pseudomonas aeruginosa. *Clin Nephrol* 66:464-467.
39. Paterson DL, Robson JM, and Wagener MM. 1998. Risk factors for toxicity in elderly patients given aminoglycosides once daily. *J Gen Intern Med* 13:735-739.
40. Sandoval RM, and Molitoris BA. 2004. Gentamicin traffics retrograde through the secretory pathway and is released in the cytosol via the endoplasmic reticulum. *Am J Physiol Renal Physiol* 286:F617-624.
41. Michel DM, and Kelly CJ. 1998. Acute interstitial nephritis. *J Am Soc Nephrol* 9:506-515.
42. Toto RD. 1990. Acute tubulointerstitial nephritis. *Am J Med Sci* 299:392-410.
43. Brewster UC, and Perazella MA. 2007. Acute kidney injury following proton pump inhibitor therapy. *Kidney Int* 71:589-593.
44. Barakat RK, Singh N, Lal R, Verani RR, Finkel KW, and Foringer JR. 2007. Interstitial nephritis secondary to bevacizumab treatment in metastatic leiomyosarcoma. *Ann Pharmacother* 41:707-710.
45. Hu D, C H, Okusa M. 2004. Polymorphoneutrophilic Infiltration in Acute Interstitial Nephritis of Sjogren's Syndrome. *The American Journal of the Medical Sciences* 237.

46. Markowitz GS, and Perazella MA. 2005. Drug-induced renal failure: a focus on tubulointerstitial disease. *Clin Chim Acta* 351:31-47.
47. Markowitz GS, Appel GB, Fine PL, Fenves AZ, Loon NR, Jagannath S, Kuhn JA, Dratch AD, and D'Agati VD. 2001. Collapsing focal segmental glomerulosclerosis following treatment with high-dose pamidronate. *J Am Soc Nephrol* 12:1164-1172.
48. Perazella MA. 1999. Crystal-induced acute renal failure. *Am J Med* 106:459-465.
49. Fogazzi GB. 1996. Crystalluria: a neglected aspect of urinary sediment analysis. *Nephrol Dial Transplant* 11:379-387.
50. Brigden D, Rosling AE, and Woods NC. 1982. Renal function after acyclovir intravenous injection. *Am J Med* 73:182-185.
51. Sawyer MH, Webb DE, Balow JE, and Straus SE. 1988. Acyclovir-induced renal failure. Clinical course and histology. *Am J Med* 84:1067-1071.
52. Keeney RE, Kirk LE, and Bridgen D. 1982. Acyclovir tolerance in humans. *Am J Med* 73:176-181.
53. Bean B, and Aeppli D. 1985. Adverse effects of high-dose intravenous acyclovir in ambulatory patients with acute herpes zoster. *J Infect Dis* 151:362-365.
54. Izzedine H, Launay-Vache, V, and Deray G. 2005. Antiviral drug-induced nephrotoxicity. *Am J Kidney Dis* 45:804-817.
55. Martinez F, Mommeja-Marin H, Estepa-Maurice L, Beaufils H, Boche, M, Daudon M, Deray G, and Katlama C. 1998. Indinavir crystal deposits associated with tubulointerstitial nephropathy. *Nephrol Dial Transplant* 13:750-753.
56. Reilly RF, Tray K, and Perazella MA. 2001. Indinavir nephropathy revisited: a pattern of insidious renal failure with identifiable risk factors. *Am J Kidney Dis* 38:E23.
57. Dlott JS, Danielson CF, Blue-Hnidy DE, and McCarthy LJ. 2004. Drug-induced thrombotic thrombocytopenic purpura/hemolytic uremic syndrome: a concise review. *Ther Apher Dial* 8:102-111.
58. Medina PJ, Sipols JM, and George JN. 2001. Drug-associated thrombotic thrombocytopenic purpura-hemolytic uremic syndrome. *Curr Opin Hematol* 8:286-293.
59. Pisoni R, Ruggenenti P, and Remuzzi G. 2001. Drug-induced thrombotic microangiopathy: incidence, prevention and management. *Drug Saf* 24:491-501.
60. Frangie C, Lefaucheur C, Medioni J, Jacquot C, Hill GS, and Nochy D. 2007. Renal thrombotic microangiopathy caused by anti-VEGF-antibody treatment for metastatic renal-cell carcinoma. *Lancet Oncol* 8:177-178.
61. Visweswaran P, Massin EK, and Dubose TD. 1997 Jun. Mannitol-induced acute renal failure. *Journal of the American Society of Nephrology* 8:1028-1033.
62. Schortgen F, Lacherade JC, Bruneel F, Cattaneo I, Hemery F, Lemaire F, and Brochard L. 2001. Effects of hydroxyethylstarch and gelatin on renal function in severe sepsis: a multicentre randomised study. *Lancet* 357:911-916.
63. Anderson RJ, Linas SL, Berns AS, Henrich WL, Miller TR, Gabow PA, and Schrier RW. 1977. Nonoliguric acute renal failure. *N Engl J Med* 296:1134-1138.
64. Corwin HL, Teplick RS, Schreiber MJ, Fang LS, Bonventre JV, and Coggins CH. 1987. Prediction of outcome in acute renal failure. *Am J Nephrol* 7:8-12.
65. Shusterman N, Strom BL, Murray TG, Morrison G, West SL, and Maislin G. 1987. Risk factors and outcome of hospital-acquired acute renal failure. Clinical epidemiologic study. *Am J Med* 83:65-71.
66. Rasmussen HH, and Ibels LS. 1982. Acute renal failure. Multivariate analysis of causes and risk factors. *Am J Med* 73:211-218.
67. SelCuk NY, Odabas AR, Cetinkaya R, Tonbul HZ, and San A. 2000. Frequency and outcome of patients with acute renal failure have more causes than one in etiology. *Ren Fail* 22:459-464.
68. Behrend T, and Miller SB. 1999. Acute renal failure in the cardiac care unit: etiologies, outcomes, and prognostic factors. *Kidney Int* 56:238-243.
69. McMurray SD, Luft FC, Maxwell DR, Hamburger RJ, Futty D, Szwed JJ, Lavelle KJ, and Kleit SA. 1978. Prevailing patterns and predictor variables in patients with acute tubular necrosis. *Arch Intern Med* 138:950-955.
70. Feest TG, Round A, and Hamad S. 1993. Incidence of severe acute renal failure in adults: results of a community based study. *Bmj* 306:481-483.
71. D'Agati V, and Appel GB. 1997. HIV infection and the kidney. *J Am Soc Nephrol* 8:138-152.
72. Liano F, Garcia-Martin F, Gallego A, Orte L, Teruel JL, Marcen,R, Matesanz R, and Ortuno J. 1989. Easy and early prognosis in acute tubular necrosis: a forward analysis of 228 cases. *Nephron* 51:307-313.
73. Morris JA Jr, Mucha P Jr, Ross SE, Moore BF, Hoyt DB, Gentilello L, Landercasper J, Feliciano DV, and Shackford SR. 1991. Acute posttraumatic renal failure: a multicenter perspective. *J Trauma* 31:1584-1590.
74. Wilkinson AH, and Cohen DJ. 1999. Renal failure in the recipients of nonrenal solid organ transplants. *J Am Soc Nephrol* 10:1136-1144.
75. McCullough PA, Wolyn R, Rocher LL, Levin RN, and O'Neill WW. 1997. Acute renal failure after coronary intervention: incidence, risk factors, and relationship to mortality. *Am J Med* 103:368-375.
76. Rosner MH, and Okusa MD. 2006. Acute kidney injury associated with cardiac surgery. *Clin. J. Am. Soc. Nephrol.* 1:19-32.

77. Gines P, Guevara M, Arroyo V, and Rodes J. 2003. Hepatorenal syndrome. *Lancet* 362:1819-1827.
78. Noel C, Hazzan M, Noel-Walter MP, and Jouet JP. 1998. Renal failure and bone marrow transplantation. *Nephrol Dial Transplant* 13:2464-2466.
79. Sandhu JS, Sood A, Midha V, Singh AD, Jain D, and Sandhu P. 2000. Non-traumatic rhabdomyolysis with acute renal failure. *Ren Fail* 22:81-86.
80. McCarthy JT. 1996. Prognosis of patients with acute renal failure in the intensive-care unit: a tale of two eras. *Mayo Clin Proc* 71:117-126.
81. Mangano CM, Diamondstone LS, Ramsay JG, Aggarwal A, Herskowitz A, and Mangano DT. 1998. Renal dysfunction after myocardial revascularization: risk factors, adverse outcomes, and hospital resource utilization. The Multicenter Study of Perioperative Ischemia Research Group. *Ann Intern Med* 128:194-203.
82. Abel RM, Buckley MJ, Austen WG, Barnett GO, Beck CH Jr, and Fischer JE. 1976. Etiology, incidence, and prognosis of renal failure following cardiac operations. Results of a prospective analysis of 500 consecutive patients. *J Thorac Cardiovasc Surg* 71:323-333.
83. Anderson LG, Ekroth R, Bratteby LE, Hallhagen S, and Wesslen O. 1993. Acute renal failure after coronary surgery--a study of incidence and risk factors in 2009 consecutive patients. *Thorac Cardiovasc Surg* 41:237-241.
84. Chertow GM, Lazarus JM, Christiansen CL, Cook EF, Hammermeister KE, Grover F, and Daley J. 1997. Preoperative renal risk stratification. *Circulation* 95:878-884.
85. McCullough PA, Adam A, Becker CR, Davidson C, Lameire N, Stacul F, and Tumlin J. 2006. Risk prediction of contrast-induced nephropathy. *Am J Cardiol* 98:27-36.
86. Rital CS, T S, Grill DE, et al. 2002. Incidence and prognostic importance of acute renal failure after pertcutaneous coronary intervention. *Circulation*:2259 -2264.
87. Thakar CV, Arrigain S, Worley S, Yared, JP, and Paganini EP. 2005. A clinical score to predict acute renal failure after cardiac surgery. *J Am Soc Nephrol* 16:162-168.
88. Fortescue EB, Bates DW, and Chertow GM. 2000. Predicting acute renal failure after coronary bypass surgery: cross-validation of two risk-stratification algorithms. *Kidney Int* 57:2594-2602.
89. Bartholomew BA, Harjai KJ, Dukkipati S, Boura JA, Yerkey MW, Glazier S, Grines CL, and O'Neill WW. 2004. Impact of nephropathy after percutaneous coronary intervention and a method for risk stratification. *Am J Cardiol* 93:1515-1519.
90. Mehran R, Aymong ED, Nikolsky E, et al. 2004. A simple risk score for prediction of contrast-induced nephropathy after percutaneous coronary intervention: development and initial validation. *J Am Coll Cardiol* 44:1393-1399.
91. Klahr S, and Miller SB. 1998. Acute oliguria. *N Engl J Med* 338:671-675.
92. Sherman DS, Fish DN, and Teitelbaum I. 2003. Assessing renal function in cirrhotic patients: problems and pitfalls. *Am J Kidney Dis* 41:269-278.
93. Bagshaw SM, and Bellomo R. 2007. The influence of volume management on outcome. *Curr Opin Crit Care* 13:541-548.
94. Rind DM, Safran C, Phillips RS, Wang Q, Calkins DR, Delbanco TL, Bleich HL, and Slack WV. 1994. Effect of computer-based alerts on the treatment and outcomes of hospitalized patients. *Arch Intern Med* 154:1511-1517.
95. Trivedi HS, Moore H, Nasr S, Aggarwal K, Agrawal A, Goel P, and Hewett J. 2003. A randomized prospective trial to assess the role of saline hydration on the development of contrast nephrotoxicity. *Nephron Clin Pract* 93:C29-34.
96. Merten GJ, Burgess WP, Gray LV et al. 2004. Prevention of contrast-induced nephropathy with sodium bicarbonate: a randomized controlled trial. *Jama* 291:2328-2334.
97. Waikar SS, and Chertow GM. 2000. Crystalloids versus colloids for resuscitation in shock. *Curr Opin Nephrol Hypertens* 9:501-504.
98. Choi PT, Y G, Quinonez LG, et al. 1999. Crystalloids versus colloids in resuscitation: a systematic review. *Crit Care Med*:200 - 210.
99. Schierhout G, and Roberts I. 1998. Fluid resuscitation with colloid or crystalloid solutions in critically ill patients: a systematic review of randomised trials. *Bmj* 316:961-964.
100. Finfer S, Bellomo R, Boyce N, French J, Myburgh J, and Norton R. 2004. A comparison of albumin and saline for fluid resuscitation in the intensive care unit. *N Engl J Med* 350:2247-2256.
101. Bunn F, Lefebvre C, Li Wan Po A, Li L, Roberts I, and Schierhout G. 2000. Human albumin solution for resuscitation and volume expansion in critically ill patients. The Albumin Reviewers. *Cochrane Database Syst Rev*:CD001208.
102. Alderson P, Schierhout G, Roberts I, and Bunn F. 2000. Colloids versus crystalloids for fluid resuscitation in critically ill patients. *Cochrane Database Syst Rev*:CD000567.
103. Berlauk JF, Abrams JH, Gilmour IJ, O'Connor SR, Knighton DR, and Cerra FB. 1991. Preoperative optimization of cardiovascular hemodynamics improves outcome in peripheral vascular surgery. A prospective, randomized clinical trial. *Ann Surg* 214:289-297; discussion 298-289.

104. Gattinoni L, Brazzi L, Pelosi P, Latini R, Tognoni G, Pesenti A, and Fumagalli R. 1995. A trial of goal-oriented hemodynamic therapy in critically ill patients. SvO2 Collaborative Group. *N Engl J Med* 333:1025-1032.
105. Myburgh JA. 2006. An appraisal of selection and use of catecholamines in septic shock - old becomes new again. *Crit Care Resusc* 8:353-360.
106. Martin C, Viviand X, Leone M, and Thirion X. 2000. Effect of norepinephrine on the outcome of septic shock. *Crit Care Med* 28:2758-2765.
107. Bellomo R, and Giantomasso DD. 2001. Noradrenaline and the kidney: friends or foes? *Crit Care* 5:294-298.
108. Meine TJ, and Washam JB. 2004. N-acetylcysteine to prevent contrast nephropathy. *Am Heart J* 147:440-441.
109. Birck R, Krzossok S, Markowetz F, Schnulle P, van der Woude FJ, and Braun C. 2003. Acetylcysteine for prevention of contrast nephropathy: meta-analysis. *Lancet* 362:598-603.
110. Burns KE, Chu MW, Novick RJ, Fox SA, Gallo K, Martin CM, Stitt LW, Heidenheim AP, Myers ML, and Moist L. 2005. Perioperative N-acetylcysteine to prevent renal dysfunction in high-risk patients undergoing cabg surgery: a randomized controlled trial. *Jama* 294:342-350.
111. Fung JW, Szeto CC, Chan WW, et al. 2004. Effect of N-acetylcysteine for prevention of contrast nephropathy in patients with moderate to severe renal insufficiency: a randomized trial. *Am J Kidney Dis* 43:801-808.
112. Kellum JA, and M Decke, J. 2001 Aug. Use of dopamine in acute renal failure: a meta-analysis. *Crit Care Med* 29:1526-1531.
113. Landoni G, Biondi-Zoccai GG, Tumlin JA, Bove T, De Luca M, Calabro MG, Ranucci M, and Zangrillo A. 2007. Beneficial impact of fenoldopam in critically ill patients with or at risk for acute renal failure: a meta-analysis of randomized clinical trials. *Am J Kidney Dis* 49:56-68.
114. Allgren RL, Marbury TC, Rahman SN, et al. 1997. Anaritide in acute tubular necrosis. *N.Engl.J.Med.* 336:828-834.
115. Kulka PJ, Tryba M, and Zenz M. 1996. Preoperative alpha2-adrenergic receptor agonists prevent the deterioration of renal function after cardiac surgery: results of a randomized, controlled trial. *Crit Care Med* 24:947-952.
116. Amano J, Suzuki A, Sunamori M, and Tofukuji M. 1995. Effect of calcium antagonist diltiazem on renal function in open heart surgery. *Chest* 107:1260-1265.
117. Weinstein JM, Heyman S, and Brezis M. 1992. Potential deleterious effect of furosemide in radiocontrast nephropathy. *Nephron* 62:413-415.
118. Duke GJ, Briedis JH, and Weaver RA. 1994. Renal support in critically ill patients: low-dose dopamine or low-dose dobutamine? *Crit Care Med* 22:1919-1925.
119. Hirschberg R, Kopple J, Lipsett P, et al. 1999. Multicenter clinical trial of recombinant human insulin-like growth factor I in patients with acute renal failure. *Kidney Int* 55:2423-2432.
120. Takala J, Ruokonen E, Webster NR, Nielsen MS, Zandstra DF, Vundelinckx G, and Hinds CJ. 1999. Increased mortality associated with growth hormone treatment in critically ill adults. *N Engl J Med* 341:785-792.
121. Ix JH, McCulloch CE, and Chertow GM. 2004. Theophylline for the prevention of radiocontrast nephropathy: a meta-analysis. *Nephrol Dial Transplant* 19:2747-2753.
122. Marenzi G, Marana I, Lauri G, Assanelli E, Grazi M, Campodonico J, Trabattoni D, Fabbiocchi F, Montorsi P, and Bartorelli AL. 2003. The prevention of radiocontrast-agent-induced nephropathy by hemofiltration. *N Engl J Med* 349:1333-1340.
123. Spargias K, Alexopoulos E, Kyrzopoulos S, et al. 2004. Ascorbic acid prevents contrast-mediated nephropathy in patients with renal dysfunction undergoing coronary angiography or intervention. *Circulation* 110:2837-2842.
124. Liss P, Persson PB, Hansell P, and Lagerqvist B. 2006. Renal failure in 57 925 patients undergoing coronary procedures using iso-osmolar or low-osmolar contrast media. *Kidney Int* 70:1811-1817.
125. Humes HD, Weinberg JM, and Knauss TC. 1982. Clinical and pathophysiologic aspects of aminoglycoside nephrotoxicity. *Am J Kidney Dis* 2:5-29.
126. Rampello E, Fricia T, and Malaguarnera M. 2006. The management of tumor lysis syndrome. *Nat Clin Pract Oncol* 3:438-447.
127. Megarbane B, Borron SW, and Baud FJ. 2005. Current recommendations for treatment of severe toxic alcohol poisonings. *Intensive Care Med* 31:189-195.
128. Ron D, Taitelman U, Michaelson M, Bar-Joseph G, Bursztein S, and Better OS. 1984. Prevention of acute renal failure in traumatic rhabdomyolysis. *Arch Intern Med* 144:277-280.
129. Homsi E, Barreiro MF, Orlando JM, and Higa EM. 1997. Prophylaxis of acute renal failure in patients with rhabdomyolysis. *Ren Fail* 19:283-288.
130. Olyaei AJ, de Mattos AM, and Bennett WM. 1999. Immunosuppressant-induced nephropathy: pathophysiology, incidence and management. *Drug Saf* 21:471-488.
131. Ladefoged SD, and Andersen CB. 1994. Calcium channel blockers in kidney transplantation. *Clin Transplant* 8:128-133.
132. Deray G. 2002 Feb. Amphotericin B nephrotoxicity. *J Antimicrob Chemother* 49 Suppl 1:37-41.

03

Renal handling of drugs and xenobiotics

Marc E. DE BROE[1] & Françoise ROCH-RAMEL[2 †]

[1]University of Antwerp, Belgium
[2]Université de Lausanne, Switzerland

Introduction

Pharmacology and clinical pharmacology define the desirable and undesirable effects of drugs and xenobiotics whereas pharmacokinetics defines the various processes that are involved in absorption - distribution - elimination of these agents. Needless to say that the former may strongly influence the latter.

The kidney and the liver have complementary functions in the elimination of drugs and xenobiotics. Lipophilic non-ionic substances of molecular weight higher than 300-500 dalton and highly bound to proteins appear to be eliminated by the liver, while the kidney prefers hydrophilic substances of molecular weight smaller than approximately 500 daltons. Metabolism occurs predominantly in the liver, transforming the original substance into more polar and more hydrophilic metabolites, which became dependent on the kidney for elimination. Consequently, the majority of all drugs and xenobiotics in one way or another have to pass through the kidney. In addition to this important "gateway" function of substances, which are not always without side-effects, the kidney itself is particularly sensitive to drugs and xenobiotics.

This susceptibility of the kidney to nephrotoxic injury has several reasons (Table 1). Renal blood flow

(25% of the resting cardiac output) exceeds 1000 ml/min = 3.5 ml/g of renal tissue/min. Compared to the majority of other tissues, except the brain, this results in a fifty times higher rate of drug delivery.

The kidney has the greatest endothelial surface per gram of tissue and possesses the highest capillary hydrostatic pressure favoring trapping of circulating antigen and *in situ* immune complexes formation. Tubular transport and other renal metabolic processes utilize considerable oxygen and are susceptible to the action of metabolic inhibitors. It is worthwhile to note that the S3-segment of the proximal tubule has the highest rate of oxygen delivery/oxygen consumption of all functional entities in the body [1]. The kidney is the only place where highly protein bound drugs dissociate, traverse the tubular cells and either accumulate within the proximal tubular epithelium and/or reach the tubular lumen. An abundance of tubular epithelial enzymes involved in the tubular transport systems can be blocked, particularly in view of the highly concentrated solutes in the tubular fluid that may reach urinary/plasma concentration ratios exceeding 1000 in some cases.

In the distal part of the nephron, urine is concentrated and the likelihood of crystalline precipitation increases substantially, particularly if urinary pH favors decreased solubility. As the urinary concentrating process also involves the counter-current mechanism, solute concentrations in the medullary interstitium can reach values several times higher than tissues elsewhere in the body. Finally during the process of renal excretion, a particular drug may undergo bioactivation resulting in reactive metabolites [2].

The kidney possesses several mechanisms for the renal handling/excretion of drugs and xenobiotics.

Table 1. Vulnerability of the kidney.

Important blood flow (1/4 cardiac output)
High metabolic activity
Largest endothelial surface by weight
Multiple enzyme systems
Transcellular transport
Concentration of substances
Protein unbinding

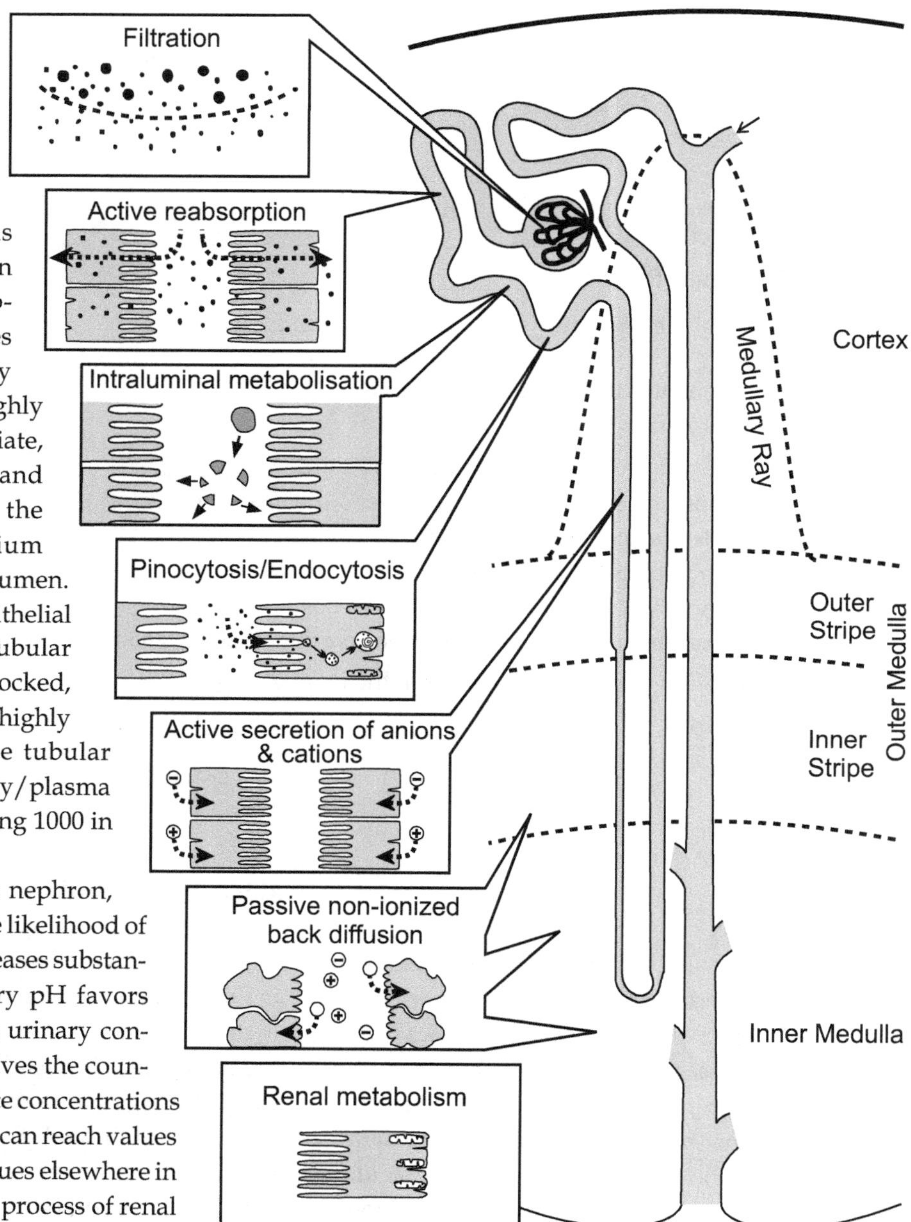

Figure 1. *Schematic representation and main localisation along the nephron of the various patterns of drug and xenobiotic handling by the kidney.*

They are listed in Figure 1 and each of them will be briefly discussed in this chapter. Numerous, if not the majority of drugs and xenobiotics, are handled-eliminated at least partly by the kidney. For their elimination by the kidney they use one, or in most cases, two or even more mechanisms (Figure 2). In addition many other polar metabolites are formed by metabolism or conjugates by the liver, which are then excreted by the kidney. The use of various *in vitro* and *in vivo* techniques as models in studying drug transport in the kidney and/or renal toxicology is well documented in the literature [3-7]. Each approach possesses its own advantages and disadvantages and all have demonstrated their usefulness and application in renal pharmacokinetics/toxicology. A representative listing of these models, summarizing their most relevant characteristics, is presented in Table 2 [6, 8].

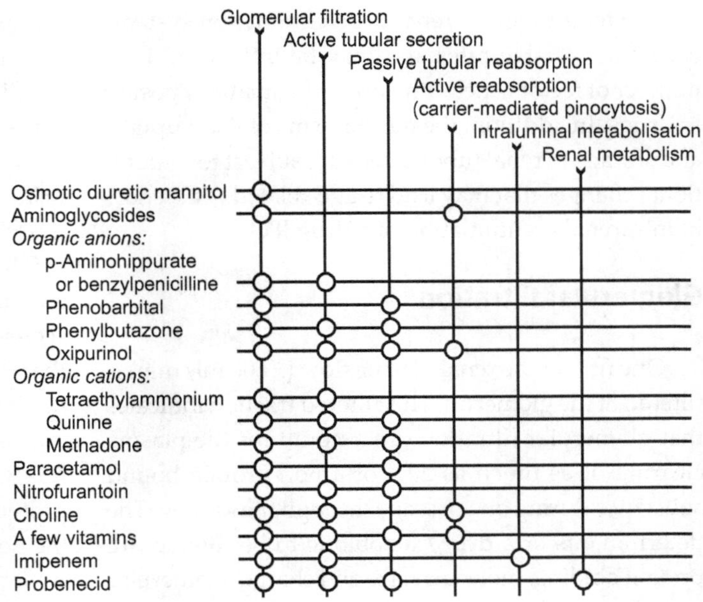

Figure 2. *Most drugs and xenobiotics have a renal handling consisting in more than one pattern.*

Table 2. *In vitro* methods for studying drug transport in the kidney

Method	Advantages	Disadvantages
Stop-flow	Easy to determine net direction of transport.	No precise anatomical localization.
Isolated perfused kidney	Morphologically identical to kidney *in vivo*. Can monitor renal function.	Short term use. In the process of degeneration.
Kidney slices	Easy technique. Good control of experimental conditions without concern for secondary effects due to hemodynamic changes.	Functional status of tubular lumen not clear. Tissue not homogenous and contains nontubular elements. Diffusion barrier for substrates to nephrons beneath the cut surface.
Micropuncture	Can study transepithelial transport in surface portions of proximal and distal tubules.	Cannot study deep segments.
Time resolved two-photon microscopy [8a,b]	Can study several segments of the nephron	Expensive methodology
Proximal tubular suspensions	Relatively homogenous cell population.	Contribution of luminal uptake is dependent on luminal openings and can vary. Short term use.
Cultures	Long-term storage. Precise control of growing environment. Cell population is relatively homogenous. Cells on filters permit study of bidirectional transport.	Dedifferentiation. Sterile conditions for culture.
Cell lines	Easily obtained and subcultured.	Origin ill-defined. Important dedifferentiation.
Primary cultures	Closely related to fresh tissue. Origin identified.	More difficult to prepare and maintain.
Vesicles	Transport in apical and basolateral membranes can be studied separately. No metabolism. No intracellular sequestration.	Membrane isolation may alter physiological function. Must correct for non-mediated transport.

Adapted from Williams & Rush [6] and Brater et al [8].

The maturation of renal drug elimination systems occurs at variable rates and may be influenced by a number of factors, including pre-or postnatal exposure to drugs. In addition, the mechanisms of drug uptake and storage in renal tubular cells are subject to maturational changes that may lead to age-related differences in intrarenal accumulation of a drug [8c].

Glomerular filtration

One fifth of the renal plasma flow (± 600 ml/min) is filtered at the glomeruli. This filtered fraction indicates that glomerular filtration can account for the plasma clearing of as much as 20% of a non-protein bound substance during one passage through the kidney. The determinants of a drug/xenobiotic to be filtered are protein binding, molecular size and charge, glomerular integrity and the number of filtering nephrons. Glomerular pores (± 75 A in diameter) allow passage of molecules up to the molecular weight of approximately 60, 000 dalton. The vast majority of drugs/xenobiotics are approximately two orders of magnitude smaller than this. For many drugs however, protein binding restricts filtration so that only the unbound fraction can be filtered (e.g. furosemide 95% and NSAID 98% bound to albumin), and in many cases depend on active tubular secretion for renal elimination. Drugs can bind to several serum proteins, however, by far the most important being albumin, followed by a α1-acid glycoprotein, an acute phase reactant. Acidic compounds preferentially bind to albumin [9] whereas for basic compounds binding to α1-acid glycoprotein is more important [10].

Nephrotic syndrome induces two important changes concerning protein binding. Hypoproteinemia causes a decrease in protein binding and the integrity of the glomerulus as a sieve is disrupted in this clinical condition. Drugs and xenobiotics can be carried with albumin into the urine enhancing renal elimination. Hypoproteinemia, however, induces simultaneously an increase in the distribution volume of numerous substances thus lowering their availability for filtration. The overall result on renal elimination being almost unperceptible.

Total plasma clearance and distribution volume of furosemide were much larger in analbuminemic rats compared to normals, whereas the urinary excretion was significantly lower. Injecting the albumin/furosemide complex markedly decreased the drug distribution volume, promoted diuresis in analbuminemic rats, in contrast to furosemide alone. Injection of the furosemide/albumin complex to furosemide resistant hypoalbuminemic nephrotic patients increased the urine volume. Another factor that may contribute to diuretic resistance in nephrotic patients is the presence of filtered albumin within the tubule lumen. Even when adequate amounts of diuretic are delivered to and secreted by the proximal tubule, much of the diuretic that reaches the lumen in a nephrotic patient will bind to filtered albumin; the protein/diuretic complex may not be effective in inhibiting the Na-K-2Cl pathway [11-14]. In rats with nephrotic syndrome, inhibitors of protein binding (warfarin and sulphisoxazole) restore the potency of furosemide [14].

Uncharged hydrophilic substances prefer glomerular filtration for their renal handling/elimination in contrast to the many ionized organic substances handled by additional nephron mechanisms, such as tubular secretion (e.g. penicillin).

Drugs and xenobiotics that have glomerular filtration as their major way of renal elimination will accumulate rapidly during acute or more chronic declines of glomerular filtration. If in addition the therapeutic/toxic window is narrow, the accumulation will result very quickly in toxic effects (e.g. aminoglycosides).

Renal tubular reabsorption

Reabsorption of weak acid and bases is generally passive, but in a few cases reabsorption can occur via facilitated reabsorption by carrier proteins or by endocytosis.

Reabsorption by simple diffusion

Passive reabsorption is driven by the progressive reabsorption of tubular fluid along the nephron. To penetrate the membranes of the tubular epithelium, whose main constituents are lipids, compounds should be liposoluble. As ionized compounds are in general hydrophilic, only the undissociated molecules of weak bases and acids will be rapidly reabsorbed by simple diffusion [15]. Consequently determinants for the rate of reabsorption are the pKa of the organic acid or base, the urinary pH, and the liposolubility of the undissociated base or acid. Another important determinant

Table 3. Drugs and xenobiotics with clinically important urine pH-dependent elimination.

Weak acids: *increased excretion at luminal pH > 7*	**Weak bases:** *increased excretion at luminal pH < 5*
Acetazolamide	Amitriptyline
Chlorthiazide	Amphetamine
Methotrexate (?)	Chloroquine
Penicillin G	Ephedrine
Phenobarbital	Imipramine
Phenylbutazone	Phencyclidine (Angel Dust)
Salicylates	Quinine
Sulfonamide derivatives	Tricyclic antidepressants

is the contact time of the solute with the epithelium. In antidiuresis, this time is prolonged compared to diuresis, and thus passive reabsorption is increased along the whole nephron, as observed for salicylate (Table 3) [16].

Alkaline diuresis will favor the excretion of weak acids (anions) such as salicylate or phenobarbital. Indeed, the more the drug is ionized, the more it is trapped in the tubular lumen and consequently is not reabsorbed, hence eliminated in the urine. This mechanism can play a role in the treatment of severe intoxications. The reverse being true for weak bases (cations) such as methadone. Acidification of the urine facilitates the reabsorption of weak acids and will retard the reabsorption of weak bases. The magnitude of the effect obtained on organic acid excretion by urinary alkalinization will be smaller than that which may be achieved for organic cation excretion by urine acidification. Indeed, the achievable urinary proton concentration is up to three orders of magnitude higher than plasma concentration (pH 4.5 versus 7.4) (Figure 3). At the other end of the pH scale urinary proton concentration cannot exceed a value of one order of magnitude lower than plasma concentration (pH 8.5 versus 7.4) (Figure 3). The effect of urinary pH on the elimination of amphetamine may be better known to abusers of these drugs or particular sport trainers than to clinicians. Since amphetamine is a weak base, alkalizing

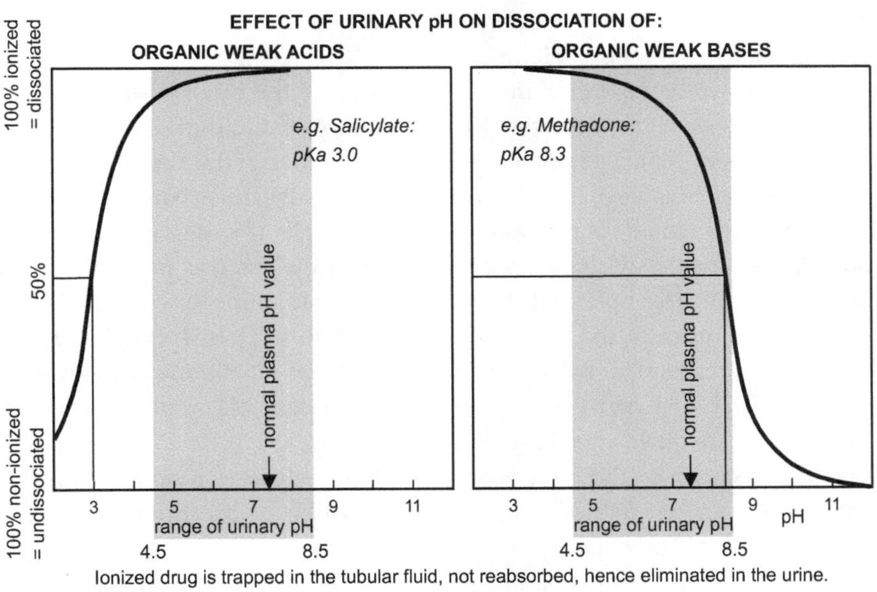

Figure 3. *Effect of urinary pH on dissociation of organic weak acids and organic weak bases. Lipid soluble compounds cross the cellular membranes preferentially in their undissociated form. The ionized form favours trapping and subsequent elimination by the kidney.*

the urine increases the non-ionized amount favoring reabsorption. Amphetamine abusers regularly ingest baking soda to prolong the "high". Therapeutically, it would be important to acidify the urine of a patient with an overdose of amphetamines or phencyclidine (angel dust) [17]. However, one has to take into account that the extent to which a change in urinary pH alters the rate of total body clearance depends on the contribution of renal clearance to the total body clearance. Weak acids like phenytoin and warfarin which are susceptible to a pH dependent elimination in the urine do not see a substantial effect of change in urinary pH on their total elimination since hepatic metabolism is the more important metabolic pathway [18].

There are examples of weak acids reabsorbed by simple nonionic diffusion which urinary excretion is not influenced by changes in urine pH. It is the case if the pKa is above or close to the upper limit of urine pH, as it is the case for barbital (pKa = 7.8), and a few other barbiturates. Also, if the pKa value is very low, such as it is the case for 2-nitroprobenecid (pKa=1.3), the acid remains mainly unionized in the physiological range of urine pH [15], and its excretion remains independent of tubular urine pH.

Reabsorption by facilitated mechanisms

A certain number of drugs and xenobiotics are reabsorbed by facilitated mechanisms. Some organic anions are transported at the apical membrane of proximal tubule by a sodium-cotransport mechanism. It is the case of vitamins, such as ascorbic acid, biotin, panthotenate, nicotinate, and pyridoxine (and its analogues) [19]. Pyrazinoate, a metabolite of pyrazinamide is reabsorbed by a sodium cotransport mechanism [20, 21], as well as by an anion-exchanger [20], which is implicated also in the reabsorption of urate. Oxypurinol, the metabolite of allopurinol might also be reabsorbed by the urate reabsorbing mechanism [22]. M-hydroxybenzoate and morphine-glucuronides are other organic anions reabsorbed by facilitated mechanisms that have yet to be identified [23, 24]. Little is known on the facilitated reabsorption of organic cations. The reabsorption of choline involved a sensitive pathway at the apical membrane [25].

Several peptide-like drugs such as β-lactam antibiotics (ceftibuten, cyclacillin) are substrates of the peptide transporters localized in the brush-border membrane, and are taken up into proximal cells. The peptide transporters mediate an electrogenic H^+-coupled cotransport of di- and tri-peptides, which is driven by the proton gradient and the negative transmembrane potential difference [26]. Two homologous peptide transporters have been identified by molecular cloning methods, PEPT1 and PEPT2. In the kidney, PEPT1 was localized to the brush-border membrane of S1 segments of proximal tubule, whereas PEPT2 was localized to the brush-border membrane of S3 segments [27]. Affinity of anionic cephalosporin without a-amino group (ceftibuten) and cyclacillin (aminopenicillin) is greater than that of aminocephalosporin, such as cephalexin, cefadroxil, cephradine. Because of their low affinity for the anionic cephalosporins PEPT1 and PEPT2, should not play a major role in cellular accumulation and potential toxicity of these cephalosporins when given at therapeutic doses. The peptide transporters might, however, be involved in the reabsorption of the nephrotoxin ochratoxin A [28]. The anticancer drug bestatin, and valacyclovir, a non-peptide antiviral agent, are also substrates for the peptide transporters [29].

The angiotensin-converting enzyme inhibitors, quinapril and enalapril, have affinity for the peptide transporters, however it is not known whether they are transported.

Endocytosis

One of the mechanisms of active reabsorption is endocytosis. Fluid phase endocytosis consists of the incorporation of fluid and solutes in vesicles formed at the base of the brush border membrane of the proximal tubular cells (Figure 1). A more efficient absorptive endocytosis involves first binding of a drug, such as the cationic aminoglycoside and/or may be cadmium [30, 31], to a carrier (phosphatidylinositol) located in the luminal membrane of the wall of the pinocytotic vesicle occurs followed by endocytosis and lysosomal fusion [32, 33].

Endocytosis is a normal mechanism for protein and insulin reabsorption at the proximal tubule of the kidney. A considerable amount of insulin (50%) is metabolized by the kidney, which may account, at least in part, for the decreased insulin requirement that occurs in diabetic patients with decreased renal function. Furthermore, this uptake process allows highly hydrophilic lipid insoluble drugs such as aminoglycosides to enter a particular intracellular compartment (lysosomes) without crossing a membrane.

Renal tubular secretion of drugs/xenobiotics

Most ionic xenobiotics are secreted by two transport mechanisms, one responsible for organic ion (or "organic acids") secretion (Table 5), the other for organic cation (or "organic bases") secretion (Table 6) [34, 35, 35a]. Despite considerable advances in the understanding of basic transport pathways and mechanisms involved in the tubular secretion of organic compounds, there is still relatively little information on the regulation of this transport [35b]. The first step of secretion, transport across the basolateral membrane, of each of the two general mechanisms is performed by several subsystems which may correspond to different carrier molecules, for which substrates of rather unspecific molecular structure may have various affinities [19, 36, 37]. The molecular structure of several isoforms of these transporters has been identified by expression cloning. They are members of a newly identified transporter family, the organic ion transporters, which comprises OAT (organic anion transporter), and OCT (organic cation transporter) isoforms [29, 38, 39].

Our understanding of the organic ion secretory mechanisms derives essentially from investigations on a few transported compounds that are considered representative of other secreted organic ions. For organic anions the classical substrate is p-aminohippurate (PAH) whereas for organic cations classical substrates are tetraethylammonium (TEA) and N_1-methylnicotinamide

Both classical transport systems are located exclusively in the proximal tubule of the nephron. Several techniques such as visual observations, stop-flow experiments, tubular micropuncture, *in vivo* and *in vitro* tubular microperfusions have demonstrated this particular transport capacity of the proximal tubular segment of the nephron [19]. Secretion entails an increase of proximal cell concentration of transported substrates that may become higher than in interstitium, and in some case may result in nephrotoxicity [40-42].

Secretion is not uniform along the proximal tubule, and may differ between superficial and juxtamedullary nephrons. This heterogeneity of secretion, varying between species and substrates, might reflect different densities of carrier molecules along the tubule [19]. Since the number of carrier molecules is limited, secretion is saturable and subject to competition between substrates. Such competition may thus result in drug interactions some of them being of clinical relevance (see below) [43].

Table 4. Transport and renal drug elimination.

Organic anion transport system (Table 5) • organic anion transport family • organic anion transporting polypeptides family
Organic cation transport system (Table 6)
ABC transporter family (Table 8) • MRP's: multi-drug resistance associated proteins family • MDR1/P-glycoprotein
Breast cancer resistance protein 1 [54a]
Multidrug and toxin extrusion transporters family (MATE) [49a,b]

The transport mechanisms of the organic ion transport systems have been characterized at both membrane sides of proximal tubule, mainly by studies in brush-border and basolateral membranes purified from homogenates of renal cortex. Since a detailed review and a critical discussion of the present knowledge in this field was published by Pritchard [44], only the main conclusions are summarized here.

Beside these classical, long recognized secretory transport systems, other transport mechanisms are involved in the renal excretion of xenobiotics [45]. They are the basolateral oxalate/sulphate exchanger and the basolateral sodium-dicarboxylate transport system [37]. These transporters were identified by expression cloning, and named SAT1 [46] and NaDC3 [47], respectively. A number of other transporters has been cloned and identified in the renal brush border, but their functional role in the kidney has yet to be defined [45]. Among them are the multidrug resistance-associated proteins MRP and MDR/P-glycoprotein, which are ATP dependent primary active transporters for organic anions and organic cations respectively [48, 49], and recently the MATE family [49a,b]. They stimulate the active efflux from cell to lumen, of various organic ions. OATP1 is another transporter that mediates the apical transport of steroid conjugates and sulphobromophtalein [50], whereas OAT-K1 and OATK2 mediate methotrexate and folate transport [51, 52]. OCTN1 [53] and OCTN2 [54] are apical multispecific organic cation transporters (Table 4).

Transport mechanisms for tubular secretion of organic anions

The transport mechanisms of organic anions have been characterized mainly for PAH (Table 5).

Owing to electro-negativity of the cell interior, resulting from Na-K-ATPase activity, a transfer of negatively charged molecules into cells occurs generally against an electrochemical gradient and requires energy ("active transport"). In contrast, efflux from cell to lumen takes place along a favorable electrochemical gradient and does not necessitate a direct energy supply. Large cell/interstitium concentration gradients, up to 40 in isolated perfused rabbit proximal tubules, can

Table 5. Organic anion transporter (OAT) and organic anion transporting polypeptide (OATP) families (from [34], with permission).

Name		Substrates	Inhibitors
OAT1 *(SLC22A6)*	Human	PAH, α-KG Drugs: anti-HIV drugs, MTX	Probenecid, urate Drugs: β-lactam antibiotics, NSAIDs, diuretics
Oat1 *(Slc22a6)*	Rat	PAH, α-KG, cAMP, cGMP, folate, ochratoxin A, PGE2, urate Drugs: beta-lactam antibiotics, anti-HIV drugs, MTX	Probenecid, glutarate Drugs: β-lactam antibiotics, NSAIDs, diuretics, antidiabetic agents
OAT2 *(SLC22A7)*	Human	PAH, α-KG, CAMP, PGE2, PGF2α Drugs: AZT, MTX	Probenecid, BSP Drugs: β-lactam antibiotics, NSAIDs
Oat2 *(Slc22a7)*	Rat	PAH, α-KG, PGE2, PGF2α Drugs: NSAIDs, AZT, MTX, zalcitabine	BSP, cholate Drugs: β-lactam antibiotics, NSAIDs, bumetanide, enalapril, glibenclamide, rifampicin, verapamil
OAT3 *(SLC22A8)*	Human	PAH, CAMP, estrone-S, E217βG, ochratoxin A, PGE2, urate Drugs: AZT, cimetidine, MTX, salicylate	Probenecid, BSP, cholate, corticosterone, TEA Drugs: B-lactam antibiotics, diuretics, NSAIDs, quinidine
Oat3 *(Slc22a8)*	Rat	PAH, estrone-S, ochratoxin A Drugs: benzylpenicillin, cimetidine	Probenecid, BSP, cholate, taurocholate Drugs: β-lactam antibiotics, diuretics, AZT, MTX, quinidine
OAT4 *(SLC22A11)*	Human	PAH, estrone-S, ochratoxin A Drugs: AZT, cimetidine, MTX	Probenecid, BSP, corticosterone Drugs: β-lactam antibiotics, diuretics, NSAIDs
Oatpl *(Slc21a1)*	Rat	LTC4, BSP, DNP-SG, aldosterone, cortisol, E217βG, estrone-S, ochratoxin A, thyroid hormones, bile acids Drugs: BQ123, dexamethasone, cardiac glycosides, enalapril. fexofenadine. pravastatin	Probenecid, steroids Drugs: atorvastatin, furosemide, lovastatin, simvastatin
Oatp3 *(Slc21a7)*	Rat	PGE2, DHEA-S, E217βG, estrone-S, LTC4, BSP, thyroid hormones, bile acids Drugs: BQ123, cardiac glycosides, fexofenadine, rocuronium	6',7'-Dihydroxybergamottin, furanocoumarins in grapefruit juice
OATP-A *(SLC21A3)*	Human	BSP, DHEA-S, E217βG, estrone-S, PGE2, thyroid hormones, ochratoxin A, bile acids Drugs: BQ123, CRC220, chlorambucil, fexofenadine, ouabain, rocuronium	Leu-Enkephalin Drugs: anti-HIV drugs, dexamethasone, erythromycin, lovastatin, naloxone, naltrindole, quinidine, verapamil
OATP-B *(SLC21A9)*	Human	Estrone-S, PGE2 Drug: benzylpenicillin	
OATP-D *(SLC21A11)*	Human	Human Estrone-S, PGE2 Drug: benzylpenicillin	
OATP-E *(SLC21A12)*	Human	Estrone-S, PGE2, taurocholate, thyroid hormones Drug: benzylpenicillin	BSP
OAT-K1 *(Slc21a4)*	Rat	DHEA-S, E217βG, estrone-S, folate, ochratoxin A, taurocholate, thyroid hormones Drugs: AZT, MTX	Probenecid, PAH, BSP, folate Drugs: NSAIDs, furosemide, valproate
Oat-k2 *(Slc21a4)*	Rat	DHEA-S, E217βG, estrone-S, PGE2, folate, ochratoxin A, taurocholate, thyroid hormones Drugs: AZT, digoxin, MTX	Probenecid, PAH, BSP, 17β-estradiol Drugs: cardiac glycosides, benzylpenicillin, dexamethasone, furosemide, indomethacin, levofloxacin, prednisolone, valproate

Abbreviations: α-KG, α-ketoglutarate; AZT, azidothymidine; BQ123, cyclo [Trp-Asp-Pro-Val-Leu]; BSP, bromosulfophthalein; DHEA-S, dehydroepiandrosterone-sulfate; DNP-SG, S-(dinitropheny1)-glutathione; E217 β G, estradiol-17 β -D-glucuronide; estrone-S, estrone sulfate; LTC4, leukotriene C4; MTX, methotrexate; PAH, p-aminohippurate; PGE2, PGF2, prostaglandin E2, F2 α; TEA, tetraethylammonium.

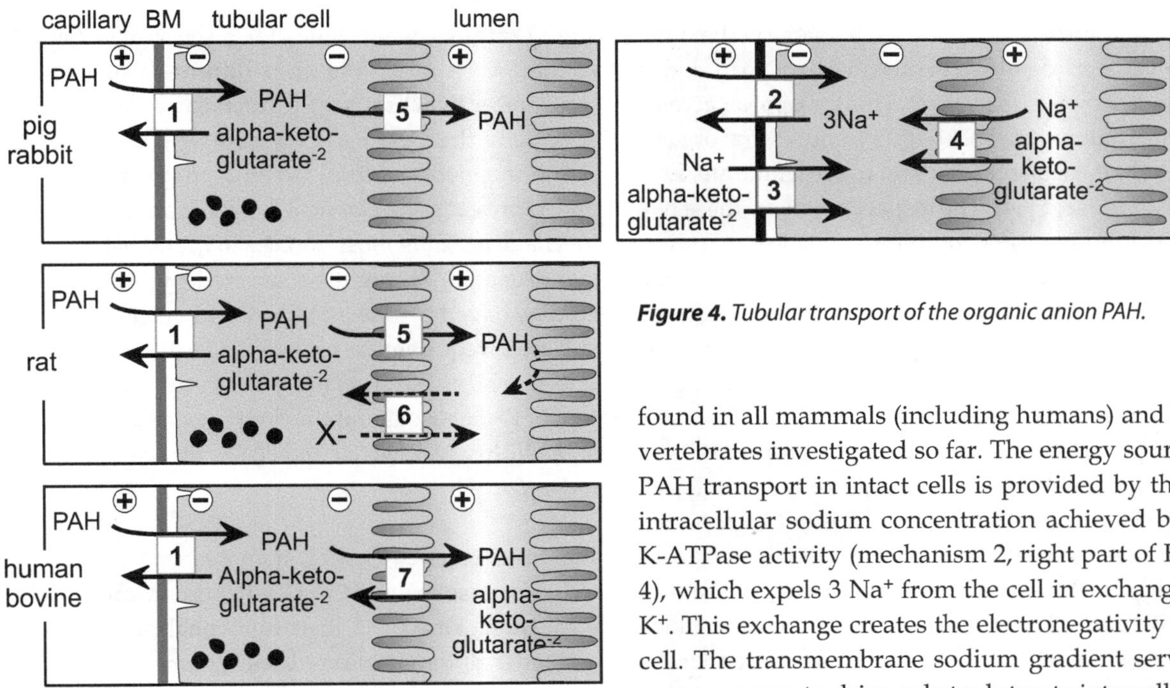

Figure 4. *Tubular transport of the organic anion PAH.*

build up during secretion [44]. However, as only part of the PAH accumulated in the cytoplasm might be free, the concentration gradient of diffusible PAH, between peritubular interstitium and cell might be lower than estimated from total concentration. There exists strong evidence that part of PAH might be sequestered in cytoplasmic organelles [55, 56].

As will be described below, the basolateral transport mechanism, which is the active step in PAH secretion, is identical in all animal species investigated so far, whereas the apical mechanism, which does not require energy, differs between animal species.

The left side of Figure 4 shows a section of proximal tubule and the PAH transport mechanisms identified in different mammalian species. On the right side of Figure 4, the mechanisms shown are indirectly implicated in PAH transport, and are common to all species.

The transport of PAH in basolateral membranes occurs through an exchange with α-ketoglutarate (mechanism 1). The molecular structure of the PAH/α-ketoglutarate exchanger has been identified. Different isoforms of this transport protein, denominated OAT1 (organic anion transporter), have been defined [38, 39] in different animal species. The specificity of the PAH/anion exchanger (OAT1) is high for α-ketoglutarate, the only natural substrate showing affinity for the antiport. This PAH basolateral transport mechanism has been found in all mammals (including humans) and lower vertebrates investigated so far. The energy source for PAH transport in intact cells is provided by the low intracellular sodium concentration achieved by Na-K-ATPase activity (mechanism 2, right part of Figure 4), which expels 3 Na^+ from the cell in exchange of 2 K^+. This exchange creates the electronegativity of the cell. The transmembrane sodium gradient serves as energy source to drive α-ketoglutarate intracellularly from peritubular interstitium (mechanism 3) as well as from tubular lumen (mechanism 4), since both basal and apical membranes possess an α-ketoglutarate-sodium cotransport mechanism. They were identified by molecular cloning and named NaDC3 [47] and NaDC1 [57], respectively. Furthermore, α-ketoglutarate can also be produced by cell metabolism. In the dog, the intracellular concentration of α-ketoglutarate from transport and cell metabolism is about 5-10 times higher than in plasma [58], and is thus not rate limiting for PAH transport. The α-ketoglutarate/PAH exchange at the basolateral membrane (mechanism 1, left side of Figure 4) allows PAH to concentrate intracellularly by a tertiary active transport.

Intracellular traffic of secreted anions appears more complex than originally thought, and might proceed through accumulation into cell organelles (black dots on the scheme), implying high local concentrations of the substrate, and involvement of a microtubular network [59, 60]. While the basolateral membrane transport system appears ubiquitous, the mechanisms involved in PAH efflux from cell to lumen differ between animal species [44]. A voltage controlled pathway (mechanism 5) and/or anion exchanger (mechanism 6 and 7) might be implicated. The former, which is present in rabbits, pigs and rats (data are lacking for dogs) [44], is facilitated transport mechanism that, because of electronegativity of the cell, should drive PAH efflux from cell to lumen. An anion exchanger, on the other hand, has been identified in rats (mechanism 6), and in dogs (not shown in the figure). This transporter accepts inorganic anions (Cl^-, HCO_3^-, OH^-), and several organic anions (X^- = lactate, succinate, α-ketoglutarate, etc.) and also uric acid [44]. The respective role of these two transport mechanisms observed in rats is not known. Indeed, in rat proximal tubule *in situ*, Ulrich did not observe any effect of changes in membrane potential on PAH cellular efflux, and did not observed any stimulation of PAH efflux by anion exchange [61]. The rat and dog anion exchanger which has affinity for urate, is most probably involved in urate reabsorption and might decrease the secretion of PAH by recycling part of it into the cell. In humans, PAH is not transported by a voltage-controlled pathway [62], nor by the anion exchanger that has urate as substrate [62]. The apical transport of PAH is by a PAH/anion exchanger, which accepts only α-ketoglutarate (mechanism 7), as it is the case in basolateral membranes [63]. The same mechanism has been found in bovine [64].

Substrate requirements for the "PAH transport mechanism".

Many studies have been devoted to the characterization of the properties of substrates for the so-called "organic anion secretory mechanism", by measuring the ability of compounds to compete for PAH transport across the basolateral membrane, the first step in secretion. In particular Ullrich et al. [61], investigated the interaction of all kinds of aliphatic and aromatic molecules on PAH influx in rat proximal tubule cells *in situ*. The findings have been reviewed by the authors, and will not be detailed here. The main findings [37], which corroborate older data [36], are that the molecular structure of the transport substrates is rather unspecific, and that substrate affinity depends on the acidity and hydrophobicity of the substrate [37]. These authors demonstrated that, unexpectedly, the ionization of the substrate is not a prerequisite for interaction with the transporter [65]. In general, most anionic xenobiotics are secreted by the PAH secretory mechanism (Table 4), and their secretion can be inhibited by probenecid. Substrates with high affinity are monovalent anions, containing a hydrophobic domain with a minimal length of about 4 A° (benzoyl derivatives). Ullrich et al. also characterized the substrate characteristics for the oxalate/sulphate transport mechanism, and the sodium-dicarboxylate cotransport mechanism, *in situ* in rat proximal tubules [37]. The oxalate/sulfate exchanger (SAT1) and the sodium-dicarboxylate transporter (NaDC3) have a much narrower substrate specificity than the PAH transporter (OAT1), which is the major basolateral organic anion transporter, and represents the classical "organic anion secretory mechanisms". Bisphosphonates [66], and in particular alendronate [67] might be secreted by SAT1. Fewer studies have been devoted to the characterization of substrate requirement for the apical PAH transport. The general substrate characteristics appear similar to that of PAH basolateral transport, i.e. hydrophobicity and acidity, and lack of molecular structure requirement [68, 69].

The molecular biology of the OAT transporter family

Several isoforms of OAT1 (rat, human, mice OAT1) have been cloned and their functional properties examined in different cultured cell systems and Xenopus oocytes. Detailed molecular structures and functional characteristics have been recently reviewed [29, 38, 39] (Figure 5). OAT1 belongs to a subgroup of a newly identified transporter family, the organic ion transporter family, which comprises other OAT isoforms, OAT2, and OAT3. These proteins possess a common structural feature, i.e. 12 putative transmembrane domains, with large hydrophobic loops between the first and second, and the sixth and seventh transmembrane domains. The organic cation transporters, OCT and OCTN are members of the same organic ion transporter family [39]. Human and rat OAT1 has been localized exclusively to the basolateral membrane of S2 segments of proximal tubules, and when transfected in cell systems such as Xenopus oocytes or epithelial cultured cells, OAT1 has the ability to transport a wide variety of organic anions which are known to be secreted *in vivo*. Transport is through an α-ketoglutarate/organic anion exchanger, which is dependent on the presence of chloride in the extracellular medium [70]. These are the same requirements than for transport trough the basolateral membrane of proximal tubules. The rat, human, or flounder OAT1 isoforms were demonstrated to transport PGE_2, cAMP, cGMP, α-ketoglutarate, estradiol 17β-D-glucuronide, nonsteroidal anti-inflammatory drugs (salicylate, acetylsalicylate, indomethacin, etc.), antiviral drugs (azidothymidine, acyclovir, etc.), diuretic (thiazide, bumetanide, ethacrynic acid, tienilic acid, and the nephrotoxin ochratoxin A [38, 39, 71-74].

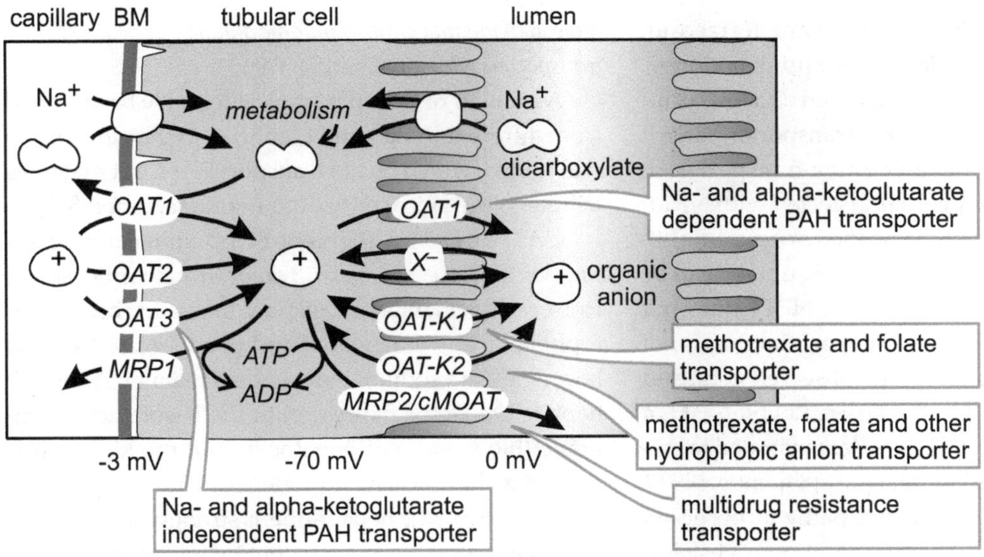

Figure 5. *Mechanisms of organic anion transport in renal tubular cells. Cellular uptake of organic anions across basolateral membranes (BM) is mediated by OAT1 (1), which is an organic anion/dicarboxylate exchanger, and by OAT2 (2) and OAT3 (3). Anionic drug conjugates with glutathione may be extruded from cells into blood by MRPI (4). Exit of cellular organic anions across brush border membranes (BBM) is mediated by unidentified transmembrane potential-dependent organic anion transporter (5) and organic anion/anion (X^-) exchanger (6). Bidirectional transport of hydrophobic anions such as methotrexate and folic acid in the brush-border membranes is mediated by OAT-K1 (7) OAT-K2 (8) may also participate in tubular reabsorption and/or secretion of hydrophobic anions such as bile acids, methotrexate. and prostaglandin E_2. MRP2/cMOAT (9) may contribute to tubular secretion of anionic conjugates of hydrophobic compounds. Adapted from [29].*

The different OAT1 isoforms have some differences in substrate affinities, which might correspond to species differences in transport. For example, urate is transported by the rat rOAT1 [75], but not by the flounder fOAT1 [76] and the human hOAT1 [77]. In human, urate is not secreted by the PAH transport mechanism [78]. This observation gives support to the role of hOAT1 in PAH secretion. Methotrexate and PGE_2 are transported by rat rOAT1 [75, 79], but they have no affinity for the human hOAT1 [80]. Probenecid is not transported by the rat and the flounder transporters despite its binding affinity [75, 79]. Because probenecid, PGE_2 and methotrexate are secreted in human and rat, this lack of transport suggests that other OAT isoforms or transport proteins are involved in their secretion.

Recently, OAT2 and OAT3, two OAT1 isoforms, have been identified. OAT2 mRNA is predominantly expressed in the liver, and weakly in the kidney. In contrast OAT3 mRNA is expressed in the kidney, as well as in the liver and the brain [80a]. The substrate spectrum of OAT2 and OAT3 is diverse like that of OAT1 [81], but in contrast to OAT1, transport is not dependent on α-ketoglutarate, and a concentration gradient is sufficient to allow transport. The nephron distribution, and the membrane localization of OAT2 and OAT3 have not been established. Rat rOAT3 mediates PAH transport [82] estrone sulfate, ochratoxin A. Substrates for human hOAT3 are still to be defined [77].

There exists clear evidences that OAT1 plays a major role in PAH and other organic anion secretion. It is localized in the basolateral membrane of proximal tubule, it has the transport characteristics of basolateral membrane transport, i.e. it is an organic anion/α-ketoglutarate exchanger, and transport is dependent on the presence of chloride in the extracellular medium. The recent observation that the expression of rat OAT1 is strongly increased at birth is compatible with the fact that the PAH secretory system develops post-natal [83].

Molecular identification of apical putative PAH transporters.

NPT1 and MPR2 are two organic anion transporters which have been identified by molecular biology techniques, and which, in the kidney, were localized to the apical membrane of proximal tubule. They might be involved in organic anion secretion.

Uchino et al. [84] cloned and characterized an apical PAH transporter isolated from human kidney, named NPT1. NPT1 was first identified as a low affinity sodium-dependent phosphate transporter, later it was characterized as an organic anion transporter. In human embryonic kidney cells transfected with NPT1, PAH, urate, benzyl penicillin, faropenem, estradiol-β-glucuronide are transported, and PAH uptake can be inhibited by various organic anions. NPT1 does not function as an organic anion exchanger, and thus is not the PAH/organic anion exchanger observed in rat and dog brush border membrane vesicles. Rabbit NPT1, a homologous of human NPT1, was demonstrated to mediate electrogenic penicillin transport [85], thus, NPT1 might be the PAH voltage sensitive pathway observed in rat and rabbit brush-border membrane vesicles. Further studies should confirm this hypothesis.

Another putative apical PAH transporter is the ATP-dependent export pump MRP2, a multidrug resistance protein isoform characterized by its apical localization in polarized cells such as hepatocytes [49]. In the kidney, MRP2 has been localized to the apical membrane of human and rat proximal tubule [86]. Substrates are anionic conjugates with glutathione (leukotriene C_4) or glucuronide (estradiol-17 β-D-glucuronide), as well as non-conjugated substrates such as probenecid, sulfinpyrazone, indomethacin, furosemide and penicillin [87]. Recently two research groups demonstrated that PAH and ochratoxin are transported substrates [88, 89]. MRP2 thus might contribute to the efflux of PAH and other organic anions at the apical membrane. MPR1 another member of the ATP-dependent export pumps that is associated with multidrug resistance in cancer cell and is expressed in a few renal tubular segments, but not in the proximal tubule [90].

Both NPT1 and MRP2 appear to be involved in the apical efflux of organic anions, the second membrane step in secretion. Transport through NPT1 occurs down an electrochemical gradient, whereas MRP2 transport is primarily active.

Recently P. Smeets et al demonstrated that in addition to MRP2, the classical ATP-dependent PAH transporter, there is another PAH transporter MRP4 with an even higher affinity for PAH compared to MRP2, and is expressed at higher levels in the kidney [90a].

Molecular identification of organic anion transporters without affinity for PAH

A number of transport molecules have been cloned from different tissues and identified in the renal proximal tubule, which do not transport PAH, but may contribute to the apical efflux of organic secretion [45].

OATP1. The S3 segment of proximal tubule expresses OATP1, an organic anion transporter cloned from rat liver, which transport bile acid, bromosulfophtalein, and conjugated and unconjugated steroid hormones, in a sodium independent manner. Although hepatic OATP1 is expressed in the basolateral membrane (blood side) of hepatocytes, in the kidney it is located in the apical membrane. In the rat renal OATP1 mRNA, but not the hepatic one, is strongly regulated by androgens and to a lesser extent by estrogens. OATP1 might play a role in the renal excretion of estrogens [50]. A homolog of OATP1, OATP3 was isolated from a rat retina and found to be expressed specifically in the retina and in the kidney. It transports taurocholate as well as thyroid hormone (T3 and T4) [91]. A homologous transporter, OATP2, a liver specific transporter, is not expressed in the kidney [91].

OAT-K1 and OAT-K2. These transporters are two homologous organic anion transporters specific to the kidney, which have been identified by molecular cloning strategy [51, 52]. In rats, OAT-K1 was localized in the apical membrane of straight proximal tubules. When expressed in cultured renal epithelial cells, OAT-K1 mediates both uptake and efflux of methotrexate through the apical membrane, and appears to be specific for methotrexate and folate [51]. Non-steroid anti-inflammatory drugs (indomethacin, ketoprofen, ibuprofen, flufenamate, phenylbutazone) inhibit methotrexate OAT-K1 mediated uptake, but are not transported themselves. OAT-K1 appears to be a site for methotrexate and non-steroidal anti-inflammatory drugs interaction [92].

In rats, OAT-K2, as OAT-K1, was localized in the apical membrane of straight proximal tubule [52]. When transfected in cultured epithelial cells, it mediates not only the apical transport of methotrexate and folate but also that of taurocholate and prostaglandin E_2. In cis-inhibition studies, steroids, bile acid analogs, and cardiac glycosides were shown to have a high affinity for OAT-K2, suggesting that it participates to the apical transport of hydrophobic anionic compounds in the kidney [52].

Conclusions

The molecular identification of various organic anion transport proteins, and the characterization of their transport mechanisms in various cell systems, gives an insight in the complexity of the renal secretion of organic anions (Figure 5). Among these numerous transport systems characterized at the molecular level, only OAT1 and OAT3 have a clearly established role, being the most likely candidates of the PAH secretory mechanism. The identification of the apical transporter for the PAH secretory mechanism remains to be established. However, in contrast to a main basolateral transporter, several apical organic anion transporters appear to facilitate the transport of the various substrates accumulated in the proximal cells by OAT1. The respective role of the apical transporters, need to be demonstrated *in situ*. *In vivo* models, such as transgenic mice, will allow the elucidation of the physiological and pharmacological roles of these transport proteins.

The proximal tubule, the nephron segment which suffers the greatest damage during renal ischemia, is essentially aerobic, with little or no glycolytic capacities in adult life, relying on Krebs cycle intermediates, including the OAT counterion, alpha-ketoglutarate. Thus, along with cellular metabolism and sodium-dicarboxylate cotransporter activity (carbon substrate influx), OAT activity (carbon substrate efflux) might be a key determinant of the metabolic health of the proximal tubule. This hypothesis suggests that circulating OAT substrates might increase the susceptibility of the proximal tubule to ischemic injury, because they are exchanged by basolateral OATs for intracellular carbon substrate. Concomitant with the transport of nephrotoxic OAT substrates (e.g. cephaloridine, cidofovir, ochratoxin) into the proximal tubular cell from blood, there is an equimolar loss of dicarboxylate, which may additionally compromise the metabolic integrity of the cell at the very time when noxious substances are increasing withing it. It is possible to imagine a vicious cycle leading to increased proximal tubule injury in such a setting [52a].

Tubular transport of organic cations

Transport mechanisms for organic cations have been investigated not only for the classical substrates, TEA and N_1-methylnicotinamide, but also for a few other organic cations, mainly drugs (Table 6).

Owing to electro-negativity of cell interior, a transfer of positively charged molecules from peritubular interstitium into cells occurs along a favorable electrochemical gradient and does not require energy. In contrast, energy is necessary for the efflux from cell to lumen which takes place against the electropositivity of the lumen. The situation is opposite to that of organic anions for which the active step is the basolateral transport. The mechanisms involved in tubular secretion of organic cations are schematically summarized in Figure 6. Transport of organic cations at the basolateral membrane occurs by a voltage sensitive pathway (mechanism 1), which was described for N_1-methylnicotinamide, TEA and/or procainamide in rats, dogs and rabbits. Because of the electronegativity of the cell this facilitated pathway drives organic cations into cells. In rabbits, an organic cation exchanger has also been observed (mechanism 2), the role of which in tubular secretion is unclear. As is described below, the molecular structure of a few isoforms of an organic cation transporter (OCT) has been defined, some of which might be the basolateral transporter of proximal tubule.

The Nernst equation predicts that because of the cell electronegativity, passive facilitated diffusion should allow a concentration ratio cell water/external medium approximating 10 to 15 at steady state. In isolated unperfused proximal tubules from rabbits, ratios exceeding 100 for TEA, have been measured [44] and one can wonder if another mechanism exists, for example a cation exchanger, as demonstrated in rabbits (mechanism 2), but which has generally not been observed in rats and dogs [44], which might be implicated in basolateral uptake. However, as reported for anions,

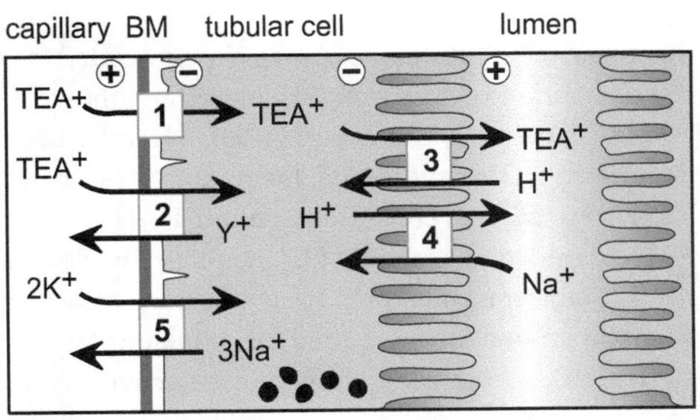

Figure 6. *Model of the organic cation tetraethylammonium transport in proximal tubule.*

Table 6. Organic cation transporter (OCT) families (from [34], with permission).

Name		Substrates	Inhibitors
OCT1 *(SLC22A1)*	Human	MPP+, TEA Drugs: acylclovir, ganciclovir	Choline, matinine, corticosterone, desipramine, dopamine, β-estradiol, nicotine, NMN, progesterone Drugs: anti-HIV drugs, acebutolol, amantadine, cimetidine, clonidine, disopyramide, midazolam, procainamide, prazosin, quinine, quinidine, vecuronium, verapamil
Oct1 *(Slc22a1)*	Rat	TEA, MPP+, NMN, monoamine neurotransmitters Drugs: AZT, cimetidine, cladribine, cytambine, D-tubocurarine	Corticosterone, guanidine, histamine, nicotine, *o*-methylisoprenaline Drugs: clonidine, desipramine, mepiperphenidol, procainamide, reserpine, quinine, quinidine
OCT2 *(SLC22A2)*	Human	TEA, MPPf, NMN, agmatine, monoamine neurotransmitters Drugs: amantadine, memantine	Corticosterone, *o*-methylisoprenaline, progesterone, SKF550 Drugs: despramine, mepiperphenidol, phenoxybenzamine, procainamide, quinine
Oct2 *(Slc22a2)*	Rat	TEA, MPP, adrenaline, agmatine, creatinine, monoamine neurotransmitters Drugs: amantadine, cimetidine, memantine	Corticosterone, dexoycorticosterone, β-estradiol, NMN, progesterone, monoamine neurotransmitters Drugs: cimetidine, cisplatin, procainamide, quinine
OCT3 *(SLC22A3)*	Human	MPP+, guanidine, monoamine neurotransmitters Drugs: cimetidine, tyramine	Corticosterone, β-estradiol, MPTP, *o*-methylisoprenaline, progesterone, SKF550 Drugs: clonidine, desipramine, imipramine, phenoxybenzamine, prazosin, procainamide
Oct3 *(Slc22a3)*	Rat	MPP+, TEA, guanidine	Monoamine neurotransmitters, corticosterone, dexoycorticosterone, β-estradiol, NMN, progesterone, testosterone Drugs: amphetamine, cimetidine, clonidine, desipramine, methamphetamine
OCTN1 *(SLC22A4)*	Human	TEA, MPP+, L-carnitine, acetyl-L-carnitine Drugs: pyrilamine, quinidine, verapamil	D-carnitine, nicotine Drugs: cephaloridine, cimetidine, procainamide, quinine
Octn1 *(Slc22a4)*	Rat	TEA, MPP+	DMA, nicotine Drugs: cirnetidine, desipramine, imipramine, procainamide, verapamil
OCTN2 *(SLC22A5)*	Human	TEA, MPP+, L, D-carnitine, acetyl-1-carnitine, betaine, choline, cysteine, lysine, methionine Drugs: pyrilamine, quinidine, valproate, verapamil	Aldosterone, corticosterone, MPTP, nicotine Drugs: cephalosporin antibiotics, cimetidine, clonidine, desipramine, emetine, procainamide, pyrilamine, quinine
Octn2 *(Slc22a5)*	Rat	L-carnitine. TEA	MPTP, nicotine Drugs: cephalosporin antibiotics, cimetidine, clonidine, despramine, procainamide

Abbreviations: AZT, azidothymidine; MPF+, 1-methyl-4-phenylpyridinium; MPTP, l-methyl-4-phenyl-l,2,3,6-tetrahydropyridine; NMN, N[1]-methylnicotinamide; SKF550, (9-fluorenyl)-N-methyl-β-chloroethylamine; TEA, tehaethylammonium.

there is evidence that part of the TEA accumulated into cells is bound to cytoplasmic organelles and that only part of TEA is freely diffusible [44, 93]. It has also been demonstrated that endosomal membrane vesicles isolated from rat renal cortex can accumulate TEA by an ATP-dependent mechanism [93]. It is conceivable that the favorable transmembrane potential is the principal or single driving force required for cellular uptake.

The efflux from cell to lumen is the active step of organic cation secretion transport being against the transmembrane potential. This active transport occurs through an exchange with protons (mechanism 3), maintained by the proton concentration gradient resulting from the Na^+/H^+ exchange at the same membrane (mechanism 4), mechanism energized itself by the low Na^+ concentration resulting from the Na-K -ATPase activity (mechanism 5). Thus, in all species investigated so far (rats, dogs, rabbits [44], pig [94], humans [95]), TEA and N_1-methylnicotinamide were demonstrated to be transported in brush-border membrane vesicles by an electroneutral organic cation exchange system where one organic cation molecule is transported against one proton. Amiloride, cimetidine, morphine, procainamide, disopyramide, gentamicin and verapamil [96] are also transported by such an electroneutral proton exchanger, in rats and/or rabbits. Larger and more hydrophobic compounds (quinidine, quinine, d-tubocurarine, vecuronium) are inhibitors of organic cation transport, but are not transported by the proton-organic cation exchanger. They are transported by another transport mechanism, probably by the MDR1/P-glycoprotein (see below).

Many studies have been performed to characterize the requirements for a substrate to be transported by the "organic cation transport mechanism" [97-100]. As for organic anions, the molecular structure of substrates is rather unspecific. Hydrophobicity and basicity are the general characteristics of substrates, but their ionization is not a prerequisite for interacting with the basolateral carrier [65]. Similar properties were found in brush border membrane [97-100]. Although the ratio of basolateral to apical membrane affinities may vary with substrates and animal species [97].

More than one organic cation/proton exchanger appears to be involved in the transport of organic cations through the apical membrane, and substrates show overlapping affinities for these different exchangers [101]. Thus, proton-stimulated guanidine uptake by brush border membrane vesicles is only minimally inhibited by TEA, N_1-methylnicotinamide and choline, whereas amiloride, clonidine, imipramine and harmaline are more potent inhibitors [101]. There are also species differences. Cephalexin, for instance, shows an affinity for the N1-methylnicotinamide or TEA transporter in human brush border membranes [95], while in rats it has no affinity for the TEA transport mechanism. At present the molecular identity of the organic cation/H^+ remains unknown, although, as discussed below, two organic cation transporters were recently identified in the kidney, which might be the apical transporters of organic cations.

Molecular Identification of putative basolateral organic cation transporter belonging to the OCT family

Expression cloning allowed the identification of several isoforms of a polyspecific organic cation transporter OCT. The molecular biology of these various OCTs have been described in detail by Koepsell et al. [108], Zhang et al. [109] and Burckardt and Wolf [76]. After the cloning of the first organic cation transporter (rOCT1) isolated from a rat kidney [110], a number of homologous cation transporters have been identified [108]. When expressed in various cell systems, OCT1 and OCT2 isoforms demonstrate a broad substrate affinities and a voltage dependent transport. These transport characteristics made them candidates to be the organic cation basolateral transporter of proximal tubule [29, 108, 111]. The HIV protease inhibitors, indinavir, nelfinavir, ritonavir, saquinavir inhibit TEA transport by hOCT1 but they are probably not transported [112]. Inhibitor potency for OCT1 and OCT2 varies with species [108, 109]. In general human hOCT1 interacts with the n-tetraalkylammonium compounds with a lower affinity than that of rats, mice, or rabbits [113]. Among OCT isoforms, rat rOCT1, rOCT2, rOCT3, human hOCT2 and hOCT3, and mice mOCT3 are involved in the renal transport of organic cations. In rats, rOCT1 and rOCT2 are expressed primarily in the kidney, and are localized in the basolateral membrane of proximal tubule [114, 115]. Both probably play a role in organic cation secretion [111]. The expression level of rOCT2 mRNA and protein in males is much higher than in females, which correlates with the higher transport of TEA in male basolateral membrane vesicles and cortical slices [116]. Because no gender differences were observed for rOCT1 expression in the kidney, rOCT2 and not rOCT1 might represent the main renal organic cation transporter in rats. Another isoform, rOCT3, which transport TEA and guanidine, is expressed in many organs including the kidney. However, because its tubular localization is still unknown, its functional role remains to be defined [117]. In the mice mOCT3 mRNA was found to be expressed in the proximal and distal tubule, but the membrane localization is unknown.

In human hOCT1 is expressed in the liver and not in the kidney, whereas hOCT2 is present predominantly in the kidney. However hOCT2, being restricted to the distal convoluted tubule, does not represent the organic cation secretory transporter in human [29](Figure 7). Human OCT3 is expressed in the kidney and also in other organs, its nephron localization has not been determined [117]. There are discrepancies between Gründeman et al. [118] and Wu et al. [117] concerning the substrate affinities for hOCT3. Wu et al demonstrated a broad substrate affinities for hOCT3, which transports various organic cations including, TEA, clonidine, imipramine, procainamide, endogenous amine, etc., whereas Gründeman et al. concluded that hOAT3 is limited to the transport of endogenous or-

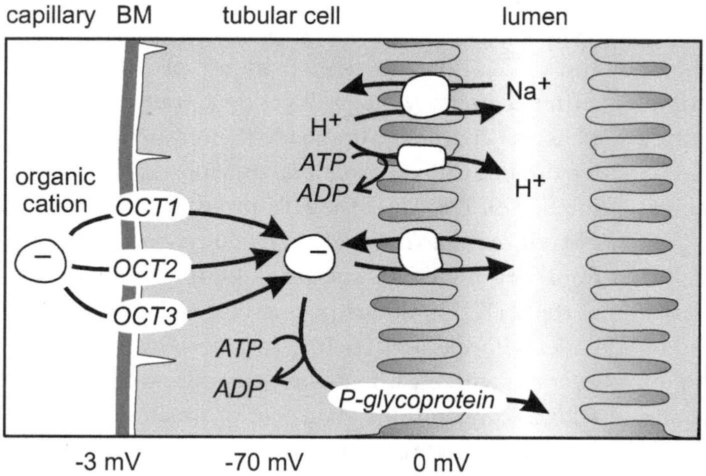

***Figure 7.** Mechanisms of organic cation transport in renal tubular cells. Cellular uptake of organic cations across the basolateral membranes (BM) is mediated primarily by membrane potential-dependent organic cation transporters such as OCT1 (1) and OCT2 (2). OCT3 (3) may contribute in part to the cellular uptake of organic cations. Exit of cellular organic cations across brush border membranes (BBM) is mediated principally by unidentified H^+/organic cation antiporter (4). P-glycoprotein (5) is involved in tubular secretion of hydrophobic drugs such as digoxin, anticancer agents, and some immunosuppressants (cyclosporine and tacrolimus). Adapted from [29].*

ganic cations, such as dopamine, histamine, and that it does not transport TEA. At present human OCT3 is the only transporter isoform that has been implicated in renal transport of organic cations. Its presence in the basolateral membrane of proximal tubule must be demonstrated before one can conclude it is the human basolateral secretory transporter of organic cations.

In conclusion, substantial evidence exist that rOCT1 and rOCT2 are involved in the secretion of organic cations in rat proximal tubule. More precise localization of transporters are needed before determining the role of rOCT3 in rats, and hOCT3 in human.

Molecular identification of putative apical organic cation transporters

A few transport mechanisms have been identified in the kidney by expression cloning, which might be involved in the apical step of organic cation secretion, although their function *in situ* has not been established.

OCTN1, OCTN2. Two organic cation transporters, OCTN1 and OCTN2, were identified in the kidney and other organs of rats, mice, rabbits and human, by their homology to the basolateral transporter OCT [53, 54, 119]. When expressed in human embryonic kidney cells and Xenopus oocytes, human OCTN1 mediates the transport of TEA in a pH dependent manner, transport being higher at neutral or alkaline pH than at acidic pH. The transport of TEA was observed to be bidirectional and inhibited by various organic cations, such as choline, clonidine, cimetidine, quinidine, verapamil, etc., and by zwitterionic compounds such as L-carnitine, cephaloridine, levoflaxin. The transport of a few of these inhibitors, quinidine, verapamil, and L-carnitine, was demonstrated [53]. In summary, OCTN1 is a multispecific, bidirectional and pH-dependent organic cation transporter, which is probably energized by a proton antiport mechanism. Although its subcellular localization in the kidney is unknown, the functional characteristics of OCTN1 suggest that it might be involved in the apical step of organic cation secretion.

In the kidney, OCTN2 is expressed predominantly in cells of proximal and distal tubules, as well as in glomeruli. OCTN2 has the same functional characteristics than OCTN1, but the substrate affinities for the transporter differ [54]. Human, rat and mouse OCTN2 has the additional peculiarity of transporting L-carnitine and other zwitterions such as cephalosporins that contain quaternary nitrogen, in a-sodium dependent manner [54, 120, 121]. Site directed mutagenesis experiments provided evidence that the transport sites for organic cations and for carnitine are distinct [122]. OCTN2 thus might play a role in organic cation secretion, and in the reabsorption of carnitine by a sodium carnitine cotransport. *In vivo* cephaloridine was reported to increase the fractional excretion of carnitine by interfering with its reabsorption [120]. The possibility exists that this type of cephalosporin might be inefficient in patients with primary carnitine deficiency, that are receiving carnitine supplementation, because of competition for carnitine transport [120]. The anionic cephalosporins are not substrates for OCTN2, but they are substrates for the peptides transporters PEPT1 and PEPT2 [45] (Table 7). Conversely, the cephalosporins, which have affinity for OCTN2, are not substrate of the peptide transporters [120].

In recent years polymorphisms of genes encoding proteins involved in the metabolism and subsequent

Table 7. Peptide transporter (PEPT) nucleoside transporter families.

Name		Substrates	Inhibitors
PEPT1 *(SLC15A1)*	Human	Glycylsarcosine, di-, tripetides Drugs: β-lactam antibiotics, cyclacillin, valacyclovir	Valine, pentaglycine Drugs: β-lactam antibiotics, bestatin, certain ACE inhibitors
Pept1 *(Slc15a1)*	Rat	Glycylsarcosine, di-, tripetides Drugs: bestatin, β-lactam antibiotics,	Drugs: β-lactam antibiotics, certain ACE inhibitors, tolbutamide, chlorpropamide
PEPT2 *(SLC15A2)*	Human	Glycylsarcosine, ALA Drugs: bestatin, cephalexin, valacyclovir	Drugs: β-lactam antibiotics
Pept2 *(SLC15a2)*	Rat	Glycylsarcosine Drug: valacyclovir	Drugs: β-lactam antibiotics, bestatin, chlorpropamide, glibenclamide, tolbutamide
CNT1 *(SLC28A1)*	Human	Adenosine, thymidine, uridine, Drugs: AZT, zalcitabine	
Cnt1 *(Slc28a1)*	Rat	Adenosine, thymidine, uridine Drug: AZT	Drugs: cytarabine, floxidine, gemcitabine, idoxuridine, zalcitabine
CNT2 *(SLC28A2)*	Human	Adenosine, uridine, inosine, thymidine Drugs: cladribine, didanosine	
Cnt2 *(Slc28a2)*	Rat	Adenosine, guanosine, inosine, thymidine, uridine Drug: didanosine	

Abbreviations: ACE, angiotensin converting enzyme; ALA, delta-aminolevulinic acid; AZT, azidothymidine

renal and/or extrarenal elimination of xenobiotics have been shown to correlate with drug sensitivity. Gain of function of an OCT relevant for drug elimination will decrease plasma levels and may prevent appropriate therapeutic effects at standard dosage. A loss-of-function polymorphism may lead to increased toxicity in affected individuals. Activation of protein kinase C leads to strong stimulation of rOCT1 expressed in human embryonic kidney cells. Protein kinase C does not only increase the maximal transport rate but it also alters the relative selectivity of the carrier. Cation transporter isoforms do not only differ in substrate affinities but also in regulation. More research correlating polymorphisms of genes encoding transport-regulating kinases with drug elimination is needed [120a].

ABC transporter family

Multidrug resistance-associated protein transporters (MRPs)

The MRP family is a subgroup of the ATP-binding cassette (ABC) transporters superfamily (Table 8). It comprises 13 members (ABCC1 to ABCC13) named MRP (1 to 9), CRTR (cystic fibrosis transmembrane conductance regulator - ABCC7), and SUR1 or 2 (sulphonylurea receptors (ABCC8 and 9). MRP mRNA is retrived from several tissues including the kidney and the transporter is located at the basolateral membrane of Henle's loop and collecting duct cells [120b,c]. MRP1 carries in an ATP-dependent manner different substrates among which are found several conjugated derivatives, sulfates, and GSH. Carrying some non-conjugated drugs necessitates an exchange with GSH. As a result, drug resistance mediated by MRP1 may be counterbalanced by GSH synthesis inhibition.

In the kidney, MRP2 (ABCC2) contributes to the detoxification of drugs and both endogenous and exogenous compounds, mainly under their conjugated form. It has been located at the brush border membrane of S1, S2 and S3 segments of proximal tubular cells [120d,e]. In the kidney, but not in the liver, 8 days following cisplatin administration MRP expression is increased. Subtotal nephrectomy induced a 200% increase in MRP2 mRNA in the remaining kidney.

In the kidney, MRP3 (ABCC3) is expressed at the basolateral membrane of distal renal tubular cells and carries glucuroconjugated compounds and other molecules from the internal tubular cell into the blood. MRP3 was shown to confer cellular drug resistance to etoposide, tenoposide and vincristine [120f,g].

MRP4 (ABCC4) mRNA has been detected in the kidney, at the brush-border membrane of proximal tubular cells. It enhances cell resistance to some antiviral agents such as adefovir and zidovudine. It also seems to play an important role in antiviral drugs renal excretion. MRP4 is also the transporter for cyclic AMP and GMP through an ATP-dependent system and it constitutes the elective excretion pathway for cyclic nucleotides in renal epithelial cells.

MRP5 (ABCC5) is widely expressed in the organism, including the kidney. It is located at the basolateral

Table 8. ABC transporter family (from [34], with permission).

Name		Substrates	Inhibitors
MRP1 *(ABCC1)*	Human	LTC_4, bilirubin-glucuronide, glutathione conjugates, GSH, PAH, fluo-3, calcein Drugs: etoposide-glucuronide, *S*-(ethacrynic acid)-glutathione, MTX	Probenecid, ochratoxin A Drugs: benzbromarone, CSA, *S*-(decyl)-glutathione, indomethacin, MK571, sufinpyrazone, valspodar
MRP1 *(Abcc1)*	Mouse	LTC_4, calcein, APA-SG Drugs: daunorubicin, vincristine	GSSG Drugs: arsenate, genistein, MK571
MRP2 *(ABCC2)*	Human	LTC_4, $E_2 17\beta G$, bilirubin-glucuronide, glutathione conjugates, GSH, PAH, ochratoxin A, fluo-3 Drugs: anti-HIV drugs, benzbromarone, furosemide, indomethacin, MTX, vinblastine	Probenecid, BSP Drugs: CSA, glibenclamide, MK571
Mrp2 *(Abcc2)*	Rat	LTC_4, LTD_4, $E_2 17\beta G$, anionic glucuronide conjugates, bilirubin-glucuronide, BSP, endothelin-1, fluo-3, folate, GSH, GSSG Drugs: cefpiramide, cefhiaxone, indomethacin, irinotecan and SN-38, MTX, pravastatin	Probenecid Drugs: CSA, glibenclamide, MK571
MRP3 *(ABCC3)*	Human	LTC_4, DNP-SG, $E_2 17\beta G$, folate, glycocholate Drug: MTX	Drugs: benzbromarone, MK571
Mrp3 *(Abcc3)*	Rat	LTC4, , bile acids Drugs: E3040-glucuronide, MTX	Anionic glucuronide / GSH conjugates
MRP4 *(ABCC4)*	Human	$E_2 17\beta G$, cAMP, cGMP Drugs: adefovir, AZTMP, MTX	Probenecid, anionic glucuronide conjugates Drugs: benzbromarone, sildenafil, trequinsin, zaprinast
MRP5 *(ABCC5)*	Human	DNP-SG, CAMP, cGMP, GSH Drugs: adefovir, 6-MP	Probenecid Drugs: benzbromarone, sildenafil, trequinsin, zaprinast
MRP6 *(ABCC6)*	Human	LTC_4, NEM-SG Drug: BQ123	Probenecid Drugs: benzbromarone, indomethacin
MDR1 *(ABCB1)*	Human	$E_2 17\beta G$, calcein, fluo-3, rhodamine 123 Drugs: cardiac glycosides, anti-HIV drugs, anticancer agents, verapamil	Progesterone Drugs: amiodarone, amitriptyline, chlorpromazine, diltiazem, dipyridamole, elacridar, fluphenazine, fucidin, lovastatin, mefloquine, phenothiazines, pimozide, propafenone, propranolol, quinine, quinidine, reserpine, simvastatin, spironolactone, staurosporin, tamoxifen, trifluoperazine, triflupromazine, valspodar
mdr1a/ mdr1b *(Abcb1)*	Rat/ Mouse	Rhodamine 123 Drugs: anti-HIV drugs, CSA, dexamethasone, digoxin, doxorubicin, fexofenadine, ivermectin, verapamil, vinblastine	

Abbreviations: APA-SG, azidophenacyl-S-glutathione; AZTMP, azidothymidine monophosphate; BQ123, (cyclo [Trp-Asp-Pro-Val-Leu]); BSP, bromosulfophthalein; CSA, cyclosporine A; DNP-SG, S-(dinitrophenyl)-glutathione; $E_2 17\beta G$, estradiol-17β-D-glucuronide; GSH, reduced glutathione; GSSG, oxidized glutathione; LTC_4/LTD_4, leukotriene C_4/D_4; MK571, 3-[3-[2-(7-chloroquinolin-2-yl)vinyl]phenyl]-(2-dimethylcarbamoyl-ethylsulfanyl) methylsulfanyl] propionic acid; 6-MP, 6-mercaptopurine; MTX, methotrexate; NEM-SG, N-ethylmaleimide glutathione; PAH, p-aminohippurate.

membrane and carries GSH.

MRP6 is expressed in the kidney, at the basolateral membrane of proximal tubular cells. It has been suggested that the loss of functional MRP6 in the kidney and the liver could induced the phenotype observed in *Pseudoxanthoma elasticum* patients.

Mutidrug transporters/P-glycoprotein (MDR or Pg)

The apical membrane of proximal tubules is particularly rich in MDR-glycoprotein ("multidrug transporter"), a membrane ATPase that mediates the active efflux of a wide variety of drugs across the plasma membrane of several cell types. This property explains the resistance of some cancer cells to hydrophobic cationic drugs [102]. It was demonstrated that MDR/P-glycoprotein can extrude many organic compounds (e.g. vinblastine, vincristine, colchicine, cyclosporine analogues) from renal proximal cell [103-105]. P-glycoprotein transport mechanism differs from the proton/organic cation exchanger since it does not transport TEA [94, 105], but the more lipophilic substrate, and vinblastine, a substrate of MDR/P-glycoprotein, is not exchanged against protons in pig brush border membrane vesicles [93].

MDR/P-glycoprotein, which transports organic cations is the analogous of MRP2, which transport lipophilic organic anions. Both are responsible for the multidrug resistances of cells to anticancer drugs. Since some substrates of the P-glycoprotein system are also transported by the proton/organic cation exchanger, it is often difficult to clearly distinguish between the two systems at the functional level. Compounds transported by both the MDR/P-glycoprotein and the organic cation transporter, include daunomycin, colchicine, verapamil, quinidine and vinblastine [106]. On the other hand, secretion of digoxin, which is not an organic cation, is restricted to P-glycoprotein only [107] (Table 8).

In the kidney, P-glycoprotein is constitutively expressed on the brush border of the proximal tubular cells and on the distal tubule [107a] and it has been suggested that P-glycoprotein may be instrumental in cyclosporine A (CsA) nephrotoxicity. CsA is a substrate of P-glycoprotein [107b] and variations in expression and/function of P-glycoprotein could lead to accumulation of CsA, along with other cytotoxic agents, within the tubular cell. An inverse relationship between CsA deposits in renal tissue and the level of P-glycoprotein expression in proximal tubular cells in animal models, suggesting that the normal P-glycoprotein response mat be defective in patients suspectible to CsA-related nephrotoxicity, leading to retention of excess amounts of CsA in the cells [107c,d]. ABCB1 polymorphism in kidney allograft donors, which is associated with decreased expression of P-glycoprotein in renal tissue, has ben shown an independent risk factor for the development of CsA-related nephrotoxicity [107e]. These findings suggest that factors that modulate P-glycoprotein-expression may have an impact on CsA-related nephrotoxicity by causing an accumulation of CsA within the renal cells.

The new immunosuppressive agent sirolimus is also a P-glycoprotein substrate [107f], although perceived as a non-nephrotoxic drug, reducing renal function when given concomitantly with CsA [107g]. Recent studies have shown that administration of sirolimus around the time of renal injury can exacerbate the injury and delay repair, an effect that may be due to a potent antiproliferative effect of sirolimus on tubular cells [107h]. Using human renal epithelial cells in primary culture it was shown that sirolimus inhibits the P-glycoprotein-mediated efflux and cellular concentration of CsA, explaining at least partly the exacerbation of CsA nephrotoxicity of sirolimus.

Effects of protein binding on organic ion secretion

It is generally recognized that the tubular secretory rate is proportional to the concentration of free drug or xenobiotic [123-126], and that plasma albumin binding is not rate limiting for tubular secretion of organic anions with high affinity for the transport system [19, 36], because the dissociation rate of the organic anion/albumin complex is much faster than the transtubular transit time [19, 127]. Such is the case for hydrochlorothiazide [36]. On the other hand, organic anions with lower affinity for the transporter (e.g. phenol red) have a reduced secretion when bound to plasma proteins [124, 128]. Although the secretion of furosemide in the perfused isolated rat kidney can be delayed by the addition of albumin to the perfusate [123], secretion in humans does not appears to be limited by protein binding. Thus, in spite of a binding of more than 95% to plasma proteins, the urinary clearance (uncorrected for plasma protein binding) of furosemide in therapeutic doses is somewhat higher than inulin clearance [36, 129, 130]. Because of the high protein binding of furosemide its filtration rate is negligible and its diuretic effect, which is related to its luminal concentration in the thick ascending limb of Henle's loop, depends on its tubular secretion. Hence, inhibition of furosemide secretion by probenecid inhibits its diuretic effect [131].

Interactions of xenobiotics/drugs for secretion

Probenecid, which was first developed to delay penicillin excretion, is now generally used (besides its use as a uricosuric) to inhibit secretion of organic anions [131a]. Thus, it is generally considered that a compound whose secretion or transport across the proximal basolateral membrane is inhibited by probenecid is a substrate of the organic anion secretory mechanism. Probenecid has also been used as a tool to investigate the role of cellular accumulation of xenobiotics in nephrotoxicity. Inhibition of basolateral uptake of cephalosporins, such as cephaloridine and cephaloglycin, by probenecid, can prevent their cellular toxicity. These cephalosporins have a low extrusion rate through the apical membrane, resulting in a rather high concentration, which is a major contributing factor to their nephrotoxicity. However, it is worth noting that cell accumulation is necessary but not sufficient for cytotoxicity, as shown by cephalexin that has a low nephrotoxic potential despite marked cortical accumulation [40] (see also chapter 9).

The nephrotoxicity of cisplatin is reduced in humans [132], mice [133] and dogs [134] by co-administration of probenecid, suggesting that cisplatin is transported by the PAH transport system. It has been proposed that platinum, like other nephrotoxic metal ions such as mercury and potassium dichromate, are taken up by tubular cells as sulphydryl conjugate through a probenecid-sensitive pathway [133]. However, cisplatin might also be transported by the organic cation transport system, since quinidine, cimetidine and ranitidine inhibited its net secretion flux in the dog kidney [134].

In human, methotrexate is largely cleared unchanged from the body by renal excretion through glomerular filtration and tubular secretion. Rises in serum methotrexate levels accompanied by life-threatening increases in methotrexate toxicity can occur if aspirin, salicylates or non-steroidal anti-inflammatory drugs are given concurrently. The increased methotrexate toxicity observed by concomitant administration of ibuprofen [135], salicylates [135], or flurbiprofen [136] might be in part the result of interaction at the basolateral membrane [137], resulting in a decrease in methotrexate renal excretion.

Excretion of digoxin is primarily renal, by glomerular filtration and tubular secretion and reabsorption. Competition studies have shown that the "classic" anion or cation transport systems are not involved. The secretory process as studied *in vivo* and in a renal epithelium *in vitro*, may be carried out by the apical membrane P-glycoprotein. It is well known clinically, that several drugs (most notably quinidine, verapamil, nifedipine, propofenone, spironolactone, and amiodarone) reduce the renal (tubular) clearance of digoxin and increase the plasma concentration and toxic risks of the cardiac glycoside [63, 138, 139]. Accordingly, these interactions may be explained by a competition at the secretory step controlled by P-glycoprotein at the luminal membrane. Such a possibility has received experimental support for several of these compounds [139-143]

Concurrent use of drugs that reduce renal blood flow in patients with renin-angiotensin prostaglandin dependent renal perfusion (e.g. NSAID), that are weak organic acids competing for tubular secretion [144] and/or nephrotoxic (cisplatin) can delay drug excretion [145] and lead to severe myelosuppression.

Interactions of cimetidine and other H_2-receptor antagonists with the renal secretion of several drugs have been repeatedly described, and comprehensively listed [146]. Thus, cimetidine inhibits renal secretion of procainamide in humans and prolongs its elimination half-life [147, 148]. Similar inhibitory effects have been shown on creatinine, ranitidine and many other cationic compounds [149].

Interactions between organic anion and organic cation secretion

Clinical significant interactions occur only when the affected transporter represents the major pathway for the overall elimination. Because of the involvement of multiple renal processes (i.e. filtration, tubular secretion, tubular reabsorption) in renal drug handling and the functional redundancy of some renal drug transporters, severe clinical drug-drug interactions at the renal level seem to be not very common. Clinical relevance of renal drug-drug interactions needs to be evaluated in the context of efficacy and safety profile of the affected drug. *In vitro* transporter interaction screening during preclinical development should be performed for all drug candidates that have a narrow therapeutic window [131a].

The lack of strict structural requirements for substrates in organic anion and cation transport systems, the prominent role of substrate hydrophobicity in the interaction with both classes of carriers, and the ability of non-ionized substrates to interact with the transporters, are all factors explaining that some substrates might be transported by both transport systems [37]. For example, the renal excretion of cimetidine and famotidine, two organic cations, is reduced by probenecid [150, 151]. *In vitro* also, cimetidine uptake by brush border membrane vesicles is inhibited by probenecid or furosemide, and cimetidine in turn can inhibit PAH uptake, demonstrating the existence of some link between organic anion and cation transport [152-155]. Such observations appear to overturn the dogma of distinct transport systems for organic ions. Some compounds have chemical characteristics ("zwitterions"), which account for their particular substrate behavior: creatinine [156], amino-cephalosporins (e.g. cephaloridine) and gyrase inhibitors [157] bear both positive and negative charges, and are therefore "bisubstrates" [37]. Cimetidine has affinity for the organic cation basolateral transporter through its imidazole group, while hydrophobicity of the molecule and electronegativity of the cyanoguanidine group explain the affinity of the drug for the organic anion transporter [158]. Famotidine and ranitidine have a guanidine group and a nucleophilic side-chain accounting for the affinity for both transport systems [158]. Clonidine and pilocarpine are other imidazole derivatives interacting with both transporters [158]. Zidovudine secretion in rats might also proceed through both transport mechanisms [159], though the anion transporter appears to predominate [160, 161]. As reported above, cisplatin also appears to be transported by both transport systems.

Many other compounds interact at the basolateral membrane with the PAH and the organic cation transport systems as was demonstrated by the systematic studies by Ullrich et al. [37].

Metabolism of drugs/ xenobiotics in the kidney

Metabolic transformation is the biological conversion of a drug to another chemical form, occurring mainly in the liver, although many other tissues, among them the kidney are also capable of drug metabolism. Microsomal enzymes are responsible for oxidation, acetylation, conjugation (acylglucuronidation, N-glucuronidation, glycination) hydrolysis of drugs and xenobiotics. The usual result of this enzymatic conversion is drug metabolites, which are more polar, and less lipid soluble than the parent compound and consequently favoring renal excretion. The same enzymatic pathways for drug metabolism present in the liver are also found in the kidney, although the specific activity of these pathways in the kidney is substantially lower than those in the liver [2, 162]. In contrast to the liver, the metabolic pathways in the kidney are not uniformly distributed throughout the kidney, they are localized to specific nephron segments (Table 4). Examples of drug metabolism by the isolated perfused kidney are oxidation of bumetanide [163], acetylation of sulphisoxazole [164], conjugation of salicylic acid [165], and esterolysis of enalapril to enalaprilat [166].

The role of renal enzyme systems involved in the metabolism of drugs and their potential nephrotoxicity is well documented in the case of analgesic mixtures containing acetylsalicylic acid, acetaminophen and/ or phenacetin combined with addicting compounds such as caffeine and codeine [167]. The kidney can metabolize acetaminophen to glucuronyl and sulphate conjugates but also to an arylating intermediate via the cytochrome P-450 mixed function oxidase system [168, 169]. The intra-renal distribution of this enzyme system explains the proximal tubular localization of acute acetaminophen toxicity [170]. Several observations in the Fischer rat suggests that this acute renal toxicity is mediated through the cytochrome P-450 mechanism [168].

Renal metabolism of isoproterenol [171], bumetanide [163], cimetidine [172] and N-methylnicotinamide [173] has been reported. Renal metabolites may have different mode of excretion [174], and may be more nephrotoxic than the original substance [175]. Renal glucuronidation may be substantial as in the case of morphine [176]. Xenobiotic glucuronidation can proceed by linkage through an ether or an ester bound. The latter process is called "acyl-glucuronide" characterized by instability under physiological conditions such that the glucuronide can deconjugate back to the parent compound (futile cycle). In patients with normal renal function, acyl-glucuronides are readily eliminated in the urine. In patients with renal insufficiency, the conjugate accumulates in plasma where it can spontaneously hydrolyse to reform the parent compound. This phenomenon, demonstrated for clofibrate [177, 178] diflunisal [179, 180] and some NSAID [181, 182], leads to a paradox in which a drug may accumulate in patients with renal insufficiency even through negligible amounts of parent drug are eliminated in the urine of patients with normal renal function.

The main role of the kidney in the process of drug metabolism consists in the excretion of the many, more or less pharmacologically active metabolites formed in the liver [8]. Needles to say that renal insufficiency may result in the accumulation of metabolites and, if pharmacological active, may result in serious side effects/ toxicity [33]. Renal metabolism of drug-xenobiotics and its contribution to elimination has been inadequately explored so that clinical implications are for the most part inferred from animal models or speculative.

The impact of knowledge of renal handling on drugs and xenobiotics on their clinical use is clearly demonstrated with the aminoglycosides (chapter 12).

References

1. Brezis M, Rosen S, Silva P, Epstein FH. Renal ischemia: a new perspective. Kidney Int 1984; 26: 374-383.
2. Rush GF, Smith JH, Newton JF, Hook JB. Chemically induced nephrotoxicity: role of metabolic activation. CRC Crit Rev Toxicol 1984; 13: 99-160.
3. Hook JB, Hewitt WR. Toxic responses of the kidney. In: Casarett & Doull's Toxicology. The basic science of poisons, 3rd edition. Klaassen CD, Amdur MO, Doull J (editors). Macmillan, New York 1986; p. 310-329.
4. Tay LK, Bregman CL, Masters BG, Williams PD. Effects of cis-diamminedichloroplatinum (II) on rabbit kidney *in vivo* and on rabbit renal proximal tubule cells in culture. Cancer Res 1988; 48: 2538-2543.
5. Williams PD. The application of renal cells in culture in studying drug-induced nephrotoxicity. *In vitro* 1989; 25: 800-805.
6. Williams PD, Rush GF. An evaluation of *in vitro* models for assessing nephrotoxicity. In: *In vitro* toxicity testing. Frazier JM (editor). Marcel Dekker Inc, New York/Basel/Hong Kong 1992; p. 85-110.
7. Kastner S, Soose M, Stolte H. Human kidney in *in vitro* pharmaco-toxicology. In: Human cells in *in vitro* pharmaco-toxicology: present status within Europe. Rogiers V, Sonck W, Shephard E, Vercruysse A (editors). VUBPress, Brussels 1993; p. 197-238.
8. Brater DC, Sokal PP, Hall SD, McKinney TD. Disposition and dose requirements of drugs in renal insufficiency. In: The kidney: physiology and pathophysiology. Seldin DW, Giebisch G (editors). Raven Press Ltd, New York 1992; p. 3671-3695.

8a. Hörbelt M, Wotzlaw C, Sutton TA, Molitoris BA, Philipp T, Kribben A, Fandrey J, Pietruck F, Pietruck F. Organic cation transport in the rat kidney *in vivo* visualized by time-resolved two-photon microscopy. Kidney Int 2007; 72: 422-429.

8b. Koepsell H, Koepsell H. *In vivo* two-photon fluorescence microscopy opens a new area for investigation of the excretion of cationic drugs in the kidney. Kidney Int 2007; 72: 387-388.

8c. John EG & Guignard JP. Development of renal excretion of drugs during ontogeny. In: Neonatal and fetal medicine. Polin RA & Fow WW Eds. Saunders WB, Philadelphia. pp 188-193, 1997.

9. Kragh-Hansen U. Molecular aspects of ligand binding to serum albumin. Pharmacol Rev 1981; 33: 17-53.
10. Routledge PA. The plasma protein binding of basic drugs. Brit J Clin Pharmacol 1986; 22: 499-506.
11. Green TP, Mirkin BL. Resistance of proteinuric rats to furosemide: urinary drug protein bindings as a determinant of drug effect. Life Sci 1980; 26: 623-630.
12. Green TP, Mirkin BL. Furosemide disposition in normal and proteinuric rats: urinary drug protein bindings as a determinant of drug excretion. J Pharmacol Exp Ther 1981; 218: 122-127.
13. Kirchner KA, Voelker JR, Brater DC. Intratubular albumin blunts the response to furosemide - a mechanism for diuretic resistance in the nephrotic syndrome. J Pharmacol Exp Ther 1990; 252: 1097-101.
14. Kirchner KA, Voelker JR, Brater DC. Binding inhibitors restore furosemide potency in tubule fluid containing albumin. Kidney Int 1991; 40: 418-424.
15. Weiner IM. Organic acids and bases and uric acid. The kidney: physiology and pathophysiology. Seldin DW, Giebisch G (editors). Raven Press Ltd, New York 1985; p. 1703-1724.
16. Roch-Ramel F, Roth L, Arnow J, Weiner LM. Salicylate excretion in the rat; free flow micropuncture experiments. J Pharmacol Exp Ther 1978; 207: 737-747.
17. Brater DC. Drugs and the kidney: renal contribution to handling of drugs. In: Handbook of renal therapeutics. Martínez-Maldonado M (editor). Plenum Medical Book Company, New York/London 1983; p. 191-206.
18. Goodman LS, Gilman A, Rall TW, Nies AS, Taylor P (editors). The pharmacological basis of therapeutics. Pergamon Press, New York 1990.
19. Roch-Ramel F, Besseghir K, Murer H. Renal excretion and tubular transport of organic anions and cations. In: Handbook of physiology, section 8: renal physiology. Windhager EE (editor). Oxford University Press, New York/Oxford 1992; p. 2189-2262.
20. Guggino SE, Aronson PS. Paradoxical effects of pyrazinoate and nicotinate on urate transport in dog renal microvillus membranes. J Clin Invest 1985; 76: 543-547.
21. Bessighir K, Roch-Ramel F. Pyrazinoate transport in the isolated perfused rabbit proximal tubule. Pflügers Arch 1986; 407: 643-648.
22. Elion GB, Yü TF, Hitchings GH. Renal clearance of oxipurinol, the chief metabolite of allopurinol. Am J Med 1968; 45: 69-77.
23. May DG, Weiner IM. The renal mechanisms for the excretion of m-hydroxybenzoic acid in cebus monkeys: relationship to urate transport. J Pharmacol Exp Ther 1971; 176: 407-417.
24. Van Crugten JT, Sallustio BC, Nation RL, Somogyi A. Renal tubular transport of morphine, morphine-6-glucuronide, and morphine-3-glucuronide in the isolated perfused rat kidney. Drug Metab Disp 1991; 19: 1087-1092.
25. Wright SH, Wunz TM, Wunz TP. A choline transporter in renal brush-border membrane vesicles - energetics and structural specificity. J Membrane Biol 1992; 126: 51-65.

26. Daniel H, Herget M. Cellular and molecular mechanisms of renal peptide transport. (review). Am J Physiol 1997; 273: F1-F8.
27. Shen H, Smith DE, Yang T, Huang YG, Schnermann JB, Brosius FCI. Localization of PEPT1 nand PEPT2 proton-coupled oligopeptide cotransporter mRNA and protein in rat kidney. Am J Physiol 1999; 276: F658-F665.
28. Keppler D, Leier I, Jedlitschky G. Transport of glutathione conjugates and glucuronides by the multidrug resistance proteins MRP1 and MRP2 (review). Biol Chem 1997; 378: 787-791.
29. Inui K, Masuda S, Saito H. Cellular and molecular aspects of drug transport in the kidney. Kidney Int 2000; 58: 944-958.
30. Foulkes EC. Transport of heavy metals by the kidney. Toxicology Letters 1990; 33: 29-31.
31. Templeton DM. Cadmium uptake by cells of renal origin. J Biol Chem 1990; 265: 21764-21770.
32. De Broe ME, Paulus GJ, Verpooten GA, Roels F, Buyssens N, Wedeen RP, Van Hoof F, Tulkens PM. Early effects of gentamicin, tobramycin and amikacin on the human kidney. A prospective, comparative study. Kidney Int 1984; 25: 643-652.
33. Laurent G, Tulkens PM. Aminoglycoside nephrotoxicity: cellular and molecular aspects. ISI Atlas of Science - Pharmacology 1987; 1: 40-44.
34. Lee W and Kim RB. Transporters and renal drug elimination. Annu Rev Pharmacol Toxicol 2004; 44: 137-66.
35. Besseghir K, Roch-Ramel F. Renal excretion of drugs and other xenobiotics. Renal Physiol 1987; 10: 221-241.
35a. Dresser, M. J., Leabman, M. K., and Giacomini, K. M. Transporters involved in the elimination of drugs in the kidney: Organic anion transporters and organic cation transporters [Review]. Journal of Pharmaceutical Sciences 90(4), 397-421. 2001.
35b. Berkhin, E. B. and Humphreys, M. H. Regulation of renal tubular secretion of organic compounds [Review]. Kidney International 59, 17-30. 2001.
36. Møller JV, Sheikh MI. Renal organic anion transport system: pharmacological, physiological, and biochemical aspects. Pharmacol Rev 1983; 34: 315-358.
37. Ullrich KJ. Specificity of transporters for organic anions and organic cations in the kidney. Biochim Biophys Acta 1994; 1197: 45-62.
38. Burckhardt G, Wolff NA. Structure of renal organic anion and cation transporters (review). Am J Physiol Renal Physiol 2000; 278(6): F853-F866
39. Sekine T, Cha SH, Endou H. The multispecific organic anion transporter (OAT) family (review). Pflügers Arch 2000; 440(3): 337-350.
40. Tune BM. Renal tubular transport and nephrotoxicity of β-lactam antibiotics: structure-activity relationships. Miner Electrolyte Metab 1994; 20: 221-231.
41. Dantzler WH, Evans KK, Groves CE, Welborn JR, North J, Stevens JL, Wright SH. Relation of cysteine conjugate nephrotoxicity to transport by the basolateral organic anion transport system in isolated S2 segments of rabbit proximal renal tubules. J Pharm Exp Ther 1998; 286: 52-60.
42. Berndt WO. The role of transport in chemical nephrotoxicity (review). Tox Pathol 1998; 26: 52-57.
43. Kosoglou T, Vlasses PH. Drug interactions involving renal transport mechanisms: an overview. CICP Ann Pharmacother 1989; 23: 116-22.
44. Pritchard JB, Miller DS. Mechanisms mediating renal secretion of organic anions and cations. Physiol Rev 1993; 73: 765-796.
45. Roch-Ramel F. Renal transport of organic anions (review). Curr Opin Nephrol Hypertens 1998; 7(5): 517-524.
46. Karniski LP, Lotscher M, Fucentese M, Hilfiker H, Biber J, Murer H. Immunolocalization of sat-1 sulfate/oxalate/bicarbonate anion exchanger in the rat kidney. Am J Physiol 1998; 275(1 Pt 2): F79-F87.
47. Wang H, Fei YJ, Kekuda R, Yang-Feng TL, Devoe D, Leibach FH, Prasad PD, Ganapathy V. Structure, function, and genomic organization of human Na^+-dependent high-affinity dicarboxylate transporter. Am J Physiol 2000; 278: C1019-C1030.
48. Klein I, Sarkadi B, Varadi A. An inventory of the human ABC proteins (review). Biochim Biophys Acta 1999; 1461: 237-262.
49. Borst P, Evers R, Kool M, Wijnholds J. A family of drug transporters: the multidrug resistance-associated proteins (review). J Nat Cancer Inst 2000; 92: 1295-1302.
49a. Masuda S, Terada T, Yonezawa A, Tanihara Y, Kishimoto K, Katsura T, Ogawa O, and Inui K. Identification and functional characterization of a new human kidney–specific H+/organic cation antiporter, kidney-specific multidrug and toxin extrusion 2. J Am Soc Nephrol 2006; 17: 2127-2135.
49b. Omote H, Hlasa M, Matsumo T et al. The MATE proteins as fundamental transporters of metabolic and xenobiotic organic cations. Trends Pharmacol Sci 2006; 27: 587-593.
50. Lu R, Kanai N, Bao Y, Wolkoff AW, Schuster VL. Regulation of renal OATP mrna expression by testosterone. Am J Physiol 1996; 270(2 Pt 2): F332-F337.
51. Masuda S, Ibaramoto K, Takeuchi A, Saito H, Hashimoto Y, Inui KI. Cloning and functional characterization of a new multispecific organic anion transporter, OAT-K2, in rat kidney. Mol Pharmacol. 1999; 55(4): 743-752
52. Masuda S, Takeuchi A, Saito H, Hashimoto Y, Inui K. Functional analysis of rat renal organic anion transporter OAT-K1: bidirectional methotrexate transport in apical membrane. FEBS Letters 1999; 459: 128-132.

52a. Eraly SA, Blantz RC, Bhatnagar V, Nigam SK. Novel aspects of renal organic anion transporters. Curr Opin Nephrol Hypertens 2003; 12: 551-558.
53. Yabuuchi H, Tamai I, Nezu J, Sakamoto K, Oku A, Shimane M, Sai Y, Tsuji A. Novel membrane transporter OCTN1 mediates multispecific, bidirectional, and pH-dependent transport of organic cations. J Pharmacol Exp Ther 1999; 289: 768-773.
54. Wu X, Huang W, Prasad PD, Seth P, Rajan DP, Leibach FH, Chen JW, Conway SJ, Ganapathy V. Functional characteristics and tissue distribution pattern of organic cation transporter 2 (OCTN2), an organic cation/carnitine transporter. J Pharmacol Exp Ther 1999; 290: 1482-1492.
54a. Huls M, Brown CD, Windass AS, Sayer R, van den Heuvel JJ, Heemskerk S, Russel FG, Masereeuw R. The breast cancer resistance protein transporter ABCG2 is expressed in the human kidney proximal tubule apical membrane. Kidney Int 2007; 73: 220-225.
55. Miller DS, Stewart DE, Pritchard JB. Intracellular compartmentation of organic anions within renal cells. Am J Physiol 1993; 264: R882-R890.
56. Masereeuw R, vandenBergh EJ, Bindels RJ. Characterization of fluorescein transport in isolated proximal tubular cells of the rat: evidence for mitochondrial accumulation. J Pharmacol Exp Ther 1994; 269: 1261-1267.
57. Pajor AM. Sequence and functional characterization of a renal sodium/dicarboxylate cotransporter. J Biol Chem 1995; 270(11): 5779-5785.
58. Lemieux G, Junco E, Perez R, Lemieux C, Allignet E. The metabolic response of the kidney to acute sodium lactate alkalosis. Can J Physiol Pharmacol 1985; 63: 687-692.
59. Miller DS, Barnes DM, Pritchard JB. Confocal microscopic analysis of fluorescein compartmentation within crab urinary bladder cells. Am J Physiol 1994; 267: R16-R25.
60. Miller DS, Pritchard JB. Nocodazole inhibition of organic anion secretion in teleost renal proximal tubules. Am J Physiol 1994; 267: R695-R704.
61. Ullrich KJ, Rumrich G. Luminal transport step of para-aminohippurate (PAH) - transport from pah-loaded proximal tubular cells into the tubular lumen of the rat kidney *in vivo*. Pflügers Arch 1997; 433(6): 735-743
62. Roch-Ramel F, Werner D, Guisan B. Urate transport in brush-border membrane of human kidney. Am J Physiol 1994; 266: F797-F805.
63. Roch-Ramel F, Guisan B, Schild L. Indirect coupling of urate and p-aminohippurate transport to sodium in human brush-border membrane vesicles. Am J Physiol 1996; 270: F165-F272.
64. Schmitt C, Burckhardt G. p-Aminohippurate/2-oxoglutarate exchange in bovine renal brush-border and basolateral membrane vesicles. Pflügers Arch 1993; 423: 280-290.
65. Ullrich KJ, Rumrich G. Renal contraluminal transport systems for organic anions (p-aminohippurate, p-aminohippurate) and organic cations (N1-methyl-nicotinamide, NMeN) do not see the degree of substrate ionization. Pflügers Arch 1992; 421: 286-288.
66. Troehler U, Bonjour JP, Fleisch H. Renal secretion of diphosphonates in rats. Kidney Int 1975; 8: 6-13.
67. Lin JH, Chen IW, Deluna FA, Hichens M. Renal handling of alendronate in rats. An uncharacterized renal transport system. Drug Metab Dispos 1992; 20: 608-613.
68. Russel FGM, Vermeulen WG. Effect of substituted benzoylglycines (hippurates) and phenylacetylglycines on p-aminohippurate transport in dog renal membrane vesicles. Pharmaceut Res 1994; 11: 1829-1833.
69. Russel FGM, Heijn M, De Laet RC, Van Ginneken CAM. Effect of substituted benzoates on p-aminohippurate transport in dog renal membrane vesicles. Naunyn-Schmiedeberg's Arch Pharmacol 1991; 343: 102-107.
70. Hosoyamada M, Sekine T, Kanai Y, Endou H. Molecular cloning and functional expression of a multispecific organic anion transporter from human kidney. Am J Physiol 1999; 276: F122-F128.
71. Van Aubel RAMH, Masereeuw R, Russel FGM. Molecular pharmacology of renal organic anion transporters (review). Am J Physiol Renal Physiol 2000; 279(2): F216-F232.
72. Uwai Y, Saito H, Hashimoto Y, Inui KI. Interaction and transport of thiazide diuretics, loop diuretics, and acetazolamide via rat renal organic anion transporter rOAT1. J Pharmacol Exp Ther 2000; 295: 261-265.
73. Wada S, Tsuda M, Sekine T, Cha SH, Kimura M, Kanai Y, Endou H. Rat multispecific organic anion transporter 1 (rOAT1) transports zidovudine, acyclovir, and other antiviral nucleoside analogs. J Pharmacol Exp Ther 2000; 294: 844-849.
74. Cihlar T, Lin DC, Pritchard JB, Fuller MD, Mendel DB, Sweet DH. The antiviral nucleotide analogs cidofovir and adefovir are novel substrates for human and rat renal organic anion transporter 1. Mol Pharmacol 1999; 56: 570-580.
75. Sekine T, Watanabe N, Hosoyamada M, Kanai Y, Endou H. Expression cloning and characterization of a novel multispecific organic anion transporter. J Biol Chem 1997; 272: 18526-18529.
76. Burckhardt BC, Wolff NA, Burckhardt G. Electrophysiologic characterization of an organic anion transporter cloned from winter flounder kidney (fROAT). J Am Soc Nephrol 2000; 11(1): 9-17.

77. Race J E, Grassl SM, Williams WJ, Holtzman EJ. Molecular cloning and characterization of two novel human renal organic anion transporters (hOAT1 and hOAT3). Biochem Biophys Res Comm 1999; 255: 508-514.
78. Boner G, Steele TH. Relationship of urate and p-aminohippurate secretion in man. Am J Physiol 19973; 225: 100-104.
79. Uwai Y, Okuda M, Takami K, Hashimoto Y, Inui K. Functional characterization of the rat multispecific organic anion transporter OAT1 mediating basolateral uptake of anionic drugs in the kidney. FEBS Letters 1998; 438: 321-324.
80. Lu R, Chan BS, Schuster VL. Cloning of the human kidney PAH transporter: narrow substrate specificity and regulation by protein kinase C. Am J Physiol 1999; 276: F295-303.
80a. Cha, S. H., Sekine, T., Fukushima, J., Kanai, Y., Kobayashi, Y., Goya, T., and Endou, H. Identification and characterization of human organic anion transporter 3 expressing predominantly in the kidney. Molecular Pharmacology 59(5), 1277-1286. 2001.
81. Sekine T, Cha S, Kanai Y, Endou H. Molecular biology of multispecific organic anion transporter family (OAT family). Clin Exp Nephrol 1999; 3: 237-243.
82. Kusuhara H, Sekine T, Utsunomiya-Tate N, Tsuda M, Kojima R, Cha SH, Sugiyama Y, Kanai Y, Endou H. Molecular cloning and characterization of a new multispecific organic action transporter from rat brain. J Biol Chem 1999; 274: 13675-13680.
83. Nakajima N, Sekine T, Cha SH, Tojo A, Hosoyamada M, Kanai Y, Yan K, Awa S, Endou H. Developmental changes in multispecific organic anion transporter 1 expression in the rat kidney. Kidney Int 2000; 57: 1608-1616.
84. Uchino H, Tamai I, Yamashita K, Minemoto Y, Sai Y, Yabuuchi H, Miyamoto K, Takeda E, Tsuji A. p-aminohippuric acid transport at renal apical membrane mediated by human inorganic phosphate transporter NPT1. Biochem Biophys Res Comm 2000; 270: 254-259.
85. Busch AE, Schuster A, Waldegger S, Wagner CA, Zempel G, Broer S, Biber J, Murer H, Lang F. Expression of a renal type I sodium/phosphate transporter (NaPi-1) induces a conductance in Xenopus oocytes permeable for organic and inorganic anions. Proc Natl Acad Sci USA 1996; 93(11): 5347-5351.
86. Schaub TP, Kartenbeck J, Konig J, Spring H, Dorsam J, Staehler G, Storkel S, Thon WF, Keppler D. Expression of the MRP2 gene-encoded conjugate export pump in human kidney proximal tubules and in renal cell carcinoma. J Am Soc Nephrol 1999; 10: 1159-1169.
87. Bakos E, Evers R, Sinko E, Varadi A, Borst P, Sarkadi B. Interactions of the human multidrug resistance proteins MRP1 and MRP2 with organic anions. Mol Pharmacol 2000; 57: 760-768.
88. Leier I, Hummel-Eisenbeiss J, Cui YH, Keppler D. ATP-dependent para-aminohippurate transport by apical multidrug resistance protein MRP2. Kidney Int 2000; 57: 1636-1642.
89. Van Aubel RAMH, Peters JGP, Masereeuw R, van Os CH, Russel FGM. Multidrug resistance protein Mrp2 mediates ATP-dependent transport of classic renal organic anion p-aminohippurate. Am J Physiol Renal Physiol 2000; 279(4): F713-F717.
90. Peng KC, Cluzeaud F, Bens M, Van Huyen JP, Wioland MA, Lacave R, Vandewalle A. Tissue and cell distribution of the multidrug resistance-associated protein (MRP) in mouse intestine and kidney. J Histochem Cytochem 1999; 47: 757-768.
90a. Smeets PH, van Aubel RA, Wouterse AC, van den Heuvel JJ, and Russel FG. Contribution of multidrug resistance protein 2 (MRP2/ABCC2) to the renal excretion of p-aminohippurate (PAH) and identification of MRP4 (ABCC4) as a novel PAH transporter. J Am Soc Nephrol 2004; 15: 2828-2835.
91. Abe T, Kakyo M, Sakagami H, Tokui T, Nishio T, Tanemoto M, Nomura H, Hebert SC, Matsuno S, Kondo H, Yawo H. Molecular characterization and tissue distribution of a new organic anion transporter subtype (oatp3) that transports thyroid hormones and taurocholate and comparison with oatp2. J Biol Chem 1998; 273: 22395-22401.
92. Masuda S, Saito H, Inui KI. Interactions of nonsteroidal anti-inflammatory drugs with rat renal organic anion transporter, OAT-K1. J Pharmacol Exp Ther 1997; 283: 1039-1042.
93. Pritchard JB, Sykes DB, Walden R, Miller DS. ATP-dependent transport of tetraethylammonium by endosomes isolated from rat renal cortex. Am J Physiol 1994; 266: F966-F976.
94. Dutt A, Heath LA, Nelson JA. P-glycoprotein and organic cation secretion by the mammalian kidney. J Pharmacol Exp Ther 1994; 269: 1254-1260.
95. Ott RJ, Hui AC, Yuan G, Giacomini KM. Organic cation transport in human renal brush-border membrane vesicles. Am J Physiol 1991; 261: F443-F451.
96. Takahashi Y, Itoh T, Kobayashi M, Sugawara M, Saitoh H, Iseki K, Miyazaki K, Miyazaki S, Takada M, Kawashima Y. The transport mechanism of an organic cation, disopyramide, by brush-border membranes: comparison between renal cortex and small intestine of the rat. J Pharm Pharmacol 1993; 45: 419-424.
97. Wright SH, Wunz TM, Wunz TP. Structure and interaction of inhibitors with the tetraethylammonium/H^+ exchanger of rabbit renal brush border membranes. Pflügers Arch 1992; 429: 313-324.
98. David C, Rumrich G, Ullrich KJ. Luminal transport system for H+/organic cations in the rat proximal tubule. Kinetics, dependence on pH; specificity as compared with the contraluminal organic cation-transport system. Pflüugers Arch 1995; 430(4): 477-492.

99. Wright S H, Wunz TM. Influence of substrate structure on turnover of the organic cation/H+ exchanger of the renal luminal membrane. Pflügers Arch 1998; 436: 469-477.

100. Wright SH, Wunz TM. Influence of substrate structure on substrate binding to the renal organic cation H+ exchanger. Pflügers Arch 1999; 437: 603-610.

101. Miyamoto Y, Tiruppathi C, Ganapathy V, Leibach FH. Multiple transport systems for organic cations in renal brush-border membranes vesicles. Am J Physiol 1989; 256: F540-F548.

102. Ford JM, Hait WN. Pharmacology of drugs that alter multidrug resistance in cancer. Pharmacol Rev 1990; 42: 156-199.

103. Speeg KV, Maldonado AL, Liaci J, Muirhead D. Effect of cyclosporine on colchicine secretion by the kidney multidrug transporter studied *in vivo*. J Pharmacol Exp Ther 1992; 261: 50-55.

104. De Lannoy IAM, Mandin RS, Silverman M. Renal secretion of vinblastine, vincristine and colchicine *in vivo*. J Pharmacol Exp Ther 1994; 268: 388-395.

105. Schramm U, Fricker G, Wenger R, Miller DS. P-glycoprotein-mediated secretion of a fluorescent cyclosporin analogue by teleost renal proximal tubules. Am J Physiol 1995; 268: F46-F52.

106. Horio M, Pastan I, Gottesma MM, Handler JS. Transepithelial transport of vinblastine by kidney-derived cell lines. Application of a new kinetic model to estimate *in situ* Km of the pump. Biochim Biophys Acta 1990; 1027: 116-122.

107. Koren G. Clinical pharmacokinetic significance of the renal tubular secretion of digoxin. Clin Pharmacokin 1987; 13: 334-343.

107a. Koziolek MJ, Riess R, Geiger H et al. Expression of multidrug resistance P-glycoprotein in kidney allografts from cyclosporine A-treated patients. Kidney Int 2001; 60: 156-166.

107b. Saeki T, Ueda K, Tanigawara Y et 01. Human P-glycoprotein transports cyclosporin A and FK506. J Biol Chem 1993; 268: 60776080.

107c. Del Moral RG, Olrno A, Osuna A et a/. Role of P-glycoprotein in chronic cyclosporine nephrotoxicity and its relationship to intrarenal angiotensin II deposits. Transplant Proc 1998; 30: 2014-2016.

107d. Garcia del Moral R, O'Valle F, Andujar M et al. Relationship between P-glycoprotein expression and cyclosporin A in kidney. An immunohistological and cell culture study. Am J Path01 1995: 146: 398-408.

107e. Hauser IA, Schaeffeler E, Gauer S et al. ABCBI genotype of the donor but not of the recipient is a major risk factor for cyclosporlne-related nephrotoxicity after renal transplantation. J Am Soc Nephrol 2005; 16: 1501-1511.

107f. Miller DS, Fricker G, Drewe J. P-Glycoprotein-mediated transport of a fluorescent rapamycin derivative in renal proximal tubule. J Pharmacol Exp Ther 1997; 282: 440-444.

107g. Kahan BD. Efficacy of sirolimus compared with azathioprine for reduction of acute renal allograft rejection: a randomised multicentre study. The Rapamune US Study Group. Lancet 2000; 356: 194-202.

107h. Pallet N, Thervet E, Le Corre D et al. Rapamycin inhibits human renal epithelial cell proliferation: effect on cyclin D3 mRNA expression and stability. Kidney Int 2005; 67: 2422-2433.

108. Koepsell H, Gorboulev V, Arndt P. Molecular pharmacology of organic cation transporters in kidney (review). J Membr Biol 1999; 167: 103-117.

109. Zhang L, Brett CM, Giacomini KM. Role of organic cation transporters in drug absorption and elimination (review). Annual Rev Pharmacol Toxicol 1998; 38: 431-460.

110. Grundemann D, Gorboulev V, Gambaryan S, Veyhl M, Koepsell H. Drug excretion mediated by a new prototype of polyspecific transporter. Nature 1994; 372: 549-552.

111. Okuda M, Urakami Y, Saito H, Inui K. Molecular mechanisms of organic cation transport in OCT2-expressing Xenopus oocytes. Biochim Biophys Acta 1999; 1417: 224-231.

112. Zhang L, Gorset W, Washington CB, Blaschke TF, Kroetz DL, Giacomini KM. Interactions of HIV protease inhibitors with a human organic cation transporter in a mammalian expression system. Drug Metab Dispos 2000; 28: 329-334.

113. Dresser MJ, Gray AT, Giacomini KM. Kinetic and selectivity differences between rodent, rabbit, and human organic cation transporters (OCT1). J Pharmacol Exp Ther 2000; 292: 1146-1152.

114. Karbach U, Kricke J, Meyer-Wentrup F, Gorboulev V, Volk C, Loffing-Cueni D, Kaissling B, Bachmann S, Koepsell H. Localization of organic cation transporters OCT1 and OCT2 in rat kidney. Am J Physiol Renal Physiol 2000; 279(4): F679-F687.

115. Sugawara-Yokoo M, Urakami Y, Koyama H, Fujikura K, Masuda S, Saito H, Naruse T, Inui K, Takata K. Differential localization of organic cation transporters rOCT1 and rOCT2 in the basolateral membrane of rat kidney proximal tubules. Histochem Cell Biol 2000; 114: 175-180.

116. Urakami Y, Nakamura N, Takahashi K, Okuda M, Saito H, Hashimoto Y, Inui K. Gender differences in expression of organic cation transporter OCT2 rat kidney. FEBS Letters 1999; 461: 339-342.

117. Wu XA, Huang W, Ganapathy ME, Wang HP, Kekuda R, Conway SJ, Leibach FH, Ganapathy V. Structure, function, and regional distribution of the organic cation transporter OCT3 in the kidney. Am J Physiol Renal Physiol 2000; 279: F449-F458.

118. Grundemann D, Liebich G, Kiefer N, Koster S, Schomig E. Selective substrates for non-neuronal monoamine transporters. Mol Pharmacol 1999; 56(1): 1-10.
119. Tamai I, Yabuuchi H, Nezu J, Sai Y, Oku A, Shimane M, Tsuji A. Cloning and characterization of a novel human ph-dependent organic cation transporter, OCTN1. FEBS Letters 1997; 419: 107-111.
120. Ganapathy ME, Huang W, Rajan DP, Carter AL, Sugawara M, Iseki K, Leibach FH, Ganapathy V. β-lactam antibiotics as substrates for OCTN2, an organic cation/carnitine transporter. J Biol Chem 2000; 275: 1699-1707.
120a. Lang F. Regulating renal drug elimination? J Am Soc Nephrol 2005; 16: 1535-1536.
120b. Zaman GJ, Versantvoort CH, Smit JJ, et al. Analysis of the expression of MRP, the gene for a new putative transmembrane drug transporter, in human multidrug resistant lung cancer cell lines. Cancer Res 1993; 53: 1747-1750.
120c. Wijnholds J, Scheffer GJ, van der Valk M, van der Valk P, Beijnen JH, Scheper RJ, Borst P. Multidrug resistance protein I protects the oropharyngeal mucosal layer and the testicular tubules against drug-induced damage. J Exp Med 1998; 188: 797-808.
120d. Peng KC, Cluzeaud F, Bens M et al. Tissue and cell distribution of the multidrug resistance-associated protein (MRP) on mouse intestine and kidney. J Histochem Cytochem 1999; 47: 757-767.
120e. Schaub TP, Kartenbeck J, Konig J, Vogel O, Witzgall R, Kriz W, Keppler D. Expression of the conjugate export pump encoded by the mrp2 gene in the apical membrane of kidney proximal tubules. J Am Soc Nephrol 1997; 8: 1213-1221.
120f. Kool M, van der Linden M, de Haas M, et al. MRP3, an organic anion transporter able to transport anti-cancer drugs. Proc Natl Acad Sci USA 1999; 96: 6914-6919.
120g. Konig J, Rost D, Cui Y, Keppler D. Characterization of the human multidrug resistance protein isoform MRP3 localized to the basolateral hepatocyte membrance. Hepatology 1999; 29: 1156-1163.
121. Wagner CA, Lukewille U, Kaltenbach S, Moschen I, Broer A, Risler T, Broer S, Lang F. Functional and pharmacological characterization of human Na^+-carnitine cotransporter hOCTN2. Am J Physiol Renal Physiol 2000; 279: F584-F591.
122. Seth P, Wu X, Huang W, Leibach FH, Ganapathy V. Mutations in novel organic cation transporter (OCTN2), an organic cation/carnitine transporter, with differential effects on the organic cation transport function and the carnitine transport function. J Biol Chem 1999; 274: 33388-33392.
123. Bowman RH. Renal secretion of [^{35}S] furosemide and its depression by albumin binding. Am J Physiol 1975; 229: 93-98.
124. Koschier FJ, Acara M. Transport of 2, 4, 5-trichlorophenoxyacetate in the isolated, perfused rat kidney. J Pharmacol Exp Ther 1979; 208: 287-293.
125. Webb DE, Edwards RM, Grantham JJ. Dependence of proximal tubule p-aminohippurate secretion on serum proteins and metabolic substrates. Am J Physiol 1986; 251: F619-F626.
126. Grantham JJ, Kennedy J, Cowley B. Tubule urate and p-aminohippurate transport: sensitivity and specificity of serum protein inhibition. Am J Physiol 1987; 252: F683-F690.
127. Rodrigues de Miranda JF, Hilbers CW. A nuclear magnetic resonance study of the kinetics of the binding of the renal contrast medium acetrizoate to albumin. Mol Pharmacol 1976; 12: 279-290.
128. Ochwadt BK, Pitts RF. Disparity between phenol red and diodrast clearance in the dog. Am J Physiol 1956; 187: 318-322.
129. Honari J, Blair AD, Cutler RE. Effects of probenecid on furosemide kinetics in man. Clin Pharmacol Ther 1977; 22: 395-401.
130. Homeida M, Roberts C, Branch RA. Influence of probenecid and spironolactone on furosemide kinetics in man. Clin Pharmacol Ther 1977; 22: 402-409.
131. Brater DC. Pharmacodynamic considerations in the use of diuretics. Annual Rev Pharmacol Toxicol 1983; 23: 45-62.
131a. Li M, Anderson GD, Wang J. Drug-drug interactions involving membrane transporters in the human kideny. Expert Opin Drug Metab Toxicol 2006; 2: 505-532.
132. Jacobs C, Kaubisch S, Halsey J, Lum BL, Gosland M, Coleman CN, Sikic BI. The use of probenecid as a chemoprotector against cisplatin nephrotoxicity. Cancer 1991; 67: 1518-1524.
133. Ban M, Hettich D, Huguet N. Nephrotoxicity mechanism of cis-plantinum (II) diamine dichloride in mice. Toxicol Letters 1994; 71: 161-168.
134. Klein J, Bentur Y, Cheung D, Moselhy G, Koren G. Renal handling of cisplatin: interactions with organic anionas and cations in the dog. Clin Inv Med 1991; 14: 388-394.
135. Tracy TS, Krohn K, Jones DR, Bradly JD, Hall SD, Brates DC. The effects of a xalicylate, ibuprofen, and naproxen on the disposition in patients with rheumatoid arthritis. Eur J Clin Pharmacol 1992; 42: 121-125.
136. Frenia ML, Long KS. Methotrexate and nonsteroidal antiinflammatory drug interactions. Ann Pharmacother 1992; 26: 234-237.
137. Nierenberg DW. Competitive inhibition of methotrexate accumulation in rabbit kidney slices by nonsteroidal anti-inflammatory drugs. J Pharmacol Exp Ther 1983; 226: 1-6.
138. Fromm MF, Kim RB, Stein CM, Wilkinson GR, Roden DM. Inhibition of P-glycoprotein-mediated drug transport - A unifying mechanism to explain the interaction between digoxin and quinidine. Circulation 1999; 99: 552-557.

139. Verschraagen M, Koks CHW, Schellens JHM, Beijnen JH. P-glycoprotein system as a determinant of drug interactions: the case of digoxin-verapamil. Pharmacol Res 1999; 40: 301-306.
140. De Lannoy IAM, Koren G, Klein J, Charuk J, Silverman M. Cyclosporin and quinidine inhibition of renal digoxin excretion - evidence for luminal secretion of digoxin. Am J Physiol 1992; 263(4 Pt 2):F613-F622.
141. De Lannoy IAM, Mandin RS, Silverman M. Renal Secretion of Vinblastine, Vincristine and Colchicine *in vivo*. J Pharmacol Exp Ther 1994; 268: 388-395.
142. Okamura N, Hirai M, Tanigawara Y, Tanaka K, Yasuhara M, Ueda K, Komano T, Hori R. Digoxin-cyclosporin A interaction: modulation of the multidrug transporter P-glycoprotein in the kidney. J Pharmacol Exp Ther 1993; 266: 1614-1619.
143. Woodland C, Verjee Z, Giesbrecht E, Koren G, Ito S. The digoxin-propafenone interaction - characterization of a mechanism using renal tubular cell monolayers. J Pharmacol Exp Ther 1997; 283: 39-45.
144. Nierenberg DW. Drug inhibition of penicillin tubular secretion: concoidance between *in vitro* and clinical findings. J Pharmacol Exp Ther 1987; 240: 712-716.
145. Dupuis L, Loren G, Shore A, Silverman ED, Laxer RM. Methotrexate non-steroidal anti-inflammatory drug interaction in children with arthritis. J Rheumat 1990; 17: 1469-1473.
146. Banditt P, Meyer FP, Walther H. Influence of cimetidine on the pharmacokinetics of other drugs. Pharmazie 1990; 45: 11-16.
147. Somogyi A, McLean A, Heinzow B. Cimetidine-procainamide pharmacokinetic interaction in man: evidence of competition for tubular secretion of basic drugs. Eur J Clin Pharmacol 1983; 25: 339-345.
148. Christian CJ, Meredith CG, Speeg KJ. Cimetidine inhibits renal procainamide clearance. Clin Pharmacol Ther 1984; 36: 221-227.
149. Van Crugten J, Bochner F, Keal J, Somogyi A. Selectivety of the cimetidine-induced alterations in the renal handling of organic substrates in humans. Studies with anionic, cationic and zwitterionic drugs. J Pharmacol Exp Ther 1986; 236: 481-487.
150. Gisclon LG, Boyd RA, Williams RL, Giacomini KM. The effect of probenecid on the renal elimination of cimetidine. Clin Pharmacol Exp Ther 1989; 45: 444-452.
151. Inotsume N, Nishimua M, Nakano M, Fujiyama S, Sato T. The inhibitory effect of probenecid on renal excretion of famotidine in young, healthy volunteers. J Clin Pharmacol 1990; 30: 50-56.
152. Hsyu PH, Gisclon LG, Hui AC, Giacomini KM. Interactions of organic anions with the organic cation transporter in renal BBMV. Am J Physiol 1988; 254: F56-F61.
153. Ott RJ, Hui C, Giacomine KM. Mechanisms of interactions between organic anions and the organic cation transporter in renal brush border membrane vesicles. Biochem Pharmacol 1990; 40: 659-661.
154. McKinney TD, Myers P, Speeg JKV. Cimetidine secretion by rabbit renal tubules *in vitro*. Am J Physiol 1981; 241: F69-F76.
155. Brandle E, Greven J. Transport of cimetidine across the basolateral membrane of rabbit kidney proximal tubules: interaction with organic anions. Pharmacology 1992; 45: 231-240.
156. Schück O. Tubular secretion of creatinine and its plasma concentration. Int J Clin Pharmacol Ther Toxicol 1990; 28: 127-128.
157. Sokol PP. Effect of DQ-2556, a new cephalosporin, on organic ion transport in renal plasma membrane vesicles from the dog, rabbit and rat. J Pharmacol Exp Ther 1990; 255: 436-441.
158. Ullrich KJ, Rumrich G, David C, Fritzsch G. Bisubstrates-substances that interact with renal contraluminal organic anion and organic cation transport systems. A. amines, piperidines, piperazines, azepines, pyridines, quinolines, imidazoles, thiazoles, guanidines and hydrazines. Pflügers Arch 1993; 425: 280-299.
159. Chatton JY, Odone M, Besseghir K, Roch-Ramel F. Renal secretion of 3'-azido-3'-deoxythymidine by the rat. J Pharmacol Exp Ther 1990; 255: 140-145.
160. Griffiths DA, Hall SD, Sokol PP. Interaction of 3'-azido-3'-deoxythymidine with organic ion transport in rat renal basolateral membrane vesicles. J Pharmacol Exp Ther 1991; 257: 149-155.
161. Griffiths DA, Hall SD, Sokol PP. Effect of 3'-azido-3'-deoxythymidine (AZT) on organic ion transport in rat renal brush border membrane vesicles. J Pharmacol Exp Ther 1992; 260: 128-133.
162. Anders MW. Metabolism of drugs by the kidney. Kidney Int 1980; 18: 636-647.
163. Bekersky I, Popick A. Metabolism of bumetanide by the isolated perfused rat kidney. Drug Metab Dispos 1983; 11: 512-513.
164. Bekersky I, Colburn WA. Acetylation of sulfisoxazole by the isolated perfused rat kidney. J Pharm Sci 1980; 69: 1359.
165. Bekersky I, Colburn WA, Fishman L, Kaplan SA. Metabolism of salicylic acid in the isolated perfused rat kidney: interconversion of salicyluric and salicylic acids. Drug Metab Dispos 1980; 8: 319-324.
166. DeLannoy IAM, Nespeca R, Pang KS. Renal handling of enalapril and enalaprilat: studies in the isolated red blood cell-perfused rat kidney. J Pharmacol Exp Ther 1989; 251: 1211-1222.
167. Elseviers MM, De Broe ME. Epidemiology of analgesic nephropathy. J Nephrol 1992; 5: 94-98.
168. McMurtry RJ, Snodgrass WR, Mitchell JR. Renal necrosis glutathione depletion and covalent binding after acetaminophen. J Toxicol Appl Pharmacol 1978; 46: 87-100.

169. Mudge GH, Gemborys MW, Duggin GG. Covalent binding of metabolites of acetaminophen to kidney protein and depletion of renal glutathione. J Pharmacol Exp Ther 1978: 206: 218-226.
170. Kleinman JG, Breitenfield RV, Roth DA. Acute renal failure associated with acetaminophen ingestion: report of a case and review of the literature. Clin Nephrol 1980; 14: 201-205.
171. Szefler SJ, Acara M. Isoproterenol excretion and metabolism in the isolated perfused rat kidney. J Pharmacol Exp Ther 1979; 210: 295-300.
172. Rennick B, Ziemniak J, Smith I, Taylor M, Acara M. Tubular transport and metabolism of cimetidine in chicken kidneys. J Pharmacol Exp Ther 1984; 228: 387-392.
173. Bessighir K, Pearce LB, Rennick B. Renal tubular transport and metabolism of organic cations by the rabbit. Am J Physiol 1981; 241: F308-F314.
174. Watrous WM, May DG, Fujimoto JM. Mechanism of the renal tubular transport of morphine and morphine ethereal sulfate in the chicken. J Pharmacol Exp Ther 1970; 172: 224-229.
175. Hook JB, MacCormack KM, Kluwe WM. Biochemical mechanisms of nephrotoxicity. In: Reviews in biochemical toxicology, vol 1. Hodgson, Bend, Philpot (editors). Elsevier/North-Holland, New York 1979; p. 53-78.
176. Jacqz E, Ward S, Johnson R, Schenker S, Gerkens J, Branch RA. Extrahepatic glucuronidation of morphine in the dog. Drug Metab Dispos 1986; 14: 627-630.
177. Meffin PJ, Zilm DM, Veendendaal JR. Reduced clofibric acid clearance in renal dysfunction is due to a futile cycle. J Pharmacol Exp Ther 1983; 227: 732-738.
178. Gugler R, Kurten JW, Jensen CJ, Klehr U, Hartlapp J. Clofigrate disposition in renal failure and acute and chronic liver disease. Eur J Clin Pharmacol 1979; 15: 341-347.
179. Verbeeck R, Tjandramaga TB, Mullie A, Verbesselt R, Verberckmoes R, De Schepper PJ. Biotransformation of diflunisal and renal excretion of its glucoronides in renal insufficiency. Brit J Clin Pharmacol 1979; 7: 273-282.
180. Eriksson LO, Wahlin-Boll E, Odar-Cederlof I, Lindholm L, Melander A. Influence of renal failure, rheumatoid arthritis and old age on the pharmacokinetics of diflunisal. Eur J Clin Pharmacol 1989; 36: 165-174.
181. Aronoff GR, Ozawa T, DeSante KA, Nash JF, Ridolfo AS. Benoxaprofen kinetics in renal impairment. Clin Phamacol Ther 1982; 32: 190-194.
182. Advenier C, Roux A, Gobert C, Massias P, Varaquaux O, Flouvat B. Pharmacokinetics of ketoprofen in the elderly. Brit J Clin Pharmacol 1983; 16: 65-70.

04

Pharmacological aspects of nephrotoxicity

Marisa D. COVINGTON and Rick G. SCHNELLMANN

Medical University of South Carolina, Charleston, SC, USA

Introduction

Because the kidney is vital to total body homeostasis, a toxic insult to the kidney can have profound effects – an insult of sufficient severity can permanently damage renal tissue, necessitating chronic dialysis or kidney transplantation. Such susceptibility to various toxicants is due to several functional properties of the kidney. First, the kidney receives approximately one-quarter of the total body blood flow to support renal function, including glomerular filtration, permitting the delivery of high levels of toxicants. The absorption of water and solutes along the nephron concentrates the tubular fluid, thereby exposing tubular epithelial cells to greater concentrations of toxicants. The high metabolic rate and work load of renal cells increases its susceptibility to toxicants. Furthermore, the kidney possesses biotransformation enzymes that can result in formation of toxic metabolites and reactive intermediates which can damage renal macromolecules. Because the nephron has specialized transporters for reabsorption and excretion, toxicants can enter and accumulate within renal cells, leading to nephrotoxicity. Finally, the unique functions of the varied segments along the nephron impart different susceptibilities to toxicants in the kidney, complicating the potential toxicities and subsequent renal damage via a variety of mechanisms. In this chapter, we will review some of these sites and mechanisms of nephrotoxicity.

Glomerulus

The glomerulus, a specialized capillary bed composed of endothelial cells, is the filtering unit of the kidney. The glomerular capillary wall forms both a charge- and size-selective barrier that prevents passage of plasma proteins and results in the formation of an ultrafiltrate. Because the glomerulus is the first structure encountered in the nephron, it is the initial site of toxicant exposure in the kidney. Nephrons are functionally integrated and as a result, toxicant-induced damage to the glomerulus not only impairs glomerular function, but also affects the function of the entire nephron.

Toxicants can decrease the glomerular filtration rate (GFR) by increasing afferent arteriolar resistance, resulting in a decrease in hydrostatic pressure. Toxicants can also decrease the glomerular surface area available for filtration by decreasing the size and number of endothelial fenestrae or altering the number of anionic charges on the glomerular structural elements, allowing passage and eventual urinary excretion of polyanionic and high-molecular weight proteins. For example, puromycin aminonucleoside exposure results in a loss of membrane anionic charges, permitting the passage of negatively charged proteins through the glomerulus, and resulting in proteinuria [1, 2]. See Figure 1 for other examples.

Chemically induced glomerular damage also can occur without significant loss of glomerular structural integrity. For example, mild renal ischemia and reperfusion results in formation of reactive oxygen species (ROS), proteinuria, and loss of charged glomerular structures with no apparent change in morphology [3].

Toxicants such as cyclosporine A and amphotericin B directly decrease renal circulation through injury of renal vessels and decrease GFR [4, 5]. Similarly, gentamicin interacts with anionic sites on the endothelial cells to decrease GFR and renal blood flow [6]. This diminished blood flow also decreases the delivery of oxygen and other critical metabolites to the tubules, further enhancing nephrotoxicity. These drugs create glomerular renal dysfunction with few morphological alterations in the glomeruli.

An important class of filtered molecules, soluble immune complexes, are generated after antibody responses to antigens which can be derived from drugs

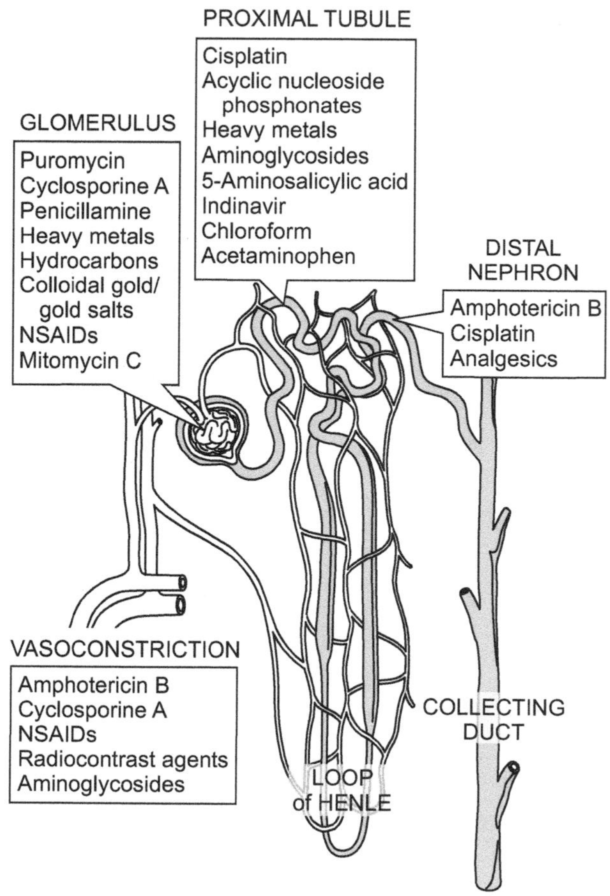

Figure 1. *Nephrotoxic targets along the nephron.*

and toxicants. Although soluble immune complexes are not always associated with pathology, some complexes can be deposited in the glomerulus and can subsequently activate complement, initiating a sequence of inflammatory events which may include recruitment of inflammatory cells, release of inflammatory mediators and enzymes, and destruction of glomerular structures. Macrophages and neutrophils are observed in the glomeruli in membranous glomerulonephritis, and the release of cytokines and ROS contribute to glomerular injury [7]. Recently, the activation and secretion of calpains, calcium-activated cysteine proteases, have been shown to participate in the development of immune glomerular injury [8].

A chemical may adhere to a native protein to produce an antigen and elicit an antibody response. For example, colloidal gold and gold salts, which are used to treat rheumatoid arthritis, induce membranous nephropathy with numerous electron-dense deposits on glomerular basement membranes [9]. Penicillamine, a drug used in chelation therapy and rheumatoid arthritis, produced similar immunoglobulin- and complement-containing deposits in glomerular basement membranes. Similarly, glomerulonephritis was observed after exposure to heavy metals, hydrocarbons, and captopril [10-13].

Proximal tubule

Proximal tubular injury is the most common toxicant-induced renal injury (see Figure 1 for examples). The proximal renal tubules are vulnerable to direct toxic effects of chemicals because of their absorption and secretion functions. Proximal tubular cells contain transporters for organic anions and cations, low-molecular weight proteins, glutathione (GSH) conjugates, and metals, which can result in the accumulation of chemicals and subsequent toxicity. Amphotericin B can bind to low-density lipoproteins and be internalized through low-density lipoprotein receptors [14]. Acyclic nucleoside phosphonates, such as cidofovir, adefovir, and tenofovir, are transported by the organic anion transporter-1 [15]. Although the inherent functionality of the kidney often means that toxicant concentrations are high in renal cells, the nephrotoxic effects are actually dependent upon the intrinsic reactivity with cellular and molecular targets.

Absorption and secretion in the nephron are functions of high energy demand; thus, these cells have elevated rates of oxidative metabolism. Therefore, chemicals that directly or indirectly disturb renal cell energy metabolism will result in cell injury and consequent renal dysfunction. For instance, heavy metals such as mercuric chloride alter mitochondrial function and morphology prior to tubular necrosis [16, 17]. Mitochondrial dysfunction is also observed with exposures to lead, aminoglycosides, and cephalosporins [17, 18]. Drugs that injure proximal tubules include 5-aminosalicylic acid (5-ASA), which is used to treat inflammatory bowel disease, and adefovir, a nucleoside reverse transcriptase inhibitor. Although the exact mechanism is unknown, 5-ASA has been shown to cause renal damage due to the uncoupling of oxidative phosphorylation and inhibition of prostaglandin synthesis [19]. Such a mechanism of action is thought to be similar to toxicities of other salicylates [20]. Adefovir has been reported to induce acute tubular necrosis and produce severe structural alterations in proximal tubular mitochondria [21]. Toxicity is thought to be mediated by direct effects on mitochondrial DNA replication, including the synthesis of cytochrome C oxidase [22], which is an important respiratory chain enzyme in the mitochondria, and its inhibition leads to mitochondrial dysfunction and loss of ATP.

As the glomerular filtrate proceeds down the tubule, the filtrate becomes increasingly concentrated and the pH of the filtrate becomes more acidic. Therefore chemicals with pH-dependent solubility have the potential to precipitate and cause tubular obstruction, resulting in local interstitial inflammation, granuloma formation, and fibrosis. Indinavir is a protease inhibitor used in the treatment of immunodeficiency virus that has been reported to cause renal toxicity. The solubility of indinavir is pH- and flow-dependent, and some patients treated with indinavir form urinary crystals that obstruct tubules, leading to inflammation or granuloma formation, resulting in renal failure [23].

Cytochrome P-450 and cysteine conjugate β-lyse are primarily localized in the proximal tubules, and these enzymes also contribute to the susceptibility of the proximal tubule to toxicant injury. Specifically, widely used industrial solvents such as chloroform produce tubular nephrotoxicity via cytochrome P-450 activation, and haloalkanes and haloalkenes (e.g. trichloroethylene) are rendered toxic by cysteine conjugate β-lyse activation [24, 24a]. In addition, overdoses of acetaminophen (APAP) cause nephrotoxicity that is characterized by proximal tubular necrosis [25]. APAP undergoes cytochrome P-450-mediated activation to produce a toxic electrophile, N-acetyl-p-benzoquinoneimine (NAPQI) [25a]. Although NAPQI is extremely reactive, it is detoxified by conjugation with reduced GSH unless NAPQI is formed in excess of the cellular capacity for GSH conjugation. The excess NAPQI is available to bind to critical cellular proteins and to induce oxidative stress, resulting in disruption of cellular homeostasis and tubular injury [26].

It is now recognized that GSH conjugation plays a critical role in chemical-induced nephrotoxicity and, in many cases, may be responsible for selective targeting and damage to the kidney versus other organ systems (Table 1). The capacity of the kidney to process and activate GSH conjugates is extensive and results in the release of toxic species within the proximal tubular cells. For example, haloalkenes and quinones are con-

Table 1. Chemicals that produce nephrotoxicity through their glutathione/cysteine conjugates.

• cisplatin
• acetaminophen
• sevoflurane
• hydroquinone
• bromohydroquinone
• cadmium
• mercury
• trichloroethylene
• tetrafluoroethylene
• hexachlorobutadiene

jugated to GSH in the liver, circulate to the kidney, and are metabolized by γ-glutamyl transpeptidase (γ-GT) to produce the cysteinyl-glycine conjugate (Figure 2) [27, 28]. The cysteinyl-glycine conjugate is further metabolized extracellularly by aminodipeptidases to cysteine conjugates [29]. The cysteine conjugates are then transported into the proximal tubule cells, where they are further metabolized into highly reactive thiols by cysteine-S-conjugate β-lyase [30]. The reactive thiols bind to cellular macromolecules, ultimately triggering cell death. In addition, the cysteine conjugates initiate oxidative stress and lipid peroxidation [31, 31a]. Similarly, the nephrotoxicity of quinone-GSH conjugates arises from their ability to undergo redox cycling [27].

Although cisplatin is not a substrate for γ-GT or cysteine-S-conjugate β-lyase, it has been shown to form GSH conjugates spontaneously in solution [32]. Cisplatin-GSH conjugates may be important in targeting cisplatin to the kidney and its resulting nephrotoxicity because γ-GT is necessary for the toxicity of the cisplatin conjugates, suggesting that metabolism of cisplatin in proximal tubule cells is required for nephrotoxicity [33, 34]. Furthermore, *in vivo* studies support the hypothesis that formation of a cisplatin-GSH conjugate is an essential component of nephrotoxicity of cisplatin [35-37].

Finally, the nephrotoxicity of inorganic mercury (i.e. mercuric chloride) has been shown to be the result of a GSH or cysteine conjugate. In a series of experiments, Zalups has shown that mercuric chloride in the blood is conjugated to cysteine and GSH as mono- or di-substituted conjugates and to serum proteins [38].

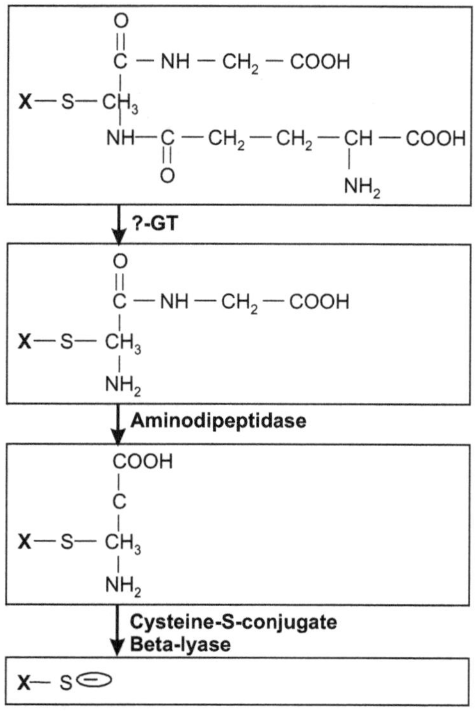

***Figure 2.** Activation of glutathione-conjugates to reactive thiols. Halogenated alkenes form glutathione-S-conjugates and are metabolized to nephrotoxins via this pathway. This pathway results in the production of unstable reactive thiols, which are toxic. The X represents the alkene.*
Adapted from Townsend et al., 2003 [34].

Uptake of these cysteine and GSH conjugates occurs across the apical membrane through Na^+-dependent and -independent amino acid transporters and across the basolateral membrane through an amino acid transporter and/or the organic anion transporter (OAT1). These examples provide strong evidence that the nephrotoxicity of numerous xenobiotics is dependent on GSH conjugation-mediated delivery to the kidney.

Distal nephron

Although most nephrotoxicity occurs in the proximal part of the nephron, some chemicals damage distal structures. The function of these structures facilitates their vulnerability to toxicants. For instance, the loop of Henle is critical to the process of urinary concentration and therefore utilizes relatively high rates of Na^+, K^+-ATPase activity and oxygen demand. This, and the fact that oxygen supply to the medulla is minimally sufficient to meet physiological needs, contributes to the susceptibility of the loop of Henle to hypoxic injury. For example, amphotericin B increases the tubular work load in the loop of Henle, intensifying hypoxic injury [39].

The final regulation of urinary volume and composition occurs in the distal tubule and collecting duct. Water permeability of the medullary collecting duct is controlled by hypertonicity and the action of antidiuretic hormone (ADH). Chemicals that increase medullary blood flow or interfere with ADH synthesis, secretion, or action will impair the concentration of urine. Drugs that have been associated with distal nephron injury impair the concentrating ability in the thick ascending limb and/or the collecting duct resulting in an ADH-resistant polyuria. The distal tubular epithelial cells are tightly bound, forming a strong barrier. Amphotericin B inhibits reabsorption in the distal nephron through its ability to form transmembrane pores and disrupt membrane permeability [40]. Cisplatin also induces polyuria , but the mechanism is not completely understood; although [41] Safirstein and Deray suggested that the polyuria arises through a vasopressin and prostaglandin inhibitor pathway.

The renal papilla is the target of analgesic abuse or the excessive ingestion of analgesics, which are often mixed with caffeine or alcohol, and results in papillary necrosis and chronic renal failure [42, 43]. Analgesics also can inhibit the vasodilatory effects of prostaglandin, predisposing the renal papillae with its already tenuous blood-supply to further ischemia and damage [44]. Because there is a high papillary concentration of toxicant, direct cellular insults of toxicants would be detrimental to the renal papilla. This is true for analgesics that cause injury by covalently binding to cells and causing oxidative damage [44].

Cellular injury

The nature and the intensity of toxicant-induced insults to the kidney determine the severity of renal damage. Most nephrotoxic chemicals target renal epithelial cells and produce cell death, which is thought to occur by apoptosis or oncosis, also known as necrotic cell death [45]. Apoptosis is a tightly controlled process in which cell death is executed through the activation of specific signaling pathways and is characterized morphologically as membrane blebbing, cell shrinking, nuclear condensation, and chromatin aggregation. Neighboring cells and macrophages rapidly digest these cellular fragments, or apoptotic bodies, without inducing inflammation or damage [46]. Apoptosis is the favored and controlled method of cell death and is vital for many processes such as organogenesis, normal cellular turnover, and the deletion of potentially neoplastic cells [47].

Apoptosis is initiated after numerous cellular insults and may proceed via an intrinsic (mitochondrial) or extrinsic (death receptor-mediated) pathway. Extrinsic apoptosis is initiated through ligand binding to one of a variety of death receptors. Tumor necrosis factor alpha (TNF-α) and FasL-induced apoptosis have been thoroughly evaluated in renal cells, and in fact, both cytokines are produced by renal epithelia and by infiltrating leukocytes [48, 49]. Nearly all renal cell types express receptors for both TNF-α and FasL, but vary in their sensitivity to these cytokines [50, 51]. Ligand binding of these lethal signaling molecules induces death receptor oligomerization, activation of caspase-8, and the downstream activation of effector caspases [49].

Apoptosis may be initiated at the level of the mitochondria or as a result of damage to an organelle, such as the endoplasmic reticulum or the nucleus. Initiation of the intrinsic or mitochondrial-mediated apoptotic program begins with the release of cytochrome c, which may be enhanced or inhibited by members of the Bcl-2 family of proteins (Bax, Bak, Bid, Bcl-2, Bcl-xL) [49]. Cytochrome c then recruits other adaptor proteins including APAF-1 and caspase 9, thereby forming what is known as the apoptosome. This cell death complex goes on to activate the effector caspase, caspase 3 [50], resulting in cell death. Although the initiation of intrinsic and extrinsic apoptotic pathways are different, they both play a role in toxicant-induced apoptotic cell death.

Oncosis/necrosis is characterized by organelle and cell swelling, cell rupture, and release of intracellular contents, which initiates an inflammatory response that is not observed in apoptosis. It is common for some toxicants to cause apoptosis at low concentrations and oncosis at high concentrations. Because apoptosis is an ATP-dependent process, nephrotoxicants that target the mitochondria and/or induce a decreased ATP predominantly cause oncosis rather than apoptosis [51, 52]. If cellular ATP levels are low and the mitochondrial membrane potential is quickly lost, then oncosis occurs. A rapid influx of Ca^{2+} into the mitochondria causes rupture of the inner and outer mitochondrial membranes resulting in a rapid loss of the mitochondrial membrane potential [53]. In contrast, if the loss of membrane potential is slow, and ATP levels are maintained, apoptosis is favored.

Toxicants that reduce ATP disrupt cell volume, ion concentrations, and cell polarity. Disruption of cell volume and ion homeostasis occurs by toxicant interaction with the plasma membrane increasing ion permeability or by attenuating energy production. ATP depletion results in a decrease in Na^+, K^+-ATPase activity, resulting in cell swelling, and ultimately cell rupture [54, 55]. The tubular epithelia are polarized cells with specific transporters on the apical and basolateral domains. When a toxicant causes ATP depletion there is a dissociation of the Na^+, K^+-ATPase from the actin cytoskeleton and a redistribution from the basolateral to apical domain in the renal proximal tubule cells [56]. The loss of polarity of the cells disrupts the adhesion complexes and loss of cell-to-cell contact that facilitates further renal damage.

Renal repair and regeneration

Although research has focused on the cellular events of nephrotoxicity, less emphasis has been placed on the mechanism of renal cell repair and regeneration after a toxic insult. Knowledge of post-injury repair/regeneration will facilitate development of new therapeutics to promote renal recovery. As a result of toxicant-induced renal injury, renal epithelial dysfunction is typically characterized by the loss of cellular apical/basal polarity, cytoskeletal redistribution, severe ATP depletion, mitochondrial dysfunction, impaired solute transport, and decreased ion pump activity including the Na^+/K^+ ATPase (Figure 3) [57, 58]. Depending on the extent of damage to the renal epithelium, cells die via necrosis or apoptosis. The remaining tubular cells survive in a sublethally injured state and undergo the complex process of regenerating the destroyed renal parenchyma [59, 60]. The standard hypothesis concerning renal cell regeneration is that sublethally injured and/or uninjured tubular cells restore cellular function, de-differentiate, proliferate, migrate, and finally re-differentiate to restore morphologic and physiologic function to the damaged nephron. Investigators have reported the presence of both endogenous renal stem cells and those originating from the bone marrow in animal models of acute renal failure [61-63]. However, the significance of these findings is still unclear, and more research in this area is needed.

In order for quiescent tubular cells of the injured nephron to carry out regeneration, gene upregulation, protein synthesis, and cell cycle entry is required. Therefore, growth factors are thought to be crucial in regenerating tubule cells, although the precise growth factors involved and their regulation are unknown [64, 65]. However, the epidermal growth factor receptor plays an important role in regulating de-differentiation, proliferation, and migration [66, 67].

There is a significant increase in cellular proliferation by surviving proximal tubular cells after renal injury in both animal models [68] and human cases of acute tubular necrosis [43] as measured by PCNA

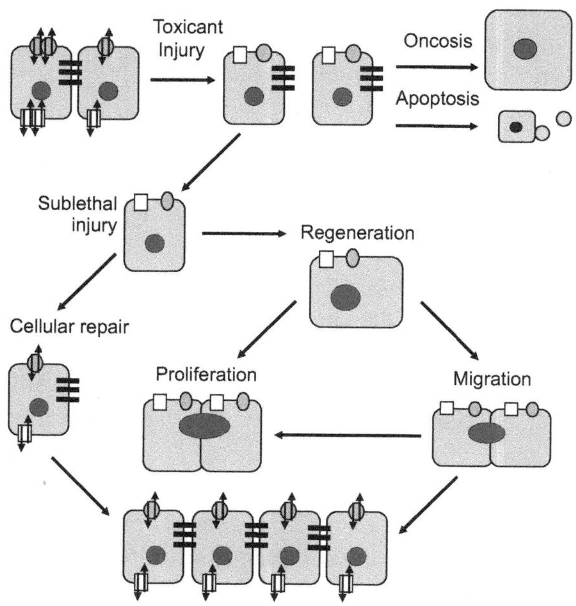

Figure 3. *Proposed mechanism of renal cell repair and regeneration. Healthy renal epithelia are differentiated, quiescent columnar epithelia. After injury, numerous renal cells die via necrosis and apoptosis depending on the level of insult. However a few cells are sublethally injured and lose cell polarity and many physiological functions. These cells can either initiate the repair process immediately or dedifferentiate into mesenchymal-like cells. Sublethally injured epithelial cells begin to migrate and proliferate to fill in denuded regions of the tubular lumen. The epithelial cells finally redifferentiate back into quiescent tubular cells and regain their polarity and physiological functions.*

staining and incorporation of [3H]thymidine into nuclear DNA. Proliferating cells resemble mesenchymal cells with flattened cell bodies, loss of a brush border, and the de-differentiated expression of embryonic proteins such as vimentin and neural cell adhesion molecule [68-70]. In many ways, dedifferentiated renal epithelial cells reiterate the cellular ontogeny of renal organogenesis. Recently more and more arguments are collected indicating that regeneration by surviving tubular epithelial cells is the predominant mechanism of repair after ischemic tubular injury in the adult mammalian kidney [71].

While the endogenous growth factors (including paracrine and autorcrine) responsible for the proliferative phase of renal cell regeneration have not been identified, numerous studies have demonstrated that exogenously administered growth factors such as epidermal growth factor (EGF), insulin-like growth factor 1 (IGF-1), hepatocyte growth factor (HGF), fibroblast growth factor (FGF), heparin-binding EGF (HB-EGF), bone morphogenic protein-7 (BMP-7), and transforming growth factor (TGF)-β promote cellular proliferation *in vitro* and enhance renal recovery after ischemia/reperfusion injury [72- 78]. While quite effective in animal models, only one of these growth factors has been evaluated in humans (IGF-1). In one clinical trial, treatment with recombinant IGF-1 did not improve renal function in subjects with comorbidities [79] while the acute renal failure was not achieved in the other clinical trial [80]. It should be noted, however, that growth factor regimens for humans would be acute in nature, to avoid potential adverse effects caused by growth factor-mediated overproduction of cells or by the stimulation of occult neoplastic cells.

Recent studies have provided evidence that repair of sublethally-injured renal tubular cells requires functional attachment of the cells to the basement membrane. It is thought that integrin ligation to collagen IV elicits signal transduction events in injured renal tubular cells that stimulate cell survival and are critical for the repair of physiological functions such as polarity and Na^+-transport [60, 81, 82]. The molecular mechanisms driving this return of function are not completely understood at the present, and greater understanding of the signaling pathways responsible for renal repair is needed before improved therapies can be developed for patients in the setting of post-ischemic renal injury.

It should be noted that nephrotoxicants can further cause renal damage by inhibiting cellular repair and regeneration, delaying or completely inhibiting recovery of normal renal function. Cisplatin and aminoglycosides have been reported to inhibit renal regeneration *in vivo* [83, 84]. In addition, mercury chloride, fumonisin B_1, and haloalkene cysteine conjugate inhibits the proliferation and migration of renal tubular cells [85]. Therefore, nephrotoxicants are capable of inhibiting the normal renal regeneration process which further contributes to renal dysfunction.

References

1. Alcorn D and Ryan GB. Distribution of anionic groups in the glomerular capillary wall in rat nephrotoxic nephritis and aminonucleoside nephrosis. Pathology 13: 37-50, 1981.
2. Kerjaschki D, Vernillo AT, and Farquhar MG. Reduced sialylation of podocalyxin--the major sialoprotein of the rat kidney glomerulus in aminonucleoside nephrosis. The American Journal of Pathology 118: 343-349, 1985.
3. Andersson M, Nilsson UA, Hjalmarsson C, Haraldsson B, and Nystrom Sorensson J. Mild renal ischemia-reperfusion reduces charge and size selectivity of the glomerular barrier. Am J Physiol Renal Physiol 292(6): F1802-9, 2007.
4. Perico N, Remuzzi A, Imberti O, Cavallotti D, Bertani T, and Remuzzi G. Morphometrical analysis of glomerular changes induced by cyclosporine in the rat. Am J Kidney Dis 17: 537-543, 1991.
5. Deray G. Amphotericin B nephrotoxicity. J Antimicrob Chemother 49 Suppl 1: 37-41, 2002.
6. Abbate GF, Alagia I, Giaquinto E, Giordano B, Leonessa V, and Altucci P. Preclinical comparative evaluation of aminoglycosides. Chemioterapia 3: 378-384, 1984.
7. Budisavljevic MN, Hodge L, Barber K, Fulmer JR, Durazo-Arvizu RA, Self SE, Kuhlmann M, Raymond JR, and Greene EL. Oxidative stress in the pathogenesis of experimental mesangial proliferative glomerulonephritis. Am J Physiol Renal Physiol 285: F1138-1148, 2003.

8. Peltier J, Bellocq A, Perez J, Doublier S, Dubois YC, Haymann JP, Camussi G, and Baud L. Calpain activation and secretion promote glomerular injury in experimental glomerulonephritis: evidence from calpastatin-transgenic mice. J Am Soc Nephrol 17: 3415-3423, 2006.
9. Davies DJ, Dowling J, and Xipell JM. Gold nephropathy. Pathology 9: 281-288, 1977.
10. Guery JC, Druet E, Glotz D, Hirsch F, Mandet C, De Heer E, and Druet P. Specificity and cross-reactive idiotypes of anti-glomerular basement membrane autoantibodies in HgCl2-induced autoimmune glomerulonephritis. European Journal of Immunology 20: 93-100, 1990.
11. Koren G. The nephrotoxic potential of drugs and chemicals. Pharmacological basis and clinical relevance. Medical Toxicology and adverse drug experience 4: 59-72, 1989.
12. Ponticelli C and Pezzagno G. Hydrocarbons and glomerulonephritis--is the definite answer in? Nephrol Dial Transplant 9: 1539-1540, 1994.
13. Textor SC, Gephardt GN, Bravo EL, Tarazi RC, Fouad FM, Tubbs R, and McMahon JT. Membranous glomerulopathy associated with captopril therapy. The American Journal of Medicine 74: 705-712, 1983.
14. Wali RK and Henrich WL. Recent developments in toxic nephropathy. Current Opinion in Nephrology and Hypertension 11: 155-163, 2002.
15. Ho ES, Lin DC, Mendel DB, and Cihlar T. Cytotoxicity of antiviral nucleotides adefovir and cidofovir is induced by the expression of human renal organic anion transporter 1. J Am Soc Nephrol 11: 383-393, 2000.
16. Weinberg JM, Harding PG, and Humes HD. Mitochondrial bioenergetics during the initiation of mercuric chloride-induced renal injury. II. Functional alterations of renal cortical mitochondria isolated after mercuric chloride treatment. The Journal of Biological Chemistry 257: 68-74, 1982.
17. Fillastre JP, Moulin B, and Josse S. Aetiology of nephrotoxic damage to the renal interstitium and tubuli. Toxicology Letters 46: 45-54, 1989.
18. Fowler BA, Kimmel CA, Woods JS, McConnell EE, and Grant LD. Chronic low-level lead toxicity in the rat. III. An integrated assessment of long-term toxicity with special reference to the kidney. Toxicology and Applied Pharmacology 56: 59-77, 1980.
19. Pardi DS, Tremaine WJ, Sandborn WJ, and McCarthy JT. Renal and urologic complications of inflammatory bowel disease. Am J Gastroenterol 93: 504-514, 1998.
20. Thuluvath PJ, Ninkovic M, Calam J, and Anderson M. Mesalazine induced interstitial nephritis. Gut 35: 1493-1496, 1994.
21. Kahn J, Lagakos S, Wulfsohn M, Cherng D, Miller M, Cherrington J, Hardy D, Beall G, Cooper R, Murphy R, Basgoz N, Ng E, Deeks S, Winslow D, Toole JJ, and Coakley D. Efficacy and safety of adefovir dipivoxil with antiretroviral therapy: a randomized controlled trial. The American Journal of Medicine 282: 2305-2312, 1999.
22. Tanji N, Tanji K, Kambham N, Markowitz GS, Bell A, and D'Agati V D. Adefovir nephrotoxicity: possible role of mitochondrial DNA depletion. Human Pathology 32: 734-740, 2001.
23. Sarcletti M, Petter A, Romani N, Lhotta K, Konig P, Maier H, and Zangerle R. Pyuria in patients treated with indinavir is associated with renal dysfunction. Clinical Nephrology 54: 261-270, 2000.
24. Monks TJ and Lau SS. The pharmacology and toxicology of polyphenolic-glutathione conjugates. Annual Review of pPharmacology and Toxicology 38: 229-255, 1998.
24a. Chen JC, Stevens JL, Trifillis AL, and Jones TW. Renal cysteine conjugate beta-lyase-mediated toxicity studied with primary cultures of human proximal tubular cells. Toxicology and Applied Pharmacology 103: 463-473, 1990.
25. Kleinman JG, Breitenfield RV, and Roth DA. Acute renal failure associated with acetaminophen ingestion: report of a case and review of the literature. Clinical Nephrology 14: 201-205, 1980.
25a. Dahlin DC, Miwa GT, Lu AY, and Nelson SD. N-acetyl-p-benzoquinone imine: a cytochrome P-450-mediated oxidation product of acetaminophen. Proceedings of the National Academy of Sciences of the United States of America 81: 1327-1331, 1984.
26. Cohen SD and Khairallah EA. Selective protein arylation and acetaminophen-induced hepatotoxicity. Drug Metabolism Review 29: 59-77, 1998.
27. Bolton JL, Trush MA, Penning TM, Dryhurst G, and Monks TJ. Role of quinones in toxicology. Chemical Research in Toxicology 13: 135-160, 2000.
28. Dekant W, Vamvakas S, and Anders MW. Formation and fate of nephrotoxic and cytotoxic glutathione S-conjugates: cysteine conjugate beta-lyase pathway. Advances in pharmacology (San Diego, Calif) 27: 115-162, 1994.
29. Hughey RP, Rankin BB, Elce JS, and Curthoys NP. Specificity of a particulate rat renal peptidase and its localization along with other enzymes of mercapturic acid synthesis. Archives of biochemistry and biophysics 186: 211-217, 1978.
30. Wolfgang GH, Gandolfi AJ, Stevens JL, and Brendel K. N-acetyl S-(1,2-dichlorovinyl)-L-cysteine produces a similar toxicity to S-(1,2-dichlorovinyl)-L-cysteine in rabbit renal slices: differential transport and metabolism. Toxicology and Applied Pharmacology 101: 205-219, 1989.

31. Groves CE, Lock EA, and Schnellmann RG. Role of lipid peroxidation in renal proximal tubule cell death induced by haloalkene cysteine conjugates. Toxicology and Applied Pharmacology 107: 54-62, 1991.

31a. Chen Q, Jones TW, Brown PC, and Stevens JL. The mechanism of cysteine conjugate cytotoxicity in renal epithelial cells. Covalent binding leads to thiol depletion and lipid peroxidation. The Journal of Biological Chemistry 265: 21603-21611, 1990.

32. Bernareggi A, Torti L, Facino RM, Carini M, Depta G, Casetta B, Farrell N, Spadacini S, Ceserani R, and Tognella S. Characterization of cisplatin-glutathione adducts by liquid chromatography-mass spectrometry. Evidence for their formation *in vitro* but not *in vivo* after concomitant administration of cisplatin and glutathione to rats anc cancer patients. Journal of Chromatography 669: 247-263, 1995.

33. Townsend DM and Hanigan MH. Inhibition of gamma-glutamyl transpeptidase or cysteine S-conjugate beta-lyase activity blocks the nephrotoxicity of cisplatin in mice. The Journal of Pharmacology and Experimental Therapeutics 300: 142-148, 2002.

34. Townsend DM, Deng M, Zhang L, Lapus MG, and Hanigan MH. Metabolism of Cisplatin to a nephrotoxin in proximal tubule cells. J Am Soc Nephrol 14: 1-10, 2003.

35. Mayer RD, Lee KE, and Cockett AT. Inhibition of cisplatin-induced nephrotoxicity in rats by buthionine sulfoximine, a glutathione synthesis inhibitor. Cancer Chemotherapy and Pharmacology 20: 207-210, 1987.

36. Mistry P, Lee C, and McBrien DC. Intracellular metabolites of cisplatin in the rat kidney. Cancer Chemotherapy and Pharmacology 24: 73-79, 1989.

37. Mayer RD, Lee KE, and Cockett AT. Improved use of buthionine sulfoximine to prevent cisplatin nephrotoxicity in rats. Journal of Cancer Research and Clinical Oncology 115: 418-422, 1989.

38. Zalups, R.K. and Diamond, G.L., Nephrotoxicity of Metals, In:Toxicology of the Kidney, Eds. J.B. Tarloff and L.H. Lash, CRC Press, 3rd edition, 2005, 937-993.

39. Brezis M, Rosen S, Silva P, and Epstein FH. Selective vulnerability of the medullary thick ascending limb to anoxia in the isolated perfused rat kidney. The Journal of Clinical Investigation 73: 182-190, 1984.

40. Bernardo JF, Murakami S, Branch RA, and Sabra R. Potassium depletion potentiates amphotericin-B-induced toxicity to renal tubules. Nephron 70: 235-241, 1995.

41. Safirstein R, Deray G. Anticancer: Cisplatin/carboplatin. In: DeBroe ME, Porter GA, Bennett WM, Verpooten GA (eds) Clinical Nephrotoxins. Renal injury from drugs and chemicals. Kluwer Academic, Dordrecht, 261–271, 1998.

42. De Broe ME, Elseviers MM. Analgesic nephropathy. N Engl J Med 1998; 338: 446-452.

43. Nadasdy T, Laszik Z, Blick KE, Johnson DL, Burst-Singer K, Nast C, Cohen AH, Ormos J, and Silva FG. Human acute tubular necrosis: a lectin and immunohistochemical study. Human Pathology 26: 230-239, 1995.

44. Silva GA, Costa LM, Brito FC, Miranda AL, Barreiro EJ, and Fraga CA. New class of potent antinociceptive and antiplatelet 10H-phenothiazine-1-acylhydrazone derivatives. Bioorganic & Medicinal Chemistry 12: 3149-3158, 2004.

45. Levin S, Bucci TJ, Cohen SM, Fix AS, Hardisty JF, LeGrand EK, Maronpot RR, and Trump BF. The nomenclature of cell death: recommendations of an ad hoc Committee of the Society of Toxicologic Pathologists. Toxicologic Pathology 27: 484-490, 1999.

46. Savill J. Apoptosis in resolution of inflammation. Kidney & Blood pressure research 23: 173-174, 2000.

47. Rich T, Allen RL, and Wyllie AH. Defying death after DNA damage. Nature 407: 777-783, 2000.

48. Ortiz A, Lorz C, Catalan MP, Danoff TM, Yamasaki Y, Egido J, and Neilson EG. Expression of apoptosis regulatory proteins in tubular epithelium stressed in culture or following acute renal failure. Kidney International 57: 969-981, 2000.

49. Ortiz A, Justo P, Catalan MP, Sanz AB, Lorz C, and Egido J. Apoptotic cell death in renal injury: the rationale for intervention. Current Drug Targets 2: 181-192, 2002.

50. Bonegio R and Lieberthal W. Role of apoptosis in the pathogenesis of acute renal failure. Current Opinion in Nephrology and Hypertension 11: 301-308, 2002.

50. Meldrum KK, Meldrum DR, Hile KL, Yerkes EB, Ayala A, Cain MP, Rink RC, Casale AJ, and Kaefer MA. p38 MAPK mediates renal tubular cell TNF-alpha production and TNF-alpha-dependent apoptosis during simulated ischemia. American Journal of Physiology 281: C563-570, 2001.

51. Kern JC and Kehrer JP. Acrolein-induced cell death: a caspase-influenced decision between apoptosis and oncosis/necrosis. Chemico-Biological Interactions 139: 79-95, 2002.

51. Lorz C, Ortiz A, Justo P, Gonzalez-Cuadrado S, Duque N, Gomez-Guerrero C, and Egido J. Proapoptotic Fas ligand is expressed by normal kidney tubular epithelium and injured glomeruli. J Am Soc Nephrol 11: 1266-1277, 2000.

52. Lash LH, Hueni SE, Putt DA. Apoptosis, necrosis, and cell proliferation induced by S-(1,2-dichlorovinyl)-L-cysteine in primary cultures of human proximal tubular cells. Toxicology and Applied Pharmacology 177: 1-16, 2001.

53. Lemasters JJ, Qian T, Elmore SP, Trost LC, Nishimura Y, Herman B, Bradham CA, Brenner DA, and Nieminen AL. Confocal microscopy of the mitochondrial permeability transition in necrotic cell killing, apoptosis and autophagy. BioFactors (Oxford, England) 8: 283-285, 1998.

54. Miller GW and Schnellmann RG. A novel low-affinity strychnine binding site on renal proximal tubules: role in toxic cell death. Life Sciences 53: 1203-1209, 1993.
55. Miller GW and Schnellmann RG. Inhibitors of renal chloride transport do not block toxicant-induced chloride influx in the proximal tubule. Toxicology Letters 76: 179-184, 1995.
56. Molitoris BA, Leiser J, and Wagner MC. Role of the actin cytoskeleton in ischemia-induced cell injury and repair. Pediatric Nephrology (Berlin, Germany) 11: 761-767, 1997.
57. Liu KD. Molecular mechanisms of recovery from acute renal failure. Critical Care Medicine 31:S572-81, 2003.
58. Bush KT, Keller SH, and Nigam SK. Genesis and reversal of the ischemic phenotype in epithelial cells. The Journal of Clinical Investigation 106: 621-626, 2000.
59. Bonventre JV. Dedifferentiation and proliferation of surviving epithelial cells in acute renal failure. J Am Soc Nephrol 14 Suppl 1: S55-61, 2003.
60. Nony PA and Schnellmann RG. Mechanisms of renal cell repair and regeneration after acute renal failure. The Journal of Pharmacology and Experimental Therapeutics 304: 905-912, 2003.
61. Lin F. Stem cells in kidney regeneration following acute renal injury. Pediatric Research 59: 74R-78R, 2006.
62. Patschan D, Plotkin M, and Goligorsky MS. Therapeutic use of stem and endothelial progenitor cells in acute renal injury: ca ira. Current Opinion in Pharmacology 6: 176-183, 2006.
63. Bussolati B, Bruno S, Grange C, Buttiglieri S, Deregibus MC, Cantino D, and Camussi G. Isolation of renal progenitor cells from adult human kidney. The American Journal of Pathology 166: 545-555, 2005.
64. Kawaida K, Matsumoto K, Shimazu H, and Nakamura T. Hepatocyte growth factor prevents acute renal failure and accelerates renal regeneration in mice. Proceedings of the National Academy of Sciences of the United States of America 91: 4357-4361, 1994.
65. Ichimura T, Maier JA, Maciag T, Zhang G, and Stevens JL. FGF-1 in normal and regenerating kidney: expression in mononuclear, interstitial, and regenerating epithelial cells. The American Journal of Physiology 269: F653-662, 1995.
66. Wang Z, Zhang B, Wang M, Carr BI. Cdc25A and ERK interaction: EGFR-independent ERK activation by a protein phosphatase Cdc25A inhibitor, compound 5. Journal of Cell Physiology 204:437-44, 2005.
67. Zhuang S, Dang Y, and Schnellmann RG. Requirement of the epidermal growth factor receptor in renal epithelial cell proliferation and migration. Am J Physiol Renal Physiol 287: F365-372, 2004.
68. Witzgall R, Brown D, Schwarz C, and Bonventre JV. Localization of proliferating cell nuclear antigen, vimentin, c-Fos, and clusterin in the postischemic kidney. Evidence for a heterogenous genetic response among nephron segments, and a large pool of mitotically active and dedifferentiated cells. The Journal of Clinical Investigation 93: 2175-2188, 1994.
69. Zhuang S, Yan Y, Han J, and Schnellmann RG. p38 kinase-mediated transactivation of the epidermal growth factor receptor is required for dedifferentiation of renal epithelial cells after oxidant injury. The Journal of Biological Chemistry 280: 21036-21042, 2005.
70. Abbate M, Brown D, and Bonventre JV. Expression of NCAM recapitulates tubulogenic development in kidneys recovering from acute ischemia. The American Journal of Physiology 277: F454-463, 1999.
71. Humphreys BD, Valerius MT, Kobayashi A, Mugford JW, Soeung S, Duffield JS, McMahon AP, Bonventre JV. Intrinsic epithelial cells repair the kidney after injury. Cell Stem Cell 2008 2: 284-291.
72. Franquesa M, Alperovich G, Herrero-Fresneda I, Lloberas N, Bolanos N, Fillat C, Rama I, Cruzado JM, Grinyo JM, and Torras J. Direct electrotransfer of hHGF gene into kidney ameliorates ischemic acute renal failure. Gene Therapy 12: 1551-1558, 2005.
73. Harris RC. Growth factors and cytokines in acute renal failure. Advances in Renal Replacement Therapy 4: 43-53, 1997.
74. Humes HD, Cieslinski DA, Coimbra TM, Messana JM, Galvao C. Epidermal growth factor enhances renal tubule cell regeneration and repair and accelerates the recovery of renal function in postischemic acute renal failure. Journal of Clinical Investigations 84: 1757-61, 1989.
75. Ichimura T, Finch PW, Zhang G, Kan M, Stevens JL. Induction of FGF-7 after kidney damage: a possible paracrine mechanism for tubule repair. American Journal of Physiology 271: F967-76, 1996.
76. Igawa T, Kanda S, Kanetake H, Saitoh Y, Ichihara A, Tomita Y, and Nakamura T. Hepatocyte growth factor is a potent mitogen for cultured rabbit renal tubular epithelial cells. Biochemical and Biophysical Research Communications 174: 831-838, 1991.
77. Miller SB, Martin DR, Kissane J, and Hammerman MR. Insulin-like growth factor I accelerates recovery from ischemic acute tubular necrosis in the rat. Proceedings of the National Academy of Sciences of the United States of America 89: 11876-11880, 1992.
78. Zeisberg M, Shah AA, and Kalluri R. Bone morphogenic protein-7 induces mesenchymal to epithelial transition in adult renal fibroblasts and facilitates regeneration of injured kidney. The Journal of Biological Chemistry 280: 8094-8100, 2005.

79. Hirschberg R, Kopple J, Lipsett P, Benjamin E, Minei J, Albertson T, Munger M, Metzler M, Zaloga G, Murray M, Lowry S, Conger J, McKeown W, O'Shea M, Baughman R, Wood K, Haupt M, Kaiser R, Simms H, Warnock D, Summer W, Hintz R, Myers B, Haenftling K, Capra W, and et al. Multicenter clinical trial of recombinant human insulin-like growth factor I in patients with acute renal failure. Kidney International 55: 2423-2432, 1999.
80. Franklin SC, Moulton M, Sicard GA, Hammerman MR, and Miller SB. Insulin-like growth factor I preserves renal function postoperatively. The American Journal of Physiology 272: F257-259, 1997.
81. Nowak G, Carter CA, and Schnellmann RG. Ascorbic acid promotes recovery of cellular functions following toxicant-induced injury. Toxicology and Applied Pharmacology 167: 37-45, 2000.
82. Nony PA and Schnellmann RG. Interactions between collagen IV and collagen-binding integrins in renal cell repair after sublethal injury. Molecular Pharmacology 60: 1226-1234, 2001.
83. Kovacs CJ, Braunschweiger PG, Schenken LL, and Burholt DR. Proliferative defects in renal and intestinal epithelium after cis-dichlorodiammine platinum (II). British Journal of Cancer 45: 286-294, 1982.
84. Leonard I, Zanen J, Nonclercq D, Toubeau G, Heuson-Stiennon JA, Beckers JF, Falmagne P, Schaudies RP, and Laurent G. Modification of immunoreactive EGF and EGF receptor after acute tubular necrosis induced by tobramycin or cisplatin. Renal Failure 16: 583-608, 1994.
85. Counts RS, Nowak G, Wyatt RD, and Schnellmann RG. Nephrotoxicant inhibition of renal proximal tubule cell regeneration. The American Journal of Physiology 269: F274-281, 1995.

05

Pharmacovigilance: from signal to action

Hubert G. LEUFKENS and Antoine C. EGBERTS

Utrecht Institute for Pharmaceutical Sciences and University Medical Centre, Utrecht, The Netherlands

Introduction

From the very beginning of modern pharmacotherapy there has been the challenge of identifying drug-induced unintended effects as soon and as comprehensive as possible. Any suspicions of an expected or a new problem with a medicine should be well reported, signalled and evaluated. Despite extensive testing of medicines before they are approved for marketing, unexpected and/or rare adverse drug reactions may occur when the medicine is used in normal daily practice. Moreover, also in case that a possible drug-induced problem is already known from the pharmacology of the medicine, e.g. so-called type A effects, it is important to quantify this risk (e.g. in terms of absolute risk, number needed to harm and risk factors), and to put into context when the product is extensively used in clinical practice. This context may include possible strategies for risk management, tailoring the treatment scenario to the individual patient in terms of choice of the medicine, dose and duration, genotyping, consideration of alternative treatments, and so on. Pre-marketing findings regarding safety of medicines are commonly based on the experience of only a few hundreds to thousand people at a maximum, who have been treated in controlled randomised trials. These trials have important limitations in terms of that they [a] usually include rather homogeneous populations (no elderly patients with other diseases, no impaired renal or liver function, etc), [b] they are too small to detect very rare events, [c] they are usual too short to detect long-term effects, [d] they are unable to predict the real world of clinical practice.

A complicating factor is that individual medicinal products are increasingly prone to extensive public debate and societal uncertainty about the safety of medicines in general. Public debate acts as a two-sided sword: attention may work out well because it sensitises patients and health care professionals to be vigilant and to report any observed event or problem related to the use of a medicine. On the other side there is the risk of differential over- and under reporting, very often resulting in biased estimates of the possible drug-induced risk. One may question whether it is still feasible to elucidate and unravel a possible drug exposure-outcome relationship in an independent, science and clinical relevance based fashion, when the debate is shaking the public and economic press, as we could witness with the COX-2 inhibitors (e.g. cardiovascular and gastrointestinal risk), the statins (e.g. myopathy and rhabdomyolysis) or the glitazones (e.g. cardiovascular, fracture risk).

Pharmacovigilance reflects a continuum

The characterization of the full safety profile of a medicine is a dynamic continuum that never ends as long as the drug is on the market. Pharmacovigilance has been defined by WHO as 'the science and activities relating to the detection, assessment, understanding and prevention of adverse effects or any other possible drug-related problems'. The context of the prescribing and usage environment may change over time leading to variations of the risk of drug-drug interactions and of adverse effects related to the patient susceptible genotype. A sudden increase in the rate of spontaneous reports always needs to be analysed in the context of these dynamics. There is increasing evidence that drug safety is a function of both molecular features and the prescribing and usage context leading to three scenarios for drug-induced risk:

- Safety issues primarily related to drug specific characteristics, e.g. type A (pharmacological) and type B (idiosyncratic) adverse reactions.
- Safety issues primarily related to patient specific characteristics e.g. underlying disease, severity of the condition or susceptible genotype, including type B (idiosyncratic) adverse reactions.
- Safety issues primarily related to errors in the prescribing, dispensing and patient usage process, e.g. prescribing-induced interactions, non-compliance with drug labelling, problems as a consequence of usage errors.

There may be some overlap between type B and risks related to patient characteristics, where the later category represents events with a known patient-related mechanism of action. Usually the mechanism of type B drug events is unknown or speculative. However as science and new insights evolve, we see a shift from type B to type A. Examples include for instance severe sensitivity reactions due to the use of abacavir, an HIV drug. This risk was already known from the beginning of clinical drug development and was classified at that time as type B reaction. Interestingly, now we have more insight in the underlying HLA-driven mechanism of this adverse effect, it is becoming more and more a type A reaction.

Another issue that needs careful consideration is that currently a number of complex safety issues cover possible drug-induced problems very close to the indication of the drug, e.g. glitazones for the treatment of diabetes and cardiovascular ADRs or antidepressants and suicide risk in children and adolescents. These cases require comprehensive methods to unravel any causality of drug and event.

To report or not to report

The basis of pharmacovigilance lies in careful watching, cross-patient thinking and the prepared mind that everything that happens in the course of a disease may be of relevance to evaluate treatment outcomes, both beneficial and adverse. Spontaneous reports represent essentially a behavioural dimension of pharmacovigilance, as doctors may be reluctant to report because they think they are too busy, they feel not responsible, or they are afraid of being held accountable or liable for any harm experienced by the patient. As the majority of medicines (between 80-90%) in most countries are prescribed in the community, an essential target of pharmacovigilance is the primary care setting. Primary care physicians are crucial to identify and communicate drug-related events with their colleagues and the competent authorities. But also in hospitals, medical specialists are in the position to link unwanted health effects to drug usage, particularly when it comes to new, specialised products, e.g. oncology drugs, immunosuppressives. Reporting of unexpected and/or adverse events to the relevant pharmacovigilance units in hospitals or to the authorities is an important responsibility of health professionals. Without these reports no functional pharmacovigilance system could exist.

Because reporting is such an explicit human activity is carries in it all the risks of selective reporting, under- or overreporting, and so on. Its power, however, lies in the nation/worldwide collection of suspicions about adverse drug reactions enabling early detection of possible drug hazards far more early than an individual professional ever could. Pharmacovigilance is essentially based on 'numbers count', although one should be careful for biased surges in reports. The literature is full of experiences where spontaneous reports were affected, both qualitative and quantitative, by publicity in the media, by publications in the medical press, or by regulatory action. In some countries there are obligatory systems of reporting of possible drug-induced problems endorsed by formal legislative systems. Many countries don't have these, and so far there is not full agreement on which of these is the best.

Methodology of pharmacovigilance

History shows that, with all the limitations, the dedicated and watchful doctor has remained the backbone for signalling any possible drug-induced problem. The act of prescribing of a medicine cannot be separated from the responsibility to follow the patient over time and to evaluate the treatment response, including any unintended effects, as detailed and prompt as possible. In virtually all countries there is some kind of a system of collecting spontaneous reports of (possible) adverse drug reactions from physicians, pharmacists, industry, nurses, and increasingly acknowledged, also from patients. Spontaneous reports from physicians heavily rely very much on careful observation and recognition of any relevant change in the clinical condition of a patient given the use of a medicine. Because such spontaneous reports can be random noise or a real signal of a clinically relevant drug-induced problem, physicians need to be trained to have an open mind towards the unexpected. Medicines may have unforeseen side effects when used in patients with multiple morbidities, impaired organ function or used in an inappropriate fashion. Determining the signal-noise ratio is a key activity in pharmacovigilance and requires a close collaboration between health professionals, patients, academia, regulatory authorities and the industry.

There is ample literature on the various methods applied in pharmacovigilance. Although there are many differences in the way the methods are implemented or adjusted for specific purpose, the underlying principles are virtually the same. Pharmacovigilance is a cyclic process of [a] signal *detection*, [b] *strengthen* them by careful analysis of background rates of the particular types of events, looking at series of reports, characteristics of the individual patients, and underlying diseases of the patients exposed to the medicine, and finally [3] *follow-up* of the signal in formal pharmacoepidemiological studies. In addition, mechanistic studies are important since they provide clues towards prevention, but have also shown to be a trigger for drug innovation. While in the detection phase there is a strong focus on qualitative issues related to a signal, e.g. quality of the report, causality assessment, the more quantitative methods are key in the strengthening, and particularly in the follow-up phase. The cyclic nature of pharmacovigilance is reflected is a constant learning loop from report-signal-data to (if needed) regulatory action-communication to patients and health professional, and back consequently back into the drug innovation process.

A first, and essential, step in signal detection of drug-induced risk is the proactive and systematic collection of spontaneous reports. After quality control of the data and exclusion of obvious unlikely associated cases from these, the question arises what the numbers say. Are 5 reports enough to raise a signal, do we need 10, 25 or more? As discussed before, a crucial limitation to detect drug-safety signals through spontaneous reports is the frequent lack of valid exposure data. How to cope with this? These are all valid questions and need to be addressed in the context of the question is the observed number more or less then expected. So we need to create an estimate of 'what could be expected', in other words what delivers a valid signal?

Overall there are two approaches to tackle this:

1. Calculation of a frequency (or rate) of the number of reports per 1000 patients, prescriptions, DDD/1000p/day or another available denominator. From there several external comparisons can be made with similar frequencies based on number of cases in an unexposed population, also coined as baseline risk or background frequency, or the number of cases in a population exposed to another medicine from the same therapeutic category. This approach is only possible when reliable denominator data are present. Moreover the head-to-head comparisons require limited under-, over- or selective reporting in the two frequencies of observed possible induced drug problems.

   Example: A study in 1,219 patients of the ATHENA (AIDS Therapy Evaluation National Centre) cohort of patients infected with HIV receiving antiretroviral therapy in the Netherlands showed a frequency of urological symptoms (including nephrolithiasis, renal colic, flank pain, hematuria, renal insufficiency, or nephropathy) of 8.3 per 100 treatment-years for indinavir compared to 0.8 per 100 treatment-years for other HIV protease inhibitors. 8.3 versus 0.8 represents a clear signal, and also a quantitative strengthening of earlier reports of indinavir-induced nephrotoxicty.

2. An alternative approach is an *internal* comparison within all collected reports assuming again limited under-, over- or selective reporting. Within all reports related to, for instance nephrotoxicity, a distribution of the different drug exposures is made. Consequently the question is addressed whether this distribution is different (disproportional) when compared with the distribution of drug exposure in all the other or a sample of all other reports. Disproportionality, evaluating more or less then expected, is a key concept in signal detection. Over the years several measures of disproportionality have been developed with all their inherent pros and contras. The most frequently used is the so-called reporting odds-ratio (ROR).
Example: In follow-up of the receipt of 7 reports acute interstitial nephritis (AIN) by the Netherlands Pharmacovigilance Centre Lareb, the databank of World Health Organisation Collaborating Centre for International Drug Monitoring in Uppsala, Sweden (containing about 3.7 million spontaneous reports from more than 80 countries worldwide) was searched for cases of AIN. A total of 150 AIN cases with recorded proton-pump inhibitors (PPI) use was found. The proportionality of PPI use within the AIN cases was compared to the same in the rest of all 3.7 million reports, resulting in a ROR of 9.4 for omeprazole.

In the strengthening and follow-up phase of pharmacovigilance we can identify a broad array of approaches including Prescription Event Monitoring (PEM), also applied successfully for signal detection, observational pharmacoepidemiological studies in automated databases (e.g. cohort, case-control and variations), and prospective randomised clinical trials. Finally we should add what all the acquired evidence of a valid signal means for regulatory action and informing prescribers and the public. It's the combination of all these activities that carry the potential, and the need, to make pharmacovigilance an important public health tool for the benefit of patient's health.

When we look at the international picture of pharmacovigilance over the last two decades (Figure 1) we may identify three important 'waves' of learning. In the mid-80s, there was growing awareness about flawed comparisons of spontaneous reports when just looking at the crude numbers without comparisons over equivalent periods of the marketing life cycles of the drugs compared. A key paper from this period showed in the case of piroxicam and the risk of gastrointestinal bleeding, perforation, and ulcer, that crude rates of spontaneous reports changed dramatically after adjustments for the heterogeneity in the underlying reporting rates over time. The importance of this learning wave was the acknowledgement of the limitations of spontaneous reports, but not to neglect them as they carry critical information items for pharmacovigilance.

The second wave of pharmacovigilance learning in the early and mid 90s coincides with the evolution of the science of pharmacoepidemiology with a strong emphasis on exposure ascertainment as a crucial factor to evaluate drug-induced effects in a valid fashion. When a surge in reports on possible drug-induced risk is observed, the proper question should be raised whether the drug is bringing the problem to the patient or the patient the problem to the drug? Very often drugs are selectively prescribed to patients with a risky profile resulting in a higher likelihood of drug-induced risk. This process of so-called drug 'channeling', also coined as confounding by indication, is important to understand and to factor in appropriated risk assessment of medicines. This concept has

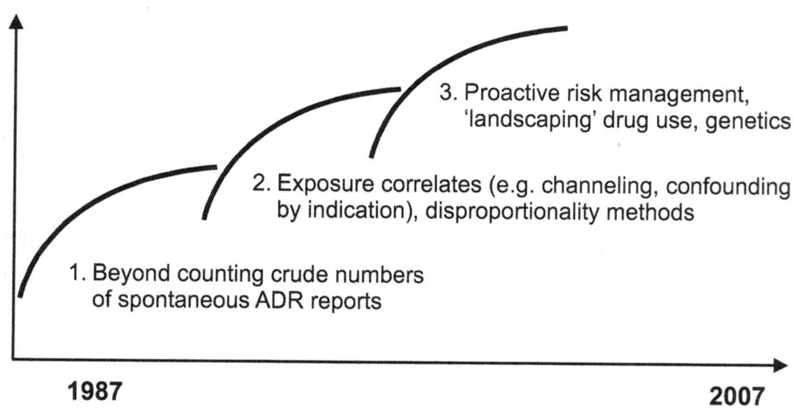

Figure 1. *Two decades of learning in pharmacovigilance.*

also been linked to the fact that aggressive marketing by the pharmaceutical industry can 'kill' important medicinal products when drugs are selectively used in high-risk patients or in an inappropriate, off-label fashion. Essentially, from a methodological point of view, channelling underpins the notion that drug prescribing is virtually never a random activity, thereby implying important challenges for studying these in an observational fashion in an unbiased way, particularly when it comes to study differential drug-induced harm related to individual drugs within drug classes. In the same period we see also a strong development in pharmacovigilance on statistical methods to support evaluation of disproportionality of rates of spontaneous reports. We now enjoy the fruits of these important methodological developments in quantifying possible signals of drug-induced harm.

In the third wave of learning in pharmacovigilance is rightly reflected by the term 'proactive'. There has been growing awareness among regulators, industry and other stakeholders that 'wait and see' is not the way we should continue in protecting individual patients and the public from unintended drug effects. This has resulted in for instance the development of comprehensive programmes for Risk Management Plans to be submitted by pharmaceutical companies as part of the dossier of new medicinal products at the level of the European regulatory system. But also in other regulatory hemispheres there is ample attention for proactive approaches for identifying, and evaluating drug-induced harm as soon as possible, including adequate risk minimisation measures, e.g. information to prescribers, precautions to be taken by patients, and the like. An important signature of these Risk Management Plans is the need to fill the gap between the first signal of drug-induced harm and scientific proof of the risk, followed by regulatory and communication action. Regulatory decision-making and timely action are often hampered by the lack of reliable data on the evidence of the risk when such evidence has to be collected in a retrospective fashion.

Another feature of this third wave of pharmacovigilance learning is the growing notion that populations exposed to certain drugs carry specific baseline risks. There is increasing evidence that the likelihood of the majority of the problems we face in pharmacovigilance is in certain patients more at risk than others. Therefore a critical part of pharmacovigilance is seen in characterizing, also coined 'landscaping', the patient population in order to identify patients and patterns of drug usage susceptible to increased risk. As part of this, pharmacogenetic biomarkers are increasingly considered as important tools to identify proactively possible non-responders in terms of safety to drug therapy. We have already pointed on the example of abacavir and more applications of pharmacogenetics are established or underway. The abacavir case is the first example of European regulatory including pharmacogenetic screening as an integral part of the drug label.

Final thoughts and integration

Pharmacovigilance has become an essential part of public health and pharmaceutical innovation. After new medicinal products have been approved for usage in normal clinical practice the real practice-based benefit-risk balance should be established. In Table 1 a number of well-known cases of drug-induced nephrotoxicity and their pharmacovigilance commonalities are listed. All the five cases show ample variety with respect to signal and exposure factors, the presence of denominator data and how confounding or effect modification might be a issue to evaluate possible drug-related risk on the renal system. This array shows the importance of integrative thinking and well-developed knowledge about the possibilities and limitations of certain approaches, from the historical case of analgesic (including phenacetin) nephropathy towards the most recent findings on gadolinium based contrast agents and nephrogenic systemic fibrosis (NSF). The prepared mind of the doctor and the awareness that reporting is always important, of course in case of newly introduced medicinal products but also with old products, makes pharmacovigilance a typical partnering activity in health care. There is no single party that can do all the work. There is no single approach that suits the solution of all problems.

By its very nature, the renal system carries a high-risk profile for drug-induced toxicity. Mechanistic and pathophysiologic thinking remains critical for a better understanding of observed harm and prediction of possible future harm. This requires at least valid data on signals, exposure, denominator and confounders. When ever possible, proactive and prospective design of the data collection is preferable, if not in many cases the only way to get reliable answers. Current international thinking on pharmacovigilance is in line with these methodological considerations, making the future of this important field in medicine and public health promising for the benefit of patients.

Table 1. Cases of drug-induced nephrotoxicity and their pharmacovigilance commonalities

	Signal factors	Exposure factors	Denominator data	Confounding factors, effect modifiers
Phenacetin	Spontaneous reports, time gap signal and use	OTC, combined with other analgesics	Poor	Co-medications, disease severity, protopatic bias
Protease inhibitors	Already known from RCTs	Combined with other drugs, dosing	Good quality, large cohorts	Previous treatment, body mass, climate
Statins	Spontaneous reports, public media effects	Shift to high potency use, class effect?	Good quality	Drug channelling, selective prescribing
Contrast agents	Problem not signalled by prescriber/radiologist	Timing of exposure, class effect?	Poor	Co-morbidity, confounding by marketing
Cyclosporine	Already known from RCTs	Dose/duration of use, long-term effects	Reasonable quality	Confounding by renal transplant indication

References

1. Bruin ML de, van Puijenbroek EP, Egberts AC, Hoes AW, Leufkens HG. Non-sedating antihistamine drugs and cardiac arrhythmias, biased risk estimates from spontaneous reporting systems? Br J Clin Pharmacol. 2002; 53: 370-4.
2. Dieleman JP, Sturkenboom MC, Jambroes M, Gyssens IC, Weverling GJ, ten Veen JH, Schrey G, Reiss P, Stricker BH; Athena Study Group. Risk factors for urological symptoms in a cohort of users of the HIV protease inhibitor indinavir sulfate: the ATHENA cohort. Arch Intern Med 2002; 162: 1493-501.
3. Egberts TC, Smulders M, de Koning FH, Meyboom RH, Leufkens HG. Can adverse drug reactions be detected earlier? A comparison of reports by patients and professionals. Br Med J 1996; 313: 530-1.
4. Härmark L, van der Wiel HE, de Groot MC, van Grootheest AC. Proton pump inhibitor-induced acute interstitial nephritis. Br J Clin Pharmacol 2007; 64: 819-23.
5. Ingelman-Sundberg M. Pharmacogenomic biomarkers for prediction of severe adverse drug reactions. N Engl J Med 2008; 358: 637-9.
6. Leufkens HG, Urquhart J. Variability in patterns of drug usage. J Pharm Pharmacol 1994; 46 Suppl 1: 433-7.
7. Maitland-van der Zee AH, de Boer A, Leufkens HG. The interface between pharmacoepidemiology and pharmacogenetics. Eur J Pharmacol 2000; 410: 121-130.
8. Meyboom RH, Edwards IR. Rosuvastatin and the statin wars--the way to peace. Lancet 2004; 364: 1997-9.
9. Meyboom RH, Lindquist M, Egberts AC, Edwards IR. Signal selection and follow-up in pharmacovigilance. Drug Saf 2002 ;25: 459-65.
10. Puijenbroek EP van, Bate A, Leufkens HG, Lindquist M, Orre R, Egberts AC. A comparison of measures of disproportionality for signal detection in spontaneous reporting systems for adverse drug reactions. Pharmacoepidemiol Drug Saf 2002; 11:3-10.
11. Rossi AC, Hsu JP, Faich GA. Ulcerogenicity of piroxicam: an analysis of spontaneously reported data. Br Med J 1987; 294:147-50.
12. Stricker BH, Psaty BM. Detection, verification, and quantification of adverse drug reactions. Br Med J 2004; 329(7456): 44-7.
13. Thomsen HS, Marckmann P, Logager VB. Nephrogenic systemic fibrosis (NSF): a late adverse reaction to some of the gadolinium based contrast agents. Cancer Imaging 2007; 7: 130-7.
14. Waller PC, Evans SJ. A model for the future conduct of pharmacovigilance. Pharmacoepidemiol Drug Saf 2003; 12:17-29.
15. WHO. The importance of pharmacovigilance. Safety monitoring of medicinal products. Geneva: World Health Organization, 2002.
16. Xiaoqing G, Chike N. How to prevent, recognize, and threat drug-induced nephrotoxicity. Cleveland Clin J Med 2002: 69: 289-12.

06

Urinary biomarkers and nephrotoxicity

William F. FINN[1] and George A. PORTER[2]

[1]University of North Carolina, Chapel Hill, North Carolina, USA
[2]Oregon Health Sciences University, Portland, Oregon, USA

Introduction

There are a number of definitions of the term "biomarker". In general, they have in common three components: [1] that they are objectively measured indicators of specific anatomic, physiologic, biochemical, or molecular events; [2] that thay are associated with normal biological processes or accompany the onset, progression and/or severity of specific pathological or toxic conditions and [3] are that they are useful for measuring the progress of injury, disease or the effects of therapeutic intervention. For example, according to the National Institutes of Health (NIH) working group, a biomarker is a characteristic that is objectively measured as an indicator of normal biological processes, pathogenic processes, or a pharmacological response to a therapeutic intervention [1].

The types of biomarkers and the purposes served vary to some extent depending on the population beng observed. For public health purposes, the requirements of useful biomarkers to protect from injurious xenobiotic exposure are three-fold: firstly, to achieve the earliest identification of the potential for health impairment; secondly, to gain insight into the mechanism(s) responsible for any adverse impact on the health of individuals or specific populations at risk; and thirdly, to help assess the effects of interventions designed to minimize the short and longterm consequences of the initial injury. Important requirments for biomarker development are a detailed understanding of biochemical pathways involved in nephrotoxicity, minimal invasiveness and capacity to screen large at-risk populations.

Those involved in individual health assessment are concerned with the early detection of specific organ kidney injury. With regard to acute kidney injury (AKI), biomarkers may serve several additional purposes. That is, they may determine AKI subtypes (prerenal, intrinisic renal, or postrenal), identify the etiology of AKI (ischemia, toxins, sepsis, or a combination), differentiate AKI from other forms of acute kidney disease (urinary tract infections, glomerulonephritis, interstitial nephritis), predict the AKI severity (risk stratification for prognostication as well as guide to therapy), monitor the course of AKI, and monitor the response to AKI interventions. For chronic kidney disease (CKD), they provide both evidence and severity of exposure and may be used to assess response to removal of offending toxin.

The pharmaceutical industry has specific interest in the development and utilization of biomarkers for evaluating and predicting the safety of drug candidates during the process of their development. In drug trials, biomarkers have been proposed for use in efficacy determination and patient population stratification, in deducing pharmacokinetic-pharmacodynamic relationships and in safety monitoring [2]. These different phases of drug development involve different functional categories of biomarkers and often involve the patterns of several biomarkers - rather than a change in a single biomarker. The effort to identify reliable biomarkers often involves the interaction of several disciplines such as genetics and epigenetics, genomics, proteomics, metabonomics and assay development [3].

Categories of biomarkers

There have been a number of attempts to formally categorize biologic markers of renal injury in order to achieve a uniform and consistent approach. This have included biomarkers related to a spcific physiologic parameter, such as markers of renal blood flow, glomerular filtration rate, or tubular function; and the chemical nature of the biomarker, such as growth factors, enzymes, adhesion molecules, inflammatory cytokines,etc. One additional classification attempts to define sequential changes in the appearance of one or more biomarkers as renal injury, either acute or chronic, progresses from the initial insult to clinical disease and includes four overlapping stages during that process [4]. These stages consider the nature and magnitude of the initial insult, its relationship to a biologically injurious stimulus, the presence of early biologic effects and eventually on alterations in the structure and/or function of the kidney. At each point along this line, individual susceptibility - which is also subject to various external factors - determines whether or not the process progresses to the development of clinical renal impairment (Figure 1).

In this schema, biomarkers are considered to fall in the three general designations. These include biomarkers of exposures, biomarkers of effect, and biomarkers of susceptibility. Each of these types of biomarkers has specific and relevant applications to the understanding of renal injury and disease. Specific and sensitive bi-

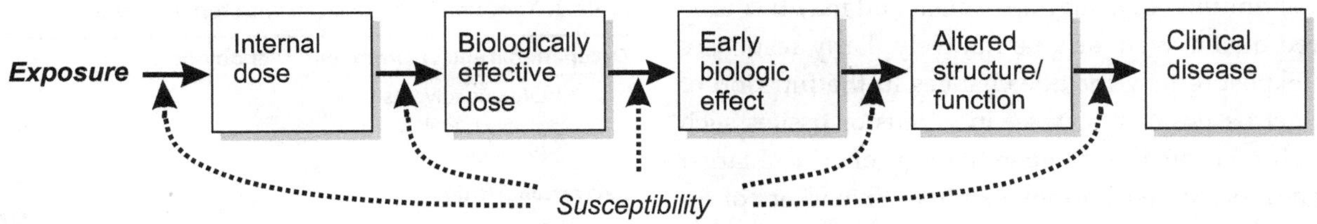

Figure 1. *Simplified flow chart of classes of biologic markers (indicated by boxes). Solid lines indicate progression, if it occurs to the next class of marker. Dashed lines indicate that individual susceptibility influences the rates of progression, as do other variables. Biologic markers represent a continuum of changes, and the classification of change might not always be distinct. (adapted from Committee on Biological Markers of the National Research Council, USA, 1987)*

omarkers constitute the missing link in the continuum of exposure to toxins and susceptibility, disease development and possible therapeutic intervention [5].

Biomarkers of exposure

Biomarkers of exposure are of greatest utility when monitoring exposure to xenobiotics, that is, various chemicals, drugs, and pollutants not naturally present in the body. A biomarker of exposure is more formally defined as "an exogenous substance or its metabolite(s) or the product of the interaction between a xenobiotic agent or other injurious stimulus and the target molecule or cell that is measured within a compartment of an organism" [4]. With regard to xenobiotics, a marker of external exposure is simply the amount of the xenobiotic to which a person is subjected, whereas a marker of internal exposure is the amount of a substance absorbed into the body. Markers of internal exposure are a more accurate means of estimating exposure than are markers of external exposure and require the analysis of biological samples.

Biomarkers of exposure are particularly important in toxicology because they are an indicator of internal dose, or the amount of chemical exposure that has resulted in absorption into the body. Biomarkers of exposure to xenobiotics causing nephrotoxicity may take one of several forms. The measurement of *blood or tissue levels* of drugs known to have adverse effects on the kidney, such as cyclosporine, aminoglycoside antibiotics, or lithium, is a standard practice. The awareness of the *total amount of drug administered* is frequently important when considering amphotericin, analgesics, and cisplatin nephrotoxicity. More difficulty is encountered with the determination of the *body burden of a toxicant,* although under certain circumstances such a value is necessary to determine the health effects of exposure to heavy metals such as cadmium and lead, and some analgesics.

Ideally, biomarkers of exposure should have a direct and quantitative relationship to the xenobiotics' *biologically effective dose.* This term refers to the internal dose of xenobiotic that produces a predictable biologic effect. To gain an understanding of the biologically effective dose, several facts are required (Table 1). These include the knowledge of the amount of xenobiotic which is present in the external environment, its route of entry and the extent of absorption, distribution and accumulation within the body, the target cell or receptor site of the xenobiotic, the route and extent of its metabolism, the modification of the effective dose by associated metabolic, physiologic and pathologic conditions, and finally the pathways of elimination.

Biomarkers of effect

A biomarker of effect is defined as "a measurable alteration of an endogenous component within an organism that, depending on magnitude, can be recognized as a potential or established health impairment or disease" [4]. Markers of effect represent points on

Table 1. Determinants of the biologically effective dose of a xenobiotic.

Amount in external environment
Route of entry
Extent of absorption, distribution and accumulation
Target cell or receptor site
Modification by associated conditions
Route and extent of metabolism
Pathways of elimination

a continuum of health impairment and may be measured qualitatively or quantitatively. Early responses to exposure may include changes in the function of target tissues or responses in organs or tissues such as chromosomal damage, mutations of critical target genes, or altered hormone status. Biomarkers of effect are classified according to their impact on health status. The utility of a biomarker of effect may range from enabling prediction of future health impairment to confirming the presence of clinical disease. The biomarker may either be an indirect manifestation of a disease process or may be a direct result of impaired organ function.

An example of an indirect marker of xenobiotic-induced renal disease is the elevated level of red cell content of either delta amino-levulinic acid dehydrase or free erythrocyte protoporphyrin in patients with lead nephrotoxicity whereas direct urinary markers of lead nephrotoxicity are capable of defining the presence of both glomerular and tubular involvement [6]. Direct examples of biomarkers of effect are dependent upon the nature of the disease process itself. To mention a few, the presence of small amounts of albumin in the urine of patients with diabetes mellitus is an early warning sign of diabetic nephropathy with an increased cardiovascular risk and impaired renal prognosis [7]. Microalbuminuria may also be found in individuals chronically exposed to cigarette smoke accompanied by elevated serum cadmium and lead levels [8]. The appearance in the urine of abnormal amounts of low molecular weight proteins such as β-2 microglobulin (β_2-m) and/or retinol binding protein have been useful in the detection and stratification of workers with industrial exposure to various heavy metals [9,10]. Abnormal patterns of urinary electrolyte excretion and impaired acidification have long been recognized in patients with amphotericin-induced renal injury [11]. Structural lesions within the kidneys may be found in certain electrolyte depletion syndromes such as in the case of the prolonged use of potassium-depleting diuretics [12]. Patients with either acute or chronic renal failure may present with many and varied manifestations of uremia. In these patients, the application of biomarkers of effect to detect clinical disease in its earliest stages is of great importance. Table 2 contains a list of various groups of xenobiotics associated with acute or chronic renal disease.

Table 2. Xenobiotics associated with renal disease.

Occupational and environmental xenobiotics	
	Organic solvents
	Heavy metals
	Pesticides
Recreational drugs	
	Heroin
	Cocaine
Diagnostic and therapeutic agents	
	Antibacterial agents
	Antiviral agents
	Antifungal agents
	Antineoplastic agents
	Immunosuppressive agents
	Non-steroidal anti-inflammatory drugs
	Osmotic agents
	Radiographic contrast material
Natural toxic compounds	
	Aflotoxins
Hemolytic agents and myotoxins	

Among the occupational and environmental xenobiotics associated with AKI are specific substances such as toluene (organic solvents), lead (heavy metals) and chlordane (pesticides). Of the diagnostic and therapeutic agents, the aminoglycosides (antibacterials), acyclovir (antivirals), amphotericin (antifungals), cisplatin (chemotherapeutic agents), cyclosporine (immunosuppressives), and contrast agents stand out. Nonselective non-steroidal anti-inflammatory drugs (NSAIDs) inhibit both cyclooxygenase (COX)-1 and COX-2 are some of the most commonly used medications worldwide. Along with the selective COX-2, these drugs continue to be associated with AKI [13,14]. Notably, high cumulative NSAID exposure is associated with an increased risk for rapid CKD progression in the elderly [15]. The parenteral administration of high doses of certain polyols (mannitol, sorbitol), sugars (glucose, fructose, sucrose, lactose), polysaccharides (inulin), and other products (e.g. radiocontrast agents) may be associated with renal injury marked by vacuolation and subsequent swelling of renal tubular epithelial cells - the so-called "resorptive vacuolation"[16]. An increasing concern is the renal dysfunction associated with the use of heroin and cocaine (recreational drugs) [17].

Some agents such as arsine may trigger a severe hemolytic reaction, causing hemoglobinuria and subsequent acute renal failure. Others may lead to the destruction of striated muscle, and myoglobinuria leading to AKI. In both cases, the consequent "pigment nephropathy" is not an uncommon cause of acute kidney injury. In sum, the most prevalent mechanisms of drug-induced acute kidney injury are vasoconstriction, altered intraglomerular hemodynamics, tubular cell toxicity due to medullary hypoxia, interstitial nephritis, crystal deposition, thrombotic microangiopathy, and osmotic nephrosis [18].

Biomarkers of susceptibility

A biomarker of susceptibility can be defined as "an indicator of an inherent or acquired limitation of an organism to respond to the challenge of exposure to a specific xenobiotic substance" [4]. These markers indicate differences in individuals or populations that affect the body's response to xenobiotic exposure. They may include variations in the balance between enzymes that detoxify or enhance the toxicity of chemicals, genetic differences in the capacity of cells to recover from injury, inherited genetic defects that increase the risk of cancer.

Perhaps the most important susceptibility marker and one quite specific to the kidney is the presence or absence of underlying CKD. It has become apparent that individuals with CKD are at increased risk for the development of more severe injury in response to either nephrotoxic or ischemic events and that the susceptibility is inversely related to the severity of the underlying renal impairment.

While it is understood that the kidneys play a major role in the excretion of drugs and has the capacity to metabolize endogenous and exogenous compounds, CKD decreases the ability of the kidney to metabolize drugs. Less understood is the fact that patients with CKD have a decrease in the nonrenal clearance of multiple drugs resulting in prolonged retention of either the unmodified toxin or its metabolic toxic residue. CKD affects the metabolism of drugs by inhibiting key enzymatic systems in the liver, intestine and kidney [19].

It should be appreciated that a major research goal is to link markers of exposure with markers of effect. Unfortunately, for the vast majority of patients with suspected toxic renal injury the precise knowledge of the offending agent is speculative and not measurable by current techniques. As a result, more is known about the risk factors associated with an adverse health effect than is known about the parameters of exposure (Table 3).

Translating this concept of progressive appearance of biomarkers from exposure to disease into actual practice remains a challenge. The dual aspects of renal function, i.e., filtration/elimination and reabsorption/secretion, assure that no single test or measure can define global renal function. Furthermore, the substantial metabolic and endocrine functions of the kidney are not considered in the classical techniques used to analyze renal function. This has led to the use of a separate category of tests designed to serve as markers of renal dysfunction or injury (Table 4). Also, considerable attention has been directed to the immunological responses that follow xenobiotic exposure. Finally, as the mechanisms responsible for cell injury,

Table 3. Some factors influencing nephrotoxicity.

Urine flow rate
Urine pH
Renal blood flow
Sodium balance
Pre-existing disease
Other drug therapy
Tolerance
Pharmacokinetic factors
Microsomal enzyme activity
Dosage and route of administration
Duration of exposure

Table 4. New parameters and techniques applicable to monitor nephrotoxicity.

Parameters	Techniques
Clearance of lithium, H_2O and N-methylnicotinamide metabolites	High pressure liquid chromatography
Enzymes and antigens	Fluorimetric and luminometric immunoassays
Microproteins	2-Dimensional electrophoresis Immunoblotting techniques Nephelometry, turbidimetry
DNA, mRNA	Southern blotting Pulse field electrophoresis Northern blotting Restricted fragment length analysis
In vivo imaging	Nuclear magnetic resonance spectroscopy
In vitro imaging	Electron probe analysis
Surface markers	Cell sorting

death and regeneration become more apparent, a new and promising set of biomarkers is emerging.

Urinalysis

Test strip screening

The examination of the urine using qualitative test strip provides an estimate of glucose, pH, hemoglobin, protein, specific gravity and a number of other substances including ketones, bilirubin, urobilinogen, leukocytes and nitrate. The degree of sophistication has progressively increased to the extent that reading of test strips with reflectometers is possible. There is a good probability that urines negative by dipstick for protein, blood, leukocytes, nitrates, glucose and ketones will be negative on microscopic examination, with only 5.3% having any abnormality. However, urines positive for one or more of these findings may not correlate well with the microscopic findings due to a number of false positive and false negative by dipsticks for red cells and leukocytes. Sensitivities for dipsticks have been reported to be 75.3% and 81.0% and specificities were 88.6% and 64.3% for red cells and leukocytes, respectively [20]. It is recommended that microscopic analysis be limited to urines in which the dipstick is abnormal. Other limitations have been identified. For example, patients with microalbuminuria or tubular proteinuria are not detected by current test strip methods. Immunological techniques, which enable the determination of specific protein molecules, may make such detection possible [21].

Urine microscopy

The microscopic examination of the urine sediment provides enhanced diagnostic efficiency. *Hematuria:* The normal number of erythrocytes in resuspended urine sediment is no more than 1 to 2 per high-powered field. When an abnormal number of erythrocytes are present it is necessary to distinguish between their origin being renal or non-renal. The simultaneous presence in the urine of casts and protein favor a renal origin. With phase-contrast microscopy, a high percentage of dysmorphic erythrocytes support a renal source of hematuria [22]. The urine should be examined immediately after voiding. Since erythrocytes may be lysed in low specific gravity urine, a concentrated sample should be used for analysis. *Pyuria:* The normal number of white blood cells in the concentrated, resuspended urine sample does not exceed 1 to 2 per high- powered field. In patients with pyelonephritis or nephrotoxic interstitial nephritis, neutrophils may be found whereas with allergic interstitial nephritis, eosinophils may appear. Macrophages and lymphocytes can be found in the urine of some patients with glomerulonephritis and be useful in monitoring the activity of the disease [23]

Tubular epithelial cells

The appearance in the urine of epithelial cells is most likely a result of tubular injury. These cells may be present alone or in casts and be indicative of either acute or chronic tubulointerstitial nephritis. Since casts may dissolve in alkaline urine, an acid urine sample is preferred for analysis.

Eosinophiluria

The finding of eosinophils in the urine with the use of Hansel's stain has been suggested to be useful in establishing the diagnosis of acute interstitial nephritis [24]. However, the positive predictive value in screening samples may be too low, and the number of false positives and negatives in selected groups may be too high for eosinophiluria to stand alone in making the diagnosis of acute interstitial nephritis [25] c. *Urinary macrophages:* The presence of macrophages in the urine of patients with glomerulonephritis reflects the pathological events in the kidney. Urinary macrophage counts increase in patients with proliferative GN, especially in the presence of active glomerular injury [26].

Visceral epithelial cells

The loss of glomerular visceral epithelial cells (podocytes) has been associated with the development of glomerular sclerosis and loss of renal function. The majority of urinary podocytes are viable, although apoptosis occurs in about one-half of the cells. Patients with active glomerular disease excrete more podocytes/mg creatinine than do healthy controls and patients with quiescent disease. It appears that the difference in growth behavior between healthy controls and subjects with active glomerular disease suggests that in active disease viable podocytes detach from the glomerular tuft due to local environmental factors rather than defects in the podocytes per se, whereas in healthy individuals, mostly senescent podocytes are shed [27].

While examination of the urinary sediment has traditionally been used to discriminate the severity of acute kidney injury and to differentiate pre-renal azotemia from established AKI or ATN, the value of this approach is imperfect. Examination of the urinary sediment may have value in critically ill patients, in particular when there is suspicion of systemic vasculitis the detection of dysmorphic red blood cells or red blood cell casts may have important diagnostic, prognostic and therapeutic value [28].

In addition, new technological evolutions have enabled creative diagnostic approaches in urinalysis. Urinary flow cytometry and automated microscopic pattern recognition are two new techniques that are characterised by a much lower imprecision and a higher throughput as compared to conventional microscopy of the urine sediment. Automated urinary test strip analysis offers analytical, clinical, and labour cost-saving advantages [29,30]. Despite these advances, for borderline results, there is no substitute for a urinalysis performed by an experienced nephrologist [31].

Blood urea nitrogen concentration and urea clearance

Urea is quantitatively the most important solute excreted by the kidney and was the first organic solute detected in the blood of patients with kidney failure [32]. Yet it is a poor marker of uremic illness. Furthermore, the blood urea nitrogen (BUN) is not a satisfactory measurement of the glomerular filtration rate. The use of urea to estimate GFR, however, is problematic due to the numerous extra-renal factors that influence its endogenous production and renal clearance, independent of GFR. First, the rate of urea production is not constant. Urea can be grossly modified by a high protein intake, critical illness (i.e. sepsis, burns, trauma), gastrointestinal hemorrhage, or drug therapy such as use of corticosteroids or tetracycline. Conversely, patients with chronic liver disease and low protein intake can have lower urea levels without noticeable changes in GFR. Second, the rate of renal clearance of urea is not constant. An estimated 40–50% of filtered urea is passively reabsorbed by proximal renal tubular cells. Moreover, in states of decreased effective circulating volume (i.e. volume depletion, low cardiac output), there is enhanced reabsorption of sodium and water in the proximal renal tubular cells along with a corresponding increase in urea reabsorption. Consequently, the serum urea concentration may increase out of proportion with changes in SCr and be underrepresentative of GFR. In addition, the urea clearance (C_{urea}) is proportional to the urine flow rate. For example, at low and high rates of urine flow, the minimal and maximal values of the C_{urea} may vary from 30% to 60% of the glomerular filtration rate. This occurs because various tubular segments are permeable to urea and allow passive reabsorption to occur under conditions of antidiuresis. The fractional excretion of urea (FE_{urea}) is calculated as [(urine urea/plasma urea)/(urine creatinine/plasma creatinine) x 100]. A low FE_{urea} may be used as an index of decreased renal perfusion [33,34].

Table 5. Reference ranges for the Scr taking into consideration differences in age and gender.

Age/Sex	Scr mg/dL	Scr µmol/L
0 - 7 d	0.6 - 1.1	53.0 - 97.2
8 d - 1 mo	0.3 - 0.7	26.5 - 61.9
1 mo - 2 yr	0.3 - 0.6	26.5 - 53.0
3 - 4 yr	0.3 - 0.7	26.5 - 61.9
5 - 9 yr	0.4 - 0.9	35.4 - 79.6
10 - 17 yr Male	0.5 - 1.1	44.2 - 97.2
10 - 17 yr Female	0.4 - 1.0	35.4 - 88.4
18 yr+ Male	0.8 - 1.4	70.7 - 123.8
18 yr+ Female	0.7 - 1.1	61.9 - 97.2

Serum creatinine concentration

Serum creatinine is an amino acid compound derived from the metabolism of creatine in skeletal muscle and from dietary meat intake [35]. The serum creatinine concentration (Scr) is a commonly used marker for the estimation of adequate renal function due to the fact that it is released into the plasma at a relatively constant rate, is freely filtered by the glomerulus, and is not metabolized nor reabsorbed by the kidney. Various 'reference ranges' for the Scr take into consideration differences in age and gender (Table 5), but fail to consider other variables such as race, body weight and muscle mass. As a result, a Scr within the 'reference range' cannot be considered to be *a priori* evidence of 'normal' renal function. For example, an estimated 10–40% of creatinine clearance occurs by tubular secretion of Scr into the urine [36]. For subjects with chronic kidney disease (CKD) there is a considerable lack of precision in accepting the Scr. SCr values may not show significant increases until approximately 50% of kidney function is lost. For individuals with glomerular filtration rate greater than 30 ml/min, the 95% confidence interval for Scr is ± 22%, whereas it is ± 13% in patients with glomerular filtration rate less than 30 ml/min [37].

The actual Scr may be increased or decreased independent of changes in the glomerular filtration rate by inhibiting or stimulating renal tubular secretion. For example, trimethoprim and/or trimethoprim/sulfamethoxazole have been demonstrated to cause a 15 to 35% increase in Scr due to an inhibition of tubular secretion [38]. The free radical scavenger, N-acetylcysteine, appears to facilitate tubular secretion in volunteers with normal renal function as judged by a fall in the Scr without a change in cystatin C levels [39], although the situation may be different in patients with stage 3 CKD [40]. In addition to trimethoprim, cimetidine and salicylates also produce elevations in the SCr by altering the normal elimination pathways of creatinine. Phenacemide has been reported to increase creatinine elimination [41].

Differences in analytical techniques may also account for variation in the reported Scr [42,43]. For example, overestimation of the Scr may occur because of interference from substances other than creatinine ("noncreatinine chromogens"), such as proteins and ketoacids, and high levels of bilirubin or glucose to cause false elevations of the Scr. Several drugs have been reported to interfere with SCr results obtained with both the Jaffé-based and enzymatic analytical assay systems by producing assay interference. When Scr samples are calibrated in a single reference laboratory, noncalibrated Scr values were greater than standardardized creatinine values [44]. The National Kidney Foundation's current practice guidelines recommend standardization of serum creatinine assay calibration to increase assay accuracy. This will result in a lower range of values being considered normal and will result in higher calculated glomerular filtration rates and creatinine clearance [45]. Recently, it has been reported that serum levels tryptophan glycoconjugate might replace inulin clearance in the clinical setting [45a]. However, because of the technical difficulty in measuring tryptophan glycoconjugate [45b] it is unlikely to gain wide-spread acceptance.

Lastly, it should be mentioned that the SCr does not depict real-time changes in GFR that occur with acute reductions in kidney function. Rather, SCr requires time to accumulate prior to being detected as abnormal, thus leading to a potential delay in the diagnosis of AKI.

Creatinine clearance

The endogenous creatinine clearance (Ccr) gives an acceptable estimate of the glomerular filtration rate and is the most widely used method in clinical practice for routine purposes. However, in normal individuals, the majority of measurements tend to yield values of Ccr that exceed the actual glomerular filtration rate by a substantial amount, owing to the fact that there is a small but significant amount of creatinine which appears in the urine as a result of tubular secretion. This problem is accentuated when the glomerular filtration rate declines. Ccr measurements may be twofold higher than the actual glomerular filtration rate because of continued tubular secretion of creatinine at a time when the rate of filtration is severely curtailed. Indeed, the amount of secreted creatinine varies inversely with the glomerular filtration rate [46,47]. An alternative method is the determination of creatinine clearance (CCr) after oral administration of cimetidine. This drug blocks tubular secretion of creatinine and CCr measured under these conditions is reported to be nearly identical to GFR in mild or severe renal failure. It has been suggestd that the measurement of CCr (without cimetidine) is an anachronism and should be abandoned [48].

Glomerular filtration rate

Estimated glomerular filtration rate

An alternative to the measurement of the Ccr is the use of either nomograms or formulae to estimate the glomerular filtration rate. The two most widely used equations are the Cockcroft-Gault and the Modification of Diet in Renal Disease (MDRD) study equations [46,47].

Cockroft and Gault, 1976 [49]:

Males:

$$\text{Ccr (ml/min)} = \frac{(140 - \text{age in years}) \times (\text{weight in kg}) \times 1.73}{72 \times \text{serum creatinine (mg/100 ml)} \times \text{body surface area (kg/m}^2)}$$

Females = males × 0.85

Modification of Diet in Renal Disease (MDRD):

Original MDRD Study equation [50]:

Estimated GFR (mL/min/1.73 m^2) =

$$186 \times (\text{Scr})^{-1.154} \times (\text{Age})^{-0.203} \times (0.742 \text{ if female}) \times (1.210 \text{ if black})$$

Reexpressed MDRD Study equation for standardized serum creatinine [51]:

Estimated GFR (mL/min/1.73m^2) =

$$175 \times (\text{standardized SCr})^{-1.154} \times (\text{Age})^{-0.203} \times (0.742 \text{ if female}) \times (1.210 \text{ if black})$$

As mentioned above, there is some degree of variability in measuring the Scr that can be corrected by standardizing the procedure [42]. When the standardized Scr is used in estimation the GFR, a slight modification in the formula occurs [51]. The National Science Foundation recommends that kidney function should be assessed and monitored using an eGFR, rather than serum creatinine concentration alone as do a number of international organizations including the National Kidney Foundation [52], using the eGFR to determine the stages of CKD according to the NKF KDOQI guidelines presented in Table 6.

In general, there is a wide degree of scatter when values of glomerular filtration rate are predicted by these equations, although the equation derived from the MDRD study provides more accurate estimates of GFR than the other formulae or measured clearances and is comparable to values obtained using iothalamate clearance. The MDRD calculation looses accuracy at eGFR > 60ml/min/1.73m^3. The variation in calculated Ccr is particularly true in the elderly or others with large decreases in muscle mass, in patients with liver disease, and individuals ingesting a high-protein diet or those receiving parenteral nutrition containing amino acid solutions. Absolute variation is also more evident at higher estimated GFR.

Measured glomerular filtration rate

Any substance used to measure glomerular filtration rate should be metabolically intact, freely filtered through the glomerular capillary wall, and be neither secreted nor reabsorbed by the tubules. Accurate plasma and urine quantitation also should be easily achievable. In addition to inulin, several compounds are useful for the measurement of glomerular filtration rate. These include the urologic contrast media, eg. diatrizoate, iohexol, other useful compounds include: ^{57}cocyanocobalamine, ^{51}Cr-ethylenediaminetetraacetic acid (EDTA) or sodium ^{125}I iodothalamate and ^{99m}Tc-diethylenetriaminepentaacetic acid (DTPA). All provide reliable measurement of glomerular filtration rate [53]. Inulin is a polymer of fructose and is an ideal glomerular filtration rate marker because it is freely filtered and neither reabsorbed or secreted by the tubules. It has been widely used as a research tool but because of a number of technical difficulties, it is rarely used in clinical settings. Isotopic methods offer a high level of reliability but the impracticality of using these methods in a clinical setting makes them unsuitable for routine use. On the other hand, Iohexol is a convenient, reliable technique for measuring GFR and has the same precision as ^{125}I-iodothalamate [54].

Table 6. Stages of CKD based on eGRF as proposed by KDOQI guidelines of NKF.

Stage of kidney disease	GFR
Stage 1	≥ 90 mL/min/1.73 M^2 and structural abnormalities
Stage 2	60-89 mL/min/1.73 M^2
Stage 3	30-59 mL/min/1.73 M^2
Stage 4	15-29 mL/min/1.73 M^2
Stage 5	<15 mL/min/1.73 M^2 or dialysis

As an alternative to the standard clearance techniques which involve the collection of urine over a known period of time plus maintaining a constant plasma level of an appropriate marker, the glomerular filtration rate can be calculated from the rate of disappearance from the plasma of any tracer, where:

$$\text{Clearance} = \frac{\text{Injected dose}}{\text{Area under plasma concentration curve}}$$

Additional techniques to obtain more reliable estimates of glomerular filtration rate without resorting to steady-state infusions involve the plotting of the declining plasma level of radio isotopic agents [55] or non-radioactive iodinated contrast agents [56] if they are cleared by glomerular filtration. The glomerular filtration rate as measured with iohexol shows excellent agreement with the values obtained using inulin and chelates throughout a wide range of kidney function. [53, 57,58]. As noted previously, in healthy adults, the endogenous creatinine clearance tends to exceed the "true" GFR as determined by inulin or iohexol clearances [59].

The "renal reserve" is determined by measuring the percentage increase in baseline dglomerular filtration rate following ingestion of a high protein meal. The failure of the glomerular filtration rate to increase in response to such a challenge suggests that underlying chronic disease and nephron atrophy has been masked by hypertrophy of other nephrons so that overall renal function seems to be well maintained. Renal function is preserved with aging in healthy subjects at the expense of elimination of the 'renal reserve" [60]. In this regard, the GFR, whether estimated or measured, is a reliable marker of susceptibity to both ischemic and nephrotixic injury - particularly when the value falls below 60 mL/min. Indeed, the susceptibility of the kidney to superimposed acute injury markedly increases as renal function declines.

Renal blood flow

If a marker is extracted from the blood exclusively by the kidney resulting in a renal venous concentration of 0% (i.e. the arterio-venous extraction fraction is 100%), then the calculated value of the clearance of the marker (Cx) is equal to renal plasma flow. In practice, a compound, such as *para*-amino hippurate (PAH) with an extraction fraction of about 87%, is used. To acknowledge the fact that there is discrepancy between the PAH clearance and renal plasma flow, the term effective renal plasma flow is used when the extraction factor is not measured. In sum, renal plasma flow = effective renal plasma flow + extraction factor and renal blood flow = effective renal plasma flow + the hematocrit.

A decrease in the PAH clearance might be due to either an actual decline in renal plasma flow or a decrease in the extraction factor of *PAH*. The latter occurs when the tubular secretion of *PAH* in proximal tubules is impaired due to tubular disease or the presence of substances, which compete with transcellular *PAH* transport. Thus, the PAH clearance cannot be considered a reliable measure of renal plasma flow, unless the extraction factor of *PAH* is measured simultaneously. This requires that a sample of renal venous blood be obtained.

Tubular function

The identification of a reliable and convenient method for the estimation of the reabsorptive and secretory capacity of the kidney has proven to be a considerable challenge to Nephrology. This is not unexpected when one considers the complex and integrated functions contributed by the various tubular segments to insure proper composition of bladder urine. General estimates of integrated tubular function include the capacity of the kidneys to concentrate or dilute the urine in response to water deprivation or administration; the ability to excrete an administered acid load; and the precision with which sodium balance is maintained. But lacking is a technique for assessing tubular function, which rivals the measurement of glomerular filtration rate.

Specific gravity and osmolality

The urinary specific gravity and osmolality are indicators of the ability of the kidney to concentrate and dilute the urine. The urinary specific gravity depends upon the size and weight of urinary solutes. The normal range is 1.003 to 1.025 whereas the possible range is 1.001 to 1.040. Osmolarity indicates the total number of solute particles per kilogram of urine water. The normal range is from 150 to 900 mosm/kg with a possible range from 50 to 1200 mosm/kg. The discovery of four major water channels in the kidney, namely aquaporins (AQP) 1, 2, 3 and 4, has allowed a substantial increase in our understanding of renal water regulation. The renal aquaporin water channels are involved in the urinary dilution and concentrating defects in cardiac failure, cirrhosis, syndrome of inappropriate hormone secretion, pregnancy, hypothyroidism, isolated glucocorticoid deficiency, isolated mineralocorticoid deficiency, primary polydipsia, acquired and genetic nephrogenic diabetes insipidus [61,62].

pH

A hydrogen ion concentration gradient of 1 to 1000 may be established across tubular cell membranes of the kidney. Since the pH is the negative logarithm of the hydrogen ion concentration, this translated into a decrease from the normal plasma pH value of 7.4 to the minimal urine pH of 4.4. The pH of urine is dependent on the time of day, the prandial state, diet, health status, and medications. Urinary pH exhibits a diurnal variation with decreased pH values at night and in the early morning (most acidic towards midnight) followed by increasing pH values upon awakening. Urine tends to become alkaline immediately after a meal because of a phenomenon known as the alkaline tide and gradually becomes acidic between meals. A high protein diet is associated with acidic urine, and a vegetarian diet typically produces more alkaline urine because of bicarbonate formation from fruits, especially citrus, and vegetables. Bacterial contamination of urine with microorganisms that split urea may yield urinary pH values > 8.0 because of bacterial decomposition of urea to ammonia. The pH values of specimens stored at -20 degrees C are relatively stable, whereas pH results > 9 develop when urine samples are stored at room temperature or higher. Degradation of nitrogenous urine analytes is most likely responsible for the noted increases in pH. [63].

Lithium clearance

The study of renal segmental tubular sodium handling by measurement of exogenous or endogenous lithium clearance has been a source of valuable information about in-vivo alterations of tubular sodium and water transport in humans The lithium clearance is a used to estimate the amount of sodium and water delivery from the pars recta of the proximal tubule into the descending limb of the loop of Henle [64]. This information may be helpful in the assessment of the state of hydration. The method is based on several assumptions the most important of which are that lithium reabsorption parallels sodium and water along the entire proximal tubule; that lithium is neither reabsorbed 'in measurable amounts beyond the pars recta of the proximal tubule; nor is it secreted by the tubular cells [65]. This technique is based on the principle that, while sodium and water are reabsorbed at several sites along the nephron, the lithium ion is taken up almost exclusively at proximal tubular sites, so that the amount of lithium escaping reabsorption at this level is quantitatively excreted in the urine. As lithium in the proximal tubule is transported by the same systems driving sodium and water, the parallel measurement of lithium, sodium and creatinine clearance may provide reasonably accurate and complete information as to the occurrence of abnormalities in sodium and water handling at different sites along the nephron.

LiCl has been used to evaluate salt and water handling in cirrhotic patients and found increased sodium reabsorption in the distal tubule accounts for the salt retention that characterizes this clinical condition [66]. Increased proximal sodium re-absorption is associated with the metabolic syndrome (MS) in white men and women. This relationship is not seen in people of African or South Asian origin, despite a greater degree of insulin resistance [67]. It appears that an alteration of renal tubular sodium handling is an important feature of MS, involving an increased rate of proximal sodium and water reabsorption with a modification of the normal pressure–natriuresis relationship [68]. Patients with ascites showed a positive correlation between lithium fractional excretion and glomerular filtration rate ($r = 0.64$, $P < 0.05$). Reduction in renal perfusion, increased filtration fraction, and Tubular-Glomerular Feedback derangement, as found in decompensated patients, are indicative of prevalent postglomerular arteriolar vasoconstriction, with ensuing stimulation of proximal tubular sodium reabsorption [69].

Proteinuria

The glomerular wall contains three layers: endothelial cells, basement membrane, and epithelial cells. Under normal circumstances, the glomerular filtration barrier restricts the transfer of high molecular weight proteins from plasma to the nephron lumen while allowing the filtration of small molecules. Much of the selectivity of filtration occurs in the basement membrane, where the barrier excludes proteins on the basis of both their size and their charge. Uncharged molecules pass through the basement membrane more readily than negatively charged proteins of a similar size. In certain pathologic states, the permselectivity of the filtration barrier changes allowing high molecular weight proteins to appear in the urine. These proteins undergo pinocytotic reabsorption in the proximal tubule creating cytoplasmic vesicles that then fuse with primary lysosomes to form secondary lysosomes. In this final form the proteins are hydrolyzed to amino acids, which are delivered into the blood stream. In contrast, under normal conditions a finite amount of low molecular weight proteins are filtered which then undergo reabsorption by proximal tubular cells. Exopeptidases situated on the brush border membrane are responsible for splitting peptides up to a molecular weight of 10,000 daltons. Following metabolic conversion, reabsorption of the amino acids or dipeptides occurs by specific sodium-dependent carriers [70]. When the reabsorptive capacity of the proximal tubular epithelium is disrupted, various low molecular weight proteins escape reabsorption and can be measured in the urine. Thus, the distinction between so-called "glomerular" proteinuria and "tubular" proteinuria is based on both the quantity and quality of the proteins measured in the urine [71] (Figure 2). A recent refinement of this differentiation in protein selectivity has been the "so-called" urine protein expert system [72,73]. This expert system, which includes total protein, albumin, β_1-microglobulin, IgG, α_2-microglobulin, NAG and creatinine, has proven to be more discriminatory in providing correct clinical diagnoses which are histologically confirmed, as compared to human expert diagnosis. Another approach to differentiating glomerular from tubular disease involves analyzing urinary proteins with the SDS-PAGE system that separates various urinary protein species. In a recent report, Lau and Woo [74] found an excellent correlation between SDS-PAGE prediction and findings on renal biopsy. In general, proteins in the urine may be classified into six main categories according to their origin (Table 7).

Measuring urinary protein excretion has been simplified by the introduction of the urine protein to creatinine ratio [U_P:U_{cr}] [75,76]. Although random spot U_P:U_{cr} ratio predicts actual 24 h protein excretion with reasonable accuracy in patients with lower levels of protein excretion but is unreliable in patients with high protein excretion and should not be used in the clinical setting unless 24 h urine collection is unavailable [77]. None-the-less, the use of spot urine U_P:U_{cr} ratio is useful as a tool in screening and monitoring proteinuria [78, 78a,78b].

Table 7. Classification of proteinuria according to site of origin.

Plasma proteins
Kidney-derived proteins
Proteins from the urogenital tract
Proteins released from tissue outside the urogenital tract
Pregnancy associated proteins
Tumor-derived proteins

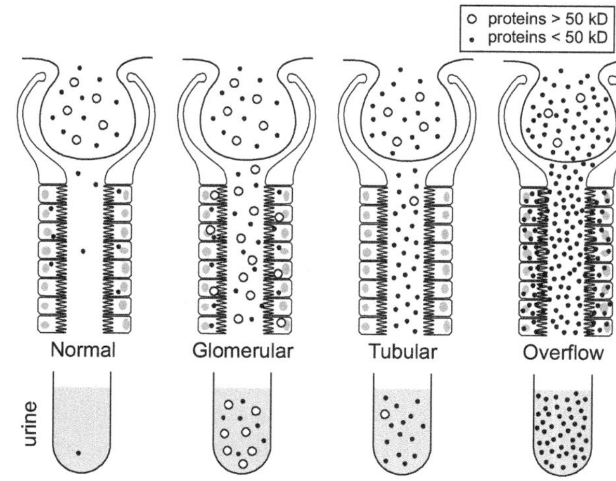

***Figure 2.** Three kinds of proteinuria.*

In addition to serving as markers of renal dysfunction, it is now evident that the filtration of abnormal amounts and/or types of proteins influences the progression of renal disease by promoting secondary injury to tubular epithelial cells and interstitial structures. Proteinuria itself has been proposed to contribute to progressive renal injury inflammation [79,80]. For example, the upregulation of various cytokines in tubular epithelial cells may contribute to the development of interstitial fibrosis and cell cycle activation leading to tubular cell proliferation and/or apoptosis [81-83]. Albumin can increase AngII production and in turn upregulate TGF-β receptor expression [84]. Other filtered components of the urine in proteinuric states, such as oxidized proteins, appear to be more potent in inducing direct injury of tubular epithelial cells and activating proinflammatory and fibrotic chemokines and cytokines. Complement and various lipoproteins are also present in the urine in proteinuric disease states and can activate reactive oxygen species [85,86]. Proteinuria may thus alter tubule cell function directly, potentially contributing to a more profibrotic phenotype, and also augment interstitial inflammation, in particular by macrophages. Proteinuria may activate many profibrotic pathways through its ability to increase NF-kB, and also by other pathways. These include, for instance, complement synthesis occurring in renal tubules [87].

Proteomics is the study of protein expression in a tissue or biological fluid. Comparison of protein patterns in biological fluids between healthy individuals and patients with disease is increasingly being used both to discover biological markers of disease and to identify biochemical processes important in disease pathogenesis. Currently available tests for urine proteins measure either the total level of urine protein or the presence of a single protein species. Emerging proteomic technologies allow simultaneous examination of the patterns of multiple urinary proteins and their correlation with individual diagnoses, response to treatment or prognosis [88,88a]. The application of proteomic methods and informatic analysis have been used to identify patterns of urine proteins that are characteristic of the nephritic syndrome resulting from FSGS, lupus nephritis, membranous nephropathy, or diabetic nephropathy. These data showed that diseases that cause nephrotic syndrome change glomerular protein permeability in characteristic patterns. The fingerprint of urine protein charge forms identifies the glomerular disease [89].

High-molecular weight proteinuria

The appearance in the urine of serum proteins with a molecular weight (MW) in excess of 40,000 to 50,000 daltons is an early marker of glomerular damage. The commonly measured high molecular weight proteinuria includes: albumin (Mr 69,000), transferrin (Mr 77,000) and IgG (Mr 146,000) (Table 8).

Albumin

Albumin is quantitatively the major urinary protein derived from plasma. Its average concentration in normal urine is at least 50 times higher than most other low molecular weight proteins. Albumin's molecular size (molecular radius: 3.6 nm) and strong negative charge, effectively retarded filtration at the glomerular barrier since the vast majority of pores perforating the glomerular filtration barrier have a radius of 2.9–3.1 nm. The loss of negative charges causes the effective small pore radius to increase to approximately 4.5 nm, which allows the passage of albumin. The small amounts of albumin that ordinarily escape into the glomerular filtrate are reabsorbed by the proximal tubule with a presumed efficiency of 99%. Transient and totally reversible increases in the albumin excretion may be observed in various "physiologic" situations that induce increases in the glomerular filtration rate such as heavy exercise, fever, or assuming an orthostatic position.

A 24 hour unine collection showing an albumin excretion at a rate of 20 to 200 μg/min or a urinary concentration of 30 to 300 mg/L measured on at least two occasions is refeerred to as microalbuminuria. Urinary albumin levels above these values are called "macroalbuminuria", or sometimes just albuminuria. To compensate for the variablility in urine concentra-

Table 8. Characteristics of urinary proteins.

Protein	Abbv.	Molecular weight kD	GSC*	Normal urinary excretion mg/mmol creatinine	Normal plasma levels mg/L
β_2-microglobulin	β_2-m	11.6	18.3 (4.4-32.2)	< 0.05	1.3
Retinol-binding protein (free)	RBP	21	13.6 (5.1-22.1)	<0.017	5.8
Thyroid-stimulating hormone	TSH	28	0.99 (0.3-1.68)	<0.05	2
α_1-microglobulin	α_1-m	31	21.1 (9.5-32.9)	<2	32
α_1-acid glycoprotein	α_1-AG	40	—	<0.02	770
Zinc-α_2-globulin	ZAG	41	—	<0.02	140
β_2-Glycoprotein I	β_2-GI	50	12.3 (6.1-18.5)	<0.03	150
Vitamin D binding protein	DBP	51.3	—	<0.01	400
Transthryetin	TTR	55	—	<0.01	300
Albumin	ALB	65.5	13.8 (6.6-21)	<0.025	45000
Transferrin	TRF	78	1.2 (0.6-1.8)	<0.19	2700
Immunoglobulin G	IgG	160	58 (34-82)	<0.2	120000

**GSC= glomerular sieving coefficient*

tion on spot check samples, it has been the practice to compare the amount of albumin in the sample against its concentration of creatinine. This is termed the albumin/creatinine ratio and microalbuminuria is defined as an albumin/creatinine ratio ≥2.5 mg/mmol (male) or ≥3.5 mg/mmol (female). However, the albumin/creatinine ratio does not appear to provide any advantage compared with the measurement of microalbuminuria alone in a spot urine sample [90]. Indeed, newer systems for microalbuminuria detection are as accurate and precise as laboratory albumin/creatine ratio estimations and an improvement over the traditional dipstick methods [91]. However it is measured, microalbuminuria may be an indicator of subclinical cardiovascular disease, a marker of vascular endothelial dysfunction and an important prognostic marker for kidney disease. Prospective and epidemiologic studies have found that microalbuminuria is predictive, independently of traditional risk factors, of all-cause and cardiovascular mortality and CVD events within groups of patients with diabetes or hypertension, and in the general population [92].

The relationship between albuminuria and risk is not restricted to the microalbuminuric range and extends to as low as 2-5 microg/min. A urinary albumin excretion above 200 microg/min (macroalbuminuria) heralds the onset of proteinuria (urinary protein excretion above 0.5 g/24 h) and progressive renal and cardiovascular disease. Proteinuria is a sign of established kidney damage and plays a direct pathogenic role in the progression of renal and cardiovascular disease as described above. Albuminuria reflects functional and potentially reversible abnormalities initiated by glomerular hyperfiltration, proteinuria, a size-selective dysfunction of the glomerular barrier normally associated with glomerular filtration rate (GFR) decline that may result in end-stage renal disease. Thus, the limit of 200 μg/min segregates patients with albuminuria or proteinuria who are at quite different risk. Among subjects with albuminuria, however, there is a continuous relationship between albumin excretion and risk and no lower bound between normal albuminuria and microalbuminuria can be identified that segregates subjects at different risk [93].

At any level, the proteinuria may be nonselective in that it contains the spectrum of molecular sizes. For example, when microalbuminuria is observed in the absence of low molecular weight proteinuria, it may be ascribed to enhanced glomerular permeability. When accompanied by an increased urinary excretion of low molecular weight proteins, microalbuminuria results wholly or partly from impaired albumin reabsorption.

Transferrin

Transferrin, the iron-transporting protein, occurs in urine at concentrations that are about 15 times lower than that of albumin. The protein has a slightly larger effective molecular radius (around 4.0 nm) than albumin (3.6 nm). Its detection in the urine allows a more sensitive indicator of early glomerular involvement in some nephropathies such as cadmium nephropathy. A strong association has been found between the presence of albumin and transferrin in the urine of patients with the nephrotic syndrome. In these patients, increased transferrin synthesis is insufficient to compensate for urinary losses and plasma levels are reduced [94].

Gamma globulins

Gamma globulins excreted in the urine include IgG, IgM, IgA, and immunoglobulin light chains. IgG and IgM are large proteins with molecular radii of 5.5 and 12 nm, respectively. The appearance in the urine of IgG indicates an increased density of large pores in the glomerular filtration barrier with a radius of 8 to 9 nm whereas the presence of IgM in the urine indicates an increased density of shunts in the glomerular capillary wall [95, 96]. Coupled with the measurement of urinary albumin concentrations, the determination of urinary levels of IgG and IgM are useful for assessing the selectivity of the glomerular-type proteinuria [97]. The urinary excretion of IgG is regarded as a reliable index of a non-selective pathway shunt through the glomerular capillary wall. In this regard, it has been reported that proteinuria in patients with type 1 diabetes mellitus is mainly due to impaired charge-selective properties of the glomerular capillary wall, while proteinuria in type 2 diabetes mellitus is predominantly caused by a decreases size selectivity of the glomerular capillary wall [98]. Moreover, proteinuric patients with a high urinary content of IgG and IgM have poor renal survival [99]. IgG, transferrin, albumin, and α_1 microglobulin were used to predict progression of renal failure and extent of tubulointerstitial disease in patients with idiopathic membranous nephropathy [100]. As a result it was found that IgG excretion has a direct, positive correlation with the extent of tubulo-interstitial disease and α_1-microglobulin excretion rates. An increased excretion of monoclonal light chains, i.e. Bence-Jones proteins, is usually the sign of an overproduction from a neoplastic origin such as multiple myeloma or Waldenstrom's macroglobulinemia.

Low-molecular weight proteinuria

In contrast, "tubular" proteinuria is often less than 1.0 g/24 hours and composed of LMW proteins. Several LMW proteins normally appear in the urine and have been evaluated as potential biomarkers of effect in renal tubular damage. Included are β_2-microglobulin (β_2-m), retinol binding protein and α-l microglobulin (α_1-m). Other LMW proteins of interest include protein 1, amylase, lysozyme, ribonuclease and cystatin C. Combining LMW proteins with prostanoids, growth factors and enzymes of renal and non-renal origin, excretory patterns have been identified which provide insight as to the site and mechanism of nephrotoxic injury.

β2-microglobulin

β2-microglobulin (β_2-m) is a low molecular weight (Mr: 11,800) globular protein located on the surface of virtually all nucleated cells. It is closely related to the class I histocompatibility antigens which consist of a heavy, variable chain and a light chain that binds to the heavy chain domain nearest to the cell membrane. The light chain consists of the β_2-m molecule. Due to its molecular weight and small radius, β_2-m is readily filtered at the glomerulus. Under normal circumstances, approximately 99.9% of the filtered β_2-m is reabsorbed by the proximal tubular epithelial cells and ultimately catabolized. A very small amount, around 70 to 80 mg/24 hours, appears in the urine. The urinary excretion of β_2-m is considerably increased in cases of renal tubular impairment. As a result, the determination of urinary β_2-m has been widely used for the screening of proximal tubular damage in the setting of industrial exposure to metals such as cadmium [101,102] and as a marker of various forms of tubulointerstitial nephritis [103-105]. A major advantage in monitoring β_2-m levels may be in the patients maintained on chronic hemodialysis therapy. In these patients β_2-m has been identified as pivotal to the pathogenesis of dialysis-related amyloidosis [106,107], as playing an important role in regulating the growth and survival of renal cell carcinoma cells [108], and as a marker for all-cause mortality. It has been suggested that measurement of β_2-m may be a useful marker to guide chronic hemodialysis therapy [109].

Lipocalins

The lipocalin superfamily of over 20 structurally related secreted proteins have been extensively used as biochemical markers of disease. Some of the more well-known lipocalins include retinol-binding protein, Protein HC (α_1-microglobulin, α_1-m), and human neutrophil lipocalin/neutrophil gelatinase-associated lipocalin (HNL/NGAL) [110].

Retinol-binding protein, (RBP, α_2-microglobulin), is a low molecular weight monomeric protein (Mr: 21,400). It is synthesized in the endoplasmic reticulum of the liver where it binds to retinol (vitamin A). It appears in the plasma bound to transthyretin (or prealbumin). Once the retinol is given up at the appropriate target tissue, RBP undergoes a conformational change and looses its affinity for transthyretin. In its new configuration, it is rapidly eliminated from plasma by glomerular filtration, then reabsorbed and catabolized by proximal tubular cells. RBP reabsorption involves megalin [111], a large glycoprotein and member of the low-density lipoprotein receptor family. Because of its stability in acid urine and since the serum level of free RBP is influenced only by renal function, the assay of urinary retinol binding protein is preferred over that of β_2-m. It has been considered a good marker of renal injury in clinical settings evaluating the potential nephrotoxic agents [112]. There has been considerable interest in the use of urinary RBP levels in diabetic patients as an early indicator of renal tubular damage with or without microalbuminuria [113] where it may serve as an independent predictor of vascular disease [114]. The urinary excretion of RBP along with other low-molecular weight proteins has been associated with cadmium and other heavy metal exposure [115,116]. Urinary retinol may also serve as a diagnostic marker of renal proximal tubule dysfunction in MM patients [117].

Alpha1-microglobulin (α_1-m), also known as protein HC (human complex-forming glycoprotein, heterogeneous in charge), is a glycosylated protein with a Mr of 27 kD. It is mainly synthesized in the liver and occurs in the serum in both a free form (free protein HC) and bound to several high molecular weight proteins such as immunoglobulin A (HC-IgA) and albumin

(HC-albumin). Normally, free α_1-m does not exceed concentrations of >60 mg/l in plasma. The renal handling of protein α_1-m is less well characterized than that of β_2-m or retinol binding protein. It has a glomerular sieving coefficient close to the benchmark separating LMW and HMW proteins. While half the amount in the plasma is complexed with immunoglobulin A, the free form is readily filtered through the glomerular basement membrane. The filtered protein is normally reabsorbed and catabolized in proximal tubular cells. In conditions with dusturbances in tubular function, reabsorption of α_1-m is reduced and increased amounts are found in the urine. The free form of this protein has been used as an indicator of proximal tubular dysfunction [118-120]. It is stable in native urine and its normal urine concentration is sufficiently high to be determined with rapid and cheap immunochemical techniques [121]. To control for variations in in urinary specific gravity or osmolality, the concentration of α_1-m should be expressed in relation to the excretion of creatinine [122]. There is also a clear diurnal variation in α_1-m excretion rate and a gender effect (higher in males). The excretion rate was higher in the daytime, with high urinary flow, compared to overnight values [123]. Notably, the decrease in urinary excretion rate of α_1-m correlates with recovery of the damaged tubular cells [124, 125]. In proteinuric glomerular disease, urinary protein α_1-m concentration correlates to the degree of IgG present in the urine [126]. It has been suggested that urinary α_1-m might be helpful for the early recognition of tubular involvement in patients with pure monoclonal light chain proteinuria [127], for the diagnosis and monitoring of tubular disorders associated with heavy metal intoxications, diabetic nephropathy, urinary outflow disorders and pyelonephritis [128].

Neutrophil gelatinase-associated lipocalin (NGAL) belongs to the lipocalin superfamily of over 20 structurally related secreted proteins [129]. It is expessed and secreted by immune cells, hepatocytes and renal tubular cells in various pathologic states. NGAL has a structural sequence similar to the lipocalin family of proteins. It acts as a growth and differentiation factor in multiple cell types, including developing and mature renal epithelia. NGAL activates nephron formation in the embryonic kidney, is markedly upregulated in response to kidney ischemic or nephrotoxic injury [130, 131] and may possess kidney-protective activity thereby limiting kidney damage. Blood, urine, and kidney NGAL levels may be real-time indicators of active kidney damage suggesting that NGAL may be an early and sensitive urinary biomarker of ischemic and nephrotoxic AKI [132].

Serum and urine NGAL values showed modest but significant increases within hours after radiocontrast exposure [133-135]. An increase in urinary NGAL levels has been found in patients with IgA Nephropathy [136]. Early elevations in urinary NGAL with IL-18 after kidney transplantation have been shown to be predictive of delayed graft function, trajectories in serum creatinine and need for renal replacement therapy during the first week following transplantation [137, 138]. Urinary concentrations of NGAL along with β_2-m, retinol-binding protein and α_1-m may allow for differentiation between stable transplants with normal tubular histology and stable transplants with subclinical tubulitis [139]. Serum and urinary NGAL levels have been found to be elevated in patients with autosomal-dominant polycystic kidney disease with a close correlation with residual renal function. That is, subjects with higher cystic growth presented higher serum and urine NGAL levels with respect to others [140]. Urinary NGAL has also been examined in patients undergoing cardiac surgery with cardiopulmonary bypass [141-143]. In children undergoing cardiopulmonary bypass, detectable increases in urinary and serum NGAL were evident within 2 h after surgery and highly predictive of subsequent AKI in the following 1–3 days [141]. In this study NGAL proved to be a powerful predictor of AKI 2 hours after bypass surgery with a sensitivity of 1.0 and a specificity of 0.98 with the threshold value set at 50 μg/L.This was an extention of there early report regarding the predicition of ATN using IL-18 [141a]. Similar postoperative increases in urinary IL-18 have now been shown in adult patients undergoing elective cardiopulmonary bypass [143]. In this study, all patients had abnormally elevated urinary NGAL values immediately following surgery. Those patients who subsequently developed AKI showed persistent and increasing values in the ensuing 3 h, whereas in those not developing AKI, urinary NGAL values started to fall by 1 h. Moreover, for those with AKI, SCr was no different from preoperative baseline levels at 24 h and did not peak until postoperative day 4.

Cystatin C is an endogenous cysteine proteinase inhibitor with practically the same Mr (13,300) as

β_2m. The cysteine proteinases are one of four major classes of endoproteinases that possess the ability to degrade intact glomerular basement membranes [144]. All nucleated cells produce cystatin at a stable rate. More than 99% is freely filtered by the glomerulus with little secretion or reabsorption. As a result, it has many of the ideal features for use as a marker of kidney function and estimate of GFR. Serum cystatin C concentrations demonstrate a good inverse correlation with radionuclide derived measurements of GFR and has been shown in several studies to be superior to creatinine and comparable to iohexol clearances in estimating eGFR [145, 146].

Cystatin C is nearly completely metabolized by proximal renal tubular cells. As a consequence, under ordinary circumstances there is little to no detectable cystatin C present in the urine. Thus, a true clearance of cystatin C cannot be determined. However, in the presence of tubular damage, cystatin C may be detected in the urine [147, 148] and may be more sensitive to early and mild changes of kidney function compared with creatinine [149, 150]. In this regard, elevation in serum cystatin C consistent with AKI, defined by at least a 50% increase from baseline, was evident 1–2 days prior to changes in SCr [151].Finally, in patients with AKI, elevated urinary cystatin C was highly predictive of subsequent need for acute renal replacement therapy and outperformed several other urinary biomarkers in some studies [152]., but not in others [152a]

Tamm-Horsfall glycoprotein

Tamm-Horsfall glycoprotein (uromodulin, THP) is a 616 amino acid, 80 kD protein with a carbohydrate component that accounts for nearly 30% of the molecular weight. It is the most abundant protein of renal origin in normal urine and is the major constituent of urinary casts. Synthesis of THP occurs in cells of the thick ascending limb of the loop of Henle where it is localized on the epithelial cell membrane. Urinary excretion occurs by proteolytic cleavage of the large ectodomain of the glycosyl phosphatidylinositol-anchored counterpart exposed at the luminal cell surface. Normally, it is excreted in the urine at a relatively constant rate up to 100 mg per day. The urinary excretion can increase following injury to the distal part of the tubule. With chronic renal disease, there may be a reduction in urinary THP excretion possibly as a result of a reduction in the number of functional distal tubular cells [153].

Viscosity of THP solutions increases markedly when the sodium chloride concentration is > 60 mM. Increasing the concentration of calcium and/.or a reduction in pH also increase viscosity and may account for the involvement of THP in the pathogenesis of cast nephropathy and tubulointerstitial nephritis. THP appears to have an inhibitory effect on urinary crystal arrgegation [154] and may play a role in preventing renal stone formation [155]. In some humans with calcium oxalate nephrolithiasis, a molecular abnormality of THP has been detected [156]. Other studies showed decreased urinary levels of THP in patients with nephrolithiasis [157, 158]. A relative deficiency in THP has been associated with impaired inhibition of crystal adhesion to renal epithelial cells instone formers [159].

Enzymuria

The acceptance by nephrologists of urinary enzyme activity as a measure of renal tubular dysfunction has been limited for several reasons. Paramount among these has been the difficulty to establish correlations between specific disease states and the presence or absence of enzymuria. In addition, a relationship between the severity of cellular injury and the magnitude or cellular source of the enzymuria has been difficult to establish. For example, enzymes that appear in the urine may originate from lysosomes, the brush-border membrane, and/or the cytoplasm of the cells. Moreover, various factors that alter urinary enzyme activity are independent of cellular integrity, i.e., urinary pH, osmolarity, and the presences of various enzyme inhibitors or activators [160].

The presumed utility and interpretation of urinary enzyme titers is founded on the premise that the sole source of high-molecular weight enzymes is damaged tubular cells [161] and that tubular enzymuria can detect tubular injury earlier than standard tests [162, 163]. In addition to normal cell shedding [164-166] enzymes also gain urinary access because of altered cell membrane permeability, increased rate of enzyme synthesis, and cell apoptosis ansd necrosis. Obviously, extraneous sources of urinary enzyme activity must be excluded including filtered plasma enzymes, cells and secretions from genitourinary tract, non-renal cells escaping into the urine, and the effect of drugs such as salicylates which can cause the desquamation of renal cells [167]. Indeed, enzymuria may reflect only mild injury that is easily reversible.

The ideal criteria for interpretation of enzymuria [168] include the following: (i) to evaluate glomerular function the enzyme should be present in blood, absent in renal tissue and have a molecular size that precludes its filtration; (ii) to evaluate tubular reabsorption the enzyme should be present in blood, absent from renal tissue, have a molecular weight that allows it to be freely filtered and be reabsorbed by the tubule; and (iii) to evaluate anatomical and functional condition of the tubular epithelium the enzyme should be restricted to the renal tissue.

The unique distribution of various enzymes along the length of the nephron provides the potential for identifying the specific injury site. Enzymes may not be uniformly distributed along or between nephrons thus the site selectivity of single enzymes is questionable, however it should be possible to localize the area of kidney damage on the basis of the pattern of enzymuria. While many urinary enzymes have been evaluated [169] as markers of damage or dysfunction of tubular epithelial cells [162, 170], only a small number are considered to be valuable as biomarkers[152].

When considering the application of urinary enzymes to monitor subtle renal dysfunction and/or to clarify mechanisms of nephrotoxicity, only a limited number of enzymes have been generally accepted as valuable urinary biomarkers. These include: lactic dehydrogenase, N-acetyl-β-D-glucosaminidase (NAG), alanine aminopeptidase (AAP), intestinal alkaline phosphatase, glutathione-S-transferase, gamma-glutamyl transferase and fructose-1,6,-biphosphatase.

The currently recommended core groups of tests for use in adult studies recommended by the US Department of Health are listed in Table 9 [171].

Lactate dehydrogenase

The use of urinary enzymes in the investigation and diagnosis of renal injury or disease was initiated by Rosalki and Wilkinson [172], who reported increased activity in the urine of patients with renal disease. However, lactate dehydrogenase soon gave way to more site-specific, easier to determine urinary enzymes.

N-acetyl-β-D-glucosaminidase

N-acetyl-β-D-glucosaminidase (NAG) is found in both the S3 segment of proximal tubular cells and the distal nephron as a lysosomal enzyme. It has its highest activity in the straight (S3) location of the proximal tubule of man, with less activity in the collecting duct portion of the distal nephron. With a molecular weight of approximately 150,000 daltons, it is normally retarded from passage through the glomerulus, and elevated urinary levels are indicative of tubular cell injury [173, 174].

The presence of NAG, an intracellular lysosomal enzyme, in the urine indicates organelle damage within the proximal tubule. In addition to occurring in the urine of individuals with tubular injury, it has also been found in the urine of patients with various forms of glomerular disease [175], obstructive uropathy and nephrosclerosis. In patients with diabetes mellitus, enzymuria has been considered a sign of tubular cell dysfunction [176] with urinary NAG excretion appearing to have the highest sensitivity and specificity compared to other markers [177]. Other non-specific increases in urinary NAG activity have been described. The enzyme activity is apparently not influenced by variations in urinary pH. Urinary NAG activities vary little throughout 24 hours if the urine creatinine concentration of the sample is used to correct the varying rates of urine flow. Thus, random samples of urine may be used for enzyme assay. Increased urinary NAG appears

Table 9. Core groups of tests for use in adult studies recommended by the US Department of Health [171].

Body fluid	Test	Functional unit tested
Serum	Creatinine	Diagnostic
Urine	Urinalysis with microscopic examinination of urine sediment	Glomerulus
	Albumin	Proximal tubule
	Retinol binding protein	Proximal tubule
	N-acetyl-β-D-glucosaminidase	Proximal tubule
	Alanine aminopeptidase	Distal tubule
	Osmolality	Control for urine concentration
	Creatinine	

to be dependent both upon the activity of the disease process and the functioning renal cell mass. Since the renal cell mass decreases in older individuals and there is lower excretion of creatinine, the relative excretion of NAG increases in individuals over 70 years of age. In animals with toxin-induced nephrotic syndrome, NAG excretion was found to be a function of proteinuria and reabsorption of proteins activating the tubular lysosomal system rather than of tubular damage *per se* [173]. To date, it is considered to be an ancillary but non-definitive marker of renal disease.

Alanine aminopeptidase

Alanine aminopeptidase is restricted to the proximal tubule. It shares with NAG great popularity as a measure of tubular injury. Increased excretion of NAG and alanine aminopeptidase has been reported in a variety of renal diseases including: pyelonephritis, glomerulonephritis, urologic cancers and renal transplant rejection. In addition, increased excretion has been reported in association with many well-defined nephrotoxins, i.e., exposure to cadmium, mercury, lead, cisplatin, aminoglycosides, cyclosporine, tacrolimus (FK-506), vancomycin, non-steroidal anti- inflammatory drugs, radiocontrast media in a number of clinical [178-187] situations and even as a marker of chronic alcohol abuse [188]. Thus, the experience with N-acetyl-β-D-glucosaminidase and alanine aminopeptidase indicates that while neither is specific with regard to discriminating between glomerular and tubular disease, they are very sensitive to acute tubular injury in which either the offending agent is known or the exposure incident is well characterized [189].

Alkaline phosphatases

Intestinal alkaline phosphatase and human tissue non-specific alkaline phosphatase are two urinary isoenzymes that have elicited interest as potential segment specific markers of the human nephron [190]. Both are members of the closely related group of alkaline phosphatases. Intestinal alkaline phosphatase is the intestinal isoenzyme that is localized on the brush border of human intestinal epithelial cells. It is also present in normal human kidney, where it is exclusively expressed on the brush border of tubulo-epithelial cells of the S3-segment of the proximal tubule. The intestinal alkaline phosphatase, which is released in urine, has its origin in the kidney. As a result, intestinal alkaline phosphatase is considered to be a specific and sensitive marker for alterations of the S3-segment of the human proximal tubule. Tissue alkaline phosphatase, in contrast, is localized on the membrane of liver cells, osteoblasts, and fibroblasts, and on the brush border all along the different segments of the proximal tubule. By measuring both enzymes, judgments as to the involvement of S1-S2 versus S3 segments can be achieved during either occupational screening [191] or when conducting clinical pharmacology studies [192]. Their usefulness as markers has been enhanced because specific monoclonal antibodies have been developed against each and because spot urine collections using appropriate preservative will remain stable for up to five months [190]. The two alkaline phosphatase isoenzymes have been validated as independent markers of proximal tubular cell alterations in over twenty occupationally exposed cohorts and clinical groups [193]. Along with N-acetyl-beta-D-glucosaminidase and gamma-glutamyl transferase, urinary alkaline phosphatase has been used to help differentiate between obstructive and nonobstructive hydronephrosis [194]

Glutathione-S-transferases

Glutathione-S-transferases (GST) are a family of enzymes that utilize glutathione in reactions contributing to the transformation of a wide range of compounds, including carcinogens, therapeutic drugs, and products of oxidative stress. These cytosolic enzymes are useful in the detoxification of endogenous compounds as well as the metabolism of xenobiotics. In addition, they serve as ideal biomarkers of organ damage as they exhibit many of the required characteristics, i.e. specific localisation, high cytosolic concentration and relatively short half-life [195]. Indeed, GSTs are very specific and sensitive biomarkers of renal tubular injury [196].

The mammalian GST super-family comprises dimeric isoenzymes of 45–55 kDa size that have been assigned to at least four generic classes: Alpha, Mu, Pi and Theta [197, 198]. In man, αGST isoform is localized to proximal tubular epithelial cells. An increased urinary excretion of αGST correlates with brush border damage and decreased αGST staining of proximal tubules [199]. Urinary αGST levels appear to correlate closely with the extent of renal injury [200, 201]. The πGST isoform is highly specific for cells of the distal tubules where it is localized in the distal convoluted tubule, the thin limb of the loop of Henle, and the collecting ducts [197, 200]. It is found in high concentrations, is readily released from injured cells into the urine and is a specific marker of distal tubule injury. In the rat, GSTYb1 replaces πGST [202] where it also serves as a uniquely specific marker of distal tubular injury.

Quantitation of αGST and πGST can be used as sensitive and relatively simple markers for early detection of toxic effects with respect to the renal tubule [203]. For example, in both human and animal studies, urinary αGST levels correlate closely with the dose of toxin [201, 204] without changes in the S_{Cr} or BUN. The unique distribution may allow renal injury to be localized to specific parts of the nephron [206] or by comparing the release of αGST and πGST in humans with αGST and GSTYb1 in rats, cross-species comparisons can be made [201, 204].

Renal papillary antigen

Renal papillary antigen 1 (RPA-1) is a protein strongly expressed and specifically found in high concentrations in the cells of the papillary collecting ducts of the rat kidney [205, 206] while renal papillary antigen 2 (RPA-2) is present in the loop of Henle. They are sensitive and specific biomarkers of injury and are released into urine upon exposure to renal toxins. RPA-1 is a potentially very useful biomarker for the serious condition of renal papillary necrosis. RPA-1 and 2 monoclonal antibodies may be identified by immunohistological procedures [205]. Urinary RPA-1 has been shown to be sensitive biomarker of renal collecting duct injury due to papillotoxins including bromoethanamine, propyleneimine and iodomethacin [206, 207].

Cytokines

Cytokines are polypeptides that affect nearly every biological process; these include embryonic development, disease pathogenesis, non-specific response to infection, specific response to antigen, changes in cognitive functions and progression of the degenerative processes of aging. In addition, cytokines are part of stem cell differentiation, vaccine efficacy and allograft rejection. They act as systemic mediators of inflammatory and immune responses, are closely involved in tissue repair, and under certain circumstances promote tissue destruction and fibrosis. The term cytokine encompasses interferons, the interleukins, the chemokine family, mesenchymal growth factors, the tumor necrosis factor family and adipokines [208]. It is now appreciated that among the mechanisms responsible for glomerular and tubulointerstitial disease, cytokines play a prominent role.

Interferons

Interferons are a group of pleiotropic cytokines with important proinflammatory functions required in defence against infections with bacteria, viruses and multicellular parasites along with fundamental functions in other processes such as cancer immunosurveillance, immune homeostasis and immunosuppression [209]. IFNs are classified into type I and type II IFNs [210]. Type I IFNs comprise multiple alpha IFNs (IFN-α), and single IFN-β, -ε, -κ, -ξ and -ω subtypes, all encoded by different genes. Type II IFN consists of a single IFN-γ gene.

The interferons are naturally protective substances. Type I IFNs are produced by most cells in response to viruses, bacteria or their products. For example, IFN-α and IFN- β are produced in response to viral infection and inhibit viral replication plus assist the induction of viral resistance. Not only do they possess antiviral activity but they also mediate the response to other infectious agents, demonstrate antitumor activity, and play a role in the regulation of growth, differentiation and development [211]. In contrast, IFN-γ has more potent immunoregulatory effects than either IFN-α or -β. Among its properties, IFN-γ is capable of activating human macrophage oxidative metabolism and microbicidal activity.

Interleukins

Interleukins are produced by a variety of cells including lymphocytes and monocytes. Originally, the term IL-1 was used to define a monocyte product and the term IL-2 was used to define a lymphocyte product. It is now appreciated that interleukins are produced by a variety of cells and are integrally involved in the function of the immune system. Most interleukins are members of three quite urelated, structural families of proteins, the representative prototypes of which are IL-1, IL-2 and IL-17 [212].

The largest family includes several sub-families. Among them are the interleukin-2 sub-family and the interleukin-10 sub-family. The interleukin-2 sub-family made up of a number of interleukins including IL-2 and IL-6. IL-2 is the only systemic treatment currently available that is capable of curing patients with metastatic renal cell carcinoma [213]. Interleukin-2 receptor antagonists have been used to decrease the incidence of acute rejection episodes following renal transplantation [214]. IL-6 is a cytokine with a wide variety of biological function. IL-6 is one of the most important mediators of fever and of the acute phase response. It is produced by both resident [215-218] and infiltrating cells [218] within the kideny. Thus, IL-6 can be measured in the urine where its presence is a reflection of local production by either glomerular mesangial cells or by cells that have infiltrated the glomeruli. Its renal expression and urinary excretion has been shown to correlate with the extent of tubulointerstitial damage and mesangial proliferation [215, 218-221]. Curiously, it is not found in the urine from patients with other types of glomerulonephritis. Urine IL-6 concentrations have been noted to markedly decrease within a few days from successful anti-rejection therapy following renal transplantation [222]. IL-6 has also been reported to be elevated in the serum of with reflux nephropathy [223].

The second largest family of the interleukins is the IL-1 family, containing IL-1α, IL-1β and IL-18. IL-1 is the first cytokine produced in the antigen recognition immune cascade and exists in two distinct forms: IL-1α and IL-1β [224]. IL-1α is predominantly a membrane- and cell-associated cytokine, while IL-1β is found free in biological fluids, including serum, urine and synovial fluid. IL-1 is expressed in the kidney during inflammatory disease. In mesangial cells, IL-1β regulates cell growth, inflammation, and extra-cellular matrix proteins [225-227]. It has been suggested that urinary IL-1β may be a useful marker for the early detection of acute pyelonephritis in febrile children and young children who are at risk for the development of renal scarring following acute pyelonephritis [228].

Interleukin-18 (IL-18), a recently described member of the IL-1 cytokine family, is now recognized as an important regulator of innate and acquired immune responses. IL-18 is a mediator of inflammation and ischemic tissue injury in many organs. IL-18 is constitutively expressed by intercalated cells of the late distal convoluted tubule, the connecting tubule, and the collecting duct of the healthy human kidney [229]. It is expressed at sites of chronic inflammation, in autoimmune diseases, in a variety of cancers, and in the context of numerous infectious diseases [230]. Experimental studies have shown IL-18, a proinflammatory cytokine and likely mediator of tubular injury, can be induced in the proximal tubule and detected in the urine in ischemic AKI [231]. The production of IL-18 increases significantly in patients with CKD [232, 233] and may play a crucial role in the process of renal tubulointerstitial fibrosis by promoting tubular proximal epithelial cell injury and activation [234]. IL-18 has been shown to be a mediator of ARI in mice, in which IL-18 was detected in the proximal tubules [235]. In patients with acute kidney injury, urinary IL-18 levels have been used for the early diagnosis and to predict the mortality of patients who have the adult respiratory distress syndrome and are in the intensive care unit [236]. IL-18 levels are elevated in urine in patients with ATN and in renal transplant recipients with delayed graft function compared with other renal diseases such as those with pre-renal azotemia, urinary tract infection, chronic kidney disease or healthy controls [237]. Elevated urinary IL-18 concentrations early after kidney transplantation have been shown as predictive of delayed graft failure [238]. Urinary levels of CXCR3-binding chemokines have been reported to correlate with biopsy proven allograft rejection [238a]. .Urinary IL-18 rises prior to SCr in non-septic critically ill children, predicts severity of AKI and is an independent predictor of mortality [239]. Elevated serum levels of IL-18 may be a predictor of future renal dysfunction in type 2 diabetic patients with normoalbuminuria [240].

The third interleukin family is the IL-17 family. Interleukin-17 is a pro-inflamatory cytokine that is primarily secreted from T-lymphocytes and whose physiological significance is only just beginning to be determined [241, 242]. Increased urinary excretion of interleukin-17 has been found in nephrotic patients [243].

Interleukin-8 (IL-8) is a potent neutrophil and lymphocyte chemotactic cytokine It is one of a family of 13 human CXC chemokines [244]. These small basic heparin binding proteins are proinflammatory and mainly involved in the initiation and amplification of acute inflammatory reactions and in chronic inflammatory processes. In the urinary tract infection model, the epithelial cells of the renal tract were shown to secrete chemokines and IL-8 was identified as the main chemokine involved in transepithelial neutrophil migration. Urinary levels of immunoreactive IL-8 may be elevated with various glomerular diseases. The glomerular production of IL-8 promotes the infiltration of leukocytes - particularly neutrophils - into glomeruli where they contribute to progressive renal injury [245]. As can be appreciated, assays for interleukins are expected to become useful for evaluating renal damage and monitoring disease activity. In addition, elevated levels of IL-8 have been reported in patients undergoing cardiac bypass surgery [246].

Tumor necrosis factor α

Tumor necrosis factor α (TNFα) is a potent proinflammatory cytokine and important mediator of inflammatory tissue damage. In addition, it has important immune-regulatory functions. Under normal physiological conditions TNF is not detectable. It is produced in response to tissue invasion by bacteria, viruses, fungi or parasitic agents. Various cells, including glomerular mesangial cells, synthesize TNF [247]. Indeed, a number of observations support a role for TNF in the pathogenesis of acute and chronic renal disease [248] including diabetic nephropathy [249]. In the mesangial cells, tumor necrosis factor may stimulate the synthesis of various prostaglandins along with platelet activating factor. It also induces cyclic AMP and cyclic GMP accumulation, promotes the generation of reactive oxygen metabolites, upregulates the expression of intercellular adhesion molecules and may have either a stimulatory or inhibitory effect on mesangial cell proliferation [250]. Some of these products, including oxygen radicals [251] and various cytokines [252] may be injurious to the mesangial cells themselves. TNF-α is cytotoxic to glomerular, mesangial and epithelial cells, and it is able to induce direct renal damage. The stimulation of mesangial cells to release and respond to TNF may accelerate the glomerular infiltration of polymorphonuclear leukocytes and monocytes. The injection of TNF enhances glomerular damage in some forms of experimental glomerulonephritis [253]. Another important target is the vascular endothelium where an increase in the local production of TNFα may result in the formation of capillary thrombi. An increase in plasma and urinary levels of two soluble tumor necrosis factor receptors has been found in patients with chronic renal failure [254].

Monocyte chemoattractant protein-1

Monocyte chemoattractant protein-1 (MCP-1) is a chemokine that plays an important role in the recruitment of monocytes/macrophages into renal tubulointerstitium [255, 256]. It is known to be produced mainly by tubular epithelial cells in kidney [257], and to contribute to renal interstitial inflammation and fibrosis [258]. Furthermore, protein overload in renal tubular cells is shown to up-regulate MCP-1 gene and its protein [259, 260]. These lines of evidence collectively suggest that increased urinary protein excretion probably aggravates renal tubular damage by enhancing MCP-1 expression in tubular cells. It has been suggested that MCP-1 expression in renal tubuli is enhanced in proteinuric states, irrespective of the types of renal disease, and that increased MCP-1 expression probably contributes to renal tubular damage in proteinuric states [261]. Urinary MCP-1 is a sensitive and specific biomarker of renal SLE flare and its severity, even in patients who receive significant immunosuppressive therapy. Persistently elevated uMCP-1 after treatment may indicate ongoing kidney injury that may adversely affect renal prognosis [262].

Cell adhesion molecules

Cell adhesion molecules (CAMs) are transmembrane glycoproteins that act at the cell surface to mediate specific binding interactions with other cell adhesion molecules on adjacent cells or with proteins in the extracellular matrix. They are responsible for the adhesion of various leukocytes with each other, with extracellular matrix and with other cell types. Several classes of molecules capable of mediating adhesion include selectins, integrins, cadherins, and immunoglobulin superfamily members [263-265]. Multiple members from every major family of cell adhesion molecules have been implicated in the development, maintenance, or repair of renal tissues

Selectins

Selectins include P-selectin (platelet selectin), E-selectin (endothelial cell selectin), and L-selectin (leukocyte selectin). *P-selectin* enables binding of platelets, polymorphonuclear leukocytes, and monocytes to activated endothelial cells and of leukocytes to activated platelets. P-selectin is expressed in the kidneys in systemic lupus erythematosis [266, 267]. The up-regulation of P-selectin expression in glomerui following binding of anti-GBM antibody may be an integral signal for neutrophile recruitment [268]. *E-selectin* is expressed only by activated endothelial cells and enables adhesion of neutrophils and monoctyes to endothelial cells. It has been suggested that in inflammatory conditions, E-selectin is involved in the development of atherosclerosis and arterial damage in patiens with end-stage renal disease [269, 270] and has been associated with the rapid progression to ESRD in IgA nephropathy [271]. *L-selectin* is expressed by leukocytes and mediates interaction of between neutrophils, monocytes, and lynphocytes with activated endothelial cells. Large numbers of L-selectin cells within glomerular and interstitial infiltrates have been found in biopsies from patients with IgA nephropathy [272] along with increased levels of circulating soluble L-selectin [273].

Cadherins

Cadherins are a gene family of membrane-anchored cell adhesion molecules which can be classified into two subfamilies, namely type I (E-cadherins, N-cadherins, P-cadherins and R-cadherins.) and type II (cadherin-5 to -12, -14 and -15) cadherins [274, 275]. They are critical for maintining intercellular connections. E-cadherin expression is restricted to the distal tubules and collecting ducts of the human kidney, whereas N-cadherin and cadherin-6 expression are found on proximal tubules [276, 277]. Cadherin-8 can only be detected on developing tubular structures. In addition to the type I and type II cadherins is cadherin-16 also known as Ksp-cadherin (kidney specific) [278, 279]. It is the only member of the cadherin family that is exclusively found in the kidney where it is found on distal tubules and collecting ducts in the later developmental stages [280]. Renal cell neoplasms are presumably derived from different cell types of the nephron. Clear cell and papillary renal cell carcinoma are thought to be of proximal tubular origin, whereas oncocytoma and chromophobe RCC are derived from intercalated cells of distal nephron. There is a high sensitivity and specificity of Ksp-cadherin for distal convoluted tubules, which can be used as adjunct for diagnosis of chromophobe renal cell carcinoma [281]. Conversely, the lack of Ksp-cadherin protein expression in clear cell carcinoma seems to be in accordance with the origin of the tumors [282].

Integrins

Integrins are a family of large integral transmembrane glycoproteins, involved in the adhesive interactions of cells [283]. They consist of two subunits, α and β chain. Each subunit is a transmembrane protein with a large extracellular domain and a small cytoplasmic domain. Integrins are classified according to the type of β-subunit. The variability in available α and β chains allows for a large family of integrins and provides cells with the ability to recognize a variety of adhesive substrates. They appear to be the primary mediators of cell adhesion to extracellular matrix adhesion and basement membranes and contribute to cell-cell adhesion and mainenance of normal tissue architecture [284]. They are thought to link the cytoskeleton of one cell with that of another or with the extracellular matrix. Integrins associate with cytoskeletal proteins viatalin, vinculin, and probably other cytoskeletal proteins [285]. Integrin-mediated signal transduction modulates the pathways controlling cell growth and survival. β1 integrins are found on mesangial cells where they appear to be the principle mediators of cell-extracellular matrix adhesion, with fibronectin, laminin and collagens as their major ligands. They are known as the very late activation antigen proteins. β2 integrins are involved in leukocyte cell-cell adhesion. Adhesion molecules may play an important role in reperfusion injury of the kidney [286, 287]. Integrins are also upregulated in models of crescentic glomerulonephritis where their role as adhesion molecules may contribute to disease [288]. It has been suggested that altered β1 integrin-mediated cell behavior may contribute to the progression of glomerulonephritis [289].

Immunoglobulin superfamily

Immunoglobulin superfamily of cell adhesion molecules are large plasma-membrane glycoproteins, which function primarily in cell-cell adhesion. For example, inflammatory systemic disorders with renal tissue damage require the adherence of polymorphonuclear leukocytes to the endothelium. This process is mediated by cell surface adhesion molecules. They include among others, intercellular adhesion molecule-1 (ICAM-1) and vascular cell adhesion molecule-1 (VCAM-1). These two members of the immunoglobulin supergene family play an important role in a variety of inflammatory and immune-mediated mechanisms, mediating both cell migration and activation. ICAM-1 is a glycoprotein expressed on endothelial cells of larger vessels, glomeruli and peritubular capillaries, epithelial, fibroblast and leukocyte cells. ICAM-2 is a glycoprotein expressed by endothelial cells, lymphocytes and some other leukocytes. VCAM-1 is a glycoprotein widely distributed on endothelial, epithelial, macrophages and dendritic cells. It supports the adhesion of eosinophils, basophiles, monocytes and lymphocytes. ICAM-1 and VCAM-1 appear to be particularly important for the firm attachment and transendothelial migration of leukocytes.

The presence of soluble forms of ICAM-1 and VCAM-1 have been confirmed in human sera and as have demonstrated increased levels of these soluble markers in patients with inflammatory diseases as well as with other immunologic mediated disorders. Changes in ICAM-1 expression have been reported in glomerulonephritis, tubulointerstitial inflammation, and renal allograft rejection. Circulating levels of ICAM-1 are elevated in some forms of glomerulonephritis [290]. Expression of VCAM-1 has been observed on proximal tubule cells in patients with vasculitis and crescentic nephritis, lupus nephritis, IgA nephropathy, and acute interstitial nephritis induced by non-steroidal anti-inflammatory drugs [291]. VCAM-1 has previously been observed to be expressed in the kidneys, both in murine and human lupus [292-294], Serum levels of soluble VCAM-1 have been found to correlate with parameters of SLE disease activity [295]. The serum level of sVCAM-1 was correlated with the SLE disease activity and decreased during remission. VCAM-1 may be a reliable urinary marker for monitoring disease activity and damage in patients with systemic lupus erythematosus nephritis [296] contributing to the ability to distinguish subjects with active renal disease from the other systemic lupus erythematosus patients [297].

Kidney injury molecule 1

Kidney injury molecule 1 (KIM-1) is a type 1 transmembrane protein with an immunoglobulin and mucin domain. The KIM-1 ectodomain is cleaved, shed from cells, detectable in urine, and reflects renal damage [298]. The cleavage of KIM-1 is mediated by ERK activation and is accelerated by p38 MAP kinase activation [299]. KIM-1 is not expressed in the normal kidney but is markedly up-regulated in renal proximal tubule cells by stimuli that promote dedifferentiation, including ischemic and toxic [300, 301] injury. Because it is expressed in proliferating and dedifferentiated epithelial cells in regenerating proximal tubules, it is thought to play an important role in the restoration of the morphological integrity and function following renal ischemic injury [302].

Extensive expression of KIM-1 has been found in proximal tubule cells in biopsies from patients with acute tubular necrosis [302]. KIM-1 is also expressed in other conditions where proximal tubules are dedifferentiated, including renal cell carcinoma [303, 304], chronic cyclosporine nephrotoxicity [305], a protein-overload model of tubulointerstitial disease [306], polycystic kidney disease [307], and contrast nephropathy. In several chronic conditions, KIM-1 has been found primarily expressed at the luminal side of dedifferentiated proximal tubules, in areas with fibrosis and inflammation. Independent of the specific disease, renal KIM-1 correlated positively with the extent of renal damage and negatively with renal function. In these patients, urinary levels of KIM-1 were and correlated positively with tissue KIM-1 and negatively with renal function. Thus, KIM-1 is upregulated in renal disease and is associated with renal fibrosis and inflammation. Urinary KIM-1 is also associated with inflammation and renal function, and reflects tissue KIM-1.

In critically ill patients with AKI, urinary KIM-1 along with N-acetyl-[beta]-(D)-glucosaminidase activity (NAG) showed increasing trends with increasing severity of illness as assessed by Acute Physiology, Age, Chronic Health Evaluation (APACHE) II and multiple organ failure scores and could be correlated to the odds for both renal replacement therapy and hospital death, suggesting these biomarkers have some predictive ability for clinical outcomes in patients with AKI [308].

It appears that the shedding of KIM-1 into the urine of patients with AKI is clinically significant, and elevated urinary KIM-1 levels are associated with adverse outcomes in this population [308]. Urinary KIM-1 serves as an earlier and more specific diagnostic indicator of kidney injury when compared with any of the conventional biomarkers (plasma creatinine, blood urea nitrogen, glycosuria, proteinuria, urinary N-acetyl--d-glucosaminidase, -glutamyltransferase, or alkaline phosphatase) [310, 311].

Miscellaneous biomarkers

Endothelins

Endothelins are a family of locally generated peptides that possess a number of biological functions [312]. In humans there are three isoforms of endothelins, called ET-1, ET-2, and ET-3, which interact with two distinct subtype receptors (ET_A and ET_B) to exert their biological effects [313]. They are potent, if not the most potent renal vasoconstrictors and stimulate vascular smooth muscle cell and mesangial cell proliferation [314]. The predominant isotype in humans is ET-1 ("classical" endothelin). Endothelial cells appear to be the primary source of ET-1 found circulating in plasma while glomerular ET is thought to arise mostly from the glomerular endothelium and from mesangial cells themselves. Endothelins often act via the intermediary of thromboxane biosynthesis, and they release platelet-derived growth factors.

The renal effects of ET-1 are in part related to the doses used and the relative concentration of the ET_A and ET_B receptors. Renal vasoconstriction may be mediated by ET_A receptor stimulation whereas ET_B receptor may be involved on maintaining a "tonic" renal vasodialtion. ET_B is the major ET receptor expressed in the renal tubules. ET-1 exerts different effects over the distinct parts of the nephron. In the proximal tubule, ET has a biphasic effect. Low concentrations increase fluid transport, whereas a high concentration of ET-1 decreases fluid transport. [315] ET inhibits chloride flux in the thick ascending limb of Henle,. [316] ET-1 inhibits Na^+ and water reabsorption in the cortical collecting duct (CCD),. ET-1 also influences salt and water homeostasis through effects on the renin-angiotensin-aldosterone system and vasopressin, thus elevating blood pressure and increasing vascular tone

It has been shown that subjects with renal diseases such as IgA nephropathy, membranous proliferative glomerulonephritis, focal sclerosis, and lupus nephritis have levels of endothelin that are significantly higher than those in healthy subjects [317]. Increased circulating ET-1 concentrations and urinary excretion of ET-1 have been observed in patients treated with the nephrotoxic immunosuppressive agent cyclosporine A and tacrolimus (FK-506) [318]. Other nephrotoxic agents, such as cisplatin, also increase urinary excretion of ET [319]. Urinary excretion of endothelin has been reported in patient following contrast media in which CIN develops despite normal plasma levels of endothelin[319a] In patients with chronic renal disease, urinary excretion of ET-1 is significantly elevated when compared to normal values. The excretion of endothelin is modulated by several mechanical and chemical stimuli such as angiotensin II, phenylephrine, radiocontrast media, cyclosporine, and cis-platin. In addition, enhanced urinary ET excretion has been found in several forms of renal failure, both acute and chronic, and in diabetes mellitus. Thus, urinary ET has the potential of serving as a marker for renal disease. [320]

Heat shock proteins

Exposure of cells to a variety of stresses induces a modification of cell metabolism called the heat shock or stress response, which is accompanied by the rapid synthesis of the so-called heat-shock proteins (Hsps). The major Hsp families have sizes of 80-90, 68-72, and 15-30 kDa. Events such as progression through the cell cycle and differentiation or environmental stresses such as heat, oxidative injury, heavy metals, inhibitors of energy metabolism, or pathological conditions such as inflammation, all result in the expression of Hsps which are considered to have essential protective functions in cells [321]. It has been suggested that Hsps may be of value as molecular biomarkers of oxidative stress associated with various renal disease states and nephrotoxicity [322]. The Hsp 70 family is the best studied class of Hsp [323]. Hsp were induced following cell exposure to ischemia-reperfusion, inflammation, amino acid analogues, tissue damage, oxidative injury, and a variety of other stimuli such as heavy metals, different pharmacological agents, and mycotoxins [324].

Small HSPs (sHSPs) beside their reported roles during stress exert multiple functions under normal conditions. sHSPs associate with nuclei, membranes and the cytoskeletal elements of eukaryotic cells and along with other chaperones, confer stability on the cell proteome by protecting diverse proteins engaged in signal transduction, metabolism, translation, transcription, migration, differentiation and other activities [325, 326]. Molecular chaperones are a large family of ubiquitous, abundant proteins that appeared early in evolution and form an effective defense system in our cells by sequestering damaged proteins and preventing their aggregation [325, 326]. Small heat shock proteins (sHSPs) function as molecular chaperones, preventing stress induced aggregation of partially denatured proteins and promoting their return to native conformations when favorable conditions pertain [327].

Clusterin

Clusterin is a disulphide-linked glycoprotein that has been isolated from several tissues including the kidney and is reported to be induced in various renal diseases, e.g. renal dysplasia, membranous glomerulonephritis, inherited polycystic renal disease and renal cell carcinoma [328-332]. The two main clusterin protein isoforms in human cells include the conventional glycosylated secreted heterodimer and a truncated nuclear form. Clusterin has been implicated in various physiological processes and in many severe physiological disturbance states including ageing, cancer progression, vascular damage, and diabetes mellitus. It is involved in the regulation of complement, and cell reproduction and aggregation [333]. Clusterin may contribute to the progression of chronic kidney disease by virtue of its role in promoting apoptosis [330, 331] - perhaps by inhibiting NF-kappaB-mediated antiapoptosis [334]. The secreted form of clusterin may be implicated in the progression of renal cell carcinoma [335].

In the kidney, clusterin is a component of immune deposits and its expression is increased after ischemia or obstruction. In gentamicin-treated rats, an increase in urinary clusterin protein may provide an early sign of nephrotoxicity [336]. In rats with unilatertral ureteral obstruction, clusterin mRNA and clusterin-beta have been detected in the kidney along with clusterin-alpha in the urine [337]. A central role for glomerular clusterin as a modulator of inflammation that potentially influences the clinical outcome in human membranous glomerulonephritis has been described [338].

Antiglomerular basement membrane antibodies

Goodpasture's disease is related to the development of an immune-type glomerulonephritis associated with the occurrence of antibodies against constituents of the glomerular basement membrane (anti-GBM antibodies). The role of anti-GBM antibodies in the pathogenesis of human glomerulonephritis was first described in 1967 in a now classic report [339]. The target antigen of the anti-GBM antibodies is the NC1 domain of a-3 type IV collagen [340].appears to be the $\alpha3$ chain in the C-terminal non-collagenous globular domain of type IV collagen [341]. An inherited susceptibility is well documented through HLA complex. The disease is known to be associated with ANCA vasculitis, Alport's syndrome, membranous nephropathy, diabetes mellitus and lymphoma.

Alport syndrome is a hereditary disorder of basement membranes that can result in hearing loss, ocular defects, and kidney failure. Following renal transplantation for Alport's Syndrome, some patients will unpredictably develop antiglomerular antibodies (anti-GBM) following renal transplantation [342]. The renal disease can appear indistinguishable from Goodpasture disease of native kidneys [343]. The collagen target of the antibody to the glomerulus [4] links these 2 disease processes. The ongoing presence of anti-GBM can affect the success of subsequent kidney transplants [344]. An appreciable percentage of patients with anti-GBM antibodies will also have antineutrophil cytoplasmic antibodies (ANCA) [345].

Antineutrophil cytoplasmic antibodies

Antineutrophil cytoplasmic antibodies (ANCA) are a class of autoantibodies with varied specificities against particular proteins in the cytoplasmic granules of neutrophils and the lysosomes of monocytes. Indirect immunofluorescence microscopy and enzyme immunoassay have defined two types of ANCA patterns: one causing cytoplasmic staining (C-ANCA) the other perinuclear staining (P-ANCA) [346]. Greater than 95% of C-ANCA antibiodies are anti-proteinase 3 antibodies (PR3-ANCA) and greater than 95% of P-ANCA antibiodies are anti-myeloperoxidase antibodies (MPO-ANCA) [347].

The high prevalence of ANCA antibodies in the serum of patients with small vessel vasculitis has been associated to some extent with disease activity [348] and as an early indicator of disease relapse [349]. In addition, both PR3-ANCA and MPO-ANCA antibodies appear to play a pathogenic role by activating neutrophils with the subsequent release of inflammatory mediators [350]. ANCA are associated with necrotizing granulomatosis and with pauci-immune necrotizing vasculitis involving many tissues and are useful for the diagnosis of Wegener's granulomatosis, microscopic polyarteritis, Churg-Strauss syndrome, systemic vasculitis and idiopathic necrotizing and crescentic glomerulonephritis. Several environmental and pharmaceutical agents have been thought to be among the factors that trigger the development of ANCA-related small vessal vasculitis [346].

Na^+/H^+ exchanger isoform 3

Na^+/H^+ exchanger isoform 3 (NHE3) are the most abundant sodium transporters within the nephron. They are located in the plasma membrane, apical membrane and recyucling endosomes of epithelial cells. They are distributed along the nephron in the proximal tubule, the thin decending limb and the thick ascending limb of Henle's Loop[351]. Du Cheyron and collegues [352] measured NHE3 protein in the urine of patients with biopsy proven ATN and compared the amount excreted, corrected for Cr content, to ICU patients with prerenal azotemia, ARF other than ATN and individuals without renal involvement. Urinary NHE3 content was significantly increased in both ATN and prerenal azotemia, however, it value was 6x greater in the ATN group without overlap. NHE3 protein proved to better discriminate between ATN and prerenal azotemia than either $FENa^+$ or Retinol-binding protein. The finding of significant increases in NHE3 in biopsy confirmed patients with ATN suggested that this biomarker maybe very useful in the early detection of significant tubular injury either in the proximal tubule or in the thick ascending limb of Henle, that site of hypoxic ischemic injury [353]. Based on this report, the authors recommend "Complementary studies in larger groups of patients using quantitative radioimmunoassay or ELISA are necessary, first to compare NHE3 with other new biomarkers and then to confirm their clinical usefulness".

References

1. Definitions Working Group: Biomarkers and surrogate endpoints: preferred definitions and conceptual framework. Clin Pharmacol Therapeut 2001; 69: 89–95.
2. Ilyin SE, Belkowski SM, Plata-Salamán CR. Biomarker discovery and validation: technologies and integrative approaches. Trends Biotechnol. 2004 ; 22: 411-6.
3. Dieterle F, Marrer E. New technologies around biomarkers and their interplay with drug development, Anal Bioanal Chem, 2007; (In press).
4. National Research Council. Commission on Life Sciences Board on Environmental Studies and Toxicology. Committee on Biological Markers, Subcommittee on Biologic Markers in Urinary Toxicology. In: Biologic Markers in Urinary Toxicology. National Academy Press, Washington DC 1995; p. 16-21.
5. Niemann CU, Serkova NJ. Biochemical mechanisms of nephrotoxicity: sapplication for metabolomics. Expert Opin Drug Metab Toxicol 2007; 3: 527-544.
6. Fels LM, C. Herbort C, Pergande M, Jung K, Hotter G, Roselló J, Gelpi E, Mutti A, De Broe M, Stolte H. Nephron target sites in chronic exposure to lead Nephrol Dial Transplant. 1994; 9: 1740-1746.
7. de Jong PE, Gansevoort RT, Bakker SJ. Macroalbuminuria and microalbuminuria: do both predict renal and cardiovascular events with similar strength? J Nephrol. 2007; 20: 375-80.
8. Cooper RG. Effect of tobacco smoking on renal function. Indian J Med Res. 2006; 124: 261-268.
9. Bernard A. Renal dysfunction induced by cadmium: biomarkers of critical effects. Biometals. 2004; 17: 519-23.
10. Roels HA, Hoet P, Lison D. Usefulness of biomarkers of exposure to inorganic mercury, lead, or cadmium in controlling occupational and environmental risks of nephrotoxicity. Ren Fail. 1999 May-Jul; 21(3-4): 251-62.
11. Fanos V, Cataldi L. Amphotericin B-induced nephrotoxicity: a review. J Chemother. 2000; 12: 463-70.
12. Widmer P, Maibach R, Künzi UP, Capaul R, Mueller U, Galeazzi R, Hoigné R. Diuretic-related hypokalaemia: the role of diuretics, potassium supplements, glucocorticoids and beta 2-adrenoceptor agonists. Results from the comprehensive hospital drug monitoring programme, berne (CHDM). Eur J Clin Pharmacol. 1995; 49(1-2): 31-6.
13. Cheng HF, Harris RC. Renal effects of non-steroidal anti-inflammatory drugs and selective cyclooxygenase-2 inhibitors. Curr Pharm Des. 2005; 11(14): 1795-804.
14. Harris RC. COX-2 and the kidney. J Cardiovasc Pharmacol. 2006; 47 Suppl 1: S37-42.
15. Gooch K, Culleton BF, Manns BJ, Zhang J, Alfonso H, Tonelli M, Frank C, Klarenbach S, Hemmelgarn BR. NSAID use and progression of chronic kidney disease. Am J Med. 2007; 120(3): 280.e1-7.
16. Perazella MA. Drug-induced renal failure: update on new medications and unique mechanisms of nephrotoxicity. Am J Med Sci. 2003 Jun; 325(6): 349-62.

17. Jaffe JA, Kimmel PL. Chronic nephropathies of cocaine and heroin abuse: a critical review. Clin J Am Soc Nephrol. 2006; 1: 655-67.
18. Schetz M, Dasta J, Goldstein S, Golper T. Drug-induced acute kidney injury. Curr Opin Crit Care. 2005; 11: 555-65.
19. Pichette V, Leblond FA. Drug metabolism in chronic renal failure. Curr Drug Metab. 2003; 4: 91-103.
20. Bonnardeaux A, Somerville P, Kaye M. A study on the reliability of dipstick urinalysis. Clin Nephrol 1994; 41: 167-172.
21. Voswinckel P. A marvel of colors and ingredients. The story of urine test strips. Kidney Int 1994; 46 (Suppl 47): S3-S7.
22. Janssens PMW. New markers for analyzing the cause of hematuria. Kidney Int 1994; 46 (Suppl 47): S111-S114.
23. Hotta O, Taguma Y, Yusa N and Ooyama M. Analysis of mononuclear cells in urine using flow cytometry in glomerular diseases. Kidney Int 1994; 46 (Suppl 47): S117-S121.
24. Nolan CR, Anger MS, Kelleher SP. Eosinophiluria--a new method of detection and definition of the clinical spectrum N Eng J Med 1986; 315: 1516-1519.
25. Ruffing KA, Hoppes P, Blend D, Cugino A, Jarjoura D, Whittier FC. Eosinophils in urine revisited. Clin Nephrol 1994; 41: 163-166.
26. Hotta O, Yusa N, Kitamura H, Taguma Y. Urinary macrophages as activity markers of renal injury. Clin Chim Acta. 2000; 297: 123-33.
27. Vogelmann SU, Nelson WJ, Myers BD, Lemley KV: Urinary excretion of viable podocytes in health and renal disease. Am J Physiol Renal Physiol 2003; 285: F40 –F48.
28. Bagshaw SM, Langenberg C, Bellomo R. Urinary biochemistry and microscopy in septic acute renal failure: a systematic review. Am J Kidney Dis 2006; 48: 695–705.
29. Delanghe J. New screening diagnostic techniques in urinalysis. Acta Clin Belg. 2007; 62: 155-61.
30. Chan RW, Szeto CC. Advances in the clinical laboratory assessment of urinary sediment. Clin Chim Acta. 2004; 340: 67-78.
31. Tsai JJ, Yeun JY, Kumar VA, Don BR. Comparison and interpretation of urinalysis performed by a nephrologist versus a hospital-based clinical laboratory. Am J Kidney Dis. 2005; 46: 820-9.
32. Meyer TW, Hostetter TH. N Engl J Med 2007; 357: 1316-1325.
33. Kaplan AA, Kohn OF. Fractional excretion of urea as a guide to renal dysfunction. Am J Nephrol 1992; 12: 49-54.
34. Carvounis CP, Nisar S, Guro-Razuman S. Significance of the fractional excretion of urea in the differential diagnosis of acute renal failure. Kidney Int 2002; 62: 2223–2229.
35. Stevens LA, Levey AS. Measurement of kidney function. Med Clin North Am 2005; 89: 457–473.
36. Shemesh O, Golbetz H, Kriss JP, Myers BD. Limitations of creatinine as a filtration marker in glomerulopathic patients. Kidney Int 1985; 28: 830–838.
37. Brochner-Mortensen J. Routine methods and their reliability for assessment of glomerular filtration rate in adults. Danish Med Bull 1978; 25: 181-202.
38. Kastrup J, Petersen P, Bartram R, Hansen JM. The effect of trimethoprim on serum creatinine. Brit J Urol 1985; 57: 265-268.
39. Hoffmann U, Fischereder M, Kruger B, Drobnik W, Kramer BK. The value of N-acetylcysteine in the prevention of radiocontrast agent-induced nephropathy seems questionable. J Am Soc Nephrol 2004; 15: 407 -410.
40. Mainra R, Gallo K, Moist L. Effect of N-acetylcysteine on renal function in patients with chronic kidney disease. Nephrology (Carlton). 2007 Oct; 12(5): 510-3.
41. Ducharme MP, Smythe M, Strohs G. Drug-induced alterations in serum creatinine concentrations. Ann Pharmacother. 1993; 27: 622-33.
42. Coresh J, Astor B, McQuillan G, et al. Calibration and random variation of the serum creatinine assay as critical elements of using equations to estimate the glomerular filtration rate.Am J Kidney Dis 2002; 39: 920-929.
43. Murthy K, Stevens LA, Stark PC, Levey AS. Variation in serum creatinine assay calibration: A practical application to glomerular filtration rate estimation. Kidney Int 2005; 68: 1884-1887.
44. Stevens LA, Manzi J, Levey AS, Chen J, Deysher AE, Greene T, Poggio ED, Schmid CH, Steffes MW, Zhang YL, Van Lente F, Coresh J. Impact of Creatinine Calibration on Performance of GFR Estimating Equations in a Pooled Individual Patient Database. Am J Kidney Dis 2007; 50: 21-35.
45. Wade WE, Spruill WJ. New serum creatinine assay standardization: implications for drug dosing. Ann Pharmacother. 2007; 41: 475-80.
45a. Trof RJ, DiMaggio F, Leemreis J, Johan-Groeneveld AB: Bimarkers of acute renal injury and renal failure. Shock 2006; 26: 245-259.
45b. Tajagura R, Yonemura K, Yonekawa O, Iwahara K, Kanno T, Fujise Y, Hishida A : Tryptophan glycoconjugate As a novel marker of renal function. Am J Med 2001; 110: 192-197.
46. Shemish O, Golbetz H, Kriss JP, Myers B. Limitations of creatinine as a filtration marker in glomerulopathic patients. Kidney Int 1985; 28: 830-838.

47. Bauer JH, Brooks CS, Burch RN. Clinical appraisal of creatinine clearance as a measurement of glomerular filtration rate. Am J Kidney Dis 1982; 2: 337-347.
48. Walser M . Assessing renal function from creatinine measurements in adults with chronic renal failure. Am J Kidney Dis 1998; 32: 23-31.
49. Cockroft DW, Gault MH. Prediction of creatinine clearance from serum creatinine. Nephron 1976; 16: 31-41.
50. Levey, AS, Bosch JP, Lewis JB, Greene T, Rogers N, Roth D. A more accurate method to estimate glomerular filtration rate from serum creatinine: a new prediction equation. Ann Intern Med 1999; 130: 461-470.
51. Levey AS, Coresh J, Greene T, Marsh J, Stevens LA, Kusek JW, Van Lente F, for Chronic Kidney Disease Epidemiology Collaboration. Expressing the Modification of Diet in Renal Disease Study Equation for Estimating Glomerular Filtration Rate with Standardized Serum Creatinine Values Clinical Chemistry 2007; 53: : 766–772.
52. National Kidney Fondation K/DOQI Clinical Practice Guidelines for Chronic Kidney Disease: Evaluation, classification, and stratification. Am J Kidney Dis 2002; 39: S1-S266.
53. Gaspari F, Perico N, Remuzzi G. Measurement of glomerular filtration rate. Kidney Int 1997; 63: S151-S154.
54. Rocco MV, Buckalew VMJr, Moore LC, Shihabi ZK. Measurement of glomerular filtration rate using nonradioactive Iohexol: comparison of two one-compartment models. Am J Nephrol 1996; 16: 138-143.
55. Maher FT, Nolan NG, Elverback LR. Comparison of simultaneous clearances of 125I-labeled sodium iothalamate and of inulin. Mayo Clin Proc 1971; 46: 690-691.
56. Gaspan F, Amuchastegui CS, Guerini E, Perico N, Mosconi L, Ruggenenti P, Remuzzi G. Plasma clearance of nonradioactive iohexol as an alternative to renal clearance of inulin for measurement of glomerular filtration rate in humans. J Am Soc Nephrol 1993; 4: 315.
57. Aurell M. Accurate and feasible measurements of glomerular filtration rate - is the iohexol clearance the answer. Nephrol Dial Transplant 1994; 9: 1222-1224.
58. Brown SCW, O'Reilly PH. Iohexol clearance for the determination of glomerular filtration rate in clinical practice: evidence for a new gold standard. J Urol 1991; 148: 675-679.
59. Sterner G, Frennby B, Mansson S, Nyman U, Vanwesten D, Almén T. Determining 'true' glomerular filtration rate in healthy adults using infusion of inulin and comparing it with values obtained using other clearance techniques or prediction equations. Scand J Urol Nephrol. 2007; 16: 1-8.
60. Esposito C, Plati A, Mazzullo T, Fasoli G, De Mauri A, Grosjean F, Mangione F, Castoldi F, Serpieri N, Cornacchia F, Dal Canton A. Renal function and functional reserve in healthy elderly individuals. J Nephrol. 2007; 20: 617-25.
61. Schrier RW. Aquaporin-related disorders of water homeostasis. Drug News Perspect. 2007; 20: 447-53.
62. Peters HP, Robben JH, Deen PM, Wetzels JF. Water in health and disease: new aspe cts of disturbances in water metabolism. Neth J Med. 2007; 65: 325-32.
63. Cook JD, Strauss KA, Caplan YH, Lodico CP, Bush DM. Urine pH: the effects of time and temperature after collection. J Anal Toxicol. 2007; 31: 486-96.
64. Thomsen K, Schou M. Renal lithium excretion in man. Am J Physiol 1968; 215: 823-827.
65. Whiting PH. The use of lithium clearance measurements as an estimate of glomerulo-tubular function. Renal Failure 1999; 21: 421-426.
66. Anastasio P, Frangiosa A, Papalia T, DeNapoli N, Capodicasa L, Loguercio C, DelVecchio BC, DeSanto NG. Renal tubular function by lithium clearance in liver cirrhosis. Sem Nephrol 2001; 21: 323-326.
67. Barbato A, Cappuccio FP, Folkerd EJ, Strazzullo P, Sampson B, Cook DG, Alberti KG. Metabolic syndrome and renal sodium handling in three ethnic groups living in England. Diabetologia. 2004; 47: 40-6.
68. Strazzullo P, Barbato A; Galletti F; Barba G; Siani A; Iacone R; D'Elia L; Russo O; Versiero M; Farinaro E; Cappuccio FP. Abnormalities of renal sodium handling in the metabolic syndrome. Results of the Olivetti Heart Study J Hypertens. 2006; 24: 1633-1639.
69. Sansoè G, Silvano S, Mengozzi G, Smedile A, Touscoz G, Rosina F, Rizzetto M. Loss of tubuloglomerular feedback in decompensated liver cirrhosis: physiopathological implications. Dig Dis Sci. 2005 May; 50(5): 955-63.
70. Guder WG, Hofman W. Markers for the diagnosis and monitoring of renal tubular lesions. Clin Nephrol 1992; 38 (Suppl 1): S3-S7.
71. Peterson PA, Evrin PE, Berggard I. Differentiation of glomerular, tubular, and normal proteinuria: determinations of urinary excretion of β-2-microglobin, albumin and total protein. J Clin Invest 1969; 48: 1189-1198.
72. Ivandic M, Hofmann W, Guder WG. Development and evaluation of a urine protein expert system. Clin Chem 1996, 42: 1214-1222.
73. Lun A, Ivandic M, Priem F, Filler G, Kirschstein M, Ehrich JH, Guder WG. Evaluation of pediatric nephropathies by a computerized Urine Protein Expert System (UPES). Ped Nephrol 1999; 13: 900-906.
74. Lau YK, Woo KT. SDS-PAGE is underutilized as a tool for investigating renal patients. Nephron 2002; 90: 227-229.

75. Ginsberg JM, Chang BS, Matarese RA, Garella S. Use of single voided urine samples to estimate quantitative proteinuria. N Engl J Med 1983; 309: 1543-1548.
76. Schwab SJ, Christensen RL, Dougherty K, Klahr S. Quantitation of proteinuria by the use of protein to creatinine ratio in single urine sample. Arch Intern Med 1987; 147: 943-949.
77. Lane C, Brown M, Dunsmuir W, Kelly J, Mangos G. Can spot urine protein/creatinine ratio replace 24 h urine protein in usual clinical nephrology? Nephrology (Carlton). 2006; 11: 245-249.
78. Leung YY, Szeto CC, Tam LS, Lam CW, Li EK, Wong KC, Yu SW, Kun EW. Urine protein-to-creatinine ratio in an untimed urine collection is a reliable measure of proteinuria in lupus nephritis. Rheumatology (Oxford). 2007; 46: 649-652.
78a. Price CP, Newall RG, Boyd JC. Use of the protein: creatinine ratio measurements on random urine samples for prediction of significant proteinuria: a systematic review. Clin Chem 2005; 51: 1577-1586.
78b. Gai M, Motta D, Giunti S, Fop F, Masini S, Mezza E, Segoloni GP, Lanfranco G. Comparison between 24-h protaeinuria, urinary protein/creatinine ratio and dipstick test in patients with nephropathy: Patterns of prolteinuia in dipstick-negative patients. Scan J Clin Lab Invest 2006; 66: 299-308.
79. Shankland SJ. The podocyte's response to injury: role in proteinuria and glomerulosclerosis. Kidney Int 2006; 69: 2131–2147.
80. Remuzzi G, Bertani T. Is glomerulosclerosis a consequence of altered glomerular permeability to macromolecules? Kidney Int 1990; 38: 384–394.
81. Bohle A, Mackensen-Haen S, von Gise H, Grund K-E, Wehrmann M, Batz Ch, Bogenschütz O, Schmitt H, Nagy J, Müller C, Müller G. The Consequences of Tubulo-Interstitial Changes for Renal Function in Glomerulopathies. A Morphometric and Cytological Analysis. Path Res Pract 1990; 186: 135-144.
82. Nath KA. Tubulointerstitial changes as a major determinant in the progression of renal damage. Am J Kidney Dis 1992; 1: 1-17.
83. Bernard A, Lauwerys RR. Proteinuria: changes and mechanisms in toxic nephropathies. Crit Rev Toxicol 1991; 21: 373-405.
84. Wolf G, Schroeder R, Ziyadeh FN, Stahl RA. Albumin up-regulates the type II transforming growth factor-beta receptor in cultured proximal tubular cells. Kidney Int 2004; 66: 1849–1858.
85. Fried LF, Orchard TJ, Kasiske BL. Effect of lipid reduction on the progression of renal disease: a meta-analysis. Kidney Int 2001; 59: 260–269.
86. Perico N, Codreanu I, Schieppati A, Remuzzi G. Pathophysiology of disease progression in proteinuric nephropathies. Kidney Int 2005 Suppl 94: S79–S82.
87. Abbate M, Zoja C, Remuzzi G. How does proteinuria cause progressive renal damage? J Am Soc Nephrol 2006; 17: 2974–2984.
88. Barratt J and Topham P. Urine proteomics: the present and future of measuring urinary protein components in disease. CMAJ. 2007; 177: 361-8.
88a. Nguyen MT, Ross, GF, Dent CL, Devarajan P. Early prediction of acute renal injury using urinary proteomics. Am. J Nephrol. 2005; 25: 318-326.
89. Varghese SA, Powell TB, Budisavljevic MN, Oates JC, Raymond JR, Almeida JS, Arthur JM. Urine biomarkers predict the cause of glomerular disease. J Am Soc Nephrol 2007; 18: 913-922.
90. Derhaschnig U, Kittler H, Woisetschläger C, Bur A, Herkner H, Hirschl MM. Microalbumin measurement alone or calculation of the albumin/creatinine ratio for the screening of hypertension patients? Nephrol Dial Transplant. 2002; 17: 81-5.
91. Sarafidis PA, Riehle J, Bogojevic Z, Basta E, Chugh A, Bakris GL. A Comparative Evaluation of Various Methods for Microalbuminuria Screening. Am J Nephrol 2007; 28: 324-329.
92. Weir MR. Microalbuminuria and cardiovascular disease. Clin J Am Soc Nephrol 2007; 2: 581-90.
93. Ruggenenti P, Remuzzi GTime to abandon microalbuminuria? Kidney Int. 2006; 70: 1214-22.
94. Prinsen BH, De Sain-Van der Velden MG, Kaysen GA, Straver HW, Van Rijn HJ, Stellaard F, Berger R, Rabelink TJ. Transferrin synthesis is increased in nephrotic patients insufficiently to replace urinary losses. J Am Soc Nephrol 2001; 12: 1017-1025.
95. Tencer J, Frick IM, Oquist BW, Alm P, Rippe B. Size-selectivity of the glomerular barrier to high molecular weight proteins: upper size limitations of shunt pathways. Kidney Int 1998; 53(3): 709-715.
96. Schurek HJ, Neuman KH, Flohr, et al: the physiological and pathophysiological basis of glomerular capillarry permeability for plasma proteins and erythrocytes. Eur J Clin Chem Clin Biochem 1992; 30: 627-633.
97. Schurek HJ, Neumann KH, Flohr H, Zeh M, Stolte H. Diagnostic and prognostic significance of proteinuria selectivity index in glomerular diseases. Clin Chim Acta 2000; 297: 73-83.
98. Bakoush O, Tencer J, Tapia J, Rippe B, Torffvit O. Higher urnary IgM excretion in type 2 diabetic nephropathy compared to type 1 diabetic nephropathy. Kidney Int 2002; 61: 203-208.
99. Tencer J, Bakoush O, Torffvit O. Diagnostic and prognostic significance of proteinuria selectivity index in glomerular diseases. Clin Chim Acta 2000; 297: 73-83.
100. Bazzi C, Petrini C, Rizza V, Arrigo G. Beltrame A, Pisano L, D'Amico G. Urinary excretion of IgG and β-1-microglobulin predicts clinical course better than extent of proteinuria in membranous nephropathy. Am J Kidney Dis 2001; 38: 240-248.

101. Bernard,A. Renal dysfunction induced by cadmium: biomarkers of critical effects. Biometals 2004; 17: 519-523.
102. Kawasaki T, Kono K, Dote T, Usuda K, Shimizu H, Dote E. Markers of cadmium exposure in workers in a cadmium pigment factory after changes in the exposure conditions. Toxicol Ind Health 2004; 20: 51-56.
103. Xu S, Venge P. Lipocalins as biochemical markers of disease. Biochim Biophys Acta. 2000; 1482: 298-307.
104. Creppy EE, Moukha S, Bacha H, Carratu MR. How much should we involve genetic and environmental factors in the risk assessment of mycotoxins in humans? Int J Environ Res Public Health 2005: 2: 185-193.
105. Dimitrov P, Tsolova S, Georgieva R, Bozhilova D, Simeonov V, Bonev A, Karmaus W. Clinical markers in adult offspring of families with and without Balkan Endemic Nephropathy. Kidney Int 2006; 69: 723-729.
106. Lee JW, Kim HJ, Sung SH, Lee SJ. A case of tubulointerstitial nephritis and uveitis syndrome with severe immunologic dysregulation. Pediatr Nephrol 2005; 20: 1805-1808.
107. Winchester JF, Salsberg JA, Levin NW. Beta-2 microglobulin in ESRD: an in-depth review. Adv Ren Replace Ther 2003; 10: 279-309.
108. Saito A, Gejyo F. Current clinical aspects of dialysis-related amyloidosis in chronic dialysis patients. Ther Apher Dial 2006; 10: 316-320.
109. Nomura T, Huang WC, Seo S, Zhau HE, Mimata H, Chung LW. Targeting beta2-microglobulin mediated signaling as a novel therapeutic approach for human renal cell carcinoma. J Ureol 2007; 178: 292-300.
110. Cheung AK, Rocco MV, Yan G, Leypoldt JK, Levin NW, Greene T, Agodoa L, Bailey J, Beck GJ, Clark W, Levey AS, Ornt DB, Schulman G, Schwab S, Teehan B, Eknoyan G. Serum beta-2 microglobulin levels predict mortality in dialysis patients: results of the HEMO study J Am Soc Nephrol 2006; 17: 546-555.
111. Marino M, Andrews D, Brown D, McLuskey RT. Trancytosis of retinol-binding protein across renal proximal tubule cells after megalin (gp 330)-mediated endocytosis. J Am Soc Nephrol 2001; 12: 637-648.
112. Camara NO, Matos AC, Rodrigues DA, Pereira AB, Pacheco-Silva A. Urinary retinol binding protein is a good marker of progressive cyclosporine nephrotoxicity after heart transplant. Transplant Proc 2001; 33(3): 2129-2131.
113. Salem MA, el-Habashy SA, Saeid OM, el-Tawil MM, Tawfik PH Urinary excretion of n-acetyl-beta-D-glucosaminidase and retinol binding protein as alternative indicators of nephropathy in patients with type 1 diabetes mellitus. Pediatr Diabetes. 2002; 3: 37-41.
114. Cabré A, Lázaro I, Girona J, Manzanares J, Marimón F, Plana N, Heras M, Masana LRetinol-binding protein 4 as a plasma biomarker of renal dysfunction and cardiovascular disease in type 2 diabetes. J Intern Med. 2007; 262: 496-503.
115. Kobayashi E, Suwazono Y, Honda R, Dochi M, Nishijo M, Kido T, Nakagawa H. Serial changes in urinary cadmium concentrations and degree of renal tubular injury after soil replacement in cadmium-polluted rice paddies. Toxicol Lett. 2007 Nov 1.
116. Bernard A. Renal dysfunction induced by cadmium: biomarkers of critical effects. Biometals. 2004 Oct; 17(5): 519-23.
117. Gavrilov V, Yermiahu T, Gorodischer R. Renal pathology and retinol status in multiple myeloma patients. Kidney Int. 2006 Jan; 69(1): 173-7.
118. Ekstrom B, Peterson PA, Berggard I. A urinary and plasma β-I-glycoprotein of low molecular weight: isolation and some properties. Biochem Biophys Res Commun 1975; 65: 1472-1535.
119. Weber MH, Verwiebe R. β1-Microglobulin (Protein HC): features of a promising indicator of proximal tubular dysfunction. Eur J Clin Chem Clin Biochem 1992; 30: 683-691.
120. Grubb A. Diagnostic value of analysis of cystatin C and protein HC in biological fluids. Clin Nephrol 1992; 38(Suppl 1): S20-S27.
121. Tencer J, Thysell H, Grubb A. Analysis of proteinuria: Reference limits for urine excretion of albumin, protein HC, immunoglobin G, k- and l-chain immunoreactrivity, orosomucoid and α1-antitrypsin. Scand J Clin Lab Invest 1996; 56: 691-700.
122. Carrieri M, Trevisan A, Bartolucci GB. Adjustment to concentration-dilution of spot urine samples: correlation between specific gravity and creatinine. Int Arch Occup Environ Health 2001; 74: 63–67.
123. Andersson L, Haraldsson B, Johansson C, Barregard L. Methodological issues on the use of urinary alpha-1-microglobuline in epidemiological studies. Nephrol Dial Transplant 2008; 23: 1252-1256.
124. Teppo AM, Honkanen E, Ahonen J, Gronhagen-Riska C. Changes of urinary β1-microglobullin in the assessment of prognosis in renal transplant recipients. Transplantation 2000; 70: 1154-1159.
125. Tsukahara H, Hiraoka M, Kuriyama M, Saito M, Morikawa K, Kuroda M, Tominaga T, Sudo M. Urinary β1-microglobulin as index of proximal tubule function in early infancy. Pediatr Nephrol 1993; 7: 199-201.
126. Bakoush O, Grubb A, Rippe B, Tencer J. Urine excretion of protein HC in proteinuric glomerular diseases correlates to urine IgG but not to albuminuria. Kidney Int 2001; 60: 1904-1909.
127. Madalena L, Facio ML, Angerosa M, Pandolfo M, Bresciani P, Alejandre M, Pizzolato M, Toblli JE. Urinary excretion of low molecular weight proteins in patients with pure monoclonal light chain proteinuria. J Nephrol. 2007 Nov-Dec; 20(6): 683-8.
128. Penders J, Delanghe JR. Alpha 1-microglobulin: clinical laboratory aspects and applications. Clin Chim Acta. 2004 Aug 16; 346(2): 107-18.

129. Mishra J, Ma Q, Prada A, et al. Identification of neutrophil gelatinase-associated lipocalin as a novel early urinary biomarker for ischemic renal injury. J Am Soc Nephrol 2003; 14: 2534–2543.
130. Mishra J, Mori K, Ma Q, et al. Neutrophil gelatinase-associated lipocalin: a novel early urinary biomarker for cisplatin nephrotoxicity. Am J Nephrol 2004; 24: 307–315.
131. Schmidt-Ott KM, Mori K, Li JY, Kalandadze A, Cohen DJ, Devarajan P, Barasch J. Dual action of neutrophil gelatinase-associated lipocalin. J Am Soc Nephrol 2007; 18: 407-413.
132. Mori K, Nakao K. Neutrophil gelatinase-associated lipocalin as the real-time indicator of active kidney damage. Kidney International 2007; doi: 10.1038/sj.ki.5002165.
133. Bachorzewska-Gajewska H, Malyszko J, Sitniewska E, et al. Neutrophil-gelatinase-associated lipocalin and renal function after percutaneous coronary interventions. Am J Nephrol 2006; 26: 287–292.
134. Bachorzewska-Gajewska H, Malyszko J, Sitniewska E, Malyszko JS, Pawlak K, Mysliwiec M, Lawnicki S, Szmitkowski M, Dobrzycki S. Could neutrophil-gelatinase-associated lipocalin and cystatin C predict the development of contrast-induced nephropathy after percutaneous coronary interventions in patients with stable angina and normal serum creatinine values? Kidney Blood Press Res 2007; 30: 408-415.
135. Hirsch R, Dent C, Pfriem H, Allen J, Beekman RH, Ma Q, Dastrala S, Bennett M, Mitsnefes M, Devarajan P. NGAL is an early predictive biomarker of contrast-induced nephropathy in children. Pediatr.Nephrol. 2007).
136. Ding H, He Y, Li K, Yang J, Li X, Lu R, Gao W. Urinary neutrophol gelatinase-associated lipocalin (NGAL) is an early biomarker for renal tubulaointerstitial injury in IgA nephropathy. Clin Immunol 2007; 123: 227-234.
137. Parikh CR, Jani A, Mishra J, Ma Q, Kelly C, Barasch J, Edelstein CL, Devarajan P. Urine NGAL and IL-18 are predictive biomarkers for delayed graft function following kidney transplantation. Am J Transplant 2006; 7: 1639-1645.
138. Mishra J, Ma Q, Kelly C, et al. Kidney NGAL is a novel early marker of acute injury following transplantation. Pediatr Nephrol 2006; 21: 856–863.
139. Schaub S, Mayr M, Honger G, Bestland J, Steiger J, Regeniter A, Mihatsch MJ, Wilkins JA, Rush D, Nickerson P. Detection of subclinical tubular injury after renal transplantation: comparison of urine protein analysis with allograft histopathologydetection of subclinical tubular injury after renal transplantation: comparison of urine protein analysis with allograft histopathology. Transplantation 2007; 84: 104-112.
140. Bolignano D, Coppolino G, Campo S, Aloisi C, Nicocia G, Frisina N, Buemi M. Neutrophil gelatinase-associated lipocalin in patients with autosomal-dominant polycystic kidney disease. Am J Nephrol 2007; 27: 373-378.
141. Parikh CR, Mishra J, Thiessen-Philbrook H, et al. Urinary IL-18 is an early predictive biomarker of acute kidney injury after cardiac surgery. Kidney Int 2006; 70: 199–203.
141a. Parikh C, Jani A, Mclnikov VY, Faubel S. Edelstein CL: Urinary interleukin-18 is a marker of human acute tubular necrosis Am. J Kid Dis. 2004; 43: 405-414.
142. Mishra J, Dent C, Tarabishi R, et al. Neutrophil gelatinase-associated lipocalin (NGAL) as a biomarker for acute renal injury after cardiac surgery. Lancet 2005; 365: 1231–1238.
143. Wagener G, Jan M, Kim M, et al. Association between increases in urinary neutrophil gelatinase-associated lipocalin and acute renal dysfunction after adult cardiac surgery. Anesthesiology 2006; 105: 485–491.
144. Baricos WH, Cortez SL, Le QC, Zhou Y, Dicarlo RM, O'Connor SE, Shah SV. Glomerular basement membrane degradation by endogenous cysteine proteinases in isolated glomeruli. Kidney Int 1990; 38: 395-401.
145. Coll E, Botey A, Alvarez L, et al. Serum cystatin C as a new marker for noninvasive estimation of glomerular filtration rate and as a marker for early renal impairment. Am J Kidney Dis 2000; 36: 29–34.
146. Jonsson AS, Flodin M, Hansson LO, Larsson A. Estimated glomerular filtration rate (eGFR(CystC)) from serum cystatin C shows strong agreement with iohexol clearance in patients with low GFR. Scand J Clin Lab Invest. 2007; 9: 1-9.
147. Herget-Rosenthal S, Feldkamp T, Volbracht L, Kribben A. Measurement of urinary cystatin C by particle-enhanced nephelometric immunoassay: precision, interferences, stability and reference range. Ann Clin Biochem 2004; 41: 111–118.
148. Herget-Rosenthal S, van Wijk JA, Brocker-Preuss M, Bokenkamp A. Increased urinary cystatin C reflects structural and functional renal tubular impairment independent of glomerular filtration rate. Clin Biochem 2007; 27 April [Epub ahead of print]. This study provides evidence for urinary cystatin C as a biomarker for tubular injury.
149. Dharnidharka VR, Kwon C, Stevens G. Serum cystatin C is superior to serum creatinine as a marker of kidney function: a meta-analysis. Am J Kidney Dis 2002; 40: 221–226.
150. Herget-Rosenthal S, Pietruck F, Volbracht L, et al. Serum cystatin C: a superior marker of rapidly reduced glomerular filtration after uninephrectomy in kidney donors compared to creatinine. Clin Nephrol 2005; 64: 41–46.
151. Herget-Rosenthal S, Marggraf G, Husing J, et al. Early detection of acute renal failure by serum cystatin C. Kidney Int 2004; 66: 1115–1122.

152. Herget-Rosenthal S, Poppenb D, Husing J, Markggraf G, Pietruck F, Jakon H-G, Phillipp T, Kribben A. Prognotic value of tubular proteinuria and enzymuria in non-oliguric renal acute tubular necrosis. Clin Chem 2004, 50: 552-558.

152a. Mazui-Sunko B, Zarkovic N, Vrkic N, Antoljak N, Beslin MB, Heitzler VN, Siranovic M, Krizmanic-Dekanic A, Klinger R: Proatrial natriuretic peptide (1-98) but not cystatin C is predictive for occurence of acute renal insufficiency in critical ill septic patients. Nephron Cloin Pract 2004; 97: c103-c107.

153. Lynn KL, Marshall RO. Excretion of Tamm-Horsfall glycoprotein in renal disease. Clin Sci 1985; 68: 253-257.

154. Serafini-Cessi F, Malagolini N, Cavallone DTamm-Horsfall glycoprotein: biology and clinical relevance. Am J Kidney Dis. 2003 Oct; 42(4): 658-76.

155. Mo L, Huang HY, Zhu XH, Shapiro E, Hasty DL, Wu XR. Tamm-Horsfall protein is a critical renal defense factor protecting against calcium oxalate crystal formation. Kidney Int. 2004 Sep; 66(3): 1159-66.

156. Hess B, Nakagawa Y, Parks JH, Coe FL: Molecular abnormality of Tamm-Horsfall glycoprotein in calcium oxalate nephrolithiasis. Am J Physiol 260: F569–F578, 1991.

157. Romero MC, Nocera S, Nesse AB: Decreased Tamm-Horsfall protein in lithiasic patients. Clin Biochem 30: 63–67, 1997.

158. Ganter K, Bongartz D, Hesse A: Tamm-Horsfall protein excretion and its relation to citrate in urine of stone-forming patients. Urology 53: 492–495, 1999.

159. Kumar V, Pena DL, Farell VG, Lieske JC: Urinary macromolecular inhibition of crystal adhesion to renal epithelial cells is impaired in male stone formers. Kidney Int 68: 1784–1792, 2005.

160. Plummer DR. Noorazar S, Obatomi DK, Haslan JD. Assessment of renal injury by urinary enzymes. Uremia Invest 1985; 9: 97-102.

161. Dubach UC, LeHir M. Conical evaluation of the diagnostic use of urinary enzymes. Contrib Nephrol 1984; 42: 74-80.

162. Scherberich JE: Urinary proteins of tubular origin: basic immunological and clinical aspects. Am J Nephrol 1990; 10: 43-51.

163. Westhuyzen J, Endre ZH, Reece G, Reith DM, Saltissie D, Morgan TJ: Measurement of tubular enzymuria facilitates early detection of acute renal impairment in the intensive care unit. Nephrol Dial Transplant 2003; 18: 543-551.

164. Mutti A. Detection of renal disease in humans. Developing markers and methods. Toxicol Lett 1989; 46: 177-191.

165. Vanderlinde RE. Urinary enzymes measurements of renal disorders. Ann Clin Lab Sci 1981; 11: 189-201.

166. Maruhn D, Fuchs I, Mues G, Bock KD. Normal limits of excretion of eleven enzymes. Clin Chem 1976; 22: 1567-1574.

167. Koenig H, Goldstone A, Hughes C. Lysosomal enzymuria in the testosterone treated mouse. Lab Invest 1978; 39: 329-341.

168. Ceriotti G. A new look at the measurement and interpretation of enzyme assays. Ann Clin Biochem 1976; 13: 345-353.

169. Dubach UC, LeHir M, Gandhi R. Use of urinary enzymes as markers of nephrotoxicity. Toxicol Lett 1988; 46: 193-196.

170. Tolkoff-Rubin NE, Rubin RH, Bonventre JV: Noninvasive renal diagnostic studies. Clin Lab Med 1988; 8: 507-526.

171. Price RG. Urinalysis to exclude and monitor nephrotoxicity. Clinica Chimica Acta 2000; 297: 173-182.

172. Rosalki SB, Wilkinson JH. Urinary lactic dehydrogenase in renal disease. Lancet 1959; 2: 327-328.

173. Bosomworth MP, Aparicio SR, Hay AWM. Urine N-acetyl-[beta]-d-glucosaminidase-a marker of tubular damage? Nephrol Dial Transplant 1999; 14: 620-626.

174. Price RG. The role of NAG (N-acetyl-beta-d-glucosaminidase) in the diagnosis of kidney disease including the monitoring of nephrotoxicity. Clin Nephrol 1992; 38: S14-S19.

175. Marchewka Z, Kuzniar J, Dlugosz A. Enzymuria and alpha-2-microalbuminuria in the assessment of the influence of proteinuria on the progression of glomerulopathies. Int Urol Nephrol 2001; 33: 673-676.

176. Ikenaga H, Suzuki H, Ishii N, Itoh H, Saruta T. Enzymuria in noninsulin dependent diabetic patients: signs of tubular cell dysfunction. Clin Sci 1993; 84: 469-475.

177. Mohammadi-Karakani A, Asgharzadeh-Haghighi S, Ghazi-Khansari M, Hosseini R. Determination of urinary enzymes as a marker of early renal damage in diabetic patients. J Clin Lab Anal. 2007; 21(6): 413-7.

178. Mattenheimer H. Enzymes in renal disease. Ann Clin Lab Sci 1977; 7: 422-432.

179. Davey PG, Cowley DM, Geddes AM, Terry J. Clinical evaluation of β2-microglobulin, murmamidase, and alanine aminopeptidase as markers of gentamicin nephroxicity. Contrib Nephrol 1984; 42: 100-106.

180. Scherberich JE, Mondorf W, Falkenberg FW, Pierard D, Scoeppe W. Monitoring drug nephrotoxicity. Contrib Nephrol 1984; 42: 81-92.

181. Mueller PW, Smith SJ, Steimberg KK, Thun MJ. Chronic renal tubular effects in relation to urine cadmium levels. Nephron 1989; 52: 45-54.

182. Porter GA. Contrast associated nephropathy. Am J Cardiol 1989; 64: E22-E26.

183. Mueller PW, Delaney V, MacNeil ML, Caudill SP, Steimberg KK. Indicators of acute renal transplant rejection in patients treated with cyclosporine. Clin Chem 1990; 36: 759-764.

184. Tataranni G, Zavagli G, Farinelli R, Malacarne F, Fiocchi O, Nunzi L, Scaramuzzo P, Scorrano R. Usefulness of the assessment of urinary enzymes and microproteins in monitoring cyclosporine nephrotoxicity. Nephron 1992; 60: 314-318.

185. Zafirovska KG, Bogdanovska SV, Marina N, Gruev T, Lozance L. Urinary excretion of three specific renal tubular enzymes in patients treated with nonsteroidal anti-inflammatory drugs (NSAID). Renal Failure 1993; 15: 51-54.

186. Donadio C, Tramont G, Giordani R, Lucchetti A, Calderazzi A, Ferrari P, Bioanchi C. Renal effects and nephrotoxicity of contrast media in renal patients. Contrib Nephrol 1993; 101: 241-250.

187. Naghibi B, Ghafghazi T, Hajhashemi V, Talebi A. Vancomycin-induced nephrotoxicity in rats: is enzyme elevation a consistent finding in tubular injury? J Nephrol. 2007; 20: 482-488.

188. Taracha E, Habrat B, Lehner M, Wislowska A, Woronowicz BT, Bogulas M, Charewicz J, Markuszewski C, Plaźnik A. Alanine aminopeptidase activity in urine: a new marker of chronic alcohol abuse? Alcohol Clin Exp Res. 2004; 28: 729-35.

188. Lauwerys RR, Bernard A. Early detection of the nephrotoxic effects of industrial chemicals: state of the art and future prospects. Am J Ind Med 1987; 11: 275-285.

189. Trof RJ, Di Maggio F, Leemreis J, Groeneveld AB. Biomarkers of acute renal injury and renal failure. Shock 206; 26: 245-253.

190. Verpooten GF, Nuyts GD, Hoylaerts MF, Nouwen EJ, Vssanyiova Z, Dlhopolcek P, De Broe ME. Immunoassay in urine of a specific marker for proximal tubular S3 segment. Clin Chem 1992; 38: 642-647.

191. Nuyts GD, Roels HA, Verpooten GF, Bernard AM, Lauwerys RR, De Broe ME. Intestinal type alkaline phosphatase in urine as an indicator of mercury induced effects on the S3 segment of the proximal tubule. Nephrol Dial Transplant 1992; 7: 225-229.

192. Verpooten GF, Nouwen EJ, Hoylaerts MF, Hendrix PG, De Broe ME. Segment specific localization of intestinal type alkaline phosphatase in human kidney. Kidney Int 1989; 36: 617-625.

193. Nouwen EJ, De Broe ME. Human intestinal versus tissue-nonspecific alkaline phosphatase as complementary urinary markers for the proximal tubule. Kidney Int 1994; 46 (Suppl 47): S43-51.

194. Taha MA, Shokeir AA, Osman HG, Abd El-Aziz Ael-A, Farahat SE. Obstructed versus dilated nonobstructed kidneys in children with congenital ureteropelvic junction narrowing: role of urinary tubular enzymes. J Urol. 2007; 178: 640-6.

195. Kilty C, Doyle S, Hassett B, Manning F.Glutathione S-transferases as biomarkers of organ damage: applications of rodent and canine GST enzyme immunoassays. Chem Biol Interact. 1998; 111-112: 123-3 5.

196. Sundberg AGM, Appelkvist E-L, Backman L, Dallner G: Quantitation of glutathione S-transferase-pi in the urine by radioimmunoassay. Nephron 1994; 66: 162-169.

197. Harrison DJ, Kharbanda R, Cunningham DS, McClellan LI, Hayes JD: Glutathione S-transferase isoenzymes in the human kidney: basis for possible markers of renal injury. J Clin Pathol 1989; 42: 624-629.

198. Hayes JD, Pulford DJ. The glutathione S-transferase supergene family: Regulation of GST and the contribution of the isoenzymes to cancer chemoprotection and drug resistance. Crit Rev Biochem Mol Biol 1995; 30: 445-600.

199. Branten AJ, Mulder TP, Peters WH, Assmann KJ, Wetzels JF. Urinary excretion of glutathione S transferase ω and pi in patients with proteinuria: reflection of the site of tubular injury. Nephron 2000; 85: 120-126.

200. Shaw M. The use of histologically defined specific biomarkers in drug development with special reference to the glutathione S-transferases. Cancer Biomark. 2005; 1: 69-74.

201. Kharasch ED, Hoffman GM, Thorning D, Hankins DC, Kilty CG. Role of renal cysteine conjugate β-lyase pathway in inhaled compound A nephrotoxicity in rats. Anesthesiology 1998; 88: 1624-1633.

202. Rozell B, Hansson HA, Guthenberg C, Tahir MK, Mannervik B. Glutathione transferases of classes alpha, mu and pi show selective expression in different regions of rat kidney. Xenobiotica (1993) 23(8): 835-849.

203. Sundberg AG, Appelkvist EL, Backman L, Dallner G. Urinary pi-class glutathione transferase as an indicator of tubular damage in the human kidney. Nephron 1994; 67: 308-316.

204. Goldberg ME, Cantillo J, Gratz I et al. Dose of compound A, not sevoflurane, determines changes in the biochemical markers of renal injury in volunteers. Anesth. Analg. (1999) 88: 437-445.

205. Falkenberg, F. et al. Papillary antigens as markers of papillary toxicity. I Identification and characterisation of rat papillary antigens with monoclonal antibodies. Arch. Toxicol. 1996; 71, 80-92.

206. Hildebrand, H. et al. Urinary antigens as markers of papillary toxicity. II Application of monoclonal antibodies for the determination of papillary antigens in rat urine. Arch. Toxicol. 1999; 73, 233-2.

207. Kilty CG, Keenan J, Shaw M Histologically defined biomarkers in toxicology. Expert Opin Drug Saf. 2007; 6: 207-215.

208. Dinarello CA. Historical insights into cytokines. Eur J Immunol. 2007; Suppl 1: S34-45.

209. Kovarik P, Sauer I, Schaljo B. Molecular mchanisms of the anti-inflammatory functions of interferons. Immunobiology. 2008; 212: 895-901.

210. Pestka S, Krause CD, Walter MR. Interferons, interferon-like cytokines, and their receptors, Immunol. Rev. 2004; 202: 8–32.

211. Baron S, Tyring SK, Fleischmann WR Jr, Coppenhaver DH, Niesel DW, Klimpel GR, Stanton GJ, Hughes TK. The interferons. Mechanisms of action and clinical applications. JAMA 1991; 266: 1375-1383.

212. Schrader JW. Interleukin is as interleukin does. Trends in Immunology 2002; 23: 573-574.

213. Rosenberg SA. Interleukin 2 for patients with renal cancer. Nature Clinical Practice Oncology 2007; 4: 497.

214. Sandrini S. Use of IL-2 receptor antagonists to reduce delayed graft function following renal transplantation: a review. Clinical Transplantation 2005; 19: 705-710.
215. Horii Y, Iwano M, Hirata E, Shiiki H, Fujii Y, Dohi K, Ishikawa H. Role of interleukin-6 in the progression of mesangial proliferative glomerulonephritis. Kidney Int 1993; 43 (Suppl 39): S71-S75.
216. Coleman D, Ruef C. Interleukin 6: an autocrine regulator of mesangial cell growth. Kidney Int 1992; 41: 604-611.
217. Frank J, Engler-Blum G, Rodemann HP, Muller GA. Human tubular cells as a cytokine source: PDGF-B, GM-CSF and iL-6 mRNA expression *in vitro*. Exp Nephrol 1993; 1: 26-35.
218. Hirano T, Akira S, Taga T, Kishimoto T. Biological and clinical aspects of interleukin 6. Immunol today 1990; 11: 443-449.
219. Fukatsu A, Matsuo S, Tamai H, Sakamoto N, Matsuda T, Hirano T. Distribution of interleukin-6 in normal and diseased human kidney. Lab Invest 1991; 65: 61-66.
220. Ohta K, Takano N, Seno A et al. Detection and clinical usefulness of urinary interleukin-6 in the diseases of the kidney and urinary tract. Clin Nephrol 1992; 38: 185-189.
221. Ranieri E, Gesualdo L, Petrarulo E, Schena FP. Urinary IL-6/EGF ratio: a useful prognostic marker of renal damage in IgA nephropathy. Kidney Int 1996; 50: 1990-2001.
222. Di Paolo S, Gesualdo L, Stallone G, Ranieri E, Schena FP. Renal expression and urinary concentration of EGF and IL-6 in acutely dysfuctioning transplanted patients. Nephrol Dial Transplant 1997; 12: 2687-2693.
223. Jutley RS, Youngson GG, Eremin O, Ninan GK. Serum cytokine profile in reflux nephropathy. Ped Surg Interna 2000; 16: 64-68.
224. Dinarello CA. Interleukin-1β. Crit. Care Med. 2005; 33: S460–62.
225. Daphna-Iken D, Morrison AR. Interleukin-1β induces interstitial collagenase gene expression, and protein secretion in renal mesangial cells. Am J Physiol Renal Fluid Electrolyte Physiol 1995; 269: F831–F837.
226. Ikeda M, Ikeda U, Oohara T, Takeda K, Kano S. Recombinant interleukin-1 inhibits the growth of rat mesangial cells in culture. Clin Exp Immunol 1991; 83: 149–153.
227. Pawluczyk IZ, Harris KP. Cytokine interactions promote synergistic fibronectin accumulation by mesangial cells. Kidney Int 1998; 54: 62–70.
228. Sheu JN, Chen MC, Cheng SL, Lee IC, Chen SM, Tsay GJ. Urine interleukin-1beta in children with acute pyelonephritis and renal scarring. Nephrology (Carlton). 2007; 12: 487-93.
229. Gauer S, Sichler O, Obermüller N, Holzmann Y, Kiss E, Sobkowiak E, Pfeilschifter J, Geiger H, Mühl H, Hauser IA. IL-18 is expressed in the intercalated cell of human kidney. Kidney Int. 2007; 72: 1081-7.
230. Gracie JA, Robertson SE, McInnes IB Interleukin-18. J Leukoc Biol. 2003; 73: 213-24.
231. Melnikov VY, Ecder T, Fantuzzi G, et al. Impaired IL-18 processing protects caspase-1-deficient mice from ischemic acute renal failure. J Clin Invest 2001; 107: 1145–1152.
232. Calvani N, Richards HB, TucciM, Pannarale G, Silvestris F. Up-regulation of IL-18 and prominence of Th1 immune response as a hallmark of lupus nephritis. Clin Exp Immunol 2004; 138: 171-178.
233. Chiang CK, hsu SP, Pai MF et al. Plasma interleukin-18 levels in chronic renal failure and continuous ambulatory peritoneal dialysis. Blood Purif 2005; 23: 144-148.
234. Liang D, Liu H-F, Yao C-W, Liu H-Y, Huang-Fu C-M, Chen X-W, Du S-H, Chen X-W. Effects of interleukin on injury and activation of human proximal tubular epithelial cells. Nephrology 2007; 12: 53-61.
235. Melnikov VY, Ecder T, Fantuzzi G. Impaired IL-18 processing protects caspase-1 deficient mice from ischemic acute renal failure. J Clin Invest 2001; 107: 1145-1152.
236. Parikh CR, Abraham E, Ancukiewicz M, Edelstein CL. Urine IL-18 is an early diagnostic marker for acute kidney injury and predicts mortality in the intensive care unit. J Am Soc Nephrol 2005; 16: 3046–3052.
237. Parikh CR, Jani A, Melnikov VY, et al. Urinary interleukin-18 is a marker of human acute tubular necrosis. Am J Kidney Dis 2004; 43: 405–414.
238. Parikh CR, Jani A, Mishra J, et al. Urine NGAL and IL-18 are predictive biomarkers for delayed graft function following kidney transplantation. Am J Transplant 2006; 6: 1639–1645.
238a. Hu H, Aizenstein BK, Puchalski Am Burmania JA, HarnawyMM, Knechtle SJ. Elevation of CXCR3-binding chemokines in urine indicated acute renal allograft rejection Am J Transpl.2004; 432-437.
239. Washburn KK, Zappitelli M, Arikan AA, Loftis L, Yalavarthy R, Parikh CR, Edelstein CL, Goldstein SL. Urinary Interleukin-18 is an Acute Kidney Injury Biomarker in Critically Ill Children. Nephrol Dial Transplant. 2007 Oct 1.
240. Araki S, Haneda M, Koya D, Sugimoto T, Isshiki K, Chin-Kanasaki M, Uzu T, Kashiwagi A. Predictive impact of elevated serum level of IL-18 for early renal dysfunction in type 2 diabetes: an observational follow-up study. Diabetologia. 2007; 50: 867-73.
241. Gaffen SL. Biology of recently discovered cytokines: Interleukin-17 – aunique inflammatory cytokine with roles in bone biology and arthritis. Arthritis Res Ther 2004; 6: 240-247.

242. Yu JJ, Gaffen SL. Interleukin-17: a novel inflammatory cytokniwe that bridges innate and adaptive immunity. Front Biosci 2008; 13: 170-177.
243. Matsumoto K, Kanmatsuse K. Increased urinary excretion of interleukin-17 in nephrotic patients. Nephron 91 : 243 –249, 2002.
244. Gomez-Chiarri M, Ortiz A, Seron D, Gonzalez E, Egido J. The intercrine superfamily and renal disease. Kidney Int 1993; 43 (Suppl 39): S81-S85.
245. Wada T, Yokoyama H, Tomosugi N, Hisada Y, Ohta S, Naito T, Kobayashi K-I, Mukaida N, Matsushima K. Detection of urinary interleukin-8 in glomerular disease. Kidney Int 1994; 46: 455-460.
246. Gormley SM, McBride WT, Armstron MA, Young IS, McClean E, MacGowna SW, Campalani G, McMurry TJ. Plasma and Urinary cytokine homeostasis and renal dysfunction during cardiac surgery. Anesthesiology 2000; 93: 1210-1216.
247. Baud L, Oudinet JP, Bens M, Noe L, Peraldi MN, Etienne J, Ardaillou R. Production of tumor necrosis factor by rat mesangial cells in response to bacterial lipopolysaccharide. Kidney Int 1989; 35: 1111-1118.
248. Baud L, Ardaillou R. Tumor necrosis factor in renal injury, Miner Electrolyte Metab 21 (1995), pp. 336–341.
249. Navarro JF, Mora-Fernández C. The role of TNF-alpha in diabetic nephropathy: pathogenic and therapeutic implications. Cytokine Growth Factor Rev. 2006; 17: 441-50.
250. Baud L, Fouqueray B, Philippe C, Amrani A. Tumor necrosis factor α and mesangial cells. Kidney Int 1992; 41: 600-603.
251. Radeke HH, Meier B, Topley N, Floge J, Habermehl GG, Resch K. Interleukin l-β and tumor necrosis factor-α induce oxygen radical formation in mesangial cells. Kidney Int 1990; 37: 767-775.
252. Zoja C, Wang JM, Bettoni S, Sironi M, Renzi D, Chiaffarino F, Abboud HE, Van Damme J, Mantovani A, Remuzzi G, Rambaldi A. Interleukin-1b and tumor necrosis factor-α induce gene expression and production of leukocyte chemotactic factors, colony-stimulating factors, and interleukin-6 in human mesangial cells. Am J Pathol 1991; 138: 991-1003.
253. Tomosugi N, Cashman S, Hay H, Pusey C, Evans D, Shaw A, Rees A. Modulation of antibodiy-mediated glomerular injury *in vivo* by bacterial lipopolysaccharide, tumor necrosis factor, and IL-l. J Immunol 1989; 142: 3083-3090.
254. Brockhaus M, Bar-Khayim Y, Gurwicz S, Frensdorff A, Haran N. Plasma tumor necrosis factor soluble receptors in chronic renal failure. Kidney Int 1992; 42: 663-667.
255. Boucher A, Droz, D, Adafer E, Noel L. Characterization of Mononuclear Cell Subsets in Renal Cellular Interstitial Infiltrates. Kidney Int 1986; 29: 1043–1049.
256. Danoff TM. Chemokines in Interstitial Injury. Kidney Int 1998; 53: 1807–1808.
257. Prodjosudjadi,W, Gerritsma JSJ, Klar-Mohamad N, Gerritsen AF, Bruijn J.A., Daha MR, Van Es LA. Production and cytokine-mediated regulation of monocyte chemoattractant protein-1 by human proximal tubular epithelial cells. Kidney Int 1995; 48: 1477–1486.
258. Lloyd CM, Minto AW, Dorf ME, Proudfoot A, Wells TNC, Salant DJ, Gutierrez-Ramos JC. RANTES and monocyte chemoattractant protein-1 (MCP-1) play an important role in the inflammatory phase of crescentic nephritis, but only MCP-1 is involved in crescent formation and interstitial fibrosis. J Exp Med 1997; 185: 1371–1380.
259. Wang Y, Chen J, Chen L, Tay Y, Rangan GK, Harris DCH. Induction of monocyte chemoattractant protein-1 in proximal tubule cells by urinary protein. J Am Soc Nephrol 1997; 8: 1537–1545.
260. Eddy, A.A.; Giachelli, C.M. Renal expression of genes that promote interstitial inflammation and fibrosis in rats with protein-overload proteinuria. Kidney Int 1995; 47: 1546–1557.
261. Morii T, Fujita H, Narita T, Koshimura J, Shimotomai T, Fujishima H, Yoshioka N, Imai H, Kakei M, Seiki Ito S. increased urinary excretion of monocyte chemoattractant protein-1 in proteinuric renal diseases. Ren Fail 2003; 25: 439-444.
262. Rovin BH, Song H, Birmingham DJ, Hebert LA, Yu CY, Nagaraja HN: Urine chemokines as biomarkers of human systemic lupus erythematosus activity. J Am Soc Nephrol 2005; 16 : 467 –473.
263. Rabb HA. Cell adhesion molecules and the kidney. Am J Kidney Dis 1994; 23: 155-166.
264. Perantoni AO. Cell adhesion molecules in the kidney: from embryo to adult. Exp Nephrol. 1999; 7: 80-102.
265. Müller GA, Müller CA, Markovic-Lipkovski J Adhesion molecules in renal diseases. Ren Fail. 1996; 18: 711-24.
266. Segawa C, Wada T, Takaeda M, Furuichi K, Matsuda I, Hisada Y, Ohta S, Takasawa K, Takeda S, Kobayashi K, Yokoyama H. 1997. *In situ* expression and soluble form of P-selectin in human glomerulonephritis. Kidney Int 1997; 52: 1054-1063.
267. Takaeda M, Yokoyama H, Segawa-Takaeda C, Wada T, Kobayashi K. 2002. High endothelial venule-like vessels in the interstitial lesions of human glomerulonephritis. Am J Nephrol. 22: 48-57.
268. Tipping PG, Huang XR, Berndt MC, Holdsworth SR. A role for P selectin in complement-independent neutrophil-mediated glomerular injury. Kidney Int. 1994; 46: 79-88.
269. Testa A, Benedetto FA, Spoto B, Pisano A, Tripepi G, Mallamaci F, Malatino LS, Zoccali CThe E-selectin gene polymorphism and carotid atherosclerosis in end-stage renal disease. Nephrol Dial Transplant. 2006; 21: 1921-6.
270. Malatino LS, Stancanelli B, Cataliotti A, Bellanuova I, Fatuzzo P, Rapisarda F, Leonardis D, Tripepi G, Mallamaci F, Zoccali C. Circulating E-selectin as a risk marker in patients with end-stage renal disease. J Intern Med. 2007; 262: 479-87.

271. Watanabe Y, Inoue T, Okada H, Kotaki S, Kanno Y, Kikuta T, Suzuki HImpact of selectin gene polymorphisms on rapid progression to end-stage renal disease in patients with IgA nephropathy. Intern Med. 2006; 45: 947-51.
272. Lai KN, Wong KC, Li PK, Lai CK, Chan CH, Lui SF, Chui YL, Haskard DO. Circulating leukocyte-endothelial adhesion molecules in IgA nephropathy. Nephron. 1994; 68: 294-300.
273. Roy-Chaudhury P, Wu B, King G, Campbell M, Macleod AM, Haites NE, Simpson JG, Power DA. Adhesion molecule interactions in human glomerulonephritis: importance of the tubulointerstitium. Kidney Int. 1996; 49: 127-34.
274. Kemler R. Classical cadherins. Semin Cell Biol 1992; 3: 149–155.
275. Nollet F, Kools P, van Roy F. Phylogenetic analysis of the cadherin superfamily allows identification of six major subfamilies besides several solitary members. J Mol Biol 2000; 299: 551–572.
276. Nouwen EJ, Dauwe S, van der Biest I, De Broe ME. Stage- and segment-specific expression of cell-adhesion molecules N-CAM, A-CAM, and L-CAM in the kidney. Kidney Int 1993; 44: 147–158.
277. Paul R, Ewing CM, Robinson JC, Marshall FF, Johnson KR, Wheelock MJ & Isaacs WB. Cadherin-6, a cell adhesion molecule specifically expressed in the proximal renal tubule and renal cell carcinoma. Cancer Res 1997; 57: 2741–2748.
278. Thomson RB, Igarashi P, Biemesderfer D, Kim R, Abu-Alfa A, Soleimani M & Aronson PS. Isolation and cDNA cloning of Ksp-cadherin, a novel kidney-specific member of the cadherin multigene family. J Biol Chem 1995; 270: 17594–17601.
279. Igarashi P. Following the expression of a kidney-specific gene from early development to adulthood. Nephron Exp Nephrol 2003; 94: e1–e6.
280. Kuehn A, Paner GP, Skinnider BF, Cohen C, Datta MW, Young AN, Srigley JR, Amin MB. Expression analysis of kidney-specific cadherin in a wide spectrum of traditional and newly recognized renal epithelial neoplasms: diagnostic and histogenetic implications. Am J Surg Pathol. 2007; 31: 1528-33.
281. Shen SS, Krishna B, Chirala R, Amato RJ, Truong LD. Kidney-specific cadherin, a specific marker for the distal portion of the nephron and related renal neoplasms. Mod Pathol. 2005; 18: 933-40.
282. Thedieck C, Kuczyk M, Klingel K, Steiert I, Müller CA, Klein G. Expression of Ksp-cadherin during kidney development and in renal cell carcinoma British Journal of Cancer. 2005; 92, 2010-2017.
283. Brady HR. Leukocyte adhesion molecules and kidney disease. Kidney Int 1994: 45: 1285-1300.
284. Bosman FT. Integrins: cell adhesives and modulators of cell function. Histochem J 1993; 25: 469-477.
285. Ruoslahti E, Noble NA, Kagami S, Border WA. Integrins. Kidney Int 1994; 45 (Suppl 44): S17-S22.
286. Burridge K, Fath K, Kelly T, Nuckolis B, Turner C. Foca adhesion: transmembrane junctions between the extracellular matrix and the cytoskeleton. Ann Rev Cell Biol 1988; 4: 487-525.
287. Kelly KJ, Williams WW Jr, Colvin RB, Bonventre JV. Antibody to intercellular adhesion molecule I protects the kidney against ischemic injury. Proc Natl Acad Sci 1994; 91: 812-816.
288. Baraldi A, Zambruno G, Furci L et al. Beta 1 and beta 3 integrin upregulation in rapidly progressive glomerulonephritis. Nephrol. Dial. Transplant. 1995; 10: 1155– 61.
289. Kagami S, Kondo S. Beta1-integrins and glomerular injury. J Med Invest. 2004; 51: 1-13.
290. Simon EE. Potential role of integrins in acute renal failure. Nephrol Dial Transplant 1994; 9 (Suppl 4): 26-33.
291. Seron D, Cameron JS, Haskard DO. Expression of VCAM-1 in the normal and diseased kidney. Nephrol Dial Transplant 1991; 6: 917-922.
292. Nakatani, K., H. Fujii, H. Hasegawa, M. Terada, N. Arita, M. R. Ito, M. Ono, S. Takahashi, K. Saiga, S. Yoshimoto, et al 2004. Endothelial adhesion molecules in glomerular lesions: association with their severity and diversity in lupus models. Kidney Int. 65: 1290-1300.
293. Seron, D., J. S. Cameron, D. O. Haskard. 1991. Expression of VCAM-1 in the normal and diseased kidney. Nephrol. Dial. Transplant. 6: 917-922.
294. Wuthrich, R. P.. 1992. Vascular cell adhesion molecule-1 (VCAM-1) expression in murine lupus nephritis. Kidney Int. 42: 903-914.
295. Ikeda Y, Fujimoto T, Ameno M, Shiiki H, Dohi K. Relationship between lupus nephritis activity and the serum level of soluble VCAM-1. Lupus. 1998; 7: 347-54.
296. Molad Y, Miroshnik E, Sulkes J, Pitlik S, Weinberger A, Monselise Y. 2002. Urinary soluble VCAM-1 in systemic lupus erythematosus: a clinical marker for monitoring disease activity and damage. Clin. Exp. Rheumatol. 20: 403-406.
297. Wu T, Xie C, Wang HW, Zhou XJ, Schwartz N, Calixto S, Mackay M, Aranow C, Putterman C, Mohan C. Elevated urinary VCAM-1, P-selectin, soluble TNF receptor-1, and CXC chemokine ligand 16 in multiple murine lupus strains and human lupus nephritis. J Immunol. 2007; 179: 7166-7175.
298. van Timmeren M.M, van den Heuvel M.C, Bailly V, Bakker S.J, van Goor H, Stegeman CA. Tubular kidney injury molecule-1 (KIM-1) in human renal disease J Pathol 2007; 212: 209-217.

299. Zhang Z, Humphreys BD, Bonventre JV. Shedding of the urinary biomarker kidney injury molecule-1 (KIM-1) is regulated by MAP kinases and juxtamembrane region. J Am Soc Nephrol. 2007; 18: 2704-14.
300. Ichimura T, Bonventre JV, Bailly V, Wei H, Hession CA, Cate RL, Sanicola M: Kidney injury molecule-1 (KIM-1), a putative epithelial cell adhesion molecule containing a novel immunoglobulin domain, is up-regulated in renal cells after injury. J Biol Chem 1998; 273: 4135–4142.
301. Ichimura T, Hung CC, Yang SA, et al. Kidney injury molecule-1: a tissue and urinary biomarker for nephrotoxicant-induced renal injury. Am J Physiol Renal Physiol 2004; 286: F552–F563.
302. Han WK, Bailly V, Abichandani R, Thadhani R, Bonventre JV. Kidney Injury Molecule-1 (KIM-1): a novel biomarker for human renal proximal tubule injury Kidney Int 2002; 62: 237-244.
303. Lin F, Zhang PL, Yang XJ, Shi J, Blasick T, Han WK, Wang HL, Shen SS, Teh BT, Bonventre JV: Human kidney injury molecule-1 (hKIM-1): A useful immunohistochemical marker for diagnosing renal cell carcinoma and ovarian clear cell carcinoma. Am J Surg Pathol 31 : 371 –381, 2007.
304. Han WK, Alinani A, Wu CL, Michaelson D, Loda M, McGovern FJ, Thadhani R, Bonventre JV: Human kidney injury molecule-1 is a tissue and urinary tumor marker of renal cell carcinoma. J Am Soc Nephrol 16 : 1126 –1134, 2005.
305. Perez-Rojas J, Blanco JA, Cruz C, Trujillo J, Vaidya VS, Uribe N, Bonventre JV, Gamba G, Bobadilla NA: Mineralocorticoid receptor blockade confers renoprotection in preexisting chronic cyclosporine nephrotoxicity. Am J Physiol Renal Physiol 292 : F131 –F139, 2007.
306. van Timmeren MM, Bakker SJ, Vaidya VS, Bailly V, Schuurs TA, Damman J, Stegeman CA, Bonventre JV, van Goor H: Tubular kidney injury molecule-1 in protein-overload nephropathy. Am J Physiol Renal Physiol 291 : F456 –F464, 2006.
307. Kuehn EW, Park KM, Somlo S, Bonventre JV: Kidney injury molecule-1 expression in murine polycystic kidney disease. Am J Physiol Renal Physiol 283 : F1326 –F1336, 2002.
308. Liangos O, Perianayagam MC, Vaidya VS, Han WK, Wald R, Tighiouart H, MacKinnon RW, Li L, Balakrishnan VS, Pereira BJ, Bonventre JV, Jaber BL. Urinary N-acetyl-beta-(D)-glucosaminidase activity and kidney injury molecule-1 level are associated with adverse outcomes in acute renal failure J Am Soc Nephrol 2007; 18: 904-912.
310. Han WK, Bailly V, Abichandani R, Thadhani R, Bonventre JV: Kidney Injury Molecule-1 (KIM-1): A novel biomarker for human renal proximal tubule injury. Kidney Int 62 : 237 –244, 2002.
311. Vaidya VS, Ramirez V, Ichimura T, Bobadilla NA, Bonventre JV: Urinary kidney injury molecule-1: A sensitive quantitative biomarker for early detection of kidney tubular injury. Am J Physiol Renal Physiol 2006; 290 : F517 –F529.
312. Feldstein C, Romero C. Role of endothelins in hypertension. Am J Ther. 2007; 14: 147-53.
313. Hoyer D, Waeber C, Palacios JM. ^{125}I endothelin-1 binding sites: autoradiographic studies in the brain and periphery of various species including humans. J Cardiovasc Pharmacol. 1989; 13(Suppl 5): S162-S165.
314. Gandhi CR, Berkowitz DE. Watkis D. Endothelins: biochemistry and pathophysiologic actions. Anesthesiology 1994; 80: 892-905.
315. Garcia NH, Garvin JL. Endothelin's biphasic effect on fluid absorption in the proximal straight tubule and its inhibitory cascade. J Clin Invest. 1994; 93: 2572-2577.
316. Plato CF, Stoos BA, Wang D, et al. Endogenous nitric oxide inhibits chloride transport in the thick ascending limb. Am J Physiol. 1999; 276: F159-F163.
317. Simonson MS, Wann S, Mene P, Dubyak M, Kester Y, Nakazato Y, Sedor JR, Dunn MJ. Endothelin stimulates phospholipase C, Na/H exchange, c-fos expression and mitogenesis in rat mesangial cells. J Clin Invest 1989; 83: 708-712.
318. Ohta K, Hirata Y, Shichiri M, Kanno K, Emori T, Tomita K, Marumo F. Urinary excretion of endothelin-1 in normal subjects and patients with renal disease. Kidney Int 1991; 39: 307-311.
319. Kon V, Sugiura M, Inagami T, Harvie BR, Ichikawa I, Hoover RL. Role of endothelin in cyclosporine-induced glomerular dysfunction. Kidney Int 1990; 37: 1487-1491.
319a. Fujisaki K, Kubo M, Masuda K, Tokumoto M, Hirakawa M, Ikeda H, Matsui R, Matsuo D, Fukada K, Kanai H. Infusion of radiocontrastagents induces exaggerated release of urinary endothelinin patients with impaired renal function. Clin. Exp Nephrol. 2003; 7: 279-283.
320. Abassi ZA, Klein H, Golomb E, Keiser HR. Urinary endothelin: a possible biological marker of renal damage. Am J Hypertens 1993; 6(12): 1046-1054.
321. Lovis C, Mach F, Donati YRA, Bonventure JV, Polla BS. Heat shock proteins and the kidney. Renal Failure 1994; 16: 179-192.
322. Muller M, Gauley J, Heikkila: Hydrogen peroxide induces heat shock protein and proto-oncogene mRNA accumulation in Xenopus laevis A6 kidney epithelial cells. Can j Physiol Pharmacol 2004; 82: 523-529.
323. Kiang JG, Tsokos GC. Heat shock protein 70 kDa: molecular biology, biochemistry, and physiology. Pharmacology and Therapeutics 1998; 80: 183-201.

324. Hassen W, Ayed-Boussema I, Bouslimi A, Bacha H. Heat shock protein (Hsp 70) response is not systematic to cell stress: case of the mycotoxin ochratoxin A. Toxicology 2007.
325. Soti C, Pal C, Papp B, Csermely P. Molecular chaperones as regulatory elements of cellular networks. Curr Opin Cell Biol 2005; 17 , pp. 210-215.
326. Sun Y, MacRae TH. Small heat shock proteins: Molecular structure and chaperone function. Cell Mol Life Sci 2005; 62 , pp. 2460-2476.
327. Sun Y, MacRae TH. The small heat shock proteins and their role in human disease. FEBS J 2005; 272 , pp. 2613-2627.
328. Dvergsten J, Manivel JC, Correa-Rotter R, Rosenberg ME. Expression of clusterin in human renal diseases. Kidney Int 1994; 45: 828-835.
329. Trougakos IP, Gonos ES. Clusterin/apolipoproyein J in human aging and cancer. Int J Biochem Cell Biol 2002; 34: 1430–48.
330. Rosenberg ME, Silkensen J. Clusterin and the kidney. Exp Nephrol 1995; 3: 9–14.
331. Rosenberg ME, Dvergsten J, Correa-Rotter R. Clusterin: an enigmatic protein recruited by diverse stimuli. J Lab Clin Med 1993; 121: 205–14.
332. Parczyk K, Pilarsky C, Rachel U, Koch-BrandtC. Gp80 (clusterin; TRPM-2) mRNA level is enhanced in human renal clear cell carcinomas. J Cancer Res Clin Oncol 1994; 120: 186–8.
333. Trougakos IP, Gonos ES. Regulation of clusterin/apolipoprotein J, a functional homologue to the small heat shock proteins, by oxidative stress in ageing and age-related diseases. Free Radic Res. 2006; 40: 1324-1334.
334. Takase O, Minto AW, Puri TS, Cunningham PN, Jacob A, Hayashi M, Quigg RJ. Inhibition of NF-kappaB-dependent Bcl-xL expression by clusterin promotes albumin-induced tubular cell apoptosis. Kidney Int. 2007 Dec 12.
335. Kurahashi T, Muramaki M, Yamanaka K, Hara I, Miyake H. Expression of the secreted form of clusterin protein in renal cell carcinoma as a predictor of disease extension. BJU International 2005; 96: 895–899.
336. Rulitzky WK, Schlegel PN. Wu D, Cheng CY, Chen C-LC, Li PS, Goldstein M, Reidenberg M, Bardin CW. Measurement of urinary clusterin as an index of nephrotoxicity. Proc Soc Exp Biol Med 1992; 199: 93-96.
337. Ishii A, Sakai Y, Nakamura A. Molecular pathological evaluation of clusterin in a rat model of unilateral ureteral obstruction as a possible biomarker of nephrotoxicity. Toxicol Pathol. 2007; 35: 376-82.
338. Tardanico R, Sanna-Cherchi S, Ferrario F, Montinaro V, Haupt R, Parodi S, Carnevali ML, Allegri L, Camussi G, Gesualdo L, Scolari F, Ghiggeri GM.Glomerular clusterin is associated with PKC-alpha/beta regulation and good outcome of membranous glomerulonephritis in humans. Kidney Int. 2006; 70: 477-85.
339. Lerner RA, Glassock RJ, Dixon FJ. The role of anti-glomerular basement membrane antibody in the pathogenesis of human glomerulonephritis. J Exp Med. 1967; 126: 989-1004.
340. Kalluri R. Goodpasture's syndrome. Kidney Int 1999; 55: 1120-2.
341. Kalluri R, Wilson CB, Eber M, Gunwar S, Chonko AM, Neilson EG, Hudson BG. Identification of the alpha 3 chain of type IV collagen as the common autoantigen in antibasement membrane doisease and Goodpasture syndrome. J Am Soc Nephrol 1995; 6: 1178-1185.
342. Kalluri R, Torre A, Shield CF III, et al. Identification of alpha3, alpha4, and alpha5 chains of type IV collagen as alloantigens for Alport posttransplant anti-glomerular basement membrane antibodies. Transplantation. 2000; 69: 679-683.
343. Brainwood D, Kashtan C, Gubler MC, Turner AN. Targets of alloantibodies in Alport anti-glomerular basement membrane disease after renal transplantation. Kidney Int. 1998; 53: 762-726.
344. Turner AN, Rees AJ. Goodpasture's disease and Alport's syndromes. Annu Rev Med. 1996; 47: 377-386.
345. Hellmark T, Niles JL, Collins AB, McCluskey RT, Brunmark C. Comparison of anti-GBM antibodies in sera with or without ANCA. J Am Soc Nephrol. 1997: 376-385.
346. ANCA-1. Bosch X, Guilabert A., Font J. Antineutrophil cytoplasmic antibodies Lancet 2006 ; 368 : 404-418 3.
347. ANCA-2. Lionaki S, Jenntte JC, Falk RJ: Antineutrophile cytoplasmic (ANCA) and anti-glomerular basement (ABM) autoantibodies in necrotizing and crescentric glomerulonephritis. Semin Immunopathol 2007; 29: 459-474 3.
348. ANCA-3. Hauer HA, Bajema IM, van Houwelingen HC, Ferrario F, Noel LH, Waldherr R, Jayne DR, Rasmussen N, Bruijn JA, Hagen BC: renal histology in ANCA-associated vasculitis: differences between diagnostic and serologic subgroups. Kidney Int 2002; 61: 80-90.
349. ANCA-4. Slot MC, Tervaert JW, Boomsma MM, Stegman CA: Positive classic antineutrophil cytoplasmic antibody (C-ANCA) titer at stitch to azathioprine therapy assoiated with repapse I proteinase 3-related vasculitis. Arthritis Rheum 51: 269-273.
350. ANCA 5. Falk RJ, Terrell RS, Charles LA, Jennette JC: Antineutrophile cytoplasmic antibodies induce neutrophils to degranulalte and produce oxygen radicals invivi. Proc Nat Acad Sci USA 1990; 87; 4115-4119.
351. Bobulescu A, DiSole F, Moe OW. Na+/H+ exchangers: physiology and link to hypertension and organ ischemia. Curr Opin Nephrol Hypertens. 2005; 14: 485-494.

352. du Cheyron D, Daubin C, Poggioli J, Ramakers M, Houillier P, Charbonneau P, Paillard M. Urinary measurement of Na+/H+ exchanger isoform 3 (NHE3) protein as new marker of tubule injury in critically ill patients with ARF. Am J. Kid Dis 2003; 42: 497-506.
353. Heyman SN, Rosenberger C, Rosen S. Regional alterations in renal hemodynamics and oxygenation: a role in contrast medium-induced nephropathy. Nephrol Dial Transpl 2005; 20(SI); i6-i11.

07

Toxin-induced immunological renal disease

Lucette PELLETIER, Abdelhadi SAOUDI and Gilbert FOURNIÉ

INSERM, Centre de Physiopathologie Purpan, University of Toulouse, France

Introduction

The last years have provided insight as to how lymphocytes respond to antigen or xenobiotics, and have increased our understanding of the pathophysiology of renal diseases. This points out new clues on the mechanisms by which chemically-induced immune response trigger immune nephropathies. We will describe the T-cell subsets including Th1 and Th2 cells that may be implicated in renal inflammation. The role of Th1 and Th2 CD4$^+$ T-cell subsets in the development of some nephropathies will be debated. Then, we will evoke the mechanism by which a drug or its metabolites may trigger autoimmunity or hypersensitivity reactions. Third, we will report nephropathies induced by xenobiotics in patients, emphasizing the possible underlying mechanisms. Fourth, we will focus on some experimental models of chemical-induced systemic autoimmune diseases that illustrate mechanisms described before. Finally, we will discuss recent insights from these models onto the genetic control of susceptibility to drug-induced immunopathology. This will allow us to introduce the impact of genetic studies in our understanding of the pathogenesis of immune nephropathies, which undoubtedly in the future will shed new light on toxin-induced nephropathies.

T cell-subsets and their role in the development of nephropathies

Characterization of T-cell subsets

CD4$^+$ T-lymphocytes are heterogeneous in terms of production of cytokines and functions [1-4]. Table 1 indicates some characteristics of these subsets. Th1 cells secrete interleukin (IL)-2, IFN-γ and lymphotoxin, which explains their role in activating macrophages and cytotoxic cells and therefore in cell-mediated immune responses. Th1 cells also help B-cells in the production of some isotypes: complement-fixing IgG2a in mice and IgG2b in rats. Th1 cells are responsible for delayed hypersensitivity reactions and are implicated in inflammatory processes with the recruitment of macrophages and neutrophils in the inflamed tissues. Th2 cells produce IL-4, IL-5, IL-6, IL-13 and IL-10 (in mice), promote IgE and IgG1 switch (in rats and mice) - IgE and IgG4 in humans; they activate eosinophils and mast cells. Th2 cells play an important role in the elimination of extracellular parasites such as helminths. In some situations, regulatory properties have been attributed to Th2 cells, owing to their capacity to produce the immunosuppressive cytokine IL-10 (in mice) and to the antagonistic effect of Th2 cytokines on the differentiation of Th1 and Th17 lymphocytes. This latter subset produces IL-17 and is involved in chronic inflammation. Th2 cells are clearly responsible for eosinophil- and mast-cell-mediated inflammation that characterizes particularly allergic asthma. Th1 and Th2-cells express different chemokine receptors [5] and display lineage specific transcription factors. c-maf, NIP-45 and GATA-3 characterize Th2 cells and control *Il4* and *Il5* gene transcription while T-bet is expressed in Th1 cells and is essential for IFN-γ expression (reviewed in [6]). The transcription factor RORγ controls IL-17 production by Th17 cells [7]. Regulatory T cells (Treg) include several types of natural and antigen-induced T

Table 1. T cell subsets.

T-cell subset	Cytokines produced	Lineage-specific transcription factor	Functions
Th1	IFN-γ, LT, TNF-α	T-bet	Eradication of intracellular pathogens, virus ... Help to CD8$^+$ T-cells, to B-cells (IgG2a, IgG3 in mice) Autoimmunity type 1 diabetes
Th17	IL-17	ROR-γ	Eradication of pathogens Chronic inflammation
Th2	IL-4, IL-5, IL-13, IL-6, IL-10	GATA-3, c-maf, NIP-45	Elimination of parasites B-cell help IgE, IgG1 Allergy (asthma)
Natural Treg	IL-10, TGF-β ? *	FOXp3	Regulation of Th1, Th17 and Th2 cells

*LT = lymphotoxin. * How regulatory T-cells control the other T-cell subsets in vivo remains unclear, especially with respect to the role of IL-10 and TGF-β.*

lymphocytes with focus on natural $CD4^+CD25^+Foxp3^+$ Treg [8] that may down-modulate pro-inflammatory Th1, Th2 and Th17 cells. The balance between these T-cell subsets conditions the immune response and eventually the features of the immune lesions in the target tissue.

Factors implicated in the differentiation of Th1 and Th2 cells

Up-to-now, there is no evidence concerning the role of Th17 cells in the development of nephropathies. Therefore, we will focus on the control of Th1/Th2 cell differentiation. Factors that influence Th1/Th2 cell polarization include the type of cytokines present during differentiation (IL-12 and IL-4 direct Th1 and Th2 maturation respectively) and the route of antigen administration [6, 9, 10]. The interactions of T-cells with dendritic cells (discussed in [11]), relating to the type and the activation status of dendritic cells, the nature of antigen and of co-stimulation, as well as the strength of TCR-peptide/MHC interaction are also important factors that direct T-cell differentiation. Thus, in the absence of IL-12 and in the presence of epithelial cell-derived thymic stromal lymphopoietin (TSLP), dendritic cells express OX40L which conduces to Th2 cell differentiation [12].

IFN-γ contributes to Th1 cell development by stabilizing the expression of the β2 chain of the IL-12 receptor (RIL-12) while IL-4 amplifies its own production. Therefore, there is a positive feedback reinforcing Th1 or Th2 cell maturation. Th1 and Th2 cell development is antagonistic. IL-4 inhibits the expression of β2RIL-12 chain and IL-10 suppresses IL-12 production. GATA-3 directly regulates *Il5* gene transcription and contributes to *Il4* gene transcription, probably by up-regulating c-maf that binds proximal *Il4* gene promoter. GATA-3 also down regulates β2RIL-12 chain expression (reviewed in [13]). The Th1 transcription factor T-bet downgrades IL-4 and IL-5 secretion.

The phenotype of differentiated Th1 and Th2 cells is stabilized after about 3-5 divisions [14]. Early in the differentiation, *Il4* and *IFNγ* loci are easily accessible; *Il4* and *IFNγ* genes are localized away from the silenced centromeric chromatin. Conversely, in Th1 cells, 52% of *Il4* alleles are reorganized in apposition to centromeric heterochromatin; and in Th2 cells 67% of *IFN-γ* alleles are directed to heterochromatic domains, which contributes to silence genes. In addition to these intra-chromosomal interactions, Spilianakis et al described in the mouse inter-chromosomal interactions between the promoter region of the IFN-gamma gene on chromosome 10 and the regulatory regions of the Th2 cytokine locus on chromosome 11 showing that genes located on separate chromosomes may associate physically in the nucleus which could favor coordinated control of cytokine gene expression [15, 16].

Role of Th1 and Th2 cell subsets cells in the development of nephropathies

Th1 cells are likely to play an important role in nephropathies associated with pauci immune deposits and with interstitial infiltrates of T-cells and macrophages (reviewed in [2]).The role of Th1 cells has been clearly demonstrated in experimental murine models of crescentic glomerulonephritis induced by immunization with sheep or goat immunoglobulins prior to injection with heterologous anti-glomerular basement membrane immunoglobulins (reviewed in [17]). Indeed kidney injury is attenuated in mice with genetically deleted Th1 cytokines (reviewed in [17]). In humans, crescentic glomerulonephritis is also presumed to be Th1-mediated [18]. C57BL/6 and BALB/c mice (that are Th1- and Th2-prone strains respectively) pre-sensitized with sheep globulin and injected with sheep anti-glomerular basement membrane develop distinct glomerulopathies. C57BL/6 mice displayed strong delayed type reactions DTH due to antigen-specific Th1-cells, glomerular accumulation of $CD4^+$ cells, macrophages and predominant IFN-γ production by antigen-specific T cells, consistent with a Th1 response. Conversely, the proteinuria in BALB/c mice resulted from an humoral response. Crescent formation was only observed occasionally in these mice in the absence of IL-12 administration (reviewed in [18]).

Th2 cells are pathogenic in gold salt-induced glomerulopathy in Brown-Norway (BN) rats (this part will be developed below). The analysis of mRNA obtained from kidneys of Buffalo/Mna rats that spontaneously develop a nephrotic syndrome associated with focal segmental glomerular sclerosis revealed an early Th2 biased profile of cytokine expression, consistent with the involvement of Th2 cells in this model of human idiopathic nephrotic syndrome [19]. In minimal change glomerulopathy, an association with atopy and IL-13 has been demonstrated (reviewed in [20]). In addition, several studies have reported an association between minimal change disease and polymorphisms in IL-4, IL-13 and STAT-6 (a transcription factor downstream of the IL-4 receptor) at least in Indonesian children [21, 22]. Th2 cells are also incriminated in human membranous glomerulopathies mainly because immune deposits contain IgG1 and IgG4 Th2- dependent isotypes.

A better understanding of the physiology of glomerular epithelial cells (podocytes) may explain the mechanisms by which Th1 and Th2 cells induce proteinuria. Proteins pass freely through the endothelium fenestrae, the principal barrier being localized at the site of the slit diaphragm between the foot processes of podocytes [23]. Interactions between integrins and extracellular matrix components transduce a signal leading to correct actin assembly and anchoring of nephrin and CD2AP to the slit diaphragm. The roles of CD2AP, nephrin, α-actinin and Rho small G proteins are supported by the fact that mice genetically knocked out for the genes encoding these proteins develop a nephrotic syndrome [24-29]. Stimuli such as TNF, aggregated IgG4, attack complex of complement (C5b-9), can trigger rearrangement of the cytoskeleton with redistribution of nephrin and CD2AP, which could result in proteinuria [30, 31]. Sub-lytic amounts of C5b-9 can activate podocytes (and tubular epithelial cells when present in the urine), resulting in the production of reactive oxygen species and of proteases such as gelatinase, in reticulum endoplasmic stress, in the reorganization of the cytoskeleton, in the production of TGF beta, and in the hyperproduction of extracellular matrix. These phenomena would contribute to proteinuria, tubulointerstitial nephrititis and renal failure which are often associated with glomerular diseases such as membranous nephropathy (discussed in [32]).

IL-4 and IL-13 by themselves could induce proteinuria since podocytes express receptors for both cytokines [33]. Alternatively, the Th2 cytokines could act on monocytes to produce vascular permeability factor(s) responsible for the nephrotic syndrome.

Role of regulatory- T cells in the outcome of nephropathies

The transfer of $CD4^+CD25^+$ regulatory T-cells markedly attenuated experimental anti-glomerular basement nephropathy. This beneficial effect is associated with prevention of T-cell-mediated renal inflammation and of glomerular injury [34]. The transfer of $CD4^+CD25^+$ Treg [35] or of $CD4^+$ T-cells transfected with Foxp-3 [36], the transcription factor expressed by Treg cells protects against the development of adriamycin-induced proteinuria and renal inflammation. Thus, Treg cells may have a therapeutic potential in the treatment of nephropathies.

General mechanisms by which xenobiotics may induce an immune response

Xenobiotics may favour the development of an inappropriate immune response by at least four mechanisms. 1) They can interfere with innate immunity resulting in the activation of antigen presenting cells, namely dendritic cells. 2) It can promote an immune response directed against an antigen modified by the toxin or its metabolites. 3) They can activate T cells through direct binding to the MHC molecules or perhaps to the T-cell receptor (TCR) itself. 4) They can induce global immune dysregulation. We will evoke how an autoimmune T-cell response may be induced, following drug exposure.

Alteration in the cross-talk between dendritic cells and T lymphocytes

The recognition of peptides/MHC complexes at the cell surface of an antigen presenting cells by a specific T lymphocyte is not sufficient for triggering an immune response. Dendritic cells need to be activated for initiating the immune response [37]. Signals delivered by pathogens through the Toll receptors at the dendritic cell surface and signals generated in injured tissues activate dendritic cells and interfere with antigen presentation [38]. For example, platelets that constitutively express CD40L can interact with CD40 expressed by dendritic cells leading to their activation in a bleeding tissue. Non immune tissue lesion leads to necrosis, release of reactive oxygen species, of heat shock proteins (HSP) and of lymphokines such as IL-1, TNFα, type I interferons, each being capable to stimulate dendritic cells. Activation of dendritic cells results in up-regulation of co-stimulatory molecules, lysosomal formation of immunogenic MHC-class II peptides complexes and redistribution of MHC class II products from intracellular compartments to the plasma membrane [38, 39]. Dendritic cell maturation is associated with down-regulation of proteins such as aquaporins involved in antigen uptake. Several groups correlate the sensitizing potential of drugs to their ability to activate dendritic cells [40]. For example, 2,4,6 trinitrobenzenesulfonic acid responsible for hypersensitivity reactions increased CD86 co-stimulatory molecule expression, decreased aquaporine 3 expression and IL-1β production [40]. The capacity of compounds to induce autoimmune reactions was also related to their capacity to activate antigen-presenting cells [41]. Many chemicals, including heavy metals, can directly activate dendritic cells [42], which certainly favours the development of a T-cell response (Figure1A-B, Figure 3). Blanca M's group compared dendritic cells from patients who have or those who have no hypersensitive reactions to amoxicillin [43]. They showed that dendritic cells from the former group only, partially maturated in the presence of the drug, resulting in an increased expression of HLA-DR, CD80 and CD86. These dendritic cells, exposed to amoxicillin activated autologous T-cells. Thus, amoxicillin appears not only to be the target of the immune response but also a stimulus for DC maturation in patients who develop hypersensitivity reactions.

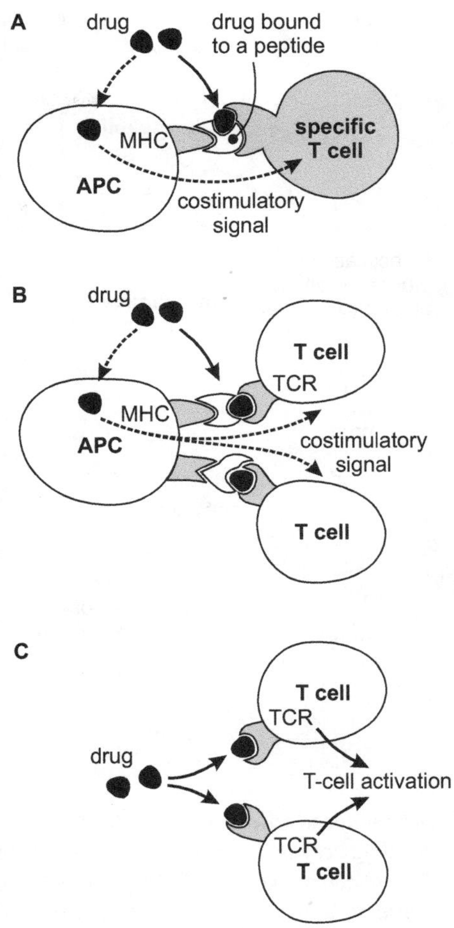

Figure 1. Drug-induced T-cell activation. A. *A drug (or its metabolite) bound to a peptide is recognized by, and activates specific T-cells.* ***B.*** *A drug interacts with MHC molecules leading to the activation of a broader number of T-cells. The drugs able to generate an immune response are able to pre-activate antigen presenting cells (APC), enhancing for example their capacity to deliver co-stimulatory signals (dotted arrows)* ***C.*** *A drug could interact with several TCR leading to T-cell activation.*

Induction of a T-cell response against an (auto)-antigen modified by the chemical

A toxin or one of its metabolites may bind to an (auto)-antigen (Figure 2A). The complex will be internalized and processed by antigen presenting cells. The peptide modified by the toxin will activate specific T-cells. This mechanism was referred to as underlying minocyclin-induced vasculitis with ANCA [44].

$HgCl_2$ binds to two cysteins in the sequence of fibrillarin, a nuclear antigen, modifying its molecular properties and inducing a T-cell response [45] (Figure 3). The fact that B10.S mice injected with $HgCl_2$ produce antibodies against toxin-modified fibrillarin with subsequent synthesis of antibodies specific for the native protein suggests that an autoimmune response may be secondary to the response against an antigen modified by the metal [46]. According to Janeway's theory [47], drug-modified determinants could stimulate specific T-cells which in turn could activate antigen presenting cells that would deliver co-stimulatory signals allowing normally silent autoreactive T-cells to be activated (Figure 2A).

Activation of T-cells by drugs

Instead of modifying nominal (auto)-antigens, chemicals may bind to immune molecules involved in the presentation process such as MHC molecules themselves [48, 49] (Figure 1B). Drugs might also activate (or perhaps inhibit) T-cells through a direct binding to

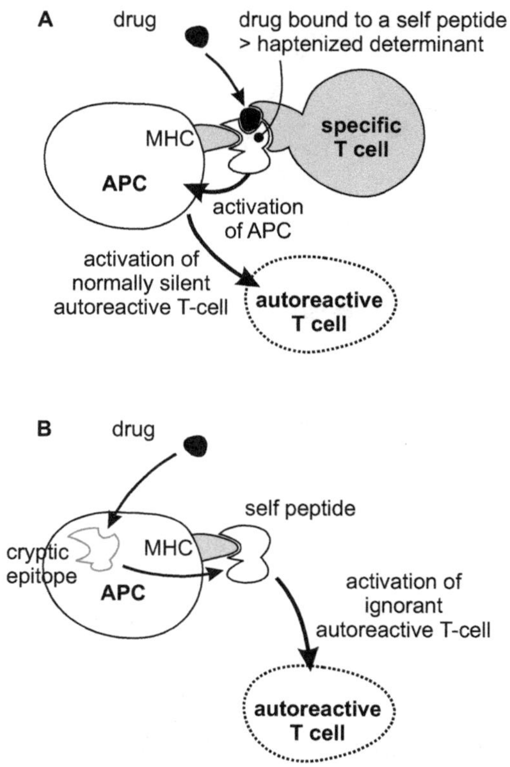

***Figure 2. Drug-induced autoreactive T-cells. A.** A self antigen modified by a drug activates specific T-cells, as a nominal antigen does. The antigen presenting cell (APC) gets activated and becomes able to activate a normally silent autoreactive T-cell specific for the native self peptide. **B.** A drug interferes with the processing/presentation process leading to the presentation of a normally cryptic self peptide at the cell surface of the APC. Autoreactive T-cells that have not been tolerized to this peptide during T-cell ontogeny get activated.*

TCRs [50] (Figure 1C). These phenomena might account for the unexpected high frequency of drug-responsive T cells [51] and explain why the rules governing drug- and antigen-induced T-cell activation are different (Table 2). Relating to this concern, new insights have been brought by the development of drug-specific T-cell hybridomas [52]. TCRs that recognize drugs are more degenerate than TCRs reacting with classical peptides,. This means than these TCR could react with a broad range of self peptides. Normally this type of signal does not lead to T-cell activation. But in some circumstances, it is possible that self peptides binding these TCR may deliver a signal similar to the one induced by the drug. This would result in breaking self-tolerance and the development of autoimmune symptoms [44].

Global immune dysregulation induced by drugs

Data showing that the T-cell membrane needs to be rearranged in order to allow full T-cell activation may provide a better understanding as to how some toxic agents induce polyclonal T-cell activation. Indeed, in normal conditions, negatively charged glycocalyx at the cell surface hampers optimal interactions between T- and antigen presenting cells [53]. Non-antigen dependent factors such as chemokines, inflammatory mediators, or factors present in lymph nodes, would play an important role in the rearrangement of surface molecules at the immune synapses referred to as the T-cell areas that contact the antigen presenting cells (reviewed in [54]). The formation of the immune synapse is likely to be Ca^{2+}-dependent [55] and requires cytoskeleton reorganization (review in [56]). Scaffold signal transducing molecules are found to be recruited at this site constituting the so-called "signalosome". Chemicals could favour or induce the organization of the signalosome. Concerning that aspect, $HAuCl_4$ and $HgCl_2$ mimic the effects of anti-TCR antibodies [57, 58]. Alternatively chemicals might act on down-stream step(s) of TCR-dependent signalling pathways.

Induction of autoreactive T-cells

Some mechanisms underlying drug-induced autoreactivity are summarized in Table 3 and Figure 2. Besides inducing autoimmunity as a consequence of an immune response against a drug-modified autoantigen, chemicals may trigger autoimmunity through

Table 2. Characterization of drug-induced T-cell activation.

Process	Characteristics of drug-induced T-cell activation
Processing	Not required : glutaraldehyde-fixed APCs may activate drug-specific T cells
Covalent binding to an antigen	Not required : Washing APCs pre-incubated with the drug prevents further T-cell activation
T-cell activation	Very fast (few minutes)
Frequency of reactive T-cells	High frequency Cross-reactive T cells, a high proportion of drug-reactive T cells being alloreactive Some drug-reactive T-cells are not MHC-restricted

From [186]. APCs = antigen presenting cells

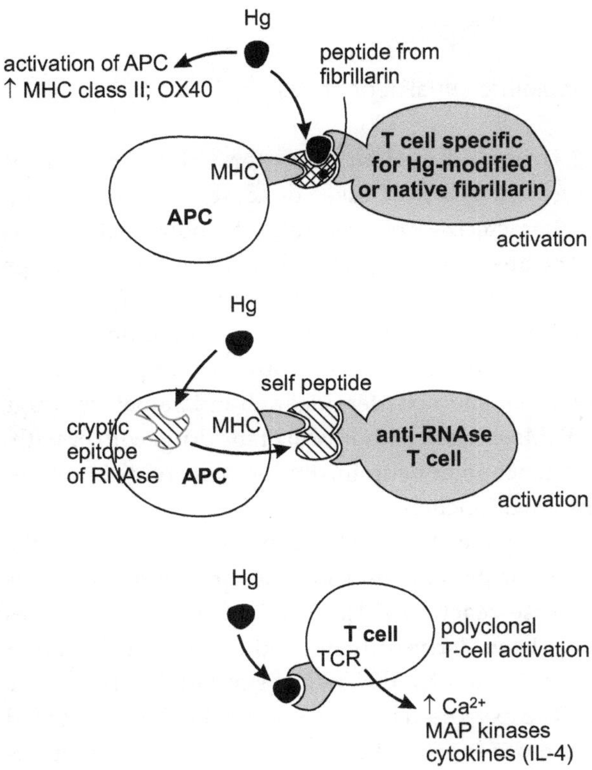

Figure 3. Effects of heavy metals (Hg and Au) on immune cells. *Hg was described as able to interact with the nuclear antigen fibrillarin which was assumed to cause a T-cell response against this modified autoantigen. True autoreactive T-cells specific for the native antigen were detected in a second time. Hg was shown to induce the expression of a normally cryptic epitope of RNAse A leading to the activation of specific T-cells. However the relevance of this mechanism in terms of induction of autoimmunity has not been demonstrated. Hg or Au have also been shown to polyclonally activate T-cells mimicking the effects of stimulation with anti-TCR antibodies. This results in an increase in intracellular Ca^{2+} concentration, MAP kinase activation and cytokine expression.*

the expression of an antigen that is normally ignored and for which no T-cell tolerance has been achieved [59-61], which could trigger immunopathological manifestations (Figure 2B). For example, $CdCl_2$ triggers HSP70 expression in SJL/J renal tubular cells, and since no tolerance towards this antigen has been acquired during ontogeny, heat shock proteins reactive-T cells are induced. The transfer of these T-cells to normal mice induces tubulointerstitial nephritis [62]. A toxin may also induce, directly or indirectly the expression of normally cryptic determinants of autoantigens. Antithyroid drugs, mainly propylthiouracil (PTU) frequently trigger ANCA autoantibodies [63] mainly against myeloperoxidase (MPO) and some patients develop vasculitis [64]. It has been proposed that PTU accumulating in neutrophils binds to MPO and induces production of cytotoxic products. The drug could induce neutrophil apoptosis, which is associated with translocation of ANCA antigens to the cell surface and could be at play in the initiation of the autoimmune response (discussed in [65]. Interestingly PTU may also induce a lupus-like disease with a spectrum of anti-nuclear auto-antibodies (anti-DNA, AHA, anti-Ro/SSA), questioning whether or not distinct mechanisms are responsible for vasculitis and lupus disease. It is also likely that genetic factors shape the type of disease. Metals including Hg and Au may induce the expression of cryptic determinants of bovine RNAse A (Figure 3) [59, 60, 66] but the role of such a phenomenon in the development of autoimmunity has not been proven. Chemicals may also act indirectly. For example, it has been reported that reactive oxygen species modify glomerular basement membrane, unmasking determinants for which there was no immune tolerance and thus leading to an autoimmune response [67]. This mechanism could be involved in some drug-induced autoimmune nephritides since drugs affecting the kidney can generate reactive oxygen species either directly or as a consequence of renal damage.

Chemicals may also cause an autoimmune kidney disease in the context of polyclonal B- and/or T-cell activation. This will lead to B-cell polyclonal activation with production of auto-antibodies since, normally

Table 3. Mechanisms responsible for drug-induced autoimmunity.

Mechanism	Drug
Breaking central T-cell-tolerance	Procainamide, Cyclosporine A
Consequence of a response against an haptenized autoantigen	Minocycline, $HgCl_2$,
Response against a normally ignored autoantigen	Anti-thyroids, $HgCl_2$, $CdCl_2$
Lowering the threshold of T-cell activation	Hydralazine, procainamide
Global immune dysregulation	$HgCl_2$, gold salts, D-penicillamine

autoreactive B-cells exist but are not activated due to a lack of T-cell help. Autoreactive T-cells with a high affinity for auto-peptides are eliminated in the thymus or at periphery while those with a low affinity for self-peptides escape deletion and emigrate to the periphery (discussed in [68] and [69]). Several mechanisms explain the absence of autoimmune disease in most of individuals. Auto-peptides do no deliver any signal (T-cells are ignorant) or are recognized by a T-cell in the absence of adequate co-stimulation (T-cells are anergic). Finally, regulatory cells exert a negative control on potentially deleterious autoreactive T-cells. In this respect, some anergic T-cells could represent a subset of regulatory T-cells due to their production of interleukin-10, an immunosuppressive cytokine [70]. In experimental models, the immunosuppressant cyclosporine A blocks T-cell signalling pathways by inhibiting the phosphatase calcineurin and may induce autoimmunity by impairing central tolerance [71] in animals in which normal regulatory T-cell (Treg) functions were defective. Normally, Treg such as $CD4^{+}CD25^{+}$ T-cells expressing the transcription factor Foxp3 are able to counteract effector Th1-or Th2-cells, a control that is overcome in immunopathological situations, Lethally irradiated mice reconstituted with bone marrow cells and treated with high doses of cyclosporine A develop inflammatory lesions in multiple organs after cyclosporine A administration has been stopped. The disease, transferable by T-cells was attributed to the fact that cyclosporine A blocks thymic negative selection. However, considering the major role of regulatory T-cells in the control of self-aggressive T cells, an impairment of regulatory T-cell differentiation/functions, induced by cyclosporine A cannot be ruled out. A toxin may also act at the periphery by lowering the threshold of T-cell activation and/or delivering co-stimulatory signals.

Immune nephropathies induced by xenobiotics in humans

The classical symptoms of drug-induced hypersensitivity reactions include fever, rashes, arthralgias, eosinophilia, eosinophiluria. Hematuria, sterile pyuria, moderate proteinuria and renal failure are observed in patients with drug-induced immune tubulointerstitial nephritis (discussed in [72]). The interstitial inflammatory cells include eosinophils, lymphocytes, monocytes, and plasma cells.

Tubulointerstitial nephritides

Drug-induced tubulointerstitial nephritides represent 1-10% of cases of acute renal failure and is characterized by infiltrates of mononuclear cells associated with tubular cell injury. A lot of drugs are incriminated, including antibiotics (β-lactams, sulfonamides, aminoglycosides, quinolones), anti-epileptic drugs, diuretics, proton pump inhibitors, foscarnet and non-steroidal anti-inflammatory drugs [73]. Most often, withdrawal of the drug, with or without concomitant administration of steroids improves the renal functions.

Drug-specific T cells have been identified in the blood of patients and persist for months after the adverse reaction [74]. Drug-specific T-cell clones have been derived; they produce IL-4, IL-5, TNF-α and inconstantly IFN-γ. The similarity between the TCRVβ expressed by drug-specific T-cells in the blood and those expressed by T-cells in the kidney biopsies strongly suggest that drug-specific T cells localize into the kidneys [74] and orchestrate inflammation.

Rifampicin-induced tubulointerstitial nephritis is interesting because, at least in some cases, a target might be identified. There is often an association between renal failure and hematological abnormalities (hemolytic anemia and thrombopenia). Antibodies directed against drug-exposed erythrocytes and platelets have been reported [75]. Patients develop rifampicin-induced IgG and IgM antibodies against the I antigen of red blood cells, which causes red blood cell lysis through interaction with the antigen on erythrocyte cell surface [76]. These antibodies, or a cell-mediated immune response could play a role in tubulointerstitial nephritis since the I antigen is also expressed on tubular epithelial cells.

Glomerulopathies

Non-steroidal anti-inflammatory drugs are known to induce a nephrotic syndrome in addition to acute tubulointerstitial nephritis (discussed in [77]). Glomerulopathies include minimal change disease, focal glomerulosclerosis that could represent a continuum with the former entity and membranous glomerulopathy. A review of 97 patients with non-steroidal anti-inflammatory drug-induced nephropathies reported the following incidence: minimal change disease (39.2%), acute tubulointerstitial nephritis (19.6%), membranous glomerulopathy (19.6%), focal glomerulosclerosis (13.4%) and others (8.2%). Lithium used to treat bipolar affective disorders [78] gold salts [79] or D-penicillamine [80] given to rheumatoid arthritis patients, or mercurials as environmental pollutant may induce minimal change disease or membranous glomerulopathy. For example, gold salts cause proteinuria in about 10% of patients due to membranous glomerulopathy (89%) or minimal change disease (10%). This indicates that the same drug may induce several types of glomerulopathies with different immunopathological mechanisms leading to proteinuria.

Genes described as implicated in drug-induced hypersensitivity reactions concern MHC, drug metabolizing enzymes, as well as genes controlling the immune response and tissue repair [81]. Thus, patients with HLA-B8 or DRW3 were at higher risk [82] for developing immune nephropathy. The role of HLA-DR3 in susceptibility to D-penicillamine-induced adverse reactions has been demonstrated since membranous glomerulopathy is 32 times more frequent in HLA-DR3 positive patients than in those who are HLA-DR3 negative [83].

Association of glomerulopathy and tubulointerstitial nephritis

An association between tubulointerstitial nephritis and minimal change disease has been reported in 18/27 patients treated with non-steroidal drugs [84].

In one case of tubulointerstitial nephritis and nephrotic syndrome induced by Triazolam, a sleep inducer numerous eosinophils [85] were found to infiltrate glomeruli and interstitium suggesting that eosinophils may be pathogenic in this situation. An association with tubulointerstitial nephritis and nephrotic syndrome has also been occasionally reported for penicillin/amoxicillin induced nephropathies [86]. Several reports have analyzed T-cells in penicillin-induced allergy. $CD4^+$ T-cells specific for penicillin may be derived from the patients and produce mainly IL-5, some of them being perforin positive with a cytolytic potential [87]. 2) β-lactam specific clones may be obtained only from patients with adverse reactions; the clones were Th2 whatever the type of clinical manifestations and whether or not specific IgE may be detected [88]; 3) Peni G impaired IFN-γ production in an antigen-independent manner [89]. These studies support the view that β-lactams induce Th2-dependent hypersensitivity reactions. Such cells may recruit eosinophils via their IL-5 production. It is also possible that direct cellular contact between activated Th2 cells and tubular epithelial cells amplifies local inflammation because IL-4 and IL-13 increase the production of RANTES, a proinflammatory mediator by tubular epithelial cells [90]. However, another group that established drug specific T-cell clones from patients with acute drug-induced acute interstitial nephritis found an absence of of Th2 or Th1-biased differentiation pattern. They conclude that drug-specific T-cells orchestrate a local inflammation in the kidney via secretion of various cytokines [74] that may influence the renal damage.

Studies of xenobiotic-induced immune dysregulation in animal models

Some drugs such as hydralazine or procainamide may induce lupus like diseases with antinuclear antibodies and proteinuria. D-Penicillamine not only causes glomerulopathy, but also myasthenia, polymyositis or lupus, suggesting that this compound provokes immune dysregulation. Gold salts are also capable of inducing various pathology including pneumonitis, anemia, thrombocytopenia and hepatitis. We shall discuss hydralazine or procainamide induced- autoimmunity as well as heavy metal-induced immunological-mediated disorders. Indeed, these compounds have been extensively studied using multiple experimental approaches and in several experimental systems and it was shown that several mechanisms may contribute to the development of autoimmunity.

Hydralazine and procainamide-induced autoimmunity

Hydralazine and procainamide have been shown to interfere with central and peripheral mechanisms of tolerance and to lower the threshold of T cell-activation, converting antigen-specific T-cells into autoreactive cells [91, 92].

Systemic injection of procainamide or its metabolites in mice does not induce any immune abnormalities. However, a metabolite of procainamide, injected into the thymus of (C57BL/6 x DBA/2) F1 mice induces the emergence of autoreactive chromatin specific T-cells and production of anti-chromatin antibodies similar to those of patients with procainamide-induced lupus. These data indicate that procainamide metabolite interferes with central tolerance mechanisms [93]. Transfer into naive mice of autoreactive peripheral T cells derived from these mice triggered autoantibody production in the recipients. This showed that procainamide injected into the thymus allowed autoreactive T cells to migrate from the thymus to the periphery. This group showed that procainamide did not reverse self-tolerance of the mature thymocyte and did not prevent deletion of high affinity autoreactive T cells in the thymus. Procainamide is likely to interfere with the establishment of tolerance to endogenous self-antigens that are normally presented by the MHC on thymic epithelial cells during the positive selection of thymocytes (reviewed and discussed in [94]).

Hydralazine and procainamide have been shown to inhibit methyl transferase activity (discussed in [95]), whereas methylation of deoxycytosine residues of gene promoters plays a major role in silencing genes during ontogeny through fixation of methylcytosine binding proteins. These changes in chromatin structures are maintained during subsequent mitoses. It was shown that antigen specific T-cell clones incubated with inhibitors of methyltransferases over-expressed LFA-1 and became able to proliferate in the presence of autologous antigen presenting cells in the absence of their nominal antigen [91, 92]. Autoreactivity is probably the consequence of the increase in LFA-1 expression since antigen specific T-cells transfected with LFA-1 also became autoreactive [96]. The injection of T-cells rendered autoreactive by incubation with procainamide and hydralazine [97] or of T-cells transfected with LFA-1 [98] into a non-irradiated syngeneic recipient triggers an autoimmune disease. This disease is characterized by anti-DNA antibody production, proliferative glomerulonephritis, pulmonary alveolitis, liver lesions resembling primary biliary cirrhosis, and histologic changes in the brain reminiscent of central nervous system lupus [99].

Histone deacetylases (HDAC) are also important with respect to the accessibility of chromatin and gene expression; acetylation of histones is required for gene expression while deacetylation correlates with inhibition of transcription. Moreover, methylcytosine binding proteins associate with histone deacetylase directing the deacetylase activity to regions destined for inactivation [100]. Numerous reports now show that targeting histone acetylation-deacetylation processes may be beneficial in inflammatory reactions as examplified in ([101] [102] [103]).

$HgCl_2$ and gold salt-induced autoimmunity

Effect of these metals in mice

Injections of susceptible murine strains including B.10S and AS.W mice with non toxic amounts of $HgCl_2$ or gold salts trigger an increase in serum IgE and IgG1 concentrations, two Th2-dependent isotypes, the induction of IgG1 anti-nucleolar antibodies mainly targeting fibrillarin and the development of immune complex-type glomerulonephritis [104, 105]. Anti-IL-4 mAb or rIL-12 administration inhibited the effect of $HgCl_2$ on serum IgE and IgG1 concentrations and induced a shift towards Th1-dependent IgG2a and IgG3 anti-nuclear antibodies without any change in the autoantibody titer [105, 106]. As discussed above, it has been put forward that drug-induced alteration of fibrillarin processing/recognition by T-cells concurs to the development of $HgCl_2$-immune disorders. However $HgCl_2$ induced a lymphoproliferation and polyclonal IgE and IgG1 production suggesting that $HgCl_2$ causes a more global immune dysregulation. In this concern, the blockade of T-cell CD28- [107] and ICOS-mediated [108] co-stimulatory pathways markedly inhibited $HgCl_2$-mediated immune disorders. Moreover administration of a blocking anti-CTLA4 antibody, that breaks an inhibitory T-cell signalling pathway, renders some normally resistant strains of mice susceptible to $HgCl_2$-induced autoimmunity [109]. Interestingly, Gleichmann's group showed that $CD4^+$ $CD25^+$ T cells recovered from mice injected with drugs such as procainamide, mercuric chloride or gold (III) are drug-specific. Indeed, the transfer of these Treg into normal syngeneic mice prevented development of anti-nuclear antibodies in the recipients treated by the same xenobiotic [110]. In contrast $CD4^+CD25^-$ T cells from the same donors were sufficient to induce autoimmunity without drug administration. Xenobiotic-primed $CD4^+CD25^+$ T cells also partially protected recipients towards autoreactivity induced by other drugs. This suggests that xenobiotic-primed regulatory T-cells can control autoreactivity.

Effect of $HgCl_2$ gold salts and D-penicillamine in rats

a) The model

Brown-Norway (BN) rats injected thrice a week with $HgCl_2$ (1 mg/kg bw, sc), $HAuCl_4$ (1 mg/kg bw, sc), aurothiopropanolsulfonate sodium salt, the gold salt used in France for rheumatoid arthritis treatment (Allochrysine ®, 20 mg/kg bw, sc) or D-penicillamine (450 mg/kg per os) develop an autoimmune disease while Lewis (LEW) rats are resistant. The disease induced by $HgCl_2$ is characterized by several phases. 1) 24 hour-$HgCl_2$ administration is sufficient for inducing αβ T-cell-independent caecal vasculitis which was shown to be mast-cell mediated [111, 112]. 2) T-cell mediated autoimmune disease develops over a period of 2-3 weeks. It is characterized by the production of numerous autoantibodies including anti-laminin, a component of the glomerular basement membrane (GBM), anti-ds DNA, anti-thyroglobulin antibodies, and an increase in serum IgE and IgG1 concentrations (reviewed in [113-115]). Glomeruli appear to be normal at the light microscopy level and some mononuclear cells with predominantly $CD4^+$ T-cells are occasionally found in the interstitium. IgG1 are first found linearly deposited along the glomerular capillary wall, with the subsequent development of a membranous glomerulopathy. Anti-laminin auto-antibodies are incriminated in both phases. The animals display heavy proteinuria. Gold salts and D-penicillamine cause a disease much less severe than $HgCl_2$ because rats treated by the former drugs do not develop significant proteinuria. 3) The disease spontaneously resolves even if drug administration is pursued and animals are resistant to a re-challenge. The long-lasting resistance is attributed to $CD8^+$ T-cells [116]. In addition, the regulation does not seem to be drug-specific. Indeed, the administration of $HgCl_2$ prevents the immune disorders induced by D-penicillamine [114] or gold salts [117]. It would be interesting to assess if drug-induced $CD4^+$ (or $CD8^+$) $CD25^+$ regulatory T-cells may be implicated in the spontaneous recovery of rats and if they can also prevent autoimmunity induced by other drugs. Low doses of D-penicillamine protected rats against the development of autoimmunity induced by higher doses which was at least partly attributed to IL-10 and TGF-β producing $CD4^+$ $CD25^+$ T cells [41, 118, 119]. Interestingly, tolerance induced by low doses of D-penicillamine was abrogated by treating the recipients with poly I-C [119], which could act by stimulating the innate immune system. Regulatory cells in this model are reminiscent of IL-10 and TGF-β producing regulatory $CD4^+$ T-cells that were identified in $HgCl_2$-injected LEW resistant rats. These T cells were shown to protect (LEW x BN) F1 rats against the development of Th2-mediated, $HgCl_2$-induced autoimmunity [120].

Whether these regulatory T cells express FOX-P3, a transcription factor that characterizes natural $CD4^+CD25^+$ Treg has to be determined.

b) $HgCl_2$-induced mast cell activation in BN rats

Oliveira et al determined that mast-cell dependent vasculitis was the earliest pathological event induced by $HgCl_2$ in BN rats [121]. Accordingly, $HgCl_2$ was shown to induce the release of reactive oxygen species (ROS) by mast cells and the administration of anti-oxidants prevent $HgCl_2$-induced vasculitis [122]. The authors presumed that NF kappa B activation induced by ROS resulted in the expression of *Il4* gene by BN mast cells [123, 124]. The eventual role of $HgCl_2$-dependent *Il4* expression by mast cells on Th2-biased cell development in BN rats remains to be investigated.

c) Non-antigen specific lymphocyte activation

$HgCl_2$ and gold salts trigger polyclonal activation of BN B- and T-cells. $HgCl_2$ does not induce the expansion of peculiar Vβ bearing cells [125], which rules out the possibility that this metal behaves as a superantigen. $HgCl_2$ and $HAuCl_4$ increase the intracellular calcium concentration in BN and LEW T-cells [58, 126, 127]. $HAuCl_4$ triggers a calcium signal in up to 100% of $CD4^+$ and $CD8^+$ T- and in 70% of purified B-cells from both BN and LEW rats. These data show that gold salts induce a pan-clonal activation of T-cells and that the resistance of LEW rats cannot be explained by an inability of metals to stimulate their lymphocytes. Stimulation of T-cells through the TCR leads to a cascade of events initiated by activation of src kinases that phosphorylate tyrosine of the ITAMs (immunoreceptor tyrosine activated motives) in the TCR/CD3 chains. This results in the phosphorylation of the tyrosine kinase ZAP-70. Multiple adapter and effector molecules are then directed to signalling complexes and are activated, including phospholipase Cγ1. The latter cleaves phosphatidylinositide 4,5 biphosphate into inositol 3, 4, 5 triphosphate and diacylglycerol. Inositol 3, 4, 5 triphosphate releases intracellular calcium stores into the cytosol with an ensuing entry of calcium responsible for a sustained increase in intracellular calcium concentration, while diacylglycerol activates protein kinases C. Finally, TCR-dependent signalling pathways converge to activate multiple transcription factors leading to proliferation, and cytokine gene transcription. The calcium response elicited by $HgCl_2$ and $HAuCl_4$ in purified T-cells is the consequence of an effect of these metals on the early steps of T-cell activation. Indeed, the metals triggered a pattern of tyrosine phosphorylation similar to the one induced by TCR ligation, and PP2, an inhibitor of src kinases, abolishes $HAuCl_4$-induced calcium signal [58].

$HAuCl_4$-induced T-cell activation resulted in early cytokine gene expression by lymphocytes from both BN and LEW rats since two to four hour incubation with the metal was sufficient to induce an increase in IL-4 and IFN-γ mRNA. Nevertheless, the expression of IL-4 predominated in BN T-cells while the expression of IFN-γ was favoured in LEW T-cells. The *in vitro* findings correlated quite well with the profile of cytokine expression in spleen cells of BN and LEW rats injected with $HAuCl_4$, which gave relevance to the *in vitro* data. The pronounced over-expression of IL-4 induced by gold in BN rats was probably related to the fact that BN rats mount preferential Th2 responses whatever the stimulus. It would be interesting to determine the frequency of IL-4 producing T-cells upon stimulation with gold and whether this phenotype concerns a peculiar T-cell subset.

It has been previously shown that $HgCl_2$ induced *Il4* gene transcription in BN but not in LEW T-cells [128]. In order to identify what are the mechanisms at play, we used IL-4 producing T-cell hybridomas, which allowed us to identify a new signalling pathway, implicating dihydropyridine receptors (DHPR) likely to be related to voltage-dependent Ca_v1 channels, classically considered as specific of excitable cells. These receptors were shown to be expressed by Th2 and not by Th1 cells [129]. DHPR antagonists currently used in the treatment of patients with high blood pressure, prevented Th2-mediated drug-induced autoimmunity [129], which is consistent with the essential role of DHPR in Ca^{2+} signalling and Th2 cytokine production. Protein kinase C [127] and cGMP-dependent protein kinase (PKG) [130] were shown to be important for controlling Ca^{2+} signalling in Th2 but not in Th1 cells, offering the possibility to develop drugs targeting these kinases to cure Th2-dependent pathology. We feel that $HgCl_2$ or $HauCl_4$ behave as polyclonal T-cell activators (Figure 3) acting on the early steps of activation and switching on the TCR-dependent signaling pathways already established in the cell studied, pathways that are already skewed to Th2 cell commitment in BN rats.

d) Mechanisms responsible for autoimmunity

The fact that normal BN T-cells incubated with $HgCl_2$ transferred the disease [131] suggested that the effect of the metal on T-cells was sufficient for the induction of autoimmunity. Figure 3 summarizes some events by which $HgCl_2$ or gold salts may induce autoreactivity.

$HgCl_2$ or gold salt-induced autoimmunity is probably not solely due to an over-expression of IL-4 since IL-4 transgenic mice have not been described as autoimmune prone except in one report [132]. $HgCl_2$ [133] and allochrysine® [134] were found to induce the emergence of autoreactive anti-class II T-cells in both BN and LEW rats. Autoreactive T-cell lines have been derived from both strains; they were Th2 only when they originated from BN rats. Furthermore, these Th2 lines that behaved as anergic cells *in vitro* transferred explosive autoimmune, inflammatory disease in $CD8^+$-cell depleted BN rats [134]. This suggests that the direct effect of metal on IL-4 gene expression certainly favours the development of autoreactive Th2 cells that are pathogenic in this model. Another interesting point is that the disease induced by the transfer of autoreactive Th2 lines was much more severe when the recipient was treated by an anti-CD8 mAb. Indeed in this case, rats displayed massive infiltration of $CD4^+$ T cells in liver, lung and kidneys. In addition, rats died from renal failure. This suggests that, in normal BN rats, $CD8^+$ cells exert some negative control on these autoreactive T-cells.

The expression of LFA-1 was increased among other markers, at the T-cell surface from BN rats injected with $HgCl_2$ [135]. This could be sufficient for inducing autoimmunity as shown by Richardson's group [99]. Roos et al also showed that $HgCl_2$ up-regulated the expression of the co-stimulatory molecule OX40 on T-cells [135], which could be important for driving Th2 cell differentiation [136].

Interestingly, neonatal administration of the drug induced tolerance but not immunopathological manifestations [137]. The tolerance to $HgCl_2$-induced autoimmunity was transferable by $CD8^+$ ($CD25^+$) spleen cells [138]. The characteristics of this tolerance differs from the one responsible for the resistance to the re-challenge with drugs (Table 4). The former was short-lived, depending upon and specific for the drug. These data suggest that drugs can induce specific-regulatory $CD8^+$ T cells in neonates, during a period known as critical for the establishment of a normal regulatory T-cell compartment [139].

The impact of genetic studies in our understanding of immunological-mediated toxic-induced renal disease

Immunological-mediated toxic-induced renal diseases are multifactorial

Like most diseases, renal diseases triggered by toxic agents are multifactorial [140, 141]. They result from complex interactions between the xenobiotic and several genes, which predispose the host to the development of the lesions. These genes as well as the toxic agent can act at two different levels, the systemic level on the one hand, and the tissue level on the other hand. At the systemic level for example, polymorphism in some genes can be involved in the xenobiotic metabolism, as shown for anti-tumour drugs [142]. Such a mechanism can indirectly trigger some systemic effect through a specific activity of some metabolic product on the immune system, as discussed previously. At the tissue level, recent works have highlighted the role of glomerular structural factors of the filtration filter in the pathophysiology of idiopathic nephrotic syndrome [143, 144]. It is highly possible that some toxic effect of xenobiotic at the tissue level, are dependent on structural specificities of the host tissues, directed by polymorphisms of genes coding different glomerular constituents, particularly of the podocytes. Such a genetic polymorphism could be implicated in a model of susceptibility to anthracycline-induced nephropathy, which has been described in the mouse [145, 146]. In this model, it is well established that direct exposure of the kidney to the drug is required for the development of nephropathy [147]. However the development of the nephropathy requires a particular genetic background. Two loci that controls the susceptibility to such drug-induced nephropathy have been localised in the mouse genome using linkage analyses in cohorts of F2 (susceptible x resistant strains) hybrids and extended haplotype analyses in a set of susceptible and resistant strains of mice [148, 149]. Identification of the genes within these loci will undoubtedly shed new light on the mechanisms involved in this model and in its human counterpart.

Such genetic approaches using a combination of strains susceptible and resistant to a particular phenotype or disease, are now widely used in mouse and rat models of various human diseases. Thus, more than 60 loci involved in the control of renal damage, renal disease susceptibility, renal function, proteinuria or albuminuria have been described in various rat models (http://mcnally.hmgc.mcw.edu/gb/gbrowse/rgd_903/?name=proteinuria). The studies we have conducted in the last ten years in the field of immunological-mediated toxic-induced renal diseases, which shed new lights in their pathophysiology are reported in the following paragraph.

Genetic control of metal-induced autoimmunity and nephropathy

An experimental model of metal-induced autoimmunity and nephropathy has been developed in the BN rat, which is genetically predisposed to develop Th2-type of immune response. In the BN rat, the injections of

Table 4. Comparison between regulatory T-cell induced during neonatal tolerance to a drug and those responsible for the resistance to drug re-challenge.

Characteristics	Neonatal tolerance	Resistance to the re-challenge *
T-cell subset responsible	$CD8^+$ ($CD25^+$)	$CD8^+$
Duration	Short-lived	Long-lasting
Specificity	Highly specific for the drug	At least partly common for $HgCl_2$, gold salt and D-penicillamine**

*$HgCl_2$, D-penicillamine and gold salts induced similar immune manifestations in BN rats although the severity varies from one compound to the other. * Rats who recovered from drug-induced autoimmunity are resistant to re-challenge with the same drug. ** These rats are also at least partially protected against the development of autoimmunity induced by the other drugs.*

gold salts such as the aurothiopropanol sulfonate (Atps - Allochrysine®) induce immune disorders [150] detailed above. These immune and nephrologic features reproduced to some extent the iatrogenic side effects observed in some patients suffering from rheumatism polyarthritis under chrysotherapy [151, 152]. Similar Th2-triggered immune features are observed in the BN rat injected with $HgCl_2$. However the kidney lesions are by far more severe under $HgCl_2$. Indeed this model is characterized by a severe proteinuria with nephrotic syndrome [153]. By contrast, the LEW rat is resistant to the immunological disorders induced by gold or mercury salts [154].

These differences between BN and LEW rats in susceptibility to metal-induced autoimmunity and nephropathy are associated with intrinsic differences in the immune system of these two strains. Indeed, from an immunological point of view, the balance between "type 1" (Th1/Tc1) and "type 2" (Th2/Tc2) cells is opposite in BN and LEW rats. BN rats are susceptible to "type 2"-mediated immunological disorders, to which the LEW strain is resistant. Conversely, "type 1"-mediated organ-specific autoimmune disease are easily induced in LEW, but not in BN rats [155]. These immunological features depend on inherent properties of T lymphocytes. *In vitro* and *in vivo* studies have shown an inherent bias in T lymphocytes (CD4 and CD8) from BN and from LEW rats to produce respectively "type 2" (IL-4, IL-5, IL-13) and "type 1" (IFN-γ cytokines [156-158]. The difference in susceptibility to metal-induced autoimmunity and nephropathy of BN and LEW strains provides a unique tool to study their genetic control.

We have studied the genetic control of the IgE response and of the nephropathy in F2 generation animals from (susceptible BN x resistant LEW) crosses, treated with Allochrysine. We identified three QTLs (quantitative trait loci) named, *Aiid1*, *Aiid2* and *Aiid3* (formerly named *Atps1*, *Atps2* and *Atps3*), respectively on chromosomes (c), 20, 10 and 9 [159-161]. *Aiid1* contains the MHC region and controls the kinetics of the IgE response, the IgG deposits in kidney arteries and the CD8 T cell population [159, 161, 162]. *Aiid2* and *Aiid3* control the intensity of the IgE response (13 and 31% of the variance, respectively) and the glomerular deposition of IgG. *Aiid2* contains a cytokine gene cluster that bears the IL-4 IL-5, IL-13, GM-CSF and IFN-regulatory factor-1 genes [163]. In human, this cluster, localized in 5q31.1, has been linked to serum IgE concentrations in families of atopic patients [164, 165]. In the mouse, the locus *Tpm1* that controls the Th1/Th2 differentiation *in vitro*, has been localized on c11, in the region syntenic to this cluster [166, 167]. Moreover, regions overlapping *Aiid1*, *Aiid2* and *Aiid3*, control the susceptibility to experimental autoimmune encephalomyelitis (EAE ; locus *Eae1*, *Eae4* and *Eae3* on respectively chromosomes 20, 10 and 9) in rat strains prone to develop Th1 reactions [168-170]. Moreover, a locus controlling the susceptibility to rat collagen-induced arthritis (*Cia15*) was identified on chromosome 9 in a region overlapping with *Aiid3* and *Eae4* [171]. Taken together these observations suggested that the loci we had identified, and particularly the locus localized on rat chromosome 9, could play an important role in the control of immune system homeostasis. This prompted us to more specifically study the genetic control of T cell function, taking advantage of the fact that, in the rat T cell cytokine profiles and functions are associated with differences in the level of expression of CD45RC on T cells [172-174]. Particularly, $CD45RC^{high}$ CD4 T cells produce preferentially IL-2 and IFN-γ and contain T cell with a pathogenic potential, while $CD45RC^{low}$ CD4 T cells produce preferentially IL-4,IL-10 and IL-13 and contain T cell with a regulatory function. Having found that the CD4 and CD8 $CD45RC^{high}$ sub-populations predominates in the LEW rat, and the CD4 and CD8 $CD45RC^{low}$ sub-populations in the BN rat, we performed linkage analyses in a new F2 (BLEW x BN) cohort. This work led us to identify two loci on chromosomes 9 (*Cec1* ; Cec: CD45RC expression in CD4 and CD8 T cells) and 20 (*Cec2*) [157, 158]. Interestingly these two loci overlapped fully with *Aiid3* and *Aiid1*.

To narrow down the genetic intervals for the further positional cloning of the genes, we have then developed c9 and c10 reciprocal congenics from the BN and LEW rats. The construction of congenic lines is a powerful approach for the dissection of polygenic diseases [175] and for ultimate gene identification in rodent models of human diseases [176-178]. Using LEW.BNc10 and BN.LEWc10 congenic lines for genetic dissection, we were able to narrow down the *Aiid2* locus from ~30 to 7 centi-Morgans, and to split it into two sub-loci named *Aiid2a* and *Aiid2b* that independently control the IgE response [160]. *Aiid2a* is syntenic to the human 5q31 region and includes the cytokine gene cluster. *Aiid2b* is syntenic to the human 17p12-p11.2 region. Therefore, the *Aiid2* locus seems to consist of at least two loci in close proximity. Such a clustering of loci controlling the same phenotype is commonly observed in murine experimental diseases [179-182]. A similar clustering could exist in humans as suggested by linkage and association analyses of lupus [183, 184] and of atopy and asthma susceptibility [185]. Results from BN.LEWc9 congenic lines, showed a major effect of this region. In these congenic lines, the gold salt-triggered IgE response was 10-fold lower than in the BN parental strain and glomerular IgG deposits that characterize Aiid were dramatically reduced [160]. Recently, using a set of congenic lines and sublines we were able to narrow *Aiid3* to a 700 kilobase interval and to show that it perfectly overlaps with *Cec1*. Moreover further studies conducted in the EAE model localized Eae4 in a one centiMorgan interval that fully includes the *Aiid3/Cec1* locus (unpublished results).

Taken together these results suggested that the control of gold salt-induced renal disease is mediated by genes localized on chromosomes 9 and 10 through immunological mechanisms and that a single gene or gene on chromosome 9 exerts a major effect. The co-localization of loci controlling different phenotypes in different strains combinations, and the functional studies conducted on $CD45RC^{high/low}$ subsets of lymphocytes led to look for the role of these loci on the control of T cell regulatory populations. By genetic dissection using the available set of reciprocal LEW/BN congenic lines and sub-lines, we were able to show that the 700 kilobase interval of the *Aiid3/Cec1* locus controls the thymic development and the pool in periphery of the $CD4^+$ $Foxp3^+$ regulatory T cell population (unpublished work).

The mechanisms by which BN and LEW rats are respectively susceptible and resistant to gold salt- and to $HgCl_2$-induced autoimmunity and nephropathy could be different. Thus, BN MHC is permissive to both types of salts, while LEW MHC is permissive to gold but not to $HgCl_2$-induced autoimmunity. Indeed BN.1L which have the same MHC as LEW rats and non MHC genes from the BN background, develop gold- but not $HgCl_2$-induced autoimmunity. Moreover gold salts but not $HgCl_2$ induce some B-cell polyclonal activation (probably under the control of Th1 cells) in LEW rats, and $HgCl_2$ but not gold salts induced IL-10 and TGF-beta producing regulatory T cells. However, the mechanism of resistance to gold salt- under the control of *Aiid3* was found likely to proceed through a general effect on the immune system homeostasis. We therefore hypothesized that the same control should be efficient on the mercury-induced autoimmunity and nephropathy. By genetic dissection using the set of reciprocal BN/LEW rats congenic for the *Aiid3* locus we were able to demonstrate that the *Aiid3/Cec1* 700 kilobase interval almost fully controls the immunological disorders and the kidney disease induced by $HgCl_2$. The identification of the gene(s) at work at this locus, and of the molecular and cellular mechanisms involved in its (their) effects are likely to shed in the near future new light on the pathophysiology of these metal-induced autoimmunity and nephropathy. This could open the way to association studies in cohorts of patients suffering from toxic-induced renal diseases with further consequences on prevention, management and treatment in human pathology.

Conclusion

There is still a long way to go before all the mechanisms responsible for drug-induced immune kidney lesions are understood. However the notion that T-cell activation, in addition to TCR-MHC interactions, also requires a tissue environment is an important concept for better understanding the immunopathogenic mechanisms. For example, the toxic effect of drugs on the kidney may initiate immune responses because they promote the presentation of haptenized determinants or even of self-peptides in inflammatory conditions. Th1 cells and probably Th2 cells can be pathogenic even if the effector mechanisms responsible for the lesions may be different. In some patients for example, eosinophils, the activation of which can be Th2-dependent, may be deleterious for the tissue. Noteworthy, drugs able to induce immune-mediated nephropathies appear capable to act on innate and adaptive immune cells on the one hand and on the renal tissue on the other one, which could be required for the development of immune aggression on predisposed genetic backgrounds. This suggests that genes of susceptibility to drug-induced immune disorders could deal with both immune and tissue-specific functions.

References

1. Rengarajan J, Szabo SJ, Glimcher LH: Transcriptional regulation of Th1/Th2 polarization. Immunol. Today 2000; 21: 479-83.
2. Tipping PG, Kitching AR: Glomerulonephritis, Th1 and Th2: what's new? Clin Exp Immunol 2005; 142: 207-15.
3. Romagnani S: Regulation of the T cell response. Clin Exp Allergy 2006; 36: 1357-66.
4. Harrington LE, Mangan PR, Weaver CT: Expanding the effector CD4 T-cell repertoire: the Th17 lineage. Curr Opin Immunol 2006; 18: 349-56.
5. MacKay CR: Follicular homing T helper (Th) cells and the Th1/Th2 paradigm. J. Exp. Med. 2000; 192: F31-F34.
6. Glimcher LH, Murphy KM: Lineage commitment in the immune system: the T helper lymphocyte grows up. Genes Dev. 2000; 14: 1693-711.
7. Ivanov, II, McKenzie BS, Zhou L, Tadokoro CE, Lepelley A, Lafaille JJ, Cua DJ, Littman DR: The orphan nuclear receptor RORgammat directs the differentiation program of proinflammatory IL-17+ T helper cells. Cell 2006; 126: 1121-33.
8. Lohr J, Knoechel B, Abbas AK: Regulatory T cells in the periphery. Immunol Rev 2006; 212: 149-62.
9. Guéry JC, Galbiati F, Smiroldo S, Adorini L: Selective development of T helper (Th)2 cells induced by continuous administration of low dose soluble proteins to normal and b2-microglobulin-deficient BALB/c mice. J. Exp. Med. 1996; 183: 485-497.
10. Foucras G, Gallard A, Coureau C, Kanellopoulos JM, Guery JC: Chronic soluble antigen sensitization primes a unique memory/effector T cell repertoire associated with th2 phenotype acquisition *in vivo*. J Immunol 2002; 168: 179-87.
11. Feili-Hariri M, Falkner DH, Morel PA: Polarization of naive T cells into Th1 or Th2 by distinct cytokine-driven murine dendritic cell populations: implications for immunotherapy. J Leukoc Biol 2005; 78: 656-64.
12. Liu YJ, Soumelis V, Watanabe N, Ito T, Wang YH, Malefyt RD, Omori M, Zhou B, Ziegler SF: TSLP: An Epithelial Cell Cytokine thaTregulates T Cell Differentiation by Conditioning Dendritic Cell Maturation. Annu Rev Immunol 2006;
13. Gomes B, Savignac M, Moreau M, Leclerc C, Lory P, Guery JC, Pelletier L: Lymphocyte calcium signaling involves dihydropyridine-sensitive L-type calcium channels: facts and controversies. Crit Rev Immunol 2004; 24: 425-48.
14. Grogan JL, Mohrs M, Harmon B, Lacy DA, Sedat JW, Locksley RM: Early transcription and silencing of cytokine genes underlie polarization of T helper cell subsets. Immunity 2001; 14: 205-15.
15. Spilianakis CG, Lalioti MD, Town T, Lee GR, Flavell RA: Interchromosomal associations between alternatively expressed loci. Nature 2005; 435: 637-45.
16. Lee GR, Kim ST, Spilianakis CG, Fields PE, Flavell RA: T helper cell differentiation: regulation by cis elements and epigenetics. Immunity 2006; 24: 369-79.
17. Tipping PG, Timoshanko J: Contributions of intrinsic renal cells to crescentic glomerulonephritis. Nephron Exp Nephrol 2005; 101: e173-8.
18. Holdsworth SR, Kitching AR, Tipping PG: Th1 and Th2 T helper cell subsets affect patterns of injury and outcomes in glomerulonephritis. Kidney Int 1999; 55: 1198-216.
19. Le Berre L, Herve C, Buzelin F, Usal C, Soulillou JP, Dantal J: Renal macrophage activation and Th2 polarization precedes the development of nephrotic syndrome in Buffalo/Mna rats. Kidney Int 2005; 68: 2079-90.
20. van den Berg JG, Weening JJ: Role of the immune system in the pathogenesis of idiopathic nephrotic syndrome. Clin Sci (Lond) 2004; 107: 125-36.
21. Wei CL, Cheung W, Heng CK, Arty N, Chong SS, Lee BW, Puah KL, Yap HK: Interleukin-13 genetic polymorphisms in Singapore Chinese children correlate with long-term outcome of minimal-change disease. Nephrol Dial Transplant 2005; 20: 728-34.
22. Acharya B, Shirakawa T, Pungky A, Damanik P, Massi MN, Miyata M, Matsuo M, Gotoh A: Polymorphism of the interleukin-4, interleukin-13, and signal transducer and activator of transcription 6 genes in Indonesian children with minimal change nephrotic syndrome. Am J Nephrol 2005; 25: 30-5.
23. Ruotsalainen V, Ljungberg P, Wartiovaara J, Lenkkeri U, Kestila M, Jalanko H, Holmberg C, Tryggvason K: Nephrin is specifically located at the slit diaphragm of glomerular podocytes. Proc Natl Acad Sci U S A 1999; 96: 7962-7.
24. Shih NY, Li J, Karpitskii V, Nguyen A, Dustin ML, Kanagawa O, Miner JH, Shaw AS: Congenital nephrotic syndrome in mice lacking CD2-associated protein. Science 1999; 286: 312-5.
25. Togawa A, Miyoshi J, Ishizaki H, Tanaka M, Takakura A, Nishioka H, Yoshida H, Doi T, Mizoguchi A, Matsuura N, Niho Y, Nishimune Y, Nishikawa Si, Takai Y: Progressive impairment of kidneys and reproductive organs in mice lacking Rho GDIalpha. Oncogene 1999; 18: 5373-80.
26. Kaplan JM, Kim SH, North KN, Rennke H, Correia LA, Tong HQ, Mathis BJ, Rodriguez-Perez JC, Allen PG, Beggs AH, Pollak MR: Mutations in ACTN4, encoding alpha-actinin-4, cause familial focal segmental glomerulosclerosis. Nat Genet 2000; 24: 251-6.
27. Pavenstadt H: Roles of the podocyte in glomerular function. Am J Physiol Renal Physiol 2000; 278: F173-9.
28. Johnson RJ: New insights into the pathogenesis of proteinuria. Am J Kidney Dis 2000; 36: 214-9.

29. Putaala H, Soininen R, Kilpelainen P, Wartiovaara J, Tryggvason K: The murine nephrin gene is specifically expressed in kidney, brain and pancreas: inactivation of the gene leads to massive proteinuria and neonatal death. Hum. Mol. Genet. 2001; 10: 1-8.
30. Koukouritaki SB, Vardaki EA, Papakonstanti EA, Lianos E, Stournaras C, Emmanouel DS: TNF-alpha induces actin cytoskeleton reorganization in glomerular epithelial cells involving tyrosine phosphorylation of paxillin and focal adhesion kinase. Mol Med 1999; 5: 382-92.
31. Doublier S, Ruotsalainen V, Salvidio G, Lupia E, Biancone L, Conaldi PG, Reponen P, Tryggvason K, Camussi G: Nephrin redistribution on podocytes is a potential mechanism for proteinuria in patients with primary acquired nephrotic syndrome. Am J Pathol 2001; 158: 1723-31.
32. Nangaku M, Shankland SJ, Couser WG: Cellular response to injury in membranous nephropathy. J Am Soc Nephrol 2005; 16: 1195-204.
33. Van Den Berg JG, Aten J, Chand MA, Claessen N, Dijkink L, Wijdenes J, Lakkis FG, Weening JJ: Interleukin-4 and interleukin-13 act on glomerular visceral epithelial cells. J Am Soc Nephrol 2000; 11: 413-22.
34. Wolf D, Hochegger K, Wolf AM, Rumpold HF, Gastl G, Tilg H, Mayer G, Gunsilius E, Rosenkranz AR: CD4+CD25+ regulatory T cells inhibit experimental anti-glomerular basement membrane glomerulonephritis in mice. J Am Soc Nephrol 2005; 16: 1360-70.
35. Mahajan D, Wang Y, Qin X, Zheng G, Wang YM, Alexander SI, Harris DC: CD4+CD25+ regulatory T cells protect against injury in an innate murine model of chronic kidney disease. J Am Soc Nephrol 2006; 17: 2731-41.
36. Wang YM, Zhang GY, Wang Y, Hu M, Wu H, Watson D, Hori S, Alexander IE, Harris DC, Alexander SI: Foxp3-transduced polyclonal regulatory T cells protect against chronic renal injury from adriamycin. J Am Soc Nephrol 2006; 17: 697-706.
37. Gallucci S, Matzinger P: Danger signals: SOS to the immune system. Curr Opin Immunol 2001; 13: 114-9.
38. Blander JM, Medzhitov R: Toll-dependent selection of microbial antigens for presentation by dendritic cells. Nature 2006; 440: 808-12.
39. Inaba K, Turley S, Iyoda T, Yamaide F, Shimoyama S, Reis e Sousa C, Germain RN, Mellman I, Steinman RM: The formation of immunogenic major histocompatibility complex class II- peptide ligands in lysosomal compartments of dendritic cells is regulated by inflammatory stimuli. J Exp Med 2000; 191: 927-36.
40. Aeby P, Wyss C, Beck H, Griem P, Scheffler H, Goebel C: Characterization of the sensitizing potential of chemicals by *in vitro* analysis of dendritic cell activation and skin penetration. J Invest Dermatol 2004; 122: 1154-64.
41. Uetrecht J: Role of animal models in the study of drug-induced hypersensitivity reactions. Aaps J 2005; 7: E914-21.
42. Manome H, Aiba S, Tagami H: Simple chemicals can induce maturation and apoptosis of dendritic cells. Immunology 1999; 98: 481-90.
43. Rodriguez-Pena R, Lopez S, Mayorga C, Antunez C, Fernandez TD, Torres MJ, Blanca M: Potential involvement of dendritic cells in delayed-type hypersensitivity reactions to beta-lactams. J Allergy Clin Immunol 2006; 118: 949-56.
44. Olsen NJ: Drug-induced autoimmunity. Best Pract Res Clin Rheumatol 2004; 18: 677-88.
45. Pollard KM, Lee DK, Casiano CA, Bluthner M, Johnston MM, Tan EM: The autoimmunity-inducing xenobiotic mercury interacts with the autoantigen fibrillarin and modifies its molecular and antigenic properties. J Immunol 1997; 158: 3521-8.
46. Kubicka-Muranyi M, Behmer O, Uhrberg M, Klonowski H, Bister J, Gleichmann E: Murine systemic autoimmune disease induced by mercuric chloride ($HgCl_2$) : Hg-specific helper T-cells react to antigen stored in macrophages. Int. J. Immunopharmac. 1993; 15: 151-61.
47. Mamula MJ, Lin R-H, Janeway Jr CA: Breaking T cell tolerance with foreign and self co-immunogens A study of autoimmune B and T cell epitopes of cytochrome c. J. Immunol. 1992; 149: 789-95.
48. Gamerdinger K, Moulon C, Karp DR, Van Bergen J, Koning F, Wild D, Pflugfelder U, Weltzien HU: A new type of metal recognition by human T cells: contact residues for peptide-independent bridging of T cell receptor and major histocompatibility complex by nickel. J Exp Med 2003; 197: 1345-53.
49. Moulon C, Choleva Y, Thierse HJ, Wild D, Weltzien HU: T cell receptor transfection shows non-HLA-restricted recognition of nickel by CD8+ human T cells to be mediated by alphabeta T cell receptors. J Invest Dermatol 2003; 121: 496-501.
50. Pichler WJ, Beeler A, Keller M, Lerch M, Posadas S, Schmid D, Spanou Z, Zawodniak A, Gerber B: Pharmacological interaction of drugs with immune receptors: the p-i concept. Allergol Int 2006; 55: 17-25.
51. Beeler A, Engler O, Gerber BO, Pichler WJ: Long-lasting reactivity and high frequency of drug-specific T cells after severe systemic drug hypersensitivity reactions. J Allergy Clin Immunol 2006; 117: 455-62.
52. Schmid DA, Depta JP, Luthi M, Pichler WJ: Transfection of drug-specific T-cell receptors into hybridoma cells: tools to monitor drug interaction with T-cell receptors and evaluate cross-reactivity to related compounds. Mol Pharmacol 2006; 70: 356-65.
53. Dustin ML, Cooper JA: The immunological synapse and the actin cytoskeleton: molecular hardware for T cell signaling. Nat Immunol 2000; 1: 23-9.
54. Cemerski S, Shaw A: Immune synapses in T-cell activation. Curr Opin Immunol 2006; 18: 298-304.

55. Revy P, Sospedra M, Barbour B, Trautmann A: Functional antigen-independent synapses formed between T cells and dendritic cells. Nat Immunol 2001; 2: 925-31.
56. Billadeau DD, Nolz JC, Gomez TS: Regulation of T-cell activation by the cytoskeleton. Nat Rev Immunol 2007; 7: 131-43.
57. Pu MY, Akhand AA, Kato M, Koike T, Hamaguchi M, Suzuki H, Nakashima I: Mercuric chloride mediates a protein sulfhydryl modification-based pathway of signal transduction for activating Src kinase which is independent of the phosphorylation/dephosphorylation of a carboxyl terminal tyrosine. J Cell Biochem 1996; 63: 104-14.
58. Savignac M, Badou A, Delmas C, Subra JF, De Cramer S, Paulet P, Cassar G, Druet P, Saoudi A, Pelletier L: Gold is a T cell polyclonal activator in BN and LEW rats but favors IL-4 expression only in autoimmune prone BN rats. Eur. J. Immunol. 2001; 31: 2266-2276.
59. Griem P, Gleichmann E: Metal ion-induced autoimmunity. Curr. Opin. Immunol. 1995; 7: 831-838.
60. Griem P, von Vultee C, Panthel K, Best SL, Sadler PJ, Shaw CF, 3rd: T cell cross-reactivity to heavy metals: identical cryptic peptides may be presented from protein exposed to different metals. Eur J Immunol 1998; 28: 1941-7.
61. Wulferink M, Dierkes S, Gleichmann E: Cross-sensitization to haptens: formation of common haptenic metabolites, T cell recognition of cryptic peptides, and true T cell cross-reactivity. Eur J Immunol 2002; 32: 1338-48.
62. Weiss RA, Madaio MP, Tomaszewski JE, Kelly CJ: T cells reactive to an inducible heat shock protein induce disease in toxin-induced interstitial nephritis. J. Exp. Med. 1994; 180: 2239-2250.
63. Pillinger MH, Staud R: Propylthiouracil and antineutrophil cytoplasmic antibody associated vasculitis: the detective finds a clue. Semin Arthritis Rheum 2006; 36: 1-3.
64. Gao Y, Chen M, Ye H, Guo XH, Zhao MH, Wang HY: The target antigens of antineutrophil cytoplasmic antibodies (ANCA) induced by propylthiouracil. Int Immunopharmacol 2007; 7: 55-60.
65. Bonaci-Nikolic B, Nikolic MM, Andrejevic S, Zoric S, Bukilica M: Antineutrophil cytoplasmic antibody (ANCA)-associated autoimmune diseases induced by antithyroid drugs: comparison with idiopathic ANCA vasculitides. Arthritis Res Ther 2005; 7: R1072-81.
66. Griem P, Panthel K, Kalbacher H, Gleichmann E: Alteration of a model antigen by Au(III) leads to T cell sensitization to cryptic peptides. EuR. J. Immunol. 1996; 26: 279-287.
67. Kalluri R, Cantley LG, Kerjaschki D, Neilson EG: Reactive oxygen species expose cryptic epitopes associated with autoimmune goodpasture syndrome. J Biol Chem 2000; 275: 20027-32.
68. Stockinger B: T lymphocyte tolerance: from thymic deletion to peripheral control mechanisms. Adv. Immunol. 1999; 71: 229-65.
69. Klein L, Kyewski B: „Promiscuous" expression of tissue antigens in the thymus: a key to T- cell tolerance and autoimmunity? J Mol Med 2000; 78: 483-94.
70. Buer J, Lanoue A, Franzke A, Garcia C, von Boehmer H, Sarukhan A: Interleukin 10 secretion and impaired effector function of major histocompatibility complex class II-restricted T cells anergized *in vivo*. J Exp Med 1998; 187: 177-83.
71. Hess AD, Thoburn CJ: Immune tolerance to self-major histocompatibility complex class II antigens after bone marrow transplantation: role of regulatory T cells. Biol Blood Marrow Transplant 2006; 12: 518-29.
72. Choudhury D, Ahmed Z: Drug-associated renal dysfunction and injury. Nat Clin Pract Nephrol 2006; 2: 80-91.
73. Markowitz GS, Perazella MA: Drug-induced renal failure: a focus on tubulointerstitial disease. Clin Chim Acta 2005; 351: 31-47.
74. Spanou Z, Keller M, Britschgi M, Yawalkar N, Fehr T, Neuweiler J, Gugger M, Mohaupt M, Pichler WJ: Involvement of drug-specific T cells in acute drug-induced interstitial nephritis. J Am Soc Nephrol 2006; 17: 2919-27.
75. Burgess JK, Lopez JA, Gaudry LE, Chong BH: Rifampicin-dependent antibodies bind a similar or identical epitope to glycoprotein IX-specific quinine-dependent antibodies. Blood 2000; 95: 1988-92.
76. De Vriese AS, Robbrecht DL, Vanholder RC, Vogelaers DP, Lameire NH: Rifampicin-associated acute renal failure: pathophysiologic, immunologic, and clinical features. Am J Kidney Dis 1998; 31: 108-15.
77. Ravnskov U: Glomerular, tubular and interstitial nephritis associated with non- steroidal anti-inflammatory drugs. Evidence of a common mechanism. Br J Clin Pharmacol 1999; 47: 203-10.
78. Markowitz GS, Radhakrishnan J, Kambham N, Valeri AM, Hines WH, D'Agati VD: Lithium nephrotoxicity: a progressive combined glomerular and tubulointerstitial nephropathy. J Am Soc Nephrol 2000; 11: 1439-48.
79. Shah P, Griffith SM, Shadforth MF, Fisher J, Dawes PT, Poulton KV, Thomson W, Ollier WE, Mattey DL: Can gold therapy be used more safely in rheumatoid arthritis? Adverse drug reactions are more likely in patients with nodular disease, independent of HLA-DR3 status. J Rheumatol 2004; 31: 1903-5.
80. Habib GS, Saliba W, Nashashibi M, Armali Z: Penicillamine and nephrotic syndrome. Eur J Intern Med 2006; 17: 343-8.
81. Pirmohamed M: Genetic factors in the predisposition to drug-induced hypersensitivity reactions. Aaps J 2006; 8: E20-6.
82. Wooley PH, Griffin J, Panayi GS, Batchelor JR, Welsh KI, Gibson TJ: HLA-DR antigens and toxic reaction to sodium aurothiomalate and D-penicillamine in patients with rheumatoid arthritis. N. Engl. J. Med. 1980; 303: 300-302.

83. Emery P, Panayi GS, Huston G, Welsh KL, Mitschell SC, Shah RR, Idle JR, Smith RL, Waring RH: D-penicillamine induced toxicity in rheumatoid arthritis : the role of sulphoxidation status and HLA-DR3. J. Rheum. 1984; 11: 626-632.
84. Pospishil YO, Antonovych TM: NSAIDs associated nephropathy. Pol J Pathol 1998; 49: 35-9.
85. Makino H, Haramoto T, Sasaki T, Hironaka K, Shikata K, Takahashi K, Ota Z: Massive eosinophilic infiltration in a patient with the nephrotic syndrome and drug-induced interstitial nephritis. Am J Kidney Dis 1995; 26: 62-7.
86. Dharnidharka VR, Rosen S, Somers MJ: Acute interstitial nephritis presenting as presumed minimal change nephrotic syndrome. Pediatr Nephrol 1998; 12: 576-8.
87. Yawalkar N, Hari Y, Frutig K, Egli F, Wendland T, Braathen LR, Pichler WJ: T cells isolated from positive epicutaneous test reactions to amoxicillin and ceftriaxone are drug specific and cytotoxic. J Invest Dermatol 2000; 115: 647-52.
88. Brugnolo F, Annunziato F, Sampognaro S, Campi P, Manfredi M, Matucci A, Blanca M, Romagnani S, Maggi E, Parronchi P: Highly Th2-skewed cytokine profile of beta-lactam-specific T cells from nonatopic subjects with adverse drug reactions. J Immunol 1999; 163: 1053-9.
89. Padovan E, von Greyerz S, Pichler WJ, Weltzien HU: Antigen-dependent and -independent IFN-gamma modulation by penicillins. J Immunol 1999; 162: 1171-7.
90. Deckers JG, De Haij S, van der Woude FJ, van der Kooij SW, Daha MR, van Kooten C: IL-4 and IL-13 augment cytokine- and CD40-induced RANTES production by human renal tubular epithelial cells *in vitro*. J Am Soc Nephrol 1998; 9: 1187-93.
91. Cornacchia E, Golbus J, Maybaum J, Strahler J, Hanash S, Richardson B: Hydralazine and procainamide inhibit T cell DNA methylation and induce autoreactivity. J. Immunol. 1988; 140: 2197-2200.
92. Quddus J, Johnson K, Gavalchin J, Amento E, Chrisp C, Yung R, Richardson B: Treating activated CD4+ T cells with either of two distinct methyltransferase inhibitors, 5-azacytidine or procainamide, is sufficient to cause a lupus-like disease in syngeneic mice. J. Clin. Invest. 1993; 92: 38-46.
93. Kretz-Rommel A, Duncan SR, Rubin RL: Autoimmunity caused by disruption of central T cell tolerance. A murine model of drug-induced lupus. J Clin Invest 1997; 99: 1888-96.
94. Rubin RL: Drug-induced lupus. Toxicology 2005; 209: 135-47.
95. Uetrecht J: Current trends in drug-induced autoimmunity. Autoimmun Rev 2005; 4: 309-14.
96. Richardson B, Powers D, Hooper F, Yung RL, O'Rourke K: Lymphocyte function-associated antigen 1 overexpression and T cell autoreactivity. Arthritis Rheum 1994; 37: 1363-72.
97. Yung RL, Quddus J, Chrisp CE, Johnson KJ, Richardson BC: Mechanisms of drug-induced lupus I. Clones Th2 cells modified with DNA methylation inhibitors *in vitro* cause autoimmunity *in vivo*. J. Immunol. 1995; 154: 3025-3035.
98. Yung R, Powers D, Johnson K, Amento E, Carr D, Laing T, Yang J, Chang S, Hemati N, Richardson B: Mechanisms of drug-induced lupus. II. T cells overexpressing lymphocyte function-associated antigen 1 become autoreactive and cause a lupuslike disease in syngeneic mice. J Clin Invest 1996; 97: 2866-71.
99. Rao T, Richardson B: Environmentally induced autoimmune diseases: potential mechanisms. Environ Health Perspect 1999; 107 Suppl 5: 737-42.
100. Nan X, Ng HH, Johnson CA, Laherty CD, Turner BM, Eisenman RN, Bird A: Transcriptional repression by the methyl-CpG-binding protein MeCP2 involves a histone deacetylase complex. Nature 1998; 393: 386-9.
101. Leoni F, Fossati G, Lewis EC, Lee JK, Porro G, Pagani P, Modena D, Moras ML, Pozzi P, Reznikov LL, Siegmund B, Fantuzzi G, Dinarello CA, Mascagni P: The histone deacetylase inhibitor ITF2357 reduces production of pro-inflammatory cytokines *in vitro* and systemic inflammation *in vivo*. Mol Med 2005; 11: 1-15.
102. Glauben R, Batra A, Fedke I, Zeitz M, Lehr HA, Leoni F, Mascagni P, Fantuzzi G, Dinarello CA, Siegmund B: Histone hyperacetylation is associated with amelioration of experimental colitis in mice. J Immunol 2006; 176: 5015-22.
103. Leng C, Gries M, Ziegler J, Lokshin A, Mascagni P, Lentzsch S, Mapara MY: Reduction of graft-versus-host disease by histone deacetylase inhibitor suberonylanilide hydroxamic acid is associated with modulation of inflammatory cytokine milieu and involves inhibition of STAT1. Exp Hematol 2006; 34: 776-87.
104. Pietsch P, Vohr HW, Degitz K, Gleichmann E: Immunopathological signs inducible by mercury compounds. II. HgCl2 and gold sodium thiomalate enhance serum IgE and IgG concentrations in susceptible mouse strains. Int. Arch. Allergy Appl. Immun. 1989; 90: 47-53.
105. Ochel M, Vohr H-W, Pfeiffer C, Gleichmann E: IL-4 is required for the IgE and IgG1 increase and IgG1 autoantibody formation in mice treated with mercuric chloride. J. Immunol. 1991; 146: 3006-11.
106. Haggqvist B, Hultman P: Effects of deviating the Th2-response in murine mercury-induced autoimmunity towards a Th1-response. Clin Exp Immunol 2003; 134: 202-9.
107. Biancone L, Andres G, Ahn H, Lim A, Dai C, Noelle R, Yagita H, De Martino C, Stamenkovic I: DistincTregulatory roles of lymphocyte costimulatory pathways on T helper type 2-mediated autoimmune disease. J. Exp. Med. 1996; 183: 1473-1481.

108. Zheng Y, Jost M, Gaughan JP, Class R, Coyle AJ, Monestier M: ICOS-B7 homologous protein interactions are necessary for mercury-induced autoimmunity. J Immunol 2005; 174: 3117-21.
109. Zheng Y, Monestier M: Inhibitory signal override increases susceptibility to mercury-induced autoimmunity. J Immunol 2003; 171: 1596-601.
110. Layland LE, Wulferink M, Dierkes S, Gleichmann E: Drug-induced autoantibody formation in mice: triggering by primed CD4+CD25- T cells, prevention by primed CD4+CD25+ T cells. Eur J Immunol 2004; 34: 36-46.
111. Kiely PD, Pecht I, Oliveira DB: Mercuric chloride-induced vasculitis in the Brown Norway rat: alpha beta T cell-dependent and -independent phases: role of the mast cell. J Immunol 1997; 159: 5100-6.
112. Vinen CS, Turner DR, Oliveira DB: A central role for the mast cell in early phase vasculitis in the Brown Norway rat model of vasculitis: a histological study. Int J Exp Pathol 2004; 85: 165-74.
113. Badou A, Saoudi A, Dietrich G, Druet E, Druet P, Pelletier L: Mercuric chloride-induced autoimmunity. Curr.Prot. Immunol. 1999; 15: 1-18.
114. Tournade H, Pelletier L, Pasquier R, Vial M-C, Mandet C, Druet P: D-penicillamine-induced autoimmunity in Brown Norway rats: similarities with $HgCl_2$-induced autoimmunity. J. Immunol. 1990; 144: 2985-2991.
115. Tournade H, Pelletier L, Guéry JC, Pasquier R, Nochy D, Hinglais N, Guilbert B, Druet P: Experimental gold-induced autoimmunity. Nephrol. Dial. Transplant. 1991; 6: 621-630.
116. Mathieson PW, Stapleton KJ, Oliveira DBG, Lockwood CM: Immunoregulation of mercuric chloride-induced autoimmunity in Brown Norway rats: a role for CD8+ T cells revealed by *in vivo* depletion studies. Eur. J. Immunol. 1991; 21: 2105-9.
117. Field AC, Bloch MF, Bellon B: Neonatal tolerance to a Th2-mediated autoimmune disease generates CD8+ Tc1 regulatory cells. J Autoimmun 2003; 21: 201-12.
118. Masson MJ, Uetrecht JP: Tolerance induced by low dose D-penicillamine in the brown Norway rat model of drug-induced autoimmunity is immune-mediated. Chem Res Toxicol 2004; 17: 82-94.
119. Seguin B, Masson MJ, Uetrecht J: D-penicillamine-induced autoimmunity in the Brown Norway rat: role for both T and non-T splenocytes in adoptive transfer of tolerance. Chem Res Toxicol 2004; 17: 1299-302.
120. Bridoux F, Badou A, Saoudi A, Bernard I, Druet E, Pasquier R, Druet P, Pelletier L: TGF-b dependent inhibition of Th2-induced autoimmunity by self MHC class II specific, regulatory CD4+ T cell lines. J. Exp. Med. 1997; 185: 1769-1775.
121. Qasim FJ, Thiru S, Mathieson PW, Oliveira DB: The time course and characterization of mercuric chloride-induced immunopathology in the brown Norway rat. J. Autoimmun. 1995; 8: 193-208.
122. Wu Z, Turner DR, Oliveira DB: Antioxidants inhibit mercuric chloride-induced early vasculitis. Int Immunol 2002; 14: 267-73.
123. Wu Z, Turner DR, Oliveira DB: IL-4 gene expression up-regulated by mercury in rat mast cells: a role of oxidant stress in IL-4 transcription. Int Immunol 2001; 13: 297-304.
124. Wu Z, MacPhee IA, Oliveira DB: Reactive oxygen species in the initiation of IL-4 driven autoimmunity as a potential therapeutic target. Curr Pharm Des 2004; 10: 899-913.
125. Fillion J, Baccala R, Kuhn J, Druet P, Bellon B: Evidence for heterogenous TCRVb expression in mercury-induced autoimmune disorders in rats. Int. Immunol. 1997; 9: 263-271.
126. Badou A, Savignac M, Moreau M, Leclerc C, Pasquier R, Druet P, Pelletier L: $HgCl_2$-induced IL-4 gene expression in T cells involves protein kinase C-dependent calcium influx through L-type calcium channels. J. Biol. Chem. 1997; 272: 32411-8.
127. Savignac M, Badou A, Moreau M, Leclerc C, Guery JC, Paulet P, Druet P, Ragab-Thomas J, Pelletier L: Protein kinase C-mediated calcium entry dependent upon dihydropyridine sensitive channels: a T cell receptor-coupled signaling pathway involved in IL-4 synthesis. Faseb J 2001; 15: 1577-9.
128. Prigent P, Saoudi A, Pannetier C, Graber P, Bonnefoy Y, Druet P, Hirsch F: Mercuric chloride, a chemical responsible for Th2-mediated autoimmunity in Brown-Norway rats, directly triggers T cells to produce IL-4. J. Clin. Invest. 1995; 96: 1484-9.
129. Savignac M, Gomes B, Gallard A, Narbonnet S, Moreau M, Leclerc C, Paulet P, Mariame B, Druet P, Saoudi A, Fournie GJ, Guery JC, Pelletier L: Dihydropyridine receptors are selective markers of Th2 cells and can be targeted to prevent Th2-dependent immunopathological disorders. J Immunol 2004; 172: 5206-12.
130. Gomes B, Savignac M, Cabral MD, Paulet P, Moreau M, Leclerc C, Feil R, Hofmann F, Guery JC, Dietrich G, Pelletier L: The cGMP/protein kinase G pathway contributes to dihydropyridine-sensitive calcium response and cytokine production in TH2 lymphocytes. J Biol Chem 2006; 281: 12421-7.
131. Pelletier L, Pasquier R, Rossert J, Vial M-C, Mandet C, Druet P: Autoreactive T cells in mercury-induced autoimmunity. Ability to induce the autoimmune disease. J. Immunol. 1988; 140: 750-4.
132. Erb KJ, Ruger B, von Brevern M, Ryffel B, Schimpl A, Rivett K: Constitutive expression of interleukin (IL)-4 *in vivo* causes autoimmune- type disorders in mice. J Exp Med 1997; 185: 329-39.
133. Rossert J, Pelletier L, Pasquier R, Druet P: Autoreactive T cells in mercury-induced autoimmunity. Demonstration by limiting dilution analysis. Eur. J. Immunol. 1988; 18: 1761-1766.

134. Saoudi A, Castedo M, Nochy D., Mandet C, Pasquier R, Druet P, Pelletier L: Self reactive anti-class II Th2 cell lines derived from gold salt-injected rats trigger B cell polyclonal activation and transfer autoimmunity in CD8-depleted normal syngeneic recipients. Eur. J. Immunol. 1995; 25: 1972-1979.
135. Roos A, Claessen N, Weening JJ, Aten J: Enhanced T lymphocyte expression of LFA-1, ICAM-1, and the TNF receptor family member OX40 in HgCl2-induced systemic autoimmunity. Scand J Immunol 1996; 43: 507-18.
136. Croft MA, Kaufman PL: Accommodation and presbyopia: the ciliary neuromuscular view. Ophthalmol Clin North Am 2006; 19: 13-24, v.
137. Field AC, Caccavelli L, Fillion J, Kuhn J, Mandet C, Druet P, Bellon B: Neonatal induction of tolerance to T(h)2-mediated autoimmunity in rats. Int Immunol 2000; 12: 1467-77.
138. Field AC, Caccavelli L, Bloch MF, Bellon B: Regulatory CD8+ T cells control neonatal tolerance to a Th2-mediated autoimmunity. J Immunol 2003; 170: 2508-15.
139. Nomura T, Sakaguchi S: Foxp3 and Aire in thymus-generated T(reg) cells: a link in self-tolerance. Nat Immunol 2007; 8: 333-4.
140. Flint J, Mott R: Finding the molecular basis of quantitative traits: successes and pitfalls. Nat Rev Genet 2001; 2: 437-45.
141. Hemminki K, Lorenzo Bermejo J, Forsti A: The balance between heritable and environmental aetiology of human disease. Nat Rev Genet 2006; 7: 958-65.
142. Johnston PG, Lenz HJ, Leichman CG, Danenberg KD, Allegra CJ, Danenberg PV, Leichman L: Thymidylate synthase gene and protein expression correlate and are associated with response to 5-fluorouracil in human colorectal and gastric tumors. Cancer Res 1995; 55: 1407-12.
143. Antignac C: Genetic models: clues for understanding the pathogenesis of idiopathic nephrotic syndrome. J Clin Invest 2002; 109: 447-9.
144. Antignac C: Molecular basis of steroid-resistant nephrotic syndrome. Nefrologia 2005; 25 Suppl 2: 25-8.
145. Sternberg SS: Cross-striated fibrils and other ultrastructural alterations in glomeruli of rats with daunomycin nephrosis. Lab Invest 1970; 23: 39-51.
146. Bertani T, Rocchi G, Sacchi G, Mecca G, Remuzzi G: Adriamycin-induced glomerulosclerosis in the rat. Am J Kidney Dis 1986; 7: 12-9.
147. Fogo AB: Animal models of FSGS: lessons for pathogenesis and treatment. Semin Nephrol 2003; 23: 161-71.
148. Zheng Z, Schmidt-Ott KM, Chua S, Foster KA, Frankel RZ, Pavlidis P, Barasch J, D'Agati VD, Gharavi AG: A Mendelian locus on chromosome 16 determines susceptibility to doxorubicin nephropathy in the mouse. Proc Natl Acad Sci U S A 2005; 102: 2502-7.
149. Zheng Z, Pavlidis P, Chua S, D'Agati VD, Gharavi AG: An ancestral haplotype defines susceptibility to doxorubicin nephropathy in the laboratory mouse. J Am Soc Nephrol 2006; 17: 1796-800.
150. Tournade H, Guéry J-C, Pasquier R, Vial MC, Mandet C, Druet E, Dansette PM, Druet P, Pelletier L: Effect of the thiol group on experimental gold-induced autoimmunity. Arthritis Rheum. 1991; 34: 1594-1599.
151. Gold therapy in rheumatoid arthritis-final report of a multi-centre controlled trial. Empire Rheumatism Council. Ann Rheum Dis 1961; 20: 315-334.
152. Fillastre JP, Mery JP, Druet P: [Drug-induced glomerular nephropathies]. Nephrologie 1983; 4: 1-9.
153. Sapin C, Druet E, Druet P: Induction of anti-glomerular basement antibodies in the Brown-Norway rat by mercuric chloride. Clin. Exp. Immunol. 1977; 28: 173-178.
154. Druet E, Sapin C, Günther E, Feingold N, Druet P: Mercuric chloride-induced anti-glomerular basement membrane antibodies in the rat. Genetic control. Eur J Immunol 1977; 7: 348-351.
155. Fournie GJ, Cautain B, Xystrakis E, Damoiseaux J, Mas M, Lagrange D, Bernard I, Subra JF, Pelletier L, Druet P, Saoudi A: Cellular and genetic factors involved in the difference between Brown Norway and Lewis rats to develop respectively type-2 and type-1 immune-mediated diseases. Immunol Rev 2001; 184: 145-60.
156. Cautain B, Damoiseaux J, Bernard I, Xystrakis E, Fournie E, van Breda Vriesman P, Druet P, Saoudi A: The CD8 T cell compartment plays a dominant role in the deficiency of Brown-Norway rats to mount a proper type 1 immune response. J Immunol 2002; 168: 162-70.
157. Subra JF, Cautain B, Xystrakis E, Mas M, Lagrange D, van Der Heijden H, van De Gaar MJ, Druet P, Fournie GJ, Saoudi A, Damoiseaux J: The balance between CD45RC(high) and CD45RC(low) CD4 T cells in rats is intrinsic to bone marrow-derived cells and is genetically controlled. J Immunol 2001; 166: 2944-52.
158. Xystrakis E, Cavailles P, Dejean AS, Cautain B, Colacios C, Lagrange D, van de Gaar MJ, Bernard I, Gonzalez-Dunia D, Damoiseaux J, Fournie GJ, Saoudi A: Functional and genetic analysis of two CD8 T cell subsets defined by the level of CD45RC expression in the rat. J Immunol 2004; 173: 3140-7.

159. Kermarrec N, Dubay C, De Gouyon B, Blanpied C, Gauguier D, Gillespie K, Druet P, Lathrop M, Hirsch F: Serum IgE concentration and other immune manifestations of treatment with gold salts are linked to MHC and IL-4 regions in the rat. Genomics 1996; 31: 111-4.
160. Mas M, Cavailles P, Colacios C, Subra JF, Lagrange D, Calise M, Christen MO, Druet P, Pelletier L, Gauguier D, Fournie GJ: Studies of congenic lines in the Brown Norway rat model of Th2-mediated immunopathological disorders show that the aurothiopropanol sulfonate-induced immunological disorder (Aiid3) locus on chromosome 9 plays a major role compared to Aiid2 on chromosome 10. J Immunol 2004; 172: 6354-61.
161. Mas M, Subra JF, Lagrange D, Pilipenko-Appolinaire S, Kermarrec N, Gauguier D, Druet P, Fournie GJ: Rat chromosome 9 bears a major susceptibility locus for IgE response. Eur J Immunol 2000; 30: 1698-705.
162. Damoiseaux JG, Cautain B, Bernard I, Mas M, van Breda Vriesman PJ, Druet P, Fournie G, Saoudi A: A dominant role for the thymus and MHC genes in determining the peripheral CD4/CD8 T cell ratio in the rat. J. Immunol. 1999; 163: 2983-2989.
163. Frazer KA, Ueda Y, Zhu Y, Gifford VR, Garofalo MR, Mohandas N, Martin CH, Palazzolo MJ, Cheng JF, Rubin EM: Computational and biological analysis of 680 kb of DNA sequence from the human 5q31 cytokine gene cluster region. Genome Res 1997; 7: 495-512.
164. Marsh DG, Neely JD, Breazeale DR, Ghosh B, Freidhoff LR, Schou C, Beaty TH: Genetic basis of IgE responsiveness: relevance to the atopic diseases. Int Arch Allergy Immunol 1995; 107: 25-8.
165. Meyers DA, Postma DS, Panhuysen CIM, Xu J, Amelung PJ, Levitt RC, Bleekers ER: Evidence for a locus regulating total serum IgE levels mapping to chromosome 5. Genomics 1994; 23: 464-70.
166. Gorham JD, Guler ML, Steen RG, Mackey AJ, Daly MJ, Frederick K, Dietrich WF, Murphy KM: Genetic mapping of a murine locus controlling development of T helper 1/T helper 2 type responses. Proc. Natl. Acad. Sci. USA 1996; 93: 12467-12472.
167. Guler ML, Gorham JD, Dietrich WF, Murphy TL, Steen RG, Parvin CA, Fenoglio D, Grupe A, Peltz G, Murphy KM: Tpm1, a locus controlling IL-12 responsiveness, acts by a cell- autonomous mechanism. J Immunol 1999; 162: 1339-47.
168. Dahlman I, Wallstrom E, Weissert R, Storch M, Kornek B, Jacobsson L, Linington C, Luthman H, Lassmann H, Olsson T: Linkage analysis of myelin oligodendrocyte glycoprotein-induced experimental autoimmune encephalomyelitis in the rat identifies a locus controlling demyelination on chromosome 18. Hum Mol Genet 1999; 8: 2183-90.
169. Roth MP, Viratelle C, Dolbois L, Delverdier M, Borot N, Pelletier L, Druet P, Clanet M, Coppin H: A genome-wide search identifies two susceptibility loci for experimental autoimmune encephalomyelitis on rat chromosomes 4 and 10. J. Immunol. 1999; 162: 1917-1922.
170. Williams RM, Moore MJ: Linkage of susceptibility to experimental allergic encephalomyelitis to the major histocompatibility locus in the rat. J Exp Med 1973; 138: 775-83.
171. Furuya T, Salstrom JL, McCall-Vining S, Cannon GW, Joe B, Remmers EF, Griffiths MM, Wilder RL: Genetic dissection of a rat model for rheumatoid arthritis: significant gender influences on autosomal modifier loci. Hum Mol Genet 2000; 9: 2241-50.
172. Powrie F, Mason D: Subsets of rat CD4+ T cells defined by their differential expression of variants of the CD45 antigen: developmental relationships and *in vitro* and *in vivo* functions. Curr Top Microbiol Immunol 1990; 159: 79-96.
173. Fowell D, McKnight AJ, Powrie F, Dyke R, Mason D: Subsets of CD4+ T cells and their role in the induction and prevention of autoimmunity. Immunol. Rev. 1991; 123: 37-64.
174. McKnight AJ, Barclay AN, Mason DW: Molecular cloning of rat interleukine 4 cDNA and analysis of the cytokine repertoire of subsets of CD4+ T cells. Eur. J. Immunol. 1991; 21: 1187-94.
175. Rogner UC, Avner P: Congenic mice: cutting tools for complex immune disorders. Nat Rev Immunol 2003; 3: 243-52.
176. Aitman TJ, Glazier AM, Wallace CA, Cooper LD, Norsworthy PJ, Wahid FN, Al-Majali KM, Trembling PM, Mann CJ, Shoulders CC, Graf D, St Lezin E, Kurtz TW, Kren V, Pravenec M, Ibrahimi A, Abumrad NA, Stanton LW, Scott J: Identification of Cd36 (Fat) as an insulin-resistance gene causing defective fatty acid and glucose metabolism in hypertensive rats. Nat Genet 1999; 21: 76-83.
177. Olofsson P, Holmberg J, Tordsson J, Lu S, Akerstrom B, Holmdahl R: Positional identification of Ncf1 as a gene thaTregulates arthritis severity in rats. Nat Genet 2003; 33: 25-32.
178. Rozzo SJ, Allard JD, Choubey D, Vyse TJ, Izui S, Peltz G, Kotzin BL: Evidence for an interferon-inducible gene, Ifi202, in the susceptibility to systemic lupus. Immunity 2001; 15: 435-43.
179. Backdahl L, Ribbhammar U, Lorentzen JC: Mapping and functional characterization of rat chromosome 4 regions that regulate arthritis models and phenotypes in congenic strains. Arthritis Rheum 2003; 48: 551-9.
180. Hattori M, Yamato E, Itoh N, Senpuku H, Fujisawa T, Yoshino M, Fukuda M, Matsumoto E, Toyonaga T, Nakagawa I, Petruzzelli M, McMurray A, Weiner H, Sagai T, Moriwaki K, Shiroishi T, Maron R, Lund T: Cutting edge: homologous recombination of the MHC class I K region defines new MHC-linked diabetogenic susceptibility gene(s) in nonobese diabetic mice. J Immunol 1999; 163: 1721-4.
181. Morel L, Blenman KR, Croker BP, Wakeland EK: The major murine systemic lupus erythematosus susceptibility locus, Sle1, is a cluster of functionally related genes. Proc Natl Acad Sci U S A 2001; 98: 1787-92.

182. Podolin PL, Denny P, Lord CJ, Hill NJ, Todd JA, Peterson LB, Wicker LS, Lyons PA: Congenic mapping of the insulin-dependent diabetes (Idd) gene, Idd10, localizes two genes mediating the Idd10 effect and eliminates the candidate Fcgr1. J Immunol 1997; 159: 1835-43.
183. Eisen MB, Spellman PT, Brown PO, Botstein D: Cluster analysis and display of genome-wide expression patterns. Proc Natl Acad Sci U S A 1998; 95: 14863-8.
184. Harley JB, Moser KL, Gaffney PM, Behrens TW: The genetics of human systemic lupus erythematosus. Curr Opin Immunol 1998; 10: 690-6.
185. Walley AJ, Wiltshire S, Ellis CM, Cookson WO: Linkage and allelic association of chromosome 5 cytokine cluster genetic markers with atopy and asthma associated traits. Genomics 2001; 72: 15-20.
186. Gerber BO, Pichler WJ: Noncovalent interactions of drugs with immune receptors may mediate drug-induced hypersensitivity reactions. Aaps J 2006; 8: E160-5.

08

Cellular mechanisms of nephrotoxicity

Istvan ARANY, Gur P. KAUSHAL, Didier PORTILLA, Judit MEGYESI, Peter M. PRICE and Robert L. SAFIRSTEIN

University of Arkansas for Medical Sciences, Little Rock, Arkansas, USA

Morphology of nephrotoxic injury

The changes in renal epithelial morphology that accompany acute kidney injury are often subtle. At least four cellular fates can be identified in acute kidney injury: cells may be necrotic; cells may become apoptotic; they may replicate and divide; or they may appear indifferent to the stress (Figure 1). Frank necrosis, as is often seen experimentally, is not prominent in the vast majority of human cases. Necrosis is usually patchy, involving small clusters of cells, sometimes resulting in small areas of denuded basement membrane. Less obvious injury is more often noted, including loss of brush borders, flattening of the epithelium, intratubular cast formation, and dilatation of the lumen. While proximal tubules show many of theses changes, injury to the distal nephron can also be demonstrated when human biopsy material is closely examined. The distal nephron is also the site of obstruction by desquamated cells and cellular debris.

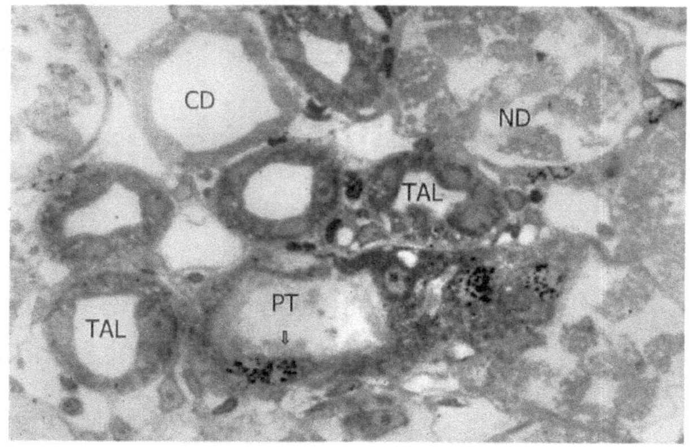

Figure 1. *Radiohistogram of outer stripe of outer medulla of rat kidney taken from animal 5 days after cisplatin, 5 mg/kg BW. Note three cell fates: 1) Necrosis (ND) of cells lining injured S3 segment; 2) apparent indifference of thick ascendary limb (TAL) and collecting duct (CD) epithelial cells; 3) cells of the proximal tubule (PT) undergoing DNA synthesis (arrow). Condensed nuclear debris may also be seen in such section indicating apoptotic bodies (not shown).*

Necrosis is a catastrophic breakdown of regulated cellular homeostasis and is accompanied by massive tissue damage leading to rapid collapse of internal homeostasis of the cell [1]. It is characterized by cell swelling with early loss of plasma-membrane integrity, major alterations of the organelles, and swelling of the nucleus with flocculation of the chromatin. Affected cells rupture and the cellular components spill into the surrounding tissue space evoking an inflammatory response. Apoptosis is also a feature of nephrotoxic injury and a distinction can be made between necrosis and apoptosis based on morphological criteria (Table 1).

In apoptosis, the most outstanding morphological and biochemical changes occur in the nucleus in which chromatin rapidly forms dense crescent-shaped aggregates lining the nuclear membrane [2-4]. The plasma membrane becomes convoluted, so that the cell separates into a cluster of membrane bound segments, "apoptotic bodies", which often contain morphologically normal mitochondria and other cellular organelles. The absence of inflammation is a crucial feature of apoptosis, and thus it permits cell death without damage to adjacent cells, and is thus advantageous for normal cell turnover, development and homeostasis of organs under physiological and

Table 1. Different characteristics between apoptosis and necrosis.

Apoptosis	Necrosis
Affects scattered individual cells	Affects massive and contiguous cells
Chromatin marginates as large crescent aggregates	Chromatin marginates as small aggregates
A ladder of DNA fragmentation (-200 bp), sometimes no fragmentation	Dominant smear pattern of DNA
Cytoplasm and cell volume decrease	Cytoplasm and cell volume increase
Organelles retain integrity	Organelles swell (mitochondria, endoplasmicreticulum)
Cell breaks into small fragments	Cell ruptures
Cell fragments are phagocytized	Cell contents released
No inflammation	Extensive inflammation

pathological conditions. This form of cell death differs from frank necrosis in that it requires the activation of a regulated program that leads to DNA fragmentation, nuclear condensation, and cell loss without causing an inflammatory response.

Proximal tubule cells may undergo necrosis or apoptosis *in vitro* depending on the severity of insult [5,6]. Much of the evidence for the role of apoptotic mechanisms in renal tubular injury relates to the demonstration of chromatin condensation, the morphological hallmark of apoptosis, and endonuclease activation resulting in oligonucleosome-length DNA fragmentation (~200 bp), considered as the biochemical hallmark for apoptosis. Thus, apoptotic bodies in renal tubules have been shown in a variety of renal injuries including ischemia/reperfusion injury *in vivo* and hypoxia/reoxygenation *in vitro*, human allografted kidney, oxidant stress and compounds such as $HgCl_2$, cisplatin, and cyclosporine. Apoptosis has been noted after the administration of bacterial cell wall constituents such as lipopolysaccharides as well.

The site and relative contribution of apoptosis to the total loss of epithelial cell integrity in nephrotoxic damage is still a matter of dispute, but a consensus is emerging that apoptosis occurs in a minority of cells (<5% of the total cells in the renal cortex) and the majority of apoptosis is confined to the distal nephron. In large part the confusion stems from an over-reliance upon the use of TUNEL staining rather than classic morphologic criteria to determine apoptosis. While endonuclease activation and resultant oligonucleosomal DNA fragments is a hallmark of apoptosis, several recent observations make equating DNA fragmentation with apoptosis problematic. Thus, chromatin condensation and DNA fragmentation are regulated by different metabolic pathways [7], apoptosis can occur without DNA fragmentation [7], and DNA fragmentation can be seen in necrotic cells. Indeed, rat renal proximal tubules subjected to hypoxia/reoxygenation result in DNA strand breaks and DNA fragmentation and, endonuclease inhibitors provided complete protection against DNA damage induced by hypoxia/reoxygenation and partial but significant protection against cell death. Iwata et al. [8] reported DNA fragmentation (indicative of endonuclease activation) *in vivo* ischemia/reperfusion injury associated with morphological features of necrosis rather than apoptosis. It is highly likely; therefore, that apoptotic and necrotic forms of cell death share many biochemical features together. The form of cell death initiated in any particular cell by a single toxin will depend on the dose of the toxin, the particular cell type, and whether the cell can mount an effective defense against the deleterious effects of the toxin (see below).

Pathophysiology of cell injury

The mechanisms of the changes in cell viability during renal injury are incompletely understood. Most of the experimental data have been derived from the ischemia-reperfusion model of acute kidney injury and have focused on necrotic cell death. Because as many as 50% of patients have ischemia-induced acute kidney injury, the observations should be relevant to a large portion of the patients at risk. Also, different stresses initiate common biochemical events, so that understanding the relevant pathways of one stress will most likely be applicable to others. What follows is a detailed analysis of some of the pathways currently thought to execute cell death in a variety of nephrotoxic insults.

Disruption of energy production

The two principal sites of energy production in proximal tubular cells reside within the mitochondria and peroxisomes. Both organelles oxidize short chain, medium chain, long chain, and very long chain fatty acids to generate ATP [9-11]. Inhibition of fatty acid oxidation represents a common pathophysiologic response of the kidney, and in particular the proximal tubule, to ischemia/reperfusion, and cisplatin-induced acute kidney injury. Ischemia/reperfusion injury and cisplatin inhibit fatty acid oxidation in mouse kidney and in proximal tubule cells in culture [12, 13]. In each of these insults there is reduced PPAR-α mediated transcription and activity. Failure to oxidize long chain fatty acids and long chain acylcarnitines during acute kidney injury results in their accumulation and cellular toxicity which further contributes to proximal tubule cell death. In the kidney PPARα activation induces the expression of genes encoding nearly every step in the cellular fatty acid utilization pathway including (i) fatty acid transport that facilitate fatty acid entry into the cell, (ii) acyl-CoA synthetases that esterify fatty acids to coenzyme A and prevent their efflux, (iii) fatty acid binding proteins that shuttle fatty acids to various cellular compartments, (iv) proteins that catalyze the import of fatty acids into the mitochondria, (v) every enzyme in the mitochondrial fatty acid β-oxidation spiral, and (vi) various accessory components of fatty acid metabolism (e.g. uncoupling proteins). Administration of PPARα ligand prior to acute kidney injury prevented the inhibition of fatty acid oxidation, the accumulation of nonesterified fatty acids and triglycerides in kidney tissue, and ameliorated apoptotic and necrotic proximal tubule cell death which resulted in significant protection of renal function only in PPARα wild type mice and not in PPARα null mice. To investigate the physiologic role of PPARα in kidney tissue and to determine whether PPARα alone without synthetic ligand was sufficient to activate fatty acid oxidation and thus prevent acute kidney injury, we generated transgenic mice that express mouse PPARα under the control of kidney androgen-regulated protein (KAP) gene promoter, which is androgen responsive. Kidney PPARα expression was detectable only in proximal tubules of female transgenic mice and could be induced by testosterone treatment. In comparison with wild type mice, up-regulation of PPARα expression by testosterone treatment in KAP2-PPARα transgenic mice prevented ischemia reperfusion and cisplatin-mediated inhibition of fatty acid oxidation and significantly ameliorated acute kidney injury.

The PGC-1α transcriptional coactivator and the control of proximal tubule energy metabolism

Transcriptional coactivators are a group of proteins that control gene expression via protein-protein interactions with DNA-bound transcription factors, including PPARα. Expression of PPAR-Gamma-Coactivator-1a (PGC-1a) was reduced by cisplatin. This latter nuclear protein has been shown to be a transcriptional co-activator of PPAR-a [22], PPAR-g [23], RXR [24], and other transcription factors like Nuclear Respiratory Factors (NRFs) that play critical roles in the regulation of oxidative metabolism, cellular respiration and adaptive thermogenesis [25,26]. *In situ* hybridization studies demonstrate the expression of PGC-1 in the mouse proximal tubule (PT) and the thick ascending limb (TAL), two nephron segments which also express high levels of PPAR-a and fatty acid oxidation enzymes and cisplatin inhibited the expression of PGC-1a in both nephron segments. The above studies suggest that the common underlying defect in proximal tubule energy production is a reduced PGC-1/PPAR-α function.

In summary, the kidney requires a continuous and abundant source of substrate to meet its high energy demands. *In situ*ations where energy needs change, such as acute kidney injury, the kidney must adapt and utilize the most efficient sources of substrate to meet its needs. PPARα and PGC-1α play a central role in this metabolic flexibility by driving robust changes in gene expression of key components of mitochondrial biogenesis and metabolism. However, it is not entirely clear whether long term PPARα-PGC-1α-mediated alterations in energy metabolism are adaptive versus maladaptive changes for chronic kidney disease and diabetic nephropathy.

Mitochondrial dysfunction in acute kidney injury

Defects in energy generation

Mitochondrial dysfunction has long been considered to play a central role in the development of cell injury during ischemia-reperfusion and hypoxia-reoxygenation [22]. Besides the inhibition of fatty acid oxidation, mitochondrial energy generation is diminished because of defects in respiratory chain function. Inhibition of the F0-F1-ATPase leading to impaired function of respiratory complex I has been observed in I/R injury. Similar to ischemia, cisplatin has been shown to affect mitochondrial respiratory complexes and function 28]. Exposure of freshly isolated porcine proximal tubules to cisplatin resulted in loss of mitochondrial membrane potential as well and this decrease preceded cell death [29]. Cisplatin specifically inhibited complexes I to IV of the respiratory chain after 20 min incubation with 50 to 500 mM, respectively. As a result intracellular ATP was decreased to 70%. A recent study in rat kidney tissue examined the *in vivo* effects of cisplatin on mitochondrial bioenergetics, redox state, and oxidative stress as well as the occurrence of cell death. Cisplatin-induced mitochondrial dysfunction was characterized by a decline in membrane electrochemical potential and a substantial decrease in mitochondrial calcium uptake. The mitochondrial antioxidant defense system was depleted, as shown by decreased GSH and NADPH levels, GSH/GSSG ratio, and increased GSSG level. Moreover, cisplatin induced oxidative damage to mitochondrial lipids, including cardiolipin, and oxidation of mitochondrial proteins, as demonstrated by a significant decrease of sulfhydryl protein concentrations and increased levels of carbonylated proteins. Additionally, aconitase activity, which is essential for mitochondrial function, was also found to be lower in the cisplatin group. Renal cell death via apoptosis was evidenced by an increased caspase-3 activity. These studies further corroborate the central role of mitochondria and the intensification of apoptosis in cisplatin-induced acute kidney injury, highlighting a number of steps that might be targeted to minimize cisplatin-induced nephrotoxicity [21].

Structural abnormalities

Two structural abnormalities in the mitochondria are considered important pathogenetic factors during ischemia. One is characterized by pore formation in the inner mitochondrial membrane and high amplitude swelling (mitochondrial permeability transition or MPT) [30, 31]. The second involves leakage of cytochrome C from the inter-membrane space into the cytosol [32]. Because of its role as an electron shuttle, dislocation of cytochrome *c* compromises respiration [33, 34], and as a cytosolic cofactor cytochrome C activates caspase 9, and triggers apoptosis [33-35] (see below).

Cytochrome C release may follow the MPT or occur independently. In a recent study of cisplatin toxicity [35] decrease in oxidative phosphorylation was due to the inhibition of mitochondrial F0-F1-ATPase activity, but the decrease in oxidative phosphorylation was accompanied by hyperpolarization of the mitochondrial membrane rather than a decrease in membrane potential that is usually associated with the MPT [36]. The studies also demonstrate a marked decrease in active Na transport and Na-K-ATPase activity that paralleled the decrease in F0-F1-ATPase activity and preceded increases in membrane potential in cisplatin treated renal proximal tubular cells. These studies would suggest that cytochrome C release into the cytoplasm and the subsequent formation of the apoptosome (see below) may occur independently of the MPT and that the initiation of cell death by disruption of energy metabolism can directly engage the caspase cascade.

Caspases and cell death

Considerable evidence is accumulating to implicate the caspase pathway in the pathophysiology of acute kidney injury. Caspases are a family of cell death proteases [37] that play an essential role in the execution phase of apoptosis and act upstream of DNA fragmentation [38-43]. The term 'caspase' for the cell death proteases embodies two distinct catalytic properties of these enzymes such that 'c' refers to the cysteine protease and 'aspase' refers to their specific ability to cleave after an Asp amino acid [37]. The role of caspases in apoptosis was first recognized in 1993 [44] when it was discovered that the cell death gene CED3 in *Caenorhabditis elegans* has sequence homology to caspase-1, which was then called interleukin-1 b converting enzyme [44].

Thus far, 14 members of caspase family have been identified from mammalian cells [38, 40, 45, 46]. They are divided into two main subfamilies based on sequence homology to caspase-1 and CED3. Caspase-8, -10, -2, and -9 have larger prodomains and are termed initiator caspases, while caspases with smaller domains, caspase-3, -7 and -6, are termed executioner caspases. Caspase-1, -4, -5, -11, -12, and -13 play a role in inflammation [39, 40, 47]. Over-expression of executioner and initiator caspases in transfected cells results in DNA fragmentation and cell death in a variety of mammalian cell lines [47-49]. Caspases share many common features, such as: i) they are synthesized as inactive proenzymes in the cytosol of living cells. Each proenzyme is composed of three structural domains: a variable prodomain, a large subunit of about 20 kDa size and a small subunit of about 10 kDa size. On receiving an apoptotic stimuli, these domains are cleaved and the large and small subunits oligomerize to form an active enzyme [38, 49], ii) they are capable of initiating an apoptotic response when transfected into recipient cells [39-41, 43, 50], iii) they are inhibited by substrate-specific synthetic peptide inhibitors and by the baculovirus protein, p35, or by the poxvirus serpin, CrmA. In cell culture, these inhibitors suppress mammalian cell apoptosis; iv) caspases are very specific proteases with an absolute requirement for cleavage after aspartic acid in the target substrates; and v) the active site contains the sequence QACxG in which C is a catalytic cysteine [38, 43, 45, 48].

At present, there are two relatively well-characterized cell death pathways that result in the activation of executioner caspases (Figure 2). One is receptor-mediated and the other is mitochondrial-dependent. On receiving an apoptotic stimulus, the receptor-dependent pathway is initiated by activation of cell death receptors such as Fas and tumor necrosis factor. The death receptor stimulation results in the formation of a death inducing signaling complex (DISC) that recruits and activates procaspase-8, which in turn cleaves and activates downstream caspases, caspases-3, -6 and -7 [51, 52]. Receptor-induced cell death and caspase-8 activation is inhibited by the cowpox virus protein Crm A [53-55] but not by Bcl-2 [50]. The other pathway is mitochondrial-dependent and is triggered by cytochrome c release from the mitochondria, which promotes the activation of procaspase-9 through Apaf-1 and dATP. Activated caspase-9 then cleaves and activates pro-caspase-3 [57-59] An active site mutant of caspase-9 is able to block activation of caspase-3 by caspase-9 [60]. Overexpression of Bcl-2/BclxL blocks cytochrome c release and the apoptosis-induced mitochondrial changes [31, 60, 61]. Recent data [62, 63] demonstrate that rat kidney cortex transcribes genes encoding caspases -1, -2, -3, -6, -8, and -9.

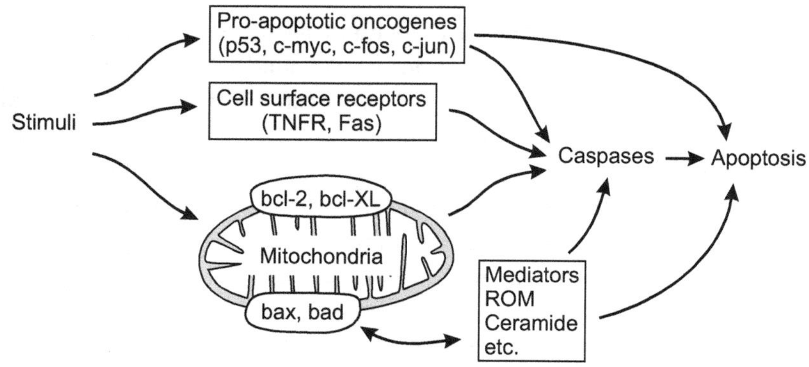

Figure 2. *Three pathways of caspases activation.*

In vitro evidence of caspase activation in cytotoxicity

In studies *in vitro*, caspases are involved in hypoxic [62, 64] injury to RTE cells. Antimycin A-induced chemical hypoxia [64] or growth under hypoxic conditions results in increased caspase activity and pancaspase inhibition prevents hypoxia-induced DNA fragmentation and cell death in RTE cells. Partial ATP depletion of MDCK cells by antimycin A was also shown to result in apoptosis with marked increase in activation of caspase-8 and inhibition of caspases provided marked protection against antimycin A-induced cell death [65]. Exposure of freshly isolated RTE to hypoxia resulted in caspase activation and cell membrane damage [66]. In a related study, activation of caspase-3 during hypoxia or ATP depletion was shown to be accompanied by bax translocation and cytochrome c release [67]. As in ischemia, cisplatin activates the caspase cascade as well. Cisplatin induces selective and differential activation of caspases including executioner caspase-3 and initiator **caspase-2,** -8 and -9 but not proinflammatory caspase-1 [76]. The activation of these caspases was markedly inhibited by their respective peptide inhibitors suggesting that these caspases may play an important role in cisplatin-induced injury to renal tubular epithelial cells. DEVD-CHO or LEHD-CHO, inhibitors of caspase-3 and caspase-9 respectively, provided partial protection against cisplatin-induced cell death and DNA damage in LLC-PK1 cells [68] indicating mechanisms other than caspase activation are also involved in cisplatin-induced cell death. Overexpression of crmA, a cowpox viral gene known to inhibit caspase-8, also provided protection against cisplatin-induced apoptosis in mouse proximal tubular cells [69] Thus, cisplatin-induced activation of caspase-8 and caspase-9 in renal proximal tubules indicate that both receptor and mitochondrial pathways participate in the activation process.

In vivo evidence of caspase activation in cytotoxicity

Renal ischemia/reperfusion injury *in vivo* activates caspase-1 and caspase-3 [62, 70]. In a murine model of ischemia/reperfusion injury, ZVAD-fmk, a pancaspase inhibitor, was shown to attenuate reperfusion-induced DNA damage (as determined by TUNEL assay) and inflammation [65]. Down-regulation of caspase-3 and caspase-8 by siRNA provided protection from acute kidney injury in a mice model of ischemia-reperfusion injury (71). Recent studies by Edelstein et al. [66, 72] help establish a link between the inflammatory aspects of the ischemic/reperfusion injury and caspase activation. In these studies it was observed that caspase 1 deficient mice were protected from ischemia-reperfusion injury. Aware that IL-18 is expressed after several cell stresses and is activated by caspase-1, the authors observed that IL-18 expression is increased in ischemia-reperfusion and caspase-1 converts IL-18 precursor to its active form. Furthermore in caspase-deficient mice the activity of IL-18 does not increase and the use of a neutralizing antibody to IL-18 offers protection in wild-type animals. The authors also demonstrate reduced leukocyte infiltration in caspase-1 deficient mice, completing a loop between cell injury, initiation of inflammation, and caspase-1 activation. Another study has demonstrated that caspase-3 activation during ischemia/reperfusion injury may be involved in the downregulation of calpastatin, an inhibitor of calpain [73] indicating a role of caspases for calpain activation during renal injury.

p53-dependent caspase activation in cisplatin injury to renal tubular epithelial cells *in vitro* and *in vivo*

Induction of p53 transcription factor in response to cisplatin has been demonstrated in renal tubular epithelial cells (RTEs) both *in vitro* [74-76] and *in vivo* [76, 77]. Similarly, activation of executioner caspases (caspase-3/7 and -6) was reported both *in vitro* [68, 78] and *in vivo* [76, 79, 80] models of cisplatin-induced acute kidney injury. Cisplatin-induced p53 activation significantly contributed to caspase-3 and caspase-2 activation in TKPTS as well as LLC-PK1 cells [76]. Down regulation of p53 by its siRNA or by p53 inhibitor pifithrin-α not only significantly blocked cisplatin-induced caspase-2 [76] and caspase-3 [74-76] activation but also cell death [74-76]. p53 is involved in cisplatin-induced activation of caspase-2 via p53-dependent PIDD induction. In RTE, the expression of the p53-responsive gene PIDD is induced by cisplatin as well as by overexpression of p53 [78] and results in activation of the Piddosome, a terniary complex required for activation of caspase-2. Caspases are also transcriptionally responsive to p53 in both *in vitro* cell cultures of RTEs and in an *in vivo* model of cisplatin nephrotoxicity (81). The executioner caspase-6 and -7 but not caspase-3 were identified as transcriptional targets of p53 [81]. p53-dependent increased production of procaspase-6 and -7 resulted in enhanced processing and activation of these caspases in cisplatin injury. Inhibition of p53 either by p53 inhibitor or using p53 (-/-) cells blocked activation of executioner caspases and provided marked protection from cisplatin-induced cell death *in vitro* in cell culture. p53 (-/-) mice ameliorated cisplatin-induced renal dysfunction and preserved kidney histology *in vivo* in cisplatin-induced acute kidney injury (81, 82). These studies suggest that p53 functions upstream of caspase-2 and -3 activation.

The Bcl-2 and the mitochondrial permeability transition: role in cell death

The essential role of cytochrome c release from injured mitochondria in the activation of caspase 9 has been alluded to above. This pathway is especially important in proapoptotic stimuli that are not initiated by surface receptors for apoptosis, such as UV irradiation, and may involve mitochondrial dependent pathways [83]. Continued respiration in the presence of an open mitochondrial pore may result in the generation of reactive oxygen species. Release of cytochrome c may be mediated by the opening of the mitochondrial PT pore, a non-selective channel whose composition is only partially defined [84]. Inhibitors of PT pore opening, such as cyclosporine, which binds to the adenine nucleotide translocator (ANT), a component of the PT pore, and bongkrekic acid, as well as Bcl-2, prevent cytochrome c release and inhibit apoptosis [85] whereas activators of the PT pore, such as atractyloside and Bax induce it [86]. Oxidants can rupture the outer membrane of mitochondria and release caspase-activating proteins [87]. Some studies have shown cytochrome c release before collapse of the mitochondrial membrane potential [83] suggesting alternate control of the PT pore. Many, but not all, of the members of the Bcl-2 family of proteins reside in the inner mitochondrial membrane, form ionic channels in lipid membranes and increase rates of proton extrusion in mitochondria [88] and thus may control the PT pore. The antiapoptotic and mitochondrial affects of Bcl-2 are independent of caspase activity as they occur in the presence of caspase inhibitors and also in yeast that lack caspases [86].

As pro- and anti-apoptotic members of the Bcl-2 family heterodimerize with each other, the relative concentration of the proapoptotic and pro-survival members may act as a rheostat for the suicide program [89]. Bax may have an independent role in apoptosis, as binding to Bcl-2 is controversial and it may damage organelles directly, a process that is inhibitable by Bcl-2 [57]. Bcl-2 has multiple antiapoptotic effects including binding to Apaf1 and preventing activation of Caspase 9 and inhibition of cytochrome c release from mitochondria [57]. The Bcl-2 proteins are regulated both transcriptionally and post transcriptionally. For example, Bad is induced transcriptionally as part of the p53-mediated damage response [90] and phosphorylated and sequestered after IL-3 addition to serum-starved hematopoietic cells. This pathway has been fully characterized and is mediated by activation of Akt/PKB [91].

The renal stress response determines whether cells survive or not

Molecular aspects

Exposure of renal cells to a hostile environment initiates a complex molecular response including the activation of phosphorylation cascades and the expression of many genes (Figure 3). Many of these molecular responses are not confined to areas of regeneration and in fact are localized to nephron segments not undergoing obvious injury or repair. For example, a typical immediate early gene response (IEG), as indicated by c-fos and c-jun activation, occurs most prominently in areas not undergoing an increase in DNA synthesis. Because the sites of increased DNA synthesis are spatially separated from those of IEG expression and many of the responses, including the expression of chemokine genes, resemble the response observed in cells exposed to adverse environmental conditions such as ionizing radiation, oxidants, and hypertonicity, the expression of these genes under these circumstances has been termed the Stress Response. ERK activation, an activator of the stress response (see below) is restricted during ischemia/reperfusion injury to surviving thick ascending limb (TAL) and not proximal tubules (PT), which undergo necrosis [92], further demonstrating the spatial separation of these responses. This response is thought to be a major determinant of whether cells survive the insult or not, and might be necessary for the repair of injured cells. Thus, the stress response may ultimately determine much of the proinflammatory, reparative, cytoreductive, and perhaps functional aspects of renal failure, as well as which cells survive the stress or not. Several elements in the stress pathway have been manipulated to effect whether cells survive a particular stress or not.

Signal transduction pathways in the stress response

At least two pathways lead to the activation of c-Jun, as outlined in a simplified form in (Figure 4). While both of these pathways converge on c-jun activation, their induction and effect on cell fate are quite different. Growth factors and phorbol esters activate c-Jun via the mitogen activated protein kinases (MAPKs), which include ERK-1 and 2. This pathway includes the activation of the MAPK kinases, MEK-1 and 2 and is most likely mediated through the activation of Ras and Raf 1. Although this cascade eventually leads to the activation of c-Jun, it does not appear to act directly on the c-Jun protein, but rather activates c-Fos, which in turn upregulates c-jun transcription via an AP-1 binding site.

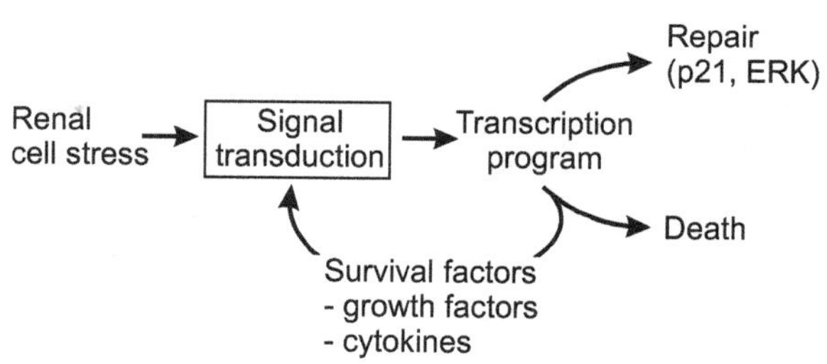

Figure 3. *Renal stress induces signal transduction and transcriptional programs that are modified by survival factors. The balance between the prosurvival or prodeath aspects of the stress response determines the ultimate fate of the cells.*

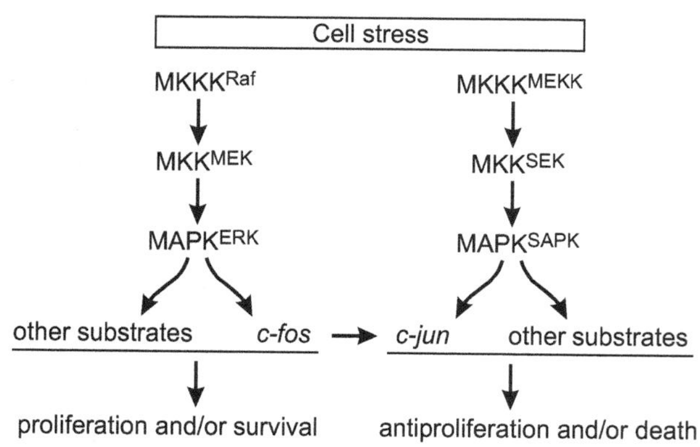

Figure 4. *Mitogen activated protein kinase pathways (MAPKs) initiated by cell stress. Note separation of MAPK^{ERK} and MAPK-^{SAPK} activation by distinct upstream kinases (see text).*

This pathway of activation is proliferative in nature. By contrast, oxidative stress and DNA damage, two stresses known to cause nephrotoxicity, increase c-fos and c-jun expression without provoking a proliferative response. The stress-associated expression of these genes is actually antiproliferative [93]. Analysis of the activation of c-Jun under these circumstances has led to the discovery of unique stress-induced protein kinases termed SAPKs (stress activated protein kinases) [94]. These kinases are comprised of the kinases JNK-1 and 2 (c-Jun N-terminal Kinase) and p38. Evidence to date suggests that the SAPKs are regulated by signal transduction paths separate from those that activate other MAPKs through distinct upstream regulators. JNK-1 and 2 have been shown to be the principal kinases responsible for c-Jun activation during oxidative stress and DNA damage while p38 seems to be the principal kinase activated by LPS and TNFa, all of which inhibit proliferation [95]. This activation of c-Jun is antiproliferative in nature and can lead to either cell survival or to cell death.

Nephrotoxicity and mitogen activated protein kinases

Kidney I/R activates ERK and SAPK [92, 93] and studies of the effect of ERK and JNK activation on renal cellular outcome have revealed that the consequence of this activation is cell type and stress specific. The activation of ERKs in oxidant stressed proximal tubules when sustained favors survival, while transient activation is not [96]. However activation of ERK provoked by cisplatin, which is sustained, is cytoreductive [97] indicating the complex nature of the response.

The epidermal growth factor receptor and survival signaling in nephrotoxicity

To gain insight into this phenomenon many laboratories have investigated the upstream regulators of the renal ERK pathway. Increased expression and activation of the epidermal growth factor receptor (EGFR) has been demonstrated after acute renal injury [98,99]. Activation of ERK can occur through the canonical EGFR-Raf-MEK kinase module [100] whereby the activated EGFR is directly connected to the Ras/Raf/MEK/ERK pathway. EGF and EGF-like ligands bind and activate the intrinsic tyrosine kinase activity of the EGF receptor and initiate autophosphorylation of various tyrosine residues. The phosphorylation creates docking sites for the recruitment of signaling mediators that are required for the activation of downstream targets such as Ras and ERK. The adaptor protein Grb2 binds to the EGFR phosphotyrosine residues and brings the SOS (son-of-sevenless) protein from the cytoplasm to the vicinity of Ras **(34)**. In addition, the Grb2/SOS complexes can be recruited to the EGFR through the Shc proteins, as well [101]. Shc binding to the receptor docking site results in its tyrosine phosphorylation and thus, provides additional docking sites for Grb2 [102]. The mammalian Shc A locus encodes three proteins, p46shc, p52shc and p66shc, respectively. All of these three Shc isoforms become phosphorylated at tyrosine residues upon activation of EGFR and form stable complexes with Grb2, an adaptor protein for the Ras exchange factor SOS [101]. The recruitment of the SOS-Grb2-Shc complex activates Ras, which initiates a cascade of downstream phosphorylation events. Ras then activates Raf-1, a serine kinase, which in turn phosphorylates and activates MEK1, which then activates ERKs. This pathway is referred to as the canonical EGFR-ERK pathway.

H_2O_2 itself induces phosphorylation of the EGFR and can initiate signaling through the Shc/Grb2/SOS complexes and the Raf-MEK module [103]. Interestingly, the duration of ERK activation was determined by ROS levels: moderate ROS (EGF or 0.5 mM H_2O_2) induced sustained ERK activation while high levels of ROS (1 mM H_2O_2).

Abrogation of EGFR-derived survival signaling by stress

Activation of proximal tubule EGFR occurs in the kidney during ischemia/reperfusion [104], yet activation of ERK or other downstream elements of the canonical pathway has not been observed in these segments following I/R injury. At least two proteins have been shown to play a role in abrogation of EGFR-derived survival signaling (Figure 5). The p66shc adaptor protein [105] is involved in signal transduction pathways that regulate cellular responses to oxidative stress and life span. Its absence increases resistance to oxidant injury and increases survival [106]. p66shc responds to increasing intracellular ROS production by changes in its phosphorylation state as well as its intracellular trafficking. Oxidative stress phosphorylates p66shc at its

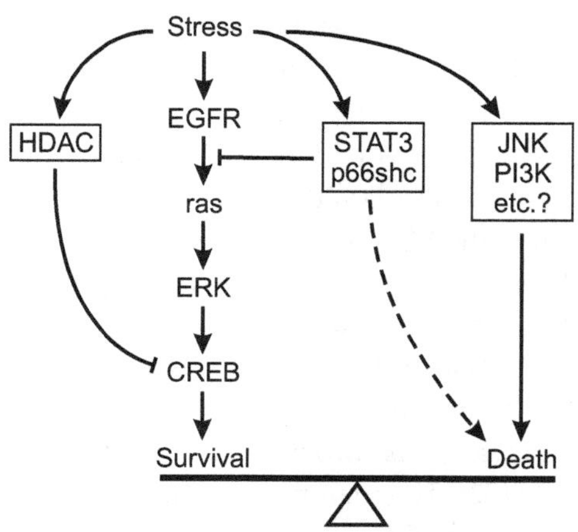

***Figure 5.** Interacting pathways that attenuate the EGFR-mediated survival signaling during stress.*

serine36 residue, which in turn terminates EGFR-mediated ERK activation by interfering with the recruitment of essential signaling proteins to the EGFR [106]. These observations suggest a central role for p66Shc in executing a death pathway by suppressing the EGFR survival signaling. Serine36 phosphorylation of p66shc occurs in both the kidney and in proximal tubule cells *in vitro* [107] during severe oxidant stress and leads to disruption of the EGFR/Grb2/SOS complex and consequent termination of ras/ERK activation [107]. Isoform specific knockdown of p66shc or mutation of the Serine36 residue to alanine but not to aspartic acid (a phosphomimetic mutant) restored ERK activation and survival of proximal tubular cells [107].

Another mechanism by which EGFR activation of ERK may be abrogated is via ROS-induced *JAK/STAT* activation [108], which has been observed in I/R injury [109]. H_2O_2 triggers STAT3 tyrosine phosphorylation and its nuclear translocation in human lymphocytes [9] and subsequent cell death. Activation of STAT3 could be mediated by the EGFR, JAK2 or ERK itself [110]. One function of STAT3 appears to be the downregulation of ERK1/2 activation [113] most probably mediated through STAT3 binding to the EGFR [112-114] and subsequent displacement of Grb2 and interruption in ERK activation after 1 mM H_2O_2 treatment.

These observations on p66Shc and Jak2/Stat3 pathways bring into focus many aspects of alternate signaling that may contribute to the death of cells undergoing severe oxidant stress even in the presence of an activated EGFR. They also suggest potential targets to restore EGFR survival signaling to improve survival of renal epithelial cells exposed to severe oxidant stress.

The cAMP responsive element binding protein, or CREB, seems to be an important downstream survival target of ERK. CREB is a transcription factor with multiple functions [115, 116] and is believed to play a key role in cell survival [117-120]. Oxidant injury regulates the activity of CREB and thus survival [121-124]. CREB activation occurs via phosphorylation at serine 133 (Ser133) by various kinases including MAPKs [115-116]: ERK phosphorylates CREB through p90rsk [117, 125]. Once activated, CREB regulates transcription of an array of genes that harbor the CREB binding site (CRE) in their promoter proximal region including those with survival function [115-116].

In vitro experiments using pharmacological inhibitors, constitutively active and dominant-negative mutants of ERK and CREB demonstrated that CREB-driven transcription is a crucial element in survival of proximal tubule cells from both oxidative and cisplatin-induced stress. Binding of phosphorylated CREB to a CREB consensus DNA element or CREB-mediated transcription was significantly decreased during oxidative injury consistent with its role in survival. I/R injury activates CREB in the surviving distal nephron segments of the kidney only [126], consistent with its pro-survival role. The identification of the key elements in CREB-driven transcription vital for survival is a fruitful area of continued research (Figure 4).

Renal stress engages the cell cycle and is a determinant of cytotoxicity

Shortly after acute kidney injury many normally quiescent kidney cells enter the cell cycle. Orderly progression through the cell cycle is regulated by sequential synthesis, activation, compartmentalization and degradation of proteins controlling both entry and exit from each of the four phases of the cycle: G1 (gap-1), S (DNA synthesis), G2 (gap-2) and M (mitosis) (Figure 6). Control of the various phases of the growth cycle is exerted by the cyclical activation and repression of the cyclin-dependent kinases. Two important regulators of the cell cycle have been now shown to participate in acute kidney injury. One family of proteins, the cyclin-dependent kinase inhibitors, which bind to and inhibit assembled cyclin kinases,

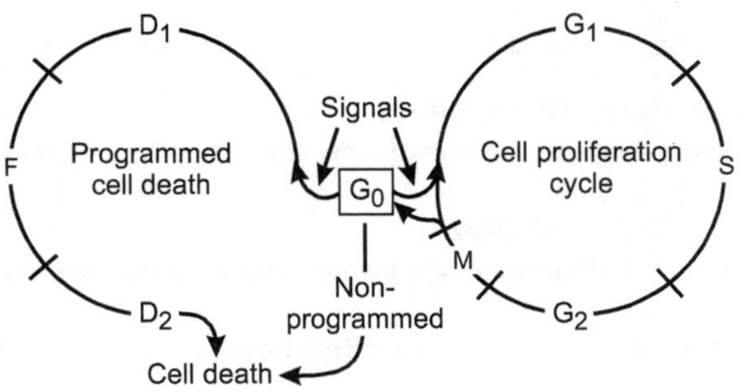

Figure 6. *The cell cycle and stress. Note proliferative and apoptotic pathways are engaged by common stresses. The link between cell stress and these two pathways is an area of intense investigation.*

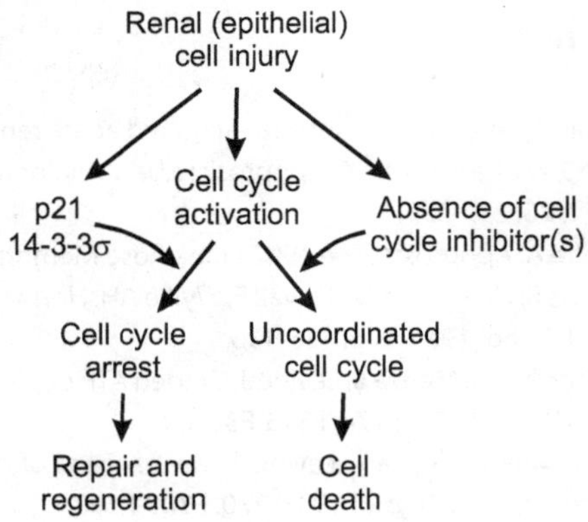

Figure 7. *Renal stress induces signal transduction and transcriptional programs that are modified by survival factors. The balance between the prosurvival or prodeath aspects of the stress response determines the ultimate fate of the cells.*

and in particular the cyclin-dependent kinase inhibitor protein p21 is expressed in all forms of renal failure studied, including ischemia-reperfusion, cisplatin and obstructive uropathy [127]. This protein controls a cell cycle checkpoint by binding the CDKs that regulate the G1/S to G2/M transition. The function of these checkpoints is to monitor the fidelity of DNA replication and other macromolecular components of the cell necessary for accurate replication. The absence of these checkpoints leads to uncoordinated replication and leads ultimately to cell death, so that the expression of p21 is antiapoptotic in most situations studied. It has been shown that mice lacking the p21 gene are more sensitive to ischemic and cisplatin nephrotoxicity [128, 129]. Similarly, antiapoptotic properties of p21 can be used to protect from renal cellular cytotoxicity, both *in vitro* and *in vivo*, by the use of p21 protein expression or by drugs that have modes of action similar to p21 [130-132]. The protective provenance of p21 was found to be solely its inhibition of cdk2, a cell cycle-associated kinase primarily active during late G1 through S phases [131]. Thus cell cycle control, initially manifested as cdk2 inhibition, is necessary for optimal recovery from acute kidney injury, and can even be used to ameliorate acute kidney injury (Figure 7). How the cell cycle machinery merges with the executioner pathways is an exciting new area of research in acute kidney injury.

Summary

Cell death, survival and repair are intimately interrelated after renal injury. Disordered energy production is common to each of the models and may be part of the stress response. Of particular interest in this regard is the inhibition of fatty acid oxidation in mitochondrial and peroxisomal compartments. The caspases seem to play a key role in executing cell death whether the outcome is necrosis or apoptosis. The stress response characterized by transduction pathways and gene transcription that serve both positive and negative aspects of cell survival is intimately involved in the outcome of ischemic and nephrotoxic damage. The cell cycle and its regulation are key components of the life and death of the stressed cells throughout the kidney. Some cells participating in this response will survive and repair, whereas others will die (Figure 7). What determines whether a cell will recover from such injury or undergo cell death by necrosis or apoptosis is probably a function of the severity of the stress, the specific changes in gene regulation that the cell is capable of mounting, and the availability of survival factors in the cell's external milieu. Augmentation of the positive aspects of the stress pathway while carefully regulating the negative ones is a reasonable approach to altering the outcome of exposure to a nephrotoxic insult.

References

1. Nolan C, Anderson R. Hospital-acquired acute renal failure. J Am Soc Nephrol 1998; 9: 710-718.
2. Kerr J, Wyllie A, Currie A. Apoptosis: a basic biological phenomenon with wide-ranging implications in tissue kinetics. Br J Cancer 1972; 26: 239-257.
3. Wyllie A. Apoptosis (The 1992 Frank Rose Memorial Lecture). Br J Cancer 2001; 67: 205-208.
4. Morris R, Hargreaves A, Duvall E, Wyllie AH. Hormone-induced cell death: surface changes in thymocytes undergoing apoptosis. Am J Pathol 1984; 115: 426-436.
5. Lieberthal W, Menza S, Levine J. Graded ATP depletion can cause necrosis or apoptosis of cultured mouse proximal tubular cells. Am J Physiol 1998; 274: F315-F327.
6. Lieberthal W, Triaca V, Levine J. Mechanisms of death induced by cisplatin in proximal tubular epithelial cells: apoptosis vs. necrosis. Am J Physiol 1996; 270: F700-F708.
7. Ueda N, Walker P, Hsu S, Shah SV. Activation of a 15-kDa endonuclease in hypoxia/reoxygenation injury without morphologic features of apoptosis. Proc Natl Acad Sci USA 1995; 92: 7202-7206.
8. Iwata M, Myerson D, Torok-Storb B, Zager RA. An evaluation of renal tubular DNA laddering in response to oxygen deprivation and oxidant injury. J Am Soc Nephrol 1994; 5: 1307-1313.
9. LeHir M, Dubach U. Distribution of two enzymes of b-oxidation of fatty acids along the rat nephron; in Anonymous Biochemistry of kidney functions. Elsevier Biochemical Press, Amsterdam 1982, 82-94.
10. LeHir M, Dubach U. Peroxisomal and mitochondrial b-oxidation in the rat kidney. Distribution of fatty acyl coenzyme A oxidase and 3-hydroxyacyl-coenzyme A dehydrogenase activities along the nephron. J Histochem Cytochem 1982; 30: 441-444.
11. Bell D, Bars R, Elcombe C. Differential tissue-specific expression and induction of cytochrome P450IVA1 and acyl-CoA oxidase. Eur J Biochem 1992; 206: 979-986.
12. Portilla D, Dai G, Peters JM, Gonzalez FJ, Crew MD, Proia AD. Etomoxir-induced PPARa-modulated enzymes protects during acute renal failure. Am J Physiol 2000; 278: F667-F675.
13. Portilla D, Dai G, McClure T, Bates L, Kurten R, Megyesi J, Price P, Li S. Alterations of PPARa and its Coactivator PGC-1 in Cisplatin-induced acute renal failure. Kidney Int 2002; 62: 1208-1218.
14. Li S, Wu P, Proia A, Megyesi J, Li S, Harris RH, Portilla D. PPARalpha ligands protect during cisplatin-induced ARF by preventing inhibition of renal FAO and PDC activity, Am J Physiol Renal Physiol. 2004 Mar;286(3):F572-80. Epub 2003 Nov 11.
15. Li S., Bhatt R., Megyesi J., Gokden N., Shah S.V., Portilla D.. PPARalpha ligand ameliorates acute renal failure by reducing cisplatin-induced increased expression of Renal Endonuclease G. Am J Physiol Renal Physiol, 2004; 286:F572-F580.
16. Li S, Gokden N, Okusa M, Bhatt R, Portilla D Anti-inflammatory effect of fibrate protects from cisplatin induced ARF. Am J of Physiol Renal Physiol, 2005; 289:F469-F480.
17. Nagothu KK, Bhatt R, Kaushal GP, Portilla D Fibrate prevents cisplatin-induced proximal tubule cell death Kid International 2005; 68: 2680-2693.
18. Portilla D, Li S, Nagothu KK, Megyesi J, Kaissling B, Schackenberg L, Safirstein RL, Beger RD Metabolomic study of cisplatin-induced nephrotoxicity Kid International,2006; 69, 2194-2204.
19. Negishi K., Noiri E., Sugaya T, Li S, Megyesi J., Nagothu KK, Portilla D. Role of L-FABP in cisplatin induced acute renal failure. Kidney Int 2007; Aug: 72(3):348-358.
20. Portilla D, Schnackenberg L, Beger R. Metabolomics as an extension of proteomic analysis: Study of acute kidney injury Seminars in Nephrology, Nov 2007; 27 (6): 609-620.
21. Santos NA, Catao CS, Martins NM, Curti C, Bianchi ML, Santos AC Cisplatin-induced nephrotoxicity is associated with oxidative stress, redox state unbalance, impairment of energetic metabolism and apoptosis in rat kidney mitochondria Arch Toxicol 2007 Jul; 81 (7):495-504.
22. Vega R, Huss J, Kelly D. the coactivator PGC-1 cooperates with peroxisome proliferator-activated receptor a in transcriptional of nuclear genes encoding mitochondrial fatty acid oxidation enzymes. Mol Cell Biol 2000; 20: 1868-1876.
23. Lemasters JJ, Nieminen AL, Qian T, Trost LC, Herman B. The mitochondrial permeability transition in toxic, hypoxic and reperfusion injury. Mol Cell Biochem 1997; 174: 159-165.
24. Kroemer G, Dallaporta B, Resche-Rigon M. The mitochondrial death/life regulator in apoptosis and necrosis. Ann Rev Physiol 1998; 60: 619-642.
25. Scarpulla R. Nuclear control of respiratory chain expression in mammalian cells. J Bioenerg Biomembr 1997;29:109-119.
26. Virbasius J, Scarpulla R. Activation of the human mitochondrial transcription factor A gene by nuclear respiratory factors: A potential regulatory link between nuclear and mitochondrial gene expression in organelle biogenesis. Proc Natl Acad Sci 1994;91:1309-1313.

27. Di Mari J, Davis R, Safirstein R. MAPK activation determines renal epithelial cell survival during oxidative injury. Am J Physiol 1999; 277:F195-F203.
28. Walker P, Shah S Hydrogen Peroxide cytotoxicity on LLC-PK1 cells: a role for iron. Kidney Int 1991;40:891-898.
29. Kruidering M, Van de Water b, de Heer E, Mulder GJ, Nagelkerke JF. Cisplatin-induced nephrotoxicity in porcine proximal tubular cells: Mitochondrial dysfunction by inhibition of complexes I to IV of the respiratory chain. J Pharmacol Exp 1997;280:638-649.
30. Gunter T, Pfeiffer D. Mechanisms by which mitochondria transport calcium. Am J. Physiol 1990; 258:C755-C786 (Abstract).
31. Lemasters JJ, Nieminen AL, Qian T, Trost LC, Herman B. The mitochondrial permeability transition in toxic, hypoxic and reperfusion injury. Mol Cell Biochem 1997; 174:159-165.
32. Kroemer G, Dallaporta B, Resche-Rigon M. The mitochondrial death/life regulator in apoptosis and necrosis. An Rev Physiol 1998; 60: 619-642.
33. Saikumar P, Dong Z, Weinberg JM, Venkatachalam MA. Mechanisms of cell death in hypoxia/reoxygenation injury. Oncogene 1998; 17: 3341-3349.
34. Varnes ME, Chiu SM, Xue LY, Oleinick NL. Photodynamic therapy-induced apoptosis in lymphoma cells: translocation of cytochrome c causes inhibition of respiration as well as caspase activation. Biochem Biophys Res Commun 1999; 255: 673-679.
35. Nowak G. Protein kinase C-a and ERK ½ mediate mitochondrial dysfunction, decreases in Active Na+ transport, and cisplatin-induced apoptosis in renal cells. J Biol Chem 2002;277:43377-43388.
36. Dzeja PP, Homuhamedov EL, Ozcan C, Pucar D, Jahangir A, Terzic A. Mitochondria: gateway for cytoprotection. Circ Res 2001;89:744-746.
37. Alnemri ES, Livingston DJ, Nicholson DW, Salvesen G, Thornberry NA, Wong WW, Yuan J. Human ICE/CED-3 protease nomenclature. Cell 1996; 87: 171.
38. Thornberry N, Lazebnik Y. Caspases: enemies within. Science 1998; 281: 1312-1316.
39. Fraser A, Evan G. A license to kill. Cell 1996; 85: 781-786.
40. Earnshaw W, Martins L, Kaufmann S. Mammalian caspases: structure, activation, substrates, and functions during apoptosis. Annu Rev Biochem 1999; 68: 383-424.
41. Cryns V, Yuan J. Proteases to die for. Genes Dev 1998; 12: 1551-1570.
42. Vaux D. Caspases and apoptosis-biology and terminology. Cell Death Differ 1999; 6: 493-494.
43. Nicholson D. Caspase structure, proteolytic substrates, and function during apoptotic cell death. Cell Death Differ 1999; 6: 1028-1042.
44. Yuan J, Shaham S, Ledoux S, Ellis HM, Horvitz HR. The C. elegans cell death gene ced-3 encodes a protein similar to mammalian interleukin-1b-converting enzyme. Cell 1993; 75: 641-652.
45 Wolf B, Green D. Suicidal tendencies: apoptotic cell death by caspase family proteinases. J Biol Chem 1999; 274: 20049-20052.
46 Ahmad M, Srinivasula SM, Hegde R, Mukattash R, Fernandes-Alnemri T, Alnemri ES. Identification and characterization of murine caspase 14, a new member of the caspase family. Cancer Res 1998; 58: 5201-5205.
47. Salvesen G, Dixit V. Caspases: intracellular signaling by proteolysis. Cell 1997; 91: 443-446.
48. Cohen G. Caspases: the executioners of apoptosis. Biochem J 1997; 326: 1-16.
49. Nicholson D, Thornberry N. Caspases: killer proteases. Trends Biochem Sci 1997; 257: 299-306.
50. Nagata S. Apoptosis by death factor. Cell 1997; 88: 355-365.
51. Boldin MP, Goncharov TM, Goltsev YV, Wallach D. Involvement of Mach, a novel MORT1/FADD-interacting protease, in Fas/APO-1 and TNF receptor-induced cell death. Cell 1996; 85: 803-815.
52. Kischkel FC, Hellbardt S, Behrmann I, Germer M, Pawlita M, Krammer PH, Peter ME. Cytotoxicity-dependent APO-1 (Fas/CD95)-associated proteins form a death-inducing signaling complex (DISC) with the receptor. EMBO J 1995; 14: 5579-5588.
53. Takahashi A, Hirata H, Yonehara S, Imai Y, Lee KK, Moyer RW, Turner PC, Mesner PW, Okazaki T, Sawai H, Kishi S, Yamamoto K, Okuma M, Sasada M. Affinity labeling displays the stepwise activation of ICE-related proteases by Fas, staurosporine, and CrmA-sensitive caspase-8. Oncogene 1997; 14: 2741-2752.
54. Tewari M, Dixit V. Fas and tumor necrosis factor-induced apoptosis is inhibited by the poxvirus crmA gene product. J Biol Chem 1995; 270: 3255-3260.
55. Miura M, Friedlander R, Yuan J: Tumor necrosis factor-induced apoptosis is mediated by a CrmA-sensitive cell death pathway. Proc Natl Acad Sci USA 1995; 92: 8318-8322.
56. Newton K, Strasser A. The Bcl-2 family and cell death regulation. Curr Opin Genet Dev 1998; 8: 68-75.
57. Green D, Reed J. Mitochondria and apoptosis. Science 1998; 281: 1309-1312.
58. Li P, Nijhawan D, Budihardjo I, Srinivasula SM, Ahmad M, Alnemri ES, Wang X. Cytochrome c and dATP-dependent formation of apaf-1/caspase-9 complex initiates an apoptotic protease cascade. Cell 1997; 91: 479-489.
59. Zou H, Henzel WJ, Liu X, Lutschg A, Wang X. Apaf-1, a human protein homologous to C. elegans CED-4, participates in cytochrome c-dependent activation of caspase-3. Cell 1997; 90: 405-413.

60. Vander Heiden MG, Chandel NS, Williamson EK, Schumacker PT, Thompson CB. Bcl-xl regulate the membrane potential and volume homeostasis of mitochondria. Cell 1997; 91: 627-637.

61 Zamzami N, Marchetti P, Castedo M, Hirsch T, Susin SA, Masse B, Kroemer G. Inhibitors of permeability transition interfere with the disruption of the mitochondrial transmembrane potential during apoptosis. FEBS Lett 1996; 384: 53-57.

62. Kaushal G, Singh A, Shah S. Identification of caspase (ICE-like proteases) gene family in rat kidney and altered expression in ischemia/reperfusion injury. Am J Physiol 1998; 274: F587-F595.

63. Kaushal G, Singh A, Shah S. Caspases in kidney: cloning, expression and alteration in ischemia/reperfusion injury. J Am Soc Nephrol 1998; 9: 579A.

64. Kaushal G, Ueda N, Shah S. Role of caspases (ICE/CED 3 proteases) in DNA damage and cell death in hypoxic injury. Kidney Int 1997;52:438-445.

65. Feldenberg LR, Thevananther S, del Rio M, de Leon M, Devarajan P. Partial ATP depletion induces Eas-and caspase-medicated apoptosis in MDCK cells. Am J Physiol 1999; 276:F837-F9846.

66. Edelstein C, Shi Y, Schrier R. Role of caspases in hypoxia-induced necrosis of rat renal proximal tubules. J Am Soc Nephrol 1999; 10: 1940-1949.

67. Saikumar P, Dong Z, Patel Y, Hall K, Hopfer U, Weinberg JM, Venkatachalam MA. Role of hypoxia-induced Bax translocation and cytochrome c release in reoxygenation injury. Oncogene 1998; 17: 3401-3415.

68. Kaushal GP, Kaushal V, Hong X, Shah SV. Role of caspases and their regulation by Akt/protein kinase B phosphorylation pathway in cisplatin-induced injury to renal tubular epithelial cells. Kidney Int 2001; 60: 1726-1736.

69. Takeda M, Kobayashi M, Shirato I, Osaki T, Endou H. Cisplatin-induced apoptosis of immortalized mouse proximal tubule cells is mediated by interleukin-1b converting enzyme (ICE) family of proteases but inhibited by overexpression of Bcl-2. Arch Toxicol 1997; 71: 612-621.

70. Daemen MA, van 't Veer C, Denecker G, Heemskerk VH, Wolfs TG, Clauss M, Vandenabeele P, Buurman WA. Inhibition of apoptosis induced by ischemia/reperfusion prevents inflammation. J Clin Invest 1999; 104: 541-549.

71. Zhang X, Zheng X, Sun H, Feng B, Chen G, Vladau C, Li M, Chen D, Suzuki M, Min L, Liu W, Garcia B, Zhong R, Min WP. Prevention of renal ischemic injury by silencing the expression of renal caspase 3 and caspase 8. Transplantation. 2006;82(12):1728-1732.

72. Melnikov VY, Ecder T, Fantuzzi G, Siegmund B, Lucia MS, Dinarello CA, Schrier RW, Edelstein CL. Impaired IL-18 processing protects caspase-1-deficient mice from ischemic acute renal failure. J Clin Invest 2001; 107: 1145-1152.

73. Shi Y, Melnikov VY, Schrier RW, Edelstein CL. Down-regulation of the calpain inhibitor protein, calpastatin, by caspases during renal ischemia. Am J Physiol 2000; 279: F509-F517.

74. Cummings BS, Schnellmann RG. Cisplatin-induced renal cell apoptosis: caspase 3-dependent and -independent pathways. J Pharmacol Exp Ther 2002; 302: 8–17

75. Jiang M, Yi X, Hsu S, Wang CY, Dong Z. Role of p53 in cisplatin-induced tubular cell apoptosis: dependence on p53 transcriptional activity. Am J Physiol Renal Physiol 2004; 287: F1140–F1147.

76. Seth R, Yang C, Kaushal V, Shah SV, Kaushal GP. p53-dependent caspase-2 activation in mitochondrial release of apoptosis-inducing factor and its role in renal tubular epithelial cell injury. J Biol Chem 2005; 280: 31230–31239.

77. Megyesi J, Udvarhelyi N, Safirstein RL, Price PM. The p53-independent activation of transcription of p21 WAF1/CIP1/SDI1 after acute renal failure. Am J Physiol 1996; 271: F1211–F1216.

78. Tsuruya K, Ninomiya T, Tokumoto M, Hirakawa M, Masutani K, Taniguchi M *et al.* Direct involvement of the receptor-mediated apoptotic pathways in cisplatin-induced renal tubular cell death. Kidney Int 2003; 63: 72–82.

79. Sheikh-Hamad D, Cacini W, Buckley AR, Isaac J, Truong LD, Tsao CC *et al.* Cellular and molecular studies on cisplatin-induced apoptotic cell death in rat kidney. Arch Toxicol 2004; 78: 147–155.

80. Faubel S, Ljubanovic D, Reznikov L, Somerset H, Dinarello CA, Edelstein CL. Caspase-1-deficient mice are protected against cisplatin-induced apoptosis and acute tubular necrosis. Kidney Int 2004; 66: 2202–2213.

81. Yang C, Kaushal V, Haun RS, Seth R, Shah SV, Kaushal GP. Transcriptional activation of caspase-6 and -7 genes by cisplatin-induced p53 and its functional significance in cisplatin nephrotoxicity. Cell Death and Dfferentiation, 2008; 15: 530–544.

82. Wei Q, Dong G, Yang T, Megyesi J, Price PM, Dong Z. Activation and involvement of p53 in cisplatin-induced nephrotoxicity. Am J Physiol Renal Physiol. 2007;293(4):F1282-91.

83. Bossy-Wetzel E, Newmeyer D, Green D. Mitochondrial cytochrome c release in apoptosis occurs upstream of DEVD-specific caspase activation and independently of mitochondrial transmembrane depolarization. EMBO J 1997; 17: 37-49.

84. Qian T, Nieminen AL, Herman B, Lemasters JJ. Mitochondrial permeability transition in pH-dependent reperfusion injury to rat hepatocytes. Am J Physiol 1997; 273: C1783-C1792.

85. Zamzami N, Susin SA, Marchetti P, Hirsch T, Gomez-Monterrey I, Castedo M, Kroemer G. Mitochondrial control of nuclear apoptosis. J Exp Med 1996; 183: 1533-1544.

86. Xiang J, Chao D, Korsmeyer S. BAX-induced cell death may not require interleukin 1 b-converting enzyme-like proteases. Proc Natl Acad Sci USA 1996; 93:14559-14563.
87. Susin SA, Zamzami N, Castedo M, Hirsch T, Marchetti P, Macho A, Daugas E, Geuskens M, Kroemer G. Bcl-2 inhibits the mtiochondrial release of an apoptogenic protease. J Exp Med 1996; 184:1331-1341.
88. Schendel SL, Xie Z, Montal MO, Matsuyama S, Montal M, Reed JC. Channel formation by antiapoptotic protein Bcl-2. Proc Natl Acad Sci USA 1997;94:5113-5118.
89. Oltvai Z, Korsmeyer S. Checkpoints of dueling dimers foil death wishes. Cell 1994; 79:189-192.
90. Han J, Sabbatini P, Perez D, Rao L, Modha D, White E. The E1B 19K protein blocks apoptosis by interacting with and inhibiting the p53-inducible and death-promoting Bax protein. Genes Dev 1996;10:461-477.
91. Cardone MH, Roy N, Stennicke HR, Salvesen GS, Franke TF, Stanbridge E, Frisch S, Reed JC. Regulation of cell death protease casepase-9 by phosphorylation. Science 1998;282:1318-1321.
92 di Mari JF, Davis R, Safirstein RL. MAPK activation determines renal epithelial cell survival during oxidative injury. American Journal of Physiology Renal Physiology 277: F195-203, 1999.
93. Park KM, Kramers C, Vayssier-Taussat M, Chen A, Bonventre JV. Prevention of Kidney Ischemia/Reperfusion-induced Functional Injury, MAPK and MAPK Kinase Activation, and Inflammation by Remote Transient Ureteral Obstruction. J Biol Chem, 2002;277: 2040-2049.
94. Blagosklonny MV. A node between proliferation, apoptosis, and growth arrest. Bioessays, 1999;21: 704-709.
95. Roovers K, Assoian RK. Integrating the MAP kinase signal into the G1 phase cell cycle machinery. Bioessays 2000;22: 818-826.
96. Arany I, Megyesi JK, Kaneto H, Tanaka S, Safirstein RL. Activation of ERK or inhibition of JNK ameliorates H2O2 cytotoxicity in mouse renal proximal tubule cells. Kidney Int, 2004;65: 1231-1239.
97. Arany I, Megyesi JK, Kaneto H *et al.* Cisplatin-induced cell death is EGFR/src/ERK signaling dependent in mouse proximal tubule cells. Am J Physiol Renal Physiol 2004; 287: F543–F549.
98. Wang Z, Chen JK, Wang SW, Moeckel G, Harris RC. Importance of functional EGF receptors in recovery from acute nephrotoxic injury. J Am Soc Nephrol, 2003;14: 3147-3154.
99. Harris RC. Potential physiologic roles for epidermal growth factor in the kidney. Am J Kidney Dis, 1991; 17: 627-630.
100. English J, Pearson G, Wilsbacher J, Swantek J, Karandikar M, Xu S, Cobb MH. New insights into the control of MAP kinase pathways. Exp Cell Res, *1999*;253: 255-270.
101. Bonfini L, Migliaccio E, Pelicci G, Lanfrancone L, Pelicci PG. Not all Shc's roads lead to Ras. Trends Biochem Sci 1996;21: 257-261.
102. Schlessinger J. How receptor tyrosine kinases activate Ras. Trends Biochem Sci 1993;18: 273-275.
103. Rao GN. Hydrogen peroxide induces complex formation of SHC-Grb2-SOS with receptor tyrosine kinase and activates Ras and extracellular signal-regulated protein kinases group of mitogen-activated protein kinases. Oncogene, 1996; 13: 713-719.
104. Safirstein R, Price PM, Saggi SJ, Harris RC. Changes in gene expression after temporary renal ischemia. Kidney Int 1990;37: 1515-1521.
105. Pellegrini M, Pacini S, Baldari CT. p66SHC: the apoptotic side of Shc proteins. Apoptosis,2005;10: 13-18.
106. Purdom S, Chen QM. p66(Shc): at the crossroad of oxidative stress and the genetics of aging. Trends Mol Med,2003;9: 206-210.
107. Arany I, Faisal A, Nagamine Y, Safirstein RL. P66SHC inhibits the pro-survival EGFR/ERK signaling during severe oxidative stress in mouse renal proximal tubule cells. J Biol Chem 2008.
108. Simon AR, Rai U, Fanburg BL, Cochran BH. Activation of the JAK-STAT pathway by reactive oxygen species. American Journal of Physiology; Cell Physiology, 1998; 275: C1640-1652.
109. Stephanou A. Role of STAT-1 and STAT-3 in ischaemia/reperfusion injury. J Cell Mol Med, 2004; 8: 519-525.
110. Vinkemeier U. Getting the message across, STAT! Design principles of a molecular signaling circuit. J Cell Biol, 2004;167: 197-201.
111. Kritikou EA, Sharkey A, Abell K, Came PJ, Anderson E, Clarkson RWE, Watson CJ. A dual, non-redundant, role for LIF as a regulator of development and STAT3-mediated cell death in mammary gland. Development, 2003;130: 3459-3468.
112. Shao H, Cheng HY, Cook RG, Tweardy DJ. Identification and characterization of signal transducer and activator of transcription 3 recruitment sites within the epidermal growth factor receptor. Cancer Res, 2003, 63: 3923-3930.
113. Xia L, Wang L, Chung AS, Ivanov SS, Ling MY, Dragoi AM, Platt A, Gilmer TM, Fu X-Y, Chin YE. Identification of Both Positive and Negative Domains within the Epidermal Growth Factor Receptor COOH-terminal Region for Signal Transducer and Activator of Transcription (STAT) Activation. J Biol Chem, 2003; 277: 30716-30723.
114. Zhang T, Ma J, Cao X. Grb2 regulates Stat3 activation negatively in epidermal growth factor signaling. Biochem J, 2003;376: 457-464.
115. Mayr B, Montminy M. Transcriptional regulation by the phosphorylation-dependent factor CREB. Nat Rev Mol Cell Biol, 2001; 2: 599-609, 2001.

116. Shaywitz AJ, Greenberg ME. CREB: a stimulus-induced transcription factor activated by a diverse array of extracellular signals. Annu Rev Biochem,1999;68: 821-861.
117. Bonni A, Brunet A, West AE, Datta SR, Takasu MA, Greenberg ME. Cell survival promoted by the Ras-MAPK signaling pathway by transcription-dependent and -independent mechanisms. Science,1999;286: 1358-1362.
118. Du K, and Montminy M. CREB Is a Regulatory Target for the Protein Kinase Akt/PKB. J Biol Chem,1998;273: 32377-32379.
119. Walton MR, and Dragunow I. Is CREB a key to neuronal survival? Trends Neurosc,2000; 23: 48-53.
120. Yamada M, Tanabe K, Wada K, Shimoke K, Ishikawa Y, Ikeuchi T, Koizumi S, Hatanaka H. Differences in survival-promoting effects and intracellular signaling properties of BDNF and IGF-1 in cultured cerebral cortical neurons. Journal of Neurochemistry,2001; 78: 940-951.
121. Crossthwaite AJ, Hasan S, Williams RJ. Hydrogen peroxide-mediated phosphorylation of ERK1/2, Akt/PKB and JNK in cortical neurones: dependence on Ca(2+) and PI3-kinase. J Neurochem,2002; 80: 24-35..
122. Ichiki T, Tokunou T, Fukuyama K, Iino N, Masuda S, Takeshita A. Cyclic AMP Response Element-Binding Protein Mediates Reactive Oxygen Species-Induced c-fos Expression. Hypertension,2003; 42: 177-183.
123. Iwata E, Asanuma M, Nishibayashi S, Kondo Y, Ogawa N. Different effects of oxidative stress on activation of transcription factors in primary cultured rat neuronal and glial cells. Brain Res Mol Brain Res,1997; 50: 213-220.
124 Pugazhenthi S, Nesterova A, Jambal P, Audesirk G, Kern M, Cabell L, Eves E, Rosner MR, Boxer LM, Reusch JE. Oxidative stress-mediated down-regulation of bcl-2 promoter in hippocampal neurons. J Neurochem,2003;84: 982-996.
125. Xing J, Ginty DD, Greenberg ME. Coupling of the RAS-MAPK pathway to gene activation by RSK2, a growth factor-regulated CREB kinase. Science,1996; 273: 959-963.
126. Arany I, Megyesi JK, Reusch JE, Safirstein RL. CREB mediates ERK-induced survival of mouse renal tubular cells after oxidant stress. Kidney Int,2005;68: 1573-1582.
127. Megyesi J, Udvarhelyi N, Safirstein RL, Price PM. 1996. p53-Independent activation of transcription of p21WAF1/CIP1/SDI1 after acute renal failure. Am. J. Physiol. 271: F1211-F1216.
128. Megyesi J, Safirstein RL, Price PM. Induction of p21 WAFI/CIP1/SDI1 in kidney tubule cells affects the course of cisplatin-induced acute renal failure. J Clin Invest 1998;101:777-782.
129. Megyesi J, Andrade L, Vieira J, Safirstein RL, Price PM. Positive effect of the induction of p21 WAF1/CIP1 on the course of ischemic acute renal failure. Kidney Int 2001;60:2164-2172.
130. Price PM, Safirstein RL, Megyesi J. Protection of renal cells from cisplatin toxicity by cell cycle inhibitors. Am. J. Physiol. Renal Physiol, 2004; 286: F378-F384.
131. Yu F, Megyesi J, Safirstein RL, Price PM. Identification of the functional domain of p21WAF1/Cip1 that protects from cisplatin cytotoxicity Am. J. Physiol. Renal Physiol. 2005; 289: F514-F520.
132. Price PM, Yu F, Kaldis P, Aleem E, Nowak G, Safirstein RL, Megyesi J. Dependence of cisplatin-induced cell death *in vitro* and *in vivo* on cyclin dependentkinase 2. J. Am. Soc. Nephrol. 2006;17: 2434-2442.

09

Animal models for the assessment of acute renal dysfunction and injury

Zoltan H. ENDRE[1] and Charles L. EDELSTEIN[2]

[1]Department of Medicine, Christchurch Hospital, University of Otago Christchurch, New Zealand
[2]Division of Renal Diseases and Hypertension, University of Colorado Health Sciences Center, Denver, USA

→

INTRODUCTION

There are a variety of experimental models of acute renal dysfunction and injury for the study of nephrotoxicity. These models include whole animals, isolated perfused kidneys, preparations for the study of the renal microcirculation (including juxtamedullary nephron preparation, hydronephrotic kidney, isolated perfused afferent arteriole, isolated perfused juxtaglomerular apparatus), isolated proximal tubules and cultured tubular cells. In this chapter, three commonly used animal models: whole animals, isolated perfused kidneys, and preparations for the study of the renal microcirculation, will be reviewed. Because the functional effect of a nephrotoxin can include vascular, intraluminal, and direct tubular cell effects, no single experimental model is ideally suited to study the pathophysiology of nephrotoxic injury. Also, each technique also has major limitations which must be appreciated when interpreting the results. However certain models are useful for studying specific types of neprotoxic injury. For example, techniques for study of the microcirculation are ideal to study drugs that cause acute renal dysfunction on a vascular basis. These drugs include prostaglandin inhibitors e.g non steroidal anti-inflammatory drugs (NSAIDs) . , direct vasoconstrictors e.g cyclosporine and angiotensin II blockers e.g. angiotensin converting enzyme (ACE) inhibitors. Each model, when appropriately applied and interpreted, produces useful information. However, it should be emphasized that complementary models and approaches need to be used to study a particular nephrotoxin. For example, tubular damage caused by intramuscular injection of glycerol is caused by heme toxicity and is due to a combination of factors that include severe intrarenal vasoconstriction, heme-mediated oxidant injury to tubular cells and obstruction of distal tubules by casts of acid hematin.

A major difficulty in interpreting *in vivo* studies of nephrotoxic acute kidney injury in whole animals is the amount and localization of nephrotoxin uptake by the kidney. It may be difficult to ascertain whether a given intervention alters pathways of nephrotoxin-mediated injury or merely the intracellular nephrotoxin burden. For example, the amount of drug which accumulates within tubular cells cannot be directly assessed because whole tissue analysis detects both intraluminal and intracellular drug content. Also, experimental conditions e.g., renal hypoperfusion, renal pedicle clamping may directly influence the amount of renal nephrotoxin uptake. Thus, a knowledge of the limitations of each *in vivo* experimental model is necessary. The use of complementary *in vitro* models e.g. isolated proximal tubules to assess direct tubular toxicity is often required.

The nature of tubular injury in AKI includes reversible sublethal injury (swelling, loss of apical brush border) and lethal injury (necrosis and apoptosis) [1-6]. In the clamp model of ischemic AKI in rats and mice, the predominant morphological change is tubular necrosis [1, 7]. However in human ischemic AKI there is less tubular necrosis but proximal tubules demonstrate degenerative changes with sloughing and simplification of the proximal tubular epithelial cells [1, 7]. Tubular cell apoptosis is present in the medullary thick ascending limb and the survival of the medullary thick ascending limb and distal tubule is critical to the recovery from AKI [8-10]. In animal models if cisplatin-induced AKI, tubular cell apoptosis is prominent [11]. The consensus among various authors is that morphology is the gold standard for detection of apoptosis and that TUNEL staining fails to discriminate between apoptosis and necrosis especially *in vivo* in the kidney in AKI [12-14]. TUNEL staining labels a high proportion of non-apoptotic nuclei and grossly overestimates apoptosis in the kidney [4, 10, 15]. In one study, the presence of TUNEL staining in ischemic AKI correlated with the expression of tubular necrosis and not apoptosis [3]. DNA fragmentation resulting from endonuclease activation can also detected in cells undergoing necrosis [16]. Thus, the nature of nephrotoxic injury, whether it is tubular dysfunction necrosis or apoptosis is also an important consideration.

1. WHOLE ANIMAL MODELS

"Knockout" mouse models

Various animal models have been used to study the pathogenesis of acute kidney injury (AKI) and develop therapeutic interventions that prevent or ameliorate the severity of tubular injury following an acute ischemic or toxic renal insult. Utilization of animal models has advantages over other *in vitro* models such as isolated perfused kidneys, isolated proximal tubules, or tubular cell culture. It reproduces the complex interactions of hemodynamics and local tubular factors seen in the whole animal with AKI.

In the early 1940s, the effect of induced ischemic myopathy on renal perfusion in the rabbit was studied. It was conclusively demonstrated in this model that there was extreme renal cortical vasoconstriction with preservation of the medullary circulation [17]. This early first demonstration of posttraumatic vasomotor nephropathy was independently confirmed 20 years later in the USA when 'preferential renal cortical ischemia' was demonstrated in acute kidney injury in man. Since then, many animals have been used to study pathogenesis of AKI. Rats and mice are the most popular experimental animals now. Dogs and rabbits are now less often used. Rats and mice are becoming more and more acceptable animals because they are easy to breed. Pigs are also being used [18, 19].

Compensatory responses

The ability to generate mice with a targeted mutation in a desired gene has made them a very attractive model. The first knockout mouse line was generated over 15 years ago. Many hundreds of genes have been targeted. In mice with a targeted mutation, it is possible to determine the function of gene product in various pathological conditions including renal ischemia. However, there may be discrepancies between results of studies in mice with a targeted mutation versus mice treated with an agent to neutralize the specific protein. For example, specific neutralization of interleukin-18 (IL-18) using anti-IL-18 antiserum, results in prolonged survival in lipopolysaccharide (LPS) lethality [20] whereas the IL-18 deficient mouse is often not protected against LPS lethality [21]. Also, neutralizing antibodies against IL-18 reduce disease severity in inflammatory bowel disease [22]. In contrast, IL-18 deficient mice exhibit enhanced disease severity [23]. In general, if neutralizing antibodies are available and if such reagents exhibit a high specificity for a particular cytokine, the use of such neutralizing antibodies is best to define the role of a cytokine compared to a deficiency of the cytokine from the time of conception as in the deficient mice. In any model involving production of several cytokines, neutralization of a single cytokine associated with a reduction in disease severity is a better test of the hypothesis because one is certain that several cytokines are produced in the wild-type mouse. In the case of the deficient mouse, one is not sure if several cytokines are produced or if some cytokines are being overproduced (compensatory). For example, it has been demonstrated in IL-18 deficient mice that levels of other cytokines such as IL-1β, IL-6 and TNFα are overproduced as compared to wild type mice [21]. A mouse deficient of a specific cytokine can be very informative and highly useful in models of spontaneous disease activity. But in the case of a specific challenge such as nephrotoxic acute kidney injury, the test of the hypothesis may be best served by specific blockade. The above principles may also apply to other proteins besides cytokines. Thus, in summary, when working with knockout animals, it is important to consider that the resultant phenotype is due to both loss of function of the targeted gene and the compensatory reaction that the animal develops to minimize that loss.

Another example of problems in interpreting results in knockout mice is demonstrated by the following: An important role of colony-stimulating factor (CSF) in hemopoiesis of myeloid lineage cells has been demonstrated. G-CSF was knocked out, animals were neutropenic and had decreased hemopoietic progenitors in bone marrow and spleen [24]. In contrast, mice with a null mutation in GM-CSF, which acts upstream to G-CSF in myeloid differentiation, demonstrated no impairment of hemopoiesis, but develop a characteristic pulmonary pathology [25]. Therefore, we have to interpret the results of our experiments with knockout mice with caution.

Strain differences

Different strains of mice have different levels of susceptibility to ischemic kidney injury. For example,

C57BL/6 mice, the major strain used in the development of genetically engineered mice, have greater susceptibility to renal ischemia/reperfusion injury than do the NIH Swiss mice [26]. The early knockout mice developed were in a mixed strain, C57BL/6 x SV129 F1. It is well known that the phenotype of a knockout mouse can depend critically on the background. For example, C57BL/6 x SV129 F1 mice have different coat colors ranging from black to white. The use of this mixed strain also runs the risk of genetic drift of background compared to the knockout mice being used. Thus, siblings from heterozygous crosses are better than "unrelated" controls. More recently, knockout mice are being "backcrossed" into the C57BL/6 background to eliminate strain differences. Rapid congenic protocols are available for the backcrossing [27, 28].

Gender differences

There are also gender differences in susceptibility to ischemic acute kidney injury in mice. Male mice may be more susceptible to renal ischemia than females [29].

Table 1 demonstrates different lines of knockout mice that have been used to study ischemic AKI. These models are of potential value in the study of nephrotoxic injury from drugs and chemicals.

Kidney Specific Gene Targeting

Conditional gene knockout has been developed in which a gene can be temporally and spatially regulated [30].The Cre/LoxP approach is widely used for conditional gene knockout. The production of tissue specific gene knockout mice requires two strains of mice. One strain of mouse expresses the Cre recombinase under the control of the promoter of a tissue specific gene. The second mouse strain contains two loxP sites flanking the DNA segment to be excised (the floxed gene). In short, the strains are crossed to produce a mouse with gene activation in a specific tissue [31]. This technique allows 1. the lack of systemic compensatory responses that are seen in global knockouts, 2. prevention of embryonic lethality that is seen when certain "essential" genes are globally knocked out. Recent studies of kidney specific gene targeting are shown in Table 2.

Table 1. Knockout mouse models of ischemic acute kidney injury.

Deficient gene	AKI model	Protection against AKI	Reference
A1 adenosine receptor	Acute radiocontrast nephropathy	Yes	[170]
A1 adenosine receptor	Bilateral renal pedicle clamping	No. Worse AKI	[171]
Proapoptotic protein Bid	Bilateral renal pedicle clamping	Yes.	[172]
Interleukin 6	Bilateral renal pedicle clamping	Yes	[173]
Interleukin 4	Bilateral renal pedicle clamping	No. Worse AKI	[174]
Interelukin 12	Bilateral renal pedicle clamping	No	[174]
Endothelial NOS	Unilateral clamp after nephrectomy	No	[175]
Poly(ADP-ribose) polymerase-1	Bilateral renal pedicle clamping	Yes	[176]
Complement factor B	Bilateral renal pedicle clamping	Yes	[177]
Na^+/Ca^{2+} exchanger	Bilateral renal pedicle clamping	Yes	[178]
Complement regulatory protein CD55	Bilateral renal pedicle clamping	No. Worse AKI	[179]
A3 adenosine receptor	Bilateral renal pedicle clamping Myoglobinuria-induced AKI	Yes	[180]
Caspase-1	Bilateral renal pedicle clamping	Yes	[181]
Caspase-1	Unilateral renal pedicle clamping	No	[182]
iNOS	Bilateral renal pedicle clamping	Yes	[183]
Interleukin-1 receptor	Bilateral renal pedicle clamping	No	[184]
ICAM-1	Bilateral renal pedicle clamping	Yes	[185]
CD4/CD8 lymphocytes	Bilateral renal pedicle clamping	Yes	[186]
Osteopontin	Bilateral renal pedicle clamping	Yes	[187]

Table 2. Kidney-specific gene targeting.

Gene	Location of knockout	Phenotype	Reference
Endothelin B	Collecting duct	Hypertension. Sodium retention	[188]
Aquaporin 2	Collecting duct	Severe urinary concentrating defect	[189]
Peroxisome proliferators-activated receptor gamma	Collecting duct	Thiazolidinedione-induced fluid retention	[190]
Endothelin 1	Collecting duct	Hypertension. Fluid retention.	[191]
Megalin	Proximal tubule	Hypocalcemia. Osteopathy.	[192]
Alpha epithelial sodium channel (αENaC)	Collecting duct	No effect on sodium and potassium balance	[193]

Types of renal injury

Ischemic, nephrotoxic, and septic rodent models of acute renal injury were developed to study mechanisms of acute kidney injury. Decreasing renal blood flow is critical in the pathophysiology of AKI in humans. Ischemic and other animal models are used to reproduce the morphological features of human disease.

Ischemic

Ischemic AKI may be induced by intrarenal norepinephrine injection or by renal artery clamping. There are similarities between these two models of ischemic renal failure. In the norepinephrine model of renal failure, as in the arterial clamping model, there is the same degree of tubular injury except for a slightly greater frequency of tubular casts at 48 hours in ischemic model [32]. In both models, calcium channel-blockers, improve renal function [33, 34]. The major difference is that in the renal artery clamping model, morphology at 48 hours showed smooth muscle necrosis in half of the resistance vessels, but in less than 10% of those in norepinephrine-induced model.

There are bilateral and unilateral models of ischemic AKI. The bilateral model is used more often because it is more similar to the pathophysiology of the syndrome of acute kidney injury in humans and the most likely to yield clinically relevant information. Moreover, uninephrectomy, immediately before renal artery occlusion may offer protection from this insult [35, 36].

It is been known that proximal tubules are damaged more severely than distal tubules in ischemic AKI and that the S3 segment of proximal tubules is more susceptible to ischemia than the S1 segment [37-40]. The greater susceptibility of the S3 segment to ischemia *in vivo* is suggested to be related to hemodynamic factors that result in persistent impaired oxygenation of the outer medulla [41]. However, the degree of damage closely correlates with the severity of renal failure. For example, as the time of vascular obstruction or the dose of a nephrotoxin increases, injury also involves both S1 and S2 segments [42, 43]. Sections of kidney, stained with hematoxylin-eosin and periodic acid Schiff (PAS), show common features of ischemic damage: loss of proximal tubular brush border, congestion of the outer medulla, interstitial edema, proximal tubular injury, cast formation and interstitial leukocyte accumulation. The distal nephron is less affected, with mild damage in the thick limb of Henle and apoptotic cells in distal tubules. In contrast, tubular necrosis is less extensive in humans with ischemic AKI than in the rodent model. Morphological injury in humans is subtle and focal, affecting both proximal and distal tubules [44, 45]. The role of apoptotic cell death and the mechanisms of induction of apoptosis in ischemic AKI have been intensively discussed for the past decade. It has become apparent that apoptosis, a form of cell death, distinct from necrosis, may contribute to ischemic AKI [46-48]. Morphological and biochemical features that distinguish apoptosis from necrosis from , as well as the role of apoptosis in ischemic AKI have been reviewed [49, 50]. Given the importance of the topic, we will again briefly summarize the features of necrosis and apoptosis and differences between them. In marked contrast to necrosis, apoptosis is an active, energy-dependent process. Even though ATP deficiency may be a signal both for apoptosis and for necrosis, cells with a rapid and severe ATP deprivation die by necrosis rather than apoptosis. Other pro-apoptotic mediators have been shown to present in AKI, such as caspase-3 activation, expression of Fas and Fas ligand in renal epithelial cells and expression of tumor necrosis factor-alpha (TNF-α) [51, 52]. The morphological characteristics of apoptosis and necrosis are quite different. The early loss of plasma membrane integrity, seen in necrosis, is associated with phospholipase with activation, oxidant injury to cellular components and cell swelling, leading to the release of proteolytic enzymes into the extracellular space and subsequent inflammatory reaction. In contrast, in apoptosis the cell becomes progressively smaller in size, nuclear chromatin becomes condensed and fragmented, while the plasma membrane retains its integrity. Later on, the apoptotic cell disintegrates into "apoptotic bodies", which are ingested by macrophages, mesangial or epithelial cells and can be easily detected by light microscopy. Apoptotic cell death almost always occurs without marked inflammation and tissue injury.

Two waves of apoptosis during the reperfusion phase after ischemic AKI have been described. The first coincides with a maximum proliferative activity that is at 2-3 days post-injury. The second occurs on day 7-8 following injury [53]. Other investigators have demonstrated that apoptosis peaks between 4 and 14 days of post-ischemia [10]. The discrepancy may be due to different methods used to detect and quantify apoptosis or different animal models of ischemic AKI.

Cell death due to apoptosis or necrosis is not the only form of tubular injury in AKI. There is also sublethal injury causing cell dysfunction. For example, alterations in proximal tubular cell polarity occur during renal ischemia. Tubule polarity is essential for its primary function of selective reabsorption of ions from the tubular fluid. Sodium-potassium-ATPase (NaK-ATPase) , the enzyme, normally localized to the basolateral membrane, maintains tubular polarity by regulation of cellular transport sodium and potassium in proximal tubules. NaK-ATPase is linked to the cytoskeleton/membrane complex by a variety of proteins including spectrin. It has been demonstrated that in early reperfusion period spectrin dissociates from the cytosleleton and NaK-ATPase moves from the basolateral membrane into the cytoplasm and apical membrane [54-58].

The loss of gate function of the renal tubular cells prevents the renal epithelium from acting as a barrier to free movement of solute and water across the tubular epithelium. Thus, "backleak" of glomerular filtrate occurs. It has been demonstrated in humans that loss of proximal tubule cell polarity for NaK-ATPase distribution is associated with enhanced delivery of filtered Na+ to the macula densa for seven days after allograft reperfusion [59].

As a result of the loss of cell-matrix adhesion, epithelial cells, normally attached to the underlying matrix, become detached from the basement membrane [60]. In the urine of patients with "acute tubular necrosis" in native and transplanted kidneys, there is significant tubular cell shedding with up to 100% viability of voided tubular cells.

Inflammation and kidney neutrophil accumulation in the post-ischemic period is another controversial issue. There is increasing evidence that leukocytes, particularly neutrophils, mediate tissue injury and play a deleterious role in the pathogenesis of renal failure [61-66]. Conversely, renal injury can occur by a neutrophil-independent pathway, as seen in neutropenic patients who develop AKI, indicating that neutrophils are not the only factor contributing to AKI. Myeloperoxidase (MPO) activity is an accepted index for assessment of leukocyte accumulation in animal model. In addition, in a mouse model of neutrophil depletion in the blood and in the kidney, the ATN score was not improved [67]. However, one should consider that hematoxylin-eosin staining (morphology of cell nucleus) remains the gold standard for identification of neutrophils. MPO assays or chloroacetate esterase staining should be regarded as tools to quantitate both neutrophils /and monocytes/macrophages [43].

It is now thought that inflammation / plays a major role in the pathophysiology of ischemic AKI [68]. CD4+ T cell and macrophages are thought to be mediators of ischemic AKI [69, 70]. Mice deficient in CD4+ T cells, are protected against ischemic AKI [71]. In a model of macrophage depletion using liposomal clodronate/, it was demonstrated that macrophages contribute to tissue damage during acute renal allograft rejection [72] and ischemic AKI [73, 74]. Gene therapy in rats expressing an amino-terminal truncated monocyte chemoattractant protein-1 (MCP-1) reduced macrophage infiltration and ATN [75]. The mechanism of macrophage-induced injury in ischemic AKI e.g. production of cytokines is currently under investigation.

In summary, loss of brush border, presence of cast formation and predominant injury of the S3 segment of proximal tubules are similar in both human and experimental AKI. Reversibility of the reduction in GFR is another important similarity. However, the clamp model of AKI in rats and mice is characterized by extensive proximal tubular necrosis, the distribution and extent of which vary with the time of clamp and time of postischemic reperfusion [7]. In contrast, tubular necrosis is much less extensive in humans with ischemic AKI [7].

In a recent American Society of Nephrology Research Report, a concern was expressed that animal models may not be applicable to the treatment of human AKI [76]. However, it was noted that humans treatments are given after the induction of AKI, whereas in most animal studies mechanisms were examined and treatments were given after induction of AKI. It was concluded that highest priority should be given to the development of complex models of AKI that better reflect the human setting

Nephrotoxic

From an epidemiological point of view, among the causes of AKI of a medical nature, drug-induced and toxic AKI are very important [77]. Nephrotoxic substances include a wide variety of compounds such as heavy metal ions, organic solvents, antibodies and natural toxins. Nephrotoxins induce AKI in humans by direct cellular toxicity, vasoconstriction, and crystal-mediated tubular obstruction. Acute interstitial inflammation is an important factor in pathogenesis of acute interstitial nephritis. In general, a decrement of GFR is the result of combination of mechanisms rather than any single mechanism.

Table 3 shows the predominant mechanism of a decrease in GFR in different animal models of nephrotoxic AKI.

Septic

Sepsis is the most frequent cause of AKI in intensive care units [78, 79]. Moreover, when sepsis is associated with AKI the mortality increases dramatically [78]. The incidence of AKI increases even further in patients with septic shock. Also, the use of nephrotoxins e.g. aminoglycosides, , amphotericin B in septic patients may precipitate or worsen the AKI.

In one prospective study, AKI occurred in 51% of septic shock patients [80]. The combination of AKI and sepsis is associated with a greater than 80% mortality [79]. Over the past 3 decades, sepsis and septic shock have been studied in various species including rats, dogs, pigs, primates. Only recently has a mouse model of septic AKI been developed. Administration of different doses of endotoxin (5-30 mg/kg intraperitoneal) to mice is associated with sepsis and septic shock, respectively [81].

The mouse peritonitis model of sepsis is also widely used. In this model, the cecum is isolated, ligated and punctured with a 25-gauge needle. The mortality, morbidity, and immunopathology in endotoxemic and peritonitis models of sepsis has been compared [82]. The models yield similar mortality and morbidity but

Table 3. Animal models of nephrotoxic AKI.

Animal model	Nephrotoxic agent	Predominant mechanism of decreased GFR	Primary site of injury	Reference
Dog	Uranyl nitrate 5-10 mg/kg	Backleak of filtrate Decreased ultrafiltration coefficient	S3 segment of proximal tubule	[194,195]
Rabbit	Glycerol 7.5g/kg	Tubular obstruction	Proximal tubules	[196]
Rat	Gentamycin 40-120 mg/kg/day	Decreased ultrafiltration coefficient Tubular obstruction	Proximal convoluted tubule	[197-199]
Dog, rats	Mercuric chloride 1-3 mg/kg	Increased preglomerular resistance Back leakage of filtrate	S3 segment of proximal tubule	[199,200]
Rat	Cisplatin 6-10 mg/kg	Renal vasoconstriction Back leakage of filtrate	S3 segment of proximal tubule	[201,202]
Mouse	Cisplatin 30 mg/kg	Apoptosis on day 2 after cisplatin ATN and neutrophil infiltration on day 3 after cisplatin Caspase-1 and 3 activation	S3 segment of proximal tubule	[203]

have significant differences in the kinetics and magnitude of cytokine production. Also, the LPS model did not accurately reproduce the cytokine profile of human sepsis. As in humans, the septic shock mouse model has a higher incidence of AKI and mortality than the normotensive sepsis model.

It has been demonstrated that the early effects of sepsis in causing AKI primarily involve renal vasoconstriction. This primary vasoconstriction can be demonstrated in the absence of sepsis-mediated hypotension. Later events include apoptosis, leukocyte infiltration and morphological evidence of coagulation (e.g. glomerular fibrin) [83-86]. There is evidence that several vasoconstrictor and vasodilator pathways are activated during sepsis in various experimental models. During septic shock a hyperdynamic state occurs in which systemic vasodilation is associated with a secondary increase in cardiac output. The rise in cardiac output, however, may not be maximal for the degree of afterload reduction because of the myocardial depressant effect of cytokines such as tumor necrosis factor alpha (TNF-α). The arterial underfilling associated with systemic arterial vasodilatation is known to activate the renin-angiotensin-aldosterone system (RAAS), the sympathetic nervous system (SNS) and the non-osmotic release of arginine vasopressin (AVP) [87-89]. While these events attenuate the degree of systemic hypotension, they also lead to renal vasoconstriction. The vasoactive events of septic shock are however more complex than initiated by arterial underfilling. The endotoxin-mediated increase in TNF-α is associated with an increase in inducible nitric oxide synthase (iNOS) [83, 90]. There is evidence in the endotoxemic rat that the increased NO which results from the upregulation of iNOS exerts a negative feedback on the endothelial NOS (eNOS) in the kidney (See Table 4). Moreover, the secondary messenger of NO, cyclic GMP, has been shown to increase in the renal cortex during the initial 16 hours of sepsis but then at 24 hours to be down-regulated in spite of continued high plasma levels of NO [81]. Both of these events, namely NO-mediated decreased eNOS and down-regulation of cyclic GMP, would impair the normal counterregulatory vasodilator pathways which attenuate the renal vasoconstriction associated with activation of the RAAS, SNS and the non-osmotic release of AVP. There is also evidence against a role of iNOS in septic AKI (See Table 4). In this study, iNOS deficient mice or mice treated with a selective iNOS inhibitor were not protected against endotoxemic AKI.

Sepsis is also associated with increased reactive oxygen species. Antioxidants and superoxide scavengers have been suggested to attenuate the renal dysfunction of sepsis [91, 92]. Recent studies have further indicated that peroxynitrite, the product of the reaction between NO and superoxide, may be responsible for the renal oxidant injury associated with endotoxemia [93].

A new rat model of sepsis-induced AKI based on cecal ligation and puncture has recently been developed [94]. This model was used to find urinary proteins that may be potential biomarkers of sepsis-induced AKI. Aged rats were treated with fluids and antibiotics after cecal ligation and puncture. There was a range of serum creatinine values at 24 h (0.4-2.3 mg/dl) and only 24% developed AKI. Histology confirmed renal injury in these rats. The mortality rate at 24 h was 27% but was increased by housing the post-surgery rats in metabolic cages. Urinary proteins were detected by difference in-gel electrophoresis (DIGE). Cecal ligation and puncture elevated interleukin (IL)-6, IL-10 nitrite compared in the blood.Changes in a number of urinary proteins including albumin, brush-border enzymes (e.g., meprin-1-alpha) and serine protease inhibitors were detected. The meprin-1-alpha inhibitor actinonin prevented AKI in aged mice.

Some animal models of sepsis are shown in Table 4.

Measurement of injury

Serum creatinine and blood urea nitrogen

Serum creatinine and blood urea nitrogen are accepted indicators of renal function in animal model of ischemic AKI, correlating well with GFR as measured by inulin clearance [95]. In the rat and mouse clamp model of ischemic AKI, the serum creatinine and BUN reach a peak in 24-48 hours of reperfusion and normalize by day 6-8 [96]. Thus, this is a reversible model of ischemic AKI.

Histology

Histologic changes remain to be an important marker of kidney injury in AKI both in human and in animals. Histological parameters of AKI include tubular necrosis, loss of proximal tubular brush bor-

Table 4. Animal models of septic (endotoxemic) AKI.

Intervention	Septic model	Protection against septic AKI	Ref.
Meprin-1-alpha inhibitor, actinonin	Rat Cecal ligation and puncture	Yes	[94]
Simvastatin	Mouse Cecal ligation and puncture	Yes	[204]
Pentoxifylline	Mouse Lipopolysaccharide 2.5mg/kg IP	Yes	[99]
Endothelial NOS deficient mice	Mouse Lipopolysaccharide 5 mg/kg IP	No. Worse AKI	[98]
Myeloid differentiation factor 88 (MyD88)	Mouse Cecal ligation and puncture	Yes. No protection against liver injury	[205]
A3 adenosine receptor deficient mice	Mouse Cecal ligation and double puncture	No. Worse AKI	[206]
CD28, a costimulatory molecule for T cell activation. CD 28 deficient mice	Lipopolysaccharide 10μg/g IP	Yes. Less T cell infiltration in kidney	[207]
Caspase-1 deficient mice	Mouse Lipopolysaccharide 2.5mg/kg IP	Yes. Protection independent of IL-1β and IL-18	[100]
ThromboxaneA(2) receptor deficient mice	Mouse Lipopolysaccharide 8.5mg/kg IP	Yes. Improved RBF and GFR	[208]
TNF inhibition (TNFsRp55)	Mouse Lipopolysaccharide 5 mg/kg IP	Yes	[209]
iNOS inhibitor (1400W)	Mouse Lipopolysaccharide 5 mg/kg IP	No	[209]
iNOS deficient mice	Mouse Lipopolysaccharide 5 mg/kg IP	No	[209]
Nonselective NOS inhibition (L-NAME)	Rat Lipopolysaccharide (0.5-50 mg/kg IP)	No	[210]
Selective iNOS inhibition (L-NIL)	Rat Lipopolysaccharide (10 mg/kg IV)	Yes	[210]
iNOS inhibition (agmatine aldehyde)	Rat Lipopolysaccharide (0.5-50 mg/kg IP)	Yes	[211]
Type IV phosphodiesterase inhibitor (RO 20-1724)	Rat Lipopolysaccharide 20 mg/kg IP	Yes	[212]
Antioxidant (Dimethylthiourea)	Rat Lipopolysaccharide (0.5 mg/100 g IV)	Yes	[213]
Antioxidant (Superoxide dismutase)	Rat Lipopolysaccharide (0.5 mg/100 g IV)	Yes	[213]
Selective endothelin B receptor antagonist (BQ-788))	Rat Lipopolysaccharide (10 mg/kg IV)	Yes	[214]
Nonselective endothelin receptor antagonist (TAK-044)	Dog Lipopolysaccharide (250 ng/kg/min for 2 hr)	Yes	[215]

der, casts in tubular lumens, neutrophil accumulation, Interstitial edema and vascular erythrocyte congestion. To assess the histological changes, a quantitative or semiquantitative approach should always be used. Areas of kidney damage such as cortex, outer or inner medulla should also be specified. Terms such as "extensive", "patchy", "widespread", "mild", or "severe" are not precise enough for evaluating the changes.

Inulin clearance

Inulin clearance has been used as the gold standard of GFR measurement. Accurate measurements of both urine and blood inulin concentrations are essential to get accurate results. Radiolabeled markers have been widely used, but they have a number of disadvantages such as cost and safety issues related to the use of radioisotopes. A new method of determining inulin clearance, representing a viable and accurate alternative to radioactive methods, has been described recently [97]. This method uses samples containing FITC-inulin that were stored between oil columns in constant-bore microcapillary tubes, which were then used as cuvettes to determine fluorescence on a microscope fluorometer. The authors report their method as simple to use, relatively inexpensive, and highly precise. The other advantage is that inulin concentration may be measured in nanoliter volumes of fluid, which make the method very important in micropuncture studies.

A novel technique using 0.75% fluorescein isothiocyanate (FITC)-inulin to measure inulin clearance in mice has recently been described [98-100]. We have determined that there is an excellent correlation between serum creatinine and inulin clearance in mice with ischemic AKI (unpublished data). We compared serum creatinine and GFR by linear regression and determined there was a highly significant negative correlation between serum creatinine and GFR, with Pearson r = -0.76 ($P = 0.004$, $n = 12$)

Molecular parameters

The effect of ischemia-reperfusion injury on activity, protein and m-RNA levels of proteins is also studied. For example, the enzymes that are involved in free radical detoxication (catalase, copper-zinc and manganese containing superoxide dismutase and glutatione peroxidase) were studied in rat kidney [101]. This study demonstrated that there was a significant decrease in the levels of m-RNA coding for all the enzymes except manganese superoxide dismutase, which remained high. There was also structural and functional damage of peroxisomes and catalase-containing subcellular organelles [102]. The authors conclude that in ischemia-reperfusion, the antioxidant enzymes, providing protection by reducing the cellular level of free radicals, were downregulated at both the transcriptional and tranclocational level and may contribute to free radical species injury of intracellular molecules critical to cell homeostasis.

Biomarkers of acute kidney injury (AKI)

In humans, serum creatinine is dependent on non renal factors independent of kidney function e.g. muscle mass, nutritional status, infection, volume of distribution. Also, serum creatinine is dependent on renal factors that are independent of function. For example, certain drugs like trimethoprim and cimetidine elevations in serum creatinine by altering the normal elimination pathways of creatinine. In addition, in humans, alterations in serum creatinine may lag several days behind actual changes in GFR. Earlier detection of AKI with a kidney specific biomarker may be essential for early and successful treatment of AKI in humans.

The study of biomarkers of kidney injury in animal models has provided important information that has led to human studies. Biomarkers of AKI in animal models is shown in Table 5.

Table 5. Biomarkers of AKI.

Biomarker	Animal Model	Detail of animal study	Reference	Human studies Reference
Urine IL-18	Mouse ischemic AKI	Massive increase in AKI	[181]	Yes [216-219]
Urine NGAL	Mouse ischemic AKI	Massive early increase in the kidney and urine	[220]	Yes [219,221]
Urine KIM-1	Mouse ischemic and cisplatin-induced AKI	Biomarker for the early detection	[222,223]	Yes [224]
Urine Cyr61	Rat and mouse ischemic AKI	Biomarker for early detection	[225]	No
Urine KC	Mouse ischemic AKI	Increase in serum and urine before serum creatinine	[226]	No

Proximal vs. distal tubular injury

The last segment of the proximal tubule the (the S3 segment) and the medullary thick ascending limb (MTAL) are both located in the outer medulla of the kidney. This region of the kidney suffers the most severe ischemic damage because of the delayed return of blood flow after ischemia. In most *in vivo* experiments, cell injury and necrosis has been shown to be more severe in proximal than distal tubules [103]. The proximal tubule is also the main site of injury in the human kidney allograft with AKI [40]. The explanation for the increased vulnerability of the S3 segment to ischemia is that proximal tubules have little capacity for glycolysis compared to distal tubules [104]. Also, it has been shown that distal tubule cells demonstrate a very well-developed response to ischemia that is characterized by an alteration in the expression of many genes, that may be adaptive and result in decreased susceptibility of this segment to injury [105, 106]. Specifically, transcriptional downregulation of epidermal growth factor (EGF) as well as the activation of the immediate early gene response characterizes this segment's response to the ischemic insult [107, 108].

Mitogen-activated protein kinase (MAPK) activation is regionally distributed in the postischemic kidney. It has been demonstrated that ischemia-reperfusion injury induces the activation of the c-Jun N-terminal kinase (JNK) that occured both in the cortex and inner stripe of the outer medulla [109, 110]. During ischemia, JNK activation has a deleterious effect and inhibition of JNK s ameliorated renal failure [109]. Proximal tubule cells are more sensitive than thick ascending limb (TAL) cells to oxidative stress as assessed by cell counting, light microscopy, propidium iodide uptake and fluorescence-activated cell sorting (FACS) analysis. Immunoprecipitation/kinase analysis revealed that JNK activation occurred in both cell types, whereas extracellular regulated kinase (ERK) activation occurred only in TAL cells. In TAL cells, ERK inhibition reduced cell survival nearly fourfold after oxidant exposure. In proximal tubule cells, activation of the ERK pathway by insulin-like growth factor I (IGF-I) increased survival by threefold and this IGF-I-enhanced cell survival was inhibited by a MAP kinase kinase (MEK)-1 inhibitor of the ERK pathway [111]. It is also possible that increased expression of some genes within the medullary thick ascending limb encode the production of paracrine growth factors that may contribute to the regenerative response in the cells of the adjacent S3 segment [105].

2. METHODS TO EVALUATE THE RENAL MICROCIRCULATION

Introduction

Studies of the pathophysiology of acute kidney injury has classically considered both tubular and vascular mechanisms [112, 113]. *In vitro* techniques isolating either the vascular or tubular components have been developed. For example, the use of isolated proximal tubules in suspension or in culture allows the study of tubular mechanisms of injury in the absence of vascular factors [114, 115]. There are both *in vitro* and *in vivo* models to study vascular injury in the kidney. *In vitro* models include the study of vascular smooth muscle cells or endothelial cells in culture. In this section, the *in vivo* methods to evaluate the renal microcirculation will be discussed. This is of relevance as many nephrotoxins exert their deleterious effects through pharmacologic actions on the resistance vasculature with parenchymal injury occurring as a consequence of ischemia. In clinical practice nephrotoxins may cause prerenal azotemia as a result of increased renal vascular resistance. Nephrotoxins that cause acute kidney injury on a vascular basis include prostaglandin inhibitors e.g. aspirin, non steroidal anti-inflammatory drugs (NSAIDs), cyclooxygenase-2 (COX-2) inhibitors, vasoconstricting drugs e.g. cyclosporine, tacrolimus, radiocontrast media and drugs that block angiotensin II e.g. angiotensin converting enzyme (ACE) inhibitors and angiotensin II receptor antagonists (ARBs) (Table 6). ACE inhibitors and ARBs are widely used for the treatment of hypertension, congestive heart failure and diabetic nephropathy. They preferentially dilate the efferent arteriole of the glomerulus and decrease intraglomerular pressure. Acute kidney injury may occur in conditions where angiotensin plays a crucial role in maintaining the glomerular filtration rate e.g. volume depletion, bilateral renal artery stenosis, diuretic-induced sodium depletion and autosomal dominant polycystic kidney disease.

Table 6. Drugs that cause acute renal dysfunction on a vascular basis.

Prostaglandin inhibitors:
Aspirin
Non-steroidal anti-inflammatory drugs (NSAIDs)
Cyclooxygenase-2 (COX-2) inhibitors
Vasoconstrictors:
Cyclosporine
Tacrolimus
Radiocontrast media
Angiotensin II blockade:
Angiotensin converting enzyme (ACE) inhibitors
Angiotensin II receptor antagonists (ARBs)

Table 7. Endogenous agents that modify vascular tone and reactivity.

Endocrine or neural:
Renal nerves
Catecholamines
Angiotensin II
Natriuretic peptides
Paracrine:
Endothelial derived e.g. nitric oxide, endothelin-1
Angiotensin II
Arachidonic acid metabolites e.g. thromboxane A2, prostaglandins, leukotrienes
Purinoreceptors and vasoactive purine agonists e.g. P1 receptors and adenosine
Dopamine and serotonin

Table 8. Techniques for study of renal microcirculation.

Juxtamedullary nephron preparation
Hydronephrotic kidney
Isolated perfused afferent arteriole
Isolated perfused juxtaglomerular apparatus
Two- photon microscopy

Control of vascular tone

Resting tone reflects basal properties intrinsic to the smooth muscle cells and the modulating influence of several well defined extrinsic factors [116]. These include the metabolic demand of the organ, neural and humoral factors, paracrine modulators and physical forces like stretch and shear. The myogenic response which increases smooth muscle tone in response to stretch is largely mediated by specialized, distinct stretch operated calcium channels [117]. The transduction of flow-related stimuli also intrinsically regulates blood vessels in the *in vivo* circulation. Flow produces shear that is readily detected by endothelial cells. Vasomotor responses to flow are predominantly dilator [118]. Nitric oxide (NO) derived from endothelial nitric oxide synthase (eNOS) [119] as well as endothelial cyclooxygenase products [120] have been implicated in the conversion of the endothelial shear response into smooth muscle relaxation. The role of NO in the resting circulation is indicated by the increases in basal vascular resistance after NOS inhibition [121]. The influence of humoral and neural factors like catecholamines, cholinergic mediators, prostanoids, angiotensin and aldosterone may be greater in stimulated or stress states than under basal conditions [116].

Vascular reactivity is the response to external and local stimuli that modify vascular tone. These factors are demonstrated in Table 7. The action of these factors varies among individual organs. For example, the kidney has greater vasoconstrictor sensitivity to endothelin-1 (ET-1) than other organs [122]. Integrity of the vascular responses is crucial in the maintenance of organ function in the face of nephrotoxins. Loss of this normal responsiveness may result in vascular injury.

Experimental models to evaluate the renal microcirculation

Techniques have been developed for study of the renal microcirculation. These techniques have distinct advantages over *in vitro* endothelial and vascular smooth muscle cell preparations. They allow study of important anatomic and physiologic relationships that are lost in isolated cell systems. For example, the effects of both pressure and flow can be determined and the spatial relationship between the endothelium and smooth muscle is maintained. These techniques permit functional assessment of the resistance micro-vasculature without destroying vessel integrity while eliminating the confounding influence of undetected circulating, neural and parenchymal factors. The techniques are demonstrated in Table 8.

In vitro perfused juxtamedullary nephron

In vivo micropuncture techniques have contributed greatly to the understanding of the forces governing glomerular hemodynamics and the ultrafiltration process [123]. The *In vitro* perfused juxtamedullary nephron first described in 1984 [124] allows study of a unique population of nephrons present in the inside cortex in apposition to the pelvic area of the kidney. These glomeruli have long afferent arterioles originating close to the main arcuate arteries. They are also located directly at the surface of the renal cortex normally covered by the pelvic mucosa. These superficial nephrons at the corticomedullary border have vascular characteristics of efferent arterioles breaking into the vasa rectae which is typical for juxtamedullary nephrons. This technique does not involve microdissection or the isolation of glomeruli and their arterioles.

Methods

The method for the *in vitro* perfused juxtamedullary nephron technique in Sprague-Dawley rats is as follows: A common dissection procedure is used to expose the arteries and related nephrons located at the inside surface of the renal cortex lining the pelvic cavity. Rats are systemically heparinized. The right kidney is removed and the left kidney is perfused with physiologic solution containing albumin. The left kidney is then decapsulated, removed from the animal and placed in a Petri dish filled with physiologic solution containing albumin at room temperature. The kidney is cut longitudinally to expose the pelvic cavity with the papilla left intact. Most of the cortical tissue is resected. The arcuate arteries are dissected and ligated with tight ligatures. A microperfusion system allows blood perfusion of the superficial nephrons via arcuate arteries.

Model

Anatomic and physiological studies can be performed in these kidneys [124]. Anatomically the models can be studied by light microscopy and scanning electron microscopy after infusion of the kidneys with resin. For physiological studies a perfusion system is used with donor blood or a cell free media. The microvasculature is viewed by videomicroscopy and vessel lumen diameters measured with a micrometer. It is also possible to simultaneously measure single nephron glomerular filtration rate or perform tubular perfusion with this technique. At a perfusion pressure of 100 mmHg, glomerular capillary pressure averaged 49 mm Hg, with most of the preglomerular pressure drop being localized to the terminal afferent arteriolar segment. Blood hematocrit can be reduced to approximately 30% with physiological solutions devoid of or containing albumin. In these conditions, the single nephron glomerular filtration rate averaged 34 nl/min (low plasma colloid osmotic pressure, PCOP) and 23.3 nl/min (maintained PCOP). Proximal tubule reabsorption ranges from 17 to 29%. In conclusion, the integrity of nephron function is maintained in this model, which provides insights into the dynamics of filtration and reabsorption processes of juxtamedullary nephrons. The procedure preserves the *in vivo* tubulovascular relationships, enables the use of a semi-microperfusion system and provides direct access to juxtamedullary nephrovascular units.

In early studies, microvascular reactivity of *in vitro* blood perfused juxtamedullary nephrons were studied in rats [125]. The effects of angiotensin II, epinephrine, and changes in perfusion pressure on glomerular capillary and afferent arteriolar pressures were assessed. At a perfusion pressure of 102 mm Hg, glomerular capillary pressure averaged 55 mm Hg. Afferent arteriolar pressure, measured at early-to-mid afferent locations, was 88 and decreased at the most terminal segments. In some nephrons, readjustments of glomerular capillary pressure occurred in response to step changes in perfusion pressure. Bolus injections of angiotensin II into the blood caused dose- dependent and reversible decreases in glomerular capillary pressure. Similar decreases in glomerular capillary pressure were observed in response to epinephrine. Epinephrine also consistently reduced afferent arteriolar pressures. In contrast, angiotensin II typically increased pressure in the early and mid segments of the afferent arteriole, but caused variable responses in the late afferent arteriole. The responses to vasoconstrictor agents were not mimicked by increases in perfusion pressure per se. This study demonstrates that the preglomerular vasculature of *in vitro* blood perfused juxtamedullary nephrons can exhibit autoregulatory behavior and is responsive to humoral vasoconstrictors.

Advantages

Advantages of the *in vitro* perfused juxtamedullary

nephron preparation are 1) preservation of the circulatory network; 2) no micro-dissection trauma to vessels; 3) the elimination of neural and hormonal influences; 4) maintenance of tubulo-vascular relationship and 5) simultaneous evaluation of both vascular and tubular effects of toxic substances.

Limitations

Limitations of the *in vitro* perfused juxtamedullary nephron preparation include 1) the availability of only a select population of juxtamedullary glomeruli near the inner surface of the kidney; 2) underestimation of the contribution of flow in large vessels to preglomerular resistance and 3) lack of characterization of tubular transport.

Studies

To date, the *in vitro* perfused juxtamedullary nephron preparation has not been used to examine the effects of nephrotoxic agents. However the preparation has been used to examine the pathophysiology of tubuloglomerular feedback. It has also been used to study the effect of mediators like adenosine, oxygen radicals and nitric oxide. Some recent studies are discussed below.

The influence of neuronal nitric oxide synthase (nNOS) on renal arteriolar tone has been studied in the perfused juxtamedullary nephron preparation [126]. Superfusion with a specific nNOS inhibitor decreased afferent and efferent arteriolar diameters, and these decreases in arteriolar diameters were prevented by interruption of distal volume delivery by papillectomy. When volume delivery to the macula densa segment was increased, afferent arteriolar vasoconstrictor responses to the nNOS inhibitor were enhanced, but this effect was again completely prevented after papillectomy. In contrast, the arteriolar diameter responses to a nonselective NOS inhibitor were only attenuated by papillectomy. Specific nNOS inhibition enhanced the efferent arteriolar vasoconstrictor response to ANG II but did not alter the afferent arteriolar vasoconstrictor responsiveness to ANG II. In contrast, non specific NOS inhibition enhanced both afferent and efferent arteriolar vasoconstrictor responses to ANG II. This study demonstrates that the modulating influence of nNOS on afferent arteriolar tone of juxtamedullary nephrons is dependent on distal tubular fluid flow and that nNOS exerts a differential modulatory action on the juxtamedullary micro- vasculature by enhancing efferent, but not afferent, arteriolar responsiveness to angiotensin II. It has also been demonstrated that superoxide inhibits nNOS influences on afferent arterioles in spontaneously hypertensive rats [127]. The role of neuronal NOS on afferent arteriolar function has been demonstrated in enhanced tubuloglomerular feedback activity [128], angiotensin II induced hypertension [129] and chronic heart failure [130].

More recently, studies have been performed to determine the responsiveness of rat juxtamedullary afferent arterioles to receptor-selective P2-purinoceptor agonists [131]. Experiments were performed *in vitro* using the blood perfused juxtamedullary nephron technique, combined with videomicroscopy. The presence of multiple P2 receptors on juxtamedullary afferent arterioles and the classification of these receptors as members of the P2X- and P2Y2 (P2U)-receptor subtypes was demonstrated. In another study, the relative contributions of adenosine A1 and A2a receptors to the responsiveness of the renal microvasculature to adenosine was investigated [132]. The presence of adenosine A1 and A2a receptors on afferent and efferent arterioles of juxtamedullary nephrons was demonstrated. Also, adenosine A2a receptor-mediated vasodilation partially buffered adenosine-induced vasoconstriction in both pre- and postglomerular segments of the renal microvasculature.

The role of the cyclooxygenase pathway interaction with nNOS [133, 134], tyrosine kinase [135]. intracellular calcium [136] and insulin-like growth factor 1 (IGF-1) [137] on afferent arteriolar function has been demonstrated in the perfused juxtamedullary nephron.

The use of knockout mice in the perfused juxtamedullary nephron model has provided much insight into the physiology of the angiotensin system on renal microcirculation. Some recent studies of the perfused juxtamedullary nephron model are shown in Table 9.

Hydronephrotic kidney

The hydronephrotic kidney was developed for *in vivo* visualization of the glomerular microcirculation, the vas afferens and the vas efferens [138]. This preparation utilizes postischemic hydronephrosis (PIH) to destroy the renal tubular system while preserving a portion of the cortex. In this preparation, glomeruli and

Table 9. Recent studies in the perfused juxtamedullary nephron.

Intervention	Findings	Reference
Angiotensin type 1A and 1B receptor double knockout (AT1 DKO) mice	Loss of angiotensin II-induced contraction, reduced vasoconstriction to norepinephrine and endothelial cell dysfunction contribute to the renal vascular phenotype of AT1 DKO mice	[227]
Angiotensin type 1A and 1B receptor knockout mice	AT(1A) and AT(1B) receptors are functionally expressed on the afferent arteriole. The efferent arteriole exclusively expresses the AT (1A) receptor	[228]
Angiotensin type 1A receptor knockout mice	AT(1A) receptors enhance tubuloglomerular feedback-mediated afferent arteriola constriction, in part by reducing the counteracting effect of nNOS	[229]
Angiotensin type 1A and 1B receptor knockout mice	Afferent arteriole vasoconstrictor responses to angiotensin II are mediated by both AT(1A) and AT(1B) receptors. Efferent arteriolar vasoconstrictor responses are mediated by only AT (1A) receptors	[230]
High salt diet in rats	The reduced vasoconstrictor response of the afferent arteriole to endothelin durining a high salt diet is mediated by endothelial endothelin (B) receptors	[231]
Hemeoxygenase (HO), nitric oxide synthase (NOS) inhibition	Endogenously produced CO does not influence afferent arteriole diameter in the presence of an intact NO system, but only when NO production is inhibited.	[232]
Reactive oxygen species (ROS) scavenger, tempol	TGF-β impairs renal autoregulation via generation of ROS	[233]
Shear stress/perfusion pressure	Increased shear stress increased NO release and simultaneously decreased endothelial cell calcium	[234]
L-type calcium channel blocker, diltiazem. T-type CCB, pimozide	Nitric oxide synthase inhibition activates L-and T-type calcium channels in afferent and efferent arterioles	[235]

associated vasculature remain intact. Observations are made with either incident light or transillumination.

Model

Briefly, the model is as follows: Rats are anesthetized, the left kidney is exposed and the ureter is permanently ligated while the artery is clamped for 60 min. The rats develop a postischemic hydronephrotic kidney in about 3 weeks. Microcirculatory experiments are begun 3 to 12 weeks after initial surgery. The animals are placed on a heated operating table. A carotid artery catheter is placed for continuous arterial blood pressure monitoring. The left hydronephrotic kidney is suffused with an isotonic and isocolloidal solution warmed to 37°C. The kidney is split at the greater curvature with a cautery knife and the halves of the kidney are visualized with transillumination and fluorescence video-microscopy. To visualize the flow velocity in single glomerular loops, fluorescent-labeled erythrocytes are injected so that only single erythrocytes pass through the glomerulus at one time. The flow velocity of fluorescent erythrocytes is monitored by analyzing sequences of single frames of video pictures. The geometry of glomerular structure is reconstructed. Capillary erythrocyte velocity and volume flow measurements are made. Blood flow velocity in afferent and efferent arterioles can be studied by the dual-slit method. Vessel internal diameter can also be measured electronically from a video image.

A high-speed video camera, recording up to 600 frames per second, can be incorporated in the set-up and erythrocyte velocity *in vivo* can be measured offline with the line-shift-diagram method [139].

Methods

In the original description of this model by Steinhausen et al, the following measurements were made: The inner diameter of the vas afferens, measured within 50 microns of the glomerular vascular pole, was 7.9 microns while that of the vas efferens was 7.7 microns. Both vessels were narrower adjacent to the glomerulus. A specialized round cell, which may act as a sphincter, was seen in the vas efferens. Blood velocity, measured in the vas afferens and efferens about 100 microns from the vascular pole, was 5.9 and 4.6 mm X sec-1, respectively. During angiotensin II infusion, the vas efferens in the vicinity of the glomerulus constricted by 22% whereas the corresponding vas afferens showed no consistent response. During angiotensin II infusion, the filtration fraction (GFR/RPF) may, therefore, be elevated by an increased resistance in the vas efferens, particularly at the outflow point of the glomerulus. Higher dosages of angiotensin II caused vasoconstriction of both vessels, especially at sites more distant from the glomerulus.

Advantages

The advantages of the hydronephrotic kidney preparation in examining the renal micro-vasculature are as follows: 1) It is possible to determine the real flow direction in both pre- as well as post-glomerular elements of the microvasculature a three-dimensional way; 2) the circulatory network is preserved such that the pressure and flow effects of changes in resistances in one vascular segment can be determined in the adjacent upstream and downstream vessels; 3) the circulation can be examined without the trauma related to microdissection; 4) both outer and inner cortical microvessels can be studied.

Limitations

Limitations of the technique include: 1) The induction of hydronephrosis may alter vasoreactivity; 2) tubular atrophy eliminates tubular influences on the microcirculation such as those observed in the tubuloglomerular feedback phenomenon and 3) intrinsic vascular resistances are higher and blood flows lower in hydronephrotic compared to normal kidneys.

Many important observations regarding segmental changes in the renal microcirculation to physiologic, pharmacologic and toxic stimuli have been made with hydronephrotic kidney preparation.

Studies

The effect of various mediators on the renal microcirculation are summarized in Table 10. The effects of various drugs, including cyclosporine nephrotoxicity, on the renal microcirculation are summarized in Table 11.

Table 10. Hydronephrotic kidney: Effects of endogenous effectors.

Agent	Effect	Reference
Angiotensin II	Efferent arteriolar vasoconstricition Blocked by saralasin	[236]
Dopamine	Afferent+efferent arteriolar vasodilation Dependence on balance of constrictors and dilators	[237]
Atrial natriuretic peptide	Reverses afferent arteriolar vasoconstriction peptide Potentiates efferent arteriolar vasoconstriction	[238,239]
Perfusion pressure	Afferent arteriole constricts. Hypertension shifts response	[240]
Sex differences	Efferent arteriole unchanged Autoregulatory response is modified by prostaglandins, especially in females	[241]
Endothelin	Decreases glomerular blood flow- dose-dependent [242] Constricts afferent and efferent arterioles. Constriction not affected by calcium channel blocker	[242,243]
Adenosine	Needs a functioning Angiotensin II receptor system for its vasoconstrictor action	[244]
Renal nerve stimulation	Afferent+efferent arteriolar constriction	[245]
Chloride channels	Ang II and NE induced afferent arteriolar Activation of voltage- dependent calcium channels	[246]
Insulin	Reverses norepinephrine/ angiotensin II vasoconstriction Effect mediated by nitric oxide	[247]
Prostaglandin E2	Vasodilatory and vasoconstrictor-afferent arteriole	[248]
Nitric oxide	Modulates myogenic vasoconstriction of afferent arteriole in spontaneously hypertensive rats	[249]

Table 11. Hydronephrotic kidney: Effects of drugs.

Drug	Effect	Reference
Cyclosporine	Interlobular, afferent and efferent arteriolar constriction Vasoconstriction due to altered NO metabolism	[250] [251]
Calcium antagonist (aranidipine)	Dilates both afferent and efferent arterioles during norepinephrine-induced constriction	[252]
Lovastatin	Vasodilatory in partial nephrectomy model	[253]
Anti-oxidant	Prevents cyclosporine induced vasoconstriction	[254]
(Lazaroids)	Improves renal blood flow during sepsis	[255]
Cobra venom	Massive constriction of the interlobar and arcuate arteries Complement activation	[256]
Angiotensin II receptor antagonist	Dilates afferent and efferent arteriole in hypertensive rats	[257]
Rho kinase inhibitor, Y-27632	Dilates the renal vasculature and inhibits autoregulation in the absence or presence of L-NAME	[258]
Na+K+2Cl- (NKCC) cotransporter inhibitors, furosemide and bumetanide.	NKCC modulation alters vasoconstrictorby a mechanism that does not involve tubuloglomerular feedback responses	[259]
Protein kinase C inhibitor, staurosporine	Enhancement of nifedipine (L-type calcium channel blocker) induced afferent arteriolar dilation in spontaneously hypertensive rats.	[260]
Staurosporine	Does not alter the effect of mibefradil (T-type calcium channel blocker) to dilate angiotensin II-induced arteriolar constriction.	[261]

Isolated renal microvessels

Methods

The isolated renal microvessel preparation was first described using adult female New Zealand White rabbits [140]. In this preparation, interlobular arteries and superficial afferent and efferent arterioles are dissected and mounted on micropipettes. Rabbits are sacrificed and the kidney is removed. The kidney is sliced along the corticomedullary axis and immediately placed in chilled artificial bath solution. A single microvessel is dissected using a sharpened forceps and transferred to a temperature-controlled chamber mounted on the stage of an inverted microscope. The vessel is viewed with a video camera fitted to the inverted microscope. Vessel lumen diameter is read directly off the video monitor. One end of the vessel is cannulated with concentric glass micropipettes. After the lumen is perfused to expel any residual erythrocytes, the other end of the vessel is occluded by sucking it into the tip of a constriction pipette. Intraluminal pressure is set with a syringe connected to the back of the perfusion pipette. Pressure is measured with a manometer or pressure transducer connected in series with the perfusion pipette. Intraluminal pressure is set at 90 mm Hg for intralobular arteries, 70 mm Hg for afferent arterioles and 20 mm Hg for efferent arterioles. After the pressure is set, the chamber temperature is gradually increased to 37°C and the vessel is allowed to equilibrate for 30-45 min before an experiment is started. Some but not all afferent and efferent arterioles develop a degree of spontaneous tone as evidenced by a sustained decrease in lumen diameter upon warming the bath from 20 to 37°C.

Model

The effect of acetylcholine, dopamine, and bradykinin on vascular tone has been examined in interlobular arteries and superficial afferent and efferent arterioles isolated from rabbit kidney [141]. Acetylcholine caused a dose-dependent relaxation of norepinephrine-induced tone in all three vessel types. Significant relaxation was observed with 10(-8) M acetylcholine and higher concentrations caused complete relaxation. In afferent and efferent arterioles dopamine caused a dose-dependent relaxation that was indistinguishable from the one caused by acetylcholine. Dopamine was much less effective on interlobular arteries. In afferent arterioles atropine blocked the effect of acetylcholine, and metoclopramide selectively inhibited dopamine-induced relaxation. Bradykinin caused a dose-dependent relaxation of norepinephrine- induced tone only in efferent arterioles. Bradykinin, either in the bath or lumen, had no effect on the preglomerular microvessels. Acetycholine and dopamine also caused relaxation of afferent arterioles with spontaneous tone while all three vasodilators relaxed efferent arterioles with spontaneous tone. This study demonstrates segmental heterogeneity for these vasodilators in the rabbit renal microvasculature, with acetylcholine causing relaxation in all three vessel types, dopamine acting primarily on the glomerular arterioles, and bradykinin affecting only the efferent arteriole.

The isolated renal vessel technique has been modified so that vessels can be isolated from rats instead of rabbits [142]. The preparation has also been modified for fluorescence measurements of cytosolic calcium in the smooth muscle cell layer [143]. Measurements of changes in smooth muscle calcium can be carried out simultaneously with determinations of changes in lumen diameters. The effects of various agonists and pressure stimulation in the presence and absence of pharmacologic agents can be determined. Angiotensin II-induced changes in lumen diameter and smooth muscle cell cytosolic calcium have been determined [121]. A maximal constricting concentration of angiotensin II caused abrupt and sustained increases in smooth muscle cell cytosolic calcium in afferent and efferent arterioles. When lumen pressure was reduced to zero, angiotensin II caused abrupt peak increases in smooth muscle cell cytosolic calcium in both afferent and efferent arterioles which declined rapidly thereafter--patterns distinctly different from pressurized vessels. With the calcium channel blocker, diltiazem in the bathing media, angiotensin II caused an abrupt rise and decline in smooth muscle cell cytosolic calcium in afferent arterioles, but a sustained elevation in efferent arterioles. This study demonstrates that maximal angiotensin II stimulates both Ca^{2+} entry and storage mobilization in afferent and efferent arterioles and that lumen pressure modifies the angiotensin II smooth muscle cell cytosolic calcium response profiles. Angiotensin II activates differing Ca^{2+} influx mechanisms in pre- and postglomerular arterioles [144]. In the afferent arteriole, angiotensin II activates dihydropyridine- sensitive L-type Ca^{2+} channels, presumably by membrane depolarization. In the efferent arteriole, Angiotensin II appears to stimulate Ca^{2+} entry via store-operated Ca^{2+} influx. Recent studies indicated that cyclic ADP-ribose (cADPR) serves as a second messenger for intracellular Ca^{2+} mobilization in a variety of mammalian cells including the renal vasculature [145]. Collectively, these studies demonstrate that the EP(4) receptor is the major receptor in preglomerular VSMC. E-prostanoid 4 receptors mediate prostaglandin E2-induced vasodilation in the rat kidney and signal through G proteins to stimulate cAMP and inhibit cytosolic calcium concentration [146].

Advantages

The advantages of the isolated vessel technique in defining microvascular physiologic and pathophysiologic mechanisms are: 1) The vessels are studied in the absence of a neurohumoral and parenchymal tissue environment, 2) it allows for direct assessment of vascular responses in defined segments, 3) transmural pressure is controlled, 4) hormones and drugs can be added to the bathing media or luminal perfusate, 5) intracellular ion concentrations can be measured by fluorescence microscopy and membrane potentials can be recorded with microelectrodes.

Limitations

The limitations of the preparation are:) autocoid production and vascular reactivity may be altered *in vitro*, 2) the absence of flow dynamics may alter endothelial cell function, 3) the small amount of tissue limits biochemical measurements, 4) isolated arterioles do not exhibit myogenic responses to changes in transmural pressure.

Studies

The isolated renal microvessel preparation demonstrates concentration-dependent sensitivity to a various constrictor and dilator substances. Early studies demonstrated the lack of an effect of atriopeptin II on rabbit arterioles [147]. In another study in rat arterioles [148], atriopeptin III dilated preconstricted afferent arterioles but constricted efferent arterioles that were either not pretreated or that were preconstricted with other agonists. The effect of atriopeptin III on preconstricted afferent arterioles did not require vasodilator prostaglandin mediation. The constrictor effect of atriopeptin III on efferent arterioles was not dependent on angiotensin, thromboxane, or alpha- adrenergic mediation.

Postsynaptic alpha-adrenoceptors have been characterized in afferent and efferent arterioles isolated from rabbit renal cortex [149]. In both the afferent and efferent arteriole selective alpha 1-adrenoceptor agonists produced concentration-dependent vasoconstrictor responses with the maximum responses being equal to that of norepinephrine. Selective alpha 2-receptor agonists had less of an effect. The alpha 1-receptor antagonist, prazosin, produced a rightward shift in the concentration-response curve to norepinephrine, while the selective alpha 2-receptor antagonist, rauwolscine had no effect on norepinephrine-mediated vasoconstriction. This study confirms the presence of alpha-adrenoceptors, exclusively of the alpha 1-subtype, on the glomerular arterioles that mediated vasoconstriction.

The influence of arachidonate cyclooxygenase products on endothelin-evoked renal vasoconstriction has been assessed [150]. In microperfused rat afferent and efferent arterioles, indomethacin had no effects on the maximal contraction by endothelin, but reduced the duration of endothelin-induced constriction in both arterioles. Endothelin infusion to rats *in vivo* resulted in a selective increase in efferent but not afferent arteriolar resistance, leading to a dramatic increase in transcapillary hydraulic pressure difference. Glomerular filtration rate, which fell progressively during infusion of endothelin alone, was markedly preserved by cyclooxygenase inhibition, but not during selective thromboxane A2 antagonism. This study provides evidence that locally released cyclooxygenase products, play a key role in sustaining endothelin-induced renal arteriolar constriction.

The role of endothelin in mediating cyclosporine A -related renal vasoconstriction has been studied [151]. Both the afferent and efferent arteriole exhibited concentration-dependent decreases in lumen diameter to increasing molar concentrations of cyclosporine A. The afferent arteriole was more sensitive to the vasoconstrictive effects of cyclosporine A than the efferent arteriole. These data suggest that cyclosporine A directly constricts renal microvessels and that this effect is mediated by endothelin in the afferent arteriole but not the efferent arteriole

Angiotensin II receptors [152], endothelin receptors [153] and vasopressin V1a receptor (V1aR) and V2 receptor (V2R) receptors [154] have been isolated in rat arterioles. In isolated rabbit arterioles, the vasoconstrictor response of angiotensin II is counteracted by vasodilatory prostaglandins and nitric oxide [155]. The calcium response to angiotensin II in the isolated rabbit afferent arteriole shows tachyphylaxis [156]. This tachyphylaxis cannot be reversed by applying increasing doses of angiotensin II, protein kinase C does not seem to be involved in the tachyphylactic phenomenon and nifedipine and NO reduced the tachyphylaxis. In another study, the afferent arteriole had a higher sensitivity to luminal than interstitial Angiotensin II in superficial but not juxtamedullary nephrons [157]. In this study, it was concluded that such heterogeneities in Angiotensin II action may be important in the control of glomerular hemodynamics under various physiological and pathological conditions.

Hydroxyeicosatetraenoic acid (HETE) release in response to angiotensin II from preglomerular microvessels in rats has recently been demonstrated [158] indicating that an angiotensin II-phospholipse C effector unit is associated with synthesis of the vasoconstrictor product, 20-HETE, in these vessels. Angiotensin II directly downregulates the expression of G proteins in young spontaneously hypertensive rats (SHR) but not in young control rat renal microvessels indicating that the diversity in its effect on G-protein expression may be important for enhanced renal sensitivity to Ang II in SHR rats [159]. Cytochrome P450 hydroxylase and cyclooxygenase arachidonic acid metabolites contribute importantly to the afferent arteriolar diameter and renal microvascular smooth muscle cell calcium responses elicited by endothelin-1 [160].

Arginine vasopressin (AVP) is a potent vasoconstrictor that preferentially reduces renal medullary blood flow through the stimulation of the vasopressin V1a receptor (V1aR). Studies have also shown that the vasopressin V2 receptor (V2R) may modulate AVP-mediated vasoconstriction. The transcriptional and translational sites of the V1aR and V2R in microdissected intrarenal vascular segments from both the cortex and medulla was studied [154]. The results indicate that V1aR mRNA and proteins are present in the isolated cortical or medullary vasculature, but the V2R mRNA and proteins were not found. This study suggests that the vasoconstrictor action of AVP within the renal medulla is mediated through the V1aR and that the modulatory V2R- mediated vasodilation is probably through the release of paracrine hormones found within the renal interstitial or tubular cells.

Bradykinin plays an important role in the regulation of renal hemodynamics. The effects of bradykinin on isolated perfused rabbit afferent arterioles and the mechanisms of action of bradykinin was studied [161].

It was concluded that 1) bradykinin has a biphasic effect on afferent arterioles; 2) both dilation and constriction may be mediated by bradykinin B2 receptors and 3) the mechanisms of vasodilation and vasoconstriction are due to cyclooxygenase products, not nitric oxide.

Isolated perfused juxtaglomerular apparatus

Tubuloglomerular feedback (TGF), which operates between the tubule and the parent glomerulus, is important to renal autoregulation and homeostasis of body fluid and electrolytes. The juxtaglomerular apparatus (JGA) which has a close anatomical relationship between the specialized tubular cells of the macula densa and the afferent and efferent arterioles, is the anatomical site of tubuloglomerular feedback. To study the function of the JGA directly, an *in vitro* preparation in which both the afferent arteriole and macula densa (MD) of a microdissected rabbit JGA are microperfused simultaneously, has recently been developed [162]. This preparation has the advantage of allowing control of both pressure in the afferent arteriole and luminal fluid concentration at the macula densa. Real time images of the afferent arteriole, including luminal diameter, can be obtained. Increasing the NaCl concentration of the macula densa perfusate constricts the afferent arteriole in the segment close to the glomerulus. This constriction is blocked by furosemide, a loop diuretic known to inhibit tubuloglomerular feedback. Microperfusion of the afferent arteriole alone showed that they constrict significantly when intraluminal pressure is elevated, the so-called myogenic response. The myogenic response is the first to respond to changes in perfusion pressure. The anatomical relationship between the myogenic response and TGF may enable the kidney to achieve its extremely efficient autoregulation. The preparation will provide important insights into the mechanism by which the macula densa controls glomerular hemodynamics. In this regard, the modulatory role of the macula densa NO pathways in tubuloglomerular feedback has been demonstrated [163]. Advantages of the preparation include [162] the following: 1) the hemodynamic influence of the larger interlobular artery can be excluded, 2) preparations from different nephron populations can be studied and 3) hormonal manipulations can easily be performed. A disadvantage of the preparation is its technical difficulty [164].

Two- photon microscopy

New advances in microscopy and optics, computer software and fluorophores to label target molecules have allowed investigators to utilize intravital two-photon microscopy to study the dynamic events within the functioning kidney. This emerging technique enables investigators to follow functional and structural alterations with subcellular resolution within the same field of view over a short period of time. This technique will enable studies of microvascular function within the kidney [165-168].

The basic methods for intravital studies using two-photon techniques are as follows: Adequate anesthesia is essential as any kidney movement limits the ability to obtain consistent data, particularly 3D and 4D data. An inverted microscope with an exteriorized left kidney (longer renal pedicle facilitates use) limits kidney movement. Maintenance of core body temperature and volume status is also essential. Only water-immersion objectives can be used, and this limits the effective magnification to approximately 60X.Three different colored fluorescent probes can be used at once with simultaneous excitation. A limitation minimizing the depth and quantitation of imaging is the loss of fluorescence due to light scatter. Under normal physiological conditions, up to 200 μm into the kidney of a rat or mouse can be visualized. This allows for visualization and quantification of superficial glomeruli in Munich-Wistar rats but does not allow for visualization of the corticomedullary regions even in mice. Image processing is a major component of digital microscopy.

Two-photon microscopy can be utilized to quantify microvascular flow rates within the kidney. Infusion of a nonfilterable intravenous fluorescent dye results in intravascular cells appearing as dark objects. Endothelial cell dysfunction within the microvasculature can be observed and quantified using the infusion of variously sized, differently colored dextrans or proteins. Movement of these molecules out of the microvasculature and accumulation within the interstitial compartment are readily observed during injury or disease.

Disadvantages of the technique include 1) Image-acquisition rates. Increasing the acquisition rate by limiting the microscopic field of study, often sacrifices other important data, 2) The depth of imaging. Although the depth is although four to five times greater than confocal imaging, it remains limited to <200 μm for the kidney, 3) The corticomedullary area of the kidney is not able to be visualized from the surface of the kidney, 4) Phototoxicity, 5) Quantification of recorded results. This is also a major area under development. Continuing improvement in software and hardware is necessary, 6) Cost remains an obstacle for the individual investigator and Core Imaging Facilities are required.

The FVB-TIE2/GFP mouse, in which the endothelium is fluorescent, has been used to study morphological changes in the renal microvascular endothelium during ischemia-reperfusion injury in the kidney [169]. Alterations in the cytoskeleton of renal microvascular endothelial cells correlated with a permeability defect in the renal microvasculature as identified using fluorescent dextrans and two-photon intravital imaging. This study demonstrates that renal vascular endothelial injury occurs in ischemic AKI and may play an important role in the pathophysiology of ischemic AKI.

3. THE ISOLATED PERFUSED KIDNEY: RAT AND MOUSE

Introduction

A huge number of studies of experimental renal injury have been performed using the isolated perfused rat kidney. Studies have explored vascular and tubular responses to toxic and hypoxic injury and to mediators thought to participate in regulation of normal renal function as well as in the biochemical and morphological changes accompanying renal injury.

Three main models have been used. The intact isolated perfused rat kidney (IPRK), is the most widely used model and first developed for the study autoregulation by Weiss et al in [262]. However, this prototype was little used initially because autoregulation and function declined after only 15-30 minutes. However, when simpler surgery and improved perfusion solutions were introduced by Ross, the model became useful for studies of renal biochemistry [263, 264]. With further improvements, including the addition of amino acids [265, 266] and sometimes erythrocytes [267-269] the model became useful for studies of physiology and pathophysiology [270-273]. Recently the technique has been adapted for use with mouse kidney (IPMK), which opens up the technique for use with many genetically modified models [274].

The second model is usually known as the hydronephrotic rat kidney model, and was developed for *in vivo* visualization of the microcirculation [275] and involves 60 min renal artery occlusion combined with 3 weeks of ligation of the ureter. Atrophy of tubular structures leaves the cortical vasculature relatively intact and visualizable using planar microscopy in an illuminated observation chamber with nerve and blood supply left intact. Absolute and relative changes in lumen diameter of the major resistance vessels-interlobular arteries, afferent and efferent arterioles can be monitored in reponse to vasoactive stimuli. This model was adapted for *in vitro* perfusion by Loutzenhiser et al [276], removing systemic neurohumoral influences.

The third model is the *in vitro* perfused juxtamedullary nephron, also developed to allow direct visualization of the renal microcirculation [277, 278]. Similarly to the IPRK, the kidney is perfused *in vitro* with albumin-containing physiological solutions with or without added erythrocytes. However, the preparation involves hemisection of the kidney, reflection of the papilla and ligation of the major branches of the renal artery until the vasculature perfusing a few glomeruli on the inner cortical surface is isolated. The microvasculature is then viewed by videomicroscopy and vessel lumen diameters measured by micrometer. Single nephron glomerular filtration rate and tubular perfusion can also be performed in this model and in contrast to the hydronephrotic model, tubuloglomerular feedback is intact in the juxtamedullary nephron preparation and can be investigated [279, 280].

Both the hydronephrotic kidney and the juxtamedullary model have been used primarily for physiological studies, including studies of drug action, whereas the IPRK has been used extensively for the studies of pathophysiology as well. Consequently the main focus of this section will be the intact IPRK, which is both the simplest and the most widely used model. The other two models will be discussed in greater detail in section 4 of this chapter.

Technique

The first useful version of the IPRK model [263,

264] recirculates Krebs bicarbonate buffer containing 6.7g% bovine serum albumin (BSA) as an oncotic agent. Glucose and amino acids are added as substrates. Two peristaltic pumps (or two passes through the same pump) are used to drive the perfusate first through in-line filters into a cascading lung oxygenator, usually gassed with 95% O_2, 5% CO_2 (Figure 1). The 5% CO_2 serves to maintain the bicarbonate buffer pH at 7.4. Prior to perfusion, the right kidney of the anesthetized rat is exposed and the ureter is cannulated using polyethylene tubing (0.28 mm (i.d.), 0.61 mm (o.d.)- known as PE10). Oxygenated and warmed perfusate is delivered into the rat kidney through a cannula introduced into the right renal artery via the mesenteric artery. The flow of warmed, oxygenated perfusate is commenced with the cannula in the mesenteric artery so that renal artery cannulation is initiated without even transient interruption of renal perfusion. After cannulation, the kidney is removed and mounted over a reservoir to collect the perfusate, which flows from the renal vein over the kidney, keeping the surface moist. The prewarmed perfusate keeps the temperature of the kidney constant, usually at 37°C. While some researchers use a constant temperature cabinet for this purpose, we have found that thermostatted tubing and glassware is simpler, reducing surface drying and making the experimental setup more mobile (Figure 1).

After 20-30 min for equilibration, perfusate samples are collected to coincide with the start of urine collections at 5 to 15 min intervals. The urine volume depends on both perfusion pressure and oncotic pressure [281]. Perfusion pressure and flow are monitored continuously. Renal function is assessed from renal vascular resistance, urine flow, the ratio of ^{14}C-inulin in urine to plasma (U/Pinulin), glomerular filtration rate (GFR as inulin clearance UV/P) and the fractional excretion of sodium (FE_{Na}) and potassium (FE_K). Inulin measurement can also be performed chemically. In some situations GFR is misleading as an index of "good function" in this model. For example, in the absence of an oncotic agent, a "reasonable" GFR is over 1 ml/g/min, however U/Pinulin is rarely more than 2, FENa is over 0.1 and histological examination shows extensive proximal necrosis within 20-40 min of intiating perfusion. It appears that in this situation the massive urine volume artefactually elevates the GFR. Similarly, dead space effects arising from urine in the renal pelvis, ureter and ureteric tubing reduce the real time relationship to a perturbation of GFR and other urine-based indices [273]. Because of these considerations, it is important to combine the various parameters of function and set minimum standards of function, which must be attained before results from individual perfused kidney experiments are utilized in data analysis (see below).

Many technical refinements have been added to this model over the years to help maintain renal physiological function as well as to assist with the technique of initiating perfusion. Technical modifications include the addition of albumin as an oncotic agent [263, 281, 282] addition of amino acids [264, 266], other substrates [283], addition of erythrocytes to improve outer medullary oxygenation [267-269], servo-control of perfusion pressure or flow [272] and ultrasonic recording of flow [272]. While incremental improvements in renal physiological function followed the various modifications mentioned, especially the addition of BSA and amino acids, the most physiological preparation with longest viability for experimental work is the model with normal concentrations of erythrocytes, albumin, globulin plus supplementation with antidiuretic hormone to preserve concentrating capacity described by Lieberthal [284]. However, because of the additional effort and expense, this model is generally avoided where the presence of erythrocytes, especially in high concentration, is not required for interpretation of the results. This seems to be the case in many studies of vascular modulation. Oxygen uptake can be measured by the Fick method [285]. During perfusion, electrodes can be inserted into the renal tissue for measurement of tissue PO_2 [286, 287, 288] and nitric oxide [289] Micropuncture studies have been applied to the IPRK [266]. At the end of perfusion the kidney can be fixed for morphological evaluation, optimally for tubular histology by perfusion with a flush solution (to remove precipitatable albumin from within the kidney) followed by fixative. Immersion fixation after sectioning may be better for assessment of vascular pathology *in vivo*. A flush solution is not essential after *in vitro* perfusion, since the vessels are already well perfused and any dilatation induced by perfusion fixation is less likely to be artefactual.

Some modifications to the perfusion circuit (Figure 1) and equipment are required for perfusion of the IPRK in high field magnets for spectroscopic analysis of compartmental biochemistry. Such studies include measurement of ATP using ^{31}P magnetic resonance spectroscopy ^{31}P (^{31}P MRS) [270, 290-293] and of cations using ^{23}Na MRS [272, 294-297] for sodium and ^{87}Rb MRS [298] for potassium. They also include using ^{1}HMR for microscopy of the intact perfused kidney [299] or a combination of both imaging and regional spectroscopy of the cortex and medulla using image-guided volume-localized magnetic resonance microspectroscopy [273, 300, 301] . Although earlier MR spectroscopy studies had yielded useful results, a major modification was required for MR microscopy to proceed, namely perfusion under buffer to eliminate air-fluid interfaces which produce magnetic susceptibility artifacts [301, 302]. This also required a reduction in rat size to allow kidneys to be perfused inside an 18 mm i.d. glass cylinder, made from a modified "20 mm" MR sample tube (Figure 1). For this it became necessary to perfuse kidneys from 130-170 gm rats, necessitating the use of smaller cannulas etc. The glass cannula originally used for renal artery cannulation limited perfusion of small kidneys from younger rats because glass cannulas have relatively large wall thickness to lumen ratios. Consequently, in our laboratory glass cannulas have been abandoned in favor of 21 to 26 gauge synthetic intravenous cannulas, which have improved and made reproducible the flow characteristics of the cannula, facilitated cannulation and reduced expense. Metal cannulas also have low wall thickness to lumen ratios, but we have avoided these since even non-magnetic metal cannulas are not usable in a strong magnetic field and our laboratory was commited to extensive application of magnetic resonance imaging and spectroscopy to the IPRK model [303]. Metal cannulas are also best avoided in studies involving free radicals including nitric oxide. Venous cannulation is usually not required and should be avoided unless

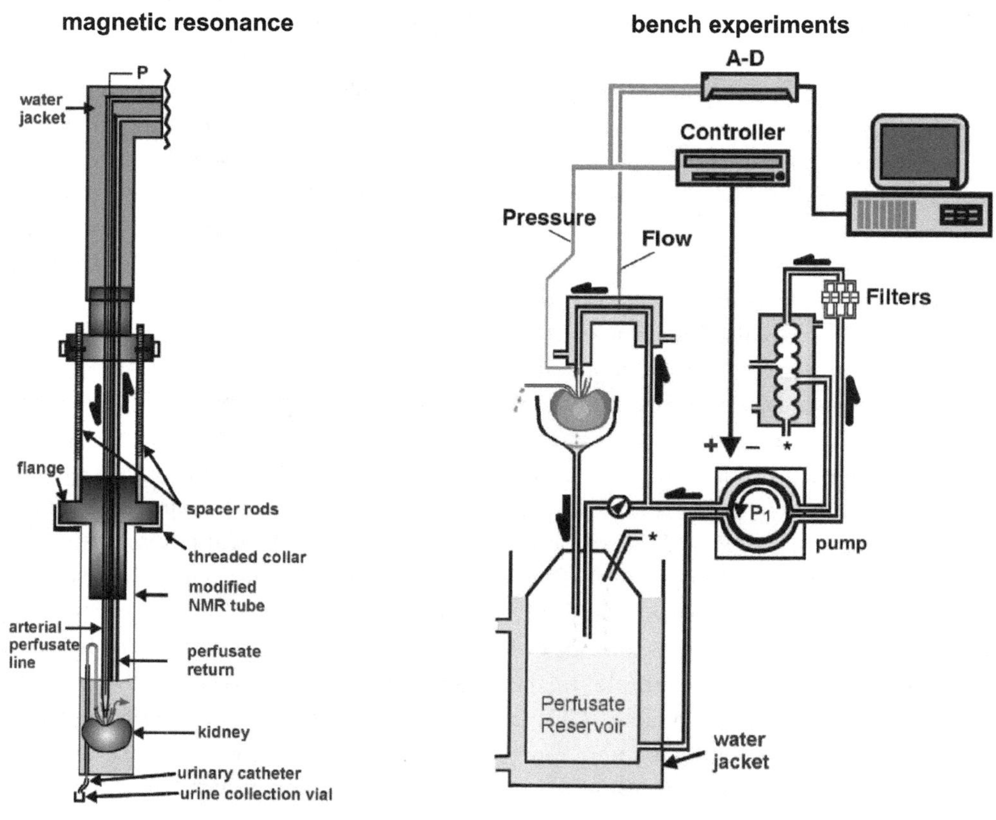

Figure 1. *The apparatus for isolated perfusion of rat kidneys is shown schematically. The typical circuit for bench experiments is shown on the right, while the extension using thermostatted tubing which is required for experiments conducted in the bore of a high field superconducting magnet for either magnetic resonance spectroscopy (MRS) or magnetic resonance microscopy is shown on the left (not to scale). Modified with permission from Endre et al [301].*

necessary since small rises in venous pressure may dramatically diminish renal function. Occassionally, venous cannulation has been used successfully, for example where observation of the renal ^{87}Rb signal was used as a K congener in MR studies of K transport [298]. In this experiment, separation of the Rb-containing venous effluent from the kidney surface was required, since the MR spectroscopy measurements averaged the whole sample and venous cannulation allowed the perfusate to be separated from a warmed Rb-free bathing solution, which was used to fill the sample space around the kidney.

Other refinements, were required to permit the 10 fold reduction in animal size required for mouse kidney perfusion [274]. The circuit, glassware and pumps used are similar to the rat kidney circuit, although modified to allow for a smaller circuit volume and improved temperature control at low flow. A 24 to 28 gauge cannula is required for direct arterial perfusion. The increased resistance produced by the reduction in internal cannula diameter produces a significant increase in circuit back pressure, which may require circuit modification. An alternative strategy is to perfuse the kidney through the aorta using a larger cannula. Depending on the species, this may require the lumbrical arteries arising from the posterior surface of the aorta to be ligated prior to en bloc removal of the kidney and aorta, which considerably complicates surgery. Aortic perfusion introduces the potential for kinking of the renal artery when the kidney is suspended over the circuit reservoir. Cannulation of the ureter is extremely difficult in the mouse and also introduces the potential problem of high resistance to urine flow if ureteric tubing sufficiently small enough to allow cannulation is used. This can be overcome by cannulation of the bladder with a wide bore (id 0.28 mm) PE tubing followed by ligation of the left ureter and urethra. Bladder cannulation is performed prior to cannulation of the renal artery. The right kidney, ureter and bladder are then removed en bloc for *in vitro* perfusion.. The IPMK model has similar advantages and limitations to the IPRK model considered below. It allows perfusion with added erythrocytes and hemodynamic monitoring [274] Hemodynamic monitoring and venous nitric oxide production has since been undertaken in the perfused mouse kidney by other groups [304-306], however as most were unable to collect urine, tubular function has not been reported.

In 1981, Alcorn et al [307] described a consistent artefact in MTAL cells in the inner stripe of the outer medulla in the cell-free perfused IPRK. This lesion was subsequently shown to be MTAL necrosis from hypoxia [308] and presumed to follow the diffusional shunting of oxygen from arterial to venous limbs of vasa recta entering the outer medulla [267]. Subsequent studies have confirmed that not only the medulla but even the cortical tissue oxygen tension (especially the medullary rays) is lower than venous PO_2 and that diffusional shunting of oxygen occurs *in vivo* as well as *in vitro* and in the presence as well as in the absence of erythrocytes [287]. Necrosis of the MTAL cells is eliminated by the presence of even low concentrations of erythrocytes under both normal [267-269], and hypoxic conditions [269]. Concentrating capacity in the IPRK falls rapidly after initiation of perfusion and is presumed to follow the loss of systemic antidiuretic hormone (vasopressin) and washout of the medullary interstitial osmotic gradient [273]. The latter presumably accompanies high perfusate flow through the renal medulla and the gradient is absent within 20 min of initiating perfusion. Low concentrations of erythrocytes eliminate histological evidence of injury to MTAL in perfused rat and mouse kidney. [274]. However, erythrocyte concentrations must be increased to near normal levels in IPRK to normalize perfusate flow to the 5-8 ml/min/g seen *in vivo* and antidiuretic hormone must be added to restore concentrating capacity [268, 284]. This observation suggested that high flow in the cell-free IPRK model was a result of low viscosity or because of near maximal-vasodilatation in response to the low oxygen concentration of cell-free perfusate or a combination of both. However, recent experiments in our laboratory suggest an additional explanation for high flow, at least in kidneys from Sprague-Dawley rats. Our data suggest that excessive renal nitric oxide production under control conditions contributes to the high flow and partially inhibits renal autoregulation [309].. Infusion of low dose angiotensin II restores autoregulation by modulating nitric oxide. The most pronounced improvements in IPRK physiological function followed the addition of erythrocytes as an oxygen carrier [89-91], although stroma-free lysates [310, 311] and alternative oxygen carriers have been used to maintain oxygenation [312, 313].

Physiological function in the cell-free IPRK shows somewhat reduced Na reabsorption, with FENa levels of 1-5% in rats larger than 200g and values up to 10% in smaller rat kidneys (eg, compare[269] with [273]). FENa in IPMK was closer to *in vivo* and as low as 0.3%, but the acual value was critically dependent on the albumin concentration and hence oncotic pressure of the perfusate [274]. GFR remains comparable to *in vivo* with values between 0.5 and 1.5 ml/gm kidney weight. Interestingly, little enhancement of physiological function accompanied elimination of the MTAL lesion under control conditions [269] suggesting that Na reabsorption in the MTAL contributes little to total Na reabsorption in this model. As highlighted already, renal vascular resistance, urine volume, FENa and the U/P inulin all need to be considered when evaluating function since GFR values may be distorted (inflated) by high urine volumes, even when extensive tubular injury is present, as in the most extreme case where kidneys are perfused with Krebs bicarbonate buffer alone. In the latter situation GFR values of 1-3 ml/gm kidney weight have often been recorded but the low oncotic pressure leads to rapid swelling of the kidney, perfusate flow rarely exceeds 10 ml/min and oxygen delivery is therefore inevitably and severely compromised. In this situation, FENa is often greater than 20-30% and histological examination reveals extensive proximal and MTAL injury within 60 to 90 min perfusion (PJ Ratcliffe, ZHEndre, JD Tange unpublished observations).

Fortunately, these limitations have not inhibited important studies of renal vascular function in the IPRK perfused without albumin or erythrocytes, often with flow fixed at very low levels, ca. 5 ml/min. Many of these studies have contributed valuable data on renal vascular regulation in normal and hypertension affected rat kidneys [314-321] and more recently in mouse kidney [306]. This highlights the apparent lack of oxygen-dependence of some of these processes and certainly demonstrates the utility of even a relatively hypoxic IPRK model in addressing vascular regulatory mechanisms embracing nitric oxide, endothelin, endothelium-derived hyperpolarizing factor and antidiuretic hormone. These albumin-free perfusion studies were driven by the need for single pass perfusion instead of recirculating perfusion to eliminate possible changes in concentration of the various agents added to the perfusate and by the high cost of purified albumin which usually makes single pass perfusion prohibitive. While such studies are valuable, it would be helpful if some were repeated under more physiological conditions to ensure the validity of the conclusions.

Applications in ischemia-reperfusion Injury

Ischemia-reperfusion injury has been studied in a number of ways using the IPRK. Studies have monitored the immediate effects of hypoxia induced by switching the gas delivered to the oxygenator from 95%O_2, 5%CO_2 to 95%N_2, 5%CO_2 [270, 272, 273, 322]. Alternatively, ischemia is produced by clamping the tubing and diverting flow over the kidney by a "Y' piece, eg, [323-325], which has the benefit of maintaining kidney temperature and avoiding dehydration. Chemical anoxia can be induced with metabolic inhibitors, eg, [326]. Alternatively, ischemia has been induced by renal artery clamping *in vivo* followed by the IPRK and IMPK monitoring of vascular and tubular function after periods of reperfusion varying from 10 minutes to 24 hours and often in the presence and absence of a therapeutic intervention [327, 328].

ATP depletion, cation shifts and oxygen-derived free radical injury

Early studies in the IPRK utilising ^{31}P magnetic resonance spectroscopy (MRS) confirmed the rapid onset of ATP depletion with induction of hypoxia [270]. These studies also demonstrated that the extent of morphological injury during perfusion at different degrees of hypoxia was proportional to the extent of ATP deletion. Later studies by Lieberthal in cultured mouse proximal tubule cells have confirmed that renal cells die after being subjected to ATP depletion; with severe ATP depletion the cells die by necrosis and with less severe ATP depletion the cells die by apoptosis [329], possibly because GTP depletion mediated activation of p53 [330].

Multinuclear MRS studies in the IPRK with ^{23}Na, ^{31}P and ^{87}Rb (a congener of potassium) MRS have demonstrated that increases in intracellular sodium and decreases in potassium accompany the decrease in ATP induced by hypoxia [331]. Multinuclear studies with ^{19}F, ^{35}Cl, ^{31}P and single, double and triple quantum ^{23}Na MR have also been performed in IPRK by the Gupta group. Brief (10 min) ischemia in an IPRK loaded with the membrane-impermeant intracellular calcium indicator, 5F-BAPTA, caused a partially reversible increase in the intracellular calcium from 256 to 660 nM as measured by ^{19}F [291]. They demonstrated that the increase in intracellular sodium approached extracellular levels after prolonged ischemia [291]. They also observed that kidneys exposed to higher (1.2 mM) extracellular $Mg2^{+}$ showed better recovery of ATP and lower accumulation of inorganic phosphate compared to kidneys exposed to low Mg^{2+} (0.3 mM) during reperfusion after a 60 min of stopped flow ischemia [297]. Measurements of the ^{23}Na TQ signal following ischemia-reperfusion revealed that kidneys exposed to 1.2 mM Mg^{2+} exhibited significantly improved maintenance of low intracellular sodium as compared to those exposed to 0.3 mM Mg^{2+}. Consistent with results in isolated proximal tubules, glycine supplementation reduced the rate of sodium accumulation in the intact hypoxic kidney [332].

Interestingly, the rate and extent of increase in total renal sodium (largely intracellular) in the IPRK was also reduced by pretreatment with dimethylthiourea (DMTU) and dimethylsulfoxide (DMSO), both scavengers of oxygen-derived free radicals (OFR) [272]. These studies supported similar indirect evidence for OFR-induced injury during reperfusion [333, 334]. The source of these radicals has been debated. Studies in the IPRK have demonstrated that activated neutrophils produce OFR mediated injury after ischemia [148, 149], while other studies in isolated proximal tubules and in the IPRK [272, 324, 325] indicated that OFR were generated and contributed to the injury process even in the absence of neutrophils. Furthermore, the role of infiltrating neutrophils in ischemia-reperfusion injury remains controversial [337, 338]. Studies in both isolated proximal tubules [339] and in the IPRK [324, 325] have identified that the specific OFR produced following ischemia-reperfusion include hydroxyl radicals and an other unidentified species, possibly an early lipid peroxidation product [325]. Pretreatment with either allopurinol, which acts both to inhibit xanthine oxidase and as an OFR scavenger, or DMTU reduced both the morphological features of injury the extent of DNA fragmentation in the MTAL [326], suggesting that hydroxyl radicals formed during reperfusion after ischemia play a significant role in both necrotic and apoptotic cell injury.

Site of renal ischemia-reperfusion injury

The target zone for hypoxic injury has also been extensively studied in the IPRK where it predominantly involves the S3 segment of the proximal tubule and distal tubules located within the outer stripe of the outer medulla and their cortical equivalent, the medullary rays. The debate over whether the proximal or distal nephron segment is the primary target for hypoxic injury has settled in favour of proximal tubule. However the distal nephron undergoes hypoxic/ischemic stimulated changes which precede but do not necessarily result in morphological apoptosis. What this combination of proximal tubular necrosis/apoptosis and distal nephron modulation reflects is that these nephron segments lie in close proximity to each other in the outer stripe of the outer medulla or in the medullary rays of cortical nephrons. These are the regions where the oxygen gradient is steep and energy expenditure is high with the result that both segments are positioned in a zone on the brink of hypoxia. As outlined below, the distal nephron survives injury because of upregulation of survival genes or other factors. Furthermore this survival may be critical for proximal tubular cell recovery, either through the paracrine effects of growth factors or other modulatory signalling emanating from surviving distal tubular cells.

Many of the morphological events in ischemic injury are model dependent as are those in the IPRK. As discussed already, the consistent artefactual necrosis of MTAL cells first described by Alcorn [307] arises as a result of the absence of an oxygen carrier during erythrocyte-free perfusion. Many studies by Brezis and his colleagues in the IPRK demonstrated that this MTAL lesion resulted from hypoxia and found that the lesion could be reduced by factors inhibiting energy consumption in the presence of substrate (oxygen) limitation, such as loop diuretics and that factors further reducing regional oxygen delivery such as the reductions in medullary blood flow produced by inhibition of prostaglandins and/or nitric oxide inhibitors would exagerrate MTAL injury [288, 308, 340, 341]. However, while aggravation of MTAL injury clearly occurs under a number of defined circumstances, particularly where multiple insults are delivered to the kidney, this usually occurs in association with increased proximal tubular injury as well [342]. Furthermore, Endre and colleagues in other studies in the IPRK showed that in the presence of erythrocytes in concentrations as low as 1%, MTAL necrosis was prevented both under control conditions with high perfusate oxygen tension and in the presence of hypoxia [269]. The proximal tubule continued to be injured by hypoxia *in vitro*, confirming that MTAL necrosis was an artefact of cell-free perfusion in this model. In IPRK perfused with normal concentrations of erythrocytes, MTAL injury was similarly absent[343] and such lesions are absent during ischemia *in vivo* [344], except perhaps where there is no recovery of the kidney after ischemic AKI such was described by Jean Oliver in post mortem kidneys suggesting a higher degree of severity of the initiating injury (R. Safirstein, personal communication). Thus, while the overwhelming data in IPRK and *in vivo* support the proximal tubule, especially the S3 segment, as the primary target for injury in hypoxia and ischemia, the broader focus on hypoxic injury in the IPRK has raised many useful questions and demonstrated that regional hypoxia in the kidney may be more widespread than previously appreciated.

A link between proximal and distal tubular injury and recovery

The studies in the IPRK and *in vivo* outlined in the previous section highlighted that both proximal straight tubules (S3) and MTAL were potential targets for hypoxic injury. The anatomical proximity of these tubular segments emphasizes the location of both segments in a region under constant threat of hypoxia. Outer medullary hyperemia is a consistent phenomenon following renal artery clamping to induce acute kidney injury first described by Mason and others [345, 346]. It was hypothesized that erythrocyte aggregation and stasis in the outer stripe was produced by oxygen-derived free radicals causing extravasation of plasma and local hemoconcentration, however free radical scavengers were of no benefit, whereas hemodilution and raised intrarterial pressure each reduced both medullary hyperemia and tubular necrosis [335]. The phenomenon of medullary hyperemia has not been as well described in the IPRK, probably because erythrocytes are usually not added to the perfusate and ischemia has been utilized by few groups in this model. When erythrocytes are present and flow is stopped for 20 min or more, a similar but less dramatic hyperemia is observable although prolonged reperfusion reduces this further. Our MR microscopy studies of the IPRK demonstrated that hypoxia rapidly reduced flow through the vascular bundles passing through the inner stripe and through their cortical equivalents, the medullary rays [299, 301]. The enlargement of the tubules in these interbundle regions accompanying the reduction in flow through the vascular bundles suggested that a simpler explanation for the parallel *in vivo* phenomenon of medullary hyperemia is cellular swelling leading to compression of the vascular bundles running between the clusters of proximal and TAL tubules. Leucocyte binding and red cell aggregation will compound any such narrowing of vascular diameter. [70, 347]. In any event, these observations in the IPRK provided anatomical support for the concept of local hypoxia in these regions.

A parallel phenomenon is the occurrence of DNA fragmentation by *in situ* end labelling (TUNEL) in MTAL cells after both brief or prolonged hypoxia in the IPRK or after brief ischemia *in vivo*, which is not accompanied by significant morphological evidence for apoptosis [325, 348]. Similarly, DNA fragmentation has been observed after 24 hours reperfusion following ischemia *in vivo* in rats, again with little or no morphological evidence of apoptosis [349]. DNA fragmentation has also been observed in human autopsy specimens after renal hypoperfusion [350]. Explanations for the dissociation between DNA fragmentation and apoptosis in MTAL cells include different pathways for these processes [351, 352] and also repair of damaged DNA and interruption of the apoptotic process. Studies by Gobé et al [349, 353] of the Bcl-2 multigene family 24 hours after 30 min bilateral arterial clamping *in vivo* have demonstrated a marked increase in expression of antiapoptotic Bcl-2 and a moderate increase in antiapoptotic Bcl-X(L) and proapoptotic Bax in distal tubules. Proximal tubules showed a marked increase in Bax expression and a moderate increase in Bcl-X(L). Twenty-four hours after expression of the Bcl-2 proteins was increased, IGF-1 and EGF protein levels were increased in the distal tubule, similar to the Bcl-2 anti-apoptotic proteins. These growth factors were also detected in the adjacent proximal tubules suggesting a paracrine action since the factors are apparently not synthesized in proximal tubules. TGF-beta expression was moderately increased in regenerating proximal tubules, but no relationship to the pattern of expression of the Bcl-2 genes was seen. To reconcile the observations of proximal cell necrosis and DNA fragmentation without apoptosis in nearby MTAL, Gobé and colleagues [349] have proposed that the distal tubule is adaptively resistant to ischemic injury via promotion of survival by anti-apoptotic Bcl-2 genes, which abort the apoptotic process in MTAL cells, leading to repair of the DNA fragmentation. Further studies by the same group [354] on the mechanism of this protection in cultured cells suggest that survival in distal tubular cells is associated with translocation of the Bcl-2 family proteins, Bcl-X(L) in the case of MDCK cells, to the mitochondrial membrane. This prevents release of cytochrome c, which precedes activation of caspase 3 in the p53 cell death pathway [355]. Additional cytoprotective reserve in MTAL cells, in contrast to proximal tubule cells against early apoptotic injury, arises through early and differential upregulation of the protective mitogen-activated kinases (MAP kinase) pathway regulated by extracellular signal kinase (ERK) [356]. Proximal tubular cells lack Bcl-2, but contain proapoptotic Bax and proceed to death by both apoptosis and necrosis. Survival of the distal tubular cells allows expression of EGF and IGF growth factors critical to the maintenance and regeneration of other distal tubular cells (autocrine action), and to survival and/or regeneration of the adjacent ischemia-sensitive proximal tubular cells (paracrine action). Since proximal cells are necrotic or have sloughed due to loss of cell adhesion, proximal recovery is delayed compared to the MTAL.

Thus studies in the IPRK have provided evidence that both ischemia and hypoxia produce reduced flow in the outer stripe of the outer medulla and that the resultant regional hypoxia affects nearby proximal and distal tubules leading to necrosis of proximal tubules and arrested apoptosis of the distal tubules. Follow up work *in vivo* and in cultured cells have suggested that the distal tubular cells are protected by Bcl-2 family and MAP Kinase upregulation and that survival of these cells allows growth factors to promote regeneration of the nearby injured proximal tubules. Interestingly these data fit with studies of localization of the early gene response and DNA synthesis in the kidney after ischemic injury. DNA synthesis occurs in the proximal tubule, whereas induction of the early gene response is restricted to the MTAL and collecting duct cells [357].

Tubuloglomerular feedback and autoregulation

Although direct observation of the microcirculation is not possible in the standard IPRK model, the use of hyperoncotic solutions to create a non-filtering kidney [358] allows a relatively clean interruption of tubuloglomerular feedback (by impairing distal tubular NaCl delivery) analogous to papillectomy in the perfused juxtamedullary nephron technique [101]. Frusemide can also be used to inhibit tubuloglomerular feedback in either preparation. This allows the interaction between tubuloglomerular feedback and autoregulation to be explored. We examined the effect of angiotensin II (Ang II), nitric oxide (NO), EDHF and prostaglandins on autoregulation of renal perfusion in the isolated perfused kidney (IPRK) from Sprague-Dawley rats during stepped increases in perfusion pressure [309]. Ang II (75–200 pM) produced dose-dependent enhancement of autoregulation whereas phenylephrine produced no enhancement and impaired autoregulation of GFR. Enhancement by Ang II was inhibited by the AT_1 antagonist, Losartan, and the superoxide scavenger, Tempol. Under control conditions nitric oxide synthase (NOS) inhibition by 10 μM N-omega-nitro-L-arginine methyl ester (L-NAME) facilitated autoregulation in the presence of non-specific cyclooxygenase (COX) inhibition by 10 μM indomethacin. Both COX and combined NOS/COX inhibition reduced the autoregulatory threshold concentration of Ang II. Facilitation by 100 pM Ang II was inhibited by 100 μM frusemide. Methacholine (50 nM) antagonized Ang II-facilitated autoregulation in the presence and absence of NOS/COX inhibition. Infusion of the NO donor, 1 μM sodium nitroprusside, inhibited L-NAME enhancement of autoregulation under control conditions and during Ang II infusion. These results suggest that an excess of NO impairs autoregulation under control conditions in the IPRK and that endogenous and exogenous NO, vasodilatory prostaglandins and endothelium-derived hyperpolarizing factor (EDHF) activity antagonise Ang II-facilitated autoregulation. Ang II also produced a counterregulatory vasodilatory response that included prostaglandin and NO release. Taken together the results suggest that Ang II facilitates autoregulation by a tubuloglomerular feedback-dependent mechanism through AT_1 receptor-mediated depletion of nitric oxide, probably by stimulating generation of superoxide.

These strategies were then applied to examine endothelial dysfunction in ischemic acute kidney injury, a dysfunction which has been attributed to both direct endothelial injury and to altered endothelial nitric oxide synthase (eNOS) activity, with either maximal upregulation of eNOS or inhibition of eNOS by excess NO derived from iNOS. We used the IPRK to investigate renal endothelial dysfunction in the intact kidney by assessing both autoregulation and endothelium-dependent vasorelaxation 24 hours after unilateral (U) or bilateral (B) renal artery occlusion for 30 or 60 minutes and in sham-operated controls [328]. The integrated response of renal endothelium was assessed from the vasodilator response to the endothelium-dependent vasodilator methacholine (MCh) after preconstriction by Ang II. Although renal failure was induced in all degrees of ischemia, neither endothelial dysfunction nor altered facilitation of autoregulation by 75pM angiotensin II was detected in U30, U60 or B30 kidneys. Baseline and angiotensin II-facilitated autoregulation were impaired, methacholine EC_{50} was increased and endothelium-derived hyperpolarizing factor (EDHF) activity preserved in B60 kidneys. Increasing angiotensin II concentration restored autoregulation and increased RVR in B60 kidneys; this facilitated autoregulation and increase in RVR was abolished by 100μM furosemide. Autoregulation was enhanced by L-NAME. Peri-ischemic inhibition of iNOS ameliorated renal failure but did not prevent endothelial dysfunction or impaired autoregulation. There was no significant structural injury to the afferent arterioles with ischemia. These results suggest tubuloglomerular feedback (TGF) is preserved in IAKI, but that excess NO and probably EDHF produce endothelial dysfunction and antagonize autoregulation. The threshold for injury producing detectable endothelial dysfunction was higher than for loss of GFR. Arteriolar endothelial dysfunction after prolonged IAKI is predominantly functional rather than structural.

Endothelin in ischemia-reperfusion injury

Many studies of endothelin action have been performed in the IPRK. The potential potent vasoconstrictor role of endothelin in acute kidney injury was first noted in the IPRK by Firth [359], who also observed that endothelin-1 mRNA was upregulated for several days after renal pedicle clamping *in vivo* [360]. *In vivo* studies suggest that this upregulation of endothelin is modestly stimulated by hypoxia alone[361-2] but that rapid and prolonged upregulation occurs after ischemia in renal medullary interstitial cells, damaged tubules at the corticomedullary junction and peritubular capillaries surrounding these damaged tubules [363-365]. IPRK studies showed that pretreatment with a selective endothelin (ETA) receptor antagonist), BQ-123, ameliorated the fall in inulin clearance and sodium transport in a renal artery clamp model of ischemic acute kidney injury [366]. The benefit of endothelin antagonists in ischemic acute kidney injury *in vivo* and *in vitro* is complicated by the different effects of ETA and ETB receptors, with protection arising from ETA antagonists and exacerbation from both non-selective and ETB-selective antagonists, the latter presumably because of impaired ETB-stimulated nitric oxide production [367].

Treatment of ischemic acute kidney injury

Many experimental treatments for acute kidney injury have been tested in the IPRK, either for efficacy or in the assessment of mechanisms leading to renal cell injury. One example leading to clinical application will be discussed. Lieberthal et al [368] observed that renal vascular resistance was increased during reflow in the isolated erythrocyte-perfused kidney subjected to 25 min of ischemia. Endothelium-independent vasodilators (atrial natriuretic factor, ANF, and sodium nitroprusside) prevented the increase. Acetylcholine and the calcium ionophore A23187, two vasodilators that act by releasing endothelium-derived relaxing factor, had no effect, while two inhibitors of EDRF, methylene blue, and gossypol, increased RVR in nonischemic kidneys by an amount comparable to that found with ischemia alone. The increase in RVR found with the combination of EDRF inhibition and ischemia was the same as that found with ischemia alone. In further studies[271], they found that ANF, administered alone after 25 min ischemia in the isolated kidney, reversed postischemic vasoconstriction but did not improve glomerular filtration rate (GFR). Mannitol alone had no effect on either renal vascular resistance or GFR. However, in isolated kidneys treated with the combination of both ANF and mannitol following reflow, GFR was markedly improved compared with GFR in the untreated ischemia group and was not different from

GFR in the nonischemic controls. Comparable results were obtained in studies performed *in vivo*, suggesting that the combination of ANF and mannitol appear to act synergistically to improve GFR following ischemic injury. These studies provided the initial experimental basis for subsequent clinical studies of ANP in acute kidney injury [369].

Nephrotoxic injury

The IPRK model has been helpful in assessing many potential nephrotoxins and in revealing mechanisms of toxicity and treatment. Given the hundreds of published studies, only selected areas will be cited. It should also be noted that many of the IPRK preparations have utilized cell-free perfusion and are therefore likely to have varying degrees of distal tubular injury. However, as already noted, this seems less of a problem where the primary interest is in vascular or proximal tubular function.

Cyclosporine

Nephrotoxicity arising from cyclosporine A has been extensively studied in the IPRK. Cyclosporine produces necrosis, vacuolization and lipid droplets of the proximal tubular cells, as well as glomerular afferent arteriolar constriction and granular juxtaglomerular cell hyperplasia. The mechanism of vasoconstriction is not well known, but there appears to be substantial impairment of endothelial cell function leading to enhanced release of vasoconstrictors such as endothelin and thromboxane [370]. L- propionylcarnitine, a potent analogue of carnitine, is able to correct and to prevent alterations in endothelial membrane permeability and has been identified in the kidney of various animal species. Pretreatment with L- propionylcarnitine before administering several doses of CyA in the IPRK reduced the vasoconstrictive effect of CyA on the glomerular and tubular capillaries and preserved the tubular epithelium both histologically and functionally with a reduction in cyclosporin-induced release of alanine aminopeptidase and N-acetyl- glucosaminidase [371].

Endothelin in hypertension and pro-atherogenic states

The role of renal endothelin receptors in diseases associated with hypertension appears to be critical. Hirata and colleagues [372] utilized the IPRK to demonstrate that ETB receptor stimulation induced release of nitric oxide. They found that ET-1 and ET-3 released nitric oxide via ETB receptors in renal vessels. ETB receptors were downregulated in deoxycorticosterone acetate (DOCA-salt) rat kidneys explaining why ETB-mediated NO release was reduced in DOCA-salt rats, an event which may modulate renal function and blood pressure regulation in DOCA-salt hypertensive rats. They subsequently observed that expression of ETB receptors in the endothelium was decreased in IPRK from 3 disease models (rats with hypertension, diabetes mellitus, and hypercholesterolemia) compared with that in the vascular smooth muscle cell[319]. Infusion of a highly selective ETB receptor agonist, BQ-3020, reduced renal perfusion pressure in Dahl salt-resistant rats but increased renal perfusion pressure in Dahl salt-sensitive rats. BQ-3020 caused a dose-dependent release of nitric oxide in both types of rats, although the level of nitric oxide release in salt-sensitive rats was lower. Similar effects of BQ-3020 were observed in streptozotocin- induced diabetic rats and diet-induced hypercholesterolemic rats. Expression of endothelial NO synthase (eNOS) decreased in salt-sensitive rats but not in diabetic or hypercholesterolemic rats. They concluded that impaired NO release in response to stimulation of ETB receptors in these pathologic states is due, at least in part, to a decrease in endothelial ETB receptors and may play a role in vascular dysfunction usually associated with arteriosclerosis-related diseases.

Radiocontrast

Studies on the mechanisms of radiocontrast nephrotoxicity have been performed in IPRK with conflicting results. While some studies provided modest support for the contrast –induced renal vasoconstriction theory, perhaps resulting from reduced nitric oxide or increased endothelin release, others demonstrated that different contrast agents had varying effects on the renal circulation. For example, pretreatment with BQ123 (a selective endothelin (ETA) receptor antagonist), but not with phosphoramidon (an endothelin-converting enzyme inhibitor), inhibited the sustained fall in renal perfusate flow produced by both iotrolan and diatrizoate. BQ123 markedly potentiated the renal vasodilatation produced by diatrizoate [373] and the AT1 receptor blocker, bosentan, prevented reduction in creatinine clearance after diatrizoate [374]. However, subsequent studies in the IPRK however suggest that NO and endothelin-mediated events are independent and not modulated by these radiocontrast agents. For example, in careful dose response studies in the IPRK, Morcos et al [375] observed that L-NAME did not interfere with the vasodilatation induced by diatrizoate in the presence of BQ123 and concluded that diatrizoate did not interfere with endothelium derived NO-dependent vasodilatation. They concluded that reduced production of NO in the vascular endothelium induced by contrast media was unlikely to play any role in the pathophysiology of the increase in renal vascular resistance produced by radiocontrast agents and specifically that the renal vasodilatation induced by diatrizoate was not dependent on endogenous production of NO. In this light it is perhaps not surprising that inhibition of ETB receptor stimulated nitric oxide release could have produced the exacerbation of radiocontrast nephrotoxicity by a non-selective endothelin antagonist in a recent prospective clinical trial [376]. Nevertheless the etiology and treatment of radiocontrast nephropathy is far from clear. Further studies will need to account, inter alia, for the exacerbation in vasoconstriction produced by prostaglandin inhibition in the IPRK [377], for the role of adenosine suggested by amelioration by theophylline [378-9] . One related experimental finding, at least, has changed clinical practice. Yoshioka et al [380] demonstrated that renal cortical antioxidant activity was reduced in water-deprived rats and that only water-deprived rats showed increased lipid peroxidation after contrast which was inhibitable by pretreatment with polyethylene glycol-coupled catalase. The link between water deprivation and, presumably free radical-mediated depletion of renal cortical oxidant activity is unclear. However, the observation has lead to the many clinical trials of prevention of contrast nephropathy by N-acetylcysteine beginning with the study of Tepel et al [381].

Mercuric chloride

A progressive fall in glomerular capillary plasma flow is observed in mercuric chloride-induced acute kidney injury although the site of the main histological lesion is the proximal tubule. Studies in the IPRK showed that intense mercuric chloride-induced vasoconstriction could be inhibited by captopril but not enalapril arguing against renin-angiotensin system involvement, with binding of free Hg by the sulphydryl group of captopril suggesting a simpler explanation and supporting possible attack by Hg to tissue thiol moieties as the mechanism for vasoconstriction [382]. However, vasoconstriction was absent in the non-filtering IPRK, suggesting that intraluminal mechanisms might be involved [169]. Adenosine analogues selective for the A1 subclass of adenosine receptors, such as N6-cyclohexyladenosine (CHA), induce vasoconstriction in the IPRK [383]. However, theophylline failed to reverse mercuric chloride-induced vasoconstriction [384]. More recent studies *in vivo* suggest that increased endothelin and reduced nitric oxide may be involved in mercuric chloride-induced vasoconstriction. Both endothelin (ET-1) and eNOS proteins are expressed in the juxtaglomerular cells of afferent arterioles. The expression of ET-1 was significantly increased after mercuric chloride-induced acute kidney injury whereas the expression of eNOS was markedly reduced[385]. Taken together, these data suggest that mercuric-chloride induced vasoconstriction is mediated by increased endothelin and reduced nitric oxide, the latter perhaps involving tubuloglomerular feedback.

Nitric oxide, endothelium-derived hyperpolarizing factor and prostaglandins

The IPRK was used to demonstrate that excess nitric oxide (NO) and possibly endothelium-derived hyperpolarizing factor (EDHF), contribute to impaired autoregulation after ischemic injury as described above [328]. A role for EDHF in renal vascular resistance and in glomerular and tubular function was first observed in the IPRK by Bhardwaj and Moore [386] and by Rademacher et al [387-8]. Others observed that manipulating NO can alter medullary oxygenation in the IPRK [288]. An increased endothelium-dependent vasodilator response to acetylcholine was observed in IPRK from cirrhotic rats [390]. Portal vein ligation also lowered renal vascular resistance that was not related to nitric oxide or prostaglandins, although increased nitric oxide production interfered with the effects of the alfa-agonist methoxamine [391], further suggesting that NO plays an important role in the modulation of the renal vascular responses to vasoconstrictors in portal hypertension. Subsequent studies by Vargas et al [392-393] in the IPRK pretreated with indomethacin and utilizing tetramethylamonium (a non-specific blocker of potassium channels that inhibits acetylcholine-induced hyperpolarization) and varying potassium concentrations suggested that both NO and EDHF are similarly involved in the endothelium-dependent vasodilatation induced by acetylcholine. Similarly, NO- and prostaglandin-independent, endothelium-dependent vasodilator responses to bradykinin are attributed to release of a hyperpolarizing factor. The contribution of K^+ channels to the renal vasodilator effect of bradykinin was assessed in the IPRK in the presence of ATP- and Ca^{2+}-activated K channel inhibitors [394-395]. These studies implicated Ca^{2+}-activated K^+ channels in the renal vasodilator response to bradykinin and similarly support a role for a hyperpolarizing factor. Other studies in IPRK have demonstrated the biological importance of S-nitrosothiols (RS-NO) in the action and metabolism of endothelium-derived relaxing factor [396].

Studies in the IPRK utilizing single-pass perfusion have demonstrated a close interaction between renal NO and the cyclo-oxygenase pathway with inhibition of prostanoid production by nitric oxide [397]. The pressor effect of L-NAME also appears to partly rely upon the vasoconstrictor effect of TxA2 and PGH2. Other studies in the recirculating IPRK have shown interactions between bradykinin and ANP on both glomerular and tubular function [398], between estrogens and calcium-modulated endothelium-dependent dilatation [399], between angiotensin II and eicosanoid release stimulated through AT2 receptors [400], and that the NO-cGMP pathway is involved in adrenomedullin induced vasorelaxation [401]. Finally, other single pass studies suggest that impaired NO release in response to stimulation of endothelin ET-B receptors may result from a decrease in endothelial ET-B receptors, which may represent a mechanism for in vascular dysfunction usually associated with arteriosclerosis- related diseases [319].

Renal and cardiac fibrosis

Short-term pirfenidone and spironolactone treatment was recently found to reverse cardiac and renal fibrosis and to attenuate increased diastolic stiffness without normalizing cardiac contractility or renal function in STZ-diabetic rats [402].

Glomerular function in the IPRK

There is a significant literature exploring many aspects of glomerular function and models of glomerular injury in the IPRK. Examples include studies of albumin excretion, protein trafficking and vasoactive modulation of glomerular permselectivity [389, 403-407]; studies of glomerular immune injury including the role of complement [408], leukotrienes [409-410], prostaglandins [411-412] and clusterin [413] and studies of glomerular hemodynamics [414].

Disadvantages of the IPRK model

In common with most isolated organs, the disadvantages of the IPRK include some physiological limitations. These can be summarized as high perfusate flow, low resistance, low filtration fraction and time-dependent deterioration of renal function, and loss of distal integrity. There is a requirement for significant technical surgical skill. The higher flow than *in vivo*, arises from relative nitric oxide excess rather than simply low perfusate viscosity[6]. The model brings with it the expense and trouble involved in preparation and use of albumin-containing solutions to achieve reasonable tubular and glomerular function and even more complexity when erythrocytes are added to preserve distal tubular integrity. Finally, despite extensive preparation and skilful handling, the model is only viable for a few hours - longer in the presence of erythrocytes, shorter in their absence. Thus, perturbations requiring longer than 2-3 hours for development can only be monitored after having first been induced *in vivo*, potentially negating at least part of the benefit of assessing some pathological or physiological events in the absence of non-renal or uncontrolled systemic influences.

Advantages of the IPRK model

The IPRK is an intact model of the kidney function, which is well suited to examining critical functions, which require an intact renal architecture but allowing simplification of complex *in vivo* responses. Such critical functions modified by the renal architecture encompass substrate delivery, including oxygen, and the links between vascular and tubular function. The model has the advantages of eliminating systemic hormonal and sympathetic nervous system influences, while still allowing tight control of pressure and flow and of permitting simultaneous measurement of renal vascular and tubular function with direct infusion of vasoactive agents into the renal artery. It allows quantifiable assessment of renal vascular, tubular and glomerular function and high quality morphological assessment. Such advantages may allow intrinsic physiological responses to be accurately defined and may provide answers opposite to conclusions drawn from models not utilizing an intact kidney, for example the renal response to changes in osmolality [305, 415] Finally the model permits more specialized assessment such as magnetic resonance microscopy and spectroscopy. With continuous modification for over 40 years, the IPRK technique has developed into a reliable and powerful method for studying many questions regarding renal physiology and function in both health and disease and utilizing most of the techniques applied *in vivo* and others that are too difficult to apply, such as magnetic resonance microscopy.

REFERENCES

1. Racusen LC: Renal histopathology and urine cytology and cytopathology in acute renal failure., chap. 9, in Acute renal failure. New concepts and therapeutic strategies, edited by Goligorsky MS, Stein JH, New York, Churchill Livingstone, 1995, p 194
2. Edelstein CL, Ling H, Schrier RW: The nature of renal cell injury. Kidney Int 51:1341-1351, 1997
3. Iwata M, Myerson D, Torok-Storb B, Zager RA: An evaluation of renal tubular DNA laddering in response to oxygen deprivation and oxidant injury. J.Am.Soc.Nephrol. 5:1307-1313, 1994
4. Nogae S, Miyazaki M, Kobayashi N, Saito T, Abe K, Saito H, Nakane PK, Nakanishi Y, Koji T: Induction of apoptosis in ischemia-reperfusion model of mouse kidney: possible involvement of Fas. J.Am.Soc.Nephrol. 9:620-631, 1998
5. Schumer M, Colombel MC, Sawczuk IS, Gobe G, Conner J, O'Toole KT, Olsson CA, Wise GJ, Buttyan R: Morphologic, biochemical and molecular evidence of apoptosis during the reperfusion phase after brief periods of renal ischemia. Am.J.Path. 140:831-838, 1992
6. Basile DP, Liapis H, Hammerman MR: Expression of bcl-2 and bax in regenerating rat tubules following ischemic injury. Am.J.Physiol. 272:640-647, 1997
7. Lieberthal W, Nigam SK: Acute renal failure:II.Experimental models of acute renal failure; imperfect but indispensable. Am J Physiol 278:F1-F12, 2000
8. Gobe G, Willgoss D, Hogg N, Schoch E, Endre Z: Cell survival or death in renal tubular epithelium after ischemia- reperfusion injury. Kidney Int 56:1299-1304, 1999
9. Gobe G, Zhang XJ, Cuttle L, Pat B, Willgoss D, Hancock J, Barnard R, Endre RB: Bcl-2 genes and growth factors in the pathology of ischaemic acute renal failure. Immunol.Cell Biol. 77:279-286, 1999
10. Gobe G, Zhang XJ, Willgoss DA, Schoch E, Hogg NA, Endre ZH: Relationship between expression of Bcl-2 genes and growth factors in ischemic acute renal failure in the rat. J Am Soc Nephrol. 11:454-467, 2000
11. Safirstein RL: Renal disease induced by anti-neoplastic agents., chap. 43, in Diseases of the Kidney and Urinary Tract., 8th ed., edited by Schrier RW, Philadelphia, Lippincott, Williams and Wilkins, 2007, pp 1068-1081
12. Andrade L, Vieira JM, Safirstein R: How Cells Die Counts. Am J Kidney Dis. 36:662-668, 2000
13. Kroemer G, Dallaporta B, Resche-Rigon M: The mitochondrial death/life regulator in apoptosis and necrosis. Annu.Rev.Physiol 60:619-642, 1998
14. Grasl-Kraupp B, Ruttkay-Nedecky B, Koudelka H, Bukowska K, Bursch W, Schulte-Hermann R: *In situ* detection of fragmented DNA (TUNEL assay) fails to discriminate among apoptosis, necrosis, and autolytic cell death: a cautionary note. Hepatology 21:1465-1468, 1995
15. De Broe ME: Apoptosis in acute renal failure. Nephrol.Dial.Transplant. 16 Suppl 6:23-26, 2001
16. Hagar H, Ueda N, Shah SV: Endonuclease induced DNA damage and cell death in chemical hypoxic injury to LLC-PK1 cells. Kidney Int 49:355-361, 1996

17. Better OS: Josep Trueta (1897-1977): military surgeon and pioneer investigator of acute renal failure. AM.J.Nephrol. 19:343-345, 1999
18. Humes HD, Fissell WH, Weitzel WF, Buffington DA, Westover AJ, MacKay SM, Gutierrez JM: Metabolic replacement of kidney function in uremic animals with a bioartificial kidney containing human cells. American Journal of Kidney Diseases 39:1078-1087, 2002
19. jayle C, Favreau F, Zhang K, Doucet C, Goujon JM, Hebrard W, Carretier M, Eugene M, Mauco G, Tillement JP, Hauet T: Comparison of protective effects of trimetazidine against experimental warm ischemia of different durations: early and long-term effects in a pig kidney model. Am.J.Physiol Renal Physiol 292:F1082-F1093, 2007
20. Netea MG, Fantuzzi G, Kullberg BJ, Stuyt RJ, Pulido EJ, McIntyre RC, Jr., Joosten LA, Van der Meer JW, Dinarello CA: Neutralization of IL-18 reduces neutrophil tissue accumulation and protects mice against lethal Escherichia coli and Salmonella typhimurium endotoxemia. J.Immunol. 164:2644-2649, 2000
21. Sakao Y, Takeda K, Tsutsui H, Kaisho T, Nomura F, Okamura H, Nakanishi K, Akira S: IL-18-deficient mice are resistant to endotoxin-induced liver injury but highly susceptible to endotoxin shock. Int Immunol. 11:471-480, 1999
22. Siegmund B, Rieder F, Lehr HA, Eigler A, Endres S, Dinarello CA: Neutralization of IL-18 exerts anti-inflammatory activity in experimental colitis in mice. Eur Cytokine Netw 11: 2000
23. Pizarro T. Differential role of IL-18 in acute versus chronic experimental colitis. 2001. Immunogenetic mechanisms of intestinal inflammation: role of cytokines and chemokines. Univ. of Virginia Health System. Ref Type: Conference Proceeding
24. Lieschke GJ, Grail D, Hodgson G, Metcalf D, Stanley E, Cheers C, Fowler KJ, Basu S, Zhan YF, Dunn AR: Mice lacking granulocyte colony-stimulating factor have chronic neutropenia, granulocyte and macrophage progenitor cell deficiency, and impaired neutrophil mobilization. Blood 84:1737-1746, 1994
25. Stanley E, Lieschke GJ, Grail D, Metcalf D, Hodgson G, Gall JA, Maher DW, Cebon J, Sinickas V, Dunn AR: Granulocyte/macrophage colony-stimulating factor-deficient mice show no major perturbation of hematopoiesis but develop a characteristic pulmonary pathology. Proc.Natl.Acad.Sci.U.S.A 91:5592-5596, 1994
26. Burne MJ, Haq M, Matsuse H, Mohapatra S, Rabb H: Genetic susceptibility to renal ischemia reperfusion injury revealed in a murine model. Transplantation 69:1023-1025, 2000
27. Markel P, Shu P, Ebeling C, Carlson GA, Nagle DL, Smutko JS, Moore KJ: Theoretical and empirical issues for marker-assisted breeding of congenic mouse strains. Nat Genet 17:280-284, 1997
28. Wakeland E, Morel L, Achey K, Yui M, Longmate J: Speed congenics: a classic technique in the fast lane (relatively speaking). Immunol Today 18:472-477, 1997
29. Park KM, Kim JI, Ahn Y, Bonventre AJ, Bonventre JV: Testosterone is responsible for enhanced susceptibility of males to ischemic renal injury. Journal of Biological Chemistry 279:52282-52292, 2004
30. Igarashi: Kidney-specific gene targeting. J.Am.Soc.Nephrol. 15:2237-2239, 2004
31. Nagy A: Cre recombinase: the universal reagent for genome tailoring. Genesis: the Journal of Genetics & Development 26:99-109, 2000
32. Conger JD, Robinette JB, Hammond WS: Differences in vascular reactivity in models of ischemic acute renal failure. Kidney Int. 39:1087-1097, 1991
33. Malis CD, Cheung JY, Leaf A, Bonventre JV: Effects of verapamil in models of ischemic acute renal failure in the rat. Am.J.Physiol. 245:F735-F742, 1983
34. Burke TJ, Arnold PE, Gordon JA, Bulger RE, Dobyan DC, Schrier RW: Protective effect of intrarenal calcium membrane blockers before or after renal ischemia. Functional, morphological, and mitochondrial studies. J Clin Invest 74:1830-1841, 1984
35. Fried TA, Hishida A, Barnes JL, Stein JH: Ischemic acute renal failure in the rat: protective effect of uninephrectomy. Am.J.Physiol 247:F568-F574, 1984
36. Nakajima T, Miyaji T, Kato A, Ikegaya N, Yamamoto T, Hishida A: Uninephrectomy reduces apoptotic cell death and enhances renal tubular cell regeneration in ischemic ARF in rats. Am J Physiol 271:F846-F853, 1996
37. Tsukamoto T, Nigam SK: Tight junction proteins form large complexes and associate with the cytoskeleton in an ATP depletion model for reversible junction assembly. J Biol.Chem. 272:16133-16139, 1997
38. Endre ZH, Ratcliffe PJ, Tange JD, Ferguson DJ, Radda GK, Ledingham JG: Erythrocytes alter the pattern of renal hypoxic injury: predominance of proximal tubular injury with moderate hypoxia. Clin.Sci. 76:19-29, 1989
39. Donohoe JF, Venkatachalam MA, Bernard DB, Levinsky NG: Tubular leakage and obstruction after renal ischemia: structural-functional correlations. Kidney Int. 13:208-222, 1978
40. Lieberthal W, Nigam SK: Acute renal failure. Relative importance of proximal vs. distal tubular injury. Am.J.Physiol. 275:F623-F632, 1998
41. Thadhani R, Pascual M, Bonventre JV: Medical progress-acute renal failure. N Engl J Med 334:1448-1460, 1996

42. Shanley PF, Rosen MD, Brezis M, Silva P, Epstein FH, Rosen S: Topography of focal proximal tubular necrosis after ischemia with reflow in the rat kidney. Am.J.Pathol. 122:462-468, 1986
43. Ysebaert DK, De Greef KE, Vercauteren SR, Ghielli M, Verpooten GA, Eyskens EJ, De Broe ME: Identification and kinetics of leukocytes after severe ischaemia/reperfusion renal injury. Nephrol.Dial.Transplant. 15:1562-1574, 2000
44. Jones DB: Ultrastructure of human acute renal failure. Lab Invest 46:254-264, 1982
45. Olsen TS, Hansen HE: Ultrastructure of medullary tubules in ischemic acute tubular necrosis and acute interstitial nephritis in man. APMIS 98:1139-1148, 1990
46. Lieberthal W, Levine JS: Mechanisms of apoptosis and its potential role in renal tubular epithelial cell injury. Am.J.Physiol 271: F477-F488, 1996
47. Daemen MARC, Van t'Veer C, Denecker G, Heemskerk VH, Wolfs TGAM, Clauss M, Vandenabeele P, Buurman W: Inhibition of apoptosis induced by ischemia-reperfusion prevents inflammation. J.Clin.Invest. 104:541-549, 1999
48. Edelstein CL: Editorial Comment: Calcium-mediated proximal tubular injury-what is the role of cysteine proteases? Nephrol.Dial. Transplant. 15:141-144, 2000
49. Lieberthal W, Koh JS, Levine JS: Necrosis and apoptosis in acute renal failure. Semin Nephrol 18:505-518, 1998
50. Lieberthal W: Biology of acute renal failure: Therapeutic implications. Kidney Int 52:1102-1115, 1997
51. Lau AH: Apoptosis induced by cisplatin nephrotoxic injury. Kidney Int 56:1295-1298, 1999
52. Kaushal GP, Singh AB, Shah SV: Identification of gene family of caspases in rat kidney and altered expression in ischemia reperfusion injury. Am.J.Physiol. 274:F587-F595, 1998
53. Shimizu A, Yamanaka N: Apoptosis and cell desquamation in repair process of ischemic tubular necrosis. Virchows Arch.B Cell Pathol.Incl.Mol.Pathol. 64:171-180, 1993
54. Molitoris BA, Geerdes A, McIntosh JR: Dissociation and redistribution of Na^+, K^+ -ATPase from its surface membrane cytoskeletal complex during cellular ATP depletion. J Clin Invest 88:462-469, 1991
55. Van Why SK, Mann AS, Ardito T, Siegel NJ, Kashgarian M: Expression and molecular regulation of NaK-ATPase after renal ischemia. Am.J.Physiol. 267:F75-F85, 1994
56. Molitoris BA: Ischemia-induced loss of epithelial polarity: potential role of the actin cytoskeleton [editorial]. Am J Physiol 260: F769-F778, 1991
57. Molitoris BA, Wilson PD, Schrier RW, Simon FR: Ischemia induces partial loss of surface membrane polarity and accumulation of putative calcium ionophores. J.Clin.Invest 76:2097-2105, 1985
58. Molitoris BA: New insights into the cell biology of ischemic acute renal failure. J Am Soc Nephrol 1:1263-1270, 1991
59. Alejandro VSJ, Nelson WJ, Huie P, Sibley RK, Dafoe D, Kuo P, Scandling JDJr, Myers BD: Postischemic injury, delayed function and NaK-ATPase distribution in the transplanted kidney. Kidney Int. 48:1308-1315, 1995
60. Racusen LC, Fivush BA, LI YL, Slatnic I, Solez K: Dissociation of tubular cell detachment and tubular cell death in clinical and experimental "acute renal failure". Lab.Invest. 64:546-556, 1991
61. Harlan JM: Neutrophil-mediated vascular injury. Acta Med.Scand.Suppl 715:123-129, 1987
62. Weiss SJ: Tissue destruction by neutrophils. N.Engl.J.Med. 320:365-376, 1989
63. Horl WH, Schafer RM, Horl M, Heidland A: Neutrophil activation in acute renal failure and sepsis. Arch.Surg. 125:651-654, 1990
64. Jennette JC, Falk RJ: Acute renal failure secondary to leukocyte-mediated acute glomerular injury. Ren Fail. 14:395-399, 1992
65. Goode HF, Webster NR: Free radicals and antioxidants in sepsis. Crit Care Med. 21:1770-1776, 1993
66. Lauriat S, Linas SL: The role of neutrophils in acute renal failure. Semin.Nephrol. 18:498-504, 1998
67. Melnikov VY, Faubel SG, Siegmund B, Lucia MS, Ljubanovic D, Edelstein CL: Neutrophil-independent mechanisms of caspase-1- and IL-18-mediated ischemic acute tubular necrosis in mice. J.Clin Invest 110:1083-1091, 2002
68. Bonventre JV, Zuk A: Ischemic acute renal failure: an inflammatory disease? Kidney Int. 66:480-485, 2004
69. Friedwald JJ, Rabb H: Inflammatory cells in ischemic acute renal failure. Kidney Int. 66:486-491, 2004
70. Ysebaert DK, De Greef KE, De Beuf A, Van Rompay AR, Vercauteren SR, Persy VP, De Broe ME: T cells as mediators in renal ischemia/reperfusion injury. Kidney Int. 66:491-495, 2004
71. Burne MJ, Daniels F, El Ghandour A, Mauiyyedi S, Colvin RB, O'Donnell MP, Rabb H: Identification of the CD4(+) T cell as a major pathogenic factor in ischemic acute renal failure. J Clin.Invest 108:1283-1290, 2001
72. Jose MD, Ikezumi Y, Van Rooijen N, Atkins RC, Chadban SJ: Macrophages act as effectors of tissue damage in acute renal allograft rejection. Transplantation 76:1015-1022, 2003
73. Day YJ, Huang L, Ye H, Linden J, Okusa MD: Renal Ischemia-Reperfusion Injury and Adenosine 2A Receptor-Mediated Tissue Protection: The Role of Macrophages. Am J Physiol Renal Physiol 288:F722-F731, 2004
74. Jo SK, Sung SA, Cho WY, Go KJ, Kim HK: Macrophages contribute to the initiation of ischemic acute renal failure in rats. Nephrol. Dial.Transplant. 21:1231-1239, 2006

75. Furuichi K, Wada T, Iwata Y, Kitagawa K, Kobayashi K, Hashimoto H, Ishiwata Y, Tomosugi N, Mukaida N, Matsushima K, Egashira K, Yokoyama H: Gene therapy expressing amino-terminal truncated monocyte chemoattractant protein-1 prevents renal ischemia-reperfusion injury. Journal of the American Society of Nephrology 14:1066-1071, 2003
76. American Society of Nephrology Renal Research Report. J.Am.Soc.Nephrol. 16, 1886-1903. 2005. Ref Type: Report
77. Ronco C, Zanella M, Brendolan A, Milan M, Canato G, Zamperetti N, Bellomo R: Management of severe acute renal failure in critically ill patients: an international survey in 345 centres. Nephrol.Dial.Transplant. 16:230-237, 2001
78. Brivet FG, Kleinknecht DJ, Loirat P, Landais PJ: Acute renal failure in intensive care units--causes, outcome, and prognostic factors of hospital mortality; a prospective, multicenter study. French Study Group on Acute Renal Failure. Crit Care Med. 24:192-198, 1996
79. Liano F, Junco E, Pascual J, Madero R, Verde E: The spectrum of acute renal failure in the intensive care unit compared with that seen in other settings. The Madrid Acute Renal Failure Study Group. Kidney Int Suppl 66:S16-S24, 1998
80. Rangel-Frausto MS, Pittet D, Costigan M, Hwang T, Davis CS, Wenzel RP: The natural history of the systemic inflammatory response syndrome (SIRS). A prospective study. JAMA 273:117-123, 1995
81. Knotek M, Esson M, Gengaro P, Edelstein CL, Schrier RW: Desensitization of soluble guanylate cyclase in renal cortex during endotoxemia in mice. J.Am.Soc.Nephrol. 11:2133-2137, 2000
82. Remick DG, Newcomb DE, Bolgos GL, Call DR: Comparison of the mortality and inflammatory response of two models of sepsis: lipopolysaccharide vs. cecal ligation and puncture. Shock 13:110-116, 2000
83. Thijs A, Thijs LG: Pathogenesis of renal failure in sepsis. Kidney Int.Suppl 66:S34-S37, 1998
84. Ortiz-Arduan A, Danoff TM, Kalluri R, Gonzalez-Cuadrado S, Karp SL, Elkon K, Egido J, Neilson EG: Regulation of Fas and Fas ligand expression in cultured murine renal cells and in the kidney during endotoxemia. Am.J.Physiol 271:F1193-F1201, 1996
85. Richman AV, Gerber LI, Balis JU: Peritubular capillaries. A major target site of endotoxin-induced vascular injury in the primate kidney. Lab Invest 43:327-332, 1980
86. Hickey MJ, Sharkey KA, Sihota EG, Reinhardt PH, MacMicking JD, Nathan C, Kubes P: Inducible nitric oxide synthase-deficient mice have enhanced leukocyte- endothelium interactions in endotoxemia. FASEB J. 11:955-964, 1997
87. Schrier RW, Abraham WT: Hormones and hemodynamics in heart failure. N.Engl.J.Med. 341:577-585, 1999
88. Schrier RW, Arroyo V, Bernardi M, Epstein M, Henriksen JH, Rodes J: Peripheral arterial vasodilation hypothesis: a proposal for the initiation of renal sodium and water retention in cirrhosis. Hepatology 8:1151-1157, 1988
89. Schrier RW: Pathogenesis of sodium and water retention in high-output and low- output cardiac failure, nephrotic syndrome, cirrhosis, and pregnancy (2). N.Engl.J.Med. 319:1127-1134, 1988
90. Khan RZ, Badr KF: Endotoxin and renal function: perspectives to the understanding of septic acute renal failure and toxic shock. Nephrol.Dial.Transplant. 14:814-818, 1999
91. Leach M, Frank S, Olbrich A, Pfeilschifter J, Thiemermann C: Decline in the expression of copper/zinc superoxide dismutase in the kidney of rats with endotoxic shock: effects of the superoxide anion radical scavenger, tempol, on organ injury. Br.J.Pharmacol. 125:817-825, 1998
92. Zacharowski K, Olbrich A, Cuzzocrea S, Foster SJ, Thiemermann C: Membrane-permeable radical scavenger, tempol, reduces multiple organ injury in a rodent model of gram-positive shock. Crit Care Med. 28:1953-1961, 2000
93. Zhang C, Walker LM, Mayeux PR: Role of nitric oxide in lipopolysaccharide-induced oxidant stress in the rat kidney. Biochem. Pharmacol. 59:203-209, 2000
94. Holly MK, Dear JW, Hu X, Schechter AN, Gladwin MT, Hewitt SM, Yuen PS, Star RA: Biomarker and drug-target discovery using proteomics in a new rat model of sepsis-induced acute renal failure. Kidney International 70:496-506, 2006
95. O'Donnel P, Burne M, Nemoto T, Keane WF, RabbH: Direct measurement of renal function in mice with ischemia-reperfusion injury; comparison of inulin clearance with serum creatinine. (abstract) J Am Soc Nephrol 11:606A, 2001
96. Chiao H, Kohda Y, McLeroy P, Craig L, Linas S, Star RA: Alpha-melanocyte-stimulating hormone inhibits renal injury in the absence of neutrophils. Kidney Int 54:765-774, 1998
97. Lorenz JN, Gruenstein E: A simple, nonradioactive method for evaluating single-nephron filtration rate using FITC-inulin. Am.J.Physiol 276:F172-F177, 1999
98. Wang W, Mitra A, Poole B, Falk S, Lucia MS, Tayal S, Schrier R: Endothelial nitric oxide synthase-deficient mice exhibit increased susceptibility to endotoxin-induced acute renal failure. American Journal of Physiology - Renal Fluid & Electrolyte Physiology 287:F1044-F1048, 2004
99. Wang W, Zolty E, Falk S, Basava V, Reznikov L, Schrier R: Pentoxifylline protects against endotoxin-induced acute renal failure in mice. American Journal of Physiology - Renal Physiology 291:F1090-F1095, 2006
100. Wang W, Faubel SG, Ljubanovic D, Mitra A, Kim J, Tao Y, Soloviev A, Reznikov L, Dinarello CA, Schrier RW, Edelstein CL: Endotoxemic acute renal failure is attenuated in caspase-1 deficient mice. Am.J.Physiol Renal Physiol 288:F997-F1004, 2005

101. Gulati S, Ainol L, Orak J, Singh AK, Singh I: Alterations of peroxisomal function in ischemia-reperfusion injury of rat kidney. Biochim.Biophys.Acta 1182:291-298, 1993

102. Gulati S, Singh AK, Irazu C, Orak J, Rajagopalan PR, Fitts CT, Singh I: Ischemia-reperfusion injury: biochemical alterations in peroxisomes of rat kidney. Arch.Biochem.Biophys. 295:90-100, 1992

103. Venkatachalam MA, Bernard DB, Donohoe JF, Levinsky NG: Ischemic damage and repair in the rat proximal tubule: differences among the S1, S2, and S3 segments. Kidney Int. 14:31-49, 1978

104. Bagnasco S, Good D, Balaban R, Burg M: Lactate production in isolated segments of the rat nephron. Am.J.Physiol 248:F522-F526, 1985

105. Witzgall R, Brown D, Schwarz C, Bonventre JV: Localization of proliferating cell nuclear antigen, vimentin, c-Fos, and clusterin in the postischemic kidney. Evidence for a heterogenous genetic response among nephron segments, and a large pool of mitotically active and dedifferentiated cells. J Clin.Invest 93:2175-2188, 1994

106. Safirstein R: Gene expression in nephrotoxic and ischemic acute renal failure [editorial]. J Am Soc Nephrol. 4:1387-1395, 1994

107. Megyesi J, Di Mari J, Udvarhelyi N, Price PM, Safirstein R: DNA synthesis is dissociated from the immediate-early gene response in the post-ischemic kidney. Kidney Int 48:1451-1458, 1995

108. Safirstein R, Price PM, Saggi SJ, Harris RC: Changes in gene expression after temporary renal ischemia. Kidney Int 37:1515-1521, 1990

109. Dimari J, Megyesi J, Udvarhelyi N, Price P, Davis R, Safirstein R: N-acetyl cysteine ameliorates ischemic renal failure. Am.J.Physiol 272:F292-F298, 1997

110. Pombo CM, Bonventre JV, Avruch J, Woodgett JR, Kyriakis JM, Force T: The stress-activated protein kinases are major c-Jun amino-terminal kinases activated by ischemia and reperfusion. J Biol.Chem. 269:26546-26551, 1994

111. di Mari JF, Davis R, Safirstein RL: MAPK activation determines renal epithelial cell survival during oxidative injury. Am.J.Physiol 277:F195-F203, 1999

112. Yaqoob M, Alkhunaizi AM, Edelstein CL, Conger JD, Schrier RW: ARF: Pathogenesis, diagnosis and management., in Renal and Electrolyte Disorders., 5 th ed., edited by Schrier RW, Philadelphia, New York, Lippincott-Raven, 1997, pp 449-506

113. Kribben A, Edelstein CL, Schrier RW: Pathophysiology of acute renal failure. J.Nephrol. 12 Suppl 2:S142-S151, 1999

114. Edelstein CL, Ling H, Wangsiripaisan A, Schrier RW: Emerging therapies for acute renal failure. Am.J.Kid.Dis. 30:S89-S95, 1997

115. Rossert J: Drug-induced acute interstitial nephritis. Kidney Int 60:804-817, 2001

116. Conger JD, Weil JU: Abnormal vascular function following ischemia-reperfusion injury. J.Invest.Med. 43:431-442, 1995

117. Harris RJ, Branston NM, Symon L, Bayhan M, Watson A: The effects of a calcium antagonist, nimodipine, upon physiological responses of the cerebral vasculature and its possible influence upon focal cerebral ischaemia. Stroke 13:759-766, 1982

118. Bevan JA, Laher I: Pressure and flow-dependent vascular tone. FASEB J. 5:2267-2273, 1991

119. Tolins JP, Palmer RM, Moncada S, Raij L: Role of endothelium-derived relaxing factor in regulation of renal hemodynamic responses. Am.J.Physiol 258:H655-H662, 1990

120. Pohl U, Holtz J, Busse R, Bassenge E: Crucial role of endothelium in the vasodilator response to increased flow *in vivo*. Hypertension 8:37-44, 1986

121. Cases A, Haas J, Burnett JC, Romero JC: Hemodynamic and renal effects of acute and progressive nitric oxide synthesis inhibition in anesthetized dogs. Am.J.Physiol Regul.Integr.Comp Physiol 280:R143-R148, 2001

122. Goetz KL, Wang BC, Madwed JB, Zhu JL, Leadley RJ, Jr.: Cardiovascular, renal, and endocrine responses to intravenous endothelin in conscious dogs. Am.J.Physiol 255:R1064-R1068, 1988

123. Blantz RC: Dynamics of glomerular ultrafiltration in the rat. Fed.Proc. 36:2602-2608, 1977

124. Casellas D, Navar LG: *In vitro* perfusion of juxtamedullary nephrons in rats. Am.J.Physiol 246:F349-F358, 1984

125. Casellas D, Carmines PK, Navar LG: Microvascular reactivity of *in vitro* blood perfused juxtamedullary nephrons from rats. Kidney Int 28:752-759, 1985

126. Ichihara A, Inscho EW, Imig JD, Navar LG: Neuronal nitric oxide synthase modulates rat renal microvascular function. Am.J.Physiol 274:F516-F524, 1998

127. Ichihara A, Hayashi M, Hirota N, Saruta T: Superoxide inhibits neuronal nitric oxide synthase influences on afferent arterioles in spontaneously hypertensive rats. Hypertension 37:630-634, 2001

128. Ichihara A, Navar LG: Neuronal NOS contributes to biphasic autoregulatory response during enhanced TGF activity. Am.J.Physiol 277:F113-F120, 1999

129. Ichihara A, Imig JD, Navar LG: Neuronal nitric oxide synthase-dependent afferent arteriolar function in angiotensin II-induced hypertension. Hypertension 33:462-466, 1999

130. Ikenaga H, Ishii N, Didion SP, Zhang K, Cornish KG, Patel KP, Mayhan WG, Carmines PK: Suppressed impact of nitric oxide on renal arteriolar function in rats with chronic heart failure. Am.J.Physiol 276:F79-F87, 1999

131. Inscho EW, Cook AK, Mui V, Miller J: Direct assessment of renal microvascular responses to P2-purinoceptor agonists. Am.J.Physiol 274:F718-F727, 1998
132. Nishiyama A, Inscho EW, Navar LG: Interactions of adenosine A1 and A2a receptors on renal microvascular reactivity. Am.J.Physiol Renal Physiol 280:F406-F414, 2001
133. Ichihara A, Imig JD, Inscho EW, Navar LG: Cyclooxygenase-2 participates in tubular flow-dependent afferent arteriolar tone: interaction with neuronal NOS. Am.J.Physiol 275:F605-F612, 1998
134. Imig JD, Deichmann PC: Afferent arteriolar responses to ANG II involve activation of PLA2 and modulation by lipoxygenase and P-450 pathways. Am.J.Physiol 273:F274-F282, 1997
135. Carmines PK, Fallet RW, Che Q, Fujiwara K: Tyrosine kinase involvement in renal arteriolar constrictor responses to angiotensin II. Hypertension 37:569-573, 2001
136. Inscho EW, Cook AK, Mui V, Imig JD: Calcium mobilization contributes to pressure-mediated afferent arteriolar vasoconstriction. Hypertension 31:421-428, 1998
137. Tonshoff B, Kaskel FJ, Moore LC: Effects of insulin-like growth factor I on the renal juxtamedullary microvasculature. Am.J.Physiol 274:F120-F128, 1998
138. Steinhausen M, Snoei H, Parekh N, Baker R, Johnson PC: Hydronephrosis: a new method to visualize vas afferens, efferens, and glomerular network. Kidney Int 23:794-806, 1983
139. De Vriese AS, Verbeuren TJ, Vallez MO, Lameire NH, De Buyzere M, Vanhoutte PM: Off-line analysis of red blood cell velocity in renal arterioles. J.Vasc.Res. 37:26-31, 2000
140. Edwards RM: Response of isolated renal arterioles to acetylcholine, dopamine, and bradykinin. Am.J.Physiol 248:F183-F189, 1985
141. Edwards RM: Response of isolated renal arterioles to acetylcholine, dopamine, and bradykinin. Am.J.Physiol 248:F183-F189, 1985
142. Yuan BH, Robinette JB, Conger JD: Effect of angiotensin II and norepinephrine on isolated rat afferent and efferent arterioles. Am.J.Physiol 258:F741-F750, 1990
143. Conger JD, Falk SA, Robinette JB: Angiotensin II-induced changes in smooth muscle calcium in rat renal arterioles. J.Am.Soc. Nephrol. 3:1792-1803, 1993
144. Loutzenhiser K, Loutzenhiser R: Angiotensin II-induced Ca(2+) influx in renal afferent and efferent arterioles: differing roles of voltage-gated and store-operated Ca(2+) entry. Circ.Res. 87:551-557, 2000
145. Li N, Teggatz EG, Li PL, Allaire R, Zou AP: Formation and actions of cyclic ADP-ribose in renal microvessels. Microvasc.Res. 60:149-159, 2000
146. Purdy KE, Arendshorst WJ: EP(1) and EP(4) receptors mediate prostaglandin E(2) actions in the microcirculation of rat kidney. Am.J.Physiol Renal Physiol 279:F755-F764, 2000
147. Edwards RM, Weidley EF: Lack of effect of atriopeptin II on rabbit glomerular arterioles *in vitro*. Am.J.Physiol 252:F317-F321, 1987
148. Lanese DM, Yuan BH, Falk SA, Conger JD: Effects of atriopeptin III on isolated rat afferent and efferent arterioles. Am.J.Physiol 261:F1102-F1109, 1991
149. Edwards RM, Trizna W: Characterization of alpha-adrenoceptors on isolated rabbit renal arterioles. Am.J.Physiol 254:F178-F183, 1988
150. Munger KA, Takahashi K, Awazu M, Frazer M, Falk SA, Conger JD, Badr KF: Maintenance of endothelin-induced renal arteriolar constriction in rats is cyclooxygenase dependent. Am.J.Physiol 264:F637-F644, 1993
151. Liu J, Hutzler M, Li C, Pechet L: Thrombotic thrombocytopenic purpura (ttp) and hemolytic uremic syndrome (hus): the new thinking. J Thromb.Thrombolysis. 11:261-272, 2001
152. Chatziantoniou C, Dussaule JC, Arendshorst WJ, Ardaillou R: Angiotensin II receptors and renin release in rat glomerular afferent arterioles. Kidney Int 46:1570-1573, 1994
153. De Leon H, Garcia R: Characterization of endothelin receptor subtypes in isolated rat renal preglomerular microvessels. Regul. Pept. 60:1-8, 1995
154. Park F, Mattson DL, Skelton MM, Cowley AW, Jr.: Localization of the vasopressin V1a and V2 receptors within the renal cortical and medullary circulation. Am.J.Physiol 273:R243-R251, 1997
155. Yoshida H, Tamaki T, Aki Y, Kimura S, Takenaka I, Abe Y: Effects of angiotensin II on isolated rabbit afferent arterioles. Jpn.J.Pharmacol. 66:457-464, 1994
156. Kornfeld M, Gutierrez AM, Persson AE, Salomonsson M: Angiotensin II induces a tachyphylactic calcium response in the rabbit afferent arteriole. Acta Physiol Scand. 160:165-173, 1997
157. Ito S, Amin J, Ren Y, Arima S, Abe K, Carretero OA: Heterogeneity of angiotensin action in renal circulation. Kidney Int Suppl 63: S128-S131, 1997

158. Croft KD, McGiff JC, Sanchez-Mendoza A, Carroll MA: Angiotensin II releases 20-HETE from rat renal microvessels. Am.J.Physiol Renal Physiol 279:F544-F551, 2000
159. Vyas SJ, Blaschak CM, Chinoy MR, Jackson EK: Angiotensin II-induced changes in G-protein expression and resistance of renal microvessels in young genetically hypertensive rats. Mol.Cell Biochem. 212:121-129, 2000
160. Imig JD, Pham BT, LeBlanc EA, Reddy KM, Falck JR, Inscho EW: Cytochrome P450 and cyclooxygenase metabolites contribute to the endothelin-1 afferent arteriolar vasoconstrictor and calcium responses. Hypertension 35:307-312, 2000
161. Yu H, Carretero OA, Juncos LA, Garvin JL: Biphasic effect of bradykinin on rabbit afferent arterioles. Hypertension 32:287-292, 1998
162. Ito S: Characteristics of isolated perfused juxtaglomerular apparatus. Kidney Int Suppl 67:S46-S48, 1998
163. Ito S, Ren Y: Evidence for the role of nitric oxide in macula densa control of glomerular hemodynamics. J.Clin.Invest 92:1093-1098, 1993
164. Ito S, Carretero OA: An *in vitro* approach to the study of macula densa-mediated glomerular hemodynamics. Kidney Int 38:1206-1210, 1990
165. Molitoris BA, Sandoval RM: Intravital multiphoton microscopy of dynamic renal processes. American Journal of Physiology - Renal Physiology 288:F1084-F1089, 2005
166. Dagher PC, Herget-Rosenthal S, Ruehm SG, Jo SK, Star RA, Agarwal R, Molitoris BA: Newly developed techniques to study and diagnose acute renal failure. Journal of the American Society of Nephrology 14:2188-2198, 2003
167. Dunn KW, Sandoval RM, Molitoris BA: Intravital imaging of the kidney using multiparameter multiphoton microscopy. Nephron Experimental Nephrology. 94:e7-11, 2003
168. Dunn KW, Sandoval RM, Kelly KJ, Dagher PC, Tanner GA, Atkinson SJ, Bacallao RL, Molitoris BA: Functional studies of the kidney of living animals using multicolor two-photon microscopy. American Journal of Physiology - Cell Physiology 283:C905-C916, 2002
169. Sutton TA, Mang HE, Campos SB, Sandoval RM, Yoder MC, Molitoris BA: Injury of the renal microvascular endothelium alters barrier function after ischemia. American Journal of Physiology - Renal Fluid & Electrolyte Physiology 285:F191-F198, 2003
170. Lee HT, Jan M, Bae SC, Joo JD, Goubaeva FR, Yang J, Kim M: A1 adenosine receptor knockout mice are protected against acute radiocontrast nephropathy *in vivo*. American Journal of Physiology - Renal Physiology 290:F1367-F1375, 2006
171. Lee HT, Xu H, Nasr SH, Schnermann J, Emala CW: A1 adenosine receptor knockout mice exhibit increased renal injury following ischemia and reperfusion. American Journal of Physiology - Renal Physiology 286:F298-F306, 2004
172. Wei Q, Yin XM, Wang MH, Dong Z: Bid deficiency ameliorates ischemic renal failure and delays animal death in C57BL/6 mice. American Journal of Physiology - Renal Physiology 290:F35-F42, 2006
173. Kielar ML, John R, Bennet M, Richardson JA, Shelton JM, Chen L, Jeyarajah DR, Zhou XJ, Zhou H, Chiquett B, Nagami GT, Lu CY: Maladaptive role of IL-6 in ischemic acute renal failure. J.Am.Soc.Nephrol. 16:3315-3325, 2006
174. Marques VP, Goncalves GM, Feitoza CQ, Cenedeze MA, Fernandes Bertocchi AP, Damiao MJ, Pinheiro HS, Antunes T, V, dos Reis MA, Pacheco-Silva A, Saraiva Camara NO: Influence of TH1/TH2 switched immune response on renal ischemia-reperfusion injury. Nephron Experimental Nephrology. 104:e48-e56, 2006
175. Yamasowa H, Shimizu S, Inoue T, Takaoka M, Matsumura Y: Endothelial nitric oxide contributes to the renal protective effects of ischemic preconditioning. Journal of Pharmacology & Experimental Therapeutics 312:153-159, 2005
176. Zheng J, Devalaraja-Narashimha K, Singaravelu K, Padanilam BJ: Poly(ADP-ribose) polymerase-1 gene ablation protects mice from ischemic renal injury. American Journal of Physiology - Renal Physiology 288:F387-F398, 2005
177. Thurman JM, Ljubanovic D, Edelstein CL, Gilkeson GS, Holers VM: Lack of a functional alternative complement pathway ameliorates ischemic acute renal failure in mice. Journal of Immunology 170:1517-1523, 2003
178. Yamashita J, Kita S, Iwamoto T, Ogata M, Takaoka M, Tazawa N, Nishikawa M, Wakimoto K, Shigekawa M, Komuro I, Matsumura Y: Attenuation of ischemia/reperfusion-induced renal injury in mice deficient in Na+/Ca2+ exchanger. Journal of Pharmacology & Experimental Therapeutics 304:284-293, 2003
179. Yamada K, Miwa T, Liu J, Nangaku M, Song WC: Critical protection from renal ischemia reperfusion injury by CD55 and CD59. Journal of Immunology 172:3869-3875, 2004
180. Lee HT, Ota-Setlik A, Xu H, D'Agati VD, Jacobson MA, Emala CW: A3 adenosine receptor knockout mice are protected against ischemia- and myoglobinuria-induced renal failure. American Journal of Physiology - Renal Physiology 284:F267-F273, 2003
181. Melnikov VY, Ecder T, Fantuzzi G, Siegmund B, Lucia MS, Dinarello CA, Schrier RW, Edelstein CL: Impaired IL-18 processing protects caspase-1-deficient mice from ischemic acute renal failure. J.Clin.Invest 107:1145-1152, 2001
182. Daemen MA, Denecker G, Van't Veer C, Wolfs TG, Vandenabeele P, Buurman WA: Activated caspase-1 is not a central mediator of inflammation in the course of ischemia-reperfusion. Transplantation 71:778-784, 2001
183. Ling H, Edelstein CL, Gengaro P, Meng X, Lucia S, Knotek M, Wangsiripaisan A, Shi Y, Schrier RW: Attenuation of renal ischemia-reperfusion injury in inducible nitric oxide synthase knockout mice. Am.J.Physiol. 277:F383-F390, 1999

184. Haq M, Norman J, Saba SR, Ramirez G, Rabb H: Role of IL-1 in renal ischemic reperfusion injury. J Am Soc Nephrol 9:614-619, 1998
185. Kelly KJ, Williams WWJr, Colvin RB, Bonventre JV: Antibody to intracellular adhesion molecule-1 protects the kidney against ischemic injury. Proc Natl Acad Sci USA 91:812-816, 1994
186. Rabb H, Daniels F, O'Donnell M, Haq M, Saba SR, Keane W, Tang WW: Pathophysiological role of T lymphocytes in renal ischemia-reperfusion injury in mice. Am.J.Physiol Renal Physiol 279:F525-F531, 2000
187. Noiri E, Dickman K, Miller F, Romanov G, Romanov VI, Shaw R, Chambers AF, Rittling SR, Denhardt DT, Goligorsky MS: Reduced tolerance to acute renal ischemia in mice with a targeted disruption of the osteopontin gene. Kidney Int 56:74-82, 1999
188. Ge Y, Bagnall A, Stricklett PK, Strait K, Webb DJ, Kotelevtsev Y, Kohan DE: Collecting duct-specific knockout of the endothelin B receptor causes hypertension and sodium retention. American Journal of Physiology - Renal Physiology 291:F1274-F1280, 2006
189. Rojek A, Fuchtbauer EM, Kwon TH, Frokiaer J, Nielsen S: Severe urinary concentrating defect in renal collecting duct-selective AQP2 conditional-knockout mice. Proceedings of the National Academy of Sciences of the United States of America 103:6037-6042, 2006
190. Zhang H, Zhang A, Kohan DE, Nelson RD, Gonzalez FJ, Yang T: Collecting duct-specific deletion of peroxisome proliferator-activated receptor gamma blocks thiazolidinedione-induced fluid retention. Proceedings of the National Academy of Sciences of the United States of America 102:9406-9411, 2005
191. Ahn D, Ge Y, Stricklett PK, Gill P, Taylor D, Hughes AK, Yanagisawa M, Miller L, Nelson RD, Kohan DE: Collecting duct-specific knockout of endothelin-1 causes hypertension and sodium retention. Journal of Clinical Investigation 114:504-511, 2004
192. Leheste JR, Melsen F, Wellner M, Jansen P, Schlichting U, Renner-Muller I, Andreassen TT, Wolf E, Bachmann S, Nykjaer A, Willnow TE: Hypocalcemia and osteopathy in mice with kidney-specific megalin gene defect. FASEB Journal 17:247-249, 2003
193. Rubera I, Loffing J, Palmer LG, Frindt G, Fowler-Jaeger N, Sauter D, Carroll T, McMahon A, Hummler E, Rossier BC: Collecting duct-specific gene inactivation of alphaENaC in the mouse kidney does not impair sodium and potassium balance. Journal of Clinical Investigation 112:554-565, 2003
194. Stein JH, Gottschall J, Osgood RW, Ferris TF: Pathophysiology of a nephrotoxic model of acute renal failure. Kidney Int 8:27-41, 1975
195. Mauk RH, Patak RV, Fadem SZ, Lifschitz MD, Stein JH: Effect of prostaglandin E administration in a nephrotoxic and a vasoconstrictor model of acute renal failure. Kidney Int 12:122-130, 1977
196. Solez K, Marel-Maroger L, Sraer J: The morphology of acute tubular necrosis in man. Analysis of 57 renal biopsies and comparison with glycerol model. Medicine (Baltimore) 58:362-376, 1979
197. Baylis C, Rennke HR, Brenner BM: Mechanisms of the defect in glomerular ultrafiltration associated with gentamicin administration. Kidney Int 12:344-353, 1977
198. Neugarten J, Aynedjian HS, Bank N: Role of tubular obstruction in acute renal failure due to gentamicin. Kidney Int 24:330-335, 1983
199. Verstrepen WA, Persy VP, Verhulst A, Dauwe S, De Broe ME: Renal osteopontin protein and mRNA upregulation during acute nephrotoxicity in the rat. Nephrol.Dial.Transplant. 16:712-724, 2001
200. Wolfert AI, Laveri LA, Reilly KM, Oken KR, Oken DE: Glomerular hemodynamics in mercury-induced acute renal failure. Kidney Int 32:246-255, 1987
201. Dobyan DC, Levi J, Jacobs C, Kosek J, Weiner MW: Mechanism of cis-platinum nephrotoxicity: II. Morphologic observations. J.Pharmacol.Exp.Ther. 213:551-556, 1980
202. Stein JH, Fried TA: Experimental models of nephrotoxic acute renal failure. Transplant.Proc. 17:72-80, 1985
203. Faubel SG, Ljubanovic D, Reznikov LL, Somerset H, Dinarello CA, Edelstein CL: Caspase-1-deficient mice are protected against cisplatin-induced apoptosis and acute tubular necrosis. Kidney Int. 66:2202-2213, 2004
204. Yasuda H, Yuen PS, Hu X, Zhou H, Star RA: Simvastatin improves sepsis-induced mortality and acute kidney injury via renal vascular effects. Kidney International 69:1535-1542, 2006
205. Dear JW, Yasuda H, Hu X, Hieny S, Yuen PS, Hewitt SM, Sher A, Star RA: Sepsis-induced organ failure is mediated by different pathways in the kidney and liver: acute renal failure is dependent on MyD88 but not renal cell apoptosis. Kidney International 69:832-836, 2006
206. Lee HT, Kim M, Joo JD, Gallos G, Chen JF, Emala CW: A3 adenosine receptor activation decreases mortality and renal and hepatic injury in murine septic peritonitis. American Journal of Physiology - Regulatory Integrative & Comparative Physiology 291:R959-R969, 2006
207. Singbartl K, Bockhorn SG, Zarbock A, Schmolke M, Van Aken H: T cells modulate neutrophil-dependent acute renal failure during endotoxemia: critical role for CD28. Journal of the American Society of Nephrology 16:720-728, 2005

208. Boffa JJ, Just A, Coffman TM, Arendshorst WJ: Thromboxane receptor mediates renal vasoconstriction and contributes to acute renal failure in endotoxemic mice. Journal of the American Society of Nephrology 15:2358-2365, 2004
209. Knotek M, Rogachev B, Gengaro P, Esson M, Edelstein CL, Dinarello CA, Schrier RW: Endotoxemic renal failure in mice:Role of tumor necrosis factor indepenent of inducible nitric oxide synthase. Kidney Int 59:2243-2249, 2001
210. Schwartz D, Mendoca M, Schwartz Y, Xia Y, Satriano J, Wilson CB, Blantz R: Inhibition of constitutive nitric oxide synthase (NOS) by nitric oxide generated by inducible NOS after lipopolysaccharide administration provokes renal dysfunction in rats. J.Clin. Invest. 100:439-448., 1997
211. Satriano J, Schwartz D, Ishizuka S, Lortie MJ, Thomson SC, Gabbai F, Kelly CJ, Blantz RC: Suppression of inducible nitric oxide generation by agmatine aldehyde: Beneficial effects in sepsis. J Cell Physiol 188:313-320, 2001
212. Carcillo JA, Herzer WA, Mi Z, Thomas NJ, Jackson EK: Treatment with the type IV phosphodiesterase inhibitor Ro 20-1724 protects renal and mesenteric blood flow in endotoxemic rats treated with norepinephrine. J Pharmacol.Exp.Ther. 279:1197-1204, 1996
213. Zurovsky Y, Gispaan I: Antioxidants attenuate endotoxin-induced acute renal failure in rats. Am J Kidney Dis. 25:51-57, 1995
214. Ruetten H, Thiemermann C: Effect of selective blockade of endothelin ETB receptors on the liver dysfunction and injury caused by endotoxaemia in the rat. Br.J Pharmacol. 119:479-486, 1996
215. Mitaka C, Hirata Y, Yokoyama K, Nagura T, Tsunoda Y, Amaha K: Improvement of renal dysfunction in dogs with endotoxemia by a nonselective endothelin receptor antagonist. Crit Care Med. 27:146-153, 1999
216. Parikh CR, Jani A, Melnikov VY, Faubel SG, Edelstein CL: Urinary interleukin-18 is a marker of human acute tubular necrosis. Am.J.Kidney Dis. 43:405-414, 2004
217. Parikh CR, Abraham E, Ancukiewicz M, Edelstein CL: Urine IL-18 is an early diagnostic marker for acute kidney injury and predicts mortality in the ICU. J.Am.Soc.Nephrol. 16:3046-3052, 2005
218. Parikh CR, Mishra J, Thiessen-Philbrook H, Dursun B, Ma Q, Kelly C, Dent C, Devarajan P, Edelstein CL: Urinary IL-18 is an early predictive biomarker of acute kidney injury after cardiac surgery. Kidney International 70:199-203, 2006
219. Parikh CR, Jani A, Mishra J, Ma Q, Kelly C, Barasch J, Edelstein CL, Devarajan P: Urine NGAL and IL-18 are predictive biomarkers for delayed graft function following kidney transplantation. American Journal of Transplantation 6:1639-1645, 2006
220. Mishra J, Ma Q, Prada A, Mitsnefes M, Zahedi K, Yang J, Barasch J, Devarajan P: Identification of neutrophil gelatinase-associated lipocalin as a novel early urinary biomarker for ischemic renal injury. Journal of the American Society of Nephrology 14:2534-2543, 2003
221. Mishra J, Dent C, Tarabishi R, Mitsnefes MM, Ma Q, Kelly C, Ruff SM, Zahedi K, Shao M, Bean J, Mori K, Barasch J, Devarajan P: Neutrophil gelatinase-associated lipocalin (NGAL) as a biomarker for acute renal injury after cardiac surgery.[see comment]. Lancet 365:1231-1238, 2005
222. Ichimura T, Bonventre JV, Bailly V, Wei H, Hession CA, Cate RL, Sanicola M: Kidney injury molecule-1 (KIM-1), a putative epithelial cell adhesion molecule containing a novel immunoglobulin domain, is up-regulated in renal cells after injury. Journal of Biological Chemistry 273:4135-4142, 1998
223. Vaidya VS, Ramirez V, Ichimura T, Bobadilla NA, Bonventre JV: Urinary kidney injury molecule-1: a sensitive quantitative biomarker for early detection of kidney tubular injury. American Journal of Physiology - Renal Physiology 290:F517-F529, 2006
224. Liangos O, Perianayagam MC, Vaidya VS, Han WK, Wald R, Tighiouart H, Mackinnon RW, Balakrishnan VS, Pereira BJ, Bonventre JV, Jaber BL: Urinary N-Acetyl-beta-(D)-glucosaminidase activity and kidney injury molecule-1 level are associated with adverse outcomes in acute renal failure. J.Am.Soc.Nephrol. 18:904-912, 2007
225. Muramatsu Y, Tsujie M, Kohda Y, Pham B, Perantoni AO, Zhao H, Jo SK, Yuen PS, Craig L, Hu X, Star RA: Early detection of cysteine rich protein 61 (CYR61, CCN1) in urine following renal ischemic reperfusion injury. Kidney Int. 62:1601-1610, 2002
226. Molls RR, Savransky V, Liu M, Bevans S, Mehta T, Tuder RM, King LS, Rabb H: Keratinocyte-derived chemokine is an early biomarker of ischemic acute kidney injury. American Journal of Physiology - Renal Physiology 290:F1187-F1193, 2006
227. Park S, Bivona BJ, Harrison-Bernard LM: Compromised renal microvacular reactivity of angiotensin type 1 double null mice. Am.J.Physiol Renal Physiol Epub ahead of print.: 2007
228. Harrison-Bernard LM, Monjure CJ, Bivona BJ: Efferent arterioles exclusively express the subtype 1A angiotensin receptor: functional insights from genetic mouse models. American Journal of Physiology - Renal Physiology 290:F1177-F1186, 2006
229. Ichihara A, Hayashi M, Koura Y, Tada Y, Sugaya T, Hirota N, Saruta T: Blunted tubuloglomerular feedback by absence of angiotensin type 1A receptor involves neuronal NOS. Hypertension 40:934-939, 2002
230. Harrison-Bernard LM, Cook AK, Oliverio MI, Coffman TM: Renal segmental microvascular responses to ANG II in AT1A receptor null mice. American Journal of Physiology - Renal Physiology 284:F538-F545, 2003
231. Schneider MP, Inscho EW, Pollock DM: Attenuated vasoconstrictor responses to endothelin in afferent arterioles during a high salt diet. Am.J.Physiol Renal Physiol 292:F1208-F1214, 2007

232. Botros FT, Navar LG: Interaction between endogenously produced carbon monoxide and nitric oxide in regulation of renal afferent arterioles. American Journal of Physiology - Heart & Circulatory Physiology 291:H2772-H2778, 2006
233. Sharma K, Cook A, Smith M, Valancius C, Inscho EW: TGF-beta impairs renal autoregulation via generation of ROS. American Journal of Physiology - Renal Physiology 288:F1069-F1077, 2005
234. Pittner J, Wolgast M, Casellas D, Persson AE: Increased shear stress-released NO and decreased endothelial calcium in rat isolated perfused juxtamedullary nephrons. Kidney International 67:227-236, 2005
235. Feng MG, Navar LG: Nitric oxide synthase inhibition activates L- and T-type Ca2+ channels in afferent and efferent arterioles. American Journal of Physiology - Renal Physiology 290:F873-F879, 2006
236. Steinhausen M, Kucherer H, Parekh N, Weis S, Wiegman DL, Wilhelm KR: Angiotensin II control of the renal microcirculation: effect of blockade by saralasin. Kidney Int 30:56-61, 1986
237. Steinhausen M, Weis S, Fleming J, Dussel R, Parekh N: Responses of *in vivo* renal microvessels to dopamine. Kidney Int 30:361-370, 1986
238. Loutzenhiser R, Hayashi K, Epstein M: Atrial natriuretic peptide reverses afferent arteriolar vasoconstriction and potentiates efferent arteriolar vasoconstriction in the isolated perfused rat kidney. J.Pharmacol.Exp.Ther. 246:522-528, 1988
239. Endlich K, Steinhausen M: Natriuretic peptide receptors mediate different responses in rat renal microvessels. Kidney Int 52:202-207, 1997
240. Hayashi K, Epstein M, Loutzenhiser R: Pressure-induced vasoconstriction of renal microvessels in normotensive and hypertensive rats. Studies in the isolated perfused hydronephrotic kidney. Circ.Res. 65:1475-1484, 1989
241. Steinhausen M, Ballantyne D, Fretschner M, Parekh N: Sex differences in autoregulation of juxtamedullary glomerular blood flow in hydronephrotic rats. Am.J.Physiol 258:F863-F869, 1990
242. Bloom IT, Bentley FR, Wilson MA, Garrison RN: *In vivo* effects of endothelin on the renal microcirculation. J.Surg.Res. 54:274-280, 1993
243. Fretschner M, Endlich K, Gulbins E, Lang RE, Schlottmann K, Steinhausen M: Effects of endothelin on the renal microcirculation of the split hydronephrotic rat kidney. Ren Physiol Biochem. 14:112-127, 1991
244. Dietrich MS, Endlich K, Parekh N, Steinhausen M: Interaction between adenosine and angiotensin II in renal microcirculation. Microvasc.Res. 41:275-288, 1991
245. Chen J, Fleming JT: Juxtamedullary afferent and efferent arterioles constrict to renal nerve stimulation. Kidney Int 44:684-691, 1993
246. Takenaka T, Kanno Y, Kitamura Y, Hayashi K, Suzuki H, Saruta T: Role of chloride channels in afferent arteriolar constriction. Kidney Int 50:864-872, 1996
247. Hayashi K, Fujiwara K, Oka K, Nagahama T, Matsuda H, Saruta T: Effects of insulin on rat renal microvessels: studies in the isolated perfused hydronephrotic kidney. Kidney Int 51:1507-1513, 1997
248. Tang L, Loutzenhiser K, Loutzenhiser R: Biphasic actions of prostaglandin E(2) on the renal afferent arteriole: role of EP(3) and EP(4) receptors. Circ.Res. 86:663-670, 2000
249. Hayashi K, Suzuki H, Saruta T: Nitric oxide modulates but does not impair myogenic vasoconstriction of the afferent arteriole in spontaneously hypertensive rats. Studies in the isolated perfused hydronephrotic kidney. Hypertension 25:1212-1219, 1995
250. Zimmerhackl LB, Fretschner M, Steinhausen M: Cyclosporin reduces renal blood flow through vasoconstriction of arcuate arteries in the hydronephrotic rat model. Klin.Wochenschr. 68:166-174, 1990
251. Bloom IT, Bentley FR, Spain DA, Garrison RN: An experimental study of altered nitric oxide metabolism as a mechanism of cyclosporin-induced renal vasoconstriction. Br.J.Surg. 82:195-198, 1995
252. Nakamura A, Hayashi K, Fujiwara K, Ozawa Y, Honda M, Saruta T: Distinct action of aranidipine and its active metabolite on renal arterioles, with special reference to renal protection. J.Cardiovasc.Pharmacol. 35:942-948, 2000
253. Glazer AA, Inman SR, Stowe NT, Novick AC: Renal microcirculatory effects of lovastatin in a rat model of reduced renal mass. Urology 50:812-817, 1997
254. Krysztopik RJ, Bentley FR, Spain DA, Wilson MA, Garrison RN: Lazaroids prevent acute cyclosporine-induced renal vasoconstriction. Transplantation 63:1215-1220, 1997
255. Krysztopik RJ, Bentley FR, Spain DA, Wilson MA, Garrison RN: Free radical scavenging by lazaroids improves renal blood flow during sepsis. Surgery 120:657-662, 1996
256. Schlottmann K, Gulbins E, Rauterberg EW, Steinhausen M: Effects of systemic complement activation on renal circulation of rats. Eur.J.Clin.Invest 24:320-330, 1994
257. Kimura K, Tojo A, Hirata Y, Hayakawa H, Goto A, Omata M: Effects of a calcium antagonist and an angiotensin II receptor antagonist on rat renal arterioles. Blood Press Suppl 5:71-74, 1994
258. Shi Y, Wang X, Chon KH, Cupples WA: Tubuloglomerular feedback-dependent modulation of renal myogenic autoregulation by nitric oxide. American Journal of Physiology - Regulatory Integrative & Comparative Physiology 290:R982-R991, 2006

259. Wang X, Breaks J, Loutzenhiser K, Loutzenhiser R: Effects of Na+/K+/2Cl- cotransporter on myogenic and angiotensin ii responses of the rat afferent arteriole. Am.J.Physiol Renal Physiol 292:F999-F1006, 2007
260. Hayashi K, Wakino S, Ozawa Y, Homma K, Kanda T, Okubo K, Takamatsu I, Tatematsu S, Kumagai H, Saruta T: Role of protein kinase C in Ca channel blocker-induced renal arteriolar dilation in spontaneously hypertensive rats--studies in the isolated perfused hydronephrotic kidney. Keio Journal of Medicine 54:102-108, 2005
261. Hayashi K, Ozawa Y, Wakino S, Kanda T, Homma K, Takamatsu I, Tatematsu S, Saruta T: Cellular mechanism for mibefradil-induced vasodilation of renal microcirculation: studies in the isolated perfused hydronephrotic kidney. Journal of Cardiovascular Pharmacology 42:697-702, 2003
262. Weiss C, Passow H, Rothstein A: Autoregulation of flow in isolated rat kidney in the absence of red cells. Am J Physiol 196:1115-1118, 1959
263 Nishiitsutsuji-Uwo JM, Ross BD, Krebs HA: Metabolic activities of the isolated perfused rat kidney. Biochem J 103:852-62, 1967
264. Ross BD, Epstein FH, Leaf A: Sodium reabsorption in the perfused rat kidney. Am J Physiol 225:1165-1171, 1973
265. Epstein FH, Brosnan JT, Tange JD, Ross BD: Improved function with amino acids in the isolated perfused kidney. Am J Physiol 243:284-92, 1982
266. Baines AD, Shaikh N, Ho P: Mechanisms of perfused kidney cytoprotection by alanine and glycine. Am.J..Physiol. 259:F80-F87, 1990
267. Schurek HJ, Kriz W: Morphologic and functional evidence for oxygen deficiency in the isolated perfused rat kidney. Lab Invest 53:145-155, 1985
268. Lieberthal W, Stephens GW, Wolf EF, Rennke HG, Vasilevsky ML, Valeri CR, Levinsky NG: Effect of erythrocytes on the function and morphology of the isolated perfused rat kidney. Ren Physiol 10:14-24, 1987
269. Endre ZH, Ratcliffe PJ, Tange JD, Ferguson DJ, Radda GK, Ledingham JG: Erythrocytes alter the pattern of renal hypoxic injury: predominance of proximal tubular injury with moderate hypoxia. Clin.Sci. 76:19-29, 1989
270. Ratcliffe PJ, Endre ZH, Scheinman SJ, Tange JD, Ledingham JG, Radda GK: 31P nuclear magnetic resonance study of steady-state adenosine 5'- triphosphate levels during graded hypoxia in the isolated perfused rat kidney. Clin.Sci. 74:437-448, 1988
271. Lieberthal W, Sheridan AM, Valeri CR: Protective effect of atrial natriuretic factor and mannitol following renal ischemia. Am J Physiol 258:1266-72, 1990
272. Cross M, Endre ZH, Stewart-Richardson P, Cowin GJ, Westhuyzen J, Duggleby RG, Fleming SJ: 23Na-NMR detects hypoxic injury in intact kidney: increases in sodium inhibited by DMSO and DMTU. Magn Reson.Med. 30:465-475, 1993
273. Cowin GJ, Crozier S, Endre ZH, Leditschke IA, Brereton IM: Cortical and medullary betaine-GPC modulated by osmolality independently of oxygen in the intact kidney. Am J Physiol 277:F338-F346, 1999
274 M. Rahgozar, Z. Guan, A. Matthias, G. C. Gobe and Z. H. Endre. Angiotensin II facilitates autoregulation in the perfused mouse kidney: An optimized *in vitro* model for assessment of renal vascular and tubular function. Nephrology (Carlton) 2004;9(5):288-96.
275. Buhrle CP, Hackenthal E, Helmchen U, Lackner K, Nobiling R, Steinhausen M, Taugner R. The hydronephrotic kidney of the mouse as a tool for intravital microscopy and *in vitro* electrophysiological studies of renin containing cells. Lab Invest 1886, 5494); 462-472.
276. Loutzenhiser R, Epstein M, Horton C: Inhibition by diltiazem of pressure-induced afferent vasoconstriction in the isolated perfused rat kidney. Am J Cardiol 59:72-75, 1987
277. Carmines PK, Morrison TK, Navar LG: Angiotensin II effects on microvascular diameters of *in vitro* blood-perfused juxtamedullary nephrons. Am J Physiol 251:610-618, 1986
278. Carmines PK, Navar LG: Disparate effects of Ca channel blockade on afferent and efferent arteriolar responses to angiotensin II. Am J Physiol 256:1015-1020, 1989
279. Moore LC, Casellas D: Tubuloglomerular feedback dependence of autoregulation in rat juxtamedullary afferent arterioles. Kidney Int 37:1402-1408, 1990
280. Ichihara A, Imig JD, Navar LG: Cyclooxygenase-2 modulates afferent arteriolar responses to increases in pressure. Hypertension 34:843-847, 1999
281. Schurek HJ, Alt JM: Effect of albumin on the function of perfused rat kidney. Am J Physiol 240:569-76, 1981
282. Bullivant M: Autoregulation of plasma flow in the isolated perfused rat kidney. J Physiol 280:141-53, 1978
283. Schurek HJ, Brecht JP, Lohfert H, Hierholzer K: The basic requirements for the function of the isolated cell free perfused rat kidney. Pflugers Arch 354:349-65, 1975
284. Lieberthal W, Vasilevsky ML, Valeri CR, Levinsky NG: Interactions between ADH and prostaglandins in isolated erythrocyte- perfused rat kidney. Am J Physiol 252:331-7, 1987
285. Silva P, Hallac R, Spokes K, Epstein FH: Relationship among gluconeogenesis, QO2, and Na^+ transport in the perfused rat kidney. Am J Physiol 11:508-513, 1982

286. Baumgartl H, Leichtweiss HP, Lubbers DW, Weiss C, Huland H: The oxygen supply of the dog kidney: measurements of intrarenal pO 2. Microvasc.Res. 4:247-257, 1972
287. Schurek HJ, Jost U, Baumgartl H, Bertram H, Heckmann U: Evidence for a preglomerular oxygen diffusion shunt in rat renal cortex. Am J Physiol 259:F910-F915, 1990
288. Brezis M, Heyman SN, Dinour D, Epstein FH, Rosen S: Role of nitric oxide in renal medullary oxygenation. Studies in isolated and intact rat kidneys. J Clin Invest 88:390-5, 1991
289. Heyman SN, Karmeli F, Rachmilewitz D, Haj-Yehia A, Brezis M: Intrarenal nitric oxide monitoring with a Clark-type electrode: potential pitfalls. Kidney Int 51:1619-23, 1997
290. Dowd T, Barac-Nieto M, Gupta RK, Spitzer A: 31P nuclear magnetic resonance and saturation transfer studies of the isolated perfused rat kidney. Ren Physiol Biochem 12:161-70, 1989
291. Gupta RK, Dowd TL, Spitzer A, Barac-Nieto M: 23Na, 19F, 35Cl and 31P multinuclear nuclear magnetic resonance studies of perfused rat kidney. Ren Physiol Biochem. 12:144-160, 1989
292. Barac-Nieto M, Gupta RK, Spitzer A: NMR studies of phosphate metabolism in the isolated perfused kidney of developing rats. Pediatr Nephrol 4:392-8, 1990
293. Barac-Nieto M, Dowd TL, Gupta RK, Spitzer A: Changes in NMR-visible kidney cell phosphate with age and diet: relationship to phosphate transport. Am J Physiol 261:153-62, 1991
294. Dowd TL, Gupta RK: Multinuclear NMR studies of intracellular cations in perfused hypertensive rat kidney. J.Biol.Chem. 267:3637-3643, 1992
295. Dowd TL, Gupta RK: NMR studies of the effect of hyperglycemia on intracellular cations in rat kidney. J Biol Chem 268:991-6, 1993
296. Dowd TL, Gupta RK: Multinuclear NMR studies of intracellular cations in the prehypertensive rat kidney. Biochim Biophys Acta 1226:83-8, 1994
297. Dowd TL, Gupta RK: NMR studies of the effect of Mg2+ on post-ischemic recovery of ATP and intracellular sodium in perfused kidney. Biochim Biophys Acta 1272:133-9, 1995
298. Endre ZH, Allis JL, Ratcliffe PJ, Radd GK: 87-rubidium NMR: a novel method of measuring cation flux in intact kidney. Kidney Int 35:1249-1256, 1989
299. Endre ZH, Solez K: Anatomical and functional imaging of transplant acute renal failure. Transplantation Review 9:147-158, 1995
300. Cowin GJ, Leditschke IA, Crozier S, Brereton IM, Endre ZH: Regional proton nuclear magnetic resonance spectroscopy differentiates cortex and medulla in the isolated perfused rat kidney. MAGMA 5:151-8, 1997
301. S. Crozier, G. Cowin and Z. Endre. MR Microscopy and Microspectroscopy of the Intact Kidney. Concepts Magnetic Resonance 2004(Part A 22A):50-9.
302. Endre ZH, Hull WE, Fichtner K-P, Werner U, Kriz W, Ritz E: Development of MR Microscopy for the functioning isolated perfused kidney, in Renal Magnetic Resonance: Experimental and Clinical Applications, edited by Endre ZH, New York, Marcel Dekker, 2002,
303. Endre ZH: Magnetic resonance imaging and spectroscopy in critical care nephrology, in Critical care nephrology, edited by C. R, Bellomo R, Dordrecht, Kluwer, 1998, pp 1517-1533
304. F. Schweda, C. Wagner, B. K. Kramer, J. Schnermann and A. Kurtz. Preserved macula densa-dependent renin secretion in A1 adenosine receptor knockout mice. Am J Physiol Renal Physiol 2003;284(4):F770-7.
305. A. Kurtz and F. Schweda. Osmolarity-induced renin secretion from kidneys: evidence for readily releasable renin pools. Am J Physiol Renal Physiol 2006;290(4):F797-805.
306. R. Takeda, H. Nishimatsu, E. Suzuki, H. Satonaka, D. Nagata, S. Oba, et al. Ghrelin improves renal function in mice with ischemic acute renal failure. J Am Soc Nephrol 2006;17(1):113-21.
307. Alcorn D, Emslie KR, Ross BD, Ryan GB, Tange JD: Selective distal nephron damage during isolated kidney perfusion. Kidney Int 19:638-647, 1981
308. Brezis M, Rosen S, Silva P, Epstein FH: Selective vulnerability of the medullary thick ascending limb to anoxia in the isolated perfused rat kidney. J Clin.Invest 73:182-190, 1984
309. Z. Guan, D. A. Willgoss, A. Matthias, S. W. Manley, S. Crozier, G. Gobe, et al. Facilitation of renal autoregulation by angiotensin II is mediated through modulation of nitric oxide. Acta Physiol Scand 2003;179(2):189-201.
310. Lieberthal W, Wolf EF, Merrill EW, Levinsky NG, Valeri CR: Hemodynamic effects of different preparations of stroma free hemolysates in the isolated perfused rat kidney. Life Sci 41:2525-33, 1987
311. Lieberthal W, Vogel WM, Apstein CS, Valeri CR: Studies of the mechanism of the vasoconstrictor activity of stroma-free hemoglobin in the isolated perfused rat kidney and rabbit heart. Prog Clin Biol Res 319:407-20, 1989

312. Baines AD, Christoff B, Wicks D, Wiffen D, Pliura D: Cross-linked hemoglobin increases fractional reabsorption and GFR in hypoxic isolated perfused rat kidneys. Am J Physiol 269:628-36, 1995
313. Baines AD, Adamson G, Wojciechowski P, Pliura D, Ho P, Kluger R: Effect of modifying O2 diffusivity and delivery on glomerular and tubular function in hypoxic perfused kidney. Am J Physiol 274:744-52, 1998
314. Hayakawa H, Hirata Y, Suzuki E, Sugimoto T, Matsuoka H, Kikuchi K, Nagano T, Hirobe M: Mechanisms for altered endothelium-dependent vasorelaxation in isolated kidneys from experimental hypertensive rats. Am J Physiol 264:1535-41, 1993
315. Hirata Y, Hayakawa H, Kakoki M, Tojo A, Suzuki E, Nagata D, Kimura K, Goto A, Kikuchi K, Nagano T, Hirobe M, Omata M: Receptor subtype for vasopressin-induced release of nitric oxide from rat kidney. Hypertension 29:58-64, 1997
316. Hirata Y, Hayakawa H, Suzuki E, Omata M: Does endothelin work as an intrarenal mechanism to alter pressure natriuresis in spontaneously hypertensive rats? J Hypertens 12:251-7, 1994
317. Hirata Y, Hayakawa H, Suzuki Y, Suzuki E, Ikenouchi H, Kohmoto O, Kimura K, Kitamura K, Eto T, Kangawa K, et al.: Mechanisms of adrenomedullin-induced vasodilation in the rat kidney. Hypertension 25:790-5, 1995
318. Hayakawa H, Raij L: Relationship between hypercholesterolaemia, endothelial dysfunction and hypertension. J Hypertens 17:611-9, 1999
319. Kakoki M, Hirata Y, Hayakawa H, Tojo A, Nagata D, Suzuki E, Kimura K, Goto A, Kikuchi K, Nagano T, Omata M: Effects of hypertension, diabetes mellitus, and hypercholesterolemia on endothelin type B receptor-mediated nitric oxide release from rat kidney. Circulation 99:1242-8, 1999
320. Kakoki M, Hirata Y, Hayakawa H, Suzuki E, Nagata D, Tojo A, Nishimatsu H, Nakanishi N, Hattori Y, Kikuchi K, Nagano T, Omata M: Effects of tetrahydrobiopterin on endothelial dysfunction in rats with ischemic acute renal failure. J Am Soc Nephrol 11:301-9, 2000
321. Kakoki M, Hirata Y, Hayakawa H, Suzuki E, Nagata D, Nishimatsu H, Kimura K, Goto A, Omata M: Effects of vasodilatory antihypertensive agents on endothelial dysfunction in rats with ischemic acute renal failure. Hypertens Res 23:527-33, 2000
322. Galat JA, Robinson AV, Rhodes RS: A model of hypoxic renal failure. J Surg Res 44:764-71, 1988
323. Kadkhodaee M, Endre ZH, Towner RA, Cross M: Hydroxyl radical generation following ischaemia-reperfusion in cell- free perfused rat kidney. Biochim.Biophys.Acta 1243:169-174, 1995
324. Kadkhodaee M, Hanson GR, Towner RA, Endre ZH: Detection of hydroxyl and carbon-centred radicals by EPR spectroscopy after ischaemia and reperfusion of the rat kidney. Free Radic.Res. 25:31-42, 1996
325. Kadkhodaee M, Gobe G, Wilgoss DA, Endre ZH: DNA fragmentation reduced by anti-oxidants following ischemia-reperfusionin the isolated perfused rat kidney. Nephrology 4:163-175, 1998
326. Brezis M, Shanley P, Silva P, Spokes K, Lear S, Epstein FH, Rosen S: Disparate mechanisms for hypoxic cell injury in different nephron segments. Studies in the isolated perfused rat kidney. J Clin Invest 76:1796-806, 1985
327. S. L. Linas, D. Whittenburg, P. E. Parsons and J. E. Repine. Mild renal ischemia activates primed neutrophils to cause acute renal failure. Kidney Int 1992;42(3):610-6.
328 Z. Guan, G. Gobe, D. Willgoss and Z. H. Endre. Renal Endothelial Dysfunction And Impaired Autoregulation After Ischemia-Reperfusion Injury result from Excess Nitric Oxide. Am J Physiol Renal Physiol 2006;Mar 28; [Epub ahead of print].
329. Lieberthal W, Menza SA, Levine JS: Graded ATP depletion can cause necrosis or apoptosis of cultured mouse proximal tubular cells. Am.J.Physiol. 274:F315-F327, 1998
330. P. C. Dagher. Apoptosis in ischemic renal injury: roles of GTP depletion and p53. Kidney Int 2004;66(2):506-9.
331. Allis JL, Endre ZH, Radda GK: 87Rb, 23Na and 31P nuclear magnetic resonance spectroscopy of the perfused rat kidney. Ren Physiol Biochem. 12:171-180, 1989
332. Endre ZH, Cowin GJ, Stewart-Richardson P, Cross M, Willgoss DA, Duggleby RG: 23Na NMR detects protection by glycine and alanine against hypoxic injury in the isolated perfused rat kidney. Biochem.Biophys.Res.Commun. 202:1639-1644, 1994
333. Paller MS, Hoidal JR, Ferris TF: Oxygen free radicals in ischemic acute renal failure in the rat. J.Clin.Invest 74:1156-1162, 1984
334. Paller MS, Hedlund BE: Role of iron in postischemic renal injury in the rat. Kidney Int 34:474-480, 1988
335. Linas SL, Whittenburg D, Repine JE: Role of neutrophil derived oxidants and elastase in lipopolysaccharide- mediated renal injury. Kidney Int 39:618-623, 1991
336. Linas SL, Shanley PF, Whittenburg D, et al.: Neutrophils accentuate ischemia/reperfusion injury in isolated perfused rat kidneys. Am J Physiol 255:F725-F733, 1988
337. Ghielli M, Verstrepen W, Nouwen E, De Broe ME: Regeneration processes in the kidney after acute injury: role of infiltrating cells. Exp Nephrol 6:502-7, 1998
338. Ghielli M, Verstrepen WA, De Greef KE, Helbert MH, Ysebaert DK, Nouwen EJ, De Broe ME: Antibodies to both ICAM-1 and LFA-1 do not protect the kidney against toxic (HgCl2) injury. Kidney Int 58:1121-34, 2000
339. Paller MS, Neumann TV: Reactive oxygen species and rat renal epithelial cells during hypoxia and reoxygenation. Kidney Int 40:1041-1049, 1991

340. Brezis M, Rosen S, Stoff JS, Spokes K, Silva P, Epstein FH: Inhibition of prostaglandin synthesis in rat kidney perfused with and without erythrocytes: implication for analgesic nephropathy. Miner Electrolyte Metab 12:326-32, 1986
341. Brezis M, Rosen S: Hypoxia of the renal medulla--its implications for disease. N.Engl.J Med. 332:647-655, 1995
342. Heyman SN, Rosen S, Darmon D, Goldfarb M, Bitz H, Shina A, Brezis M: Endotoxin-induced renal failure. II. A role for tubular hypoxic damage. Exp Nephrol 8:275-82, 2000
343. Lieberthal W, Rennke HG, Sandock KM, Valeri CR, Levinsky NG: Ischemia in the isolated erythrocyte-perfused rat kidney. Protective effect of hypothermia. Ren Physiol Biochem 11:60-9, 1988
344. Endre ZH, Ratcliffe PJ: Patterns of ischaemic renal cell injury, in Acute Renal Failure, edited by Solez K, Racusen LC, New York, Marcel Dekker, 1990, pp 173-185
345. Mason J, Welsch J, Torhorst J: The contribution of vascular obstruction to the functional defect that follows renal ischemia. Kidney Int 31:65-71, 1987
346. Wolgast M, Bayati A, Hellberg O, Kallskog O, Nygren K: Osmotic diuretics and hemodilution in postischemic renal failure. Ren Fail 14:297-302, 1992
347. H. Rabb. The T cell as a bridge between innate and adaptive immune systems: implications for the kidney. Kidney Int 2002;61(6):1935-46.
348. Beeri R, Symon Z, Brezis M, Ben-Sasson SA, Baehr PH, Rosen S, Zager RA: Rapid DNA fragmentation from hypoxia along the thick ascending limb of rat kidneys. Kidney Int. 47:1806-1810, 1995
349. Gobe G, Zhang XJ, Cuttle L, Pat B, Willgoss D, Hancock J, Barnard R, Endre RB: Bcl-2 genes and growth factors in the pathology of ischaemic acute renal failure. Immunol.Cell Biol. 77:279-286, 1999
350. Jaffe R, Ariel I, Beeri R, Paltiel O, Hiss Y, Rosen S, Brezis M: Frequent apoptosis in human kidneys after acute renal hypoperfusion. Exp Nephrol 5:399-403, 1997
351. Ueda N, Walker PD, Hsu S, Shah SV: Activation of a 15-kDa endonuclease in hypoxia/reoxygenation injury without morphologic features of apoptosis. Proc Natl Acad Sci USA 92:7202-7206, 1995
352. De Broe ME: Apoptosis in acute renal failure. Nephrol Dial Transplant 16:23-6, 2001
353. Gobe G, Willgoss D, Hogg N, Schoch E, Endre Z: Cell survival or death in renal tubular epithelium after ischemia- reperfusion injury. Kidney Int 56:1299-1304, 1999
354. Cuttle L, Zhang XJ, Endre ZH, Winterford C, Gobe GC: Bcl-X(L) translocation in renal tubular epithelial cells *in vitro* protects distal cells from oxidative stress. Kidney Int 59:1779-88, 2001
355. Li P, Nijhawan D, Budihardjo I, Srinivasula SM, Ahmad M, Alnemri ES, Wang X: Cytochrome c and dATP-dependent formation of Apaf-1/caspase-9 complex initiates an apoptotic protease cascade. Cell 91:479-489, 1997
356. J. F. di Mari, R. Davis and R. L. Safirstein. MAPK activation determines renal epithelial cell survival during oxidative injury. Am J Physiol 1999;277(2 Pt 2):F195-203.
357. Safirstein R: Renal stress response and acute renal failure. Adv.Ren Replace.Ther. 4:38-42, 1997
358. Ratcliffe PJ, Endre ZH, Nicholls LG, Tange JD, Ledingham JGG: The isolated perfused rat kidney: filtering and non-filtering models in the assessment of altered renal vascular resistance in nephrotoxicity, in Nephrotoxicity: Extrapolation from *in vitro* to *in vivo* and from animals to man., edited by Bach PH, Lock EA, New York, Plenum, 1989, pp 107-110
359. Firth JD, Ratcliffe PJ, Raine AE, Ledingham JG: Endothelin: an important factor in acute renal failure? Lancet 2:1179-82, 1988
360. Firth JD, Ratcliffe PJ: Organ distribution of the three rat endothelin messenger RNAs and the effects of ischemia on renal gene expression. J Clin Invest 90:1023-31, 1992
361. Ritthaler T, Gopfert T, Firth JD, Ratcliffe PJ, Kramer BK, Kurtz A: Influence of hypoxia on hepatic and renal endothelin gene expression. Pflugers Arch 431:587-93, 1996
362. Kramer BK, Bucher M, Sandner P, Ittner KP, Riegger GA, Ritthaler T, Kurtz A: Effects of hypoxia on growth factor expression in the rat kidney *in vivo*. Kidney Int 51:444-7, 1997
363. Wilhelm SM, Simonson MS, Robinson AV, Stowe NT, Schulak JA: Endothelin up-regulation and localization following renal ischemia and reperfusion. Kidney Int 55:1011-8, 1999
364. Forbes JM, Hewitson TD, Becker GJ, Jones CL: Ischemic acute renal failure: long-term histology of cell and matrix changes in the rat. Kidney Int 57:2375-85, 2000
365. Forbes JM, Jandeleit-Dahm K, Allen TJ, Hewitson TD, Becker GJ, Jones CL: Endothelin and endothelin a/b receptors are increased after ischaemic acute renal failure. Exp Nephrol 9:309-16, 2001
366. Chan L, Chittinandana A, Shapiro JI, Shanley PF, Schrier RW: Effect of endothelin-receptor antagonist on ischemic acute renal failure. Am.J.Physiol. 266:F135-F138, 1994
367. Forbes JM, Hewitson TD, Becker GJ, Jones CL: Simultaneous blockade of endothelin A and B receptors in ischemic acute renal failure is detrimental to long-term kidney function. Kidney Int 59:1333-41, 2001

368. Lieberthal W, Wolf EF, Rennke HG, Valeri CR, Levinsky NG: Renal ischemia and reperfusion impair endothelium-dependent vascular relaxation. Am J Physiol 256:F894-F900, 1989
369. Allgren RL, Marbury TC, Rahman SN, Weisberg LS, Fenves AZ, Lafayette RA, Sweet RM, Genter FC, Kurnik BRC, Conger JD, Sayegh MH: Anaritide in acute tubular necrosis. N Engl J Med 336:828-834, 1997
370. Perico N, Dadan J, Remuzzi G: Endothelin mediates the renal vasoconstriction induced by cyclosporine in the rat. J Am Soc Nephrol 1:76-83, 1990
371. Bertelli A, Giovannini L, Palla R, Migliori M, Panichi V, Andreini B: Protective effect of L-propionylcarnitine on cyclosporine-induced nephrotoxicity. Drugs Exp Clin Res 21:221-8, 1995
372. Hirata Y, Hayakawa H, Suzuki E, Kimura K, Kikuchi K, Nagano T, Hirobe M, Omata M: Direct measurements of endothelium-derived nitric oxide release by stimulation of endothelin receptors in rat kidney and its alteration in salt-induced hypertension. Circulation 91:1229-35, 1995
373. Oldroyd S, Slee SJ, Haylor J, Morcos SK, Wilson C: Role for endothelin in the renal responses to radiocontrast media in the rat. Clin Sci (Colch) 87:427-34, 1994
374. Oldroyd SD, Haylor JL, Morcos SK: Bosentan, an orally active endothelin antagonist: effect on the renal response to contrast media. Radiology 196:661-5, 1995
375. Morcos SK, Oldroyd S, Haylor J: Effect of radiographic contrast media on endothelium derived nitric oxide-dependent renal vasodilatation. Br J Radiol 70:154-9, 1997
376. Wang A, Holcslaw T, Bashore TM, Freed MI, Miller D, Rudnick MR, Szerlip H, Thames MD, Davidson CJ, Shusterman N, Schwab SJ: Exacerbation of radiocontrast nephrotoxicity by endothelin receptor antagonism. Kidney Int 57:1675-80, 2000
377. Cantley LG, Spokes K, Clark B, McMahon EG, Carter J, Epstein FH: Role of endothelin and prostaglandins in radiocontrast-induced renal artery constriction. Kidney Int 44:1217-23, 1993
378. Erley CM, Duda SH, Schlepckow S, Koehler J, Huppert PE, Strohmaier WL, Bohle A, Risler T, Osswald H: Adenosine antagonist theophylline prevents the reduction of glomerular filtration rate after contrast media application. Kidney Int 45:1425-31, 1994
379. Katholi RE, Taylor GJ, McCann WP, Woods WT, Jr., Womack KA, McCoy CD, Katholi CR, Moses HW, Mishkel GJ, Lucore CL, et al.: Nephrotoxicity from contrast media: attenuation with theophylline. Radiology 195:17-22, 1995
380. Yoshioka T, Fogo A, Beckman JK: Reduced activity of antioxidant enzymes underlies contrast media- induced renal injury in volume depletion. Kidney Int 41:1008-15, 1992
381. Tepel M, van der Giet M, Schwarzfeld C, Laufer U, Liermann D, Zidek W: Prevention of radiographic-contrast-agent-induced reductions in renal function by acetylcysteine. N Engl J Med 343:180-4, 2000
382. Endre ZH, Nicholls LG, Ratcliffe PJ, Ledingham JGG: Prevention and reversal of mercuric chloride-induced increase in renal vascular resistance by captopril, in Nephrotoxicity: Extrapolation from *in vitro* to *in vivo* and from animals to man., edited by Bach PH, Lock EA, New York, Plenum, 1989, pp 103-106
383. Rossi N, Churchill P, Ellis V, Amore B: Mechanism of adenosine receptor-induced renal vasoconstriction in rats. Am J Physiol 255:885-90, 1988
384. Rossi N, Ellis V, Kontry T, Gunther S, Churchill P, Bidani A: The role of adenosine in HgCl2-induced acute renal failure in rats. Am J Physiol 258:1554-60, 1990
385. Yanagisawa H, Nodera M, Kurihara N, Wada O: Altered expression of endothelin-1 and endothelial nitric oxide synthase in the juxtaglomerular apparatus of rats with HgCl2-induced acute renal failure. Toxicol Lett 98:181-8, 1998
386. Bhardwaj R, Moore PK: Endothelium-derived relaxing factor and the effects of acetylcholine and histamine on resistance blood vessels. Br J Pharmacol 95:835-43, 1988
387. Radermacher J, Forstermann U, Frolich JC: Endothelium-derived relaxing factor influences renal vascular resistance. Am J Physiol 259:9-17, 1990
388. Radermacher J, Klanke B, Kastner S, Haake G, Schurek HJ, Stolte HF, Frolich JC: Effect of arginine depletion on glomerular and tubular kidney function: studies in isolated perfused rat kidneys. Am J Physiol 261:779-86, 1991
389. Radermacher J, Klanke B, Schurek HJ, Stolte HF, Frolich JC: Importance of NO/EDRF for glomerular and tubular function: studies in the isolated perfused rat kidney. Kidney Int. 41:1549-1559, 1992
390. Garcia-Estan J, Atucha NM, Sabio JM, Vargas F, Quesada T, Romero JC: Increased endothelium-dependent renal vasodilation in cirrhotic rats. Am J Physiol 267:549-53, 1994
391. Garcia-Estan J, Atucha NM, Groszmann RJ: Renal response to methoxamine in portal hypertensive rats: role of prostaglandins and nitric oxide. J Hepatol 25:206-11, 1996
392. Vargas F, Sabio JM, Luna JD: Contribution of endothelium derived relaxing factors to acetylcholine induced vasodilatation in the rat kidney. Cardiovasc Res 28:1373-7, 1994
393. Vargas F, Osuna A, Fernandez-Rivas A: Vascular reactivity and flow-pressure curve in isolated kidneys from rats with N-nitro-L-arginine methyl ester-induced hypertension. J Hypertens 14:373-9, 1996

394. Rapacon M, Mieyal P, McGiff JC, Fulton D, Quilley J: Contribution of calcium-activated potassium channels to the vasodilator effect of bradykinin in the isolated, perfused kidney of the rat. Br J Pharmacol 118:1504-8, 1996
395. Bagate K, Grima M, Imbs JL, Jong WD, Helwig JJ, Barthelmebs M: Signal transduction pathways involved in kinin B(2) receptor-mediated vasodilation in the rat isolated perfused kidney. Br J Pharmacol 132:1735-42, 2001
396. Kaufmann MA, Castelli I, Pargger H, Drop LJ: Nitric oxide dose-response study in the isolated perfused rat kidney after inhibition of endothelium-derived relaxing factor synthesis: the role of serum albumin. J Pharmacol Exp Ther 273:855-62, 1995
397. Ziyyat A, Zhang BL, Benzoni D: Interactions between nitric oxide and prostanoids in isolated perfused kidneys of the rat. Br J Pharmacol 119:388-92, 1996
398. Boric MP, Bravo JA, Corbalan M, Vergara C, Roblero JS: Interactions between bradykinin and ANP in rat kidney *in vitro*: inhibition of natriuresis and modulation of medullary cyclic GMP. Biol Res 31:281-9, 1998
399. Rahimian R, Van Breemen C, Karkan D, Dube G, Laher I: Estrogen augments cyclopiazonic acid-mediated, endothelium-dependent vasodilation. Eur J Pharmacol 327:143-9, 1997
400. Muller C, Endlich K, Helwig JJ: AT2 antagonist-sensitive potentiation of angiotensin II-induced constriction by NO blockade and its dependence on endothelium and P450 eicosanoids in rat renal vasculature. Br J Pharmacol 124:946-52, 1998
401. Hayakawa H, Hirata Y, Kakoki M, Suzuki Y, Nishimatsu H, Nagata D, Suzuki E, Kikuchi K, Nagano T, Kangawa K, Matsuo H, Sugimoto T, Omata M: Role of nitric oxide-cGMP pathway in adrenomedullin-induced vasodilation in the rat. Hypertension 33:689-93, 1999
402. Miric G, Dallemagne C, Endre Z, Margolin S, Taylor SM, Brown L: Reversal of cardiac and renal fibrosis by pirfenidone and spironolactone in streptozotocin-diabetic rats. Br J Pharmacol 133:687-94, 2001
403. Raz E, Kaminski N, Brezis M: Effects of perfusion pressure and renal flow upon albumin excretion in isolated perfused kidneys [see comments]. Nephron 56:396-8, 1990
404. Lapinski R, Perico N, Remuzzi A, Sangalli F, Benigni A, Remuzzi G: Angiotensin II modulates glomerular capillary permselectivity in rat isolated perfused kidney. J Am Soc Nephrol 7:653-60, 1996
405. Perico N, Lapinski R, Konopka K, Aiello S, Noris M, Remuzzi G: Platelet-activating factor mediates angiotensin II-induced proteinuria in isolated perfused rat kidney. J Am Soc Nephrol 8:1391-8, 1997
406. Burne MJ, Adal Y, Cohen N, Panagiotopoulos S, Jerums G, Comper WD: Anomalous decrease in dextran sulfate clearance in the diabetic rat kidney. Am J Physiol 274:700-8, 1998
407. Eppel GA, Osicka TM, Pratt LM, Jablonski P, Howden BO, Glasgow EF, Comper WD: The return of glomerular-filtered albumin to the rat renal vein. Kidney Int 55:1861-70, 1999
408. Boyce NW, Holdsworth SR: Evidence for direct renal injury as a consequence of glomerular complement activation. J Immunol 136:2421-5, 1986
409. Fauler J, Wiemeyer A, Yoshizawa M, Schurek HJ, Frolich JC: Metabolism of cysteinyl leukotrienes by the isolated perfused rat kidney. Prostaglandins 42:239-49, 1991
410. Yared A, Albrightson-Winslow C, Griswold D, Takahashi K, Fogo A, Badr KF: Functional significance of leukotriene B4 in normal and glomerulonephritic kidneys. J Am Soc Nephrol 2:45-56, 1991
411. Jocks T, Zahner G, Helmchen U, Kneissler U, Stahl RA: Antibody and complement reduce renal hemodynamic function in isolated perfused rat kidney. Am J Physiol 270:179-85, 1996
412. Jocks T, Zahner G, Freudenberg J, Wolf G, Thaiss F, Helmchen U, Stahl RA: Prostaglandin E1 reduces the glomerular mRNA expression of monocyte- chemoattractant protein 1 in anti-thymocyte antibody-induced glomerular injury. J Am Soc Nephrol 7:897-905, 1996
413. Saunders JR, Aminian A, McRae JL, O'Farrell KA, Adam WR, Murphy BF: Clusterin depletion enhances immune glomerular injury in the isolated perfused kidney. Kidney Int 45:817-27, 1994
414. Gabbai FB, Peterson OW, Khang S, Wilson CB, Blantz RC: Glomerular hemodynamics in cell-free and erythrocyte-perfused isolated rat kidney. Am J Physiol 267:423-7, 1994
415 W. H. Beierwaltes. A different vision of the osmolar regulation of renin secretion. Am J Physiol Renal Physiol 2006;290(4):F795-6.

10

Renal cell culture models:

Contribution to the understanding of nephrotoxic mechanisms

Paul JENNINGS[1], Christian KOPPELSTÄTTER[2], Judith LECHNER[1] and Walter PFALLER[1]

[1]Dept. of Physiology and Medical Physics and [2]Dept. of Internal Medicine, Innsbruck Medical University, Austria

Introduction

The kidney represents a major target for toxic xenobiotics due to its role in the control of body fluid and electrolyte homeostasis. The high blood perfusion rate (20% of cardiac output) and the capability to extract, metabolize, secrete and concentrate toxic compounds make the kidneys extremely vulnerable to a wide variety of toxins, many of which are yet to be identified. It is estimated that therapeutic agents cause 20% of all diagnosed end stage renal disease (ESRD) and that chemicals and drugs may play a significant role in at least 50% of ESRD cases of unknown etiology [1].

Because of the functional and biochemical heterogeneity of the nephron, the susceptibility to a particular nephrotoxic insult will vary among nephron segments. The epithelial cells of the proximal nephron are target sites for a wide variety of nephrotoxic chemicals due to a large number of transport systems [2] and the presence of xenobiotic metabolizing enzymes such as cytochrome P-450, NADPH-cytochrome c reductase, glucuronyl transferase, sulfotransferases, glutathione S-transferases, cysteine conjugate β-lyase, monooxygenases and prostaglandin H synthase [3]. Another factor is the intracellular concentration of glutathione (GSH) and GSH dependent enzyme activity, which is highest in proximal tubule and decreases progressively down the nephron [4, 5]. Additionally the proximal tubule has a high requirement for oxygen which makes this area of the nepron especially sensitive to oxygen deprivation [6].

The primary means of identifying potential renal effects of drugs and chemicals involves testing in laboratory animals. However, the understanding of biochemical and cellular mechanisms together with advances in cell and tissue culture now permit the development and use of *in vitro* toxicity assays. The aim of the development of such *in vitro* tests is not only to refine, reduce and replace *in vivo* animal testing, but also to improve the relevance of data obtained for the safety evaluation in humans. The reasons for the current drive for *in vitro* assay development can be attributed to three main points: 1) Scientific experiments involving live animals are receiving bad press in recent years. Public opinion of such experiments is progressively more disapproving; and governments are listening. In 1986 the European Union issued a directive which states that animal experimentation shall not be performed if non-animal procedures are reasonable and practically available [7]. This directive is currently under revision and is requesting a greater development and use of alternatives to animal experiments than its predecessor; 2) *In vivo* test methods are expensive, time consuming and require the sacrifice of many animals. As an example, the rodent bioassay for assessing carcinogenicity costs $1-3 million and requires at least 3 years to be completed [8]. The development of reliable *in vitro* models offers potential reduction of time and cost during new product development; 3) There is often doubt concerning the relevance to humans of toxicity or lack of toxicity, of compounds tested in animals. A compound toxic in one species is not necessarily toxic in another species and vice versa. For example thalidomide only causes birth defects in humans and rabbits and not in rats or mice [9]. Another example is the herbicide acetochlor, which caused the induction of nasal adenomas in rats in 2-year feeding studies. However, after investigations including human tissue experiments it was concluded that the effects in rats were not relevant to humans [10]. Some of the species differences can be clarified; a specific isoenzyme of cytochrome P-450 found in the nasal epithelium of rat but not in humans, is thought to be responsible for the species dependent effect of acetochlor [11]. Further species variations in the expression of many Phase I and Phase II metabolizing enzymes are known [12-14]. There are, therefore, compelling ethical, financial and scientific reasons for developing *in vitro* alternatives to animal testing. The most important issue in the development of such tests is that the data produced by the test system is relevant to human risk.

Renal cell culture models

Renal cell cultures, which retain adequate renal cellular functions known to interact with xenobiotics or drugs, have the advantage of providing an experimental model that is not influenced by higher-order regulatory systems. Non cell culture based *in vitro* nephrotoxicity systems have been reviewed elsewhere [15].

Cells isolated from the kidney and successfully cultured should retain a phenotype, which preserves the key properties of the *in vivo et situ* components relevant for nephrotoxicity studies. *Glomerular microvascular endothelial cells* in culture should maintain the characteristic fenestration, the presence of Weibel-Palade bodies (both observed by transmission electron microscopy), the expression of von Willebrand factor and CD 31 (platelet-endothelial cell adhesion molecule-1) [16, 17, 23]. Microvascular endothelial cells (regardless of their organ of origin) should respond to cytokines such as tumor necrosis factor α (TNF-α), by the increased expression of cell adhesion molecules for example E-selectin and intercellular adhesion molecule-1 (ICAM-1) [17, 18]. It is advisable to not only demonstrate the presence of specific characteristics, but also the absence of non-endothelial markers such as cytokeratin-8 (epithelial cells) [19], smooth muscle α actin (smooth muscle cells) and the intermediate filament protein desmin (pericytes) [20, 21]. The morphological characterization of endothelial cells by light microscopy must be used with caution due to the marked plasticity of these cells in culture [22]. However, glomerular endothelial cells can usually be distinguished at a light microscopy level from common contaminating cells such as fibroblasts, mesangial cells and epithelial cells [17].

Glomerular visceral epithelial cells (podocytes) in culture should have retained the potency to produce basement membrane constituents (collagen IV and glycosaminoglycans) and maintain the expression of cytokeratin, synaptopodin, the membrane proteins megalin and podocalyxin and angiotensin II receptors [24-26].

Glomerular mesangial cells in culture should display the basic properties of pericytes such as the expression of the cytoskeletal filaments smooth muscle actin [27], myosin, vimentin and desmin [28] and also functional properties of their *in vivo* counterparts such as, the capability to produce extracellular matrix molecules contributing to the formation of the glomerular basement membrane [29] and response to vasoconstrictive signals [30], growth factors and mitogenic signals and display phagocytic properties [31]. Morphologically they are recognized by the formation of multilayers and hillock structure as assessed by phase contrast microscopy and bundles of microfilaments orientated parallel to the plasma membrane at an electron microscopic level [32]. The absence of expression of non-mesangial markers such as cytokeratin and von Willebrand factor will exclude the possibility of contaminants from other cell types.

Renal tubular epithelial cells in culture represent an adequate *in vitro* model for nephrotoxicity studies if they have retained: **(1)** polar architecture and junctional assembly of epithelia and correct polar distribution of membrane enzymes and transport systems, **(2)** vectorial transport of solutes and water, manifested by the formation of domes [33] and the generation of transepithelial electrophysiological properties [34, 35], **(3)** cellular uptake of xenobiotics from either the apical or basolateral side, as observed *in vivo* and **(4)** expression of nephron segment-specific characteristics, i.e. distinct antigen/enzyme differentiation markers, metabolic and transport properties, and hormone responsiveness [5, 36, 37].

Whether these requirements are better met by primary cultures or renal cell lines is still subject of debate and will depend on the type of investigation. Techniques for the isolation and culture of primary cells of the renal tubular epithelium, glomerular mesangial cells, podocytes and endothelial cells have been developed for various species including human. Although cells in primary culture tend to dedifferentiate, the characteristics of those cells are usually closer to the *in vivo* situation than are animal cell lines, at least for a limited culture period. Primary cultures have been used successfully to study the *in vitro* effects of numerous nephrotoxins including, cyclosporine A (CsA), gentamicin, mercuric chloride and Ochratoxin A [38-42].

Cell lines offer several advantages over primary cell cultures, such as an unlimited life-span and the lack of time-consuming isolation procedures. Additionally once established, they are often more stable than primary cells which are usually in a continuous state of de-differentiation. Thus, the majority of *in vitro* nephrotoxicity studies have been performed on renal epithelial cell lines. In normal somatic cells, telomeres, the tandemly repeated hexamers at the end of mammalian chromosomes, act as the cellular replicative clock [43] and shorten at each cell division. Once telomeres have exceeded a certain critical length, the so called "Hayflick limit" [44], the cell enters replicative senescence and no longer proliferates. Until recently the most widely used renal cell lines were those which arose from spontaneously acquired immortalization in culture. These cell lines include; LLC-PK_1 (Hampshire pig) [45, 46], JTC-12 (cynomolgus monkey) [47] and OK (American opossum) [48] cells, which exhibit biochemical and antigenic characteristics suggestive of proximal origin, and the MDCK (Cocker Spaniel) [49, 50], and A6 (clawed toad, Xenopus laevis) [51] cell lines which exhibit properties suggestive of distal tubule/collecting duct origin. For the majority of these cells neither the cell-type of origin, nor the agents responsible for immortalization are precisely known. Their 'origin' was merely deduced from their morphologic and functional properties, which were usually studied years after emergence resulting in an ambiguous phenotype, leaving their true origin uncertain.

The MDCK cell line, for example, is one of the most widely employed cell lines in basic renal epithelial research. MDCK cells show a hormonal profile consistent with collecting duct origin, express the furosemide-sensitive $Na^+/K^+/2Cl^-$ symporter, consistent with TAL origin, and express significant amounts of brush-border hydrolases (tnAP and LAP), consistent with PT origin [50, 52, 53]. Two cell lines that are often used as a model for the proximal nephron are the porcine cell line, LLC-PK_1 and the OK cell line from the opossum kidney. Both of these cell lines lack expression of the enzyme fructose-1, 6-bisphosphatase, rendering them incapable of gluconeogenesis, a key metabolic pathway in proximal nephron cells [5]. In addition LLC-PK1 response profile to hormones does not resemble that of the proximal tubule *in vivo* because vasopressin and calcitonin both stimulate adenylate cyclase, whereas parathyroid hormone is totally ineffective in these cells [54]. OK cells display very little γ-GT, and lack alkaline phosphatase, both considered to be markers for the proximal nephron [55].

With the advances in molecular biology it is now possible to deliberately genetically engineer cells to have extended or permanent proliferation. This is of major importance in the development of human renal cell lines, as the availability of human tissue is often the limiting factor in renal cell culture based research. Several methods exist for immortalizing mammalian cells in culture. Viral oncogenes, including Simian virus 40 (SV40) T antigen, Epstein Barr virus (EBV), Adenovirus E1A and E1B, and human papillomavirus (HPV) E6 and E7 can induce immortalization in different cell types. Viral oncogenes achieve immortalization by inactivating tumor suppressor genes, such as p53 and retinoblastoma protein, allowing cells to evade replicative senescence. Currently the most widely used human renal proximal tubular cell line, HK-2 cells, were generated by transduction of human primary proximal tubular cells with human papillomavirus (HPV) E6/E7 genes [56]. The most recently discovered approach to cell immortalization is by inducing telomerase activity by over expression of the catalytic subunit of telomerase (hTERT) [57]. Non-rodent normal somatic cells do not normally express telomerase activity and re-expression of this enzyme extends and stabilizes the telomere preventing replicative senescence. Spontaneously- and viral gene- immortalized cell lines also exhibit elevated levels of telomerase activity, demonstrating the importance of this enzyme in evading replicative senescence and subsequent immortalization. Many cancers also acquire telomerase activity which is thought to be a critical step in cancer survival and proliferation [58]. Cell lines have also been developed by transfection with both viral oncogenes and hTERT, for example human glomerular microvascular endothelial cells [59] and human proximal tubular cells [60]. Both of these cell lines retain a good differentiation status and have the added advantage that they are conditionally immortalized, thus once the oncogene has been removed the cells once again become mortal and will eventually senesce.

At present there is still a lack of well characterized and well differentiated cell lines of human origin representative of the different cell-types present in the nephron and the collecting duct system. However, once available, human immortalized cell lines of defined nephron segment origin will likely provide a welcome alternative to primary cultures for studying cell properties *in vitro* in a cell-type dependent way.

In vitro nephrotoxicity study variables

Cell culture medium

Cell cultures were originally developed for the propagation of viruses for vaccine development. Consequently, almost all of the established cell-culture methodologies, especially with respect to culture nutrients, are designed primarily for the selection of proliferating cells. This remains true for cell cultures used to study membrane trafficking, gene expression, transport, membrane electrophysiological properties, and intracellular signal cascades. The efforts undertaken to create culture media for the generation of non-proliferating, but differentiated, cells have been mostly limited to the development of serum-free media supplemented with specific hormones, growth factors or chemicals. Distinct changes in basal medium composition have been shown to produce new cell phenotypes. For example, the transient omission of glucose, but maintenance of carbon sources for nucleoside synthesis (for example, uridine or pyruvate) led to a selection of gluconeogenic phenotypes in the renal LLC-PK_1 and OK cell lines [61, 62]. Regrowth in the presence of glucose demonstrated constitutive expression of the formerly missing gluconeogenic key enzymes, fructose-1, 6-biphosphatase and phosphenol pyruvate carboxy-kinase (PEPCK) [63].

The development and use of serum free hormonally supplemented medium is, however, a step in the right direction. The application of defined medium allows a more standardized approach to cell culture delivering greater reproducibility and transferability. For renal tubular cells, defined medium supplements have been described as far back as 1982 [64], and we have successfully cultured human renal proximal tubular cells in defined medium containing EGF, hydrocortisone, insulin, transferrin and sodium selenite using DMEM-Hams F12 as the base medium [42].

Oxygen

There is often the misconception that cells in culture are exposed to higher oxygen concentrations than *in vivo* due to the use of 5% CO_2 humidified incubators balanced with air containing 21% O_2. However, in most situations the opposite is true; cells in culture suffer from hypoxic conditions. This is due to a higher oxygen consumption rate of cells at the bottom of the petri dish than the oxygen diffusion rate through the liquid column [65]. The extent of hypoxia will depend on the cell type and cell density. Renal epithelial cells are particularly responsive to alterations in oxygen tensions. Gstraunthaler et. al. demonstrated that alterations in medium volume, which effectively alters oxygen delivery rate, can also markedly affect LLC-PK1 and OK cell metabolism [66]. The problem of insufficient oxygen delivery is not easily over come in routine cultures. The use of roller bottle cultures or rocking cultures significantly improves oxygen delivery, however these systems are somewhat more laborious than conventional culture and are seldom used in modern cell culture laboratories.

Growth surface

Primary cells or cell lines can be seeded onto a variety of commercially available surfaces. Solid growth supports are made from various plastic materials (polystyrene, polycarbonate, PTFE (polymeric tetrafluoroethylene - TEFLON®), PTX (polyester) or glass. The surfaces used are usually hydrophobic and can be manipulated with regard to their surface charges by specific pretreatment. Most commonly polystyrene surfaces of cell culture platic materials are submitted to corona discharge or plasma treatment. In this context it should be kept in mind that the surface properties (hydrophilisation) produced by these measures are not permanent and thus culture dish shelf life should be controlled. The surfaces can also be coated with extracellular matrix (ECM) materials such as collagen, fibronectin or laminin or more complex matrix mixes such as Matrigel™. Epithelial cells can also be grown on microporous substrates (coated or uncoated with ECM), with nutrients supplied from both the apical and basolateral sides. Investigators have shown that renal cells cultured on microporous membranes increases polarisation and differentiation properties [67]. The distal/collecting duct cell line Madin Darby canine kidney (MDCK) cultured on microporous supports, demonstrate a more columnar organisation with an increase in cell density in comparison with cells seeded on conventional plastic substrata. After two weeks of growth on microporous supports, they generate their own basement membrane [68]. Growth of cells on filters can also result in the reversion of correct membrane targeting of proteins such as the choline carrier, which is targeted to the basolateral membrane of MDCK cells only when grown on filter supports [69]. Also the A6 cell line re-expresses functional vasopressin receptors when cultured on microporous supports [70]. The growth of renal epithelial cells on microporous supports has implications for *in vitro* toxicity studies since renal toxins *in vivo* can gain access to the cells from the blood or luminal side. It has been demonstrated that the anti-cancer agent cisplatin is more toxic to LLC-PK1 cells when applied to the basolateral side [71]. This suggests that there are specific mechanisms mediating cisplatin uptake at the basolateral membrane. Thus, renal tubular cells grown on porous supports allow access of the test compound to the basolateral side which may, depending on the compound used, influence the

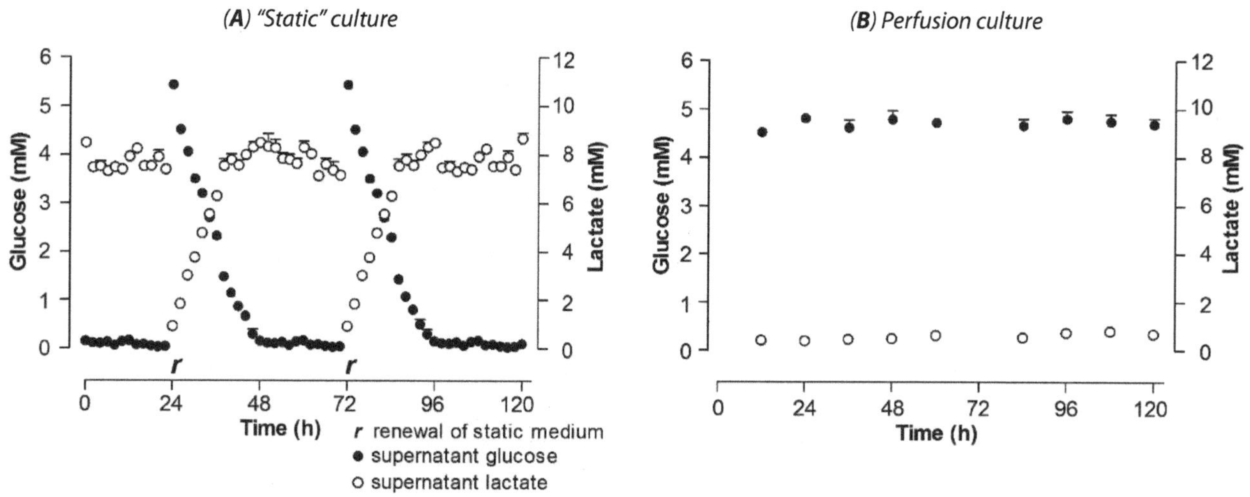

Figure 1. ***Time course of medium glucose and lactate concentrations of LLC-PK1 cells under conventional static conditions (A) and with continuous medium renewal (B).*** ***(A)*** *LLC-PK1 cells were grown to confluence and on 24 well plates, medium was removed from wells every two hours. Two medium replenishment cycles were conducted [r].* ***(B)*** *LLC-PK1 cells were cultured to confluence on micropourus filters and transferred to the EpiFlow perfusion device. Medium perfusion was 2 ml / h. Samples in the outflowing medium were collected at regular intervals. Glucose and lactate were measured using colorimetric assays. Results represent the mean ± SEM from 3 experiments. For more information see Felder et. al. 2002 [72].*

outcome of the experiment.

Medium perfusion

In conventional "static" cultures, medium composition is continuously modified by the cells, and needs replenishment at defined intervals. This condition is often referred to as feast / famine conditions. Directly after feeding, cells have a nutritious, glucose containing medium, although with no autocrine factors. At the end of the feeding cycle nutrients such as glucose are usually exhausted and metabolites such as lactate and autocrine factors are at their highest (Figure 1A) [66, 72]. Thus cells in culture must cope with a continually changing extracellular environment. This fact combined with low pericellular oxygen is thought to be the major reason for dedifferentiation of primary cell cultures. Continuous perfusion of medium solves some of these issues (Figure 1B). A number of commercial perfusion devices are now available including the Minutissue system and the EpiFlow device. Perfusion culture can also be combined with microporous supports and depending on the system used and the flow rates applied can also increase oxygen delivery. LLC-PK1 cells maintained in the EpiFlow device for five days increased their oxidative metabolism and demonstrated improved morphology [72]. However, perfusion systems are complicated and technically demanding and are not yet ready for routine cell cultures.

Co-cultures

Although generally speaking it is an advantage to have homogenous cultures of one specific cell type, sometimes the interactions between two or more cell types can bring additional and specific information. We have recently developed a co-culture model of microvascular endothelial and renal epithelial cells [73]. The peri-tubular capillary network and the proximal tubular epithelium are close collaborators in normal physiological and pathophysiological events, such as solute and water reabsorption, secretion and inflammation. We could demonstrate that microvascular endothelial cells cultured in close proximity, but without direct contact could affect specific properties of proximal tubular epithelial cells, such as gene expression and paracellular permeability. These effects were mediated by microvascular endothelial derived ECM and endothelial derived soluble factors. Additionally this method was applied to study the migration of neutrophils through epithelial and endothelial bilayers as a model of renal interstitial inflammation [74].

Endpoints for *in vitro* nephrotoxicity

Over the past decade there has been a renewed interest in the development of more specific and more sensitive endpoints for toxicity *in vitro*. Previously, the most commonly used endpoints have been the detection of cell vitality (e.g. REDOX sensitive dyes such as MTT [75]), plasma membrane integrity (e.g. the release of cytosolic enzymes such as lactate dehydrogenase [42]) and the measurement of apoptosis (e.g. DNA condensation, caspase activation [42]). The development of the three main "omics" approaches, transcriptomics (global mRNA changes), proteomics (global protein changes) and metabolomics (global metabolomic changes) presents the opportunity to search for new markers of xenobiotic induced stress in *in vitro* systems, which promise to be more specific and more sensitive. Several initiatives in the application of these technologies to *in vitro* research have been instigated by both European and American funding agencies. Once such project, the EU funded 6th framework project "Predictomics" has recently been completed. Within this project the transcriptome profiles of HK-2 cells exposed to 11 nephrotoxins have been generated and a number of potential marker genes have been identified (yet to be published).

A list of classical and novel endpoints for *in vitro* toxicity testing is given in Table 1.

Contribution of established renal cell culture models to the understanding of nephrotoxic mechanisms

In this section we provide a short review on the contribution of renal cell culture systems to the discovery of the mechanisms of the most well known

Table 1. Endpoints for assessment of nephrotoxicity on renal cell culture systems.

Cell activity modulated	Type of modulation	Detectable changes via
Gene Expression	Switching on/off genes	mRNA patterns via DNA microarrays, PCR, quantitative real time PCR
	Modulation of transcription	Transcription factor activation, e.g. NF Kappa B
	mRNA stability	Gel-electrophoresis (ethidium bromide)
Protein Expression	Global protein changes	Proteomics approaches such as 2D gel electrophoresis, HPLC and mass spectrometry
	Specific protein expression	Antibody based assays (e.g. western blots, immunohistochemistry, immunofluorescence, enzyme immune assays, protein microarrays)
	Production / Degradation	Rates of protein synthesis (e.g. ^{14}C-leucine incorporation), ubiquitinylation, myristilation, hydrolysis
Energy production and metabolism	Metabolism	Global metabolic profile via metabolomics (e.g. NMR spectroscopy, liquid chromatography–mass spectrometry (LC-MS), Lactate/pyruvate ratio, glucose and amino acid consumption, succinate dehydrogenase levels
	Respiration rate	Oxygen consumption linked to ATP production, mitochondrial membrane potential
	Redox potential	MTT assay, resazurin assay
	Oxidative stress	GSH-GSSG ratio, generation of free radical species, lipid peroxidation products and DNA strand breaks
Cell Cycle Control	Population of cells in different stages of the cell cycle	FACs analysis, p53 activity, cyclin levels (including p21)
	Senescence	Teleomere length, β-Galactosidase expression
	Apoptosis	DNA condensation, caspase 3 activation, Fas ligand expression
	Cell proliferation	Cell number and DNA synthesis (e.g. BrdU incorporation)
Morphological changes/ Motility changes	Cytoskeleton, motor proteins	Cell size and shape, actin, microtubule and mirofilament levels and organization.
Membrane activity	Ion pumps	Membrane potential, Na/K-ATPase activity, intra-cellular ion concentrations (e.g. calcium concentration).
	Membrane integrity, Integrity of cell - cell interaction (junctional complexes)	Transport of solutes and water volume regulatory properties, endo- and exocytosis, leaking of cellular constituents (e.g. LDH) transepithelial resistance and paracellular permeability

nephrotoxins.

Calcineurin inhibitors

The discovery of the potent immunosuppressive activity of the fungal metabolite Cyclosporine A (CSA) and its introduction into clinical medicine, in the 1980s, effectively revolutionized transplantation medicine. Tacrolimus (FK506) was discovered to have immunosuppressive properties towards the end of the 1980s [76, 77]. Both of these compounds are calcineurin inhibitors (CNI) and despite the discovery of several other immunosuppressive therapies, are still among the most widely used immunosuppressive agents. However, FK506 and to a greater extent CSA exhibit nephrotoxic properties. CSA, the most widely studied of the two, induces nephrotoxicity in a complex of multifactorial processes, involving the vasculature, the glomerulus, the tubular epithelium and the renal interstitium. The renal toxicity of both compounds have similarities and differences, which may or may not be related to their primary mode of action. It is difficult to delineate the mechanisms of CNI toxicity from clinical data since the majority of clinical experiences with CNI have been in renal transplant recipients. Animal models of CNI nephropathy have brought some insights; however *in vitro* cell culture techniques allow the direct determination of toxicity at a cellular and molecular level, thus allowing dissection of the effects of CNI.

Although chronic cyclosporine toxicity is mainly characterized by tubular atrophy and interstitial fibrosis, glomerular injury with expansion of mesangial matrix and sclerosis is not uncommon. CSA causes a dose and time dependent increase in contractility of cultured mesangial cells [78, 79], as measured by changes in planar cell surface area (PCSA). Since mesangial contractility, (contributing to the ultrafiltration coefficient (Kf)) is a major effector in decreased glomerular filtration rate, mesangial cell contraction is a particularly useful endpoint in the elucidation of mediators involved in this response. A number of factors have been shown *in vitro* to attenuate CSA induced increase in mesangial cell contraction including, platelet activating factor antagonists [80], the calcium channel blocker verapamil and anti-endothelin antibodies [79, 81]. CsA, also inhibited both basal and induced PGE2 synthesis in cultured rat mesangial cells [82]. In addition, CsA and to a lesser extent FK506 can induce oxygen free radicals in cultured mesangial cells [83].

TGF-beta is a potent stimulus for ECM protein synthesis in a variety of cells including tubular epithelial cells and mesangial cells and induction of the TGF-beta pathway has been proposed to be a contributing factor to both glomerulosclerosis and tubulointerstitial fibrosis [84]. While both CsA and FK506 increase TGF-beta 1 and subsequent matrix production in mesangial cells [85, 86], only CsA induces the expression of TGF-beta receptors [86]. Interestingly, CSA causes increased matrix accumulation in cultured mesangial cells isolated from mice susceptible to glomerulosclerosis, whereas in cultured mesangial cells from mice resistant to glomerulosclerosis CSA had no effect [87]. This observation suggests that genetical background may play a role in CSA-induced glomerular lesions.

The porcine proximal tubule-like cell line LLC-PK$_1$, has been the most widely utilized cell type in the study of the direct tubular effects of CNI, although a number of studies have recently been conducted in primary human proximal tubular cells and HK-2 cells. CSA induces direct toxicity to LLC-PK$_1$ cells, manifested by an increase in cell vacuolization, a decrease in cell proliferation [88] and a dose dependent decrease in overall cellular viability as measured by MTT assay and loss of membrane integrity. Such gross cell damage, with loss of membrane integrity (increased LDH release and decreases in trypan blue exclusion), is indicative of necrosis [89]. CSA has been shown to induce apoptotic cell death in LLC-PK$_1$ cells as evidenced by a decrease in cell size and an increase in cell granularity (flow cytometric analysis), externalization of phosphatidylserine (FITC-annexin V binding), DNA fragmentation (TUNEL assay) increases in Fas ligand (APO-1/CD95) expression [89] and increased caspase-3 activity [90]. CSA has also been shown to increase the tumor suppressor p53 in LLC-PK$_1$ cells with associated cell cycle arrest [91]. p53 is also a transcriptional modulator of the *bax* gene, which can under certain conditions promote apoptosis [92]. Apoptotic cell death of renal tubular epithelial cells (including DNA fragmentation, caspase 3 induction, increased p53 and bax expression, Fas ligand upregulation and decreases in Bcl-2 expression) has been associated with interstitial fibrosis in animal models of chronic CSA toxicity [93, 94]. However, in primary human proximal tubular cells and HK-2 cells no evidence of CSA induced apoptotic cell death could be demonstrated [42, 95]. These cells are nonetheless responsive to CSA and we have recently demonstrated that CSA exposure results in stress induced senescence in both HK-2 cells and primary proximal tubular cells, characterized by a reduced proliferation, a decrease in DNA synthesis, telomere attrition and p53 activation with subsequent p21 induction [42]. CsA also induced H_2O_2 production and some of the CsA induced effects were attenuated by catalase [42]. In LLC-PK1 cells, FK506 has also been shown to induce toxicity via reactive oxygen species which was attenuated by catalase [96]. A reduced ability of tubular epithelial cells to proliferate after prolonged exposure to CNIs, due to ROS induced accelerated senescence, may be a contributing factor to CNI induced tubulointerstitial fibrosis.

A number of investigations have been conducted investigating the potential of CSA to induce epithelial-mesenchymal transition (EMT). In HK-2 cells and primary proximal tubular cells CSA has been shown to cause an induction of TGF-beta 1, connective tissue growth factor (CTGF) and alpha smooth muscle actin (a myofibroblast-specific marker), as well as inducing the production of collagen IV and fibronectin [97-99]. Qiu et. al. have demonstrated in NRK-52E an activation of the TGF beta / SMAD signalling cascade (including induction of TGF-beta 1, CTGF, SMAD 3 and SMAD 7) by prolonged elevated glucose exposure [100]. Both CSA and FK506 have been shown to reduce ATP levels in LLC-PK1 cells (however this reduction is transient with FK506) [101], and CSA induces a potent and dose dependent increase in glycolysis in LLC-PK1 cells [102]. Thus it is tempting to draw a connection between CSA induction of glycolysis and CSA induction of EMT [100]. The release of CSA induced TGF-beta 1 will also likely have an effect on interstitial fibroblasts by inducing their proliferation [103] and increasing their ECM production [97]. Thus CSA can contribute to tubulointerstitial fibrosis by; (i) inducing a decreased proliferation of tubular epithelial cells and (ii) induction of tubular and mesangial TGF-beta 1 production, resulting in tubular EMT and enhanced fibroblast proliferation. The angiotensin converting enzyme inhibitor enalapril, has been shown to ameliorate the profibrotic effects of CSA by preventing CSA induced TGF-beta 1 production from renal epithelial cells [104].

LLC-PK_1 cells also respond to CSA (but not FK506) by increasing the synthesis and release of endothelin [105, 106]. These observations may implicate renal tubular cells themselves in the further contribution to CSA-induced alterations in renal and systemic hemodynamics.

Both FK506 and CSA are substrates for the P-glycoprotein [107] and both compounds can induce toxicotolerance *in vitro* by inducing this protein [108]. However, FK506 requires supratherapeutic concentrations to elicit this effect and thus this effect by FK506 may not be clinically relevant [108]. CSA also induces the expression of HSP 70 in LLC-PK_1 cells, which increases tolerance to subsequent exposure [109].

Cisplatin

Cisplatin is a widely used drug in the effective treatment of a number of human carcinomas and is a potent nephrotoxin primarily damaging the epithelial cells of the proximal tubule [110]. Recent investigations have demonstrated that this area of the kidney is susceptible to cisplatin toxicity due to the high levels of gamma-glutamyl transpeptidase (GGT) and cysteine-S-conjugate beta-lyase [111, 112]. Glutahthione and cysteine conjugates of cisplatin are more toxic to LLC-PK1 cells than cisplatin itself [111]. Additionally, inhibition of GGT prevented toxicity of the cisplatin-glutathione-conjugate but not to other cisplatin conjugates downstream of GGT (cisplatin-cysteinyl-glycine-conjugate and cisplatin-cysteine-conjugate) [111]. Inhibition of cysteine-S-conjugate beta-lyase reduced the toxicity to all conjugates. The authors conclude that cleavage of cisplatin-glutathione-conjugate to a cisplatin-cysteinyl-glycine-conjugate by GGT is the first step in the metabolism of the cisplatin-glutathione-conjugate to a nephrotoxin and that cysteine-S-conjugate beta-lyase catalyzes the final step in the pathway converting the cisplatin-cysteine conjugate to a reactive thiol. This study is supported by the fact that GGT deficient mice do not exhibit nephrotoxicity when exposed to cisplatin [112].

It has been known for some time that cisplatin is taken up preferentially by the basolateral membrane of microporous grown LLC-PK_1 cells and opossum kidney (OK) cells [71, 113]. Furthermore, cisplatin applied basolaterally was more toxic than apical exposure in LLC-PK_1 cells [113]. These studies suggest that tubular excretion of cisplatin is dominant over tubular reabsorption. More recently the transporter of cisplatin has been identified as the copper transporter, Ctr1 [114, 115]. Additionally, Ctr1 has recently been found to be expressed exclusively on the basolateral side of epithelial cells including MDCK-1 and OK cells [116].

In primary rabbit proximal tubular (RPT) cells cisplatin exposure resulted in an inhibition of DNA synthesis, which is most likely related to the primary anti-tumorigenic mechanism of this compound i.e. DNA inter and intra strand cross linking [117]. RNA and protein synthesis were decreased in RPT cells and quiescent LLC-PK_1 cells upon cisplatin exposure [117, 118]. Other effects of cisplatin on cultured RPT include a decrease in glucose uptake, an inhibition of Na^+-K^+ ATPase and alterations in total glutathione content [117]. In the normal rat kidney (NRK) cell line cisplatin (1μM for 48h) induced a marked increase in the level of lipid peroxides [119].

Cisplatin is a potent inducer of apoptosis in various proximal tubular cell models. In primary mouse proximal tubular cell cultures [120] and LLC-PK_1 cells [121], high doses of cisplatin (mM) resulted in necrosis whereas low doses (μM) caused apoptotic cell death. In mouse proximal tubular cells and normal rat kidney epithelial cells (NRK52E), cisplatin induced an increase in Fas, Fas ligand and TNF α mRNA [122]. Cisplatin induced apoptosis in LLC-PK1 cells is brought about via activation and mitochondrial translocation of the pro-apoptopic molecule Bax, which leads to release of cytochrome C into the cytosol and activation of caspase 9 [123]. The caspase 9 inhibitor LEHD-CHO could prevent cisplatin induced apoptosis in LLC-PK_1 cells whereas the caspase 8 inhibitor IETD-fmk did not [123]. Cisplatin induced apoptosis could also be inhibited by overexpresssion of crm A (a suppressor of the interleukin-1β converting enzyme family) and by over expression of bcl-2 in immortalized mouse S3 cells [124]. A recent investigation has demonstrated that hypoxic preconditioning of mouse proximal tubular cells attenuates cisplatin induced apoptosis in an HIF-1alpha-dependent fashion and increased cell proliferation as measured by BrdU incorporation [125].

Cisplatin has also been shown to induce ROS in cultured proximal tubular cells and antioxidants such as green tea tannin can dose dependently protect against cisplatin-induced nephrotoxicity *in vitro* and *in vivo* [126]. Bragado and colleagues have recently demonstrated that cisplatin-induced apoptosis requires the onset of p53-mediated p38alpha MAPK via the generation of reactive oxygen species [127].

It should be noted that cisplatin appears to inhibit the activity of LDH [128]. Thus, the use of this enzyme as a marker of cisplatin-induced toxicity should be controlled appropriately. The possible interference of test compounds with toxicity assays is not always carefully controlled, but is a prerequisite for accurate scientific evaluation.

Aminoglycosides

Aminoglycosides are antibiotics particularly active against aerobic gram-negative bacteria and certain gram-positive organisms. Aminoglycosides are used in therapy of severe infections of abdominal organs, endocarditis or sepsis. However, the clinical use is limited by severe toxic effects to the kidney and inner ear. Aminoglycoside-induced nephrotoxicity is characterized by tubular necrosis and marked decreases in glomerular filtration rate and in the ultrafiltration coefficient [129]. The mechanism of action of these antibiotics was thought to be the blockade of bacterial ribosomal protein biosynthesis. Recent studies, however, show that cationic antibiotic molecules create fissures in the outer cell membrane, resulting in the leakage of intracellular contents [130].

Gentamicin was found to induce an activation of cultured mesangial cells, as measured by contraction (PCSA) and proliferation. Since gentamicin increases the expression of inducible nitric oxide (iNOS) in these cells [131] and has been shown to elevate intracellular Ca^{2+} (via influx, and release from internal stores) [132], it is postulated that nitric oxide-induced Ca^{2+} elevation might be responsible for the observed effect. These results are in support of a mesangial cell role in the reduction of glomerular filtration rate after aminoglycoside intoxication [133, 134]. Recently it has been shown that the resveratrol, a natural hydroxystilbene and potent antioxidant could attenuate gentamycin induced mesangial cell contraction [135].

Gentamicin is more toxic to LLC-PK_1 monolayers when exposed at the apical side, indicating a preferential uptake from the luminal membrane [136]. The uptake mechanism is proposed to be via megalin mediated endocytosis, a protein which is abundantly expressed in the proximal tubule [137]. A pathway delineated in LLC-PK1 cells is proposed, whereby internalized aminoglycosides and other small molecular weight cationic compounds are transported from the early and late endosomes, through the Golgi complex, into the ER and then to the cytosol [138, 139]. Furthermore competitive inhibition of megalin via ligands such as apolipoprotein E3 have been shown to prevent gentamicin induced LLC-PK1 toxicity [140].

In LLC-PK_1 cells gentamicin induces membrane damage as shown by the loss of specific membrane enzymes (γ-glutamyl transpeptidase, alkaline phosphatase and aminopeptidase), a decrease of the lysosomal enzyme N-acetyl-β-D-glucosaminidase, an inhibition of apical Na^+-dependent glucose transporter and the basolateral Na-K-ATPase pump as well as a decrease in dome formation [141, 142]. Furthermore gentamicin results in a dose dependent decrease in intracellular ATP and cAMP [142].

Chronic gentamicin exposure of LLC-PK_1 cells (10 mM gentamicin for 15 days) resulted in an increase in cell granularity and a decrease in cell size (flow cytometric analysis), implicating enhanced rates of apoptotic cell death. Interestingly, this effect was not paralleled by an increase in Fas ligand expression [143]. LLC-PK_1 cells over expressing the anti-apoptotic protein bcl-2 were protected from gentamicin-induced apoptosis [144].

Cephalosporins

Cephalosporins are a family of β-lactam-antibiotics, which are effective bactericidal therapeutics for infections of the bloodstream, skin, respiratory and urinary tract. Renal transporters for organic anions are located in the proximal tubule segment of the nephron. The primary transporters of organic anions on the basolateral membrane of proximal tubule cells are members of the organic anion transporter (OAT) family (mainly OAT1 and OAT3) [145]. The organic anion transporter (OAT) is thought to be responsible for cephalosporin uptake from the blood for subsequent secretion into the urine. Stable transfection of OAT1 in mouse proximal tubule cells increase cephaloridine uptake and toxicity [146]. Co-incubation with probenecid, an inhibitor of organic anion transport decreased cephaloridine uptake and toxicity [146]. OAT3 has also been shown to have a high capacity to transport cephaloridine [147, 148].

OK cells, but not LLC-PK1, cells exhibit basolateral to apical unidirectional transport of p-aminohippurate (PAH) by the organic anion transport system [149]. Moreover, PAH uptake by OK cells from the basalolateral side was competitively inhibited by the beta-lactam antibiotics benzylpenicillin (PCG) and cefazolin [150]. Despite the fact that LLC-PK1 cells most likely do not contain a functional OAT transporter, most of the *in vitro* nephrotoxcity studies on cephalosporins have been conducted with these cells. Kiyomiya et al. have demonstrated that in LLC-PK_1 cells, the cytotoxic effect of cephalosporins is due to a decreased activity of cytochrome C oxidase in the mitochondria causing decreases in intracellular ATP content and consequent increases in hydrogen peroxide and lipid peroxide levels [151, 152]. Cephaloridine, ceftazidime and cefotaxime, were shown to cause direct toxicity to LLC-PK_1 monolayers, evaluated by enzyme release (brush border enzymes AP and γ-GT, cytosolic enzyme LDH and the mitochondrial enzyme glutamate dehydrogenase (GLDH)). In addition marked morphological damage was observed at both light and electron microscopic levels [153]. A decrease in transepithelial electrical resistance (TEER) was observed previous to other changes, demonstrating that TEER is a highly sensitive endpoint for LLC-PK_1 toxicity [153].

Amphotericin B

Amphotericin B (AmB) a polyene macrolide antibiotic with strong activity against a broad spectrum of fungal infections has long been identified as nephrotoxic. Nephrotoxicity includes decreased glomerular filtration rate and distal tubulopathy with urinary loss of potassium and magnesium, renal tubular acidosis and loss of urine concentrating ability [154]. The toxic mechanism is assumed to be that binding of AmB to ergosterol in the fungal cell wall results in the formation of aqueous pores, which leads to a deregulation of volume and ion concentrations within the cells [155]. In mammalian cells, AmB and other polyene antifungal antibiotics such as Nystatin, bind to cholesterol in the plasma membrane [156]. Using patch-clamp, Hsu et. al. could show that AmB, disturbs the normal ion channel function rather than forming pores in the cell membrane of MDCK cells [157].

Amp B causes mesangial cell contraction *in vitro*. This effect was related to a Ca^{2+} entry from the extracellular space through voltage-dependent calcium channels [158]. In LLC-PK_1 and renal medullary interstitial cells AmB, in therapeutic doses, induced apoptosis, which could be prevented by recombinant human insulin-like-growth-factor-1 (IGF-1) [159]. Similar results were observed in rats [159].

A number of investigations have focused to alternative chemical preparations of AmB which potentially limit its toxicity whilst maintaining antifungal activity. Liposomal preparation of AmB demonstrate reduced toxicity to LLC-PK1 cells [160]. Also, AmB bound to high-density lipoprotein (HDL) was less toxic to LLC-PK_1 cells than AmB alone or AmB bound to low-density lipoprotein (LDL), presumably due to the absence of HDL receptors in LLC-PK_1 cells [161]. Heat treated fungizone (a widely used AmB deoxycholate micellar formulation) is also less toxic to LLC-PK1 cells and HK-2 cells [162, 163]. The reduced level of heat treated fungizone toxicity is purported to be due to superaggregated of AMB following heat treatment. Liposomal, lipid-associated and heat treated AmB formulations all retain anti-fungal activity.

Cadmium

Cadmium (Cd) is a non-essensial metal used in industry as an anti-corrosive agent, and is found as a contaminant in food and also in cigarette smoke. The most serious consequence of chronic Cd poisoning is lung- and prostate cancer but the first effect during chronic intake is kidney damage, manifested by marked proteinuria [164]. Under chronic exposure, cadmium is primarily taken up by the liver, where it induces synthesis of metallothionein (MT) and induces formation of cadmium-metallothionein complexes.

Cd can be taken up by renal cells either as a free ion, a glutathione conjugate or bound to metallothionein. There is conflicting evidence in the literature as to the site of Cd uptake into the proximal tubule. Some researchers have shown that Cd uptake exhibits a slight preference (20%) at the apical side in LLC-PK1 cells due to transport via the apical inorganic anion exchange [165]. The rest of the Cd uptake was shown to show no side preference in LLC-PK1 cells [166, 167]. However, other investigations have shown that Cd is more toxic to LLC-PK1 cells and MDCK cells when applied basolaterally [168, 169]. Differences in experimental protocols most likely account for these conflicting findings.

A major route of Cd uptake *in vivo* is via the Cd-metallothionein complex. Cd-metallothionein-1, which is released from hepatic cells into the circulation, is small enough to be freely filtered by the glomerulus and then taken up by proximal tubule cells [170]. *In vitro* studies have demonstrated direct binding of metallothionein-1 to megalin [171]. Additionally, Cd-metallothionein-1 was toxic to rat proximal tubular cell cultures (WKPT-0293 Cl.2 cells), which was attenuated by co-incubation with receptor-associated protein (RAP) or IgG directed against rat megalin [172]. In contrast Cd-metallothionein was found not be toxic to LLC-PK1 cells [173]. However, in the LLC-PK1 study, FCS containing medium was used and it is likely that albumin in the FCS competes against metallothionein for megalin; given that megalin can transport albumin [174] and LLC-PK1 cells express megalin [175]. Once cadmium-metallothionein-1 has been endocytosed it is presumed to be transported through endosomal pathways to lysosomes, where the metallothionein-1 moiety is degraded by acidic proteases and Cd is liberated into the cytosol [176]. The proton-coupled divalent metal transporter DMT1, which is located in endosomes/lysosomes, is thought to be involved in the transport of Cd to the cytosol, as down regulation of this protein by RNA interference resulted in a decrease in Cd-metallothionein toxicity in WKPT-0293 Cl.2 cells [177].

Once Cd enters the cytosol it can cause cellular damage in a number of ways and a dominant role of Cd induced ROS generation and oxidative stress has been demonstrated. In LLC-PK1 cells Cd exposure leads to generation of H_20_2 and subsequent apoptosis [178, 179]. Cd toxicity can be attenuated by antioxidant supplementation such as seleneium or by induction of catalase [178, 179]. Cd has also been shown to be a specific inducer of c-fos in *mesangial cells* through activation of Erk kinase, protein kinase C and stress-activated protein kinase (SAPK) pathways [180, 181] and may therefore also play a carcinogenic role in the kidney. $CdCl_2$ also resulted in an early decrease in mitochondrial membrane potential and an increase in cytoplasmic Ca^{2+} in LLC-PK_1 cells, MDCK cells and OK cells [182]. $CdCl_2$ exposure caused a disruption in the cadherin-catenin complex resulting in reduced trans-epithelial resistance and produced alterations in the actin cytoskeleton in LLC-PK_1 cells and MDCK cells [168, 169].

Cd can also induce a number of protective mechanisms in the cell. Cd has been shown to enhance metallothionein protein and HSP70 expression in a variety of renal and non renal cell types [183, 184].

Thus pre-exposure to Cd can cause a desensitization of the cell to subsequent exposures. Continuous exposure of LLC-PK1 cells to Cd leads to the selection of cells which constitutively express high levels of metallothionein [173].

Cd can be extruded from the cell via the P-glycoprotein, as shown in LLC-PK1 cells and OK cells [185, 186]. Also there is evidence that extrusion of Cd occurs at the apical membrane [186].

Mercury

Mercury is an industrial pollutant, which can contaminate food (e.g. fish and grain) and water sources [187]. The nephrotoxic potential of mercury is related to its accumulation in the proximal tubule region and the intracellular binding to several functional groups, especially thiols, which results in inactivation of different enzymes and inhibition of protein synthesis [188]. Mercury is unique among the heavy metals in that it can exist in several physical and chemical forms, including elemental mercury, which is a liquid at room temperature. All forms of mercury have toxic effects in a number of organs, especially in the kidneys [188].

In a study of six mercury compounds, mercury chloride, mercury nitrate, sodium ethylmercurithiosalicylate, methyl mercury chloride, mercury acetate and phenylmercury acetate in MDCK cells, LLC-PK1 cells and human primary proximal tubular cells (hPTC) and non-renal cell lines (SAOS and Hep G2) it was found that all mercury compounds were toxic to all cell types as evidenced by neutral red uptake, thymidine incorporation and the MTT assay [189]. However, sodium ethylmercurithiosalicylate, methyl mercury chloride and phenylmercury acetate were one order of magnitude more toxic than the other compounds. In addition the GSH synthesis inhibitor L-buthionine sulfoximine (BSO) potentiated the toxicity of all mercury compounds [189]. In a study using primary rabbit proximal tubular cells it was also shown that methyl mercury chloride is more toxic than mercury chloride [190]. Differences in the extent and rate of metal uptake were also evident. Maximum cellular uptake of Hg^{2+} occurred within 6-24 hr after exposure and was not concentration-dependent, whereas maximum uptake of CH_3Hg^+ occurred within 3 hr of exposure and was concentration- dependent [190].

Mercury chloride exposure caused elevated c-fos mRNA levels in LLC-PK1 cells [191] and resulted in apoptosis in LLC-PK1 cells and HK-2 cells [192, 193]. In a studies using NRK52E cells it was postulated that Hg^{2+} enhances the sensitivity of kidney cells to apoptotic stimuli as a consequence of inhibition of NF-kappaB activity [194, 195].

In studies with MDCK cells transfected with the human organic anion transporter 1 (hOAT1), a role for this transporter in the basolateral uptake of cysteine-S-conjugates of inorganic mercury was established [196].

Mycotoxins

Mycotoxins are defined as mould derived secondary metabolites and include Ochratoxin A (OTA). OTA, produced by *Aspergillus ochraeus* and *Penicillium verrucosum*, can be found as a contaminant in grain, beer, coffee and meat. OTA is nephrotoxic, hepatotoxic and carcinogenic [197].

OTA is thought to be transported into the proximal tubular epithelium via organic anion transporters. In primary rabbit proximal tubule cells cultured on microporus supports; OTA was taken up from the basolateral compartment and secreted into the apical compartment. This process was sensitive to probenecid [198]. Mouse proximal tubular cells transfected with hOATs (1, 3 and 4) exhibited an enhanced uptake of OTA which was also inhibited by probenecid [199, 200]. However, it is also known that OTA has a high affinity for albumin and it has been demonstrated experimentally that human serum albumin dose dependently decreases OTA uptake via hOAT1 [201]. Whether albumin bound OTA can be transported via megalin mediated endocytosis has not been investigated.

Nanomolar concentrations of OTA resulted in the stable and irreversible dedifferentiation of MDCK-C7 cells, characterized by a distinct morphology as compared to the parent cell line (spindle-shape, pleiomorphic, narrow intercellular spaces, increased cell size), a reduced proliferation rate and numerical chromosomal aberrations [202]. Further studies could demonstrate that OTA exposure resulted in apoptosis, which was associated with induced c-jun amino-terminal-kinase (JNK) activation [203]. Long term exposure (14 days) of human proximal tubular cells to nanomolar concentrations of OTA under serum free conditions led to cell hypertrophy, NF-kappaB activation, fibronectin secretion and increases in caspase 3 activity [40].

Microarray analysis of OTA induced transcriptome alterations from primary rat proximal tubule cells demonstrated deregulation of genes involved in DNA damage response and apoptosis (upregulation of GADD 153, GADD 45, annexin V), response to oxidative stress (differential expression of hypoxia-inducible factor 1 and catalase), and inflammatory reactions (upregulation of alpha 2 macroglobulin, ceruloplasmin, and cathepsin S) [39]. Moreover these authors compared the toxicogenomic data from the *in vitro* data to data derived from rats *in vivo* and demonstrated a good correlation. There were of course differences between the two data sets. These differences were attributed to contamination of non proximal cell types in the *in vivo* samples including infiltrating immune cells and a down regulation of certain transporters and biotransformation enzymes in the *in vitro* model.

Type I interferons

Type I interferons, including IFNα, are approved for the treatment of viral, malignant and auto-immune diseases, such as hairy cell leukemia, chronic myeloid leukemia, multiple myeloma, non-Hodgkin's lymphoma, metastasizing renal cell carcinoma, malignant melanoma, hepatitis B and C, multiple sclerosis and others [204-206]. They are major immune response regulators produced and released mainly by activated monocytes/macrophages, plasmacytoid dendritic cells (also known as "natural IFN-producing cells") and virus-infected cells. They recruit and activate macrophages and natural killer cells, promote the differentiation and activation of dendritic cells and induce T-helper cell type 1 cytokine release. Type I interferons thus act as a bridge system linking innate and adaptive immunity [207]. Concomitant to their immuno-modulatory functions, type I interferons also directly affect target cells by preventing virus replication and inducing apoptotic cell death [208] thus acting as anti-viral and anti-neoplastic therapeutics. Interferon therapy is, however, accompanied by undesired side-effects limiting the benefits of high-dose interferon treatment. Besides flu-like symptoms major organ dysfunctions were attributed to IFNα therapy including renal damage. Renal impairment was observed in about 20% of the patients treated. Symptoms ranged from sub-clinical to severe dysfunction such as acute renal failure requiring dialysis [209, 210]. Clinical findings revealed tubular cell dysfunction and/or tubular cell death [210, 211]. Analysis of urinary protein revealed pathological urinary excretion of β1-microglobulin in 20% and of albumin in 15% of patients [210] and presence of urinary tubular casts [211]. Renal biopsies performed on patients with IFNα-induced acute renal failure showed diffuse interstitial edema of rapid onset, acute tubular injury characterized by tubular dilatation and sloughing of epithelial cells, signs of interstitial nephritis and/or glomerulonephritis [212-215].

Potential direct nephrotoxicity and the underlying molecular mechanisms were analyzed by *in vitro* studies in renal proximal tubular cells exposed to IFNα. IFNα was shown to induce apoptosis in LLC-PK1 renal proximal tubular like epithelium [216]. Caspase-8, a key player in death receptor signaling and caspase-9 that is involved in mitochondrial apoptosis were shown to be activated in addition to caspase-3. Furthermore, IFNα induced a breakdown of the inner mitochondrial membrane potential, further implying mitochondrial signaling in IFNα-induced apoptosis. The death receptor pathway and the mitochondrial pathway appear to both be necessary for efficient executor caspase activation by IFNα. The apoptotic signaling pathways activated by IFNα in proximal tubular cells, thus, resemble the pathways induced by IFNα in melanoma and bladder carcinoma cells [217, 218]. In addition to caspase activation, nuclear condensation, DNA fragmentation and a delayed LDH release were observed. DNA fragmentation and LDH release were partially prevented by caspase inhibition. Thus, caspase-independent death is also possible - albeit delayed and at a reduced extent [216].

IFNα was, in addition to apoptosis, found to induce a reversible decrease in transepithelial electrical resistance (TEER), dissipation of transepithelial dilution potentials, a decrease in dome formation, and an increase in paracellular permeability to fluorescent marker molecules in LLC-PK1 monolayers indicating that IFNα might interfere with tight junctional complex function [219]. Epithelial permeability was increased by IFNα independently of concomitant apoptotic cell death, since caspase inhibition did not influence permeability regulation while significantly attenuating and delaying cell death [216]. The IFNα-induced impairment of epithelial barrier function was, however, accompanied by a displacement or missorting of the junctional proteins occludin and E-cadherin as demonstrated by a prominent staining at the basal cell pole in addition to localization at the junctional region in immunofluorescence confocal microscopy. Furthermore, expression of occludin and E-cadherin was found to be induced by IFNα [219]. A mitogen-activated protein kinase (MAPK) pathway involving MEK1/2-ERK1/2 was necessary to mediate the IFNα-induced changes in epithelial barrier function since the MEK1/2 inhibitors PD98059 and U0126 were able to significantly block the observed TEER decrease [220].

The MEK1/2-ERK1/2 signaling pathway is also activated by growth factor-induced signaling via receptor tyrosine kinases, e.g. EGF receptor [221], and was found to be necessary for epithelial barrier stabilization by EGF indicated by an increased TEER in MDCK [222] and LLC-PK1 monolayers [223]. This property might contribute to repair processes, since growth factors were attributed crucial roles in renal recovery from damage [224, 225]. In animal models, functional EGF and EGF receptor were, for example, shown to be necessary for recovery from acute nephrotoxic injury [226] or from ischemia [227]. *In vitro* studies confirmed the importance of EGF in renal repair processes since EGF receptor activation was found to be required for cell proliferation and migration after mechanical damage in primary rabbit proximal tubular cells [228]. During exposure of LLC-PK1 monolayers to IFNα, however, EGF was not only unable to prevent, but even exacerbated IFNα-induced epithelial barrier destabilization [229]. ERK1/2-signaling was necessary for this effect linking it to enhanced cell proliferation. In contrast to its damage-intensifying effect, EGF accelerated epithelial barrier re-establishment when administered to LLC-PK1 monolayers after IFNα withdrawal. This action correlated with an anti-apoptotic mechanism induced by EGF and was independent of proliferation [229].

In vitro studies have revealed that nephrotoxicity of therapeutically applied IFNα might involve direct effects of IFNα on proximal tubular epithelial functions. Growth factor signaling was shown to stimulate repair processes, but -if activated during the damaging phase- may also worsen the deleterious effects induced by IFNα. A misbalanced onset of tissue repair processes by growth factors may, thus result in further exacerbation of deteriorating effects.

Hemoglobin and myoglobin

Hemoglobin (Hb) and myoglobin are also good examples of endogenous nephrotoxic substances. Hb, responsible for the transport and delivery of oxygen within the body, is composed of four globin molecules, each bound to a prosthetic iron-containing heme group. Myoglobin (consisting of one globin molecule with a prosthetic group), is an oxygen store for the muscle. When Hb as well as myoglobin are released into the extracellular compartment in large amounts due to pathological events (hemolysis, rhabdomyolysis) both will severely injure the kidney and may even lead to acute renal failure [230, 231]. Several potential mechanisms of toxicity have been proposed for these compounds such as oxidative injury by oxygen radical formation [232] and ischemic injury due to vasoconstriction and/or platelet aggregation following hemoglobin-mediated nitric oxide depletion [230].

Experimental rhabdomyolysis induced in rats by glycerol injection revealed sustained renal hypoxia and a hypoxia-induced transcriptional adaptation in proximal tubules providing evidence for a role of hypoxia in the pathophysiology of rhabdomyolysis-induced acute kidney injury [233]. Furthermore, in experimental rat models of rhabdomyolysis (by glycerol injection) or hemolysis (mimicked by intravenous infusion of Hb) iron release from the heme moiety was shown to result in hydroxyl radical formation, lipid peroxidation and renal dysfunction [234]. Hydroxyl radical scavengers or iron chelators were able to protect against injury in both models [234, 235]. *In vitro*, reactive oxygen molecules were shown to cause an early decline in ATP levels and a late response consisting of cell detachment and cell lysis in LLC-PK1, OK and NHK-C cells. Scavengers of hydroxyl radicals and iron chelators prevented these alterations [236].

Direct cytotoxicity of heme-containing molecules was, furthermore, demonstrated by exposing cells in culture to myoglobin, heme or Hb [237]. Myoglobin was shown to suppress cell proliferation and cause DNA strand breaks and suppression of protein synthesis in human proximal tubular HK-2 cells. Deferoxamine, an iron chelator, reduced myoglobin-induced cell death and also induced a growth suppressive effect [238]. Exogenous glutathione (GSH) resulted in increased myoglobin toxicity in HK-2 cells. Intracellular GSH depletion prevented this action [239]. Mitochondrial and nuclear damage induced by myolysis in rat distal tubulus was confirmed by exposing MDCK cells to heme [240]. In immortalized rat proximal tubular cells heme was shown to induce heme oxygenase-1 (HO)-dependent p21 expression, provoke cell cycle arrest, and inhibit cell growth [241]. In rats, as well as in OK cells, polymerized Hb solution increased HO activity. Inhibition of HO enzyme activity by cimetidine did not change the grade of renal injury seen with Hb infusion alone indicating that Hb-evoked renal injury was also possible by HO-independent mechanisms [242].

In summary

It is clear from the above studies that *in vitro* renal cell culture can be used successfully to study the cellular and molecular mechanisms of cell modulation by toxic compounds. Such systems allow a simple but sophisticated approach to the development of strategies to overcome nephrotoxicity of many important drugs. A cartoon summarizing the major pathways of uptake and extrusion of specific nephrotoxins and common mechanisms of cellular toxicity, derived from *in vitro* renal cell culture studies is given in Figure 2.

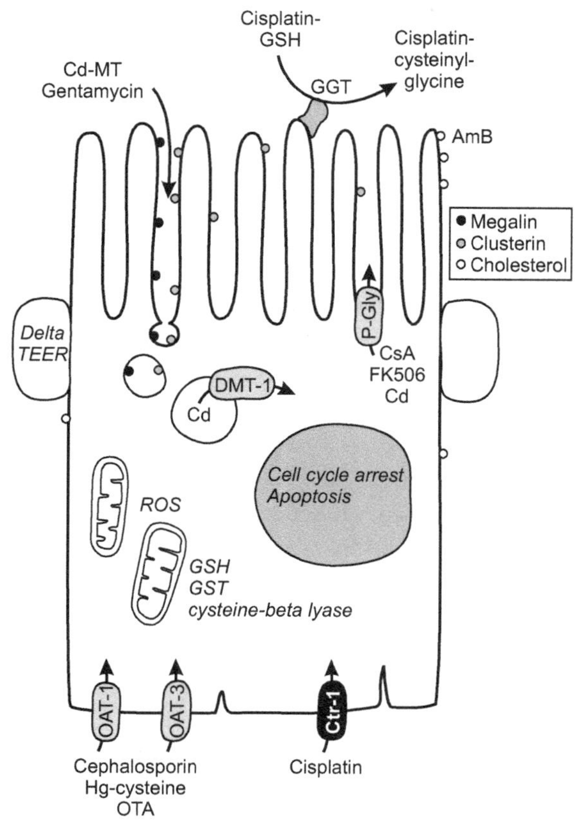

Figure 2. Contribution of renal tubular epithelial culture models to the understanding of nephrotoxin susceptibility of the proximal tubulus. *The cartoon shows the elucidated pathways of uptake and extrusion of specific nephrotoxins in the proximal tubule together with common mechanisms of cellular damage. See text for details.*

Abbreviations: P-Gly, P-glycoprotein; GGT, gamma glutamyl transpeptidase; AmB, amphotericin B; DMT1, divalent metal transporter; OAT, organic anion transporter; Ctr1, copper transporter; TEER, transepithelial electrical resistance; ROS, reactive oxygen species; GST, glutathione-S transferase; GSH, glutathione; Cd-MT, cadmium-metallothionein.

Future requirements to study nephrotoxicity *in vitro*

Renal cell cultures have an unexploited potential in the screening and evaluation of possible nephrotoxins. These systems are theoretically suited not only to short term studies but also to long term exposures and thus may be useful in the screening of compounds on a chronic basis. Predictive models of chronic renal toxicity would be a major development in the assessment of human risk to a whole range of environmental, therapeutic and industrial compounds. However, if this is to be achieved successfully a number of requirements must be met.

There is general agreement that all culture systems used for clinical risk assessment, especially when testing for long-term effects, should preferably be of human origin. Although this could be achieved by the use of primary cultures, their establishment is constantly hampered by the restriction of the availability of samples (usually from surgical sources) and by the limited life-span of cultures. In addition, the tissue used for primary culture seldom is optimum, and often is obtained from donors of advanced age or with undesirable clinical conditions such as renal carcinoma (the most common reason for nephrectomy). The limited lifespan of primary cells is an inherent mechanism of aging and replicative senescence and thus primary cells in later passages will most probably respond to stress, particularly oxidative stress, differently than younger cells in earlier passages. Furthermore, primary cell phenotypes can change rapidly, depending on the culture conditions. Alterations in primary cell phenotype are due to (a) an adaptation of the cells to their new cell culture environment (including pericellular oxygen, nutrient medium, attachment matrix, feeding cycles, lack of paracrine signalling pathways etc.), (b) artificially increased cellular proliferation and (c) accelerated aging due to increased proliferation. For these reasons, more surrogate cell lines of human origin are needed, and those that are currently available need further characterization. The use of conditional or non-conditional transfection of primary cells with hTERT to induce telomerase activity may represent a promising new strategy for this purpose.

New cell culture techniques, which may improve the applicability of renal epithelial cultures, are also required. Currently there exist two commercially available cell culture perfusion systems, which allow the continuous perfusion of culture media and optimized oxygenation [243]. These systems allow stable long-term culture of quiescent adherent cells [244]. Continuous medium perfusion furthermore may lead to the re-expression of lost functions in continuous cell lines and the maintenance of differentiated properties in primary cells. Recently our laboratory has demonstrated that LLC-PK_1 cells maintained in a newly developed perfusion system (EpiFlow®) changed from a glycolytic to a more oxidative phenotype [72]. Evidence is also available from experiments in our laboratory that this mode of cultivation helps to prolong the lifetime of primary cultures of proximal tubular cells. Combining perfusion culture with co-culture of a cell type that is an anatomical neighbour *in vivo* (e.g. epithelial with endothelial, interstitial or immune cells) may improve the state of differentiation of both partner cells and increase the complexity of autocrine and paracrine interaction [73].

The utilization of renal cell culture techniques will gain added importance in the future for screening newly synthesized drugs or environmental contaminants for adverse effects to the kidney, or to investigate mechanistic aspects leading to renal cell injury. Especially with respect to the latter, renal cultures offer the possibility of easy access to the object of interest. Cell lines can be provided in nearly unlimited amounts, and they match reasonably well their site of nephron origin. In this context continuous renal cell lines represent the current experimental system of choice. They are easy to grow, maintain and handle, they are commercially available (e.g. from the American Type Culture Collection) and retain most of the basic functions of their ancestor cell, at least in case of permanent proximal and collecting duct cells (LLC-PK_1, OK, JTC-12, HK-2, MDCK, A6). Another advantage is the enormous amount of information about culture conditions and differentiated functions, metabolism, transport, and hormone responsiveness, available from the literature [15, 33, 55, 245]. The major disadvantage is the fact that they may suffer from loss of some *in vivo et situ* functions as a result of prolonged cultivation. Under these circumstances, if the lost function is the predominant target for a nephrotoxic xenobiotic under investigation, a more laborious and difficult primary cultures should be selected. However, even primary cells may not possess the required function of the cell *in vivo* as is the case for cytochrome P450 (CYP) activity. This issue is not trivial as many compounds require phase I metabolism to exert toxic responses. In addition the complex interplay of different CYP substrate specificities makes this a challenging problem.

It is desirable that methods should be developed to re-express the "lost functions" or to tailor new cell lines more closely matching the cell type of origin in continuous cell lines. Such an enterprise may include several already available cell biology techniques. The simplest approach could be adaptation to culture conditions that more closely resemble the *in vivo* environment of the respective cell type. As already mentioned, omittance or drastic reduction of glucose and replacement against pyruvate in the media used for cultivation of LLC-PK_1 cells enables re-expression of gluconeogenesis [246]. Reintroduction of missing proteins by transfection methods may also represent a way forward [148]. These strategies should offer the possibility to establish cell lines expressing most of the important functions of human renal cells. Of course such strategies will also require a greater understanding of how compounds are taken up, metabolised and extruded by renal cells.

Last but not least there is an urgent need to "harmonize" or "standardize" all these procedures so that improved interlaboratory comparisons can be achieved. Such procedures include, cell isolation, growth substrates, cell culture media including the mode of medium application. A first initiative in this direction has been taken by ECVAM (European Center for the Validation of Alternative Methods, a section of the European Commission Institute for Health and Consumer Protection) by founding a task force dealing with the creation of guidelines for "Good Cell Culture Practice" [247, 248].

References

1. Commission of the European Communities/International Programme on Chemical Safety. Health signficance and early detection of nephrotoxicity. Proceedings of the joint CEC/IPCS Workshop. Commission of the European Communities/International Programme on Chemical Safety. Luxembourg, 26- 29 April 1988. Toxicol Lett 46: 1-306, 1989.
2. Fanos V and Cataldi L. Renal transport of antibiotics and nephrotoxicity: a review. J Chemother 13: 461-472, 2001.
3. Lohr JW, Willsky GR, and Acara MA. Renal drug metabolism. Pharmacol Rev 50: 107-141, 1998.
4. Mohandas J, Marshall JJ, Duggin GG, Horvath JS, and Tiller DJ. Differential distribution of glutathione and glutathione-related enzymes in rabbit kidney. Possible implications in analgesic nephropathy. Biochem Pharmacol 33: 1801-1807, 1984.
5. Guder WG and Ross BD. Enzyme distribution along the nephron. Kidney Int 26: 101-111, 1984.
6. Leonard MO, Kieran NE, Howell K, Burne MJ, Varadarajan R, Dhakshinamoorthy S, Porter AG, O'Farrelly C, Rabb H, and Taylor CT. Reoxygenation-specific activation of the antioxidant transcription factor Nrf2 mediates cytoprotective gene expression in ischemia-reperfusion injury. FASEB J 20: 2624-2626, 2006.
7. European Economic Community. Council Directive 86/609/EEC of 24 November on the approximation of laws, regulations, and administrative provisions of the Member States regarding the protection of animals used for experimental and other purposes. Off J Eur Commun L352: 1-29, 1986.
8. Stokes WS and Marafante E. Introduction and summary of the 13th meeting of the Scientific Group on Methodologies for the Safety Evaluation of Chemicals (SGOMSEC): alternative testing methodologies. Environ Health Perspect 106 Suppl 2: 405-412, 1998.
9. Webster WS, Brown-Woodman PD, and Ritchie HE. A review of the contribution of whole embryo culture to the determination of hazard and risk in teratogenicity testing. Int J Dev Biol 41: 329-335, 1997.
10. Ashby J, Kier L, Wilson AG, Green T, Lefevre PA, Tinwell H, Willis GA, Heydens WF, and Clapp MJ. Evaluation of the potential carcinogenicity and genetic toxicity to humans of the herbicide acetochlor. Hum Exp Toxicol 15: 702-735, 1996.
11. Green T, Lee R, Moore RB, Ashby J, Willis GA, Lund VJ, and Clapp MJ. Acetochlor-induced rat nasal tumors: further studies on the mode of action and relevance to humans. Regul Toxicol Pharmacol 32: 127-133, 2000.
12. Dybing E and Huitfeldt HS. Species differences in carcinogen metabolism and interspecies extrapolation. IARC Sci Publ: 501-522, 1992.
13. Hengstler JG, Van der Burg B, Steinberg P, and Oesch F. Interspecies differences in cancer susceptibility and toxicity. Drug Metab Rev 31: 917-970, 1999.
14. Hayes JD and Pulford DJ. The glutathione S-transferase supergene family: regulation of GST and the contribution of the isoenzymes to cancer chemoprotection and drug resistance. Crit Rev Biochem Mol Biol 30: 445-600, 1995.
15. Pfaller W and Gstraunthaler G. Nephrotoxicity testing *in vitro*--what we know and what we need to know. Environ Health Perspect 106 Suppl 2: 559-569, 1998.
16. Green DF, Hwang KH, Ryan US, and Bourgoignie JJ. Culture of endothelial cells from baboon and human glomeruli. Kidney Int 41: 1506-1516, 1992.
17. van Setten PA, van Hinsbergh VW, van der Velden TJ, van de Kar NC, Vermeer M, Mahan JD, Assmann KJ, van den Heuvel LP, and Monnens LA. Effects of TNF alpha on verocytotoxin cytotoxicity in purified human glomerular microvascular endothelial cells. Kidney Int 51: 1245-1256, 1997.
18. Haraldsen G, Kvale D, Lien B, Farstad IN, and Brandtzaeg P. Cytokine-regulated expression of E-selectin, intercellular adhesion molecule-1 (ICAM-1), and vascular cell adhesion molecule-1 (VCAM-1) in human microvascular endothelial cells. J Immunol 156: 2558-2565, 1996.
19. van Muijen GN, Ruiter DJ, and Warnaar SO. Coexpression of intermediate filament polypeptides in human fetal and adult tissues. Lab Invest 57: 359-369, 1987.
20. Diaz-Flores L, Gutierrez R, Varela H, Rancel N, and Valladares F. Microvascular pericytes: a review of their morphological and functional characteristics. Histol Histopathol 6: 269-286, 1991.
21. Herman IM and D'Amore PA. Microvascular pericytes contain muscle and nonmuscle actins. J Cell Biol 101: 43-52, 1985.
22. Hewett PW and Murray JC. Human microvessel endothelial cells: isolation, culture and characterization. *In vitro* Cell Dev Biol Anim 29A: 823-830, 1993.
23. Jennings P. Novel Approaches For *In vitro* Nephrotoxicity Testing. PhD thesis, University College Dublin Library, 2001.
24. Ronco P and Debiec H. Podocyte antigens and glomerular disease. Nephron Exp Nephrol 107: e41-46, 2007.
25. Kerjaschki D, Sharkey DJ, and Farquhar MG. Identification and characterization of podocalyxin--the major sialoprotein of the renal glomerular epithelial cell. J Cell Biol 98: 1591-1596, 1984.
26. Shankland SJ, Pippin JW, Reiser J, and Mundel P. Podocytes in culture: past, present, and future. Kidney Int 72: 26-36, 2007.

27. Johnson RJ, Iida H, Alpers CE, Majesky MW, Schwartz SM, Pritzi P, Gordon K, and Gown AM. Expression of smooth muscle cell phenotype by rat mesangial cells in immune complex nephritis. Alpha-smooth muscle actin is a marker of mesangial cell proliferation. J Clin Invest 87: 847-858, 1991.
28. Stamenkovic I, Skalli O, and Gabbiani G. Distribution of intermediate filament proteins in normal and diseased human glomeruli. Am J Pathol 125: 465-475, 1986.
29. Ishimura E, Sterzel RB, Morii H, and Kashgarian M. Extracellular matrix protein: gene expression and synthesis in cultured rat mesangial cells. Nippon Jinzo Gakkai Shi 34: 9-17, 1992.
30. Potier M, L'Azou B, and Cambar J. Isolated glomeruli and cultured mesangial cells as *in vitro* models to study immunosuppressive agents. Cell Biol Toxicol 12: 263-270, 1996.
31. Ardaillou R, Chansel D, Stefanovic V, and Ardaillou N. Cell surface receptors and ectoenzymes in mesangial cells. J Am Soc Nephrol 2: S107-115, 1992.
32. Kriz W, Elger M, Lemley K, and Sakai T. Structure of the glomerular mesangium: a biomechanical interpretation. Kidney Int Suppl 30: S2-9, 1990.
33. Gstraunthaler G and Pfaller W. Continuous renal cell lines as *in vitro* tools to study nephrotoxicity. *In vitro* Methods of Toxicology: 93-113, 1992.
34. Rabito CA. Occluding junctions in a renal cell line (LLC-PK1) with characteristics of proximal tubular cells. Am J Physiol 250: F734-743, 1986.
35. Simmons NL. Tissue culture of established renal cell lines. Methods Enzymol 191: 426-436, 1990.
36. Horster M. Primary culture of mammalian nephron epithelia: requirements for cell outgrowth and proliferation from defined explanted nephron segments. Pflugers Arch 382: 209-215, 1979.
37. Morel F. Sites of hormone action in the mammalian nephron. Am J Physiol 240: F159-164, 1981.
38. Blais A, Morvan-Baleynaud J, Friedlander G, and Le Grimellec C. Primary culture of rabbit proximal tubules as a cellular model to study nephrotoxicity of xenobiotics. Kidney Int 44: 13-18, 1993.
39. Luhe A, Hildebrand H, Bach U, Dingermann T, and Ahr HJ. A new approach to studying ochratoxin A (OTA)-induced nephrotoxicity: expression profiling *in vivo* and *in vitro* employing cDNA microarrays. Toxicol Sci 73: 315-328, 2003.
40. Schwerdt G, Holzinger H, Sauvant C, Konigs M, Humpf HU, and Gekle M. Long-term effects of ochratoxin A on fibrosis and cell death in human proximal tubule or fibroblast cells in primary culture. Toxicology 232: 57-67, 2007.
41. Springate J and Taub M. Ifosfamide toxicity in cultured proximal renal tubule cells. Pediatr Nephrol 22: 358-365, 2007.
42. Jennings P, Koppelstaetter C, Aydin S, Abberger T, Wolf AM, Mayer G, and Pfaller W. Cyclosporine A induces senescence in renal tubular epithelial cells. Am J Physiol Renal Physiol 293: F831-838, 2007.
43. Moyzis RK, Buckingham JM, Cram LS, Dani M, Deaven LL, Jones MD, Meyne J, Ratliff RL, and Wu JR. A highly conserved repetitive DNA sequence, (TTAGGG)n, present at the telomeres of human chromosomes. Proc Natl Acad Sci U S A 85: 6622-6626, 1988.
44. Hayflick L. The Limited *In vitro* Lifetime Of Human Diploid Cell Strains. Exp Cell Res 37: 614-636, 1965.
45. Gstraunthaler G, Pfaller W, and Kotanko P. Lack of fructose-1,6-bisphosphatase activity in LLC-PK1 cells. Am J Physiol 248: C181-183, 1985.
46. Hull RN, Cherry WR, and Weaver GW. The origin and characteristics of a pig kidney cell strain, LLC-PK. *In vitro* 12: 670-677, 1976.
47. Takaoka T, Katsuta H, Endo M, Sato K, and Okumura H. Establishment of a cell strain, JTC-12, from cynomolgus monkey kidney tissue. Jpn J Exp Med 32: 351-368, 1962.
48. Koyama H, Goodpasture C, Miller MM, Teplitz RL, and Riggs AD. Establishment and characterization of a cell line from the American opossum (Didelphys virginiana). *In vitro* 14: 239-246, 1978.
49. Gstraunthaler G, Pfaller W, and Kotanko P. Biochemical characterization of renal epithelial cell cultures (LLC-PK1 and MDCK). Am J Physiol 248: F536-544, 1985.
50. Gaush CR, Hard WL, and Smith TF. Characterization of an established line of canine kidney cells (MDCK). Proc Soc Exp Biol Med 122: 931-935, 1966.
51. Handler JS, Preston AS, Perkins FM, Matsumura M, Johnson JP, and Watlington CO. The effect of adrenal steroid hormones on epithelia formed in culture by A6 cells. Ann N Y Acad Sci 372: 442-454, 1981.
52. Saier MH, Jr. Growth and differentiated properties of a kidney epithelial cell line (MDCK). Am J Physiol 240: C106-109, 1981.
53. Louvard D. Apical membrane aminopeptidase appears at site of cell-cell contact in cultured kidney epithelial cells. Proc Natl Acad Sci U S A 77: 4132-4136, 1980.
54. Ausiello DA, Hall DH, and Dayer JM. Modulation of cyclic AMP-dependent protein kinase by vasopressin and calcitonin in cultured porcine renal LLC-PK1 cells. Biochem J 186: 773-780, 1980.
55. Gstraunthaler GJ. Epithelial cells in tissue culture. Ren Physiol Biochem 11: 1-42, 1988.

56. Ryan MJ, Johnson G, Kirk J, Fuerstenberg SM, Zager RA, and Torok-Storb B. HK-2: an immortalized proximal tubule epithelial cell line from normal adult human kidney. Kidney Int 45: 48-57, 1994.
57. Hong HX, Zhang YM, Xu H, Su ZY, and Sun P. Immortalization of swine umbilical vein endothelial cells with human telomerase reverse transcriptase. Mol Cells 24: 358-363, 2007.
58. Shay JW and Wright WE. Senescence and immortalization: role of telomeres and telomerase. Carcinogenesis 26: 867-874, 2005.
59. Satchell SC, Tasman CH, Singh A, Ni L, Geelen J, von Ruhland CJ, O'Hare MJ, Saleem MA, van den Heuvel LP, and Mathieson PW. Conditionally immortalized human glomerular endothelial cells expressing fenestrations in response to VEGF. Kidney Int 69: 1633-1640, 2006.
60. Kowolik CM, Liang S, Yu Y, and Yee JK. Cre-mediated reversible immortalization of human renal proximal tubular epithelial cells. Oncogene 23: 5950-5957, 2004.
61. Gstraunthaler G, Thurner B, Weirich-Schwaiger H, and Pfaller W. A novel gluconeogenic strain of OK cells with metabolic properties different from gluconegenic LLC-PK1 cells. Cell Physiol Biochem 3: 78-88, 1993.
62. Gstraunthaler G, Gersdorf E, Fischer WM, Joannidis M, and Pfaller W. Morphological and biochemical changes of LLC-PK1 cells during adaptation to glucose-free culture conditions. Ren Physiol Biochem 13: 137-153, 1990.
63. Holcomb T, Curthoys NP, and Gstraunthaler G. Subcellular localization of PEPCK and metabolism of gluconeogenic substrains of renal cell lines. Am J Physiol 268: C449-457, 1995.
64. Chung SD, Alavi N, Livingston D, Hiller S, and Taub M. Characterization of primary rabbit kidney cultures that express proximal tubule functions in a hormonally defined medium. J Cell Biol 95: 118-126, 1982.
65. Pettersen EO, Larsen LH, Ramsing NB, and Ebbesen P. Pericellular oxygen depletion during ordinary tissue culturing, measured with oxygen microsensors. Cell Prolif 38: 257-267, 2005.
66. Gstraunthaler G, Seppi T, and Pfaller W. Impact of culture conditions, culture media volumes, and glucose content on metabolic properties of renal epithelial cell cultures. Are renal cells in tissue culture hypoxic? Cell Physiol Biochem 9: 150-172, 1999.
67. Handler JS, Preston AS, and Steele RE. Factors affecting the differentiation of epithelial transport and responsiveness to hormones. Fed Proc 43: 2221-2224, 1984.
68. Cook JR, Crute BE, Patrone LM, Gabriels J, Lane ME, and Van Buskirk RG. Microporosity of the substratum regulates differentiation of MDCK cells *in vitro*. *In vitro* Cell Dev Biol 25: 914-922, 1989.
69. Zlatkine P, Moll G, Blais A, Loiseau A, and Le Grimellec C. Transport of choline by Madin-Darby canine kidney cells. Biochim Biophys Acta 1153: 237-242, 1993.
70. Lang MA, Muller J, Preston AS, and Handler JS. Complete response to vasopressin requires epithelial organization in A6 cells in culture. Am J Physiol 250: C138-145, 1986.
71. Okuda M, Tsuda K, Masaki K, Hashimoto Y, and Inui K. Cisplatin-induced toxicity in LLC-PK1 kidney epithelial cells: role of basolateral membrane transport. Toxicol Lett 106: 229-235, 1999.
72. Felder E, Jennings P, Seppi T, and Pfaller W. LLC-PK(1) cells maintained in a new perfusion cell culture system exhibit an improved oxidative metabolism. Cell Physiol Biochem 12: 153-162, 2002.
73. Aydin S, Signorelli S, Lechleitner T, Joannidis M, Pleban C, Perco P, Pfaller W, and Jennings P. Influence of microvascular endothelial cells on transcriptional regulation of proximal tubular epithelial cells. Am J Physiol Cell Physiol 294: C543-554, 2008.
74. Bijuklic K, Jennings P, Kountchev J, Hasslacher J, Aydin S, Sturn D, Pfaller W, Patsch JR, and Joannidis M. Migration of leukocytes across an endothelium-epithelium bilayer as a model of renal interstitial inflammation. Am J Physiol Cell Physiol 293: C486-492, 2007.
75. Mosmann T. Rapid colorimetric assay for cellular growth and survival: application to proliferation and cytotoxicity assays. J Immunol Methods 65: 55-63, 1983.
76. Kino T, Hatanaka H, Miyata S, Inamura N, Nishiyama M, Yajima T, Goto T, Okuhara M, Kohsaka M, Aoki H, and et al. FK-506, a novel immunosuppressant isolated from a Streptomyces. II. Immunosuppressive effect of FK-506 *in vitro*. J Antibiot (Tokyo) 40: 1256-1265, 1987.
77. Kino T, Hatanaka H, Hashimoto M, Nishiyama M, Goto T, Okuhara M, Kohsaka M, Aoki H, and Imanaka H. FK-506, a novel immunosuppressant isolated from a Streptomyces. I. Fermentation, isolation, and physico-chemical and biological characteristics. J Antibiot (Tokyo) 40: 1249-1255, 1987.
78. Potier M, Wolf A, and Cambar J. Comparative study of cyclosporin A, cyclosporin G, and the novel cyclosporin derivative IMM 125 in isolated glomeruli and cultured rat mesangial cells: a morphometric analysis. Nephrol Dial Transplant 13: 1406-1411, 1998.
79. L'Azou B, Medina J, Frieauff W, Cordier A, Cambar J, and Wolf A. *In vitro* models to study mechanisms involved in cyclosporine A-mediated glomerular contraction. Arch Toxicol 73: 337-345, 1999.
80. Rodriguez-Puyol D, Lamas S, Olivera A, Lopez-Farre A, Ortega G, Hernando L, and Lopez-Novoa JM. Actions of cyclosporin A on cultured rat mesangial cells. Kidney Int 35: 632-637, 1989.

81. L'Azou B, Lakhdar B, Potaux L, and Cambar J. Protective effect of verapamil in cyclosporin-incubated human and murine isolated glomeruli. Ren Fail 16: 665-672, 1994.
82. Stahl RA, Adler S, Baker PJ, Johnson RJ, Chen YP, Pritzl P, and Couser WG. Cyclosporin A inhibits prostaglandin E2 formation by rat mesangial cells in culture. Kidney Int 35: 1161-1167, 1989.
83. Han SY, Mun KC, Choi HJ, Kwak CS, Bae JH, Suh SI, Park SB, Kim HC, and Chang EJ. Effects of cyclosporine and tacrolimus on the oxidative stress in cultured mesangial cells. Transplant Proc 38: 2240-2241, 2006.
84. Gagliardini E and Benigni A. Therapeutic potential of TGF-beta inhibition in chronic renal failure. Expert Opin Biol Ther 7: 293-304, 2007.
85. Waiser J, Dell K, Bohler T, Dogu E, Gaedeke J, Budde K, and Neumayer HH. Cyclosporine A up-regulates the expression of TGF-beta1 and its receptors type I and type II in rat mesangial cells. Nephrol Dial Transplant 17: 1568-1577, 2002.
86. Waiser J, Dell K, Kreutzkamp J, Bohler T, Budde K, Peters H, and Neumayer HH. FK506, transforming growth factor-beta1 and mesangial matrix synthesis: parallels and differences compared with cyclosporine A. Cytokine 33: 59-65, 2006.
87. Fornoni A, Lenz O, Tack I, Potier M, Elliot SJ, Striker LJ, and Striker GE. Matrix accumulation in mesangial cells exposed to cyclosporine A requires a permissive genetic background. Transplantation 70: 587-593, 2000.
88. Becker GM, Gandolfi AJ, and Nagle RB. Effects of cyclosporin A on a kidney epithelial cell line (LLC-PK1). Res Commun Chem Pathol Pharmacol 56: 277-280, 1987.
89. Healy E, Dempsey M, Lally C, and Ryan MP. Apoptosis and necrosis: mechanisms of cell death induced by cyclosporine A in a renal proximal tubular cell line. Kidney Int 54: 1955-1966, 1998.
90. Lechner J, Malloth N, Seppi T, Beer B, Jennings P, and Pfaller W. IFN{alpha} induces barrier destabilization and apoptosis in renal proximal tubular epithelium. Am J Physiol Cell Physiol, 2007.
91. Lally C, Healy E, and Ryan MP. Cyclosporine A-induced cell cycle arrest and cell death in renal epithelial cells. Kidney Int 56: 1254-1257, 1999.
92. Miyashita T and Reed JC. Tumor suppressor p53 is a direct transcriptional activator of the human bax gene. Cell 80: 293-299, 1995.
93. Yang CW, Faulkner GR, Wahba IM, Christianson TA, Bagby GC, Jin DC, Abboud HE, Andoh TF, and Bennett WM. Expression of apoptosis-related genes in chronic cyclosporine nephrotoxicity in mice. Am J Transplant 2: 391-399, 2002.
94. Thomas SE, Andoh TF, Pichler RH, Shankland SJ, Couser WG, Bennett WM, and Johnson RJ. Accelerated apoptosis characterizes cyclosporine-associated interstitial fibrosis. Kidney Int 53: 897-908, 1998.
95. Bakker RC, van Kooten C, van de Lagemaat-Paape ME, Daha MR, and Paul LC. Renal tubular epithelial cell death and cyclosporin A. Nephrol Dial Transplant 17: 1181-1188, 2002.
96. Zhou X, Yang G, Davis CA, Doi SQ, Hirszel P, Wingo CS, and Agarwal A. Hydrogen peroxide mediates FK506-induced cytotoxicity in renal cells. Kidney Int 65: 139-147, 2004.
97. Johnson DW, Saunders HJ, Johnson FJ, Huq SO, Field MJ, and Pollock CA. Fibrogenic effects of cyclosporin A on the tubulointerstitium: role of cytokines and growth factors. Exp Nephrol 7: 470-478, 1999.
98. Slattery C, Campbell E, McMorrow T, and Ryan MP. Cyclosporine A-induced renal fibrosis: a role for epithelial-mesenchymal transition. Am J Pathol 167: 395-407, 2005.
99. McMorrow T, Gaffney MM, Slattery C, Campbell E, and Ryan MP. Cyclosporine A induced epithelial-mesenchymal transition in human renal proximal tubular epithelial cells. Nephrol Dial Transplant 20: 2215-2225, 2005.
100. Qiu J, Tu Z, Shi Y, Zhang L, Li Q, Wang W, Ye F, Wang J, and Bu H. Interference of cyclosporine on glucose metabolism: potential role in chronic transplantation kidney fibrosis. Transplant Proc 38: 2065-2068, 2006.
101. Massicot F, Martin C, Dutertre-Catella H, Ellouk-Achard S, Pham-Huy C, Thevenin M, Rucay P, Warnet JM, and Claude JR. Modulation of energy status and cytotoxicity induced by FK506 and cyclosporin A in a renal epithelial cell line. Arch Toxicol 71: 529-531, 1997.
102. Dominguez JH, Soleimani M, and Batiuk T. Studies of renal injury IV: The GLUT1 gene protects renal cells from cyclosporine A toxicity. Kidney Int 62: 127-136, 2002.
103. Strutz F, Zeisberg M, Renziehausen A, Raschke B, Becker V, van Kooten C, and Muller G. TGF-beta 1 induces proliferation in human renal fibroblasts via induction of basic fibroblast growth factor (FGF-2). Kidney Int 59: 579-592, 2001.
104. Johnson DW, Saunders HJ, Vesey DA, Qi W, Field MJ, and Pollock CA. Enalaprilat directly ameliorates *in vitro* cyclosporin nephrotoxicity in human tubulo-interstitial cells. Nephron 86: 473-481, 2000.
105. Nakahama H, Fukunaga M, Kakihara M, Horio M, Fujiwara Y, Fukuhara Y, Ueda N, Orita Y, and Kamada T. Comparative effects of cyclosporine A and FK-506 on endothelin secretion by a cultured renal cell line, LLC-PK1. J Cardiovasc Pharmacol 17 Suppl 7: S172-173, 1991.
106. Nakahama H. Stimulatory effect of cyclosporine A on endothelin secretion by a cultured renal epithelial cell line, LLC-PK1 cells. Eur J Pharmacol 180: 191-192, 1990.

107. Saeki T, Ueda K, Tanigawara Y, Hori R, and Komano T. Human P-glycoprotein transports cyclosporin A and FK506. J Biol Chem 268: 6077-6080, 1993.
108. Hauser IA, Koziolek M, Hopfer U, and Thevenod F. Therapeutic concentrations of cyclosporine A, but not FK506, increase P-glycoprotein expression in endothelial and renal tubule cells. Kidney Int 54: 1139-1149, 1998.
109. Yuan CM, Bohen EM, Musio F, and Carome MA. Sublethal heat shock and cyclosporine exposure produce tolerance against subsequent cyclosporine toxicity. Am J Physiol 271: F571-578, 1996.
110. Hanigan MH and Devarajan P. Cisplatin nephrotoxicity: molecular mechanisms. Cancer Ther 1: 47-61, 2003.
111. Townsend DM, Deng M, Zhang L, Lapus MG, and Hanigan MH. Metabolism of Cisplatin to a nephrotoxin in proximal tubule cells. J Am Soc Nephrol 14: 1-10, 2003.
112. Hanigan MH, Lykissa ED, Townsend DM, Ou CN, Barrios R, and Lieberman MW. Gamma-glutamyl transpeptidase-deficient mice are resistant to the nephrotoxic effects of cisplatin. Am J Pathol 159: 1889-1894, 2001.
113. Endo T, Kimura O, and Sakata M. Carrier-mediated uptake of cisplatin by the OK renal epithelial cell line. Toxicology 146: 187-195, 2000.
114. Kuo MT, Chen HH, Song IS, Savaraj N, and Ishikawa T. The roles of copper transporters in cisplatin resistance. Cancer Metastasis Rev 26: 71-83, 2007.
115. Ishida S, Lee J, Thiele DJ, and Herskowitz I. Uptake of the anticancer drug cisplatin mediated by the copper transporter Ctr1 in yeast and mammals. Proc Natl Acad Sci U S A 99: 14298-14302, 2002.
116. Zimnicka AM, Maryon EB, and Kaplan JH. Human copper transporter hCTR1 mediates basolateral uptake of copper into enterocytes: implications for copper homeostasis. J Biol Chem 282: 26471-26480, 2007.
117. Courjault F, Leroy D, Coquery L, and Toutain H. Platinum complex-induced dysfunction of cultured renal proximal tubule cells. A comparative study of carboplatin and transplatin with cisplatin. Arch Toxicol 67: 338-346, 1993.
118. Montine TJ and Borch RF. Quiescent LLC-PK1 cells as a model for cis-diamminedichloroplatinum(II) nephrotoxicity and modulation by thiol rescue agents. Cancer Res 48: 6017-6024, 1988.
119. Fukuishi N and Gemba M. Use of cultured renal epithelial cells for the study of cisplatin toxicity. Jpn J Pharmacol 50: 247-249, 1989.
120. Lieberthal W, Triaca V, and Levine J. Mechanisms of death induced by cisplatin in proximal tubular epithelial cells: apoptosis vs. necrosis. Am J Physiol 270: F700-708, 1996.
121. Okuda M, Masaki K, Fukatsu S, Hashimoto Y, and Inui K. Role of apoptosis in cisplatin-induced toxicity in the renal epithelial cell line LLC-PK1. Implication of the functions of apical membranes. Biochem Pharmacol 59: 195-201, 2000.
122. Tsuruya K, Ninomiya T, Tokumoto M, Hirakawa M, Masutani K, Taniguchi M, Fukuda K, Kanai H, Kishihara K, Hirakata H, and Iida M. Direct involvement of the receptor-mediated apoptotic pathways in cisplatin-induced renal tubular cell death. Kidney Int 63: 72-82, 2003.
123. Park MS, De Leon M, and Devarajan P. Cisplatin induces apoptosis in LLC-PK1 cells via activation of mitochondrial pathways. J Am Soc Nephrol 13: 858-865, 2002.
124. Takeda M, Kobayashi M, Shirato I, Osaki T, and Endou H. Cisplatin-induced apoptosis of immortalized mouse proximal tubule cells is mediated by interleukin-1 beta converting enzyme (ICE) family of proteases but inhibited by overexpression of Bcl-2. Arch Toxicol 71: 612-621, 1997.
125. Weidemann A, Bernhardt WM, Klanke B, Daniel C, Buchholz B, Campean V, Amann K, Warnecke C, Wiesener MS, Eckardt KU, and Willam C. HIF activation protects from acute kidney injury. J Am Soc Nephrol 19: 486-494, 2008.
126. Yokozawa T, Nakagawa T, Lee KI, Cho EJ, Terasawa K, and Takeuchi S. Effects of green tea tannin on cisplatin-induced nephropathy in LLC-PK1 cells and rats. J Pharm Pharmacol 51: 1325-1331, 1999.
127. Bragado P, Armesilla A, Silva A, and Porras A. Apoptosis by cisplatin requires p53 mediated p38alpha MAPK activation through ROS generation. Apoptosis 12: 1733-1742, 2007.
128. Hannemann J and Baumann K. Inhibition of lactate-dehydrogenase by cisplatin and other platinum-compounds: enzyme leakage of LDH is not a suitable method to measure platinum-compound-induced kidney cell damage *in vitro*. Res Commun Chem Pathol Pharmacol 60: 371-379, 1988.
129. Martinez-Salgado C, Lopez-Hernandez FJ, and Lopez-Novoa JM. Glomerular nephrotoxicity of aminoglycosides. Toxicol Appl Pharmacol 223: 86-98, 2007.
130. Montie T and Patamasucon P. Aminoglycosides: the complex problem of antibiotic mechanisms and clinical applications. Eur J Clin Microbiol Infect Dis 14: 85-87, 1995.
131. Rivas-Cabanero L, Rodriguez-Lopez AM, Martinez-Salgado C, Saura M, Lamas S, and Lopez-Novoa JM. Gentamicin treatment increases mesangial cell nitric oxide production. Exp Nephrol 5: 23-30, 1997.
132. Martinez-Salgado C, Rodriguez-Barbero A, Tavares P, Eleno N, and Lopez-Novoa JM. Role of calcium in gentamicin-induced mesangial cell activation. Cell Physiol Biochem 10: 65-72, 2000.

133. Klotman PE and Yarger WE. Reduction of renal blood flow and proximal bicarbonate reabsorption in rats by gentamicin. Kidney Int 24: 638-643, 1983.

134. Schor N, Ichikawa I, Rennke HG, Troy JL, and Brenner BM. Pathophysiology of altered glomerular function in aminoglycoside-treated rats. Kidney Int 19: 288-296, 1981.

135. Morales AI, Rodriguez-Barbero A, Vicente-Sanchez C, Mayoral P, Lopez-Novoa JM, and Perez-Barriocanal F. Resveratrol inhibits gentamicin-induced mesangial cell contraction. Life Sci 78: 2373-2377, 2006.

136. Kiyomiya K, Matsushita N, Matsuo S, and Kurebe M. Differential toxic effects of gentamicin on cultured renal epithelial cells (LLC-PK1) on application to the brush border membrane or the basolateral membrane. J Vet Med Sci 62: 971-975, 2000.

137. Nagai J. [Molecular mechanisms underlying renal accumulation of aminoglycoside antibiotics and mechanism-based approach for developing nonnephrotoxic aminoglycoside therapy]. Yakugaku Zasshi 126: 327-335, 2006.

138. Sandoval RM, Dunn KW, and Molitoris BA. Gentamicin traffics rapidly and directly to the Golgi complex in LLC-PK(1) cells. Am J Physiol Renal Physiol 279: F884-890, 2000.

139. Sandoval RM and Molitoris BA. Gentamicin traffics retrograde through the secretory pathway and is released in the cytosol via the endoplasmic reticulum. Am J Physiol Renal Physiol 286: F617-624, 2004.

140. Takamoto K, Kawada M, Ikeda D, and Yoshida M. Apolipoprotein E3 (apoE3) safeguards pig proximal tubular LLC-PK1 cells against reduction in SGLT1 activity induced by gentamicin C. Biochim Biophys Acta 1722: 247-253, 2005.

141. Inui K, Saito H, Iwata T, and Hori R. Aminoglycoside-induced alterations in apical membranes of kidney epithelial cell line (LLC-PK1). Am J Physiol 254: C251-257, 1988.

142. Hori R, Yamamoto K, Saito H, Kohno M, and Inui K. Effect of aminoglycoside antibiotics on cellular functions of kidney epithelial cell line (LLC-PK1): a model system for aminoglycoside nephrotoxicity. J Pharmacol Exp Ther 230: 724-728, 1984.

143. Choi KH, Kim TI, Chong DL, Lee HY, and Han DS. Gentamicin induced apoptosis of renal tubular epithelial (LLC-PK1) cells. Korean J Intern Med 15: 218-223, 2000.

144. El Mouedden M, Laurent G, Mingeot-Leclercq MP, and Tulkens PM. Gentamicin-induced apoptosis in renal cell lines and embryonic rat fibroblasts. Toxicol Sci 56: 229-239, 2000.

145. Robertson EE and Rankin GO. Human renal organic anion transporters: characteristics and contributions to drug and drug metabolite excretion. Pharmacol Ther 109: 399-412, 2006.

146. Takeda M, Tojo A, Sekine T, Hosoyamada M, Kanai Y, and Endou H. Role of organic anion transporter 1 (OAT1) in cephaloridine (CER)-induced nephrotoxicity. Kidney Int 56: 2128-2136, 1999.

147. Jung KY, Takeda M, Shimoda M, Narikawa S, Tojo A, Kim DK, Chairoungdua A, Choi BK, Kusuhara H, Sugiyama Y, Sekine T, and Endou H. Involvement of rat organic anion transporter 3 (rOAT3) in cephaloridine-induced nephrotoxicity: in comparison with rOAT1. Life Sci 70: 1861-1874, 2002.

148. Ueo H, Motohashi H, Katsura T, and Inui K. Human organic anion transporter hOAT3 is a potent transporter of cephalosporin antibiotics, in comparison with hOAT1. Biochem Pharmacol 70: 1104-1113, 2005.

149. Hori R, Okamura M, Takayama A, Hirozane K, and Takano M. Transport of organic anion in the OK kidney epithelial cell line. Am J Physiol 264: F975-980, 1993.

150. Nagai J, Takano M, Hirozane K, Yasuhara M, and Inui K. Specificity of p-aminohippurate transport system in the OK kidney epithelial cell line. J Pharmacol Exp Ther 274: 1161-1166, 1995.

151. Kiyomiya K, Matsushita N, Matsuo S, and Kurebe M. Roles of oxygen radical production and lipid peroxidation in the cytotoxicity of cephaloridine on cultured renal epithelial cells (LLC- PK1). J Vet Med Sci 62: 977-981, 2000.

152. Kiyomiya K, Matsushita N, Matsuo S, and Kurebe M. Cephaloridine-induced inhibition of cytochrome c oxidase activity in the mitochondria of cultured renal epithelial cells (LLC-PK(1)) as a possible mechanism of its nephrotoxicity. Toxicol Appl Pharmacol 167: 151-156, 2000.

153. Steinmassl D, Pfaller W, Gstraunthaler G, and Hoffmann W. LLC-PK1 epithelia as a model for *in vitro* assessment of proximal tubular nephrotoxicity. *In vitro* Cell Dev Biol Anim 31: 94-106, 1995.

154. Goldman RD and Koren G. Amphotericin B nephrotoxicity in children. J Pediatr Hematol Oncol 26: 421-426, 2004.

155. Warnock DW. Amphotericin B: an introduction. J Antimicrob Chemother 28 Suppl B: 27-38, 1991.

156. Zager RA. Polyene antibiotics: relative degrees of *in vitro* cytotoxicity and potential effects on tubule phospholipid and ceramide content. Am J Kidney Dis 36: 238-249, 2000.

157. Hsu S and Burnette RR. Characterization of the effects of amphotericin B on ion channels in MDCK cells using the patch-clamp technique. Biochim Biophys Acta 1329: 26-38, 1997.

158. Sabra R and Branch RA. Effect of amphotericin B on intracellular calcium levels in cultured glomerular mesangial cells. Eur J Pharmacol 226: 79-85, 1992.

159. Varlam DE, Siddiq MM, Parton LA, and Russmann H. Apoptosis contributes to amphotericin B-induced nephrotoxicity. Antimicrob Agents Chemother 45: 679-685, 2001.

160. Wasan KM, Rosenblum MG, Cheung L, and Lopez-Berestein G. Influence of lipoproteins on renal cytotoxicity and antifungal activity of amphotericin B. Antimicrob Agents Chemother 38: 223-227, 1994.
161. Wasan KM and Lopez-Berestein G. Modification of amphotericin B's therapeutic index by increasing its association with serum high-density lipoproteins. Ann N Y Acad Sci 730: 93-106, 1994.
162. Bartlett K, Yau E, Hartsel SC, Hamer A, Tsai G, Bizzotto D, and Wasan KM. Effect of heat-treated amphotericin B on renal and fungal cytotoxicity. Antimicrob Agents Chemother 48: 333-336, 2004.
163. Leon C, Taylor R, Bartlett KH, and Wasan KM. Effect of heat-treatment and the role of phospholipases on Fungizone-induced cytotoxicity within human kidney proximal tubular (HK-2) cells and Aspergillus fumigatus. Int J Pharm 298: 211-218, 2005.
164. Jarup L. Cadmium overload and toxicity. Nephrol Dial Transplant 17 Suppl 2: 35-39, 2002.
165. Kimura O, Endo T, and Sakata M. Comparison of cadmium uptakes from apical and basolateral membranes of LLC-PK1 cells. Toxicol Appl Pharmacol 137: 301-306, 1996.
166. Endo T, Kimura O, and Sakata M. Cadmium uptake from apical membrane of LLC-PK1 cells via inorganic anion exchanger. Pharmacol Toxicol 82: 230-235, 1998.
167. Endo T, Kimura O, and Sakata M. Further analysis of cadmium uptake from apical membrane of LLC-PK1 cells via inorganic anion exchanger. Pharmacol Toxicol 84: 187-192, 1999.
168. Prozialeck WC and Niewenhuis RJ. Cadmium (Cd2+) disrupts Ca(2+)-dependent cell-cell junctions and alters the pattern of E-cadherin immunofluorescence in LLC-PK1 cells. Biochem Biophys Res Commun 181: 1118-1124, 1991.
169. Zimmerhackl LB, Momm F, Wiegele G, and Brandis M. Cadmium is more toxic to LLC-PK1 cells than to MDCK cells acting on the cadherin-catenin complex. Am J Physiol 275: F143-153, 1998.
170. Klaassen CD, Liu J, and Choudhuri S. Metallothionein: an intracellular protein to protect against cadmium toxicity. Annu Rev Pharmacol Toxicol 39: 267-294, 1999.
171. Klassen RB, Crenshaw K, Kozyraki R, Verroust PJ, Tio L, Atrian S, Allen PL, and Hammond TG. Megalin mediates renal uptake of heavy metal metallothionein complexes. Am J Physiol Renal Physiol 287: F393-403, 2004.
172. Wolff NA, Abouhamed M, Verroust PJ, and Thevenod F. Megalin-dependent internalization of cadmium-metallothionein and cytotoxicity in cultured renal proximal tubule cells. J Pharmacol Exp Ther 318: 782-791, 2006.
173. Ishido M, Tohyama C, and Suzuki T. Cadmium-bound metallothionein induces apoptosis in rat kidneys, but not in cultured kidney LLC-PK1 cells. Life Sci 64: 797-804, 1999.
174. Zhai XY, Nielsen R, Birn H, Drumm K, Mildenberger S, Freudinger R, Moestrup SK, Verroust PJ, Christensen EI, and Gekle M. Cubilin- and megalin-mediated uptake of albumin in cultured proximal tubule cells of opossum kidney. Kidney Int 58: 1523-1533, 2000.
175. Nielsen R, Birn H, Moestrup SK, Nielsen M, Verroust P, and Christensen EI. Characterization of a kidney proximal tubule cell line, LLC-PK1, expressing endocytotic active megalin. J Am Soc Nephrol 9: 1767-1776, 1998.
176. Thevenod F. Nephrotoxicity and the proximal tubule. Insights from cadmium. Nephron Physiol 93: p87-93, 2003.
177. Abouhamed M, Wolff NA, Lee WK, Smith CP, and Thevenod F. Knockdown of endosomal/lysosomal divalent metal transporter 1 by RNA interference prevents cadmium-metallothionein-1 cytotoxicity in renal proximal tubule cells. Am J Physiol Renal Physiol 293: F705-712, 2007.
178. Liu Y, Zhang SP, and Cai YQ. Cytoprotective effects of selenium on cadmium-induced LLC-PK1 cells apoptosis by activating JNK pathway. Toxicol *In vitro* 21: 677-684, 2007.
179. Yokouchi M, Hiramatsu N, Hayakawa K, Okamura M, Du S, Kasai A, Takano Y, Shitamura A, Shimada T, Yao J, and Kitamura M. Involvement of selective reactive oxygen species upstream of proapoptotic branches of unfolded protein response. J Biol Chem 283: 4252-4260, 2008.
180. Ding W and Templeton DM. Activation of parallel mitogen-activated protein kinase cascades and induction of c-fos by cadmium. Toxicol Appl Pharmacol 162: 93-99, 2000.
181. Templeton DM, Wang Z, and Miralem T. Cadmium and calcium-dependent c-fos expression in mesangial cells. Toxicol Lett 95: 1-8, 1998.
182. Alvarez-Barrientos A, O'Connor JE, Nieto Castillo R, Moreno Moreno AB, and Prieto P. Use of flow cytometry and confocal microscopy techniques to investigate early CdCl(2)-induced nephrotoxicity *in vitro*. Toxicol *In vitro* 15: 407-412, 2001.
183. Bonham RT, Fine MR, Pollock FM, and Shelden EA. Hsp27, Hsp70, and metallothionein in MDCK and LLC-PK1 renal epithelial cells: effects of prolonged exposure to cadmium. Toxicol Appl Pharmacol 191: 63-73, 2003.
184. Urani C, Melchioretto P, Canevali C, and Crosta GF. Cytotoxicity and induction of protective mechanisms in HepG2 cells exposed to cadmium. Toxicol *In vitro* 19: 887-892, 2005.
185. Endo T, Kimura O, and Sakata M. Effects of P-glycoprotein inhibitors on cadmium accumulation in cultured renal epithelial cells, LLC-PK1, and OK. Toxicol Appl Pharmacol 185: 166-171, 2002.

186. Kimura O, Endo T, Hotta Y, and Sakata M. Effects of P-glycoprotein inhibitors on transepithelial transport of cadmium in cultured renal epithelial cells, LLC-PK1 and LLC-GA5-COL 150. Toxicology 208: 123-132, 2005.
187. Nicholson JK, Kendall MD, and Osborn D. Cadmium and mercury nephrotoxicity. Nature 304: 633-635, 1983.
188. Zalups RK. Molecular interactions with mercury in the kidney. Pharmacol Rev 52: 113-143, 2000.
189. Bohets HH, Van Thielen MN, Van der Biest I, Van Landeghem GF, D'Haese PC, Nouwen EJ, De Broe ME, and Dierickx PJ. Cytotoxicity of mercury compounds in LLC-PK1, MDCK and human proximal tubular cells. Kidney Int 47: 395-403, 1995.
190. Aleo MD, Taub ML, and Kostyniak PJ. Primary cultures of rabbit renal proximal tubule cells. III. Comparative cytotoxicity of inorganic and organic mercury. Toxicol Appl Pharmacol 112: 310-317, 1992.
191. Matsuoka M, Wispriyono B, Iryo Y, and Igisu H. Mercury chloride activates c-Jun N-terminal kinase and induces c-jun expression in LLC-PK1 cells. Toxicol Sci 53: 361-368, 2000.
192. Duncan-Achanzar KB, Jones JT, Burke MF, Carter DE, and Laird HEn. Inorganic mercury chloride-induced apoptosis in the cultured porcine renal cell line LLC-PK1. J Pharmacol Exp Ther 277: 1726-1732, 1996.
193. Sutton DJ and Tchounwou PB. Mercury induces the externalization of phosphatidyl-serine in human renal proximal tubule (HK-2) cells. Int J Environ Res Public Health 4: 138-144, 2007.
194. Dieguez-Acuna FJ, Polk WW, Ellis ME, Simmonds PL, Kushleika JV, and Woods JS. Nuclear factor kappaB activity determines the sensitivity of kidney epithelial cells to apoptosis: implications for mercury-induced renal failure. Toxicol Sci 82: 114-123, 2004.
195. Woods JS, Dieguez-Acuna FJ, Ellis ME, Kushleika J, and Simmonds PL. Attenuation of nuclear factor kappa B (NF-kappaB) promotes apoptosis of kidney epithelial cells: a potential mechanism of mercury-induced nephrotoxicity. Environ Health Perspect 110 Suppl 5: 819-822, 2002.
196. Zalups RK, Aslamkhan AG, and Ahmad S. Human organic anion transporter 1 mediates cellular uptake of cysteine-S conjugates of inorganic mercury. Kidney Int 66: 251-261, 2004.
197. O'Brien E and Dietrich DR. Ochratoxin A: the continuing enigma. Crit Rev Toxicol 35: 33-60, 2005.
198. Groves CE, Nowak G, and Morales M. Ochratoxin A secretion in primary cultures of rabbit renal proximal tubule cells. J Am Soc Nephrol 10: 13-20, 1999.
199. Babu E, Takeda M, Narikawa S, Kobayashi Y, Enomoto A, Tojo A, Cha SH, Sekine T, Sakthisekaran D, and Endou H. Role of human organic anion transporter 4 in the transport of ochratoxin A. Biochim Biophys Acta 1590: 64-75, 2002.
200. Jung KY, Takeda M, Kim DK, Tojo A, Narikawa S, Yoo BS, Hosoyamada M, Cha SH, Sekine T, and Endou H. Characterization of ochratoxin A transport by human organic anion transporters. Life Sci 69: 2123-2135, 2001.
201. Dai J, Park G, Perry JL, Il'ichev YV, Bow DA, Pritchard JB, Faucet V, Pfohl-Leszkowicz A, Manderville RA, and Simon JD. Molecular aspects of the transport and toxicity of ochratoxin a. Acc Chem Res 37: 874-881, 2004.
202. Gekle M, Gassner B, Freudinger R, Mildenberger S, Silbernagl S, Pfaller W, and Schramek H. Characterization of an ochratoxin-A-dedifferentiated and cloned renal epithelial cell line. Toxicol Appl Pharmacol 152: 282-291, 1998.
203. Gekle M, Schwerdt G, Freudinger R, Mildenberger S, Wilflingseder D, Pollack V, Dander M, and Schramek H. Ochratoxin A induces JNK activation and apoptosis in MDCK-C7 cells at nanomolar concentrations. J Pharmacol Exp Ther 293: 837-844, 2000.
204. Jonasch E and Haluska FG. Interferon in Oncological Practice: Review of Interferon Biology, Clinical Applications, and Toxicities. Oncologist 6: 34-55, 2001.
205. Kappos L, Weinshenker B, Pozzilli C, Thompson AJ, Dahlke F, Beckmann K, Polman C, McFarland H, and for the European and North American Interferon beta-1b in Secondary Progressive Multiple Sclerosis Trial Steering Committees and Independent Advisory Boards. Interferon beta-1b in secondary progressive MS: A combined analysis of the two trials. Neurology 63: 1779-1787, 2004.
206. Wadler S and Schwartz EL. New Advances in Interferon Therapy of Cancer. Oncologist 2: 254-267, 1997.
207. Belardelli F and Ferrantini M. Cytokines as a link between innate and adaptive antitumor immunity. Trends Immunol 23: 201-208, 2002.
208. Samuel CE. Antiviral Actions of Interferons. Clin Microbiol Rev 14: 778-809, 2001.
209. Izzedine H, Launay-Vacher V, and Deray G. Antiviral drug-induced nephrotoxicity. American Journal of Kidney Diseases 45: 804-817, 2005.
210. Kurschel E, Metz-Kurschel U, Niederle N, and Aulbert E. Investigations on the subclinical and clinical nephrotoxicity of interferon alpha-2B in patients with myeloproliferative syndromes. Ren Fail 13: 87-93, 1991.
211. Al Harbi A, Al Ghamdi S, Subaity Y, and Khalil A. Interferon-induced renal failure in nephrotic syndrome. Nephrol Dial Transplant 13: 1316-1318, 1998.
212. Averbuch S, Austin H, Sherwin S, Antonovych T, Bunn P, and Longo D. Acute interstitial nephritis with the nephrotic syndrome following recombinant leukocyte a interferon therapy for mycosis fungoides. N Engl J Med 310: 32-35, 1984.
213. Fahal IH, Murry N, Chu P, and Bell GM. Acute renal failure during interferon treatment. Brit medical J 306: 973., 1993.

214. Parker M, Atkins M, Ucci A, and Levey A. Rapidly progressive glomerulonephritis after immunotherapy for cancer. J Am Soc Nephrol 5: 1740-1744, 1995.
215. Rostaing L, Modesto A, Baron E, Cisterne J, Chabannier M, and Durand D. Acute renal failure in kidney transplant patients treated with interferon alpha 2b for chronic hepatitis C. Nephron 74: 512-516, 1996.
216. Lechner J, Malloth N, Seppi T, Beer B, Jennings P, and Pfaller W. IFN-{alpha} induces barrier destabilization and apoptosis in renal proximal tubular epithelium. Am J Physiol Cell Physiol 294: C153-C160 [Epub 2007, Nov 2021], 2008.
217. Chawla-Sarkar M, Lindner D, Liu Y, Williams B, Sen G, Silverman R, and Borden E. Apoptosis and interferons: role of interferon-stimulated genes as mediators of apoptosis. Apoptosis 8: 237-249, 2003.
218. Leaman DW, Chawla-Sarkar M, Vyas K, Reheman M, Tamai K, Toji S, and Borden EC. Identification of X-linked Inhibitor of Apoptosis-associated Factor-1 as an Interferon-stimulated Gene That Augments TRAIL Apo2L-induced Apoptosis. J Biol Chem 277: 28504-28511, 2002.
219. Lechner J, Krall M, Netzer A, Radmayr C, Ryan M, and Pfaller W. Effects of interferon alpha-2b on barrier function and junctional complexes of renal proximal tubular LLC-PK1 cells. Kidney Int 55: 2178-2191, 1999.
220. Lechner J and Pfaller W. Interferon alpha2b increases paracellular permeability of renal proximal tubular LLC-PK1 cells via a mitogen activated protein kinase signaling pathway. Ren Fail 23: 573-588, 2001.
221. Seger R and Krebs EG. The MAPK signaling cascade. FASEB J 9: 726-735, 1995.
222. Singh AB and Harris RC. Epidermal Growth Factor Receptor Activation Differentially Regulates Claudin Expression and Enhances Transepithelial Resistance in Madin-Darby Canine Kidney Cells. J Biol Chem 279: 3543-3552, 2004.
223. Saladik DT, Soler AP, Lewis SA, and Mullin JM. Cell Division Does Not Increase Transepithelial Permeability of LLC-PK1 Cell Sheets. Experimental Cell Research 220: 446-455, 1995.
224. Nigam SK and Lieberthal W. Acute renal failure. III. The role of growth factors in the process of renal regeneration and repair. Am J Physiol Renal Physiol 279: F3-11, 2000.
225. Schena FP. Role of growth factors in acute renal failure. Kidney Int Suppl 66: S11-15., 1998.
226. Wang Z, Chen J-K, Wang S-w, Moeckel G, and Harris RC. Importance of Functional EGF Receptors in Recovery from Acute Nephrotoxic Injury. J Am Soc Nephrol 14: 3147-3154, 2003.
227. Hammerman M. Growth factors and apoptosis in acute renal injury. Curr Opin Nephrol Hypertens 7: 419-424, 1998.
228. Zhuang S, Dang Y, and Schnellmann RG. Requirement of the epidermal growth factor receptor in renal epithelial cell proliferation and migration. Am J Physiol Renal Physiol 287: F365-372, 2004.
229. Lechner J, Malloth NA, Jennings P, Hekl D, Pfaller W, and Seppi T. Opposing roles of EGF in IFN-{alpha}-induced epithelial barrier destabilization and tissue repair. Am J Physiol Cell Physiol 293: C1843-1850 [Epub 2007, Oct 1843], 2007.
230. Rother RP, Bell L, Hillmen P, and Gladwin MT. The Clinical Sequelae of Intravascular Hemolysis and Extracellular Plasma Hemoglobin: A Novel Mechanism of Human Disease. JAMA 293: 1653-1662, 2005.
231. Sever MS, Vanholder R, and Lameire N. Management of Crush-Related Injuries after Disasters. N Engl J Med 354: 1052-1063, 2006.
232. Moore KP, Holt SG, Patel RP, Svistunenko DA, Zackert W, Goodier D, Reeder BJ, Clozel M, Anand R, Cooper CE, Morrow JD, Wilson MT, Darley-Usmar V, and Roberts II LJ. A Causative Role for Redox Cycling of Myoglobin and Its Inhibition by Alkalinization in the Pathogenesis and Treatment of Rhabdomyolysis-induced Renal Failure. J Biol Chem 273: 31731-31737, 1998.
233. Rosenberger C, Goldfarb M, Shina A, Bachmann S, Frei U, Eckardt K-U, Schrader T, Rosen S, and Heyman SN. Evidence for Sustained Renal Hypoxia and Transient Hypoxia Adaptation in Experimental Rhabdomyolysis-Induced Acute Kidney Injury. Nephrol Dial Transplant doi: 10.1093/ndt/gfm808, 2007.
234. Paller MS. Hemoglobin- and myoglobin-induced acute renal failure in rats: role of iron in nephrotoxicity. Am J Physiol Renal Physiol 255: F539-544, 1988.
235. Shah SV and Walker PD. Evidence suggesting a role for hydroxyl radical in glycerol-induced acute renal failure. Am J Physiol Renal Physiol 255: F438-443, 1988.
236. Andreoli S and McAteer J. Reactive oxygen molecule-mediated injury in endothelial and renal tubular epithelial cells *in vitro*. Kidney Int 38: 785-794, 1990.
237. Tracz MJ, Alam J, and Nath KA. Physiology and Pathophysiology of Heme: Implications for Kidney Disease. J Am Soc Nephrol 18: 414-420, 2007.
238. Iwata M and Zager R. Myoglobin inhibits proliferation of cultured human proximal tubular (HK-2) cells. Kidney Int 50: 796-804, 1996.
239. Zager R and Burkhart K. Differential effects of glutathione and cysteine on Fe2+, Fe3+, H2O2 and myoglobin-induced proximal tubular cell attack. Kidney Int 53: 1661-1672, 1998.
240. Nath K, Grande J, Croatt A, Likely S, Hebbel R, and Enright H. Intracellular targets in heme protein-induced renal injury. Kidney Int 53: 100-111, 1998.

241. Gonzalez-Michaca L, Farrugia G, Croatt AJ, Alam J, and Nath KA. Heme: a determinant of life and death in renal tubular epithelial cells. Am J Physiol Renal Physiol 286: F370-377, 2004.
242. Somers M, Piqueras AI, Strange K, Zeidel ML, Pfaller W, Gawryl M, and Harris HW. Interactions of ultrapure bovine hemoglobin with renal epithelial cells *in vivo* and *in vitro*. Am J Physiol Renal Physiol 273: F38-52, 1997.
243. Hahn H, Huck CW, Rainer M, Najam-ul-Haq M, Bakry R, Abberger T, Jennings P, Pfaller W, and Bonn GK. Analysis of glutathione in supernatants and lysates of a human proximal tubular cell line from perfusion culture upon intoxication with cadmium chloride by HPLC and LC-ESI-MS. Anal Bioanal Chem 388: 1763-1769, 2007.
244. Minuth WW, Dermietzel R, Kloth S, and Hennerkes B. A new method culturing renal cells under permanent superfusion and producing a luminal-basal medium gradient. Kidney Int 41: 215-219, 1992.
245. Gstraunthaler G, Steinmassl D, and Pfaller W. Renal cell cultures: a tool for studying tubular function and nephrotoxicity. Toxicol Lett 53: 1-7, 1990.
246. Gstraunthaler G and Handler JS. Isolation, growth, and characterization of a gluconeogenic strain of renal cells. Am J Physiol 252: C232-238, 1987.
247. Gstraunthaler G. Standardisation in Cell and Tissue Culture - The Need for Specific GLP Guidelines in the Cell Culture Laboratory (Good Cell Culture Practice - GCCP). ALTEX 23 Suppl: 274-277, 2006.
248. Balls M, Coecke S, Bowe G, Davis J, Gstraunthaler G, Hartung T, Hay R, Merten OW, Price A, Schechtman LM, Stacey G, and Stokes W. The Importance of Good Cell Culture Practice (GCCP). ALTEX 23 Suppl: 270-273, 2006.

11

Use of dialytic therapies for poisoning

James F. WINCHESTER, Nikolas HARBORD and Donald A. FEINFELD

Division of Nephrology & Hypertension,
Beth Israel Medical Center, New York, USA

Introduction

The nephrologist is often consulted in poisoning cases. Although management may involve attention to incident renal failure or electrolyte and acid-base disorders, blood purification may also be necessary [1]. The application of dialysis therapies or hemoperfusion to enhance clearance of intoxicants is an essential task for the nephrologist.

Since the first peritoneal dialysis for chlorate poisoning and the earliest hemodialysis for barbiturate intoxication in the early 1950's [2, 3], the indications for dialysis in intoxication have expanded. With the development of high-flux [4] and high-efficiency membranes [5], the introduction of convective modalities (hemofiltration and hemodiafiltration [6]), and the use of continuous treatments (CRRT) [7], dialysis technology has improved. Furthermore, improvements in sorbent technology have advanced hemoperfusion in the treatment of poisoning.

This chapter will outline the principles and use of dialysis and related procedures for the treatment of the poisoned patient. Consideration will be given to criteria for use of dialysis and related modalities, decision among available options, and recent advances. Finally, detailed discussion will follow for specific poisonings for which dialysis therapies are especially effective.

Initial approach

A standard approach is recommended for all poisoned patients and should include triage and general supportive care. Initial assessment should include evaluation and stabilization of the airway, breathing, and circulatory function. Core temperature should be assessed and hypothermia or hyperthermia appropriately corrected. Hypoglycemia should also be addressed if present. A complete physical and neurological examination should follow. Poison-specific antidotes should be administered if available [8].

Further evaluation should include a complete medical history and thorough investigation of the offending drug or chemical. Multiple drugs should be considered, especially with intentional or suicidal ingestions. Appropriate toxicology panels and laboratory studies may help with the diagnosis and identify metabolic or organ-specific dysfunction. The presence of electrolyte or acid-base disorders, elevated serum anion or osmolal gap, and crystalluria may aid diagnosis and treatment.

Previously popular, primary decontamination with gastric lavage, emetics, whole bowel irrigation and cathartics may not be effective in preventing or delaying enteric absorption of poisons [9-12]. In contrast, multiple-dose oral activated charcoal is an effective method of enteric decontamination for a wide variety of ingestions [13]. However, all enteric decontamination procedures are contraindicated in petroleum distillate and caustic ingestions.

Enhanced elimination of some drugs may also be possible through modulation of urinary pH. Among patients with preserved renal function, altering the pH of the tubular fluid can increase drug ionization, trapping the ionized species in the tubule lumen and increasing clearance. Excretion of weakly acidic drugs such as methotrexate, phenobarbital, or salicylate is increased with alkalinization to a urine pH > 7.5 [14]. Alkalinization is recommended for salicylate levels > 50mg/dl (even when alkalemia is present) and is first-line therapy when hemodialyis is not appropriate or available. As alkalinization may cause hypokalemia, alkalemia, or hypocalcemia, electrolytes and both urine and serum pH should be measured frequently. Urinary acidification is not recommended for poisoning with weakly basic drugs such as amphetamines, fenfluramine, phencyclidine (PCP), and quinine, as most patients recover with supportive care [15].

Criteria for extracorporeal removal of poisons

The decision to use an extracorporeal therapy to remove a drug or poison is dependent upon the clinical condition of the patient. Indications include abnormal vital signs suggesting airway, breathing, or circulatory instability; deterioration despite supportive treatment; mental status alteration such as confusion, lethargy, stupor, or coma; and evidence of midbrain dysfunction. Blood purification is indicated when endogenous clearance is impaired (e.g. cardiac, renal or hepatic failure) or is much slower than with extracorporeal clearance. The risk of delayed intervention among poisoned patients with severe co-morbid illness should also be considered. In addition, hemodialyis may be prescribed to rapidly correct any concomitant electrolyte or acid-base disorders. There are discrete indications to use extracorporeal techniques for poisons with delayed toxicity; including methanol and ethylene glycol. These toxins will be discussed in the final section. It should be noted that many investigators report combining different modalities in the treatment of poisoning (discussed below).

With double-lumen intravenous catheters for acute hemodialysis, hemperfusion, and plasma exchange, the most common complications are bleeding, hematomas, catheter failure, risk of infection, central vein thrombosis and stenoses, and rarely, air embolism. Femoral placement is the site associated with the fewest non-infectious complications [16]. Complications of treatment will be discussed below.

Hemodialysis, hemofiltration, and hemodiafiltration

Apparatus and principles

Hemodialysis (HD) is the method of extracorporeal drug removal most commonly used in the treatment of poisoning [1]. The apparatus consists of a blood circuit, an electronic and mechanical device (with pumps and pressure monitors), a dialyzer cartridge (containing hollow permeable fibers), and a dialysate circuit (of purified water with added electrolytes). In practice, a double-lumen catheter is first placed in a central vein.

Blood is then pumped through the dialyzer, countercurrent to the dialysate on the outside of the fibers. Poison clearance occurs by diffusion of the solute across the porous membrane and into the dialysate.

Hemofiltration (HF) is a similar modality whereby solute is removed by convection. The hemofiltration apparatus differs from HD in that no dialysate circuit is present. Rather, blood within the cartridge is subject to pressure across a high-flux (large pore) membrane creating an ultrafiltrate of solutes and water; while cells and large solutes remain in the blood and return to the circulation. Hemofiltration typically requires replacement of fluid and electrolytes lost in the ultrafiltrate.

Hemodiafiltration (HDF) is a modality in which diffusive and convective methods are combined to increase removal of large molecular weight intoxicants. If this 'ultrafiltration dialysis' is conducted at lower blood and dialysate flow rates, convection can provide equivalent total clearance with less hemodynamic perturbance and dialysate wastage.

There are several complications associated with acute dialysis and filtration. Hypotension, if present, may be multifactorial [17] and should be corrected to allow for efficient poison clearance. A syndrome of neurological deterioration (including headache, confusion, seizure and death) several hours after a treatment- known as 'dialysis dysequilibrium'- has been well described. It likely follows the rapid removal of plasma urea and subsequent development of cerebral edema due to impaired or slow egress of cerebral urea and osmosis of water into brain cells [18]. This serious complication will be of greatest concern in a poisoned and uremic patient and may be avoided by lowering the initial dialysis dose (e.g., lowering blood flow rate or shortening treatment time). Finally, hypocalcemic tetany can, in theory, follow the rapid correction of an acidosis with acute hemodialysis. Severely acidotic patients should be dialyzed with a normal or elevated calcium bath.

Factors governing drug removal (Figure 1)

The efficiency of drug removal with hemodialysis is dependent on both drug-related and dialysis-related factors. Drug factors that increase clearance include small molecular size (molecular weight <500 Da), high water solubility, low degree of protein-binding, small volume of distribution (<1 L/kg), and rapid equilibration of plasma and tissue to maintain a concentration gradient [19, 20]. Dialysis provides limited clearance of drugs that are highly lipid soluble, tightly tissue-bound, with large volumes of distribution, and slow plasma equilibration with other body compartments. However, some drugs such as salicylates are reversibly protein-bound [21] and highly dialyzable. Dialysis factors that affect clearance include access type, blood and dialysate flow rates, dialyzer properties (membrane material, surface area, and pore size), and length of treatment. The removal of drugs with larger molecular weights can be improved by increasing the dialyzer membrane surface area, pore size, and length of the treatment.

Molecular weight and protein binding are also the principal drug-related determinants of convective clearance [22]. As the molecular weight of a drug increases, membrane transport is increasingly dependent on convection exceeding diffusion [23]. With high flux membranes, convective modalities (HF and HDF) can remove solutes with molecular weight approaching

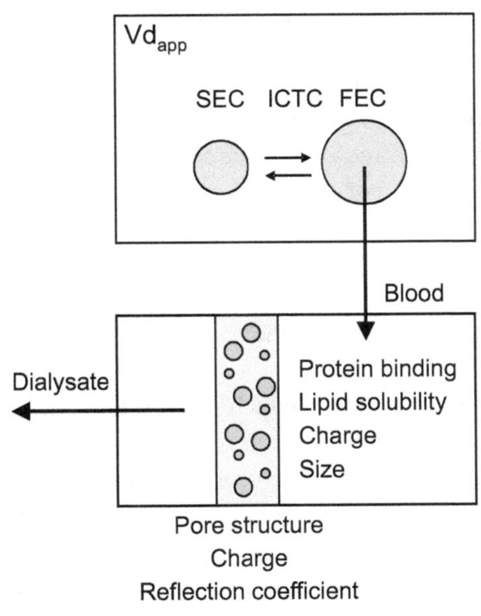

Figure 1. *Mechanisms by which drugs are removed by dialysis (indicated by dialysate) or sorbent hemoperfusion. The pore structure of dialysis membranes and sorbents is the major determinant of chemical/drug size selection.*
Abbreviations:
Vd_{app} = apparent volume of distribution, SEC = slow equilibrating compartment, ICTC = intercompartmental transfer coefficient, FEC = fast equilibrating compartment.

50, 000 Da. Clearance of middle and large molecular weight intoxicants is subsequently more efficient with hemofiltration and hemodiafiltration [24]. The degree of protein binding also influences convective clearance. As expected, increased protein binding impairs membrane transport. The ability of a molecule to pass convectively across a membrane is described by the sieving coefficient (SC). Convective clearance is equal to the sieving coefficient multiplied by the ultrafiltration rate. For molecules that pass completely (an SC of 1) the clearance is equal to the ultrafiltration rate; and increasing the rate will enhance clearance of any intoxicant with a SC greater than 0.

The utility of continuous renal replacement therapies (CRRT) such as continuous venous-venous hemodialysis (CVVHD) in the treatment of poisoning is uncertain. As CRRT provides slower clearance than conventional hemodialysis it may not be appropriate for drug removal in acute intoxications [25]. However, the lower blood flow rates and longer treatment times of continuous modalities may be desirable for vulnerable, hemodynamically unstable, patients who are not candidates for conventional hemodialysis [7]. Unlike hemodialysis, CRRT can give effective clearances in hypotensive patients. If the clinical condition of the patient requires a low intensity treatment that will necessarily decrease diffusive clearance, slow extended dialysis (SLED) or continuous treatment times with additional convective clearance (CVVHF and CVVHDF) can likely provide adequate total drug clearance [24].

Hemodialysis in poisoning

The ingestions for which conventional hemodialysis is most frequently employed are the toxic alcohols (methanol and ethylene glycol), lithium, and salicylates [26] (see section 9). As previously described, effective use of HD in the treatment of poisoning first requires assessment of the patient. In cases where poisoning is strongly suspected, early initiation of dialysis prior to exact knowledge as to the specific poison or the serum concentration may be prudent.

With known intoxicants, an understanding of the pharmacokinetics of the poison can help in the choice of modality and treatment prescription. For instance, drugs with large volumes of distribution such as lithium [27], ethchlorvynol [28], glutethimide [29] may require prolonged (or repeated) treatments to avoid large rebounds in drug concentration and relapse of intoxication [26]. If a poison is eliminated equally well with hemodialysis or hemoperfusion, hemodialysis is preferred since it is less expensive, more readily available, and can address any superimposed metabolic disorder.

Table 1 contains a list of drugs and chemicals removed with hemodialysis.

Hemofiltration and hemodiafiltration in poisoning

Data and clinical experience with hemofiltration and hemodiafiltration for blood purification are limited. This modality has been used to remove large molecule antibiotics such as aminoglycosides and vancomycin [30]. Extended treatments may be of benefit in the removal of drugs with tight tissue binding, large volumes of distribution, and slow equilibration with the plasma such as procainamide [31]. However, there is a report of the failure of continuous hemofiltration to clear the antiarrhythmic drug flecainide [32].

Hemoperfusion

Hemoperfusion is infrequently used to treat acute intoxication. A survey of major New York City hospitals showed two-thirds to be unequipped to perform acute hemoperfusion [33]. However, for some ingestions hemoperfusion provides superior drug clearance, and advances in technology may increase the utility of adsorptive clearance in the treatment of poisoning.

The hemoperfusion apparatus consists of a device (with pumps and alarms) and a blood circuit connecting the patient to and from a cartridge containing a large surface area column. The column containing sorbent particles is primed with saline and then perfused with anticoagulated blood from which solutes with molecular size between 100 and 40, 000 Da are adsorbed. Various types of natural and synthetic sorbents, with different mechanisms of adsorption, have been developed to treat of an array of illnesses. In poisoning, carbon (activated charcoal) columns have greater affinity for water-soluble molecules and are also effective at adsorbing toxins that are highly protein-bound [34]. Polymeric resins have greater affinity for lipid-soluble molecules than charcoal columns. At present, only activated charcoal columns are available in the United States.

Table 1. Drugs and chemicals removed with dialysis.

Antimicrobials/anticancer
cefaclor
cefadroxil
cefamandole
cefazolin
cefixime
cefmenoxime
cefmetazole
(cefonicid)
(cefoperazone)
ceforamide
(cefotaxime)
cefotetan
cefotiam
cefoxitin
cefpirome
cefroxadine
cefsulodin
ceftazidime
(ceftriaxone)
cefuroxime
cephacetrile
cephalexin
cephalothin
(cephapirin)
cephradine
moxalactam
amikacin
dibekacin
fosfomycin
gentamicin
kanamycin
neomycin
netilmicin
sisomicin
streptomycin
tobramycin
bacitracin
colistin
amoxicillin
ampicillin
azlocillin
carbenicillin
clavulinic acid
(cloxacillin)
(dicloxacillin)
(floxacillin)
mecillinam
(mezlocillin)
(methicillin)
(nafcillin)
penicillin
piperacillin
temocillin
ticarcillin
(clindamycin)
(erythromycin)
(azithromycin)
(clarithromycin)
metronidazole
nitrofurantoin
ornidazole
sulfisoxazole
sulfonamides
tetracycline
(doxycycline)
(minocycline)
tinidazole
trimethoprim
aztreonam
cilastatin
imipenem
(chloramphenicol)
(amphotericin)
ciprofloxacin
(enoxacin)
fluroxacin
(norfloxacin)
ofloxacin
isoniazid
(vancomycin)
capreomycin
pas
pyrizinamide
(rifampin)
(cycloserine)
ethambutol
5-fluorocytosine
acyclovir
(amantadine)
didanosine
foscarnet
ganciclovir
(ribavirin)
vidarabine
zidovudine
(pentamidine)
(praziquantel)
(fluconazole)
(itraconazole)
(ketoconazole)
(miconazole)
(chloroquine)
(quinine)
(azathioprine)
bredinin
busulphan
cyclophosphamide
5-fluorouracil
(methotrexate)

Barbiturates
amobarbital
aprobarbital
barbital
butabarbital
cyclobarbital
pentobarbital
phenobarbital
quinalbital
(secobarbital)

Nonbarbiturate hypnotics, sedatives, tranquilizers, anticonvulsants
carbamazepine
atenolol
betaxolol
(bretylium)
clonidine
(calcium channel blockers)
captopril
(diazoxide)
carbromal
chloral hydrate
(chlordiazepoxide)
(diazepam)
(diphenylhydantoin)
(diphenylhydramine)
ethiamate
ethchlorvynol
ethosuximide
gallamine
glutethimide
(heroin)
meprobamate
(methaqualone)
methsuximide
methyprylon
paraldehyde
primidone
valproic acid

Cardiovascular agents
acebutolol
(amiodarone)
amrinone
(digoxin)
enalapril
fosinopril
lisinopril
quinapril
ramipril
(encainide)
(flecainide)
(lidocaine)
metoprolol
methyldopa
(ouabain)
n-acetylprocainamide
nadolol
(pindolol)
practolol
procainamide
propranolol
(quinidine)
(timolol)
sotatol
tocainide

Alcohols
ethanol
ethylene glycol
isopropanol
methanol

Analgesics, antirheumatics
acetaminophen
acetophenetidin
acetylsalicylic acid
colchicine
methylsalicylate
(d-propoxyphene)
salicylic acid

Antidepressants
(amitriptyline)
amphetamines
(imipramine)
isocarboxazid
mao inhibitors
moclobemide
(pargylline)
(phenelzine)
tranylcypromine
(tricyclics)

Solvents, gases
acetone
camphor
carbon monoxide
(carbon tetrachloride)
(eucalyptus oil)
thiols
toluene
trichloroethylene

Plants, animals, herbicides, insecticides
alkyl phosphate
amanitin
demeton sulfoxide
dimethoate
diquat
glufosinate
methylmercury complex
(organophosphates)
paraquat
snake bite
sodium chlorate
potassium chlorate

Miscellaneous
acipimox
allopurinol
aminophylline
aniline
borates
boric acid
(chlorpropamide)
chromic acid
(cimetidine)
dinitro-o-cresol
folic acid
mannitol
methylprednisolone
4-methylpyrazole
sodium citrate
theophylline
thiocyanate
ranitidine

Metals, inorganics
(aluminum)*
arsenic
barium
bromide
(copper)*
(iron)*
(lead)*
lithium
(magnesium)
(mercury)*
potassium
(potassium dichromate)*
phosphate
sodium
strontium
(thallium)*
(tin)
(zinc)

() implies poor removal; () removed with chelating agens*
Modified from Winchester JF. Active methods for detoxification, in Clinical Management of Poisoning and Drug Overdose, Third Edition (editors LM Haddad, MW Shannon, JF Winchester), WB Saunders Co, Philadelphia

Some poisonings for which hemoperfusion is preferred are theophylline [35], lipid-soluble drugs, barbiturates [36], and other types of hypnotics/sedatives/tranquilizers. For example, the extraction ratio [inflow concentration – outflow concentration ÷ inflow concentration] of theophylline is 99 percent with hemoperfusion and only 50 percent with hemodialysis. It should be noted that high extraction ratios may not predict improved clinical outcomes, and there are no controlled studies of hemoperfusion in poisoned patients.

A significant disadvantage to hemoperfusion is that the sorbent column becomes saturated [49]; extraction ratios may progressively decline throughout a treatment. As with other modalities, "rebound" of a drug may occur after redistribution from tissue into the plasma compartment. Adverse effects of hemoperfusion, such as flushing, dyspnea, and thrombocytopenia, are less likely following changes in preparatory methods and adsorbent coating. The use of short intermittent treatments will likely provide improved clearance, less chance for saturation, less "rebound, " and fewer hematologic side effects.

Table 2 lists some drugs and chemicals removed by hemoperfusion.

Table 2. Drugs and chemicals removed with hemoperfusion

Barbiturates	**Antimicrobials/ anticancer**	**Cardiovascular**
amobarbital	(adriamycin)	atenolol
butabarbital	ampicillin	cibenzoline succinate
hexabarbital	carmustine	clonidine
pentobarbital	chloramphenicol	digoxin
phenobarbital	chloroq uine	(diltiazem)
quinalbital	clindamycin	(disopyramide)
secobarbital	dapsone	flecainide
thiopental	doxorubicin	metoprolol
vinalbital	gentamicin	n-acetylprocainamide
	ifosfamide	procainamide
Nonbarbiturate hypnotics, sedatives and tranquilizers	isoniazid	quinidine
carbamazepine	(methotrexate)	
carbromal	pentamidine	**Miscellaneous**
chloral hydrate	thiabendazole	aminophylline
chlorpromazine	(5-fluorouracil)	cimetidine
(diazepam)	vancomycin	(fluoroacetamide)
diphenhydramine		(phencyclidine)
ethchlorvynol	**Antidepressants**	phenols
glutethimide	(amitryptiline)	(podophyllin)
meprobamate	(imipramine)	theophylline
methaqualone	(tricyclics)	
methsuximide		**Solvents, gases**
methyprylon	**Plant and animal toxins, herbicides, insecticides**	carbon tetrachloride
phenytoin	amanitin	ethylene oxide
promazine	chlordane	trichloroethane
promethazine	demeton sulfoxide	xylene
valproic acid	dimethoate	
	diquat	**Metals**
Analgesics, antirheumatic	endosulfan	(aluminum)*
acetaminophen	glufosinate	(iron)*
acetylsalicylic acid	methylparathion	(thallium)
colchicine	nitrostigmine	
d-propoxyphyene	(organophosphates)	
methylsalicylate	phalloidin	
phenylbutazone	polychlorinated biphenyls	
salicylic acid	paraquat	
	parathion	

() implies poor removal; () removed with chelating agens*
Modified from Winchester JF. Active methods for detoxification, in Clinical Management of Poisoning and Drug Overdose, Third Edition (editors LM Haddad, MW Shannon, JF Winchester), WB Saunders Co, Philadelphia.

Plasma exchange and exchange transfusion

Therapeutic plasma exchange (TPE), or plasmapheresis (PP), is an extracorporeal therapy most frequently used in the treatment of hematologic disorders, and autoimmune neuropathies and vasculitides [37]. This modality occasionally is also employed in the treatment of poisoning. The apparatus involves central venous access and a blood circuit between the patient and a pheresis machine. Cytopheresis by centrifugation or filtration then separates the formed elements of blood from plasma. The cells are returned to the patient while the plasma (with the poison) is discarded. Fluid volume is typically replaced with crystalloid, colloid, or fresh frozen plasma (FFP) if clotting factor repletion is necessary.

Plasma exchange is helpful in the removal of large molecular weight substances and highly protein-bound intoxicants. Toxic ingestions of poisonous mushrooms (e.g. amanita phalloides [38, 39]) and snake-bite envenomations [40] have been effectively treated with plasma exchange. Of note, successful plasma exchange following acute cisplatin intoxication [41] has been reported. The total quantity of a drug removed can be calculated by factoring the plasma concentration by the volume of plasma removed.

Exchange blood transfusion, or 'whole blood exchange', involves repeated removal and replacement of an individuals blood with donor whole blood. It is typically employed for neonatal hyperbilirubinemia, sickle cell crisis, or massive hemolysis from drugs or malaria. However, exchange transfusion may be effective if hemolysis (e.g. sodium chlorate poisoning [42]) or methemoglobinemia (e.g. nitrobenzene [43] or dapsone [44]) complicates a poisoning. There is also a report of cyclosporine toxicity treated with whole blood exchange [45].

The use of chelators with extracorporeal therapy

Extracorporeal blood purification therapies do not efficiently remove heavy metals or their salts. Chelating agents can be combined with dialysis modalities and hemoperfusion to improve the clearance of aluminum, iron, and other metals.

Environmental and iatrogenic exposure can result in aluminum overload in dialysis patients and evident osteomalacia, anemia and dementia [46]. Furthermore, acute intoxication with aluminum can lead to encephalopathy and death [47]. Hemoperfusion, hemodialysis, or hemofiltration combined with desferoxamine (DFO) can effectively remove aluminum [48]. Hemodialysis with a high flux dialyzer and hemofiltration are likely superior to charcoal hemoperfusion [48, 49]. In aluminum intoxicated dialysis patients, improvements in osteomalacia [50], anemia [51], and dementia [52] have been demonstrated with chelation.

Iron can also be removed from patients with chronic overload using DFO and hemodialysis [53], hemofiltration [54] or hemoperfusion [55]. Clinicians should be aware that the use of DFO appears to increase the risk of mucormycosis, as chelated DFO-iron complexes may be more available as a growth factor for the rhizopus fungus [56].

There is limited evidence to recommend combined chelation and blood purification therapy for other heavy metal poisonings, such as copper, mercury, arsenic, and thallium. There are case reports, however, outlining several such attempts. Treatment of cupric sulfate ingestion by dimercaprol and penicillamine chelation followed by hemoperfusion and hemodiafiltration has been reported [57]. An interesting case of inorganic mercury poisoning treated with DMPS chelation and continuous venous-venous hemodiafiltration (CVVHDF) was also reported [58]. It should be noted that treatment continued for 14 days with a limited total removal of mercury (<13% of the ingested dose) in the ultrafiltrate; and sieving coefficients were very low and declined from the initial 0.13 [58]. Mercury chelation with dimercaprol has also been combined with plasma exchange for attempted metal removal [59].

The addition of a chelator to peritoneal dialysate was also reportedly successful in augmenting the clearance of heavy metals in PD. In particular, arsenic clearance with DMSA [60], lead clearance with EDTA [61], and aluminum clearance with DFO [62] have been reported.

Peritoneal dialysis

Peritoneal dialysis (PD) is a method of blood purification involving diffusive clearance of solute through the porous peritoneal membrane. Solute passage occurs from blood in the mesenteric vasculature into a volume of fluid dwelling in the abdominal cavity. The apparatus involves a percutaneous catheter placed through the abdominal wall and connected to a disposable tubing 'setup.' In practice, a volume of hypertonic fluid is instilled, allowed to dwell in the abdomen, and later drained. Repeat exchanges allow for cumulative solute clearance. The principal side effects relate to catheter complications and include catheter failure or fluid leakage, and risk of peritonitis or exit site infection [63]. Compared with hemodialysis, PD does not require vascular access or anticoagulation, is biocompatible, easy to perform, and inexpensive. The procedure is also well tolerated in hemodynamically unstable patients. A surgically placed flexible Tenckhoff catheter is probably the ideal catheter for prolonged acute PD, as rigid temporary catheters may require repeated replacement [64].

Isolated reports have suggested that patients with drug poisonings may be treated successfully with peritoneal dialysis. However, the use of PD solely for drug clearance is infrequent and most reports involve treatment of acute kidney injury or hypothermia/hyperthermia resulting from poisoning. Some cases involve PD use in conjunction with hemodialysis and obscure the relative efficacy of this intervention. In short, PD is much less efficient at drug removal than hemodialysis. In fact, there is little evidence to recommend PD as the initial blood purification method among poisoned patients with the hemodynamic stabilty to permit hemodialysis or hemoperfusion. PD may be indicated in remote geographic areas where HD is unavailable.

Another exception is poisoning in children, in whom PD may be a safer initial choice.

There are some poisons for which PD is likely efficacious and clearance in the dialysate demonstrated. Peritoneal clearance is established for the treatment of several ingestions including isopropyl alcohol, methanol, ethylene glycol [65], barbiturates, lithium [66] and salicylates. Of note, bismuth salt overdose (resulting in oliguric acute kidney injury) has been successfully treated with PD in an infant [67]. Chromium and chromic acid may also be cleared by PD [68, 69]. However, clinical effectiveness cannot easily be determined from individual case reports. Examples of peritoneal dialysis failing to clear poisons have also been published. A recent report suggested peritoneal dialysis was ineffective in treating the neurologic effects of baclofen overdose [70]. PD also fails to remove Fab-digoxin complexes [71] or highly-protein bound drugs such as phenytoin and quinine [72, 73].

Specific intoxicants

Lithium

Lithium is an efficacious maintenance treatment for bipolar and major affective disorders [74] and substantially decreases suicide risk among patients with these conditions [75]. Clinical utility as a "mood stabilizer" explains the persistent widespread use of lithium despite a narrow therapeutic range and well-described toxicity. Lithium is available as a carbonate (and infrequently citrate) salt; enteric absorption is complete and rapid (less than 2 hours). Sustained-release preparations of lithium carbonate may delay peak concentration to more than 4 hours post-ingestion [76, 77]. Sodium polystyrene sulfonate resin can reduce the oral bioavailability of recently ingested lithium [78] but may result in hypernatremia and hypokalemia. After absorption, the pharmacokinetics of lithium can be described by a two-compartment model of distribution: the early (alpha) phase is followed by a slower (beta) but wider distribution in almost total body water (> 0.5 liters/kg) [76]. Lithium distribution into and release from the central nervous system (CNS) is delayed due to slow passage across the blood-brain barrier [79]. As such, chronic toxicity and acute-on-therapeutic ingestion result in higher tissue concentrations and greater toxicity [80].

With the exception of very elderly patients, no toxicity is typically evident with blood levels below 1.3 mEq/L. Mild toxicity is apparent with levels between 1.5 to 2.5 mEq/L; moderate toxicity with levels of 2.6 to 3.5 mEq/L; and severe, possibly life-threatening, toxicity with levels greater than 3.6 mEq/L. With increasing blood concentrations, neurologic manifestations of toxicity progress from confusion and lethargy to stupor and coma. Motor symptoms include fine tremor, spasticity and hyperreflexia, dystonia or choreiform movements, cogwheel rigidity, and cerebellar signs. Renal effects include nephrogenic diabetes insipidus, with polyuria and polydipsia; and if water intake is insufficient, hypernatremia. Cardiovascular toxicity may result in hypotension, myocarditis, ST depression, lateral T-wave inversions, heart block, bradycardia, and premature atrial beats. Finally, gastrointestional symptoms include vomiting, diarrhea, and gastroenteritis. Cerebellar sequelae of toxicity may be permanent [81].

For lithium levels less than 2.5 mEq/L, volume expansion with isotonic fluid and diuretics (loop, amiloride, or triamterene) are usually sufficient. Extracorporeal elimination is indicated with clinically apparent toxicity or levels greater than 2.5 mEq/L [80]. Enhanced elimination may also be considered if interval levels plotted on a log-linear scale predict levels above 0.6 mEq/L at 36 hours. Hemodialysis and hemofiltration both effectively eliminate lithium. Although it is highly effective in removing lithium, serum concentrations often rebound after hemodialysis, and repeated or prolonged treatment may be necessary [80]. High-flux dialyzers likely provide clearance superior to conventional dialyzers [82]. Treatment should continue until post-dialysis levels remain below 1 mEq/L.

Salicylates

Salicylates are a subclass of non-steroidal anti-inflammatory drugs (NSAIDs) that includes acetylsalicylic acid (aspirin), salicylic acid, and methyl salicylate. They are commonly administered for analgesic, antipyretic, anti-platelet, or anti-inflammatory effects, but incautious ingestion can result in acute and chronic poisoning. Wintergreen oil, a readily available topical analgesic, contains up to 98% methyl salicylate, and ingestion may be lethal to young children in doses as small as a single teaspoon [83]. Acetylsalicylic acid

(ASA) is absorbed in the jejunum within 90 minutes although delayed gastric emptying from ingested food and enteric coating may prolong absorption time by many hours [84].

Clinical features of acute intoxication may include tinnitus and occasionally deafness [85]. Gastrointestinal irritation and likely decreased production of prostaglandins can cause mucosal ulceration while stimulation of the chemoreceptor trigger zone in the medulla may result in nausea and vomiting. Activation of medullary respiration frequently results in hyperventilation and a respiratory alkalosis. The uncoupling of mitochondrial oxidation can lead to hyperthermia, diaphoresis, flushing, and lactic acidosis. The typical acid-base disorder is respiratory alkalosis or mixed respiratory alkalosis-metabolic acidosis but respiratory acidosis may result from severe toxicity and respiratory collapse. Respiratory alkalosis is uncommon in younger children. Pulmonary edema may be evident. Central nervous system impairment results from cerebral edema, salicylate penetration, and acidemia and may include agitation or lethargy, and seizure.

Gastrointestinal decontamination with multiple dose activated charcoal is recommended for recent acute ingestion [86] and may be most effective (along with cathartics) for enteric coated salicylate preparations. Induction of emesis with ipecac is no longer recommended [86]. Alkalinization of the urine is recommended for patients with preserved renal function who are unsuitable or do not meet criteria for dialysis [87] and may be of benefit during preparation for hemodialysis.

Hemodialysis is recommended for acutely poisoned patients with salicylate levels greater than 80-100mg/dL, acidosis, CNS dysfunction, or pulmonary edema. Chronic intoxication with levels >60 mg/dL is a further indication. While hemoperfusion is also effective, hemodialysis is preferred to correct acid-base and electrolyte disturbances.

Methanol

Ingestion of methanol (or methyl alcohol) has been reported among alcoholics, following exposure to industrial solvents [88], and in counterfeit or bootleg 'wood alcohol' poisoning outbreaks [89]. Poisoning may infrequently follow inhalation or skin absorption. Methanol absorption from an empty stomach follows ingestion by less than 5 minutes, and the volume of distribution is greater than 0.7 L/kg [90]. Only 5% of ingested methanol is typically excreted unchanged in the urine, as methanol undergoes biotransformation in the liver and kidneys: first, to formaldehyde by the action of alcohol dehydrogenase (ADH) and subsequently to formic acid by aldehyde dehydrogenase. These metabolites are principally responsible for methanol toxicity, and enzyme inhibition is instrumental to prevention of toxic sequelae.

Intoxication may present as inebriation and drowsiness similar to ethanol use. Other symptoms are vomiting, diarrhea, delirium and agitation, back and abdominal pain, and clammy skin. Toxic effects usually follow a latent period of several hours. Formate inhibits mitochondrial cytochromes resulting in neurotoxicity. Ocular signs include blurred vision, dilated pupils, and direct retinal toxicity with optic disc hyperemia and ultimately permanent blindness [91]. Cerebral hemorrhagic necrosis has been reported [92]. Severe poisoning may result in Kussmaul respiration, inspiratory apnea, coma, and death. Urine samples may have the characteristic smell of formaldehyde. An elevated serum osmolal gap from methanol will be evident early in presentation but may disappear after approximately 12 hours. At this time, an elevated anion gap metabolic acidosis from retained formate may be evident.

Treatment begins with supportive care, and enteric suction is useful only if recent ingestion or retained gastric methanol is suspected. To prevent formation of toxic metabolites, fomepizole (4-methyl pyrazole or 4-MP) or ethanol to inhibit ADH should be administered. Fomepizole is preferred over ethanol if available [93]. It is well tolerated and may improve initial visual defects [94]. Mild methanol poisoning with levels below 20 mg/dL can likely be treated with fomepizole only and bicarbonate; however a methanol elimination half-life of over 50 hours with fomepizole requires prolonged infusion and monitoring [95]. Folic or folinic acid should be administered to promote conversion of formate to water and carbon dioxide [96].

Hemodialysis corrects any metabolic acidosis while removing methanol and formate [97]; and should be considered with evidence of organ toxicity, presence of acidosis, and methanol levels greater than 50 mg/dL. Fomepizole is dialyzable (see next section). Closure of the osmolal gap correlates with methanol removal and can be followed if methanol levels are unavailable or delayed [98]. Rebound of methanol concentration may follow dialysis and treatment should continue until levels fall and remain below 20 mg/dL.

Ethylene glycol

Ethylene glycol is another alcohol with fatal toxic potential. Ingestion is most frequently related to suicide attempts and misguided alcohol abuse. Ethylene glycol is available as an industrial solvent or as 'antifreeze' fluid for car radiators and de-icing solutions. It is commonly mixed with sodium fluorescein dye for identification but may be ingested by children and pets attracted to its sweet taste. Peak levels of ethylene glycol have been demonstrated in blood by 1-hour post-ingestion [99]. Ethylene glycol alcohol undergoes biotransformation into toxic metabolites more rapidly than with methanol [100]. Alcohol dehydrogenase (ADH) converts ethylene glycol to glycoaldehyde, and subsequent metabolism yields glycolic acid, glyoxylic acid, and oxalic acid [101].

Intoxication may present with stuporous inebriation (without the odor of ethanol) from 30 minutes to 12 hours post ingestion; caused by ethylene glycol and glycoaldehyde. After 12 to 14 hours post-ingestion, the deposition of birefringent calcium oxalate crystals leads to characteristic tissue destruction. Neurological symptoms include focal seizures, cranial nerve paralyses, and coma following cerebral edema and crystal deposition in meningeal blood vessels [102]. Liver deposition may result in acute toxic hepatitis. Congestive heart failure with pulmonary edema and circulatory collapse may occur in severe poisoning without demonstrable myocardial crystal deposition. A late phase of toxicity involves oliguric acute kidney injury with tubular epithelial vacuolization and interstitial inflammation following renal tubular oxalate deposition [103, 104].

Early laboratory findings include a high serum osmolal gap from the ethylene glycol. An extreme metabolic acidosis with greatly elevated anion gap follows, principally from glycolic acid [100]. Hypocalcemia and hyperkalemia may be evident and urinalysis may reveal calcium oxalate crystalluria, hematuria, and proteinuria.

Treatment should include correction of metabolic acidosis, inhibition of ethylene glycol metabolism; and if necessary, extracorporeal elimination of the parent alcohol and metabolites. Acidemia likely increases tissue penetration of toxic metabolites and hinders renal clearance. Although evidence is lacking, bicarbonate administration should be given to correct acidemia. Although more expensive, fomepizole is preferred to ethanol for ADH inhibition due to proven efficacy, predictable pharmacokinetics, and lack of adverse effects [105]. Inhibition of ADH with fomepizole prevents formation of toxic metabolites and renal injury, and improves acid-base status [106]. Elimination half-life of ethylene glycol with fomepizole in patients with preserved renal function is approximately 20 hours [107]. Pyridoxine and thiamine should be administered to promote glyoxylic acid conversion less toxic metabolites than oxalate [108].

Hemodialysis removes ethylene glycol and metabolites, and further corrects metabolic acidosis by administering bicarbonate. Dialysis is indicated when there is evidence of organ toxicity or acidosis; and although not evidence-based, when ethylene glycol levels are greater than 50mg/dL. Again, levels should be monitored to avoid rebound and treatment should continue until levels remain below 20 mg/dL. During hemodialysis, the fomepizole dosing interval should be decreased to every four hours because the drug is dialyzable.

References

1. Watson WA, Litovitz TL, Rodgers Jr. GC, et al. 2004 Annual report of the American Association of Poison Control Centers Toxic Exposure Surveillance System. *Am J Emerg Med.* 2005;23:589-666
2. Linquette, Goudemande, Warot, et al. Acute poisoning by sodium chlorate; anuria; exchange transfusions and peritoneal dialysis. *Echo Med Nord.* 1950;21:269-276.
3. Brown IA. The use of hemodialysis in the treatment of barbiturate intoxication *Minn Med.* 1954;37:650-652
4. Peces R, Fernandez EJ, Regidor D, et al. Treatment of acute lithium intoxication with high-flux haemodialysis membranes. *Nefrologia.* 2006;26:372-378
5. Palmer BF. Effectiveness of hemodialysis in the extracorporeal therapy of phenobarbital overdose. *Am J Kidney Dis.* 2000;36:640-643
6. Wrathall G, Sinclair R, Moore A, et al. Three case reports of the use of haemodiafiltration in the treatment of salicylate overdose. *Hum Exp Toxicol.* 2001;20:491-495
7. Feinfeld DA, Rosenberg JW, Winchester JF. Three controversial issues in extracorporeal toxin removal. *Semin Dial.* 2006;19:358-362
8. Betten DP, Vohra RB, Cook MD, et al. Antidote use in the critically ill poisoned patient.*J Intensive Care Med.* 2006;21:255-277
9 Vale JA, Kulig K. Position paper: gastric lavage. *J Toxicol Clin Toxicol.* 2004;42:933-943
10. Position paper: Ipecac syrup. *J Toxicol Clin Toxicol.* 2004;42:133-143
11. Position paper: whole bowel irrigation. *J Toxicol Clin Toxicol.* 2004;42:843-854
12. Position paper: cathartics. *J Toxicol Clin Toxico*l. 2004;42:243-253
13. Chyka PA, Seger D, Krenzelok EP, et al. Position paper: Single-dose activated charcoal. *Clin Toxicol (Phila).* 2005;43:61-87
14. Proudfoot AT, Krenzelok EP, Vale JA, et al. Position Paper on urine alkalinization. *J Toxicol Clin Toxicol.* 2004;42:1-26
15. Garrettson LK; Geller RJ. Acid and alkaline diuresis. When are they of value in the treatment of poisoning? *Drug Saf.* 1990;5:220-232
16. El Minshawy O, Abd El Aziz T, Abd El Ghani H. Evaluation of vascular access complications in acute and chronic hemodialysis. *J Vasc Access.* 2004;5:76-82
17. Sulowicz W, Radziszewski A. Pathogenesis and treatment of dialysis hypotension. *Kidney Int Suppl.* 2006;104:S36-39
18. Silver SM. Cerebral edema after rapid dialysis is not caused by an increase in brain organic osmolytes. *J Am Soc Nephrol.* 1995;6:1600-1606
19 Maher JF.Principles of dialysis and dialysis of drugs. *Am J Med.* 1977;62:475
20. Gibson TP, Atkinson AI. Effect of changes in intercompartment rate constants on drug removal during hemoperfusion. *J Pharm Sci.* 1978; 67:1178
21. Furst DE, Tozer TN, Melmon KL. Salicylate clearance, the resultant of protein binding and metabolism. *Clin Pharmacol Ther.* 1979;26:380-389
22. Vincent HH, Vos MC, Akcahuseyin AE, et al. Drug clearance by continuous haemodiafiltration. Analysis of sieving coefficients and mass transfer coefficients of diffusion. *Blood Purif.* 1993;11:99-107
23. Depner T, Garred L. Solute transport mechanisms in dialysis. in *Replacement of Renal Function by Dialysis*, 5th edition, editors Horl W, Koch KM, Lindsay RM, Ronco C, Winchester JF. Kluwer Academic Publishers, Dordrecht, 2004:73-93
24. Liao Z, Zhang W, Hardy PA. Kinetic comparison of different acute dialysis therapies. *Artif Organs.* 2003;27:802-807
25. Goodman JW, Goldfarb DS. The role of continuous renal replacement therapy in the treatment of poisoning. *Semin Dial.* 2006;19:402-407
26. Pond SM. Extracorporeal techniques in the treatment of poisoned patients. *Med J Aust.* 1991;154:617-622
27. Jaeger A, Sauder P, Kopferschmitt J. When should dialysis be performed in lithium poisoning? A kinetic study in 14 cases of lithium poisoning. *J Toxicol Clin Toxicol.* 1993;31:429-447
28. Winek CL, Wahba WW, Winek CL Jr. Body distribution of ethchlorvynol. *J Forensic Sci.* 1989;34:687-690
29. Thompson TA, Vermeulen JD, Wagner WE Jr., et al. Aminoglutethimide bioavailability, pharmacokinetics, and binding to blood constituents. *J Pharm Sci.* 1981;70:1040-1043
30. Akil IO, Mir S. Hemodiafiltration for vancomycin overdose in a patient with end-stage renal failure. *Pediatr Nephrol.* 2001;16:1019-1021
31. Domoto DT, Brown WW, Bruggensmith P. Removal of toxic levels of N-acetylprocainamide with continuous arteriovenous hemofiltration or continuous arteriovenous hemodiafiltration. *Ann Intern Med.* 1987;106:550-552
32. Borgeat A, Biollaz J, Freymond B, et al. Hemofiltration clearance of flecainide in a patient with acute renal failure. *Intensive Care Med.* 1988;14:236-237

33 Shalkham AS, Kirrane BM, Hoffman RS, et al. The availability and use of charcoal hemoperfusion in the treatment of poisoned patients. *Am J Kidney Dis.* 2006;48:239-241
34. Kawasaki CI, Nishi R, Uekihara S, et al. How tightly can a drug be bound to a protein and still be removable by charcoal hemoperfusion in overdose cases? *Clin Toxicol.* 2005;43:95-99
35. Shannon MW. Comparative efficacy of hemodialysis and hemoperfusion in severe theophylline intoxication. *Acad Emerg Med.* 1997;4:674-678
36. Bouma AW, van Dam B, Meynaar IA, et al. Accelerated elimination using hemoperfusion in a patient with phenobarbital intoxication. *Ned Tijdschr Geneeskd.* 2004;148:1642-1645
37. Yeo FE, Bohen EM, Yuan CM, et al. Therapeutic plasma exchange as a nephrological procedure: a single-center experience. *J Clin Apher.* 2005;20:208-216
38. Jander S, Bischoff J. Treatment of Amanita phalloides poisoning: I. Retrospective evaluation of plasmapheresis in 21 patients. *Ther Apher.* 2000;4:303-307
39. Jander S, Bischoff J, Woodcock BG. Plasmapheresis in the treatment of Amanita phalloides poisoning: II. A review and recommendations.*Ther Apher.* 2000;4:308-312
40. Yildirim C, Bayraktaroglu Z, Gunay N, et al. The use of therapeutic plasmapheresis in the treatment of poisoned and snake bite victims: an academic emergency department's experiences. *J Clin Apher.* 2006;21:219-223
41. Choi JH, Oh JC, Kim KH, et al: Successful treatment of cisplatin overdose with plasma exchange. *Yonsey Med J.* 2002;43:128-132
42. Steffen C, Seitz R. Severe chlorate poisoning: report of a case. *Arch Toxicol.* 1981;48:281-288
43. Martinez MA, Ballesteros S, Almarza E, et al. Acute nitrobenzene poisoning with severe associated methemoglobinemia: identification in whole blood by GC-FID and GC-MS. *J Anal Toxicol.* 2003;27:221-225
44. Southgate HJ, Masterson R. Lessons to be learned: a case study approach: prolonged methaemoglobinaemia due to inadvertent dapsone poisoning; treatment with methylene blue and exchange transfusion. *J R Soc Health.* 1999;119:52-55
45. Kwon SU, Lim SH, Rhee I, et al: Successful whole blood exchange by apheresis in a patient with acute cyclosporine intoxication without long-term sequelae. J *Heart Lung Transplant.* 2006;25:483-485
46. Becaria A, Campbell A, Bondy SC, et al. Aluminum as a toxicant. *Toxicol Ind Health.* 2002;18:309-320
47. Berend K, van der Voet G, Boer WH. Acute aluminum encephalopathy in a dialysis center caused by a cement mortar water distribution pipe. *Kidney Int.* 2001;59:746-753
48. Weiss LG, Danielson BG, Fellstrom B, et al. Aluminum removal with hemodialysis, hemofiltration and charcoal hemoperfusion in uremic patients after desferrioxamine infusion. A comparison of efficiency. *Nephron.* 1989;51:325-329
49. Bouchard NC, Malostovker I, Harbord N, et al. Acute aluminum encephalopathy: aluminum extraction with high flux hemodialysis is superior to charcoal hemoperfusion (abstract). *Clin Toxicol.* 2005;43:677-678
50. Rapoport J, Chaimovitz C, Abulfil A, et al. Aluminum-related osteomalacia: clinical and histological improvement following treatment with desferrioxamine (DFO). *Isr J Med Sci.* 1987;23:1242-1246
51. Bia MJ, Cooper K, Schnall S, et al. Aluminum induced anemia: pathogenesis and treatment in patients on chronic hemodialysis. *Kidney Int.* 1989;36:852-858
52. McCarthy JT, Milliner DS, Johnson WJ, et al. Clinical experience with desferrioxamine in dialysis patients with aluminium toxicity. *Q J Med.* 1990;74:257-276
53. Baker LR, Barnett MD, Brozovic B, et al. Hemosiderosis in a patient on regular hemodialysis: treatment by desferrioxamine. *Clin Nephrol.* 1976;6:326-328.
54. McCarthy JT, Libertin CR, Mitchell JC 3rd, et al. Hemosiderosis in a dialysis patient: treatment with hemofiltration and deferoxamine chelation therapy. *Mayo Clin Proc.* 1982;57:439-441
55. Chang TM, Barre P. Effect of desferrioxamine on removal of aluminum and iron by coated charcoal haemoperfusion and haemodialysis. *Lancet.* 1983;2:1051-1053
56. Boelaert JR, Van Cutsem J, de Locht M, et al. Deferoxamine augments growth and pathogenicity of Rhizopus, while hydroxypyridinone chelators have no effect. *Kidney Int.* 1994;45:667-671
57. Takeda T, Yukioka T, Shimazaki S. Cupric sulfate intoxication with rhabdomyolysis, treated with chelating agents and blood purification.*Intern Med.* 2000;39:253-255
58. Dargan PI, Giles LJ, Wallace CI, et al. Case report: severe mercuric sulphate poisoning treated with 2, 3-dimercaptopropane-1-sulphonate and haemodiafiltration. *Crit Care.* 2003;7:R1-6.
59. Yoshida M, Satoh H, Igarashi M, et al. Acute mercury poisoning by intentional ingestion of mercuric chloride. *Tohoku J Exp Med.* 1997;182:347-352
60. Hantson P, Haufroid V, Buchet JP, et al. Acute arsenic poisoning treated by intravenous dimercaptosuccinic acid (DMSA) and combined extrarenal epuration techniques. *J Toxicol Clin Toxicol.* 2003;41:1-6

61. Roger SD, Crimmins D, Yiannikis C, et al. Lead intoxication in an anuric patient: management by intraperitoneal EDTA. *Aust N Z J Med.* 1990;20:814-817
62. Mactier RA. Aluminum and deferoxamine kinetics in CAPD. *Adv Perit Dial.* 1991;7:26-29
63. Rinaldi S, Sera F, Verrina E, et al. Chronic peritoneal dialysis catheters in children: a fifteen-year experience of the Italian Registry of Pediatric Chronic Peritoneal Dialysis. *Perit Dial Int.* 2004;24:481-486
64. Wong SN, Geary DF. Comparison of temporary and permanent catheters for acute peritoneal dialysis. *Arch Dis Child.*1988;63:827-831
65. Vale JA, Prior JG, O'Hare JP, et al. Treatment of ethylene glycol poisoning with peritoneal dialysis. *Br Med J (Clin Res Ed).* 1982;284:557
66. Islek I, Uysal S, Gok F, et al. Reversible nephrotoxicity after overdose of colloidal bismuth subcitrate. *Pediatr Nephrol.* 2001;16:510-514
67. Hansen HE, Amdisen A. Lithium intoxication. (Report of 23 cases and review of 100 cases from the literature). *Q J Med.* 1978;47:123-144.
68. Schiffl H, Weidmann P, Weiss M, et al. Dialysis treatment of acute chromium intoxication and comparative efficacy of peritoneal versus hemodialysis in chromium removal. *Miner Electrolyte Metab.* 1982;7:28-35
69. Kobayashi T, Unishi G, Matsuzaki S, et al. A survival case of acute chromic acid poisoning treated by peritoneal dialysis. *Nippon Jinzo Gakkai Shi.* 1984;26:1259-1261
70. Lois F, Wallemacq P, de Tourtchanninoff M, et al. Prolonged unconsciousness in a patient on automated peritoneal dialysis. *Eur J Emerg Med.* 2006;13:361-363
71. Berkovitch M, Akilesh MR. Acute digoxin overdose in a newborn with renal failure: use of digoxin immune Fab and peritoneal dialysis. *Ther Drug Monit.* 1994;16:531-533
72. Czajka PA, Anderson WH, Christoph RA, et al. A pharmacokinetic evaluation of peritoneal dialysis for phenytoin intoxication. *J Clin Pharmacol.* 1980;20:565-569
73. Sabto JK, Pierce RM, West RH, et al. Hemodialysis, peritoneal dialysis, plasmapheresis and forced diuresis for the treatment of quinine overdose. *Clin Nephrol.* 1981;16:264-268
74. Burgess S, Geddes J, Hawton K, et al. Lithium for maintenance treatment of mood disorders. *Cochrane Database Syst Rev.* 2001;(3): CD003013.
75. Baldessarini RJ, Tondo L, Davis P, et al. Decreased risk of suicides and attempts during long-term lithium treatment: a meta-analytic review. *Bipolar Disord.* 2006;8:625-639
76. Arancibia A, Corvalan F, Mella F, et al. Absorption and disposition kinetics of lithium carbonate following administration of conventional and controlled release formulations. *Int J Clin Pharmacol Ther Toxicol.* 1986;24:240-245
77. Heim W, Oelschlager H, Kreuter J, et al. Liberation of lithium from sustained release preparations. A comparison of seven registered brands. *Pharmacopsychiatry.* 1994;27:27-31
78. Belanger DR, Tierney MG, Dickinson G. Effect of sodium polystyrene sulfonate on lithium bioavailability. Ann Emerg Med. 1992 Nov; 21(11):1312-1315
79. Plenge P, Stensgaard A, Jensen HV, et al. 24-hour lithium concentration in human brain studied by Li-7 magnetic resonance spectroscopy. *Biol Psychiatry.* 1994;36:511-516
80. Waring WS. Management of lithium toxicity. *Toxicol Rev.* 2006;25:221-230
81. Niethammer M, Ford B. Permanent lithium-induced cerebellar toxicity: Three cases and review of literature. *Mov Disord.* 2007;22:570-573
82. Peces R, Fernandez EJ, Regidor D, et al. Treatment of acute lithium intoxication with high-flux haemodialysis membranes. *Nefrologia.* 2006;26:372-378
83. Davis JE. Are one or two dangerous? Methyl salicylate exposure in toddlers. *J Emerg Med.* 2007;32:63-69
84. Bochner F, Somogyi AA, Wilson KM. Bioinequivalence of four 100 mg oral aspirin formulations in healthy volunteers. *Clin Pharmacokinet.* 1991;21:394-399
85. Wecker H, Laubert A. Reversible hearing loss in acute salicylate intoxication. *HNO.* 2004;52:347-351
86. Chyka PA, Erdman AR, Christianson G, et al. Salicylate poisoning: an evidence-based consensus guideline for out-of-hospital management. *Clin Toxicol (Phila).* 2007;45:95-131
87. Proudfoot AT, Krenzelok EP, Vale JA. Position Paper on urine alkalinization. *J Toxicol Clin Toxicol.* 2004;42:1-26
88. Davis LE, Hudson D, Benson BE, et al. Methanol poisoning exposures in the United States: 1993-1998. *J Toxicol Clin Toxicol.* 2002;40:499-505
89. Paasma R, Hovda KE, Tikkerberi A, et al. Methanol mass poisoning in Estonia: outbreak in 154 patients. *Clin Toxicol (Phila).* 2007;45:152-157
90. Graw M, Haffner HT, Althaus L, et al. Invasion and distribution of methanol. *Arch Toxicol.* 2000;74:313-321

91. Onder F, Ilker S, Kansu T, et al. Acute blindness and putaminal necrosis in methanol intoxication. *Int Ophthalmol.* 1998-1999;22:81-84
92. Hsu HH, Chen CY, Chen FH, et al. Optic atrophy and cerebral infarcts caused by methanol intoxication: MRI. *Neuroradiology.* 1997;39:192-194
93. Megarbane B, Borron SW, Faud FJ. Current recommendations for treatment of severe toxic alcohol poisonings. *Intensive Care Med.* 2005;31:189-195
94. Brent J, McMartin K, Phillips S, et al. Fomepizole for the treatment of methanol poisoning. *N Engl J Med.* 2001;344:424-429
95. Hovda KE, Andersson KS, Urdal P, et al. Methanol and formate kinetics during treatment with fomepizole. *Clin Toxicol (Phila).* 2005;43:221-227
96. Moore DF, Bentley AM, Dawling S, et al. Folinic acid and enhanced renal elimination in formic acid intoxication. *J Toxicol Clin Toxicol.* 1994;32:199-204
97. Hantson P, Haufroid V, et al. Formate kinetics in methanol poisoning. *Hum Exp Toxicol.* 2005;24:55-59
98. Hunderi OH, Hovda KE, Jacobsen D. Use of the osmolal gap to guide the start and duration of dialysis in methanol poisoning. *Scand J Urol Nephrol.* 2006;40:70-74
99. Vasavada N, Williams C, Hellman RN, et al. Ethylene glycol intoxication: case report and pharmacokinetic perspectives. *Pharmacotherapy.* 2003;23:1652-1658
100. Jacobsen D, McMartin KE. Methanol and ethylene glycol poisonings. Mechanism of toxicity, clinical course, diagnosis and treatment. *Med Toxicol.* 1986;1:309-334
101. Leth PM, Gregersen M. Ethylene glycol poisoning. *Forensic Sci Int.* 2005;155:179-184
102. Froberg K, Dorion RP, McMartin KE. The role of calcium oxalate crystal deposition in cerebral vessels during ethylene glycol poisoning. *Clin Toxicol (Phila).* 2006;44:315-358
103. Stokes MB. Acute oxalate nephropathy due to ethylene glycol ingestion. *Kidney Int.* 2006;69:203
104. Meier M, Nitschke M, Perras B, et al. Ethylene glycol intoxication and xylitol infusion--metabolic steps of oxalate-induced acute renal failure. *Clin Nephrol.* 2005;63:225-258
105. Barceloux DG, Krenzelok EP, Olson K, et al. American Academy of Clinical Toxicology Practice Guidelines on the Treatment of Ethylene Glycol Poisoning. Ad Hoc Committee. *J Toxicol Clin Toxicol.* 1999;37:537-560
106. Brent J, McMartin K, Phillips S, et al. Fomepizole for the treatment of ethylene glycol poisoning. Methylpyrazole for Toxic Alcohols Study Group. *N Engl J Med.* 1999;340:832-838
107. Sivilotti ML, Burns MJ, McMartin KE, et al. Toxicokinetics of ethylene glycol during fomepizole therapy: implications for management. For the Methylpyrazole for Toxic Alcohols Study Group. *Ann Emerg Med.* 2000;36:114-125
108. Lheureux P, Penaloza A, Gris, et al. Pyridoxine in clinical toxicology: a review. *Eur J Emerg Med.* 2005;12:78-85

B

SPECIFIC DRUGS

12

Aminoglycosides and vancomycin

Brian S. DECKER and Bruce A. MOLITORIS

Indiana University School of Medicine, Indianapolis, USA

Aminoglycoside nephrotoxicity

Introduction

Since the discovery of streptomycin in 1944, aminoglycosides have endured as indispensable agents in the antimicrobial armamentarium. This is despite their well described potential for serious nephrotoxicity and otoxicity and the emergence of other classes of antibiotics with similar antibacterial spectrums. The major aminoglycoside antibiotics in clinical use worldwide include gentamicin, tobramycin, amikacin, netilmicin, neomycin, isepamicin and arbekacin. These agents remain in clinical use against gram negative infections largely because of their dependable efficacy. Several attributes render these antibiotics particularly effective. First, aminoglycosides exhibit a concentration-dependent bactericidal activity [1, 2]. Unlike the β-lactams, the bactericidal activity of aminoglycosides depends more on their concentration rather than the duration of antimicrobial exposure. Further, the bactericidal efficacy increases with increasing aminoglycoside concentration. Aminoglycosides also exhibit a post-antibiotic effect meaning they continue to kill bacteria even after the aminoglycoside concentration has fallen below the bacterial minimum inhibitory concentration. Another useful attribute of aminoglycosides is their synergism with antibiotics that inhibit bacterial cell wall biosynthesis, such as β-lactams and vancomycin. Finally, aminoglycosides have relatively predictable pharmacokinetic characteristics that allow them to be dosed to minimize their inherent toxicities. However, despite this predictable pharmacokinetic profile, aminoglycosides always retain their potential for serious toxicity. Moreover, aminoglycoside toxicity can occur despite the maintenance of serum levels in the therapeutic range. The purpose of this section is to describe the nephrotoxicity associated with the clinical use of aminoglycoside antibiotics.

Epidemiology of aminoglycoside nephrotoxicity

Numerous individual studies and meta-analyses have shown the incidence of aminoglycoside nephrotoxicity is quite variable with a reported range of from 0 to 50% [3-24]. There are several explanations for this marked variability in incidence. First, the various studies differed in the parameters used to define nephrotoxicity. Some studies used increases of serum creatinine as the threshold for nephrotoxicity; others used a percentage increase of serum creatinine from a baseline value as the guide. In addition, not all of the studies used the same aminoglycosides or treated similar patient populations. This is significant since aminoglycosides differ in their nephrotoxic potential. Smith et al. noted renal impairment in 26% of patients who received gentamicin, but only 12% of patients who received tobramycin [11]. Not surprisingly, an elderly cohort of patients with extensive co-morbid disease or the critically ill had a much greater incidence of nephrotoxicity as compared to a cohort of healthier subjects [19, 20, 95]. The studies reviewed also differed in the type of infections treated and the duration of aminoglycoside therapy administered [4]. Finally, whether a study utilized a conventional pharmacokinetic monitoring program or a once daily aminoglycoside (ODA) regimen was important since ODA programs may attenuate the risk of nephrotoxicity [3]. Despite this variability, however, an overall incidence of nephrotoxicity of from 5 to 10% of patient courses has been reported in the majority of studies [19, 95].

Risk factors for aminoglycoside nephrotoxicity

Several risk factors can predispose a patient to nephrotoxicity after an aminoglycoside is administered. Aminoglycosides differ in their inherent nephrotoxic potential, so the choice of a specific agent can be clinically important. This inherent aminoglycoside nephrotoxicity appears to be related to the degree to which an aminoglycoside concentrates in the renal cortex after administration. Streptomycin does not concentrate in the renal cortex and is the least nephrotoxic aminoglycoside. Conversely, neomycin concentrates to the greatest degree in the renal cortex and is the most nephrotoxic [2]. As a result, neomycin is not used as a systemic agent. Differences in the nephrotoxicity of gentamicin and tobramycin remain controversial. However, one early study demonstrated less nephrotoxicity with tobramycin as compared to gentamicin [11]. In contrast, amikacin appears to have similar nephrotoxic potential as gentamicin [17]. Netilmicin has been shown to have less nephrotoxic potential than tobramycin [26]. When considered as a group, gentamicin appears to have the greatest nephrotoxic potential followed in decreasing order of nephrotoxicity by tobramycin, amikacin and netilmicin [30].

Other aminoglycoside-related factors that have been shown to predispose patients to nephrotoxicity include prolonged duration of therapy and elevated serum aminoglycoside levels [9, 20, 21, 22, 29]. Studies have shown that patients treated with aminoglycosides for longer than one week have a greater incidence of nephrotoxicity. In one study, 3.9% of elderly patients treated for seven or fewer days developed nephrotoxicity compared to 30% of patients treated for 8 to 14 days and 50% treated for more than 14 days [22]. Both elevated peak and serum trough levels have been shown to increase the incidence of nephrotoxicity. Koo et al demonstrated that a peak serum level of greater than 12mg/dL increased the incidence of nephrotoxicity in elderly patients [9]. A trough greater than 2.5 mg/dL was also shown to be an important cause of nephrotoxicity in another study of elderly patients [21].

Patient-related factors can have a significant impact on the risk of aminoglycoside nephrotoxicity. Bertino et al. observed that advanced age, ascites, male gender, hypoalbuminemia and leukemia were significant risk factors for aminoglycoside nephrotoxicity [20]. However, in another study female gender was shown to be a risk factor for nephrotoxicity [28]. Medications used concurrently with aminoglycosides can contribute greatly to nephrotoxic risk. Clindamycin, vancomycin, piperacillin, cephalosporins and angiotensin converting enzyme inhibitors have all been implicated as risk factors for nephrotoxicity [20, 23]. Not surprisingly, specific nephrotoxic agents such as cyclosporine, intravenous iodinated contrast, furosemide, cisplatinum increase the risk for aminoglycoside nephrotoxicity [28,30]. Co-morbid diseases also are an important risk factor for aminoglycoside nephrotoxicity. Researchers have demonstrated that co-morbid diseases such as diabetes mellitus and pneumonia increase the risk for nephrotoxicity [21,23]. In addition, aminoglycosides given to hypotensive or intravascularly depleted patients confers an increased risk; in one study it had an additive effect [4, 29]. Not unexpectedly, patients with baseline chronic kidney disease have been shown to be at increased risk for nephrotoxicity with aminoglycosides [28]. Interestingly, other researchers found that patients with high initial creatinine clearances were at increased risk for nephrotoxicity [4, 28, 29]. This may be secondary to the increased ability of normally functioning kidneys to concentrate the aminoglycoside in the renal cortex as compared to lesser functioning kidneys. Finally, electrolyte abnormalities such as hypokalemia, hypomagnesemia and hypercalcemia have been shown to increase the risk of aminoglycoside nephrotoxicity [30].

Aminoglycoside pharmacokinetics

The pharmacokinetics of aminoglycosides ascribes to an interrelated two or three compartment model. The three compartment model comprises three phases, an α or distributive phase, and two elimination phases, β and γ. After administration of an intravenous dose in the three compartment model, the aminoglycoside first enters the α or distributive phase [33]. During this initial phase, the aminoglycoside is transported from the vascular to the extracellular compartment. The β or elimination phase represents the elimination of the aminoglycoside from the plasma and extravascular compartments [33]. The third or γ phase corresponds to the protracted elimination of the aminoglycoside from the deep-tissue compartment. The two compartment pharmacokinetic approach omits the γ slow elimination phase from its model. Though the two and three compartment model provide a more accurate description of aminoglycoside pharmacokinetics, a one compartment model is used clinically for reasons of ease and practicality. In clinical practice, accurate pharmacokinetic dosing of aminoglycosides can be achieved if the aminoglycoside serum concentration is obtained after the α or distribution phase [34].

Absorption

The aminoglycosides are highly polar cations and poorly absorbed from the gastrointestinal tract. A scant 0.3 to 1.5% of an orally or rectally administered dose appears in the urine [31, 2, 32]. However, there are case reports of aminoglycoside toxicity in patients with poor renal function on long-term oral or rectal aminoglycoside therapy. Similarly, patients with gastrointestinal diseases such as ulcers and inflammatory bowel disease have demonstrated increased absorption of aminoglycosides from the gastrointestinal tract. Though absorption is minimal on intact skin, applying aminoglycosides transdermally for extended periods can result in toxicity when given to patients with renal insufficiency and cutaneous ulcers, burn injuries or large wounds. In contrast, owing to robust blood perfusion peritoneal absorption of aminoglycosides is rapid and complete. Finally, diffusion of aminoglycosides into pleural and synovial fluid is relatively slow by comparison. With repeated administrations, however, aminoglycoside concentrations in pleural and synovial fluid can approximate the plasma concentration.

The most common route of administration of aminoglycosides is intravenous, though aminoglycosides can be given intramuscularly. After an intravenous infusion of an aminoglycoside, the peak serum concentration occurs after 30 minutes. Peak serum concentrations for intramuscular injections occur after 30 to 90 minutes. An intravenous dose of 1.5 mg/kg of gentamicin, tobramycin or netilmicin will result in a peak serum concentration of from 4 to 12 ug/ml; a 7.5 mg/kg dose of amikacin will produce a peak serum concentration of 20 to 35 ug/ml.

Distribution

As a result of their high cationic polarity, aminoglycosides do not distribute intracellularly and concentrations in secretions and tissues are minimal [2, 31, 32]. Furthermore, aminoglycosides do not cross the blood-brain barrier into the central nervous system or penetrate the vitreous humor of eye. Aminoglycosides can cross the placenta, however, and achieve fetal serum concentrations that are 21 to 37% or maternal serum concentrations. Moreover, high concentrations of aminoglycosides can be found in the renal cortex and the endolymph and perilymph of the inner ear owing to active uptake systems for these compounds. These high concentrations likely contribute to the nephrotoxicity and ototoxicity seen with this class of antibiotics. Aminoglycosides do not avidly bind to albumin. With the exception of streptomycin, binding to albumin is less than 10%. As a result, the apparent volume of distribution of aminoglycosides is 25% of lean body weight and approximates the volume of the extracellular fluid.

Elimination

Aminoglycosides antibiotics are primarily eliminated unchanged in the urine following glomerular filtration [31, 32]. Elimination of aminoglycosides by the kidney accounts for approximately 85 to 95% of the dose administered which results in urinary concentrations of 50 to 200 ug/ml. In patients with normal renal function, the elimination half-life of aminoglycosides ranges from 2 to 3 hours. For patients with renal insufficiency such as the elderly, the elimination half-life can be greatly prolonged due to the attenuated glomerular filtration rate [35]. There is some active secretion of the aminoglycosides hepatically into the bile, but this is considered an extremely minor elimination route. Interestingly, renal clearance of aminoglycosides is approximately two-thirds of the simultaneous creatinine clearance suggesting a significant element of tubular reabsorption. Furthermore, 24 to 48 hours after a dose of aminoglycoside is given, plasma clearance exceeds renal elimination by 10 to 20%. Subsequently, an amount approaching 100% is recovered in the urine. This initial lag period likely represents the saturation of aminoglycoside binding in the peripheral tissue compartment. The elimination of aminoglycosides from this deep peripheral tissue compartment can be exceedingly protracted with an estimated half-life ranging from 30 to 700 hours.

Renal transport of aminoglycosides

Cortical uptake

After parenteral administration, aminoglycosides distribute to a compartment approximately equivalent in volume to the extracellular fluid [36]. Though most of the aminoglycoside is eliminated by glomerular filtration and appears unchanged in the urine, a significant portion of the parenteral dose (5-10%) is retained in the renal cortex where it achieves concentrations markedly exceeding the concurrent serum concentration [2, 37, 38, 39, 40, 42]. Within the renal cortex, pioneering autoradiographic studies demonstrated that aminoglycosides accumulate chiefly in the pars recta of the proximal tubule [40, 41, 42, 43, 44]. A subsequent study revealed that the accumulation is confined to the S1 and S2 segments of the proximal tubule [41]. However, in a study of renal ischemia gentamicin achieved elevated intracellular concentrations in the S1, S2 and S3 segments [45, 46, 82]. In addition, within the S3 cells a portion of the intracellular gentamicin localized in abnormal intracellular structures. These abnormal intracellular structures which were composed primarily of internalized microvilli did not develop in the S1 and S2 cells. This may explain the increased sensitivity of S3 cells to ischemic injury [45].

Proximal tubule cell transport

The multiple amino groups on an aminoglycoside molecule confer polybasic and polycationic properties at physiologic pH [43, 47]. Not surprisingly, the initial renal cortical binding sites for the aminoglycosides were found to be the acidic, anionic phospholipids within the plasma membrane on the apical and basolateral surfaces of the proximal tubule cell (PTC) [39, 42, 43, 47]. Specifically, aminoglycosides bind to these sites on the plasma membrane of the PTC secondary to a saturable, electrostatic charge interaction between the cationic aminoglycoside and the anionic phospholipid. The unique phospholipids within the PTC that participate in this charge interaction are phosphatidic acid, phosphatidyl serine, phosphatidylinositol, phosphatidylinositol 4-monophoshate and phosphatidyl 4,5-diphosphate [45]. Though these acidic phospholipids are integral components of the plasma membranes of most other organ systems, there is a higher concentration of phosphatidylinositols in the kidney and the inner ear compared to other tissues.

This higher concentration of phosphatidylinositols is likely an important component in the pathogenesis of the selective impairment of these tissues observed with aminoglycoside toxicity. Moreover, the relative affinity of a specific aminoglycoside for the PTC membrane binding site has been shown to correlate with their inherent nephrotoxic potential [51]. Neomycin has the highest affinity for the renal membrane binding site and has the greatest nephrotoxicity of the aminoglycosides. After neomycin, tobramycin and gentamicin have less, but similar binding affinities conferring decreased nephrotoxicity. Amikacin binds to the renal membrane binding site with reduced relative affinity than tobramycin or gentamicin which results in less nephrotoxic potential. Streptomycin which has the least binding affinity for the renal binding site has the least nephrotoxicity of the aminoglycosides. This trend in relative binding affinities also correlates well with the nephrotoxicity observed with the aminoglycosides used in clinical practice [11, 17, 26].

Role of megalin in aminoglycoside transport, RAP and cubilin

After the initial binding to the anionic phospholipids of the PTC, the aminoglycoside molecule is quickly transferred to the transmembrane protein megalin and endocytosed [42, 43, 48-50, 52-59, 66-68, 72, 73]. Aminoglycosides enter the PTC on either the apical or basolateral plasma membrane via receptor-mediated endocytosis. and are ultimately sequestered in the same endosomal compartment [68]. In an experiment with LLC-PK1 cells, Ford et al. demonstrated that aminoglycosides were internalized equally across the apical and basolateral membranes by receptor-mediated endocytosis. This was followed by colocalization within the lysosomal compartment and similar magnitudes of cellular dysfunction [68].

Megalin is a 600 kD type 1 cell surface receptor and a member of the supergene family of the low-density lipoprotein (LDLR). It is also referred to as LDL-receptor-related protein-2 or LRP-2 [43, 50]. Megalin is most abundantly expressed in the renal proximal tubule, but it is also found in many other tissues including glomerular podocytes, type II pneumocytes, ependymal cells, parathyroid-hormone secreting cells, retinal cells, and ciliary and inner ear epithelium [43, 46, 55]. Megalin functions as a transmembrane endocyctic receptor for a broad and diverse range of ligands and has been termed a scavenger receptor [50]. It has a high affinity for proteins with regions of positively charged amino acids. As a result of their polycationic charge at physiological pH, aminoglycosides avidly bind to megalin.

Closely associated with megalin and other members of the LDL-receptor family are the 40 kD receptor-associated protein (RAP) and the 460 kD endocytic receptor protein cubilin [50, 52, 60-64]. Through a high-affinity association with megalin, RAP serves as a chaperone or escort protein for megalin. Specifically, RAP functions as a receptor antagonist protecting newly synthesized megalin from premature binding of ligands as the megalin is transported to the cell surface. It may also function to ensure proper folding and post-translational modification such as disulfide bridge formation and glycosylation of the megalin receptor after its synthesis. In contrast, cubilin is a multiligand endocyctic receptor found in the yolk sac, ileal enterocytes, renal proximal tubule brush border and intracellular endocytic compartments [52, 62, 63, 64]. It is a peripheral membrane protein with a glycophoshatidylinositol anchor, but lacks a transmembrane domain [50, 52, 65]. Cubilin requires megalin for its internalization and binds to megalin through a calcium-dependent high affinity bond [50, 52, 62, 64, 65]. Though cubilin does not play a direct role in aminoglycoside transport, cubilin binds several ligands including RAP and interacts with megalin in a dual-receptor complex [64, 65]. In this dual-receptor complex, megalin and cubilin are important endocyctic receptors involved in the reabsorption of protein, primarily albumin, in the proximal tubule cells [50, 52, 62-65].

Post-endocytotic transport of aminoglycosides

After megalin-mediated endocytosis, the endosomes containing the aminoglycosides are transported through the endocytic system where they ultimately fuse with lysosomes [41, 44, 68-70]. Within these lysosomes, the aminoglycosides are sequestered resulting in a protracted renal cortical half-life and a markedly high intra-lysosomal concentration [37, 41, 44, 71]. This is not the only metabolic endpoint for aminoglycosides, however. Extensive in-vitro and in-vivo studies performed by Sandoval et al. have identified an important second intracellular fate for the aminoglycosides. The revelation of this second intracellular pathway began with an early cell culture experiment using porcine kidney proximal tubule cells (LLC-PK1) and a fluorescently-labeled gentamicin. This in-vitro study demonstrated co-localization of the gentamicin not only to the lysosome, as expected, but also to the Golgi complex [70]. Subsequent in-vivo work in rats corroborated the earlier cell culture study also demonstrating the localization of the fluorescently-labeled gentamicin to the Golgi complex [74]. Interestingly, a related study revealed increased trafficking of gentamicin to the Golgi complex in renal ischemia which may explain why certain subpopulations of patients with hypotension are more susceptible to aminoglycoside nephrotoxicity [79]. Additional cell culture studies showed that the trafficking of the gentamicin to the Golgi complex occurs rapidly, within 15 to 30 minutes, and accounts for approximately 5-10% of the total cellular accumulation of gentamicin [70, 75]. Finally, similar to the mechanism by which several toxins such as the Shiga toxin exert their deleterious cytotoxic effect, gentamicin was shown to traffic in a retrograde fashion through the Golgi complex to the endoplasmic reticulum (ER) [76, 77, 78, 80] (Figure 1). The researchers further demonstrated that after this retrograde transport to the ER, gentamicin was released to the cytosol and distributed throughout the cell accumulating in subcellular organelles such as the mitochondria and the nucleus [78] (Figure 2, 3, 4). This last body of work provided the greatest insight and most likely mechanism for intracellular organelle distribution and the detrimental effects observed in the PTC and subcellular organelles after aminoglycoside administration.

Prior to these studies fully delineating the secondary intracellular pathway for gentamicin, researchers believed that PTC toxicity was secondary to aminoglycoside accumulation in the lysosomes followed by lysosomal rupture, release and association with the protein-synthetic machinery. However, it has been shown that the attenuation in protein synthesis occurs rapidly after aminoglycoside administration and thus could not be attributed solely to lysosomal rupture which occurs later in the time-course of aminoglycoside nephrotoxicity [81]. The relatively quick trafficking of the aminoglycoside to the Golgi complex after administration with the subsequent disruption of protein sorting and synthesis is more consistent to what is observed and a more plausible explanation for the early damage that is observed in the PTC. Further, the observed co-localizations of the aminoglycoside to the mitochondria and nuclei after the retrograde transport to the ER and cytosolic release explains the perturbations in mitochondrial potential and protein synthesis within the PTC observed with aminoglycoside nephrotoxicity [78].

Morphological pathology of aminoglycoside nephrotoxicity

Studies of the morphological changes observed in aminoglycoside nephrotoxicity using animal models found that epithelial cell damage was progressive with time and confined to the S1 and S2 segments of the proximal tubule [83, 84]. In one early study, seven days of continuous high dose gentamicin administration demonstrated minimal light microscopic (LM) alterations of the renal epithelium [83]. Electron microscopic (EM) studies at this time point, however, were more revealing. The superficial cortex revealed vacuoliza-

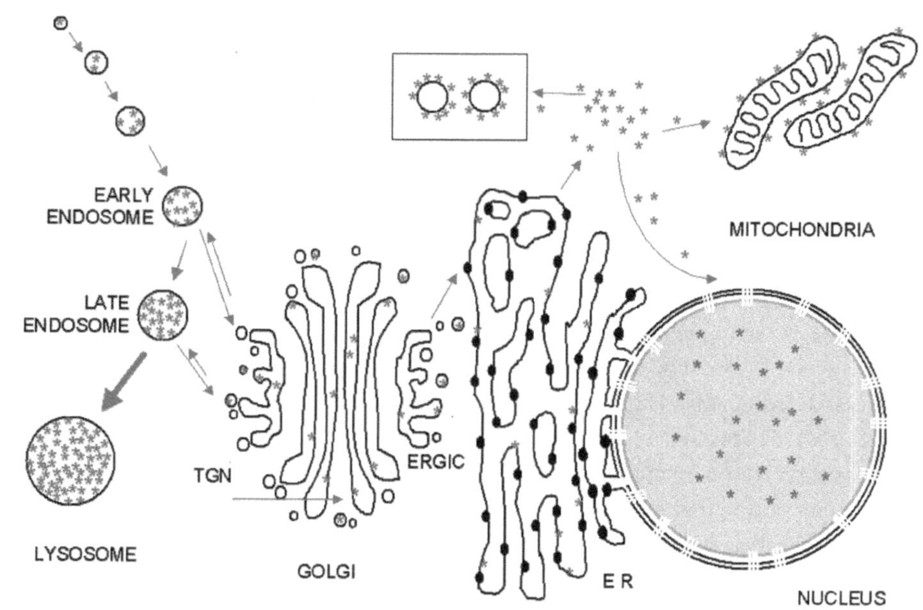

***Figure 1.** Retrograde trafficking of gentamicin along the endocytic pathway in LLC-PK1 cells [78].*

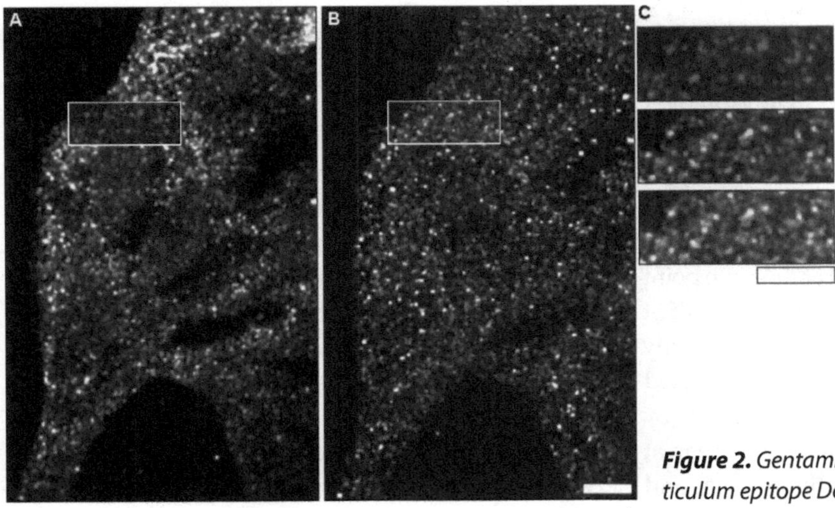

Figure 2. *Gentamicin co-localizes with the endoplasmic reticulum epitope Dolichos phosphate mannose synthase [78].*

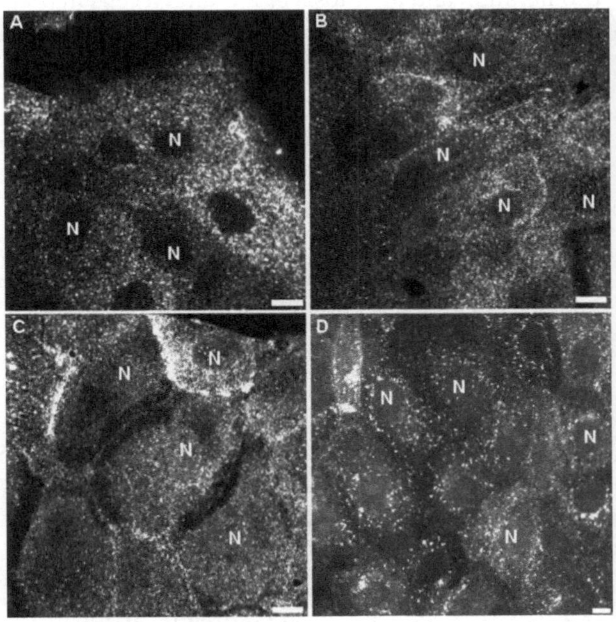

Figure 3. *Exposure to native gentamicin resulted in cytosolic release and nuclear accumulation in LLC-PK1 cells [78].*

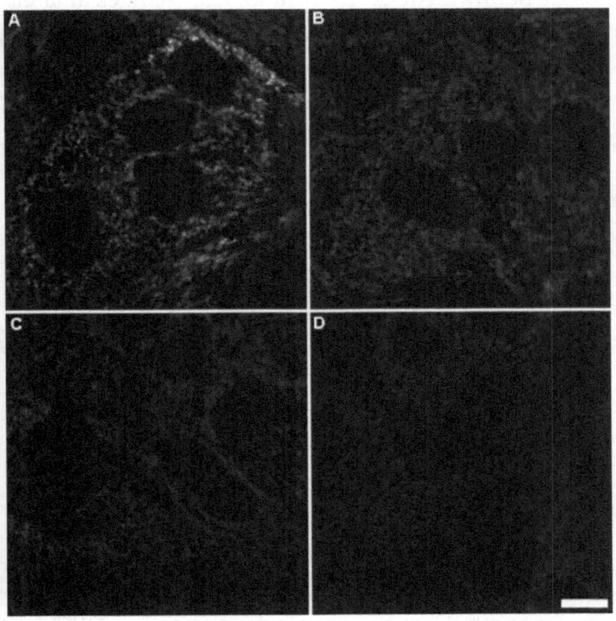

Figure 4. *LLC-PK1 cells exposed continuously to gentamicin exhibit a decrease in mitochondrial potential [78].*

tion of the proximal tubular epithelium. In addition, most of the proximal tubule cells contained enlarged nuclei and prominent areas of aggregated chromatin; mitoses were rare. Furthermore, nearly all of the proximal tubule epithelial cells contained large, irregular dense lysosomes [83]. There was also an increase in the size and number of the secondary lysosomes or cytosegrosomes [84]. Secondary lysosomes are primary lysosomes that have fused with endocytic or autophagic vacuoles [84]. Found within these secondary lysosomal structures were unicentric and multicentric myeloid bodies [41, 42, 83, 84]. These myeloid bodies are electron-dense lamellar structures of concentrically arranged and densely packed membranes. They likely represent sequestration of fragments of membranes and organelles which were damaged in the evolving toxicity. Within the secondary lysosomes, these cellular membrane and organelle fragments are undergoing processing and digestion. Of interest, aminoglycoside nephrotoxicity in humans also produced these same lysosomal morphological alterations [85]. Moreover, the myeloid bodies occasionally appeared in the cytoplasm without surrounding lysosome membranes; sometimes they were present in small, tightly packed aggregates in the lumina of the proximal tubules. The mitochondria also appeared damaged at this time point appearing swollen and vacuolated in the basal half of the cells. Cisternae of the rough ER were markedly dilated. Interestingly, the glomeruli, distal convoluted tubules and collecting tubules appeared normal by light and EM. Another morphological change seen at this early time point is a decrease in the number and height of microvillae of the brush border membrane.

Attesting to the progressive nature of aminoglycoside nephrotoxicity, morphological changes at later time points were more striking. At ten days, proximal tubule epithelial necrosis and desquamation was apparent by LM. Many epithelial cells were vacuolated and appeared to be undergoing granular disintegration. By EM, mitochondria were markedly swollen with attenuated, distorted cristae and matrix loss. Generally, lysosomes and myeloid bodies were less conspicuous at 10 days than they were at 7 days. Both proximal and distal tubules were filled with eosinophilic, granular material which by EM was comprised of cytoplasmic debris, membrane fragments and myeloid bodies.

Regeneration of proximal tubule cells was observed even while the aminoglycoside was still being administered [83, 97]. At ten days of gentamicin therapy, two types of squamoid cells which could be distinguished by EM on the basis of cellular differ-entiation. The less differentiated cell type was identified as regenerating proximal tubule cells. These cells were taller with less organized cytoplasm and many ribosomes. Occasionally these cells were observed insinuating themselves between the damaged cells and the basement membrane. After the aminoglycoside is discontinued, renal recovery progresses and by four weeks most areas of the kidney regain normal architecture comparable to controls. However, residual scarring containing collections of collapsed atrophic tubules was observed in focal areas of the cortex.

Apoptosis and aminoglycoside nephrotoxicity

An intriguing subset of the morphological changes seen in aminoglycoside nephrotoxicity is the increase in apoptosis of the proximal tubule cells observed with gentamicin exposure. Unlike the previous studies these apoptotic changes can occur at much lower aminoglycoside concentrations. Mouedden et al. was able to demonstrate increased apoptosis with proximal tubule cells in rats given gentamicin at low multiples of the usual clinical doses (10mg/kg) [86]. Coincident apoptosis and necrosis of proximal tubule cells occurred when this dose was doubled. A later cell culture study by Mouedden et al. corroborated these in-vivo findings. For this study, two renal cell lines from different species, LLC-PK1 and MDCK, and rat embryonic fibroblasts were used [87]. Each of these cell lines demonstrated increased apoptosis with gentamicin exposure. In a combined in-vitro and in-vivo study, Martinez-Selgado et al. demonstrated increased proliferation and apoptosis of mesangial cells in both cultured rat mesangial cells exposed to gentamicin and in rats given 100 mg/kg of gentamicin [91].

They were also able to show that reactive oxygen species (ROS) may mediate gentamicin induced apoptosis in the cultured mesangial cells [91]. Servais et al. was able to describe a potential pathway for the gentamicin-mediated apoptosis of the PTC that included initial lysosomal disruption and mitochondrial dysfunction in LLC-PK1 cells [69]. Disruption of lysosomal membranes has been shown to be an effective inducer of apoptosis. Similarly, mitochondrial dysfunction by gentamicin with the subsequent and partial release of intra-granular cytochrome c has also been shown to be a potent inducer of apoptosis. More recent work by Servais et al. with LLC-PK1 cells corroborated their earlier finding [88]. Moreover, the discovery of the retrograde transport of gentamicin through the secretory pathway and its release to the cytosol by the ER established a plausible route for the mitochondrial dysfunction and subsequent apoptosis. Intriguingly, the authors proposed that lysosomes may initially provide a protective function from general cellular toxicity by sequestering large amounts of gentamicin. This protective effect is lost and cell death is precipitated, however, once the gentamicin is released as a consequence of lysosomal disruption. The lysosomal integrity can be disrupted by a diversity of pathways including drug and phospholipid overloading, direct permea-bilization of the lysosomal membrane, interference with proteins that stabilize the lysosomal membrane or retrograde trafficking through the Golgi complex and ER [69, 70, 75,

78, 88-90].

Biochemical pathology of aminoglycoside nephrotoxicity

In addition to the morphological and apoptotic changes, diverse biochemical derangements also occur that contribute to the pathology of aminoglycoside nephrotoxicity. The apical membrane, the initial interface between the aminoglycoside and the PTC, is the site where the biochemical alterations first manifest. Aminoglycosides have been shown to attenuate apical membrane transport of organic base, glucose and low-molecular weight protein [105, 114, 115]. These decrements in molecular transport coupled with loss of brush border enzymes and phospholipids in the urine results in altered phospholipid composition early in the course of aminoglycoside administration. Aminoglycosides also cause a variety of functional derangements in the basolateral membrane. Specifically, there is reduced transport of organic base and the ions, Ca^{2+}, Na^{+}, and K^{+}. Conversely, organic acid transport is increased. [84, 105]. Of interesting note, research by Adams et al revealed that gentamicin, kanamycin and streptomycin increased Ca^{2+} efflux from isolated vascular smooth muscle resulting in a reduced contractile response [155]. This may explain the occasional in-vivo cardiovascular depression that has been observed after the administration of streptomycin [156]. In addition, aminoglycosides can cause decrements in enzymes reducing the activity of Na^{+}- K^{+} ATPase and adenylate cyclase [84, 105]. The phospholipid composition of the basolateral membrane is also altered by aminoglycosides; calcium bound to the phospholipids is displaced [84]. Many of these biochemical changes are evident within 90 minutes of a single injection of aminoglycoside.

Another pathological finding associated with aminoglycoside nephrotoxicity is apparent morphologically in the form of lysosomal myeloid bodies. Numerous studies have documented that gentamicin exposure induces a phospholipid accumulation within the lysosomes resulting in phospholipidosis and the myeloid-body morphology [74, 84, 92, 93, 94, 95]. However, El Mouedden et al. were not able to demonstrate this phospholipidosis in LLC-PK1 cells exposed to gentamicin, though lysosomal phospholipidosis may develop in LLC-PK1 cells if incubation is prolonged [87, 98]. Later work in this area showed that the phospholipidosis occurs secondary to the inhibition of phospholipase A1, A2 and C and sphingomyelinase by gentamicin [92, 94, 96]. Interestingly, these lysosomal ultrastructural changes were not associated with cell death and can exist without a decrement in renal function. Research by Giurgea-Marion et al, though, demonstrated decrements in lysosomal-endocytic vesicle fusion in rats given gentamicin which may inhibit the efficient processing of cellular membranes and toxic phospholipids [93]. Currently, a direct causal link between lysosomal phospholipidosis and apoptosis remains elusive, however. It is reasonable to postulate, though, that to the extent that phospholipidosis contributes to lysosomal instability and promotes disruption, phospholipidosis may be an important early component of aminoglycoside-induced apoptosis [87, 89].

The mitochondria are another important subcellular site where aminoglycoside-induced morphological and biochemical alterations are observed. Morphologically, aminoglycoside exposure has diverse effects on mitochondria resulting in a composite of contracted, enlarged and ruptured mitochondria. The enlarged mitochondria contain granular inclusions and myeloid bodies [99]. Biochemically, gentamicin can inhibit oxidative phosphorylation in the renal cortical mitochondria. Furthermore, these specific biochemical effects occur before any functional or morphological evidence of renal injury. This early injury to the mitochondria is supported by the recent elucidation of a pathway to the Golgi complex and mitochondria that occurs rapidly after gentamicin administration [78]. Gentamicin has also been shown to compete and displace Mg^{2+} at the inner mitochondrial membrane [100, 101]. This displacement of Mg^{2+} by gentamicin could then allow cations such as Na^{+} and K^{+} to interact with the mitochondrial membrane components. This could conceivably result in altered cation transport and diminished maximal electron transport potential due to the association between the cation and electron transport properties of the mitochondrial membrane. [101]. In addition, another study utilizing proteomic analysis identified more than 20 proteins that could serve as putative biomarkers for gentamicin nephrotoxicity of the rat kidney cortex [113]. Many of these were mitochondrial proteins involved with either the citrate cycle or fatty acid biosynthesis [113]. Aminoglycoside-mitochondrial interactions have also been implicated in promoting apoptosis. Mather et al. has identified a pathway where aminoglycoside toxicity causes mitochondria to release proapoptotic, soluble intermembrane proteins (SIMP), such as cytochrome c and adenylate kinase 2 [102]. Finally, aminoglycosides have also been shown to promote the release of free radicals such as hydrogen peroxide, hydroxyl and reactive iron species from the renal cortical mitochondria [103, 104].

Aminoglycosides also cause biochemical derangements merely as an extension of their primary mechanism of action. Therapeutically, aminoglycosides act by inhibiting bacterial protein synthesis [106, 107]. Aminoglycosides accomplish this by binding to the prokaryotic ribosomes thereby blocking the ribosomal initiation complex or by causing mistranslation [108, 110]. However, aminoglycosides have also been shown to cause similar actions in eukaryotic ribosomes [109, 111, 112]. *In vivo* studies have shown that protein synthesis is reduced within one to two days after gentamicin administration [74]. This inhibition is also progressive with a 50% decrement at three days [74]. These reductions in protein synthesis occurred before gross morphological cellular alterations were apparent. Similarly, Bennett et al. were able to demonstrate attenuated microsomal protein synthesis in renal tubular cells obtained from rats given gentamicin for two days [81]. This observation of early disruption in protein synthesis is consistent with the discovery of the rapid trafficking of gentamicin to the Golgi complex after administration [78].

Immunologic pathology of aminoglycoside nephrotoxicity

Acute kidney injury (AKI) is associated with increased mortality in critically-ill patients and commonly occurs in concert with the serious infections observed in sepsis [152-154, 168, 165, 166]. AKI in sepsis is believed to be secondary to the activation of systemic and local immune responses, though a complete understanding of the underlying mechanism has remained elusive. Recent research with the toll-like receptors (TLR), however, is elucidating more of this pathophysiology. The TLR are the critical, initial recognition molecules that alert a host that a microbial pathogen has breached the integument or mucous membrane defenses [165, 166, 169]. They are a growing family of currently 11 transmembrane glycoproteins of the innate immune system that bind a diverse group of pathogen and non-pathogen-associated ligands such as endotoxin, lipopolysaccharide (LPS), lipoteichoic acid, and viral double-stranded RNA and DNA [158, 165, 166, 169]. Once a TLR binds a specific ligand, a signaling cascade is activated that induces the synthesis of a diverse group of proinflammatory and effector molecules. For example, the interaction between TLR4 and the LPS of gram negative bacteria can trigger the release of various cytokines and chemokines initiating a cascade that results in the systemic inflammation of sepsis [159, 166, 167]. In contrast, TLR3 and TLR9 recognize viral double-stranded RNA and double-stranded DNA ligands, respectively. Once activated, these TLR3 and TLR9 induce the production of anti-viral interferons that activate natural killer cells [161].

A substantial body of nephrology research has been performed with TLR4 in the setting of sepsis. It is known that during experimental sepsis, TLR4 is expressed in a wide anatomic distribution in the kidney. TLR4 is found on the glomeruli, proximal and distal convoluted tubules and peritubular capillaries [166]. Furthermore, El-Achkar et al demonstrated that during sepsis, the expression of TLR4 in the kidney is markedly increased [167]. Also, Zager et al demonstrated increased TLR4 fragments in urine, reduced proximal tubule TLR4 content, but increased renal cortical TLR4 mRNA in rats subjected to hypoxic and toxic renal injury [158]. The increase in TLR4 shedding in this experiment was speculated to be a beneficial response, attenuating the hyper-reactive TLR4-ligand pathway in AKI [158]. Other early work by Zager et al refined our current understanding of the pathophysiology of TLR4 and AKI and subsequent research showed a possible role for gentamicin as well. Zager et al. demonstrated that in experimental AKI, there is an increased release of TLR-dependent inflammatory mediators, such as tumor necrosis factor-alpha (TNF-α) and monocyte chemotactic protein-1 (MCP-1) when a TLR-4 (endotoxin, LPS) or a TLR2 (lipoteichoic acid) ligand is administered [162, 163, 164]. This led the researchers to conclude that when an acutely damaged kidney is challenged with proinflammatory TLR ligands, it responds by releasing cytokines that worsens systemic inflammation, multiorgan failure and mortality. Recently, Zager et al showed a possible role for gentamicin in this process. Zager et al observed that a single day of gentamicin treatment augmented LPS-mediated TNF-α generation [160]. Specifically, gentamicin pretreated mice given LPS manifested a two-fold higher concentration of TNF-α than controls just given LPS [160]. MCP-1 also appeared to participate in this phenomenon. Levels of MCP-1 were three-fold higher in gentamicin-LPS mice than in mice given only LPS. These observations suggested that gentamicin may impact both renal and extra-renal inflammatory responses and serve to explain why in the setting of endotoxemia, hypotension and renal ischemia, gentamicin exacerbates renal injury [160].

Conventional and once-daily aminoglycoside dosing regimens

Conventional pharmacokinetic dosing

Pharmacokinetic aminoglycoside dosing programs were first developed to reduce the risk of nephrotoxicity and ototoxicity. Several studies have evaluated these programs as to patient outcome, incidence of toxicity and cost-benefit. Though some of the individual studies have shown improved efficacy and reduced toxicity with pharmacokinetic dosing, others have shown no clinical advantage. Whipple et al determined that individualized pharmacokinetic dosing based on aminoglycoside levels achieved significantly improved survival without nephrotoxicity compared to the traditional approach of determining a dose and interval based on patient weight and estimates of renal function [116]. The improved survival was attributed to attaining therapeutic peak serum concentrations earlier in the course of infection and by administering more total aminoglycoside without increasing toxicity. Bartal et al. also demonstrated that a cohort of patients receiving pharmacokinetic dosing of aminoglycosides had less nephrotoxicity than the control group which received a single, daily, weight-based dose of an aminoglycoside without pharmacokinetic monitoring [117]. Cost-benefit analyses performed by Destache et al and Burton et al showed similar trends with shorter hospitalizations, improved clinical response, and a trend toward less toxicity in the pharmacokinetically monitored cohort relative to the physician-directed dosing group [118, 119]. In contrast, Kemme et al. did not show a major clinical benefit of individualized pharmacokinetic dosing program as compared to the physician dosing method in terms of clinical benefit or incidence of nephrotoxicity [120]. Similarly, work by Leehey et al. did not find any reduction in the incidence of nephrotoxicity in a cohort of patients who received individualized pharmacokinetic dosing [121]. Research by Dillon et al with amikacin showed no clinical advantage, but a decreased risk of toxicity with pharmacokinetic dosing versus standard physician-directed dosing [122]. Resolving these disparate results requires a closer reappraisal of what constitutes the accepted therapeutic and toxic aminoglycoside serum levels and whether these levels are rigorously supported by science. McCormack et al critically evaluated a large series of pharmacokinetic studies of aminoglycosides and discovered that the accepted therapeutic levels were derived from a relatively small number of inadequately controlled studies [123]. In addition, our understanding of what constitutes a toxic aminoglycoside level may need revision. The emergence of the ODA regimen and the associated supratherapeutic aminoglycoside levels it produces casts sufficient doubt whether a high peak level is associated with toxicity. Moreover, an elevated aminoglycoside serum trough level has long been accepted as a cause of nephrotoxicity attributable to its longer renal residence time and increased renal cortical uptake. However, in their critique McCormack et al did not find a direct or causal relationship between any specific serum aminoglycoside serum level, peak or trough, and the development of nephrotoxicity [123]. Unfortunately, the studies evaluated used variable criteria for defining renal toxicity and in many cases the increased aminoglycoside concentrations were measured after the declines in renal function had already occurred. Thus, it was not possible to determine whether a aminoglycoside concentration was elevated before or after the increase in serum creatinine. In essence, increasing trough serum concentrations may be due solely to reductions in drug clearance secondary to nephrotoxicity rather than the cause of nephrotoxicity. This is significant because an elevated aminoglycoside trough level may merely indicate a reduced glomerular filtration rate (GFR) which would result in less aminoglycoside available to damage proximal tubule cells. In support of this, researchers have shown that an increased creatinine clearance paradoxically causes more aminoglycoside-induced nephrotoxicity [4, 28, 29]. Despite the uncertainty and limitations in our current understanding of both aminoglycoside therapy and toxicity, monitoring programs remain useful providing they achieve the following goals. Monitoring programs should ensure that patients with relative contraindications receive less toxic antibiotics and that adequate doses are given early in therapy. Furthermore, the inherent limitations of estimating a patient's GFR by the available formulas and the clinical urgency that often precludes a more accurate 24 hour urine collection for creatinine clearance mandates the monitoring of aminoglycoside levels. Patients should also be evaluated regularly for signs and symptoms of ototoxicity and nephrotoxicity and the aminoglycoside therapy should be discontinued as soon as clinically possible.

Once daily aminoglycoside dosing

In ODA therapy, a much larger loading dose of an aminoglycoside is given much less frequently such as every 24-48 hours or even longer. The frequency of dosing in an ODA program is based on a serum aminoglycoside level typically drawn 6-14 hours after the dose is given. In contrast, conventional aminoglycoside dosing programs administer a scheduled dose of aminoglycoside two to three times a day with subsequent dosing based on pharmacokinetic monitoring of both serum peak and trough aminoglycoside levels. Generally, fewer serum aminoglycoside levels are needed in an ODA program to appropriately monitor therapy than in a conventional dosing program. The impetus for the development of the ODA programs was based on insights into the unique pharmacodynamic attributes of aminoglycosides, specifically their concentration-dependent bactericidal activity and post-antibiotic effect. Clinicians wanted to exploit these favorable pharmacodynamic properties to improve aminoglycoside efficacy and reduce toxicity. Subsequent clinical studies of ODA programs have largely supported this rationale. A study of 2184 patients treated in an ODA program demonstrated both excellent clinical effectiveness and a remarkably low rate of nephrotoxicity (1.2%) [3]. The researchers of this study also cited a pharmacoeconomic benefit of their ODA program. With fewer doses of aminoglycoside to prepare and administer, and less serum aminoglycoside levels to determine, there was a significant reduction in workload [3]. A later pharmacoeconomic study that compared conventional aminoglycoside dosing with an ODA program quantified this pharmacoeconomic benefit. These researchers discovered their ODA program achieved a 58% reduction in aminoglycoside-associated hospital cost and a savings of 70% per patient in nephrotoxicity management costs [27]. Other researchers have further corroborated the clinical superiority of ODA programs. Prins and Buller compared two similar groups of patients randomly assigned to receive either once daily (OD) or a multiple dose (MD) of aminoglycoside [16]. Clinical efficacy was equivalent in both groups, but the incidence of nephrotoxicity was only 5% in the OD group compared to 24% in the MD group [16]. Finally, several meta-analyses of studies that compared ODA programs to conventional aminoglycoside dosing demonstrated that ODA programs confer equal clinical efficacy and less or a trend toward less nephrotoxicity [12, 13, 14, 24, 25].

Though the data largely appears to support ODA programs, they may require modification or avoidance in certain patient populations. A comparison of a once daily program and conventional aminoglycoside dosing in an elderly patient population demonstrated equal clinical efficacy and nephrotoxicity [9]. However, in a subgroup analysis of the ODA cohort in this study, a much higher incidence of nephrotoxicity (60%) was observed when serum peak concentration was greater than 12.0 mg/dL than when less than 12.0mg/dL (8.3%). The authors recommended that high serum peak concentrations of aminoglycosides be specifically avoided in elderly patients. In addition, ODA programs are not considered appropriate for patients with advanced chronic kidney disease (CKD) [157]. For this patient population, non-aminoglycoside antibiotics should be sought to reduce the risk of further renal damage and the need for renal replacement therapy. However, if an aminoglycoside is clinically necessary, then strategies to minimize aminoglycoside nephrotoxicity should be utilized (Table 1).

Similar to the conventional dosing program, controversy also exists regarding the pharmacokinetic monitoring of aminoglycosides in ODA programs. Like the conventional dosing regimen, there is a dearth of scientific evidence in the ODA literature pertaining to what specific aminoglycoside level produces clinical efficacy or toxicity [124]. ODA regimens frequently use a target peak of 20 mg/L to achieve a minimum inhibitory concentration that is ten times that of their most troublesome pathogen. However, there is no evidence that achieving this peak level improves patient outcome. Others recommend establishing a

Table 1. Strategies to prevent aminoglycoside-induced nephrotoxicity.

1. Select least nephrotoxic aminoglycoside
2. Correct hypokalemia and hypomagnesemia
3. Avoid use if possible in high-risk patients
4. Adjust dose for renal function
5. Limit duration of therapy to 7-10 days
6. Avoid concomitant nephrotoxic medications
7. Pharmacokinetically monitor drug levels
8. Use once-daily aminoglycoside regimen

dosing interval to achieve a trough level of less than 0.5 mg/ml for at least 4 hours. Most recommend a trough concentration less than 2 mg/L. Each of these trough level recommendations is not based on any clinical evidence, but rather expert opinion. Unfortunately, until more studies are done to refine our understanding of aminoglycoside clinical therapeutics and toxicity, expert opinion and careful clinical observation must serve as the guide to ODA therapies.

Prevention of aminoglycoside nephrotoxicity

A wide variety of agents have been evaluated for their potential to prevent aminoglycoside nephrotoxicity targeting specific aspects of its pathogenesis. Polyamino acids are a group of compounds that have been extensively studied and been shown to be quite effective in preventing aminoglycoside nephrotoxicity in laboratory animals. Importantly, these agents were renal protective without altering the antimicrobial activity of the aminoglycoside [132]. The two polyamino compounds most often cited are poly-$_L$-aspartic (PAA) and poly-$_L$-glutamic acid (PGA) [42, 125-131]. Similar to aminoglycosides, PAA and PGA are polycations and bind to the same anionic phospholipids of the PTC plasma membrane. Furthermore, in their pioneering work Williams et al showed that PAA and PGA markedly inhibit gentamicin binding at the renal brush border [129]. As a result, the mechanism of action of the polyamines was initially believed to be secondary to an inhibition of aminoglycoside binding at the PTC plasma membrane [129,131]. This would suggest that in PAA-treated animals renal cortical concentrations of aminoglycoside would be lower than in animals not given PAA. However, studies performed by Gilbert et al. showed that PAA actually enhanced renal cortical uptake of aminoglycoside. They found renal gentamicin levels that were approximately ten times that of rats given gentamicin alone [132]. Other researchers independently corroborated this renal cortical aminoglycoside accumulation in PAA and gentamicin treated rats [126, 133]. Later studies revealed that PAA reduced the lysosomal derangements induced by aminoglycoside exposure. Both Beuchamp and Kishore et al. were able to show a reduction in lysosomal enlargement, deposition of myeloid bodies and lysosomal phospholipidosis in rats given PAA and gentamicin [126, 117, 130]. Kishore et al. was able to show that PAA binds gentamicin optimally at pH 5.4 which is equal to the intra-lysosomal pH [134]. PAA also was shown to displace gentamicin from negatively charged lysosomes [134]. These subsequent findings led researchers to postulate that PAA may afford renal protection by binding to gentamicin directly or by displacing it from negatively charged lysosomes, thus preventing the development of lysosomal phospholipidosis [134].

Several antioxidant agents have been investigated as potential compounds to ameliorate aminoglycoside nephrotoxicity. Some of the candidate antioxidant agents were deferrioxamine, methimazole, vitamin E, vitamin C and selenium [32, 125, 144]. Each of these was shown to be beneficial in preventing gentamicin nephrotoxicity. Other antioxidants proven effective include superoxide dismutase, dimethyl-sulphoxide (DMSO), lipoic acid, N-acetylcysteine and melatonin [125, 136-141]. Interestingly, the beta blocker carvedilol and the antihyperlipidemic probucol were also shown to be effective in preventing free radical mediated gentamicin nephrotoxicity [142,143].

Calcium has also been proven an effective prophylactic agent in gentamicin nephrotoxicity. Early work by Bennett et al. demonstrated that dietary calcium loading in rats given gentamicin delayed the onset and reduced the magnitude of nephrotoxicity [145]. Later work by Quarum et al. and Humes et al. also showed that dietary calcium supplements moderated gentamicin-induced nephrotoxicity [146, 147]. The renal protective effect of Ca^{2+} is thought to be similar to PAA. Not only does Ca^{2+} inhibit the binding of gentamicin at the PTC brush border, it also has been shown to prevent critical gentamicin-membrane interactions within the renal tubular cell [147].

Despite the promise shown by these agents in preventing aminoglycoside-induced nephrotoxicity, they all await further evaluation and adoption in the clinical setting. However, a gentamicin congener that does not have the nephrotoxic liability and yet retains its antimicrobial efficacy has recently been discovered that may make these various interventions ultimately unnecessary. Commercially available gentamicin is not a homogeneous compound, but a variable composite of four different congeners of gentamicin, C_1, $C_{1a,}$ C_2 and C_{2a}. Moreover, each of these congeners differs in its ability to cause nephrotoxicity [149]. The earlier work by Kohlhepp et al which evaluated the C_1, C_{1a} and C_2 congeners was hindered by the technical limitations of HPLC at the time and likely cross-contamination of their C_2 sample with C_{2a}. As a result, these earlier workers erroneously attributed the nephrotoxicity of gentamicin to the C_2 congener. The recent study by Sandoval et al served to expand and refine this previous research by Kohlhepp et al [148]. Sandoval et al were able to show that the C_2 congener actually caused minimal renal cellular toxicity and retained its bactericidal properties [149]. Furthermore, they demonstrated that the C_{2a} congener was responsible for a high level of renal cellular toxicity. Finally, with immunofluorescent techniques, Sandoval et al were able to show that the C_2 congener did not induce the typical intracellular trafficking abnormalities of the Golgi complex and lysosomes that were observed with the cytotoxic congeners and native gentamicin. This is the likely the reason why the C_2 congener lacks significant renal cellular toxicity. Given the established and reliable clinical utility of aminoglycosides in an increasingly antibiotic resistant milieu, the clinical potential of an aminoglycoside that is efficacious and lacks nephrotoxicity is readily apparent.

Though the renal-protective interventions and the C_2 gentamicin congener have yet to be proven clinically effective and adopted as standards of care, there are established clinical strategies to reduce the incidence of aminoglycoside-induced nephrotoxicity (Table 1). The selection of the least toxic aminoglycoside when possible is important as these agents differ in their relative nephrotoxicities (Table 2). Of the aminoglycosides used systemically, gentamicin is considered the most nephrotoxic, followed in decreasing order of nephrotoxicity by tobramycin, amikacin, netilmicin and streptomycin [30]. Other effective strategies include correcting hypokalemia and hypomagnesemia, avoiding aminoglycosides in patients at high-risk for acute kidney injury, adjusting the dose for renal function, limiting duration of therapy to seven to 10 days and minimizing concomitant administration of other nephrotoxic medications [30, 150, 151]. There is currently scant evidence supporting what is clinically accepted as the therapeutic and toxic aminoglycoside serum level; however the goals previously described support continuing pharmacokinetic monitoring. Finally, secondary to evidence of increased clinical efficacy and less toxicity, utilization of a once daily dosing regimen in selected patients should be the preferred approach over conventional multiple dose regimens [12-14, 24, 25, 150, 151].

Table 2. Most to least nephrotoxic of systemically used aminoglycosides.

1. Gentamicin
2. Tobramycin
3. Amikacin
4. Netilmicin
5. Streptomycin

Vancomycin nephrotoxicity

Introduction

Vancomycin is a complex, tricyclic glycopeptide produced by *Streptococcus orientalis* with a molecular mass of approximately 1,500 D [170-172]. It was first discovered in 1956 and then utilized clinically a relatively short time later in 1958 [172]. Vancomycin given intravenously is primarily active against gram positive bacteria and is bactericidal for dividing microorganisms in concentrations of 5 to 10 ug/ml with the notable exception of *Enterococci* for which it is bacteriostatic [170-172]. It is also synergistic *in vitro* with gentamicin and streptomycin against *Enterococcus faecium* and *Enterococcus faecalis*. In its oral formulation, vancomycin is used to treat the colitis caused by *Clostridium difficile.* Vancomycin exerts its main bactericidal effect by inhibiting the biosynthesis of peptidoglycan, the major structural polymer of the bacterial cell wall [172]. Similar to the aminoglycosides, vancomycin also exhibits a post-antibiotic effect. *In vitro,* the post-antibiotic effect has a duration of approximately 1.5 to 3 hours against *Staphylococcus aureus* [172]. Vancomycin also exhibits concentration-independent killing when serum concentrations exceed the minimal bactericidal concentration or are approximately 4 to 5 times the minimum inhibitor concentration (MIC). As a result, greater serum concentrations of vancomycin do not increase its antibacterial activity; achieving high initial serum concentrations would provide little clinical benefit for most infections [172].

Clinical interest and use of vancomycin has followed a bimodal distribution. Vancomycin was first used heavily after its discovery to treat the increasingly prevalent penicillin-resistant *Staphylococcal* bacteria. After the introduction of the seminsynthetic antistaphylococcal penicillins and the toxicity encountered with the early impure vancomycin preparations, clinical use of vancomycin waned. However, the subsequent emergence of the increasingly resistant gram positive bacteria, especially methicillin resistant *Staphylococcus aureus* (MRSA), resulted in a resurgence of clinical interest and use of vancomycin. More recently, though, the clinical use of vancomycin has declined due to the emergence of vancomycin-resistant gram positive bacteria such as the vancomycin-resistant *Enterococci* (VRE).

Vancomycin exhibits predictable pharmacokinetic properties and its clinical use has been guided by the pharmacokinetic monitoring of serum levels to determine the dose and frequency of administration. Pharmacokinetic monitoring of vancomycin, however, has become increasingly controversial given the improved safety of this antibiotic and the lack of data to support what are considered the therapeutic and toxic serum levels. Historically, the most severe toxicities of vancomycin were ototoxicity and nephrotoxicity. The incidence of nephrotoxicity has declined since its introduction possibly due to the availability of purer forms of the antibiotic. Ototoxicity has always been a rare adverse event of vancomycin, but it has been observed with excessively high concentrations of the drug in plasma [170-172]. The purpose of this section is to describe the nephrotoxicity associated with the clinical use of vancomycin.

Pharmacokinetics of vancomycin

Absorption

Vancomycin is poorly absorbed after oral administration. However, in patients with normal renal function, low concentrations of vancomycin have been demonstrated in the urine indicating some systemic absorption even by this route. For systemic gram positive infections, vancomycin is administered intravenously. The peak serum levels of vancomycin are approximately proportional to the dose given. For example, intravenous administration of 500 mg of vancomycin to normal volunteers resulted in serum levels of 2 to 10 mg/L two hours after the dose. After 1000 mg or 2000 mg of vancomycin are given, two hour serum levels approximate 25 mg/L and 45 mg/L, respectively [184].

Distribution

Vancomycin is approximately 30 to 55% bound to plasma proteins. Its distribution after intravenous administration proceeds as a biphasic process and is consistent with a two or three compartment model. The half-life of the first distributive phase is approximately 0.4 hour in patients with normal renal function; the second distributive phase is approximately 1.6 hours [172]. Consistent with its multicompartment pharmacokinetic modeling, vancomycin is widely distributed and penetrates into many different body fluids and tissues including the cerebrospinal fluid (CSF). With inflamed meninges, vancomycin achieves CSF levels that are 7 to 30% of the simultaneous serum levels. Vancomcyin also penetrates into bile, and pleural, pericardial, synovial and ascitic fluids [170-172, 174, 184]. This wide distribution results in a total volume of distribution (Vd) of vancomycin that ranges from of 0.5 to 0.9 L/kg [31, 172, 184]

Elimination

In patients with normal renal function, 70 to 90% of an intravenous dose of vancomycin is excreted in the urine unchanged by glomerular filtration. The serum elimination half-life in patients with normal renal function is variable, but averages 6 hours [171]. However, terminal half-lives ranging from 3 to 11 hours have been observed [184]. In anuric patients, the serum half-life increases markedly to 6 to 10 days [171]. The liver may also be involved in the disposition of vancomycin as dose adjustments have been required in patients with severe liver dysfunction [172]. An interesting study by Golper et al that compared systemic vancomycin clearance simultaneously with the renal clearances of vancomycin, creatinine, inulin and para-aminohippurate demonstrated a substantial non-renal clearance of vancomycin of 30%. In addition, the researchers found that the non-renal clearance of vancomycin was concentration dependent with a 10% greater clearance at serum concentrations of 14 mg/ml as compared to 7 mg/ml [185].

Renal transport of vancomycin

Despite the known renal disposition and nephrotoxicity of vancomycin, elucidation of its renal transport pathway remains incompletely defined. Early research by Sokol in rabbits demonstrated that vancomycin enters the proximal tubule cell across the basal lateral membrane via the organic acid transport system [186]. In addition, Sokol showed that vancomycin remains sequestered and concentrates inside the PTC. Vancomycin was found to enter the tubular lumen only by the much slower transport pathway of simple diffusion; a secretory pathway was not found. This data would suggest that this renal transport pathway is a potential mechanism of vancomycin nephrotoxicity. However, there is not yet data that associates the PTC sequestration of vancomycin with nephrotoxicity or whether there is renal accumulation of vancomycin in humans [189]. Work by Rodvold et al which revealed substantial tubular secretion of vancomycin in a human study of vancomycin pharmacokinetics and renal dysfunction also confounds an understanding of the vancomycin renal transport [187]. Finally, a study by Yano et al found that vancomycin enhanced the binding of tobramycin to the rat renal brush border at the apical surface [188]. This may be a potential mechanism for the increased incidences of nephrotoxicity seen when vancomycin and an aminoglycoside are used concomitantly. More importantly, though, the existence of this deleterious drug interaction may suggest some magnitude of interaction of vancomycin at the apical surface of the PTC. It is readily apparent that more research is needed before a complete understanding of the complex renal transport of vancomycin is known.

Epidemiology of vancomycin nephrotoxicity

The early formulations of vancomycin, termed "Mississippi mud" because of its brownish color, were replete with impurities. Fever, hypotension and severe dose-limiting phlebitis were frequently seen in the patients first treated with vancomycin and were attributed to these impurities and pyrogens in these early preparations of vancomycin. In addition, the nephrotoxicity and ototoxicity first seen with vancomycin was also attributed to these impure formulations. Since its introduction, however, preparations of vancomycin have consistently improved achieving 92 to 95% purity since 1980 and the incidence of nephrotoxicity and ototoxicity has attenuated [172, 174]. The incidence of nephrotoxicity associated with vancomycin is wide ranging with reports ranging from 0 to 44% in several prospective studies [174-178]. However, obtaining an accurate estimate of the incidence of nephrotoxicity from these studies is hindered by the variable purity of the vancomycin preparations administered, the different endpoints used to define nephrotoxicity, the presence of severe comorbid disease and the concomitant use of nephrotoxic medications in many of the study patients [174]. More recent reviews of the more contemporary vancomycin formulations place the overall incidence of nephrotoxicity of from 0 to 5% [183, 184].

Risk factors for nephrotoxicity

Despite the relative uncertainty regarding the actual incidence of vancomycin-associated nephrotoxicity, studies have revealed various factors that place a patient at increased risk. Elderly patients appear to be at increased risk for nephrotoxicity from vancomycin therapy. This is likely secondary to their age-related decline in GFR which reduces vancomycin clearance and places them at risk for drug accumulation [179]. Vance-Bryan et al demonstrated that in a cohort of hospitalized patients greater than 60 years of age, the incidence of nephrotoxicity of 18.9%. However, in a similar cohort less than 60 years of age, the incidence of nephrotoxicity was only 7.8% [175]. Using an aminoglycoside with vancomycin is also a risk factor for nephrotoxicity as shown in several studies [178, 180-182]. In a study by Wood et al, vancomycin alone and with tobramycin was administered to rats. Tobramycin in isolation was nephrotoxic, vancomycin was not. However, concomitant use of tobramycin and vancomycin resulted in earlier and more severe nephrotoxicity [180]. Rybak et al showed similar results in a prospective evaluation of patients receiving vancomycin alone or in combination with an aminoglycoside [178]. Only 5% of patients receiving vancomycin alone developed nephrotoxicity compared to 11% receiving only gentamicin and 22% receiving both vancomycin and gentamicin [178]. These previous results were corroborated by a meta-analysis of seven studies which found the incidence of nephrotoxicity of vancomycin with an aminoglycoside was 13.3% greater than vancomycin alone and 4.3% greater than aminoglycoside alone [181]. Other cited risk factors include a supratherapeutic peak and trough levels, prolonged therapy greater than 21 days and preexisting CKD [174, 183].

Therapeutic drug monitoring of vancomycin

Due to the risks of serious adverse events such as nephrotoxicity and ototoxicity observed when systemic vancomycin was first used, therapeutic drug monitoring programs (TDM) for vancomycin were developed. To ameliorate the risk of toxicity, clinicians have historically targeted a peak vancomycin serum concentration of 30 to 40 mg/L and a trough serum concentration of 5 to 10 mg/L. However, there is a notable lack of reliable data to show that these target serum concentrations improve clinical outcome or avoid toxicity [173, 184, 190-196]. Ototoxicity is the only clinical endpoint that has been shown to be associated with a specific vancomycin serum concentration, observed in patients with vancomycin serum concentrations greater than 40 to 50 mg/L. A critical review by Cantu et al of several studies involving systemic vancomycin therapy found no evidence that adherence to specific ranges of serum vancomycin concentrations was clinically beneficial or avoided nephrotoxicity [190]. Furthermore, it is widely believed that maintaining an elevated vancomycin trough serum concentration (>10 ug/ml) is associated with nephrotoxicity. However, any interpretation of a potential nephrotoxic event associated with vancomycin is inherently confounded since vancomycin is dependent on glomerular filtration for elimination. As a result, an observed decline in renal function from any etiology will increase vancomycin serum concentrations and lead to the possibly erroneous association of an elevated vancomycin serum concentration and nephrotoxicity.

The relative paucity of clinical data to support the target serum concentrations of vancomycin and the associated medical expenses of therapeutic monitoring programs has led many researchers to question the necessity of monitoring vancomycin therapy. In addition, there is the perception that serious vancomycin toxicity has attenuated with the improved formulations. Freeman et al in their critical analyses and review state that in a majority of patients routine therapeutic monitoring of vancomycin is unnecessary. Vancomycin dosing can be done empirically based on the age, size and estimate of the renal function of the patient as with other antibiotics [192]. Conversely, Welty et al found that TDM of vancomycin was a significant clinical benefit for the patient [197]. Freeman et al conclusions may prove true; however, there is a significant subset of patients for which it would be clinically prudent to monitor vancomycin serum concentrations despite the uncertainties regarding efficacy and toxicity. The first group would be patients receiving vancomycin and another nephrotoxin such as an aminoglycoside. Though it remains unresolved whether monitoring serum vancomycin concentrations prevents nephrotoxicity, increasing vancomycin serum concentrations may be a harbinger of nephrotoxicity. The increasing concentrations could serve to alert the clinician that dosing adjustments may be needed in both the vancomycin and the nephrotoxin. Patients receiving hemodialysis also could benefit from the monitoring of vancomycin serum concentrations [191]. Given the prolonged vancomycin elimination half-life in anuria, hemodialysis patients receive vancomycin infrequently. In addition, there is significant vancomycin removal that occurs with each hemodialysis session. As a result, hemodialysis patients are at risk of having a prolonged sub-therapeutic vancomycin serum concentration and ineffective antibiotic therapy. Another group of patients that could benefit from the TDM of vancomycin are patients receiving a higher-than-usual dose of vancomycin. This has been increasingly observed in the treatment of bacterial meningitis from penicillin-resistant pneumococci. Standard doses of vancomycin have been shown to be inadequate for meningitis given the uncertainty of penetration into the CSF; treatment failures have occurred [191]. Monitoring serum concentrations of vancomycin would be another guide for the clinician and provide a degree of assurance that the patient is receiving adequate therapy. Burn patients and the morbidly obese would also derive benefit from monitoring vancomycin serum concentrations given the pharmacokinetic uncertainty regarding dosing in these patient populations. Monitoring vancomycin serum concentrations may also be reasonable in patients with rapidly changing renal function. It may be more efficient to monitor serum levels than repeatedly adjusting the vancomycin regimen on the basis of nomograms or other formulae [191]. Finally, immunocompromised patients with hematologic malignancies should receive monitoring of vancomycin serum concentrations. In a study by Fernandez de Gatta et al this patient group achieved a cost-effective, clinical benefit from the TDM of vancomycin.

Prevention of vancomycin nephrotoxicity

Interventions to ameliorate the nephrotoxicity observed with vancomycin have largely been confined to the laboratory and have focused on attenuating oxidative stress. Oxidative stress has been postulated as the primary mechanism in the pathogenesis of vancomycin-induced nephrotoxicity [200]. A study by Ocak et al tested a diverse group of antioxidants that included caffeic acid phenethyl ester (CAPE), vitamin C, vitamin E and N-acetylcysteine [198]. Each of these agents were administered to rats given a seven day course of vancomycin. Evaluation of the renal tissue of the control group that received only vancomycin demonstrated tubular cell degenerations with interstitial edema, epithelial vacuolization and desquamation; the glomeruli appeared normal. Ockak et al demonstrated that all of the agents attenuated the vancomycin-induced tubular injury in the rats. However, the rats given vitamin E had the least degree of vancomycin-induced tubular damage. This was followed in order of increasing tubular damage by vitamin C, N-acetylcysteine and CAPE [199]. Similar decrements in vancomycin-induced renal injury were achieved in another study by Nishino et al using hexamethyl-enediamine-conjugated superoxide dismutase (AH-SOD). This compound rapidly accumulates in the renal proximal tubule cells and has been shown to ameliorate free radical injury. Histological examination of the kidneys of rats given vancomycin alone revealed marked destruction of glomeruli and necrosis of proximal tubules. In contrast, the rat cohort given vancomycin and AH-SOD did not exhibit these renal pathological changes [199]. Finally, in two different studies, Oktem et al using the antioxidant erdosteine and Celik et al using the antioxidants α-lipoic, Gingko biloba extract, melatonin and amrinone reduced oxidative injury in rats with vancomycin-induced nephrotoxicity [200, 201].

Alternative gram positive antibiotics

Interventions to reduce the risk of vancomycin-induced nephrotoxicity have not yet been translated to the clinical setting. As a result, alternative antibiotics provide the most viable option to avoid the potential toxicities of vancomycin. Teicoplanin is a glycopeptide antibiotic that has a similar antimicrobial spectrum of activity as vancomycin and is better tolerated; reports of nephrotoxicity and ototoxicity are uncommon. Teicoplanin can also be administered less frequently than vancomycin and does not require TDM [202]. Two other antibiotics that are finding increasingly greater clinical application are linezolid and quinupristin-dalfopristin [203-206]. These antibiotics target drug-resistant gram positive cocci including vancomycin-resistant *Enterococci* (VRE) and methicillin-resistant *Staphylococcus aureus* (MRSA). Though each has its own specific adverse event profile, none of them are currently associated with nephrotoxicity. Daptomycin is the first of the class of cyclic lipopeptides. It has bactericidal activity against gram positive bacteria including MRSA and has not been associated with nephrotoxicity. There are reports, however, of creatine kinase elevations with its clinical use which could conceivably place a patient at risk for myoglobinuric acute kidney injury [206]. Finally, tigecycline is the first available member of the glycylcylines, another new class of antimicrobial agents [208]. Tigecycline has a much broader spectrum of activity that includes gram positive, gram negative and anaerobic bacteria [208]. Of the gram positive bacteria, tigecycline has activity against MRSA and glycopeptide-intermediate and resistant *Staphylococcus aureus* and VRE. Currently there have been no reports of nephrotoxicity associated with clinical use of this agent.

Though each of these antibiotics meets or exceeds many of the clinical attributes of vancomycin, it remains to be seen where these new agents will ultimately be placed in the antibiotic armentarium or whether they will fully replace vancomycin in clinical use. As a result, these newer antibiotics should be reserved for patients who have either acquired a vancomycin-resistant infection or cannot tolerate vancomycin.

References

1. Vackulenko SB, Moashery S, Versatility of aminoglycosides and prospects for their future, Clinical Microbiology Reviews, 2003; 16(3): 430-50.
2. Chambers HF, Chapter 45 Aminoglycosides In Goodman and Gilman's The Pharmacological Basis of Therapeutics, 11 edition, editors Hardman JG, Limbird LE, Molinoff PB, Ruddon RW, Goodman Gilman A, 2006, McGraw-Hill New York.
3. Nicolau DP, Freeman CD, Belliveau PP, Experience with once-daily aminoglycoside program administered to 2184 adult patients, Antimicrob Agents Chemother, 1995; 39(3): 650-55.
4. Smith CR, Moore RD, Lietman PS, Studies of risk factors for aminoglycoside nephrotoxicity, Am J Kidney Dis, 1986; 8(5): 308-13.
5. Schentag JJ, Cerra FB, Plaut ME, Clinical and pharmacokinetic characteristics of aminoglycoside nephrotoxicity in 201 critically ill patients, Antimicrob Agents Chemother, 1982; 21(5): 721-26.
6. Beauchamp D, Labrecque G, Aminoglycoside nephrotoxicity: do time and frequency of administration matter?, Current opinion in critical care, 2001; 7: 401-08.
7. English WP, Williams MD, Should aminoglycoside antibiotics be abandoned?, Am J Surg, 2000; 180:512-16.
8. Hou SH, Bushinsky DA, Wish JB, Cohen JJ, Harrington JT, Hospital-acquired renal insufficiency: a prospective study, Am J Med, 1983; 74: 243-48.
9. Koo J, Tight R, Rajkumar V, Hawa Z, Comparison of once-daily versus pharmacokinetic dosing of aminoglycosides in elderly patients, Am J Med, 1996; 101: 177-83.
10. Rybak MJ, Abate BJ, Kang SL, Ruffing MJ, Lerner SA, Drusano GL, Prospective evaluation of the effect of an aminoglycoside dosing regimen on rates of observed nephrotoxicity and ototoxicity, Antimicrob Agents Chemother, 1999; 43(7): 1549-55.
11. Smith CR, Lipsky JJ, Laskin OL, Hellmann DB, Mellits ED, Longstreth J, Lietman PS, Double-blind comparison of the nephrotoxicity and auditory toxicity of gentamicin and tobramycin, New Engl J Med, 1980; 302 (20): 1106-1109.
12. Munckhof WJ, Grayson ML, Turnidge JD, A meta-analysis of studies on the safety and efficacy of aminoglycosides given either once daily or as divided doses, J Antimicrob Chemother, 1996; 37: 645-63.
13. Hatala R, Dinh T, Cook DJ, Once-daily aminoglycoside dosing in immunocompetent adults, Ann Int Med, 1996; 124(8): 717-25.
14. Ferriols-Lisart R, Alos-Alminana M, Effectiveness and safety of once-daily aminoglycosides: a meta-analysis, Am J Health Syst Pharm, 1996; 53(10): 1141-50.
15. Barza M, Ioannidis JP, Capelleri JC, Lau J, Single or multiple daily doses of aminoglycosides: a meta-analysis, BMJ, 1996; 312(7027): 338-44.
16. Prins JM, Buller HR, Once versus daily gentamicin in patients with serious infections, Lancet, 1993; 341: 335-39.
17. Smith CR, Baughma KL, Edwards CQ, Rogers JF, Lietman PS, Controlled comparison of amikacin and gentamicin, New Engl J Med, 1977; 296 (7): 349-53.
18. Klkeinknecht D, Landais P, Goldbarb B, Pathophysiology and clinical aspects of drug-induced tubular necrosis in man, Contr Nephrol, 1987; 55: 145-58.
19. Lane AZ, Wright GE, Blair DC, Ototoxicity and nephrotoxicity of amikacin, Am J Med, 1977; 62: 911-18.
20. Bertino JS, Booker LA, Franck PA, Jenkins PL, Franck KR, Nafziger AN, Incidence of and significant risk factors for aminoglycoside-associated nephrotoxicity in patients dosed by using individualized pharmacokinetic monitoring, J Inf Dis, 1993; 167:173-79.

21. Raveh D, Kopyt M, Hite Y, Rudensky B, Sonnenblick M, Yinnon AM, Risk factors for nephrotoxicity in elderly patients receiving once-daily aminoglycoside, Q J Med, 2002; 95: 291-97.
22. Galloe AM, Graudal N, Christensen HR, Kampmann JP, Aminoglycosides: single or multiple daily dosing, Eur J Pharmacol, 1995; 48: 39-43.
23. Paterson DL, Robson JM, Wagener MM, Risk factors for toxicity in elderly patients given aminoglycosides once daily, J Gen Intern Med, 1998; 13: 735-39.
24. Baciewicz AM, Sokos DR, Cowan RI, Aminoglycoside-associated nephrotoxicity in the elderly, Ann Pharmacother, 2003; 37: 182-6.
25. Bailey TC, Little JR, Littenberg B, Reichhley RM, Dunagan WC, A meta- analysis of extended-interval dosing versus multiple daily dosing of aminoglycosides, Clin Infect Dis, 1997; 24: 786-95.
26. Lerner AM, Reyes MP, Cone LA, Blair DC, Jansen W, Wright GE, Lorber RR, Randomised, controlled trial of the comparative efficacy, auditory toxicity and nephrotoxicity of tobramycin and netilmicin, Lancet, 1983; 1123-25.
27. Hitt CM, Klepser ME, Nightingale CH, Quintiliani R, Nicolau DP, Pharmacoeconomic impact of once-daily aminoglycoside administration, Pharmacotherapy, 1997; 17(4): 810-14.
28. Moore RD, Smith CR, Lipsky JJ, Mellits ED, Lietman PS, Risk factors for nephrotoxicity in patients treated with aminoglycosides, Ann Int Med, 1984; 100: 352-57.
29. Sawyers CL, Moore RD, Lerner SA, Smith CR, A model for predicting nephrotoxicity in patients treated with aminoglycosides, J Infect Dis, 1986; 153(6): 1062-68.
30. Humes, HD, Aminoglycoside nephrotoxicity, Kidney Int; 1988; 33: 900-11.
31. Burton ME, Shaw LM, Schentag JJ, Evans WE, Applied pharmacokinetics and pharmacodynamics: principles of therapeutic drug monitoring, 4th ed, 2006, Lippincott Williams and Wilkins, Baltimore, MD, Philadelphia PA.
32. Ali BH, Gentamicin nephrotoxicity in humans and animals: some recent research, Gen Pharmac, 1995; 26(7): 1477-87.
33. Shargel L, Multi-compartment models, In: Applied biopharmaceutics and pharmacokinetics, Shargel L, Wu Pong S, Yu A, editors, McGraw-Hill, New York, 2005.
34. McNamara DR, Nafziger AN, Menhinick AM, Bertino JS, A dose-ranging study of gentamicin pharmacokinetics: implications for extended interval aminoglycoside therapy, J Clin Pharm, 2001; 41: 374-77.
35. Triggs E, Charles B, Pharmacokinetics and therapeutic drug monitoring of gentamicin in the elderly, Clin Pharmacokinet, 1999; 37(4): 331-41.
36. Laurent G, Kishore B, Tulkens PM, Aminoglycoside-induced renal phospholipidosis and nephrotoxicity, Biochem Pharm, 1990; 40(11): 2383-92.
37. Fabre J, Rudhardt M, Blanchard P, Regamey C, Persistence of sisomicin and gentamicin in renal cortex and medulla compared with other organs and serum of rats, Kidney Int, 1976; 10: 444-49.
38. Giuliano RA, Paulus GJ, Verpooten GA, Pattyn VM, Pollet DE, Nouwen EJ, Laurent G, Carlier MB, Maldague P, Tulkens PM, De Broe ME, Recovery of cortical phospholipidosis and necrosis after acute gentamicin loading in rat, Kidney Int, 1984; 26: 838-47.
39. Giuliano RA, Verpooten GA, Verbist L, Wedeen RP, DeBroe ME, *In vivo* Uptake kinetics of aminoglycosides in the kidney cortex of rats, J Pharmacol Exp Ther, 1985; 236 (2): 470-75.
40. Vandewalle A, Farman N, Morin JP, Fillastre JP, Hatt PY, Bonvalet JP, Gastineau M, Wanstok F, Gentamicin incorporation along the nephron: autoradiographic study on isolated tubules, Kidney Int, 1981; 19: 529-39.
41. Wedeen RP, Batuman V, Cheeks C, Marquet E, Sobel H, Transport of gentamicin in rat proximal tubule, 1983, Lab Invest, 1983; 48(2): 212-23.
42. Mingeot-Leclercq MP, Tulkens PM, Aminoglycosides: nephrotoxicity, Antimicrob Agents Chemotherap, 1999; 43(5): 1003-1012.
43. Nagai J, Takano M, Molecular aspects of renal handling of aminoglycosides and strategies for preventing the nephrotoxicity, Drug Metab Pharmacokinet, 2004; 19(3): 159-70.
44. Silverblatt FJ, Kuehn C, Autoradiography of gentamicin uptake by the rat proximal tubule cell, Kidney Int, 1979; 15: 335-45.
45. Molitoris, BA, Meyer C, Dahl R, Geerdes A, Mechanism of ischemia-enhanced aminoglycoside binding and uptake by proximal cells, Am J Physiol, 1993; F907-916.
46. Spiegel DM, Shanley PF, Molitoris BA, Mild ischemia predisposes the S3 segment to gentamicin toxicity, Kidney Ing, 1990, 38: 459-64.
47. Sastrasinh M, Knauss TC, Weinberg JM, Humes HD, Identification of the aminoglycoside binding site in rat renal brush border membranes, J Pharmacol Ext Ther, 1982; 22(2): 350-58.
48. Moestrup SK, Cui S, Vorum H, Bregengard C, Bjorn SE, Norris K, Gliemann J, Christensen EI, Evidence that epithelial glycoprotein 330/megalin mediates uptake of polybasic drugs, J Clin Invest, 1995; 96: 1404-13.
49. Hammond TG, Majewski RR, Kaysen JH, Goda FO, Navar GL, Pontillon F, Verroust PJ, Gentamicin inhibits rat renal cortical homotypic endosomal fusion: role of megalin, Am J Physiol, 1997; 272 (41): F117-23.

50. Christensen EI, Birn H, Megalin and cubilin: multifunctional endocytic receptors, Nature Reviews: Molecular Biology, 2002; 3: 258-68.
51. Williams PD, Bennett DB, Gleason CR, Hottendorf GH, Correlation between renal membrane binding and nephrotoxicity, Antimicrob Agents Chemotherap, 1987; 31(4): 570-74.
52. Christensen EI, Birn H, Megalin and cubilin: synergistic endocytic receptors in renal proximal tubule, Am J Physiol, 2001; 280: F562-73.
53. Christensen EI, Willnow TE, Essential role of megalin in renal proximal tubule for vitamin homeostasis, J Am Soc Nephrol, 1999; 10: 2224-36.
54. Kerjaschki D, Fahquhar MG, The pathogenic antigen of Heymann nephritis is a membrane glycoprotein of the renal proximal tubule brush border, Proc Nat Acad Sci, USA, 1982; 79: 5557-61.
55. Lundgren S, Carling T, Hjalm G, Juhlin C, Rastad J, Pihlgren U, Rask L, Akerstrom G, Hellman P, Tissue distribution of human gp330/megalin, a putative calcium-sensing protein, J Histochem Cytochem, 1997; 45(3): 383-92.
56. Schmitz C, Hilpert J, Jacobsen C, Boensch C, Christensen EI, Luft FC, Willnow TE, Megalin deficiency offers protection from renal aminoglyside accumulation, J Biol Chem, 2002; 277 (1): 618-22.
57. Cui S, Verroust PJ, Moestrup SK, Christensen EI, Megalin/gp330 mediates uptake of albumin in the renal proximal tubule, Am J Physiol, 1996; 271: F900-907.
58. Nagai J, Tanaka H, Nakanishi N, Murakami T, Takano M, Role of megalin in renal handling of aminoglycosides, Am J Physiol, 2001; 281: F337-44.
59. Christensen EI, Birn H, Verroust P, Moestrup SK, Membrane receptors for endocytosis in the renal proximal tubule, Int Rev Cytol, 1998, 237-84.
60. Willnow TE, Receptor-associated protein (RAP): a specialized chaperone for endocytic receptors, Biol Chem, 1998; 379: 1025-31.
61. Birn H, Vorum H, Verroust PJ, Moestrup SK, Christensen EI, Receptor- associated protein is important for normal processing of megalin in kidney proximal tubules, J Am Soc Nephrol, 2000; 11: 191-202.
62. Zhai, XY, Nielsen R, Birn H, Drumm K, MildenbergerS, Freudinger R, Moestrup SK, Verrouost PJ, Christensen EI, Gekle M, Cubilin and megalin- mediated uptake of albumin in cultures proximal tubule cells of opossum kidney, 2000, 58: 1523-33.
63. Birn H, Fyfe JC, Jacobsen C, Mounier F, Verroust PJ, Orskov H, Willnow TE, Moestrup SK, Christensen EI, Cubilin is an albumin binding protein important for renal tubular albumin reabsorption, J Clin Invest, 2000; 105: 1353-61.
64. Koryraki R, Cubilin, a multifunctional epithelial receptor: an overview, J Mol Med, 2001; 79: 161-67.
65. Verroust PJ, Birn H, Nielsen R, Kozyraki R, Christensen EI, The tandem endocytic receptors megalin and cubilin are important proteins in renal pathology, Kidney Int, 2002; 62: 745-56.
66. Bennett WM, Mechanisms of aminoglycoside nephrotoxicity, Clin Exp Pharm Physiol, 1989; 16: 1-6.
67. Olbricht CJ, Fink M, Gutjahr E, Alterations in lysosomal enzymes of the proximal tubule in gentamicin nephrotoxicity, Kidney Int, 1991; 39: 639-46.
68. Ford, DM, Dahl RH, Lamp CA, Molitoris BA, Apically and basolaterally internalized aminoglycosides colocalize in LLC-PK1 lysosomes and alter cell function, Am J Physiol, 1994; 266: C52-57.
69. Servais H, Van Der Smissen P, Thirion G, Van Der Essen, G, Van Bambeke F, Tulkens PM, Mingeot-Leclercq M, Gentamicin-induced apoptosis in LLC-PK1 cells: involvement of lysosomes and mitochondria, Toxicol Appl Pharmacol, 2005; 206: 321-33.
70. Sandoval R, Leiser J, Molitoris BA, Aminoglycoside antibiotics traffic to the Golgi complex in LLC-PK1 cells, J Am Soc Nephrol, 1998; 9: 167-74.
71. Tulkens P, Trouet A, The uptake and intracellular accumulation of aminoglycoside antibiotics in lysosomes of cultured rat fibroblasts, Biochem Pharm, 1977; 27: 415-24.
72. Takano M, Ohishi Y, Okuda M, Yasuhar M, Hori R, Transport of gentamicin and fluid-phase endocytosis markers in the LLC-PK1 kidney epithelial cell line, J Pharmacol Exp Therap, 1993, 268(2): 669-74.
73. Hori R, Okuda M, Ohisi Y, Masato Y, Takano M, Surface binding and intracellular uptake of gentamicin in the cultured kidney epithelial cell line (LLC-PK1), J Pharmacol Exp Therap, 1992, 261(3): 1200-05.
74. Sundin DP, Sandoval R, Molitoris BA, Gentamicin inhibits renal protein and phospholipid metabolism in rats: implications involving intracellular trafficking, J Am Soc Nephrol, 2001, 12: 114-23.
75. Sandoval R, Dunn KW, Molitoris BA, Gentamicin traffics rapidly and directly to the Golgi complex in LLC-PK1 cells, Am J Physiol, 2000, 279: F884-890.
76. Sandvig K, Ryd M, Garred O, Schwea E, Holm PK, van Deurs B, Retrograde transport from the Golgi complex to the ER of both Shiga toxin and the nontoxic Shiga B-fragment is regulated by butyric acid and cAMP, J Cell Biol, 1994, 126: 53-64.
77. Lord JM, Roberts LM, Toxin entry: retrograde transport through the secretory pathway, J Cell Biol, 1998, 140: 733-36.

78. Sandoval RM, Molitoris BA, Gentamicin traffics retrograde through the secretory pathway and is released in the cytosol via the endoplasmic reticulum, Am J Physiol, 2004, 286: F617-24.
79. Sandoval RM, Bacallao RL, Dunn KW, Leiser JD, Molitoris BA, Nucleotide depletion increases trafficking of gentamicin to the Golgi complex in LLC-PK1 cells, Am J Physiol, 2002, 283: F1422-29.
80. Sandvig K, Garred O, van Helvoort A, van Meer G, Van Deurs B, Importance of glycolipid synthesis for butyric acid-induced sensitization to Shiga toxin and intracellular sorting of toxin in A431 cells, Mol Biol Cell, 1996; 7: 1391-1404.
81. Bennett WM, Mela-Riker LM, Houghton DC, Gilbert DN, Buss WC, Microsomal protein synthesis inhibition: an early manifestation of gentamicin nephrotoxicity, Am J Physiol, 1988; 24: F265-69.
82. Zager RA, Gentamicin nephrotoxicity in the setting of acute renal hypoperfusion, Am J Physiol, 1988; 23: F574-81.
83. Houghton DC, Hartnett M, Campbell-Boswell M, Porter G, Bennett W, A light and electron microscopic analysis of gentamicin nephrotoxicity in rats, Am J Pathol, 1976, 82: 589-612.
84. Humes HD, Weinberg JM, Knauss TC, Clinical and pathophysiologic aspects of aminoglycoside nephrotoxicity, Am J Kidney Dis, 1982; 2(1): 4-29.
85. Kosek JC, Mazze RI, Cousins MJ, Nephrotoxicity of gentamicin, Lab Invest, 1974, 30(1): 48-57.
86. El-Mouedden M, Laurent G, Mingeot-Leclercq MP, Taper HS, Cumps J, Tulkens PM, Apoptosis in renal proximal tubules of rats treated with low doses of aminoglycosides, Antimicrob Agents Chemotherap, 2000, 44(3): 665-75.
87. El-Mouedden M, Laurent G, Mingeot-Leclercq MP, Tulkens PM, Gentamicin- induced apoptosis in renal cell lines and embryonic rat fibroblasts, Toxicol Sci, 2000, 56:229-39.
88. Servais H, Jossin Y, Van Bambeke F, Tulkens PM, Mingeot-Leclercq MP, Gentamicin causes apoptosis at low concentrations in renal LLC-PK1 cells subjected to electroporation, Antimicrob Agents Chemotherap, 2006, 50(4): 1213-21.
89. Laurent G, Kishore BK, Tulkens PM, Aminoglycoside-induced renal phospholipidosis and nephrotoxicity, Biochem Pharmacol, 1990, 40(11): 2383-92.
90. Miyazaki T, Sagawa R, Honma T, Noguchi S, Harada T, Komatsuda A, Ohtani H, Wakui H, Sawada K, Otaka M, Watanabe S, Jikei M, Ogawa N, Hamada F, Itoh H, 73-kDa molecular chaperone HSP73 is a direct target of antibiotic gentamicin, J Biol Chem, 2004; 279(17): 17295-17300.
91. Martinez-Salgado C, Eleno N, Morales AI, Perez-Barriocanal F, Arevalo M, Lopez-Novoa JM, Gentamicin treatment induces simultaneous mesangial proliferation and apoptosis in rats, Kidney Int, 2004, 65: 2161-71.
92. Laurent G, Carlier MB, Rollman B, Van Hoof F, Tulkens P, Mechanism of aminoglycoside-induced lysosomal phospholipidosis: *in vitro* and *in vivo* studies with gentamicin and amikacin, Biochem Pharmac, 1982, 31(23): 3861-70.
93. Giurgea-Marin L, Toubeau G, Laurent G, Heuson-Stiennon JA, Tulkens PM, Impairment of lysosome-pinocytotic vesicle fusion in rat kidney proximal tubules after treatment with gentamicin at low doses, Toxicol Appl Pharmacol, 1986, 86: 271-85.
94. Hostetler KY, Hall LB, Inhibition of kidney lysosomal phospholipases A and C by aminoglycoside antibiotics: possible mechanism of aminoglycoside toxicity, Proc Nat Acad Sci, 1982, 79: 1663-67.
95. Appel GB, Aminoglycoside nephrotoxicity, Am J Med, 1990, 88:16S-20S.
96. Schwertz DW, Kreisberg JI, Venkatachalam, Effects of aminoglycosides on proximal tubule brush border membrane phosphatidylinositol-specific phospholipase C, J Pharmac and Exp Therap, 1984, 231(1): 48-55.
97. Sundin DP, Meyer C, Dahl R, Geerdes A, Sandoval R, Molitoris BA, Cellular mechanism of aminoglycoside tolerance in long-term gentamicin treatment, Am J Physiol, 1997, 272: C1309-18.
98. Schwertz DW, Kreisberg JI, Venkatachalam, Gentamicin-induced alterations in pig kidney epithelial (LLC-PK1) cells in culture, 1985, 236(1): 254-62.
99. Simmons CF, Bogusky RT, Humes HD, Inhibitory effects of gentamicin on renal mitochondrial oxidative phosphorylation, J Pharmac Ext Therap, 1980, 214(3): 709-15.
100. Weinberg, JM, Harding PG, Humes HD, Mechanisms of gentamicin-induced dysfunction of renal cortical mitochondria: effects on mitochondrial monovalent cation transport, Arch Biochem Biophys, 1980, 205(1): 232-39.
101. Weinberg, JM, Humes HD, Mechanisms of gentamicin-induced dysfunction of renal cortical mitochondria: effects on mitochondrial respiration, Arch Biochem Biophys, 1980, 205(1): 222-31.
102. Mather M, Rottenberg H, Polycations induce the release of soluble intermembrane mitochondrial proteins, Biochim Biophys Acta, 2001, 1503: 357-68.
103. Walker PD, Shav SV, Evidence suggesting a role for hydroxyl radical in gentamicin-induced acute renal failure in rats, J Clin Invest, 1988, 81: 334-41.
104. Ueda N, Guidet B, Shah SV, Gentamicin-induced mobilization of iron from renal cortical mitochondria, Am J Physiol, 1993, 34: F435-39.
105. Kaloyanides GJ, Aminoglycoside-induced functional and biochemical defects in the renal cortex, Toxicol Sci, 1984, 4(6): 930-43.

106. Weisblum B, Davies J, Antibiotic inhibitors of the bacterial ribosome, Bacteriol Rev, 1968, 32(4): 493-528.
107. Davies, J, Gorini L, Davis BD, Misreading of RNA codewords induced by aminoglycoside antibiotics, Mol Pharmacol, 1965, 1: 93-106.
108. Tai PC, Davis BD, Triphasic concentration effects of gentamicin activity on misreading in protein synthesis, Biochem, 1979, 18(1): 193-98.
109. Clark JM, Chang AY, Inhibitors of the transfer of amino acids from aminoacyl soluble ribonucleic acid to proteins, J Biol Chem, 1965, 240(12): 4734-39.
110. Kuhberger R, Piepersberg W, Petzet A, Buckel P, Bock A, Alteration of ribosomal protein L6 in gentamicin-resistant strains of Escherichia coli: effects on fidelity of protein synthesis, Biochem, 1979, 18(1): 187-92.
111. Wilhelm JM, Jessop JJ, Pettitt SE, Aminoglycoside antibiotics and eukaryotic protein synthesis: stimulation of errors in the translation of natural messengers in extracts of cultured human cells, Biochem, 1978, 17(7): 1149-53.
112. Moskowitz M, Kelker N, Sensitivity of cultured mammalian cells to streptomycin and dihydrostreptomycin, Science, 1963, 141: 647-48.
113. Charlwood J, Skehel JM, King N, Camilleri P, Lord P, Bugelski P, Atif U, Proteomic analysis of rat kidney cortex following treatment with gentamicin, J Proteom Res, 2002, 1(1): 73-82.
114. Moriyama T, Nakahama H, Fukuhara Y, Horio M, Yanase M, Orita Y, Kamada T, Kanashiro M, Miyake Y, Decrease in the fluidity of brush border membrane vesicles induced by gentamicin, Biochem Pharmac, 1989, 38(7): 1169-74.
115. Inui K, Saito H, Iwata T, Hori R, Aminoglycoside-induced alterations in apical membranes of kidney epithelial cell line (LLC-PK1), Am J Physio, 254: C251-57.
116. Whipple JK, Ausman RK, Franson T, Quebbeman EJ, Effect of individualized pharmacokinetic dosing on patient outcome, Crit Care Med, 1991, 19(12): 1480-85.
117. Bartal C, Danon A, Schlaffer F, Reisenberg K, Alkan M, Smoliakov R, Sidi A, Almog Y, Pharmacokinetic dosing of aminoglycosides: a controlled trial, Am J Med, 2003, 114: 194-98.
118. Destache CJ, Meyer SK, Bittner MJ, Hermann KG, Impact of clinical pharmacokinetic service on patients treated with aminoglycosides: a cost-benefit analysis, Ther Drug Mon, 12: 419-26.
119. Burton ME, Ash CL, Hill DP, Handy R, Shepherd MD, Vasko MR, A controlled trial of the cost benefit of computerized Bayesian aminoglycoside administration, Clin Pharmacol Ther, 49: 685-94.
120. Kemme DJ, Daniel CI, Aminoglycoside dosing: a randomized prospective study, South Med J, 1993, 86(1): 46-51.
121. Leehey DJ, Braun MI, Tholl DA, Chung LS, Gross CA, Roback JA, Lentino JR, Can pharmacokinetic dosing decrease nephrotoxicity associated with aminoglycoside therapy?, 1993, J Am Soc Nephrol, 1993, 4: 81-90.
122. Dillon KR, Dougherty SH, Casner P, Polly S, Individualized pharmacokinetic versus standard dosing of amikacin: a comparison of therapeutic outcomes, J Amtimicrob Chemo, 1989, 24: 581-89.
123. McCormack JP, Jewesson PJ, A critical reevaluation of the "therapeutic range" of aminoglycosides, Clin Infect Dis, 1992, 14: 320-39.
124. McCormack JP, An emotional-based medicine approach to monitoring once- daily aminoglycosides, Pharmacother, 2000, 20(12): 1524-27.
125. Ali BH, Agents ameliorating or augmenting experimental gentamicin nephrotoxicity: some recent research, Food Chem Toxicol, 2003, 41: 1447-52.
126. Beauchamp D, Laurent G, Maldague P, Abid S, Kishore BK, Tulkens PM, Protection against gentamicin-induced early renal alterations (phospholipidosis and increased DNA synthesis by coadministration of poly-L-aspartic acid, J Pharmacol Exp Therap, 1990, 255(2): 858-66.
127. Kishore BK, Lambricht P, Laurent G, Maldague P, Wagner R, Tulkens PM, Mechanism of protection afforded by polyaspartic acid against gentamicin- induced phospholipidosis. II. Comparative in-vitro and in-vivo studies with poly-L-aspartic, poly-L-glutamic and poly-D-glutamic acids, J Pharmacol Exp Therap, 1990, 255(2): 875-85.
128. Ramsammy LS, Josepovitz C, Lane BP, Kaloyanides, Polyaspartic acid protects against gentamicin nephrotoxicity in the rat, J Pharmacol Exp Therap, 1989, 250(1): 149-53.
129. Williams PD, Hottendorf GH, Bennett DB, Inhibition of renal membrane binding and nephrotoxicity of aminoglycosides, J Pharmacol Exp Therap, 1986, 237(3): 919-25.
130. Kishore BK, Ibrahim S, Lambricht P, Laurent G, Maldague P, Tulkens PM, Comparative assessment of poly-L-aspartic and poly-L-glutamic acids as protectants against gentamicin-induced renal lysosomal phospholipidosis, phospholipiduria and cell proliferation in rats, J Pharmacol Exp Therap, 1992, 262(1): 424-32.
131. Josepovitz C, Pastorzia-Munoz E, Timmerman D, Scott M, Feldman S, Kaloyanides GJ, Inhibition of gentamicin uptake in rat renal cortex *in vivo* by aminoglycosides and organic polycations, J Pharmacol Exp Therap, 1982, 223(2): 314-21.

132. Gilbert DN, Wood CA, Kohlhepp SJ, Kohnen PW, Houghton DC, Finkbeiner HC, Lindsley J, Bennett WM, Polyaspartic acid prevents experimental aminoglycoside nephrotoxicity, J Infect Dis, 1989, 159(5): 945-53.
133. Swan SK, Gilbert DN, Kohlhepp SJ, Leggett JE, Kohnen PW, Bennett WM, Duration of the protective effect of polyaspartic acid on experimental gentamicin nephrotoxicity, Antimicrob Agents Chemother, 1992, 36(11): 2556-58.
134. Kishore BK, Kallay Z, Lambricht P, Laurent G, Tulkens PM, Mechanism of protection afforded by polyaspartic acid against gentamicin-induced phospholipidosis I. polyaspartic acid binds gentamicin and displaces it from negatively charged phospholipid layers *in vitro*, J Pharmacol Exp Therap, 1990, 255(2): 867-74.
135. Mingeot-Leclercq, MP, Glupczynski Y, Tulkens PM, Aminoglycosides: activity and resistance, Antimicrob Agents Chemother, 1999, 43(4): 727-37.
136. Ali BH, Bashir AK, Effect of superoxide dismutase treatment on gentamicin nephrotoxicity in rats, Gen Pharmac, 1996, 27(2): 349-53.
137. Ali BH, Mousa HM, Effect of dimethyl sulfoxide on gentamicin-induced nephrotoxicity in rats, Hum Exp Toxicol, 2001, 20: 199-203.
138. Sandya P, Mohandass S, Varalakshmi P, Role of DL a-lipoic acid in gentamicin induced nephrotoxicity, Mol Cell Biochem, 2005, 145(1): 11-17.
139. Mazzon E, Britti D, De Sarro A, Caputi AP, Cuzzocrea S, Effect of N-acetylcysteine on gentamicin-mediated nephropathy in rats, Eur J Pharmacol, 2001, 424: 75-83.
140. Reiter RJ, Tan D, Sainz RM, Mayo JC, Lopez-Burillo S, Melatonin: reducing the toxicity and increasing the efficacy of drugs, J Pharm Pharmacol, 2002, 54: 1299-1321.
141. Ozbek E, Turkoz Y, Sahna E, Ozugurlu F, Mizrak B, Ozbek M, Melatonin administration prevents the nephrotoxicity induced by gentamicin, BJU Int, 2000, 85: 742-46.
142. Kumar KV, Shifow AA, Naidu MR, Ratnaker KS, Carvedilol: a betablocker with antioxidant property protects against gentamicin-induced nephrotoxicity in rats, Life Sci, 2000, 26: 2603-11.
143. Kumar KV, Naidu MR, Shifow AA, Ratnakar KS, Probucol protects against gentamicin-induced nephrotoxicity in rats, Ind J Pharmacol, 2000, 32: 108-13.
144. Ben-Ismail TH, Ali BH, Bashir AA, Influence of iron, deferoxamine and ascorbic acid on gentamicin-induced nephrotoxicity in rats, Gen Pharmacol, 1994, 25(6): 1259-52.
145. Bennett WM, Elliott WC, Houghton DC, Gilbert DN, DeFehr J, McCarron DA, Reduction of experimental gentamicin nephrotoxicity in rats by dietary calcium loading, Antimicrob Agents Chemotherap, 1982, 22(3): 508-12.
146. Quarum ML, Houghton DC, Gilbert DN, McCarron DA, Bennett WM, Increasing dietary calcium moderates experimental gentamicin nephrotoxicity, J Lab Clin Med, 1984, 103(1): 104-14.
147. Humes HD, Sastrasinh M, Weinberg JM, Calcium is a competitive inhibitor of gentamicin-renal membrane binding interactions and dietary calcium supplementation protects against gentamicin nephrotoxicity, J Clin Invest, 1982, 73: 134-47.
148. Kohlhepp SJ, Loveless MO, Kohnen PW, Houghton DC, Bennett WM, Gilbert DN, Nephrotoxicity of the constituents of the gentamicin complex, J Infect Dis, 149(4): 605-14.
149. Sandoval RM, Reilly JP, Running W, Campos SB, Santos JR, Phillips CL, Molitoris BA, A non-nephrotoxic gentamicin congener that retains antimicrobial efficacy, J Am Soc Nephrol, 17: 2697-2705.
150. Guo X, Nzerue C, How to prevent, recognize and treat drug-induced nephrotoxicity, Clev Clin J Med, 2002, 69(4): 289-312.
151. Martin JE, Commentary: once-daily aminoglycoside dosing: where are we now?, J Crit Care, 2003, 18(2): 107-13.
152. Loef BG, Epema AH, Smilde TD, Henning RH, Ebels T, Navis G, Stegeman CA, Immediate postoperative renal function deterioration in cardiac surgical patients predicts in-hospital mortality and long-term survival, J Am Soc Nephrol, 2005, 16: 195-200.
153. Lassnigg A, Schmidlin D, Mouhieddine M, Bachman LM, Druml W, Bauer P, Hiesmayr M, Minimal changes of serum creatinine predict prognosis in patients after cardiothoracic surgery: a prospective cohort study, J Am Soc Nephrol, 2004, 15: 1597-1605.
154. Chertow GM, Burdick E, Honour M, Bonventre JV, Bates DW, Acute kidney injury, mortality, length of stay and costs in hospitalized patients, J Am Soc Nephrol, 2005, 16: 3365-70.
155. Adams HR, Goodman FR, Weiss GB, Alteration of contractile function and calcium ion movement in vascular smooth muscle by gentamicin and other aminoglycoside antibiotics, Antimicrob Agents Chemotherap, 1974, 5(6): 640-46.
156. Cohen LS, Wechsler AS, Mitchell JH, Glick G, Depression of cardiac function by streptomycin and other antimicrobial agents, Am J Cardiol, 1970, 26: 505-11.
157. Mosenkis A, Kirk D, Berns JS, When chronic kidney disease becomes advanced, Postgrad Med, 2006, 119(1): 83-104.
158. Zager RA, Johnson AC, Lund S, Randolph-Habecker J, Toll-like receptor (TRL4) shedding and depletion: acute proximal tubular cell responses to hypoxic and toxic injury, Am J Physiol, 2007, 292: F304-312.
159. Hopkins P, Cohen J, Toll-like receptors: the key to the stable door?, Crit Care, 2002, 6: 99-101.

160. Zager RA, Subclinical gentamicin nephrotoxicity: a potential risk factor for exaggerated endotoxin-driven TNF-α production, Am J Physiol, 2007, 293: F43-49.
161. Tabeta K, Georgel P, Janssen E, Du X, Hoebe K, Crozat K, Mudd S, Shamel L, Sovath S, Goode J, Alexopoulou L, Flavell RA, Beutler B, Toll-like receptors 9 and 3 as essential components of innate immune defense against mouse cytomegalovirus, Proc Nat Acad Sci USA, 101(10): 3516-21.
162. Zager RA, Johnson AC, Lund S, Hanson S, Acute renal failure: determinants and characteristics of the injury-induced hyperinflammatory response, Am J Physiol, 2006, 291: F546-56.
163. Zager RA, Johnson AC, Lund S, Endotoxin tolerance: TNF-α hyper-reactivity and tubular cytoresistance in a renal cholesterol loading state, Kidney Int, 2007, 71: 496-503.
164. Zager RA, Johnson AC, Hanson SY, Lund S, Ischemic proximal tubular injury primes mice to endotoxin-induced TNF-α generation and systemic release, Am J Physiol, 2005, 289: F289-97.
165. Anders HJ, Banas B, Schlondorff D, Signaling danger: toll-like receptors and their potential roles in kidney disease, J Am Soc Nephrol, 2004, 15: 854-67.
166. El-Achkar T, Dagher PC, Renal toll-like receptors: recent advances and implications for disease, Nat Rev Neph, 2(10): 568-81.
167. El-Achkar T, Huang X, Plotkin Z, Sandoval RM, Rhodes GJ, Dagher PC, Sepsis induces changes in the expression and distribution of toll-like receptor 4 in the rat kidney, Am J Physiol, 2005, 290: F1034-43.
168. Chertow GM, Levy EM, Hammermeister KE, Grover F, Daley J, Independent association between acute renal failure and mortality following cardiac surgery, Am J Med, 1998, 104(4): 343-48.
169. Opal SM, Huber CE, Bench-to-bedside review: toll-like receptors and their role in septic shock, Crit Care, 2002, 6: 125-36.
170. Chambers HF, Chapter 46, Protein synthesis inhibitors and miscellaneous antibacterial agents, In Goodman and Gilman's The Pharmacological Basis of Therapeutics, 11 edition, editors Hardman JG, Limbird LE, Molinoff PB, Ruddon RW, Goodman Gilman A, 2006, McGraw-Hill New York.
171. Chambers HF, Chapter 43, Beta-lactam and other cell wall and membrane-active antibiotics, In Basic and clinical pharmacology, 10th edition, editors Katzung B, 2006, McGraw-Hill Medical, New York.
172. Wilhelm MP, Estes L, Vancomycin, Mayo Clin Proced, 1999, 74: 928-35.
173. Elting LS, Rubenstein EB, Kurtin D, Rolston KV, Fangtang J, Martin CG, Raad II, Whimbley EE, Manzullo E, Bodey GP, Mississippi mud in the 1990s, risks and outcomes of vancomycin-associated toxicity in general oncology practice, Cancer, 1998, 83: 2597-607.
174. Chow AW, Azar RM, Glycopeptides and nephrotoxicity, Inten Care Med, 1994, 20: S23-29.
175. Vance-Bryan K, Rotschafer JC, Gilliland SS, Rodvold KA, Fitzgerald CM, Guay DR, A comparative assessment of vancomycin-associated nephrotoxicity in the young versus the elderly hospitalized patient, J Antimicrob Chemother, 1994, 33: 811-21.
176. Downs NJ, Neihart RE, Dolezal JM, Hodges GR, Mild nephrotoxicity associated with vancomycin use, Arch Intern Med, 1989, 149: 1777-81.
177. Gudmundsson GH, Jensen LJ, Vancomycin and nephrotoxicity, Lancet, 1989, Mar 18: 625.
178. Rybak MJ, Albrecht LM, Boike SC, Chandrasekar PH, Nephrotoxicity of vancomycin, alone and with an aminoglycoside, J Antimicrob Chemotherap, 25(4): 679-87.
179. Cutler NR, Narang PK, Lesko LJ, Ninos M, Power M, Vancomycin disposition: the importance of age, Clin Pharmcol Ther, 1984, 36(6): 803-10.
180. Wood CA, Kohlhepp SJ, Kohnen PW, Houghton DC, Gilbert DN, Vancomycin enhancement of experimental nephrotoxicity, Antimicrob Agent Chemother, 1986, 30(1): 20-24.
181. Goetz MB, Sayers J, Nephrotoxicity of vancomycin and aminoglycoside therapy separately and in combination, J Antimicrob Chemother, 1993, 32: 325-34.
182. Cimino MA, Rotstein CR, Slaughter RL, Emrich LJ, Relationship of serum antibiotic concentrations to nephrotoxicity in cancer patients receiving concurrent aminoglycoside and vancomycin therapy, Am J Med, 1987, 83: 1091-97.
183. Farber BF, Moellering RC, Retrospective study of the toxicity of preparations of vancomycin from 1974 to 1981, Antimicrob Agent Chemother, 1983, 23(1): 138-41.
184. Moellering RC, Pharmacokinetics of vancomycin, J Antimicrob Chemother, 1984, 14: 43-52.
185. Golper TA, Noonan HM, Elzinga L, Gilbert D, Brummett R, Anderson JL, Bennett WM, Vancomycin pharmacokinetics, renal handling and nonrenal clearances in normal human subjects, Clin Pharmacol Ther, 1988, 43(5):565-70.
186. Sokol, PP, Mechanism of vancomycin transport in the kidney: studies in rabbit renal brush border and basolateral membrane vesicles, Am J Kidney Dis, 1991, 259(3): 1283-87.
187. Rodvold KA, Blum RA, Fischer JH, Zokufa HZ, Rotschafer JC, Crossley KB, Riff LJ, Vancomycin pharmacokinetics in patient with various degrees of renal function, Antimicrob Agent Chemother, 1988, 32(6): 848-52.

188. Yano Y, Hiraoka A, Oguma T, Enhancement of tobramycin binding to rat renal brush border membrane by vancomycin, J Pharmacol Exp Ther, 1995, 274: 695-99.
189. Appel GB, Given DB, Levine LR, Cooper GL, Vancomycin and the kidney, Am J Kidney Dis, 1986, 8: 75-80.
190. Cantu TG, Yamanaka-Yuen NA, Lietman PS, Serum vancomycin concentrations: reappraisal of their clinical value, Clin Infect Dis, 1994, 18: 533-43.
191. Moellering RC, Editorial: monitoring serum vancomycin levels: climbing the mountain because it is there?, Clin Infect Dise, 1994, 18: 544-46.
192. Freeman CD, Quintiliani R, Nightingale CH, Vancomycin therapeutic drug monitoring: is it necessary?, Ann Pharmacother, 1993, 27: 594-98.
193. Fernanez de Gatta, M, Calvo V, Hernanadez JM, Caballero D, San Miguel JF, Dominguez-Gil A, Cost-effectiveness analysis of serum vancomycin concentration monitoring in patients with hematologic malignancies, Clin Pharmacol Ther, 1996, 60: 332-40.
194. Leader WG, Chandler MH, Castiglia M, Pharmacokinetic optimization of vancomycin therapy, Clin Pharmacokinet, 1995, 28(4): 327-42.
195. Karam CM, McKinnon PS, Neuhauser MM, Rybak MJ, Outcome assessment of minimizing vancomycin monitoring and dosing adjustments, Pharmacother, 1999, 19(3), 257-266.
196. Darko W, Medicis JJ, Smith A, Guharoy R, Lehmann DF, Mississippi mud no more: cost-effectiveness of pharmacokinetic dosage adjustment of vancomycin to prevent nephrotoxicity, Pharmacother, 2003, 23(5): 643-50 197.
197. Welty TE, Copa AK, Impact of vancomycin therapeutic drug monitoring on patient care, Ann of Pharmacother, 1994, 28: 1335-39.
198. Ocak S, Gorur S, Hakverdi S, Celik S, Erdogan S, Protective effects of caffeic acid phenethyl ester, vitamin C, vitamin E and N-acetylcysteine on vancomycin- induced nephrotoxicity in rats, Basic Clin Pharmacol Toxicol, 2007, 100: 328-333.
199. Nishino Y, Takemura S, Minamiyama Y, Hirohashi K, Ogino T, Inoue M, Okada S, Kinoshita H, Targeting superoxide dismutase to renal proximal tubule cells attenuates vancomycin-induced nephrotoxicity in rats, Free Rad Res, 2003, 37(4): 373-79.
200. Oktem F, Arslan MK, Ozguner F, Candir O, Yilmaz HR, Ciris M, Uz E, *In vivo* evidences suggesting the role of oxidative stress in pathogenesis of vancomycin- induced nephrotoxicity: protection by erdosteine, Toxicol, 2005, 215: 227-33.
201. Celik I, Cihangiroglu M, Ilhan N, Akpolat N, Akbulut HH, Protective effects of different antioxidants and amrinone on vancomycin-induced nephrotoxicity, Basic Clin Pharmacol Toxicol, 2005, 97: 325-32.
202. Wood MJ, The comparative efficacy and safety of Teicoplanin and vancomycin, J Antimicrob Chemother, 1996, 37: 209-22.
203. Rehm SJ, Two new treatment options for infections due to drug-resistant gram- positive cocci, Clev Clin J Med, 2002, 69(5): 397-413.
204. Schmidt-Ioanas M, de Roux A, Lode H, New antibiotics for the treatment of severe staphylococcal infection in the critically ill patient, Curr Op Crit Care, 2005, 11: 481-86.
205. Delgado G, Neuhauser MM, Bearden DT, Danziger LH, Quinupristin- Dalfopristin: an overview, Pharmacother, 2000, 20(12): 1469-85.
206. Akins RL, Haase KK, Gram positive resistance: pathogens, implications and treatment options, Pharmaother, 2005, 25(7): 1001-10.
207. French GL, Bactericidal agents in the treatment of MRSA infections—the potential role of daptomycin, J Antimicrob Chemother, 2006, 58: 1107-17.
208. Rose WE, Rybak MJ, Tigecycline: first of a new class of antimicrobial agents, Pharmacother, 2006, 26(8): 1099-1110.
209. Mercier RC, Kennedy C, Meadows C, Antimicrobial activity of tigecycline (GAR-936) against Enterococcus faecium and Staphylococcus aureus used alone and in combination, Pharmacother, 2002, 22(12): 1517-23.

13

Beta-lactam antibiotics

Constantin COJOCEL†

Kuwait University, Kuwait

Constantin Cojocel passed away in 2007.
This chapter was updated by the editors.
The editors wish to dedicate this chapter to his memory.

Introduction

The large family of β-lactams comprises penicillins, cephalosporins, cephamycins, monobactams, carbacephems and carbapenems and are so named since they all containing the β-lactam moiety.

Penicillin was the first β-lactam antibiotic and was discovered in 1928 by Sir Alexander Fleming at St. Mary's Hospital, London [1]. The β-lactam chemical structure for penicillin was first proposed by Abraham and Chain in 1943 and finally established in 1945 by X-ray crystallographic analysis. In the same year, Giuseppe Brotzu, a Sardinian professor of bacteriology, isolated *Cephalosporium acremonium* from the sea near a sewage outfall at Cagliari, which produced antibiotic material with a broad spectrum of activity. It was almost eight years later in 1953 when Newton and Abraham, while studying the production of antibiotics by Brotzu's Cephalosporium, that they discovered a penicillin-like substance providing resistance to hydrolysis by penicillinases which was named cephalosporin C.

By 1959, Rolinson and coworkers completed the isolation of the penicillin nucleus, 6-aminopenicillanic acid, (Figure 1) in quantity. At about the same time the β-lactam-dihydrothiazine structure for the cephalosporin C was proposed [2] and confirmed subsequently by X-ray crystallographic analysis. In 1962, Morin and coworkers established a chemical method for the production of 7-aminocephalosporanic acid (Figure 1) from cephalosporin C in quantity. These developments opened the way to the preparation of a large number of semi-synthetic *cephalosporins* with hopes of being used as therapeutic agents. Cephalothin was prepared in 1962 and was the first semi-synthetic cephalosporin to find extensive clinical use in the 1960s. Cephalothin was followed by cephaloridine, in which the acetoxy group at C-3′ of cephalothin was replaced by a pyridinium group (Figure 2). These cephalosporins were followed by four generation of cephalosporins that are now categorized based on their spectrum of activity.

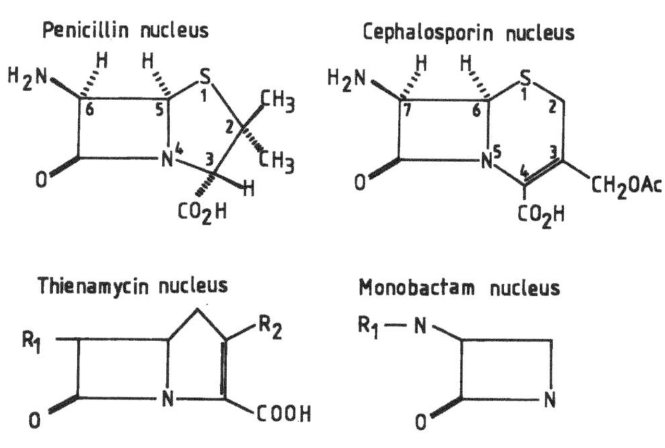

Figure 1. *Core structure of penicillins, cephalosporins, carbapenems and monobactams.*

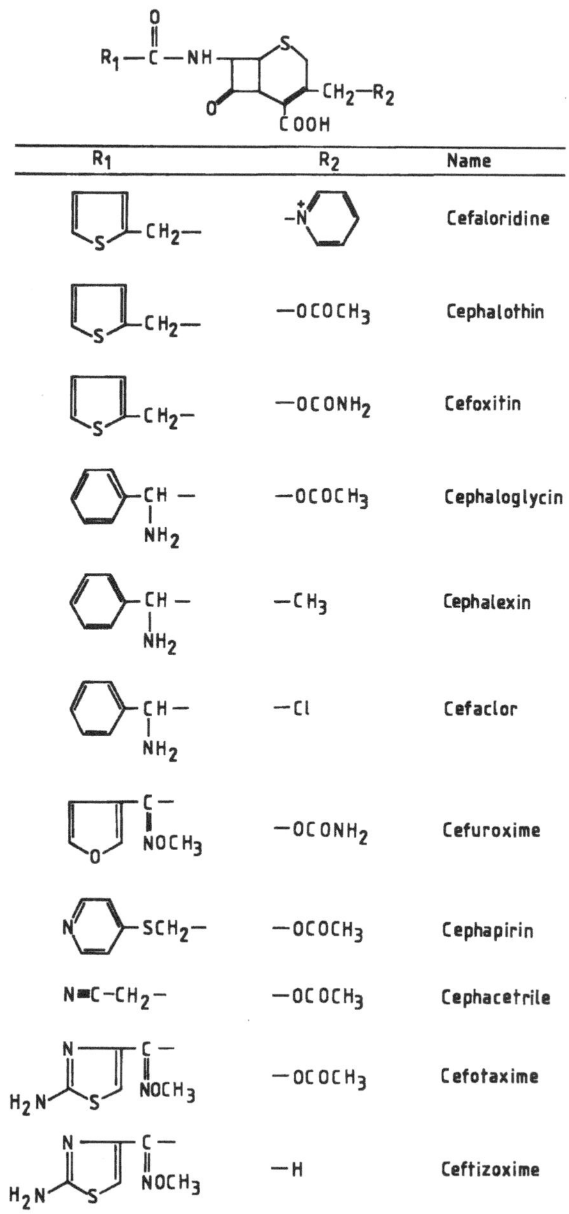

Figure 2. *Various side chains attached to the β-lactam nucleus, which are involved in renal toxicity.*

Cephamycins, including cefoxitin, cefotetan, cefmetazole and moxalactam (latamoxef), are related to cephalosporins but contain a metoxy group rather than a hydrogen at the 7-position on the β-lactam ring of the cephalosporin nucleus [3]. Cefoxitin (Figure 2) is the best known semi-synthetic cephamycin antibiotic derived from cephamycin C, a substance produced by *Streptomyces lactamdurans*. Molecular alterations such as an exchange of oxygen for sulfur at the S1 position in the dihydrothiazine ring resulted in the development of moxalactam, which is an oxa-β-lactam rather than a cephalosporin. Moxalactam is stable to β-lactamases due to the presence of a 7-methoxy group in its chemical structure. It is highly active and has a broad spectrum of activity except against *Pseudomona aeruginosa*.

Clavulanic acid was discovered in 1976 and is a β-lactam antibiotic with low antibiotic activity, but does protect β-lactamase-sensitive compounds of high intrinsic activity such as benzylpenicillin, ampicillin, and amoxicillin from β-lactamase destruction. Subsequently other β-lactamase inhibitors such as sulbactam and tazobactam were developed [4].

Carbacephems are structurally related to cephalosporins [5]. Loracarbef, the first this new class of β-lactam antibiotics, is a carbacephem analog of cefaclor (Figure 2) in which the sulfur atom in the dihydrothiazine ring has been replaced by a methylene group. Carbacephems have greater chemical stability than cephalosporins. Loracarbef has *in vitro* activity against most pathogenes responsible for upper respiratory tract infections. It is active *in vitro* against *Streptococcus pneumoniae* and has activity against most strains of *Staphylococcus aureus*.

Carbapenems, which are β-lactam antibiotics (penems) that are neither penicillins (penams) nor cephalosporins (cephems), proved to be of clinical significance and scientific interest. The first compound of this new type of β-lactam class was thienamycin [6]. Replacing the sulfur atom with a carbon atom altered the penem ring of thienamycin. All biologically active members of the class contain the unsaturated carbapen-2-em carboxylic acid nucleus (Figure 1). The carbapenem derivatives of thienamycin such as imipenem and panipenem showed exceptional activity against a wide range of bacteria including strains of *Pseudomona aeruginosa* and are high resistance to hydrolysis by β-lactamases. Imipenem is a semi-synthetic β-lactam antibiotic and is the N-formidoyl derivative of thienamycin, a carbapenem antibiotic produced by *Streptomyces cattleya*. The derivative imipenem is formulated in combination with cilastatin, which prolongs the half-life of imipenem by preventing its inactivation by dehydropeptidases in the kidney. Meropenem and biapenem are newer carbapenems, which show stability to renal hydrolysis and do not need to be combined with cilastatin [7].

From the *monobactam* group, aztreonam is a monocyclic β-lactam antibiotic (Figure 1), which is produced by *Chromobacterium violaceum*. Aztreonam has a high activity against gram-negative aerobic bacteria including *Pseudomona aeruginosa*, but it is virtually inactive against gram-positive bacteria and anaerobes. Aztreonam shows a high degree of stability to a wide range of both plasmid- and chromosomally-mediated β-lactamases comparable to the third-generation cephalosporins [8].

Recent adaptations in Gram-negative have made them more resistance to the broad spectrum β-lactam antibiotics. In particular the emergence of extended-spectrum β-lactamases, plasmid-mediated AmpC enzymes, and carbapenem-hydrolyzing β-lactamases, have lead to the use of more combination therapy in order to overcome this resistance [8a]. Unfortunately, combining β-lactam antibiotics with aminoglycosides, as is commonly done, is associated with a greater risk of nephrotoxicity. In the analysis reported by Zhang et al [8b] the rate of nephrotoxicity for cephalosporins was 2.37%, 4.55% for aminoglycosides and 8.64% for combined treatment, a highly significant increased risk for pediatric patients being treated with combination therapy.

Nephrotoxic beta-lactams

Beta-lactams such as cephaloridine, cephalothin, cefotiam and imipenem have been associated with nephrotoxicity in humans and experimental animals [9]. An understanding of their nephrotoxicity mechanisms may provide valuable information for elucidation of the biochemical mechanisms of newer β-lactam nephrotoxicity. Similarly to cephaloridine, third- generation cephalosporins such as ceftazidime and cefsulodin and fourth-generation cephalosporins such as cefpirome and cefepime possess a quaternary nitrogen attached to the dihydrothiazine ring which may impart nephrotoxic potential [10]. Clinical and animal studies carried out with β-lactams, such as cephaloglycin, cephaloridine, cephalothin or imipenem, indicated that they show a differential accumulation at the site of their toxicity, the renal cortex [11]. Elucidation of the mechanism of toxic action of these model β-lactams has become the focus of several research efforts [12-16].

Penicillins

Penicillins are β-lactam antimicrobials, which have a 4-membered β-lactam ring that is fused to a 5-membered thiazolidine ring, thus forming the penam nucleus (Figure 1). Modifications of the parent compound can alter the bacterial spectrum of these β-lactams. The natural penicillins, penicillins G and V, remain the drugs of choice for infections caused by S. pyrogens, Peptococcus, Treponema and other organisms. The penicillinase resistant drugs such as methicillin and oxacillin are primarily used for staphylococcal infections. Whereas aminopenicillins such as amoxicillin and ampicillin are effective against E. coli, Proteus, Salmonella and Shigella, the extended spectrum penicillins such as tircarcillin and carbecillins are active against Enterobacteriaceae and Pseudomonas.

When 1500 mg/kg ampicillin was administered to female rabbits as a single dose, there was no evidence of nephrotoxicity judged by the absence of tubular necrosis 48 hours after administration [17]. In the other hand, carbenicillin, methicillin and ampicillin have been associated with acute interstitial nephritis (AIN) [18-20].

AIN is characterized by fever, eosinophilia, hematuria, mild proteinuria and skin rash occur an average of 15 days after exposure (range 2-40). Rising serum creatinine concentration and acute renal failure with oliguria develop in about 50% of AIN cases, especially in older patients. Histologically, interstitial granulomas and variable degrees of tubular necrosis may be seen on renal biopsy.

Benzylpenicillin is a β-lactam with low or no renal toxicity [21]. However, when administered in large doses, benzylpenicillin or amoxicillin [22] have the potential to induced nephrotoxicity. Acute interstitial nephritis and disturbances of blood electrolytes have also been reported [23]. By comparison, dicloxacillin induced a pathological increase of creatinine, while cloaxicillin had only a marginal effect on the renal function [24].

The peroxidative potential of mezlocillin was determined by measuring both the generation of superoxide and malondialdehyde (MDA). The results showed that the amount of generated superoxide was almost equal to that produced by cefsulodin, under the same experimental conditions, while the amount of MDA was about 50% of that generated by cefsulodin [10]. After incubation of renal cortical slices with mezlocillin there was no change in the accumulation of the organic anion para-aminohippurate (PAH) in slices when compared to control whereas a significant decrease in the accumulation of the cation tetraethylammonium (TEA) occurred [10], suggesting a preferential sensitivity of organic cation transporter.

Cephalosporins and cephamycins

Therapeutic demands for new antimicrobial antibiotics arise from the emergence and dissemination of new opportunistic pathogens, especially in a expanding immune system-debilitated host population. As the number of β-lactams, and especially of cephalosporins, continues to expand, the need for classification increases. Changing the molecular environment of the β-lactam ring resulted in the development of β-lactam antibiotics possessing a penam or cephem nucleus known as "classical β-lactams" and of those with an unusual nucleus as "non-classical β-lactams" such as carbapenems (Figure 1). The introduction of specific side chains to the penam ring or cephem ring has resulted in a variety of changes in biological properties of these drugs: expansion of the antibacterial spectrum, increase in stability against β-lactamase and improved pharmacokinetic properties, slower elimination allowing longer dosage intervals and lower toxicity, especially nephrotoxicity [25, 26].

Cephalosporins are β-lactam antibiotics in which the β-lactam ring is fused to a 6-membered dihydrothiazine ring, thus forming the cephem nucleus. To differentiate between the successive waves of cephalosporins that have appeared since 1975, the introduction of the term "generations" served for separate one cephalosporin group from another. Cephalosporins have been classified as belonging to a first-, second-, third- or fourth-generation on the basis of their biological characteristics and clinical use for management of specific infections [25].

First-generation cephalosporins are mainly active against gram-positive cocci (except enterococci) and numerous Enterobacteriaceae. First generation cephalosporins (cephalothin, cephaloridine, cefazolin, cephalexin, cephapirin) have limited activity against gram-negative bacteria although some strains of *Escherichia coli, Klebsiella pneumoniae, Proteus mirabilis,* and Shigella may be inhibited *in vitro* by these drugs. However, gram-negative bacteria, which possess β-lactamases, are able to hydrolyze these cephalosporins partially or totally. Cefazolin has a substantially longer half-life and reaches much higher serum concentrations than other members of this group.

The nephrotoxicity of β-lactams, such as cephaloridine, is characterized by decreased glomerular filtration rate, proteinuria, enzymuria, urinary granular casts, impaired ability of renal cortical slices to accumulate organic ions and to synthesize glucose [27].

Ultrastructural changes of proximal tubular cells occur as early as 1 hour after cephaloridine administration to rabbits and are characterized by loss of brush border, less elongated mitochondria and disappearance of structures associated with endocytosis. Later ultrastructural changes include disorganization of lateral interdigitations of plasma cell membrane and mitochondrial swelling [28,29].

Treatment of rabbits [30] or rats [31] with inhibitors of renal organic anion transport, such as probenecid, decreases renal cortical accumulation of cephaloridine and its nephrotoxicity. This correlates with the results of more recent studies, which indicate that cephaloridine, is actively transported into proximal tubular cells by a renal organic anion transporter 1 [32, 33]. Results from numerous *in vitro* and *in vivo* animal studies using real cortical slices, isolated tubule fragments and renal cortical microsomes [26, 31, 34-41] as well as *in vitro* studies using human renal cortical slices and human renal microsomes [9] revealed marked cephaloridine-induced lipid peroxidation. Cephaloridine-induced oxidative stress caused a significant decrease in renal accumulation of organic anions and cations, plus significantly impairing the ability of the renal cortical tissue to synthesize glucose [26, 31, 36, 37, 39, 42]. Similar results were obtained with cephalothin, which was less nephrotoxic than cephaloridine; cefazolin-induced lipid peroxidation was substantially less than that caused by cephalothin and did not affect the renal cortical accumulation of the cation tetraethylammonium (TEA) or gluconeogenesis [26]. It appears that cephaloridine-induced lipid peroxidation antedates the inhibition of organic ion accumulation [37]. Furthermore, species differences in cephaloridine- [9, 42] or cephalothin-induced nephrotoxicity have been reported [43]. Selenium deficiency potentiated cephaloridine nephrotoxicity [35, 44]. In contrast to selenium deficiency, copper deficiency did not increase cephaloridine-induced nephrotoxicity [44].

Second-generation cephalosporins (cefuroxime, cefotiam, cefonicid, cefaclor, cefamandole) differ from the first generation in that they are generally less active against staphylococci and streptococci, may have more resistance to β-lactamases and have greater *in vitro* activity against gram-negative bacteria than the first generation cephalosporins. Cefuroxime and cefamandole have enhanced activity against most strains of *Haemophilus influenzae* and some Enterobacteriaceae. Second generation cephalosporins are inactive against methicillin-resistant Staphylococci and enterococci. The N-methyl-tetrazole-thiol (NMTT) side chain in position 3 of the cephem nucleus confers epileptogenic activity, disulfiram-like activity and hypoprothrombinemia to cephamandole and cefotiam [26, 45].

Histochemistry and electron microscopy of rabbit kidneys treated with large doses of cefotiam revealed both loss of microvilli and the presence of degenerative processes in the proximal tubule [46]. When compared to the first-generation cephalosporin cephazolin, cefotiam has a comparable peroxidative potential but greater nephrotoxicity [26].

Third-generation cephalosporins (cefotaxime, cefodizime, ceftizoxime, cefixime, ceftriaxone, ceftazidime, cefsulodin, cefoperazone) have an expanded spectrum of activity against gram-negative bacteria compared with the first- and second-generation compounds. They are very resistent to β-lactamases, high potency against Enterobacteriaceae and some activity against *Pseudomona aeruginosa* and *Bacteroides fragilis.* However, they are usually less active *in vitro* against susceptible staphylococci than the first generation cephalosporins.

Cefoperazone, like cefamandole, has the ability to induce epileptogenic activity, disulfiram-like activity, and hypoprothrombinemia. It appears that hypothrombinemia occurs more frequently with cefoperazone than with other cephalosporins [45].

Two clinical studies indicated a small but significant decrease in glomerular filtration rate during ceftazidime therapy [47, 48]. A significant elevation in the excretion of alanine aminopeptidase was also observed [48]. Although cefotaxime and cefoperazone have peroxidative potential, they do not affect TEA accumulation and glucose synthesis by renal cortical slices [26]. Results of studies conducted with renal cortical microsomes showed that cefsulodin, when compared with ceftazidime and cefotaxime, was the most potent cephalosporin, causing superoxide production and induction of lipid peroxidation [10]. In studies conducted with renal cortical slices, ceftazidime induced the greatest decrease in PAH accumulation when compared to cefotaxime and cefsulodin but all three decreased TEA accumulation to a similar extent [10].

Fourth-generation cephalosporins such as cefpirome, cefepime, cefoselis, cefluprenam and cefclidin are zwitterionic 7-methoxyimino cephalosporins, which are active *in vitro* and *in vivo* against both gram-negative and gram-positive bacteria. These zwitterionic β-lactams remain active against some, but not all, ceftazidime-resistant Enterobacteriaceae. Antipseudomonas activities are generally similar to that of ceftazidime except for cefclidin which is more active. However, these cephalosporins are not active against *Bacteroides fragilis*.

The nephrotoxic potential of the fourth-generation cefpirome and of two third-generation cephalosporins, cefotaxime and ceftazidime was compared using both *in vitro* and *in vivo* studies with renal cortical slices [49]. While cefpirome and cefotaxime did not have an effect on gluconeogenesis, ceftazidime caused a significant decrease. Furthermore cefpirome and ceftazidime decreased TEA accumulation whereas cefotaxime showed no effect [49]. These differences may be explained, at least in part, by the zwitterionic structure of cefpirome and ceftazidime as opposed to cefotaxime which lacks a pyridinium ring. Other factors besides peroxidative injury may play a role in the decrease of TEA accumulation caused by ceftazidime and cefpirome. Little or no evidence is yet available concerning the nephrotoxic potential of other fourth-generation cephalosporins.

Cephamycins include β-lactam such as cefoxitin, cefotetan, cefmetazole and latamoxef (moxalactam). Cephamycins are active against anaerobic bacteria, are less active against gram-positive cocci and, have no activity against methicillin-resistant staphylococci and enterococci. Cephamycin antibiotics such as cefotetan and latamoxef have a side chain called the methylthiotetrazole group (MTT), which predisposes to hypothrombinemia and bleeding, and alcohol intolerance by causing a disulfiram reaction.

The nephrotoxicity of cefotetan in rabbits was considerably less than that of cefazolin [50]. When compared to cefotiam, cefoxitin appears to be better tolerated by the kidney since the cefotiam-induced decrease of TEA accumulation and the decrease of gluconeogenesis in renal cortical slices was 2-3 times greater than with cefoxitin [26].

Carbacephems and carbapenems

Chemically, *carbacephems* differ from cephalosporin antibiotics in the dihydrothiazine ring where a methylene group has been substituted for the sulfur group (Figure 1). Loracarbef is the carbacephem analog of cefaclor. Loracarbef has been shown to be active against gram-positive aerobes such as *Staphylococcus pneumoniae* and gram-negative aerobes such as *Escherichia coli* and *Haemophilus influenzae*. When administered to female rabbits (1500 mg/kg) cefaclor and its carbacephem analog loracarbef differentiate in their nephrotoxicity with loracarbef showing a greater potential to cause tubular necrosis than cefaclor [17]. A case of acute interstitial nephritis associated with loracarbef resulting in end-stage renal failure has been described [51].

Carbapenems are a relatively new class of β-lactam antibiotics (penems) with a remarkably broad spectrum. These antibiotics have potent activity against gram-positive cocci including enterococci, and potent activity against gram-negative organisms, including *Pseudomonas aeruginosa*. Carbapenems also display high activity against gut anaerobes.

When given as a large single dose, imipenem can produce acute proximal tubular necrosis in experimental animals [52]. Imipenem has an unsaturated ring adjacent to the β-lactam ring, which is normally hydrolyzed by dehydropeptidase-1, a renal tubular brush border enzyme [53]. Cilastatin, a specific inhibitor of dehydropeptidase-1, blocks the inactivation of imipenem, resulting in high imipenem urinary concentrations and reduced nephrotoxicity. The nephroprotective effect of cilastatin is due to the inhibition of the contraluminal imipenem transport reducing the intracellular accumulation and preventing high tissue concentrations and nephrotoxicity [52]. Newer carbapenems such as meropenem are stable to the hydrolytic action of dehydropeptidase-1, without combination with cilastatin, and are well tolerated in elderly and renal impaired patients [54,55].

In an earlier study of the effects of imipenem in the rabbit kidney it was shown that imipenem caused a significant decrease of mitochondrial respiration, depletion of reduced glutathione, increased production of oxidized glutathione and lipid peroxidation [56]. However, these effects were less than those produced by a comparable nephrotoxic dose of cephaloridine [56]. Panipenem induced nephrotoxicity at a dose of 200 mg/kg, i.v., but this was less severe than that caused by a single dose of imipenem [57]. Simultaneous administration of β-mipron (N-benzoyl-3-propionic acid) with imipenem and panipenem reduced the nephrotoxicity of these carbapenems by inhibiting the active transport of carbapenems in the renal cortex [57].

In a more recent study, peroxidative and nephrotoxic injuries induced by meropenem and imipenem/cilastatin in rat and human cortical slices and microsomes were compared to those induced by cephaloridine [9]. While meropenem and imipenem/cilastatin did produce lipid peroxidation and depressed PAH accumulation and gluconeogenesis in rat and human renal cortex, the effect was substantially less than with cephaloridine [9]. The human renal cortical tissue appears to be less susceptible to β-lactam induced lipid peroxidation than the rat renal cortical tissue; with meropenem showed lower renal toxicity then imipenem/cilastatin [9].

Monocyclic beta-lactams

Aztreonam, a *monobactam*, is a useful alternative for patients with aerobic gram-negative infections who are allergic to penicillins, but has no activity against anaerobes. Aztreonam appears to be the only β-lactam antibiotic that can be safely administered to penicillin-allergic patients [58]. Aztreonam has a spectrum of activity that is comparable to the aminoglycosides but it is less nephrotoxic in patients [59] and it appears to be well tolerated in infants and children [60].

Results of *in vitro* experiments carried out with rat renal microsomes and renal cortical slices showed that aztreonam has a low potential to induce reactive oxygen species and lipid peroxidation [10]. However, aztreonam caused a decrease in renal cortical accumulation of PAH comparable to that of paraquat without a significant decrease in TEA accumulation [10]. Therefore, it appears that the nephrotoxic activity of aztreonam may be not directly related to the superoxide generation and lipid peroxidation.

Relationship between beta-lactam structure and renal toxicity

A consequence of the development of the large number of cephalosporins is that the molecular structures have become more and more complex. Alterations in the cephalosporin molecule have resulted in differences between cephalosporins in spectrum of activity, protein binding, peak serum level, serum half-life, route of excretion, cerebrospinal fluid levels and toxicity. Cephalosporins are semi-synthetic antibiotics derived from 7-aminocephalosporanic acid, which is also called the cephalosporin nucleus. The cephem ring ("nucleus") is composed of a β-lactam ring fused with a dihydrothiazine ring (Figure 1).

Cephalosporins differ in the substituents attached to the 3 and/or 7 positions of the cephem ring. Usually ***modifications at position 7*** influences the antibacterial spectrum and resistance against β-lactamases (Figure 2). For example, the presence of a methoxyimino group at the position 7 as found in cefuroxime, cefotaxime, ceftizoxime and ceftriaxone, confers enhanced β-lactamase stability with some loss of gram-positive activity. Addition of an aminothiazolyl side chain, as found in all the above except cefuroxime, provides unusually high affinity for the penicillin binding proteins found in gram-negative bacteria. Ceftazidime has a propylcarboxyl group at this location, which produces superior Pseudomonas activity but markedly reduces effectiveness against gram-positive organisms. The presence of a methoxy group at position 7 of the cephamycins cefoxitin and cefotetan, by steric hindrance, confers resistance to gram-negative β-lactamases, although it also reduces affinity for penicillin binding proteins [61].

Substitutions at position 3 of the dihydrothiazine ring play a major role in the overall pharmacokinetic properties and toxicity. For example, the unusually long half-life of ceftriaxone appears to be caused by the presence of a triazine substituted at this position [62]. Cephalosporins such as cephalothin, cephaloglycin, cephapirin, cephacetrile and cefotaxime share an acetoxymethyl group at the position 3 (Figure 2) and are all metabolically converted to desacetyl derivatives and to the antibacterially inactive lactone of these substances.

With increasing complexity of the molecular structure it seems inevitable that the ***toxic profile will be altered***. The most striking example of the effect of chemical alterations on the safety profile of β-lactams is the 3-methylthiotetrazole (MTT) side ring attached in position 3 of the cephem nucleus (Figure 3) The MTT side ring is present in many cefamycins (cefotetan, moxalactam) and cephalosporins (cefmenoxime, cefoperazone and cefamandole) and confers epileptogenic activity, disulfiram-like activity and reduced synthesis of prothrombin. Hypoprothrombinemia and bleeding complications during therapy with these drugs occurred in geriatric, debilitated, or other patients with vitamin K deficiency or in patients with severe renal failure or following radical gastrointestinal surgery [63]. The substitution of the MTT side chain and the presence of the 2-methyl-1,3,4-thiodiazole-5-thiole (MTD) side ring in position 3 of the cephem nucleus of cefotiam, cefonicid and cefazolin (Figure 3) induces weaker but similar effects to those caused by the MTT side ring. It appears that the ionization of the N-dimethylaminoethyl group attached to the N-methyl-tetrazole-thiol (NMTT) side chain of cefotiam enhances its secretory transport in kidney epithelial cells [64].

Cephalosporins such as cephaloglycin, cephalexin and cefaclor have in common a ***D-phenylglycyl side chain at C-7′*** but they differ in the side chain on the C-3′ of the cephem nucleus (Figure 2). While cephaloglycin possess an acetoxymethyl group at C-3 and a high intrinsic nephrotoxic potential, cephalosporins such as cephalexin and cefaclor, which in place of the acetoxymethyl group contain a methyl group or a chloride, respectively, are basically not nephrotoxic [11].

While the D-phenylglycyl side chain is not totally responsible for nephrotoxic potential of the β-lactam molecule, it does increase the nephrotoxic potential of the β-lactam if other molecular components are not metabolically detoxified or if renal metabolism occurs at a slow rate, as in the case of cephaloglycin [65].

However, the ***acetoxymethyl side chain in position*** 3 of the cephem ring may confer nephrotoxic potential as in the case of cephaloglycin [11] and cephalothin [43] but not with cefotaxime (Figure 2) [26]. It is likely that the presence of D-phenylglycyl side chain in the cephaloglycin molecule and its global molecular configuration insures that the acetoxymethyl side chain will be metabolized at a slower rate by the renal enzymes. This leads to an intracellular accumulation of the intact cephaloglycin sufficient to reach threshold nephrotoxic concentration [64]. Thus, these results suggest that the presence of the acetoxymethyl group on the position 3 of the cephem ring does not lead to inevitable renal damage and thus cannot be solely responsible for the occurrence of nephrotoxicity. The difference between cephaloglycin and cefotaxime is due to the presence on the position 7 of the cephem nucleus of the D-phenylglycyl side chain for cepha-

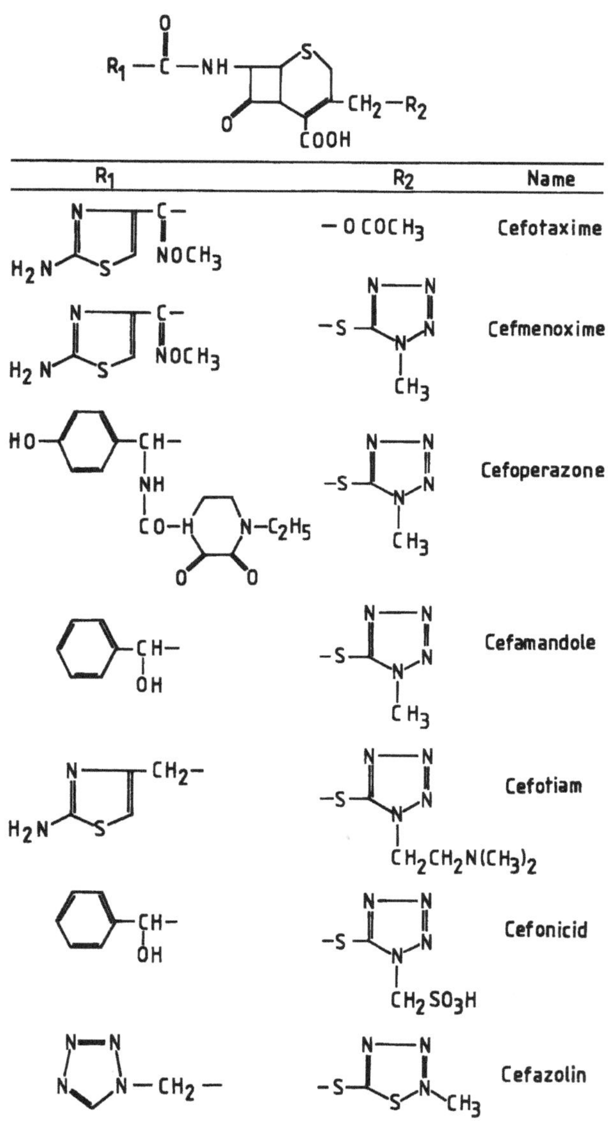

Figure 3. *Side chains attached to the cephem nucleus, which have a toxic potential.*

loglycin and of the ***aminothiazolyloximino side ring*** for cefotaxime. The lack of the nephrotoxic potential of the aminothiazolyloximino side chain is proven by the molecular structure of ceftizoxime, which has only a hydrogen atom on the position 3 of cephem nucleus (Figure 2).

More interesting, the presence of the ***thiophene ring in position*** 7 of the cephem nucleus (Figure 2) has been associated with nephrotoxic effects in the case of cephaloridine and cephalothin and to a lesser extent in the case of the cephamycin cefoxitin [26, 66]. When compared to cephalothin, small alterations of the cefoxitin molecule in positions 3 and 7 of the cephem nucleus, such as replacement of the methyl group with

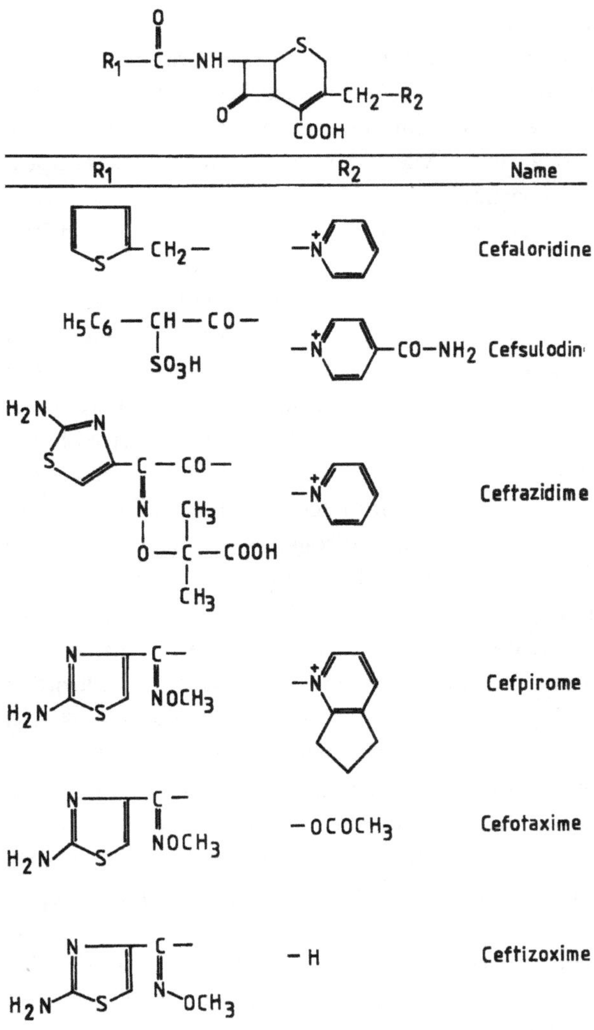

Figure 4. *Cephalosporins containing the pyridinium ring attached to the cephem nucleus.*

an amino group and addition of the methoxy group respectively, reduced its nephrotoxic potential [66]. The aminoacetoxy side chain of cefoxitin that is also present in the molecule of cefuroxime (Figure 2), did not, by itself, confer a nephrotoxic potential to these two β-lactams.

The presence of other structures in position 7 of the cephem nucleus, such as the aminothiazolyloximino side ring of cefotaxime, ceftizoxime and cepirome (Figure 4) or the corresponding complex structure of cefoperazone (Figure 3), does not confer a nephrotoxic potential to these β-lactams [26, 49]. Furthermore, the results of various studies suggested that the ***pyridinium ring when attached at position*** 3 to the cephem nucleus could be implicated in the nephrotoxic effects seen with cephaloridine, cefsulodin and ceftazidime [10, 26, 34]. The concomitant presence of the thiophene ring and pyridinium ring in the molecule (Figure 4) creates the most nephrotoxic cephalosporin to date, cephaloridine. The presence of an acetoxymethyl side chain instead of the pyridinium ring resulted in the reduction of the nephrotoxic potential of cephalothin by about 30-50% when compared to cephaloridine [9, 26].

However, β-lactams such as cefotiam or imipenem which contain neither a D-phenylglycyl nor a pyridinium ring in their molecule act as nephrotoxicants [9, 26, 67]. Imipenem induces acute proximal tubular necrosis in monkeys [68] and rabbits [56] similar to that produced by cephaloridine. Both impairment of mitochondrial respiration and oxidative injury appear to be involved in the nephrotoxic action of imipenem [35, 69]. Nephrotoxic cephalosporins have an active leaving group in their C-3 side chain and cause mitochondrial injury by acylating and inactivating the mitochondrial receptors [11]. Although imipenem does not have any leaving group, it also causes similar nephrotoxicity [56].

The differences in nephrotoxicity of carbapenems are due to the different structural features, especially the physicochemical properties. The structure of meropenem differs from the structure of imipenem and panipenem due to the presence of a 1β-methyl group and the lesser basicity of the amino group in the C-2 side chain. The basicity of meropenem is much lower than that of imipenem and panipenem [70]. The reduced meropenem nephrotoxicity is not related to the presence of the 1β-methyl group. However, the basicity of the C-2 side chain of carbapenems is important for the occurrence of nephrotoxicity [70].

The strained structure of carbapenems confers a higher reactivity to the carbapenem skeleton than that of cephalosporin skeleton. It has been suggested that both β-lactam ring and the basicity of C-2 side play a major role in carbapenem-induced nephrotoxicity [70].

To summarize, the nephrotoxic potential of β-lactams is not solely due to the presence of a specific side chain in the molecule, but rather, the entire molecular structure determines the nephrotoxic action.

Effects on plasma cell membrane and subcellular organelles

Plasma cell membrane

The cell membrane serves as a protective barrier in renal cells. It is the initial site which β-lactams encounter in their journey to the cellular environment from the blood or tubular fluid. β-lactams may disrupt the functional organization of the membrane through peroxidation of membrane lipids, which, in turn, leads to the inability of membrane to serve as an osmotic barrier and causes the cytosol contents to leak. As a result of the cephalosporins disruptive effect on cell membrane, increased leakage of the cytosolic enzyme lactate dehydrogenase (LDH) occurs. The increased LDH concentration was from the cytosol of the renal cortex [49,71] or from isolated proximal and distal tubular cells [39] or in the urine of experimental animals [39]. The results of these studies indicate that plasma membrane became permeable to large molecules such as LDH. After cephalosporin treatment, cephaloridine caused the greatest decrease of LDH concentration in cytosol [49]. Whereas, cephaloridine induced a greater release of LDH from proximal tubular cells than cephalothin and cephalexin, distal cells were not affected by any of these cephalosporins [38,39].

Endoplasmatic reticulum

The major intracellular source of reactive oxygen species such as superoxide anion and hydrogen peroxide are the cytochrome P-450 system of the endoplasmatic reticulum and mitochondria.

The endoplasmic reticulum is a continuous anastomosing network of lipoprotein membranes extending from plasma membrane to nucleus and mitochondria. The microsomal fraction derived from endoplasmatic reticulum consists of membranous vesicles. Microsomal cytochromes P-450 are a superfamily of hemoproteins that play a central role in the metabolism of a large variety of xenobiotics plus synthesis and catabolism of endogenous compounds. Results of studies using nephron fragments have shown that cytochrome P-450 was localized exclusively in the proximal tubule [72] whereas NADPH-cytochrome c reductase was distributed along the entire nephron [73]. The average concentration of cytochrome P450 in unstimulated renal cortex microsomal membranes is about 0.150 nmol/mg protein in rats while in humans it amounts to about 0.050 nmol/mg protein [73, 74].

The renal cytochrome P-450 enzyme system is involved in oxidative reactions in which an atom of molecular oxygen is inserted in an organic molecule. The flavoprotein NADPH-cytochrome P-450 reductase is an essential component of the mixed-function oxidase systems (MFO). Microsomal membranes appear to be particularly subject to attack by reactive oxygen radicals due to their high content of unsaturated fatty acids and the presence of the cytochrome P-450 system [40]. Cephaloridine-induced peroxidation of membrane lipids is decreased by the cytochrome P-450 inhibitor cobalt chloride [31], suggesting a role for a cytochrome P-450 reductase in the β-lactam-induced generation of reactive oxygen species and subsequent peroxidation products.

Cephaloridine-induced reactive oxygen species such as superoxide, hydrogen peroxide, and hydroxyl radical could, in addition to inducing peroxidative damage of membrane lipids [40], destroy and/or inactivate renal cortical membrane proteins and enzymes [75,77]. Treatment of rats with cephaloridine (CPH) caused an *in vivo* depletion of the microsomal cytochrome P-450 and b5 as well as induction of a polypeptide of molecular weight 44,000. SDSD-gel electrophoresis and phenobarbital induction studies indicated that the two depleted polypeptides were cytochrome P-450 isoenzymes [74]. The *in vivo* depletion of renal cortical cytochrome P-450 by CPH was dose-dependent. It is worth noting that statistically significant depletion of cytochrome P-450 occurred at relatively low dosage. More interestingly, the time course of CPH-induced decrease in renal cortical content of cytochrome P-450 isoenzymes indicates that a significant depletion occurred as early as 3 h after a single dose of 1200 mg/kg CPH [74].

An almost complete depletion of cytochrome P450 was measured at 12 and 24 hours after CPH treatment followed by a slow recovery of the cytochrome P-450 content over 48 to 72 hours despite continuing CPH-treatment (1200 mg/kg/d). Measurement of MDA content in the same alloguate of renal cortex and microsomes showed that a significant increase in CPH-induced lipid peroxidation occurred 24 hours after administration of 1200 mg/kg/d CPH [74]. The time course of these biochemical events indicates that the onset of CPH-induced cytochrome P-450 loss distinctly precedes the onset of CPH-induced lipid peroxidation.

After intravenous treatment of rats with 1200 mg/kg/d CPH for 3 days, homogenates of the renal cortex were separated into subcellular fractions and their protein composition analyzed. The results of the SDS-gel electrophoresis of the renal cortical subfractions showed significant alterations of the polypeptide pattern in the microsomal fraction. The analysis of the polypeptide composition of the microsomal fraction indicated that paralleling to the depletion of cytochrome P-450 isoenzymes in the molecular weight range 50-53,000 was the induction of a polypeptide of molecular weight 44,000 [74].

The question rose whether the CPH-induced 44,000 molecular weight polypeptide is a cytochrome P450-isoenzyme. Thus, induction experiments were carried out in which saline-treated rats were compared with phenobarbital- and CPH-treated rats. Analysis of the polypeptide composition of the microsomal fraction from the phenobarbital group indicated a significant increase of polypeptides in the 50-53,000 molecular weight (P-450 region), but no increase in 44,000 molecular weight polypeptides [75]. However, in the renal cortical microsomes from the CPH treated rats (1200 mg/kg/d for 3 days), there was a time- and dose-dependent increase in the amount of the 44,000 molecular weight polypeptide with a simultaneous depletion of the 50-53,000 molecular weight polypeptides from the cytochrome P-450 region. These results suggest that the 44,000 renal microsomal polypeptide induced by CPH-treatment is not a cytochrome P-450 isoenzyme nor is it the result of degradation of high molecular weight proteins by CPH [75].

Solubilization experiments revealed that the CPH-induced 44,000 molecular weight polypeptide is a peripheral rather than an integral membrane protein [75]. The precise function of the inducible 44,000 molecular weight microsomal protein is not known at the present time. However, data showing an increase in the enzymatic activities of drug metabolizing enzymes such as renal cortical microsomal GSH-S-transferase (3.5-fold) suggest that the CPH-induced 44,000 polypeptide is an enzyme of the endoplasmatic reticulum involved in the detoxification of the reactive species evolving from intracellular bioactivation of CPH [74, 75].

CPH-treatment of rats (1200 mg/kg/d for 2 d) induced the enzymatic activities of other renal cortical drug-metabolizing enzymes such as 7-ethoxy-coumarine-O-deethylase and cytosolic GSH-S-transferase whereas the enzymatic activities of aniline hydroxylase and aminopyrine-N-demethylase were simultaneously decreased or remained unchanged, respectively (Table 1) [74]. Treatment of male and female rats with cephaloridine (750 mg/kg/d) for two weeks to three

Table 1. Effects of cephaloridine on the activity of drug metabolizing enzymes from rat renal cortex microsomes.

Enzymes	Control rats	Treated rats	% of control
NADPH-cytochrome-c-reductase (nmoles/mg protein/min)	13.64 ± 2.81	11.65 ± 2.03	85.2
Aminopyrine-N-demethylase (nmoles/mg protein/min)	0.81 ± 0.12	0.82 ± 0.07	101.2
Anilline hydroxylase (nmoles/mg protein/min)	0.330 ± 0.02	0.018 ± 0.003*	5.5
7-Ethoxycoumarin-O-deethylase (nmoles/mg protein/min)	0.095 ± 0.02	0.130 ± 0.07*	136.8
Glutathione-S-transferase (nmoles/ mg protein/min):			
I. **Microsomal**	9.8 ± 1.6	35.0 ± 1.8*	357.1
II. **Cytosolic**	94.75 ± 7.4	298.62 ± 11.3*	315.2

*Cephaloridine was administered for 2 days (1200 mg/kg/d, i.v.). Results are mean ± SD from 5 different preparations. * Values are significant at P< 0.05.*

months resulted in a 2-fold increase of glutathione-S-transferase activity in the renal cortex [76]. These results suggest an adaptive response to cephaloridine subchronic treatment.

Renal brush border

The effects of CPH-treatment of rats (1200 mg/kg/d for 3d) on the polypeptide composition of renal brush border from the proximal tubule cells; enzymatic activities and transport systems of the brush border membrane vesicles (BBMV) were investigated [77]. The results of these studies showed that CPH-treatment induces a 20-30% decrease in the specific activities of renal brush border enzymes leucine aminopeptidase and -glutamyltransferase. SDS-gel electrophoresis showed that CPH-treatment induced a decrease of the intensity of 3 brush border polypeptides of molecular weights of 72,000, 58,000 and 39,000 [77].

Lysosomes

Cephaloridine has been shown to interact with lysosome phospholipids; this reaction is, in part, hydrophobic in nature [78]. High cephaloridine concentrations have a disruptive effect on lysosomes whereas at low concentrations cephaloridine has a stabilizing effect on the lysosomal membrane system [78,79]. The stabilizing effect is greater with cefazolin and cephaloridine than with ampicillin [80]. This membrane stabilizing effect could be due to the cephaloridine inhibition of the lysosomal membrane bound phospholipase 2 [78].

Treatment of rats with latamoxef (2000 mg/g day) for 5 days induced an insignificant increase in the release of N-acetyl-β-D-glucosaminidase from lysosomes, when compared to control rats [81]. After intravenous treatment of rats with 1200 mg/kg/d CPH for 3 days, homogenates of the renal cortex were separated into subcellular fractions and their protein composition was analyzed. The results of the SDS-gel electrophoresis of the renal cortical subfractions showed no relevant alterations of the polypeptide pattern in the lysosomal fraction [75].

Mitochondria

Administration of cephaloridine induces mitochondria elongation followed by mitochondria swelling [28, 29] which lead to mitochondrial dysfunction. Cephaloridine and other β-lactams decreased mitochondrial respiration significantly, suggesting a loss of mitochondrial integrity [35,56]. It has been suggested that mitochondrial damage may mediate, at least in part, the nephrotoxicity of some β-lactams. Nephrotoxic β-lactams (cephaloridine, cephaloglycin, imipenem) cause similar patterns of respiratory depression whereas non-nephrotoxic β-lactams do not alter mitochondrial function [67]. It is also possible that intracellular accumulation of the nephrotoxic β-lactams cause disruption of lysosomal membrane, release of lysosomal hydrolases which inflict mitochondrial membrane injuries and mitochondrial dysfunction. Structural damage, which can be observed by light microscopy usually, means that the β-lactam-induced toxicity is severe. Under this conditions it may be difficult to decide whether or not the mitochondrial effects are the cause of renal toxicity or are secondary to the death of the cell. Many studies have shown that the β-lactam-induced injuries are early indications of cell injuries. However, some caution must be observed in interpreting the data as mitochondria can undergo reversible changes in conformation, which may reflect changes in osmolality of the cell rather than a direct mitochondrial inhibition.

Mechanisms of action

High intracellular concentration

Contraluminal uptake of organic ions from blood along with the luminal secretion and/or uptake of organic ions plays a crucial role in the renal handling of organic ions, especially β-lactams [82, 83].

Cephalosporins such as cephalothin and cephaloridine interact with both the anionic (p-aminohippurate, PAH) and cationic (tetraethylammonium, TEA or N-methylnicotinamid, NMN) transport systems [31, 67, 85]. β-lactams have been shown to be secreted by the S2 segment of the proximal tubule via the PAH transport system [85]. Cephalothin inhibited the transport of PAH in rabbit basolateral and in brush border membrane vesicles [84] while cephaloridine inhibited the transport of PAH and TEA and in rat renal cortical slices [26, 77] and of PAH [77, 84] or NMN [84] in rat brush border membrane vesicles (BBMV).

Cephaloridine-induced nephrotoxicity is not restricted to the S2 segment but also involves the S3 segment of the proximal tubule [86]. More recent studies suggest that the rat renal organic anion transporter 1 (OAT1) located in the renal basolateral cell membrane, is the major transporter responsible for the renal secretion of antibiotics, especially that of β-lactams [32, 33]. The luminal secretion of β-lactam across brush-border membrane into urine has also thought to be carrier-mediated. The multispecific organic anion transporter, multidrug resistance-associated protein 2 (MRP2), is localized to the luminal membrane of all proximal tubule segments [87] and mediates the efflux of anionic lipophilic compounds such as glucuronides and glutathione conjugates from the cell. MRP2 or MRP2 isoforms are possible carrier candidates for the luminal secretion of organic anions such as β-lactams.

Apart from the secretion mechanisms, brush border membrane also contains transport systems for reabsorption of compounds from the luminal urine. Treatment of rats with 1200 mg/kg/d cephaloridine greatly reduced the uptake of cephalexin and cefotiam into BBMV whereas the posttreatment uptake of cephaloridine by the BBMV remained unaffected [77]. The unaffected uptake of cephaloridine into BBMV from cephaloridine treated rats indicates that cephaloridine is transported by a transport system, which is different from the dipeptide transporter. OCTN2 is an organic cation/carnitine transporter, which can transport not only organic cations but also of the zwitterions cephaloridine, carnitine and acylcarnitins [88]. Cephaloridine and other β-lactams with quaternary nitrogen such as cefoselis and cefepime are recognized by OCTN2 as transportable substrates [88]. β-lactams that do not contain a quaternary nitrogen but possess an -amino group are recognized as transportable substrates by the peptide transporters PEPT1 and PEPT2 [89]. PEPT2 has a much higher affinity for β-lactams such as cephadroxil and amoxicillin [89], which do not contain a quaternary nitrogen but posses an -amino group in the penam or cephem nucleus. Available evidence indicates that PEPT2 mediates H^+-peptide cotransport from the luminal urine across brush-border membrane into the proximal tubule cells [90].

Available experimental data indicates that cephaloridine-induced nephrotoxicity is dependent upon its renal cortical concentration [67]. Experimental data showed that probenecid, 2-4-dinitrophenol, ouabain and anoxia decreased the renal cortex accumulation of cephaloridine and cephalexin [91]. Concomitant exposure of renal cortical slices to cephaloridine and probenecid decreased cephaloridine-induced nephrotoxicity as shown by TEA accumulation in renal cortical slices [35]. Since inhibitors of organic ion transport prevent both transport and nephrotoxicity of cephaloridine, it could be concluded that the nephrotoxicity of cephaloridine is related to high intracellular concentrations resulting from active transport [67, 91] and bioactivation within kidney cells [34, 40].

Cytochrome P-450 and renal bioactivation

Kidneys are able to carry out extensive oxidation, reduction hydrolysis and conjugation reactions. The attractive hypothesis that cephaloridine is metabolized prior to producing nephrotoxicity [92] was not substantiated by experimental data. However, pretreatment of rats with 60 mg/kg cobalt chloride decreased cephaloridine-induced lipid peroxidation in renal cortical slices [31]. These results suggest that prior to producing nephrotoxicity, cephaloridine is taken up into renal cells, where, with the involvement of cytochrome P-450, it induces peroxidation of cell membrane lipids.

Whereas many cephalosporins such as cefaclor, cefadroxil, cefonicid, ceforanide, ceftazidime, ceftizoxime, cefuroxime, cephalexin, and cephradine are not metabolized, cefamandole naftate is rapidly hydrolyzed in plasma to cefamandole, which has greater antibacterial activity than the parent compound. Ceftriaxone is metabolized to a small extent to microbiologically inactive metabolites in the intestines after biliary excretion. Cefuroxime axetil is rapidly hydrolyzed to cefuroxime, the microbiologically active form of the drug, by nonspecific esterases in the intestinal mucosa and blood following oral administration. The axetil moiety is further metabolized to acetaldehyde and acetic acid [93].

Desacetylation of cephalosporins occurs in liver and kidney via the activity of acetylesterases. Desacetylated cephalosporins all maintain some antibacterial activity. Desacetylcefotaxime penetrates well extravascular body sites, achieves high tissue concentrations and acts synergistically with cefotaxime [94, 95]. Desacetylation of cephaloglycin, cephalothin and cephapirin resulted in formation of less active desacetyl forms [94] and less toxicity [64]. About 50% of cephaloglycin is metabolized to desacetylcephloglycin, which is less nephrotoxic at equal dosage [17]. Thus, desacetylation appears to be a detoxification mechanism for toxic cephalosporins such as cephaloglycin and cephalothin [64, 96].

Reactivity of the beta-lactam nucleus

The central β-lactam nucleus is involved in the molecular events leading to renal toxicity. Among other factors reactivity of the central β-lactam core contributes to the antimicrobial potency of these compounds. In the bacterial cell wall β-lactams form covalent complexes with membrane bound proteins (acylation), thus blocking cell wall formation and bacterial proliferation. The ability of a variety of penicillins and cephalosporins to acylate bacterial cell wall proteins was ranked as following: ceftazidime > cefaclor > cephaloglycin > cephalothin > or = cephaloridine > or = cefazolin >> penicillins > cephalexin and other 3-methyl-cephalosporins [97]. It appears that there is a partial correlation between β-lactam acylation potency and their nephrotoxicity which ranked as following: cephaloglycin > cephaloridine > cephalothin > cefazolin > cefaclor > penicillins, cephalexin, ceftazidime and cefotaxime [26, 67]. Moreover, cefaclor which appears to have high acylation potential has low renal toxicity.

Further, cephaloridine with moderate acylating activity is one of the most nephrotoxic cephalosporins. It was speculated that this discrepancy may be due to the presence of the cationic nitrogen group near to the carboxyl group of cephaloridine; this could limit cephaloridine access to the anionic targets and thus requiring high intracellular concentration to induce nephrotoxicity [67]. Whereas experimental evidence supports the concept that some β-lactams may induce acylation of mitochondrial substrate carries, little is known about the functional consequences of acylation of other cellular proteins [67].

Mitochondrial dysfunction

It has been suggested that mitochondrial injury may mediate, at least in part, the nephrotoxicity of some β-lactams [67]. Mitochondrial respiration with and uptake of succinate after exposure to toxic doses of cephaloridine, cephaloglycin, or imipenem [98] showed significant reduction of both functions. Cephalexin did not affect either the mitochondrial uptake or respiration with succinate. Depressed mitochondrial respiration secondary to acylation of the mitochondrial transporter for succinate appears to be implicated in renal toxicity caused by cephalosporins and carbapenems [98]. The organic anion fluorescein accumulates in mitochondria of renal proximal tubular cells [99, 100]. Valproate, indometacin, and salicylate induced a significant inhibition of fluorescein [101]. However, cephaloglycin and cephaloridine did not inhibited the fluorescein uptake. This is contrast with the results of previous studies in which an activation of the mitochondrial transporter was described [56]. This discrepancy between the results of these studies may be explained by the involvement of other carrier systems and/or species differences.

Using t-butyl hydroperoxide as a model hydroperoxide, the temporal sequence of cellular events leading to renal proximal tubular cell death was determined [102]. The results of the *in vitro* studies using rabbit isolated tubule suspensions showed that lipid peroxidation and glutathione oxidation are the initial events in t-butyl hydroperoxide-induced toxicity followed by mitochondrial dysfunction and cell death [102]. The temporal sequence of cellular events causing functional impairment and cell death was determined after exposure of rat renal cortical slices or suspensions of rabbit renal cortical tubules to cephaloridine [37, 38]. The results of these studies indicate that GSH depletion and lipid peroxidation are initial events, which precede mitochondrial dysfunction, impairment of the cellular uptake of organic ions and cell death. Moreover, supplementation of GSH to the incubation medium containing renal cortical microsomes significantly reduced cephaloridine-induced lipid peroxidation within the first 3 minutes after onset of incubation [36].

Glutathione and glutathione transferases

Reduced glutathione is the most important non-protein thiol present in animal cells [103]. Most of the intracellular GSH is found in the cytosol. However, a minor mitochondrial pool of GSH contributes to the total cellular pool of glutathione [102, 104, 105].

GSH transferases are inducible enzymes with overlapping substrate specificity [73]. They are also found in renal cells as cytosolic enzymes or as membrane-bound microsomal transferases. GSH conjugates are usually less toxic than their parent compounds and are readily excreted in the bile and in the urine as their corresponding mercapturic acids. However, evidence is accumulating that GSH conjugates and/or their corresponding cysteine conjugates are nephrotoxic [106, 107].

Moreover, intracellular accumulation and cytochrome P450 catalyzed bioactivation of β-lactams such as cephaloridine overwhelms of the GSH redox cycle by inhibiting glutathione reductase activity [35, 56], depletion of GSH and accumulation of GSSG [35, 42, 49, 56]. Most of GSSG formed is subsequently reduced by glutathione reductase and GSH is regenerated with concomitant oxidation (consumption) of NADPH to $NADP^+$ [104].

Depletion of GSH by cephaloridine [34, 35, 56], cephaloglycin and imipenem [56]) was accompanied by a significant rise of GSSG concentration of the renal cortex. GSH depletion in renal cortex was dose-dependent and was greatest in rabbits, intermediate in rats and least in mice [42]. This pattern is consistent with the species susceptibility to cephaloridine nephrotoxicity. Further *in vitro* studies [36-38] using kidney slices and renal proximal tubule suspension were aimed at establishing the temporal sequence of biochemical events leading to cell death. The results of these studies showed that GSH depletion and lipid peroxidation were the earliest measurable events (0.25 to 1.5 hours) occurring after exposure of the renal tissue to cephaloridine [36-38].

These results correlate with the *in vivo* studies where a significant GSH depletion was measured 1 h after treating animals with cephaloridine, cephaloglycin or imipenem [42, 56].

Modulation of GSH level in cells (inhibition or stimulation) prior to treatment with different compounds affects the cellular response and drug toxicity [42,104,109]. Pretreatment of mice with buthionine sulfoximine enhanced peroxidative injury and trichloroethylene-mediated nephrotoxicity [109]. Similarly, diethylmaleate significantly depleted GSH in the rat renal cortex and potentiated cephaloridine-induced nephrotoxicity [42]. GSH synthesis may be stimulated by the drug oxothiazolidine-4-carboxylate (OTZ). After uptake in the cell, OTZ is enzymatically decarboxylated to yield cysteine, which is then used to synthesize GSH and thus increasing cellular GSH levels [110]. Another way of increasing cellular and tissue GSH levels is by use of GSH esters. The ester group attached to GSH facilitates penetration through the cell membrane inside the cell, where esterases hydrolyze the ester group to yield free GSH.

Reactive oxygen species and lipid peroxidation

It has been shown that the renal bioactivation of xenobiotics such as the herbicides paraquat and diquat [10, 111, 112], and of β-lactams such as cephaloridine and cefsulodin [10, 40, 41] or the antitumor agent adriamycin [113, 114] can induce the generation of reactive oxygen species (oxidative stress) which can be involved in alterations of the structure and functions of cell membranes, cytoskeletal injury, mutagenicity, carcinogenicity, and cell necrosis [115-117].

Reactive oxygen species

Although the mechanism(s) of β-lactam-induced nephrotoxicity is not fully elucidated, there is growing evidence that for some of the β-lactams, oxidative stress plays a pivotal role in the chain of events leading to nephrotoxicity and cell death [10, 34, 40].

The univalent reduction during redox cycling of compounds such as paraquat or cephaloridine, after exposure to renal microsomes, leads to production of the superoxide anion radical (Figure 5) [10, 40, 112]. Recent *in vitro* studies utilizing renal microsomes demonstrate that cephaloridine-induced reactive oxygen species readily oxidized porphyrinogens to porphyrin [118]. Results of *in vivo* studies in rats show that treatment with cephaloridine (10-500 mg/kg) produced a dose-dependent increase in urine concentration of the total porphyrin levels [118]. These results support cephaloridine-induced production of reactive oxygen species, *in vivo*. Pyridinium ring containing cephalosporins such as cephaloridine, cefsulodine and ceftazidime as well as other β-lactams such as mezlocillin and aztreonam, which do not contain a pyridinium ring, also induce superoxide production in the presence of rat renal microsomes and NADPH [10].

The capacity to generate, and the amount of superoxide produced by a *in vitro* renal microsome system is dependent on the molecular structure of the specific β-lactam. Superoxide production is a function of exposure time and β-lactam concentration (Figure 5). The rank order of the magnitude of superoxide production by β-lactams *in vitro* is as follows: cephaloridine > cefsulodin > mezlocillin > aztreonam > ceftazidime > cefotaxime [10].

The magnitude of renal damage caused by oxygen reactive species will also be influenced by the presence or absence of transition metals. Addition of $FeCl_2$ to a renal microsomes system increased cephaloridine-induced peroxidation of membrane lipids in a concentration-dependent manner [36]. These data are relevant to *in vivo* conditions where the availability of physiological concentrations of iron is critical. Ferritin, which is present at the subcellular level in the cytosol and endoplasmatic reticulum, appears to be the source for ferric iron *in vivo* [119].

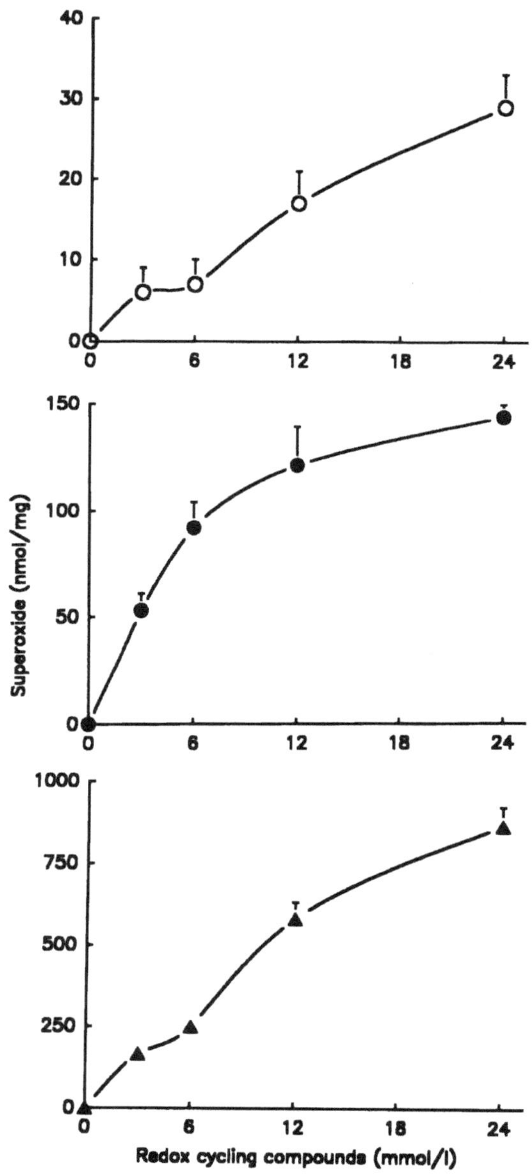

Figure 5. *Concentration-dependent production of superoxide induced by paraquat (•), cephaloridine (●) and ceftazidime (○).*

Superoxide generated by xanthine oxidase or in the redox cycling of paraquat can cause the reductive release of $F3^+$ from ferritin, a process that is dependent on the activity of microsomal NADPH-cytochrome P-450 reductase [119]. Iron appears to be an essential component in the formation of reactive species such as superoxide and hydroxyl radical via redox cycling of cephaloridine. Addition of EDTA or of the specific iron chelator desferrioxamine to an incubation system containing renal cortex microsomes and cephaloridine depressed cephaloridine-induced peroxidation of microsomal lipids significantly; EDTA showed a weaker effect than desferrioxamine at equimolar concentrations. By chelating $F3^+$ preferentially [120], desferrioxamine reduced the availability of $F2^+$ produced by the iron redox cycle and decreased cephaloridine-stimulated peroxidation of membrane lipids [36, 37].

Previous studies have shown that renal cortical microsomes are able to catalyze the reduction of cephaloridine in the presence of NADPH with subsequent formation of superoxide and hydrogen peroxide [40]. The divalent reduction of oxygen or the univalent reduction of superoxide yields non-radical species that are protonated at physiological pH to give hydrogen peroxide in a concentration-dependent manner (Figure 6). Hydrogen peroxide, which is a long-lived and membrane permeable species can diffuse and cause injury of cell macromolecules at considerable distances from its generation site.

Beta-lactam-induced generation of superoxide and hydrogen peroxide triggers formation of further highly

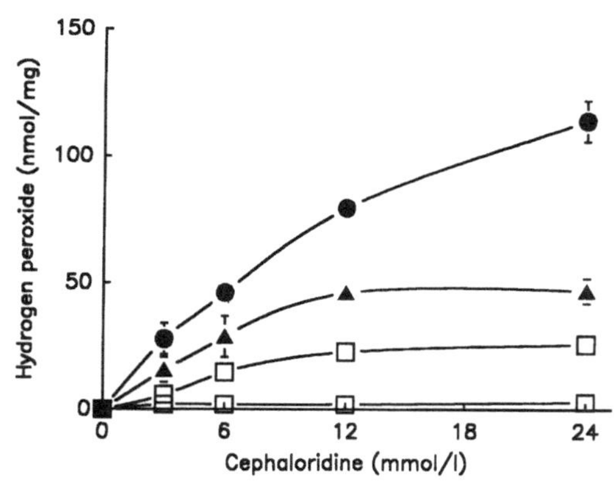

Figure 6. *Concentration-dependent hydrogen peroxide production induced by cephaloridine: 3-24 mmol/l (●), cephaloridine and catalase: 60 µg/ml (▲), cephaloridine and catalase: 120 µg/ml (❑), cefotaxime: 3-24 mmol/l (❑).*

reactive and cytotoxic oxygen species such as hydroxyl radical. Hydroxyl radical can further contribute in the presence of iron salts, to the decomposition of hydrogen peroxide and formation of additional reactive oxygen species such as singlet oxygen [40]. Kohda and Gemba [120a] have assessed the participation of reactive oxygen species (ROS) generation on cephaloridine nephrotoxicity in rats. Based on chemiluminescence and protein kinase C activity, they detected enhanced ROS generation in mitochondria at both 1.5 and 3.5 hours after cephaloridine administration which preceded histologic damage as assessed by electromicroscopy. They speculate that enhanced PKC and subsequent ROS generation precede changes in plasma parameters and histologic changes characteristic of cephaloridine toxicity. In addition these same authors recently reported a renoprotective effect of a serum thymic factor, FTS, when rats were administered nephrotoxic doses of cephaloridine [120b].

Beta-lactam induced lipid peroxidation

Free radical chain reactions, which occur during lipid peroxidation, lead to formation of lipid hydroperoxides that decompose to several types of secondary free radicals and a large number of secondary reactive compounds, such as aldehydes, all resulting in the destruction of cellular membranes and other cytotoxic responses.

Under *in vivo* conditions, liver and kidney microsomal NADPH-cytochrome P-450 reductases are also able of initiating peroxidation reactions resulting in the breakdown of polyunsaturated fatty acids to short-chain products. Uncontrolled, these peroxidation reactions can cause disorganization of membrane structure, leading to the inactivation of membrane-associated enzymes, membrane leakage and cell death. Activated oxygen species resulting from bioactivation of paraquat and β-lactams react with polyunsaturated fatty acids to cause peroxidation of the cell membrane lipids and subsequent nephrotoxicity [10, 34, 37, 39, 40, 56]. Among the more stabile end products of lipid peroxidation are compound such as malondialdehyde (MDA), ethane, pentane, and hydroxy-trans-neonal. Generation of conjugated dienes, MDA and pentane have been frequently used to demonstrate *in vivo* induction of β-lactam peroxidative damage in the kidney [34, 37, 56, 109].

Because NADPH-cytochrome P-450 reductase activity is highest in the cortex [77,121] and medullary microsomes lack cytochrome P450 [121], renal cortical tissue was used to investigate peroxidative injury caused by β-lactam accumulation in the kidney. Renal cortical microsomes, slices, tubule and cell suspensions, primary cultured renal cells and established kidney cell lines were exposed to β-lactams with the aim to investigate the subcellular mechanism of the nephrotoxic injury.

Studies conducted with renal cortical slices from pig, rabbit and rat revealed that slices from rabbit and rat renal cortex are more susceptible to β-lactam induced peroxidative injury [43]. Comparing the peroxidative potential of cephalosporins of different generations revealed that not only first-generation cephalosporins, but also second-generation cephalosporins such as cefotiam and third- and fourth-generation cephalosporins (Table 2) can produce a significant increase of lipid peroxidation measured as MDA production [10,26,49].

Table 2. Malondialdehyde (MDA) content and gluconeogenesis as a function of the cephalosporin concentration in the incubation medium.

	MDA (nmol/h/g tissue)					**Gluconeogenesis** (µmol/h/g tissue)				
Cephalosporin (mg/ml)	**0**	**1.25**	**2.5**	**5**	**10**	**0**	**1.25**	**2.5**	**5**	**10**
Cephaloridine	36.0 ±6.2	48.4 ±5.5	65.5* ±3.1	96.4* ±2.0	111.2* ±2.5	26.7 ±1.7	18.8* ±2.1	16.2* ±1.3	5.4* ±1.9	4.4* ±1.2
Ceftazidime	38.0 ±3.6	41.5 ±3.4	44.4* ±1.4	48.6* ±0.4	57.4* ±2.3	26.9 ±2.4	28.8 ±1.3	8.2* ±3.3	13.8* ±2.8	2.8* ±0.7
Cefpirome	41.2 ±3.1	46.5 ±4.1	45.2 ±1.2	47.3 ±4.0	58.3* ±3.1	25.6 ±3.3	25.7 ±1.9	21.2 ±2.9	18.9 ±3.9	23.0 ±3.5
Cefotaxime	41.3 ±2.9	42.8 ±2.4	41.3 ±1.9	46.6 ±3.6	55.4* ±4.2	25.5 ±1.6	25.3 ±2.7	24.3 ±4.1	25.7 ±1.6	26.8 ±1.3

Data represent mean ± SD from at least 4 rats. Values are significant at P< 0.05.*

Exposure of renal cortical microsomes or primary renal epithelial culture cells to different type of antibiotics led to a significant increase in production of superoxide and MDA after cephaloridine and mezlocillin [10, 40] but not after gentamicin [40, 122].

Significant increase in the cephaloridine-induced MDA generation was manifest in the proximal tubule suspensions while incubation of distal tubules with cephaloridine failed to increase MDA production tubule cell toxicity [36, 41, 50]. Exposure of rabbit and rat isolated proximal tubules or rat renal cortical slices to cephaloridine caused a time- and concentration-dependent generation of MDA [37, 38, 40, 41]. Inhibition of cephaloridine uptake into kidney slices [40] or isolated proximal tubules by 1.0 and 2.0 mM probenecid reduced MDA production in a concentration-dependent manner [39]. These results provide indirect evidence that biochemical processes leading to MDA production do not occur in the incubation medium but within the cortical cells after an obligatory uptake process across the cell membrane. Furthermore, pretreatment of rats with 60 mg/kg cobalt chloride significantly decreased cephaloridine-induced lipid peroxidation in renal cortical slices [31]. Addition of $FeCl_2$ to the incubation medium of renal cortical microsomes caused a significant stimulation of the cephaloridine-induced lipid peroxidation [36, 37]. Collectively, these results are indicative of the cytochrome P450 involvement in the intracellular bioactivation of cephaloridine and its subsequent peroxidative and nephrotoxic action [123]. However, it appears that β-lactams are nephrotoxic through more than one molecular mechanism.

Dr Cojocel's final publication defined the use of +cynidanol-3 and Vitamin E to protect the kidney against cephalosporin induced lipid peroxidation [123a]. Together with his co-authors he reported that, when animals were pretreated with either vitamin E or cyanidanol E , the cephalosporin-induced lipid peroxidation was significantly reduced and the renal cortical PAH uptake improved indicating a renoprotective effect against cephalosporin toxicity.

Protection by antioxidants and radical scavengers

Under normal physiological conditions the liver and the kidney cells appear to possess adequate defense mechanisms against lipid peroxidation. The most crucial intracellular components of the antiperoxidant defense system are glutathione and the glutathione-dependent enzymes.

The use of the detoxifying enzymes superoxide dismutase and catalase to suppress formation of superoxide and hydrogen peroxide, respectively, as well as specific radical scavengers for the hydroxyl radical and singlet oxygen such as mannitol, (+)-cyanidanol-3, thiourea, sodium benzoate, N-acetyl tryptophan and histidine, effectively decreased paraquat- or cephaloridine-induced peroxidation of microsomal lipids *in vitro* [15, 40, 41]. The chelation of iron should inhibit the production of hydroxyl radical and therefore mitigate the lipid peroxidation. Deferoxamine, a specific iron chelator, significantly inhibited peroxidation and protects against nephrotoxicity [36, 37]. Moreover, nonspecific antioxidants such as vitamin E, N,N'-diphenyl-phenylenediamine, promethazine, probucol or reduced glutathione significantly depressed cephaloridine-induced peroxidation of lipids in renal cortical slices and microsomes [37, 40, 41, 124]. Intracellular signaling pathways of cAMP and protein kinase C (PKC) have been reported to modulate cephaloridine-induced free radicals and nephrotoxicity. [72, 125]. Phorbol myristate acetate (PMA) enhancement of cephaloridine-induced lipid peroxidation and cell injury was blocked by a PKC inhibitor [71].

Alterations of cellular biochemical processes

Various β-lactam antibiotics such as cephalosporins and guanylureido penicillins may cause nonimmunologic nephrotoxic effects. The elucidation of the precise biochemical mechanisms involved in nephrotoxicity of β-lactams is of obvious importance for their rational and efficient utilization in the clinical management of infectious disease and for development of future cephalosporins.

Renal transport systems

For the zwitterion cephaloridine (CPH) a quantitative correlation between CPH-concentration and the degree of nephrotoxicity has been found [126]. CPH is taken up from blood into the proximal tubule cells and it was assumed that CPH uptake across the basolateral membrane occurs by the transport systems for PAH [127, 128]. However, it was also shown that zwitterionic β-lactams such as CPH can interact with the cation transport systems [82].

Because rats treated with CPH had altered protein composition and enzymatic activities of membranes from endoplasmic reticulum membranes [74, 75] and since intracellular CPH accumulation and nephrotoxicity was ascribed to relative impermeability of the luminal membrane for CPH [129], the effects of CPH-treatment on transport systems located in the brush border membrane were investigated [77].

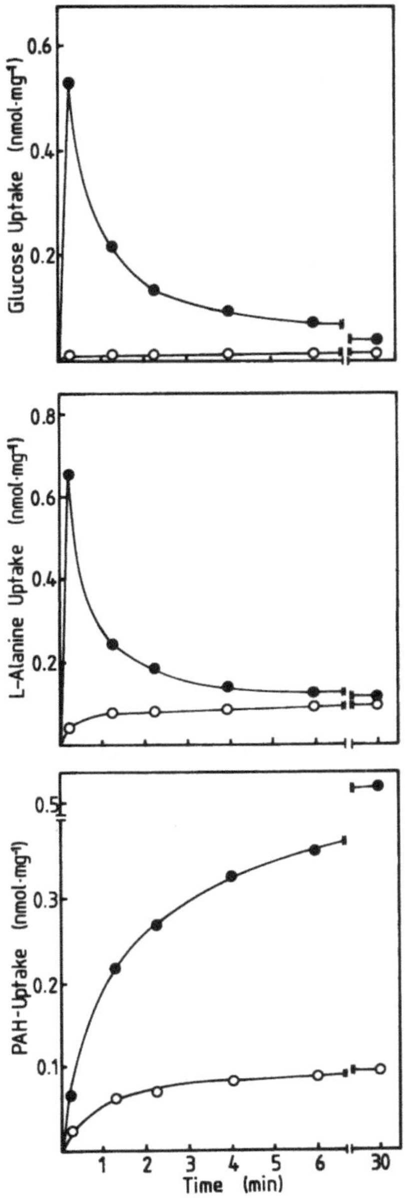

Figure 7. *Time-dependent uptake of PAH, L-alanine and glucose by renal brush border membrane vesicles. (●), control rats; (○), rats treated with cephaloridine (1200 mg/kg for 3 days).*

The uptake of *D-glucose* into renal brush border vesicles (BBMV) from control rats is a Na+-dependent transport process which demonstrates an overshoot phenomenon. After treatment of rats with CPH, the D-glucose transport into renal BBMV shows neither a Na^+-dependency nor an overshoot phenomenon (Figure 7). Furthermore, the equilibrium values for D-glucose uptake were reduced to 35% of controls in these studies. Similar results were obtained with BBMV from small intestine after treatment of animals with the anticancer drug mitomycin C [130, 131] but the equilibrium uptake values for D-glucose remained unchanged.

The effect of CPH-treatment upon the Na^+-dependent transport of the amino acid *L-alanine* was investigated [75]. The results of these studies showed that Na+-dependent transport of L-alanine was also reduced by the treatment with CPH and the overshoot phenomenon completely eliminated (Figure 7). In contrast to D-glucose, the equilibrium uptake values for L-alanine remained unchanged. Weinberg and colleagues [132] found that alanine and glycine can be protective against injury associated with increases in cytosolic free Ca^{2+}, reactive oxygen species, ATP depletion, and Na-K-ATPase inhibition in isolated kidney tubule cells in culture. Thus, the cephaloridine-induced decrease of alanine transport at the luminal cell membrane would diminish the cell defense ability against the toxic injuries caused by oxygen reactive species resulting from intracellular bioactivation of accumulated cephaloridine.

The carrier-mediated uptake of *p-aminohippuric acid* (PAH) into BBMV (Figure 7) and PAH accumulation by renal cortical slices [69,77] were also significantly reduced by CPH treatment (1200 mg/kg/d for 3d). Furthermore, the transport of other cephalosporins across the renal brush border membrane is also affected by CPH-treatment; the uptake of cephalexin and cefotiam into BBMV was greatly reduced whereas the uptake of CPH remained unaffected [77]. Secretion of cephalosporins across the brush border membrane is assumed to occur by the PAH-system as well as by the organic cation/H+-antiporter [127, 133]. Reabsorption of many cephalosporins is performed by the dipeptide transport system [69, 133]. The unaffected uptake of CPH into BBMV from CPH-treated rats indicates that CPH is transported by a system different from the dipeptide transporter. This is in agreement with results of other studies [82, 127] indicating that CPH interacts with transport systems for organic cations and anions in the brush border membrane. The similar uptake values for CPH in renal BBMV from untreated and CPH-treated rats do not support the previous hypothesis that the brush border membrane is impermeable for CPH [129].

Since cephalexin is transported by the dipeptide transport system [75, 133], the question arose whether or not the reduction of cephalexin transport activity following CPH treatment could be caused by either reduction in the number of transport sites or an impairment of the transport system for β-lactam antibiotics and dipeptides [77]. Using photoaffinity labeling, two membrane polypeptides of brush border membrane of molecular weight of 130,000 and 95,000 were identified as constituents of the dipeptide transport system [77]. The results of this study demonstrated that CPH-treatment of rats greatly reduced the photoaffinity labeling of the binding protein for β-lactam antibiotics and dipeptides with apparent molecular weight 130000. The labeling of the polypeptide of 95000 molecular weight was almost completely depressed [77]. The decrease in labeling intensity of the putative dipeptide transporter is suggestive for a reduction in the number of transport sites following CPH treatment. These results provide further evidence to elucidate the biochemical mechanism by which cephaloridine-induced oxidative injuries alter cell membrane permeability. Recent reports from Endou laboratory in Japan [133a,b,c] have provided insight as to the transport of cephalosporin antibiotics into proximal tubular cells. Both rat and human organic anion transporters (OAT) E have been shown to be involved in the transcellular transport. In particular, human OAT-1 and OAT-3 mediate the basal uptake of cephalosporins from the plasma, while OAT-4 is responsible for the apical transfer. Based in the difference in Ki values between hOAT-4 and hOAT-1, Takeda et al [133b] speculate that hOAT-4 limits the efflux of cephaloridine and contributes to it mechanism of nephrotoxicity.

Gluconeogenesis

Gluconeogenesis is an important metabolic function of the kidney [134]. Renal cortical slices from nive rats exposed to cephalosporins *in vitro* or renal cortical slices from animals treated with cephaloridine showed a time- and dose-dependent decrease of renal gluconeogenesis [26, 37, 49]. Glucose synthesis occurred in the proximal but not in the distal tubule suspensions [36]. Inhibition gluconeogenesis within 5 minutes of drug treatment may be an early event in cephaloridine-induced renal toxicity occurring prior to the onset of lipid peroxidation in renal cortical slices [135]. However, decreased gluconeogenesis should not cause cellular necrosis. Interestingly, antioxidants used to protect against cephaloridine-induced inhibition of organic ion accumulation do not block inhibition of gluconeogenesis by cephaloridine [135]. Cephaloridine-induced decrease in gluconeogenesis has been shown to be related to a simultaneous inhibition of the microsomal bound enzyme glucose-6-phosphatase activity in the renal cortex [135]. In contrast, the activity of another rate-limiting enzyme of gluconeogenesis, fructose-1,6-diphosphatase, was not inhibited by cephaloridine [12].

Renal lipid metabolism and protein degradation

Penicillin treatment of rabbit neonates (90,000 IU for 2d) altered *lipid metabolism in vivo* by significantly increasing serum concentration of non-esterified fatty acids and decreasing renal triglyceride content [136]. It appears that penicillin was either decreasing the utilization of non-esterified fatty acids or increasing release. The decrease of renal triglyceride content could be the result of the inhibition of the triglyceride synthesis or penicillin might have increased the utilization of this substrate.

Cephaloridine contains a quaternary nitrogen, exists as a zwitterion under physiological conditions and has structural similarities with carnitine. Proximal tubule cells are the internal sites of carnitine acylation [137]. Cephalosporin and carbapenem antibiotics inhibit carnitine tubular reabsorption [68, 138] and mitochondrial uptake of acylcarnitine leading to massive acylcarnitinuria [67]. Newer β-lactam such as cefepime and cefoselis, which possess a quaternary nitrogen as does carnitine, may also inhibit carnitine tubular reabsorption [88].

In order to be metabolized, long-chain fatty acids must first undergo conjugation to carnitine for transport by the acylcarnitine-carnitine carrier across the mitochondrial inner membrane [139]. Short-chain fatty acids enter the mitochondria through monocarboxylic acid transporters [139]. Studies were carried out to assess the effects cephaloridine, cephaloglycin and cephalexin on the mitochondrial oxidative metabolism of fatty acids such as butyrate and palmitate [67].

The results of these studies showed significant inhibition of palmitoylcarnitine-mediate respiration by cephaloridine *in vitro*, whereas cephaloglycin, which lacks structural homology with carnitine, caused a greater inhibition of the mitochondrial transport and oxidation of butyrate than cephaloridine. It is possible that the mitochondrial uptake of butyrate was not affected by cephaloridine maybe because the pyridinyl nitrogen hinders its attack on the monocarboxylate receptors. Cephalexin induced only mild *in vitro* toxicity to the mitochondrial uptake and oxidation of butyrate and palmitate [67].

Cephaloridine effect on the intracellular *renal protein degradation* was investigated using the labeled low molecular weight protein, ^{125}I-lysozyme. Treatment of rats with cephaloridine for 5 days was followed by administration of ^{125}I-lysozyme one hour prior sacrifice. Release of trichloroacetic acid (TCA) soluble radioactivity into incubation medium from renal cortical slices was used to quantify lysosomal degradation of lysozyme [141].

The results of these experiments showed that cephaloridine caused a dose-dependent decrease of intracellular protein degradation thus impairing the renal metabolism of endogenous and exogenous peptides and proteins taken up by the renal cells.

Clinical toxicity of beta-lactam antibiotics

Cephalosporins are the 16th most frequent cause of adverse drug reactions in hospitals in the United States [141a]. Their importance as a cause of nephrotoxicity was recently confirmed by meta-analysis [141b]. Usually β-lactam induced adverse reactions are readily recognized by the clinician. On the other hand, the relationship between antimicrobial activity and the development of a drug-initiated adverse effect can be very subtle and elude the most astute clinician. If a β-lactam is uniquely advantageous for a patient, a carefully controlled rechallenge can be considered to more precisely identify a cause-effect relationship. With appropriate clinical management renal failure caused by β-lactams is often reversible. Identification and elimination of the risk factors associated with β-lactam nephrotoxicity is essential to the prevention of nephrotoxicity. Of these factors, correction of volume depletion and/or congestive heart failure and reversing diminished renal perfusion are of primary importance. While fluid resuscitation can limit the renal damage caused by nephrotoxic β-lactams, there is a risk of overhydration if renal failure develops. Monitoring of serum drug concentration should be helpful to confirm β-lactam-induced renal toxicity, especially when drug interactions are involved.

Interaction with other nephrotoxic drugs

Beta-lactam induced renal toxicity can results from their use in monotherapy or when used in combination with other nephrotoxic drugs such as aminoglycosides, amphotericin B, cisplatin, cyclosporine, furosemide, ifosfamide, vancomycin and nephrotoxic β-lactams. While the risk of nephrotoxic injury from monotherapy with β-lactams is relatively low, this risk is substantially increased when multiple drug combinations are required.

Benzylpenicillin and ureidopenicillins such as piperacillin and mezlocillin appear to have a little or no nephrotoxic potential when administered alone or in combination with other drugs.

Rats treated with piperacillin (1600 mg/kg) and furosemide (100 mg/kg) have elevation blood urea nitrogen (BUN) and creatinine concentration, and mild histologic degeneration of the proximal tubules. These alterations were similar to those observed in rats treated with furosemide alone [142].

The combination of cephalothin with an aminoglycoside was more nephrotoxic than methicillin plus aminoglycoside [143]. There is good evidence that concurrent administration of cephalothin and gentamicin are additive nephrotoxins in humans, especially in patients over 60 years of age as wells as in rabbits [144], and renal injuries are intensified in the presence of mild renal ischemia or endotoxemia [108]. The results of prospective randomized comparative studies of the combination mezlocillin/cefotaxime versus gentamicin/cefoxitin showed that the concurrent administration of mezlocillin/cefotaxime has low renal toxicity and can be recommended for the rational and empirical treatment of serious systemic infections [145].

Results from animal studies indicate that while furosemide enhanced cephaloridine nephrotoxicity no increased renal toxicity was observed by combining of piperacillin with furosemide [142]. Latamoxef and flomoxef may decrease nephrotoxicity of vancomycin by inhibiting its uptake into the kidney [146, 147]. The results of a retrospective study including renal transplant patients indicate that aztreonam can be safely administered with cyclosporine [148]. Combination therapy with ampicillin/aztreonam in neonates showed a lower renal toxicity than in the group with concurrent administration of oxacillin/amikacin [149].

New lactam antibiotics

There is a continuous need for new antibiotics to overcome resistance. However, in the case of β-lactams there is a need to inhibit β-lactamase enzymes, which hydrolyze, and thereby inactivate β-lactam antibiotics. Novel tricyclic carbapenems (trinems) and 2-naphtylcarbapenems have broad spectrum and showed potent activities against gram-negative bacteria [150, 151] including methicillin-resistant *Staphylococcus aureus* (MRSA). The γ-lactams may be less susceptible to degradation by hydrolases. A number of compounds containing the γ-lactam (pyrrolidin-2-one) moiety show interesting biological and pharmaceutical activities. Some novel monocyclic thienyl γ-lactams are reported to show moderate to high antibacterial activity against gram-positive and gram-negative bacteria [152].

Prevention of clinical toxicity of beta-lactam antibiotics

Adverse drug effects represent a major source of morbidity and mortality and must be considered in the differential diagnosis for patients who are experiencing new medical problems or whose clinical status is worsening. Familiarity with β-lactam induced adverse reactions can improve antibiotic selection and reduce adverse events. Before antibiotic therapy is started, the potential benefits and the possible adverse effects should be investigated in light of each patient's situation. Prevention should be considered in the first place, but if adverse events do occur, they must be recognized and corrected promptly.

The most important approach to decreasing β-lactam nephrotoxicity is judicious use of these drugs. If a β-lactam is uniquely advantageous for a patient, a carefully controlled rechallenge can be considered to more precisely identify a cause-effect relationship. When β-lactams are used in neonates, accurate determination of the dosage is required, especially for compounds with low therapeutic index and in patients with renal failure.

Occurrence of acute renal failure from β-lactam treatment may be prevented by early treatment of serious infections, together with maintenance of hemodynamic stability, renal perfusion, and urinary solute excretion. The β-lactam induced renal failure has a time course comparable to acute tubular necrosis of other origins. While there is no firm evidence that dialysis will speed up renal recovery, clinical stability and good nutrition are likely to improve recovery, as it is also the case with other types of renal failure.

Concomitant administration of piperacillin and cephaloridine to rabbits resulted in a significant protective effect against cephaloridine nephrotoxicity [153]. Cephaloridine nephrotoxicity can be prevented by administration of other cephalosporins or penicillins that produce little or no reduction of the cortical concentration of cephaloridine [154]. However, ceftriaxone protects against tobramycin nephrotoxicity by reducing the intracortical accumulation of tobramycin [155]. Combination of tobramycin with latamoxef protects the rat kidney from tobramycin nephrotoxicity, and the protective effect may be partially due to suppression of intrarenal accumulation of tobramycin by latamoxef. This suppression of nephrotoxicity is roughly dependent on the latamoxef dosage [81, 156].

Methimazole (1-methylimidazole-2-thiol) protects against cephaloridine-induced nephrotoxicity when was given 30 min prior cephaloridine administration to rats [157]. Furthermore, cephaloridine transport and accumulation in the kidney was not affected by methimazole [157].

Comparison of cephaloridine-induced nephrotoxicity in normoglycemic and diabetic rats showed lower renal toxicity in diabetic rats than normoglycemic rats. This is apparently due to the fact that the diabetic renal tissue accumulated less cephaloridine than the tissue from normoglycemic rats [158].

Acknowledgements

Supported by Kuwait University.

References

1. Fleming A. On the antibacterial action of cultures of Penicillium with special reference to their use in the isolation of *B.influemzae*. Brit J Exper Pathol 1929; 10: 228-236.
2. Abraham EP, Newton GGF. The structure of cephalosporin C. Biochem J 1961; 79: 377-393.
3. Nagarajan R, Boeck LD, Gorman M, Hamil RC, Higgens CE, Hoehn MM, Stark WM, Whitney, JG. β-lactam antibiotics from Streptomyces. J Am Chem Soc 1971; 93: 2308-2310.
4. Page MG. B-Lactamase inhibitors. Drug Resist Updat 2000; 3(2): 109-125.
5. Cooper RD. The carbacephems: a new β-lactam antibiotic class. Am J Med 1992; 92(6A): 2S-6S.
6. Tally FP, Jacobus NV, Gorbach SL. *In vitro* activity of thienamycin. Antimicrob Agents Chemother 1978; 14 (3): 436-438.
7. Sader HS, Gales AC. Emerging strategies in infectious diseases: new carbapenem and trinem antibacterial agents. Drugs 2001; 61(5): 553-564.
8. Cimarusti CM, and Sykes RB. Monocyclic β-lactam antibiotics. Med Re. Rev 1984; 4(1): 1-24.

8a. Jacoby GA and Munoz-Price LS. The new β-lactamases. New Eng J Med 2005;352:380-391

8b. Zhang Q, Matsumura Y, Teratani T, Yoshimoto S, Mineno T, Nakagawa K, Nagahama M, Kuwata S, Takeda H. The application of an institutional clinical data warehouse to the assessment of adverse drug reactions (ADRs). Methods Inf Med 2007;46:516-522

9. YousifT, Pooyeh S, Hannemann J, Baumann J, Tauber R, Baumann K. Nephrotoxic and peroxidative potential of meropenem and imipenem/cilastatin in rat and human renal cortical slices. Inter. J Clin Pharmacol Therap 1999; 10: 475-486.
10. Duwe J, Cojocel C, Baumann K. Effect of paraquat-like substances and cephalosporins on accumulation of p-aminohippurate and tetraethylammonium in rat renal cortical slices, and on lipid peroxidation in rat renal microsomes and cortical alices. In: Nephrotoxicity. Mechanisms, early diagnosis, and therapeutic management. Bach PH, Gregg NJ, Wilks MF, Delacruz L (editors). Marcel Dekker Inc, New York 1991; p. 13-17.
11. Tune BM. The nephrotoxicity of cephalosporin antibiotics-structure-activity relationships. Comm Toxicol 1986; 1(2): 145-170.
12. Goldstein RS, Smith PF, Tarloff, JB, Contardi L, Rush GF, Hook JB. Biochemical mechanisms of cephaloridine nephrotoxicity. Life Sci 1988; 42(19): 1809-1916.
13. Kaloyanides GJ. Metabolic interactions between drugs and renal tubulo-interstitial cells. Role in nephrotoxicity. Kidney Int 1991; 39: 531-540.
14. Schnellmann RG, Griner RD. Mitochondrial mechanisms of tubular injury. In: Mechanisms of injury in renal disease and toxicity. Goldstein RS, Editor.CRC Press Inc, Boca Raton, Florida, USA 1994; p. 247-265.
15. Tomita M, Okuyama T, Watanabe S, Watanabe H. Quantitation of the hydroxyl radical adducts of salicylic acid by micellar electrokinetic capillary chromatography: oxidizing species formed by a Fenton reaction. Arch Toxicol 1994; 68: 428 - 433.
16. Tomita M., and Okuyama T. Effect of paraquat on the malondialdehyde level in rat liver microsomes (*in vitro*). Arch. Toxicol 1994; 68: 187-192.
17. Tune BM, Hsu C-H, Fravert D. Cephalothin and carbacephem nephrotoxicity. Role of tubular cell uptake and acylating potential. Biochem Pharmacol 1996; 51: 557-561.
18. Roselle GA, Clyne DH, Kaufman CA. Carbenicillin nephrotoxicity. South Med J 1978; 71(1): 84-86.
19. Elis D, Fried WA, Yunis EJ, Blau EB. Acute interstitial nephritis in children: a report of 13 cases and review of the literature. Pediatrics 1981; 67(6): 862-870.
20. Pommer W, Offerman G, Schultze G, Krause PH, Molzhan M. Acute interstitial nephritis caused by drugs. Dtsch Med Wochenschr 1983; 108(20): 783-788.
21. Browning MC, Tune BM. Reactivity and binding of β-lactam antibiotics in rabbit renal cortex. J Pharmacol. Exp Ther 1983; 226(3): 640-644.
22. Geller RJ, Chevalier RL, Spyker DA. Acute amoxicillin nephrotoxicity following an overdose. J. Toxicol Clin Toxicol 1986; 24(2): 175-182.
23. Schellie SF, Groshong T. Acute interstitial nephritis following amoxicillin overdose. Mo Med 1999; 96(6): 209-211.
24. Hedstrom SA, Hybbinette CH. Nephrotoxicity in isoxazolylpenicillin prophylaxis in hip surgery. Acta Orthop Scand 1988; 59(2): 144-147.
25. Dunn GL. Ceftizoxime and other third-generation cephalosporins: Structure activity relationships. J Antimicrob Chemother 1982; 10: 1-10.
26. Cojocel C, Goettsche U., Toelle K-L., Baumann, K. Nephrotoxic potential of first-, second-, and third-generation cephalosporins. Arch Toxicol 1988; 62: 458-464.
27. Fillastre JP, Kleinknecht D. Acute renal failure associated with cephalosporin therapy. Am Heart J 1975; 89(6): 809-810.
28. Silverblatt F, Turck M, Bulger R. Nephrotoxicitydue to cephaloridine: a light- and electron-microscopy study in rabbits. J Infect Dis 1970; 122(1): 33-44.

29. Yamada Y. Studies on the mechanisms of renal damage induced by nephrotoxic compounds. Nippon Hoigaku Zasshi 1995; 49(6): 447-457.
30. Tune BM. Effect of organic transport inhibitors on renal uptake and proximal tubular toxicity of cephaloridine. J Pharmacol Exper Therap 1972; 181: 250-256.
31. Cojocel C, Laeschke KH, Insellman G, Baumann K. Inhibition of cephaloridine-induced lipid peroxidation. Toxicology 1985; 35(4): 295-305.
32. Takeda M, Tojo A, Sekine T, Hosoyamada M, Kanai Y, Endou H. Role of organic anion transporter 1 (OAT1) in cephaloridin (CER)-induced nephrotoxicity. Kidney Int 1999; 56: 2128-2136.
33. Jariyawat S, Sekine T, Takeda M, Apiwattanakul N, Kanai Y, Sophasan S, Endou H. The interaction and transport of β-lactam antibiotics with the cloned rat renal organic anion transporter 1. J Pharmacol Exp Ther1999; 290 (2): 672-677.
34. Kuo C-H, Maita, K, Sleight SD, Hook JB. Lipid peroxidation: a possible mechanism of cephaloridine-induced nephrotoxicity. Toxicol Appl Pharmacol 1983; 67: 78-88.
35. Tune B, Fravert D, Hsu C-Y. Oxidative and mitochondrial toxic effects of cephalosporin antibiotics in the kidney. A comparative study of cephaloridine and cephloglycine. Biochem Pharmacol 1989; 38(3): 795-802.
36. Cojocel C, Mayer D. Protection by glutathione and antioxidants against cephaloridine-induced lipid peroxidation. Biochem. Pharmacol (Life Sci Adv) 1991; 10: 41-51.
37. Goldstein RS, Pasino DA, Hewit WR, Hook JB. Biochemical mechanisms of cephaloridine nephrotoxicity: time and concentration dependence of peroxidative injury. Toxicol Appl Pharmacol 1986; 83: 261-270.
38. Rush GF, Ponsler GD. Cephaloridine-induced biochemical changes and cytotoxicity in suspensions of rabbit isolated proximal tubules. Toxicol Appl Pharmacol 1991; 109: 314-326.
39. Rush GF, Heim RA, Ponsler GD, Engelhardt J. Cephaloridine-induced renal pathological and biochemical changes in female rabbits and isolated proximal tubules in suspension. Toxicol Pathol 1992; 20(2): 155-168.
40. Cojocel C, Hannemann J, Baumann K. Cephaloridine-induced lipid peroxidation initiated by reactive oxygen species as a possible mechanism of cephaloridine nephrotoxicity. Biochim Biophys Acta 1985; 834: 402–410.
41. Suzuki Y, Sudo J. Lipid peroxidation and generation of oxygen radicals induced by cephaloridine im renal cortical microsomes of rats. Jpn J Pharmacol 1990; 52(2): 233-243.
42. Kuo C-H, Hook JB. Depletion of renal gluthathione content and nephrotoxicity of cephaloridine in rabits, rats, and mice. Toxicol Appl Pharmacol 1982; 63: 292-302.
43. Cojocel C, Inselmann G, Laeschke KE, Baumann K. Species differences in cephalosporin-induced lipid peroxidation. Drugs Exptl Clin Res 1984; 10(11): 781-784.
44. Kays SE, Crowell WA, Johnson MA. Cephaloridine nephrotoxicity is potentiated by selenium deficiency but not by copper deficiency in rats. J Nutr 1992; 122: 1232-1241.
45. Alitalo R, Ruutu M, Valtonen V, Lehtonen T, Pentkäinen PJ. Hyoprothrombinaemia and bleeding during administration of cefamandole and cefoperazone. Ann Clin Res 1985; 17: 116-119.
46. Wachsmuth ED. Nephrotoxicity of cefotiam (CGP 14221/E) in rats and rabbits. Arch Toxicol 1996; 48: 135-156.
47. Norrby SR, Burman LA, Linderhol H, Trollfors B. Ceftazidime: pharmakokinetics in patients and effects on renal function. J Antimicrob Chemother 1982; 10(3): 199-206.
48. Alestig K, Trollfors B, Andersson R, Oolaison L, Suurkula M, Norrby SR. Ceftazidime and renal function. J Antimicrob Chemother 1984; 13(2): 177-181.
49. Cojocel C. Biochemical aspects of the renal tolerance for cefpirome and other cephalosporins. rzneimittelforschung 1990; 40(10):1140-1144.
50. Suzuki H, Imamura K, Yoshida T, Shibata M, Matsuzawa T, Ozaki H, Sakai T, Shiobara Y, Tachibana A, Yanko K. Animal pharmacokinetis and toxicology of cefotetan - a new cephamycin antibiotic. J Antimicrob Chemother 1983; 11(Suppl): 179-183.
51. Thieme RE, Caldwell SA, Lum GM. Acute interstitial nephritis associated with loracarbef therapy. J Pediatr 1995; 127(6): 997-1000.
52. Birnbaum J, Kahan FM, Kropp H, Macdonald JS. Carbapenems, a new class of β-lactam antibiotics: discovery and development of imipenem/cilastatin. Am J Med 1985; 78(Suppl 6A): 3-21.
53. Kropp H, Sundelof JG, Hajdu R, Kahan FM. Metabolism of thienamycin and related carbapenem antibiotics by the renal dipeptidase, dehydropeptidase-1. Antimicrob Ag Chemother 1982; 22: 62-70.
54. Cunha BA. Meropenem in elderly and renally impaired patients. Int J Antimicrob Agents 1988; 10: 107-117.
55. Asbel LE, Levison ME. Cephalosporins, carbapenems, and monobactams. Infect Dis Clin North Am 2000; 14(2): 435-437.
56. Tune BM., Fravert D, Hsu C-Y. Thienamycin nephrotoxicity. Mitochondrial injury and oxidative effects of imipenem in the rabbit kidney. Biochem Pharmacol 1989; 38(21): 3779-3783.

57. Hirouchi Y, Naganuma H, Kawahara Y, Okada R, Kammiya A, Inui K, Hori R. Preventive effect of ßmipron on nephrotoxicity and uptake of carbapenems in rabbit renal cortex. Jpn J Pharmacol 1994; 66(1): 1-6.
58. Cunha BA. Aztreonam. Urology 1993; 41(3): 249-258.
59. Moore RD, Lerener SA, Levine, DP. Nephrotoxicity and ototoxicity of aztreonam versus aminoglycoside therapy. J Infect Dis 1992; 165(4): 683-688.
60. Chartrand SA. Safety and toxicity profile of aztreonam. Pediatr Infect Dis J 1989; 8(Suppl 9): 120-123.
61. Ohya S, Yamazaki M, Sugawara S. Effect of 7 α substitution of cephems on their β-lactamase stability and affinity for penicillin-binding proteins in Morganella morganii. Antimicrob Agents Chemother 1983; 23(4): 522-525.
62. Patel IH, Kaplan SA. Phrmacokinetic profile of ceftriaxone in man. Am J Med 1984; 77(4C): 17-25
63. Sattler FR, Weitekamp MR, Ballard JO. Potential for bleeding with the new β-lactam antibiotics. Ann Intern Med 1986; 105(6): 924-931.
64. Goto K, Oda M, Saitoh H, Nishida M, Takada M. Effect of side chains including N-methyl-tetrazole-thiol group of β-lactam antibiotics on transport in cultured kidney epithelial cells LLC-PK1. Biol Pharm Bull 1988; 21(10): 113-116.
65. Williams PD, Laska DA, Tay LK, Hottendorf, GH. Comparative toxicities of cephalosporin antibiotics in a rabbit kidney cell line (LLC-RK1). Antimicrob Agents Chemother 1988; 32(3): 314-318.
66. Viotte G, Morin GP, Godin M, Fillastre JP. Chamges in the renal function of rats treated with cefoxitin and a comparison with other cephlosporins and gentamicin. J Antimicrob Chemother 1981; 7(5): 537-550
67. Tune BM. The renal toxicity of β-lactam antibiotics: mechanism and clinical impications. In: Clinical nephrotoxins – renal injury from drugs and chemicals. 1st Ed.. De Broe ME, Porter GA, Bennett WM, Verpooten GA (editors). Kluwer Academic Publ, Dordrecht, 1998; p. 121-134.
68. Topham JC, Murgatroyd LB, Johns DV, Goonetilleke UR, Wright J. Safety evaluation of meropenem in animals: studies on the kidney. J Antimicrob Chemother 1989; 24(Suppl A): 287-386.
69. Harrison MP, Jones DV, Pickford RJ, Wilson ID. ß-Hydroxybutyrate: a urinary marker of imipenem induced nephrotoxicity in the cynomolgus monkey detected by high field spectroscopy. Biochem Pharmacol 1991; 41(12): 2045-2049.
70. Nouda H, Matsumura H, Tanio T, Sunagawa M. Structural feature of carbapenem compounds or nephrotoxicity: effect of C-2 side chain. J Antibiotics 1996; 49(6): 603-606.
71. Kohda Y, Gemba M. Modulation by cyclic AMP and phorbol myristate acetate of cephaloridine-induced injury in rat renal cortical slices. Jpn J Pharmacol 2001; 85(1): 54-59.
72. Cojocel C, Maita K, Pasino DA, Kuo, C-H, Hook J B. Metabolic heterogeneity of proximal and distal tubules. Life Sci 1983; 33: 855-861.
73. Lock EA. Renal drug-metabolizing enzymes in experimental animals and humans. In: Mechanisms of injury in renal disease and toxicity. Goldstein R S (editor). CRC Press Inc, Boca Raton, Florida 1994; p. 173-206.
74. Cojocel C, Kramer W, Mayer D. Depletion of cytochrome P450 and alterations in activities of drug metabolizing enzymes induced by cephaloridine in rat kidney cortex. Biochemical Pharmacol 1988; 37(19): 3781-3785.
75. Kramer W, Cojocel C, Mayer D. Specific alterations of rat renal microsomal proteins induced by cephaloridine. Biochem Pharmacol 1988; 37 (21): 4135-4140.
76. Olivier MF, Dutertre-Catella H, Thevenin M, Martin C, Warnet JM, Claude JR. Increased reduced glutathione and glutathione S-transferase activity in chronic cephaloridine nephrotoxicity studies in the rat. Drug Chem Toxicol 1990; 13(1-2): 209-219.
77. Kramer W, Cojocel C, Mayer D. Effect of cephaloridine treatment on transport systems of the rat renal brush border membrane. Biochem Pharmacol (Life Sci Adv) 1990; 9: 127-133.
78. Fry M, Plummer DT. The interaction of cephaloridine with model membrane systems and rat kidney lysosomes. Chem Biol Interact 1979; 25(1): 113-124.
79. Ngaha EO. Further studies on the *in vivo* effect of cephaloridine on the stability of rat kidney lysosomes. Biochem Pharmacol 1982; 31(10): 1843-1847.
80. Yamagouchi A, Hiruma R, Sawai T. Phospholipid bilayer oermeability of β-lactam antibiotics. J Antibiot (Tokyo) 1982; 35(12): 1692-1696.
81. Kojima R, Ito M, Suzuki Y. Studies on the nephrotoxicity of aminoglycoside antibiotics and protection from these effects (4). Effects of tobramycin alone and in combination with latamoxef on the stability of rat kidney lysosomal membranes. Jpn J Pharmacol 1987; 43(1): 73-80.
82. Ullrich KJ, Rumrich G, Kloss S. Contraluminal organic anion and cation transport in the proximal renal tubule: V. Interaction with sulfamoyl- and phemoxy diuretics, and with β-lactam antibiotics. Kidney Int 1989; 36(1): 78-88.
83. Van Aubel RAMH, Masereeuw R, Russsel FGM. Molecular pharmacology of renal organic anion transporters. Am J Physiol Renal Physiol 2000; 279(2): F216-F232.

84. Williams PD, Hitchcock MJ, Hottendorf GH. Effect of cephalosporins on organic ion transport in renal membrane vesicles from the rat and rabbit kidney cortex. Res Commun Chem Pathol Pharmacol 1985; 47(3): 357-371.
85. Ullrich KJ, Rumrich G, Wieland T, Dekant W. Contraluminal para-aminohippurate (PAH) transport in the proximal tubule of the rat kidney. VI. Specificity: amino acids, their N-methyl-, Nacetyl- and N-benzoylderivatives; glutathione- and cysteine conjugates, di- and oligopeptides. Pflügers Arch 1989; 415(3): 342-350.
86. Atkinson RM, Curie LP, Prat PAH, Sharpe HM, Tomich EG. Acute toxicity of cephaloridine, an antibiotic derived from cephalosporin C. Toxicol Appl Pharmacol 1966; 8(3): 398-406.
87. Schaub TP, Kartenbeck J, König J, Spring H, Dorsam J, Sthaeler G, Störkel S, Thon WF, Keppler D. Expression of the MRP2 gene-encoded conjugate export pump in human kidney proximal tubule and in renal carcinoma. J Am Soc Nephrol 1999; 10(6): 1159-1169.
88. Ganapathy ME, Huang W, Rajan DP, Carter AL, Sugawara M, Iseki K, Leibach FH, Ganapathy V. β-lactam antibiotics as substrates for OCTN2, an organic cation/carnitine transporter. J Biol Chem 2000; 275(3): 1699-1707.
89. Terada T, Saito H, Mukai M, Inui K-I. Recognition of β-lactam antibiotics by rat peptide transportrers, PEPT1 and PEPT2 in LLC-Pk1 cells. Am J Physiol Renal Physiol 1997; 273(42): F706-F711.
90. Daniel H, Herget M. Cellular and molecular mechanisms of renal peptide transport. Am J Physiol Renal Physiol 1987; 273:F1-F8.
91. Hori R, Ishikawa Y, Takano M, Okano T, Kitazawa S, Inui K. The interaction of cephalosporin antibiotics with renal cortex of rats: accumulation to cortical slices and binding to purified plasma membranes. Biochem Pharmacol 1982; 31(13): 2267-2272.
92. McMurty RJ, Mitchell JR. Renal and hepatic necrosis after metabolic activation of 2-sustituted furans and thiophenes, including furosemide and cephaloridine. Toxicol Appl Pharmacol 1977; 42: 285-300.
93. Spurling NW, Harcourt RA, Hyde JJ. An evaluation of the safety of cefuroxime axetil during six months oral administration to beagle dogs. J. Toxicol Sci 1986; 11(4): 237-277.
94. Johns RN. A review of cephalosporin metabolism: a lesson to be learned for future chemotherapy. Diagn. Microbial Infect Dis 1989; 12(1): 25-32.
95. Marone P, Navarra A, Monzillo V, Traverso A. Antibacterial activity of combined cefotaxime and desacetyl-cefotaxime against aerobic gram-negative bacilli. Drugs Exp Clin Res 1990; 16(12): 629-633.
96. Hottendorf GH, Laska DA, Williams PD, Ford SM. Role of desacetylation in the detoxification of cephalothin in renal cells in culture. J Toxicol Environ Health 1987; 22(1): 101-111.
97. Indelicato JM, Dinner A, Peters LR, Wilham WL. Hydrolysis of 3-chloro-3-cephems. Intramolecular nucleophilic attack in cefaclor. J Med Chem 1977; 20: 961-963
98. Tune BM, Hsu C-Y. The renal mitochondrial toxicity of β-lactam antibiotics: *In vitro* effects of cephaloglycin and imipenem. J Amer Soc Nephrol 1990; 1(5): 815-821.
99. Masereeuw R, van den Bergh EJ, Bindels RJ, Russel Fg. Characterization of fluorescein transport in isolated proximal tubular cells of the rat: Evidence for mitochondrial accumulation. J Pharmacol Exp Ther 1994; 269: 1261-1267.
100. Miller DS, Stewart DE, Pitchard JB. Inracellular compartimentation of organic anions within renal cells. Am J Physiol 1993; 264: R882-R890.
101. Terlouw SA, Tanriseven O, Russel FGM, Masereeuw R. Metabolite anion carriers mediate the uptake of the anion drug fluorescein in renal cortical mitochondria. J Pharmacol Exp Ther 2000; 293(3): 968-973.
102. Schnellmann R G, Gilchrist S M, Mandel L J. Intracellular distribution and depletion of glutathione in rabbit renal proximal tubules. Kidney Int 1988; 34: 229-233.
103. Meister A, Anderson M A. Glutathione. Annu Rev Biochem 1985; 52: 711-760.
104. Reed D J. Regulation of reductive processes by glutathione. Biochem Pharcol 1986; 35(1): 7-13.
105. Moldeus P, Quanguang J. Importance of the glutathione cycle in drug metabolism. Pharmacol Ther 1987; 33: 37-40.
106. Elfarra AA, Anders MW. Renal processing of glutathione conjugates. Role in nephrotoxicity. Biochem Pharmacol 1984; 33(23): 3729-3732.
107. Beuter W, Cojocel C, Muller W, Donaubauer HH, Mayer D. Peroxidative damage and nephrotoxicity of dichlorovinylcysteine in mice. J Appl Toxicol. 1989; 9(3): 181-186.
108. Tune BM, Hsu C-Y, Fravert D. Mechanisms of bacterial endotoxin-cephaloridine toxic synergy and the protective effects of saline infusion in the rabbit kidney. J Pharmacol Exp Ther 1988; 244(2): 520-525.
109. Cojocel C, Beuter W, Müller W, Maye, D. Lipid peroxidation: a possible mechanism of trichloroethylene-induced nephrotoxicity. Toxicology 1989; 55: 131-141.
110. Mitchell JB, Biaglow JE, Russo A. Role of glutathione and other endogenous thiols in radiation protection. Pharmacol Ther 1988; 39(1-3): 269-274.
111. Bus JS, Gibson JE. Paraquat: model for oxidant-initiated toxicity. Environ Health Persp 1984; 55: 37-46.

112. Tomita M. Comparison of one-electron reduction activity against the bipyridylium herbicides, paraquat and diquat, in microsomal and mitochondrial fractions of liver, lung and kidney (*in vitro*). Biochemical Pharmacol 1991; 42(2): 303-309.
113. Gianni L, Zweier JL, Levy A, Mayers CE. Characterisation of the cycle of iron-mediated electron transfer from adriamycin to molecular oxygen. J Biol Chem 1985; 260(11): 6820- 6826.
114. Mimnaugh EG. Potentiation by reduced glutathione of adriamycin-stimulated lipid peroxidation in kidny microsomes. Biochem Pharmacol 1986; 35(23): 4337-4339.
115. Fridovich I. Biological effects of the superoxide radical. Arch Biochem Biophys 1986; 247: 1-11.
116. Halliwell B, Gutteridge JMC. Oxygen free radicals and iron in relation to biology and medicine: some problems and concepts. Arch Biochem Biophys 1986; 246: 501-514.
117. Li W, Zhao Y, Chou IN. Paraquat-induced cytoskeletal injury in cultured cells. Toxicol Appl Pharmacol 1987; 91: 96-106.
118. Miller DM, Woods JS. Urinary porphyrins as biological indicators of oxidative stress in the kidney. Interaction of mercury and cephaloridine. Biochem Pharmacol 1993; 46 (12): 2235-2241.
119. Thomas CE, Aust SD. Reductive release of iron from ferritin by cation free radicals of paraquat and other bipyridils. J Biol Chem 1986; 261(28): 13064-13070.
120. Minotti G, Aust SD. The role of iron in the initiation of lipid peroxidation. Chem Phys Lipids 1987; 44(2-4): 191-208.
120a. Kohda Y, Gemba M. Enhancement of protein kinase C activity and chemiluminescence intensity in mitochondria isolated from the kidney cortex of rats treated with cephaloridine. Biochem Pharmacol 2002;64:543-549.
120b. Kohda Y, Matsunaga Y, Katsuya Y, Yoshiko K, Aways A, Gemba M. Protective effect of serum thymic factor, FTS, on cepholridine-induced nephrotoxicity in rats. Biol Pharm Bull 2005;28:2087-2091.
121. Zenser TV, Mattammal MB, Davis BB. Differential distribution of the mixed-function oxidase activities in rabbit kidney. J Pharmacol Exp Ther 1978; 207(3): 719-725.
122. Swann JD, Acosta D. Failure of gentamicin to elevate cellular malondialdehyde content or increase generation of intracellular reactive oxygen species in primary cultures of renal cortical epithelial cells. Biochem Pharmacol 1990; 40(7): 1523-1526.
123. Tune BM, Kuo CH, Hook JB, Hsu CY, Fravert D. Effects of piperonyl butoxide on cephalosporin nephrotoxicity in the rabbit. An effect on cephaloridine transport. J Pharmacol Exp Ther 1983; 224(3): 520-524.
123a. Cojocel C, Tolle K-L, El-Hajj H, Baumann K. Protection against cephalosporin-induced lipid peroxidation and nephrotoxicity by (+)-cyanidanol-3 and vitamin E. Brazilian J Med Biol Res. 2007;40:867-875.
124. Roy K, Saha A, De K, Sengupta C. Ceftriaxone induced lipid peroxidation and its inhibition with various antioxidants: Part II. Evaluation of glutathione and probucol as antioxidants. Acta Pol Pharm 2000; 57(5): 385-390.
125. Kawai Y, Gemba M. Amelioration by cAMP of cephaloridine-induced injury in the porcine kidney cell line LLC-PK1. Jpn J Pharmacol 1996; 72(1): 67-70.
126. Tune BM, Wu KY, Longerbeam DF, Kempson RL. Transport and toxicity of cephaloridine in the kidney. Effect of furosemide, p-aminohippurate and saline diuresis. J Pharmacol Exp Ther 1977; 202(2): 472-478.
127. Kasher JS, Holohan PD, Ross CR. Na+ gradient-dependent p-aminohippurate (PAH) transport in rat basolateral membrane vesicles. J Pharmacol Exp Ther 1983; 227(1): 122-129.
128. Tune BM, Fernholt M. Relationship between cephaloridine and p-aminohippurate transport in the kidney. Am J Physiol 1973; 225(5): 1114-1117.
129. Tune BM, Fernholt M, Schwartz A. Mechanism of cephaloridine transport in the kidney. J Pharmacol Exp Ther 1974; 191(2): 311-317.
130. Mizuno M, Hamaura T, Hashida M, Sezaki H. Changes in D-glucose uptake by brush-border vesicles from small intestine of rats treated with mitomycin C. Biochem Pharmacol 1986; 35(7): 1153-1158.
131. Mizuno M, Yoshino H, Hashida M, Sezaki H. Decreased transport of D-glucose and L-alanine across brush-border membrane vesicles from small intestine of rats treated with mitomycin C. Biochim Biophys Acta 1987; 902(1): 93-100.
132. Weinberg JM, Venkatachalam MA, Roeser NF, Davis JA, Varani J, Johnson KJ. Amino acid protection of cultured kidney tubule cells against calcium ionophore-induced lethal cell injury. Lab Invest 1991; 65: 671-678.
133. Inui K, Saito H, Takano M, Okano T, Kitazawa S, Hori R. Enzyme activities and sodium-dependent active D-glucose transport in apical membrane vesicles isolated from kidney epithelial cell line (LLC-PK1). Biochim Biophys Acta 1984; 769(2): 514-518.
133a. Jung KY, Takeda M, Shimoda M, Narikawa S, TojoA, Kim DK, Chairoungdua A, Choi BK, Kusuhara H, SugiyamaY, Sekine T, Endou H. Involvement of rat organic anion transporter 3 (rOAT3) in cephaloridine-induced nephrotoxicity: in comparion with rOAT1. Life Sci 2002;70:1861-1874
133b. Takeda M, Babu E, Narikawa S, Endou H. Interaction of human organic anion transporters with various cephalosporin antibiotics. Eur J Pharmacol 2002;438:137-142.

133c. Khamdang S, Takeda M, Babu E, Noshiro R, Onozato ML, Tojo A, Enomoto A, Huang XL, Narikawa S, Anzai N, Piyachaturawat P, Endou H. Interaction of human and rat organic anion transporter 2 with various cephalosporin antibiotics. Eur J Pharmacol 2003;465:1-7.
134. Cersosimo E, Garlick P, Ferretti J. Renal substrate metabolism and gluconeogenesis during hypoglycemia in humans. Diabetes 2000; 49: 1186-1193.
135. Goldstein RS, Contardi LR, Pasino DA,Hook JB. Mechanisms mediating cephaloridine inhibition of renal gluconeogenesis. ToxicolApplPharmacol 1987; 87: 297-305.
136. Stroo WE, Hook JB. Dissociation of renal organic anion transport from renal lipid metabolism. I. Endogenous nonesterified fatty acids (NEFA) as determinants of transport. J Pharmacol Exp Ther 1983; 227(1): 55-59.
137. Wagner S, Deufel T, Guder WG. Carnitine metabolism in isolated rat kidney cortex tubules. Biol Chem Hoppe Seyler 1986; 367(1): 75-79.
138. Arrigoni-Martelli E, Caso V. Carnitine protects mitochondria and removes toxic acyls from xenobiotics. Drugs Exp Clin Res 2001; 27(10): 27-49.
139. Bieber LL, Farel SS. Carnitine acyl transferases. Enzymes 1983; 16: 624-644.
140. Ramsay RR, Gandour RD, van der Leij FR. Molecular enzymology of carnitine transfer and transport. Biochem Biophys Acta 2001; 1546(1): 21-43.
141. Cojocel C, Smith JH, Maita K, Sleight SD, Hook JB. Renal protein degradation: a biochemical target of specific nephrotoxicants. Fund Appl Toxicol 1983; 3: 278-284.
141a. Bond CA and Raehl CL. Adverse drug reactions in United States hospitals. Pharmacother 2006;26:601-608
141b. Falagas ME, Matthaiou DK, Karveli EA, Peppas G. Meta-analysis: randomized controlled trials of clindamycin/aminoglycoside vs. β-lactam monotherapy for the treatment of intra-abdominal infections. Aliment Pharmacol Ther. 2007;25:537-556.
142. Hori R, Shimakura M, Aramata Y, Kizawa K, Nozawa I, Takahata M, Minami S. Nephrotoxicity of piperacillin combined with furosemide in rats. Jpn J Antibiot 2000; 53(8): 582-591.
143. Wade JC, Smith CR, Petty BG, Lipski JJ, Conrad G, Ellner J, Lietman PS. Nephrotoxicity of piperacillin combined with furosemide in rats. Jpn J Antibiot 2000; 53(8): 582-591.
144. Bendirdjian JP, Prime DJ, Browning MC, Hsu CY, Tune BM. Additive nephrotoxicity of cephalosporins and aminoglycosides in the rabbit. J Pharmacol Exp Ther 1981; 218(3): 681-685.
145. Kosmidis J, Daikos GK. Prospective randomized comparative studies of mezlocillin/cefotaxime vs. gentamicin/cefoxitin. J Antimicrob Chemother 1983; 11(Suppl C): 91-95.
146. Itoh F, Sato K, Harauchi T, Hirata M, Mizushima Y. Modification of vancomycin nephrotoxicity by other antibiotics in rats. Jpn J Antibiot 1995; 48(3): 380-388.
147. Toyoguchi T, Nakagawa Y. Nephrotoxicity and drug interaction of vancomycin (2). Nippon Yakurigaku Zasshi 1996; 107(5): 225-235.
148. Reitbroeck RC, Hoitsma AJ, Koene RA. Aztreonam can be safely used with cyclosporin without aggravating nephrotoxicity. Transpl Int 1989; 2(4): 232-234.
149. Fanos V, Musap M, Verlato G, Plebani M, Padovani EM. Evaluation of the antibiotic-induced nephrotoxicity in preterm neonates by determining urinary a1-microglobulin. Pediatr Nephrol 1996; 10: 645-647.
150. Greenlee ML, DiNinno F, Herrmann JJ, Jaworsky C, Muthard DA, Salzmann TN. 2-Naphthylcarbapenems: broad spectrum antibiotics with enhanced potency against MRSA. Bioorg Med Chem Lett 1999; 9(19): 2893-2896.
151. Kanno O, Shimoji Y, Ohya S, Kawamoto I. Synthesis and biological evaluation of novel tricyclic carbapenems (trinems). J Antib (Tokyo) 2000; 53(4): 404-414.
152. Kar GK, Roy BC, Adhikari SD, Ray JK, Brahama NK. Synthesis of some thieno γ lactam monocyclic acids with high antibacterial activity: a new look at an old molecular system. Bioorg Med Chem 1998; 6(12): 2397-2402.
153. Hayashi T, Watanabe Y, Kumano K, Kitayama R, Yasuda T, Saikawa I, Katahira J, Kumada T, Shimizu K. Protective effect of piperacillin against nephrotoxicity of cephaloridine and gentamicin in animals. Antimicrob Agents Chemother 1988; 32(6): 912-918.
154. Tune BM, Browning MC, Hsu CY, Fravert D. Prevention of cephalosporin nephrotoxicity by other cephalosporins and by penicillins without significant inhibition of renal cortical uptake. J Infect Dis 1982; 145(2): 174-180.
155. Beauchamp D, Theriault G, Grenier L, Gourde P, Perron S, Bergeron Y, Fontaine L, Bergeron MG. Ceftriaxone protects against tobramycin nephrotoxicity. Antimicrob Agents Chemother 1994; 38(4): 750-756.
156. Kojima R, Ito M, Suzuki Y. Studies on the nephrotoxicity of aminoglycoside antibiotics and protection from these effects (3). Protective effect of latamoxef against tobramycin nephrotoxicity and its protective mechanism. Jpn J Pharmacol 1986; 42(3): 397-404.
157. Sausen PJ, Elfarra AA, Cooley AJ. Methimazole protection of rats against chemically induced kidney damage *in vivo*. J Pharmacol Exp Ther 1992; 260(1): 393-401.

158. Valentovic M, Ball JG, Rogers BA, Meadows MK, Harmon RC, Moles J. Cephaloridine *in vitro* toxicity and accumulation in renal slices from normoglycemic and diabetic rats. Fundam Appl Toxicol 1997; 38(2): 184-190.

14

Amphotericin B

Nathalie K. ZGHEIB[1], Blair CAPITANO[1] and Robert A. BRANCH[1]

[1]University of Pittsburgh, Pittsburgh, Pennsylvania, USA

Introduction

In recent years, systemic mycoses have become a prominent cause of disease particularly in severely ill and immunocompromised patients. The factors contributing to the increased prevalence of fungal infections are related to larger number of patients with underlying immunosuppression, for example the acquired immunodeficiency syndrome (AIDS), more aggressive cancer chemotherapy, increase in transplantation, greater number of other immunocompromised patients, and more frequent use of prosthetic devices [1]. There have been a number of recent surveys, which illustrate the extent of this problem. The Center for Disease Control reported that among 51 USA hospitals, candidiasis was the eighth most common infection, accounting for 5% of the isolates [1, 2]. This value can be considerably higher in certain specific patient groups. The National Cancer Institute estimated that 43% of patients dying with acute leukemia had systemic fungal infection at autopsy [3]. In patients with AIDS, the most common fungal infection is oropharyngeal candidiasis. However, in these patients, the fungal infection with the highest mortality rate is cryptococcosis. It is evident that systemic fungal infection is an important consideration in the treatment of a severely ill, immunosuppressed patients [4].

Amphotericin B (AmB) has remained a mainstay of therapy for serious fungal infections since its introduction in 1956, owing to its broad spectrum of reliable activity and lack of availability of equally efficacious alternative agents [5]. The usefulness of this agent, however, is limited by the frequent occurrence of several acute and chronic adverse effects that often necessitate changes in, or premature discontinuation of, therapy. These include fever, chills, nausea, vomiting, anorexia, headache, bronchospasm, hypotension, anaphylaxis, and bone marrow suppression. The most limiting adverse effect, however, is nephrotoxicity [6-11]. Several novel antifungal agents, found to be equally efficacious and less toxic as compared to AmB in clinical trials, have been introduced over the past several years. Thus, the role of AmB as the "gold standard" in the treatment of serious fungal infections is likely to be challenged and re-defined in the next decade [12].

AmB is a member of the polyene macrolide class of antibiotics. The molecule consists of a large macrolide lactone ring of 37 carbon atoms, one side of which is composed of a rigid lipophilic chain of seven conjugated double bonds, and the opposite side of a similar number of hydrophilic hydroxylated carbon atoms (Figure 1). Thus, the molecule is amphipathic, and this feature of its structure is believed to be important in its mechanism of action [13]. The major action of AmB is believed to be on the cell membrane of fungal and mammalian cells. It is generally accepted that the drug binds to sterols in the cell membrane and induces formation of aqueous pores, which result in impairment of barrier function and loss of protons and cations from the cell. At low concentrations, the increased permeability is restricted to small molecules or cations such as sodium and potassium. At higher concentrations or after prolonged exposure, other cell constituents are lost and this leads to metabolic disruption and even cell death [13].

The cellular events that follow this membrane effect are complex and depend on a variety of factors, such as the growth phase of the cells, the dose, and the mode of AmB administration [14]. Some studies suggest that cell mortality is not simply a consequence of changes in permeability of membranes, and that formation of active oxygen species may play a role in the lytic or lethal actions of AmB [15, 16].

Clinical manifestations of nephrotoxicity

The most restrictive adverse effect associated with AmB therapy is its potential to induce nephrotoxicity, manifested as disturbances in both glomerular and tubular function. The clinical manifestations usually include azotemia, renal tubular acidosis, decreased concentrating ability of the kidney, and electrolyte disturbances such as urinary potassium wasting leading to hypokalemia, and magnesium wasting to result in hypomagnesemia [17].

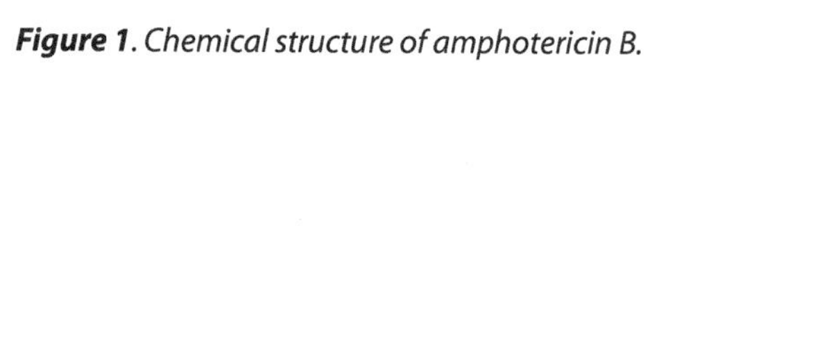

***Figure 1**. Chemical structure of amphotericin B.*

Incidence and risk factors

The incidence of AmB-induced renal impairment is highly variable depending on the definition of nephrotoxicity and upon the presence of underlying risk factors. Following AmB introduction, a survey of 56 patients treated between 1956 and 1963 confirmed that 93% of patients developed values of BUN exceeding 200 mg/L, and 83% had serum creatinine levels greater than 15 mg/L [18]. A more recent report indicates that in almost every patient treated with AmB, the glomerular filtration rate (GFR) falls approximately 40% within the first 2 to 3 weeks of therapy, stabilizes at 20% to 60% of normal and remains at this level throughout the course of treatment [19]. Clements and Peacock [8] reported an incidence for azotemia of 60% in a retrospective analysis conducted between 1984 and 1987. In general, the incidence of azotemia due to AmB in the literature ranges between 50-90%. This variability may reflect various factors, among which are the definition used for nephrotoxicity, the dose of AmB, concomitant administration of other nephrotoxic agents, and the presence or absence of other proposed risk factors. In general, azotemia is transient and limited to the duration of therapy; renal function usually returns to pretreatment levels after discontinuation of the drug. In many cases, cessation of therapy for a few days allows renal function to recover enough to permit administration of the full course of therapy. In rare cases, however, permanent renal damage persists after cessation of therapy.

The relationship of the cumulative dose of AmB to the development of nephrotoxicity is controversial. Earlier studies suggested that greater cumulative doses of AmB (e.g. 3-4 g) were associated with a greater risk of nephrotoxicity [20]. This implies that the likelihood of a rise in the serum creatinine concentration increases in proportion to the length of therapy. However, we observed patients who developed azotemia at doses ranging from 100 mg to 1.5 g, with no significant increase in frequency as the cumulative dose increased. Our experience indicated that the frequency of nephrotoxicity did not increase with extended therapy over this dose range (Figure 2) [21]. With larger cumulative doses, renal impairment may be irreversible, as reported by Winn [22] who found persistent renal impairment in 88% of patients who had received cumulative doses exceeding 5 g.

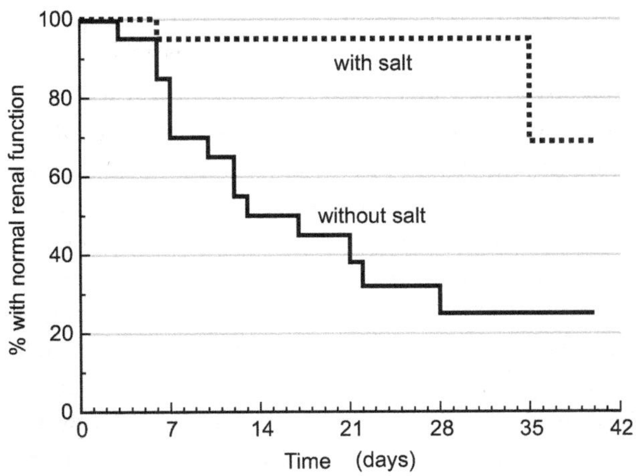

Figure 2. *Estimated proportion of patients retaining normal renal function during therapy with amphotericin B. Patients received amphotericin B with (dotted line, n=17) or without (solid line, n=21) parenteral salt supplementation due to co-administration of ticarcillin. (Used with permission from [21])*

The clinical utility of a risk factor such as cumulative dose to identify patients at risk of nephrotoxicity is limited since knowledge of this parameter is unavailable prior to the commencement of treatment. The rate of infusion of AmB and the frequency of dosing have also been found to impact the likelihood of nephrotoxicity in that use continuous infusion or administration of drug on alternate days reduces the incidence of nephrotoxicity [23, 24].

Several clinical assessments have identified additional characteristics that may be used to identify patients at increased risk for AmB nephrotoxicity such as abnormal baseline renal function, dehydration, older age [10, 20], diuretic use, pre-existing atherosclerosis, diabetes and heart failure [25].

In a multivariate risk factor assessment, Luber et al. [9] demonstrated that the AmB nephrotoxicity incidence varied with the definition used for renal impairment. Among 178 patients a change in creatinine of >46 µmol/L over baseline occurred in 50%; a doubling of creatinine over baseline in 49%; a change in creatinine of >92 µmol/L in 29%; a doubling and/or a change in creatinine of >92 µmol/L in 49%; and an increase in creatinine to >230 µmol/L in 8%. In this study, nephrotoxicity was associated with a greater cumulative dose of AmB and concomitant nephrotoxic drugs for all definitions. In those patients who experienced severe nephrotoxicity (creatinine increased to >230 µmol/L), concomitant cyclosporine therapy was the most significant risk factor (odds ratio 18.8, P= 0.022).

Harbarth and colleagues conducted a 9 year retrospective epidemiological assessment of AmB nephrotoxicity in 494 patients who received ≥ 2 doses in attempt to clarify discrepancies in the literature regarding the incidence and influence of specific risk factors, including AmB dose and duration. The results yielded 5 categorical risk factors for nephrotoxicity including an average daily dose of ≥ 35 mg, male sex, weight ≥ 90 kg, chronic renal disease and use of amikacin or cyclosporine. The incidence of moderate to severe nephrotoxicity, defined as doubling of the serum creatinine level to ≥ 2.0 mg/dl, was 4% (6/137) in patients with none of these risk factors, 8% (14/181) in those with 1 risk factor and 29% (21/117) in those with ≥ 3 risk factors. Based on these data, the authors proposed that patients identified with ≥ 2 of identified risk factors or a "risk score" of ≥2 to be candidates for alternative therapy. A limitation of this study was lack of information as to whether patients received hydration or sodium load prior to AmB administration, a method known to reduce nephrotoxicity [11]. Girmania and colleagues tested the utility of Harbath's risk score in 46 consecutive patients who received AmB at 1 mg/kg over 2 hours with hydration of at least 1 L/m^2 containing at least 1 L of 0.9% saline solution. The rate of moderate to severe nephrotoxicity was 0% (0/12) in patients with 1 risk factor, 6.3% in patients with 2 (1/16) and 11.1% (2/18) in patients with 3 risk factors. The overall rate of AmB induced nephrotoxicity in this study was lower than that observed in the previous study (13% vs. 28%, respectively). Although the population was small, the results found the risk scores to be predictive of patients at risk of moderate to severe nephrotoxicity. The authors concluded that adequate hydration and sodium loading should be employed prior to AmB administration to reduce the incidence of nephrotoxicity [26]. Consistent with previous data, a retrospective analysis of a homogenous population of 69 bone marrow or peripheral blood stem cell transplant recipients with multiple myeloma revealed baseline estimated creatinine clearance, use of cyclosporine or receipt of multiple nephrotoxic agents within 30 days of starting AmB to be significantly predictive of nephrotoxicity in this patient population [27].

Wasan and colleagues have conducted a series of studies evaluating the association of AmB with plasma lipoproteins demonstrating that less damage to renal cells is evoked when the drug associates with high density lipoproteins (HDL) as compared to low density proteins (LDL). Their work continues in order to determine whether measurement of plasma HDL and LDL concentrations may be used to identify patients more likely to experience AmB nephrotoxicity. Although very interesting, at this time, no clinically applicable conclusions may be extrapolated from the data [28-31].

Urinary concentration defects

Many studies have shown that AmB can induce a loss of concentrating ability of the kidney [18, 32, 33]. This abnormality is almost invariably present and occurs early (1-2 weeks) in the course of therapy. The impairment in concentrating ability probably reflects direct tubular toxicity since it occurs in the absence of a decrease in GFR, and is temporally unrelated to azotemia. Barbour et al. [34] reported a study of 3 patients whose inability to concentrate the urine was associated with a defect in free water reabsorption even under maximal stimuli, and concluded that a tubular functional abnormality was induced because of the failure of the vasopressin response in the medullary collecting tubule.

Electrolyte disturbances

Electrolyte disorders secondary to renal wasting of potassium and magnesium are commonly encountered adverse effects in patients receiving AmB [17, 35]. Although hypokalemia has been emphasized in prior studies, its impact on patient management and on the course of other manifestation of AmB nephrotoxicity has not been well examined. In addition to its known systemic effects (muscle weakness, fatigue, cramps, rhabdomyolysis and myoglobinuria), potassium depletion may alter renal function causing further impairment of concentrating ability, urinary acidification, renal insufficiency and abnormal sodium reabsorption [36]. It is conceivable that these effects may influence or contribute to the nephrotoxicity of AmB.

Approximately 75% of patients develop hypokalemia during the course of treatment with AmB [37] However, a need for potassium supplementation to maintain a normal plasma level of potassium can be regarded as an objective parameter of a potassium losing diathesis. Using this criterion, the incidence is as high as 90% or more [8, 38]. The maintenance of normokalemia requires up to 300 mEq of potassium chloride replacement a day. These patients are often severely ill and unable to tolerate oral supplementation, so prolonged (6-7 hours) of administration of large intravenous doses of potassium chloride with appropriate and careful monitoring may be necessary. The logistics of such continuous intravenous maintenance infusions can create problems in timely administration [8].

Some investigators consider hypokalemia a dose-dependent response, although the mechanism of urinary potassium wasting is unclear. A recent study has shown that AmB affects sodium flux in both the distal and transverse human colon, suggesting a change in sodium/potassium exchange to result in potassium loss [39]. Selective renal distal tubular epithelial toxicity seems to be, at least in part, responsible for the profound potassium wasting. The magnitude of urinary potassium loss increases in the presence of a high sodium chloride intake. If potassium depletion is allowed to occur with AmB, a vicious circle is created which further enhances the tubular toxicity and contributes to overall changes in renal function [40].

Magnesium wasting has also been reported as a consequence of AmB administration [41, 42]. A negative magnesium balance probably occurs in all patients, but clinically relevant magnesium depletion only occurs when the urinary loss is high and not replaced. In the study by Barton et al [41] the lowest serum level and the largest fractional excretion of magnesium were observed by the fourth week of AmB therapy, after a cumulative dose of approximately 500 mg. This abnormality was fully reversible, evidenced by the normal serum and urinary magnesium levels measured 1 year after discontinuation of therapy. As in the case of potassium depletion, if magnesium depletion is evaluated by measurement of magnesium balance rather than by the serum level, the incidence of magnesium depletion is high. In a recent study, a marked change in the urinary excretion of magnesium occurred after a cumulative AmB dose of only 150 mg, suggesting some degree of magnesium depletion, although serum magnesium levels remained in the low normal range [38].

The mechanisms for the observed AmB induced renal magnesium wasting remain unclear. Increased urinary excretion of magnesium, despite a reduced filtered load, suggests a tubular defect in magnesium reabsorption [41]. When magnesium and potassium wasting occur concomitantly, potassium replacement may not be successful unless magnesium deficiency is corrected first.

Renal tubular acidosis

Chronic features of renal tubular acidosis can be anticipated in patients receiving total doses of AmB of 0.5-1 g or more, and are generally reversible after therapy is discontinued [5]. In our experience this is one of the earlier manifestations of tubular toxicity, since all patients developed an acidification defect in response to an acid load after 2 weeks of therapy and a cumulative dose of 300 mg of AmB [38]. This defect appears to be a specific tubular effect of AmB, since impairment in acid secretion has been demonstrated in the isolated turtle bladder and attributed to increased passive permeability of the luminal membrane to hydrogen ions [43, 44], plus the impaired excretion of titratable acids is greater than can be accounted for by depression of GFR [45, 46]. It is also thought that distal renal tubular acidosis is a contributing pathogenic mechanism for urinary losses of potassium and magnesium [37, 45, 46].

Pathological findings

Despite the almost universal changes in renal function, histological changes associated with AmB therapy are minimal and occur in both glomerulus and renal tubule. Tubular damage primarily involves the distal convoluted tubule and the ascending limb of the loop of Henle [41]. Morphologic changes include fragmentation and thickening of basement membranes, necrosis and vacuolization of distal tubular epithelium and nephrocalcinosis [18, 32, 46, 47]. Glomerular changes include calcific foci, along with hypercellularity and vacuolization of smooth-muscle cells in small arteries and arterioles [33, 46]. In studies conducted in rats, cortical changes associated with AmB were restricted to the medullary ray, an area that is vulnerable to hypoxia, and consisted of focal rupture and calcification of the thick ascending limbs [48]. Calcification was also detected in the macula densa, an area rich in oxygen. Administration of AmB to salt depleted rats

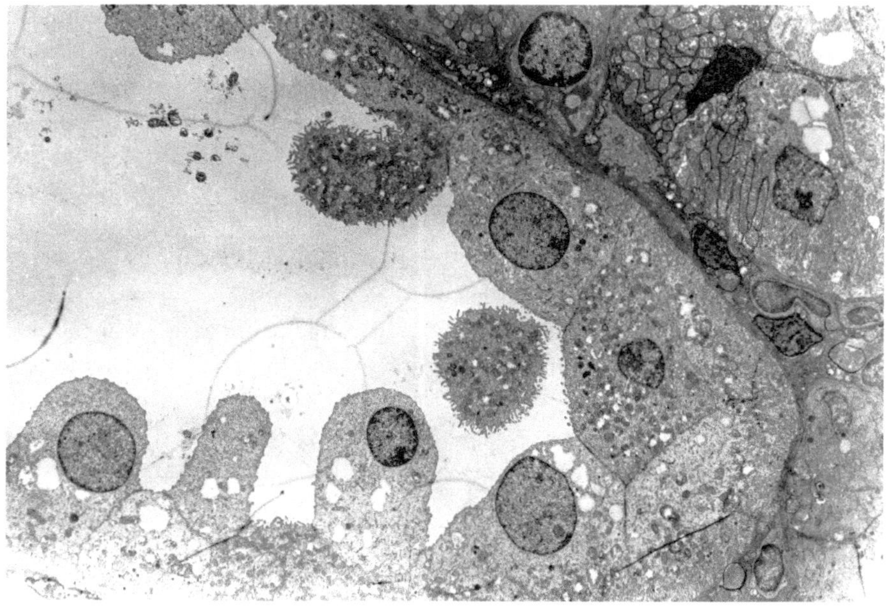

Figure 3. *Distal tubulus of rat kidney after 14 days of AmB administration. Electron microscopy shows intratubular casts and debris, loss of brush border, tubular cell vacuolization, and protrusion of cells into the tubulus lumen. Magnification 3600x. With permission from [49].*

resulted in an extension of these changes to the area rich in vascular tissue between the medullary rays and to atrophic changes in the thick ascending limb in the inner stripe [49] (Figure 3).

Mechanisms of nephrotoxicity

Before mechanisms can be proposed to account for renal cell injury, the possible sites of nephron involvement should be identified based upon structural and functional changes [50]. AmB is known to cause acute renal vasoconstriction and to preferentially damage the distal tubular epithelium, but the exact mechanisms mediating its nephrotoxicity have not been clearly defined. The initial event is thought to involve binding of AmB to membrane sterols in the renal vasculature and epithelial cells causing an alteration in membrane permeability. This interaction may then trigger other cellular events that result in activation of second messenger systems, release of mediators or activation of renal homeostatic mechanisms. It is, therefore, possible that the membrane effect per se is not the sole factor that determines the extent of change in renal function.

Effects on cell membranes

It is generally accepted that AmB-induced injury to cells is due to its binding to sterols in the cell membrane: ergosterol in the case of fungal cells and cholesterol in mammalian cells [14]. This binding is more avid to ergosterol than to cholesterol, which explains AmB's relatively selective toxicity to fungal cells [51, 52].

In the early 1960s, studies showed that polyene antibiotics induced changes in cellular permeability that resulted in the leakage of important cellular constituents, followed by lysis and death [53-57] it was also discovered that the toxic effect of the drugs on cells was dependent on the presence of sterols in the cell membranes, and that addition of sterols to the growth media of certain fungi prevented the polyene-induced inhibition of growth and permeability changes [53, 58, 59]. This increased permeability has been documented in both artificial and natural membranes [60]. It has been proposed that AmB, acting as a pseudophospholipid, interacts with sterol molecules to cause formation of aqueous pores, which consist of an annulus of polyene and sterol, in which the hydrophilic region of the drug molecule faces the interior of the pore (Figure 4) [60-62]. Among the documented effects of AmB on living tissues are increased permeability of the toad urinary

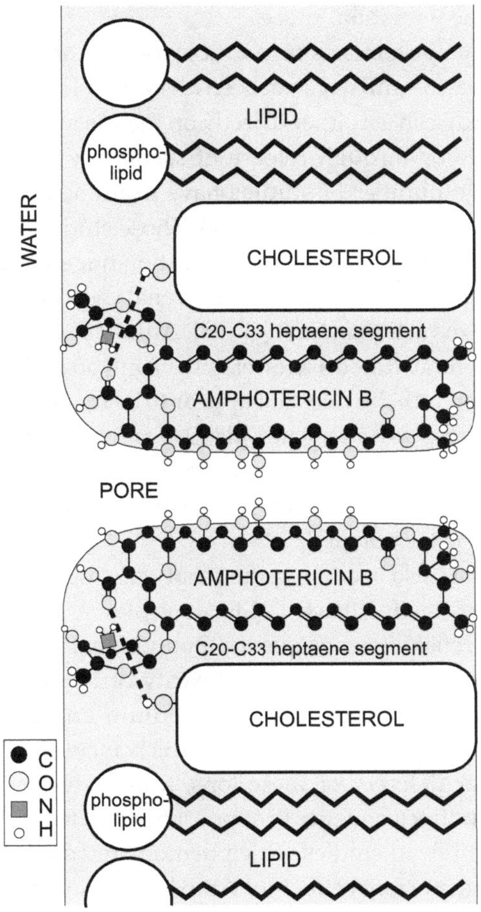

Figure 4. *Proposed partial model for the AmB-induced pore in the cell membrane. The drug acts as a counterfeit phospholipid, with the C_{15} hydroxyl, C_{16} carboxyl, and C_{19} mycosamine groups situated at the membrane-water interface, and the C_1 to C_{14} and C_{20} to C_{33} chains aligned in parallel within the membrane. The heptaene chain will seek a hydrophobic environment while the hydroxyl groups will seek a hydrophilic environment. Thus, a cylindrical pore will be formed, the inner wall of which consists of the hydroxyl-substituted carbon chains of the AmB molecules, and outer wall of which is formed by the heptaene chains of the molecules and by sterol nuclei. (Used with permission from [60]).*

bladder to urea, potassium and chloride ions [63-65], of erythrocytes and liposomes to potassium ions [66, 67], and of erythrocytes to sodium and chloride ions [68, 69]. It also alters the permeability of the turtle bladder and of purified renal brush border membrane vesicles to sodium and hydrogen ions [43, 70-72].

Considering the renal tubular effects of AmB observed in clinical practice, it is reasonable to suggest that part or all of these effects may be explained by a direct effect on tubular cell membranes. In support of this suggestion is the *in vivo* finding that while AmB binds to sterols in most tissues, the highest level documented is in the kidney [73]. Furthermore, binding of AmB to the cell membrane appears to be necessary for its toxic effect, since inhibition of sterol synthesis by ketoconazole reduces the binding of AmB as well as the permeability changes induced by AmB in a parallel fashion [71, 74]. In agreement with these suggestions is the finding of increased tubular permeability to inulin *in vivo* in rats following acute or chronic administration of AmB, resulting in back-leak of inulin [75].

Further evidence to support a direct toxic effect of AmB on renal cells is the demonstration of increased apoptosis in proximal tubular and medullary interstitial cell lines [76]. The occurrence of apoptosis has also been confirmed in an in-vivo model in rats in which AmB administration also caused hypokalemia, loss of concentrating ability and dehydration. Interestingly, prevention of apoptosis by recombinant human insulin growth factor-1 (rhIGF-1) ameliorated the tubular toxicity indicating the importance of apoptosis in AmB-induced renal tubular toxicity process. A possible mechanism for this action is suggested by a recent study that has demonstrated that AmB exposure increases cellular ceramide as well as sphingomyelin levels in proximal tubular cells [77]. It is noteworthy that ceramide has been postulated to play a role in inducing apoptosis in several cell types [78]. Although the role of these changes in nephrotoxicity is still uncertain, these findings suggest that the interaction of AmB with cell membranes is not limited to a physicochemical interaction with sterols leading to pore formation and changes in permeability, but may also involve other complex effects that lead to alteration in production or function of membrane associated signaling molecules.

An alternative postulated mechanism of AmB induced cell damage involves oxidative stress with the formation of free radical intermediates [15, 16, 79]. Evidence against this hypothesis has been provided by recent studies that evaluated the anti- or pro-oxidant effects of AmB by examining its effects on phospholipid pattern in aortic smooth muscle cells [80] as well as on lipid-peroxidation of cis-Parinaric acid in liposomes [81]. These studies provided evidence for an antioxidant role for AmB rather than a pro-oxidant role and suggesting that oxidative stress is not involved in AmB-induced toxicity.

In addition, alternative factors may modulate the direct cellular toxicity of AmB. For example, maintaining kidney epithelial cells in an acidic environment enhances the permeability changes induced by AmB in an irreversible fashion [82]. This suggests that the low pH characteristic of the distal tubule makes those cells more vulnerable to the toxic effects of AmB, and may explain the protective effect of alkalinizing agents [45].

Effects on physiological parameters: whole animal studies

Acute studies (Single dose)

Infusions of AmB, intravenously or into the renal artery, induce short-term reduction in renal blood flow (RBF) and GFR, and an increase in renal vascular resistance, in both rats and dogs [83-85]. The effects of short term infusions of AmB on the renal microcirculation in rats revealed that the single nephron GFR was decreased by 2 mechanisms (Table 1): 1) a decrease in single nephron plasma flow, due to vasoconstriction of the afferent and efferent arterioles, and 2) a reduction in the glomerular capillary ultrafiltration coefficient (Kf), an effect probably mediated by mesangial cell contraction [86]. Previous micropuncture studies demonstrated a similar vasoconstriction of the afferent arteriole but also an increased permeability of the tubular epithelium to inulin [75]. Thus, the reduction in GFR after acute AmB infusions can be attributed to contraction of afferent smooth muscle cells, efferent smooth muscle cells and glomerular mesangial cells, as well as increased tubular permeability with back-leak into the interstitial space.

The mechanisms responsible for the contractile responses to AmB have not been identified. Theoretically, the drug can act either directly on the vascular smooth muscle or through release of secondary mediators. A large number of studies have examined putative indirect mechanisms of action. Those studies have revealed that neither renal denervation nor angiotensin II receptor blockade prevent the renal vasoconstriction or the reduction in GFR [87, 88]. Although Cutaia et al [89] demonstrated a toxic effect of AmB on endothelial cells, endothelin does not appear to be involved in the acute responses to AmB [88, 90] and reduced nitric oxide synthesis, consequent to endothelial injury is not involved in modulation of AmB-induced renal vasoconstriction [88].

It has also been suggested that activation of tubuloglomerular feedback (TGF) may play a role in the acute renal effects of this compound. That hypothesis suggested that the tubular toxicity of AmB resulted in impaired reabsorption of sodium and chloride ions by the proximal tubule, which increased distal tubular delivery of these ions, thus activating TGF [91]. Indirect evidence in support of a role for TGF was derived from studies which demonstrated inhibition of the acute renal effects of AmB by physiological and pharmacological interventions that also blocked TGF, namely, salt loading, and administration of furosemide, theophylline or calcium channel blockers [84-86, 92-99]. Finally, some studies suggested a protective effect of pentoxiphylline, a vascular decongestant and antagonist of tumor necrosis factor-alpha (TNF) and interleukin-1alpha, against AmB-induced acute and

Table 1. Effect of amphotericin B infusions (0.05 mg/kg/min i.a.) on systemic glomerular hemodynamic parameters.

	Before	After	p-value
Mean arterial pressure (mmHg)	114 ± 5	117 ± 4	NS
Renal plasma flow (ml/min)	4.69 ± 0.35	2.82 ± 049	< 0.025
Glomerular filtration rate (ml/min)	1.03 ± 0.65	0.70 ± 0.09	< 0.005
Single nephron glomerular filtration rate (ml/min)	35.5 ± 2.2	22.8 ± 2.8	< 0.0005
Plasma flow (ml/min)	142 ± 12	89 ± 14	< 0.005
Single nephron filtration fraction	0.26 ± 0.03	0.27 ± 0.04	NS
Afferent arteriolar resistance (10^{10} dyn.sec.cm^{-5})	1.91 ± 0.17	3.95 ± 0.38	< 0.01
Efferent arteriolar resistance (10^{10} dyn.sec.cm^{-5})	1.30 ± 0.10	2.08 ± 0.12	< 0.01
Glomerular capillary ultrafiltration coefficient [n/(sec.mmHg)]	0.043 ± 0.008	0.032 ± 0.009	< 0.005

chronic nephrotoxicity, suggesting a role for these factors in the renal effects of the drug [100, 101].

More recent studies provided evidence against a role for TGF in acute AmB nephrotoxicity. In contrast to its inhibition of TGF activity, theophylline prevented the acute renal responses to AmB by a mechanism unrelated to adenosine receptor antagonism [102]. Furthermore, micropuncture studies revealed that the AmB-induced reduction in single nephron GFR was the same irrespective of whether TGF was active or interrupted (by measuring GFR from distal and proximal tubular collections, respectively) [96]. The latter study also showed that distal tubular chloride ion concentrations were not increased by AmB, which indicated that the signal for TGF was unchanged.

A direct effect of AmB on cell function was suggested by *in vitro* experiments, which demonstrated a vasoconstrictor action of AmB in perfused afferent arterioles and isometrically contracting rings of rabbit aorta or renal artery, effects which were prevented in Ca^{++}-free medium and by Ca^{++} channel blockers or theophylline [103]. Thus, AmB-induced reductions in RBF or GFR are not secondary to activation of TGF, but due to its direct vasoconstrictor effect. A role for thromboxane A_2 has also been suggested based upon partial inhibition of the AmB-induced vasoconstriction and reduction in GFR by pretreatment with ibuprofen or a thromboxane receptor antagonist [104].

The results obtained in isolated vessels are consistent with findings in cultured glomerular mesangial cells where AmB caused a concentration-dependent increase in intracellular calcium levels ($[Ca^{++}]i$), an effect almost completely inhibited when either Ca^{++} or Na^+ ions were omitted from the cell medium (Figure 5) [105]. Diltiazem (20 μM) also suppressed the AmB-induced rise in $[Ca^{2+}]i$. These results indicated that the reduction in K_f observed *in vivo* was most likely due to contraction of mesangial cells. Thus, the contractile effects of AmB in the nephron are probably due to a direct interaction with cell membranes, leading to formation of pores. One possibility is that these pores allow entry of Na^+ ions into the cells along the electrochemical gradient leading to depolarization-induced opening of voltage-dependent calcium channels and contraction.

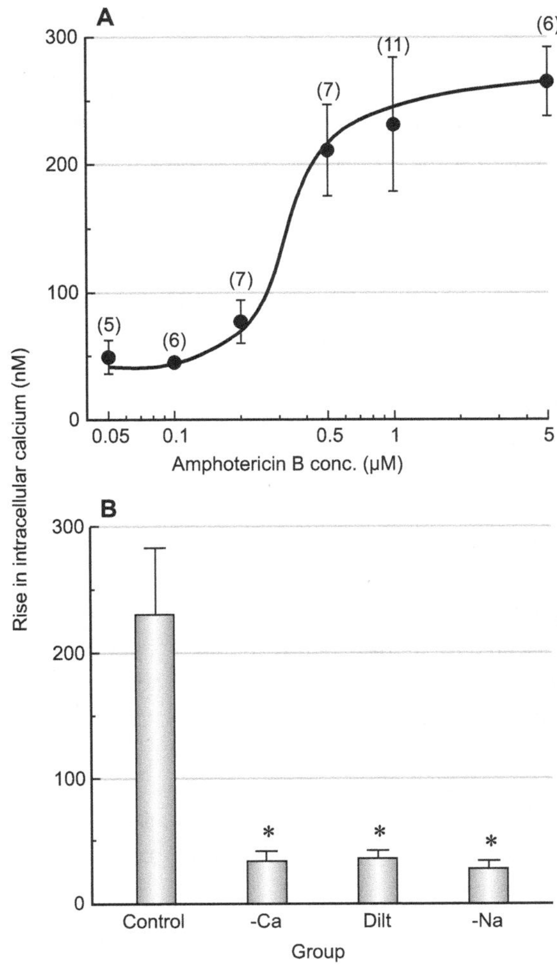

Figure 5. *Concentration dependent increase in intracellular calcium levels in cultured glomerular mesangial cells (A) and its inhibition by removal of Ca^{++} and Na^+ ions from the medium (-Ca and -Na, respectively), and by addition of 20 μM diltiazem (Dilt) (B). (Used with permission from [105]).*

Chronic studies (Multidose)

Animal models of chronic nephrotoxicity have also shown that certain interventions can modify the nephrotoxicity of AmB. Rats co-treated with sodium bicarbonate sustain smaller reductions in GFR compared with rats treated with AmB alone for 3 weeks [45]. Oral NaCl supplementation also attenuates the decrease in GFR and the elevation in renovascular resistance induced by daily administration of AmB over 3 weeks [96, 98]. In addition, renal impairment following a 7-day course of AmB in rats was less severe when theophylline was co-administered [99]. These interventions also attenuate the acute renal responses to AmB, suggesting that similar mechanisms contribute to its chronic nephrotoxicity. Similar logic would suggest that salt supplementation and theophylline are protecting the kidney by a mechanism unrelated to TGF. It is, however, possible that the latter does contribute to AmB nephrotoxicity but only at later stages of therapy, when severe damage to the tubules may have taken place. Interestingly, the protection by salt loading is associated with lower concentrations of drug in the kidney despite similar concentrations in plasma and liver tissue [96]. This raises an alternative possible mechanism of protection by salt loading involving a pharmacokinetic interaction with AmB, which limits its uptake into the kidney.

Studies on the effects of chronic administration of calcium channel blockers on chronic AmB induced nephrotoxicity have been discordant. Nifedipine does not offer a significant protective effect [106], but diltiazem blunts the increase in serum creatinine and the decreases in GFR and RPF [97]. It is possible that these differences relate to the heterogeneity of calcium channels and the differential activity of calcium channel blockers on them. However, no specific studies have addressed this question.

The co-administration of 5-flucytosine with AmB, which is commonly used clinically to obtain a synergistic antifungal effect, protects against acute and chronic nephrotoxicity [107]. The mechanisms by which flucytosine influences the renal response to AmB are not clear but may relate to (i) its administration in 0.9% NaCl, which itself is protective, (ii) a renal vasodilator effect of flucytosine that antagonizes AmB-induced vasoconstriction, and (iii) reduction in renal uptake of AmB [107].

Cell death induced by AmB in the medullary thick ascending limb is prevented by ouabain [108]. A reasonable explanation for this observation is that ouabain, by inhibiting transport, decreases the oxygen demand of an area of the nephron that already has a limited oxygen supply. This is consistent with the observation that AmB exhibits preferential damage to the medullary ray, an area that is vulnerable to hypoxic injury [48]. It is also conceivable that AmB-induced renal vasoconstriction and ischemia to this section of the nephron enhances cell death produced by a direct toxic action. Thus, any maneuver that improves renal perfusion, or decreases oxygen demand, would be expected to be protective. This may explain the salutary effect of salt loading, theophylline, calcium channel blockers, pentoxiphylline, dopamine or dopamine pro-drugs such as fenoldopam on AmB nephrotoxicity [102-104]. All these interventions can be expected to improve renal perfusion. Furosemide protection could be explained on a basis that it not only inhibits solute transport in the thick ascending limb to reduce oxygen demand, but also enhances renal perfusion to increase oxygen supply.

Measures to reduce nephrotoxicity

Despite being considered one of the most toxic antimicrobial drugs in use today [109], AmB remains a primary choice for the treatment of otherwise uniformly fatal systemic fungal infections [4, 5]. Consequently, it will remain in use despite the predictable occurrence of severe systemic and renal toxicity. Therefore, therapeutic interventions that decrease AmB toxicity assume critical importance. Among the early interventions that were examined was the administration of mannitol. Studies suggested a protective effect of mannitol in dogs and renal transplant recipients [110-112]. Unfortunately, these were either case-reports or poorly controlled since later reports failed to detect any protective effect of mannitol in dogs, and ascribed the protective findings to the lower doses of AmB used [113]. In addition, a small controlled trial of mannitol co-administration in humans failed to document any beneficial effect [33]. A more recent intervention is the use of spironolactone which has been suggested as adjuvant therapy with AmB, a combination that prevented hypokalemia in neutropenic patients, but this has not been pursued [114].

Theoretically, any of the protective interventions mentioned in the previous section may be applicable to a clinical setting, but few have actually been studied, in some instances, because there are practical limitations to their use. For example, the duration of protection conferred by furosemide is brief, being confined to the time furosemide is present in the renal tubule. Furosemide would exacerbate electrolyte imbalance by causing sodium and potassium depletion, which, if not adequately monitored and replaced, would be expected to potentiate AmB-induced nephrotoxicity. Furthermore, none of the advocated drug interventions are innocuous. Of all the alternatives, manipulation of sodium status or of the method of administration offer simple interventions that can be readily and usually safely be introduced into clinical practice [91]. The use of continuous infusion or administration of drug on alternate days has been found to reduce the incidence of nephrotoxicity [23, 24, 115]. An alternative approach is to use a lipid formulation of amphotericin B (LFAB) or other antifungal agents.

Salt supplementation

The demonstration of a renal protective effect of salt loading on AmB-induced nephrotoxicity in animal models has provided a rational basis to evaluate this simple intervention in patients. Clinical evidence supporting the ability of sodium loading to attenuate AmB-induced nephrotoxicity is derived from three sources: case reports, retrospective studies and prospective studies.

One of the earliest case reports was by Butler and colleagues who reported a patient in whom a low sodium diet (9 mEq/d) exacerbated renal dysfunction, increased urinary sodium loss, and caused postural hypotension [18]. Administration of supplemental oral sodium chloride promptly reversed the defect within 12 hours. These abnormalities were confirmed on rechallenge during treatment, but were absent 13 months after completion of AmB therapy.

In a subsequent study, 5 patients were receiving AmB in clinical situations where salt-conserving states could be identified. These included dietary salt restriction, vomiting, diuretic therapy, Addison's disease and cirrhosis with ascites. In each patient sustained increases in BUN and serum creatinine levels were observed within 6 to 12 days after starting AmB [116]. Four to 12 days after liberalization of dietary sodium intake, administering intravenous saline, and/or discontinuation of diuretic therapy, renal function improved in all patients. Improvement was sustained and the full course of AmB was successfully completed after a brief interruption (range: 1 to 5 days), without permanent renal impairment. A retrospective study revealed that only two of 17 patients (12%) receiving ticarcillin (with its obligatory sodium load of 150 mEq/day) had a nephrotoxic response to AmB, compared with 14 of 21 patients (67%) not receiving ticarcillin (Figure 2) [21]. Anecdotally, withdrawal of ticarcillin in patients continuing to receive AmB led to deterioration of renal function over a one-week period. In a companion study, the benefit of routine intravenous saline (1 L of 0.9% saline) was assessed prospectively in leukemic patients receiving a 28-day course of AmB for persistent fever of unknown origin. Only two of 20 patients (10%) developed mild renal dysfunction, which, however, did not necessitate interruption of therapy. Furthermore, a recent medical record review for 573 extremely low birth weight infants born at Michigan State University revealed that combining conventional AmB with adequate hydration and higher amounts of sodium (>4 mEq/kg/day) is renoprotective [117].

The question of the influence of salt supplementation was addressed using a prospective, randomized, placebo controlled trials of the influence of salt supplementation on the course of renal function during therapy with AmB [38, 118]. In Llanos et al's study, AmB administration was preceded by 1 liter of either 0.9% saline or 5% dextrose in water administered i.v. over 4 hours. While the mean serum creatinine increased over time in the dextrose group, it remained unchanged in the saline group. Similarly, creatinine clearance decreased in the dextrose group, but remained unchanged in the saline group. The beneficial effect of salt loading however occurred at the expense of greater hypokalemia, since the saline group required significantly higher amounts of potassium supplementation to maintain a normal serum K level (Figure 6). Therefore, based upon these studies, it is reasonable to recommend routine salt supplementation with administration of AmB, with special attention being paid to maintaining potassium balance [38].

More recently, Mayer and coworkers [119] have expanded the notion that early introduction of potassium and magnesium supplements in equal amounts to that lost through the kidneys results in decreased incidence of AmB infusion-related side effects and decreased frequency of an increase in serum creatinine. This study provided further evidence to support that sufficient hydration and timely supplementation of sodium, potassium and magnesium reduces the renal toxicity of AmB. This has also been supported by further recent evidence from Oto et al in patients with febrile neutropenia and fungal infections [120]. Interestingly, a prospective trial has shown that oral rehydration solution (ORS) is more effective in preventing hypokalemia when compared to intravenous saline solution (SS) [121].

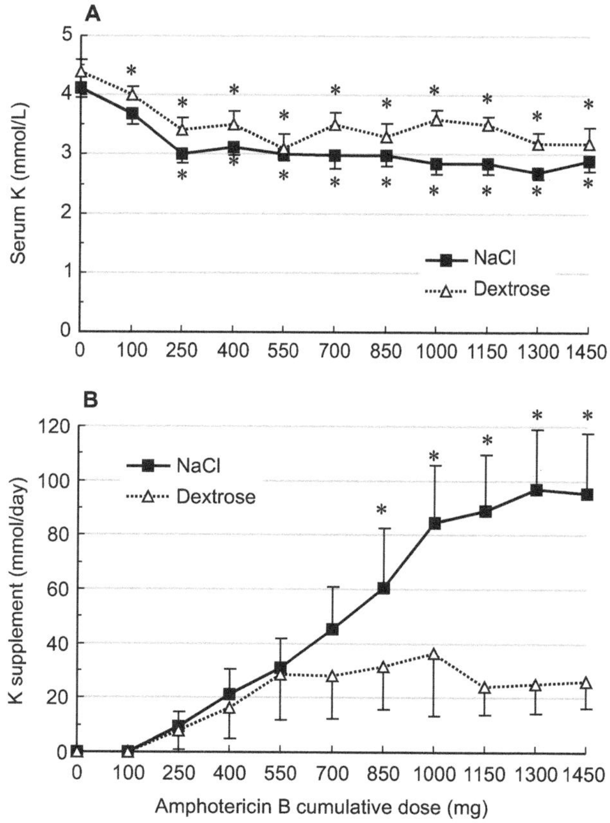

***Figure 6**. Serum K levels (A) and K supplements given to maintain serum K levels at or above 3 mmol/l (B) in patients receiving AmB with either 1 liter of 0.9% NaCl (solid line) or 1 liter of 5% dextrose in water (dotted line). Notice the difficulty in maintaining serum K levels despite significantly higher amounts of supplements in the former group. *: P<0.05 compared with baseline. (Used with permission from [38]).*

Continuous Infusion

AmB deoxycholate is usually administered slowly over a 2 to 6 hours. However, administration of the dose using a 24-hour continuous infusion has been found in several small studies to be better tolerated and associated with a lower incidence of nephrotoxicity, without an apparent impact on efficacy [115, 122-124].

As previously discussed, pretubular nephrotoxic effects of AmB are said to be caused by a dose dependent vasoconstriction of renal arterioles and consequent reduction in renal blood flow ultimately leading to a lower glomerular filtration rate which is reflected as a reduced creatinine clearance. Tubular toxic effects are caused by disruption of the renal tubular cell membrane by the drug which results in electrolyte abnormalities such as hypokalemia and hypomagnesemia [85]. Administration of AmB by a 24 hour continuous infusion resulted in significantly less impairment of creatinine clearance, as compared to rapid infusion over 4 hours, in a randomized controlled study involving 80 patients with suspected or proven invasive fungal infection. However, electrolyte abnormalities, including hypokalemia and hypomagnesemia, were observed in both patient groups with no significant difference found between groups. These data indicate a non-significant impact on of AmB administered by continuous infusion on creatinine clearance; therefore, it was concluded that administration by continuous infusion reduces, specifically, pretubular nephrotoxicity. Continuous infusion was also better tolerated than the more rapid infusion, resulting in less infusion related adverse effects. Although the study population was too small to assess efficacy, a significantly higher overall and 3 month mortality was observed, respectively, in the rapid infusion group [115]. The authors of this study hypothesized that continuous infusion results in a reduction of toxicity based on a slower delivery of AmB to tissue, similar to that realized with delivery of AmB via a lipid formulation. In fact, several investigators have offered that the incidence of infusion related and nephrotoxic adverse effects observed with continuous infusion appears to be similar to that reported with the lipid formulations of AmB. Thus, this administration technique may offer a less expensive alternative as compared to the lipid formulations [122-124].

The area of antifungal pharmacodynamics (PD) is not well defined in humans; however, animal infection models indicate that AmB exhibits concentration dependent activity whereby a higher rate and extent of kill is afforded with higher peak drug concentrations. This fact raises concern with regard to the administration by continuous infusion where peak concentrations are minimized [125, 126]. Lewis and colleagues pointed out the fact that many in-vitro and in-vivo PD data for AmB were derived without consideration of the presence of human serum albumin, a factor that impacts protein binding which is likely to occur in the treatment of human infection. To address this, they conducted an in-vitro PD assessment to compare the activity of AmB administered as a rapid and continuous infusion against various Candida species in the presence and absence of human serum albumin. The results showed that the PD of AmB changed in the presence of human serum albumin and continuous infusion exhibited similar antifungal activity to rapid infusion [127].

Large, controlled randomized clinical trials are needed to establish the efficacy of continuous infusion in patients; nevertheless, these data perhaps provide insight into the observations made in small clinical studies where a sacrifice of efficacy is not readily apparent with use of continuous infusion. In addition to the need for more efficacy data, other concerns that prevent the general adoption of continuous infusion as standard of care include the requirement for dedication of venous access solely for AmB administration due to it incompatibility with other agents and the general belief that AmB is a concentration dependent killing agent.

Other formulations: lipid formulation of amphotericin B (LFAB)

The narrow therapeutic index of conventional AmB led to the development of new formulations of the drug that utilize either liposomes or complex phospholipids as drug carriers to decrease untoward effects, enhance activity and to provide site specific delivery of doses of this drug [128, 129].

Despite not being strictly a lipid formulation, data for the preparation of amphotericin B in fat emulsion (Intralipid) instead of 5% glucose is controversial, and its use is currently not recommended. Although several studies have shown that its use is associated with decreased nephrotoxicity when compared to amphotericin in 5% dextrose [130-135], others did not reveal any significant advantage over the conventional formulation [136, 137]. Furthermore, a safety and efficacy review for AmB in Intralipid has been conducted by Sievers TM et al and revealed no advantages for its use in systemic fungal infections [138]. Finally, a randomized study has been prematurely stopped due to pulmonary toxicity [133].

Liposomes are microscopic vesicles consisting of one or more phospholipid membranes surrounding a discrete water compartment. The lipid layer is composed of amphipathic phospholipids whose hydrophobic tails associate, while the polar hydrophilic heads align toward the bulk of the water phase. A variety of liposomes with unique physical and chemical structure can be manufactured by altering non-polar and polar groups. Excellent reviews have been recently published [12, 129, 139, 140].

Different mixtures using several lipoproteins and combined in different ratios have appeared during the last decade. At least 5 formulations have been tested in man. They include dimyristoyl phosphatidylcholine (DMPC) / phosphatidylglycerol (DMPG) liposomes, amphotericin B in lipid complex (ABLC; Abelcet, The Liposome Company, Princeton, NJ), intralipid AmB, AmB colloidal dispersion (ABCD; Amphotec, Alza Corporation, Palo Alto, CA), and amphotericin B liposome (L-Amph; AmBisome, Fujisawa Healthcare, Deerfield, IL) (Table 2). In the last decade, these preparations have been extensively examined *in vitro*, whole animal and clinical studies [28, 128, 141-165]. When conventional AmB is used as a frame of reference, it is clear that there are substantial differences in the pharmacokinetic disposition between these formulations. However, for equally effective doses, the toxicity profile is disappointingly similar (Table 2). ABLC was the first agent approved by the FDA. ABLC consist of two phospholipids in a 1:1 drug-to-lipid

Table 2(a). Comparative pharmacokinetics of amphotericin B and liposomal formulations.

Agent	AmB	L-AmB	ABLC	ABCD
Distribution compared to AmB:				
in liver:		higher	higher	higher
in lungs:		similar	higher	similar
in kidney:		similar	similar	similar
Cmax	2.9 mcg/ml	higher	lower	lower
Vd	4 L/kg ml/min.kg	lower	similar	higher
Cl	0.43 mcg.h/ml	lower	higher	similar
AUC	8.6 mcg.h/ml	higher	lower	lower

2(b). Adverse events - percentage of population with response.

	AmB	L-AmB	ABLC	ABCD
mg/kg/day:	1.5-6	5	4-6	0.8-1
Chills	53	48	18	77
Hypokalemia	20	43	5	17
Nausea	6	40	9	8
Vomiting	6	32	8	9
Dyspnea	4	23	7	8
Creatinine increase	28	22	11	20
Hyperbilirubinemia	17	18	4	16
Hypotension	6	14	8	12
Hypertension	6	8	5	6

molar ratio. Electron microscopy reveals ribbon-like, macromolecular structures, ranging from 2 to 5 microns in diameter L-Amph is a unilamellar liposomal preparation, consisting of phosphatidylcholine, cholesterol, distearoylphosphatidylglycerol and AmB in a 2:1:0.8:0.4 molar ratio; with an average diameter of 60 to 70 nm. Amphotec is created by complexing amphotericin B with cholesteryl sulfate in a 1:1 molar ratio to form a colloidal suspension in aqueous solution. The two components form a bilayer in a disk shape, with amphotericin B forming a shield at the disk edges. The disk size is uniform (about 115 nm in diameter and 4 nm thick) and very stable, with the lyophilized form retaining stability for months to years.

To evaluate whether incorporation of AmB into lipid formulations reduces nephrotoxicity, any comparison of conventional AmB with a new formulation of the drug should address the following questions: 1) do the different formulations have the same or different actions? 2) if they have the same action, what is the dose ratio between antifungal and toxic effects, especially nephrotoxicity? and 3) is there a selective advantage in the dose ratios indicating a wider therapeutic margin, i.e., is the dose ratio of lipid formulation of AmB/ AmB lower for the antifungal effect compared to the nephrotoxic effect?

Collective evidence in the literature suggests that LFAB and conventional AmB have a similar action on fungal and mammalian cells. Very few studies, however, have established a dose ratio for antifungal and nephrotoxic effects. In most, only one aspect of the activity or only one formulation was studied. Thus, comparisons between studies are difficult, and inferences should be made with caution. There is evidence that the fungicidal activity of lipid formulations of AmB is influenced by several properties of the liposomes including lipid composition, physical size, the molar ratio of lipids, and the presence or absence of sterols [143-145]. Furthermore, the tests used to assess *in vivo* toxicity have rarely examined renal function adequately. The testing of new formulations by obtaining the acute LD_{50} of the drug, does not necessarily relate to the nephrotoxic potential of chronic therapy [144, 146-148]. Finally, Phase II-III studies in man are complicated by difficulties in the diagnosis of fungal infection, the underlying clinical condition of the patients, and frequent concomitant use of other nephrotoxic agents.

Cell studies

The binding of AmB to various compounds or formulations may result in reduced bioavailability of free AmB with a consequent reduction in toxicity to mammalian and /or fungal cells. Thus, the different formulations may act as a reservoir for free AmB. Since it is recognized that AmB has a higher affinity for ergosterol (the main sterol in fungal cell membranes) than for cholesterol (that is found in human cells) it is possible that the reduced amounts of free AmB is sufficient to be toxic to fungal cells and not to mammalian cells. A selective rate of transfer may be related not only to changes in the sterol components of cell membranes but also to different level of expression of lipoprotein receptors in the target cells.

Much has been learned from *in vitro* studies focused to address the relationship between either free AmB or lipid formulations of AmB with both high- and low-density lipoproteins (HDLs, LDLs). In a series of elegant studies by Lopez-Berenstein and coworkers, it was shown that AmB predominantly associates with HDL and that this effect is enhanced when it is incorporated into positively and negatively charged liposomes [29, 166] These investigators have evaluated the influence of HDLs and LDLs on the toxicity of AmB to fungal and renal cells and observed a selective protective effect of HDL associated AmB for mammalian cells. The minimum inhibitory concentration of AmB and DMPC:DMPG liposome on Candida albicans fungal cells was not modified whether or not HDLs or LDLs were added to the incubation plates. However, HDL-associated AmB was less toxic than free AmB to LLC-PK1 cells, while LDL-associated AmB was as toxic as free AmB. In addition, DMPC:DMPG liposomes and both HDL- and LDL-associated DMPC:DMPG liposomes were less toxic to LLC-PK1 cells than was AmB [166]. Examination of HDL and LDL receptors in the LLC-PK1 cells revealed a high-affinity and low-affinity LDL receptors but only a low-affinity HDL receptor. After trypsinization of the LLC-PK1 renal cells to reduce the LDL receptor, LDL associated AmB was also less toxic than free AmB. Thus, the reduced level of toxicity of HDL-associated AmB and of DMPC:DMPG may be explained by the low level of expression of HDL receptors in LLC-PK1 [166]. Taking this information into account, it appears that AmB in lipid formulations may exist in a complex system that includes free drug, lipoprotein-bound drug and liposomal bound drug (Figure 7). Since the dynamic of the equilibrium is not known, it is difficult to conclude whether doses of AmB in lipid formulations result in comparable free drug concentration as the conventional preparation. These results also support the notion that the relative distribution of AmB among the serum lipoproteins is a major factor influencing the therapeutic index of AmB incorporated into liposomes.

Ralph et al. demonstrated that DMPC:DMPG is generally less active than AmB on yeast cells, and has a slower onset of action [149]. The authors suggest that this lipid formulation of AmB acts as a reservoir for free AmB, which is the active moiety. Others found either an equivalent or 3-4 fold less efficacy for a lipid-complexed form of AmB [144, 147, 150]. These differences may be attributed to the different preparations used and/or to the different strains of fungi examined.

An *in vitro* evaluation of a therapeutic ratio between mammalian and fungal cells serves as a basis of comparison to a ratio of dose required to induce *in vivo* renal toxicity to determine if nephrotoxicity is selectively diminished by the incorporation of AmB into liposomes. One study has calculated a concentration ratio for the actions of lipids formulation of AmB and conventional AmB on mammalian and fungal cells. Juliano et al. compared the in-vitro toxicity of AmB and LFAB to Candida albicans and mammalian erythrocytes [145]. While the two formulations were equipotent in their effects on ion fluxes in yeast cells (indicating formation of membrane pores), only AmB induced such an effect in erythrocytes, despite achieving concentrations of LFAB that were 10 to 20-fold higher than those of AmB. The time required to achieve this effect in fungi was the same for the two formulations, which suggested that LFAB did not constitute a slow-release form of the drug.

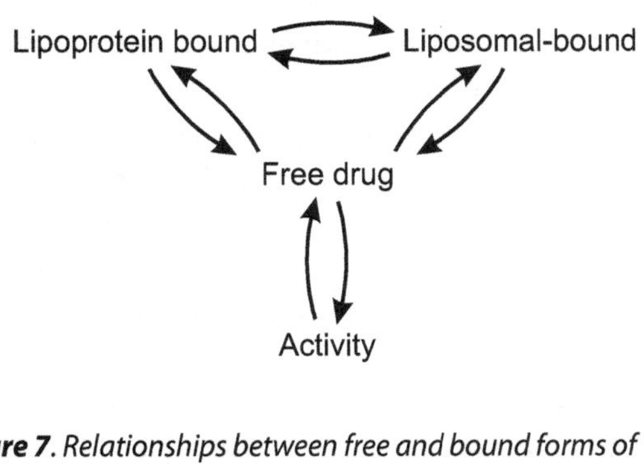

***Figure 7**. Relationships between free and bound forms of amphotericin B to activity.*

The reason for the reduced toxicity of LFAB in mammalian cells was proposed to be preferential transfer of AmB from liposomes to fungal cells compared with its transfer to mammalian cells.

Other studies have also directly compared the antifungal and toxic effects of the two formulations to confirm a wider therapeutic index. A greater toxicity to kidney epithelial cell structures of AmB was apparent when compared with AmB in DMPC:DMPG liposomes. LLC-PK1 renal cells, exposed to short exposure times (2 hours), with different formulations of DMPC:DMPG liposomes, exhibited different EC_{50}'s, the most potent having an EC_{50} 13 times that of AmB [151]. Taken in concert with previous studies [159], this indicates that the renal epithelial cell toxic concentration ratio of DMPC:DMPG liposomes/AmB (13-20:1) is higher than its antifungal concentration ratio (1:1). Further confirmation of differential toxicity was provided by the acute administration of liposomal AmB to primary cultures of rabbit proximal tubule cells and to LLC-PK1 cells (a kidney epithelial cell line) [151]. Joly et al. suggested that higher concentrations of AmB combined to liposomes did not induce the changes elicited by smaller concentrations of conventional AmB. Evidence used to support this was increased K^+ efflux and LDH release with AmB but not LFAB despite achieving 4 to 8 fold higher concentrations of the latter [141]. Unfortunately, antifungal activity was not assessed in this study and no dose ratio can be calculated.

Acute studies require cautious interpretation as chronic exposure of LLC-PK1 cells to LFAB (1-2 days), which is more representative of events that occur clinically, resulted in profound toxic effects at concentrations similar to those of AmB (LFAB/AmB =1:1), manifested by changes in cellular transport processes and in morphology [151]. This finding raises questions as to the applicability and relevance of results derived from short-term in-vitro experiments to whole animal or clinical situations.

Whole animal studies

Animal studies suggest that lipid formulations of AmB are effective in the treatment of fungal infections, but usually require higher doses than AmB [143, 146, 147, 154, 155, 163, 164]. The lack of concomitant assessment of renal function in many of these studies makes it impossible to determine a dose ratio, although most reports confirm that the drug was well tolerated. As mentioned previously, AmB can be distributed in the tissue and serum as free drug, protein-bound drug and liposome-bound drug (Figure 7). However, most studies have not discriminated between these components, so interpretation of serum and tissue concentrations of the drug remains uncertain. This is further complicated by the fact that in ex vivo blood samples, a significant proportion of the total AmB concentration in blood settles as a sediment during the centrifugation process [139]. Thus, it is difficult to interpret the measured free AmB fraction in serum, which may differ between formulations due to physicochemical characteristics of the mixture or to artifactual processes involved after blood sampling.

Detailed pharmacokinetic studies confirm the tissue distribution and pharmacokinetics of LFAB differ from the conventional drug formulation [139, 148, 167] (Table 2a). In general, a greater volume of distribution and greater systemic clearance is apparent when AmB is incorporated into liposomes, suggesting substantial penetration into many organs. After parenteral administration, the total concentration in liver and spleen were higher for the lipid formulations than with conventional AmB due to accumulation in the tissues of the reticuloendothelial system [168]. In contrast, concentrations of AmB in the kidney are lower at equivalent doses. For both AmBisome and ABLC, the results of the biodistribution multidose studies are consistent with reduced kidney toxicity of these formulations [148, 167]. Higher doses of AmBisome (5 mg/kg) and ABLC (10 mg/kg), are required to result in comparable kidney concentrations of AmB to that obtained after 1 mg/kg of conventional AmB.

The acute nephrotoxicity of the two formulations has been examined in rabbits, where AmB induced a fall in GFR and a rise in urinary sodium and potassium excretion rates, while LFAB, at 2.5 times the dose, did not affect these parameters [152]. Here again, antifungal activity was not assessed. Unexpectedly, however, and in contrast to AmB, LFAB increased the excretion of N-acetylglucosaminidase in these animals indicating renal tubular toxicity. The authors suggested that increased delivery of AmB to renal tubular cells by the liposomes led to an interaction with lysosomes and provided an additional mechanism of injury. In support of this conclusion is the finding that the tubular toxicity induced by repeated administration of AmB and LFAB over 5 days was similar when a high enough dose of LFAB (2.4 times that of AmB) was used [153].

A clear reduction in the single dose toxicity for AmBisome and ABLC has been described. The LD_{50} of AmBisome in mice was found to be greater than 175 mg/kg compared to 2.3 mg/kg for the conventional preparation. In rats the LD_{50} was more than 30 fold greater than the value of 1.6 mg/kg for Fungizone [148]. Similarly ABLC could be successfully administered up to 10 mg/kg whereas the maximum non-lethal dose that could be administered to normal mice was 1 mg/kg of Fungizone.

Recently AmB and ABCD were administered in rats, and both drugs showed no decrease in glomerular function; they however caused damage to renal tubuli. Toxicity was more pronounced with AmB than ABCD [169, 170].

Human studies

Similar findings have been reported in patients, with several studies showing that in patients who failed to respond to conventional AmB, or develop nephrotoxicity, had either a complete or partial responders to lipid formulation of AmB, without associated deterioration in renal function [128, 156-159, 161, 162, 164], and recently it has been shown that induction of human monocytes by AmB, ABCD, ABLC and L-Amph leads to a differential expression of cytokines and chemokines. This differential inflammation could be contributing to the difference in efficacy and toxicity of AmB and its related lipid based formulations [171].

All of the three lipid formulations of amphotericin B available in North America and Western Europe, in controlled trials, have demonstrated significantly lower nephrotoxicity than amphotericin B [172]. Differences in biochemical, pharmacokinetic and pharmacodynamic properties among the lipid products have been documented (Table 2). Although the clinical significance of pharmacokinetic differences between lipid preparations is not well known, data generated from many observational as well as controlled trials comparing LFAB use to AmB in the treatment of documented fungal disease and empirical therapy suggest that LFAB confers equal and sometimes superior efficacy when compared to conventional AmB, with the definite advantage of less nephrotoxicity risk. Administration of lipid formulations of AmB are associated with fewer adverse effects, and are generally well-tolerated [25, 173-179].

The clinical experience with these products has been mainly in patients with intolerance to conventional AmB. To date, there is no convincing evidence that any of the lipid-based formulations confers superior efficacy when prospectively compared with AmB in the treatment of documented fungal infections. Therefore the US Food and Drug Administration (FDA) has approved ABCD (recommended dose: 3-4 mg/kg/d) and ABLC (recommended dose: 5 mg/kg/d) for fungal infections in patients who were refractory or intolerant to AmB [180, 181].

L-Amph (recommended dose: 3 mg/kg/d) was the only lipid soluble formulation well studied in empiric therapy and hence it has been FDA approved for presumed fungal infection in fever and neutropenia [182]. In a randomized double blind clinical trial comparing ABCD to AmB in the empiric treatment of fever and neutropenia, ABCD was found to be significantly less nephrotoxic; however it was also associated with a higher incidence of infusion related toxic events [183]. The National Institute of Allergy and Infectious Diseases Mycoses Study Group reported their head to head comparison of L-Amph against conventional AmB in a randomized, double-blind multicenter study in 344 patients with persistent fever and neutropenia as empiric therapy for occult invasive fungal infections [184]. As in previous trials, efficacy was similar with respect to survival (93% vs. 90%, respectively) and resolution of fever during neutropenia (58% vs. 58%, respectively). Discontinuation of therapy due to drug related side effects was also similar (14% vs 19%, respectively). However, the liposomal preparation had a lower rate of increase serum creatinine by two times upper limit of normal (19% vs. 34%, respectively and infusion related fever (17% vs 44%, respectively). In this study, the authors noted a significantly lower frequency of breakthrough fungal infections (3% vs. 8%, respectively $p<0.009$). This same multicenter research team also undertook a subsequent comparison of L-Amph in comparison to voriconazole in 837 patients with the same entry criteria [185]. In that study, voriconazole proved equally effective to L-Amph, but less toxic with respect to nephrotoxicity and fever. However, it had a higher CNS toxicity causing visual disturbances and hallucinations. The ability to administer voriconazole both parenterally and orally did confer an advantage in allowing somewhat earlier patient discharge. Interestingly, this study suggested a lower documented breakthrough with voriconazole having a breakthrough rate of 2% while L-Amph had a breakthrough rate of 5% ($p=0.02$). This latter rate is higher than in the first study and not very different from conventional AmB, thus the relatively small numbers in each study with breakthrough are too small to provide confidence in our ability to discriminate differences.

Experience of using L-Amph in pyrexia of unknown origin has been extended to children and to considering the dose of L-Amph required in a further randomized study of 134 adults and 204 children from the Royal Free Hospital in London [186]. In this study, a low dose L-Amph arm (1 mg/kg/day) was compared to the same dose used in prior studies (3 mg/kg/day). In this study, efficacy was observed in 49% with conventional AmB, 58% with low-dose L-Amph and 64% with high dose L-Amph. A difference was also observed for adverse events, for example doubling of serum creatinine occurred in 24% on conventional AmB versus a 10% and 12% in the two L-Amph arms. A high frequency of fever and rigors with conventional AmB was not observed with L-Amph, but rare cases of CNS toxicity (encephalopathy and seizures) only occurred in L-Amph group. These authors concluded the L-Amph does offer a therapeutic advantage over conventional amphotericin, and that the reduced toxicity profile is particularly valuable in children. Walsh et al have previously conducted an open-label clinical trial showing that ABLC is safe in pediatric patients of all ages including less than 6 months old [187]. Pediatric data is controversial for ABCD: One study suggested it to be safe while another had been prematurely stopped due to infusion related toxicity [188, 189]. ABLC and L-Amph have not been compared in this special population.

L-Amph is also approved for Cryptococcal meningitis in AIDS patients (recommended dose: 6 mg/kg/d), and in the treatment of other fungal infections with patients who were refractory and or intolerant to AmB or with baseline renal impairment (recommended dose: 3-5 mg/kg/d) [182, 190]. Different dose of ABLC have been compared to AmB in the treatment of cryptococcal meningitis; however the risk of nephrotoxicity with ABLC was not convincingly lower than that with AmB [191].

It appears that most studies have focused on L-Amph. There was not much enthusiasm for ABCD because of its infusion related toxicity. This effect is more frequent during the first infusion and decreases with continuation of therapy [180, 183, 189]. The use of ABLC has been recently extensively investigated in 4 observational (both retrospective and prospective) studies in heterogenous patient populations. Two confirmed that ABLC infrequently causes renal toxicity [192, 193], and more interestingly, two have suggested that ABLC is probably safe to be administered to patients with pre-existing renal impairment as well as patients with increased risk for renal toxicity [194, 195].

Currently, there are only few studies comparing ABLC and L-Amph, and all but one suggested a similar renal safety profile. For instance, Wingard et al [196] have compared the safety of two lipid formulations of amphotericin B in febrile neutropenic patients. Subjects were randomized to receive amphotericin B lipid complex (ABLC) at a dose of 5 mg/kg/d (n=78), liposomal amphotericin B (L-Amph) at a dose of 3 mg/kg/d (n=85), or L-Amph at a dose of 5 mg/kg/d (n=81). They found that the incidence of nephrotoxicity (doubling of the baseline serum creatinine concentration) was 42% in the group of patients that received ABLC, 15% in the group that received L-Amph at a dosage of 3 mg/kg/d, and 14% in the group that received L-Amph at a dose of 5 mg/kg/d. A further multicenter, randomized study comparing amphotericin B lipid complex with conventional amphotericin B (AmB) as empiric therapy for febrile neutropenic patients, found a similar incidence of nephrotoxicity (defined as a doubling of the baseline serum creatinine concentration) and infusion-related reactions (fever and chills) in both treatment arms [197]. Furthermore, a prospective and retrospective study compared a heterogenous group of patients who received L-Amph or ABLC and showed similar efficacy and toxicity rates [198]. Finally, Miller et al assessed renal function in Stem cell transplant patients, and reported that renal function improves with L-Amph or ABLC when given as initial therapy as compared to secondary therapy to AmB [199].

Subsequent studies have questioned the nephroprotective effect for therapeutic equivalent doses of LFAB and conventional AmB; For instance, Carriagan [172] suggested in a commentary that if ABLC therapy is administered at higher doses than recommended by the Food and Drug Administration (5 mg/kg/day) then a similar degree of nephrotoxicity to conventional AmB can be anticipated. However recently, data has shown that similar efficacy but less toxicity can be maintained with ABLC at both intermediate doses as well as doses as low as 1mg/Kg/d [200, 201]. Furthermore, a case report described absence of nephrotoxicity in a 9 year old boy who underwent allogenic bone marrow transplantation and received a prolonged and very high cumulative dose of L-Amph [202].

It is challenging to compare rates of toxicity because of different patient populations, different methods of measured infusion related toxic effects, and different dose scheduling. Two systematic reviews have evaluated the efficacy and tolerability of AmB lipid formulations. In July 2000, Johansen and Gotzche published a Cochrane collaboration review on patients with cancer and neutropenia [203]. This review has been updated to include a data search up to July 2004. Several open label and comparative trials have been identified but only 12 fit the selection criteria (1895 patients). Meta-analysis showed that Intralipid, ABLC, ABCD and L-Amph were not associated with decreased mortality when compared to AmB. They however decreased invasive fungal infection with L-Amph being the most effective (RR 0.63). They were all four associated with less nephrotoxicity when compared to AmB (RR 0.45); however the authors argued that AmB was not administered under optimal circumstances and hence a definite conclusion cannot be reached. Barret et al analyzed the results of seven studies (8 publications) in order to evaluate mortality, efficacy and tolerability of ABCD, ABLC and L-Amph compared to AmB in the treatment of suspected or confirmed fungal infections [204]. Meta-analysis showed that all three lipid formulations were associated with a significantly less renal toxicity when compared to AmB. There was no significant difference in efficacy; however LFAB significantly decreased all cause mortality. Both systematic reviews suggested the need for larger well designed comparative trials of LFAB with conventional AmB given with adequate premedication, hydration and electrolytes management, and hence neither recommended the use of lipid formulations as initial therapy. Ostrosky-Zeichner et al have recently reviewed eight open-label studies and 10 major controlled studies to evaluate efficacy and toxicity of LFABs in both proven fungal disease and empiric therapy. The authors suggested that LFABs were clearly superior to conventional AmB, and it is about "time for a new Gold Standard" [205]. This conclusion however stimulated a lot of interesting correspondence discussing several issues. The main points were that it is not "time for a new Gold Standard" until adequate pharmacoeconomic analyses prove cost -effectiveness for the very costly LFABs when compared to the much cheaper AmB. Again it has been pointed out that treatment with AmB was suboptimal and hence comparisons were inadequate [206-209].

Given the relative rather than absolute differences in nephrotoxic potential between formulations that have equal efficacy, it becomes relevant to weigh the benefits of decreased nephrotoxicity against the cost of therapy. This differential persists although L-Amph cost has decreased over time. Currently, the cost for a prescription of 50mg AmB is $5, while the cost for ABLC is about $200 and $500 for L-Amph depending on the institutional accounts. Cost therefore raises the question of the relative value between the alternative therapies.

Some pharmacoeconomic studies analyzed the effect of amphotericin induced nephrotoxicity on mortality and length of stay. This analysis was however complicated by the fact that very sick patients sometimes die early and hence dilute the results. Furthermore, most studies did not consider predisposing factors for renal failure independently of treatment with AmB. Nevertheless, two retrospective studies evaluated the cost-effectiveness of conventional AmB in a heterogenous patient population and concluded that AmB nephrotoxicity leads to high incidence of mortality and increases length of stay [210, 211]. In addition, Chen et al conducted a multicenter prospective study evaluating the treatment outcomes with AmB. They showed that AmB accelerates mortality and increases length of stay [212]. There has also been a trial comparing the use of conventional AmB to LFABs in 4 European countries. The authors confirmed that AmB use causes more nephrotoxity which is associated with prolongation of stay in the hospital and increased cost [213].

The cost issue has probably been best explored by Cagnoni et al [214] in a randomized, double-blind, comparative, multicenter trial in persistently febrile neutropenic patients treated as first-line empirical therapy with either liposomal versus conventional AmB. By using itemized hospital billing data on 414 patients, hospital costs from the time of first dose to discharge were significantly higher for all patients who received liposomal AmB ($48, 962 vs. $43, 183; p=0.022) without any difference in clinical outcome assessed by major clinical events [215]. In the opinion of these authors, until superior efficacy is clearly shown (for proved infections) or pharmacoeconomic analyses document the value of these drugs, current use of such expensive agents should be restricted to patients with preexisting renal dysfunction, patients who do not respond clinically to AmB, or in patients who have a significant decrease in their renal function while receiving conventional formulations AmB.

In addition to the controversial cost issue, it is important to note that although lipid formulations have been shown, most of the times, to have less nephrotoxicity than AmB, they are not free of toxicity, and each has its clinically relevant adverse profile. Therefore, it is currently not the "standard of care" to start all patients on LFABs, especially if patients are considered low risk. For instance Roberto Berdicheski et al have recently shown that AmB is safe in hemodynamically stable subjects with initial normal renal function and who were given adequate saline loading. They concluded that treatment of low risk patients with the expensive LFAB therapy is not warranted [216].

Alternative agents

Despite its unfavorable adverse effect profile, AmB has remained the gold standard antifungal treatment of choice for the management of a broad range of serious fungal infections for over 40 years. Although less toxic agents were introduced over the past few decades, their antifungal spectrum was not as broad and clinical efficacy not as reliable as that of AmB in both non-neutropenic and neutropenic patient populations. Thus, the management of serious invasive fungal infections required, in most cases, use of AmB as either the conventional deoxycholate or lipid formulation. The pharmaceutical industry addressed this problem with the development and introduction of 5 novel antifungal agents that have become licensed over the past 6 years, including a new class of agents, the echinocandins.

The echinocandins, caspofungin (2001), micafungin (2005) and anidulafungin (2006), exert antifungal activity through binding to the enzyme 1, 3-β-glucan synthase to inhibit formation of 1, 3-β-glucan, a vital component of the fungal cell membrane. The target site of action for the echinocandins does not exist in human cells; therefore, these agents are associated with very few and rare adverse effects. The echinocandins display activity against several fungal pathogens. Caspofungin, the first available agent of this class, has been found to be equally efficacious in the treatment of invasive candidiasis to AmB. Caspofungin is recommended as a primary treatment option for the management of candidemia in neutropenic or non-neutropenic patients according to the 2004 Infectious Diseases Society of America clinical practice guidelines for the treatment of candidiasis. As these guidelines were created prior to the release of the newer echinocandins, micafungin and anidulafungin, the updated version may also include these agents as a primary treatment choice. The echinocandins offer a safer and equally effective alternative to AmB in the primary management of candidiasis [12, 217-219].

Voriconazole (2002) and posaconazole (2006) are novel triazole antifungals that display a very broad spectrum of antifungal activity against both yeasts and molds. These are better tolerated as compared to AmB exhibiting a favourable adverse effect profile. Voriconazole has replaced AmB as the treatment of choice in the management of invasive aspergillosis based on superior efficacy and survival that was demonstrated in a large randomized clinical trial. Due to its recent Food and Drug Administration approval, the place in therapy of posaconazole has not yet been well established [12, 220].

Clinical use

General underlying condition of the patient

The indication for AmB is the presence of proved or suspected systemic fungal disease. As previously mentioned, patients who receive AmB are usually immunocompromised and severely ill, with some degree of malnutrition, multiple organ failure and life threatening infections. The clinical condition of these patients may, therefore, confer an increased risk of nephrotoxicity. Once the decision to implement AmB has been made, an algorithm can be used to optimize therapy (Figure 8) [91]. The first step is to assess renal function, the sodium status of the patient, and to correct overt sodium depletion. It is important to realize that milder sodium depleted states which are not clinically apparent can substantially enhance the nephrotoxic potential of AmB. It is, therefore, important to assess whether the patient can tolerate sodium supplementation in addition to a normal salt intake. Otherwise healthy subjects usually tolerate a supplement of 150 mEq/d over and above the normal sodium intake of 150 to 200 mEq/d without difficulty. Increased sodium intake, however, may exacerbate cardiac failure, cirrhosis with ascites, or renal failure.

Another factor to consider is whether the patient will receive sodium supplementation as a consequence of concomitant antibiotic therapy (e.g., ticarcillin). When the opportunity to choose among several antibiotics arises, the alternative with the highest obligatory sodium load should be selected whenever possible.

Finally, it is prudent to check for the presence of potassium and magnesium deficits prior to therapy since AmB will invariably cause loss of these electrolytes during therapy. Correction of these abnormalities, before or concomitantly with the start of therapy, should delay or avoid the early development of electrolyte disturbances and possible additional toxicity (e.g., arrhythmia, rhabdomyolysis) that sometimes necessitate the early discontinuation of therapy.

In our opinion, the elective use of LFAB at the outset should be restricted to only those patients who have impaired renal function, who have clinical contraindications to salt supplementation or who are children. Otherwise, the use of AmB is generally advocated.

Amphotericin B administration

AmB therapy is recommended to be initiated with a low dose, gradually escalating to a full therapeutic dose according to patient tolerance. However, severe life-threatening infections require rapid dose escalation as tolerated by the patient. Traditionally AmB has been administered as an IV infusion over 4-6 hours as recommended in the insert package. However, continuous infusion over 24 hours provides a reasonable alternative as it induces fewer side effects and significantly decreases nephrotoxicity [115].

If a 4-hour infusion is to be used in conjunction with ticarcillin, we advocate administration between doses of ticarcillin. If ticarcillin is not indicated, we advocate that AmB should be given between two 30-min infusions of 0.5 L normal saline, intravenously. This amount of supplementation is based on empiric observation, and further studies are needed to ascertain whether lower amounts confer an equivalent degree of protection. If vomiting occurs, sodium supplementation should be increased.

Concomitant use of nephrotoxic drugs

If AmB is to be used in conjunction with another nephrotoxic agent, several measures can be taken in order to minimize the potential synergistic toxicity of amphotericin B. For example, if an aminoglycoside or cyclosporine is to be used, monitoring of their serum concentrations will help avoid toxic levels. It is also imperative to evaluate electrolyte losses closely and be aggressive in their replacement, since cyclosporine A nephrotoxicity may be exacerbated by dehydration [221], and to follow magnesium levels closely since both drugs cause hypomagnesemia.

Potassium and magnesium supplementation

Urinary potassium and magnesium losses are anticipated consequences of AmB therapy. Some of the losses can be compensated for with increased dietary intake, while others will require oral or intravenous replacement. It should be recognized that the serum levels of these ions do not necessarily correlate with the total deficit, as the plasma levels tend to be conserved while cellular stores are becoming depleted. In general, potassium and magnesium supplements should be given to all patients and the amounts increased if the

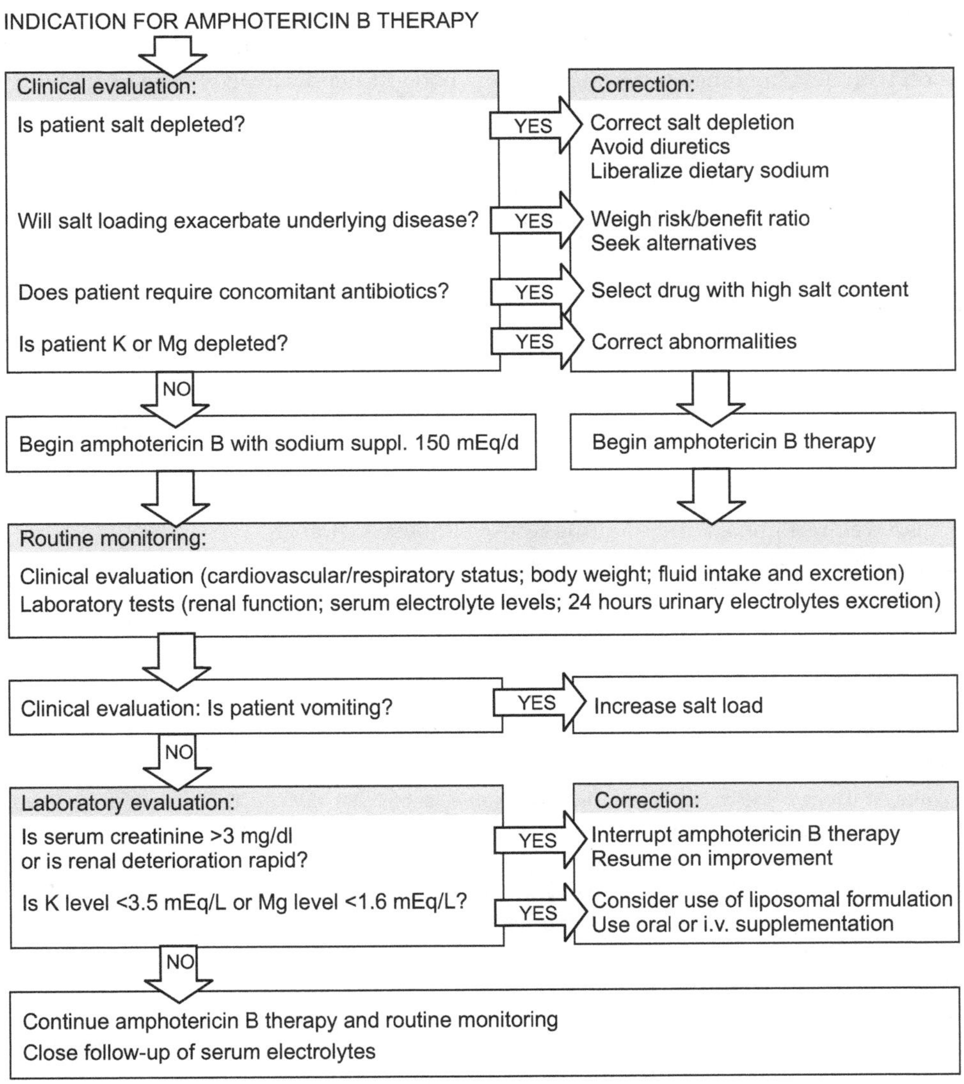

Figure 8. *Proposed approach for management of amphotericin B therapy*

potassium level falls below 3.5 mEq/l or the magnesium level falls below 1.6 mEq/l, with either dietary or pharmacological supplementation. Amiloride, in low doses, is an alternative therapy in patients who need high dose intravenous potassium replacement [222].

Frequent monitoring of serum electrolytes (potassium and magnesium) with adequate hydration and ion supplementation corresponding to amounts lost by kidneys concomitant to AmB therapy provides an effective intervention for prophylaxis of AmB-induced renal toxicity [119].

Follow-up

In patients with mild renal dysfunction prior to AmB therapy, sodium supplementation has proved to be safe and effective. In patients not receiving sodium supplementation who develop renal impairment during AmB therapy, initiation of sodium supplementation may permit continued therapy with AmB. However, if renal function continues to deteriorate, or if the rate of deterioration is rapid, temporary discontinuation of AmB therapy may be required. Therapy can be resumed in rehydrated patients when serum creatinine concentrations begin to return toward baseline values or LFAB can be used in place of AmB.

Conclusion

AmB remains a very effective antifungal agent. Nephrotoxicity is a well-recognized dose-limiting complication, leading to interruption or discontinuation of the therapy. It is commonly expressed as azotemia and decreased GFR; however tubular abnormalities are also important. The underlying mechanisms include direct vasoconstrictor effects and direct cytotoxicity, as a reflection of its action on cell membranes leading to alteration of cell permeability. These effects are amenable to modulation. In the clinical setting, the use of salt supplementation lowers incidence and severity of nephrotoxicity; however, requires careful attention to potassium and magnesium replacement. The information accumulated to this date support the notion that LFABs confer equal and sometimes superior efficacy when compared to conventional AmB with the definite advantage of less nephrotoxicity risk; however due to their high cost, it is currently recommended to restrict their use to special situations only. Use of continuous infusion offers another approach to decrease the likelihood of nephrotoxicity. The availability of safer antifungal agents with equivalent or superior antifungal activity will likely challenge the position of AmB as the "gold standard" within the next decade.

Acknowledgements

The research work presented in this chapter was supported by United States Public Health Service grant GM43263 and United States National Institute of Health grant 1U54RR023506-01. This is an update and revision of the book chapter originally written by Jose F. Bernardo, Ramzi Sabra, Subhash J. Vyas and Robert A. Branch.

References

1. Denning DW. Epidemiology and pathogenesis of systemic fungal infections in the immunocompromised host. J Antimicrob Chemother 1991;28 Suppl B:1-16.
2. Horan TC, White JW, Jarvis WR, et al. Nosocomial infection surveillance, 1984. MMWR CDC Surveill Summ 1986;35:17SS-29SS.
3. Bodey GP. Fungal infections complicating acute leukemia. J Chronic Dis 1966;19:667-87.
4. Hay RJ. Overview of the treatment of disseminated fungal infections. J Antimicrob Chemother 1991;28 Suppl B:17-25.
5. Gallis HA, Drew RH, Pickard WW. Amphotericin B: 30 years of clinical experience. Rev Infect Dis 1990;12:308-29.
6. Wingard JR, Kubilis P, Lee L, et al. Clinical significance of nephrotoxicity in patients treated with amphotericin B for suspected or proven aspergillosis. Clin Infect Dis 1999;29:1402-7.
7. Pathak A, Pien FD, Carvalho L. Amphotericin B use in a community hospital, with special emphasis on side effects. Clin Infect Dis 1998;26:334-8.
8. Clements JS, Jr., Peacock JE, Jr. Amphotericin B revisited: reassessment of toxicity. Am J Med 1990;88:22N-7N.
9. Luber AD, Maa L, Lam M, Guglielmo BJ. Risk factors for amphotericin B-induced nephrotoxicity. J Antimicrob Chemother 1999;43:267-71.

10. Stein RS, Albridge K, Lenox RK, et al. Nephrotoxicity in leukemic patients receiving empirical amphotericin B and aminoglycosides. South Med J 1988;81:1095-9.
11. Harbarth S, Pestotnik SL, Lloyd JF, et al. The epidemiology of nephrotoxicity associated with conventional amphotericin B therapy. Am J Med 2001;111:528-34.
12. Kleinberg M. What is the current and future status of conventional amphotericin B? Int J Antimicrob Agents 2006;27 Suppl 1:12-6.
13. Warnock DW. Amphotericin B: an introduction. J Antimicrob Chemother 1991;28 Suppl B:27-38.
14. Brajtburg J, Powderly WG, Kobayashi GS, Medoff G. Amphotericin B: current understanding of mechanisms of action. Antimicrob Agents Chemother 1990;34:183-8.
15. Brajtburg J, Elberg S, Schwartz DR, et al. Involvement of oxidative damage in erythrocyte lysis induced by amphotericin B. Antimicrob Agents Chemother 1985;27:172-6.
16. Sokol-Anderson ML, Brajtburg J, Medoff G. Amphotericin B-induced oxidative damage and killing of Candida albicans. J Infect Dis 1986;154:76-83.
17. Sabra R, Branch RA. Amphotericin B nephrotoxicity. Drug Saf 1990;5:94-108.
18. Butler WT, Bennett JE, Alling DW, et al. Nephrotoxicity of amphotericin B; early and late effects in 81 patients. Ann Intern Med 1964;61:175-87.
19. Medoff G, Kobayashi GS. Strategies in the treatment of systemic fungal infections. N Engl J Med 1980;302:145-55.
20. Miller RP, Bates JH. Amphotericin B toxicity. A follow-up report of 53 patients. Ann Intern Med 1969;71:1089-95.
21. Branch RA, Jackson EK, Jacqz E, et al. Amphotericin-B nephrotoxicity in humans decreased by sodium supplements with coadministration of ticarcillin or intravenous saline. Klin Wochenschr 1987;65:500-6.
22. Winn WA. Coccidioidomycosis and amphotericin B. Med Clin North Am 1963;47:1131-48.
23. Littman ML, Horowitz PL, Swadey JG. Coccidioidomycosis and its treatment with amphotericin B. Am J Med 1958;24:568-92.
24. Rubin SI, Krawiec DR, Gelberg H, Shanks RD. Nephrotoxicity of amphotericin B in dogs: a comparison of two methods of administration. Can J Vet Res 1989;53:23-8.
25. Saliba F. Antifungals and renal safety--getting the balance right. Int J Antimicrob Agents 2006;27 Suppl 1:21-4.
26. Girmenia C, Cimino G, Micozzi A, et al. Risk Factors For Nephrotoxicity Associated With Conventional Amphotericin B Therapy. The American Journal of Medicine 2002;113:351.
27. Gubbins PO, Penzak SR, Polston S, et al. Characterizing and predicting amphotericin B-associated nephrotoxicity in bone marrow or peripheral blood stem cell transplant recipients. Pharmacotherapy 2002;22:961-71.
28. Wasan KM, Brazeau GA, Keyhani A, et al. Roles of liposome composition and temperature in distribution of amphotericin B in serum lipoproteins. Antimicrob Agents Chemother 1993;37:246-50.
29. Wasan KM, Rosenblum MG, Cheung L, Lopez-Berestein G. Influence of lipoproteins on renal cytotoxicity and antifungal activity of amphotericin B. Antimicrob Agents Chemother 1994;38:223-7.
30. Wasan KM, Conklin JS. Enhanced amphotericin B nephrotoxicity in intensive care patients with elevated levels of low-density lipoprotein cholesterol. Clin Infect Dis 1997;24:78-80.
31. Wasan KM, Wong J, Corr T. Role of plasma lipids and lipoproteins in predicting amphotericin B-induced nephrotoxicity in pediatric oncology patients. Cancer Chemother Pharmacol 2006;57:120-4.
32. Holeman CW, Jr., Einstein H. The toxic effects of amphotericin B in man. Calif Med 1963;99:90-3.
33. Bullock WE, Luke RG, Nuttall CE, Bhathena D. Can mannitol reduce amphotericin B nephrotixicity? Double-blind study and description of a new vascular lesion in kidneys. Antimicrob Agents Chemother 1976;10:555-63.
34. Barbour GL, Straub KD, O'Neal BL, Leatherman JW. Vasopressin-resistant nephrogenic diabetes insipidus. A result of amphotericin B therapy. Arch Intern Med 1979;139:86-8.
35. Fisher MA, Talbot GH, Maislin G, et al. Risk factors for Amphotericin B-associated nephrotoxicity. Am J Med 1989;87:547-52.
36. Rose BD. Hypokalemia. In: Rose BD, ed. Clinical Physiology of Acid-Base and Electrolyte Disorders. McGraw Hill, Inc., 1989:715-56.
37. Burgess JL, Birchall R. Nephrotoxicity of amphotericin B, with emphasis on changes in tubular function. Am J Med 1972;53:77-84.
38. Llanos A, Cieza J, Bernardo J, et al. Effect of salt supplementation on amphotericin B nephrotoxicity. Kidney Int 1991;40:302-8.
39. Sellin JH, De Soignie R. Ion transport in human colon *in vitro*. Gastroenterology 1987;93:441-8.
40. Bernardo JF, Murakami S, Branch RA, Sabra R. Potassium depletion potentiates amphotericin-B-induced toxicity to renal tubules. Nephron 1995;70:235-41.
41. Barton CH, Pahl M, Vaziri ND, Cesario T. Renal magnesium wasting associated with amphotericin B therapy. Am J Med 1984;77:471-4.
42. Douglas JB, Healy JK. Nephrotoxic effects of amphotericin B, including renal tubular acidosis. Am J Med 1969;46:154-62.

43. Steinmetz PR, Lawson LR. Defect in urinary acidification induced *in vitro* by amphotericin B. J Clin Invest 1970;49:596-601.
44. Gil FZ, Malnic G. Effect of amphotericin B on renal tubular acidification in the rat. Pflugers Arch 1989;413:280-6.
45. Gouge TH, Andriole VT. An experimental model of amphotericin B nephrotoxicity with renal tubular acidosis. J Lab Clin Med 1971;78:713-24.
46. McCurdy DK, Frederic M, Elkinton JR. Renal tubular acidosis due to amphotericin B. Clin Res 1964;12:471.
47. Takacs FJ, Tomkiewicz ZM, Merrill JP. Amphotercin B Nephrotoxicity with Irreversible Renal Failure. Ann Intern Med 1963;59:716-24.
48. Heyman SN, Stillman IE, Brezis M, et al. Chronic amphotericin nephropathy: morphometric, electron microscopic, and functional studies. J Am Soc Nephrol 1993;4:69-80.
49. Mayer J, Doubeck M, Doubeck J, et al. Reduced nephrotoxicity of conventional amphotericin B therapy after minimal nephroprotective measures: animal experiments and clinical study. J Am Soc Nephrol 2002.
50. Porter GA. Extrapolation of animal data to man: the concordance between toxicity screening and clincial consequence. In Nephrotoxicity in the experimental and clinical situation Part 2. Martinus Nijhoff Publishers. 1987. Ref Type: Music Score
51. Gruda I, Nadeau P, Brajtburg, Medoff G. Application of different spectra in the UV-visible region to study the formation of amphotericin. Biochem Biophys Res Commun 1980.
52. Vertut-Croquin A, Bolard J, Chabbert M, Gary-Bobo C. Differences in the interaction of the polyene antibiotic amphotericin B with cholesterol- or ergosterol-containing phospholipid vesicles. A circular dichroism and permeability study. Biochemistry 1983;22:2939-44.
53. Caltrider PG, Gottlieb D. Capacidin: a new member of the polyene antibiotic group. Antribiot Chemother 1961.
54. Kinsky SC. The effect of polyene antibiotics on permeability in Neurospora crassa. Biochem Biophys Res Commun 1961;4:353-7.
55. Kinsky SC. Alterations in the permeability of Neurospora crassa due to polyene antibiotics. J Bacteriol 1961;82:889-97.
56. Marini FP, Arnow P, Lampen JO. The effect of monovalent cations on the inhibition of yeast metabolism by nystain. J General Microbiol 1961.
57. Sutton DD, Arnow PM, Lampen JO. Effect of high concentrations of nystatin upon glycolysis and cellular permeability in yeast. Proc Soc Exp Biol Med 1961;108:170-5.
58. Gottlieb D, Carter HE, Sloneker JH, Ammann A. Protection of fungi against polyene antibiotics by sterols. Science 1958;128:361.
59. Kotler-Brajtburg J, Price HD, Medoff G, et al. Molecular basis for the selective toxicity of amphotericin B for yeast and filipin for animal cells. Antimicrob Agents Chemother 1974;5:377-82.
60. Andreoli TE. On the anatomy of amphotericin B-cholesterol pores in lipid bilayer membranes. Kidney Int 1973;4:337-45.
61. DeKruijiff B, Demel RA. Polyene antibiotic-sterol interactions in membranes of Acholeplesma laidlawii cells and lecithin liposomes. III. Molecular structure of the polyene antibiotic-cholesterol complexes. Biochem Biophys Acta 1974;339:57-70.
62. Holz RW. The effects of the polyene antibiotics nystatin and amphotericin B on thin lipid membranes. Ann N Y Acad Sci 1974;235:469-79.
63. Gatzy JT, Reuss L, Finn AL. Amphotericin B and K+ transport across excised toad urinary bladder. Am J Physiol 1979;237:F145-F156.
64. Lichtenstein NS, Leaf A. Effect of amphotericin B on the permeability of the toad bladder. J Clin Invest 1965;44:1328-42.
65. Lichtenstein NS, Leaf A. Evidence for a double series permeability barrier at the mucosal surface of the toad bladder. Ann N Y Acad Sci 1966;137:556-65.
66. Teerlink T, de Kruijff B, Demel RA. The action of pimaricin, etruscomycin and amphotericin B on liposomes with varying sterol content. Biochim Biophys Acta 1980;599:484-92.
67. Butler WT, Alling DW, Cotlove E. Potassium loss from human erythrocytes exposed to amphotericin B. Proc Soc Exp Biol Med 1965;118:297-300.
68. Kinsky SC. Comparative responses of mammalian erythrocytes and microbial protoplasts to polyene antibiotics and vitamin A. Arch Biochem Biophys 1963;102:180-8.
69. Kinsky SC, Avruch J, Permutt M, Rogers HB. The lytic effect of polyene antifungal antibiotics on mammalian erythrocytes. Biochem Biophys Res Commun 1962;9:503-7.
70. Finn JT, Cohen LH, Steinmetz PR. Acidifying defect induced by amphotericin B: comparison of bicarbonate and hydrogen ion permeabilities. Kidney Int 1977;11:261-6.
71. Capasso G, Schuetz H, Vickermann B, Kinne R. Amphotericin B and amphotericin B methylester: effect on brush border membrane permeability. Kidney Int 1986;30:311-7.

72. Schell RE, Tran NV, Bramhall JS. Amphotericin B-induced changes in renal membrane permeation: a model of nephrotoxicity. Biochem Biophys Res Commun 1989;159:1165-70.
73. Hoeprich PD. Chemotherapy of systemic fungal diseases. Annu Rev Pharmacol Toxicol 1978;18:205-31.
74. Joly V, Saint-Pierre-Chazalet M, Saint-Julien L, et al. Inhibiting cholesterol synthesis reduces the binding and toxicity of amphotericin B against rabbit renal tubular cells in primary culture. J Infect Dis 1992;165:337-43.
75. Cheng JT, Witty RT, Robinson RR, Yarger WE. Amphotericin B nephrotoxicity: increased renal resistance and tubule permeability. Kidney Int 1982;22:626-33.
76. Varlam DE, Siddiq MM, Parton LA, Russmann H. Apoptosis contributes to amphotericin B-induced nephrotoxicity. Antimicrob Agents Chemother 2001;45:679-85.
77. Zager RA. Polyene antibiotics: relative degrees of *in vitro* cytotoxicity and potential effects on tubule phospholipid and ceramide content. Am J Kidney Dis 2000;36:238-49.
78. Hannun YA, Luberto C. Ceramide in the eukaryotic stress response. Trends Cell Biol 2000;10:73-80.
79. Lamy-Fruend MT, Ferreira VFN, Schreier S. Mechanism of inactivation of the polyene antibiotic amphotericin B. J Antibiot (Tokyo) 1985.
80. Osaka K, Tyurina YY, Dubey RK, et al. Amphotericin B as an intracellular antioxidant: protection against 2, 2'-azobis(2, 4-dimethylvaleronitrile)-induced peroxidation of membrane phospholipids in rat aortic smooth muscle cells. Biochem Pharmacol 1997;54:937-45.
81. Osaka K, Ritov VB, Bernardo JF, et al. Amphotericin B protects cis-parinaric acid against peroxyl radical-induced oxidation: amphotericin B as an antioxidant. Antimicrob Agents Chemother 1997;41:743-7.
82. Walev I, Bhakdi S. Possible reason for preferential damage to renal tubular epithelial cells evoked by amphotericin B. Antimicrob Agents Chemother 1996;40:1116-20.
83. Butler WT, Hill GJ, Szwed CF, Knight V. Amphotericin B renal toxicity in the dog. J Pharmacol Exp Ther 1964;143:47-56.
84. Gerkens JF, Heidemann HT, Jackson EK, Branch RA. Aminophylline inhibits renal vasoconstriction produced by intrarenal hypertonic saline. J Pharmacol Exp Ther 1983;225:611-5.
85. Heidemann HT, Gerkens JF, Jackson EK, Branch RA. Effect of aminophylline on renal vasoconstriction produced by amphotericin B in the rat. Naunyn Schmiedebergs Arch Pharmacol 1983;324:148-52.
86. Sabra R, Takahashi K, Branch RA, Badr KF. Mechanisms of amphotericin B-induced reduction of the glomerular filtration rate: a micropuncture study. J Pharmacol Exp Ther 1990;253:34-7.
87. Tolins JP, Raij L. Adverse effect of amphotericin B administration on renal hemodynamics in the rat. Neurohumoral mechanisms and influence of calcium channel blockade. J Pharmacol Exp Ther 1988;245:594-9.
88. Sabra R, Zeinoun N, Sharaf LH, et al. Role of humoral mediators in, and influence of a liposomal formulation on, acute amphotericin B nephrotoxicity. Pharmacol Toxicol 2001;88:168-75.
89. Cutaia M, Bullard SR, Rudio K, Rounds S. Characteristics of amphotericin B-induced endothelial cell injury. J Lab Clin Med 1993;121:244-56.
90. Heyman SN, Clark BA, Kaiser N, et al. In-vivo and in-vitro studies on the effect of amphotericin B on endothelin release. J Antimicrob Chemother 1992;29:69-77.
91. Branch RA. Prevention of amphotericin B-induced renal impairment. A review on the use of sodium supplementation. Arch Intern Med 1988;148:2389-94.
92. Schnermann J. Regulation of single nephron filtration rate by feedback-facts and theories. Clin Nephrol 1975;3:75-81.
93. Thurau K. Modification of angiotensin-mediated tubulo-glomerular feedback by extracellular volume. Kidney Int Suppl 1975;S202-S207.
94. Wright FS, Schnermann J. Interference with feedback control of glomerular filtration rate by furosemide, triflocin, and cyanide. J Clin Invest 1974;53:1695-708.
95. Gerkens JF, Branch RA. The influence of sodium status and furosemide on canine acute amphotericin B nephrotoxicity. J Pharmacol Exp Ther 1980;214:306-11.
96. Ohnishi A, Ohnishi T, Stevenhead W, et al. Sodium status influences chronic amphotericin B nephrotoxicity in rats. Antimicrob Agents Chemother 1989;33:1222-7.
97. Tolins JP, Raij L. Chronic amphotericin B nephrotoxicity in the rat: protective effect of calcium channel blockade. J Am Soc Nephrol 1991;2:98-102.
98. Tolins JP, Raij L. Chronic amphotericin B nephrotoxicity in the rat, protective effect of prophylactic salt loading. Am J Kidney Dis 1988;11:313-7.
99. Heidemann HT, Bolten M, Inselmann G. Effect of chronic theophylline administration on amphotericin B nephrotoxicity in rats. Nephron 1991;59:294-8.

100. Wasan KM, Vadiei K, Lopez-Berestein G, et al. Pentoxifylline in amphotericin B toxicity rat model. Antimicrob Agents Chemother 1990;34:241-4.
101. Luke DR, Wasan KM, Verani RR, et al. Attenuation of amphotericin-B nephrotoxicity in the candidiasis rat model. Nephron 1991;59:139-44.
102. Kuan CJ, Branch RA, Jackson EK. Effect of an adenosine receptor antagonist on acute amphotericin B nephrotoxicity. Eur J Pharmacol 1990;178:285-91.
103. Sawaya BP, Weihprecht H, Campbell WR, et al. Direct vasoconstriction as a possible cause for amphotericin B-induced nephrotoxicity in rats. J Clin Invest 1991;87:2097-107.
104. Hardie W, Ebert J, Takahashi K, Badr KF. Thromboxane A2 receptor antagonism reverses amphotericin B-induced renal vasoconstricition in the rat. Prostaglandins 2007.
105. Sabra R, Branch RA. Effect of amphotericin B on intracellular calcium levels in cultured glomerular mesangial cells. Eur J Pharmacol 1992;226:79-85.
106. Soupart A, Decaux G. Nifedipine and amphotericin B nephrotoxicity in the rat. Nephron 1989;52:278-80.
107. Heidemann HT, Brune KH, Sabra R, Branch RA. Acute and chronic effects of flucytosine on amphotericin B nephrotoxicity in rats. Antimicrob Agents Chemother 1992;36:2670-5.
108. Brezis M, Rosen S, Silva P, et al. Polyene toxicity in renal medulla: injury mediated by transport activity. Science 1984;224:66-8.
109. UTZ JP. Chemotherapy of the systemic mycoses. Med Clin North Am 1982;66:221-33.
110. Hellesbusch AA, Salama F, Eadie E. The use of mannitol to reduce the toxicity of amphotericin B. Surg Gynecol Obstet 1972.
111. Olivero JJ, Lozano-Mendez J, Ghafary EM, et al. Mitigation of amphotericin B nephrotoxicity by mannitol. Br Med J 1975;1:550-1.
112. Rosch JM, Pazin GJ, Fireman P. Reduction of amphotericin B nephrotoxicity with mannitol. JAMA 1976;235:1995-6.
113. Said R, Marin P, Anicama H, et al. Effect of mannitol on acute amphotericin B nephrotoxicity. Res Exp Med (Berl) 1980;177:85-9.
114. Ural AU, Avcu F, Cetin T, et al. Spironolactone: is it a novel drug for the prevention of amphotericin B-related hypokalemia in cancer patients? Eur J Clin Pharmacol 2002;57:771-3.
115. Eriksson U, Seifert B, Schaffner A. Comparison of effects of amphotericin B deoxycholate infused over 4 or 24 hours: randomised controlled trial. BMJ 2001;322:579-82.
116. Heidemann HT, Gerkens JF, Spickard WA, et al. Amphotericin B nephrotoxicity in humans decreased by salt repletion. Am J Med 1983;75:476-81.
117. Holler B, Omar S, Farid M, Patterson Jevitz M. Effect of Fluid and Electrolyte Management on Amphotericin B-Induced Nephrotoxicity Among Extremely Low Birth Weight Infants. Pediatrics 2004;113.
118. Girmenia C, Cimino G, Di CF, et al. Effects of hydration with salt repletion on renal toxicity of conventional amphotericin B empirical therapy: a prospective study in patients with hematological malignancies. Support Care Cancer 2005;13:987-92.
119. Mayer J, Doubek M, Vorlicek J. Must we really fear toxicity of conventional amphotericin B in oncological patients? Support Care Cancer 1999;7:51-5.
120. Oto OA, Paydas S, Disel U, et al. Amphotericin B deoxycholate (d-AMB) use in cases with febrile neutropenia and fungal infections: lower toxicity with suitable premedication. Mycoses 2007;50:135-9.
121. Echevarria J, Seas C, Cruz M, et al. Oral rehydration solution to prevent nephrotoxicity of amphotericin B. Am J Trop Med Hyg 2006;75:1108-12.
122. Speich R, Dutly A, Naef R, et al. Tolerability, safety and efficacy of conventional amphotericin B administered by 24-hour infusion to lung transplant recipients. Swiss Med Wkly 2002;132:455-8.
123. Uehara RP, Sa VH, Koshimura ET, et al. Continuous infusion of amphotericin B: preliminary experience at Faculdade de Medicina da Fundacao ABC. Sao Paulo Med J 2005;123:219-22.
124. Furrer K, Schaffner A, Vavricka SR, et al. Nephrotoxicity of cyclosporine A and amphotericin B-deoxycholate as continuous infusion in allogenic stem cell transplantation. Swiss Med Wkly 2002;132:316-20.
125. Andes D, Stamsted T, Conklin R. Pharmacodynamics of amphotericin B in a neutropenic-mouse disseminated-candidiasis model. Antimicrob Agents Chemother 2001;45:922-6.
126. Andes D. Clinical pharmacodynamics of antifungals. Infect Dis Clin North Am 2003;17:635-49.
127. Lewis RE, Wiederhold NP, Prince RA, Kontoyiannis DP. *In vitro* pharmacodynamics of rapid versus continuous infusion of amphotericin B deoxycholate against Candida species in the presence of human serum albumin. J Antimicrob Chemother 2006;57:288-93.
128. Lopez-Berestein G, Fainstein V, Hopfer R, et al. Liposomal amphotericin B for the treatment of systemic fungal infections in patients with cancer: a preliminary study. J Infect Dis 1985;151:704-10.
129. Gates C, Pinney RJ. Amphotericin B and its delivery by liposomal and lipid formulations. J Clin Pharm Ther 1993;18:147-53.

130. Chavanet PY, Garry I, Charlier N, et al. Trial of glucose versus fat emulsion in preparation of amphotericin for use in HIV infected patients with candidiasis. BMJ 1992;305:921-5.
131. Barquist E, Fein E, Shadick D, et al. A randomized prospective trial of amphotericin B lipid emulsion versus dextrose colloidal solution in critically ill patients. J Trauma 1999;47:336-40.
132. Nucci M, Loureiro M, Silveira F, et al. Comparison of the toxicity of amphotericin B in 5% dextrose with that of amphotericin B in fat emulsion in a randomized trial with cancer patients. Antimicrob Agents Chemother 1999;43:1445-8.
133. Caillot D, Reny G, Solary E, et al. A controlled trial of the tolerance of amphotericin B infused in dextrose or in Intralipid in patients with haematological malignancies. J Antimicrob Chemother 1994;33:603-13.
134. Friedlich PS, Steinberg I, Fujitani A, deLemos RA. Renal tolerance with the use of intralipid-amphotericin B in low-birth-weight neonates. Am J Perinatol 1997;14:377-83.
135. Sorkine P, Nagar H, Weinbroum A, et al. Administration of amphotericin B in lipid emulsion decreases nephrotoxicity: results of a prospective, randomized, controlled study in critically ill patients. Crit Care Med 1996;24:1311-5.
136. Nath CE, Shaw PJ, Gunning R, et al. Amphotericin B in children with malignant disease: a comparison of the toxicities and pharmacokinetics of amphotericin B administered in dextrose versus lipid emulsion. Antimicrob Agents Chemother 1999;43:1417-23.
137. Torre D, Banfi G, Tambini R, et al. A retrospective study on the efficacy and safety of amphotericin B in a lipid emulsion for the treatment of cryptococcal meningitis in AIDS patients. J Infect 1998;37:36-8.
138. Sievers TM, Kubak BM, Wong-Beringer A. Safety and efficacy of Intralipid emulsions of amphotericin B. J Antimicrob Chemother 1996;38:333-47.
139. Janknegt R, de Marie S, Bakker-Woudenberg IA, Crommelin DJ. Liposomal and lipid formulations of amphotericin B. Clinical pharmacokinetics. Clin Pharmacokinet 1992;23:279-91.
140. Gregoriadis G. Overview of liposomes. J Antimicrob Chemother 1991;28 Suppl B:39-48.
141. Joly V, Saint-Julien L, Carbon C, Yeni P. Interactions of free and liposomal amphotericin B with renal proximal tubular cells in primary culture. J Pharmacol Exp Ther 1990;255:17-22.
142. Colette C, Van Der Auwerz P, Lopez P, et al. Tissue concentrations and bioactivity of amphotericin B in cnacer patients treated with amphotericin B. Antimicrob Agents Chemother 1989.
143. Payne NI, Cosgrove RF, Green AP, Liu L. In-vivo studies of amphotericin B liposomes derived from proliposomes: effect of formulation on toxicity and tissue disposition of the drug in mice. J Pharm Pharmacol 1987;39:24-8.
144. Szoka FC, Jr., Milholland D, Barza M. Effect of lipid composition and liposome size on toxicity and *in vitro* fungicidal activity of liposome-intercalated amphotericin B. Antimicrob Agents Chemother 1987;31:421-9.
145. Juliano RL, Grant CW, Barber KR, Kalp MA. Mechanism of the selective toxicity of amphotericin B incorporated into liposomes. Mol Pharmacol 1987;31:1-11.
146. Clemons KV, Stevens DA. Comparative efficacy of amphotericin B colloidal dispersion and amphotericin B deoxycholate suspension in treatment of murine coccidioidomycosis. Antimicrob Agents Chemother 1991;35:1829-33.
147. Hostetler JS, Clemons KV, Hanson LH, Stevens DA. Efficacy and safety of amphotericin B colloidal dispersion compared with those of amphotericin B deoxycholate suspension for treatment of disseminated murine cryptococcosis. Antimicrob Agents Chemother 1992;36:2656-60.
148. Proffitt RT, Satorius A, Chiang SM, et al. Pharmacology and toxicology of a liposomal formulation of amphotericin B (AmBisome) in rodents. J Antimicrob Chemother 1991;28 Suppl B:49-61.
149. Ralph ED, Khazindar AM, Barber KR, Grant CW. Comparative *in vitro* effects of liposomal amphotericin B, amphotericin B-deoxycholate, and free amphotericin B against fungal strains determined by using MIC and minimal lethal concentration susceptibility studies and time-kill curves. Antimicrob Agents Chemother 1991;35:188-91.
150. Anaissie E, Paetznick V, Proffitt R, et al. Comparison of the *in vitro* antifungal activity of free and liposome-encapsulated amphotericin B. Eur J Clin Microbiol Infect Dis 1991;10:665-8.
151. Krause HJ, Juliano RL. Interaction of liposome-incorporated amphotericin B with kidney epithelial cell structures. Mol Pharmacol 1987.
152. Joly V, Dromer F, Barge J, et al. Incorporation of amphotericin B (AMB) into liposomes alters AMB-induced acute nephrotoxicity in rabbits. J Pharmacol Exp Ther 1989;251:311-6.
153. Longuet P, Joly V, Amirault P, et al. Limited protection by small unilamellar liposomes against the renal tubular toxicity induced by repeated amphotericin B infusions in rats. Antimicrob Agents Chemother 1991;35:1303-8.
154. Gondal JA, Swartz RP, Rahman A. Therapeutic evaluation of free and liposome-encapsulated amphotericin B in the treatment of systemic candidiasis in mice. Antimicrob Agents Chemother 1989;33:1544-8.
155. Lopez-Berestein G, Mehta R, Hopfer RL, et al. Treatment and prophylaxis of disseminated infection due to Candida albicans in mice with liposome-encapsulated amphotericin B. J Infect Dis 1983;147:939-45.

156. Lopez-Berestein G, Bodey GP, Frankel LS, Mehta K. Treatment of hepatosplenic candidiasis with liposomal-amphotericin B. J Clin Oncol 1987;5:310-7.
157. Lopez-Berestein G. Liposomes as carriers of antifungal drugs. Ann N Y Acad Sci 1988;544:590-7.
158. Lopez-Berestein G, Bodey GP, Fainstein V, et al. Treatment of systemic fungal infections with liposomal amphotericin B. Arch Intern Med 1989;149:2533-6.
159. Meunier F, Sculier JP, Coune A, et al. Amphotericin B encapsulated in liposomes administered to cancer patients. Ann N Y Acad Sci 1988;544:598-610.
160. Llanos-Cuentas, A., Chang J, Cieza J, Echevarria J, Garcia P, and Lentnek A. Safety and tolerance of amphotericin B lipid complex vs Fungizone in patients with mucocuntaneous leishmaniasis. Antimicrob Agents Chemother. 1990. Ref Type: Electronic Citation
161. Meunier F, Prentice HG, Ringden O. Liposomal amphotericin B (AmBisome): safety data from a phase II/III clinical trial. J Antimicrob Chemother 1991;28 Suppl B:83-91.
162. Ringden O, Meunier F, Tollemar J, et al. Efficacy of amphotericin B encapsulated in liposomes (AmBisome) in the treatment of invasive fungal infections in immunocompromised patients. J Antimicrob Chemother 1991;28 Suppl B:73-82.
163. Taylor RL, Williams DM, Craven PC, et al. Amphotericin B in liposomes: a novel therapy for histoplasmosis. Am Rev Respir Dis 1982;125:610-1.
164. Meunier F. New methods for delivery of antifungal agents. Rev Infect Dis 1989;11 Suppl 7:S1605-S1612.
165. Graybill JR, Craven PC, Taylor RL, et al. Treatment of murine cryptococcosis with liposome-associated amphotericin B. J Infect Dis 1982;145:748-52.
166. Wasan KM, Lopez-Berestein G. Modification of amphotericin B's therapeutic index by increasing its association with serum high-density lipoproteins. Ann N Y Acad Sci 1994;730:93-106.
167. Olsen SJ, Swerdel MR, Blue B, et al. Tissue distribution of amphotericin B lipid complex in laboratory animals. J Pharm Pharmacol 1991;43:831-5.
168. Poste G. Liposome targetting *in vivo*: problems and opportunites. Biol Cell 1983.
169. Doubek M, Mayer J, Lauschova I, et al. Comparison of the effect of amphotericin B desoxycholate and amphotericin B colloidal dispersion on renal functions and renal morphology in rats. Nephrology (Carlton) 2005;10:57-62.
170. Krejcirova L, Lauschova I, Horky D, et al. Influence of amphotericin B deoxycholate or amphotericin B colloidal dispersion on renal tubule epithelium in rat. Biomed Pap Med Fac Univ Palacky Olomouc Czech Repub 2004;148:221-3.
171. Simitsopoulou M, Roilides E, Dotis J, et al. Differential expression of cytokines and chemokines in human monocytes induced by lipid formulations of amphotericin B. Antimicrob Agents Chemother 2005;49:1397-403.
172. Carriagan C, Hanf-Kristufek. Comparison of amphotericin B products. BMJ 2001.
173. Lemke A, Kiderlen AF, Kayser O. Amphotericin B. Appl Microbiol Biotechnol 2005;68:151-62.
174. Wong-Beringer A, Jacobs RA, Guglielmo BJ. Lipid formulations of amphotericin B: clinical efficacy and toxicities. Clin Infect Dis 1998;27:603-18.
175. Deray G. Amphotericin B nephrotoxicity. Journal of Antimicrobial Chemotherapy 2002;49:37-41.
176. Hann IM, Prentice HG. Lipid-based amphotericin B: a review of the last 10 years of use. Int J Antimicrob Agents 2001;17:161-9.
177. Costa S, Nucci M. Can we decrease amphotericin nephrotoxicity? Curr Opin Crit Care 2001;7:379-83.
178. Blau IW, Fauser AA. Review of comparative studies between conventional and liposomal amphotericin B (Ambisome) in neutropenic patients with fever of unknown origin and patients with systemic mycosis. Mycoses 2000;43:325-32.
179. Veerareddy PR, Vobalaboina V. Lipid-based formulations of amphotericin B. Drugs Today (Barc) 2004;40:133-45.
180. Bowden R, Chandrasekar P, White MH, et al. A double-blind, randomized, controlled trial of amphotericin B colloidal dispersion versus amphotericin B for treatment of invasive aspergillosis in immunocompromised patients. Clin Infect Dis 2002;35:359-66.
181. Anaissie EJ, Vadhan-Raj S. Is it time to redefine the management of febrile neutropenia in cancer patients? Am J Med 1995;98:221-3.
182. Leenders AC, Daenen S, Jansen RL, et al. Liposomal amphotericin B compared with amphotericin B deoxycholate in the treatment of documented and suspected neutropenia-associated invasive fungal infections. Br J Haematol 1998;103:205-12.
183. White MH, Bowden RA, Sandler ES, et al. Randomized, double-blind clinical trial of amphotericin B colloidal dispersion vs. amphotericin B in the empirical treatment of fever and neutropenia. Clin Infect Dis 1998;27:296-302.
184. Walsh TJ, Finberg RW, Arndt C, et al. Liposomal amphotericin B for empirical therapy in patients with persistent fever and neutropenia. National Institute of Allergy and Infectious Diseases Mycoses Study Group. N Engl J Med 1999;340:764-71.
185. Walsh TJ, Pappas P, Winston DJ, et al. Voriconazole compared with liposomal amphotericin B for empirical antifungal therapy in patients with neutropenia and persistent fever. N Engl J Med 2002;346:225-34.
186. Prentice HG, Hann IM, Herbrecht R, et al. A randomized comparison of liposomal versus conventional amphotericin B for the treatment of pyrexia of unknown origin in neutropenic patients. Br J Haematol 1997;98:711-8.

187. Walsh TJ, Seibel NL, Arndt C, et al. Amphotericin B lipid complex in pediatric patients with invasive fungal infections. Pediatr Infect Dis J 1999;18:702-8.
188. Sandler ES, Mustafa MM, Tkaczewski I, et al. Use of amphotericin B colloidal dispersion in children. J Pediatr Hematol Oncol 2000;22:242-6.
189. Timmers GJ, Zweegman S, Simoons-Smit AM, et al. Amphotericin B colloidal dispersion (Amphocil) vs fluconazole for the prevention of fungal infections in neutropenic patients: data of a prematurely stopped clinical trial. Bone Marrow Transplant 2000;25:879-84.
190. Johnson JR. Voriconazole versus liposomal amphotericin B for empirical antifungal therapy. N Engl J Med 2002;346:1745-7.
191. Sharkey PK, Graybill JR, Johnson ES, et al. Amphotericin B lipid complex compared with amphotericin B in the treatment of cryptococcal meningitis in patients with AIDS. Clin Infect Dis 1996;22:315-21.
192. Chandrasekar P. The experience is CLEAR. Int J Antimicrob Agents 2006;27 Suppl 1:31-5.
193. Slain D, Miller K, Khakoo R, et al. Infrequent occurrence of amphotericin B lipid complex-associated nephrotoxicity in various clinical settings at a university hospital: a retrospective study. Clin Ther 2002;24:1636-42.
194. Aguado JM, Lumbreras C, Gonzalez-Vidal D. Assessment of nephrotoxicity in patients receiving amphotericin B lipid complex: a pharmacosurveillance study in Spain. Clin Microbiol Infect 2004;10:785-90.
195. Alexander BD, Wingard JR. Study of renal safety in amphotericin B lipid complex-treated patients. Clin Infect Dis 2005;40 Suppl 6:S414-S421.
196. Wingard JR, White MH, Anaissie E, et al. A randomized, double-blind comparative trial evaluating the safety of liposomal amphotericin B versus amphotericin B lipid complex in the empirical treatment of febrile neutropenia. L Amph/ABLC Collaborative Study Group. Clin Infect Dis 2000;31:1155-63.
197. Winston DJ, Schiller GJ. Controlled trials of amphotericin B lipid complex and other lipid-associated formulations. Clin Infect Dis 2000;30:236-7.
198. Cannon JP, Garey KW, Danziger LH. A prospective and retrospective analysis of the nephrotoxicity and efficacy of lipid-based amphotericin B formulations. Pharmacotherapy 2001;21:1107-14.
199. Miller CB, Waller EK, Klingemann HG, et al. Lipid formulations of amphotericin B preserve and stabilize renal function in HSCT recipients. Bone Marrow Transplant 2004;33:543-8.
200. Subira M, Martino R, Gomez L, et al. Low-dose amphotericin B lipid complex vs. conventional amphotericin B for empirical antifungal therapy of neutropenic fever in patients with hematologic malignancies--a randomized, controlled trial. Eur J Haematol 2004;72:342-7.
201. Martino R, Cortes M, Subira M, et al. Efficacy and toxicity of intermediate-dose amphotericin B lipid complex as a primary or salvage treatment of fungal infections in patients with hematological malignancies. Leuk Lymphoma 2005;46:1429-35.
202. Cesaro S, Zignol M, Burlina AB, et al. Assessment of nephrotoxicity of high-cumulative dose of liposomal amphotericin B in a pediatric patient who underwent allogenic bone marrow transplantation. Pediatric Transplantation 2006;10:255-8.
203. Johansen HK, Gotzsche PC. Amphotericin B lipid soluble formulations vs amphotericin B in cancer patients with neutropenia. Cochrane Database Syst Rev 2000;CD000969.
204. Barrett JP, Vardulaki KA, Conlon C, et al. A systematic review of the antifungal effectiveness and tolerability of amphotericin B formulations. Clin Ther 2003;25:1295-320.
205. Ostrosky-Zeichner L, Marr KA, Rex JH, Cohen SH. Amphotericin B: time for a new "gold standard". Clin Infect Dis 2003;37:415-25.
206. Johnson JR. Reduction of nephrotoxicity associated with amphotericin B deoxycholate. Clin Infect Dis 2004;38:303-7.
207. Schneemann M, Bachli EB. Continuous infusion of amphotericin B deoxycholate: a cost-effective gold standard for therapy of invasive fungal infections? Clin Infect Dis 2004;38:303-4.
208. Spellberg B, Witt MD, Beck CK. Amphotericin B: is a lipid-formulation gold standard feasible? Clin Infect Dis 2004;38:304-5.
209. Powers JH, Albrecht R. Lipid amphotericin B formulations as comparators in clinical trials. Clin Infect Dis 2004;38:305-6.
210. Bates DW, Su L, Yu DT, et al. Mortality and costs of acute renal failure associated with amphotericin B therapy. Clin Infect Dis 2001;32:686-93.
211. Harbarth S, Burke JP, Lloyd JF, et al. Clinical and economic outcomes of conventional amphotericin B-associated nephrotoxicity. Clin Infect Dis 2002;35:e120-e127.
212. Chen CY, Kumar RN, Feng YH, et al. Treatment outcomes in patients receiving conventional amphotericin B therapy: a prospective multicentre study in Taiwan. J Antimicrob Chemother 2006;57:1181-8.
213. Ullmann AJ, Sanz MA, Tramarin A, et al. Prospective study of amphotericin B formulations in immunocompromised patients in 4 European countries. Clin Infect Dis 2006;43:e29-e38.
214. Cagnoni PJ, Walsh TJ, Prendergast MM, et al. Pharmacoeconomic analysis of liposomal amphotericin B versus conventional amphotericin B in the empirical treatment of persistently febrile neutropenic patients. J Clin Oncol 2000;18:2476-83.

215. Harbarth S, Burke JP, Lloyd JF, et al. Clinical and economic outcomes of conventional amphotericin B-associated nephrotoxicity. Clin Infect Dis 2002;35:e120-e127.
216. Berdichevski RH, Luis LB, Crestana L, Manfro RC. Amphotericin B-related nephrotoxicity in low-risk patients. Braz J Infect Dis 2006;10:94-9.
217. Mora-Duarte J, Betts R, Rotstein C, et al. Comparison of caspofungin and amphotericin B for invasive candidiasis. N Engl J Med 2002;347:2020-9.
218. Walsh TJ, Teppler H, Donowitz GR, et al. Caspofungin versus liposomal amphotericin B for empirical antifungal therapy in patients with persistent fever and neutropenia. N Engl J Med 2004;351:1391-402.
219. Enoch DA, Ludlam HA, Brown NM. Invasive fungal infections: a review of epidemiology and management options. J Med Microbiol 2006;55:809-18.
220. Herbrecht R, Denning DW, Patterson TF, et al. Voriconazole versus amphotericin B for primary therapy of invasive aspergillosis. N Engl J Med 2002;347:408-15.
221. Gerkens JF, Bhagwandeen SB, Dosen PJ, Smith AJ. The effect of salt intake on cyclosporine-induced impairment of renal function in rats. Transplantation 1984;38:412-7.
222. Smith SR, Galloway MJ, Reilly JT, Davies JM. Amiloride prevents amphotericin B related hypokalaemia in neutropenic patients. J Clin Pathol 1988;41:494-7.

15 Sulfonamides, sulfadiazine, trimethoprim-sulfamethoxazole, pentamidine, pyrimethamine, dapsone, quinolones

Gabriel N. CONTRERAS, Cristiane MOCELIN CARVALHO,
Jorge M. DIEGO, Decio CARVALHO and Isabel ESPINAL

University of Miami, Florida, USA

Introduction

A number of drugs of miscellaneous class are capable of producing various degrees of renal damage and will be reviewed in this Chapter. Some have been used extensively in the past for the treatment of general infections (sulfonamides), others have had specific indications (pentamidine, dapsone), and others such as quinolones are of more recent application. Many of these, however, are of current interest because of their use in treating the complications occurring in patients with acquired immunodeficiency syndrome (AIDS).

Sulfonamides

These compounds were extensively used in the 40's through the 60's to treat pulmonary and other systemic infections. Reports of acute kidney injury, secondary to crystalluria were common [1-3]. Rarely, the sulfonamides can cause acute interstitial nephritis, necrotizing arteritis or hemoglobinuric acute kidney injury due to massive acute hemolytic anemia [4-6].

Data from the decade of 1940-1950 reviewed by Simon *et al* [7]in 1990 indicate an incidence of crystalluria of 0.4 to 49%, hematuria (with or without flank pain) of 1 to 32%, oliguria, anuria, or azotemia of 0.4 to 29%, and renal stones of 0.4 to 20%, for an overall incidence of renal toxicity (excluding crystals) between 1 and 32%. For a number of reasons detailed elsewhere [7], these early data are difficult to assess. However, even with the use of preventive measures such as urine alkalinization, renal toxicity was 2% [7], and the incidence of gross hematuria and microscopic hematuria despite high fluid intake were 2-3% and 24%, respectively [8]. A major limiting factor in the use of the sulfonamides was their limited solubility and the need of relatively large dosage, both favoring crystallization. This complication of sulfonamide therapy was well known at the time. In the ensuing decades more soluble sulfa compounds became available and the appearance of effective antibiotics resulted, with few exceptions, (i.e., sulfadiazine), in the replacement of the older sulfas as chemotherapeutic agents. Thus, the notion of the possibility of sulfonamide-induced nephrotoxicity was somewhat lost or became a rarity. The emerging use over the last 20 years of two sulfa compounds, sulfadiazine and trimethoprim-sulfamethoxazole, in the treatment of opportunistic infections of AIDS, has again brought to the attention of nephrologists and physicians the "old and perhaps forgotten" problem of sulfa nephrotoxicity. The review of the potential nephrotoxicity of sulfasalazine (5-aminosalicylic acid and sulfapyridine), a drug extensively used in patients with inflammatory bowel disease can be found in Chapter 13. Aside from the renal failure associated with sulfasalazine attributed initially to the intratubular precipitation of sulfapyridine crystals [9], currently sulfasalazine toxicity is considered secondary to its 5-aminosalicylic moiety.

Sulfadiazine

A large bibliography exists from the 1940's related to crystalluria and acute kidney injury associated with the use of sulfadiazine [1, 10, 11]. Sulfadiazine disappeared from clinical use for a long time until it re-emerged again in the AIDS era. More recently, the number of reports in adults and children has increased substantially because of the use of sulfadiazine and pyrimethamine, as the treatment of choice for cerebral toxoplasmosis associated with AIDS, other immunosuppressive states or specific infections [7, 12-35]. Acute kidney injury secondary to sulfadiazine crystalluria has been also reported in renal transplant patients[36, 37].

It is apparent that most recent cases of sulfadiazine-induced nephrotoxicity are not prospectively reported, thus the current incidence of sulfadiazine nephrotoxicity is unknown. In 1987, a study of 57 patients with AIDS treated for toxoplasma encephalitis indicated a renal toxicity of 6% [26]. A more recent international bibliographic search (1987 to 1995) reported 35 patients with AIDS and toxoplasma encephalitis with sulfadiazine nephrotoxicity [27]. In that study, the patients with AIDS who received sulfadiazine for toxoplasmosis were compared to those who received sulfadiazine in the 1940's and 1950's. The prevalence of sulfadiazine nephrotoxicity was 1.9 to 7.5% in the AIDS group and 1 to 4% in the non-AIDS patients. On average, renal dysfunction was evident after three weeks of treatment in the AIDS patients who received the larger cumulative dose of sulfadiazine (84 g) compared to the control group (40 g). Renal densities or stones were found by ultrasonography in 77% of the AIDS patients. The majority of the patients recovered rapidly (median of 6 days) with appropriate treatment.

Sulfadiazine is a short-acting sulfonamide derivative that undergoes acetylation in the liver to a variable degree (10-40%). The acetylation product has no antibacterial activity but retains its toxic potential. Indeed, the acetylated forms of older sulfas are less soluble and thus, more prone to crystalluria. About 30 to 55% of the drug is protein bound, and the binding decreases in renal failure. The kidney is the major route of excretion. Both, the free (60-85%) and acetylated (15-40%) forms are rapidly excreted in the urine in high concentration. Alkalinization increases the excretion of both forms by diminishing their tubular reabsorption. Because of the rapid excretion, large doses are required for the treatment of toxoplasmosis: 1 to 1.5 g every 6 hours if renal function is normal; reduction in dosage is necessary if renal function is impaired [25].

Sulfadiazine, like other sulfas, has a low urinary solubility, particularly in acid urine. When the urine is alkalinized and pH rises above 7.15, the drug ionizes and forms a soluble salt that is excreted avoiding crystallization. It has been estimated that at a pH of 5.5 about 16 liters of urine will be needed to insure that the sulfadiazine is soluble when excreted following a dose of 4 g per day [5]. Indeed, the urinary solubility of sulfadiazine and its major metabolite, acetylsulfadiazine, are many times higher at a pH of 7.5 than at a pH of 6.5 (sulfadiazine 200 and 28 mg/dl, acetylsulfadiazine 512 and 75 mg/dl, respectively) [30]. The crystals of sulfadiazine and acetylsulfadiazine can be recognized by examining the urine sediment, where they resemble characteristic "sheaves of wheat" [3]. As the crystals transit

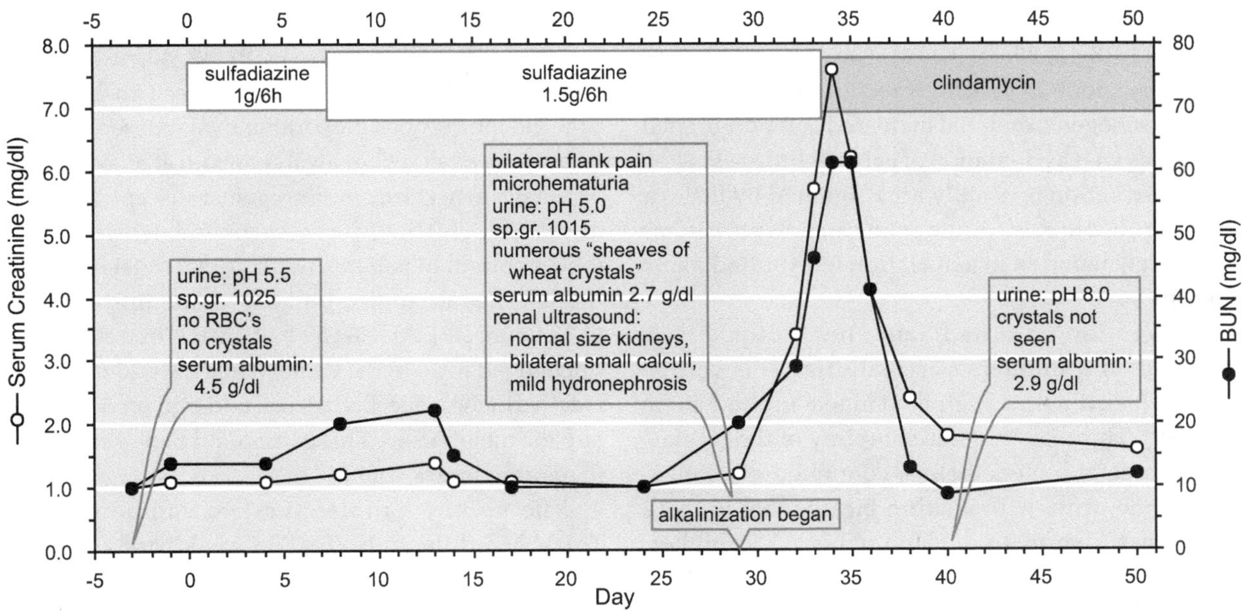

***Figure 1**. Sulfadiazine nephrotoxicity (crystalluria and acute renal failure). 35 year old man with AIDS and cerebral toxoplasmosis treated for 33 days with 4-6 g/day of sulfadiazine.The patient received oral hydration and possibly had an episode of transient renal impairment during days 8-13. By day 29 of treatment, crystalluria, hematuria, flank pain, renal calculi, and acute renal failure developed. Urine was alkalinized late in the course.*

through the tubular lumen they cause local abrasion and chemical irritation of the collecting duct epithelium and the lining of the urinary tract. There is peritubular hemorrhage, infiltration by white cells, necrosis, and calcium deposition. The crystals can form local concretions or small calculi leading to obstruction at any level from the collecting ducts to the bladder. This explains the clinical manifestations of the crystalluria and its associated renal pathology: asymptomatic crystalluria, microhematuria, gross hematuria, renal colic, oliguria, acute urinary tract obstruction, and acute kidney injury. An example of reversible sulfadiazine nephrotoxicity in a patient with AIDS and toxoplasma encephalitis is illustrated in Figure 1.

The risk factors for sulfadiazine nephrotoxicity in patients with AIDS include: (a) more prolonged courses of therapy as compared to those for community-acquired infections in normal hosts; (b) difficulty in maintaining high oral fluid intake in patients with toxoplasma encephalitis because of chronic illness, anorexia, and altered mental status; (c) concurrent fluid loses due to diarrhea; (d) levels of plasma creatinine within the range of "normal" despite impaired renal function due to AIDS-associated muscle wasting, thus masking renal insufficiency; (e) the presence of hypoalbuminemia and competition for the albumin binding sites of other antibiotics concomitantly administered, increasing the concentration of free-drug and the risk of crystalluria; and (f) the possibility of preexisting AIDS or non AIDS-related renal disease. It should be remembered that in patients with severe renal failure the serum half-life of sulfadiazine is prolonged from a normal value of 8 to 17 hours to 22 to 34 hours resulting in acetylation of sulfadiazine and a marked decrease in the active form of the drug with increase in the acetylated form, less soluble and more prone to crystallization [38]. Dosing recommendations for patients with renal failure can be found in recent reviews [39, 40].

The appearance of microhematuria or gross hematuria in a patient receiving sulfadiazine should raise the suspicion of crystalluria. The recognition of classical sulfadiazine crystals in the urine sediment does not confirm renal toxicity; but this finding should increase concern regarding its impending appearance. Unfortunately, urinalyses are not done regularly in these patients; therefore, the possibility of missing early microhematuria associated with sulfa crystals is real. Sulfadiazine stones are radiolucent and nicely demonstrated by ultrasonography [11, 15-17, 27, 28, 32-34]. The renal ultrasound findings include hyperechoic foci in the renal parenchyma, echogenic material in dilated and non-dilated calyces as well as dilatation of calyces and pelvis [28, 29]. Obstruction is usually accompanied by little or no hydronephrosis. Acute interstitial nephritis has been rarely reported in association with sulfadiazine therapy [42].

Prevention of sulfadiazine nephrotoxicity is centered in minimizing crystalluria. This can be accomplished with a high fluid intake (up to 3 liters per day). This may increase solubility of the crystals up to threefold. Nonetheless, continued alkalinization of the urine with sodium bicarbonate (6 to 12 g/day), assuring that the urine pH is 7.5 or higher, can increase solubility several fold and is very effective. As always, awareness of the possibility of this complication is the best form of prevention.

Treatment of sulfadiazine nephrotoxicity consists in stopping sulfadiazine or decreasing its dosage. The acute kidney injury, however, may resolve despite continuation of the treatment [41]. Hydration and especially alkalinization are the basis for the treatment. Urinary tract obstruction may require placement of ureteral stents [13] or nephrostomy [33]. This complication is essentially reversible and dialysis is rarely needed [27].

With increasing frequency, clindamycin in combination with pyrimethamine is been used as the replacement drug for sulfadiazine in the treatment of cerebral toxoplasmosis. Perhaps this new combination again may send sulfadiazine nephrotoxicity into "oblivion". Nevertheless, until this possibility occurs, primary care physicians should be aware that sulfadiazine can cause renal toxicity and that effective preventive measures are available.

Trimethoprim-sulfamethoxazole (cotrimoxazole)

The synergistic combination of trimethoprim (TMP), and sulfamethoxazole (SMZ), both folic acid antagonist antibacterial agents, was introduced over 30 years ago for its effect against a variety of infective organisms, including *Pneumocystis carinii (PC)*. Prior to the AIDS era, TMP-SMZ, also referred as cotrimoxazole, was used predominantly for the treatment of respiratory and urinary tract infections, including PC pneumonia (PCP) [42, 43, 47].

The fixed 1:5 TMP-SMZ ratio used in both the oral and intravenous preparations was chosen because it provides peak serum levels of about 1:20, which are optimally synergistic *in vitro* against susceptible pathogens [38]. TMP is 45% protein bound, whereas SMZ is 60% bound. In patients with normal renal function, the half-lifes are similar for both compounds- about 8 to 12 hours [47]. At least 50% of TMP is excreted as an unchanged form in the urine, while only 20% of SMZ is active in the urine. Both drugs undergo predominant hepatic metabolism. This compound penetrates body fluids and tissues well.

The kidney handles the two components of TMP-SMZ differently: TMP (a weak base with pKa of 7.3) is transported across the tubules by nonionic diffusion and is secreted into the urine [48], whereas SMZ undergoes glomerular filtration and tubular reabsorption [49]. Trimethoprim dissociation increases as pH falls. The unchanged base is more lipid-soluble and crosses cell membranes more readily than cations. Accordingly, TMP base diffuses passively from the peritubular fluid (pH 7.4) into the acidic urine via the tubular epithelium, and, thus, is excreted [48]. Their renal tubular accumulation is also different: In the rat [49], TMP, given alone [49, 50] or in combination with SMZ [49] achieves concentrations that are several folds greater in the renal cortex than in the serum or medium [51]. In contrast, the renal tissue concentration of SMZ is much less; SMZ concentration, when the agent is administered either alone or in combination with TMP is lower in the cortex, medulla and papilla than in the serum. Similar results were obtained in rhesus monkeys [52]. Trottier *et al* [49] have suggested that the "trapping" of TMP, in the acid tubular fluid environment, contributes to the high renal tissue accumulation of TMP. In contrast, SMZ, a weak acid with a pKa of 5.6 undergoes tubular reabsorption. Furthermore, the tissue concentrations and interactions of TMP and SMZ cannot be ascertained from their respective serum and urine levels [49]. Sulfamethoxazole is more soluble than older sulfonamides, and used at a lower dosage, resulting in a likelihood of crystalluria that is much smaller than with sulfadiazine and older sulfas.

It has been suggested by Berglund *et al* [53]

that TMP interferes with the tubular secretion of creatinine resulting in mild increases in its serum concentration and consequently decreases in the creatinine clearance (Ccr), whereas the glomerular filtration rate simultaneously measured with I131 iothalamate remains unchanged. This view was challenged by Shouval *et al* [54] who using the true creatinine method (Hare and Hare) for measuring Ccr found only very mild decreases in Ccr in normal subjects suggesting that the laboratory assay method used to measure creatinine may determine the variation of its serum levels. Nevertheless, there is convincing evidence to support the contention that the mild increase (about 15-20%) in serum creatinine (and the corresponding decrease in Ccr) reported in patients with normal renal function receiving TMP-SMZ is due to TMP interference with the tubular secretion of creatinine, as shown by simultaneous measurements of GFR by Ccr and independent methods (inulin, I131 iothalamate, and ^{51}Cr-EDTA) [53, 55-57]. Berglund *et al* [53] also suggested that the effects of TMP resulted from organic base inhibition of creatinine secretion. There was no evidence that SMZ affects creatinine transport [53]. Furthermore, *in vitro* studies in the rat strengthened the hypothesis that TMP inhibits creatinine secretion via the organic cation transport system [58]. The effect of TMP on serum creatinine is more pronounced in patients with decreased renal function [59, 60].

The dosage of TMP-SMZ should be reduced in patients with renal failure because the half-life of TMP becomes prolonged when GFR decreases below 30 ml/min [61], and in addition, there may be accumulation of the metabolite N-acetyl-SMZ [61, 62]. The latter may be associated with rare hypersensitivity reactions [63]or crystallization [64]. Dosing recommendations for patients with impaired renal function can be found in recent reviews [39, 40]. Because of effective removal of TMP-SMZ in patients with end-stage renal disease during hemodialysis, 50% of its maintenance dose should be supplemented after each dialysis [65]. Overall, it appears that TMP-SMZ can be given safely to patients with reduced renal function provided that the dosage is carefully reduced. Most problems arise when TMP-SMZ is given at its usual or larger dosage to patients with decreased function (serum creatinine above 2 mg/dl [59]), due to preexisting renal disease, presence of severe dehydration, or in association with other nephrotoxins [53, 66].

The clinical evaluation of the nephrotoxic effects of TMP-SMZ, notably much less frequent than other side effects of the drug (skin, gastrointestinal) and very rarely of a serious nature (hematological, dermatological), requires keeping in mind the already described effects of TMP on serum creatinine. In practical terms, an increase in serum creatinine concentration not accompanied by increases in blood urea nitrogen concentration or other data supporting a decrease in GFR, does not indicate renal dysfunction.

In view of the extensive use of this compound around the world for the treatment of urinary tract infections, renal adverse reactions are extremely rare. Indeed, in 1982 the Boston Collaborative Drug Surveillance Program reporting on data obtained from 1966 through 1980 on 1121 hospitalized patients receiving TMP-SMZ described an overall incidence of adverse effects of 8%[67]. The most common were gastrointestinal (3.9%), and dermatological (3.3%). Four patients with elevations of serum creatinine (0.4%), and one patient with transient renal tubular acidosis were reported. Unfortunately, given the nature of this study (many hospitals, many physicians reporting) the exact causal role, rarely could be established with certainty. Nevertheless, this report emphasizes the extreme rarity of the association of renal toxicity with TMP-SMZ therapy.

The risk of developing serious renal toxicity in people receiving TMP-SMZ, TMP alone, or cephalexin was also estimated in a large British population, and found to be extremely low [68]. Only five cases of acute parenchymal renal disease occurred in the almost 700,000 subjects evaluated, suggesting that none was likely to be caused by the study drugs. Nonetheless, since in these patients TMP-SMZ manifests considerable extrarenal toxicity, reduction of dosage according to GFR, Ccr or to measured blood levels should be considered in patients with impaired renal function.

In accordance with the better urinary solubility of SMZ, in comparison to older sulfas or sulfadiazine, reports of renal dysfunction secondary to crystalluria are extremely rare [69-71]. Even this theoretical risk inherited from the experience with older sulfas and sulfadiazine, can be avoided by providing adequate hydration.

When the drug is given intravenously a potential problem due to fluid volume load may arise. Because TMP-SMZ is relatively unstable in solution, it is the recommendation of the manufacturers that each ampule of TMP-SMZ (80 mg of TMP and 400 mg of SMZ) be dissolved in 75 to 125 ml of 5% dextrose in water. This relatively large water load may lead to hyponatremia, particularly in predisposed patients, such as those with impaired renal function, borderline cardiorespiratory status, AIDS with increased AVP levels, and in those treated with high dose TMP-SMZ [71-73]. The use of a smaller volume (50 ml) of isotonic sodium chloride solution as diluent for TMP-SMZ should mitigate this potential problem [74].

Non-oliguric acute tubular necrosis associated with interstitial edema and cellular infiltration was described in two patients treated with TMP-SMZ reported by Kalowski *et al* [59]. The same group [75] reported four patients with underlying renal disease and a hypersensitivity rash who developed acute kidney injury when treated with TMP-SMZ. Two patients died, and in two, the renal biopsy showed acute interstitial nephritis with prominent eosinophilic infiltrates. Recurrent acute kidney injury secondary to acute interstitial nephritis with mononuclear cell and eosinophilic infiltrates was described in a patient treated with TMPSMZ but also receiving penicillin-type drugs and gentamicin [66]. Other cases of acute interstitial nephritis have been reported, including those presenting in children [76-79]and in renal transplant recipients [80]. It should be noted, that many of the patients described with renal impairment were elderly [59], had preexisting renal dysfunction, were receiving other drugs with nephrotoxic potential or received large doses, or doses inappropriate for the level of renal function. As noted, before the AIDS era, TMP-SMZ was considered a safe drug, even when administered for prolonged periods [44], or in patients with renal impairment if the daily dose is appropriately adjusted [45, 81, 82].

Rare life-threatening multisystemic reactions to TMP-SMZ with severe skin lesions and progressive renal, hepatic, and cardiac damage appearing immediately or weeks after the drug was discontinued have been described [83, 84]. In these patients the renal lesion was interstitial nephritis, and thus, the clinical picture may represent an extension of the more limited forms of hypersensitivity reactions. These severe lesions have been tentatively attributed to an inherent defect in mechanisms normally responsible for inactivating or detoxifying sulfonamide metabolites (i.e., hydroxylamine metabolite of SMZ), resulting in both direct cytotoxicity and an immune hypersensitivity reaction [85].

There are two groups of patients that currently are of particular interest to the nephrologists with respect to potential TMP-SMZ nephrotoxicity: transplant recipients and patients with AIDS. In these two groups, TMP-SMZ is usually used either for the treatment of infections or for the long-term prophylaxis against opportunistic infections. In addition, TMP-SMZ is concomitantly used with other potentially nephrotoxic drugs in these two patients' groups.

As noted before, renal biopsy documented acute interstitial nephritis has been described in few transplant patients treated with TMP-SMZ prior to the cyclosporine era, usually for urinary tract infection or PC pneumonia [59, 80]. Reports of synergistic renal toxicity between TMP-SMZ and cyclosporine also appeared [86-89]. Thompson and co-workers [86] reported that transplant recipients receiving cyclosporine developed a marked impairment in renal function when treated with TMP or TMP-SMZ, the majority for asymptomatic bacteremia. Renal dysfunction reversed with discontinuation of the sulfa compound. A graft renal biopsy was performed in one patient, and revealed mild focal mononuclear cell infiltration in the interstitium. Five patients received TMP alone, including the one who was biopsied. In another case series, Josephson and co-workers reported five renal transplant recipients with acute renal allograft dysfunction or delayed allograft function in which the renal biopsies showed histopathologic features of drug-induced interstitial nephritis without evidence of acute rejection, calcineurin inhibitor nephrotoxicity, or both. All the patients were receiving TMP-SMZ and other drugs associated with acute interstitial nephritis [90]. The renal biopsy findings in these patients revealed focal interstitial infiltrates of primarily mononuclear inflammatory cells with prominent involvement at the corticomedullary junction and clusters of eosinophils within the infiltrates, typical features of drug-induced acute interstitial nephritis [91].

A prospective randomized-double-blind study of prophylaxis of infections with oral TMP-SMZ in renal transplant recipients concluded that long-term prophylaxis (average 8.9 months) conferred significant protection against infection after transplantation [92]. The sulfa compound was very well tolerated by the 66 patients randomized to receive the drug, and no patient developed hypersensitivity reactions, perhaps due to the concomitant immunosuppressive therapy. Serum creatinine levels were 15% higher in the patients receiving TMP-SMZ, whereas no such increase was observed in the control group. Nevertheless, GFR measured with ^{99m}Tc-DTPA showed no change in a crossover study performed in 17 of the patients studied with TMP-SMZ. Furthermore, the authors demonstrated that the differences in serum creatinine were not due to interference of TMP-SMZ, cyclosporine or both with the method used for the measurement of creatinine (automated Jaffe reaction). Moreover, TMP-SMZ did not influence the pharmacokinetics of cyclosporine or result in decreased immunosuppression or increased incidence of rejection. Sulfamethoxazole may interfere with the measurement of cyclosporine by high-pressure liquid chromatography but not by radioimmunoassay [92] resulting in higher levels [93]. On the basis of their experience, the authors cautioned about the reports of putative toxicity in renal transplant patients receiving oral TMP-SMZ therapy simultaneously with cyclosporine. The prophylactic treatment was effective, safe, and cost effective [92]. The effect of larger intravenous dosage has not been studied.

The evaluation of the possible renal toxicity of TMP-SMZ or other drugs in patients with AIDS is compounded by the many factors that can cause renal dysfunction in these patients. These include preexisting renal disease, including HIV-related nephropathy [94-97], frequent dehydration or marked hypoalbuminemia resulting in severe volume contraction, and the concomitant or sequential use of drugs with known nephrotoxic potential. On the other hand, severe muscular wasting, by decreasing the body pool of creatinine, results in lower serum creatinine levels, thereby masking the presence of renal impairment. Of interest is the observation that the incidence of hypersensitivity reactions to drugs might be less in AIDS patients due to their immunodeficient state [92].

Prior to the recognition of AIDS as a major health problem, immunosuppressed patients with PCP (children with immune deficiency disorders or patients receiving cytotoxic or immunosuppressive drugs for lymphoreticular malignancies or organ transplantation) were treated with TMP-SMZ and/or pentamidine with varied success, depending in great measure on the underlying condition [98, 99]. Currently, in most patients with AIDS, TMP-SMZ represents the treatment of choice for PCP. Although, an increase in the incidence of side effects attributable to TMP-SMZ particularly dermatologic, hematologic, and hepatic toxicities has been recognized in patients with AIDS when compared to patients without AIDS, no increase in nephrotoxicity was reported [100, 101].

When compared to pentamidine, TMP-SMZ has been associated with a lesser degree of renal impairment in the treatment of opportunistic infections in AIDS. In a prospective, randomized study of patients with AIDS, Wharton *et al* [102] reported major adverse renal reactions characterized by an increase in serum creatinine of ≥ 3.0 mg/dl in 1 of 32 patients treated with intravenous TMP-SMZ in comparison to 2 of 32 patients receiving pentamidine. Lesser increases in serum creatinine (levels between 1.5 to 3.0 mg/dl) occurred in 11 of 32 (34%) and 19 of 32 (59%), respectively. Sattler *et al* [103] in a prospective, randomized noncrossover study found elevations of serum creatinine in 21 of 34 (64%) patients receiving intravenous pentamidine for about 16 days. The average increase in creatinine above baseline (1.0±0.1 mg/dl) was 1.6±1.1 mg/ dl; in four patients the peak serum creatinine ranged from 4.1 to 6.6 mg/dl. By contrast, in the 36 patients receiving TMP-SMZ, creatinine concentration increased only in five (14%), a value significantly different from that of the pentamidine group ($p < 0.0001$). The known effect of TMP on the tubular secretion of creatinine may have been in part responsible for the latter changes. Gordin *et al* [104] in a retrospective study reported no renal abnormalities with TMP/SMZ in 37 patients, whereas elevations in serum creatinine occurred in 6 of 30 patients treated with pentamidine. Overall, however, the incidence of non-renal side effects was higher with TMP-SMZ.

Zuñiga et al retrospectively evaluated renal function in 38 patients (mean age 38±2 years) [105]with AIDS and PCP who were treated with intravenous TMP-SMZ for 5 to 24 days (average of 10±1 days). The dose of TMP was 19±2 (SE) and that of SMZ 95±5 mg/kg day. Risk factors for nephrotoxicity were identified: volume depletion (47%), preexisting renal dysfunction (11%), sepsis (13%), and concomitant use of known nephrotoxic agents (18%). Nephrotoxicity was defined as an increase in serum creatinine concentration of at least 0.5 mg/dl above baseline. In only three patients did serum creatinine increase above baseline. In two of these, other risk factors for nephrotoxicity were present (volume depletion, gentamicin, and amphotericin B). Thus, in only one of 38 patients (2.6%) was the renal dysfunction attributable to TMP-SMZ. Estimated creatinine clearance in 22 patients (Cockcroft and Gault formula) remained stable: at baseline, 107±10 ml/min; at peak change, 106±11 ml/min, and at end of treatment 101±9 ml/min. In four patients who have elevated serum creatinine levels at baseline, the values declined toward normal despite continuing TMP-SMZ administration (Figure 2). There was no relationship between the duration of treatment and the change in serum creatinine. From these data we can conclude that TMP-SMZ is a safe drug for the treatment of PCP in patients with AIDS. Even in the presence of compounding risk factors for nephrotoxicity, the risk seems very low.

These findings are in accordance with Chua et al study in the volume depleted female Sprague-Dawley rat [106]. Rats were injected intramuscularly with five times the human dose of TMP-SMZ (100/500 mg/kg/ day) for nine days. Prior to treatment, the animals were placed in a low sodium diet for seven days and salt depleted by means of administration of furosemide (2 mg/kg/day) for the first three days. At baseline, experimental and control (glucose given instead of TMP-SMZ) groups have similar GFR, serum creatinine, and hematocrit and were conserving sodium maximally. Nine days of TMP-SMZ did not affect GFR, serum creatinine or electrolyte levels. Loss of body weight and anemia only developed in the rats treated with TMP-SMZ. In this study performed in female rats, known to have a lower tubular secretion of creatinine [107, 108], TMP did not appear to decrease the tubular secretion of creatinine.

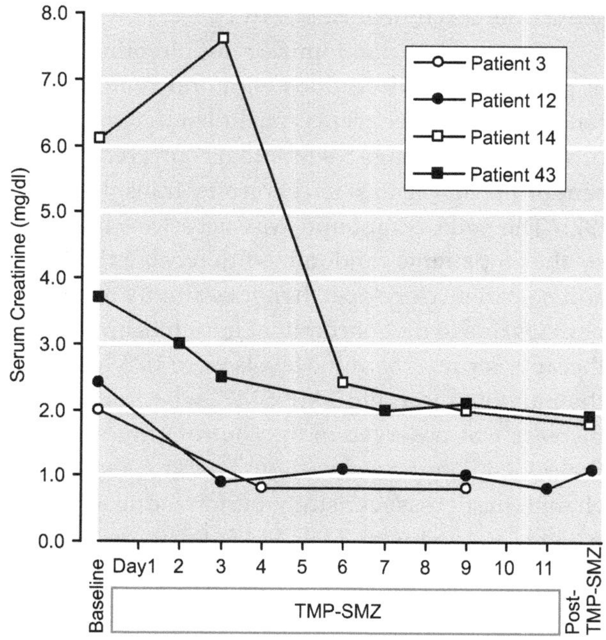

Figure 2. *Effect of intravenous TMP-SMZ in four patients with AIDS and PCP and prior impaired renal function. Patients received 20 mg of SMZ per Kg body weight per day for 9 to 11 days given intravenously. Data from Zúñiga et al [105].*

In HIV-infected patients, nephrotoxicity from oral TMP-SMZ in long-term prophylaxis against opportunistic infections is not seen or is notably much less frequent than other side effects of the drug (dermatological, gastrointestinal, and hematological). Bozzette *et al* [109] in a randomized trial reported no renal abnormalities with TMP-SMZ in 276 patients with a total 690 person-years of follow-up. Similarly, in another randomized trial of TMP-SMZ used as primary prophylaxis for PCP, Para *et al* [110] did not report renal abnormalities, however, 33% of study subjects discontinued TMP-SMZ due to non-renal-limiting adverse effects. Most of these treatment-limiting reactions occurred within the first four weeks of beginning therapy, and the gradual initiation of TMP-SMZ was associated with significantly fewer adverse drug reactions.

Although, the nephrotoxicity from the use of TMP-SMZ alone for long-term seems rare, TMP-SMZ can potentiate the renal toxic effects of other drugs concomitantly used in HIV-infected patients. In one retrospective study by Boubaker et al [111], 18.6% of HIV-infected patients treated with indinavir and TMP-SMZ had a sustained elevation of creatinine associated with leukocyturia and renal parenchymal abnormalities attributed to indinavir-induced crystal nephropathy. Nephrolithiasis is the most common serious adverse effect reported in 4%-9% of HIV-infected patients treated with indinavir [112] [113]. In Boubaker et al study [111], the prolong use of TMP-SMZ for more than 160 weeks increased indinavir nephrotoxicity risk by 4.7 folds (95% CI, 1.2-19.2) independently of other predictors. These findings are in accordance with Araujo and Seguro study in male Wistar rats [114]. In that study, rats in six groups received for 15 days by gavage: 1) vehicle-control; 2) indinavir 80 mg/kg; 3) TMP-SMZ 100 mg of TMP/kg; 4) the combination of indinavir and TMP-SMZ; 5) nelfinavir 75 mg/kg; 6) the combination of nelfinavir and TMP-SMZ. At baseline, all the groups had similar characteristics. At follow-up, no changes were observed in body weight, urine volume and blood pressure. TMP-SMZ induced a small non-significant decrease in inulin clearance (0.72 ± 0.03 mL/min/100 g BW) without alterations of tubular functions. Indinavir decreased significantly inulin clearance (indinavir: 0.48 ± 0.04 vs. control: 0.93 ± 0.08 mL/min/100 g BW, $p < 0.001$) and renal blood flow (indinavir: 6.2 ± 0.2 vs. control: 8.0 ± 0.3 mL/min, $p < 0.05$). Indinavir renal adverse effects, inulin clearance (indinavir+TMP-SMZ: 0.39 ± 0.03 vs. control: 0.93 ± 0.08 mL/min/100 g BW, $p < 0.001$) and renal blood flow (indinavir+TMP-SMZ: 3.8 ± 0.4 vs. control: 8.0 ± 0.3 mL/min, $p < 0.05$) were potentiated by the concomitant use of TMP-SMZ. Nelfinavir alone or in combination with TMP-SMZ effects on inulin clearance and renal blood flow were not different from controls. In summary, these resuts suggest that indinavir nephrotoxicity in rats is potentiated by TMP-SMZ. The mechanism involved in this enhanced nephrotoxicity could be related to metabolism or to excretion interactions between both drugs. Drug interactions with TMP-SMZ can occur via the inhibition of hepatic metabolism by the cytochrome p450 enzyme system. Also, TMP is a known inhibitor of renal tubular secretion and indinavir and TMP are both weak bases that could compete for the same carrier proteins of the organic renal transport system in the proximal tubule. Currently availability of various protease inhibitors allows better tailoring of treatment in patients receiving TMP-SMZ. The increased risk of indinavir nephrotoxicity when used with TMP-SMZ for long-term should make clinicians choose an alternative protease inhibitor to minimize renal adverse effects.

The use of TMP-SMZ has been associated with the appearance of *hyperkalemia*. In one study, patients with underlying renal filtration dysfunction receiving large dose of TMP-SMZ were particularly susceptible to hyperkalemia [73]. In other studies, patients either had AIDS and were receiving large doses of TMP-SMZ for the treatment of PCP [115-117] or were elderly subjects without either AIDS or PCP treated for respiratory or urinary tract infections with standard doses [118-120]. The hyperkalemia is usually mild (rarely exceeding 6.5 mEq/L) and reversible on discontinuation of the drug. It appears that in patients without renal dysfunction, AIDS, or advance age hyperkalemia must be very rare since no case of hyperkalemia was reported in 649 patients treated with standard doses of TMP-SMZ [121]. Indeed in Chua et al experimental study no changes in serum potassium occurred in rats treated with TMP-SMZ for nine days [106]: baseline, 5.24±0.06 mEq/L; day 5, 5.14±0.13 mEq/L; day 9, 5.23±0.12 mEq/L; n=7. Initially, in the patients with AIDS, the hyperkalemia was attributed to adrenal insufficiency or the syndrome of hyporeninemic hypoaldosteronism [122-124]. Velazquez and coworkers [125] reported 30 consecutive hospitalized patients with PCP during treatment with high dose TMP-SMZ or TMP-dapsone and noted that 27 of the 30 patients exhibited a rise in serum potassium. Fifteen of these patients developed a peak serum potassium concentration greater than 5 mEq/L, while two reached a potassium concentration more than 6 mEq/L. Seven patients were studied in detail. Among these patients, urinary potassium concentrations averaged 11.3±5.8 mEq/L, urinary sodium averaged 103±65 mEq/L, and the average transtubular potassium concentration gradient was 1.9±1.1. Three patients restudied after discontinuation of TMP-SMZ showed normalization of their transtubular potassium concentration gradients. Their renal function was within normal limits and serum cortisol, plasma renin activity and plasma aldosterone concentrations were also normal or high during hyperkalemia. It has been suggested that TMP, even at lower dosage, has an effect similar to amiloride, inhibiting apical sodium channels in the distal nephron and effectively reducing the transepithelial voltage that favors potassium secretion in a dose-dependent fashion [117, 125, 126]. A patient with renal tubular acidosis associated with TMP administration has been described suggesting also an abnormal proton excretion due to the altered transepithelial voltage in the distal nephron [127].

In summary, taken as a whole, the clinical and experimental data indicated that TMP-SMZ when used intravenously for the treatment of infections or orally for long-term prophylaxis against opportunistic infections is safe, and it is accompanied by very low incidence of nephrotoxicity. The risk factors associated with nephrotoxicity are preexisting renal dysfunction, concomitant use of other drugs potentially nephrotoxic, advanced age, volume depletion, dose inappropriately adjusted for the level of renal function, and sepsis. When TMP-SMZ toxicity occurs pathways of nephrotoxicity are tubulo-obstructive, tubulotoxic, and immunologic.

Pentamidine

Pentamidine is a diamidine compound developed more than five decades ago [128]. Initially, it was only used for its antiprotozoal properties against African trypanosomiasis [129], and visceral leishmaniasis [130]. Subsequently, its use was extended to the treatment and prophylaxis of PCP in immunosuppressed patients [131-133]. The use of pentamidine, which was rare in countries without tropical diseases, increased notably because of the high incidence of PCP observed in patients with AIDS [72, 97, 134-136]. Until 1984, pentamidine distribution in the USA was restricted; indeed it was only available through the Center for Disease Control. Although TMP-SMZ is regarded as the preferred treatment for PCP [102, 103], pentamidine or less frequently used combinations (trimetrexate/leucovorin, clindamycin/primaquine [137]) are reasonable alternatives when TMP-SMZ is not tolerated or is without effect [138].

The pharmacological properties of pentamidine have been studied for decades [139] and the development of high-performance liquid chromatographic and biological assays has permitted studies of the distribution and pharmacokinetics of this medication [140]. For a number of reasons detailed elsewhere [141], the true half-life of pentamidine is difficult to measure in humans. Pentamidine is largely bound to plasma proteins, [134] has a high volume of distribution, a long elimination half life (4 to > 12 days), [142, 143]is mainly metabolized by the liver (with interindividual differences in metabolism rates) [144] and has a low renal excretion of 5-12% of the administered dose [142]. Conte et al studied the pharmacokinetics of intravenous pentamidine during multiple dosing [145] in patients with AIDS with normal renal function and in those receiving hemodialysis [141, 145]. In their study, the true-elimination (slowest) half-life ranged from 29 hours (3 mg/kg dose) for the patients with normal renal function to 73 to 118 hours for the patients on maintenance hemodialysis (3 or 4 mg/kg dose). Conte estimated that renal clearance accounted for about 2% of the plasma clearance in patients with normal renal function, and that renal excretion increases with repeated dosing. The complete absence of renal function resulted in an increased drug disposition or ultimate total-body pentamidine burden.

Experiments utilizing clinically relevant multiple dosing regimens of pentamidine (10 mg/kg for 14 days) in rats showed that following the initial injection, pentamidine appears in the urine in small amounts; however, with each subsequent injection, there is a progressive increase in the urinary excretion of pentamidine, whereas fecal excretion did not increase in a similar manner. Plasma levels of pentamidine were very low, the drug accumulated in several tissues, with the kidney achieving the highest concentration, followed by the lungs, spleen, pancreas, stomach, and lesser levels in the liver, heart, and other organs [146]. Similar results have been found in the dog [147]. In the rat, fat and muscle did not contain much pentamidine raising the possibility, contrary to common belief, that metabolism of pentamidine may occur *in vivo* [148].

Interestingly, it was shown that pentamidine slowly accumulates in and is slowly excreted from the major human organs; detectable levels of pentamidine are present in some tissues as late as one year after the last dose. Tissue levels of pentamidine obtained in autopsy specimens from AIDS patients revealed that tissue accumulation was usually greater in liver, kidneys, adrenal glands, and spleen than in the lung. Nevertheless, there is no correlation between tissue levels and renal dysfunction, as measured by serum creatinine levels [149].

Poola et al studied the renal excretion of pentamidine in the isolated perfused rat kidney, which is an established model to study the renal disposition of drugs and that correlates with *in vivo* disposition. The data showed that a combination of filtration, active secretion and passive reabsortion are involved in the renal disposition of pentamidine [150].

Prior to the AIDS epidemic, the incidence of acute kidney injury associated with intravenous pentamidine administration for the treatment of PCP was between 19 to 23% [132, 134]. During the 1980's the number of reported cases increased (Table 1). The average incidence of nephrotoxicity, the most frequent systemic adverse effect, was 41%, ranging from 20 to 94% as reported in 475 patients [102-104, 137, 151-155]. If other risk factors for renal impairment are not present the majority of the cases reported are mild (see below). The acute kidney injury is usually of the nonoliguric variety. There is mild proteinuria, glycosuria, pyuria, and granular casts. Gross hematuria can occur [156], as well as myoglobinuria [157]. Renal failure usually appears within the second week of treatment, and the recovery begins within few days after discontinuation of pentamidine. Nevertheless, it may take several weeks before renal function returns to baseline. Dialysis support may be necessary [39]. Nephrotoxicity can occur after repeated treatment courses with pentamidine [137].

From October 1988 to January 1989, Chua et al undertook a retrospective analysis of 33 consecutive patients with AIDS who received intravenous pentamidine isethionate for at least seven days for the treatment of PCP [154]. Nephrotoxicity was defined as a rise in serum creatinine greater than 0.5 mg/dl above baseline. Nephrotoxicity developed in 33%; it was mild and reversible in the majority of patients. Only one patient developed severe acute kidney injury. Comparison of patients who developed nephrotoxicity (n=11) with those without renal impairment (n=22) revealed similar age, body weight, initial serum creatinine concentration, and total dose of pentamidine received. Particular attention was given to the presence of other risk factors for the development of nephrotoxicity, such as: volume depletion, sepsis, preexisting renal dysfunction, and recent or concomitant use of other nephrotoxic agents (aminoglycosides, radiocontrast, and non-steroidal anti-inflammatory agents). The risk of nephrotoxicity during pentamidine treatment was directly related to the number of risk factors present (r=0.93; p=0.02). Ten of 11 patients with pentamidine nephrotoxicity (91%) had additional risk factors. In contrast, 13 of 22 patients without nephrotoxicity (59%) had no risk factors (X^2; p <0.02). The clinical data as well as experimental results in rats [158] suggest that pentamidine has a relatively low toxicity index, and that concomitant risk factors, particularly, volume depletion are of importance in determining the appearance

Table 1. Clinical studies reporting on adverse effects of pentamidine in patients with AIDS (1984-1997).

Authors (Reference)	Nº of patients	Nº and (%) of patients with any adverse effect[a]	Nº and (%) of patients with nephrotoxicity[b]
Gordin et al [104]	30	13 (43%)	6 (20%)
Andersen et al [151]	24	20 (83%)	6 (25%)
Wharton et al [102]	32	32 (100%)	21 (65%)
Waskin et al [152]	164	94 (57%)	38 (23%)
Lachaal et al [153]	16	15 (94%)	5 (94%)
Sattler et al [103]	33	NA	21 (64%)
Chua et al [154]	33	NA	11 (33%)
Briceland et al [155]	37	NA	27 (73%)
O'Brien et al [137]	106	76 (72%)	48 (45%)[c]
Total	**475**	**250 (67%)**	**193 (41%)**

[a] *These include immediate reactions (hypotension, nausea/vomiting, arrythmias, etc.), local reactions (pain at injection site, phebitis, urticaria, etc.), and systemic adverse effects (hematologic, fever, liver, renal dysfunction, and electrolyte abnormalities).*

[b] *Nephrotoxicity defined as increase in serum creatinine concentration: >30% above baseline [104]; increase of 0.5 mg/dL or 50% above baseline [103, 137, 153-155], or not specified [102,151].* [c] *In 54% of these patents nephrotoxicity was associated with the concurrent use of other nephrotoxic agents.*

NA = not available

of nephrotoxicity in patients with AIDS. This is supported by the suggestion that patients receiving pentamidine as outpatients may have a greater risk of nephrotoxicity than those treated under inpatient conditions, perhaps because the intravenous fluid therapy that they receive is less aggressive [159]. In a recent retrospective review [137] the most significant risk factor for adverse pentamidine reactions was an increased number of concomitant medications, non-white ethnicity, concomitant use of nephrotoxic drugs, and daily cumulative dose of pentamidine.

Antoniskis et al reported four cases of reversible acute kidney injury in patient with AIDS who received both intravenous pentamidine (for PCP) and amphotericin B (for systemic mycoses). Of note, nephrotoxicity did not develop in three AIDS' patients treated with both TMP-SMZ and amphotericin B or in two patients who concomitantly received inhaled pentamidine and amphotericin B [160]. Reports of renal damage in patients receiving parenteral pentamidine for the treatment of non-HIV diseases continue. Reversible acute kidney injury and nephrotic syndrome were documented in a young child given pentamidine mesylate and an antimonial salt for the treatment of visceral leishmaniasis [161]. In Africa (Kenya) patients with visceral leishmaniasis have developed renal toxicity during prolonged treatment (1 to 10 months) with pentamidine [162].

Currently, pentamidine in the form of aerosol is used for the prophylaxis of PCP with apparent success [163-166]. Initially no renal side effects were described with its use. However, two reports of acute renal dysfunction raised the possibility of a systemic absorption of aerosolized pentamidine [167, 168]. One of the patients received a previous large dose of TMP-SMZ and the other appears to have had concomitant volume depletion caused by severe diarrhea while an elevation of serum creatinine occurred. We have been unable to find additional reports of renal toxicity associated with aerosol pentamidine administration[169]. Likewise, no renal side effects were reported with the use of aerosolized pentamidine for the prophylaxis of PCP in patients who received bone marrow, renal or hepatic transplants [165, 166]. Although the use of aerosolized pentamidine may be associated with renal dysfunction, this seems much less frequent compared to the parenteral administration of this drug.

Early experimental studies of pentamidine renal toxicity in animals were limited to few sheep, goats [170] and rabbits [171] given rather large doses of pentamidine (up to 40 mg/kg). The results of these studies, although indicating some degree of renal toxicity, are difficult to interpret because of the small number of animals employed, the large doses of pentamidine used, and the absence of controls or detailed renal function studies.

The exact mechanism of pentamidine renal toxicity is unknown. Early on, Makula et al suggested that renal toxicity may result from the ability of pentamidine to react with and form insoluble precipitates with nucleotides, leading to depletion of the nucleotide pool (e.g. ATP) necessary for various energy-dependent functions; inhibition of DNA, RNA and protein synthesis. In addition, the complexes could be deposited in the kidney impairing the normal filtration process [172].

A study explored in rats, some possible pathogenetic mechanisms for pentamidine nephrotoxicity [171]. The authors measured the urinary loss of tubular cells, malate dehydrogenase activity, and creatinine clearance after five daily injections of pentamidine. The tubular toxicity of pentamidine was dose-related (1, 10, or 20 mg/day/ 5 days) and reversible. As expected, tobramycin, amphotericin B, and cyclosporine increased pentamidine nephrotoxicity. On the other hand, fosfomycin (an inhibitor of cell wall synthesis) and D-glucoro-1, 5-lactam (an inhibitor of lysosomal β-glucuronidase) ameliorated the renal dysfunction, and both verapamil and enalapril increased creatinine clearance reversing the effect of pentamidine. The authors suggested that pentamidine may share some of the mechanisms of tubular toxicity attributed to the aminoglycosides. Furthermore, they proposed that drugs that stabilize lysosomal membranes, inhibit lysosomal enzymes' activity or change renal hemodynamics may decrease pentamidine nephrotoxicity.

Poola et al studied pentamidine toxicity in the isolated perfused rat kidney evaluating the effects of dosing and co-administration of tetraethylammonium [150]. They also found that tubulotoxicity of pentamidine is dose-related and attributed to its degree of kidney sequestration caused by either the administration of a high dose of drug or by decreased tubular transport as caused by tetraethylammonium. Important for clinical practice is the possibility that medications that are substrates for the luminal organic cation transporter can alter the renal disposition of pentamidine, increasing the risk of nephrotoxicity. Although not examined in this study, it was suggested that lysosomal accumulation could be involved in the mechanism of toxicity.

Chua et al investigated the effects of volume depletion and blockade of prostaglandin synthesis on pentamidine nephrotoxicity in the female Sprague-Dawley rat treated for a prolonged period, similar to that used in clinical protocols [158]. First, intact animals were injected for 14 days with subcutaneous pentamidine given at daily doses of 4, 10, or 20 mg/kg. With this protocol no changes in serum creatinine were observed. To mimic the state of volume depletion commonly seen in patients with AIDS, sequentially studied groups of rats were placed in a low sodium diet one week prior to injections. In addition, all groups received daily injections of indomethacin while receiving pentamidine (20 mg/kg/ day) for 14 days. The creatinine clearance decreased 35% ($p<0.03$) only in the group treated with salt restriction plus indomethacin and pentamidine, and this difference appeared after the first week of pentamidine administration. The changes in the other three groups (normal salt intake + indomethacin and pentamidine; normal salt + indomethacin; and low salt + indomethacin) were minimal or not statistically significant. From this study it can be concluded that at least in the intact female Sprague-Dawley rat, pentamidine alone, even at a large dose appears to have minimal nephrotoxic effect. A state of sodium/volume depletion and of inhibition of prostaglandin synthesis may be necessary to reduce renal function in the rat[158].

It has been recommended that the dosing interval of pentamidine be extended to 48 hours for patients with a GFR less than 10 ml/min [173] and that there is no need for dosing after hemo or peritoneal dialysis. However, Conte in his report [141], suggested that dose reduction of pentamidine for renal impairment is unnecessary and noted that while his patients had mild to moderate PCP, it remains unknown whether the pharmacokinetics of pentamidine might be altered in more severely ill patients.

The plasma and tissue concentrations of pentamidine associated with toxicity in man remain unknown and it seems there is no correlation between tissue levels and renal dysfunction, as measured by serum creatinine levels [149]. It has been shown that there is minimal transfer of pentamidine to the human fetus and significant concentration of the drug in placental tissue [174]. The last mentioned finding raises an important question about placental toxicity.

Perturbations in mono- and divalent cation renal handling have been reported in association with pentamidine administration. Several reports of *hyperkalemia* in association with pentamidine therapy have been published [153, 155, 157, 158, 175, 176]. Lachaal and Venuto [153] in a retrospective review reported a very high incidence of hyperkalemia (5.1 to 8.7 mEq/ L) in 19 of 20 patients (95%). This incidence was greater than the 5% reported earlier [132], or the 24% reported subsequently [155] in 37 patients with AIDS, and was challenged as a possible overestimation [177]. The hyperkalemia usually correlates with the presence of decreased GFR [153, 155]. In Chua et al clinical study [154] the mean serum potassium concentration tended to be higher in the AIDS patients that developed pentamidine nephrotoxicity than in those that did not (5.0 ± 0.3 vs 4.3 ± 0.2, respectively, $p<0.055$). In this study, no patient, had a serum potassium concentration higher than 6.0 mEq/L. Arrhythmias can occur during the use of pentamidine [178], but they are mainly reported to be a consequence of prolongation of the QT interval [179], although there is a report in which the authors attributed a cardiac arrest to hyperkalemia [180]. The hyperkalemia usually reversed on discontinuation of pentamidine, and although most patients required only conservative measures, occasionally dialysis was necessary [153].

The exact mechanism of the pentamidine-induced hyperkalemia has not yet been defined. Many different mechanisms can impair the renal handling of potassium and thus favor hyperkalemia in patients with AIDS. These include: decreased renal function secondary to volume depletion, presence of underlying renal disease, including tubular dysfunction with the possibility of hyporeninemic hypoaldosteronism, hypoadrenalism, and the administration of drugs with potential for impairing renal potassium excretion (nonsteroidal anti-inflammatory agents, ACE inhibitors, potassium-sparing diuretics,

B-blockers, TMP-SMZ). In Chua et al study regarding pentamidine nephro-toxicity in the rat, however, there were no statistically significant differences observed in the potassium level among any of the groups receiving pentamidine concomitant to low versus high salt intake and or indomethacin [158], suggesting the possibility that extrarenal mechanisms or a more severe degree of renal dysfunction may be necessary to induce hyperkalemia. Recent *in vivo* experiments [181], however, have shown that the application of pentamidine to amphibian or mammalian distal nephron cells results in inhibition of amiloride-sensitive sodium channels and sodium reabsorption, and decrease in the electrochemical gradient that drives secretion of distal potassium into the urine. In isolated perfused rat kidney pentamidine also inhibited reabsorption of sodium ions by blocking the luminal sodium ion channels [139, 150]. This renal tubular effect of pentamidine may be the mechanisms for the induced hyperkalemia. In a recent study performed on Sprague-Dawley rats, Gabriels et al observed dose-dependent decrease in the excretion of potassium and decreased of GFR (by 43,5% at the dose of 10mg/kg) [182].

Symptomatic *hypocalcemia* and *hypomagnesemia with renal magnesium wasting* associated with pentamidine therapy was described in a patient with AIDS [183]. Three other cases have been reporte [184-186].

Another previous report [187] described severe hypocalcemia with tetany in patients with AIDS concomitantly receiving pentamidine and foscarnet. The hypocalcemia, however, was attributed to the administration of foscarnet. Despite magnesium replacement, magnesium wasting may persist up to two months after the discontinuation of pentamidine, suggesting that anatomic renal tubular injury may be responsible [183, 185]. Both abnormalities developed within 6 to 10 days of pentamidine administration. Because life-threatening arrhythmias can develop, especially at serum magnesium levels less than 1.6 mg/dl, early replacement therapy is clinically warranted.

Perturbations in insulin regulation both resulting in *hypoglycemia* and *diabetes mellitus* have been shown in patients treated with pentamidine [188-192]. This is not surprising considering that pentamidine accumulates in the pancreas [149], and that in 1948 the drug was considered for use as an antihypoglycemic agent [128]. The overall incidence of hypoglycemia with AIDS is several folds higher (27 to 40%) [190, 191] than previously reported for patients with other immunocompromising diseases treated with pentamidine [98]. The incidence of nephrotoxicity in patients who developed hypoglycemia was 100% [191]. The hypoglycemia, which appears early (within a week) after commencing pentamidine therapy, is associated with inappropriately high levels of insulin in the postabsorptive state [188]. The appearance of diabetes mellitus is usually delayed by several weeks. It has been suggested that pentamidine can induce hypoglycemia because of an early cytolytic release of insulin, and then diabetes mellitus because of B cell destruction and insulin deficiency [153].

In summary, parenteral pentamidine administration for the treatment of PCP can be associated with the development of usually mild, reversible acute kidney injury. Compounding risk factors, of which volume depletion is the most important, are found in the majority of cases of pentamidine nephrotoxicity. There is no convincing evidence that the aerosol route of pentamidine administration for PCP prophylaxis results in nephrotoxicity. Hypocalcemia and hypomagnesemia with renal magnesium wasting, and particularly, hyperkalemia are seen with pentamidine therapy.

Pyrimethamine

Pyrimethamine is a folic acid antagonist that for many years has been used as an antimalarial drug [193-195], specially for chloroquine-resistant *P. falciparum*. Due to its synergistic activity, pyrimethamine also has been used, in combination with sulfadiazine or dapsone for the treatment or prophylaxis of cerebral toxoplasmosis or PCP in patients with AIDS [196].

Pyrimethamine does not belong to the group of known nephrotoxic agents [39]. Because pyrimethamine and trimethoprim have a similar 2, 4-diaminopyrimidine molecular structure, Opravil *et al* [197] reported a similar handling of tubular secretion of creatinine. In six healthy volunteers and nine patients with AIDS, pyrimethamine caused a reversible, small to moderate, similar between the two groups, but statistically significant increase (26%) in serum creatinine concentration with a concomitant decrease in creatinine clearance compared to baseline values. Of importance, these changes occurred without a decrease in the simultaneously measured inulin clearance. The authors concluded that pyrimethamine like trimethoprim and other compounds (cimetidine, probenecid), reversibly and mildly (at least in patients with normal renal function) inhibits renal tubular secretion of creatinine without affecting the glomerular filtration rate. Thus, physicians using this medication should be aware of the possibility of pyrimethamine elevating serum creatinine concentration.

Different from trimethoprim, pyrimethamine does not induce hyperkalemia, as it does not affect urinary sodium and potassium excretion [182].

Pyrimethamine has a long half-life (83±14 hours) [197] with only a small fraction been excreted during the first days of administration, but drug and metabolites will appear slowly in the urine for one to two months [39]. Dosage adjustment is usually not recommended for patients with renal failure. It is not known, however, if metabolite accumulation with potential hematologic toxicity may occur with the prolonged use of pyrimethamine in patients with cerebral toxoplasmosis at doses higher than dose employed for prophylaxis of malaria[39]. It appears that dialytic removal of pyrimethamine must be small because of its high protein binding (85-90%) and large volume of distribution [194, 195].

Dapsone

Dapsone, a sulfone with chemical similarities to sulfapyridine, has been used for over 50 years. It is the most widely used drug for the treatment of of leprosy, and it is used for quinine-resistant *Plasmodium falciparum* malaria. Dapsone is currently used for the primary treatment of dermatitis herpetiform, chronic bullous dermatosis and can be replaced by sulfapyridine in patients with intolerance to the sulfone [198]. Dapsone in combination with trimethoprim is also used for the treatment of mild to moderate first episodes of PCP, or alone for PCP prophylaxis [115, 198]. The most frequent adverse events are dose related metheglobinemia and hemolytic anemia. Since multi-drug therapy began to be used in leprosy patients, an increasing number of a rare, idiosyncratic reaction with multiorgan involvement called dapsone hypersensitivity syndrome have been reported [199-201].

Dapsone is well absorbed when given by the oral route, is extensively protein (70-90% of the drug, 99% of its metabolite monoacetyl dapsone) and tissue bound, and is metabolized by N-oxidation and acetylation in the liver. The serum half-life averages 24 to 28 hours, and the kidneys will excrete about 5 to 15% of the dose [202]. No specific guidelines for dosage modifications in patients with renal failure are available [39, 203]. When dapsone and trimethoprim (with SMZ) are used together, higher plasma levels of both drugs are achieved, than when either drug is used alone [204].

In the study of Opravil *et al* [197], administration of dapsone alone to healthy volunteers or to patients with AIDS did not result in changes in renal function. Likewise, dapsone alone did not cause hyperkalemia in patients with AIDS treated for PCP [115]. Nevertheless, renal adverse effects attributable to dapsone have been reported [199-201, 205-209]. A single case of nephrotic syndrome following a three-week course of treatment with dapsone at 100 mg daily for a pruritic rash was reported [205]. Although a causative effect for dapsone seemed plausible, no renal histology or long-term follow-up was available. Bilateral renal cortical necrosis developed in a patient treated for dermatitis herpetiform for several years with large doses of dapsone [206]. He had hemolytic anemia and normal G6PD levels. Two fatal cases of acute kidney injury associated with intravascular hemolysis secondary to G6PD deficiency were described in Indian patients treated with dapsone [207]. Acute kidney injury associated with massive dapsone overdose also was reported [210]. Renal involvement as part of the unusual dapsone hypersensitivity syndrome has been reported and include a case of frank hematuria[200], and cases of acute kidney injury, some of which required dialytic therapy [201, 208, 211]. Lau reported the finding of tubulointerstitial nephritis in post-mortem pathology evaluation [209]. Alves-Rodrigues et al reported the case of a patient with biopsy proven vasculitis that required short term dialytic therapy. The histopathological analysis revealed an interstitial perivascular lymphocytic infiltrate affecting the media of arched and interlobular arteries, composed of T cells. Direct immunofluorescence of the glomeruli was negative for IgA, IgD, IgE, IgG, IgM, C3, C1q and fibrin [199].

The treatment of choice for acute dapsone intoxication is the oral administration of activated charcoal and its efficacy is fully comparable to that of hemodialysis in increasing dapsone rate of elimination [212]. Endre et al reported a case of massive dose dapsone ingestion, presenting with metheglobinemia, hemolysis and progressive clinical deterioration despite standard therapy with gastric lavage, activated charcoal and methylene blue. The patient was also treated .with charcoal hemoperfusion and sequential dialysis. Assessment of the differential effects of the two different modalities on dapsone clearance was evaluated by simultaneously drawing blood from three sites in the circuit; before and after the charcoal column and after the dialyser. Succesful accelerated dapsone removal occurred and as expected, with the predominant fall in concentration across the charcoal column, reducing its half-life to approximately 90 minutes. The authors concluded that charcoal hemoperfusion is a safe, simple procedure in clearing dapsone from the circulation and that as dapsone is poorly dialyzable, this procedure is unnecessary [213].

It appears that dapsone is a safe drug when used in standard dosage. Perhaps, renal involvement should be watched for when administering dapsone to patients with G6PD deficiency that could develop hemolytic complications [207] and in patients that present with dapsone hypersensitivity syndrome.

Quinolones

The quinolones are an important and widely prescribed class of antibiotics with broad-spectrum activities against both gram-negative and gram-positive bacteria. They have proved to be effective against infections in the urinary tract, respiratory tree, gastrointestinal tract, as well as skin, soft tissue and bone, and for sexually transmitted bacterial diseases [214]. Nalidixic acid introduced in 1962, was the first in this series of agents [215]. Subsequently, many 4-fluoroquinolones have been introduced into clinical practice including ciprofloxacin, ofloxacin, lomefloxacin, gemifloxacin norfloxacin, enoxacin, gatifloxacin, moxifloxacin, trovafloxacin, sparfloxacin, and grepafloxacin. Several others are already in use or undergoing trials [214]. We will consider ciprofloxacin as the prototypical agent for the new 4-fluoroquinolones.

Nalidixic acid

Nalidixic acid is a highly protein bound oral quinolone (>90%), that undergoes major hepatic metabolism (80%) to active (hydroxynalidixic acid) and inactive metabolites [216]. The parent drug and its metabolites are rapidly excreted in the urine [217]. Most of the antibacterial effect is due to the biologically active hydroxynalidixic acid, which is 16 times more active than the parent compound. Nalidixic acid has a terminal half-life of about two hours. The drug does not accumulate in tissues even after prolonged administration; the kidney is the only organ in which this may occur. Furthermore, nalidixic acid does not diffuse into prostatic fluid [214].

This drug is essentially devoid of renal toxicity. Although increased toxicity has not been reported in patients with renal failure given the usual dosage, nalidixic acid, preferably, should not be used in patients with a decreased GFR (less than 50 ml/min) or in patients with liver disease, because of the risk of enhancing gastrointestinal or dermatological adverse-effects [214]. Overdosage with nalidixic acid induces metabolic acidosis [218]. In the past the use of this drug was limited to treatment of urinary tract infections. Currently, other newer quinolones, as well as other chemotherapeutic agents, have replaced nalidixic acid.

Ciprofloxacin

Ciprofloxacin is arguably the most effective antipseudomonal fluoroquinolone and is undoubtedly the most thoroughly studied of the newer oral quinolones, is rapidly absorbed from the gastrointestinal tract. A parenteral preparation is also available. Protein binding is low, about 35%, and the serum half-life is 3-4.5 hours. About 30-60% of the active drug and 10% of its metabolites are excreted in the urine during 24 hours; 15% appears in the feces, and less than 1% in the bile [219, 220]. Table 2 illustrates that the newer quinolones exhibit differences sometimes important in their pharmacokinetics, which might affect their individual behavior. The quinolones undergo hepatic metabolism and renal excretion. Hepatic metabolism includes conjugation with glucuronic acid as well as carboxylation, hydroxylation, and demethylation.

Tissue penetration, particularly in the kidneys and prostate, is excellent (Table 2). Those quinolones with longer half-life have smaller penetration ratios [220]. Available studies suggest that penetration of the newer quinolones into all extravascular sites (large-volume spaces i.e., ascites, pleural fluid, etc.), secretory fluids (urine, prostatic secretions, sputum, etc.), barrier fluids (CSFL), and whole tissues is high relative to the penetration reported for most other categories of antimicrobial agents, particularly, the penicillins, cephalosporins, and aminoglycosides [221]. Renal elimination is by glomerular filtration and active tubular secretion, which can be blocked by probenecid. As noted in Table 2, urinary recovery of the quinolones is variable. The antibacterial activity of these compounds is reduced at low urinary pH [215].

The bioavailability of oral or parenterally administered ciprofloxacin was not affected in patients and rats with renal insufficiency [222]. The renal clearance of the quinolone, however, was reduced resulting in a prolonged half-life [223-225]. Thus, a reduction of 50% in the dose of ciprofloxacin has been recommended when the creatinine clearance is between 10 and 30 ml/ min/1.73 m^2 [224]. Of interest, it has been suggested that there may be a compensatory transintestinal elimination of ciprofloxacin in patients and rats with reduced renal function [224, 225].

A study of the pharmacokinetics of orally administered ciprofloxacin in elderly (63-76 years) and young volunteers (22-34 years) without renal impairment, revealed in the elderly group a decreased renal clearance of the quinolone with no differences detected in the terminal half-life (3.5 hours). This was accompanied, however, by a surprising increase in the absolute availability of the drug [226]. The authors cautioned about the need for a reduction of oral dosage of ciprofloxacin in the elderly population.

The newer fluoroquinolones (ciprofloxacin, norfloxacin, enoxacin, pefloxacin, gatifloxacin and moxifloxacin) have similar toxicities and incidence of adverse effects. In general, compared to other antibiotics, these are relatively safe agents [214]. Gastrointestinal side-effects are the most common (0.8 to 6.8% of patients), followed by central nervous system manifestations (0.9 to 1.8%), and skin reactions (0.6 to 2.4%). Rare cases of increased serum creatinine levels have been reported [227]. Indeed, in a study of 133 febrile episodes in neutropenic patients comparing the effectiveness and safety of high-dose oral ciprofloxacin versus azlocillin and netilmicin, there were no renal adverse effects reported in the quinolone group, whereas nephrotoxicity developed in 3% of the patients treated with the combination azlocillin/netilmicin [228]. Ball [229] described only one case of acute kidney injury in his review of almost 6,000 patients worldwide. In another review of 2,829 patients, minor increases in serum creatinine and blood urea nitrogen were reported, but only one patient each with acute kidney injury and interstitial nephritis were described [230]. Thus, initially

Table 2. Pharmacokinetics of selected newer quinolones after single oral dosage*.

Drug	Half-life (h)		Urinary Excretion (%)		Tissue Penetration**		Removal by dialysis	
	NRF	ESRD	Unchanged	Metabolites	Kidney	Prostate	HD (%)	PD (%)
Ciprofloxacin	3-4.5	6-9	30-60	10	5+	3+	<10	<10
Enoxacin	4-6	NA	50-55	15	4+	2+	<5	NA
Fleroxacin	9-13	21-28	70	NA	NA	NA	NA	NA
Lomefloxacin	8	44	70	10	NA	NA	<10	NA
Norfloxacin	3-4.5	8	20-40	20	5+	2+	<10	NA
Ofloxacin	5-6	28-37	70-90	5-10	5+	4+	10-30	2-10
Pefloxacin	10-11	12-15	5-15	55	NA	NA	NA	NA
Sparfloxacin	15-20	38.5	10	NA	NA	NA	NA	NA

* *Adapted from references [203, 214 and 216].*
** *Scale of 1+ to 5+.*
NRF= normal renal function; ESRD= end-stage renal disease; NA = not available; HD = Hemodialysis; PD = Peritoneal dialysis.

it was thought that ciprofloxacin was almost devoid of renal toxicity. Nevertheless, since 1987 many case reports and case series of patients with acute kidney injury and a clinical presentation compatible with acute interstitial nephritis have been reported [231-263]. The diagnosis has been confirmed by renal biopsy in 15 patients [232, 238, 241, 242, 246, 248-259], and by postmortem examination in one[236]. The age of the patients ranged from 11 to 88 (data on 25 patients) with an average of 59 years. There was a predominance of elderly patients (48% were 65 or older), and, of note, 58% were women (ages 21 to 88).

The nonoliguric variety of acute kidney injury was common (76%), but oliguria (23%) or anuria were also observed. The average duration of quinolone therapy prior to the recognition of nephrotoxicity was seven days. In the 20 patients reviewed by Lo et al [247], skin rashes were uncommon, five patients had eosinophiluria, six had eosinophilia, abnormal urinary sediment was not always present, and the duration of therapy with the quinolone prior to the diagnoses of renal failure ranged from 3 to 18 days. In only six of the 20 patients (30%) was ciprofloxacin the only drug given with the potential for causing renal dysfunction. The majority of the patients received a variety of other medications with nephrotoxic potential: aminoglycosides in six, penicillins-cephalosporins in five, amphotericin B, cisplatin andnon-steroidal anti-inflammatory agents in two each, and others. Thus, although the chronological sequence of events and the observed improvement after stopping the quinolone strongly favors a causative role for ciprofloxacin, it is not possible to be absolute certain about the cause of the nephrotoxicity. Renal function improved in 14 patients after discontinuation of ciprofloxacin therapy. It is not possible to evaluate the beneficial effect of prednisone, which was given to only 4 of 21 patients. Only one patient required dialytic support [247].

Although the pathogenesis of ciprofloxacin-induced acute interstitial nephritis is not clear, it has been attributed to an inflammatory interstitial response secondary to the crystalluria associated with the quinolone (foreign body response) [232, 238, 248]. Crystalluria and the presence of crystals of ciprofloxacin in the renal tissue have been shown in animal experiments. The species studied (rats, monkeys, dogs), however, have alkaline urine, and because the quinolone solubility is poor at a neutral or alkaline pH, crystallization may occur under those circumstances, with ciprofloxacin precipitating in the tubular lumen with magnesium and protein but only in an alkaline urine. Indeed, at an acid pH crystallization does not occur [264]. It has been argued, however, that only uncommonly and intermittently, is the human urine highly alkaline [265]. *By* supplementing the diet of normal volunteers with sodium bicarbonate it was possible to demonstrate crystals of ciprofloxacin in the urine of individuals who received large doses of the quinolone; nevertheless, no adverse renal effects developed [266]. Because the majority of the patients with acute interstitial nephritis secondary to ciprofloxacin are assumed to or have acid urine, it has been suggested that an idiosyncratic reaction rather than intratubular crystallization, might be involved in the pathogenesis of acute interstitial nephropathy [238]. Of importance, a report on four cases of acute interstitial nephritis and two cases of hepatitis induced by quinolone [260], revealed by immunoblotting analysis that all sera from these patients contained autoantibodies that recognize a 65-kDa protein expressed in normal human kidney and liver microsomes. Only 6% of sera from healthy individuals who did not ingest quinolone recognized the same protein. These findings suggest that a modification of microsomal proteins by quinolone itself or by a metabolite could generate an autoimmune response, and that the presence of autoantibodies could be used as a sensitive marker.

Patients who received bone marrow [267] and heart transplants [268] did not show any evidence of nephrotoxicity when receiving ciprofloxacin. Contrary to previous preliminary findings [253, 269], more recent data suggest lack of relevant pharmacokinetic interaction of ciprofloxacin with cyclosporine[268]. Similar preliminary claims of norfloxacin [270], ofloxacin [271], and pefloxacin-cyclosporine [272] interactions have been made.

Other quinolones

Early reports of acute interstitial nephritis [273] and of acute tubular necrosis [274] associated with the use of *piromidic acid* (a non-fluorinated quinolone available in Europe) have been published. At large dosage, crystals of *norfloxacin* can be occasionally seen in freshly voided urine, this, however, does not occur when low doses are used [220]. One patient treated with norfloxacin developed acute kidney injury compatible with allergic interstitial nephritis [275]. Exceptional cases of Levofloxacin associated nephrotoxicity, purpura/vasculitis and granulomatous interstitial nephritis have been reported [276-279]. A unique case of acute kidney injury probably induced by prulifloxacin in an elderly woman was recently published by Galleli et al [263]. No crystalluria or crystal formation was reported in acute toxicity studies with *temafloxacin* in mice, rats, or dogs. Furthermore, no nephrotoxicity was observed in rats, or dogs, when temafloxacin was administered orally for six months [280]. Finally, pre-marketing data obtained in 5,300 patients revealed no crystalluria or clinically important nephrotoxicity with the use of temafloxacin [281]. However, prior to its withdrawal from the world market, temafloxacin was associated with a syndrome of immune hemolytic anemia and renal failure based on 95 spontaneous reports of hemolysis sent to the Food and Drug Administration. New- onset renal dysfunction was noted in 54 cases (57%), and dialysis was required in 34 cases (63%) [259]. Pre-marketing animal and clinical studies with *ofloxacin* revealed the absence of renal toxicity [282]. Likewise, no adverse renal effects were reported in a comparative study of *lomefloxacin* with TMP-SMZ [283]. The renal handling of *flexoracin, a* trifluorinated quinolone, in humans occurs by glomerular filtration, and both renal tubular secretion and reabsorption [284]. Animal studies indicated that the tubular transport processes of some of the quinolones have a considerable species dependency [284].

It is reasonable to conclude that in general, quinolones are safe drugs from the renal point of view. It is often difficult, however, to ascertain the exact causative role of these agents in the appearance of nephrotoxicity. Judging by the recent accumulated experience with ciprofloxacin, physicians using quinolones should be alert for the development of acute interstitial nephritis leading to renal failure. This concern should be extended to the other newer fluoroquinolones despite the paucity of reports dealing with nephrotoxicity.

Acknowledgements

Parts of the work described in this chapter were supported by designated VA Research funding and grants from the Kidney Foundation of South Florida, U.S.A. The authors thank Ms. Esther Márquez for her skilled secretarial help.

References

1. Dowling HF LM. Toxic reactions following therapy with sulfapyridine, sulfa-thiazole and sulfadiazine. JAMA. 1943;121:1190-4.
2. Vilter CF BM. Toxic reactions of the newer sulfonamides. JAMA. 1944;126:691-5.
3. Lehr D. Clinical toxicity of sulfonamides. Annals of the New York Academy of Sciences. 1957 Oct 12;69(3):417-47.
4. Weinstein L, Madoff MA, Samet CM. The sulfonamides. The New England journal of medicine. 1960 Nov 3;263:900-7 contd.
5. Dorfman LE, Smith JP. Sulfonamide crystalluria: a forgotten disease. The Journal of urology. 1970 Sep;104(3):482-3.
6. Appel GB, Kunis C.L.. Acute interstitial nephriitis. In: Cotran RS BB, Stein JH, ed. *Tubulointerstitial nephropathies.* New York: Churchill 1983:151-85.
7. Simon DI, Brosius FC, 3rd, Rothstein DM. Sulfadiazine crystalluria revisited. The treatment of Toxoplasma encephalitis in patients with acquired immunodeficiency syndrome. Archives of internal medicine. 1990 Nov;150(11):2379-84.
8. Nissen NI, Aagaard K, Flindt-Hansen E. Sulfonamide hematuria; frequency of injury to the urinary tract as estimated on the basis of 6,084 cases treated with different sulfonamide preparations. Acta medica Scandinavica. 1950;138(4):301-14.
9. Dwarakanath AD, Michael J, Allan RN. Sulphasalazine induced renal failure. Gut. 1992 Jul;33(7):1006-7.
10. Finland M SE, Peterson O.L. Sulfadiazine: therapeutic evaluation and toxic effects in four hundred and forty-six patients. Jama. 1941;16:2641-7.
11. Fox CLJ, Jensen OJ Jr, Mudge G.H. The prevention of renal obstruction during sulfadiazine therapy. Jama. 1943;121:1147-50.
12. Yap HK, Yip WC, Tay JS, Tan SH, Lee BW. Reversible ultrasound findings in the kidneys of a patient with sulphonamide induced obstructive uropathy. The Journal of the Singapore Paediatric Society. 1984;26(1-2):105-6.
13. Goadsby PJ, Donaghy AJ, Lloyd AR, Wakefield D. Acquired immunodeficiency syndrome (AIDS) and sulfadiazine-associated acute renal failure. Annals of internal medicine. 1987 Nov;107(5):783-4.

14. Sahai J, Heimberger T, Collins K, Kaplowitz L, Polk R. Sulfadiazine-induced crystalluria in a patient with the acquired immunodeficiency syndrome: a reminder. The American journal of medicine. 1988 Apr;84(4):791-2.
15. Ventura MG, Wybran J, Farber CM. Sulfadiazine revisited. The Journal of infectious diseases. 1989 Sep;160(3):556-7.
16. Carbone LG, Bendixen B, Appel GB. Sulfadiazine-associated obstructive nephropathy occurring in a patient with the acquired immunodeficiency syndrome. Am J Kidney Dis. 1988 Jul;12(1):72-5.
17. Christin S, Baumelou A, Bahri S, Ben Hmida M, Deray G, Jacobs C. Acute renal failure due to sulfadiazine in patients with AIDS. Nephron. 1990;55(2):233-4.
18. Antopol W RH. Urolithiasis and renal pathology after oral administration of 2-sulfanilylamino (sulfapyridine).. Proc Soc Exp Biol Med. 1939;40:428-30.
19. Molina JM, Belenfant X, Doco-Lecompte T, Idatte JM, Modai J. Sulfadiazine-induced crystalluria in AIDS patients with toxoplasma encephalitis. AIDS (London, England). 1991 May;5(5):587-9.
20. Filks I.N FCR, Barbas Filho J.V, Kairalla R.A, Oliveira-Vianna E dos S, Stavale ML, de Carvalho C.R. Kidney Failure as a Complication of the treatment of pulmonary paracoccidioidomycosis. Rev Hosp Clin Fac Med Sao Paulo. 1992;47:103-5.
21. Marques LP, Silva MT, Madeira EP, Santos OR. Obstructive renal failure due to therapy with sulfadiazine in an AIDS patient. Nephron. 1992;62(3):361.
22. De Jaureguiberry JP RP, Vey N, Jaubert D. Acute renal failure caused by sulfadiazine crystalluria in AIDS. An historical resurgent iatrogenic complication. Ann Med Interne. 1992;143:218-9.
23. Corbella X MJ, Santin M, Carratala J. Insuficiencia renal aguda por sulfadiazina en el tratamiento de una toxoplasmosis cerebral. Rev Clin Esp. 1992;190:330-1.
24. Farinas MC, Echevarria S, Sampedro I, Gonzalez A, Perez del Molino A, Gonzalez-Macias J. Renal failure due to sulphadiazine in AIDS patients with cerebral toxoplasmosis. Journal of internal medicine. 1993 Apr;233(4):365-7.
25. Hein R, Brunkhorst R, Thon WF, Schedel I, Schmidt RE. Symptomatic sulfadiazine crystalluria in AIDS patients: a report of two cases. Clinical nephrology. 1993 May;39(5):254-6.
26. Haverkos HW. Assessment of therapy for toxoplasma encephalitis. The TE Study Group. The American journal of medicine. 1987 May;82(5):907-14.
27. Becker K, Jablonowski H, Haussinger D. Sulfadiazine-associated nephrotoxicity in patients with the acquired immunodeficiency syndrome. Medicine. 1996 Jul;75(4):185-94.
28. Kane D, Murphy JM, Keating S, Wilson GF, Mulcahy FM. Renal ultrasonic findings in sulphadiazine-induced renal failure. The British journal of radiology. 1996 Oct;69(826):925-8.
29. Colebunders R, Depraetere K, De Droogh E, Kamper A, Corthout B, Bottiau E. Obstructive nephropathy due to sulfa crystals in two HIV seropositive patients treated with sulfadiazine. Jbr-Btr. 1999 Aug;82(4):153-4.
30. Goodman LS GA. The Pharmacological Basis of Therapeutics. 8th Ed ed. New York: McGraw Hill 1991:1047.
31. Diaz F, Collazos J, Mayo J, Martinez E. Sulfadiazine-induced multiple urolithiasis and acute renal failure in a patient with AIDS and Toxoplasma encephalitis. The Annals of pharmacotherapy. 1996 Jan;30(1):41-2.
32. de Sequera P, Albalate M, Hernandez J, Vazquez A, Abad J, Ramiro E, et al. Acute renal failure due to sulphadiazine crystalluria in AIDS patients. Postgraduate medical journal. 1996 Sep;72(851):557-8.
33. Mir N, O'Farrell N, Creagh TA, Knowles C. Obstructive renal failure requiring surgical intervention in an AIDS patient being treated with sulphadiazine. International journal of STD & AIDS. 1997 Jan;8(1):61-2.
34. Dong BJ, Rodriguez RA, Goldschmidt RH. Sulfadiazine-induced crystalluria and renal failure in a patient with AIDS. The Journal of the American Board of Family Practice / American Board of Family Practice. 1999 May-Jun;12(3):243-8.
35. Crespo M, Quereda C, Pascual J, Rivera M, Clemente L, Cano T. Patterns of sulfadiazine acute nephrotoxicity. Clinical nephrology. 2000 Jul;54(1):68-72.
36. Portoles J, Torralbo A, Prats D, Blanco J, Barrientos A. Acute renal failure and sulphadiazine crystalluria in kidney transplant. Nephrol Dial Transplant. 1994;9(2):180-1.
37. Guitard J, Kamar N, Mouzin M, Borde JS, Tran-Van T, Durand D, et al. Sulfadiazine-related obstructive urinary tract lithiasis: an unusual cause of acute renal failure after kidney transplantation. Clinical nephrology. 2005 May;63(5):405-7.
38. Bergan T, Brodwall EK, Vik-Mo H, Anstad U. Pharmacokinetics of sulphadiazine, sulphamethoxazole and trimethoprim in patients with varying renal function. Infection. 1979;7 Suppl 4:S382-7.
39. Berns JS, Cohen RM, Stumacher RJ, Rudnick MR. Renal aspects of therapy for human immunodeficiency virus and associated opportunistic infections. J Am Soc Nephrol. 1991 Mar;1(9):1061-80.
40. Swan S.K BW, . Use of drugs in patients with renal failure. In: Schrier R.W GCW, ed. *Diseases of the Kidney*. 6th Ed. ed. Boston: Little, Brown & Co. 1996:1061-80.
41. Oster S, Hutchison F, McCabe R. Resolution of acute renal failure in toxoplasmic encephalitis despite continuance of sulfadiazine. Reviews of infectious diseases. 1990 Jul-Aug;12(4):618-20.

42. Robson M, Levi J, Dolberg L, Rosenfeld JB. Acute tubulo-interstitial nephritis following sulfadiazine therapy. Israel journal of medical sciences. 1970 Jul-Aug;6(4):561-6.
43. Nanra RS, Anderton JL, Evans M, Fairley KF, Kincaid-Smith P. The use of trimethoprim and sulphamethoxazole in the management of chronic and recurrent upper and lower urinary tract infection. The Medical journal of Australia. 1971 Jan 2;1(1):25-7.
44. Rosenfeld JB, Najenson T, Grosswater Z. Effect of long-term co-trimoxazole therapy on renal function. The Medical journal of Australia. 1975 Oct 4;2(14):546-8.
45. Bennett WM, Craven R. Urinary tract infections in patients with severe renal disease. Treatment with ampicillin and trimethoprim-sulfamethoxazole. Jama. 1976 Aug 23;236(8):946-8.
46. Lawson DH, Paice BJ. Adverse reactions to trimethoprim-sulfamethoxazole. Reviews of infectious diseases. 1982 Mar-Apr;4(2):429-33.
47. Foltzer MA, Reese RE. Trimethoprim-sulfamethoxazole and other sulfonamides. The Medical clinics of North America. 1987 Nov;71(6):1177-94.
48. Bergan T, Brodwall EK. Kidney transport in man of sulfamethoxazole and trimethoprim. Chemotherapy. 1972;17(5):320-33.
49. Trottier S, Bergeron MG, Lessard C. Intrarenal distribution of trimethoprim and sulfamethoxazole. Antimicrobial agents and chemotherapy. 1980 Mar;17(3):383-8.
50. Tu YH, Allen LV, Jr., Fiorica VM, Albers DD. Pharmacokinetics of trimethoprim in the rat. Journal of pharmaceutical sciences. 1989 Jul;78(7):556-60.
51. Cacini W, Myre SA. Uptake of trimethoprim by renal cortex. Biochemical pharmacology. 1985 Oct 1;34(19):3483-8.
52. Craig WA, Kunin CM. Distribution of trimethoprim-sulfamethoxazole in tissues of rhesus monkeys. The Journal of infectious diseases. 1973 Nov;128:Suppl:575-9 p.
53. Berglund F, Killander J, Pompeius R. Effect of trimethoprim-sulfamethoxazole on the renal excretion of creatinine in man. The Journal of urology. 1975 Dec;114(6):802-8.
54. Shouval D, Ligumsky M, Ben-Ishay D. Effect of co-trimoxazole on normal creatinine clearance. Lancet. 1978 Feb 4;1(8058):244-5.
55. Brautigam M FP, Baethke R, Kessel M. Zur kreatininaus scheidung beim Menschen nach Gabe von cotrimoxazole. Klin Wochenschr. 1979;57:95-6.
56. Trollfors B, Wahl M, Alestig K. Co-trimoxazole, creatinine and renal function. The Journal of infection. 1980 Sep;2(3):221-6.
57. Kainer G, Rosenberg AR. Effect of co-trimoxazole on the glomerular filtration rate of healthy adults. Chemotherapy. 1981;27(4):229-32.
58. Lee J, Hollyer R, Rodelas R, Preuss HG. The influence of trimethoprim, sulfamethoxazole, and creatinine on renal organic anion and cation transport in rat kidney tissue. Toxicology and applied pharmacology. 1981 Apr;58(2):184-93.
59. Kalowski S, Nanra RS, Mathew TH, Kincaid-Smith P. Deterioration in renal function in association with co-trimoxazole therapy. Lancet. 1973 Feb 24;1(7800):394-7.
60. Myre SA, McCann J, First MR, Cluxton RJ, Jr. Effect of trimethoprim on serum creatinine in healthy and chronic renal failure volunteers. Therapeutic drug monitoring. 1987 Jun;9(2):161-5.
61. Paap CM, Nahata MC. Clinical use of trimethoprim/sulfamethoxazole during renal dysfunction. Dicp. 1989 Sep;23(9):646-54.
62. Siber GR, Gorham CC, Ericson JF, Smith AL. Pharmacokinetics of intravenous trimethoprim-sulfamethoxazole in children and adults with normal and impaired renal function. Reviews of infectious diseases. 1982 Mar-Apr;4(2):566-78.
63. Eknoyan. Acute renal failure associated with tubulointerstitial nephropathies. In: Brenner BM LJ, ed. *Acute Renal Failure*. 2nd ed. New York: Churchill Livingstone 1988:491-534.
64. Siegel WH. Unusual complication of therapy with sulfamethoxazole-trimethoprim. The Journal of urology. 1977 Mar;117(3):397.
65. Nissenson AR, Wilson C, Holazo A. Pharmacokinetics of intravenous trimethoprim-sulfamethoxazole during hemodialysis. American journal of nephrology. 1987;7(4):270-4.
66. Saltissi D, Pusey CD, Rainford DJ. Recurrent acute renal failure due to antibiotic-induced interstitial nephritis. British medical journal. 1979 May 5;1(6172):1182-3.
67. Jick H. Adverse reactions to trimethoprim-sulfamethoxazole in hospitalized patients. Reviews of infectious diseases. 1982 Mar-Apr;4(2):426-8.
68. Jick H, Derby LE. A large population-based follow-up study of trimethoprim-sulfamethoxazole, trimethoprim, and cephalexin for uncommon serious drug toxicity. Pharmacotherapy. 1995 Jul-Aug;15(4):428-32.
69. Hanley. The synergy of trimethoprim and sulfonamides. Postgraduate medical journal. 1969;45(Suppl):85.
70. Buchanan N. Sulphamethoxazole, hypoalbuminaemia, crystalluria, and renal failure. British medical journal. 1978 Jul 15;2(6131):172.
71. Ahn YH, Goldman JM. Trimethoprim-sulfamethoxazole and hyponatremia. Annals of internal medicine. 1985 Jul;103(1):161-2.

72. Wofsy CB. Use of trimethoprim-sulfamethoxazole in the treatment of Pneumocystis carinii pneumonitis in patients with acquired immunodeficiency syndrome. Reviews of infectious diseases. 1987 Mar-Apr;9 Suppl 2:S184-94.
73. Mori H, Kuroda Y, Imamura S, Toyoda A, Yoshida I, Kawakami M, et al. Hyponatremia and/or hyperkalemia in patients treated with the standard dose of trimethoprim-sulfamethoxazole. Internal medicine (Tokyo, Japan). 2003 Aug;42(8):665-9.
74. Deans KW, Lang JR, Smith DE. Stability of trimethoprim-sulfamethoxazole injection in five infusion fluids. American journal of hospital pharmacy. 1982 Oct;39(10):1681-4.
75. Richmond JM, Whitworth JA, Fairley KF, Kincaid-Smith P. Co-trimoxazole nephrotoxicity. Lancet. 1979 Mar 3;1(8114):493.
76. Kraemer MJ, Kendall R, Hickman RO, Haas JE, Bierman CW. A generalized allergic reaction with acute interstitial nephritis following trimethoprim-sulfamethoxazole use. Annals of allergy. 1982 Dec;49(6):323-5.
77. Chandra M, Chandra P, McVicar M, Susin M, Teichberg S. Rapid onset of co-trimoxazole induced interstitial nephritis. The International journal of pediatric nephrology. 1985 Oct-Dec;6(4):289-92.
78. Payne FE, Jr., Giesecke TF. Multiple system reaction to trimethoprim-sulfamethoxazole. Southern medical journal. 1987 Feb;80(2):275-6.
79. Dutertre JP, Despert F, Jonville AP, Autret E, Nivet H. Acute tubular necrosis during a treatment with Bactrim. Archives francaises de pediatrie. 1991 Jun-Jul;48(6):441-2.
80. Smith EJ, Light JA, Filo RS, Yum MN. Interstitial nephritis caused by trimethoprim-sulfamethoxazole in renal transplant recipients. Jama. 1980 Jul 25;244(4):360-1.
81. Tasker PR, MacGregor GA, de Wardener HE. Use of co-trimoxazole in chronic renal failure. Lancet. 1975 May 31;1(7918):1216-8.
82. Bourgault AM, Van Scoy RE, Brewer NS, Rosenow EC. Trimethoprim with sulfamethoxazole for treatment of infection with Pneumocystis carinii in renal insufficiency. Chest. 1978 Jul;74(1):91-2.
83. Brockner J, Boisen E. Fatal multisystem toxicity after co-trimoxazole. Lancet. 1978 Apr 15;1(8068):831.
84. Finlayson WB, Johnson G. Multisystem toxicity after co-trimoxazole. Lancet. 1978 Sep 23;2(8091):682-3.
85. Epstein M, Wright JM. Severe multisystem disease caused by trimethoprim-sulfamethoxazole: possible role of an *in vitro* lymphocyte assay. The Journal of allergy and clinical immunology. 1990 Sep;86(3 Pt 1):416-7.
86. Thompson JF, Chalmers DH, Hunnisett AG, Wood RF, Morris PJ. Nephrotoxicity of trimethoprim and cotrimoxazole in renal allograft recipients treated with cyclosporine. Transplantation. 1983 Aug;36(2):204-6.
87. Ringden O, Myrenfors P, Klintmalm G, Tyden G, Ost L. Nephrotoxicity by co-trimoxazole and cyclosporin in transplanted patients. Lancet. 1984 May 5;1(8384):1016-7.
88. Berg KJ, Nordby G, Rootwelt K, Djoseland O, Fauchald P, Mehl A, et al. Effects on renal function of combined treatment with trimethoprim and cyclosporine A in kidney transplant patients. Transplantation proceedings. 1988 Jun;20(3):413-5.
89. Sen S, Bayrak R, Ok E, Basdemir G. Drug-induced acute interstitial nephritis and vasculitis or vasculary rejection in renal allografts. Am J Kidney Dis. 2001 Jan;37(1):E4.
90. Josephson MA, Chiu MY, Woodle ES, Thistlethwaite JR, Haas M. Drug-induced acute interstitial nephritis in renal allografts: histopathologic features and clinical course in six patients. Am J Kidney Dis. 1999 Sep;34(3):540-8.
91. Colvin RB FL. Interstitial Nephritis. In: Tisher CC BB, ed. *Renal Pathology*. 2nd ed. Philadelphia: Lippincott 1994:723-68.
92. Maki DG, Fox BC, Kuntz J, Sollinger HW, Belzer FO. A prospective, randomized, double-blind study of trimethoprim-sulfamethoxazole for prophylaxis of infection in renal transplantation. Side effects of trimethoprim-sulfamethoxazole, interaction with cyclosporine. The Journal of laboratory and clinical medicine. 1992 Jan;119(1):11-24.
93. Kimmelt MS PT, Kramer NC, Thompson AM. *In vitro* and *in vivo* interaction of sulfamethoxazole with cyclosporin A measurement by high-pressure liquid chromatography (HRLC). Kidney international. 1985;27:343A.
94. Bourgoignie JJ. Renal complications of human immunodeficiency virus type 1. Kidney international. 1990 Jun;37(6):1571-84.
95. Rao TK, Friedman EA. Renal syndromes in the acquired immunodeficiency syndrome (AIDS): lessons learned from analysis over 5 years. Artificial organs. 1988 Jun;12(3):206-9.
96. Humphreys MH, Schoenfeld PY. Renal complications in patients with the acquired immune deficiency syndrome (AIDS). American journal of nephrology. 1987;7(1):1-7.
97. Bourgoignie J. J O-BC, Green DF, Pardo V. Renal Disease and AIDS. In: Broder S MTJ, Bolognesi D, ed. *Textbook of AIDS Disease*. Baltimore: Williams and Wilkins 1993:597-608.
98. Walzer PD, Perl DP, Krogstad DJ, Rawson PG, Schultz MG. Pneumocystis carinii pneumonia in the United States. Epidemiologic, diagnostic, and clinical features. Annals of internal medicine. 1974 Jan;80(1):83-93.
99. Glatt AE, Chirgwin K. Pneumocystis carinii pneumonia in human immunodeficiency virus-infected patients. Archives of internal medicine. 1990 Feb;150(2):271-9.
100. Kovacs JA, Hiemenz JW, Macher AM, Stover D, Murray HW, Shelhamer J, et al. Pneumocystis carinii pneumonia: a comparison between patients with the acquired immunodeficiency syndrome and patients with other immunodeficiencies. Annals of internal medicine. 1984 May;100(5):663-71.

101. Wolfsy. Use of trimethoprim-sulfamethoxazole in the treatment of Pneumocystis carinii pneumonitis in patients with acquired immunodeficiency syndrome. Reviews of infectious diseases. 1987;9:S184-94.
102. Wharton JM, Coleman DL, Wofsy CB, Luce JM, Blumenfeld W, Hadley WK, et al. Trimethoprim-sulfamethoxazole or pentamidine for Pneumocystis carinii pneumonia in the acquired immunodeficiency syndrome. A prospective randomized trial. Annals of internal medicine. 1986 Jul;105(1):37-44.
103. Sattler FR, Cowan R, Nielsen DM, Ruskin J. Trimethoprim-sulfamethoxazole compared with pentamidine for treatment of Pneumocystis carinii pneumonia in the acquired immunodeficiency syndrome. A prospective, noncrossover study. Annals of internal medicine. 1988 Aug 15;109(4):280-7.
104. Gordin FM, Simon GL, Wofsy CB, Mills J. Adverse reactions to trimethoprim-sulfamethoxazole in patients with the acquired immunodeficiency syndrome. Annals of internal medicine. 1984 Apr;100(4):495-9.
105. Zuniga CA Chua A, Alpert H, Vaamonde CA. Trimethoprim-sulfamethoxazole nephrotoxicity in patients with AIDS. Nat Kidney Found 1990;20:A29(abstract).
106. Chua A ZC, Alpert H, Vaamonde CA. Trimethoprim-sulfametoxazole nephrotoxicity in the sodium-depleted rat. J Am Soc Nephrol. 1990;1:608(abstract).
107. Harvey AM, Malvin RL. Comparison of creatinine and inulin clearances in male and female rats. The American journal of physiology. 1965 Oct;209(4):849-52.
108. Gouvea W, Vaamonde CM, Owens B, Alpert H, Pardo V, Vaamonde CA. The protection against gentamicin nephrotoxicity in the streptozotocin-induced diabetic rat is not related to gender. Life sciences. 1992;51(22):1747-58.
109. Bozzette SA, Finkelstein DM, Spector SA, Frame P, Powderly WG, He W, et al. A randomized trial of three antipneumocystis agents in patients with advanced human immunodeficiency virus infection. NIAID AIDS Clinical Trials Group. The New England journal of medicine. 1995 Mar 16;332(11):693-9.
110. Para MF, Finkelstein D, Becker S, Dohn M, Walawander A, Black JR. Reduced toxicity with gradual initiation of trimethoprim-sulfamethoxazole as primary prophylaxis for Pneumocystis carinii pneumonia: AIDS Clinical Trials Group 268. Journal of acquired immune deficiency syndromes (1999). 2000 Aug 1;24(4):337-43.
111. Boubaker K, Sudre P, Bally F, Vogel G, Meuwly JY, Glauser MP, et al. Changes in renal function associated with indinavir. AIDS (London, England). 1998 Dec 24;12(18):F249-54.
112. Kopp JB, Miller KD, Mican JA, Feuerstein IM, Vaughan E, Baker C, et al. Crystalluria and urinary tract abnormalities associated with indinavir. Annals of internal medicine. 1997 Jul 15;127(2):119-25.
113. Valencia ME J-NI, Rodriguez-Rosado R, Soriano V, Carrillo de Albornoz ML, Gonzalez Lahoz J. Incidence of nephrolithiasis in HIV infected patients under indinavir treatment. [abstract 448]. Sixth European Conference on Clinical Aspects and Treatment of HIV Infection; October 1997; Hamburg; October 1997.
114. de Araujo M, Seguro AC. Trimethoprim-sulfamethoxazole (TMP/SMX) potentiates indinavir nephrotoxicity. Antiviral therapy. 2002 Sep;7(3):181-4.
115. Medina I, Mills J, Leoung G, Hopewell PC, Lee B, Modin G, et al. Oral therapy for Pneumocystis carinii pneumonia in the acquired immunodeficiency syndrome. A controlled trial of trimethoprim-sulfamethoxazole versus trimethoprim-dapsone. The New England journal of medicine. 1990 Sep 20;323(12):776-82.
116. Greenberg S, Reiser IW, Chou SY, Porush JG. Trimethoprim-sulfamethoxazole induces reversible hyperkalemia. Annals of internal medicine. 1993 Aug 15;119(4):291-5.
117. Choi MJ, Fernandez PC, Patnaik A, Coupaye-Gerard B, D'Andrea D, Szerlip H, et al. Brief report: trimethoprim-induced hyperkalemia in a patient with AIDS. The New England journal of medicine. 1993 Mar 11;328(10):703-6.
118. (a) Modest GA PB, Mascoli N; (b) Pennypacker LC, Mintzer J, Pitner J; (c) Canaday DH, Johnson JR; (d) Reiser IW, Chou SY (e) Velazquez H, Ellison DH. Hyperkalemia in elderly patients receiving standard doses of trimethoprim-sulfametoxazole. . Annals of internal medicine. 1994;120:437-8(letters).
119. Perazella MA. Hyperkalemia and trimethoprim-sulfamethoxazole: a new problem emerges 25 years later. Connecticut medicine. 1997 Aug;61(8):451-8.
120. Funai N, Shimamoto Y, Matsuzaki M, Watanabe M, Tokioka T, Sueoka E, et al. Hyperkalaemia with renal tubular dysfunction by sulfamethoxazole-trimethoprim for Pneumocystis carinii pneumonia in patients with lymphoid malignancy. Haematologia. 1993;25(2):137-41.
121. Lawson DH, Jick H. Adverse reactions to co-trimoxazole in hospitalized medical patients. The American journal of the medical sciences. 1978 Jan-Feb;275(1):53-7.
122. Kalin MF, Poretsky L, Seres DS, Zumoff B. Hyporeninemic hypoaldosteronism associated with acquired immune deficiency syndrome. The American journal of medicine. 1987 May;82(5):1035-8.
123. Guy RJ, Turberg Y, Davidson RN, Finnerty G, MacGregor GA, Wise PH. Mineralocorticoid deficiency in HIV infection. BMJ (Clinical research ed. 1989 Feb 25;298(6672):496-7.

124. Murphy CE, Ratnavel RG, Davidson AC. Mineralocorticoid deficiency in HIV infection. BMJ (Clinical research ed. 1989 Apr 29;298(6681):1181.
125. Velazquez H, Perazella MA, Wright FS, Ellison DH. Renal mechanism of trimethoprim-induced hyperkalemia. Annals of internal medicine. 1993 Aug 15;119(4):296-301.
126. Schlanger LE, Kleyman TR, Ling BN. K(+)-sparing diuretic actions of trimethoprim: inhibition of Na+ channels in A6 distal nephron cells. Kidney international. 1994 Apr;45(4):1070-6.
127. Murphy JL. Renal tubular acidosis in children treated with trimethoprim-sulfamethoxazole during therapy for acute lymphoid leukemia. Pediatrics. 1992 Jun;89(6 Pt 1):1072-4.
128. Schoenbach EB GE. The pharmacology, mode of action, and therapeutic potentialities of stilbamidine, pentamidine, propamidine and other aromatic diamidines. A review. Medicine. 1948;27:327-77.
129. Van Hoof L HC, Peel E. Pentamidine in the prevention and treatment of trypanosomiasis. Trans Roy Soc Trop Med Hyg. 1944;37:271-80.
130. Napier LE SGP. The treatment of kala-azar with diaminodiphenoxypentane. Preliminary observations on the treatment of 32 cases. Indian Med Gaz. 1943;78:177-83
131. Ivady G, Paldy L, Koltay M, Toth G, Kovacs Z. Pneumocystis carinii pneumonia. Lancet. 1967 Mar 18;1(7490):616-7.
132. Western KA, Perera DR, Schultz MG. Pentamidine isethionate in the treatment of Pneumocystis carinii pneumonia. Annals of internal medicine. 1970 Nov;73(5):695-702.
133. Hughes WT, Feldman S, Chaudhary SC, Ossi MJ, Cox F, Sanyal SK. Comparison of pentamidine isethionate and trimethoprim-sulfamethoxazole in the treatment of Pneumocystis carinii pneumonia. The Journal of pediatrics. 1978 Feb;92(2):285-91.
134. Sands M, Kron MA, Brown RB. Pentamidine: a review. Reviews of infectious diseases. 1985 Sep-Oct;7(5):625-34.
135. Pearson RD, Hewlett EL. Pentamidine for the treatment of Pneumocystis carinii pneumonia and other protozoal diseases. Annals of internal medicine. 1985 Nov;103(5):782-6.
136. Haley. Pentamidine in Pneumocystis carinii pneumonia. Microlink Update. 1987;3:1-4.
137. O'Brien JG, Dong BJ, Coleman RL, Gee L, Balano KB. A 5-year retrospective review of adverse drug reactions and their risk factors in human immunodeficiency virus-infected patients who were receiving intravenous pentamidine therapy for Pneumocystis carinii pneumonia. Clin Infect Dis. 1997 May;24(5):854-9.
138. Sattler FR, Frame P, Davis R, Nichols L, Shelton B, Akil B, et al. Trimetrexate with leucovorin versus trimethoprim-sulfamethoxazole for moderate to severe episodes of Pneumocystis carinii pneumonia in patients with AIDS: a prospective, controlled multicenter investigation of the AIDS Clinical Trials Group Protocol 029/031. The Journal of infectious diseases. 1994 Jul;170(1):165-72.
139. Waalkes TP, Denham C, DeVita VT. Pentamidine: clinical pharmacologic correlations in man and mice. Clinical pharmacology and therapeutics. 1970 Jul-Aug;11(4):505-12.
140. Bernard EM, Donnelly HJ, Maher MP, Armstrong D. Use of a new bioassay to study pentamidine pharmacokinetics. The Journal of infectious diseases. 1985 Oct;152(4):750-4.
141. Conte JE, Jr. Pharmacokinetics of intravenous pentamidine in patients with normal renal function or receiving hemodialysis. The Journal of infectious diseases. 1991 Jan;163(1):169-75.
142. Bronner U, Gustafsson LL, Doua F, Ericsson O, Miezan T, Rais M, et al. Pharmacokinetics and adverse reactions after a single dose of pentamidine in patients with Trypanosoma gambiense sleeping sickness. British journal of clinical pharmacology. 1995 Mar;39(3):289-95.
143. Vohringer HF AK. Pharmakokinetik von Pentamidin bei knochenmarktransplantierten und AIDS-patienten. In: Gruyter Wd, ed. *Pneumocystis-carinii-Pneumonie bei Immunsuppression* Berlin, New York 1991:25-32.
144. Lidman C, Bronner U, Gustafsson LL, Rombo L. Plasma pentamidine concentrations vary between individuals with Pneumocystis carinii pneumonia and the drug is actively secreted by the kidney. The Journal of antimicrobial chemotherapy. 1994 Apr;33(4):803-10.
145. Conte JE, Jr., Upton RA, Phelps RT, Wofsy CB, Zurlinden E, Lin ET. Use of a specific and sensitive assay to determine pentamidine pharmacokinetics in patients with AIDS. The Journal of infectious diseases. 1986 Dec;154(6):923-9.
146. Berger BJ, Hall JE, Tidwell RR. The distribution of multiple doses of pentamidine in rats. Pharmacology & toxicology. 1990 Mar;66(3):234-6.
147. Navin TR, Dickinson CM, Adams SR, Mayersohn M, Juranek DD. Effect of azotemia in dogs on the pharmacokinetics of pentamidine. The Journal of infectious diseases. 1987 May;155(5):1020-6.
148. Berger BJ, Lombardy RJ, Marbury GD, Bell CA, Dykstra CC, Hall JE, et al. Metabolic N-hydroxylation of pentamidine *in vitro*. Antimicrobial agents and chemotherapy. 1990 Sep;34(9):1678-84.
149. Donnelly H, Bernard EM, Rothkotter H, Gold JW, Armstrong D. Distribution of pentamidine in patients with AIDS. The Journal of infectious diseases. 1988 May;157(5):985-9.

150. Poola NR, Kalis M, Plakogiannis FM, Taft DR. Characterization of pentamidine excretion in the isolated perfused rat kidney. The Journal of antimicrobial chemotherapy. 2003 Sep;52(3):397-404.
151. Andersen R, Boedicker M, Ma M, Goldstein EJ. Adverse reactions associated with pentamidine isethionate in AIDS patients: recommendations for monitoring therapy. Drug intelligence & clinical pharmacy. 1986 Nov;20(11):862-8.
152. Waskin H, Stehr-Green JK, Helmick CG, Sattler FR. Risk factors for hypoglycemia associated with pentamidine therapy for Pneumocystis pneumonia. Jama. 1988 Jul 15;260(3):345-7.
153. Lachaal M, Venuto RC. Nephrotoxicity and hyperkalemia in patients with acquired immunodeficiency syndrome treated with pentamidine. The American journal of medicine. 1989 Sep;87(3):260-3.
154. Chua A BJ, Alpert H, Vaamonde CA. Risk factors for pentamidine nephrotoxicity in AIDS patients. Nat Kidney Found. 1989;19:A5 (abstract).
155. Briceland LL, Bailie GR. Pentamidine-associated nephrotoxicity and hyperkalemia in patients with AIDS. Dicp. 1991 Nov;25(11):1171-4.
156. Shuster M, Dunn M. Pentamidine and hematuria. Annals of internal medicine. 1986 Jul;105(1):146.
157. Sensakovic JW, Suarez M, Perez G, Johnson ES, Smith LG. Pentamidine treatment of Pneumocystis carinii pneumonia in the acquired immunodeficiency syndrome. Association with acute renal failure and myoglobinuria. Archives of internal medicine. 1985 Dec;145(12):2247.
158. Chua A BJ, Papendick R, Alpert H, Vaamonde CA. Pentamidine nephrotoxicity in the rat. Kidney international. 1990;37:478A.
159. Stehr-Green JK, Helmick CG. Pentamidine and renal toxicity. The New England journal of medicine. 1985 Sep 12;313(11):694-5.
160. Antoniskis D, Larsen RA. Acute, rapidly progressive renal failure with simultaneous use of amphotericin B and pentamidine. Antimicrobial agents and chemotherapy. 1990 Mar;34(3):470-2.
161. Morin D, Dumas ML, Valette H, Dumas R. Transitory acute kidney insufficiency and insulin-dependent after treatment of kala-azar with pentamidine and N-methylglucamine antimony. Archives francaises de pediatrie. 1991 May;48(5):349-51.
162. Bryceson AD, Chulay JD, Mugambi M, Were JB, Gachihi G, Chunge CN, et al. Visceral leishmaniasis unresponsive to antimonial drugs. II. Response to high dosage sodium stibogluconate or prolonged treatment with pentamidine. Transactions of the Royal Society of Tropical Medicine and Hygiene. 1985;79(5):705-14.
163. Golden JA, Chernoff D, Hollander H, Feigal D, Conte JE. Prevention of Pneumocystis carinii pneumonia by inhaled pentamidine. Lancet. 1989 Mar 25;1(8639):654-7.
164. Jensen BN, Nielsen TL, Lerche B, Jensen TH, Backer V, Mathiesen L, et al. Prevention of Pneumocystis carinii pneumonia relapse by aerosolised pentamidine, 60 mg biweekly, using an Acorn System 22 nebuliser. Scandinavian journal of infectious diseases. 1990;22(5):533-6.
165. Link H, Vohringer HF, Wingen F, Bragas B, Schwardt A, Ehninger G. Pentamidine aerosol for prophylaxis of Pneumocystis carinii pneumonia after BMT. Bone marrow transplantation. 1993 May;11(5):403-6.
166. Saukkonen K, Garland R, Koziel H. Aerosolized pentamidine as alternative primary prophylaxis against Pneumocystis carinii pneumonia in adult hepatic and renal transplant recipients. Chest. 1996 May;109(5):1250-5.
167. Miller RF, Delany S, Semple SJ. Acute renal failure after nebulised pentamidine. Lancet. 1989 Jun 3;1(8649):1271-2.
168. Chapelon C, Raguin G, De Gennes C. Renal insufficiency with nebulised pentamidine. Lancet. 1989 Oct 28;2(8670):1045-6.
169. Soo Hoo GW, Mohsenifar Z, Meyer RD. Inhaled or intravenous pentamidine therapy for Pneumocystis carinii pneumonia in AIDS. A randomized trial. Annals of internal medicine. 1990 Aug 1;113(3):195-202.
170. French MH MA. Some metabolic disturbances in domestic stock following injection of 4:4′-diamidine 1:5 diphenoxypentane. Vet Rec. 1941;53:413-6.
171. Wien R FW, Scotcher NM. The metabolic effects produced by certain aromatic diamidines. Ann Trop Med Parasitol. 1943;37:19-33.
172. Makulu DR, Waalkes TP. Interaction between aromatic diamidines and nucleic acids: possible implications for chemotherapy. Journal of the National Cancer Institute. 1975 Feb;54(2):305-9.
173. Gambertoglio JG AF, Blythe WB. Use of drugs in patients with renal failure. In: Schrier R.W GCW, ed. *Diseases of the Kidney*. 5th ed. Boston: Little, Brown and Co 1993:3211-68.
174. Fortunato SJ, Bawdon RE. Determination of pentamidine transfer in the *in vitro* perfused human cotyledon with high-performance liquid chromatography. American journal of obstetrics and gynecology. 1989 Mar;160(3):759-61.
175. DeVita VT, Emmer M, Levine A, Jacobs B, Berard C. Pneumocystis carinii pneumonia: successful diagnosis treatment of two patients with associated malignant processes. The New England journal of medicine. 1969 Feb 6;280(6):287-91.
176. Peltz S, Hashmi S. Pentamidine-induced severe hyperkalemia. The American journal of medicine. 1989 Dec;87(6):698-9.
177. Buff DD, Aboal AA. Pentamidine-associated renal dysfunction and hyperkalemia. The American journal of medicine. 1990 May;88(5):552.

178. Bibler MR, Chou TC, Toltzis RJ, Wade PA. Recurrent ventricular tachycardia due to pentamidine-induced cardiotoxicity. Chest. 1988 Dec;94(6):1303-6.
179. Owens RC, Jr., Nolin TD. Antimicrobial-associated QT interval prolongation: pointes of interest. Clin Infect Dis. 2006 Dec 15;43(12):1603-11.
180. Balslev U, Berild D, Nielsen TL. Cardiac arrest during treatment of Pneumocystis carinii pneumonia with intravenous pentamidine isethionate. Scandinavian journal of infectious diseases. 1992;24(1):111-2.
181. Kleyman TR, Roberts C, Ling BN. A mechanism for pentamidine-induced hyperkalemia: inhibition of distal nephron sodium transport. Annals of internal medicine. 1995 Jan 15;122(2):103-6.
182. Gabriels G, Stockem E, Greven J. Potassium-sparing renal effects of trimethoprim and structural analogues. Nephron. 2000 Sep;86(1):70-8.
183. Shah GM, Alvarado P, Kirschenbaum MA. Symptomatic hypocalcemia and hypomagnesemia with renal magnesium wasting associated with pentamidine therapy in a patient with AIDS. The American journal of medicine. 1990 Sep;89(3):380-2.
184. Burnett RJ, Reents SB. Severe hypomagnesemia induced by pentamidine. Dicp. 1990 Mar;24(3):239-40.
185. Gradon JD, Fricchione L, Sepkowitz D. Severe hypomagnesemia associated with pentamidine therapy. Reviews of infectious diseases. 1991 May-Jun;13(3):511-2.
186. Mani S. Pentamidine-induced renal magnesium wasting. AIDS (London, England). 1992 Jun;6(6):594-5.
187. Youle MS, Clarbour J, Gazzard B, Chanas A. Severe hypocalcaemia in AIDS patients treated with foscarnet and pentamidine. Lancet. 1988 Jun 25;1(8600):1455-6.
188. Bouchard P, Sai P, Reach G, Caubarrere I, Ganeval D, Assan R. Diabetes mellitus following pentamidine-induced hypoglycemia in humans. Diabetes. 1982 Jan;31(1):40-5.
189. Sharpe SM. Pentamidine and hypoglycemia. Annals of internal medicine. 1983 Jul;99(1):128.
190. Murdoch JK KJ. Pentamidine and hypoglycemia Annals of internal medicine. 1983;99:879 (letter).
191. Stahl-Bayliss CM, Kalman CM, Laskin OL. Pentamidine-induced hypoglycemia in patients with the acquired immune deficiency syndrome. Clinical pharmacology and therapeutics. 1986 Mar;39(3):271-5.
192. Collins J, Pien FD, Houk JH. Insulin-dependent diabetes mellitus associated with pentamidine. The American journal of the medical sciences. 1989 Mar;297(3):174-5.
193. Hitchings G. The use of an antimetabolite in chemotherapy of malaria and other infections. Clin Pharm Ther. 1960;1:570-89.
194. Ritschel WA, Hammer GV, Thompson GA. Pharmacokinetics of antimalarials and proposals for dosage regimens. International journal of clinical pharmacology and biopharmacy. 1978 Sep;16(9):395-401.
195. White N. Clinical pharmacokinetics of antimalarial drugs. Clinical pharmacokinetics. 1985;10(3):187-215.
196. Opravil M, Heald A, Lazzarin A, Hirschel B, Luthy R, and the Swiss Group for Clinical Studies in AIDS. . Combined prophylaxis of pneumocystis carinii pneumoniae and toxoplasmosis: dapsone+pyrimethamine vs aerolized pentamidine. AIDS (London, England). 1992;6:S8.
197. Opravil M, Keusch G, Luthy R. Pyrimethamine inhibits renal secretion of creatinine. Antimicrobial agents and chemotherapy. 1993 May;37(5):1056-60.
198. Paniker U, Levine N. Dapsone and sulfapyridine. Dermatologic clinics. 2001 Jan;19(1):79-86, viii.
199. Alves-Rodrigues EN, Ribeiro LC, Silva MD, Takiuchi A, Fontes CJ. Dapsone syndrome with acute renal failure during leprosy treatment: case report. Braz J Infect Dis. 2005 Feb;9(1):84-6.
200. Sener O, Doganci L, Safali M, Besirbellioglu B, Bulucu F, Pahsa A. Severe dapsone hypersensitivity syndrome. J Investig Allergol Clin Immunol. 2006;16(4):268-70.
201. Bucaretchi F, Vicente DC, Pereira RM, Tresoldi AT. Dapsone hypersensitivity syndrome in an adolescent during treatment during of leprosy. Revista do Instituto de Medicina Tropical de Sao Paulo. 2004 Nov-Dec;46(6):331-4.
202. Zuidema J, Hilbers-Modderman ES, Merkus FW. Clinical pharmacokinetics of dapsone. Clinical pharmacokinetics. 1986 Jul-Aug;11(4):299-315.
203. Aronoff GR BJ, Brier ME, Golper TA, Morrison G, Singer I, Swan SK, Bennett WM. Drug Prescribing in Renal Failure. Dosing Guidelines for Adults. 4th Ed ed. Philadelphia 1999:48.
204. Lee BL, Medina I, Benowitz NL, Jacob P, 3rd, Wofsy CB, Mills Jt. Dapsone, trimethoprim, and sulfamethoxazole plasma levels during treatment of Pneumocystis pneumonia in patients with the acquired immunodeficiency syndrome (AIDS). Evidence of drug interactions. Annals of internal medicine. 1989 Apr 15;110(8):606-11.
205. Belmont A. Dapsone induced nephrotic syndrome. Jama. 1967;200:262-3.
206. Hoffbrand BI. Dapsone and renal papillary necrosis. British medical journal. 1978 Jan 14;1(6105):78.
207. Chugh KS, Singhal PC, Sharma BK, Mahakur AC, Pal Y, Datta BN, et al. Acute renal failure due to intravascular hemolysis in the North Indian patients. The American journal of the medical sciences. 1977 Sep-Oct;274(2):139-46.

208. Alves-Rodrigues EN, Ribeiro LC, Silva MD, Takiuchi A, Rabel-Filho OC, Martini-Filho D, et al. Renal hypersensitivity vasculitis associated with dapsone. Am J Kidney Dis. 2005 Oct;46(4):e51-3.
209. Lau G. A fatal case of drug-induced multi-organ damage in a patient with Hansen's disease: dapsone syndrome or rifampicin toxicity? Forensic science international. 1995 May 22;73(2):109-15.
210. Kenner DJ, Holt K, Agnello R, Chester GH. Permanent retinal damage following massive dapsone overdose. The British journal of ophthalmology. 1980 Oct;64(10):741-4.
211. Higuchi M, Agatsuma T, Iizima M, Yamazaki Y, Saita T, Ichikawa T, et al. A case of drug-induced hypersensitivity syndrome with multiple organ involvement treated with plasma exchange. Ther Apher Dial. 2005 Oct;9(5):412-6.
212. Neuvonen PJ, Elonen E, Haapanen EJ. Acute dapsone intoxication: clinical findings and effect of oral charcoal and haemodialysis on dapsone elimination. Acta medica Scandinavica. 1983;214(3):215-20.
213. Endre ZH, Charlesworth JA, Macdonald GJ, Woodbridge L. Successful treatment of acute dapsone intoxication using charcoal hemoperfusion. Australian and New Zealand journal of medicine. 1983 Oct;13(5):509-12.
214. Hooper D. Quinolones. In: Mandel GL BJ, Dolin R, ed. *Principles and practice of infectious diseases*. New York: Churchill Livingstone 1995:364-76.
215. Lesher GY, Froelich EJ, Gruett MD, Bailey JH, Brundage RP. 1,8-Naphthyridine Derivatives. a New Class of Chemotherapeutic Agents. Journal of medicinal and pharmaceutical chemistry. 1962 Sep;91:1063-5.
216. Fluoroquinolones U. USPDI: Fluoroquinolones. In: The United States Pharmacopeial Convention IDIftHCP, ed. 14th ed. Rockville 1994:1392-401.
217. Ferry N, Cuisinaud G, Pozet N, Zech PY, Sassard J. Nalidixic acid kinetics after single and repeated oral doses. Clinical pharmacology and therapeutics. 1981 May;29(5):695-8.
218. Portmann GA, McChesney EW, Stander H, Moore WE. Pharmacokinetic model for nalidixic acid in man. II. Parameters for absorption, metabolism, and elimination. Journal of pharmaceutical sciences. 1966 Jan;55(1):72-8.
219. Porter G. Antimicrobial nephrotoxicity. In: Massry SG GR, ed. *Textbook of Nephrology*. Baltimore: Williams & Wilkins 1989:812-8.
220. Bergan T. Pharmacokinetics of fluorinated quinolones. In: VT A, ed. *The Quinolones*. London: Academic Press 1988:119-54
221. Gerding DN, Hitt JA. Tissue penetration of the new quinolones in humans. Reviews of infectious diseases. 1989 Jul-Aug;11 Suppl 5:S1046-57.
222. Plaisance KI, Drusano GL, Forrest A, Weir MR, Standiford HC. Effect of renal function on the bioavailability of ciprofloxacin. Antimicrobial agents and chemotherapy. 1990 Jun;34(6):1031-4.
223. Drusano GL. An overview of the pharmacology of intravenously administered ciprofloxacin. The American journal of medicine. 1987 Apr 27;82(4A):339-45.
224. Rohwedder R, Bergan T, Thorsteinsson SB, Scholl H. Transintestinal elimination of ciprofloxacin. Chemotherapy. 1990;36(2):77-84.
225. Nouaille-Degorce B, Veau C, Dautrey S, Tod M, Laouari D, Carbon C, et al. Influence of renal failure on ciprofloxacin pharmacokinetics in rats. Antimicrobial agents and chemotherapy. 1998 Feb;42(2):289-92.
226. Ljungberg B, Nilsson-Ehle I. Pharmacokinetics of ciprofloxacin in the elderly: increased oral bioavailability and reduced renal clearance. Eur J Clin Microbiol Infect Dis. 1989 Jun;8(6):515-20.
227. R Stahlmann HL. The Quinolones. In: VT A, ed. *Safety overview: Toxicity, adverse events, and drug interactions*. London: Academic Press 1988:201-33.
228. Johnson PR, Liu Yin JA, Tooth JA. A randomized trial of high-dose ciprofloxacin versus azlocillin and netilmicin in the empirical therapy of febrile neutropenic patients. The Journal of antimicrobial chemotherapy. 1992 Aug;30(2):203-14.
229. Ball P. Ciprofloxacin: an overview of adverse experiences. The Journal of antimicrobial chemotherapy. 1986 Nov;18 Suppl D:187-93.
230. Arcieri G, Griffith E, Gruenwaldt G, Heyd A, O'Brien B, Becker N, et al. Ciprofloxacin: an update on clinical experience. The American journal of medicine. 1987 Apr 27;82(4A):381-6.
231. Gerritsen WR, Peters A, Henny FC, Brouwers JR. Ciprofloxacin-induced nephrotoxicity. Nephrol Dial Transplant. 1987;2(5):382-3.
232. Rippelmeyer DJ, Synhavsky A. Ciprofloxacin and allergic interstitial nephritis. Annals of internal medicine. 1988 Jul 15;109(2):170.
233. Lee CW, Fialkow RZ, Van Wyck D. Adverse effects associated with the newer fluoroquinolones. Am J Kidney Dis. 1989 Jun;13(6):510-1.
234. Hootkins R, Fenves AZ, Stephens MK. Acute renal failure secondary to oral ciprofloxacin therapy: a presentation of three cases and a review of the literature. Clinical nephrology. 1989 Aug;32(2):75-8.
235. Ying LS, Johnson CA. Ciprofloxacin-induced interstitial nephritis. Clinical pharmacy. 1989 Jul;8(7):518-21.
236. Helmink R, Benediktsson H. Ciprofloxacin-induced allergic interstitial nephritis. Nephron. 1990;55(4):432-3.

237. Rastogi S, Atkinson JL, McCarthy JT. Allergic nephropathy associated with ciprofloxacin. Mayo Clinic proceedings. 1990 Jul;65(7):987-9.
238. Allon M, Lopez EJ, Min KW. Acute renal failure due to ciprofloxacin. Archives of internal medicine. 1990 Oct;150(10):2187-9.
239. Murray KM, Wilson MG. Suspected ciprofloxacin-induced interstitial nephritis. Dicp. 1990 Apr;24(4):379-80.
240. Hatton J, Haagensen D. Renal dysfunction associated with ciprofloxacin. Pharmacotherapy. 1990;10(5):337-40.
241. Simpson J, Watson AR, Mellersh A, Nelson CS, Dodd K. Typhoid fever, ciprofloxacin, and renal failure. Archives of disease in childhood. 1991 Sep;66(9):1083-4.
242. Arvieux C, Charasse C, Guilhem I, Rivalan J, Le Pogamp P, Ramee MP. Acute kidney failure due to tubulo-interstitial nephropathy after treatment with ciprofloxacin. Presse Med. 1991 Oct 26;20(34):1686.
243. Gonski PN. Ciprofloxacin-induced renal failure in an elderly patient. The Medical journal of Australia. 1991 May 6;154(9):638-9.
244. George MJ, Dew RB, 3rd, Daly JS. Acute renal failure after an overdose of ciprofloxacin. Archives of internal medicine. 1991 Mar;151(3):620.
245. Andersen I, Sjostrom P. Ciprofloxacin can cause allergic interstitial nephritis with acute renal failure. Lakartidningen. 1991 Apr 3;88(14):1298-9.
246. Bailey JR, Trott SA, Philbrick JT. Ciprofloxacin-induced acute interstitial nephritis. American journal of nephrology. 1992;12(4):271-3.
247. Lo WK, Rolston KV, Rubenstein EB, Bodey GP. Ciprofloxacin-induced nephrotoxicity in patients with cancer. Archives of internal medicine. 1993 May 24;153(10):1258-62.
248. Lien YH, Hansen R, Kern WF, Bangert J, Nagle RB, Ko M, et al. Ciprofloxacin-induced granulomatous interstitial nephritis and localized elastolysis. Am J Kidney Dis. 1993 Oct;22(4):598-602.
249. Reece RJ, Nicholls AJ. Ciprofloxacin-induced acute interstitial nephritis. Nephrol Dial Transplant. 1996 Feb;11(2):393.
250. Rosado LJ, Siskind MS, Copeland JG. Acute interstitial nephritis in a cardiac transplant recipient receiving ciprofloxacin. The Journal of thoracic and cardiovascular surgery. 1994 May;107(5):1364; author reply -6.
251. Shih DJ, Korbet SM, Rydel JJ, Schwartz MM. Renal vasculitis associated with ciprofloxacin. Am J Kidney Dis. 1995 Sep;26(3):516-9.
252. Dharnidharka VR, Nadeau K, Cannon CL, Harris HW, Rosen S. Ciprofloxacin overdose: acute renal failure with prominent apoptotic changes. Am J Kidney Dis. 1998 Apr;31(4):710-2.
253. Avent CK, Krinsky D, Kirklin JK, Bourge RC, Figg WD. Synergistic nephrotoxicity due to ciprofloxacin and cyclosporine. The American journal of medicine. 1988 Sep;85(3):452-3.
254. Anand A. Ciprofloxacin nephrotoxicity. Archives of internal medicine. 1993 Dec 13;153(23):2705-6.
255. Raja N, Miller WE, McMillan R, Mason JR. Ciprofloxacin-associated acute renal failure in patients undergoing high-dose chemotherapy and autologous stem cell rescue. Bone marrow transplantation. 1998 Jun;21(12):1283-4.
256. Yew WW, Chau CH, Wong PC, Choi HY. Ciprofloxacin-induced renal dysfunction in patients with mycobacterial lung infections. Tuber Lung Dis. 1995 Apr;76(2):173-5.
257. Hadimeri H, Almroth G, Cederbrant K, Enestrom S, Hultman P, Lindell A. Allergic nephropathy associated with norfloxacin and ciprofloxacin therapy. Report of two cases and review of the literature. Scandinavian journal of urology and nephrology. 1997 Oct;31(5):481-5.
258. Ortiz A, Plaza JJ, Egido J. Ciprofloxacin-associated tubulointerstitial nephritis with linear tubular basement membrane deposits. Nephron. 1992;60(2):248.
259. Blum MD, Graham DJ, McCloskey CA. Temafloxacin syndrome: review of 95 cases. Clin Infect Dis. 1994 Jun;18(6):946-50.
260. Gauffre A, Mircheva J, Glotz D, Fillastre JP, Simon P, Beaune PH, et al. Autoantibodies against a kidney--liver protein associated with quinolone-induced acute interstitial nephritis or hepatitis. Nephrol Dial Transplant. 1997 Sep;12(9):1961-2.
261. Moffett BS, Rosenstein BJ, Mogayzel PJ, Jr. Ciprofloxacin-induced renal insufficiency in cystic fibrosis. J Cyst Fibros. 2003 Sep;2(3):152-4.
262. Bald M, Ratjen F, Nikolaizik W, Wingen AM. Ciprofloxacin-induced acute renal failure in a patient with cystic fibrosis. The Pediatric infectious disease journal. 2001 Mar;20(3):320-1.
263. Gallelli L, Gallelli A, Vero G, Roccia F, Pelaia G, De Sarro G, et al. Acute renal failure probably induced by prulifloxacin in an elderly woman: a first case report. Clinical drug investigation. 2006;26(1):49-53.
264. Schluter G. Ciprofloxacin: Review of potential toxicologic effects. The American journal of medicine. 1987;82:S91-3.
265. Christ W, Lehnert T, Ulbrich B. Specific toxicologic aspects of the quinolones. Reviews of infectious diseases. 1988 Jan-Feb;10 Suppl 1:S141-6.
266. Thorsteinsson SB, Bergan T, Oddsdottir S, Rohwedder R, Holm R. Crystalluria and ciprofloxacin, influence of urinary pH and hydration. Chemotherapy. 1986;32(5):408-17.

267. Kruger HU, Schuler U, Proksch B, Gobel M, Ehninger G. Investigation of potential interaction of ciprofloxacin with cyclosporine in bone marrow transplant recipients. Antimicrobial agents and chemotherapy. 1990 Jun;34(6):1048-52.
268. Robinson JA, Venezio FR, Costanzo-Nordin MR, Pifarre R, O'Keefe PJ. Patients receiving quinolones and cyclosporine after heart transplantation. The Journal of heart transplantation. 1990 Jan-Feb;9(1):30-1.
269. Elston RA, Taylor J. Possible interaction of ciprofloxacin with cyclosporin A. The Journal of antimicrobial chemotherapy. 1988 May;21(5):679-80.
270. Thomson DJ, Menkis AH, McKenzie FN. Norfloxacin-cyclosporine interaction. Transplantation. 1988 Aug;46(2):312-3.
271. Vogt P, Schorn T, Frei U. Ofloxacin in the treatment of urinary tract infection in renal transplant recipients. Infection. 1988 May-Jun;16(3):175-8.
272. Gluckman E, Devergie A, Lokiec F, Traineau R, Cosset JM, Lemercier N, et al. Role of immunosuppressive drugs for prevention of graft-v-host disease after human HLA matched bone marrow transplantation. Transplantation proceedings. 1987 Dec;19(6 Suppl 7):61-5.
273. Rossi E, Silvestri MG, Manari A, Savazzi G, Migone L. Acute renal failure and piromidic acid. Nephron. 1982;32(1):80-2.
274. Godin M, Ducastelle T, Bercoff E, Dubois D, Fillastre JP, Bourreille J. Renal failure and quinolone. Nephron. 1984;37(1):70-2.
275. Boelaert J, de Jaegere PP, Daneels R, Schurgers M, Gordts B, van Landuyt HW. Case report of renal failure during norfloxacin therapy. Clinical nephrology. 1986 May;25(5):272.
276. Famularo G, De Simone C. Nephrotoxicity and purpura associated with levofloxacin. The Annals of pharmacotherapy. 2002 Sep;36(9):1380-2.
277. Zaigraykin N, Kovalev J, Elias N, Naschitz JE. Levofloxacin-induced interstitial nephritis and vasculitis in an elderly woman. Isr Med Assoc J. 2006 Oct;8(10):726-7.
278. Ramalakshmi S, Bastacky S, Johnson JP. Levofloxacin-induced granulomatous interstitial nephritis. Am J Kidney Dis. 2003 Feb;41(2): E7.
279. Wood ML SS. Levaquin induced acute tubulointerstitial nephritis--two case reports. J Miss State Med Assoc. 2002;43(4):116-7.
280. Krasula RW, Pernet AG. Comparison of organ-specific toxicity of temafloxacin in animals and humans. The American journal of medicine. 1991 Dec 30;91(6A):38S-41S.
281. Norrby SR, Pernet AG. Assessment of adverse events during drug development: experience with temafloxacin. The Journal of antimicrobial chemotherapy. 1991 Dec;28 Suppl C:111-9.
282. Davis GJ, McKenzie BE. Toxicologic evaluation of ofloxacin. The American journal of medicine. 1989 Dec 29;87(6C):43S-6S.
283. Mouton Y, Ajana F, Chidiac C, Capron MH, Home P, Masquelier AM. A multicenter study of lomefloxacin and trimethoprim/sulfamethoxazole in the treatment of uncomplicated acute pyelonephritis. The American journal of medicine. 1992 Apr 6;92(4A):87S-90S.
284. Shiba K, Saito A, Shimada J, Hori S, Kaji M, Miyahara T, et al. Renal handling of fleroxacin in rabbits, dogs, and humans. Antimicrobial agents and chemotherapy. 1990 Jan;34(1):58-64.

16

Antiviral agents

Jeffrey S. BERNS, Alden DOYLE and Nishaminy KASBEKAR

University of Pennsylvania School of Medicine, Philadelphia, Pennsylvania, USA

Introduction

The ability to prevent viral infections is becoming an increasingly important part of clinical medicine. The interest in the development of new antiviral agents and new uses of these medications is driven in large part by the treatment of human immunodeficiency virus (HIV) and growth of the field of transplantation. Although most of the use of these antiviral agents is well-tolerated by patients, there are a variety of potential kidney toxicities that should be appreciated. The most important of these toxicities is acute kidney injury (AKI), which is the main focus of this chapter. We will also consider fluid and electrolyte complications observed with these medications as well as other direct toxic effects on the kidneys. For information regarding clinical pharmacokinetics of antiviral agents and dosing guidelines for their use in patients with kidney injury, which are not discussed in detail here, the reader is referred to several recent reviews [1-5]. This discussion is limited to antiviral agents that are administered orally or parenterally only; topical and intraocular applications are not addressed. The nephrotoxicity of immunomodulatory agents that have anti-viral properties *in vivo* such as interferon alpha are discussed elsewhere.

Acyclovir

Acyclovir is a cyclic analogue of deoxyguanosine, with activity against herpes viruses. Acyclovir diffuses freely into cells, where its subsequent activation and accumulation is dependent upon a herpes virus-specific thymidine kinase. *In vitro*, acyclovir has its greatest action against herpes simplex viruses (HSV) 1 and 2, compared to varicella-zoster virus (VZV), Epstein-Barr virus, and cytomegalovirus (CMV), which are less sensitive. Intravenous acyclovir is the drug of choice for treating serious infections caused by herpes simplex virus or varicella-zoster virus, especially in immunocompromised hosts. Oral acyclovir is used to treat less serious herpes simplex infections and for suppression of herpes simplex virus recurrences.

Evidence for significant nephrotoxicity of acyclovir was apparent from preclinical toxicological studies, in which large parenteral doses resulted in the deposition of acyclovir crystals in distal kidney tubules and collecting ducts of animals, causing acute kidney dysfunction due to tubular obstruction [6]. Numerous reports have documented acyclovir nephrotoxicity in humans [7-17]. In a review by Brigden et al., of 354 immunocompromised patients with life-threatening herpes infections treated with intravenous acyclovir, 58 developed AKI [7]. Keeney and colleagues, in reviewing the early British experience with intravenous bolus acyclovir, reported that 10.3% of adults and 11.5% of children developed azotemia [9]. In another study, up to 48% of outpatients receiving high-dose intravenous therapy developed elevations in the serum creatinine concentration [10].

The decline in kidney function usually occurs within the first few days of therapy, and may be detected after only a few doses or, more rarely, later in the course of treatment [7-17]. Patients may be asymptomatic, but nausea, vomiting, and abdominal, back, or flank pain are common, while oliguria is uncommon. The rise in the serum creatinine concentration is usually modest, and dialysis has only rarely been necessary [18, 19] Most patients recover kidney function within 3 to 14 days of stopping acyclovir therapy, reducing the dose, or increasing hydration [7, 8, 10-17, 20]. Chronic renal dysfunction has been only rarely attributed to oral acyclovir use Urinalysis usually shows mild proteinuria, microscopic hematuria, and variable degrees of pyuria. Birefringent needle-shaped crystals may be seen either free or within white blood cells in the urine sediment [17]. It should be noted, however, that acyclovir crystalluria has also been found in patients without acute kidney failure [21]. Kidney tissue from one autopsy specimen demonstrated crystal deposits in distal tubules [7]. In other cases, however, kidney biopsies from patients with acute AKI attributed to acyclovir failed to detect such crystals [12, 14]. Instead, tubulointerstitial injury with necrosis and mitotic figures, proteinaceous tubular casts, interstitial infiltration by lymphocytes, plasma cells, and eosinophils, and occasional granulomata were seen.

In an *in vivo* animal study, at doses not causing crystalluria or tissue crystal deposition, short term exposure to acyclovir caused increased renal vasoconstriction and an associated fall in renal blood flow and single nephron plasma flow [22]. Longer-term treatment resulted in a fall in glomerular ultrafiltration coefficient. Thus, it is not clear whether the pathogenesis of acyclovir-induced AKI in humans reflects an obstructive nephropathy from intratubular precipitation of acyclovir, a hemodynamic response, or a type of toxic, immunologic, or hypersensitivity reaction. It is also possible that more than one process may be involved.

The most important risk factors for acyclovir nephrotoxicity are intravascular volume contraction, preexisting kidney desease, and the use of a high-dose, rapid bolus intravenous infusion [7] Nephrotoxicity with oral acyclovir has been reported only rarely [23]; The main non-renal toxicities of acyclovir are gastrointestinal and neurologic side effects, which primarily occur in patients on high-dose intravenous acyclovir. As acyclovir is primarily cleared by the kidney, lower intravenous doses and even oral administration can lead to neurotoxicity in patients with decreased kidney function from either CKD or AKI [15, 17, 24, 25].

Valacyclovir

Valacyclovir is the L-valyl ester of acyclovir, with oral bioavailability three to five times that of oral acyclovir. Following ingestion, it is rapidly converted by intestinal and hepatic hydrolases to acyclovir. Valacyclovir has gastrointestinal and neurological side effects similar to those seen with acyclovir. To date, significant nephrotoxicity and crystalluria as seen with acyclovir has only rarely been reported with valacyclovir, perhaps because of more conscientious dose adjustments in high-risk patients and avoidance of the very high peak blood levels seen with intravenous acyclovir [26]

A thrombotic microangiopathic anemia (TMA) syndrome with renal involvement and other clinical features similar to thrombotic thrombocytopenic purpura (TTP) has been reported rarely among patients with HIV infection enrolled in a clinical trial of CMV prophylaxis and in one additional case report [27, 28]. A similar syndrome, with a microangiopathic hemolytic anemia and features of TTP or hemolytic uremic syndrome (HUS) has also been well described in HIV-infected patients not receiving valacyclovir [29, 30]. In the clinical trial, which compared high-dose valacyclovir and two doses of acyclovir, the risk of developing TTP was greater among valacyclovir-treated patients (14 of 523) than acyclovir-treated patients (4 of 704) [27]. Many of the patients had anemia and thrombocytopenia for several weeks to months prior to the onset of kidney disease. Kidney injury, which varied from mild to severe, was present at the time of diagnosis or developed shortly thereafter in all but one of the patients. Kidney biopsies showed evidence of a TMA in four of five patients. A more gradual onset than is seen with idiopathic or HIV-related TTP, a generally poor response to therapy, including plasmapheresis, and a poor prognosis was described. Death was attributed to HUS, TTP, or kidney injury in half the patients. In more than half of the cases, the diagnosis of TMA was not made until valacyclovir had already been discontinued, and on some of the patients, it was felt that other infectious processes could have accounted for the hematologic and kidney manifestations [27]. Thus, the precise role of valacyclovir and the relative risk of developing TMA with lower doses of valacyclovir remain unclear.

Ganciclovir

Ganciclovir is an acyclic nucleoside analogue of guanine that is structurally similar to acyclovir, but is more effective in the treatment and prophylaxis of severe cytomegalovirus infection in immunocompromised hosts. Ganciclovir is myelotoxic, but has no significant nephrotoxicity [22]. It does, however, require dose adjustment for patients with reduced kidney function.

Valganciclovir

Valganciclovir is a pro-drug that is rapidly converted to ganciclovir in the body. It has higher oral bioavailability than ganciclovir and is used for both prophylaxis and treatment of CMV. Like ganciclovir, it requires dose adjustment for decreased kidney function and is generally not recommended for those on dialysis. Also similar to ganciclovir, there has not been any reported kidney toxicity with this medication.

Famciclovir & penciclovir

Penciclovir is an acyclic guanine analogue similar to ganciclovir, with *in vitro* activity against the herpes viruses and hepatitis B virus. Poor oral availability limits it use to topical applications. Famciclovir is an analogue of penciclovir with a similar spectrum of antiviral activity that is well absorbed following oral administration. As a pro-drug, famciclovir is rapidly metabolized to penciclovir. To date, there has not been significant kidney toxicity reported with either famciclovir or penciclovir.

Cidofovir

Cidofovir is an acyclic nucleotide analogue of the monophosphate of cytosine. When phosphorylated by host cellular enzymes, the active compound cidofovir diphosphate has broad activity against the herpes viruses, including CMV, HSV 1 and 2, VZV, Epstein-Barr virus, and the BK polyomavirus. Cidofovir has primarily been used in the treatment of CMV retinitis in patients who have failed treatment with ganciclovir or foscarnet and in acyclovir-resistant herpes simplex infections. More recently, there is also a growing experience with the use of this medication in kidney transplant patients who have BK virus-associated nephropathy [31], although this interest has been dampened by significant toxicity and only modest clinical activity [32]

Nephrotoxicity was found in preclinical studies to be the major toxicity of cidofovir, associated with histologic evidence of damage to proximal tubule epithelial cells [33]. Dose- and schedule-dependent nephrotoxicity is also the treatment limiting toxicity of cidofovir in humans [34-37]. Cidofovir is thought to be concentrated by a basolateral membrane organic anion transporter in proximal tubule epithelial cells [38]. Probenecid, an inhibitor of organic anion transport, ameliorates kidney toxicity of cidofovir by reducing cellular uptake [33, 39, 40]. *In vitro*, toxicity of cidofovir has been conveyed into mammalian cells by transfection with a gene for a human renal organic anion transporter, and correlates with concomitant intracellular accumulation of the drugs [412]. Renal clearance of cidofovir exceeds creatinine clearance, suggesting that active tubular secretion contributes to renal clearance [34, 39]. At cidofovir doses of 3 mg/kg, probenecid does not appear to affect cidofovir pharmacokinetics, while at higher doses, tubular secretion and kidney clearance of cidofovir are reduced [39].

Experience from clinical trials suggest that twenty five percent or greater of patients receiving intravenous doses of cidofovir of 3 mg/kg or more develop AKI. This is often associated with a Fanconi syndrome, with tubular proteinuria and evidence of proximal tubular dysfunction, with glucosuria, hypophosphatemia, and urinary bicarbonate wasting, and evidence of proximal tubular injury on kidney biopsy [34-37, 42]. Volume expansion with isotonic saline and administration of probenecid substantially reduces this risk. Probenecid is routinely given along with each administration of cidofovir. Preexisting kidney insufficiency, recent use of other nephrotoxic agents, and the development while on therapy of proteinuria or other tubular abnormalities predispose patients to risk of severe AKI with cidofovir, which should be avoided or discontinued in these settings. Kidney injury from cidofovir can be severe enough to result in the need for dialysis. Both the kidney injury and proximal tubule dysfunction associated with cidofovir may be only partially reversible or even completely irreversible [43, 44, 45], despite discontinuation of therapy and pretreatment with intravenous saline and probenecid. Nephrogenic diabetes insipidus has also been described during therapy with cidofovir [46]. Kidney injury attributed to topical cidofovir has also been reported [47].

Foscarnet

Foscarnet (trisodium phosphonoformate) is an inorganic pyrophosphate analog, which inhibits many DNA polymerases, retroviral reverse transcriptase, and some RNA polymerases, and has antiviral activity against all of the herpes viruses and HIV. Foscarnet has been used primarily for the treatment of serious cytomegalovirus infection.

Foscarnet competitively inhibits Na^+-P_i cotransport in animal and human kidney proximal tubule brush border membrane vesicles, reversibly inhibiting sodium-dependent phosphate transport [48, 49]. Renal cortical Na-K-ATPase and alkaline phosphatase activity are not inhibited by foscarnet, nor is proline, glucose, succinate, or Na^+ transport [48, 49]. Foscarnet induces isolated phosphaturia without hypophosphatemia in thyroparathyroidectomized rats maintained on a low phosphorus diet, without affecting glomerular filtration rate, urinary adenosine 3′5′-cyclic monophosphate (cAMP) activity, or urinary calcium, sodium or potassium excretion [48, 50]. Sodium-P_i cotransport in brush border membrane vesicles from human renal cortex was reported to be even more sensitive to inhibition by foscarnet than in rat renal brush border membrane vesicles [49].

Acute kidney injury can be severe with foscarnet. Some degree of kidney injury has been reported to occur in as many as two-thirds of patients treated with foscarnet and has been a dose-limiting toxicity in 10-20% of cases [51-56]. Despite dose reduction or discontinuation of foscarnet, azotemia typically progresses for at least a few days before resolving. It may be possible to continue foscarnet at reduced doses in some patients with mild azotemia. Foscarnet-induced AKI is usually reversible, although temporary dialysis may be required [57]. Recovery may be slow, particularly in patients with preexisting kidney insufficiency. Elevated serum creatinine concentrations may persist for several months after discontinuation of foscarnet. Foscarnet nephrotoxicity may be also associated with mild proteinuria. Volume expansion with isotonic saline was effective in reducing the incidence of foscarnet nephrotoxicity to 13%, compared to 66% in non-hydrated historical controls, and allowed patients with prior kidney insufficiency to receive foscarnet without further reduction of kidney function [54, 58]. Intermittent, rather than continuous, infusion of foscarnet may also reduce the incidence of nephrotoxicity [52].

Acute tubular necrosis, tubulointerstitial nephritis, and glomerulonephritis have been described in patients with foscarnet-induced acute kidney injury [54, 59-62]. Kidney biopsy specimens from patients who had received foscarnet have, in several reports, shown the presence of crystals within glomerular capillaries and tubules [59, 61-64]. These crystals have had an appearance similar to that of crystalline foscarnet. In addition to trisodium foscarnet, crystals have also been identified as being mixed sodium-calcium and rarely pure calcium salts of foscarnet [63, 64].The pathophysiologic role of these crystals is uncertain, as they are not seen in all patients with foscarnet-induced AKI. Disruption of glomerular basement membrane by these crystals has been suggested as a cause of non-immune glomerulonephritis seen in some foscarnet-treated patients [61, 62, 64]. Interestingly, crystalluria has not been seen in patients receiving foscarnet [65].

Nephrogenic diabetes insipidus has been described in patients receiving foscarnet, either alone or associated with a distal renal tubular acidosis [66, 67, 68]. In fact, a recent review cited foscarnet as the second most common reported cause of drug-induced diabetes insipidus, second only to lithium [69]. In experiments using toad urinary bladders [70], serosal application of foscarnet enhanced water flow in the presence of submaximal ADH concentrations, but did not affect water transport in the absence of ADH or when maximal concentrations of ADH were used. Mucosal foscarnet did not affect water transport. Further studies are needed to clarify the mechanisms for altered water handling by the kidneys with foscarnet.

Hypo- and hypercalcemia, hypo- and hyperphosphatemia, and hypomagnesemia have all been described in patients receiving foscarnet [56, 71-73]. Hypocalcemia is the most common and serious of these electrolyte disturbances. Severe symptomatic hypocalcemia with paresthesias, accompanied by Chvostek's and Trousseau's signs and fatal hypocalcemia have occurred with foscarnet [71]. Jacobson et al. systematically evaluated changes in the serum calcium and phosphate concentrations occurring during single and repeated doses of foscarnet [72]. Ionized calcium levels fell below the lower limit of normal in all patients receiving an infusion of 120 mg/kg and 66% of those who received 90 mg/kg. No changes in total calcium or phosphate concentrations were found. Despite normal total serum calcium concentrations, symptoms compatible with hypocalcemia occurred in two patients. No significant changes in serum phosphate, magnesium, ionized or total calcium, parathyroid hormone, or 1, 25-$(OH)_2$ vitamin D levels were found after a 14 day course of therapy, although increases in parathyroid hormone and vitamin D levels have been reported [53]. Likewise, urinary calcium, phosphorus, magnesium, and potassium excretion were unchanged during 14 days of foscarnet. *In vitro* studies showed an inverse relationship between serum or plasma foscarnet concentrations and ionized calcium concentration, but not with total calcium or phosphate concentrations [72].

Foscarnet is a phosphate analog, and can chelate calcium, as well as other metal ions [74] As studies have not demonstrated an increase calcium binding to plasma proteins, some authors have concluded that ionized hypocalcemia was primarily a result of foscarnet complexing with ionized calcium [72]. In another study, total calcium concentrations declined during and after foscarnet infusion, with ionized calcium concentrations falling to an even greater extent than total calcium [73]. Total magnesium levels also declined, with ionized magnesium concentrations falling to a greater extent. These data also suggest that foscarnet lowers calcium and magnesium levels primarily by binding to calcium and magnesium ions, respectively. Intravenous magnesium ameliorates the fall in ionized magnesium levels with foscarnet, but not the fall in calcium levels [75]. An experimental liposome-encapsulated foscarnet preparation did not reduce plasma calcium levels in animals [76].

Antiretroviral agents

Nucleoside reverse transcriptase inhibitors

Nucleoside reverse transcriptase inhibitors (NRTIs) were the first class of medications approved for the management of HIV infection. They are structural analogues of nucleic acids. They undergo intracellular phosphorylation to a triphosphate metabolite and it is this metabolite that is pharmacologically active against reverse transcriptase. Drugs in this class include abacavir, adefovir, didanosine, emtricitabine, lamivudine, stavudine, tenofovir, and zidovudine.

Despite their widespread clinical use, direct nephrotoxicity has not been reported with zidovudine, emtricitabine or didanosine. Electrolyte disorders have been described but are uncommon. Hypokalemia was reported in didanosine treated patients, which may have been related to HIV infection or didanosine related diarrhea; in somes though, hypokalemia occurred without diarrhea [77]. Symptomatic hypocalcemia, without changes in serum magnesium, phosphorus, parathyroid hormone, and vitamin D levels (or findings of pancreatitis, a known adverse effect of didanosine) has also been seen with didanosine [78]. Asymptomatic hyperuricemia may be seen in didanosine treated patients, particularly at higher dosages. This occurs as a result of metabolism of didanosine (a purine analogue) to hypoxanthine and eventually uric acid [79-81]. Reduction of the didanosine dose and increased hydration usually correct the hyperuricemia, which has not been associated with the development of gout. Hyperuricemia is not a complication of treatment with zidovudine, a pyrimidine analogue.

Lamivudine, a weak inhibitor of organic cation transport by renal tubule epithelial cells [82], has also not been associated with significant nephrotoxicity.

Acute kidney injury with eosinophilic interstitial nephritis was attributed to abacavir in one patient with HIV infection who also had what appeared to be "classic" FSGS on renal biopsy [83]. The serum creatinine returned to baseline levels after treatment with prednisone and discontinuation of abacavir.

Adefovir is an acyclic analogue of adenosine monophosphate. When phosphorylated by host enzymes, it is a potent inhibitor of hepatitis B Virus (HBV) DNA polymerase, including reverse transcriptase. Adefovir was initially studied in the management of HIV infection. Large doses that were required to achieve anti-HIV activity were associated with dose-limiting nephrotoxicity. Adefovir is currently only FDA approved in lower dosages for the management of HBV infection as at a dose of 10 mg/day adefovir has not been found to be nephrotoxic in randomized controlled trials.

As seen with cidofovir, adefovir is conveyed into mammalian cells by a human renal organic anion transporter; *in vitro* toxicity correlates with intracellular accumulation of the drug [41]. Probenecid as well as nonsteroidal anti-inflammatory drugs reduce the cellular uptake and *in vitro* cytotoxicity of adefovir [84]. Patients treated with high doses adefovir commonly experience proximal tubule dysfunction and AKI, which may take weeks to resolve after drug discontinuation. [85, 86]. A role for depletion of proximal tubule cell mitochondrial DNA has been suggested as a possible cause of adefovir-related AKI [87]. Adefovir has similar pharmacokinetic properties as cidofovir, suggesting that the kidney toxicity of these drugs may be similar. Adefovir is currently only FDA approved in lower dosages for the management of HBV infection as at a dose of 10 mg/day adefovir has not been found to be nephrotoxic in randomized controlled trials.

Reports of a myopathy developing in patients with AIDS being treated with zidovudine led to the observation that this drug and others in this class could cause mitochondrial toxicity related to effects on mitochondrial DNA [88-91]. Myopathies and other neuromuscular and systemic manifestations occur in a variety of circumstances as a consequence of mutations in mitochondrial nuclear DNA. Mitochondria have their own extrachromosomal DNA that is distinct from nuclear DNA and encode proteins for four of the five complexes involved in oxidative phosphorylation and for structural and transfer RNA's required for mitochondrial translation of the protein-encoding genes. Mutations occur more frequently in mitochondrial DNA than nuclear DNA, and have been found in each of the mitochondrial DNA genes. Phenotypically, these mutations are associated most commonly with neuromuscular syndromes, but virtually any organ system can be affected [92-94]. Kidney manifestations include Fanconi syndrome most commonly, but nephrotic syndrome (usually with focal and segmental glomerular sclerosis), chronic kidney disease with interstitial fibrosis and tubular atrophy and lactic acidosis have also been described [95]. Other significant toxicities include peripheral neuropathy, pancreatitis and hepatic steatosis with liver failure.

Subsequent reports described a syndrome of type B lactic acidosis in patients treated with zidovudine and other nucleoside reverse transcriptase inhibitors, including stavudine, lamivudine, and didanosine which has also been attributed to mitochondrial DNA toxicity [95-106]. There are five types of DNA polymerase in human cells that catalyze the synthesis of new complementary DNA from the original DNA template (HIV encodes a reverse transcriptase DNA polymerase which uses RNA as the template). The active triphosphate metabolites of zidovudine, didanosine, and stavudine inhibit DNA polymerase gamma in mitochondria, block the elongation of mitochondrial DNA, and deplete mitochondrial DNA [91-93, 101, 105-108]. The link between NRTI effects on mitochondrial DNA and lactic acidosis is not entirely clear but is most likely related to disturbances of oxidative phosphorylation and impaired pyruvate metabolism leading to lactate accumulation.

Perhaps one of the most dramatic examples of hepatic failure and lactic acidosis associated with nucleoside analogues occurred with an investigational nucleoside analogue, fialuridine. This occurred during early clinical trials evaluating fialuridine for the treatment of chronic hepatitis B [109]. Seven of fifteen study patients developed progressive liver failure and lactic acidosis. Five of the patients died with severe lactic acidosis; two patients underwent emergency liver transplantation and survived. Severe mitochondrial toxicity was proposed as the mechanism for this injury, based in part on the similarity of this presentation to that seen in individuals with inherited disorders of mitochondrial DNA and the presence of histopathological evidence of mitochondrial injury [107-109].

The lactic acidosis seen with these drugs has ranged from mild and chronic to acute, severe, and fatal [95-106]. The acidosis generally develops after several months of therapy. Patients with NRTI-associated lactic acidosis present with symptoms of nausea, vomiting and abdominal pain. Other features often include elevated liver enzymes, hepatic steatosis, pancreatitis and elevated creatinine kinase with evidence of a myopathy, and liver failure. The lactic acidosis may persist for many weeks despite discontinuation of the NRTI [95-106]. NRTI-related mitochondrial toxicity may also present with rhabdomyolysis and acute kidney failure [110]. Mortality related to NRTI-induced acute lactic acidosis is high, in the range of 50% to 100%, despite drug discontinuation.

In addition to discontinuation of the NRTI, L-carnitine, riboflavin, and thiamine have been used in isolated reports but with unclear therapeutic role [106, 111-113] Many of these patients have been treated with high-dose intravenous sodium bicarbonate. Hemodialysis [114] and continuous venovenous hemodiafiltration [85] have been used to reduce the lactic acidosis, even in the absence of significant kidney injury. Lactic acidosis transiently and modestly improved after administration of dichloroacetate in one report [99]. The benefit of any of these therapies remains unclear.

A Fanconi syndrome with nephrogenic diabetes insipidus was reported in a patient with AIDS who was receiving didanosine (and other medications) [115] and also in a patient treated with stavudine and lamivudine [116]. The metabolic acidosis in this case was partly due to lactic acidosis, perhaps related to mitochondrial dysfunction. Abacavir was recently implicated as a cause of biopsy-proven interstitial nephritis in a patient with AKI [117, 118]. Structurally similar to adefovir and cidofovir, tenofovir has also been associated with several kidney syndromes such as the development of AKI with acute tubular necrosis, Fanconi syndrome, and nephrogenic diabetes insipidus [119-123]. Tenofovir has also been associated with hypokalemia [124] and fatal lactic acidosis [122]. In the majority of patients, tenofovir induced kidney impairment was described as reversible, however glomerular filtration rates did not always return to baseline values [124 a, b]. The exact mechanism for the development of tenofovir toxicity remains unknown, however suggested mechanisms include epithelial cell mitochondrial DNA depletion and direct tubular cytotoxicity which were mechanisms associated with adefovir and cidofovir toxicity. [41, 87]. Drug interactions that occur when tenofovir is given concomitantly with other medications in the treatment of HIV infection have also been suggested as a proposed mechanism for tenofovir toxicity [124 a].

Non-nucleoside reverse transcriptase inhibitors

Medications in this class include delavirdine, efavirenz, and nevirapine. Similar to the NRTIs, these agents bind to viral reverse transcriptase and block DNA polymerase activity. A key difference is that NNRTIs do not require intracellular phosphorylation and are not incorporated into viral DNA. Clinically significant kidney toxicities or specific fluid-electrolyte complications have not been reported with this class of agents. In the rat model, efavirenz was associated with a species specific dependent kidney toxicity which occurred secondary to the development of a unique glutathione conjugate produced as a metabolite of efavirenz associated with renal tubular epithelial cell necrosis [125-126]. This toxicity has not been observed in humans. One patient was recently reported to have reversible nephrotic-range proteinuria attributed to efavirenz use, in which a kidney biopsy showed diffuse podocyte foot process effacement [127]. Another report noted the development of rhabdomyolysis and acute tubular necrosis as a result of a drug interaction between delavirdine and atorvastatin [128]. Kidney toxicity due to nevirapine has not been reported.

Protease inhibitors

This class of agents affects a later part of the HIV cycle, by inhibiting the protease enzyme and leading to impaired assembly of mature HIV virions. Examples include amprenavir, atazanavir, darunavir, fosamprenavir indinavir, lopinavir, nelfinavir, ritonavir, and saquinavir. There have been no published reports of AKI or other direct kidney toxicity due to amprenavir, darunavir, fosamprenavir, and lopinavir.

Indinavir has been associated with development of crystalluria and nephrolithiasis, which was recognized during initial clinical trials. [129]. Urinary excretion accounts for up to 20% of an indinavir dose and the urinary solubility is pH dependent, with greater solubility occurring at lower pH [130]. Ten to twenty percent of individuals receiving indinavir may develop indinavir crystalluria, even in the absence of any symptoms [131-137]. In one large series, about 8% of indinavir-treated patients had symptoms related to crystal or stone formation; about two-thirds had crystalluria associated with dysuria, urinary urgency, and/or back or flank pain and about one-third had nephrolithiasis [131]. In another retrospective series, 12.4% of patients receiving indinavir developed nephrolithiasis [132]. A prospective study recently evaluated the incidence of urinary abnormalities in a cohort of 54 HIV infected individuals. Patients were evaluated during the first year of indinavir treatment and were specifically instructed to maintain a high fluid intake, evaluated with monthly urinalyses [133]. Crystals first began to appear in urine samples after 1 to 2 weeks of indinavir, beyond which time about 25% of urine specimens contained crystals. Crystals were seen in at least one urine sample from two-thirds of patients. Hypovolemia, a concentrated urine and a high urinary pH (>6) appear to be risk factors for indinavir crystalluria and nephrolithiasis [134, 135].

Patients with indinavir crystalluria may be asymptomatic or can develop clinical symptoms such as flank pain, back pain, dysuria, urinary urgency, fever, nausea, and vomiting. Pyuria and hematuria (commonly microscopic) may also be seen [131-133, 135-137, 138]. Indinavir crystals (Figure 1) are variable in their appearance by microscopy, usually with needle-shaped, plate-like, fan-shaped, or starburst-like appearances [131, 133]. Ultrasound imaging is emerging as imaging modality of choice and may be more

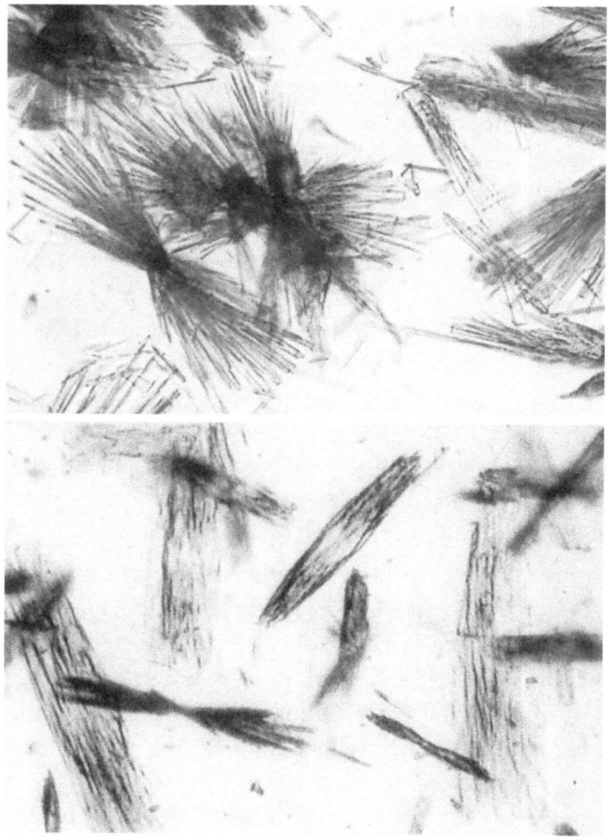

Figure 1. *Photomicrograph of unstained urine sediment showing indinavir crystals (orig. magn. x50). Reproduced with permission from [133].*

diagnostically helpful than abdominal radiographs, intravenous urography or CT [139]. Fewer than 30% of these stones are radiopaque on plain radiographs [139]. Renal parenchymal defects can sometimes be noted on contrast enhanced CT scans of the kidneys [131]. Using ultrasound, the development of sludge in the renal collecting system and hydronephrosis may be seen. The crystals are composed primarily of indinavir [131, 138]. Calcium oxalate and calcium phosphate have also been identified. These latter crystals may coexist with indinavir and, at times, can serve as a nidus for the formation of indinavir crystals [138, 140]. Urologic intervention may be required for removal of stone or relief of urinary tract obstruction and associated AKI [131, 132, 139-142]. After temporary discontinuation of indinavir and volume repletion, many patients are able to resume treatment with indinavir, although recurrence may occur. Patients receiving indinavir should be instructed to maintain a high fluid intake (approximately 48 ounces per day). Renal calculi have also been described in single case reports with saquinavir [143], nelfinavir (with 99% of the stone composed of nelfinavir) [144], and atazanavir [145]

Interstitial nephritis has been found in kidney biopsies in patients treated with indinavir [146-151]. Some of these cases have described eosinophiluria and crystals (assumed to be indinavir) associated with histiocytes and giant cells in the renal tubules. Some of these patients were asymptomatic, while others reported classic symptoms of nephrolithiasis. Cortical atrophy was found in some patients, suggesting the progression from acute injury towards chronic kidney disease [152].

Other protease inhibitors have also been rarely associated with kidney injury. A single case of interstitial nephritis and reversible AKI in a patient treated with atazanavir has also been reported [153] Acute kidney injury attributed to ritonavir has been reported in several patients [154-157], the majority of whom were receiving concomitant nephrotoxic medications, while others had preexisting kidney disease or were volume depleted. In several patients, AKI recurred upon ritonavir rechallenge. Kidney biopsies were not performed, so histopathologic correlates and etiology of kidney injury were not precisely defined.

Fusion Inhibitors

Fusion inhibitors are a new class of agents approved in the management of HIV infection. They bind to surface proteins on T-lymphocytes and prevent entry of the HIV virus. The only fusion inhibitor currently approved for use is enfuvirtide. Nephrotoxicity has not been reported with enfuvirtide, however, one patient with a previous history of proteinuria and hematuria was described to have developed membranoproliferative glomerulonephritis [158]. The cause and effect relationship of this event and the use of the fusion inhibitor remain unclear.

Amantadine hydrochloride and rimantadine

Amantadine and rimantadine are tricyclic aliphatic primary amines, active only against influenza A virus Both agents are utilized for the treatment and prophylaxis of influenza A infections, outbreaks or as pandemic control. Amantadine has also been noted to have an effect on catecholamines resulting in amelioration of symptoms associated with Parkinson's disease or extrapyramidal reactions. Nephrotoxicity with amantadine has not been described, although prolonged use has occasionally been associated with orthostatic hypotension. Acute overdose of amantadine has been associated with urinary retention and kidney injury on that basis. Severe neurologic reactions to amantadine have been reported in patients with reduced kidney function [159, 160]. Rimantadine is structurally similar to amantadine, and has a similar spectrum of antiviral activity. To date, nephrotoxicity has not been described with rimantadine.

Neuraminidase inhibitors

Two agents, oseltamivir and zanamivir, are approved for the management of Influenza A and B infection. Both are potent neuraminidase inhibitors responsible for inhibiting viral replication. These agents differ in their structural compounds, enabling oseltamavir to have greater bioavailability and be the only oral option. There have been no reports of nephrotoxicity with the use of either agent.

Ribavirin

Ribavirin is a synthetic guanosine analogue, with *in vitro* activity against a broad spectrum of DNA and RNA viruses and retroviruses, including HIV. Ribavirin has been used for treatment of a variety of viral infections, including respiratory syncytial virus, chronic hepatitis C, influenza types A and B, viral hemorrhagic fevers, and others. For the management of hepatitis C infection, ribavirin is combined with interferon alpha. Ribavirin is primarily excreted in the urine with approximately 30% eliminated as unchanged drug. It is contraindicated in patients with advanced chronic kidney disease secondary to a significant risk of anemia that it may cause. Cases of direct nephrotoxicity related to ribavirin have not been reported.

Conclusion

There is an increasing array of both the number of available antiviral agents and the clinical indications for their use. With this growth in the use of antiviral therapy have come increasing reports of a variety of significant kidney toxicities including acute and chronic kidney injury, nephrolithiasis, glomerulonephrities, as well as a variety of fluid and electrolyte disorders. Despite these reports of adverse events, most of these agents can be used safely if close attention is paid to dose adjustments for diminished kidney function, maintenance of ideal patient volume status, and a keen awareness of the interactions of these agents with other medications. These precautions are especially important in patients with solid organ transplants and those with HIV disease, as they often have multiple overlapping co-morbidities and routinely receive a complex medley of pharmacologic agents

References

1. Jayasekara D, Aweeka FT, Rodriguez R, Kalayjian RC, Humphreys MH, Gambertoglio JG: Antiviral therapy for HIV patients with renal insufficiency. JAIDS 1999; 21: 384-395.
2. Aronoff GR, Berns JS, Brier ME, Golper TA, Morrison G, Singer I, Swan SK, Bennett WM. Drug prescribing in renal failure. In: Dosing guidelines for adults, 4th edition. Philadelphia: American College of Physicians, 1999.
3. Berns JS, Cohen RM, Stumacher RJ, Rudnick MR. Renal aspects of therapy for human immunodeficiency virus and associated opportunistic infections. J Am Soc Nephrol 1991; 1: 1061-1080.
4. Izzedine H, Launay-Vacher V, Baumelou A, Deray G. An appraisal of antiretroviral drugs in hemodialysis. Kidney Int 2001; 60: 821-830.
5. Berns JS, Kasbekar N. Highly active antiretroviral therapy and the kidney: An update on antiretroviral medications for nephrologists. Clin J Am Soc Nephrol 2006;1:117-129.
6. Tucker WE. Preclinical toxicology profile of acyclovir: an overview. Am J Med 1982; 73: 27-30.
7. Brigden D, Rosling AE, Woods NC. Renal function after acyclovir intravenous injection. Am J Med 1982; 73: 182-185.
8. Selby PJ, Powles RL, Jameson B, Kay HEM, Watson JG, Thornton R, Morgenstern G, Clink HM. Parenteral acyclovir therapy for herpes virus infections in man. Lancet 1979; 2: 1267-1270.
9. Keeney RE, Kirk LE, Brigden D. Acyclovir tolerance in humans. Am J Med 1982; 73: 171-181.
10. Bean B, Aeppli D. Adverse effects of high dose intravenous acyclovir in ambulatory patients with acute herpes zoster. J Infect Dis 1985; 151: 362-365.
11. Spiegal D, Lau K. Acute renal failure and coma secondary to acyclovir therapy. JAMA 1986; 255: 1882-1883.
12. Sawyer MH, Webb DF, Balow JE, Straus SE. Acyclovir induced renal failure: clinical course and histology. Am J Med 1988; 84: 1067-1071.
13. Giustina A, Romanelli G, Cimino A, Brunori G. Low dose acyclovir and acute renal failure. Ann Intern Med 1988; 108: 312.
14. Rashed A, Azadeh B, Abu-Romeh SH. Acyclovir-induced acute tubulo-interstitial nephritis. Nephron 1990; 56: 436-438.
15. Eck P, Silver SM, Clark EC. Acute renal failure and coma after a high dose of oral acyclovir. N Engl J Med 1991; 325: 1178-1179.
16. Bianchetti M, Roduit C, Oetliker OH. Acyclovir-induced renal failure: course and risk factors. Pediatr Nephrol 1991; 5: 238-239.
17. Becker BN, Fall P, Hall C, Milam D, Leonard J, Glick A, Schulman A. Rapidly progressive acute renal failure due to acyclovir: Case report and review of the literature. Am J Kid Dis 1993; 22(4): 611-615.
18. Hsu CC, Lai TL, Lien WC, Chen WJ, Fang CC. Emergent hemodialysis for acyclovir toxicity.Am J Emerg Med, 2005; 23(7); 899-900.
19 Khajehdehi P, Jamal JA, Bastani B. Removal of acyclovir during veno-venous hemodialysis and hemodiafiltration with high-efficiency membranes. Clin Nephrol 2000; 54(4): 351-5.
20. Sodhi PK, Ratan SK. Case of chronic renal dysfunction following treatment with oral acyclovir. Scand J Infect Dis 2003; 35(10):770-2.
21. Potter JL, Krill CE. Acyclovir crystalluria. Pediatr Infect Dis 1986; 5: 710-712.
22. DosSantos MDeFF, DosSantos OFP, Boim MA, Razvickas CV, DeMoura LAR, Ajzen H, Schor N. Nephrotoxicity of acyclovir and ganciclovir in rats: evaluation of glomerular hemodynamics. J Am Soc Nephrol 1997; 8: 361-367.
23. Yavuz BB, Cankurtaran M, Halil M, Dagli N, Kirkpantur A. Renal dysfunction after oral acyclovir in a geriatric woman: a case report. Scand J Infect Dis 2005; 37(8):611-613.
24. MacDiarmaid-Gordon AR, O'Connor M, Beaman M, Ackrill P. Neurotoxicity associated with oral acyclovir in patients undergoing dialysis. Nephron 1992; 62: 280-283.
25 Almond MK, Fan S, Dhillon S, Pollock AM, Raftery MJ. Avoiding acyclovir neurotoxicity in patients with chronic renal failure undergoing hemodialysis. Nephron 1995; 69: 428-432.

26. Catalano C, Conforto L. Valacyclovir-related neuro- and nephrotoxicity in two geriatric patients. G Ital Nefrol (Italian) 2005; Suppl 31: S132-4.
27. Bell WR, Chulay JD, Feinberg JE. Manifestations resembling thrombotic microangiopathy in patients with advanced human immunodeficiency virus (HIV) disease in a cytomegalovirus prophylaxis trial (ACTG 204). Medicine 1997; 76: 369-380.
28. Rivaud E, Massiani M-A, Vincent F, Azoulay E, Couderc L-J. Valacyclovir hydrochloride therapy and thrombotic thrombocytopenic purpura in an HIV-infected patient. Arch Int Med 2000; 160: 1705-1706.
29. Leaf AN, Laubenstein LJ, Raphael B, Hochster H, Baez L, Karpatkin S. Thrombotic thrombocytopenic purpura associated with human immunodeficiency virus type 1 (HIV-1) infection. Ann Intern Med 1988; 109: 194-197.
30. Berns J. Hemolytic uremic syndrome and thrombotic thrombocytopenic purpura associated with HIV infection. In: Renal and Urologic Aspects of HIV Infection. Kimmel PL, Berns JS (editors). Churchill Livingstone, Inc., Philadelphia, PA 1995; p. 111-133.
31. Kuypers DR, Vandooren AK, Lerut E, Evenepoel P, Claes K, Snoeck R, Naesens L, Vanrenterghem Y. Adjuvant low-dose cidofovir therapy for BK polyomavirus interstitial nephritis in renal transplant recipients. Am J Transplant 2005; 5:1997-2004.
32. Trofe J, Hirsch HH, Ramos E. Polyomavirus-associated nephropathy: update of clinical management in kidney transplant patients. Transpl Infect Dis 2006;8:76-85.
33. Lacy SA, Hitchcock MJ, Lee WA, Tellier P, Cundy KC. Effect of oral probenecid coadministration on the chronic toxicity and pharmacokinetics of intravenous cidofovir in cynomolgus monkeys. Toxicol Sci 1998; 44: 97-106.
34. Lalezari JF, Drew WL, Glutzer E, James C, Miner D, Flaherty J, Fisher PE, Cundy K, Hannigan J, Martin JC, Jaffe HS. (S)-1-[3-hydroxy-2-(phosphonylmethoxy)propyl] cytosine (Cidofovir): results of a phase I/II study of a novel antiviral nucleotide analogue. J Infect Dis 1995; 171: 788-796.
35. Lalezari JP, Stagg RJ, Kuppermann BD, Holland GN, Kramer F, Ives DV, Youle M, Robinson MR, Drew WL, Jaffe HS. Intravenous cidofovir for peripheral cytomegalovirus retinitis in patients with AIDS. A randomized, controlled trial. Ann Intern Med 1997: 126: 257-263.
36. Polis MA, Spooner KM, Baird BF, Manischewitz JF, Jaffe HS, Fisher PF, Falloon J, Davey RT Jr, Kovacs JA, Walker RE, Whitcup SM, Nussenblatt RB, Lane HC, Masur H. Anticytomegaloviral activity and safety of cidofovir in patients with human immunodeficiency virus infection and cytomegalovirus viremia. Antimicrob Agents Chemother 1996; 39: 882-886.
37. Lalezari JP, Holland GN, Kramer F, McKinley GF, Kemper CA, Ives DV, Nelson R, Hardy WD, Kupperman BD, Northfelt DW, Youle M, Johnson M, Lewis RA, Weinberg DV, Simon GL, Wolitz RA, Ruby AE, Stagg RJ, Jaffe HS. Randomized, controlled trial of the safety and efficacy of intravenous cidofovir for the treatment of relapsing cytomegalovirus retinitis in patients with AIDS. J AIDS Hum Retrovirol 1998;17: 339-344.
38. Cihlar T, Lin DC, Pritchard JB, Fuller MD, Mendel DB, Sweet DH. The antiviral nucleotide analogs cidofovir and adefovir novel substrates for human and rat renal organic anion transporter 1. Mol Pharmcol 1999; 56: 570-580.
39. Cundy KC, Petty BG, Flaherty J, Fisher PE, Polis MA, Wachsman M, Lietman PS, Lalezari JP, Hitchcock MJM, Jaffe HS. Clinical pharmacokinetics of cidofovir in human immunodeficiency virus-infected patients. Antimicrob Agents Chemother 1995; 39: 1247-1252.
40. Hitchcock MJM, Jaffe HS, Martin JC, Stagg RJ. Cidofovir, a new agent with potent anti-herpes virus activity. Antiviral Chem Chemother 1996; 7: 115-127.
41. Ho ES, Lin DC, Mendel DB, Cihlar T. Cytotoxicity of antiviral nucleotides adefovir and cidofovir is induced by the expression of human renal organic anion transporter 1. J Am Soc Nephrol 2000; 11: 383-393.
42. Ljungman P, Deliliers GL, Platzbecker U, Matthes-Martin S, Bacigalupo A, Einsele H, Ullmann J, Musso M, Trenschel R, Ribaud P, Bornhauser M, Cesaro S, Crooks B, Dekker A, Gratecos N, Klingebiel T, Tabliaferri E, Ullmann AJ, Wacker P, Cordonnier C. Cidofovir for cytomegalovirus infection and disease in allogeneic stem cell transplant recipients. Blood 2001; 15: 388-392.
43. Kay TD, Hogan PG, McLeod SE, Johnson DW. Severe irreversible proximal renal tubular acidosis and azotaemia secondary to cidofovir. Nephron 2000; 86: 348-349.
44. Vandercam B, Moreau M, Goffin E, Marot JC, Cosyns JP, Jadoul M. Cidofovir-induced end-stage renal failure. Clin Infect Dis 1999; 29: 948-949.
45. Meier P, Dautheville-Guibal S, Ronco PM, Rossert J. Cidofovir-induced end-stage renal failure. Nephrol Dial Transplant 2002; 17: 148-149.
46. Schliefer K, Rockstroh JK, Spengler U, Sauerbruch T. Nephrogenic diabetes insipidus in a patient taking cidofovir. Lancet 1997; 350: 413-414.
47. Bienvenu B, Martinez F, Devergie A, Rybojad M, Rivet J, Ballenger P, Morel P, Gluckman E, Lebbe C. Topical use of cidofovir induced acute renal failure. Transplantation 2002; 73: 661-662.
48. Szczepanska-Konkel M, Yusufi ANK, VanScoy M, Webster SK, Dousa TP. Phosphonocarboxylic acids as specific inhibitors of Na^+-dependent transport of phosphate across renal brush border membrane. J Biol Chem 1986; 261: 6375-6383.

49. Yusufi ANK, Szczepanska-Konkel M, Kempson SA, McAteer JA, Dousa TP. Inhibition of human renal epithelial Na^+/P_i cotransport by phosphonoformic acid. Biochem Biophys Res Comm 1986; 139: 679-686.
50. VanScoy M, Loghman-Adham M, Onsgard M, Szcepanska-Konkel M, Homma S, Knox FG, Dousa TP. Mechanism of phosphaturia elicited by administration of phosphonoformate *in vivo*. Am J Physiol 1988; 255: F984-F994.
51. Ringden O, Lonnqvist B, Paulin T, Ahlmen J, Klintmalm G, Wahren B, Lernestedt J-O. Pharmacokinetics, safety and preliminary clinical experiences using foscarnet in the treatment of cytomegalovirus infections in bone marrow and renal transplant recipients. J Antimicrob Chemother 1986; 17: 373-387.
52. Jacobson MA, O'Donnell JJ, Mills J. Foscarnet treatment of cytomegalovirus retinitis in patients with the acquired immunodeficiency syndrome. Antimicrob Agents Chemother 1989; 33: 736-741.
53. Cacoub P, Deray G, Baumelou A, Le Hoang P, Rozenbaum W, Gentilini M, Soubrie C, Rousselie E, Jacobs C. Acute renal failure induced by foscarnet: 4 cases. Clin Nephrol 1988; 29: 315-318.
54. Deray G, Martinez F, Katlama C, Levaltier B, Beaufils H, Danis M, Rozenheim M, Baumelou A, Dohin E, Gentilini M, Jacobs C. Foscarnet nephrotoxicity: mechanism, incidence, and prevention. Am J Nephrol 1989; 9: 316-321.
55. Jacobson MA. Review of the toxicities of foscarnet. J AIDS 1992; 5(Suppl 1): S11-S17.
56. Chatelain E, Deminiere C, Lacut JY, Potaux L. Severe renal failure and polyneuritis induced by foscarnet. Nephrol Dial Transplant 1998; 13: 2368-2369.
57. Deray G, Cacoub P, Le Hoang P, Baumelou A, Soubrie C, Rousselie F, Morer I, Jacobs C. Foscarnet-induced acute renal failure and effectiveness of haemodialysis. Lancet 1987; 2: 216.
58. Deray G, Katlama C, Dohin E. Prevention of foscarnet nephrotoxocity. Ann Intern Med 1990; 113: 332.
59. Beaufils H, Deray G, Katlama C, Dohin E, Henin D, Sazdovitch V, Jouanneau C. Foscarnet and crystals in glomerular capillary lumens. Lancet 1990; 336: 755.
60. Nyberg G, Svalander C, Blohme I, Persson H. Tubulointerstitial nephritis caused by the antiviral agent foscarnet. Transplant Int 1989; 2: 223-227.
61. Zanetta G, Maurice-Estepa L, Mousson C, Justrabo E, Daudon M, Rifle G, Tanter Y. Foscarnet-induced crystalline glomerulonephritis with nephrotic syndrome and acute renal failure after kidney transplantation. Transplantation 1999; 67: 1376-1378.
62. Trolliet P, Dijoud F, Cotte L, Cahen R, Francois B, Trepo C, Patricot LM. Crescentic glomerulonephritis and crystals within glomerular capillaries in an AIDS patient treated with foscarnet. Am J Nephrol 1995; 15: 256-259.
63. Maurice-Estapa L, Daudon M, Katlama C, Jouanneau C, Sazdovitch V, Lacour B, Beaufils H. Identification of crystals in kidneys of AIDS patients treated with foscarnet. Am J Kid Dis 1998; 32: 392-400.
64. Justrabo E, Zanetta G, Martin L, Assem M, Mousson C, Maurice-Estepa L, Rifle G, Tanter Y. Irreversible glomerular lesions induced by crystal precipitation in a renal transplant after foscarnet therapy for cytomegalovirus infection. Histopathology 1999; 34: 365-369.
65. Goldfarb DS, Coe FL. Foscarnet crystal deposition and renal failure. Am J Kid Dis 1998; 32: 519-520.
66. Farese RV Jr, Schambelan M, Hollander H, Stringari S, Jacobson MA. Nephrogenic diabetes insipidus associated with foscarnet treatment of cytomegalovirus retinitis. Ann Intern Med 1990; 112: 955-956.
67. Conn J, Colman P, Brown G, Street A, Bate K. Nephrogenic diabetes insipidus associated with foscarnet – a case report. J Antimicrob Chemother 1996; 37: 1180-1181.
68. Navarro JP et al. Nephrogenic diabetes insipidus and renal tubular acidosis secondary to foscarnet therapy. Am J Kidney Dis. 1996; 27(3):431-4.
69. Bendz H, Aurell M. Drug-induced diabetes insipidus: incidence, prevention and management. Drug Saf 1999; 2: 449-456
70. Hoch, BS, Shahmehdi SJ, Louis BM, Lipner HI. Foscarnet alters antidiuretic hormone-mediated transport. Antimicrob Agents Chemother 1995; 39: 2008-2012.
71. Youle MS, Clarbour J, Gazzard B, Chanas A. Severe hypocalcemia in AIDS patients treated with foscarnet and pentamadine. Lancet 1988; 1: 1455-1456.
72. Jacobson MA, Gambertoglio JG, Aweeka FT, Causey DM, Portale A. Foscarnet-induced hypocalcemia and effects of foscarnet on calcium metabolism. J Clin Endocrinol Metab 1991; 72: 1130-1135.
73. Noormohamed FH, Youle MS, Tang B, Martin-Munley S, Gazzard BG, Lant AF. Foscarnet-induced changes in plasma concentrations of total and ionized calcium and magnesium in HIV-positive patients. Antivir Ther 1996; 1: 172-179.
74. Perrin DD, Stunzi H. Viral chemotherapy: antiviral actions of metal ions and metal-chelating agents. Pharmac Ther 1981; 12: 255-297.
75. Huycke MM, Naguib MT, Stroemmel MM, Blick K, Monti K, Martin-Munley S, Kaufman C. A double-blind placebo-controlled crossover trial of intravenous magnesium sulfate for foscarnet-induced ionized hypocalcemia and hypomagnesemia in patients with AIDS and cytomegaloviral infection. Antimicrob Agents Chemother 2000; 44: 2143-2148.

76. Omar RF, Dusserre N, Desormeaux A, Poulin L, Tremblay M, Beauchamp D, Bergeron M. Liposomal encapsulation of foscarnet protects against hypocalcemia induced by free foscarnet. Antimicrob Agents Chemother 1995; 39: 1973-1978.
77. Katlama C, Tubiana R, Rosenheim M, Valantin MA, Caumes E, Bricaire F, Gentilini M. Dideoxyinosine-associated hypokalaemia. Lancet 1991; 337: 183.
78. Connolly KJ, Allan JD, Fitch H, Jackson-Pope L, McLaren C, Canetta R, Groopman JE. Phase I study of 2'-3'-dideoxyinosine administered orally twice daily to patients with AIDS and AIDS-related complex and hematologic intolerance to zidovudine. Am J Med 1991; 91: 471-478.
79. Yarchoan R, Pluda JM, Thomas RV, Mitsuya H, Brouwers P, Wyvill KM, Hartman N, Johns DG, Broder S. Long-term toxicity/activity profile of 2', 3'-dideoxyinosine in AIDS or AIDS-related complex. Lancet 1990; 336: 526-529.
80. Lambert JS, Seidlin M, Reichman RC, Plank CS, Laverty M, Morse GD, Knupp C, LcLaren C, Pettinelli C, Valentine FT, Dolin R. 2', 3'-dideoxyinosine (ddI) in patients with the acquired immunodeficiency syndrome or AIDS-related complex. N Engl J Med 1990; 322: 1333-1340.
81. Richardson D, Liou SH, Kahn JO. Uric acid and didanosine compliance in AIDS clinical trials: an analysis of AIDS clinical trials group protocols 116A and 116B/117. J AIDS 1993; 6: 1212-1223.
82. Takubo T, Kato T, Kinami J, Hanada K, Ogata H. Effect of lamivudine on uptake of organic cations by rat renal brush-border and basolateral membrane vesicles. J Pharm Pharmacol 2000; 52: 569-575.
83. Krishnan M, Nair R, Haas M, Atta MG. Acute renal failure in an HIV-positive 50- year old man. Am J Kidney Dis 2000; 36: 1075-1078.
84. Mulato AS, Ho ES, Cihlar T. Nonsteroidal anti-inflammatory drugs efficiently reduce the transport and cytotoxicity of adefovir mediated by the human renal organic anion transporter 1. J Pharmacol Exp Ther 2000; 295: 10-15.
85. Fisher E, Brosgart C, Cohn D, Chaloner K, Pulling C, Semetter B, Alston B, El-Sadr W, CPCRA 039 Team. Safety of adefovir dipivoxil (ADV) and incidence of proximal tubular disorders (PRTD) in a placebo-controlled trial in patients with advanced HIV disease. 6th Conference on Retroviruses and Opportunistic Infections, Chicago 1999 (abstract 678).
86. Kahn J, Lagakos S, Wulfsohn M, Cherng D, Miller M, Cherrington J, Hardy D, Beall G, Cooper R, Murphy R, Basgoz N, Ng E, Deeks S, Winlsow D, Toole JJ, Coakley D. Efficacy and safety of adefovir dipivoxil with antiretroviral therapy. JAMA 1999; 282: 2305-2312.
87. Tanji N, Tanji K, Kambham N, Markowitz GS, Bell A, D'agati VD. Adefovir nephrotoxicity: possible role of mitochondrial DNA depletion. Hum Pathol 2001; 32: 734-740.
88. Arnaudo E, Dalakas M, Shanske S, Morales CT, DiMauro S, Schon EA. Depletion of muscle mitochondrial DNA in AIDS patients with zidovudine-induced myopathy. Lancet 1991; 337: 508-510.
89. Chen SC, Barker SM, Mitchell DH, Stevens SM, O'Neill P, Cunningham AL. Concurrent zidovudine-induced myopathy and hepatotoxicity in patients treated for human immunodeficiency virus (HIV) infection. Pathology 1992; 24: 109-111.
90. Dalakas MC, Illa I, Pezeshkpour GH, Laukaitis JP, Cohen B, Griffin JL. Mitochondrial myopathy caused by long-term zidovudine therapy. N Engl J Med 1990; 322: 1098-1105.
91. Chen CH, Vazquez-Padua M, Cheng YC. Effect of anti-human immunodeficiency virus nucleoside analogs on mitochondrial DNA and its implication for delayed toxicity. Mol Pharmacol 1991; 39: 625-628.
92. Zeviani M, Tiranti V, Plantadosi C. Reviews in molecular medicine. Medicine 1999; 77: 59-72.
93. Johns DR. Mitochondrial DNA and disease. N Engl J Med 1995; 33(10):638-644.
94. Niaudet P, Rotig A. The kidney in mitochondrial cytopathies. Kidney Int 1997; 51: 1000-1007.
95. Sundar K, Suarez M, Banogon PE, Shapiro JM. Zidovudine-induced fatal lactic acidosis and hepatic failure in patients with acquired immunodeficiency syndrome: report of two patients and review of the literature. Crit Care Med 1997;25: 1425-1430.
96. Gopinath R, Hutcheon M, Cheema-Dhadli S, Halperin M. Chronic lactic acidosis in a patient with acquired immunodeficiency syndrome and mitochondrial myopathy: biochemical studies. J Am Soc Nephrol 1992; 3: 1212-1219.
97. Chattha G, Arieff AI, Cummings C, Tierney LM Jr. Lactic acidosis complicating the acquired immunodeficiency syndrome. Ann Intern Med 1993; 118: 37-39.
98. Haupt MT, Carlson RW, Fulop M, Coyle T, Chariot P, Baram D, Chattha G. Lactic acidosis and AIDS. Ann Intern Med 1993;119: 343-345.
99. Shaer A, Rastegar A. Lactic acidosis in the setting of antiretroviral therapy for the acquired immunodeficiency syndrome. Am J Nephrol 2000; 20: 332-338.
100. Bleeker-Rovers CP, Kadir SW, vanLeusen R, Richter C. Hepatic steatosis and lactic acidosis caused by stavudine in an HIV-infected patient. Neth J Med 2000; 57: 190-193.
101. Bartley PB, Westacott L, Boots RJ, Lawson M, Potter JM, Hyland VJ, Woods ML. Large hepatic mitochondrial DNA deletions associated with L-lactic acidosis and highly active antiretroviral therapy. AIDS 2001; 15: 419-420.

102. Mokrzycki MH, Harris C, May H, Laut J, Palmisano J. Lactic acidosis associated with stavudine administration: a report of five cases. Clin Infect Dis 2000; 30: 198-200.
103. John M, Moore CB, James IR, Nolan D, Upton RP, McKinnon EJ Mal SA. Chronic hyperlactatemia in HIV-infected patients taking antiretroviral therapy. AIDS 2001; 15: 717-723.
104. Miller KD, Cameron M, Wood LV, Dalakas MC, Kovacs JA. Lactic acidosis and hepatic steatosis associated with use of stavudine: report of four cases. Ann Intern Med 2000; 133: 192-196.
105 Brinkman K, terHofstede HJ, Burger DM, Smeitink JA, Koopmans PP. Adverse effects of reverse transcriptase inhibitors: mitochondrial toxicity as common pathway. AIDS 1998; 12: 1735-1744.
106. Moyle G. Clinical manifestations and management of antiretroviral nucleoside analog-related mitochondrial toxicity. Clin Ther 2000; 22: 911-936.
107. Swartz M. Mitochondrial toxicity – new adverse drug effects. N Engl J Med 1995; 333: 1146-1148.
108. Côté HCF, Brumme ZL, Craib KJP, Alexander CS, Wynhoven B, Ting L, Wong H, Harris M, Harrigan PR, O'Shaughnessy MV, Montaner JSG. Changes in mitochondrial DNA as a marker of nuceloside toxicity in HIV-infected patients. New Engl J Med 2002; 346: 811-820.
109. McKenzie R, Fried M, Sallie R, Conjeevaram H, DiBisceglie AM, Park Y, Savarese B, Kleiner D, Tsokos M, Luciano C, Pruett T, Stotka JL, Straus SE, Hoofnagle JH. Hepatic failure and lactic acidosis due to fialuridine (flau), an investigational nucleoside analogue for chronic hepatitis B. N Engl J Med 1995; 333: 1099-1105.
110. Chariot P, Ruet E, Authier FJ, Levy Y, Gherardi R. Acute rhabdomyolysis in patients infected by human immunodeficiency virus. Neurology 1994; 44: 1692-1696.
111. Foulty B, Frerman F, Reves R. Riboflavin to treat NRTI-induced lactic acidosis. Lancet 1999; 352: 291-292.
112. Luzzati R, DelBravo P, DiPerri G, Luzzani A, Concia E. Riboflavine and severe lactic acidosis. Lancet 1999; 353: 901-902.
113. Claessens YE, Cariou A, Chiche JD, Dauriat G, Dhainaut JF. L-carnitine as a treatment of life-threatening lactic acidosis induced by nucleoside analogues. AIDS 2000; 14: 472-473.
114. Chodock R, Eleftherios M, Shemin D, Valgerdur R, Yodice P, Renzi R, Tashima K, Towe C, Rich J. Survival of a human immunodeficiency patient with nucleoside-induced lactic acidosis – role of haemodialysis treatment. Nephrol Dial Transplant 1999; 14: 2484-2486.
115. Crowther MA, Callaghan W, Hodsman AB, Mackie ID. Dideoxyinosine-associated nephrotoxicity. AIDS 1993; 7: 131-132.
116. Morris AAM, Baudouin SV, Snow MH. Renal tubular acidosis and hypophosphataemia after treatment with nucleoside reverse transcriptase inhibitors. AIDS 2001; 15: 140-141.
117. Krishnan M, Nair R, Haas M, Atta MG. Acute renal failure in an HIV-positive 50-year-old man. Am J Kidney Dis 2000; 36: 1075-1078.
118. Ahmad M. Abacavir -induced reversible Fanconi syndrome with nephrogenic diabetes insipidus in a patient with acquired immunodeficiency syndrome. J Postgrad Med. 2006; 52(4): 296-7.
119. Coca S, Perazella MA. Acute renal failure associated with tenofovir: evidence of drug-induced nephrotoxicity. Am J Med Sci 2002; 324: 342-344.
120. Verhelst D, Monge M, Meynard J-L, Fouqueray B, Mougenot B, Girard P-M, Ronco P, Rossert J. Fanconi syndrome and renal failure induced by tenofovir: a first case report. Am J Kidney Dis 2002; 40: 1331-1333
121. Malik, A, Abraham P, Malik N. Acute renal failure and Fanconi syndrome in an AIDS patient on tenofovir treatment – case report and review of the literature. J Infection 2005; 51:e61-65.
122. Murphy MD, O;Hearn M, Chou S. Fatal lactic acidosis and acute renal failure after addition of tenofovir to an antiretroviral regimen containing didanosine. Clin Infect Dis 2003; 36:1082-5.
123. Rollot F, Nazal EM, Chauvelot-Moachon L et al. Tenofovir-related fanconi syndrome with nephrogenic diabetes insipidus in a patient with acquired immunodeficiency syndrome: the role of lopinavir-ritonavir-didanosine. Clin Infect Dis 2003; 37:e174-6.
124. Cirino CM, Kan VL. Hypokalemia in HIV patients on tenofovir. AIDS 2006; 20(12):1671-1673.
124a. Zimmerman AE, Pizzoferrato T, Bedford J et al. Tenofovir - associated acute and chronic kidney disease: A case of multiple drug interactions. Clin Infect Dis 2006;42:283-90.
124b. Vidal F, Domingo JC, Guallar J. et al. *In vitro* Cytotoxicity and Mitochondrial toxicity of tenofovir alone and in combination with other antiretrovirals in human renal proximal tubule cells. Antimic Agents Chemother 2006; 50(11): 3824-3832.
125. Mutlib AE, Chen H, Nemeth GA, Markwalder JA, Seitz SP, Gan LS, Christ DD. Identification and characterization of efavirenz metabolites by liquid chromatography/mass spectrometry and high field NMR: species differences in the metabolism of efavirenz. Drug Metab Dispos 1999; 27: 1319-1333.
126. Mutlib AE, Gerson RJ, Meunier PC, Haley PJ, Chen H, Gan LS, Davies MH, Gemzik B, Christ DD, Krahn DF, Markwalder JA, Seitz SP, Robertson RT, Miwa GT. The species dependent metabolism of efavirenz produces a nephrotoxic glutathione conjugate in rats. Toxicol Appl Pharmacol 2000; 169: 102-113.

127. Barbour TD. Furlong TJ, Finlayson RJ. Efavirenz-associated podocyte damage. AIDS. 2007; 21(2):257-8.
128. Castro JG, Gutierrez L. Rhabdomyolysis with acute renal failure probably related to the interaction of atorvastatin and delavirdine. Am J Med 2002; 112:505.
129. Olyaei AJ, deMattos AM, Bennett WM. Renal toxicity of protease inhibitors. Curr Opin Nephrol Hypertens 2000; 9: 473-476.
130. Balani SK, Woolf EJ, Hoagland VL, Sturgill MG. Disposition of indinavir, a potent HIV-1 protease inhibitor, after an oral dose in humans. Drug Metab Dispos 1995; 24: 1389-1394.
131. Kopp JB, Miller KD, Mican JM, Feuerstein IM, Vaughan E, Baker C, Pannell LK, Falloon J. Crystalluria and urinary tract abnormalities associated with indinavir. Ann Intern Med 1997; 127: 119-125.
132. Reiter WJ, Pernerstorfer-Schon H, Dorfinger K, Hofbauer J, Marberger M. Frequency of urolithiasis in individuals seropositive for human immunodeficiency virus treated with indinavir is higher than previously assumed. J Urol 1999; 161: 1082-1084.
133. Gagnon, RF, Tecimer SN, Watters, AK, Tsoukas CM. Prospective study of urinalysis abnormalities in HIV-positive individuals treated with indinavir. Am J Kid Dis 2000; 36: 507-515.
134. Brodie SB, Keller MJ, Ewenstein BM, Sax PE. Variation in incidence of indinavir-associated nephrolithiasis amount HIV-positive patients. AIDS 1998; 12: 2433-2437.
135. Trainor LD, Steinberg JP, Austin GW, Solomon HM. Indinavir crystalluria: identification of patients at increased risk of developing nephrotoxicity. Arch Pathol Lab Med 1998; 122: 256-259.
136. Padberg J, Fritsche L, Bergmann F, Schurmann D, Suttorp N. Nephropathy and renal colic in patients treated with indinavir, ritonavir plus indinavir or ritonavir plus saquinavir. AIDS 1999; 13: 2173-2174.
137. Bonfanti P, Valsecchi L, Parazzini F, Carradori S, Pusterla L, Furtuna P, Timillero L, Alessi F, Ghiselli G, Gabbuti A, DiCintio E, Martinelli C, Faggion I, Landonio S, Quirino T. Incidence of adverse reactions in HIV patients treated with protease inhibitors: a cohort study. Coordinamento Italiano Studio Allergia e Infezione da HIV (CISAI) group. J AIDS 2000; 23: 236-245.
138. Herman JS, Ives NJ, Nelson M, Gazzard BG, Easterbrook PJ. Incidence and risk factors for the development of indinavir-associated renal complications. J Antimicrob Chemother 2001; 48: 355-360.
139. Schwartz, BF, Schenkman N, Armenakas NA, Stoller ML. Imaging characteristics of indinavir calculi. Am J Urol 1999; 161: 1085-1087.
140. Kohan AD, Armenakas NA, Fracchia JA. Indinavir urolithiasis: an emerging cause of renal colic inpatients with human immunodeficiency virus. J Urol 1999; 161: 1765-1768.
141. Berns JS, Cohen RM, Silverman M, Turner J. Acute renal failure due to indinavir crystalluria and nephrolithiasis: report of two cases. Am J Kid Dis 1997; 30: 558-560.
142. Kalaitzis C. Dimitriadis G. Tsatidis T. Kuntz R. Touloupidis S. Kelidis G. Treatment of indinavir sulfate induced urolithiasis in HIV-positive patients. Int Urol Nephrol 2002; 34(1):13-5.
143. Green ST, McKendrick MW, Schmid ML, Mohsen AH, Prakasam SF. Renal calculi developing de novo in a patient taking saquinavir. Int J STD AIDS 1998; 9: 555.
144. Engeler DS, Hubert J, Rentsch KM, Ruef C, Oertle D, Suter S. Nelfinavir urinary stones. J Urol 2002; 167: 1384-1385.
145. Pacanowski J, Poirer JM, Petit I, Meynard JL, Girard PM. Atazanavir urinary stones in an HIV-infected patient. AIDS 2006; 20(16):2131.
146. Tashima KT, Horowitz JD, Rosen S. Indinavir nephropathy. N Engl J Med 1997; 336: 138-139.
147. Sarcletti M, Petter A, Zangerle R. Indinavir and interstitial nephritis. Ann Intern Med 1998; 128: 320-322.
148. Grabe DW, Eisele G, Miller C, Singh J, Stein D. Indinavir-induced nephropathy. Clin Nephrol 1999; 51: 181-183.
149. Perazella MA, Kashgarian M, Cooney E. Indinavir nephropathy in an AIDS patient with renal insufficiency and pyuria. Clin Nephrol 1998; 50: 194-196.
150. Jaradat M, Phillips C, Yum MN, Cushing H, Moe S. Acute tubulointerstitial nephritis attributable to indinavir therapy. Am J Kid Dis 2000; 35: 1-5.
151. Marroni M, Gaburri M, Mecozzi F, Baldellli F. Acute interstitial nephritis secondary to the administration of indivavir. Ann Pharmocother 1998; 32: 843-844.
152. Hanabusa H, Tagami H, Hataya H. Renal atrophy associated with long term treatement with indinavir. New Engl J Med 1999; 340: 392-393.
153. Brewster UC, Perazella MA. Acute interstitial nephritis associated with atazanavir, a new protease inhibitor. Am J Kidney Dis 2002; 40:1331-3.
154. Duong M, Sgro C, Grappin M, Biron F, Boibieux A. Renal failure after treatment with ritonavir. Lancet 1996; 348: 693-694.
155. Witzke C, Plentz A, Schafers RF, Reinhardt W, Heemann U, Philipp T. Side effects of ritonavir and its combination with saquinavir with special regard to renal function. AIDS 1997; 11: 836-838.
156. Bochet MV, Jacquiaud C, Valantin MA, Katlama C, Deray G. Renal insufficiency induced by ritonavir in HIV-infected patients. Am J Med 1998; 105: 457.

157. Chugh S, Bird R, Alexander EA. Ritonavir and renal failure. N Engl J Med 1997; 336: 138.
158. Lalezari JP, Henry K, O'Hearn M et al. Enfuvirtide, an HIV-1 fusion inhibitor, for drug resistant HIV infection in North and South America. N Engl J Med 2003; 348:2175-2185.
159. Ing TS, Daugirdas JT, Soung LS, Klawans HL, Maharker SD, Hayashi JA, Geis WP, Hong JE. Toxic effects of amantadine in patients with renal failure. Can Med Assoc J 1979; 120: 695-698.
160. Ing TS, Rahn AC, Armbruster KFW, Oyama JH, Klawans HL. Amantadine accumulation in renal failure. N Engl J Med 1974; 291: 1257.

17

Analgesics and 5-aminosalicylic acid

Monique M. ELSEVIERS and Marc E. DE BROE

University of Antwerp, Belgium

Introduction

Classic analgesic nephropathy is a slowly progressive disease resulting from the daily use for many years of analgesic mixtures containing at least two antipyretics, anilides and salicylates, and usually caffeine or codeine (or both). The nephropathy is characterized by renal papillary necrosis/calcifications and chronic interstitial nephritis, with an insidious progression to renal failure, sometimes in association with transitional-cell carcinoma of the uroepithelium [1-10]. This type of nephropathy has never been described after the intake of single analgesic substances. Analgesic nephropathy is a facultative part of a broad spectrum of clinical findings that is summarized as 'analgesic syndrome' (see below). Historically, these analgesic mixtures most frequently contained phenacetin in combination with a further analgesic and a centrally acting agent such as caffeine or codeine, which may lead to psychological dependence [11-15].

In addition to the classical picture of analgesic nephropathy, epidemiological observations revealed that excessive exposure to analgesics and NSAIDs may contribute to the progression of a chronic renal disease of whatever etiology towards end-stage renal failure [16-21]. In all these epidemiological studies, however, it is impossible to rule out bias caused by the consumption of these analgesics for symptoms of the conditions that predisposed patients to renal failure.

Renal failure induced by abuse of analgesic mixtures, was identified as a serious problem in several countries in the second part of the 20th century. The initial reports [1, 22-24], observing that phenacetin was present in most abused analgesics, held this substance solely responsible for the development of what was called "phenacetin nephritis". In the late 1970's, it became apparent that the abuse of different kinds of analgesic mixtures might induce renal damage, whether they contained phenacetin or not. Consequently, the disease was more appropriately named 'analgesic nephropathy'.

Apart from classic analgesic nephropathy, this chapter will also handle the possible nephrotoxic role of 5-aminosalicylic acid (5-ASA) used in patients with chronic inflammatory bowel disease (IBD). During the last decade, 5-ASA replaced sulfasalazine as first-line therapy for mildly to moderately active IBD. For decades, sulphasalazine, an azo-compound derived from sulphapyridine and 5-aminosalicylic acid (5-ASA), has been the only valuable non-corticosteroid drug in the treatment of inflammatory bowel disease. Azad Kahn et al. [25] showed that the pharmacologically active moiety in sulphasalazine for the treatment of these diseases was 5-ASA. Consequently, this resulted in a number of new 5-ASA formulations (mesalazine, olsalazine, balsalazine) for topical and oral use. Since the metabolite sulphapyridine was largely responsible for the side effects of sulfasalazine, the primary advantage of the newer 5-ASA agents is their improved adverse effect profile.

In recent years, however, several case reports have been published, suggesting an association between the use of 5-ASA and the development of a particular type of chronic tubulo-interstitial nephritis, characterized by an important cellular infiltration of the interstitium [26, 27]. In some cases, it was shown that this cellular infiltration was not disappearing upon arrest of the drug, even after a period of more than one year [28]. Although acute renal failure under non-steroidal anti-inflammatory drugs (NSAID) is well documented, the risk for developing chronic lesions remains controversial.

Chronic renal effects associated to the use of non-steroidal anti-inflammatory drugs (NSAID) is discussed in chapter 18.

Analgesics

Epidemiological observations

Association between analgesic abuse and analgesic nephropathy

Clinical evidence linking the abuse of analgesic mixtures with the development of renal failure was well documented from the 1960's on. There are numerous reports demonstrating a high incidence of heavy analgesic consumption in patients with renal failure or papillary necrosis [14]. Also the observed deterioration of renal function in patients with analgesic nephropathy who continued their abuse, and in contrast the stabilization of renal function after discontinuation of the abuse, is in favor of this association [29-32].

Epidemiological evidence of the overall association between analgesic abuse and the development of renal impairment is documented in nine case-control studies [16-18, 20-21, 33-34, 36-38], two prospective cohort studies [39, 40] and two observational cohort studies [41, 42] published in the last decades (Figure 1). It is inherent to epidemiological studies however, that the observed association between chronic renal failure and analgesic consumption does not establish cause and effect. Moreover, serious flaws in study design and analysis of the data have to be considered and were discussed in several reviews (Table 1) [7, 43,44,45].

In the case-control studies, the overall risk after any analgesic consumption with a minimum between 217 g and 7000 pills, ranged from 1.02 (95%, CI 0.8-1.3) to 17.2 (95%, CI 8,5-34,7). Four out of six case-control studies reporting the consumption of 'any analgesic', showed an increased risk for the development of renal failure. The studies of Sandler, Pommer and Morlans [16, 36, 18] resulted in comparable odds ratios between 2 and 3, despite the differences in study design. McCredie's study showed a considerable higher odds ratio by using the more specific lesion of renal papillary necrosis as disease under study [33].

The most solid demonstration of the association between analgesic abuse and renal failure has been provided by the two prospective controlled cohort studies performed in Switzerland and Belgium with a follow-up of 10 and 6 years, respectively [39, 40]. Although both studies differed substantially with respect to study populations, analgesics consumed and length of follow-up, reported odds ratio's were

A

Case-control studies	Cases	Controls	Lifetime dose
McCredie et al, Australia, 1982 [33]	80 women with RPN	80 healthy women	3 units/week for one year
Murray et al, USA, 1983 [34]	527 p. with ESRD	1047 hospitalized p.	almost daily for 30 days
Sandler et al, USA, 1989+1991 [16,17]	554 p. with newly diagnosed CRF	516 population based	daily for one year
Pommer et al, West Berlin, 1989 [36]	517 p. with ESRD	517 outpatient clinic p.	15 units/month for one year
Morlans et al, Barcelona, 1990 [18]	340 p. with ESRD	673 hospitalized p.	15 units/month for 30 days
Perneger et al, USA, 1994 [20]	716 p. with ESRD	361 population based	daily for one year
Fored et al, Sweden, 2001 [21]	926 p. with newly diagnosed CRF	998 population based	twice a week for 2 months
Ibanez et al, Barcelona, 2005 [37]	583 p. with ESRD	1190 hospitalized p.	15 units/month for 30 days
Van der Woude et al, Austria, Germany, 2007 [38]	907 p. with ESRD	3622 population based, no fenacetine intake	1 unit per month; no phenacetin intake
Prospective controlled cohort studies			
Dubach et al, Switzerland, 1983 [39]	623 healthy women; followed for 10 years, outcome decreased eGFR	621 healthy women	urine positive for paracetamol
Elseviers and De Broe, Belgium, 1995 [40]	200 healthy subjects; followed for 7 years, outcome decreased eGFR	200 healthy subjects	daily for 1 year with total > 1000 units
Observational cohort studies			
Kurth et al, USA, 2004 [41]	4494 healthy male physicians, aged 40-84, followed for 15 years, outcome decreased eGFR		all kinds of analgesics, daily aspirin intake
Curhan et al, USA, 2004 [42]	1697 healthy female nurses, aged 30-55, followed for 12 years, outcome decreased eGFR		all kinds of analgesics

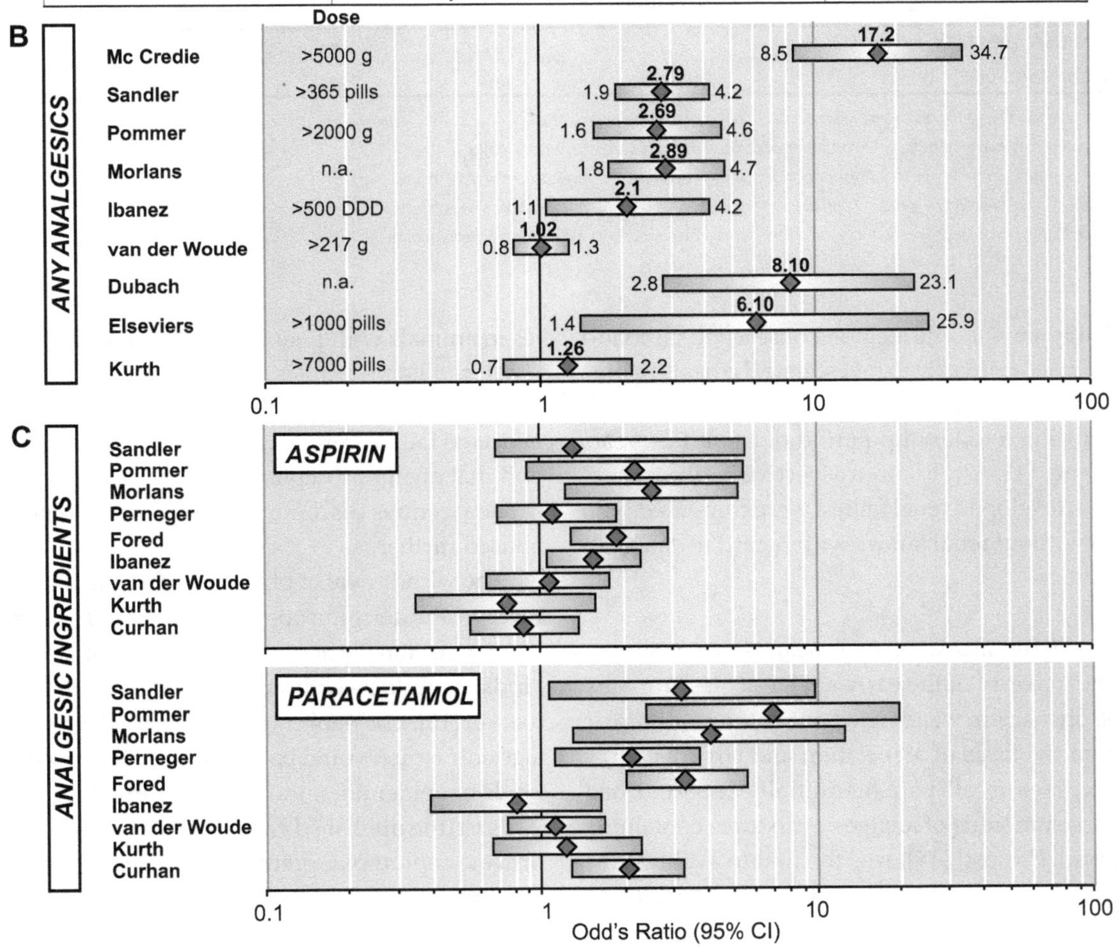

Figure 1. ***Overview of epidemiological studies investigating the renal risk of analgesic consumption. A.*** *Description of methodological details used in the included studies.* ***B.*** *Presentation of the overall risk (odds ratio with 95% confidence interval) associated to the consumption of 'any analgesic' exceeding the mentioned dose.* ***C.*** *Presentation of the odds ratios with 95% confidence interval published in the included epidemiological studies focussing separately on the ingredients aspirin and paracetamol.*

Table 1. Sources of bias in the epidemiological studies.

	Selection bias	Information bias	Indication or protopathic bias	Ingredient bias	Dose bias
Case-control studies					
McCredie et al, Australia, 1982 [33]	yes	no	yes	yes	no
Murray et al, USA, 1983 [34]	yes	no	yes	yes	yes
Sandler et al, USA, 1989+1991 [16,17]	no	yes	yes	yes	no
Pommer et al, West Berlin, 1989 [36]	no	no	yes	no	no
Morlans et al, Barcelona,1990 [18]	yes	no	no	yes	yes
Perneger et al, USA,1994 [20]	yes	yes	yes	yes	no
Fored et al, Sweden, 2001 [21]	no	no	no	yes	yes
Ibanez et al, Barcelona, 2005 [37]	yes	no	no	yes	yes
Van der Woude et al, Austria, Germany, 2007 [38]	yes	no	no	no	yes
Prospective controlled cohort studies					
Dubach et al, Switzerland, 1983 [39]	no	yes	yes	yes	no
Elseviers and De Broe, Belgium, 1995 [40]	no	no	yes	no	no
Observational cohort studies					
Kurth et al, USA, 2004 [41]	no	yes	yes	yes	no
Curhan et al, USA, 2004 [42]	no	yes	yes	yes	no

Selection bias = random selection of controls failed or the chosen control population is biased.
Information bias = methods used to obtain information about analgesic consumption were doubtful.
Indication (protopathic) bias = failure to control for analgesic intake preceding the development of renal failure.
Ingredient bias = failure to entangle the use of particular ingredients either as single analgesic or as one of the ingredients of analgesic mixtures.
Dose bias = definition of analgesic use far below the amount consumed by patients with analgesic nephropathy.

remarkably similar. The included observational cohort studies aimed primarily to investigate the health status of a large cohort of US male physicians and US female nurses during a follow-up period of 14 and 11 years respectively [41, 42]. In a retrospective analysis, subjects who developed renal failure were compared with controls without renal failure with regard to analgesic consumption.

Nephrotoxicity of different kinds of analgesic mixtures

In the majority of the early analgesic nephropathy reports, phenacetin was singled out as the nephrotoxic culprit on the basis of association and circumstantial evidence. Nearly all patients initially reported had taken large amounts of analgesic mixtures containing phenacetin. Prescott [14], was the first to evaluate the nephrotoxic role of phenacetin and other analgesics. He stated that in the past insufficient attention had been given to the possible nephrotoxicity of the other analgesics invariably taken with phenacetin, and that the common belief that phenacetin is the primary cause of analgesic nephropathy can be challenged on many counts. He argued that numerous chronic toxicity studies in animals with phenacetin have failed to produce renal papillary necrosis, that the removal of phenacetin in some countries has not been followed by the expected fall in mortality from analgesic nephropathy and that analgesic nephropathy has a poor prognosis if phenacetin is discontinued but other analgesics are abused further.

The withdrawal of phenacetin from analgesic mixtures in Western Europe and the United States, gave rise to question the nephrotoxic potency of the different kinds of products without phenacetin, available on the market [10]. The nephrotoxic potency of the newer analgesic mixtures could be demonstrated using different kinds of epidemiological observations [46].

First, the published case-control studies could confirm the nephrotoxic potency of analgesic mixtures and the different substances worked-up in these mixtures (Figure 1). Interpretation of the presented odds ratios per substance however, remains difficult since they were seriously influenced by the additional effect of other substances invariably taken together. Most case-control studies suffered from ingredient bias and were not able to evaluate the nephrotoxic effect of different combinations separately (Table 1). The only study that carefully avoid this bias, used too low doses to achieve trustful risk estimates [38]. Only Pommer attempted to entangle thoroughly the influence of different substances worked up in analgesic mixtures, showing an increased risk for phenacetin, paracetamol and phenazone containing analgesic mixtures controlled for the use of other combinations [36]. In the prospective controlled cohort studies, the study design and the limited number of cases with renal failure did not allow to study the nephrotoxic effect of different substances used [39, 40].

Moreover, a cohort of 226 patients with a clear diagnosis of analgesic nephropathy was investigated regarding their analgesic consumption. Patients were recruited within the framework of diagnostic criteria studies in Belgium (n=130) and eleven other European countries (n=96) [50, 51]. In all patients, analgesic nephropathy was diagnosed using the same validated renal imaging criteria with high diagnostic performance [51, 52]. In all included patients, the history of abuse was documented by the same methodology using the same structured questionnaire accompanied by a color picture book showing the analgesics with a high sales volume in each particular country. Results clearly showed that analgesic nephropathy was associated with the abuse of different kind of analgesic mixtures mostly containing phenacetin. However, 46 out of the 226 patients never consumed phenacetin-containing analgesics. Their documented analgesic nephropathy was associated with the abuse of the following combinations: aspirin and acetaminophen, aspirin and a pyrazolone, acetaminophen and a pyrazolone, and two pyrazolones all of which were combined with caffeine, codeine or both. Additionally, the minimal analgesic consumption for developing analgesic nephropathy could be defined as a daily consumption for at least five years. None of the subjects with a daily use of analgesic mixtures for less than 5 years (n=16) or those with a weekly but not a daily consumption for more than 5 years (n=19) met the renal imaging criteria of analgesic nephropathy [53].

Furtheron, a broad range of other clinical and epidemiological observations is in support with the previous results. For single analgesics, abuse is only poorly documented and the nephrotoxic potency of single analgesics can be considered as minimal. Even in patients with rheumatoid arthritis in which high dose salicylate therapy was the mainstay of treatment, analgesic nephropathy seldom developed [14]. For single analgesics combined with caffeine/codeine, the example of Sweden is of particular interest. Although, Sweden has a high sales volume of this type of analgesics (40% of the total volume), prevalence of analgesic nephropathy remained at the low level of 1-2% during the last decade [54]. Moreover, it is of interest to note that in countries with a low prevalence of analgesic nephropathy such as Sweden and France, analgesic mixtures containing two analgesic substances combined with caffeine/codeine are not available (Sweden) or not sold (France), despite the fact that in both countries the total volume of analgesics sold is higher than in Belgium.

Nephrotoxicity of single analgesics

The most important clinical question remains to evaluate the nephrotoxic potential of different analgesic ingredients, when used as single substance.

Particularly, the potential nephrotoxicity of paracetamol used as single analgesic remains a matter of debate. Case-control studies as well as observational cohort studies have controversial results, with 6 studies showing an increased risk and 3 studies that did not (Figure 1). Since most studies are not able to distinguish between paracetamol used as single analgesic and in combinations, presented risk ratios do not answer the question of nephrotoxicity when used as single analgesic (ingredient bias, see Table 1).

The renal safety of aspirin used as single ingredient is easier to evaluate. From the seven case-control studies, only 3 showed an increased risk. All 3 suffered from the same ingredient bias as previously mentioned for paracetamol. In contrast however, both observational studies reported a robust, slightly decreased, odds ratio for the use of aspirin (Figure 1). In both studies, calculated odds ratio's were based on hundreds of regular users of aspirin [41, 42].

Quantification of the problem

Detailed information concerning the extent of the problem of analgesic nephropathy is limited, particularly for recent years. National annual data were collected in Australia/New Zealand by the Australian and New Zealand Dialysis and Transplant Registry (ANZDATA) [51] and in the United States by the United States Renal Data System (USRDS) [52]. In Europe, the registration system of the European Dialysis and Transplant Association (EDTA) [53] published regularly incidence and prevalence data of analgesic nephropathy for all European countries in the past.

Australian incidence rates showed a significant decline after the restriction of over-the-counter analgesic sales in 1979. During the 1970's, Australia had the highest incidence rate in the world (up to 22%). The incidence declined to 15% in 1985 and to 11% in 1990 [58, 59]. In recent years the incidence remained at a level of 4%, decreasing earlier and faster among younger patients [55]. In Flanders, a region with well-documented high incidence of analgesic nephropathy in end stage renal failure patients, the incidence fell from 17% in the mid eighties to 3-4% in recent years (Figure 2).

In the United States the national prevalence of analgesic nephropathy is not well documented. In the 1980's, local studies showed incidences, ranging from 1.7 in Philadelphia and 2.8% in Washington D.C. to 10% in Northwest North Carolina [34, 60,61]. According the USRDS annual data report, incidence of analgesic nephropathy remained at the very low level of 0.2% for patients starting renal replacement therapy in the last decade (USRDS 2005) [56]. In Canada 2.5% of dialysis patients had analgesic nephropathy in 1976. The recent prevalence can be expected to be low [62]. In South Africa in the early eighties, 33% of the white patients starting chronic renal replacement therapy in Durban were diagnosed with analgesic nephropathy [63]. In Kuala Lumpur, Malaysia, 8% of the 180 dialysis patients had consumed excessive quantities of analgesics and in 4% signs of renal papillary necrosis were observed [64]. More recently high analgesic abuse of 7-10% in rural areas was reported [65]. Incidence of analgesic nephropathy in ESRD population of Thailand is however unknown.

On the other hand, Central and Eastern European countries were confronted in the 1990s with an increasing incidence of the disease partly due to the increasing number of older patients accepted for renal replacement therapy. In 1992, Matousovic et al. [66] measured an incidence rate of 9.1% of analgesic nephropathy in the Czech and Slovak Republics using renal imaging criteria [67]. The same methodology was used in Hungary where an incidence up to 13% was noted in 1996 [68]. In contrast, in the southwest region of Poland not any case of analgesic nephropathy could be identified in the period 1991-1992. The investigators concluded, however, that a reassessment of the incidence after 5-10 years should be mandatory because in the early 1990's only 40% of (younger) ESRD patients received dialysis treatment [69].

Pathophysiology

The exact pathophysiological mechanism(s) of analgesic nephropathy is unknown. The disease is characterized by capillary sclerosis of the vessels of the renal pelvis and ureteral mucosa, renal papillary necrosis and calcification, interstitial infiltration fibrosis, progressive cortical atrophy next to zones with hypertrophy of the remaining nephrons, aspecific glomerular changes. The main pathological lesion strongly indicates the more distal parts of the nephron as the predilected target for analgesic toxicity (Figure 3).

The potentiating effect of aspirin with both phenacetin and acetaminophen may be related to two factors:

- Acetaminophen undergoes oxidative metabolism by prostaglandin H synthase to reactive quinoneimine that is conjugated to glutathione. If acetaminophen is present alone, there is sufficient glutathione generated in the papillae to detoxify the reactive intermediate. However, if acetaminophen is ingested with aspirin, the aspirin is converted to salicylate, which becomes highly concentrated and depletes glutathione in both the cortex and papillae of the kidney. With the cellular glutathione depleted, the reactive metabolite of acetaminophen then produces lipid peroxides and arylation of tissue proteins, ultimately resulting in necrosis of the papillae [9, 70].
- Aspirin and NSAID suppress prostaglandin production by inhibiting cyclooxygenase enzymes. Renal blood flow, particularly within the renal medulla, is highly dependent upon systemic and local production of vasodilatory prostaglandins. Thus, this region, in the setting of combined aspirin and NSAID use, is more prone to ischemic damage. Loss of proteoglycans and glycosaminoglycans, essential constituents of medullary matrix may occur.

Clinical aspects

Clinically, analgesic nephropathy is characterized

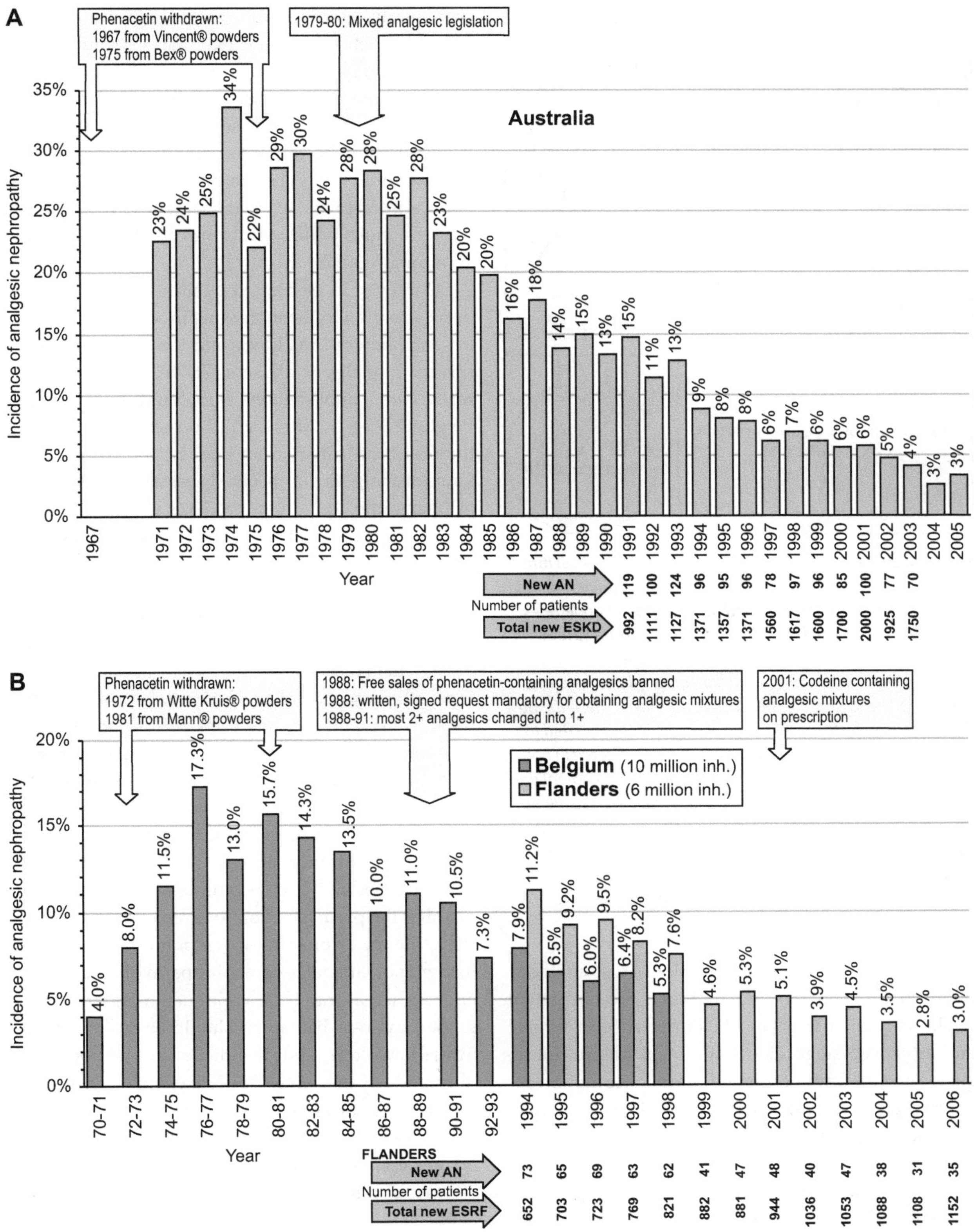

Figure 2. *. Incidence of analgesic nephropathy (AN) in Australia 1971-2005.* ***B.*** *Incidence of AN in Belgium 1970-1998 and in Flanders 1994-2006. At the bottom, absolute numbers of new AN.*

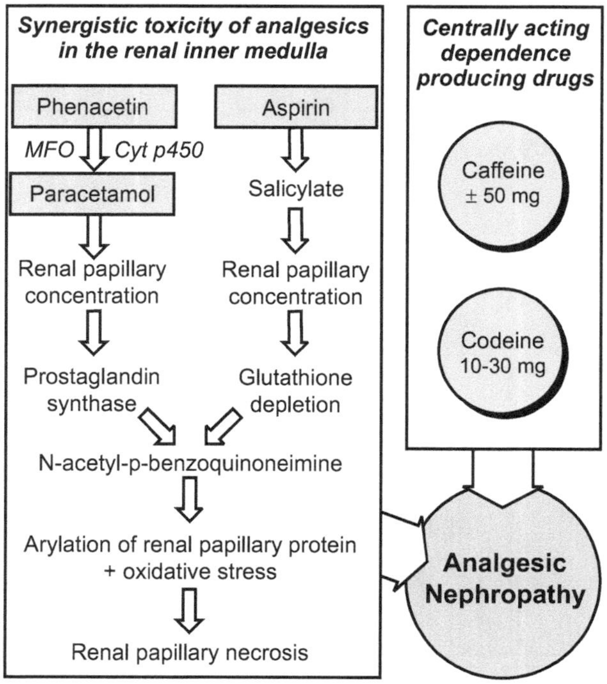

Figure 3. Synergistic toxicity of analgesics in the renal inner medulla and centrally acting dependence-producing drugs leading to analgesic nephropathy. *Paracetamol undergoes oxidative metabolism by prostaglandin H synthase to reactive quinoneimine that is conjugated to glutathione. If paracetamol is present alone, there is sufficient glutathione generated in the papillae to detoxify the reactive intermedicate. If the paracetamol is ingested with aspirin, the aspirin is converted to salicylate and salicylate becomes highly concentrated in both the cortex and papillae of the kidney. Salicylate is a potent depletory of glutathione. With the cellular glutathione depleted, the reactive metabolite of paracetamol then produces lipid peroxides and arylatyion of tissue proteins, ultimately resulting in necrosis of the papillae.*
[Reproduced with permission from refs. 5 and 9].

by its slow and stealthy progression. Most analgesic nephropathy patients only attended the outpatient nephrology clinic when renal failure reached a chronic and advanced stage. End-stage renal failure due to analgesic abuse was observed after consumption for approximately 20 years and most patients with analgesic nephropathy entered renal replacement therapy in their fifth-sixth decade.

An increased occurrence of anemia and an increased risk of developing vascular diseases and ischemic heart disease are mentioned in patients with analgesic nephropathy [71]. Gastrointestinal manifestations occur in more than half of analgesic abusers and particularly gastric ulcerations are frequently reported [72, 73]. Psychological and psychiatric manifestations are common in analgesic abusers and this is reflected in the frequency of associated addictive habits such as smoking, alcoholism and the excessive use of psychotropic drugs. Also the prematurely aged appearance of these patients has been emphasized. These observations pointed to the fact that analgesic nephropathy is part of a much wider syndrome called "the analgesic syndrome" [30, 74, 75].

Moreover, in 1965 a first publication from Sweden drew attention to the increasing incidence of tumoral degeneration of the kidney and the urinary tract observed in analgesic abusers [76-78]. Additional case reports were published in Switzerland, Australia, and Belgium [79-81]. Although, the risk for developing tumors of the urinary tract after the abuse of different kinds of analgesics is not clearly established, the abuse of phenacetin containing products showed a four-to tenfold increased risk [84]. The tumors generally become apparent after 15 to 25 years of analgesic abuse [82], usually but not always in patients with clinically evident analgesic nephropathy [83]. Most patients are still taking the drug at the time of diagnosis, but clinically evident disease can first become apparent several years after cessation of analgesic intake and even after renal transplantation has been performed [82]. It is presumed that the induction of malignancy results from the intrarenal accumulation of N-hydroxylated phenacetin metabolites that have potent alkylating action [83]. Because of urinary concentration, the highest concentration of these metabolites will be in the renal medulla, ureters, and bladder, possibly explaining the predisposition to carcinogenesis at these sites. The major presenting symptom of urinary tract malignancy in analgesic nephropathy is microscopic or gross hematuria. Thus, continued monitoring is essential, and new hematuria should be evaluated with urinary cytology, and, if indicated, cystoscopy with retrograde pyelography [78]. It may also be prudent to obtain yearly urine cytology for the first several years if analgesics are discontinued or indefinitely if drug intake persists. The incidence of urothelial carcinoma after renal transplantation in patients with analgesic nephropathy is comparable to the general incidence of up to 10% of urothelial carcinomas in end-stage renal failure patients with analgesic nephropathy. Removal of the native kidneys prior to renal transplantation has

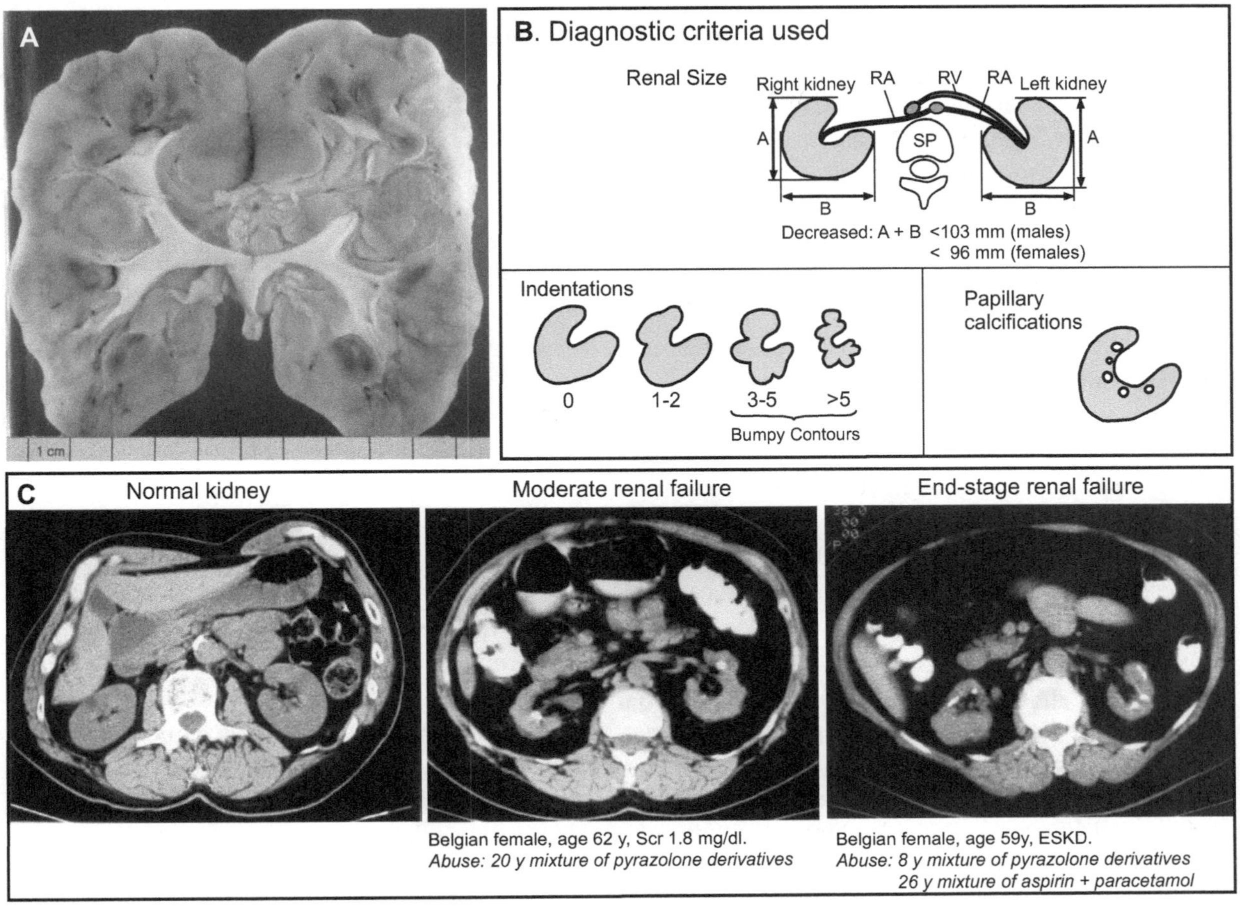

Figure 4. Diagnostic criteria of analgesic nephropathy. A. *Macroscopic aspect of an analgesic nephropathy kidney from an ESKD patient.* ***B.*** *Diagnostic criteria used.* ***C.*** *CT scans without contrast material of subject with normal kidneys, and patients with analgesic nephropathy with CKD3 and ESKD.*

also been suggested, but the efficacy of this regimen has not been proven [82].

Diagnosis

Until recently, the diagnosis of analgesic nephropathy was difficult to obtain. The disease is associated with a large number of mainly aspecific clinical symptoms [80]. Renal papillary necrosis, considered as the hallmark of analgesic nephropathy, can only be directly demonstrated by autopsy, after nephrectomy or in the exceptional case of a patient eliminating a papilla [85]. In a large part of cases, the diagnosis was mainly based on a documented history of abuse after a process of exclusion of other causes of renal failure. Since, furthermore, several authors [86, 87] have noted that a clear history of abuse is difficult to obtain, the need for diagnostic criteria with a well-defined performance became mandatory.

In Belgium, a prospective controlled multicentre study started in 1988, aiming to select diagnostic criteria for analgesic nephropathy with well-defined performance in patients with end-stage renal failure. In a cohort of 60 analgesic abusers and 188 controls, all starting renal replacement therapy, a large number of clinical, laboratory and radiological signs reported to be associated with analgesic nephropathy were tested. It was found that renal imaging investigations (sonography and tomography) demonstrating a decrease in length of both kidneys combined with either bumpy contours or signs of renal papillary necrosis were the only ones which showed a high sensitivity and specificity for diagnosing the disease. Other signs frequently mentioned such as hypertension, anemia, sterile pyuria and bacteriuria showed low sensitivity and/or specificity [51].

In a separate study, the diagnostic value of CT scan without contrast media was compared to the previously used renal imaging techniques (sonography and tomography) (Figure 4). A cohort of 40 analgesic abusers (= daily use of mixtures during at least 5 years) and 40 controls, all end-stage renal failure patients without a clear renal diagnosis were investigated with sonography, tomography and CT scan without contrast, searching for the renal imaging signs of analgesic nephropathy. Using CT scan the renal size and contour could be evaluated with comparable results while this technique scored better for the detection of papillary calcifications (Figure 4) [50, 67].

In an additional controlled study, the diagnostic performance of CT scan in patients with incipient/moderate renal failure was studied. In a cohort of 53 analgesic abusers with a serum creatinine between 1.5 and 4 mg/dl and in the absence of a clear renal diagnosis, a CT scan was performed. It was found that the renal image of analgesic nephropathy on CT scan in an early stage of renal failure is comparable with the observations made in end-stage renal failure patients (Figure 4). Especially the demonstration of bilateral papillary calcifications showed a high sensitivity of 92% with a specificity of 100% for the early diagnosis of analgesic nephropathy (Figure 4) [50].

The diagnostic value of CT-scan in the case of AN in ESKD patients was validated using all CT-scan documents (N=67) performed within the framework of the ANNE study in seven renal units. The renal imaging criteria were validated by a radiologist not involved in the process of data collection, and without knowledge of a possible history of abuse. His validation consisted of a blind re-examination of the CT-scans, accepting or rejecting the diagnosis of AN based on the observation of a decrease in renal volume plus either bumpy contours and or papillary calcifications. Afterwards, these results were compared with the history of AN use/abuse. This blind re-examination resulted in a comparable number of patients in whom the diagnosis of AN was accepted or rejected. The overall accordance of 94% was obtained between the original examination and the blind re-examination [50].

Several studies using this validated diagnostic test showed either the absence or low prevalence of AN [69], others confirmed the underestimation of AN in their country showing that within the cohort of patients with "unknown aetiology", or chronic interstitial nephritis a substantial number of patients with AN were detected [66, 68]. A recent study in ESKD patients (NANS-study) in the US evaluated the value of the non-contrast-enhanced computerized tomography as diagnostic test for AN [88]. It turned out that in contrast to previous studies [66, 68, 69], the sensitivity of the non contrast CT-scan for the detection of analgesic associated kidney injury was too low to be used as a test system. A specificity of more than 95% was found, being comparable with the earlier reports [51]. This overall result is not surprising since the low prevalence of AN (clearly below 5%) found in the US precludes clinically relevant sensitivity of the test.

Prevention

Analgesic nephropathy is one of the few renal diseases currently suitable for primary prevention.

Informative campaigns focused on the population at risk did not solve the problem of analgesic nephropathy. In Belgium, it was clearly demonstrated that in most abusers, sustained analgesic consumption was no longer related to a physical complaint but analgesics were mainly taken for their mood-altering capacities. Most analgesic abusers admitted to having been informed of the health risks related to long-standing analgesic abuse and even if renal impairment occurred, only a part of the cases stopped their analgesic abuse [89].

Also the withdrawal of phenacetin from analgesic mixtures did not solve the problem. When phenacetin was withdrawn from most analgesic mixtures in Australia (1970's), no decline in the occurrence of analgesic nephropathy could be observed [80, 85]. A declining incidence rate was only observed after restriction of the over-the-counter sales of all analgesic mixtures in 1979-1980 [59, 55, 90]. Some countries in Europe, particularly Sweden, have succeeded in controlling the disease after legislative measures were taken. As early as the sixties, Sweden elaborated legislation that only a few years later became very effective. The legislation was simple and clear: all analgesic containing, even the slightest dose of phenacetin became prescription limited. This resulted in a prescription status of almost all combined analgesics, hence a dramatic drop in their sale. In spite of the substantial total increase of consumption of single analgesics between 1980-1990, analgesic nephropathy belongs nowadays to the history of medicine-nephrology (< 1% of Swedish dialysis population) [54].

In contrast, in many other European countries, no effective legislative measurements were taken. In Belgium, Germany and Switzerland, the pharmaceutical industry spontaneously removed phenacetin from their products. Phenacetin was replaced by another analgesic substance such as pyrazolone maintaining a high volume of analgesic mixtures still containing two or more analgesic substances. In Belgium, the Ministry of Health decided in 1988 that when obtaining analgesic mixtures in the pharmacy users had to sign a request and received an information sheet warning for possible renal consequences of extensive analgesic consumption. This resulted obviously in a fall of the sale/consumption of analgesic mixtures. Although these measures were only effective during one year, their long-term and indirect effect was more important. After 1988, several pharmaceutical companies modified their analgesic products, resulting in a reduction of the mixtures from two analgesic components to one analgesic plus caffeine and/or codeine.

Analgesic nephropathy gained recognition in recent years in several Central and Eastern European countries. Abuse of analgesic mixtures is also reported in several third world countries without any knowledge about the extent of the problem of analgesic nephropathy. Moreover, in many countries there are no legislative limitations to introduce analgesic mixtures containing two analgesic substances combined with caffeine/codeine onto the market.

In view of prevention, it would be advisable to obtain legislative measures worldwide in order to limit the over-the-counter availability of all analgesics containing two analgesic components plus caffeine/codeine. This is formally asked in Europe [8] as well as in the United States [7] by a large group of investigators active in the field.

5-Aminosalicylic acid

Epidemiological observations

Case reports

The association between the use of 5-aminosalicylic acid (5-ASA) and the development of chronic tubulointerstitial nephritis in patients with inflammatory bowel disease (IBD) gained recognition in the 1990s by the publication of several case reports [26, 28, 92-99] (Figure 5). Reported cases are summarized in Table 2. The disease was more prevalent in males with a male/female ratio of 16:3. The age of reported cases ranged from 14 to 45 years. In contrast with analgesic nephropathy where renal lesions were only observed after several years of analgesic abuse, interstitial nephritis associated to 5-ASA was already observed during the first year of treatment in 8 out of 19 reported cases. Most cases started 5-ASA therapy with a documented normal renal function. Complete recovery upon arrest of the drug however, was only observed in 6 out of 19 published cases and dependent on the degree of renal damage at diagnosis. In a recent review article, case reports of IBD patients showing renal disease associated with 5-ASA treatment, increased to a total of 46 reported cases [100].

Retrospective study

A retrospective study was performed aiming to obtain more insight in the frequency of this disease [27]. Nephrologists of Belgium, France and the Netherlands were asked to report all cases of inflammatory bowel disease (IBD) showing signs of renal impairment associated or not with 5-ASA therapy. Questionnaires were completed and returned by 71 nephrologists. Among them, 44 reported that they had no such cases. The remaining 27 nephrologists sent detailed information on 40 cases of IBD with renal failure. Among 40 reported cases 26 used 5-ASA including 15 with biopsy proven interstitial nephritis (Figure 5). It is worthwhile to notice that on the one hand a few cases with chronic tubulointerstitial nephritis never used 5-ASA and on the other hand some cases with 5-ASA therapy showed renal failure diagnosed as glomerulonephritis or amyloidosis.

A recent investigation performed by a written questionnaire sent to all gastro-enterologists and nephrologists in the United Kingdom confirmed these observations. Retrospectively, a total of 202 cases of 5-ASA nephrotoxicity were identified during the preceeding 10 years. On drug withdrawal, complete renal recovery was only observed in 25% of the patients [101].

Prospective studies

Until now, the risk ratio of 5-ASA associated renal failure in patients with inflammatory bowel disease is not known. It will be rather difficult to obtain more

Table 2. Published case reports of interstitial nephritis in patients with inflammatory bowel disease using 5-ASA.

Reference	Sex	Age	5-ASA use duration (months)	Creatinine clearance (ml/min) onset therapy	Creatinine clearance (ml/min) lowest level	Follow-up upon arrest 5-ASA (months)	Recovery ?
von Mühlendal [92]	m	14	5	?	31*	1	complete
Henning [92]	m	31	42	normal	17	4	partial
Ruf-Ballauf [94]	m	45	7	80*	33	12	complete
Mehta [95]	m	29	5	normal	38	2	complete
Masson [96]	m	26	18	normal	55*	3	complete
Thulavath [97]	m	28	26	normal	45	3	no
	m	24	36	121*	47	>12	no
Smilde [98]	m	42	20	90	18	54	partial
	f	37	5	51	25	?	complete
	m	25	26	78	14	12	partial
	m	30	5	116	54	36	no
	m	34	8	73	13	5	no
World [26]	m	31	42	?	33	2	no
	m	43	28	?	25	12	no
	m	24	22	?	17	27	no
	f	30	3	?	<10*	44	no
Stolear [28]	m	24	23	104*	11*	27	partial

*:calculated creatinine clearance

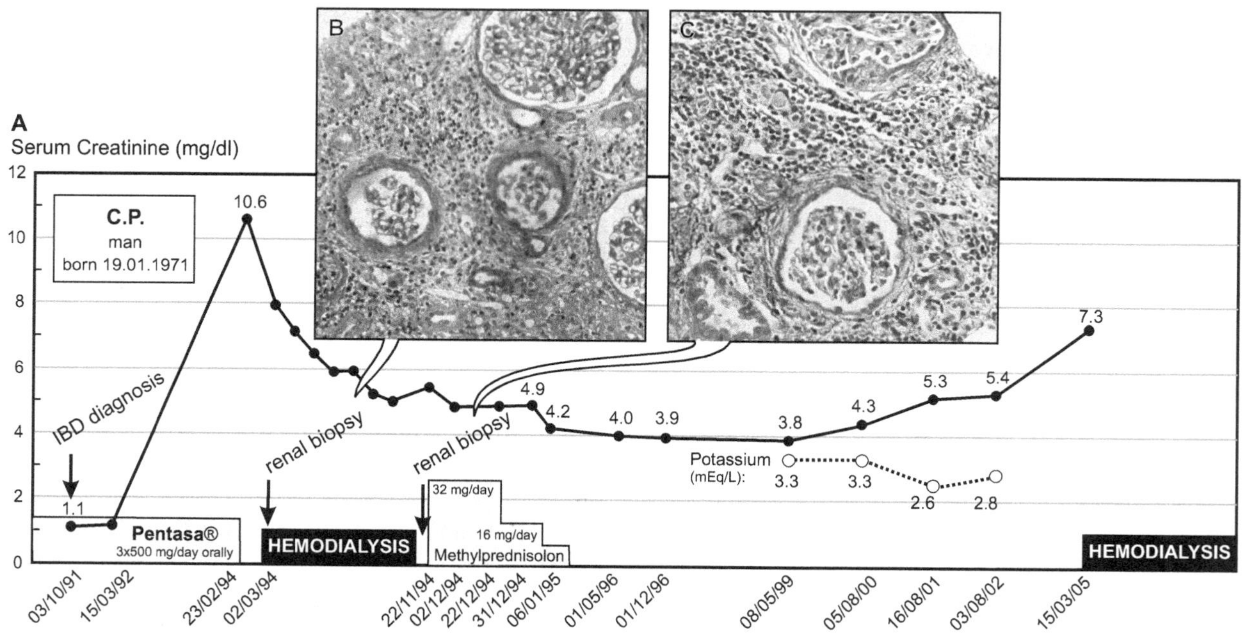

Figure 5. Case report of nephrotoxicity of 5-aminosalicylic acid (5-ASA) in inflammatory bowel disease.
A. Evolution of renal failure. B. First renal biopsy. C. Second renal biopsy. Note the important cellular infiltration in both biopsies. Normal aspect of glomeruli. B-C: H&E staining, orig. magn. x350.

insight in this risk. Drug usage in these patients is irregular and acute episodes of inflammation result in either increasing drug regimen and/or increasing number of drugs prescribed, including some with known nephrotoxic potential. Furthermore, the kidney is an extra-intestinal target of the disease as shown in Table 2.

In recent years several attempts were made to measure early signs of renal impairment in patients with IBD treated with 5-ASA. Schreiber et al. [102] investigated 223 IBD patients using sensitive markers of glomerular and tubular dysfunction. Patients receiving high amounts of 5-ASA showed an increased prevalence of tubular proteinuria. He concluded that the possibility exists that high doses of 5-ASA may be associated with proximal tubular proteinuria but that his study design was not able to dissect the possible impact of chronic inflammation on the development of renal impairment. In contrast, K.R. Herlinger et al. [103] performed an investigation on 95 IBD patients carefully assessing disease activity. They concluded that tubular proteinuria occurred in the majority of IBD patients and was related to disease activity rather than to 5-ASA treatment. Their observations were confirmed by A.C. Poulou et al [104] in a prospective study of 86 IBD patients, showing that the observed microproteinuria was mainly associated with IBD activity but not affected by 5-ASA

A European prospective study aiming to register all IBD patients with renal impairment and to control for a possible association with 5-ASA therapy was performed [105, 106]. During a one-year observation period, gastroenterologists of Belgium, France, Italy, Republic of Macedonia and Yugoslavia registered 1529 patients with IBD seen at their outpatient clinic. At the start of the study a questionnaire was filled in focused on medical and drug history. Additional data were collected at baseline, after 6 months and after 12 months, including activity of IBD, actual medication and results of the serum creatinine determination. Only 34 patients (2.2%) showed at least once a decreased creatinine clearance. Consecutive decreased creatinine clearances were observed in 13 patients (0.9%). Dehydration due to low body mass combined with active IBD was the main reason for an intermittent decrease in renal function in most of these patients. Particularly, the observation of 5-ASA therapy in 5 patients with sustained renal impairment of unknown origin is suggestive for a possible etiological role of 5-ASA. Comparing patients with and without renal impairment, the presence of a stoma revealed the highest increased risk.

The number of renal impairment cases observed in this prospective study is highly comparable with the estimations made by World et al. 5 years ago. They stated that the available evidence suggested that renal impairment of any severity may occur in up to one in 100 patients, but clinically significant interstitial nephritis occurs in less than one in 500 patients [26]. The more recent experience of 5-ASA nephrotoxicity in the United Kingdom led to an estimated incidence of clinical nephrotoxicity of only one in 4000 patients/year [101].

Pathophysiology

This particular form of chronic tubulo-interstitial nephritis is characterized by an important cellular infiltration of the interstitium with macrophages, T-cells but also B-cells. Furthermore, after arrest of the drug, there is improvement of the renal function in some cases [26, 93]. In those in which there is a delayed diagnosis of renal damage, recovery of renal function does not occur. Instead, several of those patients needed one or another form of renal replacement therapy. An important aspect of this type of toxic nephropathy is the documented persistence of the inflammation of the renal interstitium even several months after arrest of drug intake [28].

The molecular structure of 5-ASA is very close of that of salicylic acid, phenacetin and aminophenol, drugs with a well-documented nephrotoxic potential (Figure 6). In rats, it is demonstrated that after a single intravenous injection of 5-ASA, at doses of 1.4, 2.8, 5.7 mM per kg body weight (high pharmacological doses), necrosis of the proximal convoluted tubules and papillary necrosis developed [107].

The mechanism of renal damage caused by 5-ASA may be analogue to that of salicylates by inducing hypoxia of renal tissues either by uncoupling oxidative phosphorylation in renal mitochondria, by inhibiting the synthesis of renal prostaglandins, or by rendering the kidney susceptible to oxidative damage by a reduc-

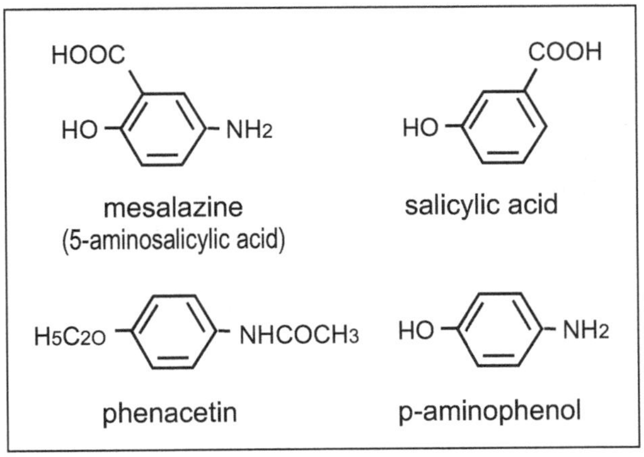

Figure 6. *Molecular structure of 5-aminosalicylic acid, salicylic acid, phenacetin and p-aminophenol.*

ing renal glutathione concentration after inhibition of the pentose phosphate shunt.

5-ASA is taken up by the gastrointestinal tract, particularly in the acetylated form and eliminated as such in the urine. The colon is the predilected place for this acetylation since in the small bowel there is a lack of the responsible bacterial flora. Hence, there is a limited readily absorption of 5-ASA as such in the small bowel. How far this may form a rationale for a possible difference in nephrotoxicity for the different preparations remains to be determined. Indeed, experimental evidence has shown that free 5-ASA is more nephrotoxic than the acetylated form [108, 109].

Clinical aspects

A typical case report is shown in Figure 5.

An association between the use of 5-ASA in patients with chronic inflammatory bowel disease and the development of a particular type of chronic tubulo-interstitial nephritis is difficult to interpret since renal involvement in chronic inflammatory bowel disease may be an extra-intestinal manifestation of the underlying disease [110]. Extra-intestinal manifestations of chronic inflammatory bowel disease are well recognized. The most frequent renal complications are oxalate stones and their consequences such as pyelonephritis, hydronephrosis and on the long-term amyloidosis [111, 112]. As for many drugs, reversible acute interstitial nephritis has been described [90].

Glomerulonephritis may be associated with chronic inflammatory bowel disease and has a heterogeneous expression [113]. Minimal change glomerulonephritis, membranous, membranoproliferative, focal glomerulosclerosis, and proliferative crescentic glomerulonephritis have been described and a summary of these case reports is available in the paper of Wilcox et al. [114]. In almost half of these cases, there was no relationship with drug intake such as sulphasalazine or 5-ASA.

That 5-ASA seems to be implicated in the generation/development/maintenance of this particular reaction at the level of the kidney however, is supported by a large number of case reports appearing in recent literature of patients with IBD using 5-ASA as the only medication, the improvement at least partial of the impaired renal function arrest of the drug and a worsening after resuming 5-ASA use [87, 100, 101].

Prevention

The efficacy of 5-ASA as first-line treatment for IBD is clearly documented and generally accepted [115, 116]. Preventive measures need to be taken into consideration however, in order to avoid nephrotoxic adverse effects. Although the incidence and risk ratio's of 5-ASA associated chronic tubulo-interstitial nephritis are not well known, the link established by case reports and the demonstration that recovery of renal function was observed only in patients with limited renal damage necessitates preventive measures [26]. The experience in the United Kingdom confirmed that the improvement of renal function for patients with nephrotoxicity treated for less than one year was significantly better than those on treatment for much longer [101].

Patients receiving 5-ASA should be screened regularly in order to detect signs of renal impairment. It is suggested that serum creatinine concentration should be measured each month for the first 3 months of treatment, three monthly for the remainder of the first year and annually thereafter [26]. The use of concurrent immunosuppressive therapy may necessitate extension to the period of intensive monitoring. Moreover, it is shown that IBD patients with a stoma and patients with extreme dehydration are more susceptible to develop renal impairment (Table 3).

Table 3. Risk factors for renal impairment in inflammatory bowel disease patients.

	Risk ratio (95% CI)
Stoma	6.2 (1.8-20.9)
Male sex	3.1 (1.1-8.6)
Duration of IBD symptoms (weeks)	1.06 (1.01-1.12)

References

1. Spuehler O, Zollinger HU. Die chronisch-interstitielle Nephritis. Zeitschr Klin Medizin 1953; 151: 1–50.
2. Gloor F. Die doppelseitige chronische nichtobstruktive interstitielle Nephritis. Ergebnisse der allgemeinen Pathologie und Pathologischen Anatomie 1961; 41: 63–207.
3. Burry AF, de Jersey P, Weedon D. Phenacetin and renal papillary necrosis: results of a prospective autopsy investigation. Med J Australia 1966; 53: 873–879.
4. Kincaid-Smith P. Pathogenesis of the renal lesion associated with the abuse of analgesics. Lancet 1967; i: 859–862.
5. Kincaid-Smith P, Nanra RS. Lithium-induced and analgesic-induced renal diseases. In: Diseases of the kidney, 5th edition. Schrier RW, Gottschalk CW (editors). Little Brown, Boston 1993; p. 1099-1129.
6. Mihatsch MJ, Torhorst J, Amsler B, Zollinger HU. Capillarosclerosis of the lower urinary tract in analgesic (phenacetin) abuse. Virchows Archiv A. Pathol Anat Histol 1978; 381: 41–47.
7. Henrich WL, Agodoa LE, Barrett B, Bennett WM, Blantz RC, Buckalew VM Jr, D'Agati VD, De Broe ME, Duggin GG, Eknoyan G. Analgesics and the kidney: summary and recommendations to the Scientific Advisory Board of the National Kidney Foundation from an Ad Hoc Committee of the National Kidney Foundation. Am J Kidney Dis 1996; 27(1): 162-165.
8. De Broe ME, Elseviers MM, Bengtsson U, Mihatsch MJ, Molzahn M, Pommer W, Ritz E, Schwarz A. Analgesic nephropathy. Nephrol Dial Transplant 1996; 11: 2407-2408.
9. Duggin GG. Combination analgesic-induced kidney disease: the Australian experience. Am J Kidney Dis 1996; 28 (suppl 1): S39-S47.
10. De Broe ME, Elseviers MM. Analgesic nephropathy. N Engl J Med 1998; 338: 446-452.
11. Haschek H (editor). International symposium on problems of phenacetin abuse. Egermann, Vienna 1973.
12. Gsell O. Nephropathie durch Analgetika. Ergebnisse der inneren Medizin und Kinderheilkunde 1974; 35: 68–175.
13. Carro-Ciampi G. Phenacetin abuse: a review. Toxicology 1978; 10: 311–339.
14. Prescott LF. Analgesic nephropathy: a reassessment of the role of phenacetin and other analgesics. Drugs 1982; 23: 75-149.
15. Kincaid-Smith P. Effects of non-narcotic analgesics on the kidney. Drugs 1986; 42(4): 109-128.
16. Sandler DP, Smith JC, Weinberg CR, Buckalew VM Jr, Dennis VW, Blythe WB, Burgess WP. Analgesic use and chronic renal disease. N Engl J Med 1989; 320(19): 1238-1243.
17. Sandler DP, Burr FR, Weinberg CS. Nonsteroidal anti-inflammatory drugs and the risk for chronic renal disease. Ann Int Med 1991; 115(3): 165-172.
18. Morlans M, Laporte JR, Vidal X, Cabeza D, Stolley PD. End-stage renal disease and non-narcotic analgesics: a case-control study. Br J Clin Pharmacol 1990; 30(5): 717-723.
19. Pommer W. Clinical presentation of analgesic-induced nephropathy. In: Analgesic and NSAID-induced kidney disease. Stewart JH (editor). Oxford University Press, Oxford 1993; p. 108-118.
20. Perneger TV, Whelton PK, Klag MJ. Risk of kidney failure associated with the use of acetaminophen, aspirin, and nonsteroidal antiinflammatory drugs. N Engl J Med 1994; 331: 1675–1679.
21. Fored CM, Ejerblad E, Lindblad P, Fryzek JP, Dickman PW, Signobello LB, Lipworth L, Elinder CG, Blot WJ, McLaughlin JK, Zack MM, Nyrén O. Acetaminophen, aspirin, and chronic renal failure. N Engl J Med 2001; 345: 1801-1808.
22. Larsen K, Moller CE. A renal lesion caused by abuse of phenacetin. Acta Med Scand 1959; 164: 53-71.
23. Jacobs LA, Morris JG. Renal papillary necrosis and the abuse of phenacetin. Med J Australia 1962; 2(14): 531-538.
24. Grimlund K. Phenacetin and renal damage at a Swedish factory. Acta Med Scan 1963; 174 (suppl 405): 1-26.
25. Azad Khan AK, iris J, Truelove SC. An experiment to determine the active therapeutic moiety of sulphasalazine. Lancet 1977; 1: 892-895.
26. World MJ, Stevens PE, Ashton MA, Rainford DJ. Mesalazine-associated interstitial nephritis. Nephrol Dial Transplant 1996; 11: 614-621.
27. De Broe ME, Stolear JC, Nouwen EJ, Elseviers MM. 5-Aminosalicylic acid (5-ASA) and chronic tubulo-interstitial nephritis in patients with chronic inflammatory bowel disease: is there a link ? Nephrol Dial Transplant 1997; 12: 1839-1841.
28. Stolear JC, Georges B, Gossun A, Ros Ph, Nouwen EJ, De Broe ME. Néphrite interstitiëlle associée à la Mésalazine. Confrontations anatomo-cliniques en pathologie renale et vasculaire; Hôpital Tenon, Paris, 10 Janvier 1996.
29. Murray RM. Analgesic nephropathy: removal of phenacetin from proprietary analgesics. Brit Med J 1972; 4: 131-132.
30. Nanra RS, Stuart-Taylor J, De Leon AH, White KH. Analgesic nephropathy: etiology, clinical syndrome, and clinicopathologic correlation in Australia. Kidney Int 1978; 13: 79-92.
31. Schwarz A, Kunzendorf U, Keller F, Offerman G. Progression of renal failure in analgesic-associated nephropathy. Nephron 1989; 53: 244-249.

32. Hauser AC, Derfler K, Balcke P. Progression of renal insufficiency in analgesic nephropathy: Impact of continuous drug abuse. J Clin Epidemiol 1991; 44: 53-56.
33. McCredie M, Stewart JH, Mahony JF. Is phenacetin responsible for analgesic nephropathy in New South Wales ? Clin Nephrol 1982; 17(3): 134-140.
34. Murray TG, Stolley PD, Anthony JC, Schinnar R, Hepler-Smith E, Jeffreys JL. Epidemiologic study of regular analgesic use and end-stage renal disease. Arch Intern Med 1983; 143: 1687-1693.
35. Pommer W, Glaeske G, Molzahn M. The analgesic problem in the Federal Republic of Germany: analgesic consumption, frequency of analgesic nephropathy and regional differences. Clin Nephrol 1986; 26: 273-278.
36. Pommer W, Bronder E, Greiser E, Helmert U, Jesdinsky HJ, Klimpel A, Borner K, Mohlzahn M. Regular analgesic intake and the risk of end-stage renal failure. Am J Nephrol 1989; 9: 403-412.
37. Ibáñez L, Morlans M, Vidal X, Martínez MJ, Laporte JR. Case-control study of regular analgesic and nonsteroidal anti-inflammatory use and end-stage renal disease. *Kidney Int* 2005; **67**(6): 2393-8.
38. van der Woude FJ, Heinemann LA, Graf H, Lewis M, Moehner S, Assmann A, Kuhl-Habich D. Analgesics use and ESRD in younger age: a case-control study. *BMC Nephrol* 2007; **8**(1): 15.
39. Dubach UC, Rosner B, Pfister E. Epidemiologic study of abuse of analgesics containing phenacetin. Renal morbidity and mortality (1968-1979). N Engl J Med 1983; 308: 357-362.
40. Elseviers MM, De Broe ME. A long-term prospective controlled study of analgesic abuse in Belgium. Kidney Int 1995; 48: 1912-1919.
41. Kurth T, Glynn RJ, Walker AM, Rexrode KM, Buring JE, Stampfer MJ, Hennekens CH, Gaziano JM. Analgesic use and change in kidney function in apparently healthy men. *Am J Kidney Dis* 2003; **42**(2): 234-44.
42. Curhan GC, Knight EL, Rosner B, Hankinson SE, Stampfer MJ. Lifetime nonnarcotic analgesic use and decline in renal function in women. Arch Intern Med 2004; **164**(14):1519-24.
43. McLaughlin JK, Lipworth L, Chow W-H, Blot WJ. Analgesic use and chronic renal failure: A critical review of the epidemiologic literature. Kidney Int 1998; 54: 679-686.
44. Delzell E, Shapiro S. A review of epidemiologic studies of nonnarcotic analgesics and chronic renal disease. Medicine 1998; 77(2): 102-121.
45. Buckalew VM, Schey HM. Renal disease from habitual antipyretic analgesic consumption: an assessment of the epidemiologic evidence. Medicine 1986, 11: 291-303.
46. Elseviers M.M., De Broe M.E. Analgesic nephropathy: Is it caused by multi-analgesic abuse or single substance use ? Drug Safety 1999; 20(1): 15-24.
47. Gates TN, Temple AR. Analgesic use and chronic renal disease. N Engl J Med 1989; 321: 1125.
48. McCredie M. Analgesic use and chronic renal disease. N Engl J Med 1989; 321: 1125.
49. Elseviers MM, De Broe ME. Epidemiology of analgesic nephropathy. J Nephrol 1992; 5: 94-98.
50. Elseviers MM, De Schepper A, Corthouts R, Bosmans JL, Cosyn L, Lins RL, Lornoy W, Matthys E, Roose R, Van Caesbroeck D, Waller I, Horackova M, Schwarz A, Svrcek P, Bonucchi D, Franek E, Morlans M, De Broe ME. High diagnostic performance of CT scan for analgesic nephropathy in patients with incipient to severe renal failure. Kidney Int 1995; 48: 1316-1323.
51. Elseviers MM, Bosteels V, Cambier P, De Paepe M, Godon JP, Lins R, Lornoy W, Matthys E, Moeremans C, Roose R, Theelen B, Van Caesbroeck D, Verbanck J, De Broe ME. Diagnostic criteria of analgesic nephropathy in patients with end-stage renal failure: results of the Belgian study. Nephrol Dial Transplant 1992; 7: 479-486.
52. Elseviers MM, Waller I, Nenov D, Levora J, Matousovic K, Tanquerel T, Pommer W, Schwarz A, Keller E, Thieler H, Köhler H, Lemoniatou H, Cresseri D, Bonucchi D, Fiocchi O, Jordans J, Franek E, Silva FJ, Fernandez Ruiz EJ, Morlans M, Hellström M, Wauters JP, Felle D, Cassi HV, De Broe ME. Evaluation of diagnostic criteria for analgesic nephropathy in patients with end-stage renal failure: results of the ANNE study. Nephrol Dial Transplant 1995; 10: 808-814.
53. Elseviers MM, De Broe ME. Combination analgesic involvement in the pathogenesis of analgesic nephropathy. Am J Kidney Dis 1996; 28(6): 958-962 (letter to the editor).
54. Noels LM, Elseviers MM, De Broe ME. Impact of legislative measures on the sales of analgesics and the subsequent prevalenceof analgesic nephropathy: a comparative study in France, Sweden and Belgium. Nephrol Dial Transplant 1995; 10: 167-174.
55. Chang SH, Mathew TH, McDonald SP. Analgesic Nephropathy and Renal Replacement Therapy in Australia: Trends, Comorbidities and Outcomes. Clin J Am Soc Nephrol 2008; 3: 768-776.
56. U.S. Renal Data System, USRDS 2007 Annual Data Report: Atlas of Chronic Kidney Disease and End-Stage Renal Disease in the United States, National Institutes of Health, National Institute of Diabetes and Digestive and Kidney Diseases, Bethesda, MD, 2007.
57. Wing AJ, Brunner FP, Geerlings W, Broyer M, Brynger H, Fassbinder W, Rissoni G, Selwood NH, Tufveson G. Contribution of toxic nephropathies to end-stage renal failure in Europe: a report from the EDTA-ERA Registry. Toxicol Lett 1989; 46: 281-292.

58. Nanra RS. Analgesic nephropathy in the 1990's: an Australian perspective. Kidney Int 1993; 42 (suppl 44): 86-92.
59. Stewart JH, McCredie M, Disney APS, Mathew TH. Trends in incidence of end-stage of end-stage renal failure in Australia, 1972-1991. Nephrol Dial Transpl 1994; 9: 1377-1382.
60. McAnally JF, Winchester JF, Schreiner GE. Analgesic nephropathy. An uncommon cause of end-stage renal disease. Arch Intern Med 1983; 143: 1897-1899.
61. Gonwas TA, Hamilton RW, Buckalew VM. Chronic renal failure and end-stage renal disease in Northwest North Carolina. Importance of analgesic-associated nephropathy. Arch Intern Med 1981; 141: 462-465.
62. Wilson DR, Gault MH. Declining incidence of analgesic nephropathy in Canada. Can Med Assoc J 1982; 127: 500-503.
63. Seedat YK, Naicker S, Rawat R, Parsoo I. Racial differences in the causes of end-stage renal failure in Natal. S Afr Med J 1984; 65: 956-958.
64. Segasothy M, Suleimam AB, Puvaneswary M, Rohana A. Paracetamol: a cause for analgesic nephropathy and end-stage renal disease. Nephron 1988; 50: 50-54.
65. Kantachuvesiri S, Kaojarern S, Kitayaporn D, Phanichphant S, Sumethkul V, Wananukul W, Pongskul C, Arkaravichien W, Jankriengkri S, Chanchairujira T. Risk factors between analgesic use and chronic nephropathy in Thailand. Southeast Asian J Trop Med Public Health 1996; 27(2): 350-355.
66. Matousovic K, Elseviers MM, Devecka D, Horackova M, Turek T, De Broe ME, and the Group of Czech and Slovak Nephrologists. Incidence of analgesic nephropathy among patients undergoing renal replacement therapy in Czech republic and Slovak republic. Nephrol Dial Transplant 1996; 11: 1048-1051.
67. Elseviers MM, De Broe ME. Is analgesic nephropathy still a problem in Belgium ? Nephrol Dial Transplant 1988; 2: 143-149.
68. Matyus J, Ujhelyi L, Karpati I, Ben T, Kakuk G. Increase in the incidence of analgesic nephropathy in Hungary. Nephrol Dial Transplant 1997; 12(8): 1774-1775.
69. Franek E, Kokot F, Grzeszczak W, Gajos L. Is analgesic nephropathy a problem in the South-West Region of Poland ? Nephron 1996; 72: 353 (letter to the editor).
70. Bennett WM, De Broe ME. Analgesic nephropathy – a preventable renal disease. N Engl J Med 1989; 320: 1269-1271.
71. Mihatsch MJ, Staehelin HB, Musfeld D, Perret E, Oberholzer M. Phenacetin-Abusus: Kardiovaskuläre Risikofactoren. Nieren Hochdruck 1983; 3: 83-92.
72. Ivey KJ. Gastrointestinal intolerance and bleeding with non-narcotic analgesics. Drugs 1986; 32(suppl 4): 71-89.
73. Laporte J-R, Carne X, Vidal X, Moreno V, Juan J. Upper gastrointestinal bleeding in relation to previous use of analgesics and non-steroidal anti-inflammatory drugs. Lancet 1991; 337: 85-89.
74. Mihatsch MJ. Empfohlene Massnahmen zur Bekampfung des Analgetikamisbrauchs. In: Das Analgetikasyndrom. Mihatsch MJ (editor). George Theme Verlag, Stuttgart 1986; p. 134-135.
75. Stewart JH. The analgesic syndrome. In: Analgesic and NSAID-induced kidney disease. Stewart JH (editor). Oxford University Press, Oxford 1993; p. 58-66.
76. Hultengren N, Lagergren C, Ljungqvist A. Carcinoma of the renal pelvis in renal papillary necrosis. Acta Chir Scand 1965; 130: 314-320.
77. Bengtsson U, Johansen S, Angervall L. Malignancies of the urinary tract and their relation to analgesic abuse. Kidney Int 1978; 13: 107-113.
78. Kliem V, Thon W, Krautzig S, Kolditz M, Behrend M, Pichlmayr R, Koch KM, Frei U, Brunkhorst R. High mortality from urothelial carcinoma despite regular tumor screening in patients with analgesic nephropathy after renal transplantation. Transpl Int 1996; 9: 231-235.
79. Mihatsch MJ, Manz T, Knüsli C, Hofer HO, Rist M, Guetg R, Rutishauser G, Zollinger HU. Phenacetinabusus III. Maligne Harnwegtumoren bei Phenacetinabusus in Basel 1963-1977. Schweiz Med Wschr 1980; 110: 255-264.
80. McCredie M, Ford JM, Stuart Taylor J, Stewart JH. Analgesics and cancer of the pelvis in New South Wales. Cancer 1982; 49: 2617-2625.
81. Lornoy W, Becaus I, Morelle V, Fonteyne E. Néphropathies chroniques par abus d'analgésiques: fréquence, pathogenèse, aspects cliniques, développement de tumeurs malignes. In: Séminaires d'uro-néphrologie. Chatelain C (editor). Masson, Paris 1988; p. 99-105.
82. Blohme I, Johansson S. Renal pelvic neoplasms and atypical urothelium in patients with end-stage analgesic nephropathy. Kidney Int 1981; 20(5): 671-675.
83. McCredie M, Stewart JH, Carter JJ, Turner J, Mahony JF. Phenacetin and papillary necrosis: independent risk factors for renal pelvic cancer. Kidney Int 1986; 30(1): 81-84.
84. Kincaid-Smith P. Renal toxicity of non-narcotic analgesics. At-risk patients and prescribing applications. Med Toxicol 1986; 1 (suppl 1): 14–22.

85. Gloor FJ. Changing concepts in pathogenesis and morphology of analgesic nephropathy as seen in Europe. Kidney Int 1978; 13: 27-33.
86. Murray RM. Genesis of analgesic nephropathy in the United Kingdom. Kidney Int 1978; 13: 50-57.
87. Schwarz A, Faber U, Borner K, Keller F, Offerman G, Molzahn M. Reliability of drug history in analgesic users. Lancet 1984; 2:1163-1164.
88. Henrich WL, Clark RL, Kelly JP, Buckalew VM, Fenves A, Finn WF, Shapiro JI, Kimmel PL, Eggers P, Agodoa LE, Porter GA, Shapiro S, Toto R, Anderson T, Cupples LA, Kaufman DW. Non-contrast-enhanced computerized tomography and analgesic-related kidney disease: report of the national analgesic nephropathy study. *J Am Soc Nephrol* 2006; **17**(5):1472-80.
89. Elseviers MM, De Broe ME. Analgesic nephropathy in Belgium is related to the sales of particular analgesic mixtures. Nephrol Dial Transplant 1994; 9: 41-46.
90. Kincaid-Smith P. Analgesic nephropathy in Australia. Contrib Nephrol 1979; 16: 57-64.
91. Nanra RS, Kincaid-Smith P. Experimental evidence for nephrotoxicity of analgesics. In: Analgesic and NSAID-induced kidney disease. Stewart JH (editor). Oxford University Press, Oxford 1993, p. 17-31
92. von Mühlendahl KE. Nephritis durch 5-aminosolicylsäure. Deutsch Med Wschr 1989; 114: 236.
93. Henning HV, Meinhold J. Chronische interstitielle nephritis durch 5-aminosalicylsäure ? Deutsch Med Wsch 1989; 114: 1091.
94. Ruf-Ballauf W, Hofstädter F, Krentz K. Acute interstitielle nephritis durch 5-aminosalicylsäure ? Internist 1989; 30: 262-264.
95. Mehta RP. Acute interstitial nephritis due to 5-aminosalicylic acid. Can Med Assoc J 1990; 143(10): 1031-1032.
96. Masson EA, Rodhes JM. Mesalazine associated nephrogenic diabetes insipidus presenting as weight loss. Gut 1992; 33: 563-4.
97. Thuluvath PJ, Ninkovic M, Calam J, Anderson M. Mesalazine induced interstitial nephritis. Gut 1994; 35: 1493-1496.
98. Smilde TJ, van Liebergen FJHM, Koolen MI, Gerlag PGG, Assmann KJM, Berden JHM. Tubulo-interstitiële nefritis door mesalazine (5-ASA)-preparaten. Ned Tijdschr Geneesk 1994; 138: 2557-2561
99. Calvino J, Romero R, Pintos E, Losada E, Novoa D, Güimil D, Mardaras J, Sanchez-Guisande D. Mesalazine-associated tubulo-interstitial nephritis in inflammatory bowel disease. Clin Nephrol 1998; 49(4): 265-257.
100. Gisbert JP, Gonzalez-Lama Y, Maté J. 5-Aminosalicylates and renal function in inflammatory bowel disease: a systematic review. Inflamm Bowel Dis 2007; 13(5): 629-638.
101. Muller AF, Stevens PE, Mcintyre AS, Ellison H, Logans RF. Experience of 5-aminosalicylate nephrotoxicity in the United Kingdom. Aliment Pharmacol Ther 2005; 21: 1217-1224.
102. Schreiber S, Hämling J, Zehnter E, Howaldt S, Daerr W, Raedler A, Kruis W. Renal tubular dysfunction in patients with inflammatory bowel disease treated with aminosalicylate. Gut 1997; 40: 761-766.
103. Herrlinger KR, Noftz MK, Fellermann K, Schmidt K, Steinhoff J, Stange EF. Minimal renal dysfunction in inflammatory bowel disease is related to disease activity but not to 5-ASA use. Aliment Pharmacol Ther 2001; 15: 363-369.
104. Poulou AC, Goumas KE, Dandakis DC, Tyrmpas I, Panagiotaki M, Georgouli A, Soutos D, Archimandritis A. Microproteinuria in patients with inflammatory bowel disease: is it associated with the disease activity or the treatment with 5-aminosalicylic acid? World J Gastroenterol 2006; 12(5): 739-746
105. Elseviers M.M., De Broe M.E., the 5-ASA-Study Group. Risk of chronic interstitial nephritis in patients with inflammatory bowel disease treated with 5-ASA therapy. J Am Soc Nephrol 11: 128A, 2000.
106. Elseviers MM, D'Haens G, Lerebours E, Plane C, Stolear JC, Riegler G, Capasso G, Van Outryve M, Mishevska-Mukaetova P, Djuranovic S, Pelckmans P, De Broe ME, for the 5-ASA study group. Renal impairment in patients with inflammatory bowel disease: association with aminosalicylate therapy? Clin Nephrol 2004; 61(2): 83-91.
107. Calder IC, Funder CC, Green CR, Ham KN, Tange JD. Nephrotoxic lesions from 5-aminosalicylic acid. Brit Med J 1972; 1: 152-154.
108. Calder IC, Funder CC, Green CR, Ham KN, Tange JD. Comparative toxicity of aspirin and phenacetin derivatives. Brit Med J 1971; 4: 518-521.
109. Dwarakanath AD, Michael J, Allan RN. Sulphasalazine induced renal failure. Gut 1992; 33: 1006-1007
110. Izzedine H, Simon J, Piette AM, Lucsko M, Baumelou A, Charitanski D, Kernaonet E, Baglin AC, Deray G, Beaufils H. Primary chronic interstitial nephritis in Crohn's disease. Gastroenterology 2002; 123(5): 1436-1440.
111. Glickman RM. Inflammatory bowel disease (ulcerative colitis and Crohn's disease). In: Harrison's Principles of Internal Medicine (13th edition, volume 2). Isselbacher KJ, Braunwald E, Wilson JD, Martin JB, Fauci AS, Kasper DL (editors). McGraw-Hill, In, New York, p. 1403-1417.
112. Greenstein AJ, Janowitz HD, Sachar DB. The extra-intestinal complications of Crohn's disease and ulcerative colitis: a study of 700 patients. Medicine 1976; 55(4): 401-412.
113. Moayyedi P, Fletcher S, Harnder P, Axon ATR, Brownjohn A. Mesangiocapillary glomerulonephritis associated with ulcerative colitis: case report of two patients. Nephrol Dial Transplant 1995; 10: 1923-1924.
114. Wilcox GM, Aretz HT, Roy MA, Roche JK. Glomerulonephritis associated with inflammatory bowel disease. Gastroenterology 1990; 98: 786-791.

115. Järnerot G. New salicylates as maintenance treatment in ulcerative colitis. Gut 1994; 35: 1155-1158.
116. Clemett D, Markham A. Prolonged-release mesalazine: a review of its therapeutic potential in ulcerative colitis and Crohn's disease. Drugs 2000; 59(4): 929-956.

18

Non-steroidal anti-inflammatory drugs

Ali J. OLYAEI[1], Andrew WHELTON[2], Til STURMER[3] and George A. PORTER[1]

[1]Oregon Health Science University, Portland, Oregon, USA
[2]Universal Clinical Research Center and Johns Hopkins University, Baltimore, Maryland, USA
[3]German Centre for Research on Ageing, Heidelberg, Germany

Introduction

The discovery and commercialization of asprin over 100 years ago, and the introduction of other non-steroidal anti-inflammatory drugs (NSAIDs) have had a profound impact on the practice of medicine and the treatment of the inflammatory conditions. Widespread access and over-the-counter availability of these agents has lead to the impression that these drugs are safe and relatively void of toxicity. NSAID use can pose substantial risks to patients, especially when used chronically. Gastrointestinal (GI) complications associated with NSAID use are the most common serious adverse drug reaction reported in the United States. Additionally, aspirin is extensively used as an anti-platelet agent, as well as an analgesic agent. Aspirin, as well as other non-specific NSAID's have a demonstrated risk of gastrointestinal hemorrhage.

NSAIDs are frequently used to treat chronic inflammatory conditions and for the amelioration of acute and chronic pain. Unfortunately, to report a reliable numerical frequency to the renal functional disorders induced by non-steroidal anti-inflammatory drugs (NSAID) is next to impossible. This is due, in part, to the heterogeneity of the individuals who consume these agents and the variability in social customs that strongly influence the per capita ingestion of analgesic-anti-inflammatory drugs. Nonetheless, in most unselected populations in developed countries who seek care from their family physicians, approximately 1-3% of persons ingesting a NSAID will manifest one of a variety of renal functional abnormalities typically requiring physician intervention [1-5]. Although this percentage is relatively low, the number of "at risk" individuals are very high because of the current use-profile of NSAIDs and their availability either by prescription or as over-the-counter medications. In view of the enormous number of patients consuming these compounds, the frequency with which patients expected to develop some variety of renal functional abnormality is substantial.

Over 30 billion tablets of non-steroidal anti-inflammatory drugs (NSAID) were dispensed in the United States in 2000; approximately 16% represent prescriptions for NSAIDs [1]. One in seven inhabitants of the North American (~ 50 million) is likely to be treated with an NSAID for a rheumatologic disorder in any given year [3]. In 2004 nearly 112 million prescriptions were written for NSAIDs of which almost half, 50+ million were for COX-2 inhibitors [3A]. These compounds enjoy a remarkable benefit/risk ratio when used in the treatment of acute self-limited pain syndromes. Unfortunately, when taken for prolonged periods of time, either by the elderly or individuals with certain co-morbid conditions, the frequency of adverse reactions rises dramatically.

The NSAID-induced abnormalities of renal function, in descending order of clinical frequency, are (i) fluid and electrolyte disturbances; (ii) destabilization of controlled hypertension (iii) decompensated congestive heart failure; (iv) acute deterioration of renal function; (v) nephrotic syndrome with interstitial nephritis; and (vi) chronic renal failure/papillary necrosis [1, 3-5].

Most of the renal abnormalities that are clinically encountered as a result of NSAIDs can be attributed to the inhibitory action of these compounds upon prostaglandin production within the kidney. Hence, a brief overview of the influence of prostaglandins on renal function will be presented, followed by an analysis of the pathophysiologic mechanisms involved in the induction of renal disturbances, the clinical manifestations of these abnormalities, the patient risk factors involved and the preventive approaches to NSAID related renal syndromes.

Prostaglandins and renal function

The prostaglandin pathway

Renal prostaglandins serve a critical role in regulating both glomerular hemodynamics and tubular function [6]. For this process to occur, an intact arachidonic acid cascade is crucial. Prostaglandins are derived from deacylated arachidonic acid derived from cell membranes (Figure 1). The cellular release of arachidonic acid is controlled by a variety of vasoactive hormones including: norepinephrine, angiotensin, bradykinin and vasopressin [7, 8]. Once released, cyclooxygenase [COX-1 and -2] facilitates the addition of molecular oxygen to arachidonic acid creating endoperoxide PGG_2. The key role that COX's occupies in the cascade revolves around the regulation of the rate and amount of prostaglandin precursors that is converted to prostacyclin, prostaglandin and thromboxane (Figure 1).

Prostaglandins are ubiquitous substances that influence renal function along with the function of other body systems [6, 8]. Prostaglandins are local hormones or 'autocoids' because they act in a paracrine or autocrine fashion. Biologic activity is characteristically limited to their site of production and interaction with the associated prostanoid receptors (Figure 1), the latter being responsible for activating the cellular response mechanisms. Because of the short circulatory half-life of prostaglandins, they are without significant systemic effect. In addition, prostaglandins are not stored in tissue but, rather, are synthesized on demand.

Arachidonic acid can also be metabolized to a variety of mediators, depending on the cell type. For example, lipoxygenase catalyzes the production of leukotrienes, and mixed-function oxygenases catalyze the production of epoxyeicosatrienoic acids. Collectively, these oxygenated metabolites may play a critical role in NSAID-induced nephrotic syndrome by shunting arachidonic acid metabolism from prostaglandins to lipoxygenase products, a shift that favors production of eicosanoid, an endogenous product that increase capillary permeability [9]. Prostaglandins act as autocoids at either cortical and medullary sites of renal production [10]. Prostaglandins produced in the renal cortex modulate vascular resistance [RVR] and renin secretion, while those produced in the medulla have a major influence on salt and water balance. The major prostaglandins with renal action include: PGE_2, PGI_2 and TxA_2. PGE_2, produced in the greatest amounts, is found in both tubular and interstitial cells. Prostaglandins undergo rapid local metabolized to inactive products by a 15-prostaglandin dehydrogenase [7].

Renal prostanoid receptors

Four EP receptor sub-types have been identified (table 1) [11]. Since prostaglandins are autocoids with a short half-life, interaction with specific EP receptors within the nephron activates the biologic effect of PGE_2. Three of the four E-prostanoid receptors, EP2, EP3, and EP4, exert their biologic effect by the coupling of G proteins to cAMP, whereas, EP1 receptor action is coupled by increasing intracellular calcium. The existence of EP2 receptor in the kidney remains to be confirmed. Breyer et al. [11] has recently reviewed the distribution of the EP receptors known to exist in the kidney. EP4, IP, and possible EP2 are located in the glomerular area. IP and EP4 probably mediate afferent arteriolar dilatation, while EP4 is involved with renin release. EP3 in the mTAL is thought to modify intense active Cl transport and reduce NaCl reabsorption. EP1, EP3, EP4 coexist in the both the cortical collecting duct (CCD) and medullary collecting duct (MCD). EP3 inhibits basolateral water reabsorption, while EP1 inhibits basolateral Na reabsorption. EP4, which is located at both the luminal and basolateral cell surfaces, stimulates water reabsorption. The relative expression

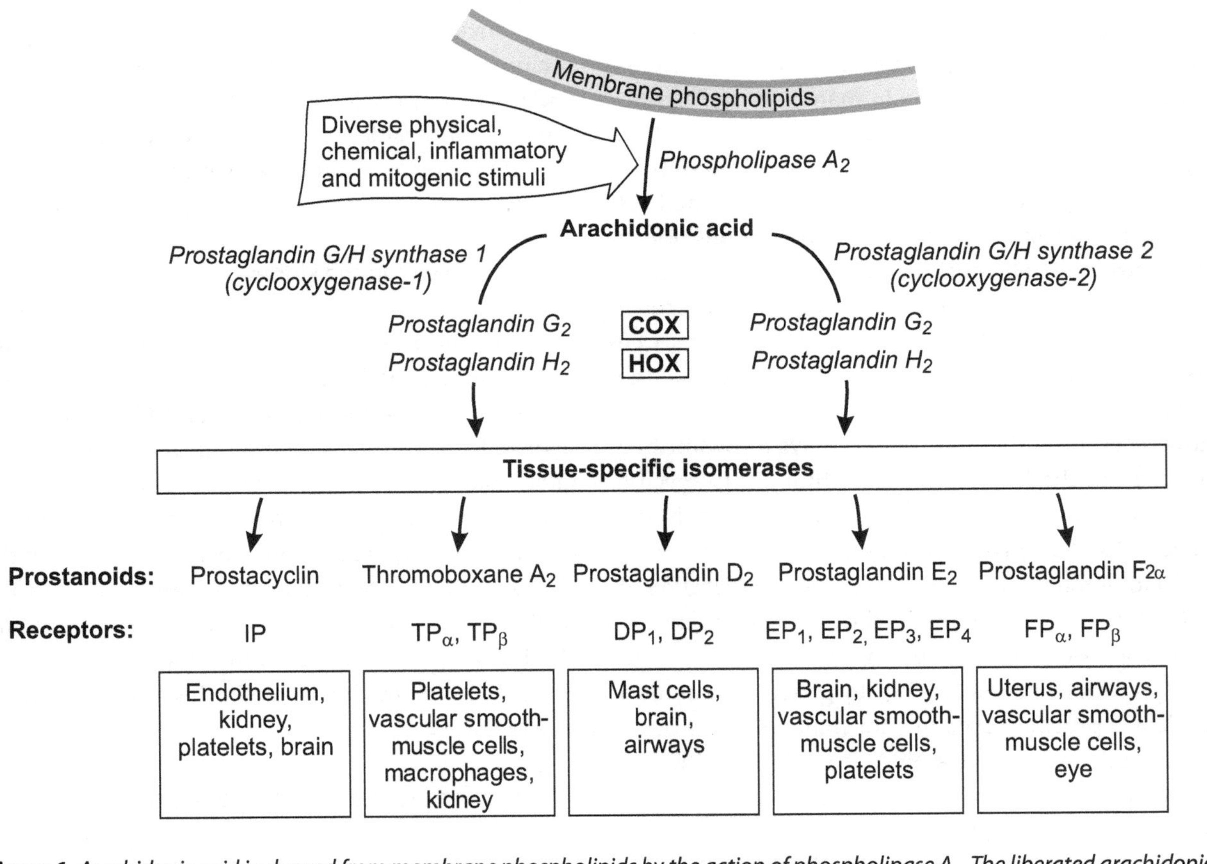

Figure 1. *Arachidonic acid is cleaved from membrane phospholipids by the action of phospholipase A_2. The liberated arachidonic acid is then acted upon by prostaglandin G/H synthase to produce the unstable intermediate PGH2. PGH2 is converted to the multiple prostanoids shown by tissue specific isomerases. The resulting prostanoids then activate cell-membrane receptor which couple G proteins leading to the terminal effect designated in each of the boxes (with permission from [8]).*

Table 1. E-prostanoid (EP) receptor characteristics.

E-receptor	Function	Signal	mRNA
EP1	Contracts	IP3/DAG/PKC	CD/musc. Mucosa
EP2	Relaxes	↑ cAMP	Utreus Arteries
EP3	Contracts	↓ cAMP	CD/cTal Stomach
EP4	Dilates	↑ cAMP	Kidney Bladder

Adapted from Breyer et al. [14]

of each of the receptors at the various intrarenal sites will determine the extent of the biologic modulation induced by local prostaglandin production.

Cyclooxygenase isoforms

Factors regulating isoform expression

Two isoforms of human cyclooxygenase (COX-1 and -2), possessing similar molecular weights (70-kDa) have been cloned, sequenced, and identified as being expressed in various human cells and tissues but possessing different mechanisms of regulation [6, 12]. COX-1 has been referred to as a constitutive enzyme, responsible for maintenance of normal cellular processes such as platelet function, protection of the gastrointestinal mucosa, and renal function under conditions of hemodynamic stress or decreased renal perfusion [13]. COX-2 was initially thought to be solely an inducible enzyme, activated to mediate the inflammatory response and pain perception [14]. It is now recognized that COX-2 also plays a constitutive role within the kidney [15, 16] although its specific functions have yet to be fully characterized. Nonetheless, COX-2 appears to play an important role in regulating renal salt and water homeostasis and renal hemodynamics and is induced during the inflammatory response thus contributing to the development of interstitial fibrosis [17-19]. In general, inhibition of COX-2 probably accounts for many of the desired therapeutic abilities of a NSAID while inhibition of COX-1 explains many of the undesirable gastrointestinal side effects of a NSAID.

The relative proportion of COX-1/COX-2 inhibition exhibited by both non-selective and selective NSAID has become an important clinical issue since the selective inhibition of the COX-2 isoforms offers the opportunity for a drug that possesses exclusive anti-arthritic therapeutic benefit without the drawback of gastric and renal side effects. Recently, FitzGerald and Patrono [8] have summarized the *in vitro* COX-1/COX-2 IC-50 inhibitory actions of a variety of NSAIDs. While the whole-blood assay for COX inhibitory action has improved the predictability of a similar result in human applications, the ultimate test remains the clinical trial. In this regard several large efficacy and safety trials have been conducted using the COX-2 inhibitors, celecoxib, rofecoxib and valdecoxib, and these are reviewed in detail later in this chapter.

The results of whole-blood assays identify indomethacin as the most potent inhibitor of cyclooxygenase-1, being 60 times more potent against this isoform than against cyclooxygenase-2 [20]. Aspirin was 166 times more active against cyclooxygenase-1 than cyclooxygenase-2, but was less potent than indomethacin on each of the isoforms. Acetaminophen was only a weak inhibitor of both isoforms. Some of the NSAIDs were virtually equally potent in their effects upon cyclooxygenase-1 and cyclooxygenase-2 (ibuprofen and naproxen). Of the once available COX-2 inhibitors, rofecoxib and valdecoxib are the most potent inhibitor of cyclooxygenase-2 and also demonstrated the greatest selectivity for cyclooxygenase-2 inhibition [21].

Distribution within the kidney

Distribution of the COX-2 isoform in the adult human kidney is based upon *in-situ* hybridization and immunolocation studies [11]. COX-2 has been detected in both the macula densa and medullary interstitial cells in patients with Bartter's syndrome and congestive heart failure [22] as well as in elderly patients. COX-1, in addition to being expressed in the glomerulus, is constitutively expressed in both the cortical and medullary collecting ducts [15, 16] (Figure 2). The exact role of the duel expression of both COX isoforms in the medullary collecting duct remains to be elucidated.

Mechanism of action of NSAIDs

All NSAIDs act by inhibiting COX and thereby preventing prostaglandin synthesis[5]. The interaction between aspirin and cyclooxygenase (acetylation) is irreversible, whereas with other NSAIDs this binding is reversible. Traditional NSAIDs are non-selective blockers of both the COX-1 and COX-2 isoforms, whereas celecoxib, rofecoxib, lumaricoxib and valdecoxib are specific inhibitors of COX-2 [21].

The kidney is a frequent target of adverse effects from NSAIDs use [1-5, 9]. Much of this relates to the pharmacological action of NSAIDs in the presence of a stimulated endogenous prostaglandin system. NSAIDs therapeutic action derives from the 70-95% inhibition of the key regulatory enzyme COX. This inhibition has a profound effect on renal function since it eliminates the possible production of compensatory prostaglandins. This is especially true for the hemodynamically stressed individual where compensatory prostaglandin production acts to preserve renal function in the face of a systemic reduction in blood flow. Renal blood flow [RBF] is regulated by changes in RVR, which ultimately is determined by the balance between the amount of vasodilatory PGE_2 and PGI_2 and vasoconstrictive vasopeptides, e.g. TxA_2, angiotensin II, endothelin [4, 5]. Glomerular filtration rate (GFR) also responds to these prostaglandins, increasing with PGE_2 and PGI_2 and declining with TxA_2. Because of the reduction in RVR, which follows vasodilatation, prostaglandins can directly influence renin secretion, with PGI_2, PGE_2 increasing it, and TxA_2 either without effect or decreasing it. Medullary salt and water regulation are strongly influenced by PGE_2, which has both a natriuretic and diuretic action, while PGI_2 action is limited to natriuresis [23].

Renal prostaglandin production is minimal during non-stress conditions, and thus do not play a significant role in the maintenance of renal function under normal conditions. However, their production and release are substantially increased during hemodynamic instability being called forth to preserve both glomerular perfusion and tubular function [1]. A reduction in effective blood volume initiates secretion of the various vasoconstrictive peptides, which can initiate arachidonic acid release from the membrane (Figure 1). If, during such a stimulated state, NSAIDs are administered a marked reduction in production of vasodilatory prostaglandins PGE_2 and PGI_2 will result in a predictable imbalance causing a decreased renal perfusion and an increased tubular sodium reabsorption. Interruption of PG's production by NSAIDs is manifested by a variety of renal syndromes [1-3, 3-5, 24].

Renal syndromes associated with NSAIDs

Several renal syndromes can complicate NSAID use [1-3, 3-5, 24]. Generally, individuals who have normal renal function and are properly hydrated, are not at risk for developing adverse renal effects [1]. NSAID-induced deterioration in renal function depends on the specific drug, the dose and duration of pharmacologic effect and the state of health of the recipient [25]. Patients who have prostaglandin-dependent states associated with co-morbid diseases, such as high renin states or chronic renal insufficiency, are especially susceptible

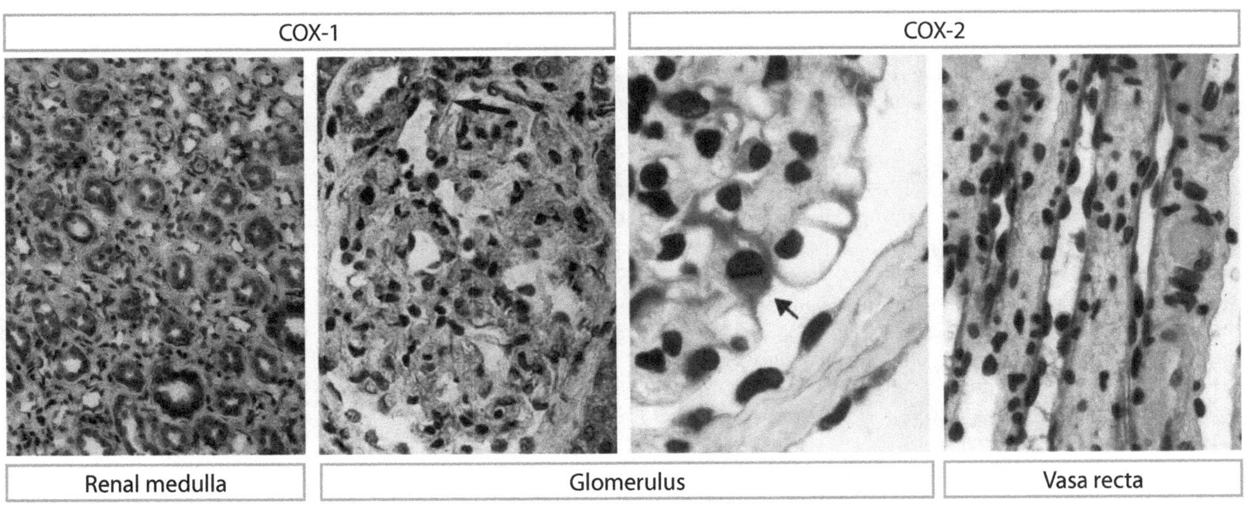

Figure 2. *Localization of COX-1 and COX-2 immunoreactive protein in adult and fetal human kidney (reproduced with permission from [15].*

to NSAID-induced renal toxicities. Renal prostaglandins, by initiating counterregulatory vasodilation, are crucial in maintaining perfusion in 1) individuals with parenchymal renal disease and renal impairment, and 2) when circulating volume is decreased, such as in dehydrated patients or in individuals with a decrease in their "effective" circulating volume such as CHF or significant liver disease associated with ascites [1, 3]. The renal syndromes associated with NSAIDs can be predicted based upon inhibition of COX, which modifies the compensatory actions of prostaglandins. These modifications lead to a fall in both RBF and GFR with concomitant abnormal water and electrolyte excretion [24]. In addition, nephrotic syndrome, papillary necrosis and chronic tubulo-interstitial disease can complicate NSAIDs use [2]. These syndromes are summarized on table 2.

Acute deterioration of renal function

NSAID-induced acute renal deterioration occurs in the setting of severe vasoconstrictive renal ischemia and can be attributed to interruption of the delicate balance between hormonally mediated pressor mechanisms and prostaglandin-associated vasodilatory effects (Figure 3). During NSAID inhibition of renal prostaglandin synthesis, unopposed vasoconstriction occurs by eliminating crucial counter-regulatory vasodilation [4, 5]. Similar to traditional NSAIDs, all COX-2 specific agents, celecoxib, rofecoxib, lumaricoxib and valdecoxib have been shown to reduce renal prostaglandin synthesis [19, 26-28]. High-risk individuals (Table 3) can develop AKI within days of starting traditional NSAID therapy. Fortunately, the incidence of such an event is low, ranging from 0.5% to 1.0% of patients [3].

There is an apparent association between the relatively rapid onset of AKI and ingestion of NSAIDs with short half-lives (e.g. ibuprofen) [29]. In a crossover study, involving 11 days of active treatment, renal decompensation appeared within a few days of initiation of ibuprofen therapy, whereas no evidence of AKI was reported from NSAIDs with prolonged half-lives (e.g. sulindac and piroxicam) [29]. Although NSAIDs do not reduce glomerular filtration in normal individuals [30, 31], they are capable of induce acute renal decompensation in "at risk" patients with various renal and extrarenal clinical conditions that cause a decrease in blood perfusion to the kidney (Table 3). Renal prostaglandins play an important role in the maintenance of homeostasis in these patients, so disruption of counter-regulatory mechanisms can produce clinically impor-

Table 2. Effects of NSAIDs on the kidney (adapted from Whelton [125]).

Syndrome	Mechanism	Risk factors	Treatment
Sodium retention and edema	↓ PG, ↓ RBF, ↓ GFR, ↑ chloride absorption	NSAID use, hepatic disease, renal disease, HTN, DM, diuretic use, circulatory compromise, dehydration, advanced age	Discontinue NSAID
Hyperkalemia	↓ PG, ↓ RAA axis activity, ↓ K+ delivery to renal tubule	Renal disease, CHF, type 2 DM, multiple myeloma, use of K^+ supplements, K^+ sparing diuretics, ACE inhibitors	Discontinue NSAID, avoid indomethacin in patients at risk
Acute renal failure	↓ PG, ↓ RBF, ↓ GFR Hemodynamic disruption	CHF, renal disease, hepatic disease, diuretic use, advanced age, dehydration, SLE, shock, sepsis, hyperreninemia, hyperaldosteronemia	Discontinue NSAID, support with dialysis and steroids, if needed
Proteinuria/ Interstitial nephritis*	↑ recruitment and activation of lymphocytes, likely through leukotriene formation, affecting glomerular and peritubular permeability	Fenoprofen use, possibly female gender, advanced age	Discontinue NSAID, support with dialysis and steroids, if needed
Renal papillary necrosis*	Direct toxicity ↓ PG	Massive NSAID ingestion Dehydration	Discontinue NSAID Rehydrate

Abbreviations: NSAID = nonsteroidal anti-inflammatory drugs, PG = prostaglandin, RBF = renal blood flow, GFR = glomerular filtration rate, HTN = hypertension, DM = diabetes mellitus, K^+ = potassium, RAA = renin-angiotensin- aldosterone, CHF = congestive heart failure, ACE = angiotensin-converting enzyme, SLE = systemic lupus erythematosis.
**: distinctly unusual*

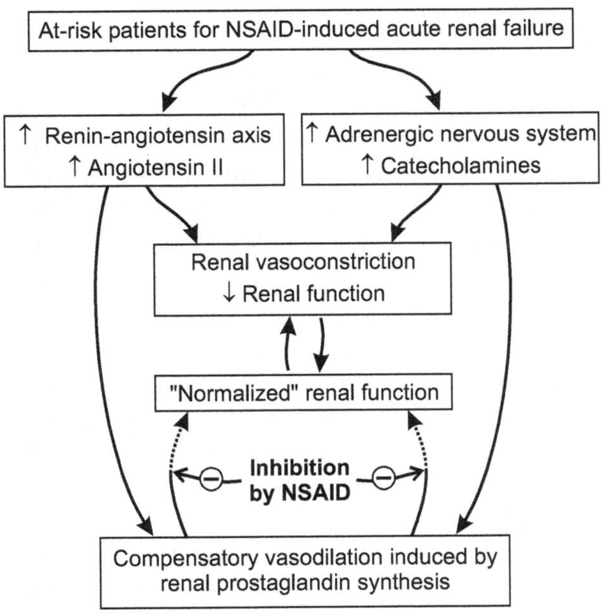

Figure 3. *Mechanism by which NSAIDs disrupt the compensatory vasodilation response of renal prostaglandins to vasoconstrictor hormones in patients with prerenal conditions.*

tant and even severe deterioration in renal function [4, 5]. Typically, the addition of a NSAID increases the risk of hemodynamically mediated ischemic damage to the kidney by removing the protective effects of vasodilatory prostaglandins and allowing unopposed vasoconstriction. In the hemodynamically stressed patient a reduction in effective arterial blood volume initiates a neuroendocrine cascade, which has both renal and extrarenal consequences that require intact prostaglandin production [3].

Fortunately, the AKI usually reverses once the NSAID is stopped but in the high risk patient, can occur with any COX inhibitor.

Epidemiology and Incidence

Recently, Perez Gutthann et al. [32] evaluated the incidence of NSAID-induced AKI from a population-based, case control study using data from Canada. Over 200, 000 health plan members were included because they had filled at least 1 prescription for NSAIDs during the 5-year interval. The crude incidence for AKI requiring hospitalization was 1.7/100, 000 persons. Current NSAID use increased risk of AKI 4 fold, a risk that equaled the risk associated with other known nephrotoxins, e.g. aminoglycosides, contrast media. The risk of AKI was especially high

Table 3. "At risk" patients for NSAID-induced acute renal failure.

Severe heart disease (congestive heart failure)
Severe liver disease (cirrhosis)
Nephrotic syndrome (low oncotic pressure)
Chronic renal disease
Elderly population (age 80 or >)
Dehydration (protracted - several days)

during the first month of NSAID therapy and a direct dose relationship was observed. While the incidence of AKI is low as compared to other clinical settings, the outcome is serious since nearly half the patients died. Confirmation of the increased incidence of AKI during the first 30 days of NSAID use comes from the recent publication of Schneider et al [32A]. Using a population-based, nested case-control analysis of 121, 722 new NSAID users older then 65 years of age, they identified 4228 cases of AKI and 84540 age and followup time matched controls. Current users (30 days from index date) had an adjusted rate ratio of 2.05 (CL_{95} 1.61-2.60). The risk declined with continued use. In addition they calculated the AKI risk for specific NSAID's. For conventional NSAID's:2.30 (1.60-3.32); Rofecoxib: 2.31(1.73-3.08); Naproxen: 2.42 (1.52-3.85); Celecoxib: 1.54(1.14-2.09). In addition, the average incidence of AKI was 1.48 cases/100 person-years and remained stable during the study period. AKI cases were more likely to be male and have hypertension, diabetes and preexisting renal disease. Patients using more than one NSAID during the 30 day interval had a doubling of the risk ratio, 4.65 (2.31-9.37). They also noted a dose dependence with regard to AKI when higher doses of Rofecoxib, Naproxen and Celecoxib were used. The authors conclude "Compared with the other NSAIDs, celecoxib tended to have a better renal safety profile, particularily at a dose of 200 mg/day or less." Finally, this same group of authors has published on the incidence of NASID associated acute myocardial infarction in the same cohort (162) and found that the incidence of AKI was 50% higher. The adverse effect of multiple NSAIDs on renal outcomes was confirmed by the recent report of Clinard et al [32B] who found that the Odd Ratio for adverse drug reactions involving the kidney, liver or GI tract increase between 50 and 100%. For AKI this increased from 3.2 (CL_{95} 2.5-4.1) to 4.8 (2.6-8.8).

Evans et al. [33] conducted a case-control study involving a population base of 420, 600 individuals searching for any relationship between AKI and NSAID ingestions. AKI was confirmed by analysis of individual hospital charts. These authors found that the risk of AKI was doubled for patients who ingested NSAIDs within 90 days of hospitalization for AKI and also for patients taking therapeutic doses of Aspirin. Interestingly, they could not identify any interaction between NSAID use in patients with chronic renal failure and subsequent hospitalization for AKI.

Griffin et al. [34] reported a nested, case-control study involving 1799 AKI cases compared to 9899 controls. Chart survey was used to confirm both the diagnosis of AKI and the use of NSAIDs. 18.1% of the AKI patients were NSAID-users compared to only 11.3% of the controls (OR 1.58; 1.34-1.86). They estimated that NSAID-use was associated with 25 excess hospitalizations/10, 000 years of use. The NSAIDs with odds ratio that were significantly correlated with AKI included ibuprofen, piroxicam, fenoprofen, and indomethacin. Based on these finding and the results of three other case-control studies, they concluded that the odds ratio significantly favored a direct relationship between NSAID ingestion and AKI, especially in the elderly.

The more recent case-control study is that reported by Huerta et al [34A] using the General Practice Research Database from the United Kingdom. They confirmed that current use of NSAID increased the relative risk of AKI by 3.2 fold over non-users. They also identified significant increase in the relative risk of AKI when NSAID were combined with either diuretics (RR 11.6 (CL_{95} 4.2-32.2)) or calcium channel blockers (RR 7.8 (3.0-20.5)). In addition, they provided analysis of individual NSAID relative risk. Diclofenac 3.12 (1.38-7.05), Ibuprofen 2.64 (1.01-6.88), Meloxicam 8.05 (1.98-32.81), Naproxen 2.98 (0.62-14.21). In patients with congestive heart failure the combination of current use of NSAIDs increased their RR from 2.82 (1.05-7.57) to 7.63 (2.7-21.56), while for patients with hypertension the RR increased from 2.09 (0.87-5.02) to 6.12 (2.54-14.78). It is noteworthy that the incidence of AKI in this study, 1.1 cases/10, 000, is 100 times less than that reported by Schneider et al [32A] using a population based approach.

To summarize, the risk characteristics, based upon these epidemiological studies include: 1) Patients taking NSAIDs develop AKI 2 to 4 times more frequently than non-users; 2) AKI is more common within the first month of starting NSAIDs; 3) Elderly patients and patients taking ibuprofen, diclofenac, naproxen, meloxicam, piroxicam, fenoprofen, indomethacin, and rofecoxib are at greater risk of developing AKI. 4) Patient taking more that one NSAID simultaneously are at greater risk of AKI, as are patients taking diuretics and calcium channel blockers in concert with their NSAID. However, these case control studies have methodological limitations. Limitations include: confounding by indication for the drug use, the bias introduced by difficulty in establishing the time-order of exposure, and, in some cases, the bias introduced by recall. While Evans and co-workers [33] failed to demonstrate an increased risk of NSAID-induced AKI in patients with pre-existing renal impairment, Schneider et al [32A] did report pre-existing renal failure as a risk factor and should prompt a more focused study of this selected risk category.

Clinical features of NSAID-induced acute kidney injury

At onset, NSAID-induced renal impairment is of moderate severity and is characterized by increasing blood urea nitrogen, serum creatinine, serum potassium, and weight with variable decrease in urinary output. With early detection and drug discontinuation, this form of NSAID-induced acute kidney injury is usually reversible over 2-7 days. Indomethacin-induced acute kidney injury may take longer to reverse following drug discontinuation, but reversal is the rule [29]. If NSAID-induced renal failure is not recognized early, severe morbid consequences occur. Continued NSAID therapy in the setting of deteriorating renal function may advance rapidly to the point wherein dialysis support is needed [35]. While this profound level of renal failure is often designated as "acute tubular necrosis", it often is only the extreme end of the spectrum of a hemodynamic insult and probably does not deserve identification as a separate clinical entity. Fortunately, even this profound level of renal functional impairment will nonetheless recover several days to weeks after discontinuation of the NSAID.

A possible relationship between the parenteral administration of the NSAID, ketorolac, and AKI has been evaluated in a multi-center study by Feldman et al. [36]. These authors found no difference in the frequency of AKI for patients receiving either ketorolac or morphine sulfate during the first 5 post-operative days; however, a significant, preferential increase in AKI frequency occurred when ketorolac treatment was extended beyond 5 days.

Clinical risk factors for acute kidney injury

A tabulation of patients at risk for NSAID induced AKI is presented on Table 3. Thus, conditions associated with reduced RBF, e.g. CHF, cirrhosis, shock, and volume contraction, triggers pressor responses via adrenergic and renin-angiotensin pathways that is referred to as the neuro-endocrine cascade. The risk of NSAID-induced acute renal deterioration is greatest in patients with liver disease, pre-existing renal impairment including the nephrotic syndrome, cardiac failure, volume contraction due to protracted intercurrent dehydration or diuretic therapy, and old age. For example, NSAID-induced renal decompensation has been well documented in patients with cirrhosis, particularly when ascites is present [7]. This sensitivity can be traced to increased urinary excretion of prostaglandin E_2, prostacyclin metabolites, and thromboxane A_2 in these patients [37, 38]. An analogous prostaglandin dependent renal function exists in patients with underlying congestive heart failure [39], nephrotic syndrome [40, 41], or lupus nephritis [42, 43]. A drug-drug interaction to be aware of is that combining NSAIDs with triameterene which significantly increases the risk of AKI [44].

Patients with chronic renal impairment because of diminished renal prostaglandin production may also be at increased risk of NSAID-induced renal failure. NSAID-induced acute kidney injury has been documented in patients with asymptomatic, but mild chronic renal failure, defined as a recruitment serum creatinine between 133 μmol/L and 265 μmol/L (1.5 and 3.0 mg/dl) [45]. Baseline excretion of urinary prostaglandin E_2 and 6-keto-prostaglandin $F_{1\alpha}$ was quantitatively lower in the individuals who developed NSAID-induced renal decompensation than in those who did not. Upon initiation of ibuprofen, urinary prostaglandin excretion fell in all patients, but trough concentrations were quantitatively lower in the subset of patients who experienced acute kidney injury.

Volume contraction due to diuretic therapy or an intercurrent disease represents another important risk factor for the development of NSAID-induced acute deterioration of renal function [1, 3, 33]. Elderly patients are also at increased risk. It is estimated that, in the absence of other disease entities, the age of 80 years or greater is an independent risk factor since 50% of the population at age 80 have a 50% loss of glomerular function primarily as a result of the progression of arteriolonephrosclerosis [46].

To summarize patient a risk of NSAID-induced AKI. Frequency will be greater in patient populations with restricted renal blood flow, e.g. CHF, cirrhosis, nephrotic syndrome, shock. However, for absolute numbers, the elderly are probably most at risk since they are the primary group who take NSAIDs for relieve rheumatic complaints [3].

Hyperkalemia/Hyporenin-Hypoaldosteronism sydrome

Hyperkalemia is an unusual complication of NSAID ingestion, presumably because of the multiplicity of factors that are capable of maintaining potassium homeostasis, even in the absence of prostaglandins. However, NSAID-induced hyperkalemia can occurs in up to 46% of high-risk individuals, but is reversible upon cessation of therapy [47]. Patients at risk to develop hyperkalemia include those with: pre-existing renal impairment [48, 49], cardiac failure [50], diabetes [50], multiple myeloma [51], concomitant potassium supplementation [52], potassium-sparing diuretic therapy [53] or taking an angiotensin converting enzyme inhibitor [3]. The interaction of NSAIDs with ACE inhibitors is an important and common form of drug-drug interaction. In particular, this interaction must be recognized when an arthritic patient, who is receiving long term NSAID treatment, develops hypertension that requiring drug therapy. If, in addition, the patient has mild renal impairment, our experience suggests that a baseline serum creatinine value of 180 μmol/L or greater (2.0 mg/dl or >) at least doubles their risk for NSAID related acute deterioration of renal function. In this clinical situation the angiotensin converting enzyme (ACE) inhibitor-NSAID drug combination should be avoided because of the potential for the development of both hyperkalemia and acute renal injury [3, 45]. The general interaction of NSAIDs with antihypertensive drugs will be addressed later in this chapter.

Indomethacin appears to be the NSAID most frequently associated with the development of hyperkalemia, including patients without apparent risk factors [54]. In addition to the known effects of NSAIDs on potassium delivery to the distal tubule and their inhibition of the renin-angiotensin and aldosterone pathways, indomethacin may have a direct effect to limit cellular uptake of potassium [55].

As noted above, hyperkalemia often complicates the NSAID-induced acute renal deterioration. However, the severity of hyperkalemia can be disproportionate to the degree of renal impairment. Tan et al. [56] have reported a patient who had a serum potassium level of 6.2 mEq/L in spite of only mildly abnormal renal function. In this patient, plasma renin and aldosterone levels were suppressed and failed to respond to furosemide or postural changes. Urinary prostaglandin E_2 was also suppressed. Discontinuation of indomethacin resulted in normalization of potassium, prostaglandin E_2, and a rebound of renin and aldosterone.

The COX-2 inhibitor, Celecoxib, appears to have little effect on serum potassium, even in patients receiving diuretic therapy [57-59] and similarly, there does not appear to be any significant effect of rofecoxib on serum potassium.

In conclusion, hyperkalemia associated with the use of traditional NSAIDs or the coxibs becomes a clinical risk in individuals with significantly decreased renal function and/or in those with the combination of decreased renal function and use of an ACE inhibitor.

Pharmacodynamic and pharmacokinetic relationships in NSAID-induced acute kidney injury

NSAID-induced acute renal decompensation is a pharmacologically predictable phenomenon that possesses a dose-dependent component. In a triple-crossover study of 12 females with mild renal failure, ibuprofen (800 mg three times daily) was discontinued in 3 patients after 8 days because of worsening renal function (> 133 µmol/L - > 1.5 mg/dl increase in serum creatinine) or hyperkalemia (potassium > 6 mmol/ml). When these 3 patients were rechallenged at a 50% lower dose of ibuprofen, two developed evidence of acute renal deterioration [45].

An additional important finding from this study was the time of onset of acute renal decompensation. Ibuprofen-induced renal failure occurred rapidly (within 8 days), but piroxicam and sulindac were not associated with any deterioration of renal function during the 11-day treatment period [39]. A pharmacokinetic analysis of the drugs used in these patients suggested the following: Ibuprofen, which has a short elimination half-life, reached maximum serum concentrations quickly; in contrast, piroxicam and sulindac have longer half-lives and continued to accumulate throughout the treatment period. These findings are consistent with basic pharmacologic principles and suggest that NSAIDs having short elimination half-lives will reach steady-state and exert maximum pharmacologic effects before this occurs with NSAIDs having longer half-lives.

Salt and water retention

Electrolyte abnormalities

NSAID, by inhibiting both cortical and medullary prostaglandin production, cause a variety of electrolyte abnormalities include sodium, potassium and water retention [24, 60, 61]. While sodium retention is usually transient with escape after several days, occasionally a patient will develop significant edema [62]. Water retention secondary to NSAIDs is manifest as hyponatremia [63] and occurs when the basal prostaglandin antagonism of antidiuretic hormone is removed, allowing unmodified water reabsorption in the collecting duct of the kidney. When this action is coupled with the NSAID-induced enhanced sodium chloride reabsorption in the thick ascending limb of Henle, free water clearance is virtually eliminated causing even more profound hyponatremia.

Edema Formation

Edema due to NSAIDs induced sodium and fluid retention usually occurs in susceptible individuals within the first week of therapy. Furthermore, these effects are reversible when the drug is discontinued. Clinically evident peripheral edema occurs in up to 5% of patients [3], likely as a result of decreased renal blood flow, possible redistribution of intrarenal blood flow, and increased reabsorption of sodium chloride in the thick ascending loop of Henle. In elderly patients this increased sodium chloride reabsorption coupled with increased water reabsorption is more likely to result in the edema.

Diuretics and NSAIDs

The renal saluretic response to loop diuretics is partially dependent on intact intrarenal prostaglandin production in the thick ascending loop of Henle. The decrease in the response to loop diuretics is mediated both by removing the inhibition of sodium chloride reabsorption and an increase in renal medullary blood flow causing a reduction in renal concentrating capacity. The net result is that the concurrent use of a NSAID may blunt the diuresis induced by loop diuretics.

For the practicing physician, this interaction is not of major clinical importance since either increasing the diuretic dose or, if possible, discontinuation of the NSAID will permit reinstitution of the desired diuretic response. In patients who are well controlled on a stable regimen of chronic loop diuretics use, the intercurrent need for long term use of an NSAID will typically lead to increasing the dosage of the loop agent, or the addition of a diuretic that acts in the distal nephron.

Thiazide diuretics do not stimulate or require prostaglandins to produce their desired effect and they do not directly interact with NSAIDs. The magnitude of increased risk of NSAID-induced AKI with concomitant triamterene cannot be estimated based on sporadic case reports [44].

Antihypertensive drugs and NSAIDs

Four recent reports have provided insight regarding the interaction between antihypertensive therapy and NSAIDs. The first is a case control study by Gurwitz et al. [64] involving 9411 medicare patients and examined the frequency with which antihypertensive therapy was required following initiation of NSAID therapy. Based on odds ratio, NSAID users were nearly 70% more likely to require antihypertensive drugs and this requirement correlated with the NSAID dose. The need for antihypertensive treatment was evident within the first 3 months of NSAID administration. Two study of interest are both meta-analysis of NSAIDs effect on blood pressure. Pope et al. [65] included 54 short-term studies encompassing 1324 patients, 92% being hypertensive. The adverse influence of NSAIDs on blood pressure (3.5 mm Hg - 6.2 mm Hg increase) was limited to hypertensive patient taking indomethacin, naproxen or piroxicam. These authors could not eliminate the confounding effect of dietary sodium. The meta-analysis reported by Johnson et al. [66] included 50 clinical trials encompassing 771 patients only 80% of who were hypertensive. NSAID administration resulted in a mean increase in blood pressure of 5 mmHg in the hypertensive patients, but no significant increase in the normotensive patients. A more recent meta-analysis was conducted by Aw et al [66A] comparing the effect of selective COX2 inhibitors vs. non-specific NSAIDs on blood pressure. They included 19 randomized control trials and used weighted mean differences and the Der Simonian and Laird method of pooled results to obtain relative risk of developing hypertension. COX-2 inhibitors were associated with a non-significantly higher RR of 1.61 (CL_{95} 0.91-2, 84) compared to placebo, and a non-significantly higher RR of 1.25 (0.87-1.78) when compared to non-selective NSAIDs. In a recent review of analgesics and hypertension, Graziano [66B] concluded that while acute changes in BP following the introduction of NSAID therapy seem well established, the long term impact on NSAIDs on blood pressure is less certain. While NSAIDs antagonized the antihypertensive action of b-blockers =ace-inhibitors > vasodilators > diuretics = calcium channel blockers, significant alteration of body weight, daily urinary sodium excretion, creatinine clearance, plasma renin activity, or the urinary excretion of either PGE_2 or 6-keto-PGF_1 were absent. Thus, in hypertensive patients, especially the elderly, NSAIDs will interfere with antihypertensive treatment especially if β-blockers, ACE inhibitors or angiotensin receptor blockers [67] are the principle drugs used. The interaction between NSAIDs and antihypertensive medications is likely due to the fact that certain antihypertensive medications exert a substantial part of their therapeutic effect via prostaglandin-mediated mechanisms [68]. Calcium channel blockers are not dependent on the prostaglandin pathway however, b-blockers, vasodilators, and ACE inhibitors seem to be particularly affected by NSAID therapy [4]. The lack of an interaction between chronic NSAID-treatment and the anti-hypertensive action of CCB's has been confirmed by a large prospective study [69]. Regarding the likelihood of developing new onset hypertension with COX2 inhibitors vs. NSAIDs, Wang et al [69A]) conducted a cohort study using secondary data from GE Centricity Electronic Medical Record database involving a sample of 51444 patients of whom 17148 were receiving celecoxib and 34296 were receiving non-specific NSAIDs. Relative to non-specific NSAIDs users, celecoxib users had a similar rate of post-exposure hypertension with the hazard rate of 1.013 (CL_{95} 0.862-1.190). Thus there was no difference in the risk of developing new onset hypertension when comparing specific COX2 inhibitors with traditional NSAIDs.

Proposed mechanism of blood pressure destabilization

Prostaglandins, in concert with nitric oxide, act as a renal vasodilator-natriuretic system [70] whose action is to offset the vasoconstrictive-sodium retaining effects of the renin-angiotensin system. Because of these interactions, significant destabilization of blood pressure control can occur during systemic administration of NSAIDs. PGE_2 and PGI_2 possess both prohypertensive and antihypertensive actions on blood pressure [68]. The prohypertensive actions involve increasing renin release and raising cardiac output. The antihypertensive action includes vasodilatation, reversing vasopeptide-induced vasoconstriction and inducing a negative sodium balance. Recent evidence has identified a decline in nitric oxide availability in both elderly [71] and hypertensive patients [72]. In addition, the plasma nitric oxide response to alterations in dietary sodium intake is distinctly abnormal in elderly salt-sensitive hypertensive patients [73]. When these observations are combined with the recent studies of Perinotto et al. [74], which confirmed that endogenous prostaglandin will counteract the renal actions of endogenous angiotensin II in the face of NO inhibition, a mechanistic explanation for NSAIDs-induced hypertension can be formulated. The speculation involves the following: The decline in NO production in elderly, hypertensive patients puts additional requirement on the endogenous renal PG to counteract the intrinsic action of the RAS. When NSAIDs are given, the vasodilator-natriuretic action of PG is removed and thus the RAS is unopposed leading to destabilization of BP control.

The interaction between sodium intake, blood pressure and NSAIDs has been studied by Mulkerrin et al. [75]. These authors measured the change in blood pressure and sodium excretion in five young normotensive females and five elderly females to an intravenous saline load before and after 1800 mg of ibuprofen was given for 3 days. Saline loading induced a consistent 25mmHg rise in systolic pressure with or without ibuprofen in the elderly patients, while ibuprofen alone caused a 14mmHg rise from baseline in the elderly patients before saline. The naturiesis associated with saline loading in both groups was significantly blunted in the elderly after treatment with ibuprofen. They concluded that aging increases the susceptibility to salt retention and hypertension from NSAIDs. This may well be due to unmasking the diminished activity of nitrous oxide synthetase, which characterizes elderly patients who are salt sensitive.

Alam et al. [76] used chronic salt loading to examine the interaction between blood pressure, salt and NSAIDs. Thirty-one healthy individuals, age 60 or more, were enrolled in a randomized, placebo-controlled, crossover study. Patients were stratified as to normotensive or isolated systolic hypertension based on their blood pressure response after 6 weeks of a controlled 150 mEq/d sodium diet. Crossover involved a two-week interval receiving either low sodium (90 mEq/d) diet or high sodium diet (240 mEq/d) diet and placebo or indomethacin 75 mg/d. For all patients, high salt diet was associated with a 6mmHg rise in systolic pressure and 3 mmHg in diastolic pressure. Indomethacin administration increased systolic but not diastolic pressure. High salt diet and indomethacin had an additive effect on blood pressure, but failed to demonstrate any interaction. Indomethacin significantly elevated the blood pressure in normotensive individuals but did not in patients classified as salt-sensitive. They concluded that salt-sensitive patients with isolated systolic hypertension were resistant to the pressor effect of indomethacin but normotensive elderly patients were not.

The duration and magnitude of salt loading between these two studies may account for the different conclusion reached by each set of authors.

The concept of "renal sparing" NSAIDs

While all NSAIDs have the potential for inducing renal failure, there has been speculation of quantitative differences among the individual NSAIDs. Sulindac was thought to be renal sparing, possibly because of its unusual metabolic pathway [29, 77-79]. The parent compound, sulindac sulphoxide, is an inactive prodrug, which undergoes hepatic metabolism to sulindac sulphide, the metabolite responsible for its anti-inflammatory activity. Sulindac sulphoxide is also metabolized to a much lesser extent to an inactive metabolite, sulindac sulphone. It was hypothesized that, within the human kidney, sulindac sulphide was reversibly oxidized to the inactive parent compound, sulindac sulphoxide, with the result that renal prostaglandin production was not perturbed [29, 78].

In clinical studies, urinary prostaglandin levels and renal effects were unchanged in patients with normal renal function [29, 30] and patients with proteinuria [79]. However, the duration of sulindac exposure in these studies may not have been sufficient to allow the full pharmacologic effect of sulindac. Also, NSAID-induced changes may not have been detectable because of the presence of only very mild renal impairment or the absence of co-existing renal failure in this study [80]. Longer courses of sulindac in patients with slightly more severe renal impairment have been associated with statistically significant reductions in urinary prostaglandins [45, 80] and GFR [81].

The ability of sulindac to inhibit prostaglandin synthesis and impair renal function has been confirmed in a different high-risk group, namely patients with hepatic cirrhosis and ascites [82]. We have also identified the development of profound acute kidney injury in risk prone patients who received sulindac for several days to weeks. Collectively, these studies suggest caution in accepting any NSAID as being "renal sparing".

Nephrotic syndrome with interstitial nephritis

This rare complication of NSAID use may develop at any time during treatment, but typically occurs months to years after therapy has been initiated, and generally resolves upon discontinuation of therapy [1, 83].

Fenoprofen, on a per capita use basis, has been associated with interstitial nephritis more frequently than other traditional NSAIDs [83, 84]. To date, there have been three reports of coxib-induced acute interstitial nephritis [85-87]. All were biopsy proven and cleared after stopping the coxib.

Clinical presentation

The features of this NSAID-induced renal syndrome are somewhat variable. The patient may experience edema, oliguria, and clinical signs indicative of significant proteinuria [88, 89]. Systemic signs of allergic interstitial nephritis such as fever, drug rash, peripheral eosinophilia, and eosinophiluria are typically absent. The urine sediment contains microscopic hematuria and cellular elements reported as pyuria [9, 89]. In a recent discussion of NSAID-induced acute interstitial nephritis, Rossert [83] confirmed that proteinuria, usually in the nephrotic range, occurs in 70% of cases [84]. The occurrence of acute kidney injury parallels the nephrotic syndrome. For patients without the nephritic syndrome the functional extent of renal deterioration can range from minimal to requiring hemodialysis. The onset of NSAID-induced nephrotic syndrome is usually delayed, having a mean time of onset of 5.4 months after initiation of NSAID therapy and ranging from 2 weeks to 18 months [9, 88]. NSAID-induced nephrotic syndrome is usually reversible between 1 month and 1 year after discontinuation of NSAID therapy. During the recovery period, some 20% of patients require dialysis. Steroids have been used empirically, but it is not certain that they hasten recovery. If proteinuria is not significantly reduced within two weeks of discontinuation of the putative NSAID, we recommend a standard 2-month trial of corticosteroids as would be employed in an adult patient with idiopathic minimal change glomerulonephritis. While pyuria and eosinophiluria develop in ~40% of patients who present with nephrotic syndrome, gross hematuria occurs in less than 10% of patients [83].

Histologic features of NSAID-induced nephrotic syndrome

NSAID-induced acute interstitial nephritis is a recognized cause of AKI [17], the frequency of which appears to be increasing [90]. In a recent series reported by Schwarz [90] of 64 biopsy-proven cases of acute interstitial nephritis, 85% were drug induced. The responsible drugs included: antibiotics, analgesics, NSAIDs and diuretics. Characteristically, the histology of this form of NSAID-induced nephrotic syndrome consists of minimal change glomerulonephritis with tubulo-interstitial nephritis. This is an unusual combination of findings and, when noted in the clinical setting of protracted NSAID use, is virtually pathognomic of NSAID-related nephrotic syndrome. Nephrotic syndrome without apparent interstitial disease has been reported in a handful of patients taking fenoprofen, sulindac, or diclofenac. Conversely, interstitial disease without nephrosis has been reported in a few patients, but this may, possibly, represent allergic interstitial nephritis [89].

In spite of the nephrotic range proteinuria, the most impressive histopathologic findings in NSAID-induced nephrotic syndrome involve the interstitium and tubules [91]. A focally, diffuse inflammatory infiltrate can be found around the proximal and distal tubules. While this infiltrate consists primarily of cytotoxic T lymphocytes, it also contains other T cells, some B cells, and plasma cells [92]. Changes in the glomeruli in these patients were minimal and resembled those of classic minimal change glomerulonephritis with marked epithelial-foot process fusion. These findings are consistent with reports by other investigators [8, 35, 36, 93].

Of the 14 cases of biopsy proven drug-induced allergic nephritis reported by Shibasaki et al. [94], 4 were ascribed to NSAIDs; while in the series reported by Schwarz et al. [90], 16 of 68 biopsies were ascribed to NSAIDs. While 3 of the patients had taken the offending agent for less than 1 week, the forth had received aspirin for 3 months. All presented with oliguric renal failure without systemic signs of rash or fever. Positive 67Ga scintigrams were obtained in both patients in whom it was performed. In 3 of the 4 patients serum creatinine returned to normal range at follow-up. The authors conclude that 67Ga scintigram combined with a lymphocyte stimulation test can confirm a diagnosis of suspect drug-induced allergic nephritis without resorting to a renal biopsy.

NSAID induced nephrotic syndrome is suspected of being immunologically mediated and idiosyncratic. It has a distinct presentation when compared to that ascribed to acute interstitial nephritis. The nephrotic syndrome is not associated with hemodynamically stressed patients. Recently Radford et al. [95] published a retrospective study of NSAIDs induced membranous nephropathy using the Mayo Clinic biopsy registry. They reported that >10% of biopsy proven membranous glomerulonephritis [stage I/II] was attributable to NSAIDs. They summarized the clinical features of NSAID-induced nephrotic syndrome as having no consistent clinical predisposition, with a median duration of 43 weeks of drug ingestion, and nephrotic range proteinuria that was present for <8 weeks but reversed with discontinuation of the drug. The clinical features, absence of risk factors, and pathophysiology distinguish this from other NSAID-induced renal syndromes and from classic drug-induced allergic interstitial nephritis.

Risk factors for NSAID-induced nephrotic syndrome

The risk factors associated with NSAID-related nephrotic syndrome are not well identified. Underlying renal impairment does not appear to be a risk factor. Old age has been identified as a risk factor [33, 88], but this may also be a reflection of the usual candidate for chronic NSAID therapy. The syndrome has been more frequently reported with fenoprofen, so the actual NSAID itself may be critical. However, the syndrome has been attributed to virtually all NSAIDs, including those from structurally distinct classes [8, 35, 88, 89, 89].

Mechanism of NSAID-induced nephrotic syndrome

The mechanism of NSAID-induced nephrotic syndrome has not been fully characterized, but some likely contributing mechanisms are under evaluation. While the mechanism of toxicity is unknown, it is theorized to be the result of leukotrienes, which are formed from arachidonic acid via the lipooxygenase pathway when the cyclooxygenase pathway is blocked [89]. Leukotrienes increase glomerular and peritubular permeability, which may lead to the induction of interstitial nephritis and proteinuria. The association of this syndrome with structurally distinct NSAIDs suggests a common pathophysiologic denominator [91]. It is conceivable that T lymphocytes function as immune mediators instead of the humoral factors that are responsible for classic drug-induced allergic interstitial nephritis. In keeping with this hypothesis, NSAID-induced prostaglandin inhibition may play an indirect role. By inhibiting cyclooxygenase, NSAIDs may promote metabolism of arachidonic acid to non-prostaglandin eicosanoids. Indeed, leukotrienes, the products of the interaction between lipoxygenase and arachidonic acid, are known to recruit T lymphocytes and promote the inflammatory process. As noted above, leukotrienes may contribute to proteinuria by increasing vascular permeability [8, 88, 89].

Chronic renal failure/papillary necrosis

Epidemiology

There is limited information regarding any link between long-term NSAIDs ingestion and development of chronic renal failure. In the case control study reported by Perneger et al. [96], individuals judged to be taking an average annual dose of NSAID were not at additional risk of developing ESRD (adjusted RR 1.0, 95% CI 0.5 to 2.0). However, the relative risk of ESRD was concluded to be 8.8 for individuals who took in excess of 5000 doses of NSAID. On the other hand, in a multicenter case control study conducted by Sandler et al. [97], the relative risk of chronic renal failure was found to be 2.1 (95% CI 1.1 to 4.1) with one year's use of daily NSAIDs. Fields et al. [98] enrolled 4099 patients 70 years or older in a cross-sectional analysis. The serum creatinines were separated into quartiles and chronic NSAIDs users were significantly more prevalent in the highest quartile (Scr ≥ 1.4mg/dl or 124 mmol/L), OR 1.7 (95% CI 1.3 to 2.3). More recently, Sturmer et al. [99] conducted a cross-sectional study of 802 patients regarding the association between NSAIDs and impaired renal function. Detailed questionnaires were used to define NSAID use and renal function measurements included serum creatinine and calculated creatinine clearance. Overall, while impaired renal function was slightly more common in NSAID users than non-users (16% vs. 14%), the difference was not significant. However, individuals who used longer half-life NSAIDs (> 4 hours) had a significantly greater prevalence of impaired renal function. Interestingly, diuretics were associated with a significant incidence of renal impairment, OR 3.5 (95% CI 1.6 to 7.6), but no additional interaction with NSAIDs could be identified [100]. No significant interaction between ACE inhibitors and NSAIDs was evident from their data. The authors concluded that elderly patients taking long half-life NSAIDs are at increased risk for impaired renal function. While the information to date is suggestive of an association between high dose and/or long duration NSAID use and ESRD, additional epidemiological studies are needed [99].

Three observational studies using national cohorts have examimed the risk of deteriorating renal function with chronic NSAID exposure. Two of the reports involvedata from the Physician Health Study [99A, 99B] while the third involved the nurses from the National Health Survey [99C]. After adjusting for confounding risk factors none of the studies identified an increase risk of loss of renal function with moderate NSAID intake. More recently Ibanez et al [99D] conducted a 2 year case control study regarding the relative risk of ESRD associated with NSAIDs. They reported a Odd Ratio of 1.22 (CL_{95} 0.89-1.66) for the risk of ESRD associated with NSAIDs.

Calvo-Alen et al. [101] evaluated creatinine clearance, osmolar clearance, free water clearance, sodium excretion and urinalysis in 104 arthritic patients whose treatment with NSAIDs exceeded 2 years compared to 123 health controls. The major abnormal finding was restrict to impaired renal concentrating capacity in the arthritic patients as manifested by a decreased osmolar clearance, increased free water clearance and a decreased urinary density. Compared to controls, no significant differences in either sodium excretion or creatinine clearance were recorded. However, Murray et al. [25] determined the incidence and risk factors for ibuprofen-associated renal impairment by analyzing 1908 computerized patient records. Multivariable analysis of the 343 patient records with renal impairment identified: age, prior renal insufficiency, coronary artery disease, male gender, elevated systolic blood pressure and diuretic use as risk factors. Only two subsets of at risk patients, age > 65 and coronary artery disease, were at greater risk to develop renal insufficiency when compared to acetaminophen.

The observation by Schwarz et al. [90] are germane to the influence of NSAID-induced AKI on the development of chronic renal failure. While NSAIDs accounted for only 20% of the cases of acute interstitial nephritis [90], nearly 2 out of every 3 patients from the NSAID subgroup was found to have permanent renal impairment at follow-up which represented the greatest frequency of any of the drug-induced acute interstitial nephritis.

Papillary necrosis

In a prospective study by Segasothy et al. [102] conducted over 11 years, IVP confirmed NSAID-induced papillary necrosis was reported to occur in 27% of heavy analgesic users. In over half of the cases (55%), the offending analgesic was excess NSAIDs consumption more often a single type rather than multiple agents. In over 80% of the cases the NSAID was prescribed for an arthritic condition, with male: female ratio of 1.9:1. Coexisting additive behavior was rare in the patients include in this study. Because of the wide differences in relative risk noted in these limited studies, plus questions that have been raised as to their validity [9], a precise risk cannot be stated. Papillary necrosis is the least common type of NSAID-induced renal toxicity, but unlike the other types, it is irreversible. Volume depleted patients who ingest large quantities of NSAIDs may be at higher risk for developing papillary necrosis and parenchymal damage is permanent [103-105]. Its cause is likely a combination of decreased renal papillary perfusion and excessive papillary parenchymal NSAID and NSAID-metabolite concentrations.

Definition and differentiation of acute versus chronic papillary necrosis lesion

By definition, papillary necrosis represents the development of irreversible damage within the parenchyma of the renal papillae. The papillae of the kidney contain the tip portions of the long loops of Henle, together with the terminal portions of the collecting duct complexes, which open in to the minor calyces. The minor calyces of the kidneys representing the first location in the upper renal outflow tract into which urine is collected before it travels into the renal pelvis and into the urinary bladder via the ureters.

The mechanism of NSAID-induced acute papillary necrosis is often not clear and the causative role of the NSAID in question may be difficult to delineate because of the presence of confounding factors such as underlying disease, urinary tract infection, and/or concomitant medications. Selected NSAIDs may exert a direct toxic effect on renal papillae and may become highly concentrated in the medullary-papillary region of the kidney. Aspirin depletes cellular glutathione, which would otherwise neutralize the acetaminophen metabolite, N-acetyl-benzo-quinoneimine. Without glutathione, this highly reactive metabolite could lead to cell death [106]. Prostaglandin inhibition may also play a role [9]. Medullary ischemia, a possible precipitating factor in development of papillary necrosis, results from NSAID-induced reduction of blood into the renal medulla in experimental models [107, 108].

The development of acute papillary necrosis, as a consequence of the use of a single NSAID, at recommended dosing levels, is an extremely rare event. In preclinical studies, nearly all of the NSAIDs produced papillary necrosis in experimental animal models. Although, as already identified, clinical toxicity is exceedingly rare it has been reported for ibuprofen [103], phenylbutazone [109, 110], fenoprofen [105], and mefenamic acid [104] and, according to prescribing information, several other NSAIDs.

The chronic progression of events that lead to NSAID/analgesic related papillary necrosis are well known since the days of the first descriptions of chronic combined analgesics abuse nephropathy and the subsequent extensive investigations which defined the consequences of chronic (5-20 years) exposure of the kidney to high doses of analgesic combinations such as salicylate and acetaminophen (the metabolite of phenacetin) often with the addition of caffeine [106]. Fortunately, the incidence of this form of chronic analgesic abuse nephropathy has diminished because of a better understanding of the drugs involved, patient education, and in some countries thanks to efficient regulatory measures. The topic of chronic papillary necrosis related to analgesic-NSAID mixtures is reviewed in detail elsewhere in the text and will not be further discussed here.

The clinical circumstances that lead to chronic "analgesic abuse" nephropathy [111] are quite distinct to the rare occurrence of acute papillary necrosis associated with exposure of the patient to a single NSAID and often with only a short period of drug exposure. In these acute circumstances, the patient will typically present clinically with gross hematuria and may have flank pain suggestive of ureteric obstruction consequent to the passage of a sloughed papilla.

Other NSAID-induced renal syndromes

Phenylbutazone, suprofen, and benoxaprofen produce unique renal syndromes that are of historic interest. Fortunately, the use of phenylbutazone use has diminished because of the availability of safer drugs, and suprofen and benoxaprofen have been voluntarily removed from the market.

Two mechanisms responsible for phenylbutazone-induced acute oligo-anuric renal failure include: 1) inhibition of uric acid reabsorption, leading to hyperuricosuria and, ultimately, bilateral ureteral obstruction due to uric acid stones [112]; 2) an idiosyncratic reaction has been reported that results in acute tubular injury without uric acid precipitation [113].

Suprofen-induced AKI is characterized by acute flank and/or abdominal pain. In series of 16 patients, Hart et al. [114] described that the mean peak serum creatinine was 3.6 mg/dl (range: 2 to 8 mg/dl), which returned to normal limits at follow-up. Suprofen is know to have uricosuric activity leading Hart and colleagues [114] to suggest that this renal syndrome may have resulted from ureteral or tubular precipitation of uric acid.

Benoxaprofen, an NSAID with a very long half-life, was removed from the market in the early 1980s because of severe hepatic toxicity that occasionally resulted in death; however, renal failure was a contributing factor. Risk factors for benoxaprofen-induced toxicity were old age, concomitant diuretic therapy, and likely excessive drug administration.

Renal effects of COX-2 inhibitors

Vane published the seminal work on the mechanism of action of aspirin-like drugs in the early 1970's [115]. Since that time, the goal in NSAID research has been to formulate agents with increased potency and limited toxicity. The elderly comprise the majority of patients who use high doses of NSAIDs for their analgesic and anti-inflammatory effects. However, the gastrointestinal toxic effects of the traditional NSAIDs and underlying disease states, such as hypertension and congestive heart failure (CHF), may preclude their use. Hence, these agents must be used cautiously in this population.

The most recent advance in NSAID pharmacology are agents that specifically block the cyclooxygenase-2 (COX-2) isoform while sparing the effect of COX-1 related activities [116] (Figure 4). These drugs have been designated by the WHO as a new pharmacology category of NSAIDs, namely the 'coxibs' [117]. By blocking COX-2, the intent is to spare toxicity in organs such as the gut and kidney, thereby increase their utility, especially in elderly patients. All of the currently available COX-2 specific inhibitors, i.e. celecoxib, rofecoxib and valdecoxib, have established their safety advantage with respect to clinically important reductions in gastrointestinal toxicity and platelet-sparing characteristics [28, 116-123]. Bleeding complications as seen with aspirin and traditional NSAIDs have essentially been eliminated. However, the clinical impact of the coxibs upon renal and cardiovascular function is an area of evolving information, especially now that it is known that the COX-2 isoenzyme is expressed within the human kidney [15, 17, 124]. The nephrotoxic effects of traditional NSAIDs are well recognized and have been the subject of extensive reviews [4, 125].

Effects on renal function: GFR/ urinary sodium excretion

The effect of COX-2 specific inhibitors on renal function, including sodium excretion, has been assessed in prostaglandin dependent patients. Catella-Lawson et al. [26] enrolled 36 healthy elderly patients for her study, which evaluated not only sodium excretion and glomerular filtration rates, but also changes in body weight, blood pressure and the urinary metabolites of thromboxane. Patients were randomized to either rofecoxib, indomethacin or placebo while receiving a isocaloric diet containing 200 mEq of sodium. Both NSAIDs induced a significant, but transient, decrease in sodium excretion during the first 72 hours of ingestion. Following this sodium excretion returned to pretreatment levels despite continued administration of the NSAIDs. Only indomethacin caused a significant reduction in GFR after 14 days of treatment. Body weight and blood pressure did not change significantly for any of the treatment groups. Inhibition of platelet thromboxane synthesis was limited to indomethacin treated patients, while both rofecoxib and indomethacin were associated with a significant reduction in urinary excretion of the prostacyclin metabolite, 2, 3-dinor-6-keto prostaglandin F_1 . Because of the later finding, the possibility of a prothrombotic state resulting from the administration of coxibs was suggested by these authors. The basis for the speculation is as follows: Activation of platelet aggregation is thromboxane dependent and under the control of the COX-1 isoform. Production of prostacyclin by vascular endothelium is a COX-2 dependent step. By inhibiting the production of prostacyclin, a anti-platelet aggregation factor, this would leave thromboxane mediated platelet aggregation unopposed and could result in a prothrombotic state. However, the anti-platelet aggregation action of endothelin would be unaffected during COX-2 inhibition [8].

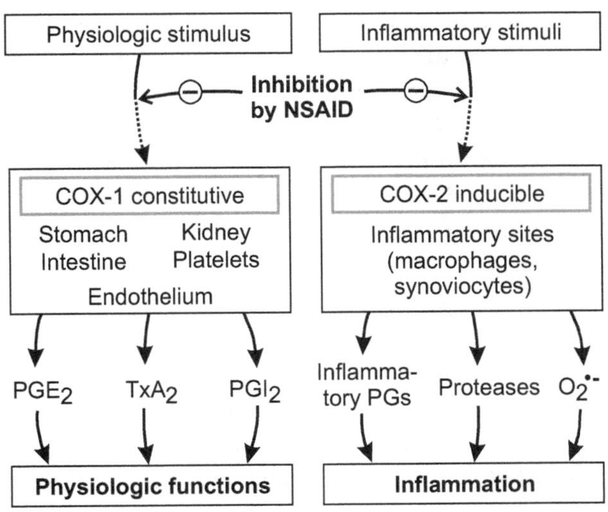

Figure 4. *Different functions of COX-1 and COX-2 in prostag-*

Rossat et al. [126] conducted their renal assessment of COX-2 inhibition using health male volunteers rendered prostaglandin-dependent by a combination of low salt diet and administration of a loop diuretic. Their trial consisted of a parallel, randomized study involving giving either celecoxib, 200 mg bid or 400 mg bid, naproxen 500 mg bid or placebo for seven days. Blood pressure, renal hemodynamics, urinary salt and water excretion were measured before and 3 hours after ingestion of the test drug. The urinary excretion of sodium, potassium, lithium, and water were significantly decreased on both day one and day seven at the second and third hour after administration of either celecoxib or naproxen. Accumulative sodium excretion was significantly reduced during the first 3 days of NSAID dosing, but then subjects escaped from the effect. Glomerular filtration rates were transiently decreased following the 800 mg dose of celecoxib on day one, and the naproxen dose on day seven. These same authors confirmed that lack of an effect of celecoxib on platelet thromboxine synthesis. They concluded that COX-2 inhibition in salt-depleted subjected induced retention of sodium and potassium.

Whelton et al. [19] enrolled 29 healthy elderly individuals in a single blind, randomized, cross-over study to determine the effects of celecoxib on prostaglandin dependent renal function. Either celecoxib or naproxen was given for 10 days followed by a 7 day washout period and then 10 days of the alternate drug. During the first 5 days, celecoxib 200 mg bid was given, then the dose was increased to 400 mg bid for the final 5 days of the trial. Naproxen dose as 500 mg bid throughout the 10 days. Only the –7.5 ml/min/1.73 m^2 decrease in GFR on day 6 of naproxen proved to be significant. Transient sodium retention was noted with both celecoxib and naproxen treatments, returning to baseline within the first 3 days. Both NSAIDs caused a significant reduction in urinary PGE_2 and 6-keto-PGF-$_1$ throughout the 10 days of administration. The authors concluded that, like conventional NSAIDs, celecoxib effects the urinary excretion of both sodium and prostaglandin E2. However, in elderly patients, unlike conventional NSAIDs, celecoxib spares renal hemodynamics.

Swan et al. [127] conducted a multi-center that involved both a randomized, single-dose crossover study and a randomized, parallel group, multidose study involving elderly, salt-depleted subjects. The single dose study involved 15 subjects who where crossed over between rofecoxib 250 mg or indomethicin 75 mg. For the multidose trial 60 subjects received either rofecoxib 12.5 or 25 mg/d, indomethacin 150 mg/d, or placebo for 6 days, with measurement performed during the last 6 hours of study day 6. Peak GFR, measured by either inulin or iothalamate clearance, fell by nearly 40% following acute administration of either rofecoxib or indomethacin. For the multidose trial, the reduction in GFR, while still significant, was less than 10%. While sodium excretion was reduced by both drug following acute administration, only 12.5 mg rofecoxib was associated with significant sodium retention after 6 days of drug. These author concluded that the effects of rofecoxib on renal function resembled nonselective NSAIDs and that COX-2 plays an important role in human renal function.

Collectively, these studies suggest that COX-2 plays a dominate role in the regulation of salt and water excretion in prostaglandin dependent patient, while the role of COX-1 seems to involve the regulation of renal hemodynamics, including GFR. The Swan et al. [127] study suggests that COX-2 may also play a role in regulating GFR; however, the combination of elderly patients who are salt depleted may have provided a more severe hemodynamic stress than was present in the other three studies.

Incidence of adverse cardio-renal events

Serum electrolytes and creatinine

In the recent 8000-patient celecoxib long-term arthritis safety study [118], significantly more patients receiving traditional NSAIDs (ibuprofen or diclofenac) experienced clinically significant elevations in serum creatinine and/or serum urea nitrogen levels when compared to celecoxib. This was confirmed in a follow-up study using the same data base [118A]. In patients defined as having pre-existing uremia, when these patients received either diclofenac or ibuprofen, the had significantly greater increases in serum creatinine than patients receiving celecoxib. In an equally large gastrointestinal safety trial with rofecoxib, the incidence of adverse effects related to renal function for rofecoxib was similar to naproxen (1.2% versus 0.9%, respectively) [119]. When rofecoxib and celecoxib were directly evaluated in elderly hypertensive OA patients who manifested "normal" serum creatinine at the time of study recruitment, the overall incidence of clinically significant increases in serum creatinine, blood urea nitrogen, and serum potassium was 1.5% for both agents [128]. In post-marketing surveillance, AKI has been reported for both coxib compounds. Uniformly, this complication has been reported in patients with significant pre-existing renal impairment (serum creatinine ≥ 3.0 mg/dl [250 mmol/L] prior to coxib treatment). Details of 4 cases of AKI associated with COX-2 specific inhibitor use have been reported in the literature [129, 130]. In each of these cases, creatinine clearances returned to baseline after cessation of COX-2 specific inhibitor therapy. Ahmad et al [131], reported 264 cases of renal failure due to either celecoxib or rofecoxib based on voluntary reported submitted to the FDA AER system. 122 cases occurred with celecoxib and 142 with rofecoxib. Hypertension, diabetes, congestive heart failure and renal insufficiency were shared risk factors for both drugs. However, concomitant use of diuretics, ACE inhibitors and other NSAID's occurred more frequently in patients with renal failure attributed to rofecoxib. No correlation with dose was evident. In of the 122 cases of celecoxib associated renal failure initial renal function was normal, while in 12 of 142 cases of rofecoxib initial renal function was reported to be normal. Zhao et al [132] compared the renal-related adverse drug reactions between rofecoxib and celecoxib as reported to WHO Safety Monitoring Center. The center uses a statistical parameter, e.g. information component (IC), from a Bayesian confidence propagation neural network method to calculate each drug-ADR combination. When the IC values for rofecoxib were compared to celecoxib, an statistically significant adverse renal impact of rofecoxib was present for: water retention (R 1.97 vs. C 1.18, $p<0.01$), abnormal renal function (R 2.38 vs. C 0.70, $p<0.01$), renal failure (R 2.22 vs. C 1.09, $p<0.01$), cardiac failure (R 2.39 vs. 0.48, $p<0.01$), hypertension (R 2.15 vs. C 1.33, $p<0.01$). As with the report of Ahmad et al [131], information as to dosage is missing.

Peripheral edema

In a post-hoc analysis of over 9500 patients with osteoarthritis (OA) or rheumatoid arthritis (RA) enrolled in 12 well-controlled trials, the incidence of celecoxib-induced edema was similar to that observed with the traditional NSAIDs (2.1%) and significantly different from placebo (1.1%) [57]. No correlation was evident between weight gain or blood pressure increase and peripheral edema. There was also no evidence of a dose-related increase in the frequency of edema with celecoxib. No clinically important differences in peripheral edema incidence were found between OA and RA patients who received celecoxib 100-400 mg twice daily (BID) [57]. Unlike celecoxib, the incidence of lower extremity edema with rofecoxib appears to be dose-related. In OA clinical trials to determine the general safety of rofecoxib 50 mg once daily (QD), the incidence of lower extremity edema was 6.3% compared to 3.7% at the recommended OA doses of 12.5 mg and 25 mg QD. In a six-weeks study of 810 older, stable hypertensive patients with OA, those treated with rofecoxib 25 mg QD had significantly more edema than patients treated with celecoxib 200 mg QD (9.5% versus 4.9%; $p = 0.014$) [128]. Similar results were observed in a recent study of the same design in over 1100 patients [133].

Hypertension

Traditional NSAIDs are well known to cause peripheral edema and increases in blood pressure [65, 66, 76]. Two large meta-analyses found increases in mean arterial pressure of 3.5 mm Hg to 6.2 mm Hg [65, 66]. However, the same meta-analyses have concluded that NSAID-induced changes in blood pressure are almost exclusively limited to patients with pre-existing hypertension. This concept may have to change following the report of Dedier et al. [134]. These authors accumulated 381, 078 patient years over an 8 year follow-up to determine if non-narcotic analgesic use was associated with the development of hypertension. Over 10, 000 incident cases of hypertension were identified. Analgesic use was determined by questionnaire. After adjusting for potential confounders, significantly high frequency of hypertension occurred in women taking aspirin 1.21 (95% CI, 1.13 to 1.30); acetaminophen 1.20 (95% CI 1.08 to 1.33); and NSAID's 1.35 (95% CI, 1.25 to 1.46). In addition they identified an increased risk of hypertension with increasing frequency of analgesic use ($p<0.001$). A prolonged increase in diastolic blood pressure of 5-6 mm Hg has been associated with a 67% increased risk of stroke and a 15% increased risk of coronary heart disease [135]. Less well established are the cardiovascular effects on the COX-2 specific inhibitors (celecoxib and rofecoxib), and how they may differ from each other and from traditional NSAIDs. Recent data suggest, however, that there may be differences.

In CRECENT study, patients were randomized to 200 mg of celecoxib once daily (n = 136), 25 mg of rofecoxib once daily (n = 138), or 500 mg of naproxen twice daily (n = 130) for 12 weeks[136]. Twenty-four-hour ambulatory BP monitoring was performed at weeks 6 and 12 of treatment. In this study, the mean 24-hour systolic BP following 6 weeks of therapy was significantly higher for rofecoxib group (from 130.3 +/- 1.2 to 134.5 +/- 1.4 mm Hg; P < .001) compared to celecoxib (132.0 +/- 1.3 to 131.9 +/- 1.3 mm Hg; P = .54) or naproxen (133.7 +/- 1.5 to 133.0 +/- 1.4 mm Hg; P = .74). The BP difference between rofecoxib to celecoxib and naproxen were 3.78 mm Hg (P = .005) and 3.85 mm Hg (P = .005) respectively. Although significantly higher in rofecoxib treated patients, but destabilization of blood pressure occurred in all treatment groups.

In two other clinical studies directly compared celecoxib and rofecoxib in large (> 800 patients), well-controlled trials in older hypertensive subjects with OA increases in blood pressure were observed in 17% of rofecoxib and 11% of celecoxib treated individuals [128]. Similar increases in blood pressure, i.e. Rofecoxib > celecoxib were observed in a recent study of the same design including over 1100 patients [133].

No significant change in blood pressure was noted in a study of 36 healthy normotensive older adults on a fixed-sodium diet when rofecoxib was compared with indomethacin and placebo [68]. Similarly, no effect on systolic or diastolic blood pressure was observed in another study (n=67) of healthy normotensive elderly volunteers that compared in-house administration of celecoxib 400 mg QD, rofecoxib 25 mg QD, and naproxen 500 mg BID for 14 days under a strict weight-maintaining isocaloric diet. Finally, two studies compared the COX-2 specific inhibitors with traditional NSAIDs, one in hypertensive subjects [58] and one in normal subjects. In summary, rofecoxib, unlike celecoxib, is associated with dose-related increases in blood pressure (12.5-25 mg incidence rate = 3.5 %; 50 mg incidence rate = 8.2%)[57]. This differential effect of rofecoxib on blood pressure may be traced to elimination of the diurnal dip. Reitblat et al. [137] compared the effect of rofecoxib and nabumetone on diurnal blood pressure patterns in OA patients with stable hypertension. Nabumetone induced a moderate increase in both day and night blood pressure without changing the biological diurnal variation. Rofecoxib, on the other hand, had no effect on daytime blood pressure but raised nighttime systolic BP +15.7 and diastolic BP +8.5, thus eliminating the biologic diurnal variation.

As noted above, it is suggested from the results of the two large comparator studies in higher risk individuals, that patients who receive celecoxib 200 mg QD will experience significantly less edema and less destabilization of SBP than patients receiving rofecoxib 25 mg QD [128, 133]. The design of these studies mimicked real life conditions (i.e. involving doses commonly prescribed for the management of OA, blood pressure was measured by standard cuff methodology, and there was no control of diet or sodium intake other than that recommended by the treating physician). In contrast, a placebo-controlled study in 67 healthy elderly, normotensive volunteers that compared in-house administration of celecoxib 400 mg QD, rofecoxib 25 mg QD, and naproxen 500 mg BID for 14 days under a strict weight-maintaining isocaloric diet, found no difference among groups in systolic or diastolic blood pressure changes, and reported no incidences of edema. Recently, Dilger et al [138] compared the effects of celecoxib vs. diclofenac on blood pressure and renal function in young and elderly normotensive patients. Using standard arthritic doses of each, they were unable to demonstrate any adverse effect of either drug on blood pressure or renal function on either age group during the 15 days of treatment.

Two studies that compared the interaction of celecoxib with ACE inhibitors found no difference in blood pressure effects compared to placebo [58, 59]. In one study (n=359), the blood pressure (systolic and diastolic) effects of celecoxib 200 mg BID and nabumetone 1 g BID were found to be similar to placebo, but significantly different from ibuprofen 800 mg TID [58]. In the second study (n=178), the effects of celecoxib 400 mg daily and placebo on 24-hour blood pressure in hypertensive patients controlled on lisinopril 10-40 mg daily was evaluated [59]. No difference between groups was observed in 24-hour ambulatory SBP. The difference between groups in 24-hour diastolic BP was only 1.4 mm Hg. The change from baseline in 24-hour blood pressure (1.8 mm Hg/1.4mm Hg) is less than what has been the effect of NSAIDs on the SBP (defined as an increase >20 mm Hg with an absolute value of >140 mm Hg) reported for traditional NSAIDs in ACE inhibitor-treated patients. On the other hand, co-administration of rofecoxib 25 mg daily with benazepril 10-40 mg for 4 weeks in patients with mild to moderate hypertension was associated with a 3 mm Hg increase in mean arterial pressure.

These changes take on significance since one out of every 4 adults has hypertension, and only 27% of this group is on anti-hypertensive medication and have well-controlled blood pressure [139]. The remaining 73% of patients are either unaware of their hypertension, are not taking medication, or are uncontrolled on their current medication [139]. Nearly 50% of people who have a first heart attack and 66% of those who have a first stroke have blood pressures > 160/95 mm Hg [139].

Elevated SBP has been shown to be associated with an increased risk of stroke, CHF, myocardial infarction and death [140, 141]. The authors of the ALLHAT study suggested that a 3 mm Hg increase in SBP could explain a 10% to 20% increase in the incidence of CHF [142]. In a meta-analysis of 15, 693 older patients with isolated systolic hypertension from 8 trials, a 10 mmHg higher initial SBP was associated with relative hazard rates of 1.26 (p=0.001) for total mortality, 1.22 (p=0.007) for cardiovascular mortality, and 1.22 (p=0.02) for stroke [143]. The recent meta-analysis by Aw et al [66A] involving 45451 patients found that rofecoxib was associated with a higher risk of developing hypertension compared to celecoxib.

It has been estimated that approximately 20 million Americans are currently taking concomitant NSAIDs and anti-hypertensive medications [144]. Thus, the potential for destabilization of controlled hypertension or worsening hypertension in those already uncontrolled is of great public health concern.

Cardiovascular diseases

The past few years have been a confusing and frustrating time for many healthcare providers for trying to choose the best therapeutic modality for the treatment of inflammatory conditions. Use of non-selective NSAIDs and COX-2 selective NSAIDS has been under spotlight and investigation by medical community, media, pharmaceutical companies and regulatory agencies. Is there any evidence to support the higher incidence of cardiovascular disease with the use of selective COX-2 inhibitors compared to non-slective NSAIDs? There is no short or simple answer to this question. A review of data reveals that all NSAIDs may cause an increased risk of serious cardiovascular thrombotic events, myocardial infarction, and stroke, which can be fatal. All NSAIDs may have a similar risk. It seems that this risk may increase with dose and duration of usage. Patients with cardiovascular disease or risk factors for cardiovascular disease may be at greater risk.

In Sept. 30, 2004, Merck & Co. Inc. unexpectedly announced a worldwide voluntary worldwide withdrawal of rofecoxib.[145] This action was promoted based on APPROVe (Adenomatous Polyp Prevention on VIOXX) trial.[146] APPROVe study was a three-year, prospective, randomized, placebo-controlled clinical trial in preventing recurrence of colorectal polyps in patients with a history of colorectal adenomas. In this study, patients (n=2586) were randomized to rofecoxib 25 mg daily or placebo. After 18 months of there was an increased relative risk for confirmed cardiovascular events, in the patients randomized to rofecoxib compared to the placebo arm (Serious thrombotic events; HR 1.92 or 1.5%/year). The result of this study was consistent with VIGOR study (Vioxx Gastrointestinal Outcome Research Trial) [119]. The incidents of myocardial infarction, cerebrovascular accidents and deaths were significantly greater with the rofecoxib treatment group versus the naproxen treatment group in the VIGOR trial. The overall incidences of serious adverse events - including myocardium infraction, stroke and death - were significantly greater, and the increased rate was noted to be statistically significant (RR 2.4 $p < 0.001$). Initially, it was suggested that the differing incidence of serious cardiovascular adverse events was most likely due to a cardiovascular protective effect of naproxen. In 2002, Ray and his coworkers investigated in a retrospective observational study whether non-asprin, non-selective NSAIDs provide a cardio-protective effect. This study was conducted by reviewing Tennessee Medicaid data that included cardiovascular risk factor status, prescription data, hospital and outpatient admissions and visits, and death certificate information. This study concluded that the overall rate of cardiac death, hospitalization and admissions rate ratios in the naproxen (both low and high doses) were not significantly different from those of controls. This study clearly demonstrates the lack of any cardioprotective effect of naproxen even in a high-risk population. Ray, et al. published a follow up study in 2002 which further confirms his original study. Initially, it was postulated that he cardiovascular implications of rofecoxib including thrombotic myocardium infraction cerberovasculay events and death, are caused by prostaglandin inhibition and the activation of thromboxane A2 (TXA2) from selective inhibition of COX-2 enzyme. Therefore, inhibition of COX-2 selectively may increase the risk of cardiovascular events. It is critical to know the COX-2 enzyme is constitutively expressed and regulates important physiological functions in the kidney and vascular beds. The new clinical date does not validate this hypothesis any more. When Hunagh and coworkers examined the cardiovascular toxicity of 4 commonly used NSAIDs, no significant differences in the risk for cardiovascular was noted between etodolac, nabumetone, ibuprofen, or naproxen or celecoxib[147, 148]. In TARGET study (n=18, 000 over 12 monthss), patients randomized to the ibuprofen had more cardiovascular events compared to lumiracoxib (2.14% vs. 0.25%, p=0.038) [149] The overall rate of events was similar in the naproxen treated patients compared to lumiracoxib (1.58% vs. 1.48%, p=0.899). The incidence of new onset heart failure also was documented in ibuprofen group than lumiracoxib (1.28% vs. 0.14%; p=0.031). The latest date suggest that patients with preexisting medical conditions appeared to have a significantly higher risk for cardiovascular events associated with the use of all NSAIDs and celecoxib compared with patients without these conditions. The overall instance of hypertension, edema and cardiovascular events is significantly higher for rofecoxib compared to other traditional NSAIDs.

The majority of the evidence against use of COX-2 selective agents and increased risk of cardiovascular events has been derived from three gastrointestinal clinical trails. In Adenoma Prevention with Celecoxib (APC) and Prevention of colorectal Sporadic Adenomatous Polyps (PreSAP) studies approximately 3000 patients with previously documented colorectal adenoma were randomized to high dose celecoxib (400 mg vs 800 mg) and placebo [150]. The objectives of these studies were to assess the efficacy (the recurrence of adenomata) and safety of celecoxib (substantial overdose) at 5 years. After mean period of 33 months, both studies were discontinued due to increase risk of cardiovascular events in the celecoxib recipients' patients.

In APC study, a total of 2035 patients were randomized to celecoxib 200 mg twice a day (400 mg daily) or celecoxib 400 mg twice a day (800 mg daily) or placebo[151]. Patients were closely monitored for recurrence of adenomata and serious cardiovascular events. The recurrence of adenomata was reduced by 29% and 38% in celecoxib 400 and 800 mg daily, respectively compared to placebo group, an increase risk of cardiovascular events noted in both arms of celecoxib groups.

In patients with established cardiovascular disease prior to enrollment to the study, 8.8% experience cardiovascular events compared to 3% of patients in the placebo arm. In patients without established past medical cardiovascular disease, only 2.2% had a cardiovascular events which was lower than patients with past medical history significant for cardiovascular events and were randomized to placebo arm.

In the PreSAP study a total of 1738 patients received either celecoxib 400 mg daily or placebo[152]. Like APC study, patients were closely monitored for recurrence of adenomata and serious cardiovascular events. The recurrence of adenomata was reduced by 32%, but increase risk of cardiovascular events were noticed in this study. Like ACP study, high-risk patients whom randomized to celecoxib 400 mg daily for 33 months had higher incidence of events compared to placebo.

In fact, the result of these studies indicated that low risk of gastrointestinal ulcers or hemorrhages in patients randomized to celecoxib over the placebo group in non-aspirin treated patients. Even in aspirin treated patients only a small but non-significant increase risk of gastrointestinal ulcers or hemorrhages were noted in the celecoxib treated patients compared to the placebo group. In addition, the result of these studies suggests that the dose 800 mg/day should be avoided for long-term use in patients in most patients. Finally in patients with ischemic heart disease celecoxib should be used with caution like most commonly used NSAIDs.

The Alzheimer's Disease Anti-inflammatory Prevention Trial (ADAPT) was another well designed quality clinical study that point toward increase risk of cardiovascular disease associated with the long term use of naproxen compared to placebo group.[153] ADAPT was a randomized, parallel, placebo-controlled, multicenter trial intended to study the efficacy of a naproxen (220 mg po twice a day) and celecoxib (200 mg po twice a day) vs. placebo. A total of 2, 625 dementia-free patients over age of 70 years were enrolled.. These data showed an apparent increase in cardiovascular and cerebrovascular events among patients taking a low dose of naproxen when compared with the placebo arm. In spite of these finds related to naproxen, ADAPT study was discontinued early.

Conversely, in this study no significant increase in risk for cardiovascular event was noted in the celecoxib treated patients compared to placebo arm of the study. Since, it was not clear at that time that all NSAIDS share this risk of cardiovascular disease number of investigators recently have examined the risk of cardiovascular disease among all NSAIDs (non-selective and selective) users.

Schlienger et al. conducted a retrospective case control study from 1992-1997 to investigate if NSAIDs had the same cardiovascular benefit in prevention of AMIs.[154] A total of 3, 319 cases with first time AMIs were determined and matched with 13, 139 controls based on age, gender, and practice and calendar time. After adjustment for other risk factors like smoking, BMI, HRT and aspirin, there was a trend towards increased risk of AMI in NSAID users. The higher doses of NSAIDs were associated with significantly increased risk of MI as much as doubled. The authors concluded that NSAIDs was associated with an increased risk of AMI and no cardioprotection was observed with use of NSAIDs.

In a similar study, Mamdani et al. conducted a retrospective cohort study from 1998- 2001 with NSAID naïve elderly patients who had either celecoxib, rofecoxib, naproxen, or other non-naproxen NSAIDs.[155] Prior to adjusting compared to the community group there was a significant increased risk of AMIs for all NSAIDs except naproxen which only trended towards an increase. But once the values were adjusted for comparison to their controls none of the groups had an increased risk that was significantly different than the controls. This study was designed to determine if naproxen had would decrease the risk of AMIs and they concluded that naproxen has no cardioprotective properties. This study also showed an increased risk of AMI for high dose ibuprofen.

Kimmel et al. preformed an observational case-control study (telephone interviews) to compare the effect the COX-2 inhibitors, non-selective NSAIDs, and concomitant aspirin use on risk of nonfatal myocardial infarction[156]. Information was obtained by telephone interviews and included patients from 36 hospitals from 5 counties who were between the ages of 40 to 75 years (average = 57.4 years). The study group was patients hospitalized for primary nonfatal AMI between May 1998 and December 2002 and the control group was from the community without a history of AMI. The study group included subjects taking rofecoxib, celecoxib non-selective NSAIDs or those not taking NSAIDs . This study suggested that cardiovascular risk factors such as higher BMI and low levels of physical activity were more likely to occur in subjects taking COX-2 inhibitors in comparison to non-users of NSAIDs. Patients who took celecoxib had lower risk for AMI than rofecoxib users (0.43, 95% CI 0.23 to 0.79). Overall, this study lacked an association between COX-2 inhibitor use and non-fatal AMI. The authors concluded that there are differences between the COX-2 inhibitors regarding odds of AMI and more research is necessary. Finally, celecoxib use was not associated with increased risk of nonfatal AMI risk in comparison to NSAID non-users.

Graham DJ et al conducted a nested case-control cohort study to determine the risk of COX-2 inhibitor or non-selective NSAID use for the risk of serious coronary heart disease[157]. Information was obtained from the Kaiser Permanente database and telephone interviews in California, and included patients who had filled at least one prescription for a COX-2 inhibitor or a non-selective NSAID between Jan 1, 1999 and Dec 31, 2001. The study group (n=4669) and control group (n=18, 720) patients were between the ages of 18 to 84 years (average = 66.9 years). This study indicated that rofecoxib significantly increases the risk for developing serious cardiovascular events and high-dose (> 25mg) rofecoxib was associated with higher risk for cardiovascular events when compared to remote NSAID or celecoxib use. The cardiovascular event may occur early (mean= 112.5 days) after the initiation of standard or high dose rofecoxib. In regard to celecoxib a slightly lower risk of cardiovascular events was observed in subjects were taking celecoxib compared to other non-selective NASIDs and naproxen. Naproxen was also associated with a increased risk of serious coronary disease. The authors concluded that rofecoxib and most NSAIDs were associated with an increased risk for cardiovascular events and that celecoxib was associated with insignificant risk of cardiovascular events. In addition naproxen is not cardioprotective agents and was associated with a increased risk of serious cardiovascular disease.

Using the QRESEARCH database Hippisley-Cox et

al identified 9218 cases with a first AMI in a UK general practices over 16 years.[158] Each case of AMI was matched up to 10 controls by age, sex, calendar time, and practice, for a total of 86, 349 control patients. The odds ratios for AMI were derived for each of the class and specific drug and adjusted for possible confounding effects [smoking, comorbidity, diabetes, obesity, socioeconomic deprivation, and concomitant drug use (aspirin, tricyclics, SSRIs, and statins)]. This study revealed that NSAIDs use may increase the risk of AMI. In regard to specific agents, a significantly increased risk of AMI in patients taking rofecoxib, diclofenac, and ibuprofen was noted ($p < 0.01$).

In another observational case-control study, investigators were interested to determine the first-time AMI risk upon the discontinuation of NSAIDs. Information for the study was collected from a British research database and included 8688 study subjects and 33923 matched case subjects.[159] Case subjects were less than 90 years of age who had a first-time AMI between 1995 and 2001. The results of this study are as follows: 1) patients discontinuing NSAID therapy had an increased risk of developing a first-time AMI, 2) subjects using NSAIDs on a long-term basis were more at risk for first-time AMI than patients taking short-term NSAIDs, 3) there is an increased risk of first-time AMI in patients with underlying inflammatory diseases such as RA or SLE, 4) RA and SLE are independent risk factor for new onset cardiovascular events.

Johnsen and coworkers [160] conducted another observational population-based case-control study to identify the risk of AMI in patients who used non-aspirin non-selective and COX-2 specific NSAIDs. Information for the study was collected from hospital discharge databases in Denmark and included 10, 280 cases of first-time hospitalization for AMI and 102, 797 matched controls without a history of AMI. Data was obtained for patients with a mean age of 69.6 years. There was a significantly higher incidence of serious cardiovascular events (AMI) in those whom were taking rofecoxib in comparison to subjects not taking NSAIDs (nonusers). Same observation was noted in the celecoxib, other COX-2 selective inhibitors, naproxen, and other non-selective NSAIDs groups, although to a lesser extent than for rofecoxib. In this study, celecoxib was associated with the lowest risk of AMI when compared to rofecoxib and the other non-selective NSAIDs. The authors concluded that caution should be used with the use of COX-2 inhibitors as well as for the non-selective NSAIDs due to the possible increased risk of MI. Levesque et al [161] conducted a population-based, retrospective, nested case-control cohort study to evaluate the risk of having a first AMI in patients using various types of specific and non-specific COX-2 NSAIDs. Information from the study was collected from computerized health insurance and vital statistic databases from Canada and included elderly population without having a previous AMI, and who were newly treated with an NSAID. The mean age of the patients was 75.2 years. The control group consisted of 56, 880 patients. Current use rofecoxib was associated with increased risk of AMI, and especially at doses ≥ 25mg per day compared with those did not have exposure to NSAIDs. This increased risk of AMI was observed even in elderly populations with a relatively low risk of cardiovascular events. The use of celecoxib or the non-selective NSAIDs was not associated with increased risk for first-time AMI. The authors conclude that using caution is extremely important in high and low risk patients taking rofecoxib or other COX-2 selective inhibitors with equal or greater potency. The increased risk of AMI with rofecoxib is expected due to its pharmacodynamic differences when compared to other NSAIDs.

Same authors investigated time-matched, nested case-control cohort to confirm the risk of AMI in patients taking COX-2 inhibitors (rofecoxib and celecoxib) [162]. Information for this study was collected from Jan 1999 to Jun 2002 from Quebec's computerized health database. The results of this study confirmed that first-time use of rofecoxib was associated with the greatest increased risk of an AMI with a median time frame of 9 days after receiving the prescription (the period of highest risk is within two weeks of obtaining the prescription). This risk was reduced for rofcoxib as drug was taken for a longer duration of time. The overall risk of AMI from rofecoxib returned to baseline shortly after the drug was discontinued. The first-time use of celecoxib was not associated with increased risk of an AMI. The authors concluded that only rofecoxib was associated with a higher risk of cardiovascular events, and celecoxib with notably lower risk of AMI. The authors found similar results to other literature regarding the COX-2 inhibitors and risk of AMI.

Helin-Salmivaara et al. conducted a retrospective study in Finland with case control matches from

2000-2003 [163]. A total of 33, 309 patients had an AMI, while 138, 949 controls were matched for age, gender, hospital. People were broken into groups that were current users (medication started before and ended after the MI) of NSAIDs prior to their AMI or recent users (1-30 days) or past users (31 days-2 years). There were differences between the cases and their controls in the amount of DM, hypertension, and CAD. Current use of any NSAIDs was associated with a significantly higher risk of AMIs regardless choice of the agent. Of the current users, the duration of therapy also carried increased risk of AMI, this was true NSAIDs as a class and when broken into conventional, semi-selective and selective agents. Authors concluded that all current NSAIDs use can modestly increase a person's risk for their first AMI.

Rahme and Nedjar conducted a retrospective study from 1999-2002, of people over 65 years old of which were 158, 910 acetaminophen users, 55, 867 rofecoxib users, 81, 932 celecoxib users, 102, 021 non-selective NSAIDs users, 14, 843 rofecoxib and aspirin users, 20, 421 celecoxib and aspirin users, 22, 374 non-selective NSAIDs and aspirin users, and 54, 503 acetaminophen and aspirin users. Again the risk of cardiovascular disease was noted in all patients taking NSAIDs but the combination of rofecoxib and aspirin pose the greatest risk of AMI for users.

Spalding et al. conducted a retrospective analysis of data from private medical and pharmacy claims involving 31, 743 patients and their risk for cardiovascular events while using anti-inflammatory medications [164]. Of the entire cohort, rofecoxib users were the only group to have a statistically significant increased risk for cardiovascular events over celecoxib, non-selective NSAIDs or non-users. When the groups were broken into normotensive versus hypertensive user groups, again, only rofecoxib hypertensive persons had a significantly higher chance of cardiovascular events than the other hypertensive users and normotensive users. This study suggests that rofecoxib may destabilize blood pressure as a possible and most likely mechanism of increased cardiovascular events.

Hawkey et al. ran a prospective case control study with a total of 205 cases and 258 community controls (those with the same from the same general area, same gender, and age +/- 5 years) and 205 hospital controls (admitted at the same time) to investigate the association between the first AMI and use of NSAIDs and/or aspirin[165]. The final conclusion of the authors was that selective or non-selective NSAIDs were associated with an increased risk of MI and that using aspirin and NSAIDs.

A systematic review and meta-analysis of controlled observational studies was undertaken to compare the risks of serious CV events with nonselective NSAIDs and COX-2 inhibitors. Reported papers on cardiovascular events with selective COX-2 inhibitor and/or nonselective NSAID use, with nonuse/remote were reviewed. The data presented in the study support one more time supported COX-2 selectively and use of celecoxib is associated with similar relative cardiovascular risk to other NSAIDs (Table 4)[166].

Finally, Lee and coworkers reported a higher risk of cardiovascular events with the NSAID use, however most likely to a better pain management , the use of NSAID was associated with lower mortality.[167] In this nested case-control study in a cohort of US veterans (n=500, 000) with a diagnosis of osteoarthritis, the adjusted odds ratios for cardiovascular or cerebrovascular events for any NSAID were 1.14 (95% confidence interval [CI], 1.08-1.21), however, treatment with NSAIDs was associated with a decreased risk of all-cause mortality in both the low (0.72, 95% CI, 0.68-0.77) and high risk (0.79, 95% CI, 0.73-0.86) groups. This study highlights the importance of NSAIDs use in patients with osteoarthritis.

In summary, it is clear that clinical research validates the point that rofecoxib is associated with an

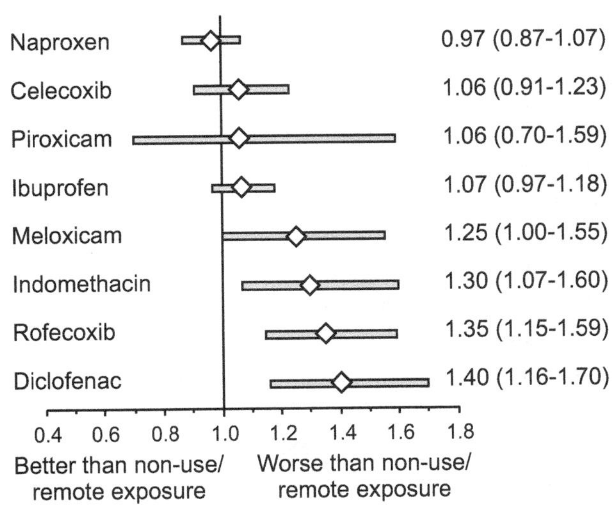

Figure 5. *Meta-analysis of observational studies and overall risk (95% CI) of cardiovascular events [166].*

increased risk of cardiovascular events (Figure 5). Celecoxib is only minimally associated with cardiovascular events (in most cases not statistically significant), but most likely close to naproxen. Although the studies conflict regarding the interaction between aspirin and all NSAIDs, a number of studies has confirmed the interactions between ibuprofen and aspirin. All NSAIDs should be used with cautions in patients with risk of cardiovascular disease [168, 169] (Figure 5).

Congestive Heart Failure

When the NSAID induced decrease of therapeutic efficacy of diuretics is combined with NSAID-induced retention of salt and water, the development of CHF is promoted. Patients with a history of CHF are particularly prone to worsening heart failure when taking traditional NSAIDs. Hospitalizations due to CHF were increased 2-fold in elderly patients who reported concomitant use of diuretics and NSAIDs when compared to those taking diuretics alone [170]. A second study also found a 2-fold increased risk of hospitalization for CHF among elderly patients reporting use of traditional NSAIDs within the week prior to admission [171]. Thus, in susceptible patients, high doses of traditional NSAIDs with prolonged half-lives were associated with increased risk of developing CHF. However, both reports [170, 171] have been criticized for not excluding pre-existing ventricular dysfunction as a risk factor. Feenstra et al. [172], using the Rotterdam population based cohort, conducted a prospective 6½ year study of both 1) the association of NSAID treatment and initial hospitalization for heart failure and 2) the risk of subsequent cardiac decompensation and hospitalization when NSAID are used. These authors could not confirm NSAID-induced heart failure in patients without co-existing ventricular dysfunction. However, in patients with prevalent heart failure, the use of NSAIDs was associated with a significant risk of relapse, adjusted relative risk 9.9 (95% CI, 1.7-57.0). While NSAIDs were not associated with increased heart failure incidence, in heart failure patients, NSAIDs substantially increased the risk of relapse.

In the 6-week comparative study of rofecoxib and celecoxib in elderly hypertensive patients with OA, 4 patients (1.0%) in the rofecoxib group and none in the celecoxib group developed CHF during the study [128].

The purpose of another population-based retrospective cohort study was to determine the risk of heart failure in elderly patients taking non-selective NSAIDs compared to COX-2 inhibitors.[173] The information was obtained through accessing health information databases in Canada and included patients over the age of 65 years (mean=76.1 years) who were prescribed study drugs from April 17, 2000 to March 31, 2001.The study group consisted of patients taking rofecoxib (n=14, 583), celecoxib (n=18, 908), or non-selective NSAIDs (n=5, 391). The matched control group (n=100, 000) had not taken NSAIDs. The results indicate that 1) non-selective NSAIDs and rofecoxib increase the risk for hospital admissions for CHF, while celecoxib did not, and 2) rofecoxib was associated with a higher risk of hospital admissions for CHF in comparison to the non-selective NSAID group, 3) patients who had previously been admitted to the hospital for CHF (within the previous 3 years of the study) had a higher risk of readmission for CHF after taking rofecoxib or non-selective NSAIDs compared to patients non-NSAID users, 4) patients taking the study drugs had a higher risk for primary initiation of therapy for CHF and hypertension. The authors concluded that their results agree with other studies and that differences in cardiovascular risk exist between the NSAIDs. Hudson and coworkers reviewed 8, 512 cases of new onset heart failure and 34, 048 controls. The overall risk factor and patient demographic were similar. The odds ratio for hospital readmit for heart failure was significantly higher the indomethacin treated patients (odds ratio [OR] 2.04, CI 1.16-3.58) and rofecoxib (OR 1.58, CI 1.19-2.11) compared with celecoxib. Authors concluded that there was no difference between naproxen, diclofenac, and ibuprofen compared with celecoxib, however, higher incidence of heart failure admission for the indomethacin and rofecoxib groups [174].

Concurrent use of an oral synthetic prostaglandin analog with a NSAID

The synthetic prostaglandin E1 analogue, misoprostal, has been used in combination with NSAIDs to prevent the NSAID-induced complication of gastric ulcers. It is well tolerated in patients with rheumatologic conditions and does not interfere with NSAID anti-inflammatory activity. Misoprostol appears to exert renal vasodilatory effects in experiment models and in humans. In experimental models, exogenously administered prostaglandin E_1 has renal effects comparable to those of prostaglandin E_2, a potent vasodilatory prostaglandin [175-178]. In rats, misoprostol has mitigated cyclosporine-induced acute nephrotoxicity [179], which is thought to be mediated partly by prostaglandins. Misoprostol minimized NSAID-induced reductions in GFR in a double-blind, crossover study [180]. Six of 12 females with normal renal function experienced at least a 10% decrease in GFR following a 3-day course of indomethacin (25 mg four times daily) ($p<0.05$). When misoprostol was added, four of these six NSAID-sensitive patients experienced no change in GFR. Misoprostol also blunted indomethacin-induced decreases in creatinine clearance and natriuresis in another at-risk group, patients with alcoholic cirrhosis and ascites [181].

In contrast to the above results, Boers and colleagues [182] failed to detect any beneficial effects of misoprostol in a double-blind, crossover study of diclofenac-treated patients with renal insufficiency (creatinine clearance < 80 ml/min/1.73 m^2). Renal prostaglandin production was not measured in this study, which precludes any conclusions regarding the interactions between misoprostol and NSAID on prostaglandins. It is conceivable that the dose of misoprostol (200 μg three times daily) used was inadequate to prevent NSAIDs from suppressing renal prostaglandin production. Alternatively, the dose (50 mg three times daily) and duration (14 to 21 days) of diclofenac may not have been sufficient to suppress urinary prostaglandins or renal function. Furthermore, as noted by the authors of this study, NSAID therapy was not withdrawn, so the effect of diclofenac on renal function is unclear.

Two prospective, crossover, placebo controlled, double-blind evaluations of the nephroprotective role of misoprostol in patients with mild stable chronic renal failure, taking either ibuprofen or indomethacin have been reported [183]. The mean baseline GFR of the patients at the time of entry into the study was 53 ml/min (misoprostol)/55 ml/min (placebo), and 57 ml/min (misoprostol)/57 ml/min (placebo) in Study I (ibuprofen) and Study II (indomethacin) respectively. At this level of renal functional impairment, the use of the non-selective NSAIDs did not produce additional significant impairment of renal function, hence a renal protective role for misoprostol could not be demonstrated. The findings from study I indicate that a numerically small, but significant, improvement in serum creatinine took place during the first week of the study when misoprostol treatment was compared with placebo. A similar trend was noted for the GFR and effective RPF results, but it was not significant.

Wiegmann and colleagues have reported that misoprostol does have a potential nephroprotective effect in patients undergoing radiocontrast procedures [184].

In the setting of chronic renal failure in which NSAIDs are being intercurrently used, we conclude that the nephroprotective role of misoprostol has not yet been satisfactorily resolved and additional controlled trial of misoprostol-NSAID effect in patients with more pronounced chronic renal failure could resolve this quandary.

Conclusions and future challenges

The NSAIDs are considered safe and effective therapeutic agents for the management of a variety of acute and chronic conditions. The risk of inducing acute deterioration renal function after the initiation of any given NSAID is low, nonetheless, the number of at-risk patients is high because of the widespread use of these drugs. Similarly, the risk of inducing other renal syndromes, such as the nephrotic syndrome, is rare, but in view of the massive number of individuals who consume NSAIDs the associated must always be considered in the evaluation of new onset nephrotic range proteinuria.

When selecting a NSAID, it is prudent to consider the potential effect of seemingly minor elevations in SBP. In the one study of elderly treated hypertensive patients with OA, a 3.1 mm Hg increase in mean SBP was measured after 6 weeks of therapy in a rofecoxib-treated group compared to a celecoxib-treated group [128]. Russell et al. estimated the impact of this increase in mean SBP on the occurrence and associated costs of coronary heart disease (CHD) and stroke over a 4-year period [185]. They estimated that a 3.07 mm Hg increase in mean SBP might be associated with 21, 800 additional CHD events and 22, 100 additional stroke events. Treating patients with these events was estimated to cost US$650 million.

Risk factors have been identified for most NSAID-induced renal syndromes (Table 3). It is prudent to avoid high-dose, chronic NSAID therapy in patients with underlying renal impairment (Scr > 1.5 mg/dl), congestive heart failure, cirrhosis, volume contraction due to aggressive diuretic therapy or prolonged dehydration associated with intercurrent illnesses. Unfortunately, this is not always possible. If NSAIDs are necessary in these high-risk groups or in elderly patients, the patient serum creatinine and potassium should be monitored closely and receive appropriate counseling. Monitoring should begin within a week after initiation of a short-acting NSAID such as ibuprofen and continue indefinitely for signs of syndromes having a more delayed onset, such as the nephrotic syndrome with interstitial nephritis.

In the event of NSAID-induced renal failure, the NSAID should be discontinued promptly. The patient should receive supportive care, including temporary dialysis if needed. Beware that after stabilization of renal function, rechallenge with the same or even a structurally different NSAID is likely to reproduce the undesirable side effect. Hence, if anti-inflammatory therapy is essential, underlying risk factors should be identified and eliminated. If this is not possible, as in the case of old age or chronic kidney or liver failure, the patient may require alternative therapy using corticosteroids or other supportive drugs, such as acetaminophen and/or opioids.

In summary, it is clear that massive amounts of traditional NSAIDs and COX-2 specific inhibitors will continue to be consumed worldwide. Because these agents inhibit renal prostaglandin synthesis, they affect salt and water homeostasis and renal hemodynamics. This inhibition will have little clinical effect in the majority of patients, who are well-hydrated, have good renal function, and no concomitant disease states. However, both traditional NSAIDs and COX-2 specific inhibitors must be used judiciously in patients with compromised renal blood flow and cardiovascular events. In general, non-selective NSAIDs and the COX-2 specific inhibitors are well tolerated by the kidney and it is only in the clinical setting of significant pre-existing renal impairment that these agents should be avoided or at least used with very careful monitoring of renal function. With respect to destabilization of blood pressure in treated hypertensive patients or the development of edema in susceptible older individuals, these agents should be used with some caution. Seemingly minor elevations in SBP caused by these agents can potentially have catastrophic cardiovascular complications. Prior to initiation of therapy, each patient should be carefully assessed, weighing the benefit of using these agents against their risks. Thereafter, patients should be closely followed so that appropriate preventive clinical therapeutic strategies can be instituted. Future studies will need to clarify the inherent mechanistic differences that seem to account for the differentiation of cardiorenal safety profiles of the currently available traditional NSAIDs and COX-2 specific inhibitors.

Table 4. Relative risk and odds ratio are given with 95% confidence interval between brackets.

Type of Study	Primary endpoint	Study Population	Increased Risk
Levesque et al. [161] 2005			
Retrospective, population-based, nested, matched, case-control	1st hospitalization with a diagnosis of acute MI, nonfatal or fatal	113927 elderly persons without previous MI & newly treated w/ an NSAID	**Relative Risk:** Rofecoxib 1.24 (1.05-1.46)(more pronounced at higher doses) No increased risk with celecoxib RR 0.99 (0.85-1.16) compared to other NSAIDS. Increased risk for fatal and non-fatal MI in elderly patients without a hx of MI when using rofecoxib. No evidence of increased risk with other NSAIDs (including celecoxib).
Fischer et al.[159] 2004			
Retrospective case-control analysis	First time acute MI	8688 patients 88 years or younger, with first time acute MI and 33923 subjects matched to age, sex, calendar time, general practice attendance	**Odds Ratio :** Cessation of NSAIDs prior to index date with adjustment for risk factors 1.52 (1.33-1.74). Current NSAID use 1.07 (0.96-1.19). Past NSAID use 1.05 (0.99-1.12) Risk of first-time AMI increased for several weeks after the cessation of long-term NSAID use, especially in those with underlying inflammatory diseases. Increased risk not significant of first-time AMI in current NSAID users
Johnsen et al.[160] 2005			
Population-based case-control	First-time hospitalization for MI	10280 cases of first time hospitalization for MI and 102797 sex and age matched controls	**Adjusted Relative Risk:** Rofecoxib 1.8 (1.47-2.21) Celecoxib 1.25 (0.97-1.62) Other Cox-2 inhibitors 1.45 (1.09-1.93) Naproxen 1.5 (0.99-2.29) Conventional NSAIDS 1.68 (1.52-1.85) Increased risk of MI with the use of selective and non-selective NSAIDs. Most risk of MI with use of rofecoxib, and the least risk with celecoxib. Highest risk among the new users of all studied NSAIDs.
Hippisley-Cox et al.[158] 2005			
Nested case control	First ever adverse upper GI outcome and those with first ever recorded	4436 patients with an adverse upper GI event aged 25 years or more at diagnosis. 88867 controls matched by age, calendar time, sex, and practice	**Adjusted Odds Ratios:** Naproxen 2.12 (1.73-2.58). Diclofenac 1.96 (1.78-2.15) Rofecoxib 1.56 (1.30-1.87). Celecoxib 1.11 (0.87-1.41) Other Cox-2 inhibitors 1.75 (1.41-2.15). Other non-selective NSAIDS 1.67 (1.43-1.94)
Kimmel et al.[156] 2005			
Case-control, non-matched	Non-fatal MI's	1718 Case-patients with a first, nonfatal MI admitted to 36 hospitals in a 5-county area. 6800 random controls from same counties.	**Adjusted Odds Ratio:** Non-selective NSAIDS 0.61 (0.52-0.71). All Cox-2 inhibitors 0.73 (0.49-1.07) Rofecoxib 1.16 (0.70-1.93). Celecoxib 0.43 (0.23-0.79) Overall, no association between Cox-2 inhibitor use and non-fatal MI. Different Cox-2 inhibitors differ in cardiovascular effects. More non-fatal MI risk with rofecoxib vs celecoxib.
Mamdani et al.[155] 2004			
Population-based retrospective cohort study	Hospitalization for AMI	593808 Canadian residents of Ontario, 66 years and older. 1000 control subjects matched by age & sex	Overall, no association between Cox-2 inhibitor use and non-fatal MI
Schlienge at al.[154] 2002			
Population based case-control analysis	First-time AMI Free patients, but all tables listed Adjusted odds ratio according to first-time AMI	3315 patients 75 years or less free of metabolic or cardiovascular diseases. 13139 controls matched by age, sex, practice attended, and calendar	**Adjusted Odds Ratios:** Long-term NSAID use relative risk 1.21 (0.94-1.55) Current NSAID use 1.17 (0.99-1.37). Current high dose NSAID use 1.29 (1.05-1.58) No increased risk of first-time AMI (in patients without clinical risk factors for AMI) with current and long-term use of NSAIDs. Increased risk in those using high doses of NSAIDs. *Questionable study.*
Kimmel et al.[186] 2004			
Case-control	First non-fatal MI admitted to hospital	1718 case-patients, 40-75 years of age. 6800 random controls from same countries	**Adjusted Odds Ratios:** Non-selective NSAID use 0.61 All Cox-2 inhibitors 0.73 Rofecoxib only 1.16. Celecoxib only 0.43

Table 4 (continued)

Type of Study	Primary endpoint	Study Population	Increased Risk
Graham et al.[157] 2005			
Nested case-control	Incidence of serious coronary heart disease, defined as acute MI requiring admission or sudden cardiac death	8143 individuals 18-84 years who filled at least one prescription for a Cox-2 selective or non-selective NSAID. 31496 matched by date of the case event, birth year, sex and health plan region	**Adjusted Odds Ratio:** Current use: Celecoxib 0.84 (0.67-1.04). Ibuprofen 1.06 (0.96-1.17). Naproxen 1.14 (1.00-1.30) Rofecoxib all doses 1.34 (0.98-1.82) Rofecoxib (<25mg/day) 1.23 (0.89-1.71). Rofecoxib (>25mg/day) 3.00 (1.09-8.31) Other NSAIDS 1.13 (1.01-1.27) Increased risk of coronary heart disease with all studied doses of rofecoxib (less than celecoxib). No protection against coronary heart disease with naproxen.
Mamdani et al.[173] 2004			
Population-based retrospective cohort	Primary diagnosis of CHF	38882 individuals 66 years and older who were prescribed study and 100000 randomly selected non-NSAID users matched by sex and age	**% study cohort w/ admission procedures for CHF in past 5 years:** Non-NSAID 4% (4475/100000). Celexocib 6% (1170/18908) Rofecoxib 6% (857/14583). Non-selective NSAIDS 5% (542/11606) **Adjusted Rate Ratio:** Rofecoxib relative to celecoxib for admission for CHF 1.8 (1.4-2.4) Non-selective NSAIDs relative to celecoxib for admission for CHF 1.4 (1.0-1.9) and (rofecoxib users relative to non-NSAID users. Additional analysis with age-matched and sex-matched controls showed similar patterns. Increased risk of CHF in elderly patients when using rofecoxib and non-selective NSAIDs (but not celecoxib)
Brophy et al.[187] 2006			
Population-based, retrospective, matched, nested case-control	First hospitalization of acute MI, non-fatal or fatal	3423 individuals with a mean age of 75.3 years. 68456 controls matched on month and year of cohort entry and age, randomly selected from the case's risk-set and assigned the same index date	3, 423 of 122079 were hospitalized for MI during study Period (2.8%) **Adjusted Rate Ratios:** NSAIDs 1.00 (0.75-1.34) No previous MI 1.01 (0.74-1.38) Previous MI 0.95 (0.44-2.04) Naproxen 1.24 (0.83-1.84) No previous MI 1.18 (0.75-1.84) Previous MI 1.56 (0.68-3.58) Rofecoxib 1.28 (1.10-1.49) No previous MI 1.23 (1.05-1.45) Previous MI 1.59 (1.15-2.18) Celexocib 1.08 (0.94-1.25) No previous MI 1.03 (0.88-1.20) Previous MI 1.40 (1.06-1.84) Meloxicam 0.78 (0.36-1.68) No previous MI 0.88 (0.41-1.91) Previous MI no data Increased risk for MI in patients taking rofecoxib without having a previous MI, and especially in those previously having MI (risk doubles). Increased risk of MI when taking celecoxib only in patients having a previous MI.
Helin-SaLmivaara et al.[163] 2006			
Population-based, matched case-control study	First MI requiring hospitalization	33309 cases and 138949 controls matched for age, sex, hospital catchment area	**Adjusted Odds Ratios among current users days 1-14 (study also assessed risk by proximity and category of latest prescription):** Any NSAID 1.39 (1.23-1.58) Conventional (diclofenac, ibuprofen, naproxen…) 1.37 (1.17-1.60) Semi-selective (etodolac, nabumetone, meloxicam) 1.56 (1.18-2.05) Cox-2 selective 1.32 (0.88-1.96) Increased, modest, and similar risk of first-time MI in patients taking conventional, semi-selective, and Cox-2 selective NSAIDs.
Rodriguez, Varas-Lorenzo et al.[188] 2004			
Nested case-control cohort	MI associated with NSAID use	404183 subjects 50-84 years old. 20000 Controls were randomly sampled and frequency was matched to cases by age, sex, and calendar year.	**Multivariate Adjusted Odds ratio:** Current NSAID use vs nonuse 1.07 (0.95-1.20) Previous CHD History 1.12 (0.91-1.38) Incidence rate of MI was slightly higher among people with history of CHD. Estimates for Naproxen, ibuprofen, and diclofenac were comparable with no major effects on the risk of MI.
Rahme et al.[189] 2007			
Population-based retrospective cohort study	First hospitalization for AMI or GI bleeding	510871 patients ≥65 years old.	**Adjusted Hazard Ratio of Hospitalization for AMI/GI vs the Acetaminophen (with no aspirin) Group:** *Aspirin Non-users:* Rofecoxib 1.27 (1.13-1.42) Celecoxib 0.93 (0.83-1.03) Naproxen 1.59 (1.31-1.93) Diclofenac 1.17 (0.99-1.38) Ibuprofen 1.05 (0.74-1.51) *Aspirin users:* Rofecoxib 1.73 (1.52-1.98) Celecoxib 1.34 (1.19-1.52) Naproxen 1.35 (0.97-1.88) Diclofenac 1.69 (1.35-2.10) Ibuprofen 1.51 (0.95-2.41) Acetaminophen 1.29 (1.17-1.42) Naproxen is associated with the highest risk of AMI/GI events in those not taking aspirin. Celecoxib and acetaminophen AMI/GI risk is similar and less than the other NSAIDs (selective and non-selective). Celecoxib and naproxen are the least toxic in comparison to the other NSAIDs in those using aspirin.

Table 4 (continued)

Type of Study	Primary endpoint	Study Population	Increased Risk
Levesque et al.[162] 2006			
Time-matched, nested case-control cohort study	First hospital admission with a discharge diagnosis of acute fatal or non-fatal MI anytime after study entry	113927 patients ≥66 years old without a previous MI	**Adjusted Relative Risk:** Rofecoxib current use 1.24 (1.05-1.46) Rofecoxib first-time use 1.67 (1.21-2.30) Celecoxib current use 0.99 (0.85-1.16) Celecoxib first-time use 1.29 (0.90-1.83) Rofecoxib is associated with a higher risk of MI, and especially within a few weeks of receiving a first prescription (median of 9 days). Celecoxib was not associated with an increased risk of MI
Gislason, et al.[190] 2006			
Case-crossover analysis.	Death from MI and re-hospitalization for AMI	58432 study subjects ≥30 years old hospitalized with first-time AMI	**Hazard Ratio:** Rofecoxib 2.80 (2.41-3.25) Celecoxib 2.57 (2.15-3.08) Ibuprofen 1.50 (1.36-1.67) Diclofenac 2.40 (2.09-2.80) Other NSAIDs 1.29 (1.16-1.43) Increased risk of death with use of all dosages of Cox-2 selective NSAIDs in those with previous MI. Increased risk of death with use of high dose non-selective NSAIDS in those with previous MI. Increased risk of re-hospitalization for MI for all NSAIDs in patients who previously have had MI.
Spalding et al.[164] 2007			
Population-based, retrospective cohort study	AMI and stroke	31, 743 study subjects with arthritis ≥18 years old (including 8579 control subjects, or non-users)	**Hazard Ratio:** *Normotensive:* Non-selective NSAIDS 0.91 (.68-1.21) Rofecoxib 1.05 (0.61-1.80) Celecoxib 1.19 (0.86-1.66) *Hypertensive:* Non-selective NSAIDs 1.21 (0.88-1.67) Rofecoxib 2.16 (1.51-3.09) Celecoxib 1.18 (0.89-1.57) Increased risk for AMI and stroke is not class specific but specific in patients with hypertension. Increased risk of thromboembolic CV events with use of rofecoxib when compared to non-selective NSAIDs and non-users, and especially in patients with hypertension.

References

1. Bennett WM, Henrich WL, Stoff JS, Bennett WM, Henrich WL, Stoff JS. The renal effects of nonsteroidal anti-inflammatory drugs: summary and recommendations. American Journal of Kidney Diseases 1996;28: S56-S62.
2. Bennett WM, Porter GA, Bennett WM, Porter GA. Analgesic nephropathy and the use of nonsteroidal anti-inflammatory drugs in renal patients: new insight. Journal of Nephrology 1998;11: 70-75.
3. Whelton A, Hamilton CW, Whelton A, Hamilton CW. Nonsteroidal anti-inflammatory drugs: effects on kidney function. Journal of Clinical Pharmacology 1991;31: 588-598.

3A. Source: IMS Health, IMS National Prescription Audit PLUS (TM), 3/2007, used with permission

4. Whelton A, Whelton A. Nephrotoxicity of nonsteroidal anti-inflammatory drugs: physiologic foundations and clinical implications. American Journal of Medicine 1999;106: 13S-24S.
5. Brater DC, Brater DC. Anti-inflammatory agents and renal function. Seminars in Arthritis & Rheumatism 2002;32: 33-42.
6. Breyer MD, Hao C, Qi Z, Breyer MD, Hao C, Qi Z. Cyclooxygenase-2 selective inhibitors and the kidney. Current Opinion in Critical Care 2001;7: 393-400.
7. Oates JA, FitzGerald GA, Branch RA et al. Clinical implications of prostaglandin and thromboxane A2 formation (2). New England Journal of Medicine 1988;319: 761-767.
8. FitzGerald GA, Patrono C, FitzGerald GA, Patrono C. The coxibs, selective inhibitors of cyclooxygenase-2. New England Journal of Medicine 2001;345: 433-442.
9. Clive DM, Stoff JS, Clive DM, Stoff JS. Renal syndromes associated with nonsteroidal antiinflammatory drugs. New England Journal of Medicine 1984;310: 563-572.
10. Stokes JB, Stokes JB. Effect of prostaglandin E2 on chloride transport across the rabbit thick ascending limb of Henle. Selective inhibitions of the medullary portion. Journal of Clinical Investigation 1979;64: 495-502.
11. Breyer MD, Zhang Y, Guan YF et al. Regulation of renal function by prostaglandin E receptors. Kidney International - Supplement 1998;67: S88-S94.

12. O'Banion MK, Winn VD, Young DA, O'Banion MK, Winn VD, Young DA. cDNA cloning and functional activity of a glucocorticoid-regulated inflammatory cyclooxygenase. Proceedings of the National Academy of Sciences of the United States of America 1992;89: 4888-4892.
13. Crofford LJ, Crofford LJ. COX-1 and COX-2 tissue expression: implications and predictions. Journal of Rheumatology - Supplement 1997;49: 15-19.
14. Hla T, Neilson K, Hla T, Neilson K. Human cyclooxygenase-2 cDNA. Proceedings of the National Academy of Sciences of the United States of America 1992;89: 7384-7388.
15. Komhoff M, Grone HJ, Klein T et al. Localization of cyclooxygenase-1 and -2 in adult and fetal human kidney: implication for renal function. American Journal of Physiology 1997;272: F460-F468.
16. Harris RC, McKanna JA, Akai Y et al. Cyclooxygenase-2 is associated with the macula densa of rat kidney and increases with salt restriction. Journal of Clinical Investigation 1994;94: 2504-2510.
17. Whelton A, Whelton A. Renal aspects of treatment with conventional nonsteroidal anti-inflammatory drugs versus cyclooxygenase-2-specific inhibitors. American Journal of Medicine 2001;110 Suppl 3A: 33S-42S.
18. Blume C, Heise G, Muhlfeld A et al. Effect of flosulide, a selective cyclooxygenase 2 inhibitor, on passive heymann nephritis in the rat. Kidney International 1999;56: 1770-1778.
19. Whelton A, Schulman G, Wallemark C et al. Effects of celecoxib and naproxen on renal function in the elderly. Archives of Internal Medicine 2000;160: 1465-1470.
20. Mitchell JA, Akarasereenont P, Thiemermann C et al. Selectivity of nonsteroidal antiinflammatory drugs as inhibitors of constitutive and inducible cyclooxygenase. Proceedings of the National Academy of Sciences of the United States of America 1993;90: 11693-11697.
21. McMurray RW, Hardy KJ, McMurray RW, Hardy KJ. Cox-2 inhibitors: today and tomorrow. American Journal of the Medical Sciences 2002;323: 181-189.
22. Harris RC, Harris RC. Cyclooxygenase-2 in the kidney. Journal of the American Society of Nephrology 2000;11: 2387-2394.
23. Stokes JB, Kokko JP, Stokes JB, Kokko JP. Inhibition of sodium transport by prostaglandin E2 across the isolated, perfused rabbit collecting tubule. Journal of Clinical Investigation 1977;59: 1099-1104.
24. Schlondorff D, Schlondorff D. Renal complications of nonsteroidal anti-inflammatory drugs. Kidney International 1993;44: 643-653.
25. Murray MD, Brater DC, Tierney WM et al. Ibuprofen-associated renal impairment in a large general internal medicine practice. American Journal of the Medical Sciences 1990;299: 222-229.
26. Catella-Lawson F, McAdam B, Morrison BW et al. Effects of specific inhibition of cyclooxygenase-2 on sodium balance, hemodynamics, and vasoactive eicosanoids. Journal of Pharmacology & Experimental Therapeutics 1999;289: 735-741.
27. Van HA, Schwartz JI, Depre M et al. Comparative inhibitory activity of rofecoxib, meloxicam, diclofenac, ibuprofen, and naproxen on COX-2 versus COX-1 in healthy volunteers. Journal of Clinical Pharmacology 2000;40: 1109-1120.
28. Ormrod D, Wellington K, Wagstaff AJ, Ormrod D, Wellington K, Wagstaff AJ. Valdecoxib. . Drugs 2002;62: 2059-2071.
29. Sedor JR, Williams SL, Chremos AN et al. Effects of sulindac and indomethacin on renal prostaglandin synthesis. Clinical Pharmacology & Therapeutics 1984;36: 85-91.
30. Berg KJ, Berg KJ. Acute effects of acetylsalicylic acid on renal function in normal man. European Journal of Clinical Pharmacology 1977;11: 117-123.
31. Donker AJ, Arisz L, Brentjens JR et al. The effect of indomethacin on kidney function and plasma renin activity in man. Nephron 1976;17: 288-296.
32. Perez GS, Garcia Rodriguez LA, Raiford DS et al. Nonsteroidal anti-inflammatory drugs and the risk of hospitalization for acute renal failure.. Archives of Internal Medicine 1996;156: 2433-2439.
32A. Schneider V, Levesque LE, Zhang B, Hutchinson T, Brophy JM. Association of selective and conventional nonsteroidal antiinflammatory drugs with acute renal failure: A population-based, nested case-control analysis. Am J Epidemiol 2006;164:881-889.
32B. Clinard F, Sgro C, Bardou M, HillonP, Dumas M, Kreft-Jais C, Escousse A, Bonithon-Kopp C. Association between concomitant use of several systemic NSAIDs and an excess risk of adverse drug reaction. A case/non-case study from the French pharmacovigilance system database. Eur J Clin Pharamcol. 2004;60:279-283
33. Evans JM, McGregor E, McMahon AD et al. Non-steroidal anti-inflammatory drugs and hospitalization for acute renal failure. Qjm 1995;88: 551-557.
34. Griffin MR, Yared A, Ray WA, Griffin MR, Yared A, Ray WA. Nonsteroidal antiinflammatory drugs and acute renal failure in elderly persons. American Journal of Epidemiology 2000;151: 488-496.
34A. Huerta C, Castellsague J, Varas-Lorenzo C, Gracia-Rodriguez LA. Nonsteroidal anti-inflammatory drugs and the risk of ARF in the general population. Am J Kid Dis 2005;45:;531-542

35. Blackshear JL, Napier JS, Davidman M et al. Renal complications of nonsteroidal antiinflammatory drugs: identification and monitoring of those at risk. Seminars in Arthritis & Rheumatism 1985;14: 163-175.
36. Feldman HI, Kinman JL, Berlin JA et al. Parenteral ketorolac: the risk for acute renal failure.. Annals of Internal Medicine 1997;126: 193-199.
37. Zipser RD, Hoefs JC, Speckart PF et al. Prostaglandins: modulators of renal function and pressor resistance in chronic liver disease. Journal of Clinical Endocrinology & Metabolism 1979;48: 895-900.
38. Zipser RD, Radvan GH, Kronborg IJ et al. Urinary thromboxane B2 and prostaglandin E2 in the hepatorenal syndrome: evidence for increased vasoconstrictor and decreased vasodilator factors. Gastroenterology 1983;84: 697-703.
39. Walshe JJ, Venuto RC, Walshe JJ, Venuto RC. Acute oliguric renal failure induced by indomethacin: possible mechanism. Annals of Internal Medicine 1979;91: 47-49.
40. Arisz L, Donker AJ, Brentjens JR et al. The effect of indomethacin on proteinuria and kidney function in the nephrotic syndrome. Acta Medica Scandinavica 1976;199: 121-125.
41. Kleinknecht C, Broyer M, Gubler MC et al. Irreversible renal failure after indomethacin in steroid-resistant nephrosis. New England Journal of Medicine 1980;302: 691.
42. Kimberly RP, Gill JR, Jr., Bowden RE et al. Elevated urinary prostaglandins and the effects of aspirin on renal function in lupus erythematosus. Annals of Internal Medicine 1978;89: 336-341.
43. Fong HJ, Cohen AH, Fong HJ, Cohen AH. Ibuprofen-induced acute renal failure with acute tubular necrosis. American Journal of Nephrology 1982;2: 28-31.
44. Favre L, Glasson P, Vallotton MB, Favre L, Glasson P, Vallotton MB. Reversible acute renal failure from combined triamterene and indomethacin: a study in healthy subjects. Annals of Internal Medicine 1982;96: 317-320.
45. Whelton A, Stout RL, Spilman PS et al. Renal effects of ibuprofen, piroxicam, and sulindac in patients with asymptomatic renal failure. A prospective, randomized, crossover comparison.. Annals of Internal Medicine 1990;112: 568-576.
46. Whelton A, Whelton A. Renal effects of over-the-counter analgesics. Journal of Clinical Pharmacology 1995;35: 454-463.
47. Perazella MA, Perazella MA. Drug-induced hyperkalemia: old culprits and new offenders. American Journal of Medicine 2000;109: 307-314.
48. Galler M, Folkert VW, Schlondorff D, Galler M, Folkert VW, Schlondorff D. Reversible acute renal insufficiency and hyperkalemia following indomethacin therapy. JAMA 1981;246: 154-155.
49. Findling JW, Beckstrom D, Rawsthorne L et al. Indomethacin-induced hyperkalemia in three patients with gouty arthritis. JAMA 1980;244: 1127-1128.
50. Nicholls MG, Espiner EA, Nicholls MG, Espiner EA. Indomethacin-induced azotaemia and hyperkalaemia: a case study. New Zealand Medical Journal 1981;94: 377-379.
51. Paladini G, Tonazzi C, Paladini G, Tonazzi C. Indomethacin-induced hyperkalemia and renal failure in multiple myeloma. Acta Haematologica 1982;68: 256-260.
52. Akbarpour F, Afrasiabi A, Vaziri ND, Akbarpour F, Afrasiabi A, Vaziri ND. Severe hyperkalemia caused by indomethacin and potassium supplementation. Southern Medical Journal 1985;78: 756-757.
53. Mor R, Pitlik S, Rosenfeld JB, Mor R, Pitlik S, Rosenfeld JB. Indomethacin- and Moduretic--induced hyperkalemia. Israel Journal of Medical Sciences 1983;19: 535-537.
54. Goldszer RC, Coodley EL, Rosner MJ et al. Hyperkalemia associated with indomethacin. Archives of Internal Medicine 1981;141: 802-804.
55. MacCarthy EP, Frost GW, Strokes GS, MacCarthy EP, Frost GW, Strokes GS. Indomethacin-induced hyperkalaemia. Medical Journal of Australia 1979;1: 550.
56. Tan SY, Shapiro R, Franco R et al. Indomethacin-induced prostaglandin inhibition with hyperkalemia. A reversible cause of hyporeninemic hypoaldosteronism. Annals of Internal Medicine 1979;90: 783-785.
57. Whelton A, Maurath CJ, Verburg KM et al. Renal safety and tolerability of celecoxib, a novel cyclooxygenase-2 inhibitor. American Journal of Therapeutics 2000;7: 159-175.
58. Palmer RH, Haig AE, Flavin SK, Lyengaer NK. Effects of Ibuprofen, nabumetone and celecoxib on blood pressure control in hypertensive patients on ACE inhibitors. American Journal of Hypertension 2001;14: 85A.
59. White WB, Kent J, Taylor A et al. Effects of celecoxib on ambulatory blood pressure in hypertensive patients on ACE inhibitors. Hypertension 2002;39: 929-934.
60. Orloff J, Handler Js, Bergstrom S, Orloff J, Handler Js, Bergstrom S. Effect Of prostaglandin (PGE-1) on the permeability response of toad bladder to vasopressin, theophylline and adenosine 3', 5'-monophosphate. Nature 1965;205: 397-398.
61. Anderson RJ, Berl T, McDonald KD et al. Evidence for an *in vivo* antagonism between vasopressin and prostaglandin in the mammalian kidney. Journal of Clinical Investigation 1975;56: 420-426.

62. Schooley RT, Wagley PF, Lietman PS, Schooley RT, Wagley PF, Lietman PS. Edema associated with ibuprofen therapy. JAMA 1977;237: 1716-1717.
63. Blum M, Aviram A, Blum M, Aviram A. Ibuprofen induced hyponatraemia. Rheumatology & Rehabilitation 1980;19: 258-259.
64. Gurwitz JH, Avorn J, Bohn RL et al. Initiation of antihypertensive treatment during nonsteroidal anti-inflammatory drug therapy. JAMA 1994;272: 781-786.
65. Pope JE, Anderson JJ, Felson DT, Pope JE, Anderson JJ, Felson DT. A meta-analysis of the effects of nonsteroidal anti-inflammatory drugs on blood pressure. Archives of Internal Medicine 1993;153: 477-484.
66. Johnson AG, Nguyen TV, Day RO, Johnson AG, Nguyen TV, Day RO. Do nonsteroidal anti-inflammatory drugs affect blood pressure? A meta-analysis.. Annals of Internal Medicine 1994;121: 289-300.
66A. Aw TJ, Haas SJ, Liew D, Krum H. Meta-analysis of Cyclooxygenase -2 inhibitors and their effects on blood pressure. Arch Intern Med 2005; 165:490-496
66B. Gaziano JM. Nonnarcotic analgesics and hypertension. Am J Cardiol 2006; 97(suppl):10E-16E.
67. Fogari R, Zoppi A, Carretta R et al. Effect of indomethacin on the antihypertensive efficacy of valsartan and lisinopril: a multicentre study. Journal of Hypertension 2002;20: 1007-1014.
68. Ruoff GE, Ruoff GE. The impact of nonsteroidal anti-inflammatory drugs on hypertension: alternative analgesics for patients at risk. Clinical Therapeutics 1998;20: 376-387.
69. Celis H, Thijs L, Staessen JA et al. Interaction between nonsteroidal anti-inflammatory drug intake and calcium-channel blocker-based antihypertensive treatment in the Syst-Eur trial. Journal of Human Hypertension 2001;15: 613-618.
69A. Wang J, Mullins CD, Mamdani M, Rublee DA, Shaya FT. New diagnosis of hypertension among celecoxib and nonselective NSAID users: A population-based cohort study. Ann Pharmacother 2007;41:937-43.
70. Raij L, Baylis C, Raij L, Baylis C. Glomerular actions of nitric oxide. Kidney International 1995;48: 20-32.
71. Taddei S, Virdis A, Mattei P et al. Aging and endothelial function in normotensive subjects and patients with essential hypertension. Circulation 1995;91: 1981-1987.
72. Forte P, Copland M, Smith LM et al. Basal nitric oxide synthesis in essential hypertension.. Lancet 1997;349: 837-842.
73. Campese VM, Amar M, Anjali C et al. Effect of L-arginine on systemic and renal haemodynamics in salt-sensitive patients with essential hypertension. Journal of Human Hypertension 1997;11: 527-532.
74. Perinotto P, Biggi A, Carra N et al. Angiotensin II and prostaglandin interactions on systemic and renal effects of L-NAME in humans. Journal of the American Society of Nephrology 2001;12: 1706-1712.
75. Mulkerrin EC, Clark BA, Epstein FH, Mulkerrin EC, Clark BA, Epstein FH. Increased salt retention and hypertension from non-steroidal agents in the elderly. Qjm 1997;90: 411-415.
76. Alam S, Purdie DM, Johnson AG, Alam S, Purdie DM, Johnson AG. Evaluation of the potential interaction between NaCl and prostaglandin inhibition in elderly individuals with isolated systolic hypertension. Journal of Hypertension 1999;17: 1195-1202.
77. Brater DC, Anderson S, Baird B et al. Effects of ibuprofen, naproxen, and sulindac on prostaglandins in men. Kidney International 1985;27: 66-73.
78. Bunning RD, Barth WF, Bunning RD, Barth WF. Sulindac. A potentially renal-sparing nonsteroidal anti-inflammatory drug. JAMA 1982;248: 2864-2867.
79. Ciabattoni G, Cinotti GA, Pierucci A et al. Effects of sulindac and ibuprofen in patients with chronic glomerular disease. Evidence for the dependence of renal function on prostacyclin. New England Journal of Medicine 1984;310: 279-283.
80. Klassen DK, Stout RL, Spilman PS et al. Sulindac kinetics and effects on renal function and prostaglandin excretion in renal insufficiency. Journal of Clinical Pharmacology 1989;29: 1037-1042.
81. Mistry CD, Lote CJ, Currie WJ et al. Effects of sulindac on renal function and prostaglandin synthesis in patients with moderate chronic renal insufficiency. Clinical Science 1986;70: 501-505.
82. Quintero E, Gines P, Arroyo V et al. Sulindac reduces the urinary excretion of prostaglandins and impairs renal function in cirrhosis with ascites. Nephron 1986;42: 298-303.
83. Rossert J, Rossert J. Drug-induced acute interstitial nephritis. Kidney International 2001;60: 804-817.
84. Porile JL, Bakris GL, Garella S, Porile JL, Bakris GL, Garella S. Acute interstitial nephritis with glomerulopathy due to nonsteroidal anti-inflammatory agents: a review of its clinical spectrum and effects of steroid therapy. Journal of Clinical Pharmacology 1990;30: 468-475.
85. Rocha JL, Fernandez-Alonso J, Rocha JL, Fernandez-Alonso J. Acute tubulointerstitial nephritis associated with the selective COX-2 enzyme inhibitor, rofecoxib.. Lancet 2001;357: 1946-1947.
86. Henao J, Hisamuddin I, Nzerue CM et al. Celecoxib-induced acute interstitial nephritis.. American Journal of Kidney Diseases 2002;39: 1313-1317.
87. Alper AB, Jr., Meleg-Smith S, Krane NK, Alper ABJ, Meleg-Smith S, Krane NK. Nephrotic syndrome and interstitial nephritis associated with celecoxib. American Journal of Kidney Diseases 2002;40: 1086-1090.

88. Abraham PA, Keane WF, Abraham PA, Keane WF. Glomerular and interstitial disease induced by nonsteroidal anti-inflammatory drugs. American Journal of Nephrology 1984;4: 1-6.
89. Levin ML, Levin ML. Patterns of tubulo-interstitial damage associated with nonsteroidal antiinflammatory drugs. Seminars in Nephrology 1988;8: 55-61.
90. Schwarz A, Krause PH, Kunzendorf U et al. The outcome of acute interstitial nephritis: risk factors for the transition from acute to chronic interstitial nephritis.. Clinical Nephrology 2000;54: 179-190.
91. Ravnskov U, Ravnskov U. Glomerular, tubular and interstitial nephritis associated with non-steroidal antiinflammatory drugs. Evidence of a common mechanism. British Journal of Clinical Pharmacology 1999;47: 203-210.
92. Bender WL, Whelton A, Beschorner WE et al. Interstitial nephritis, proteinuria, and renal failure caused by nonsteroidal anti-inflammatory drugs. Immunologic characterization of the inflammatory infiltrate. American Journal of Medicine 1984;76: 1006-1012.
93. Stachura I, Jayakumar S, Bourke E, Stachura I, Jayakumar S, Bourke E. T and B lymphocyte subsets in fenoprofen nephropathy. American Journal of Medicine 1983;75: 9-16.
94. Shibasaki T, Ishimoto F, Sakai O et al. Clinical characterization of drug-induced allergic nephritis. American Journal of Nephrology 1991;11: 174-180.
95. Radford MG, Jr., Holley KE, Grande JP et al. Reversible membranous nephropathy associated with the use of nonsteroidal anti-inflammatory drugs. JAMA 1996;276: 466-469.
96. Perneger TV, Whelton PK, Klag MJ, Perneger TV, Whelton PK, Klag MJ. Risk of kidney failure associated with the use of acetaminophen, aspirin, and nonsteroidal antiinflammatory drugs. New England Journal of Medicine 1994;331: 1675-1679.
97. Sandler DP, Burr FR, Weinberg CR, Sandler DP, Burr FR, Weinberg CR. Nonsteroidal anti-inflammatory drugs and the risk for chronic renal disease.. Annals of Internal Medicine 1991;115: 165-172.
98. Field TS, Gurwitz JH, Glynn RJ et al. The renal effects of nonsteroidal anti-inflammatory drugs in older people: findings from the Established Populations for Epidemiologic Studies of the Elderly. Journal of the American Geriatrics Society 1999;47: 507-511.
99. Sturmer T, Elseviers MM, De Broe ME, Sturmer T, Elseviers MM, De Broe ME. Nonsteroidal anti-inflammatory drugs and the kidney. . Current Opinion in Nephrology & Hypertension 2001;10: 161-163.
99A. Rexrode KM, Buring JE, Glynn RJ, Stampfer MJ, Youngman LD, Gaziano JM. Analgesic use and renal function in men. JAMA 2001;286:315-321.
99B. Kurth T, Glynn RJ, Walker AM, Rexrode KM, Buring JE, Stampfer MJ, Hennekens CH, Gaziano JM. Analgesic use and change in kidney function in apparently healthy men. Am J Kid Dis 2003;42:234-244.
99C. Curhan GC, Knight EL, Rosner B, Hankinson SE, Stampfer MJ. Lifetime nonnarcotic analgesic use and decline in renal function in women.Arch Intern Med 2004;164:1519-1524
99D. Ibanez, L, Morlans M, Vidal X, Martinez MJ, Laporte JR. Case-control study of regular analgesic and nonsteroidal anti-inflammatoryuse and end-stage renal disease. Kid Internal 2005;67:2393-2398.
100. Sturmer T, Erb A, Keller F et al. Determinants of impaired renal function with use of nonsteroidal anti-inflammatory drugs: the importance of half-life and other medications. American Journal of Medicine 2001;111: 521-527.
101. Calvo-Alen J, De Cos MA, Rodriguez-Valverde V et al. Subclinical renal toxicity in rheumatic patients receiving longterm treatment with nonsteroidal antiinflammatory drugs. Journal of Rheumatology 1994;21: 1742-1747.
102. Segasothy M, Chin GL, Sia KK et al. Chronic nephrotoxicity of anti-inflammatory drugs used in the treatment of arthritis. British Journal of Rheumatology 1995;34: 162-165.
103. Shah GM, Muhalwas KK, Winer RL, Shah GM, Muhalwas KK, Winer RL. Renal papillary necrosis due to ibuprofen. Arthritis & Rheumatism 1981;24: 1208-1210.
104. Robertson CE, Ford MJ, Van S, V et al. Mefenamic acid nephropathy. Lancet 1980;2: 232-233.
105. Husserl FE, Lange RK, Kantrow CM, Jr., Husserl FE, Lange RK, Kantrow CMJ. Renal papillary necrosis and pyelonephritis accompanying fenoprofen therapy. JAMA 1979;242: 1896-1898.
106. Kincaid-Smith P, Kincaid-Smith P. Effects of non-narcotic analgesics on the kidney. Drugs 1986;32 Suppl 4: 109-128.
107. Kirschenbaum MA, White N, Stein JH et al. Redistribution of renal cortical blood flow during inhibition of prostaglandin synthesis. American Journal of Physiology 1974;227: 801-805.
108. Stein JH, Fadem SZ, Stein JH, Fadem SZ. The renal circulation. JAMA 1978;239: 1308-1312.
109. Lourie SH, Denman SJ, Schroeder ET, Lourie SH, Denman SJ, Schroeder ET. Association of renal papillary necrosis and ankylosing spondylitis. Arthritis & Rheumatism 1977;20: 917-921.
110. Morales A, Steyn J, Morales A, Steyn J. Papillary necrosis following phenylbutazone ingestion. Archives of Surgery 1971;103: 420-421.
111. Fored CM, Ejerblad E, Lindblad P et al. Acetaminophen, aspirin, and chronic renal failure.. New England Journal of Medicine 2001;345: 1801-1808.
112. Weisman J, Bloom B. Anuria folloing phenylbutazone therapy. NEJM 1955;252: 1086-1087.

113. Lipsett M, Goldman R. Phenylbutazone toxicity:report of a case of acute renal failure. Annual of Internal Medicine 2007;41: 1075-1079.

114. Hart D, Ward M, Lifschitz MD, Hart D, Ward M, Lifschitz MD. Suprofen-related nephrotoxicity. A distinct clinical syndrome. Annals of Internal Medicine 1987;106: 235-238.

115. Vane JR, Vane JR. Inhibition of prostaglandin synthesis as a mechanism of action for aspirin-like drugs. Nature - New Biology 1971;231: 232-235.

116. Verburg KM, Maziasz TJ, Weiner E et al. Cox-2-specific inhibitors: definition of a new therapeutic concept. American Journal of Therapeutics 2001;8: 49-64.

117. Lipsky LP, Abramson SB, Crofford L et al. The classification of cyclooxygenase inhibitors. Journal of Rheumatology 1998;25: 2298-2303.

118. Silverstein FE, Faich G, Goldstein JL et al. Gastrointestinal toxicity with celecoxib vs nonsteroidal anti-inflammatory drugs for osteoarthritis and rheumatoid arthritis: the CLASS study: A randomized controlled trial. Celecoxib Long-term Arthritis Safety Study.. JAMA 2000;284: 1247-1255.

118A.Whelton A, Lefkowith JL, West CR, Verburg KM. Cardiorenal effects of celecoxib as compared with the nonsteroidal anti-inflammatory drugs diclofenac and ibuprofen. Kid Internal 2006;70:1495-1502

119. Bombardier C, Laine L, Reicin A et al. Comparison of upper gastrointestinal toxicity of rofecoxib and naproxen in patients with rheumatoid arthritis. VIGOR Study Group.. New England Journal of Medicine 2002;343: 1520-1528.

120. Goldstein JL, Silverstein FE, Agrawal NM et al. Reduced risk of upper gastrointestinal ulcer complications with celecoxib, a novel COX-2 inhibitor. American Journal of Gastroenterology 2000;95: 1681-1690.

121. Leese PT, Hubbard RC, Karim A et al. Effects of celecoxib, a novel cyclooxygenase-2 inhibitor, on platelet function in healthy adults: a randomized, controlled trial. Journal of Clinical Pharmacology 2000;40: 124-132.

122. 127. Gastroenterology 2007.

123. Langman MJ, Jensen DM, Watson DJ et al. Adverse upper gastrointestinal effects of rofecoxib compared with NSAIDs.. JAMA 1999;282: 1929-1933.

124. O'Neill GP, Ford-Hutchinson AW, O'Neill GP, Ford-Hutchinson AW. Expression of mRNA for cyclooxygenase-1 and cyclooxygenase-2 in human tissues. FEBS Letters 1993;330: 156-160.

125. Whelton A, Whelton A. Renal and related cardiovascular effects of conventional and COX-2-specific NSAIDs and non-NSAID analgesics. American Journal of Therapeutics 2000;7: 63-74.

126. Rossat J, Maillard M, Nussberger J et al. Renal effects of selective cyclooxygenase-2 inhibition in normotensive salt-depleted subjects. Clinical Pharmacology & Therapeutics 1999;66: 76-84.

127. Swan SK, Rudy DW, Lasseter KC et al. Effect of cyclooxygenase-2 inhibition on renal function in elderly persons receiving a low-salt diet. A randomized, controlled trial.. Annals of Internal Medicine 2000;133: 1-9.

128. Whelton A, Fort JG, Puma JA et al. Cyclooxygenase-2--specific inhibitors and cardiorenal function: a randomized, controlled trial of celecoxib and rofecoxib in older hypertensive osteoarthritis patients. American Journal of Therapeutics 2001;8: 85-95.

129. Perazella MA, Eras J, Perazella MA, Eras J. Are selective COX-2 inhibitors nephrotoxic?. American Journal of Kidney Diseases 2000;35: 937-940.

130. Wolf G, Porth J, Stahl RA, Wolf G, Porth J, Stahl RA. Acute renal failure associated with rofecoxib. Annals of Internal Medicine 2000;133: 394.

131. Ahmad SR, Kortepeter C, Brinker A et al. Renal failure associated with the use of celecoxib and rofecoxib. Drug Safety 2002;25: 537-544.

132. Zhao SZ, Reynolds MW, Lejkowith J et al. A comparison of renal-related adverse drug reactions between rofecoxib and celecoxib, based on the World Health Organization/Uppsala Monitoring Centre safety database. Clinical Therapeutics 2001;23: 1478-1491.

133. Whelton A, White WB, Bello AE et al. Effects of celecoxib and rofecoxib on blood pressure and edema in patients > or =65 years of age with systemic hypertension and osteoarthritis.. American Journal of Cardiology 2002;90: 959-963.

134. Dedier J, Stampfer MJ, Hankinson SE et al. Nonnarcotic analgesic use and the risk of hypertension in US women. Hypertension 2002;40: 604-608.

135. Collins R, Peto R, Godwin J et al. Blood pressure and coronary heart disease. Lancet 1990;336: 370-371.

136. Sowers JR, White WB, Pitt B et al. The Effects of cyclooxygenase-2 inhibitors and nonsteroidal anti-inflammatory therapy on 24-hour blood pressure in patients with hypertension, osteoarthritis, and type 2 diabetes mellitus. Archives of Internal Medicine 2005;165: 161-168.

137. Reitblat T, Zamir D, Estis L et al. The different patterns of blood pressure elevation by rofecoxib and nabumetone. Journal of Human Hypertension 2002;16: 431-434.

138. Dilger K, Herrlinger C, Peters J et al. Effects of celecoxib and diclofenac on blood pressure, renal function, and vasoactive prostanoids in young and elderly subjects. Journal of Clinical Pharmacology 2002;42: 985-994.
139. Heart and Stroke Statistics Upate. American Heart Association 2000.
140. Prevention of stroke by antihypertensive drug treatment in older persons with isolated systolic hypertension. Final results of the Systolic Hypertension in the Elderly Program (SHEP). SHEP Cooperative Research Group.. JAMA 1991;265: 3255-3264.
141. Staessen JA, Fagard R, Thijs L et al. Randomised double-blind comparison of placebo and active treatment for older patients with isolated systolic hypertension. The Systolic Hypertension in Europe (Syst-Eur) Trial Investigators. Lancet 1997;350: 757-764.
142. Major cardiovascular events in hypertensive patients randomized to doxazosin vs chlorthalidone: the antihypertensive and lipid-lowering treatment to prevent heart attack trial (ALLHAT). ALLHAT Collaborative Research Group. JAMA 2000;283: 1967-1975.
143. Staessen JA, Gasowski J, Wang JG et al. Risks of untreated and treated isolated systolic hypertension in the elderly: meta-analysis of outcome trials. Lancet 2000;355: 865-872.
144. Houston MC, Houston MC. Nonsteroidal anti-inflammatory drugs and antihypertensives. American Journal of Medicine 1991;90: 42S-47S.
145. Trying times for painkiller choices. Vioxx, Bextra, and Celebrex can increase the risk for heart attack and other cardiovascular problems. So can the old standbys, like ibuprofen and acetaminophen. Harvard Heart Letter 2006;17: 1-3.
146. Bresalier RS, Sandler RS, Quan H et al. Cardiovascular events associated with rofecoxib in a colorectal adenoma chemoprevention trial. New England Journal of Medicine 2005;352: 1092-1102.
147. Rocca B, Davi G. Should patients with osteoarthritis be treated with COX2 inhibitors rather than traditional NSAIDs? Nat Clin Pract Rheumatol. 2007 Apr 3; [Epub ahead of print] No abstract available. Nat Clin Pract Rheumatol 2007 Apr 3; [Epub ahead of print] No abstract available 2007;4.
148. Huaang WF, Hsiao FY, Wen YW, Tsai YW. Cardiovascular events associated with the use of four nonselective NSAIDs (etodolac, nabumetone, ibuprofen, or naproxen) versus a cyclooxygenase-2 inhibitor (celecoxib): a population-based analysis in Taiwanese adults. Clinical Therapeutics 2007;28: 1827-1836.
149. Farkouh ME, Greenberg JD, Jeger RV, Rammanathan K, Verheugt FW. Cardiovascular outcomes in high-risk patients with osteoarthritis treated with Ibuprofen, Naproxen, or Lumiracoxib. Ann Rheum Dis 2007;5: [Epub ahead of print].
150. Solomon SD, Pfeffer MA, McMurray JJ et al. Effect of celecoxib on cardiovascular events and blood pressure in two trials for the prevention of colorectal adenomas. Circulation 2006;114: 1028-1035.
151. Bertagnolli MM, Eagle CJ, Zauber AG et al. Celecoxib for the prevention of sporadic colorectal adenomas.. New England Journal of Medicine 2006;355: 873-884.
152. Arber N, Eagle CJ, Spicak J et al. Celecoxib for the prevention of colorectal adenomatous polyps.. New England Journal of Medicine 2006;355: 885-895.
153. ADAPT Research Group. Cardiovascular and Cerebrovascular Events in the Randomized, Controlled Alzheimer's Disease Anti-Inflammatory Prevention Trial (ADAPT). WWW Plosclinicaltrials org 2007;e33: 001-010.
154. Schlienger RG, Jick H, Meier CR, Schlienger RG, Jick H, Meier CR. Use of nonsteroidal anti-inflammatory drugs and the risk of first-time acute myocardial infarction. British Journal of Clinical Pharmacology 2002;54: 327-332.
155. Mamdani M, Rochon P, Juurlink DN et al. Effect of selective cyclooxygenase 2 inhibitors and naproxen on short-term risk of acute myocardial infarction in the elderly. Archives of Internal Medicine 2003;163: 481-486.
156. Kimmel SE, Berlin JA, Reilly M et al. Patients exposed to rofecoxib and celecoxib have different odds of nonfatal myocardial infarction. Annals of Internal Medicine 2005;142: 157-164.
157. Graham DJ, Campen D, Hui R et al. Risk of acute myocardial infarction and sudden cardiac death in patients treated with cyclo-oxygenase 2 selective and non-selective non-steroidal anti-inflammatory drugs: nested case-control study.. Lancet 2005;365: 475-481.
158. Hippisley-Cox J, Coupland C, Hippisley-Cox J, Coupland C. Risk of myocardial infarction in patients taking cyclo-oxygenase-2 inhibitors or conventional non-steroidal anti-inflammatory drugs: population based nested case-control analysis.. BMJ 2005;330: 1366.
159. Fischer LM, Schlienger RG, Matter CM et al. Discontinuation of nonsteroidal anti-inflammatory drug therapy and risk of acute myocardial infarction. Archives of Internal Medicine 2004;164: 2472-2476.
160. Johnsen SP, Larsson H, Tarone RE et al. Risk of hospitalization for myocardial infarction among users of rofecoxib, celecoxib, and other NSAIDs: a population-based case-control study. Archives of Internal Medicine 2005;165: 978-984.
161. Levesque LE, Brophy JM, Zhang B, Levesque LE, Brophy JM, Zhang B. The risk for myocardial infarction with cyclooxygenase-2 inhibitors: a population study of elderly adults. Annals of Internal Medicine 2005;142: 481-489.
162. Levesque LE, Brophy JM, Zhang B, Levesque LE, Brophy JM, Zhang B. Time variations in the risk of myocardial infarction among elderly users of COX-2 inhibitors.. CMAJ Canadian Medical Association Journal 2006;174: 1563-1569.

163. Helin-Salmivaara A, Risto VesalainenJuha M.Grönroos, Juha M.Grönroos. NSAID use and the risk of hospitalization for first myocardial infarction in the general population: a nationwide case–control study from Finland. 27, 1657-1663. 2006.
164. Spilding WM, Reeves MJ, Whelton A. Thromboembolic Cardiovascular Risk Among Arthritis Patients Using Cyclooxygenase-2-Selective Inhibitor or Nonselective Cyclooxygenase Inhibitor Nonsteroidal Anti-inflammatory Drugs. American Journal of Therapeutics 2007; 3-12.
165. Hawkey CJ, Hawkey GM, Everitt S et al. Increased risk of myocardial infarction as first manifestation of ischaemic heart disease and nonselective nonsteroidal anti-inflammatory drugs. British Journal of Clinical Pharmacology 2006;61: 730-737.
166. McGettigan P, Henry D, McGettigan P, Henry D. Cardiovascular risk and inhibition of cyclooxygenase: a systematic review of the observational studies of selective and nonselective inhibitors of cyclooxygenase 2. JAMA 2006;296: 1633-1644.
167. Lee TA, Bartle B, Weiss KB, Lee TA, Bartle B, Weiss KB. Impact of NSAIDS on mortality and the effect of preexisting coronary artery disease in US veterans. American Journal of Medicine 2007;120: 98-16.
168. Stillman MJ, Stillman MT. Appropriate use of NSAIDs: considering cardiovascular risk in the elderly. Geriatrics 2007;62: 16-21.
169. Stillman MJ, Stillman MT. Choosing nonselective NSAIDs and selective COX-2 inhibitors in the elderly. A clinical use pathway. Geriatrics 2007;62: 26-34.
170. Heerdink ER, Leufkens HG, Herings RM et al. NSAIDs associated with increased risk of congestive heart failure in elderly patients taking diuretics. Archives of Internal Medicine 1998;158: 1108-1112.
171. Page J, Henry D, Page J, Henry D. Consumption of NSAIDs and the development of congestive heart failure in elderly patients: an underrecognized public health problem.. Archives of Internal Medicine 2000;160: 777-784.
172. Feenstra J, Heerdink ER, Grobbee DE et al. Association of nonsteroidal anti-inflammatory drugs with first occurrence of heart failure and with relapsing heart failure: the Rotterdam Study. Archives of Internal Medicine 2002;162: 265-270.
173. Mamdani M, Juurlink DN, Lee DS et al. Cyclo-oxygenase-2 inhibitors versus non-selective non-steroidal anti-inflammatory drugs and congestive heart failure outcomes in elderly patients: a population-based cohort study. Lancet 2004;363: 1751-1756.
174. Hudson M, Rahme E, Richard H, Piloate L. Risk of congestive heart failure with nonsteroidal antiinflammatory drugs and selective Cyclooxygenase 2 inhibitors: A class effect? Arthritis & Rheumatism 2007;29: 516-523.
175. Johnston HH, Herzog JP, Lauler DP, Johnston HH, Herzog JP, Lauler DP. Effect of prostaglandin E1 on renal hemodynamics, sodium and water excretion. American Journal of Physiology 1967;213: 939-946.
176. Fulgraff G, Brandenbusch G, Fulgraff G, Brandenbusch G. Comparison of the effects of the prostaglandins A1, E2, and F2alpha on kidney function in dogs. Pflugers Archiv - European Journal of Physiology 1974;349: 9-17.
177. Chang LC, Splawinski JA, Oates JA et al. Enhanced renal prostaglandin production in the dog. II. Effects on intrarenal hemodynamics. Circulation Research 1975;36: 204-207.
178. Strandhoy JW, Ott CE, Schneider EG et al. Effects of prostaglandins E1 and E2 on renal sodium reabsorption and Starling forces. American Journal of Physiology 1974;226: 1015-1021.
179. Paller MS, Paller MS. The prostaglandin E1 analog misoprostol reverses acute cyclosporine nephrotoxicity. Transplantation Proceedings 1988;20: 634-637.
180. Weir MR, Klassen DK, Hall PS, Schubert C. Minimization of indomethacin-induced reduction in renal function by misoprostol. Journal of Clinical Pharmacology 1989;31: 729-735.
181. Pincus T, Koch GG, Sokka T, et al. A randomized, double-blind crossover clinical trial of diclofenac versus misoprostol versus acetaminophen in patients with osteoarthritis of the knees or hip. Arthritis Rheum 2001;44:1587–98.
182. Boers M, Dijkmans BA, Breedveld FC et al. No effect of misoprostol on renal function of rheumatoid patients treated with diclofenac. British Journal of Rheumatology 1991;30: 56-59.
183. Whelton A, Scott H, Stout RL. Effects of Misoprostol on Nonsteroidal Anti-Inflammatory Drug-Induced Renal Insufficiency in Patients with Stable Chronic Renal Failure: A Double-Blind, Crossover Study. American Journal of Therapeutics 1995;2: 858-863.
184. Gurkowski L, Macdougal M, Weigmann t. Effects of Misoprostol on Contrast-Induced Renal Dysfunction. American Journal of Therapeutics 1995;2: 837-842.
185. Singh G, Miller JD, Huse DM, et al. Consequences of increased systolic blood pressure in patients with osteoarthritis and rheumatoid arthritis.
186. Kimmel SE, Berlin JA, Reilly M et al. Patients exposed to rofecoxib and celecoxib have different odds of nonfatal myocardial infarction. Annals of Internal Medicine 2005;142: 157-164.
187. Brophy JM, Levesque LE, Zhang B. The coronary risk of cyclo-oxygenase-2 inhibitors in patients with a previous myocardial infarction. Heart 2007;93: 189-194.
188. Garcia Rodriguez LA, Varas-Lorenzo C, Maguire A et al. Nonsteroidal antiinflammatory drugs and the risk of myocardial infarction in the general population. Circulation 2004;109: 3000-3006.
189. Rahme E, Nedjar H. Risks and benefits of COX-2 inhibitors vs non-selective NSAIDs: does their cardiovascular risk exceed their gastrointestinal benefit? A retrospective cohort study. Rheumatology 2007;46: 435-438.

190. Gislason GH, Jacobsen S, Rasmussen JN et al. Risk of death or reinfarction associated with the use of selective cyclooxygenase-2 inhibitors and nonselective nonsteroidal antiinflammatory drugs after acute myocardial infarction. Circulation 2006;113: 2906-2913

19

Gold salts, D-penicillamine and allopurinol

Shiro UEDA[1] and George A. PORTER[2]

[1]Chiba University, Chiba, Japan
[2]Oregon Health Sciences University, Portland, Oregon, USA

Gold nephropathy

Introduction

Gold salts have been used in the treatment of patients with rheumatoid arthritis since 1927 [1]. After a controlled study, the Empire Rheumatism Council [2], confirmed the effectiveness of gold salts for the treatment of rheumatoid arthritis. Even today, chrysotherapy has remained one of the major therapeutic modalities in the second line treatment of progressive rheumatoid arthritis. Gold salts are also used in the treatment of pemphigus vulgaris [3] and bronchial asthma [4]. Before the introduction of an orally administered gold compound, auranofin (triethylphosphine gold tetra-acetyl glycopyranoside), to clinical use [5-7], parenterally administered gold salts, such as sodium aurothiomalate and gold thioglucose comprised chrysotherapy. The frequency and severity of the side effects for patients treated with parenteral gold versus those given oral gold preparations are significantly different [8-10]. With introduction of newer parental DMARDs, toxicity has been reduced using combination therapy [10a, 10b].

Parenterally administered gold

Despite the efficiency of injectable gold salts in the treatment of rheumatoid arthritis, they are associated with a variety of adverse effects, such as skin rashes [11-13], thrombocytopenia [14, 15], granulocytopenia [11, 16], aplastic anemia [17, 18], interstitial pneumonitis [19, 20], gastrointestinal side effects [11, 21], chrysiasis of cornea and lens [12], and proteinuria and nephrotic syndrome [11, 22, 23]. One or more of these adverse reactions have been reported in approximately one-third of patients treated with gold salts [12]. Proteinuria, including nephrotic syndrome, is the commonest manifestation of gold-induced nephropathy, occurring in 2% to 10% in patients receiving chrysotherapy [10, 22-24]. However, the decreased frequency of proteinuria has paralleled the reduction in dosage of injectable gold salts, prolonging the interval between injections and the introduction of several new disease modifying agents. The risk of proteinuria is increased at higher doses [26] and in the patients with HLA DR3 [27-30]. In one-third to half of the patients, the proteinuria is accompanied by microscopic hematuria [31, 32]. The severity of the proteinuria varies greatly and does not correlate with the duration of treatment or the total dose of gold received [31, 33]. The peak incidence of proteinuria occurs after four to six months of treatment [33], but it may develop at any time from 1 week to 39 months after the start of treatment [33, 34]. Complete resolution of gold-induced proteinuria occurs in all patients 3 years after cessation of therapy, however, one-third of patients had resolved their proteinuria in 6 months after stopping therapy [34a]. Progressive loss of renal function following withdrawal of gold therapy is rare [34b]. Furthermore, reinstitution of gold therapy at a lower dose in patients with prior history of gold-induced proteinuria without recurrence suggests that the proteinuria may have a dose dependency [34c]. Renal function is usually normal to minimal impairment in these proteinuric patients.

Histopathology of glomerular lesions

Histopathological examinations of the renal biopsy specimens from patients with proteinuria show predominantly membranous glomerulopathy [10, 22, 31-40]. Electron microscopy of renal tissue usually demonstrates subepithelial electron dense deposits (especially when the disease is of short duration) [22, 32-40], intramembranous electron dense deposits [32, 34, 40], and fusion and increased density of foot processes of epithelial cells [22, 32, 35-40]. Light microscopy occasionally discloses varying degrees of uniform thickening of the glomerular basement membrane. Small, fuchsinophilic deposits with associated spike like extensions of the basement membrane may be identified on trichrome-stained sections. Immunofluorescent study of the renal tissues with subepithelial electron dense deposits reveals granular deposition of IgG, IgM and/or complements [10, 33, 34, 37, 39]. In addition to membranous glomerulonephritis, there are reports of minimal change glomerulonephritis [32, 41], focal segmental glomerulonephritis [32], and mesangioproliferative glomerulonephritis with immune complex deposition in mesangial areas [10, 31, 40]. Skrifvars et al. [42] reported a highly unusual fatal renal complication induced by sodium aurothiomalate. This complication was characterized by microhematuria, impaired renal function and by a granulomatous glomerulonephritis.

Histopathology of interstitial lesions

In addition to the glomerular lesions mentioned above, focal tubular atrophy of variable severity is a feature of the majority of biopsy specimens of gold induced nephropathy [32, 37, 39, 43]. Interstitial fibrosis can be recognized in many of the specimens (Figure 1), and the degree of fibrosis tends to parallel the severity and extent of the tubular atrophy. However, interstitial inflammation is not usually prominent [32]. Electron microscopy reveals the existence of characteristic filamentous, electron dense cytoplasmic inclusions in various renal cells at high frequency [22, 37-39, 44, 45]. These filamentous inclusions may be complexes containing gold and other molecules [52, 50, 53]. The inclusions are concentrated in proximal tubular epithelial cells, interstitial macrophages, but rarely occur in mesangial cells and visceral epithelial cells, and spare the basement membrane or subepithelial space. They are much more prominent in patients who have received large doses of gold [22]. There may be a significant association between the degree of histological interstitial changes and the number of gold inclusions. Cramer et al. [43] reported a patient who suffered from chronic interstitial nephritis after receiving large quantities of aurothioglucose for rheumatoid arthritis. Gold deposition was seen by electron microscopy and confirmed by microprobe X-ray analysis within both tubular epithelial cells and interstitial macrophages but not the interstitium. They hypothesized that the administration of massive amounts of gold salts resulted in these depositions and the subsequent interstitial nephritis [43]. Lesato et al. [46] reported a high incidence of subtle renal tubular dysfunction in rheumatoid arthritis patients receiving gold treatment, demonstrating tubular proteinuria and the urinary excretion of large amounts of renal tubular epithelial antigen, tubular basement membrane (TBM) antigen, and β2-microglobulin. However, the amounts of these proteins in urine did not correlate with the total dose of gold [46]. Renal tubular dysfunction has been induced in Hartley guinea pigs by the injection of sodium aurothiomalate, as manifested by the urinary excretion of tubular basement membrane and renal tubular epithelial antigens and tubular proteinuria. Excretion of these proteins tended to be dose dependent [47]. Following the tubular dysfunction, autoimmune tubulointerstitial nephritis with anti-TBM antibodies developed in the animals [47].

Pathogenesis

There are mainly two types of gold-induced nephropathy, one being immune complex type glomerulonephritis and the other limited to tubular lesions. The latter may be induced by the direct toxic action of gold, and this toxicity seems to be dose dependent. The morphological changes in the tubules usually involve gold inclusions [22, 37, 39, 44-46]. Nagi et al. [48] using large doses of sodium aurothiomalate (1 mg/week) produced renal tubular necrosis in rats, characterized by degenerative changes of the cytoplasmic contents of epithelial cells of proximal convoluted tubules. The ultracellular structure changes involved swollen mitochondria that had lost their shape. Eiseman et al. [49]

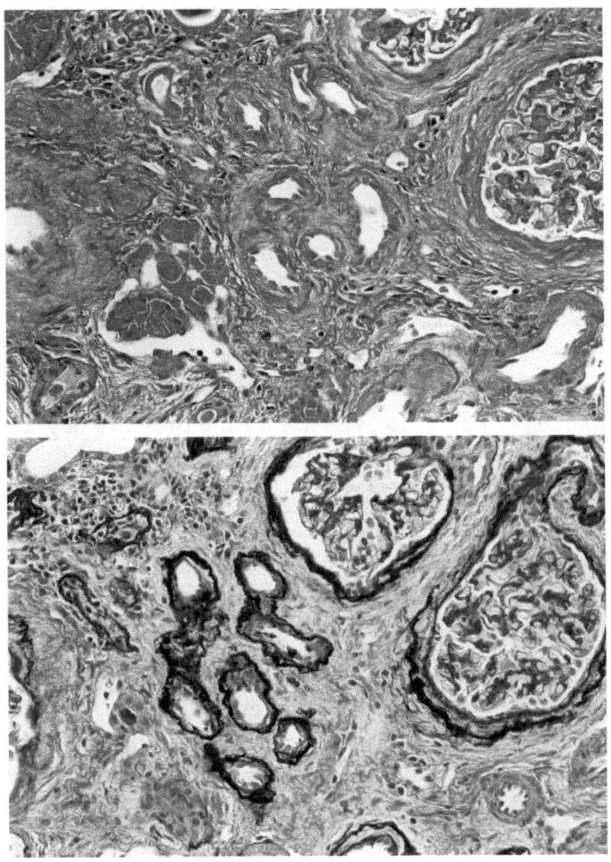

Figure 1. *Photomicrographs of the kidney from a rheumatoid arthritis patient with gold nephropathy, demonstrating prominent interstitial fibrosis and tubular cell degeneration (magn. x340). Above: Masson's trichrome staining; below: PAM staining.*

reported morphofunctional and biochemical changes in rat kidneys following a single ip injection of a high dose (75 mg/kg) of gold sodium thiomalate. This included severe coagulative necrosis of the proximal tubular epithelium at one day, followed by epithelial regeneration by day 4 and nearly complete resolution by day 8. Alternations in renal heme biosynthesis and drug metabolism paralleled the morphological changes [49]. Tubular dysfunction has also been reported in rheumatoid arthritis patients receiving gold treatment [46] and in animals being treated with low doses of gold salts [47, 48].

The pathogenesis of immune complex type glomerular lesions associated with chrysotherapy remains unclear. To clarify the pathogenesis of this nephropathy, it is necessary to confirm the specificity of the antigens and antibodies responsible for the immune complex of the glomerular lesions. Gold salts may act as a hapten, and specific IgE antibodies against gold salts have been detected in the sera of rheumatoid arthritis patients with mucocutaneous and hematologic adverse reaction to gold salts [50, 51]. A positive lymphocyte transformation test to gold salts has been reported in some rheumatoid arthritis patients with hematologic side effects after chrysotherapy [52]. Derot et al. [53] reported a rare case of fatal acute tubular necrosis due to gold induced nephropathy. Allergic reaction to gold salts might have been responsible for the development of this nephritis; however, such immunological phenomena are rarely seen in the patients with gold-induced nephropathy [50, 51]. To date, no evidence for the presence of gold in renal immune deposits has been reported.

It is difficult to confirm that gold is the causal antigen or hapten in gold-induced immune complex nephropathy. Palosuo et al. [54] demonstrated a circulating antigen in a patient with gold-induced nephropathy before and after the development of nephropathy, which shared immunological determinants with tissue antigens extracted with deoxycholate from microsomal fractions of various organs including human liver, human kidney, and rat liver. Precipitating antibodies against this circulating antigen were found in the serum sample pre-dating diagnosis. This serum reacted with various tissue antigens extracted from human organs, but not with kidney specific antigen [54]. In an experimental rat model, Nagi et al. [48] reported the successful induction of slowly progressive immune complex nephropathy by weekly injections of small doses of sodium aurothiomalate (0.0025 mg/week), suggesting the important pathogenetic role of renal tubular antigen released from damaged tubular epithelial cells (Figure 2). Skrifvars [55] also emphasized the possible role of autoimmunization secondary to released tubular antigens in the pathogenesis of gold-induced glomerular lesions. In the guinea pig model, renal dysfunction was also induced by injections of sodium aurothiomalate, as manifested by the urinary excretion of renal tubular antigens including renal tubular epithelial and tubular basement membrane antigens. Following the tubular dysfunction, immune complex nephropathy with circulating anti-renal tubular epithelial antibody, including deposition of renal tubular epithelial antigen in the glomerular immune complexes, developed in the animals [47]. Thus, shed renal tubular antigens from damaged tubular epithelium may play an important role in the pathogenesis of gold-induced immune complex nephropathy. There are many drugs that injure the renal tubular epithelium, but rarely induce immune complex nephropathy. Thus, in addition to tubular damage, there must be other factors that promote the development of gold nephropathy. Other tissue autoantigens released and/or altered by the effect of gold and heterogeneous antigens may also participate in the pathogenetic mechanisms.

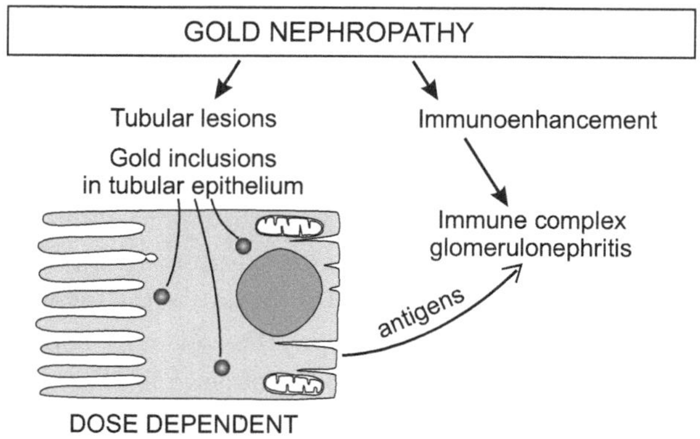

Figure 2. *An illustration of possible mechanisms in the pathogenesis of gold nephropathy.*

That gold salts possess immunosuppressive effects has been demonstrated by both *in vivo* and *in vitro* studies [56-59]. In addition, they also have an immunoenhancing effect on the immune response of mice, depending on dosage [60]. BALB/c mice are highly susceptible to autoimmune interstitial nephritis, while C57BL/6 mice are genetically resistant to this nephritis when immunized with tubular basement membrane antigen with adjuvant [61]. When both strains of mice are following pretreated with appropriate doses of sodium aurothiomalate immunization with tubular basement membrane antigen with adjuvant, BALB/c mice become resistent to the development of nephritis, but nephritis is induced in the genetically resistant C57BL/6 mice. Thus, gold salts may depress the activity of all T cells, and the phenotypical effect of gold salts on the immune response to some antigens may depend on the character of the dominant T cells [62]. Selective *in vitro* inhibition of T cells has also been shown in patients receiving chrysotherapy [63]. There must be other, as yet defined factors that are involved in the development of gold nephropathy.

Therapy and prognosis

Proteinuria is usually slow to resolves after withdrawal of the drug. In 1970, Vaamonde et al. [31] reviewed 19 case reports of nephrotic syndrome associated with chrysotherapy. In 17 patients whose outcomes were known, 13 recovered in 3 months to 7 years. Hall et al. [33] reported a long-term study of 21 patients with rheumatoid arthritis who developed proteinuria during treatment with sodium aurothiomalate. Ten patients developed proteinuria after 6 months' of treatment, 15 after 12 months, and 18 after 24 months. When chrysotherapy was stopped the proteinuria had reached a median peak of 2.1 g/day (range 0.7-30.7 g/day) at two months (range 1-13 months) before resolving spontaneously, in 8 patients by 6 months, in 13 by 12 months, and in 18 by 24 months. All patients were free of proteinuria after 39 months, the median duration being 11 months after withdrawal. Renal function did not deteriorate, and no patient died from or needed treatment for renal failure. HLA-B8 and/or DR3 alloantigens were identified in seven of the patients [33].

Newton et al. [64] studied 27 patients with gold-induced proteinuria, and provided guidelines as to when gold should be permanently stopped in these patients. They demonstrated that proteinuria of up to 2 g/L is compatible with continued gold therapy, since the low risk of more serious nephropathy developing was low. They concluded: 1) mild proteinuria (less than 0.4 g/L) is common in rheumatoid arthritis patients on gold, and such a level may not even be related to this drug. It usually disappears spontaneously without alteration of therapy, but rarely can proceed to more serious problems. 2) moderate proteinuria (0.4-2.0 g/L) should be treated more seriously. Gold injections should be stopped. If the urine clears within three months, then further treatment with gold may be given without precipitating heavy proteinuria. 3) none of their subjects have sustained permanent renal impairment [66]. The advice of Howard-Lock et al about D-penicillamine therapy may also be suitable for gold therapy. They advocate withholding the drug if there is (1) proteinuria of 2^+ on the dipstick, (2) persistent (longer than 3 weeks) proteinuria of 1^+, (3) if there are red cell casts, white cell casts, or hyaline casts present, or (4) if red cells >10 per high power field are present. For patients whose disease has improved but who developed proteinuria of between 300 to 1, 000 mg/day but without other renal abnormality, they suggest continuing the drug cautiously at a reduced dose with close monitoring. If the proteinuria exceeds 2 g/day or the glomerular filtration rate falls, the drug should be discontinued immediately [65]. Manthorpe et al. reported a successful one year treatment with auranofin (6 mg/day) in 7 rheumatoid arthritis patients with previous proteinuria associated with parenterally injected gold salts [66].

Prediction, prevention and monitoring of development of gold nephropathy

To predict the adverse effects of gold, the association with HLA antigen has been studied [27, 28, 67-69]. A genetic predisposition to gold toxicity was first suggested by Panayi et al. [67]. Wooley et al. [68] investigated the possible relation between HLA antigens and toxicity of D-penicillamine and sodium aurothiomalate in rheumatoid arthritis patients. Nineteen of 24 patients in whom proteinuria developed were positive for HLA-B8 and DRw3 antigens. Furthermore, all 13 episodes of proteinuria exceeding 2 g/day occurred in patients with DRw3. Several investigators confirmed the association between gold-induced proteinuria and DR3 [27-30] and B8 [30], but others were unable to confirm it [70]. Conversely, DR3 patients tended to exhibit a better therapeutic response to sodium aurothiomalate than patients with DR4 [28]. DR4 and/or DR2 positive patients may have some degree of protection against gold toxicity [28, 29]. Given the uncertainty about HLA types and toxic reactions, together with the suggestion that patients with DR3 respond better than the more numerous DR4, and taking into account the cost involved, any suggestion of using HLA typing as a guide to therapy seems premature [71]. While Van Riel et al. [72] reported the predictive value of serum IgA for gold toxicity, the study of Ostuni et al., involving a larger population, concluded that the monitoring of serum IgA was not useful in predicting gold toxicity [73]. Recently, Ayesh et al. [74] reported the predictive efficacy of the prior measurement of sulphoxidation capacity. A patient with poor sulphoxidation capacity had a nine-fold greater risk of developing gold-induced adverse reactions including nephropathy. Hopefully this will be confirmed by prospective studies involving various races and a large population. To date, there is no confirmed method for predicting gold toxicity including nephropathy, thus it is essential to monitor patients closely for any appearance of nephropathy. However, Shah et al [74a] have evaluated the association between gold ADR's (thrombocytopenia or proteinuria) and HLA-DR3 status. Based on a cohort of 41 patients they concluded that patients with nodular disease were more likely to develop ARDs (51.3% vs. 25.6%, OR= 3.0, p=0.02 and also more likely to be HLA-DR3 positive (41.2% vs. 17.6%, OR= 3.0, p= 0.045. The authors suggest that nodular patients with HLA-DR3 should not receive parenteral gold as their primary treatment for RA.

The decline in the number of reports of parenterally administered gold-induced nephropathy may indicate that the dose of gold salts used per injection is decreased and intervals between injections are being extended to prevent adverse reactions. Furthermore, introduction of methotrexate therapy, along with several biological agents, for rheumatoid arthritis, has contributed to decreased reliance on gold salts. However, intriguing reports using nanotechnology gold in treatment of malignancies has renewed interest in gold as a therapeutic agent [74b, c].

Auranofin nephropathy

Auranofin, a unique gold compound, has been available for clinical use for 25 years after it proved to be one of the most potent oral antiarthritic compounds among alkylphosphine gold coordination complexes [75]. Initial clinical studies suggested that this compound was therapeutically active when taken by mouth, with no renal adverse effects in any of the 32 patients studied [5-7]. Subsequently, the therapeutic benefits and toxicity of auranofin have been evaluated [24, 76], compared with placebo [9, 77, 78], sodium aurothiomalate [8-10, 79], and D-penicillamine [80-82]. The incidence of proteinuria in a world-wide trial was 3% for auranofin [10, 24]. The risk of developing proteinuria with auranofin therapy is significantly less than with parenteral gold [9, 24], or D-penicillamine [82]. Histopathological findings in renal biopsy specimens from patients with moderate to heavy proteinuria are consistent with the membranous nephropathy similar to injectable gold nephropathy [33, 83, 84]. Heuer et al. [10] reported a total of 3, 475 rheumatoid arthritis patients receiving auranofin therapy in 27 countries. Proteinuria developed in 3% of the patients, resulting in drug withdrawal in 0.9%, compared with 4% proteinuria in patients receiving injectable gold, with 0.8% being withdrawn. Katz et al. [24] evaluated proteinuria in 1800 rheumatoid arthritis patients given chrysotherapy. Three percent (41 cases) of 1283 auranofin-treated patients had an abnormal 24-hour urine protein level: 15 had mild (0.15 to 1 g/day), 17 had moderate (1 to 3.5 g/day), and 9 had heavy (>3.5 g/day) proteinuria. Permanent renal impairment did not occur in any patient. In 36 patients with long-term follow-up after drug withdrawal, proteinuria cleared in 31 patients within 1 week to 24 months. Seven of 8 patients who were rechallenged once the proteinuria had cleared were able to continue treatment without recurrent episodes [24].

Pathogenic mechanism of auranofin-induced nephropathy resemble those of parenteral gold-induced nephropathy. The reason for the reduced risk of proteinuria with auranofin compared to parenteral gold salts is not known. However, differences in the pharmacokinetics of the two types of gold preparations may be important. In rats treated with auranofin or sodium aurothiomalate for one year, renal gold concentrations were 33 times higher with the latter formulation [85]. Renal elimination of an orally administered dose of auranofin in human is less than 15%, compared with greater than 70% for parenterally administered sodium aurothiomalate [86].

D-penicillamine

Introduction

D-penicillamine is so named because it was first isolated as an amine, from the degradation products of penicillin by Abraham et al [87]. Later studies showed the characteristic chemical behavior of D-penicillamine which involves three types of reactions, formation of disulphide links, formation of thiazolidine rings, and formation of metal complexes and chelates [67]. It was first used in 1956 in the treatment of Wilson's disease [88]. D-penicillamine has since been used in the treatment of many diseases, such as cystinuria [89], rheumatoid arthritis [90-92], systemic sclerosis [93], primary biliary cirrhosis [94], heavy metal poisoning due to lead [95], cadmium [96], and mercury [97], and hyperviscosity syndrome [99]. In rheumatoid arthritis, D-penicillamine has been widely accepted as an effective second line treatment. Despite of its effectiveness, it causes many adverse effects, such as skin rashes [99, 100], taste abnormalities [100, 101], hepatic dysfunction [102-104], gastrointestinal toxicity [99, 105], proteinuria [100, 106], hematuria [107, 108], thrombocytopenia [92, 109], aplastic anemia [110], lupus-like syndrome [111, 112], Goodpasture's-like pulmonary renal syndrome [113-115], vasculitis [116, 117], myasthenia gravis [118-122], polymyositis [123, 124], and dermatomyositis [125]. One or more of these adverse reactions was recorded in nearly 60% of patients treated with D-penicillamine [100, 126-129]. Among these adverse reactions, nephropathy developed in patients with proteinuria, hematuria, lupus-like syndrome, Goodpasture's-like pulmonary renal syndrome, and vasculitis.

Proteinuria

Proteinuria, including nephritic syndrome, is the commonest manifestation of nephropathy, reported as occurring in between 2 and 32% of patients [100, 101, 109, 124, 126-130]. The risk of proteinuria is increased at higher doses [100, 131-133], in patients with HLA B8 and/or DRW3 antigens [68], and in patients with previous gold toxicity [134, 135]. However, others have not confirmed the relationship to the drug dosage [136], duration of therapy [137], or HLA antigens [70]. In the majority of patients, proteinuria is accompanied by microscopic hematuria [100, 127]. The peak incidence of proteinuria occurs in the second six months of treatment, but it may develop at any time from 6 weeks to 74 months [107, 101, 138]. Proteinuria may be persistent or may slowly progress to nephrotic syndrome if therapy is continued. Up to 1/3 of the patients with significant proteinuria progress to nephrotic syndrome if therapy is continued [106]. Renal function is normal to minimal impairment in patients with isolated proteinuria.

Histopathology

Histopathological examination of renal biopsy specimens from the patients with isolated proteinuria due to D-penicillamine shows predominant membranous glomerulopathy [139-141]. Electron microscopy of renal tissue usually demonstrates subepithelial electron dense deposits and fusion of epithelial foot processes [139-141]. The deposits on the epithelial side of the glomerular basement membrane appear to be slowly covered and later incorporated into the basement membrane. With time the deposits become fainter and move towards the endothelial side of the basement membrane [142]. Immunofluorescent study may demonstrate granular deposits of IgG and C3 in the capillary wall. These changes in glomerular histology can persist for at least a year after the withdrawal of the drug [139]. Sellars et al. [143] reviewed the renal biopsies of 30 patients with rheumatoid arthritis and clinical evidence of renal disease. They reported all 9 patients with membranous glomerulonephritis but only 6 of 13 with mesangial change had received D-penicillamine or gold. Besides membranous glomerulonephritis, there are reports of minimal change glomerulonephritis [144, 145], mild mesangioproliferative glomerulonephritis without crescent [110, 142, 146], or IgM nephropathy [147, 148] associated with D-penicillamine induced proteinuria.

Therapy and prognosis of proteinuria

Proteinuria usually resolves slowly after withdrawal of the drug. Hall et al. [149] reported a long-term study of 33 patients with rheumatoid arthritis who developed proteinuria during treatment with D-penicillamine. Of these, fourteen patients developed proteinuria within 6 months after the start of treatment and 27 within 12 months. When treatment was stopped, the proteinuria reached a median peak of 4.2 g/day (range 0.3-15 g/day) at one month (range 0-7 months) before resolving spontaneously by six months in 12 patients, 12 months in 21, and 21 months in all. In all their patients whose nephropathy was due to D-penicillamine the proteinuria resolved completely when the drug was withdrawn; renal function did not deteriorate, and corticosteroids were unnecessary [149]. Jaffe [150] reported that reintroduction of D-penicillamine in patients with drug induced proteinuria, starting with a daily dose of 250 mg, was usually followed by a return of proteinuria at about the same time and at about the same cumulative dose as on the first occasion. However, Hill et al. [133] reported successful reintroduction and continuation for a minimum of 13 months in 5 rheumatoid arthritis patients who developed proteinuria during the first course of the drug. They instituted the "go slow, go low" method of Jaffe [151], starting with a daily dose of 50 mg and increasing by monthly increment of 50 mg to a maintenance dose of 150 mg daily. The dose was held at 150 mg/day for 4 months and thereafter increased by 50 mg at 3-months intervals if disease remained active. Proteinuria did not recur, and improvement of disease was shown in all 5 patients [133]. Howard-lock et al. [65] advocated withholding D-penicillamine if there is (1) proteinuria of 2+ on the dipstick, (2) persistent (longer than 3 weeks) proteinuria of 1+ (3) if there are red cell casts, white cell casts, or hyaline casts present, or (4) if red cells > 10 per high power field are present. For patients whose disease has improved but who developed proteinuria between 300 to 1, 000 mg/day, but without other renal abnormality, they suggest the continued use of the drug cautiously at a reduced dose with close monitoring. If proteinuria exceeds 2 g/day or the glomerular filtration rate falls, the drug should be discontinued immediately.

Goodpasture's-like syndrome

Besides the benign proteinuria mentioned above, proliferative glomerulonephritis with fulminant renal failure has also occurred with D-penicillamine therapy. One is Goodpasture's-like syndrome, which is characterized by pulmonary hemorrhage and rapidly progressive glomerulonephritis. Goodpasture's -like syndrome associated D-penicillamine treatment has been reported in patients with Wilson's disease [113], rheumatoid arthritis [114, 115, 152, 153], primary biliary cirrhosis [154], and progressive systemic sclerosis [155]. D-penicillamine was given for at least 7 months (range: 7-84 months), and at a daily dose higher than 750 mg (range: 750-2, 000 mg) preceding the onset of symptoms. Pulmonary X-rays showed bilateral extensive infiltrates in all 10 cases. Lung hemorrhage was the principle cause of death in 3 cases [113].

The histopathology of renal specimens usually showed proliferative glomerulonephritis with crescent formation in 30 to 100% of the glomeruli. Direct immunofluorescent study failed to show linear IgG deposition along the glomerular basement membrane, but granular deposition of IgG and/or C3 were present along the glomerular capillary walls in 5 of 6 patients. Subepithelial electron dense deposits were observed in 3 of 4 patients tested. Circulating anti-glomerular basement membrane antibody was not detected in any of the cases tested. In Brown Norway rats, the administration of D-penicillamine induced antinuclear antibodies and significantly high concentrations of immune complexes. Iin these animals there was no granular deposition of IgG, but linear deposition of IgG along the glomerular basement membrane. IgG eluted from diseased kidneys bound both *in vitro* and *in vivo* to the kidney basement membrane [156]. HLA-DR2 antigen was absent in the 2 cases where HLA phenotype was determined, whereas there is a strong association between HLA-DR2 and antibody-mediated Good-pasture's syndrome [157]. Anti-nuclear antibodies have been detected both before [115, 156] and after initiation of the drug [152, 115]. Although this syndrome is potentially life-threatening, aggressive treatment with plasmapheresis, steroids, immunosuppressive drugs such as azathioprine and cyclophosphamide, and mechanical ventilation with PEEP may be life saving [113, 152-155]. Derk and Jimenez [155a] recently reviewed the case for Goodpasture-like syndrome occurring in systemic sclerosis patients treated with penicillamine. Basically they describe rapidly progressive glomerulonephritis without anti-GBM antibiodies, but with linear or granular glomerular deposits. While they raise the possibility of pausi-immune GN this could not be confirmed since ANCA was not tested in their patient. Despite their conclusions, the case report by Bienaime et al ([155b] makes a compelling case for penicillamine induced ANCA associated RPGN in a patient with Wilson Disease. Since Wilson Disease has never been associated with pauci-immune GN, the authors are confident that penicillamine is capable of inducing ANCA associated RPGN, To date all patients with suspected pauci-immune GN have tested positive for anti-MPO antibodies. Since this observation was limited to a patient with Wilson Disease, it remains to be confirmed that patients with systemic sclerosis or rheumatoid arthritis receiving penicillamine who develop the Goodpasture-like syndrome described as a complication of penicillamine treatment should be classified as pauci-immune GN with anti-MPO antibodies.

Renal vasculitis

Extracapillary glomerulonephritis with renal vasculitis is also been reported as a rare complication of D-penicillamine therapy [117, 126, 156]. Necrosis of interlobular arteries with glomerular crescent [117] and necrotic and occluded periglomerular arterioles [156] have been reported. Aggressive treatment with pulse steroid, anticoagulants, and antiplatelet agents may be beneficial. The two patients with renal vasculitis, whose outcome was known, died from bacterial infection within ten months after the onset of the disease [117, 156]. These cases mostly likely represent pauci-immune GN as reviewed in the preceding paragraph.

Systemic lupus erythematosus syndrome

A drug-induced systemic lupus erythematosus (SLE) with proliferative glomerulonephritis has also been described in patients treated with D-penicillamine [111, 157]. Systemic lupus erythematosus syndrome is induced in approximately 2% of patients treated with D-penicillamine [112, 158]. Unlike other forms of drug-induced systemic lupus erythematosus, anti-double-strand DNA antibodies and/or hypocomplementemia are seen in D-penicillamine-induced systemic lupus erythematosus syndrome [111, 156]. Nephropathy is rare in D-penicillamine-induced systemic lupus erythematosus syndrome [111]. Walshe [112] reported that 8 patients developed the serological change of systemic lupus erythematosus of 120 patients with Wilson's disease treated with D-penicillamine, but none of them showed nephropathy.

Chalmers [111] reported 6 rheumatoid arthritis patients with D-penicillamine-induced systemic lupus erythematosus syndrome. All patients had previous mucocutaneous reactions to chrysotherapy. Manifestations included pleurisy in 5 of 6 patients, rashes in 3, and nephritis in 2. LE cells were present in 5 patients, anti nuclear antibodies in all 6, anti-double-strand DNA in 3, 3 were Coomb's test positive, and low C4 complement in 5 of the 6 [111]. Results of a renal biopsy from a patient with nephritis showed diffuse endocapillary proliferative glomerulonephritis with focal crescent formation and vasculitis. Electron microscopy showed scattered subendothelial deposits, and immunofluorescent study revealed granular deposition of IgG, IgM, C3 complement and C1q. The patient was successfully treated with prednisolone and azathioprine [112]. Ntoso et al. [156] reported penicillamine-induced rapidly progressive glomerulonephritis in two patients with progressive systemic sclerosis. Anti nuclear antibodies, anti-Sm antibody, and Coomb's antibodies were positive in both patients. Renal biopsies from the two patients demonstrated a diffuse, predominantly extracapillary, proliferative glomerulonephritis with crescents and focal necrosis, and by immunofluorescence, focal areas of IgG, C3, and fibrinogen were observed in areas of glomerular necrosis. Subendothelial and mesangial deposits were observed by electron microscopy. Both patients responded to pulse methylprednisolone and subsequent daily steroids [156].

Pathogenesis of D-penicillamine-induced nephropathy

Deposition of immune complexes in the glomerular basement membrane may play an important role in the pathogenesis of D-penicillamine-induced nephropathy, such as isolated proteinuria, Goodpasture's-like syndrome, and nephritis associated with D-penicillamine-induced systemic lupus erythematosus rheumatoid arthritis syndrome. Immunofluorescent study show predominantly granular deposition of IgG and/or C3, and electron microscopy revealed subepithelial or subendothelial electron dense deposits. In rheumatoid arthritis patients, D-penicillamine alters the circulating immune complexes [159]. D-penicillamine has the capacity to convert large complexes into small ones *in vitro* and there has been speculation that similar mechanisms *in vivo* could explain the deposition of complexes and renal damage [160]. Small immune complexes deposit in the glomeruli easier than big ones.

In addition to penicillamine nephropathy, other side effects of the drug may be related to the widespread deposition of immune complexes (Figure 3). Dense, granular immunoglobulin deposits have been identified at the epidermodermal junction in 4 rheumatoid arthritis patients who developed toxic reactions, such as severe rashes, thrombocytopenia, aplastic anemia, and proteinuria. Three of 4 penicillamine-induced systemic lupus erythematosus syndrome patients had similar findings on skin biopsy [161].

Besides immune complex deposition, autoantibodies against several autoantigens are frequently detected in patients treated with D-penicillamine, leading to autoimmune diseases. The exact mechanism by which this drug induces autoimmunity remains to be investigated. It may directly stimulate oligoclonal B cell activity, upset the balance between T cell subsets, or alter antigens by hapten formation. D-penicillamine can bind with various proteins, and may change the antigenicity of these proteins as a hapten. However, to date, no evidence for the presence of penicillamine in renal immune deposits has been reported. Nagata et al. [162] reported that D-penicillamine can act as a hapten for specific T cells when presented on the surface of appropriate stimulator cells, and suggested that the adverse immunological side effects of this drug in patients may have a pathogenesis similar to graft-versus-host reaction.

The possibility of ANCA associated vasculitis, as described in the case report of Bienaime et al [155b], raises an alternate explanation for the pathogenesis of penicillamine-induced vasculitis. Since all of the ANCA associated GN due to penicillamine have had anti-MPO antibodies, this suggests that an interaction with MPO is critical in triggering the ANCA induced vasculitis. However, it is not clear that penicillamine induces autoimmunity, thus the exact mechanism remains to be elucidated, although both humoral and cellular immunity are thought to play significant roles [162a].

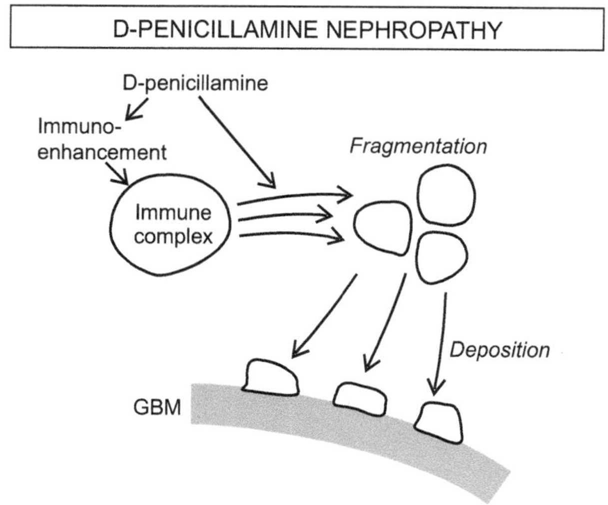

Figure 3. *An illustration of the pathogenesis of D-penicillamine induced nephropathy.*

Prediction and monitoring of development of D-penicillamine nephropathy

To predict D-penicillamine side effects, the association between side effects and various factors, such as HLA antigens [68, 70, 128, 130, 163, 164], autoantibodies [165, 166], and previous gold toxicity [101, 138, 167, 168] has been studied. Wooley et al. [68] investigated the possible interaction between HLA antigens and toxicity of D-penicillamine and sodium aurothiomalate in rheumatoid arthritis patients. Nineteen of 24 patients in whom proteinuria developed were positive for HLA-B8 and DRw3 antigens. Furthermore, all 13 episodes of proteinuria exceeding 2 g/day occurred in patients with DRw3 [68]. There is also a strong association between idiopathic membrane nephropathy and HLA-DRw3, B8 and B18 [169]. Other investigators have confirmed the association between D-penicillamine-induced proteinuria and DR3 [128, 130, 164] and B8 [70, 128, 130]. However, other investigators could not confirm a significant association between D-penicillamine proteinuria and HLA-DR3 [70, 170]. In addition to HLA antigens, Emery et al. [163] emphasized the sulphoxidation status of patients as a new predictor of outcome of drug toxicity.

Moutsopoulos et al. [165, 166] reported that anti-Ro (SSA) positive Greek rheumatoid arthritis patients experienced a significantly high frequency of side effects from D-penicillamine. Despite their dissimilar chemical structures, the thiol compounds, sodium aurothiomalate and D-penicillamine, have remarkably similar clinical effects, and this similarity extends to the incidence and type of adverse effects [138, 167]. Several investigators have noted the association between prior gold nephropathy and D-penicillamine. Billingsley and Stevens reported the significant correlation of D-penicillamine-induced proteinuria to a previous history of gold nephropathy [134]. Patients with gold-induced proteinuria are at a higher risk for the development of proteinuria during D-penicillamine therapy ($p<0.001$), and this occurs within the first six months of treatment [138]. All six patients who developed systemic lupus erythematosus syndrome while being treated with D-penicillamine had previous mucocutaneous reactions to chrysotherapy [114]. Dood et al. [165] noted that all patients who took D-penicillamine within six months after an adverse reaction to gold developed side effects from D-penicillamine, and recommended an interval exceeding six months between treatment with gold and treatment with D-penicillamine in patients who have developed adverse reactions to gold, to reduce the risk of adverse reactions to D-penicillamine, Kean et al. [101] analyzed the influence of previous sodium aurothiomalate therapy on the toxicity pattern of D-penicillamine, but could not confirm a synergistic effect of D-penicillamine and sodium aurothiomalate leading to increased adverse reaction in patients with rheumatoid disease [101].

Although there are several predictors of adverse reactions, the most useful clinical predictor is urinalysis. Patients on D-penicillamine therapy should be closely monitored for evidence of proteinuria as the first sign of penicillamine induced nephropathy [170a].

Allopurinol

Introduction

Allopurinol (4-hydroxypyrazolo [3, 4-d] pyrimidine) is an inhibitor of xanthine oxidase that was successfully introduced in the treatment of primary gout about 45 years ago [171]. Allopurinol continues to be accepted as standard therapy in the treatment of primary and secondary hyperuricemia. Adverse reactions occur in about 10% of patients treated with allopurinol and are relatively mild and self-limited [171, 172]. A mild maculopapular eruption or gastrointestinal disorders are usually noted, which promptly regress with cessation of therapy. Isolated instances of allopecia [173], bone marrow depression [174], ocular lesions [175], acute cholangitis [176], various types of hepatic injuries [177, 178] temporal arthritis [179], and xanthine stones [180] have been reported. Recently, LaRosa et al [180a] have reported a case of xanthine nephropathy during treatment of childhood T-cell ALL. Xanthine nephropathy has been reported in tumor lysis syndrome (TLS) in patients with hypoxanthine-guanine phosphoribosyl transferase (HGPRT) enzyme deficiency [180b], however, this patients' cultured fibroblasts yielded normal levels of HGPRT enzyme. Allopurinol pretreatment allows the build up of both xanthine and hypoxanthine which, in the absence of HGPRT, cannot be recycled and thus xanthine supersaturation in the urine resulting in xanthine stones with subsequent obstructive renal failure.

In 1970, reports began to appear of systemic, severe, prolonged hypersensitivity reactions occurring in patients during treatment with allopurinol, now known as allopurinol hypersensitivity syndrome (AHS) [182]. These reactions are characterized by fever, chills, malaise, generalized dermatitis, eosinophilia, abnormalities of liver function tests, and rapidly progressive renal failure [181-188]. Allopurinol-induced nephropathy is usually reported as a part of these reactions. In 1979, Gorge et al. [186] reported 3 cases of such reactions and reviewed 38 patients including their 7 patients. The average dose of the drug in these patients was 300 mg/day. The average time from initiation of the therapy to onset of the reaction was 3.8 weeks. The most common type of dermatitis was a pruritic, diffuse, erythematosus, maculopapular eruption noted in over 60% of the patients. Toxic epidermal necrosis, Stevens-Johnson syndrome, and exfoliative dermatitis were also noted in some patients. Exfoliative dermatitis has also been reported in a patient with metabolic syndrome as a delayed skin reaction heralding the onset of AHS [188a]. The presence of eosinophilia (4-53%) was noted in all but two patients. Thirty-one of 32 patients (97%) had documented impaired renal function prior to allopurinol therapy. Following the onset of the hypersensitivity reaction, further deterioration of renal function occurred in 30 of 32 patients [186]. In 1986, Singer et al. [188] reported 8 additional patients with such reactions and reviewed an additional 72 patients described in the literature. Forty of 80 patients (50%) had impaired renal function prior to allopurinol therapy. Further deterioration of renal function was found in 48 of 80 patients. Underestimation of the presence of impaired renal function in hospitalized patients with gout was recently highlighted by the findings of Petersel and Schlesinger [188b]. Based on a two year retrospective review of records of hospitalized patients with acute gout they found renal failure (serum creatinine > 1.5

mg/dL) in 65% and a decreased eGRF in 73%. CKD III was present in 47%, CKD IV in 20% and CKD V in 5%. Combination therapy with Colchicine and NSAIDs was used in over 80% of the patients with renal failure and gout. Only 27% of the patients admitted with gouty arthritis were receiving allopurinol prophylaxis. In patients receiving allopurinol prophylaxis as outpatient treatment, one quarter do not have their serum creatinine monitored [188c].

Histopathology

Histopathological examination of renal biopsy or autopsy specimens revealed renal vasculitis [181], focal segmental glomerulonephritis [184], and acute interstitial nephritis [185, 187, 189, 190]. Jarzobski et al. [181] reported a case of the hypersensitivity type of vasculitis with fibrinoid necrosis and eosinophilic reaction, involving multiple organs, especially the kidney, resulting in uremia and death. Boyer et al. [191] also reported 3 cases of the same type including the efficacy of prednisolone in treating this type of disease. Kantor et al. [182] reported a case of glomerulonephritis associated with allopurinol-hypersensitivity. Linear deposition of IgG and complement along the glomerular basement membrane were demonstrated, and a necrotizing, hemorrhagic pneumonitis was also reported. However, no circulating anti-glomerular basement membrane antibody was detected. Acute interstitial nephritis has also been reported associated with by the administration of allopurinol [185, 187, 189, 190]. Gelbart et al. [185] reported a case of allopurinol-induced interstitial nephritis with extensive infiltration of lymphocytes, plasma cells and tubular damage. No immunoglobulins, complement, or fibrin were evident in the tubular basement membrane. This patient also had other typical symptoms of hypersensitivity reactions. Grussendrof et al. [187] also reported a case of acute interstitial nephritis with circulating anti-tubular basement membrane antibody and granular C3 deposition on the tubular basement membrane. The interstitium was diffusely widened, edematous and infiltrated with lymphocytes, plasma cells, histiocytes and numerous eosinophils. The nephritis was induced by controlled re-exposure to allopurinol in a patient who had two successive severe hypersensitivity reactions to this drug. More recently, Morel et al [191a] reported a case of allopurinol hypersensitivity reaction with renal failure on admission, in which skin manifestations and renal failure recurred after initial recovery. The case was considered unique due to the presence of an ANA titer or 1:2000 on admission. Treatment consisted of intravenous and oral steroids with residual renal impairment after 7 months of therapy. A renal biopsy, at the time of recurrence, yielded deposits of C3 complement in the vessel walls. A previous skin biopsy on admission yielded leukocytoclastic, non-specific vasculitis. The authors concluded that the "findings suggested the participation of ribonucleotide alterations in the pathophysiology of allopurinol hypersensitivity syndrome".

Pathogenesis

The pathogenesis of nephropathy associated with allopurinol-induced hypersensitivity reactions is unclear. However, pathogenic role of the immune reactions against allopurinol or its metabolites has not been excluded. Emmerson et al. [192] studied the lymphocyte reactivities to allopurinol and its active metabolite, oxypurinol, in 9 patients with previous documented adverse reactions to allopurinol. They suggested that some adverse reactions to allopurinol represented delayed type hypersensitivity to oxypurinol, but not to allopurinol. Allopurinol is oxidized by xanthine oxidase to oxypurinol, which is also an inhibitor of the enzyme (Figure 4). Allopurinol plasma half life is less than 2 hours due to rapid renal clearance and oxidation to oxypurinol [193]. Oxypurinol, because of its reabsorbance by the renal tubules, has a plasma half-life of 18 to 30 hours. The clearance of oxypurinol is diminished in renal insufficiency [194]. In addition, thiazide diuretics might be expected to cause accumulation of oxypurinol since its renal handling is similar to that of uric acid [195]. Hypersensitivity syndrome has been found to occur most frequently when allopurinol is given with thiazides or in patients with renal insufficiency [184, 188]. The immune reactions to oxypurinol may play an important role in the pathogenesis of the syndrome, including being dose dependent. The serum concentration of oxypurinol has been monitored to prevent adverse reactions [195, 196]. Recommended plasma oxypurinol concentrations are below 100 μmol/L [196]. Several authors [195, 196] reported that no adverse reactions have occurred in patients with lower plasma oxypurinol levels; how-

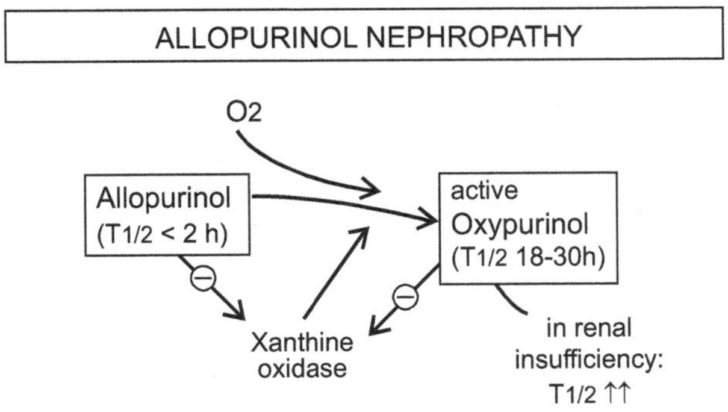

Figure 4. *Suggestion of reactions leading to allopurinol nephropathy.*

ever, hypersensitivity syndrome occasionally develops in patients with a therapeutic plasma oxypurinol concentration [197]. In addition to plasma oxypurinol concentration, other factors probably contribute to the development of the syndrome.

Human herpes virus 6 (HHV 6) infection is recently attracted a great deal of attention as a possible cause of drug-induced hypersensitivity. Suzuki et al reported a case of allopurinol-induced hypersensitivity syndrome with dramatically increased anti-HHV 6 IgG antibodies. They also demonstrated the presence of HHV 6 in the skin of this patient using a polymerase chain reaction and *in situ* hybridization [198]. Thus, drug-induced hypersensitivity syndrome may not be a simple allergic reaction to drug. Further investigations regarding the relation of HHV 6 infection and drug-induced hypersensitivity syndrome may provide insight to the pathogenesis of allopurinol-induced hypersensitivity syndrome.

Therapy, prognosis, and prevention

Withdrawal of the drug and the prolonged administration of systemic steroids are beneficial for the hypersensitivity syndrome with renal involvement. Initial dose of steroid should be 1 to 2 mg/kg/day of methylprednisolone, with careful gradual tapering of steroids required in the majority of patients. The recovery time ranged from 1 week to 11 months. Mortality from this syndrome is high, with twenty-one of 80 patients died as a result of the syndrome [188]. In fulminant cases, such as acute renal failure complicating toxic epidermal necrosis or Stevens-Johnson syndrome, methylprednisolone 'pulse' therapy might be beneficial. Patients with HHV 6 infection also require prednisolone therapy.

To prevent unnecessary morbidity and mortality due to the allopurinol hypersensitivity, Singer et al. [188] recommended the indications for allopurinol as follow: 1) tophaceous gout; 2) major uric acid overproduction (urinary excretion of more than 900 mg of uric acid/day on a diet with rigid purine restriction); 3) frequent gouty attacks unresponsive to prophylactic colchicines, when uricosuric agents cannot be used due to intolerance, lack of efficacy, renal insufficiency, or poor patient compliance; 4) recurrent uric acid renal calculi; 5) recurrent calcium oxalate renal calculi when associated with hyperuricosuria; or 6) prevention of acute urate nephropathy in patients receiving cytotoxic therapy for malignancies. The tumor lysis syndrome (TLS) has come under increased scrutiny with the more aggressive chemotherapeutic management of both hemopoeitic and solid tumor malignancies. Because of the massive release of purine nuceloties, pretreatment with allopurinol often is inadequate to control the hyperuricemia and acute uric acid nephropathy develops [198a]. To overcome this deficiency of allopurinol protection, febuxostat, a more prowerful xanthine oxidase inhibitor has been developed. However, in criticizing a recent clinical trial comparing febuxostat with allopurinol [198b], Gelber [198c] wrote "caution, however, needs to be exercise in as much as the reported frequency of adverse events leading to discontinuation of the drug occurred two and three times as often in the low-dose and high-dose febuxostat group, respectively, as in the allopurinol group". Rasburicase is a urate oxidase that converts uric acid to allantoin which is much more soluble thus precluding acute urate nephropathy in TLS [198d, h]. A combination of rasburicase and allopurinol has been successfully used in preventing hyperuricemia of TLS [198i]. While Rasburicase has been shown to be successful in preventing the hyperuricemia of TLS [198e, f, g] it should not be given to patients with G6PD deficiency, methemaglobinemia and history of anaphalaxis [198e]. Also, concern has been raised about the high immunogenicity of rasburicase and native uricase since antibodies to the drug occurred in 14% of patient in a clinical trial of TLS [198a]. There is disagreement regarding the value of allopurinol treatment for asymptomatic hyperuricemia, uncomplicated gout, and acute gouty attacks which Singer et al [188] consider counter- indicated while Kelley [199] advised allopurinol therapy for asymptomatic hyperuricemia, but only when it is truly severe (serum uric acid level > 13 mg/dl and 24-hour urine excretion > 1,100 mg). For the treatment of acute hyperuricemia with renal insufficiency Ronco and coworkers [198g] present compelling data supporting the use of rasburicase. The allopurinol hypersensitivity syndrome occurs most frequently when the drug is given with diuretics or in patients with renal insufficiency. CKD patients on allopurinol therapy should be closely monitored especially within the first several weeks after initiating administration of the drug. If the AHS develops, allopurinol should be withdrawn but may be reintroduced using a gradually increasing dosage schedule [200]. Finally, patients at high risk for developing hyperuricemia should start the therapy with lower dose of allopurinol. Indications for chronic treatment of symptomatic gout in high risk patients using either rasburicase or febuxostat needs to be confirmed by clinical trials.

References

1. Lande K. Die gunstige Beeinflussung schleichender Dauerinfekte durch Solganal. Munchen Med Wochenshr 1927; 74: 1132-1134.
2. The Research Sub-Committee of the Empire Rheumatism Council. Gold therapy in rheumatoid arthritis. Final report of a multicenter controlled trial. Ann Rheum Dis 1961; 20: 315-333.
3. Penneys NS, Eaglestein WH, Frost P. Management of pemphigus with gold compounds. Arch Dermatol 1976; 112: 185-187.
4. Muranaka M, Miyamoto T, Shida T, Kabe J, Makino S, Okumura H, Takeda K, Suzuki S, Horiuchi Y. Gold salt in the treatment of bronchial asthma - a double blind study. Ann Allergu 1978; 40: 132-137.
5. Finkelstein AE, Walz DT, Batista V, Mizrazi M, Roisman F, Misher A. Auranofin – new oral gold compound for treatment of rheumatoid arthritis. Ann Rheum Dis 1976; 35: 251-257.
6. Berglof FE, Berglof K, Walz DT. Auranofin: an oral chrysotherapeutic agent for the treatment of rheumatoid arthritis. J Rheumatol 1978; 5: 68-74.
7. Weisman MH, Hannifin DH. Management of rheumatoid arthritis with oral gold. Arthritis Rheum 1979; 22: 922-925.
8. Davis P, Menard H, Thompson J, Harth M, Beaudet F. One-year comparative study of gold sodium thiomalate and auranofin in the treatment of rheumatoid arthritis. J Rheumatol 1985; 12: 60-67.
9. Ward JR, Williams HJ, Egger MJ, Reading JC, Boyce E, Altz-Smith M, Samuelson CO, Willkens RF, Solsky MA, Hayes SP, Blocka KL, Weinstein A, Meenan RF, Guttadauria M, Kaplan SB, Klippel J. Comparison of auranofin, gold sodium thiomalate and placebo in the treatment of rheumatoid arthritis: A controlled clinical trial. Arthritis Rheum 1983; 26: 1303-1315.
10. Heuer MA, Pietrusko RG, Morris RW, Scheffler BJ. An analysis of worldwide safety experience with auranofin. J Rheumatol 1985; 12: 695-699.

10a. O'Dell JR, Petersen K, Leff R, Palmer W, Schned E, Blakely K, Haire C, Fernandez A. Etanercept in combination with sulfasalaazine, hydroxychloroquine, or gold in the treatment of rheumatoid arthritis. J Rheumatol 2006;33:213-218.

10b. Rau R, Schleusser B, Herborn G, Karger T. Longterm combination therapy of refractory and destructive rheumatoid arthritis with methotrexate (MTX) and intramuscular gold or other disease modifying antirheumatic drugs compare to MTX monotherapy. J Rheumatol 1998;25:1485-1492.

11. Hartfall SJ, Garland HG, Goldie W. Gold treatment of arthritis. A review of 900 cases. Lancet 1937; 9: 838-842.
12. Gibbons RB. Complication of chrysotherapy. A review of recent studies. Arch Intern Med 1979; 139: 343-346.
13. Penneys NS, Ackerman AB, Gottlieb NL. Gold dermatitis. Arch Dermatol 1979; 109: 372-376.
14. Benson WG, Moore N, Tugwell P, D, Souza M, Singal DP. HLA antigens and toxic reactions to sodium aurothiomalate in patients with rheumatoid arthritis. J Rheumatol 1984; 11: 358-361.
15. Adachi JD, Bensen WG, Singal DP, Powers PJ. Gold-induced thrombocytopenia: platelet associated IgG and HLA typing in three patients. J Rheumatol 1984; 11: 355-357.
16. Gottlieb NL, Gray RG. Diagnosis and management of adverse reaction from gold compounds. J Analytic Toxicol 1978; 2: 173.
17. Baldwin JL, Storb R, Thomas ED, Mannik M. Bone marrow transplantation in patients with gold-induced marrow aplasia. Arthritis Rheum 1977; 20: 1043-1048.
18. Gibson J, McGirr EE, York J, Kronenberg H. Aplastic anemia in association with gold therapy for rheumatoid arthritis. Aust NZ J Med 1983; 13: 130-135.
19. Winterbauer RH, Wilske KR, Wheelis RF. Diffuse pulmonary injury associated with gold treatment. N Engl J Med 1976; 294: 919-921.

20. Partanen J, van Assendelft AHW, Koskimies S, Forsberg S, Hakala M, Ilonen J. Patients with rheumatoid arthritis and fold-induced pneumonitis express two high-risk major histocompatibility complex patterns. Chest 1987; 92: 277-281.
21. Fam AG, Paton TW, Shamess CJ, Lewis AJ. Fulminant colitis complicating gold therapy. J Rheumatol 1980; 7: 479-485.
22. Silverberg DS, Kidd EG, Shnitka TK, Ulan RA. Gold nephropathy. A clinical and pathological study. Arthritis Rheum 1970; 13: 812-825.
23. Kean WF, Anastassiades TP. Long-term chrysotherapy. Incidence of toxicity and efficacy during sequential time periods. Arthritis Rheum 1979; 22: 495-501.
24. Katz WA, Blodgett RC Jr, Pietrusko RG. Proteinuria in gold treated rheumatoid arthritis. Ann Intern Med 1984; 101: 176-179.
25. Brock H, Han MT. Gold nephrosis. N Engl J Med 1966; 274: 210-211.
26. Furst DE, Levine S, Srinivasan R, Metzger L, Bangert R, Paulus E. A double-blind trial of high versus conventional dosages of gold salts for rheumatoid arthritis. Arthritis Rheum 1977; 20: 1473-1480.
27. Gran JT, Husby G, Thorsby E. HLA DR antigens and gold toxicity. Ann Rheum Dis 1983; 42: 63-66.
28. Bensen WG, Moore N, Tugwell P, D Souza M, Singal DP. HLA antigens and toxic reactions to sodium aurothiomalate in patients with rheumatoid arthritis. J Rheumatol 1984; 11: 358-361.
29. Barger BO, Acton RT, Koopman WJ, Alarcon GS. DR antigens and gold toxicity in white rheumatoid patients. Arthritis Rheum 1984; 27: 601-605.
30. Hakala M, van Assendelef AHW, Ilonen J, Jalava S, Tiilikainen A. Association of different HLA antigens with various toxic effects of gold salts in rheumatoid arthritis. Ann Rheum Dis 1986; 45: 177-182.
31. Vaamaonde CA, Hunt FR. The nephritic syndrome as a complication of gold therapy. Arthritis Rheum 1970; 13: 826-834.
32. Francis KL, Jenis EH, Jensen GE, Calcagno PL. God-associated nephropathy. Arch Pathol Lab Med 1984; 108: 234-238.
33. Hall CL, Fothergill NJ, Blackwell MM, Harrison PR, MacKenzie JC, MacIver AG. The natural course of gold nephropathy: long term study of 21 patients. Br Med J 1987; 295: 745-748.
34. Tornroth T, Skrifvars B. Gold nephropathy. Prototype of membranous glomerulonephritis. Am J Med 1974; 75: 573-590
34a. Hall CL. Gold nephropathy. Nephron 1988;50:265-272.
34b. Hall CL, The natural course of gold and penicillamine nephropathy. A longterm study of 54 patients. Adv. Exp Med Biol 1989;252:247-256/
34c. Klinkhoff AV, Teufel A. Reinstitution of gold after gold induced proteinuria. J Rheumatol 1997;24:1277-1279.
35. Lee JC, Dushinkin M, Eyring EJ, Engleman EP, Hopper JR. Renal lesions associated with gold therapy. Light and electron microscopic studies. Arthritis Rheum 1965; 8: 1-13.
36. Mattson JC. Glomerular diseases as a complication of gold therapy. Lab Invest 1974; 30: 383.
37. Katz A, Little AH. Gold nephropathy. An immunopathologic study. Arch Pathol 1973; 96: 133-136.
38. Watanabe I, Whitter FC, Moore J, Cuppage FE. Gold nephropathy. Ultrastructural fluorescent and microanalytic study of two human cases. Arch Path Lab Med 1976; 100: 632-635.
39. Davies DJ, Dowling J, Xipell JM. Gold nephropathy. Pathology 1977; 9: 281-288.
40. Skrifvars BV, Tornroth TS, Tallqvist GN. Gold-induced immune complex nephritis in seronegative rheumatoid arthritis. Ann Rheum Dis 1977; 36: 549-556.
41. Wolters J, Frederik P, van Rie H, Zeppenfeldt E. Minimal change nephropathy during gold treatment. A case with unusual histopathological and immunopathological features. Netherland J Med 1987; 31: 234-240.
42. Skirfvars B, Tornroth T, Flalck HM. Granulomatous glomerulonephritis in a patient with rheumatoid arthritis treated with gold salts. Scand J Rheumatol 1979; 8: 234-240.
43. Cramer CR, Hagler HK, Silva FG, Eigenbrodt EH, Meltzer JI, Pirani CL. Chronic interstitial nephritis associated with gold nephropathy. Arch Path Lab Med 1983; 107: 258-263.
44. Tubbs RR, Valenzuela R, McGorman LJ, Pohl MA, Barenberg S. Gold nephropathy. New Eng J Med 1977; 296: 1413-1414.
45. Yarom R, Stein H, Peter PD, Slavin S, Hall TA. Nephrotoxic effect of parenteral and intraarticular gold. Ultrastructural and electron microprobe examination of clinical and experimental materials. Arthritis Rheum 1975; 99: 36-43.
46. Iesato K, Mori Y, Ueda S, Wakashin Y, Wakashin M, Matsui N, Inoue S, Okuda K. Renal tubular dysfunction as a complication of gold therapy in patients with rheumatoid arthritis. Clin Nephrol 1982; 17: 46-52.
47. Ueda S, Wakashin M, Wakashin Y, Yoshida H, Iesato K, Mori T, Mori Y, Akikusa B, Okuda K. Experimental gold nephropathy in guinea pigs: Detection of autoantibodies to renal tubular antigens. Kidney Int 1986; 29: 539-548.
48. Nagi AH, Alexander F, Barabas AZ. Gold nephropathy in rats. Light and electron microscopic studies. Exp Molec Path 1971; 15: 354-362.
49. Eiseman JL, Ribas JL, Knight E, Alvares AP. Acute nephropathy induced by gold sodium thiomalate: Alterations in renal heme metabolism and morphology. Toxicol Appl Pharmacol 1987; 91: 193-203.

50. Bretza J, Wells I, Novey HS. Association of IgE antibodies to sodium aurothiomalate and adverse reactions to chrysotherapy for rheumatoid arthritis. Am J Med 1983; 74: 945-950.
51. Davis P, Ezeoke A, Munro J, Hobbs JR, Hughes GRV. Immunological studies on the mechanism of gold hypersensitivity reactions. Br Med J 1973; 3: 676-678.
52. Denman EJ, Denman AM. The lymphocyte transformation test and gold hypersensitivity. Ann Rheum Dis 1968; 27: 582-588.
53. Derot M, Kahn J, Mazalton A, Peyrafort J. Fatal anuric nephritis with associated chrysocyanosis following gold therapy. Bull Soc Med Hop Paris 1954; 70: 234-239.
54. Palosuo T, Provast TT, Milgrom F. Gold nephropathy. Serologic data suggesting an immune complex disease. Clin Exp Immunol 1976; 25: 311-318.
55. Skirfvars B. Hypothesis for the pathogenesis of sodium aurothiomalate induced immune complex nephritis. Scand J Rheumatol 1979; 8: 113-118.
56. Jessop JD, Vernon-Roberts B, Harris J. Effects of gold salts and prednisolone on inflammatory cells. I. Phagocytic activity of macrophages and polymorphs in inflammatory exudates studied by a 'skin-window' technique in rheumatoid and control patients. Ann Rheum Dis 1973; 32: 294-300.
57. Vernon-Roberts B, Jessop JD, Dore J. Effects of gold salts and prednisolone on inflammatory cells. II. Suppression of inflammation and phagocytosis in the rat. Ann Rheum Dis 1973; 32: 301-307.
58. Panush RS. Effects of certain antirheumatic drugs on normal human peripheral blood lymphocytes. Inhibition of mitogen- and antigen- stimulated incorporation of tritiated thymidine. Arthritis Rheum 1976; 19: 907-917.
59. Harth M, Stiller CR, Sinclair C, Evans J, McGirr D, Zuberi R. Effects of a gold salt on lymphocyte responses. Clin Exp Immunol 1977; 27: 357-364.
60. Measel W. Effects of gold on the immune response of mice. Infect Immunity 1975; 11: 350-354.
61. Ueda S, Wakashin M, Wakashin Y, Yoshida H, Azemoto R, Iesato K, Mori T, Mori Y, Ogawa M, Okuda K. Autoimmune interstitial nephritis in inbred mice. Analysis of mouse tubular basement membrane antigen and genetic control of immune response to it. Am J Pathol 1988; 132: 304-318.
62. Ueda S, Wakashin Y, Yoshida H, Mori T, Mori Y, Azemoto R, Ogawa M, Kato I, Wakashin M. Gold nephropathy - effect of gold on immune response to renal tubular basement membrane (TBM) antigen in mice. In: Nephrotoxicity. *In vitro* to *in vivo*, animals to man. Bach BH, Lock EA, editors. Plenum, New York 1989; p. 139-145.
63. Lorber A, Kunishima D, Simon T. Selective inhibition of T suppressor lymphocytes during chrysotherapy [Abstract]. Clin Pharmacol Ther 1983; 303: 300-302.
64. Newton O, Swinburn WR, Swinson DR. Proteinuria with gold nephropathy: When should gold be permanently stopped? Br J Rheumatol 1983; 22: 11-17.
65. Howard-Lock HE, Lock CJL, Mewa A, Kean WF. D-penicillamine; Chemistry and clinical use in rheumatic disease. Sem Arthritis Rheum 1986; 15: 261-281.
66. Manthorpe R, Bendixen G. Auranofin in rheumatoid arthritis: Use in patients with side-effect or lack of effect to gold sodium thiomalate or gold thioglucose and/or D-penicillamine. Scand J Rheumatol 1988; 17: 401-405.
67. Panayi GS, Wooley P, Batchelor JR. Genetic basis of R.A. HLA antigen, disease manifestations and toxic reactions to drugs. Br Med J 1978; 11: 1326-1328.
68. Wooly PH, Griffen J, Panayi GS, Batchelor JR, Welsh KI, Gibson TJ. HLA-DR antigens and toxic reaction to sodium aurothiomalate and D-penicillamine in patients with rheumatoid arthritis. N Engl J Med 1980; 303: 300-302.
69. Bardin T, Legrand L, Naveau B, Marcelli-Barge A, Debeyre N, Lathrop GM, Poirier JC, Schmid M, Ryckewaert A, Dryll A. HLA antigens and seronegative rheumatoid arthritis. Ann Rheum Dis 1985; 44: 50-53.
70. Dequeker J, Van Wanghe P, Verdickt W. A systematic survey of HLA-A, B, C, and D antigens and drug toxicity in rheumatoid arthritis. J Rheumatol 1984; 11: 282-286.
71. Ford PM. HLA antigens and drug toxicity in rheumatoid arthritis. J Rheumatol 1984; 11: 269-261.
72. Van Riel PL, Van de Putte LB, Gribnau FW, de Waal RM. Serum IgA and gold induced toxic effects in patients with rheumatoid arthritis. Arch Intern Med 1984; 144: 1401-1403.
73. Ostuni PA, Simioni M, Marson P, Travaglia P, Volante D, Gambari PF. Serum IgA and gold toxicity in rheumatoid arthritis: lack of predicting value. Clin Exp Rheumatol 1986; 4: 359-362.
74. Ayesh R, Mitchell SC, Waring RH, Withrington RH, Seifert MH, Smith RL. Sodium aurothiomalate toxicity and sulphoxidation capacity in rheumatoid arthritis patients. Br J Rheumatol 1987; 26: 197-201.
74a. Shah P, Griffith SM, Shadforth MF, Fisher J, Dawes PT, Poulton KV, Thomson W, Ollier WE, Mattey DL. Can gold ltherapy be used more safely in rheumatoid arthritis? Adverse drug reactions are more likely in patients with nodular disease, independent of HLA-DR3 status. J Rheumatol 2004;31:1903-1905.

74b. Pissuwan D, Vlaenzuela SM, Cortie MB. Therapeutic possibilities of plasmonicall heated gold nanoparticles. Trends in Biotech. 2006;24:62-67
74c. Zharov VP, Galitovskaya EN, Johnson C, Kelly T. Synergistic enhancement of selective nanophotothermolysis with gold nanoclusters: Potential for cancer therapy. Lasers in Surg Med. 2005;37:219-226.
75. Blodgett RC Jr, Heuer MA, Pietrusko RG. Auranofin: a unique oral chrysotherapeutic agent. Semin Arthritis Rheum 1984; 13: 255-273.
76. Bandilla K, Gross D, Gross W, Herrlinger J-D, Kriegel W, Muller W, Siegmeth W, Tausch G, Thumb N, Wagenhauser J. Oral gold therapy with auranofin (SK&F39162). J Rheumatol 1982; 9 (Suppl 8): 154-159.
77. Katz W, Alexander S, Bland J, Blechman W, Bluhm GB, Bonebrake Ra, Falbo A, Greenwald RA, Hartman S, Hobbs T, Indenbaum S, Lergier JE, Lanier BG, Lightfoot RW, Phelps P, Sheon RP, Torretti D, Wenger ME, Wilske K. The efficacy and safety of auranofin compared to placebo in rheumatoid arthritis. J Rheumatol 1982; 9 (Suppl 8): 173-178.
78. Wenger ME, Alexander S, Bland JH, Blechman WJ. Auranofin versus placebo in the treatment of rheumatoid arthritis. Am J Med 1983; 75: 123-127.
79. Menard HA, Beaudet F, Davis O, Harth M, Percy JS, Russell AS, Thompson M. Gold therapy in rheumatoid arthritis. Interim report of the Canadian multicentre prospective trial comparing sodium aurothiomalate and auranofin. J Rheumatol 1982; 9: 179-183.
80. Felix-Davies DD, Stewart AM, Wilkinson BR, Bateman JR, Delamere JP. A 12-month comparative trial of auranofin and D-penicillamine in rheumatoid arthritis. Am J Med 1983; 75(6A): 138-141.
81. Manthrope R, Horbov S, Sylvest J, Vinterberg H. Auranofin versus penicillamine in rheumatoid arthritis. One-year results from a prospective clinical investigation. Scand J Rheumatol 1986; 15: 13-22.
82. Hochberg MC. Auranofin or D-penicillamine in the treatment of rheumatoid arthritis. Ann Intern Med 1986; 105: 528-535.
83. Revach M, Freed RL, Ehrlich GE. Reversible proteinuria as a complication of oral gold therapy [Letter]. Arthritis Rheum 1979; 22: 1417-1418.
84. Plaza JJ, Herrero G, Barat A, Loutaif JJ, Hernando L, Vallado P, Oliva H. Membranous glomerulonephritis as a complication of oral gold therapy [Letter]. Ann Intern Med 1982; 97: 563-564.
85. Gottlieb NL. Comparative pharmacokinetics of parenteral and oral gold compounds. J Rheumatol 1982; 9 (Suppl 8): 99-109.
86. Blocka K. Auranofin versus injectable gold: Comparison of pharmacokinetic properties. Am J Med 1983; 75(6A): 114-122.
87. Abraham EP, Chain E, Baker W, Robinson R. Penicillamine, a characteristic degradiation product of penicillin. Nature 1943; 151: 107.
88. Walshe JM: Penicillamine. A new oral therapy for Wilson's disease. Am J Med 1956; 2: 487-495.
89. Drawhall JC, Scowen EF, Watts RWE. Effects of penicillamine on cystinuria. Br Med J 1963; 1: 588-590.
90. Jaffe IA. Intra-articular dissociation of the rheumatoid factor. J Lab Clin Med 1962; 60: 409-421.
91. Jaffe IA. The effect of penicillamine in the laboratory parameters in rheumatoid arthritis. Arthritis Rheum 1965; 8: 1064-1078.
92. Multicenter trial group. Controlled trial of D-penicillamine in severe rheumatoid arthritis. Lancet 1973; 1: 275-280.
93. Steen VD, Medsger TA, Rodnan GP. D-penicillamine therapy in progressive systemic sclerosis (scleroderma). A retrospective analysis. Ann Intern Med 1982; 97: 652-659.
94. Jain S, Scherer PJ, Samourian S. A controlled trial of D-penicillamine therapy in primary biliary cirrhosis. Lancet 1977; 1: 831-834.
95. Goldberg Am Smith JA, Lochhead AC. Treatment of lead poisoning with oral penicillamine. Br Med J 1963; 1: 1270-1275.
96. Freeman HC, Huq F, Stevens GN: Metal binding by D-penicillamine: Crystal structure of D-penicillamine cadmium (II) hydrate. J Chem Soc Chem Commun 1976; 90-91.
97. Tamir M, Boustein B, Behar M, Chwat M. Mercury poisoning from an unsuspected source. Br J Ind Med 1968; 21: 299-303.
98. Deutsch MF, Morton JI. Dissociation of human serum macroglobulins. Science 1957; 125: 600-601.
99. Kean WF, Dwosh JL, Anastassiades TP, Ford PM, Kelly HG. The toxicity pattern of D-penicillamine therapy. A guide to the use in RA. Arthritis Rheum 1980; 23: 158-165.
100. Stein HB, Patterson AC, Offer RC, Atkins CJ, Teufel A, Robinson HS. Adverse effects of D-penicillamine in rheumatoid arthritis. Ann Intern Med 1980; 92: 24-29.
101. Kean WF, Lock CJL, Howard-Lock HE, Buchanan WW. Prior gold therapy does not influence the adverse effects of D-penicillamine in rheumatoid arthritis. Arthritis Rheum 1982; 25: 917-922.
102. Wollheim FA, Lindstrom CG. Liver abnormalities in penicillamine treated patients with rheumatoid arthritis. Scand J Rheumatol 1979; 28 (Suppl):100-107.
103. Barzilai D, Dickstein G, Enat R, Bassan H, Lichtig C, Gellei B. Cholestatic jaundice caused by D-penicillamine. Ann Rheum Dis 1978; 37: 98-100.
104. Multz CV. Cholestatic hepatitis caused by penicillamine. JAMA 1981; 246: 674-675.
105. Hickling P, Fuller J. Penicillamine causing acute colitis. Br Med J 1979; 2: 367.

106. Crawhall JC. Proteinuria in D-penicillamine-treated rheumatoid arthritis. J Rheumatol 1981; 8: 161-163.
107. Davison AM, Day AT, Golding JR, Thomson D. Effect of penicillamine on the kidney. Proc R Soc Med 1977; 70: 109-113.
108. Barraclough D, Cunningham TJ, Muirden KD. Microscopic haematuria in patients with rheumatoid arthritis on D-penicillamine. Aust NZ J Med 1981; 11: 706-708.
109. Singh G, Fries JF, Williams CA, Zatarain E, Spitz P, Bloch DA. Toxicity profiles of disease modifying antirheumatic drugs in rheumatoid arthritis. J Rheumatol 1991;18: 188-194.
110. Weiss AS, Markenson JA, Weiss MS, Kammerer WH. Toxicity of D-penicillamine in rheumatoid arthritis. A report of 63 patients including two with aplastic anemia and one with the nephritic syndrome. Am J Med 1978; 64: 114-120.
111. Chalmers A, Thompson D, Stein HE, Reid G, Patterson HC. Systemic Lupus Erythematosus during penicillamine therapy for rheumatoid arthritis. Ann Intern Med 1982; 97: 659-663.
112. Walshe JM. Penicillamine and the SLE syndrome. J Rheumatol 1981; 8 (Suppl 7): 155-160.
113. Sternlieb I, Bennet B, Scheinberg IH. D-penicillamine induced Goodpasture's syndrome in Wilson's disease. Ann Intern Med 1975; 82: 673.
114. Gibson T, Barry HC, Ogg C. Goodpastures' syndrome and D-penicillamine. Ann Intern Med 1976; 84: 100.
115. Gavaghan TE, McNaught PJ, Ralston M, Hayes JM. Penicillamine-induced 'Goodpasture's syndrome'; successful treatment of a fulminant case. Aust NZ J Med 1981; 11: 261-265.
116. Jaffe IA. The treatment of rheumatoid arthritis and necrotizing vasculitis with penicillamine. Arthritis Rheum 1970; 13: 436-443.
117. Banfi G, Imbasciati E, Guerra L, Mihatsch MJ, Ponticelli C. Extracapillary glomerulonephritis with necrotizing vasculitis in D-penicillamine treated patients with rheumatoid arthritis. Nephron 1983; 33: 56-60.
118. Torres CF, Griggs RC, Baum J, Penn AS. Penicillamine induced myasthenia gravis in progressive sclerosis. Arthritis Rheum 1980; 23: 505-508.
119. Dawkins RL, Garlepp MJ, McDonald BL, Williamson J. Myasthenia gravis and D-penicillamine. J Rheumatol 1981; 8 (Suppl 7): 169-174.
120. Vincent A, Newsom-Davis J. Acetylcholine receptor antibody characteristic in myasthenia gravis. Patients with penicillamine-induced myasthenia or idiopathic myasthenia of recent onset. Clin Exp Immunol 1982; 49: 266-272.
121. Bever CT, Chang HW, Penn AS, Jaffe IA, Bock E. Penicillamine induced myasthenia gravis. Effects of penicillamine on acetylcholine receptor. Neurology 1982; 32: 1077-1082.
122. Bocanegra T, Espinoza LR, Vassey FB, Germain BF. Myasthenia gravis in penicillamine treatment of RA. JAMA 1980; 244: 1822-1823.
123. Cucher BG, Goldman AL. D-penicillamine induced polymyositis in RA. Ann Intern Med 1976; 85: 615-618.
124. Schreider PL, Peters HA, Dahl DS. Polymyositis and penicillamine. Arch Neurol 1972; 27: 456-457.
125. Wojnarowska F. Dermatomyositis induced by penicillamine. J R Soc Med 1980; 73: 884.
126. Halverson PB, Kozin F, Bernhard GC, Goldman AL. Toxicity of penicillamine. A serious limitation to therapy in rheumatoid arthritis. JAMA 1978; 240: 1870-1871.
127. Steen VD, Blair S, Medsger TA. The toxicity of D-penicillamine in systemic sclerosis. Ann Intern Med 1986; 104: 699-705.
128. Moens HJB, Ament BJW, Feltkamp BW, Korst JK. Longterm followup of treatment with D-penicillamine to rheumatoid arthritis: effectivity and toxicity in relation to HLA antigens. J Rheumatol 1987; 14: 1115-1119.
129. Shiokawa Y, Horiuchi Y, Honma M, Kageyama T, Okada T, Azuma T. Clinical evaluation of D-penicillamine by multicentric double blind comparative study in chronic rheumatoid arthritis. Arthritis Rheum 1977; 20: 1464-1472.
130. Stockman A, Zilko PJ, Major GAC, Tait BD, Property DN, Mathews JD, Hannah MC, McCluskey J, Muirden KD. Genetic markers in rheumatoid arthritis-Relationship of toxicity from D-penicillamine. J Rheumatol 1986; 13: 269-273.
131. Hill HFH, Hill AGS, Day AT, Brown RM, Golding JR, Lyle WH. Maintenance dose of penicillamine in rheumatoid arthritis: A comparison between standard and a response-related flexible regimen. Ann Rheum Dis 1979; 38: 429-433.
132. Williams HJ, Ward JR, Reading JC, Egger MJ, Grandone JT, Samuelson CO, Furst DE, Sullivan JM, Watson MA, Guttadauria M, Cathcart ES, Kaplan SB, Halla JT, Weinstein A, Plotz PH. Low dose D-penicillamine treatment of R.A. A controlled double blind clinical trial. Arthritis Rheum 1983; 26: 581-592.
133. Hill H, Hill A, Davison M. Resumption of treatment with penicillamine after proteinuria. Ann Rheum Dis 1979; 38: 229-231.
134. Billingsley LM, Stevens MB. The relationship between D-penicillamine-induced proteinuria and prior gold nephropathy. Johns Hopkins Med J 1981; 148: 64-67.
135. Halla JT, Cassidy J, Hardin JG. Sequential gold and penicillamine therapy in rheumatoid arthritis. Am J Med 1982; 72: 423-426.
136. Ross JH, McGinty F, Brewer DG. Penicillamine nephropathy. Nephron 1980; 26: 184-186.
137. Dische FE, Swinson DR, Hamilton EBD, Parsons V. Immunopathology of penicillamine-induced glomerular disease. J Rheumatol 1976; 3: 145-154.

138. Halla JT, Cassidy J, Hardin JG. Sequential gold and penicillamine therapy in rheumatoid arthritis. Am J Med 1982; 72: 423-426.
139. Bacon PA, Tribe CR, MacKenzie JC, Jones JV, Cumming RH, Amer B. Penicillamine nephropathy in rheumatoid arthritis. Q J Med 1976; 45: 661-684.
140. Jaffe IA, Treser G, Suzuki Y, Ehrenreich T. Nephropathy induced by D-penicillamine. Ann Intern Med 1968; 69: 549-556.
141. Swinson DR, Hamilton EBD, Dische FE. Penicillamine nephropathy [letter]. Ann Rheum Dis 1975; 34: 544.
142. Neild GH, Gartner HV, Bohle A. Penicillamine induced membranous nephritis. Scand J Rheumatol 1979; 28: 79-90.
143. Sellars L, Siamopoulos K, Wilkinson R, Leohapand T, Morley AR. Renal biopsy appearances in rheumatoid disease. Clin Nephrol 1983; 20: 114-120.
144. Herve JP, Leguy P, Cledes J, Leroy JP. Nephrotic syndrome with minimal glomerular lesions during treatment with D-penicillamine. Nouv Press Med 1980; 9: 2847.
145. Kitazawa K, Ohseto Y, Kawazumi H, Saito K, Shibata T, Uchida J, Yonekura M, Schiwachi S, Ito S, Sugisaki T. D-penicillamine induced lipoid nephrosis in a patient with scleroderma. Ryumachi 1982; 22: 397-403.
146. Hayslett JP, Bensch KG, Kashgarian MZ, Rosenberg LE. Focal glomerulitis due to penicillamine. Lab Invest 1968; 19; 376-381.
147. Rehan A, Johnson K. IgM Nephropathy associated with penicillamine. Am J Nephrol 1986; 6: 71-74.
148. Liao K, Huang CC, Ho HH, Wu CH, Hsueh S. IgM nephropathy after D-penicillamine therapy: Report of a case. J Formosan Med Assoc 1987; 86: 906-909.
149. Hall CL. Jawad S, Harrison PR, MacKenzie JC, Bacon PA, Klouda PT, MacIver AG. Natural course of penicillamine nephropathy: A long-term study of 33 patients. Br Med J 1988; 296: 1083-1086.
150. Jaffe IA. D-penicillamine. Bull Rheum Dis 1977-8; 28: 948-952.
151. Jaffe IA. Penicillamine in rheumatoid disease with particular reference to the rheumatic factor. Postgrad Med J 1968 (suppl): 34-40.
152. Swainson CP, Thompson D, Short AIK, Winney RJ. Plasma exchange in the successful treatment of drug-induced renal disease. Nephron 1982; 30: 244-249.
153. Peces R, Rivera JR, Arboleya LR, Lopez-Larrea C, Alvarez J. Goodpasture's syndrome in a patient receiving penicillamine and carbimazole. Nephron 1985; 45: 316-320.
154. Matloff DS, Kaplan MM. D-penicillamine-induced Goodpasture's-like syndrome in primary biliary cirrhosis: successful treatment with plasmapheresis and immunosuppressives. Gastroenterology 1980; 78: 1046-1049.
155. Devogelaer J-P, Pirson Y, Vandenbroucke J-M, Cosyns J-P, Brichard S, Deuxchaisnes CN. D-penicillamine induced crescentic glomerulonephritis: Report and review of the literature. J Rheumatol 1987; 14: 1036-1041.
155a. Derk CT & Jimenez SA. Goodpasture-like syndrome induced by d-penicillamine in a patient with systemic sclerosis: Report and review of the literature. J. Rheumatol 2003;30:1616-1620.
155b. Bienaime G, Clerbaux G, Plaisier E, Mougenot B. Ronco P, Rougier JP. D-penicillamine-induced ANCA-associated crescentic glomerulonephritis in Wilson disease. Am J Kid Dis 2007;50:821-825.
156. Falck HM, Tornooth T, Kock B, Wegelius O. Fatal renal vasculitis with minimal change glomerulonephritis complicating treatment with penicillamine. Acta Med Scand 1979; 205: 133-138.
157. Ntoso KA, Tomaszewski JE, Jimenez SA, Neilson DG. Penicillamine-induced rapidly progressive glomerulonephritis in patients with progressive systemic sclerosis: Successful treatment of two patients and review of the literature. Am J Kidney Dis 1986; 8: 159-163.
158. Camus J-P, Homberg JC, Crouzet J, Mery C, Delrieu F, Massias P, Abuaf N. Autoantibody formation in D-penicillamine treated rheumatoid arthritis. J Rheumatol 1981; 7 (suppl): 80-83.
159. Mohammed I, Barraclough D, Holborrow EJ, Ansell BM. Effect of D-penicillamine therapy on circulating immune complexes in rheumatoid arthritis. Ann Rheum Dis 1976; 35: 458-462.
160. Aarden LA. Pathogencity of immune complexes. In: Non-articular forms of rheumatoid arthritis. Feltkamp TEW, editor. Stafleu's Scientific Publishing Co, Leyden 1977; 15.
161. Kirby JD, Dieppe PA, Huskisson EC, Smith B. D-penicillamine and immune complex deposition. Ann Rheum Dis 1979; 38: 344-346.
162. Nagata N, Hurtenbach U, Gleichmann E. Specific sensitization of Lyt-$1^{+}2^{-}$stereoisomer. J Immunol 1986; 136: 136-142.
162a. Doyle MK and Cuellar ML. Drug-induced vasculitis. Expert Opin Drug Saf. 2003;2:401-409.
163. Emery P, Panayi GS, Huston G, Welsh KI, Mitchell SC, Shah RR, Idle JR, Smith RL, Waring RH. E-penicillamine induced toxicity in rheumatoid arthritis: the role of sulphoxidation status and HLA-DR3. J Rheumatol 1984; 11: 626-632.
164. Speerstra F, Reekers P, van de Putte LBA, Vandenbroucke JP, Rasker JJ, de Rooij DJRAM. HLA-DR antigens and proteinuria induced by aurothioglucose and D-penicillamine in patients with rheumatoid arthritis. J Rheumatol 1983; 10: 948-953.

165. Moutsopoulos HM, Skopouli FN, Sarras AK, Tsampoulas C, Mavridis AK, Constantopoulos SH, Maddison PJ. Anti-Ro(SSA) positive rheumatoid arthritis: a clinicoserological group of patients with high incidence of D-penicillamine side effects. Ann Rheum Dis 1985; 44: 215-219.
166. Moutsopoulos HM, Giotaki H, Maddison PJ, Mavridis AK, Drosos AA, Skopouli FN. Antibodies to cellular antigens in Greek patients with autoimmune diseases: anti-Ro(SSA) antibody a possible marker of D-penicillamine intolerance. Ann Rheum Dis 1984; 43: 285-287.
167. Dodd MJ, Griffiths ID, Thomson M. Adverse reaction to D-penicillamine after gold toxicity. Br Med J 1980; 26: 1498-1500.
168. Webley M, Coomes EN. Is penicillamine therapy in RA. influenced by previous gold ? Br Med J 1978; 2: 91.
169. Klouda PT, Manos J, Acheson EJ, Dyer PA, Goldby FS, Harris R, Lawler W, Mallick NP, Williams G. Strong association between idiopathic membranous nephropathy and HLA-DRW3. Lancet 1979; 2: 770-771.
170. Swiss Federal Commission for the rheumatic diseases, Subcommission for Research. HLA-DR antigens in rheumatoid arthritis –A Swiss collaborative study; final report. Rheumatol Int 1986; 6: 89-92.
170a. Schiff MH and Whelton A. Renal toxicity associated with disease-modifying antirheumatic drugs used for the treatment of rheumatoid arthritis. Semin Arthritis Rheum 2000; 30:196-208.
171. Rundles RW, Wyngaarden JB, Hitchings GH, Elison B, Silberman HR. Effects of a xanthine oxidase inhibitor on thiopurine metabolism, hyperuricemia, and gout. Trans Assoc Am Physicians 1963; 76: 126-140.
172. Rundles RW, Metz EN, Silberman HR. Allopurinol in the treatment of gout. Ann Intern Med 1966; 64: 229-258.
173. Auerbach R, Orentrich N. Alopecia and ichthyosis secondary to allopurinol. Arch Dermatol 1968; 98: 104.
174. Boston Collaborative Drug Surveillance Program. Allopurinol and cytotoxic drugs. JAMA 1974; 227: 1036-1040.
175. Pinnas G. Possible association between macular lesions and allopurinol. Arch Ophthalmol 1968; 79: 786-787.
176. Korting HC, Lesch R. Acute cholangitis after allopurinol treatment. Lancet 1978; 1: 275-276.
117. Boyer TD, Sun N, Reynolds TB. Allopurinol-hypersensitivity. Vasculitis and liver damage. West J Med 1977; 126: 143-147.
178. Raper R, Barnes P, Ibels L, Lunzer M, Lauer C. Fulminant hepatic failure due to allopurinol. Aust NZ J Med 1984; 14: 63-65.
179. Bailey RR, Neale TJ, Lynn KL. Allopurinol-associated arteritis. Lancet 1976; 2: 907.
180. Greene ML, Fujimoto WY, Seegmiller JE. Urinary xanthine stones, a rare complication of allopurinol therapy. N Eng J Med 1969; 280: 426-427.
180a. LaRosa C, McMullen L, Bakdash S, Ellis D, Krishnamurti L, Wu HY, Mortiz ML. Acute renal failure from xanthine nephropathy during management of acute leukemia. Pediatr Nephrol 2007;22:132-135
180b. Rebentisch G, Stolz s, Muche J. Xanthinuria with xantine lithiasis in a patient with Lesch-Nyhan syndrome under allopurinol therapy. Aktuelle Urol. 2004;215-221.
181. Jarzobski J, Ferry J, Womboldt D, Fitch DM, Egan JD: Vasculitis with allopurinol therapy. Am Heart J 1970; 79: 116-121.
182. Kantor GC. Toxic epidermal necrolysis, azotemia, and death after allopurinol therapy. JAMA 1970; 212: 478-479.
183. Mills RM. Severe hypersensitivity reactions associated with allopurinol. JAMA 1971; 216: 799-802.
184. Young JC, Boswell RB, Niles AS: Severe allopurinol hypersensitivity. Arch Intern Med 1974; 134: 553-558.
185. Gelbart DC, Weinstein AB, Fajardo CF. Allopurinol-induced interstitial nephritis. Ann Intern Med 1977; 86: 196-198.
186. Lupton GP, Odom RB. The allopurinol hypersensitivity syndrome. J Am Acad Dermatol 1979; 1(4): 365-374.
187. Grussendorf M, Andrassy K, Waldherr R, Ritz E. Systemic hypersensitivity to allopurinol with acute interstitial nephritis. Am J Nephrol 1981; 1: 195-109.
188. Singer JZ, Wallace SL. The allopurinol hypersensitivity syndrome. Unnecessary morbidity and mortality. Arthritis Rheum 1986; 29: 82-87.
188a. Tausche AK, Aringer M, Schroeder HE, Bornstein SR, Wunderlich C, Wozel G. The janus faces of allopurinol – Allopurinol Hypersensitivity Syndrome. Am J Med. 2008;121:e3-e4.
188b. Petersel D, Schlesinger N. Treatment of acute gout in hospitalized patients. J. Rheumatol 2007;34:1566-1568.
188c. Raebel MA, McClure DL, Simon SR, Chan KA, Feldstein AC. Gunter MJ, Lafata JE, Harrold L, Nelson WW, Platt R. Frequency of serum creatinine monitoring during allopurinol therapy in ambulatory patients. Ann Pharmacother 2006;40:386-391.
189. McMenamie RA, Davies LM, Crasswell OW. Drug induced interstitial nephritis, hepatitis and exfoliative dermatitis. Aust NZ J Med 1976; 6: 583-587.
190. McKendrick MW, Geddes AM. Allopurinol hypersensitivity. Br J Med 1979; i: 988.
191. Boyer TD, Sun N, Reynolds TB. Allopurinol-hypersensitivity. Vasculitis and liver damage. West J Med 1977; 126: 143-147.
191a. Morel D, Cuez S, Merville P, Deminiere C, Tamisier JM, Potaux L. Recurrent renal failure associated with hypersensitivity to allopurinol. Nephrol Dial Transplant 1999;14:780-781.
192. Emmerson BT, Hazelton RA, Frazer IH. Some adverse reactions to allopurinol may be mediated by lymphocyte reactivity to oxypurinol. Arthritis Rheum 1988; 31: 436-440.

193. Elion GB, Kovensky A, Hitchings GH. Metabolic studies of allopurinol, an inhibitory of xanthine oxidase. Biochem Pharmacol 1965; 15: 863-880.
194. Elion GB, Yu TF, Gutman AB, Hitchings GH. Renal clearance of oxypurinol, the chief metabolite of allopurinol. Am J Med 1968; 45: 69-77.
195. Hande KR, Noone RM, Stone WJ. Severe allopurinol toxicity. Description and guidelines for prevention in patients with renal insufficiency. Am J Med 1984; 76: 47-56.
196. Simmonds HA, Cameron JS, Morris GS, Davies PM. Allopurinol in renal failure and the tumor lysis syndrome. Clin Chim Acta 1986; 31: 189-195.
197. Puig JP, Casas EA, Ramos TH, Michan AA, Mateos FA. Plasma oxypurinol concentration in a patient with allopurinol hypersensitivity. J Rheumatol 1989; 16: 842-844.
198. Suzuki Y, Inagi R, Aono T, Yamanishi K, Shihara T. Human herpesvirus 6 infrction a risk factor for the development of severe drug-induced hypersensitivity syndrome. Arch Dermatol 1998; 134: 1108-1112.
198a. Tiu RV, Mountantonakis SE, Dunbar AJ, Schreiber MJ Jr. Tumor lysis syndrome. Semin Thromb Hemost. 2007;33:397-407.
198b. Becker MA, Schumacher R Jr., Wortmann RL, MacDonald PA, Eustace D, Palo WA, Streit J, Joseph-Ridge N. Febuxostat compared with allopurinol in patients with hyperuricemia and gout. N Eng J Med 2005;353:2450-2461.
198c. Gelber AC. Febuxostat versus allopurinol for gout. N Engl J Med 2006;354:1532-1533.
198d. Stamp L, Searle M, O'Donnell J, Chapman P. Gout in solid organ transplantation; A challenging clinical problem. Drugs 2005;65:2593-2611.
198e. Sood AR, Burry LD, Cheng DKF. Clarifying the role of rasburicase in tumor lysis syndrome. Pharmacother 2007;27:11-=121.
198f. Bessmertny O, Robitaille LM, Cairo MS. Rasburicase: a new approach for preventing and/or treating tumor lysis syndrome. Current Pharmaceutical Design. 2005;11:4177-4185.
198g. Ronco C, Inguaggiato P, Bordoni V, DeCal M, Bonello M, Andrikos E, Assuman Y, Rattanarat R, Bellomo R. Rasburicase therapy in acute hyperuricemia and renal dysfunction. Contrib Nephrol 2005;147:115-123.
198h. Suh WM, Wainberg ZA, deVos S, Cohen AH, Kurtz I, Nguyen MK. Acute lymphoblastic leukemia presenting as acute renal failure. Naature Clin Pract. Nephrology 2007;3:106-110.
198i. DeAngelis S, Noce A, DiRenzo L, Cianci R, Naticchia A, Giarrizzo GR, Giordano F, Tozzo C, Splendiani G, DeLorenzo A. Is rasburicase an effective alternative to allopurinol for the management of hyperuricemia in renal failure patients/ A double –blind randomized study. Euro Rev Med Pharmacol Sci. 2007;11:179-184.
199. Kelley WN. Gout and related disorders of purine metabolism. In: Textbook of Rheumatology (1st edition). Kelly WN, Harris Jr ED, Sledge CB, editors. WB Saunders, Philadelphia 1981; p. 1397-1437.
200. Fam AG. Gout in the elderly. Drug & Aging. 1999;13:229-243.

20 Angiotensin I converting enzyme inhibitors and angiotensin II receptor antagonists

Paul E. DE JONG

University of Groningen, The Netherlands

Introduction

Over the last decade, the treatment of hypertension has changed dramatically from the concept of stepped care, advocated in the 1970's, to the more individualized care preferred nowadays. This phenomenon was largely due to the recent development of new classes of antihypertensives, which made it possible to adequately lower blood pressure in most patients with only one or two antihypertensive drugs, thus avoiding the need for a combination of multiple drugs. One of these new drug classes, the angiotensin I converting enzyme inhibitors (ACEI), drew a lot of attention since these were aimed at inhibiting the formation of angiotensin II, a hormone thought to be involved in the origin of systemic hypertension.

However, some major concerns appeared to restrict the widespread use of these drugs, including both renal histological changes such as a membranous glomerulopathy and an acute interstitial nephritis associated with ACEI, and functional changes such as an ACEI-induced fall in glomerular filtration rate (GFR) in some specified risk groups. Interestingly, although this fall in GFR was initially a reason for concern, after further studies that increased our understanding of the causes of this fall, some possible clinical uses of this phenomenon were recognized. Among these was the use of ACEI to improve the diagnostic armamentarium for renovascular hypertension, to treat urinary protein leakage in patients with the nephrotic syndrome, and most importantly, to preserve renal function in patients with progressively declining renal function.

M.E. De Broe & G.A. Porter (Editors). Clinical Nephrotoxins, 3rd Edition, 481-494

In this chapter we first will discuss the undesirable aspects of these effects of ACEI and will show how most of these effects may be prevented by cautious use of the agents. Since the mechanisms of the ACEI-induced membranous glomerulopathy and interstitial nephritis are different from those causing the fall in GFR, we will discuss each separately.

Captopril-associated membranous glomerulopathy

Proteinuria in association with membranous glomerulopathy has been described during the use of captopril [1-3]. Because of the similar pattern of these side effects to that of other agents containing a sulfhydryl group, like penicillamine, it was suspected that the sulfhydryl moiety of the captopril molecule was involved in the genesis of these effects, either by a direct toxic action or by an immunological mechanism [4]. It was feared that this would seriously limit the use of captopril and future sulfhydryl-containing angiotensin I converting enzyme inhibitors [5]. However, Lewis et al. reported that only 1.1% of 4878 patients treated with captopril exhibited increased proteinuria, with an incidence of nephrotic range proteinuria (more than 3 grams per 24 hours) of 0.8%. Analysis of these cases revealed that more than half of these patients had pre-existing renal disease, and many were taking doses in excess of 450 mg per day [6]. Furthermore, in studies in which doses of captopril of 37.5 to 150 mg per day were used, no increased incidence of proteinuria was detected as compared to placebo [7]. Lewis even questioned whether the occurrence of proteinuria during ACEI is related to the sulfhydryl moiety of captopril, since proteinuria has also been demonstrated during treatment with the non-sulfhydryl containing enalapril [8]. However, no data are available on biopsy-documented membranous glomerulopathy in relation to enalapril or other ACEI.

The causal role of captopril in the pathogenesis of membranous glomerulopathy has been questioned by the finding of glomerular abnormalities suggestive for membranous glomerulopathy in biopsies of hypertensive patients that had not received the ACEI. In both captopril- and non-captopril-treated patients, spherical dense bodies were found within the glomerular capillary wall with vascular and mesangial deposits of immunoglobulins and C3 that in the early reports were suspected to represent a captopril-induced membranous glomerulopathy [6, 9, 10]. Taken together, data lead us to conclude that proteinuria due to membranous glomerulopathy during captopril treatment seems to be restricted to patients with pre-existing renal disease who use high doses of the drug.

Angiotensin I converting enzyme inhibitor-induced acute interstitial nephritis

Acute interstitial nephritis during treatment with an ACEI has been observed in very few instances. Luderer et al. described a patient with skin rash, Coombs positive hemolytic anemia, eosinophilia, and acute kidney injury with eosinophiluria seven weeks after the start of captopril (300 mg per day). An allergic interstitial nephritis was suspected, but unfortunately no renal biopsy was performed and the patient moreover also received furosemide and aspirin [11]. Renal function improved after discontinuation of captopril. Cahan described two patients, one with a biopsy-proven acute eosinophilic interstitial nephritis (together with a membranous glomerulopathy) and the other with chronic interstitial nephritis during treatment with captopril [12]. Since again, both of these patients were also receiving furosemide, the development of interstitial nephritis could not definitely be attributed to captopril. In both patients the nephrotic range proteinuria persisted despite discontinuation of captopril and treatment with prednisolone [12]. Four other cases of acute interstitial nephritis with eosinophils have been described, mostly after usual doses of captopril (50-125 mg) given for a few days or weeks [13-16]. In one patient renal interstitial granulomas were also found [15]. In these cases renal function improved promptly after discontinuation of the drug. Another case report described a hypertensive patient presenting with a generalized maculopapular rash after three weeks of captopril therapy [17]. Eosinophilia was present without eosinophiluria. The renal biopsy showed acute tubular necrosis, however without evidence of allergic interstitial nephritis. Renal function improved promptly after discontinuation of captopril. Although a rash and eosinophilia have also been described during enalapril treatment, no data are available on the occurrence of acute interstitial nephritis in patients on enalapril. Moreover, in one of the above-mentioned case reports, captopril rechallenge, but not enalapril, caused renal functional deterioration [14].

Finally, functional tubular changes have also been described. Renal glycosuria, either with [18] or without [19] a fall in GFR has been found during treatment with captopril. In both cases the abnormality disappeared after withdrawal of the drug.

Thus far, no reports have been published on membranous glomerulopathy or acute interstitial nephritis in relation to the use of angiotensin II receptor antagonists. Whether this is due to the relatively short experience with these agents, or the fact that these ACEI-induced side effects are specific for ACEI and thus not related to the interference in the renin angiotensin system in general, cannot be concluded as yet.

Angiotensin I converting enzyme inhibitor-induced fall in GFR

In order to understand the ACEI-induced fall in GFR, it is important to begin with a basic understanding of the physiological role of the renin-angiotensin system in the regulation of renal hemodynamics (Figure 1). When renal perfusion pressure drops, renin is released into the plasma and lymph by the juxtaglomerular cells of the kidney. This enzyme cleaves angiotensinogen to form angiotensin I, which is further cleaved by converting enzyme to form angiotensin II, the primary effector molecule in this system. Angiotensin II participates in GFR regulation in at least two ways. First, angiotensin II increases arterial pressure, directly and acutely by causing vasoconstriction, and indirectly and more chronically by increasing body fluid volumes through stimulation of renal sodium retention (both indirectly via aldosterone and through a direct effect on the tubules), as well as by stimulating thirst. Second, angiotensin II preferentially constricts the efferent arteriole, thus helping to preserve glomerular capillary hydrostatic pressure and, consequently, GFR. Although the renin-angiotensin system is now known to be much more complicated than originally thought, including the likelihood that it serves paracrine and autocrine functions as well as endocrine functions, the simplified description above still holds true. As shown in figure 1, angiotensin I converting enzyme or kininase II also interferes in the breakdown of bradykinins, which may contribute to the vasodilation of ACE-inhibitors.

Under conditions in which arterial pressure or body fluid volumes are sensed as subnormal, the renin-angiotensin system will be activated and plasma renin activity and angiotensin II levels will be elevated. These conditions include dietary sodium restriction or sodium depletion (such as during diuretic therapy), renal artery stenosis, and congestive heart failure. In each case, fluid and sodium will be retained until the pressure and volume are again sensed as normal. Note

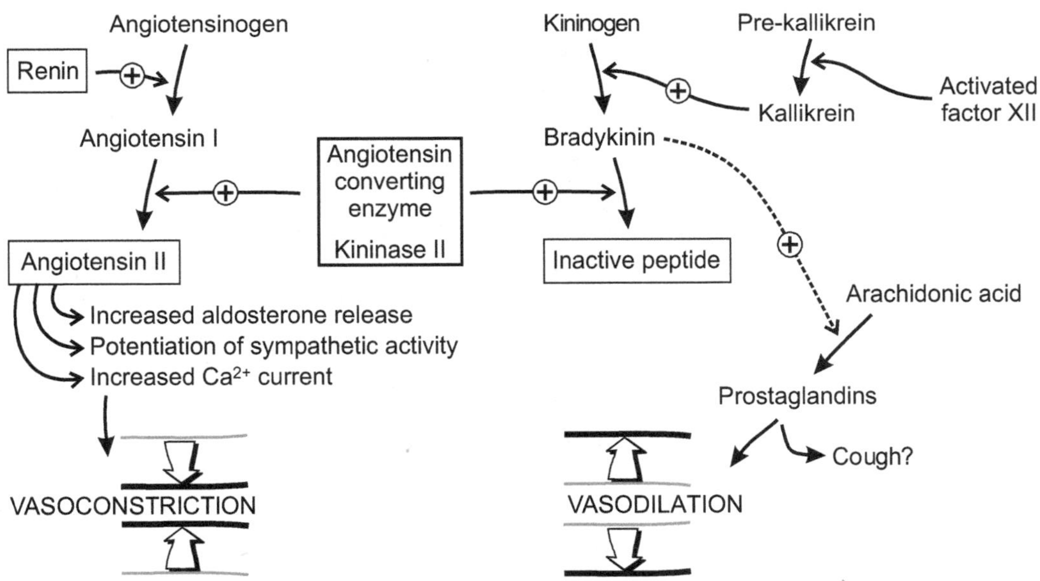

Figure 1. *Inhibition of the angiotensin converting enzyme, or kininase II.*

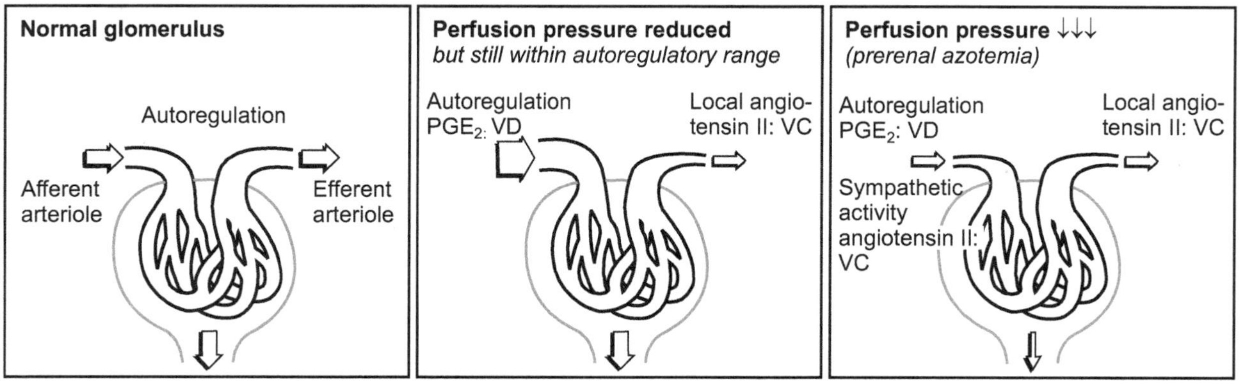

Figure 2. *Renal hemodynamics in normal and hypoperfusion conditions.*
PGE_2= prostaglandin E_2; VD= vasodilatation; VC= vasoconstriction.

that it is possible for the pressure and/or volume to actually be greater than normal but sensed as normal or subnormal, as in the case of congestive heart failure or renovascular hypertension. In conditions in which the renin-angiotensin system is activated, this system becomes especially important in maintenance of GFR, and the kidney becomes more sensitive to the effects of blockade with an ACEI or angiotensin II receptor antagonist.

The phenomenon of constant GFR and plasma flow during changes in renal arterial pressure is known as autoregulation, which under normal conditions is not renin angiotensin dependent (Figure 2). In case of renal arterial pressures below a certain value (about 80 mmHg), the renin-angiotensin system becomes involved. Its importance in this response has been demonstrated by Hall et al., who showed that intrarenal infusion of an angiotensin II antagonist impaired GFR autoregulation but not renal blood flow autoregulation, and that the impairment was more pronounced in sodium-depleted dogs [20]. During angiotensin II receptor antagonism, filtration fraction and efferent arteriolar resistance progressively fell at all renal arterial pressures below control. These investigators also showed that administration of captopril to sodium-depleted dogs impaired autoregulation of GFR but not of renal blood flow when renal perfusion pressure was reduced [21]. Both GFR and renal blood flow were returned to control values when angiotensin II was infused during captopril administration and aortic constriction. Calculated afferent and efferent resistances suggested that an angiotensin-stimulated increase in efferent resistance is important for efficient autoregulation of GFR when renal arterial pressure is clearly reduced. Thus, these investigators have provided strong evidence that an intact renin-angiotensin system is required for maintenance of GFR when renal perfusion pressure falls, and that angiotensin II participates in this GFR autoregulation by preferentially constricting the efferent arteriole.

Although generally accepted to be true, it is actually not known whether the renal hemodynamic effects of ACEI are necessarily due to blockade of the renin-angiotensin system. Acute kidney injury has not been seen after administration of other antihypertensive agents that do not interfere with the renin-angiotensin system, suggesting that it is blockade of this system, which is responsible for the acute kidney injury. However, angiotensin-converting enzyme is identical to kininase II, the enzyme responsible for degradation of kinins, so that administration of ACEI causes a buildup of vasodilator kinins (e.g. bradykinin) as well as depletion of angiotensin II. Thus, an excess of vasodilator kinins could theoretically contribute to the fall in GFR during ACEI. However, the finding of Hall et al. that an angiotensin receptor antagonist has similar effects to captopril or renin depletion on GFR autoregulation [20], and that the effects of captopril can be reversed by an infusion of angiotensin II [21], would suggest that changes in the kinin system play a minor role, if any, in the effects of ACEI on renal hemodynamics.

In patients in whom the renin-angiotensin system is activated, one would expect that efferent arteriolar resistance is maintained at least in part by circulating and/or intrarenal angiotensin II. If angiotensin II preferentially constricts the efferent vessels, then administration of an ACEI should preferentially dilate these vessels, thus causing a fall in glomerular hydrostatic pressure and a fall in GFR. This would be expected to occur even if renal perfusion pressure was unchanged. Moreover, a captopril-induced fall in systemic arterial pressure (and therefore renal artery pressure), together with impairment of GFR autoregulatory capability, would further contribute to a reduction in GFR.

These predictions from a basic understanding of the physiology of the renin-angiotensin system are upheld by clinical findings. Specifically, in some pathophysiological conditions in which maintenance of GFR is highly dependent on an angiotensin II-mediated efferent vasoconstriction, ACEI may result in an acute and pronounced fall in GFR. This is true for patients with bilateral renal artery stenosis or renal artery stenosis in a solitary kidney, for patients with congestive heart failure, and for patients with severe renal failure, especially when they are volume depleted. We will discuss the effect of ACEI in these three patient groups separately.

Renal artery stenosis

Shortly after the introduction of ACEI in clinical practice, attention was given to the acute and severe fall in GFR that may be encountered with these drugs in patients with bilateral renal artery stenosis and artery stenosis of a solitary kidney, the latter for example in patients with a renal allograft. In the first report to document such a GFR decline it was suggested to be due to a direct nephrotoxicity of the ACEI [22]. It soon became clear, however, that the fall in filtration was the consequence of renal ischemia, possibly related to the fall in blood pressure and thus in perfusion pressure in the post-stenotic kidney.

In one of the earliest reports it was shown that not only captopril but also minoxidil caused GFR to decrease in a patient with a transplant renal artery stenosis [23], suggesting that it was the fall in blood pressure itself, which caused the reduced GFR. However, in other studies it was found that GFR decreased only during treatment with captopril and enalapril [24] whereas a fall in blood pressure during sodium nitroprusside [25] or minoxidil [26, 27], which do not directly interfere with the renin-angiotensin system, did not result in a decline in GFR. Furthermore, studies from Anderson et al. indicated that during infusion of an ACEI in the renal artery, in doses low enough not to cause any systemic blood pressure effect, an efferent vasodilation occurs resulting in a lowering of filtration pressure in the post-stenotic kidney [28]. The same authors showed that the recovery of GFR that is normally observed after the induction of a renal artery stenosis in dogs is prevented by enalapril treatment [29]. Thus it appears that it is not the fall in systemic blood pressure *per se* that causes GFR to decrease after captopril in a renal artery stenosis patient.

Whatever the precise mechanism may be, the fall in intraglomerular capillary pressure in the post-stenotic kidney may lead to a severe decrease in GFR, even up to total loss of filtration. This is reflected by an acute rise in serum creatinine in patients with bilateral stenosis or stenosis in a solitary kidney [24, 30]. With the contralateral kidney intact however, changes in overall GFR tend to be small and variable, due to compensation by the non-stenotic kidney. Wenting et al., in their elegant study [31] showed not only that captopril greatly reduced the extraction ratio of sodium iodohippurate and iothalamate in the poststenotic kidney in half of the patients with unilateral renal artery stenosis, but also that such a fall in GFR could easily be detected on renal scintigraphy with 99mTc-diethylenetriamine-penta-acetic acid (DTPA), whereas DTPA-uptake had not diminished in the kidney of patients with essential hypertension (Figure 3). Since in patients with a unilateral renal artery stenosis a fall in filtration in the poststenotic kidney may not be detected by a rise in serum creatinine, they concluded that radioisotope renography thus should be performed after beginning captopril treatment in patients with renal artery stenosis [31]. In case of a fall in tracer uptake after captopril the drug should be withdrawn and the physician should aim at a curative approach if possible.

As predicted by our understanding of the basic physiology, the fall in filtration after ACEI in a patient with renal artery stenosis is dependent upon the prevailing sodium status of the patient [27, 32-34]. The critical role of sodium balance in this fall in GFR during ACEI has been nicely documented in a case report by Hricik [34], who showed that GFR decreased more markedly in a patient with a transplant renal artery stenosis when captopril was given in a sodium depleted as compared to a sodium replete situation (Table 1). Moreover, Andreucci et al. reported that intravenous infusion of saline could reverse the fall in creatinine clearance or rise in serum creatinine during captopril administration [35].

Since the fall in GFR after ACEI is reversible immediately after withdrawal of the drug [27, 30-32, 36], some authors concluded that its use in patients with renal artery stenosis is relatively safe [37, 38].

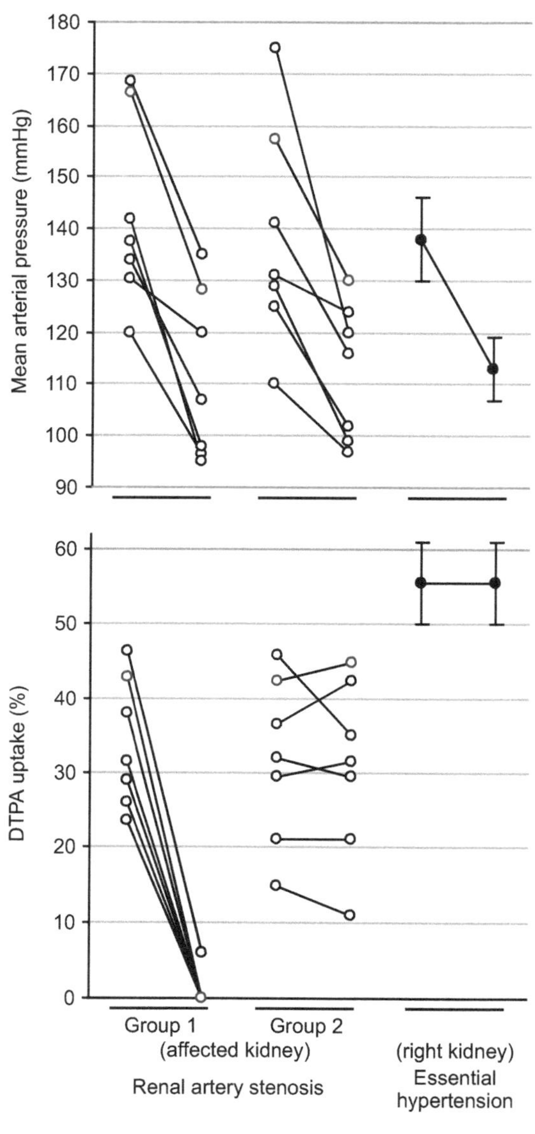

Figure 3. *Effect of long-term captopril 150 mg daily on blood pressure and single kidney uptake of 99mTc-DTPA in 14 patients with unilateral renal artery stenosis and 17 patients with essential hypertension. Note that DTPA uptake diminished impressively in half of the poststenotic kidneys in patients with renovascular hypertension, whereas it did not change in another half of the post-stenotic kidneys and in the kidneys of essential hypertensive patients. Reproduced with permission from [31].*

However, both animal data and human experience suggests that after continued treatment with an ACEI, atrophy of the stenosed kidney (Figure 4) [39] or complete obstruction of the artery with ischemia of the poststenotic kidney may occur [40, 41]. Whether these effects are directly related to the ACEI or to the natural history of the disease has yet to be established. Another argument against using ACEI in patients with renovascular hypertension, is the fact that in a number of these patients therapy (either transluminal angioplasty, stenting or operative procedures) that will directly address the primary problem is frequently available. The fact that renal function does not worsen during treatment with an ACEI should be evaluated against an expected improvement in renal function after correction of the stenosis.

Congestive heart failure

A fall in GFR may also be encountered if ACEI are given to patients with congestive heart failure. In a double blind study, Cleland found GFR to decrease from 53 to 48 ml/min (although not a statistically significant fall) during long-term treatment with captopril in 14 patients with congestive heart failure [42]. This fall in renal function, however, is not observed in all patients [43], and may also be different during the different stages of treatment [44]. Packer et al. showed that creatinine clearance worsened only in one third of the patients with severe chronic heart failure during treatment with captopril or enalapril, whereas creatinine clearance remained stable or improved in the other two thirds of the patients during ACEI [43]. The patients that demonstrated worsening of renal function had a lower central venous pressure and used more diuretics prior to the start of the ACEI. They exhibited a greater

Table 1. The effect of sodium intake on the renal response to captopril in a patient with a transplant renal artery stenosis.

	Sodium deplete		Sodium replete	
Captopril:	–	+	–	+
Body weight (kg)	73.6	73.9	75.2	76.8
Blood pressure (mmHg)	150/96	121/71	130/75	131/83
Serum creatinine (mg/dl)	1.5	3.6	1.6	1.6
Inulin clearance (ml/min)	73	37	62	53

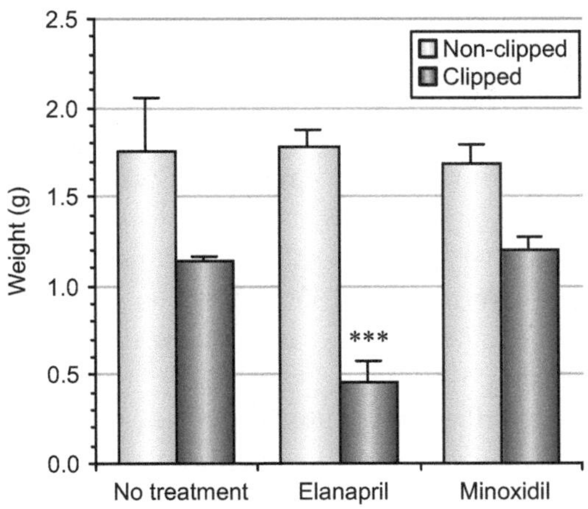

***Figure 4.** Weight of the clipped and nonclipped kidneys of two-kidney one-clip rats with Goldblatt's hypertension after 12 months of no treatment, enalapril, or minoxidil treatment. *** p<0.001 compared with no treatment group. Reproduced with permission from [39].*

fall in mean arterial pressure and left ventricular filling pressure than the patients in whom renal function remained stable or improved (Table 2). These authors also showed that the drug-induced azotemia resolved after a reduction in the dose of the diuretics, despite unaltered treatment with captopril or enalapril [43]. When instituting a patient with congestive heart failure on an ACEI, renal function should be monitored closely, at least during the first one to two weeks, especially since a decline in renal function may be transient. Mujais et al. showed GFR to decrease the first days after start of the angiotensin I converting enzyme inhibitor, but to improve again during the next days [44]. They interpreted this difference in response during different stages of treatment to reflect the balance between the different mechanisms influencing kidney hemodynamics in heart failure and their alteration by ACEI.

Renal failure

Patients with pre-existing renal failure are also at risk of developing an acute fall in GFR after ACEI [45-48]. Such a fall in GFR again appears to occur especially *in situ*ations of a concomitant volume depletion, such as during strict diuretic treatment, diarrhea, or during lithium therapy [49]. Since most ACEI are eliminated via renal excretion it should be emphasized that the dose of the drug has to be adjusted for renal function. In patients with renal failure the ACEI should be started at very low doses and should be titrated only gradually. Since GFR may return to pretreatment levels after withdrawal of the ACEI, it can be concluded that the deleterious effect of ACEI on renal function is the consequence of a functional response, i.e. an efferent renal vasodilation which in the presence of an impaired renal perfusion pressure may result in a severe fall in intraglomerular capillary pressure.

This acute and sometimes severe fall in GFR during ACEI-treatment in patients with renal disease should be considered separately from the expected beneficial effects of ACEI to prevent the progressive renal function decline so commonly observed in patients with renal disease (see later). In this respect the study of Speirs et al. is of interest [50]. They reported on a postmarketing surveillance of enalapril. For that purpose they evaluated the reports of more than 15,000 patients that had been instituted on enalapril (mostly in a clinical setting) and of whom a prescription event monitoring report had been received. 1098 of these patients had died. Reports of these patients were evaluated for the cause of death and the possible role of enalapril in the death. It was found that enalapril

Table 2. Renal function and hemodynamics during long term angiotensin I converting enzyme inhibition (ACEI) in severe chronic heart failure. The patients are divided in a group with stable renal function (n=70) and a group with worsening renal function (n=34) [from ref. 43].

	Stable renal function		Worsening renal function	
	ACEI –	ACEI +	ACEI –	ACEI +
Serum creatinine (mg/dl)	1.8 ± 0.1	1.7 ± 0.1	1.6 ± 0.1	2.2 ± 0.2
Creatinine clearance (ml/min)	42.7 ± 3.7	50.9 ± 2.0	49.6 ± 5.1	31.2 ± 2.8
Mean arterial pressure (mmHg)	83.9 ± 1.7	69.9 ± 2.0	83.1 ± 2.6	62.1 ± 2.8
Left ventricular filling pressure (mmHg)	27.1 ± 0.6	18.7 ± 1.0	26.0 ± 0.9	11.4 ± 1.4

appeared to have contributed to a decline in renal function and subsequent death in 10 of these patients. These patients shared some characteristics, i.e. old age, the use of high dose diuretics and/or potassium sparing diuretics, pre-existing renal disease and concomitant use of non-steroidal anti-inflammatory drugs [50].

Risk for combined treatment

In the previous paragraphs it has already been stressed that a decline in GFR during ACEI occurs predominantly *in situ*ations that the ACEI is combined with a diuretic regimen. As also mentioned before, the combination of an ACEI with a non-steroidal anti-inflammatory drug should be avoided, especially in patients with a pretreatment impaired GFR [50-52]. In such a situation the combination of afferent vasoconstriction (due to the prostaglandin synthesis inhibition) and efferent vasodilation (due to the ACEI) will result in a further fall in GFR, as has also been shown in patients with nephrotic range proteinuria [53, 54]. During these combined treatment regimens the patient is also at greater risk for the development of hyperkalemia.

Angiotensin I converting enzyme inhibitor-induced fetal nephrotoxicity

Although it is always difficult to prove that a certain drug or drug class induces fetal toxicity, the reports on ACEI-induced fetal renal damage are substantial. The most commonly reported fetal side effect of ACEI is second to third trimester onset of oligohydramnios and growth restriction, followed by delivery of an infant whose neonatal course is complicated by prolonged and often profound hypotension and anuria [55]. Most cases have been described in association with the use of enalapril, captopril and lisinopril (the earliest registered compounds), but there is no reason to expect that the other ACEI should not have the same risk [56]. These side effects have not been described with the use of angiotensin II receptor antagonists. As these drugs have not been used so long to date, it is to early to conclude whether the ACEI fetopathy is limited to the specific characteristics of ACEI or to the interference in the renin angiotensin system in general.

Histological studies of the kidney in ACEI-exposed fetuses show renal tubular dysgenesis [57-59]. Besides, delayed development of the calvaria and persistence of a patent ductus arteriosus has been described [60]. The true incidence of the fetal adverse effects of ACEI is not to determine, but in a series of 31 pregnancies exposed to an ACEI two ended with a miscarriage and three with stillbirth. Preterm delivery occurred in 12, and 6 out of the 26 liveborn babies were small for gestational age. Two infants with patent ductus arteriosus were reported [61]. There is no evidence that the use of ACEI causes harm in the first trimester of pregnancy [60].

The described renal tubular dysgenesis is characterized by dilatation of Bowman's space and of the tubules, diminished to absent differentiation of proximal convoluted tubules, and increased cortical and medullary mesenchyme and later fibrosis (Figure 5) [60]. These abnormalities are compatible with ischemic injury, and it has been argued that the mechanism by which ACEI affect development of the fetal kidney is through decreased renal blood flow [62, 63]. In fact, a similar histological pattern of renal tubular dysgenesis has also been reported in association with exposure to nonsteroidal anti-inflammatory agents [64-68], arguing that these abnormalities are not specific for ACEI exposure.

The vulnerability of nephrogenesis to ACEI extends after birth. When newborn rats were exposed during postnatal days 0-12 to enalapril medullary tubulogenesis was perturbed, as indicated by tubular dilatation and lack of E cadherin expression in these tubules. In the medulla of these enalapril treated rats ED2+, ED1+ and CD4+ T-cells were upregulated, accompanied by an increased TNF-alpha expression [69].

Based upon the available evidence it is advised not to use ACEI during pregnancy. In the case of an ACEI-exposed fetus, the pediatrician should be notified of the potential for neonatal hypotension and anuria.

Lessons to be learned from these side effects

Interestingly, in contrast to the situation with many other drugs, the documentation of these severe unwanted side effects did not lead to the withdrawal of these agents from the market. It of course is mandatory to constantly be aware of these potential risks. However, once the possible physiologic mechanisms of these side effects had been elucidated, it became increasingly clear that these effects could also be used to extend the diagnostic and therapeutic armamentarium of today's medicine.

Angiotensin I converting enzyme inhibition renography

Although it is a simple screening method for renal artery stenosis, until recently renography alone did not appear to be sufficiently sensitive for this purpose. This is thought to be at least partly due to the fact that the stenotic kidney is able to maintain adequate filtration and blood flow through systemic and local angiotensin II effects, thus obscuring the typical differences in tracer handling between the stenotic and non-stenotic side. The deleterious effects of an ACEI on flow and filtration in the poststenotic kidney in a patient with a renal artery stenosis are currently of use to improve the sensitivity of renography techniques in detecting the presence of a renal artery stenosis. It indeed has been shown, both in animal [70, 71] and human [72, 73] studies that the uptake and/or excretion of the tracer is more impaired in the post-stenotic kidney after ACEI as compared to the situation prior to the administration of the ACEI. This phenomenon appears to contribute to the alleged improvement of renography sensitivity during ACEI for the detection of renal artery stenosis. At present however, ACEI-renography is not so much advocated anymore, due to the high costs of the test in view of the suboptimal sensitivity.

Antiproteinuric effects and renal function preservation

The renal hemodynamic effects of ACEI in patients

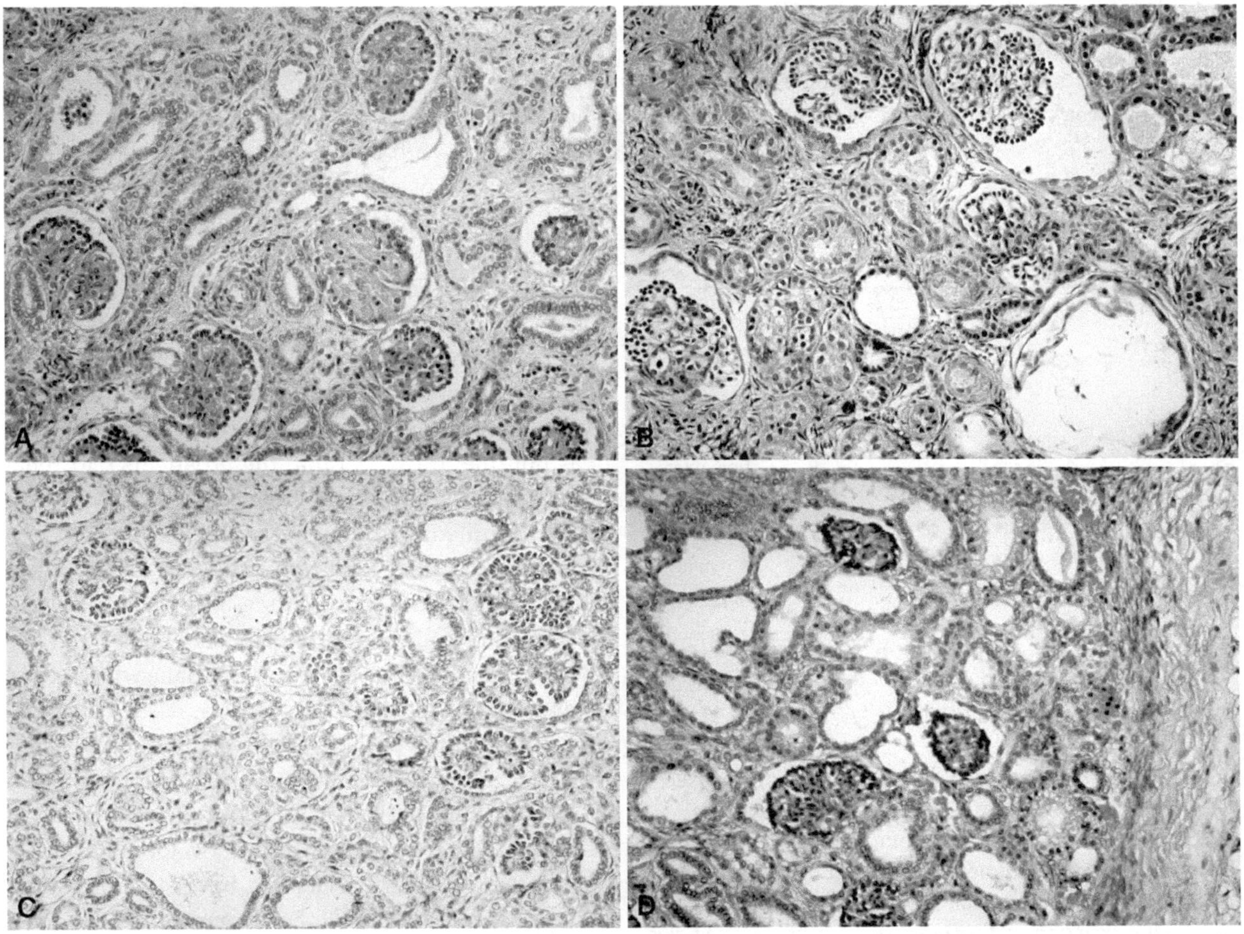

Figure 5. *Renal tubular dysgenesis in four different cases of ACI-induced fetopathy; note particularly the ductular ectasia, dilatation of Bowman's space, and poor to no differentiation of proximal convoluted tubules. Reprinted by permission of M. Barr [60] and Wiley-Liss, Inc., a subsidiary of John Wiley & Sons, Inc.*

with renal parenchymal disease and renal function impairment deserves particular attention. Also in these patients renal plasma flow generally will increase during ACEI [74, 75]. The response of GFR again is dependent upon the prevailing sodium balance and the dose of the ACEI (Figure 6) [76, 77]. In contrast to the more acute and severe fall in GFR as discussed before, the fall in filtration in this patient group generally is rather small, and mostly not diagnosed as such if only changes in serum creatinine are used as diagnostic criterium. However, using more accurate measurements of renal function, such as the clearance of inulin or radioisotope labeled tracers, a fall in filtration rate generally can be demonstrated. This fall in filtration reflects a fall in intraglomerular capillary pressure. Since in animal experiments a rise in intraglomerular capillary pressure was found to be associated with a rise in urinary protein loss [78] and a progressive glomerulosclerosis and renal failure [79], it followed that ACEI were used in an attempt to lower proteinuria and to prevent progressive renal function decline. ACEI indeed have been found to lower urinary protein excretion in patients with renal disease of various origins. Both in patients with asymptomatic proteinuria and in patients with frank nephrotic syndrome a fall in proteinuria with a rise in serum albumin has been described [74-76, 80, 81]. It has been argued that this improvement in the urinary protein leakage is the consequence of the renal hemodynamic effect of the ACEI, since blood pressure lowering with other antihypertensives does not result in a fall in proteinuria [75, 76]. In addition, the effects of ACEI or angiotensin II receptor antagonism to block the growth-promoting capacity of angiotensin-II adds to the beneficial effects of RAS blockade. In the last years the beneficial effects of both ACEI and angiotensin II receptor antagonists to prevent the progressive renal function decline in both type I [82] and type II [83, 84, 86, 87] diabetic nephropathy as well as in nondiabetic nephropathies [87-90] has been well documented.

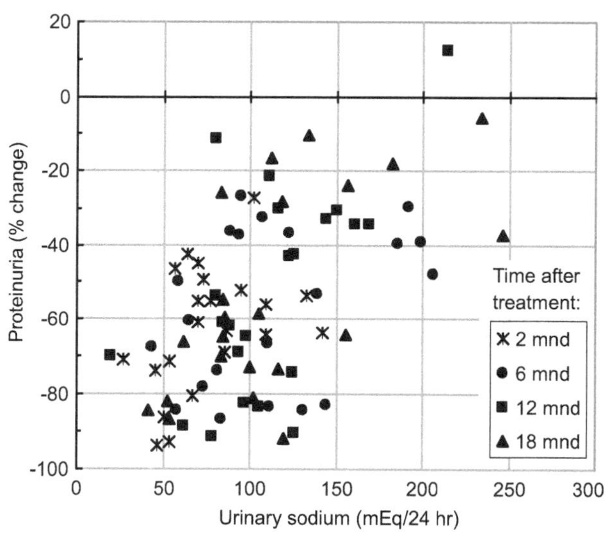

Figure 6. *Correlation between the antiproteinuric response (% change compared to baseline) and the urinary sodium excretion in 22 patients with proteinuria due to non-diabetic renal disease during treatment with the ACE inhibitor lisinopril (r-0.54; p<.001). Each data point represents the antiproteinuric and sodium excretion value of one individual at the time point of 2 months (*), 6 months (l), 12 months (n) or 18 months (p) after start treatment. Reproduced with permission from [76].*

It is well known for long time already that GFR may fall shortly after start of ACEI. This acute change in GFR in fact predicts a long-term stability of GFR on treatment [91]. The last years however, various reports showed that long-term treatment with ACEI may also be associated with a worse renal survival. In a long-term follow up of subjects with diabetic nephropathy it was found that the risk to reach end stage renal failure was greater in the subjects that were treated with ACE inhibitors than subjects that had been treated with other antihypertensives [92]. A similar warning was also derived from a report that renal function improved in some patients in whom after longstanding use of ACEI these drugs were discontinued, a finding that was not due to the fact that these patients had renal artery stenosis, and that moreover was not due to the short term hemodynamic response [93]. It has been suggested that such long-term unfavourable effects of ACEI are not found during long-term treatment with an angiotensin II receptor antagonist [94].

There is some experimental data, which could explain why some patients in the long-term may experience such unfavourable effects of ACEI. In a Fisher to Lewis rat model of chronic renal transplant failure treatment with either an ACEI or an angiotensin II receptor antagonist prevented the development of proteinuria and glomerulosclerosis, but not of interstitial damage. Moreover both these agents enhanced the development of intimal hyperplasia and reduced renal function [95]. This data was further corroborated when the same group showed that ACEI both in healthy rats as well as in adriamycin nephrotic rats induced an increase in the total medial area of afferent arterioles in combination with tubulo-interstitial damage especially in salt depleted, but not, or much less pronounced, in salt replete animals [96]. To define the impact of these clinical and experimental data for long-term renal protection needs further studies. At present, the evidence for this unfavourable effect is that sparse that there is no reason to abandon the long term use of ACEI as a tool to renoprotection. Good monitoring of renal function and proteinuria during treatment however, remains crucial.

Summary

Soon after the introduction of ACEI much attention was given to their renal side effects. This initiated a lot of research, especially because hypertension frequently is present in patients with renal vascular and/or parenchymal disease and the use of ACEI therefore was prompted in such patient groups. In the early eighties nephrotic syndrome due to a membranous glomerulopathy was described in association with the use of captopril. Further detailed studies showed this side effect to be related to the very high doses that at that time were used in patients with renal disease. More common is the acute renal functional deterioration that may occur during ACEI in certain groups, such as in patients with renovascular hypertension, in patients with severe heart failure and in patients with severe renal failure, especially in case of volume depletion. However, this fall in filtration is reversible after withdrawal of the drug or after volume repletion. This finding of a renal hemodynamically mediated fall in intraglomerular capillary pressure prompted studies that provided evidence of an antiproteinuric and renoprotective effect of this class of drugs. Close monitoring of side effects of drugs such as ACEI along with a basic understanding of the role of the renin angiotensin system in patients with renal diseases opens new perspectives for the treatment of such patients.

References

1. Hoorntje SJ, Kallenberg CGM, Weening JJ, Donker AJM, The TH, Hoedemaeker PJ. Immune complex glomerulopathy in patients treated with captopril. Lancet 1980; 1: 1212-1214.
2. Prins EJL, Hoorntje SJ, Weening JJ, Donker AJM. Nephrotic syndrome in a patient on captopril. Lancet 1979; 2: 306.
3. Sturgill BC, Shearlock KT. Membranous glomerulopathy and nephrotic syndrome after captopril therapy. JAMA 1983; 250: 2343-2345.
4. Kallenberg CGM, van der Laan S, de Zeeuw D. Captopril and the immune system. Lancet 1981; 2: 92.
5. Captopril: benefits and risks in severe hypertension. Editorial. Lancet 1980; 2: 129-130.
6. Lewis EJ and the Captopril Collaborative Study Group. Proteinuria and abnormalities of the renal glomerulus in patients with hypertension. Clin Exp Pharmacol Physiol 1982; 7: 105-115.
7. Veterans Administration Cooperative Study Group on Antihypertensive Agents. Low-dose captopril for the treatment of mild to moderate hypertension. Arch Intern Med 1984; 144: 1947-1953.
8. Lewis EJ. Captopril and membranous glomerulopathy. JAMA 1984; 252; 7: 900.
9. Captopril Collaborative Study Group. Does Captopril cause renal damage in hypertensive patients ? Report from the Captopril Collaborative Study Group. Lancet 1982; 1: 988-990.
10. Smit AJ, Hoorntje SJ, Weening JJ, Donker AM, Hoedemaeker PJ. Unilateral membranous glomerulopathy during captopril treatment. Neth J Med 1985; 28: 23-27.
11. Luderer JR, Schoolwerth AC, Sinicopre RA, Ballard JO, Lookingbill DP, Hayes AH. Acute renal failure, hemolytic anemia and skin rash associated with captopril therapy. Am J Med 1981; 71: 493-496.
12. Cahan DH, Ucci AA. Acute renal failure, interstitial nephritis, and nephrotic syndrome associated with captopril. Kidney Int 1984; 25: 160.
13. Chauveau P, Rouveix B, Kleinknecht D. Insuffiscance rénale aiguë d'origine immuno-allergique apres captopril. Néphrologie 1985; 6: 193-194.
14. Hooke D, Walker RG, Walter NMA, D'Apice AJF, Whitworth JA, Kincaid-Smith P. Repeated renal failure with use of captopril in a cystinotic renal allograft recipient. Brit Med J 1982; 285: 1538.
15. Islam S, Dubigeon MP, Guenel J. Néphropathie interstitielle granulomateuse aiguë et réversible apres traitement par le captopril. Rev Méd Interne (Paris) 1990; 11: 231.

16. Smith WR, Neill J, Cusham WC, Butkus DE. Captopril associated acute interstitial nephritis. Am J Nephrol 1989; 9: 230-235.
17. Steinman TI, Silva P. Acute renal failure, skin rash, and eosinophilia associated with captopril therapy. Am J Med 1983; 75: 154-151.
18. Cressman MD, Vidt DG, Acker C. Renal glucosuria and azotaemia after enalapril maleate. Lancet 1982; 2: 440.
19. Jójárt GY, Sonkodi S. Does captopril induce glucosuria ? Brit Med J 1984; 288: 368.
20. Hall JE, Guyton AC, Jackson TE, Coleman TG, Lohmeier TE, Trippodo NC. Control of glomerular filtration rate by renin-angiotensin system. Am J Physiol 1977; 233: F366-F372.
21. Hall JE, Coleman TG, Guyton AC, Kastner PR, Granger JP. Control of glomerular filtration rate by circulating angiotensin II. Am J Physiol 1981; 241: R190-R197.
22. Woodhouse K, Farrow PR, Wilkinson R. Reversible renal failure during treatment with captopril. Brit Med J 1979; 2: 1146-1147.
23. Collste P, Haglund K, Lundgren G, Magnusson G, Östman J. Reversible renal failure during treatment with captopril. Brit Med J 1979; 2: 612-613.
24. Hricik DE, Browning PJ, Kopelman R, Goorno WE, Madias NE, Dzau VJ. Captopril-induced functional renal insufficiency in patients with bilateral renal artery stenoses or renal artery stenosis in a solitary kidney. N Engl J Med 1983; 308: 373-376.
25. Textor SC, Tarazi FM, Novick AC, Bravo EL, Fouad FM. Regulation of renal hemodynamics and glomerular filtration in patients with renovascular hypertension during converting enzyme inhibition with captopril. Am J Med 1984; 76 (suppl): 29-37.
26. Mason JC, Hilton PJ. Reversible renal failure due to captopril in a patient with transplant artery stenosis: case report. Hypertension 1983; 5: 623-627.
27. van Son WJ, Donker AJM, Van der Woude FJ, Meijer S, Slooff MJH, Tegzess AM, Van der Slikke LB. Deterioration of renal function after converting enzyme inhibition in a patient with renal artery stenosis after transplantation. Neth J Med 1984; 27: 10-13.
28. Anderson WP, Korner PI, Johnston CI, Angus JA, Casley DJ. Intrarenal actions of angiotensin II in restoring renal artery pressure after acute renal artery stenosis. Clin Exp Pharmacol Physiol 1978; 5: 529-533.
29. Anderson WP, Denton KM, Woods RL, Alcorn D. Angiotensin II and the maintenance of GFR and renal blood flow during renal artery narrowing. Kidney Int 1990; 38 (suppl 30): 109-113.
30. Curtis JJ, Luke RG, Whelchel JD, Diethelm AG, Jones P, Dustan HP. Inhibition of angiotensin converting enzyme in renal transplant recipients with hypertension. N Engl J Med 1983; 308: 377-381.
31. Wenting GJ, Tan-Tjiong HL, Derckx FHM, de Bruyn JHB, Man in 't Veld AJ, Schalekamp MADH. Split renal function after captopril in unilateral renal artery stenosis. Brit Med J 1984; 288: 886-890.
32. Hollenberg NK. Renal hemodynamics in essential and renovascular hypertension. Influence of captopril. Am J Med 1984; 76 (suppl 5B): 22-28.
33. Watson ML, Bell GM, Muir AL, Buist TAS, Kellett RJ, Padfield PL. Captopril/diuretic combinations in severe renovascular disease: a cautionary note. Lancet 1983; 2: 404-405.
34. Hricik DE. Captopril-induced renal insufficiency and the role of sodium balance. Ann Intern Med 1985; 103: 222-223.
35. Andreucci VE, Conte G, Dal Canton A, Di Minno G, Usberti M. The causal role of salt depletion in acute renal failure due to captopril in hypertensive patients with a single functioning kidney and renal artery stenosis. Renal Failure 1987; 10: 9-20.
36. Jackson B, McGrath BP, Matthews PG, Wong C, Johnston CI. Differential renal function during angiotensin converting enzyme inhibition in renovascular hypertension. Hypertension 1986; 8: 650-654.
37. Reams GP, Bauer JH, Gaddy P. Use of the converting enzyme inhibitor enalapril in renovascular hypertension. Hypertension 1986; 8: 290-297.
38. Franklin SS, Smith RD. A comparison of enalapril plus hydrochlorothiazide with standard triple therapy in renovascular hypertension. Nephron 1986; 44 (suppl 1): 73-82.
39. Jackson B, Franze L, Sumithran E, Johnston CI. Pharmacologic nephrectomy with chronic angiotensin converting enzyme inhibitor treatment in renovascular hypertension in the rat. J Lab Clin Med 1990; 115: 21-27.
40. Hoefnagels WHL, Thien T. Renal artery occlusion in patients with renovascular hypertension treated with captopril. Brit Med J 1986; 292: 24-25.
41. Hodsman GP, Brown JJ, Cumming AMM, Davies DL, East BW, Lever AF, Morton JJ, Murray GD, Robertson JIS. Enalapril in treatment of hypertension with renal artery stenosis. Am J Med 1984; 77 (2A): 52-59.
42. Cleland JGF, Dargie HJ, Gillen G, Robertson I, East BW, Ball SG, Morton JJ, Robertson JIS. Captopril in heart failure: a double blind study of the effects on renal function. J Cardiovasc Pharmacol 1986; 8: 700-706.
43. Packer M, Lee WH, Medina N, Yushak M, Kessler PD. Functional renal insufficiency during long-term therapy with captopril and enalapril in severe chronic heart failure. Ann Intern Med 1987; 106: 346-354.
44. Mujais SK, Fouad FM, Textor SC, Tarazi RC, Bravo EL, Hart N, Gifford RW. Transient renal dysfunction during initial inhibition of converting enzyme in congestive heart failure. Brit Heart J 1984; 52: 63-71.
45. Verbeelen DL, de Boel S. Reversible acute on chronic renal failure during captopril treatment. Brit Med J 1984; 289: 20-21.

46. Murphy BF, Whitworth JA, Kincaid-Smith P. Renal insufficiency with combinations of angiotensin converting enzyme inhibitors and diuretics. Brit Med J 1984; 288: 844-845.
47. Brivet F, Roulot D, Poitrine A, Dormont J. Reversible acute renal failure during enalapril treatment in patient with chronic glomerulonephritis without renal artery stenosis. Lancet 1985; 1: 1512.
48. Chapman AB, Gabow PA, Schrier RW. Reversible renal failure associated with angiotensin converting enzyme inhibitors in polycystic kidney disease. Ann Intern Med 1991; 115: 769-773.
49. Navis GJ, de Jong PE, de Zeeuw D. Volume homeostasis, angiotensin converting enzyme inhibition, and lithium therapy. Am J Med 1989; 86: 621.
50. Speirs CJ, Dollery CT, Inman WHW, Rawson NSB, Wilton LV. Postmarketing surveillance of enalapril. II: Investigation of the potential role of enalapril in deaths with renal failure. Brit Med J 1988; 297: 830-832.
51. Packer M. Why do the kidneys release renin in patients with congestive heart failure ? A nephrotic view of converting enzyme inhibition. Am J Cardiol 1987; 60: 179-184.
52. Seelig CB, Maloley PA, Campbell JR. Nephrotoxicity associated with concomitant ACE inhibitor and NSAID therapy. Sth Med J 1990; 83: 1144-1148.
53. Heeg JE, de Jong PE, Vriesendorp R, de Zeeuw D. Additive antiproteinuric effect of the NSAID indomethacin and the ACE inhibitor lisinopril. Am J Nephrol 1990; 10 suppl 1: 94-97.
54. Heeg JE, de Jong PE, de Zeeuw D. Additive antiproteinuric effect of angiotensin converting enzyme inhibition and non-steroidal anti-inflammatory drug therapy: a clue to the mechanism of action. Clin Science 1991;81:367-372.
55. Rosa FW, Bosco LA, Fossum-Graham C, Milstien JB, Dreis M, Creamer J. Neonatal anuria with maternal angiotensin-converting enzyme inhibition. Obstet Gynecol 1989; 74: 371-374.
56. Brent RL, Beckman DA. Angiotensin-converting enzyme inhibitors, an embryopathic class of drugs with unique properties: information for clinical teratology counsellors. Teratology 1991: 43: 543-546.
57. Knott PD, Thorp SS, Lamont CAR. Congenital renal dysgenesis possibly due to captopril. Lancet 1989; 1: 451.
58. Cunnif C, Jones KL, Philipson K, Short S, Wujek J. Oligohydramnios and renal tubular malformation associated with maternal enalapril use. Am J Obstet Gynecol 1990; 162: 187-189.
59. Pryde PG, Sedman AB, Nugent CE, Barr M. Angiotensin-converting enzyme inhibitor fetopathy. J Am Soc Nephrol 1993; 3: 1575-1582.
60. Barr M Jr. Teratogen Update: Angiotensine-Converting Enzyme Inhibitors. Teratology 1994; 50: 399-409.
61. Kreft-Jais C, Plouin C, Tchobroutsky C, Boutroy MJ. Angiotensin-converting enzyme inhibitors during pregnancy: A survey of 22 patients given captopril and nine give enalapril. Br J Obstet Gynaecol 1988; 95: 420-422.
62. Martin RA, Jones KL, Mendoza A, Barr M, Benirschke K. Effect of ACE inhibition on the fetal kidney: decreased renal blood flow. Teratology 1992; 46: 317-321.
63. Landing BH, Ang SM, Herta N, Larson EF, Turner M. Labeled lectin studies of renal tubular dysgenesis and renal tubular atrophy of postnatal renal ischemia and end-stage kidney disease. Pediatr Pathol 1994; 14: 87-99.
64. Simeoni U, Messer J, Weisburd P, Haddad J, Willard D. Neonatal renal dysfunction and intrauterine exposure to prostaglandin synthesis inhibitors. Eur J Pediatr 1989; 149: 371-373.
65. Restaino I, Kaplan BS, Kaplan P, Rosenberg HK, Witzleben C, Roberts N. Renal dysgenesis in a monozygotic twin: Association with in utero exposure to indomethacin. Am J Med Genet 1991; 39: 252-257.
66. Bavoux F. Toxicite foetal des anti-inflammatoires non steroidiens. Presse Med 1992; 21: 1909-1912.
67. Buderes S, Thomas B, Fahnenstich H, Kowalewski S. Renal failure in two preterm infants: toxic effect of prenatal maternal indomethacin treatment. Br J Obstet Gynaecol 1993; 100: 97-98.
68. Voyer LE, Drut R, Mendez JH. Fetal renal maldevelopment with oligohydramnios following maternal use of piroxicam. Pediatr Nephrol 1994; 8: 592-594.
69. Lasaitiene D, Chen Y, Guron G, Marcussen N, Tarkowski A, Telemo E, Friberg P. Perturbed medullary tubulogenesis in neonatal rat exposed to renin-angiotensin system inhibition. Nephrol Dial Transplant 2003; 18: 2534-2541
70. Nally JV Jr, Clarke HS Jr, Grews GP, Saunders M, Gross ML, Potvin WJ, Windham JP. Effect of captopril on 99mTc-diethylenetriaminepentaacetic acid renograms in two-kidney, one clip hypertension. Hypertension 1986; 8: 685-693.
71. Jonker GJ, de Zeeuw D, Huisman RM, Piers DA, Beekhuis H, van der Hem GK. Angiotensin converting enzyme inhibition improves diagnostic procedures for renovascular hypertension in dogs. Hypertension 1988; 12: 411-419.
72. Geyskes GG, Oei HY, Puylaert CBAJ, Dorhout Mees EJ. Renovascular hypertension identified by captopril-induced changes in the renogram. Hypertension 1987; 9: 451-458.
73. Kremer Hovinga TK, de Jong PE, Piers DA, Beekhuis H, van der Hem GK, de Zeeuw D. Diagnostic use of ACE inhibitors in radioisotope evaluation of unilateral renal artery stenosis. J Nucl Med 1989; 30: 605-614.

74. Reams GP, Bauer JH. Effect of enalapril in subjects with hypertension associated with moderate to severe renal dysfunction. Arch Intern Med 1986; 146: 2145-2148.
75. Heeg JE, de Jong PE, van der Hem GK, de Zeeuw D. Reduction of proteinuria by angiotensin converting enzyme inhibition. Kidney Int 1987; 32: 78-83.
76. Heeg JE, de Jong PE, van der Hem GK, de Zeeuw D. Efficacy and variability of the antiproteinuric effect of ACE inhibition by lisinopril. Kidney Int 1989; 36: 272-279.
77. Gansevoort RT, de Zeeuw D, de Jong PE. Long-term benefits of the antiproteinuric effect of angiotensin-converting enzyme inhibition in nondiabetic renal disease. Am J Kidney Dis 1993; 22: 202-206.
78. Pelayo JC, Quan AH, Shanley PF. Angiotensin II control of the renal microcirculation in rats with reduced renal mass. Am J Physiol 1990; 258: F414-F422.
79. Anderson S, Meyer TW, Rennke HG, Brenner BM. Control of glomerular hypertension limits glomerular injury in rats with reduced renal mass. Clin Invest 1985; 76: 612-619.
80. Taguma Y, Kitamoto Y, Futaki G, Ueda H, Monma H, Ishazaki M, Takahashi H, Sekino H, Sasaki Y. Effect of captopril on heavy proteinuria in azotemic diabetes. N Engl J Med 1985; 313: 1617-1620.
81. Bjorck S, Mulec H, Johnsen SA, Nyberg G, Aurell M. Contrasting effects of enalapril and metoprolol on proteinuria in diabetic nephropathy. Brit Med J 1990; 300: 904-907.
82. Lewis EJ, Hunsicker LG, Bain RP, Rohde RD. The effect of angiotensin-converting-enzyme inhibition on diabetic nephropathy. N Engl J Med 1993; 329: 1456-1462.
83. Brenner BM, Cooper ME, de Zeeuw D, Keane WF, Mitch WE, Parving HH, Remuzzi G, Snapinn SM, Zhang Z, Shahinfar S, for the RENAAL Study Investigators. Effects of losartan on renal and cardiovascular outcomes in patients with type 2 diabetes and nephropathy. N Engl J Med 2001; 345: 861-869.
84. Lewis EJ, Hunsicker LG, Clarke WR, Berl T, Pohl MA, Lewis JB, Ritz E, Atkins RC, Rohde R, Raz I, for the Collaborative Study Group. Renoprotective effect of the angiotensin-receptor antagonist irbesartan in patients with nephropathy due to type 2 diabetes. N Engl J Med 2001; 345: 851-859.
85. Parving HH, Lehnert H, Bröchner-Mortensen, Gomis R, Andersen S, Arner P. The effect of irbesartan on the development of diabetic nephropathy in patients with type 2 diabetes. N Eng J Med 2001; 345: 870-878.
86. Brenner BM, Cooper MA, de Zeeuw D, Keane WF, Mitch WE, Parving HH, Remuzzi G, Snapinn S, Zhang Z, Shahinfar S. Effects of losartan on renal and cardiovascular outcomes in patients with type 2 diabetes and nephropathy. N Engl J Med 2001; 345: 861-869.
87. Maschio G, Alberti D, Janin G, Locatelli F, Mann JF, Motolese M, Ponticelli C, Ritz E, Zucchelli P. Effect of the angiotensin-converting-enzyme inhibitor benazepril on the progression of chronic renal insufficiency. N Engl J Med 1996; 334: 939-945.
88. The GISEN Group (Gruppo Italiano di Studi Epidemiologici in Nefrologia). Randomised placebo-controlled trial of effect of ramipril on decline in glomerular filtration rate and risk of terminal renal failure in proteinuric, non-diabetic nephropathy. Lancet 1997; 349: 1857-1863.
89. Ruggenenti P, Perna A, Gherardi G, Garini G, Zoccali C, Salvadori M., Scolari F, Schena FP, Remuzzi G. Renoprotective properties of ACE-inhibition in non-diabetic nephropathies with non-nephrotic proteinuria. Lancet 1999; 354: 359-364.
90. Jafar T, Schmid C, Landa M, Giatras I, Toto R, Remuzzi G, Maschio G, Brenner BM, Kamper A, Zucchelli P, Becker G, Himmelmann A, Bannister K, Landais P, Shahinfar S, de Jong PE, de Zeeuw D, Lau J, Levey A, for the ACE-inhibition in progressive renal disease Study Group. Angiotensin-converting enzyme inhibitors and progression of nondiabetic renal disease: a meta-analysis of patient-level data. Ann Intern Med 2001; 135: 73-87.
91. Apperloo AJ, de Zeeuw D, de Jong PE. A short-term antihypertensive treatment induced fall in glomerular filtration rate reflects long-term stability of renal function. Kidney Int 1997; 51: 793-797
92. Suissa S, Hutchinson T, Brophy JM, Kezouh A. ACE-inhibitor use and the long-term risk of renal failure in diabetes. Kidney Int 2006; 69: 913-919
93. Onuigbo MA, Onuigbo NT. Late onset renal failure from angiotensin blockade: a prospective thirty-month Mayo Health System clinic. Med Sci Monit 2005; 11: CR462-469
94. Woo KT, Lau YK, Wong KS, Chan CM. ACE inhibitor use and the long-term risk of renal failure in diabetes. Kidney Int 2006; 70: 1376-1377 Letter
95. Smit-van Oosten A, Navis GJ, Stegeman CS, Joles JA, Klok PA, Kuipers F, Tiebosch ATMG, van Goor H. Chronic blockade of angiotensin II action prevents glomerulosclerosis, but induces graft vasculopathy in experimental kidney transplantation. J Pathol 2001; 194: 122-129
96. Hamming I, Navis G, Kocks MJA, van Goor H. ACE inhibition has adverse renal effects during dietary sodium restriction in proteinuric and healthy rats. J Pathol 2006: 209: 129-139

21

Diuretics and alcohol ingestion

Sheldon C. CHAFFER and Jules B. PUSCHETT

Department of Internal Medicine, Texas A&M University, Temple, Texas, USA

Introduction

Diuretics are among the most frequently prescribed drugs for the treatment of both edematous and non-edematous states. With respect to the latter category, they are most often utilized in the therapy of hypertension. They may injure the kidney either reversibly or irremediably, a distinction which often depends upon whether they have induced functional or anatomic damage. Ordinarily, the former type of disorder reverses more rapidly than the latter. However, anatomical lesions, for example those that may be associated with acute kidney injury, may also respond to the removal of the offending agent.

Functional abnormalities

Effects on renal hemodynamics

Diuretics may cause reductions in glomerular filtration rate (GFR) either by a direct constriction of the renal arterial network, or secondary to their induction of extracellular fluid (ECF) volume contraction. Listed in Table 1 are the renal hemodynamic alterations induced in the experimental animal or in man by the most commonly prescribed, currently available diuretic agents. Acetazolamide, a proximally active agent and the prototypical carbonic anhydrase inhibitor (Figure 1), consistently reduces renal blood flow (RBF) by

25-37% and GFR by 10 to 46% [1]. This phenomenon is thought to result from the effect of the drug on the "tubulo-glomerular feedback" (TGF) mechanism. Tubulo-glomerular feedback denotes the process through which a change in tubular flow from the proximal to the distal tubule at the level of the macula densa is able to affect the function of the glomerular microvasculature [2-5]. Feedback regulation maintains relatively constant tubular flow rate under the local or regional influence of multiple effectors including angiotensin II [6], nitric oxide [7] and COX-2 [8-10]. Thus, if diuretics inhibit sodium and fluid transport proximal to the distal convolution leading to increased fluid delivery to the distal nephron, the glomeruli will respond with reduced function. While the loop of Henle agents such as furosemide would be expected to have similar effects, these drugs appear to inhibit the TGF system, thus preventing a decrease in GFR [11-16]. However, in those studies with loop diuretics in which ECF was substantially contracted, GFR (and single nephron glomerular filtration rate, SNGFR) fell [14, 15, 17, 18].

In most studies in which it has been investigated, ethacrynic acid administration results in a marked reduction in renal vascular resistance [13, 19-21]. However, this effect is nullified, as in the case with furosemide, by the superimposition of volume depletion [20-22]. Studies of bumetanide in the experimental animal have generally shown no change in GFR or renal plasma flow (RPF) [23, 24] except for transient acute increases in the latter which approximated 27 to 40%, declining later in the experiments to only modest elevations or to control levels [25, 26]. In man, bumetanide is associated with either no change [27, 28] or a 12 to 16% increase in effective renal plasma flow and glomerular filtration rate [29].

The thiazides, especially the most extensively studied of this group of agents, chlorothiazide, are stated to either reduce both RBF and GFR or to cause no change in these parameters [1]. When a reduction does occur, it may be the result of volume contraction

Table 1. Renal hemodynamic effects of diuretics according to nephron site of action[a,b].

Drug	Experimental model(s)	Effect on RBF or RPF	Effect on GFR	Mechanism of observed alterations in hemodynamics
Proximal tubule				
Acetazolamide	rat, dog, man	RBF ↓ ~25-37%	↓ ~10-46%	Activation of TGF
Benzolamide	rat	undetermined, but nephron plasma ↓ ~35%	↓ ~18-21%	Activation of TGF, probably mediated by angiotensin II
Loop of Henle				
Furosemide	rat, dog, rabbit, man	↑ 25-30%[c], or no change	no change[c]	Inhibits TGF mediated ↓ SNGFR, which would otherwise be expected because of ↑ distal delivery
Ethacrynic acid	dog, man	↓ 28-47%[c], or no change	no change[c]	Does not alter TGF, renal vasodilatory effects may be effected by volume depletion
Bumetanide	dog, man	↓ ≤ 40%[c], or no change	↑, or no change[c]	Effects on TGF similar to furosemide
Early distal convoluted tubule				
Chlorothiazide	rat, dog, man	↓, or no change	↓, or no change	Decline in SNGFR, when it occurs, may be related to ↑ proximal intratubular pressure, volume contraction or afferent arteriolar vasodilation
Metolazone	dog, man	no change	no change	
Indapamide	dog, man	no change	no change	
Late distal convoluted tubule and collecting duct				
Spironolactone	man	no change	no change	
Triamterene	man	no change[d]	no change[d]	
Amiloride	rat, dog, man	no change	no change	
Eplerenone	rat, man	no change	no change	

[a]Reproduced with permission of the editor from Puschett JB, Winaver J. Effects of diuretics on renal function. In: Handbook of physiology. Section 8 renal physiology. Windhager EE (editor). Oxford Press, New York 1992; p. 2335-406.
[b]Abbreviations: renal blood flow (RBF), renal plasma flow (RPF), glomerular filtration rate (GFR), single nephron glomerular filtration rate (SNGFR), tubuloglomerular feedback (TGF).
[c]Effects of the drug on RBF and GFR are related to alterations in in extracellular fluid volume induced by the agent.
[d]Large doses (300 mg/day) have been reported to reduce effective RPF and GFR.

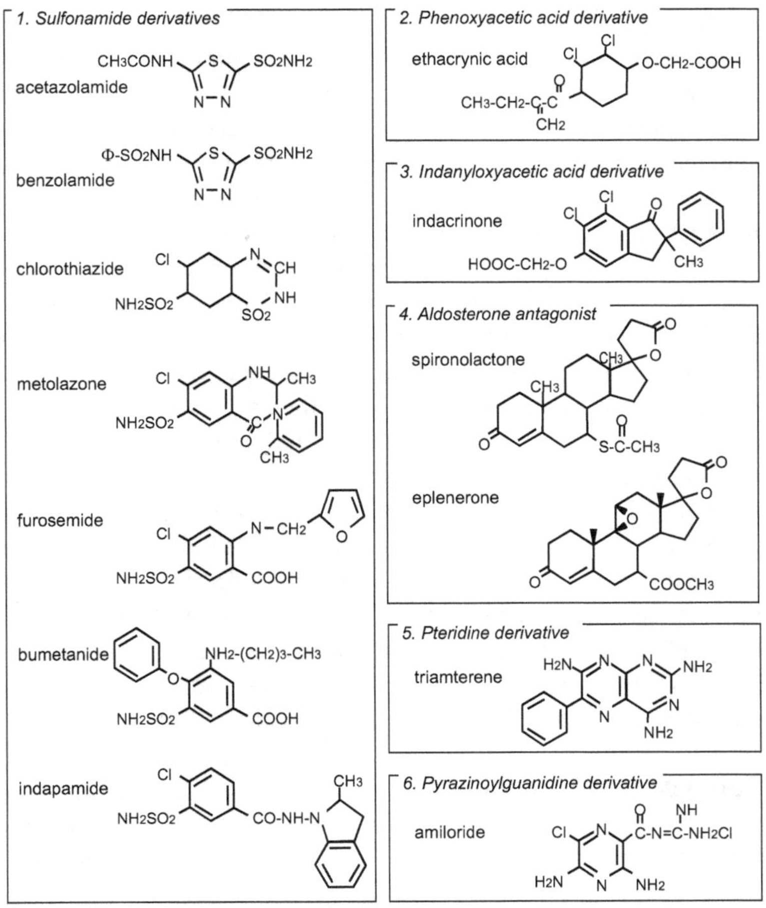

Figure 1. *Chemical structures of the commonly utilized diuretic agents grouped according to drug class.*

[30] (as outlined above), an increase in proximal tubular pressure [31], or a vasodilatory effect of the drug on the post-glomerular vasculature [32]. Effects of the thiazide-like agent, metolazone, and another sulfonamide derivative, indapamide, have been studied in the experimental animal and in man. In general these drugs likewise cause no consistent alterations in either RBF or GFR unless volume contraction occurs [1].

Clinically, volume depletion manifests itself in one of two patterns related to alterations in serum chemistry values: either there is an elevation in the blood urea nitrogen (BUN) with no increase in serum creatinine, or both are elevated but the BUN proportionately more so than the creatinine. This phenomenon, which has been termed "prerenal azotemia", results from reduced flow through the nephron and increased contact time between the tubular contents and the epithelium of the collecting duct. Urea is a small, non-charged moiety, which is transported much more easily than is creatinine (a much larger, usually charged molecule). Ordinarily, prerenal azotemia and reductions in GFR can be reversed with cessation of the diuretic and liberalization of sodium in the diet. In severe cases, however, the infusion of saline may be necessary, assuming the patient does not have co-morbid conditions which prevent expansion of the extracellular volume.

There have been reports of oliguric acute kidney injury with high doses (>200 mg/day) of the osmotic diuretic mannitol, which responded to hemodialysis [33-41]. The rapid and dramatic improvement of renal function with hemodialysis suggests functional abnormalities. However, anatomic changes such as vacuolization and swelling of the renal proximal tubular cells with substantial reduction of the adjacent tubular lumen (osmotic nephropathy) have been reported in individuals with normal renal function [42, 43]. Low dose mannitol has been shown to produce renal vasodilation whereas high doses appear to induce vasoconstriction [40, 44-46]. It has been proposed that the large solute loads that are delivered to the macula densa during high dose mannitol therapy may activate TGF causing afferent arteriole vasoconstriction producing a marked drop in GFR [35]. Some data also support a direct vasoconstrictive effect of mannitol on the renal artery [46].

The potassium-sparing agents, spironolactone, triamterene, amiloride and eplerenone appear to cause no consistent primary changes in RBF or GFR. Increased recognition of the importance of aldosterone in the the pathophysiologic changes seen in hypertensive heart disease [47-49], ischemic cardiomyopathy [50, 51], stroke [52] and kidney damage [53] has led to increased utilization of the potassium-sparing agents spironolactone and eplerenone owing to their aldosterone receptor blocking action. However, in the setting of impaired glomerular hemodynamics, hyperfiltration and non-selective proteinuria secondary to underlying pathology, spironolactone and eplerenone have been shown to reduce proteinuria and slow decline in renal function, in part related to reductions in effective RPF and GFR [54-57]. Triamterene, when used in large doses, 300 mg per day or more, has been reported to reduce both effective RPF and GFR.

Renal parenchymal lesions

Interstitial nephritis

Following Councilman's classic description of acute interstitial nephritis in 1898 [58], similar histopathology has been described in a variety of drug classes. Early recognition of sulfonamide [59] and penicillin [60] associated cases has expanded to include additional etiologic agents. Interstitial nephritis accounts for as many as 15% of biopsies indicated for unexplained acute kidney injury [61]. Renal biopsy characteristically reveals an intense interstitial infiltrate comprised primarily of lymphocytes and plasma cells, with variable number of neutrophils, eosinophils and histiocytes. A retrospective review of 1068 biopsies from 1968 to 1997 by Schwartz et al. revealed acute interstitial nephritis in 6.5% of cases. Drugs were implicated in 85% of these cases, with 7.8% being diuretic related [62].

Acute interstitial nephritis was described by Lyons et al. in four patients with idiopathic interstitial nephritis, evidenced by peripheral eosinophilia, skin rash in two patients, and moderate to severe renal failure. Biopsies in all cases revealed dense interstitial infiltrate consisting predominantly of lymphocytes, tubular degenerative changes and interstitial edema with early fibrosis. In each case, withdrawal of furosemide or or thiazide and administration of prednisone resulted in reversal of renal failure [63]. Though specific immunologic evidence for diuretic as the inciting agent was not available, rechallenge of one patient with furosemide (and azathioprine) resulted in recurrence of anuria, fever and erythema multiforme. Likewise, each case was noted to have pre-existing proliferative glomerulonephritis, raising the possibility that the development of acute interstitial nephritis was related to the use of sulfonamide derivative diuretics in combination with underlying glomerular disease [63]. Three cases of acute kidney injury with pathologic changes consistent with acute interstitial nephritis were also described by Magil et al. 5 to 10 weeks following initiation of combination hydrochlorothiazide and triamterene (Dyazide®). Withdrawl of the medication resulted in restoration of normal renal function in two patients and near normal function in the third [64]. In each case, no evidence of glomerular pathology was found histologically or ultrastructurally. Infiltrates were noted to be primarily composed of lymphocytes, monocytes and macrophages with one biopsy also revealing occasional, moderately well defined, non-necrotizing granulomas suggestive of delayed-type hypersensitivity. A clear etiologic role for hydrochlorothiaze was not possible in these cases due to the concomitant use of triamterene, which has also been reported in association with cases of interstitial nephritis [65, 66]. In a blinded crossover study of 26 hypertensive patients taking hydrochlorothiazide, the effects of triamterene and amiloide were evaluated in a blinded examination of urinary sediment [67]. No difference was found between the amiloride period and the triamterene period with respect to serum creatinine, BUN, protein excretion or creatinine clearance. However, 14 of 26 urine samples taken during the triamterene period revealed reddish brown crystals with casts, consistent with triamterene related casts. No similar casts or crystals were seen during the amiloride period. Case reports of the development of acute interstitial nephritis have also been described in association with the administration of chlorthalidone [68, 69], tienilic acid [70], indapamide [71], and other thiazides administered alone [72] or simultaneously with triamterene [73, 74].

Interstitial nephritis with accelerated deterioration of renal function may present in a more subacute form, including chronic tubulointerstitial nephritis

(CTIN). Clinical manifestations of CTIN commonly include acidification and concentrating defects, non-nephrotic range proteinuria, microscopic hematuria, pyuria and glycosuria [75]. Park et al. have reported a biopsy proven case of interstitial nephritis in association with high dose furosemide (up to 1.2 grams per day) with biopsy revealing tubular cell atrophy with flattened epithelial cells, interstitial fibrosis and areas of mononuclear interstitial infiltrates [76]. Findings suggestive of cell-mediated delayed-type hypersensitivity have been previously reported by Magil et al. These include diuretic associated cases of interstitial nephritis and possibly CTIN, and may represent a delayed type hypersensitivity response. However, it remains unclear whether this represents a direct effect or a combination of factors.

Finally, vasculitis has been reported with the administration of thiazide diuretics [77-82], and metolazone [83]. Larsson and collegues found high titers of antibodies against myeloperoxidase and cardiolipin in a patient treated with a thiazide diuretic. When the drug was stopped, progression of the renal insufficiency also abated and the antibodies disappeared [77].

Nephrolithiasis and nephrocalcinosis

Diuretics have been shown to have variable effects in relationship to urinary calcium excretion and supersaturation, most notably including loop diuretic induced hypercalciuria and attenuation of urinary calcium excretion by thiazide diuretics. The factors contributing to nephrotoxicity are most commonly associated with multiple factors that favor calcium salt or uric acid deposition at the tubulo-interstitial level. Management of renal stone formation and nephrocalcinosis therefore presents a unique clinical challenge, balancing factors that increase risk for abnormal calcium salt deposition or crystallization, and factors that reduce this risk.

Hyperuricemia and resultant increases in urinary supersaturation for uric acid, are common consequences of diuretic therapy [84]. Several factors are related to development of hyperuricemia, including: (1) the thiazides and other diuretics compete for the uric acid secretory pathway in the proximal tubule; (2) volume contraction reduces renal blood flow, leading to reduced delivery of diuretic to the secretory site; and (3) as a result of volume contraction, proximal tubular reabsorption of sodium and urate are increased [85, 86]. A dose-dependent increase in serum uric acid has been documented with the administration of both bendrofluazide [87] and hydrochlorothiazide [88].

Whether hyperuricemia leads to the development of uric acid nephrolithiasis and/or urate nephropathy, or even predisposes to the development of these lesions, is unknown [89]. The likelihood that patients with hyperuricemia will undergo silent renal damage related to the development of gouty nephropathy is considered to be small [90]. Hall et al, reporting data from the Framingham study, found that only 12 of 240 patients with a serum uric acid level exceeding 7 mg/dL had renal disease. In 5 of the 12, this was preexistent, and the nature of the renal impairment in the other 7 patients was undetermined [90]. Guman and Yü found that clearances of inulin, creatinine and p-aminohippurate were normal in 13 hyperuricemic but asymptomatic relatives of patients with gout [91]. Fessel et al., could find no statistically significant differences in mean serum creatinine levels in a group of patients before and 4 years after the onset of hyperuricemia [92]. In a subsequent study, Fessel reported that mild azotemia developed in 1.8% (2/113) of patients with asymptomatic hyperuricemia followed for 8 years, but also in 2.1% (4/193) of normouricemic control subjects [93]. In 168 patients with gout followed for 10 years, azotemia was also mild, did not significantly correlate with serum uric acid level, and the risk of uric acid nephrolithiasis was small: one stone episode per 295 patients per year in asymptomatic hyperuricemic patients, one per 852 patients per year in normouricemic controls, and one per 114 patients per year in patients with gout. Azotemia of clinical importance did occur when serum uric acid level exceeded 13 mg/dl in men and 10 mg/dl in women. However, the risk of development of uric acid nephrolithiasis was so low that the author suggested that hyperuricemia should probably not be treated prophylactically until a patient experienced his/her first stone episode [94]. Although these findings highlight the small risk for decline in glomerular filtration rate in asymptomatic hyperuricemia, evidence of renal tubular dysfunction was found by Klinenberg et al. In 5 of 19 subjects studied, abnormalities in maximal urinary concentrating capacity were found and in 5 of 6 patients tested, total acid and titratable acid excretion were reduced by 15-20% [94].

In contrast to asymptomatic patients, prevention of

further deterioration of renal function by treating hyperuricemia in patients with gouty nephropathy may be beneficial [95]. However, as pointed out by Berger and Yü, long-term follow-up of patients with primary gout revealed that hyperuricemia was not associated with consistent reductions in renal function [96]. Furthermore, Rosenfeld has demonstrated that normalizing serum uric acid is ineffective in improving glomerular filtration rate in normotensive as well as hypertensive patients, with or without impaired renal function [97]. Finally, with respect to the production of uric acid nephrolithiasis by diuretics, Steele et al. have noted that hyperuricemia associated with diuretic usage results in decreased uric acid excretion, and therefore tends to minimize stone formation [98].

Loop diuretic therapy has been implicated in the development of renal calcifications in both preterm and full-term infants [99-105]. In a study by Jacinto et al., nephrocalcinosis occurred in 20 of 31 (64%) of premature infants with birth weights less than 1500 g, with 65% of affected infants having received furosemide [103]. Nephrocalcinosis was found in 14% of full-term infants with congestive heart failure receiving long-term furosemide therapy [104]· Furosemide may induce high urinary calcium excretion rates and low urinary citrate to creatinine ratio, risk factors for renal calcification [106].

Dose and length of therapy with loop diuretics may predict the likelihood of developing calcium deposits in the renal parenchyma. Ten premature infants developed nephrocalcinosis after receiving furosemide at a dose of at least 2 mg/kg per day for 12 days [102]. In a study by Saarela et al, infants who developed renal calcifications were receiving higher daily doses of furosemide than infants who had not developed this complication (1.9 ± 0.6 vs. 1.3 ± 0.4 mg/kg per day; p value-0.01) [104]. Calcifications were diagnosed within a few months of initiating furosemide.

Spontaneous resolution of nephrocalcinosis usually occurs within 6 months after discontinuation of loop diuretic therapy [106], but may persist for greater than 1 year [100, 104]. Measurement of serum calcium-to-creatinine ratio may be predictive of resolution when nephrocalcinosis is first diagnosed. Premature infants with unresolved nephrocalcinosis had mean calcium-to-creatinine ratios upon initial diagnosis that were approximately five-fold greater than ratios in infants with resolved nephrocalcinosis (2.23 ± 0.99 vs. 0.34 ± 0.18; p value <0.005) [106].

Since unresolved nephrocalcinosis may lead to residual abnormalities in the kidney including microscopic hematuria, hypercalcemia, and impaired tubular function [100, 104, 105], renal ultrasonography within a few months of initiating loop diuretics may be warranted [100 104]. If long-term diuretic therapy is needed, a thiazide diuretic alone or in combination with furosemide may reduce the risk of renal calcifications by decreasing urinary calcium and oxalate excretion [100, 102, 104, 107, 108]. However, two studies of premature infants failed to show a reduction in either urinary oxalate or calcium excretion when thiazides were added to furosemide therapy [107, 109].

Functional and anatomic lesions

Hypokalemic nephropathy

Diuretics commonly cause hypokalemia [110]. The more effective these drugs are in inducing natriuresis, the more likely is the development of hypokalemia [111]. This is the case for the following reasons: (1) with the exception of the potassium-sparing agents, diuretics inhibit transport of sodium upstream of the $Na+/K+/H+$ exchange sites (site 4, Figure 2). Accordingly, they cause the presentation of increased amounts of sodium to these antiporters for exchange with potassium and hydrogen ions [112]. Furthermore, because of the volume depletion that they induce, the diuretics cause the activation of the angiotensin-renin-aldosterone axis. The latter phenomenon stimulates the distal nephron exchange just described, resulting in the excretion of increased urinary potassium excretion. (2) Potassium is virtually completely reabsorbed by the time tubular fluid reaches the end of the loop of Henle and enters the distal convoluted tubule [113] Accordingly, any drug that impairs transport at sites in the nephron where significant amounts of potassium reabsorption occurs (the proximal tubule, site 1 and the loop of Henle, site 2, Figure 2) has the potential to interfere with potassium reabsorption. This increased distal delivery of potassium has limited opportunity for reabsorption and thus allows increased potassium excretion. If potassium excretion exceeds intake, negative potassium balance results, inducing hypokalemia and decreased total body potassium content. This phenomenon is most frequently seen in edematous states

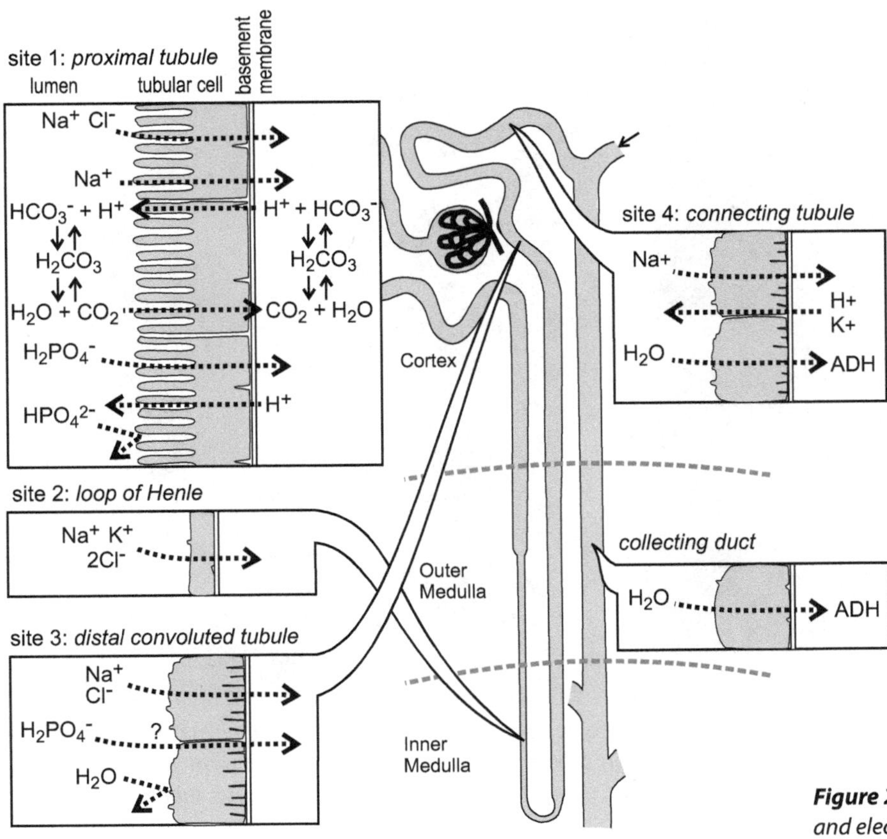

Figure 2. *Sites of tubular transport of water and electrolytes throughout the nephron.*

when vigorous diuresis has been performed. On the other hand, the employment of diuretics for the treatment of hypertension, the most common use of the these drugs, generally results in only modest decline in serum potassium levels. These are usually diagnosed and treated. It is only in those cases of chronic potassium depletion that hypokalemic nephropathy occurs. Although limited data are available as to the incidence of this complication following diuretic administration, it appears to be rare, and seems to require long-term, substantial depletion of total body potassium [114-116]. Given recent emphasis on potassium replacement and use of lower doses of diuretics than were previously employed for the treatment of hypertension [117], hypokalemic nephropathy is generally seen only in the setting of diuretic and/or laxative abuse [116, 118].

Both functional abnormalities and anatomic damage result from chronic hypokalemia and severe potassium depletion. Chronic tubulointerstitial changes have been described as developing slowly over the period of 5-10 years [117]. Changes include initial vacuolization in the proximal convoluted tubular cells [119], marked interstitial inflammatory infiltrate with mononuclear cells and tubular atrophy [117, 120] (Figure 3). The most commonly noted functional abnormalities are polyuria and an impairment in urinary concentrating ability [120, 121]. While the exact mechanism of this functional abnormality is not known, it appears to relate to decreased expression of aquaporin-2, independent of interstitial tonicity [122] and impaired responsiveness at the collecting duct level to the influence of vasopressin due either to the release of prostaglandins, or some other interference with the generation or action of cyclic adenosine-3′,5′-monophosphate [123, 124]. The latter nucleotide serves as the second message that transduces the action of vasopressin into permeability of the collecting duct epithelium to tubular water [125]. Metabolic alkalosis is commonly seen, as is a decrement in ammonium excretion [120], causing a persistently alkaline urine.

Alcohol ingestion

Acute alcohol intoxication present varied diagnostic and therapeutic challenges, owing largely to differences in toxicity of the principle agent and/or

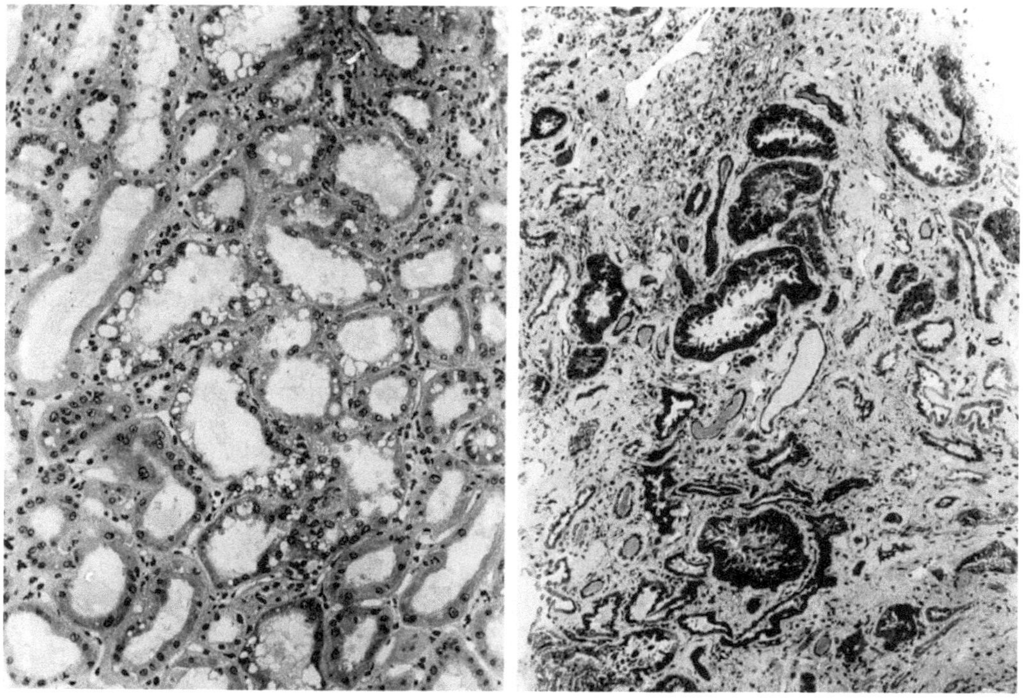

***Figure 3.** Sequential renal biopsies, separated by 10 years, in a patient with hypokalemia related to chronic diuretic abuse. Initial biopsy (on the left) shows proximal tubular cell vacuolization and mild interstitial inflammation. The subsequent examination (on the right) demonstrates marked interstitial fibrosis, tubular atrophy and dropout.*

Reproduced with permission: Bennett WM. Diuretic toxicity and drug interactions. In: Diuretics: physiology, pharmacology and clinical use. Dirks JH, Sutton RAL (editors). Saunders, Philadelphia 1986; p. 362-373.

metabolites. Nephrotoxicity may represent a consequence of other organ dysfunction, renal tubular or interstitial pathology or obstructive uropathy related to metastatic deposition of calcium salts.

Isopropyl alcohol (2-propanol, isopropanol) is widely available as a cleaning agent including window cleaner and deicing agent, as a solvent and sterilizing agent used in the home and in industrial settings, as rubbing alcohol and in topical preparations including aftershave, skin lotions and hair tonics. A limited number of case reports have cited isopropanol in association with renal pathology [126]. As much as 20% of isopropanol is excreted unchanged in the urine [127]. Approximately 80% of isopropanol is metabolized to acetone in the liver, resulting in ketonuria, a key clinical feature differentiating it from methanol or ethylene glycol ingestion and potentially leading to misdiagnosis of diabetic ketoacidosis or ethanol intoxication. Since isopropanol and its metabolic products are not organic acids, metabolic acidosis is an uncommon finding, seen only in extremis associated with hypoperfusion lactic acidosis [128]. Doses of 150 to 250 mL may be fatal, and as is the case with nephrotoxicity, primarily related to hypotensive shock in association with central nervous system and myocardial depression [129]. Elevation in colorimetric serum creatinine level has been described as "pseudo" renal failure due to interference of acetone with the assay [130].

Methanol is most commonly used as commercial and industrial solvent, antifreeze, windshield-washing fluid, as an adulterating agent in ethyl alcohol when produced as a cleaning agent [131] and is also used as a warming agent and as fuel in small model engines [132]. Methanol is rapidly absorbed from the gastrointestinal tract and converted by the action of alcohol dehydrogenase and acetaldehyde dehydrogenase, primarily in the liver, into the toxic metabolites formaldehyde and formic acid. Toxicity is mediated by the formation of formic acid, which is responsible for metabolic acidosis, and brain and optic nerve pathology [133]. Elevation in the osmolal gap, as with ethanol, isopropyl alcohol and ethylene glycol, are dependent on the presence of the parent alcohol. Therefore, even in the setting of significant ingestion, elevated osmolal gap may be insufficiently sensitive to exclude clinically important toxicity [134-136]. Clinical pathology correlates with serum and tissue levels of fomic acid, rather than methanol levels [137]. Fatalities have been reported involving doses between 60 and 240 mL, or 15 to 30 mL of a 40% solution [138].

Acute kidney injury has been reported in association with a limited number of methanol intoxication cases [139-143]. As in previously reported cases, Verhelst et al reported a case series of 15 patients with acute kidney injury within 48 hours of methanol ingestion, 11 patients with laboratory evidence of hemolysis, 8 patients with significant myoglobinuria without elevated serum creatinine phosphokinase levels and 7 patients with both hemolysis and myoglobinuria [134]. In comparison to 11 patients presenting with acute methanol intoxication without acute kidney injury (0 deaths), mortality was significantly increased in the acute kidney injury group (6 deaths). Renal histological samples were available in 5 patients, 2 post-mortem, revealed hydropic changes in the proximal tubule of nearly all nephrons visualized with no evidence of glomerular pathology. It remains unclear whether pathologic findings were related to a direct toxic consequence of methanol metabolites. Additionally, co-morbid events including hypotension requiring pressor therapy in 6 of the 15 patients with acute kidney injury, as well as osmotic changes related to requirement for ethanol infusion could also have been involved. In a report of successful renal transplantation of 4 deceased donor renal allografts from 2 patients with brain death following acute methanol intoxication, post-revascularization biopsy in one patient revealed no vacuolization or hydropic changes [143]. This report supports previous anecdotal findings, suggesting that renal impairment following methanol intoxication may be mediated by other organ dysfunction, prerenal hemodynamic influences and/or osmotic perturbations related to the ethanol infusion utilized as treatment.

Ethylene glycol, most commonly used as an antifreeze agent, de-icing agent, and fabric cleaner [144, 145] presents a multifactorial interplay of renal pathology mediated by four toxic metabolites (glycoaldehyde, glycolate, glyoxalate and oxalate). In both experimental and human studies, the metabolism of glycolic acid to glyoxalate represents the rate limiting step [146, 147]. In species that preferentially metabolize ethylene glycol to oxalate, including humans, urinary oxalate

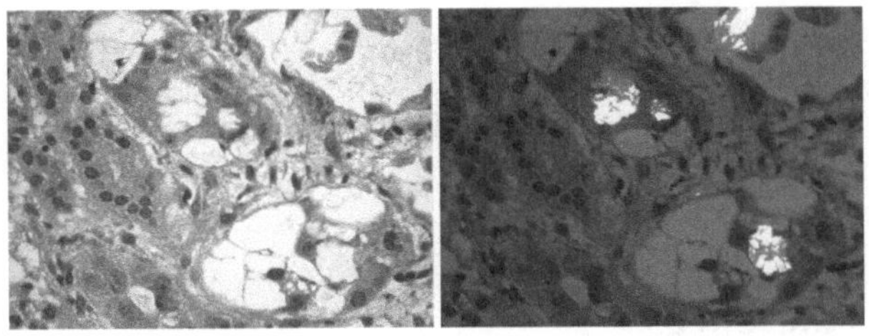

Figure 4. *Renal histopathology following acute ethylene glycol ingestion resulting in oxalate nephropathy. Tubular epithelium shows 'ballooning degeneration' with large cytoplasmic vacuolization (on the left) and calcium oxalate inclusions by polarized microscopy (on the right).*

Adapted by permission from Macmillan Publishers Ltd: Stokes MB. Acute oxalate nephropathy due to ethylene glycol ingestion. Kidney Int 2006; 69:203.

crystals including calcium oxalate monohydrate and calcium oxalate dihydrate are the primary mediators of renal damage as a result of tubular obstruction and interstitial crystal deposition [132, 148-150] (Figure 4). McMartin et al. have utilized isolated rat proximal tubular mitochondria to suggest that cellular toxicity may by related to a loss of ATP production and eventual cell death via transformation of the inner mitochondrial membrane, whereby it becomes permeable to small solutes [151]. No signs of renal injury have been noted at initial plasma glycolic acid concentrations of up to 10.1 mM (76.7 mg/dl) or at initial plasma ethylene glycol levels of up to 3.2 mM (20 mg/dl) [152]. Doses of 100 mL for a 70 kg adult is sufficient to produce toxicity, though with appropriate treatment survival has been noted at much higher doses [146]. Standard treatment of ethylene glycol poisoning has focused on the prevention of ethylene glycol metabolism to toxic metabolites. Standard treatment strategies have utilized ethanol [153], sodium bicarbonate [154] and hemodialysis [155].

Fomepizole has proven effective in the treatment of both methanol and ethylene glycol poisoning through its competitive inhibition of hepatic oxidation via alcohol dehydrogenase and therefore, decreased generation of toxic metabolites for both toxicities [146, 156-158]. In the setting of methanol intoxication, excretion is shifted primarily to pulmonary and renal routes and is slowed significantly (half-life, 48-54 hours) [146]. Moreover, excretion of formic acid is partially dependent on tetrahydrofolate, and therefore potentially accelerated by the administration of folic acid [159]. In the setting of ethylene glycol intoxication, excretion following fomepizole administration is primarily renal (half-life, 17-20 hours) [160]. Further studies have suggested that in the subset of patients with ethylene glycol toxicity, normal renal function and acid-base status, fomepizole alone may be a sufficient antidote, obviating the need for hemodialysis [158, 161].

References

1. Puschett JB, Winaver J. Effects of diuretics on renal function. In: Handbook of physiology. Section 8 renal physiology. Windhager EE (editor). Oxford Press, New York 1992; p. 2335-406.
2. Thomson SC, Blantz RC. Homeostatic efficiency of tubuloglomerular feedback in hydropenia, euvolemia, and acute volume expansion. Am J Physiol 1993; 264(6 Pt 2):F930-6.
3. Thomson SC, Blantz RC, Vallon V. Increased tubular flow induces resetting of tubuloglomerular feedback in euvolemic rats. Am J Physiol 1996; 270(3 Pt 2):F461-8.
4. Schnermann J, Wright FS, Davis JM, Stackerberg WV, Grill G. Regulation of superficial nephron filtration rate by tubuloglomerular feedback. Pflugers Arch 1970; 318:147-75.
5. Thurau K, Schnermann J, Nagel W, Horster M, Wahl M. Composition of tubular fluid in the macula densa segment as a factor regulationg the function of the juxtaglomerular apparatus. Circ Res 1967; 20-21 (Suppl 2):79-90.
6. Tucker BJ, Steiner RW, Gushwa LC, Blantz RC. Studies on the tubulo-glomerular feedback system in the rat. The mechanism of reduction in filtration rate with benzolamide. J Clin Invest 1978; 62:993-1004.
7. Harris RC, Cheng H, Wang J, Zhang M, McKanna JA. Interactions of the renin-angiotensin system and neuronal nitric oxide synthase in regulation of cyclooxygenase-2 in the macula densa. Acta Physiol Scand 2000; 168:47-51.
8. Harris RC, McKanna JA, Akai Y, Jacobson HR, Dubois RN, Breyer MD. Cyclooxygenase-2 is associated with the macula densa of rat kidney and increases with salt restriction. J Clin Invest 94(6):2504-10, 1994
9. Jensen BL, Kurtz A. Differential regulation of renal cyclooxygenase mRNA by dietary salt intake. Kidney Int 1997; 52(5):1242-9.
10. Yang T, Singh I, Pham H, Daqing S, Smart A, Schnermann JB, Briggs JP. Regulation of cyclooxygenase expression in the kidney by dietary salt intake. Am J Physiol 1998; 274(3 Pt 2):F481-89.
11. Puschett JB, Goldberg M. The acute effects of furosemide on acid and electrolyte excretion in man. J Lab Clin med 1968; 71:666-677.
12. Burke TJ, Duchin KL. Glomerular filtration during furosemide diuresis in the dog. Kidney Int 1979; 16:672-680.
13. Hook JB, Blatt AH, Brody MJ, Williamson HE. Effects of several saluretic-diuretic agents on renal hemodynamics. J Pharmacol Exp Ther 1966; 154:667-673.
14. Vander AJ, Carlson J. Mechanism of the effects of furosemide on renin secretion in anesthetized dogs. Circ Res 1969; 25:145-152.
15. Tucker BJ, Blantz RC. Effect of furosemide administraton on glomerular and tubular dynamics in the rat. Kidney Int 1984; 26:112-121.
16. Meyer P, Menard J, Papanicolaou N, Alexandre JM, Devaux C, Milliez P. Mechanism of rennin release following furosemide diuresis in the rabbit. Am J Physiol 1968; 215:908-915.
17. Brenner BM, Keimowitz RI, Wright FS, Berliner RW. An inhibitory effect of furosemide on sodium reabsorption by the proximal tubule of the rat nephron. J Clin Invest 1969; 48:290-300.
18. Burke TJ, Robinson RR, Clapp JR. Determinants of the effect of furosemide on the proximal tubule. Kidney Int 1972; 1:12-18.
19. Birtch AG, Zakheim RM, Jones LG, Barger AC. Redistribution of renal blood flow produced by furosemide and ethacrynic acid. Cir Res 1967; 21:869-878.
20. Dluhy AG, Wolf GL, lauler DP. Vasodilator properties of ethacrynic acid in the perfused dog kidney. Clin Sci 1970; 38:347-357.
21. McNay JL, Kishimoto T. Selective renal vascular effects of ethacrynic acid. J Pharmacol Exp Ther 1970; 174:159-168.
22. Early LE, Friedler RM. Tubular effects of ethacrynic acid. J Clin Invest 1964; 43:1495-1506.
23. Olsen UB. Indomethacin inhibition of bemetanide diuresis in dogs. Acta Pharmacol Toxicol 1975; 37:65-78.
24. Puschett JB, Sylk D, Teredesai PR. Uncoupling of proximal sodium bicarbonate from sodium phosphate transport by bumetanide. Am J Physiol 1978; 235 (Renal Fluid Electrolyte Physiol 4):F403-F405.
25. Olsen UB. Prostaglandin/kinin activity related to changed renal compliance after bumetanide in dogs. Acta Pharmacol Toxicol 1977; 40:430-438.
26. Olsen UB, Ahnfelt-Ronne I. Renal cortical blood redistribution after bumetanide related to hterogenicity of cortical prostaglandin metabolism in dogs. Acta Physiol Scand 1976; 97:251-257.

27. Bourke E, Asbury MJA, O'Sullivan S, Gatenby PBB. The sites of action of bumetanide in man. Eur J Pharmacol 1973; 23:283-289.
28. Karlander S-G, Henning R Lundvall O. Renal effects of bumetanide, a new saluretic agent. Eur J Clin Pharmacol 1973; 6:220-223.
29. Jayakumar S, Puschett JB. Study of the sites and mechanism of action of bumetanide in man. J Pharmacol Exp Ther 1977; 201:251-258.
30. Walter SJ, Laycock JF, Shirley DG. A micropuncture study of proximal tubular function after acute hydrochlorothiazide administration to Brattleboro rats with diabetes insipidus. Clin Sci 1979; 57:427-434.
31. Krause HH, Dume T, Koch KM, Ochwadt B. Intratubularer druck, glomerularer capillardruck und glomerulumfiltrat nach furosemid und hydrochlorothiazide. Pflugers Arch 1967;295:80-89.
32. Cassin S, Vogh B. Effect of hydrochlorothiazide on renal blood flow and clearance of para-aminohippurate and creatinine. Proc Soc Exp Biol Med 1966; 122:970-973.
33. Gadllah MF, Lynn M, Work J. Case Report: Mannitol nephrotoxicity syndrome: role of hemodialysis and postulate of mechanisms. Am J Med Sci 1995; 309(4):219-222.
34. Better OS, Rubinstein I, Winaver JM, Knochel JP. Mannitol therapy revisited (1940-1997). Kidney Int 1997; 51:886-894.
35. Goldwasser P, Fotino S. Acute renal failure following massive mannitol infusion: Appropriate response of tubuloglomerular feedback? Arch Intern Med 1984; 144:2214-2216.
36. Whelan TV, Bacon ME, Madden M, Patel TG, Handy R. Acute renal failure associated with mannitol intoxication. Arch Intern Med 1984; 144:2053-2055.
37. Horgen KJ, Ottaviano YL, Watson AJ. Acute renal failure due to mannitol intoxication. Am J Nephrol 1989; 9:106-109.
38. Rello J, Trigner C, Sanchez JM, Net A. Acute renal failure following massive mannitol infusion. Nephron 1989; 53:377-378.
39. Weaver A, Sica DA. Mannitol-induced acute renal failure. Nephron 1987;45:233-235.
40. Rabetoy GM, Fredericks MR, Hostetteler CF. Where the kidney is concerned, how much mannitol is too much? Ann Pharmacother 1993;27:25-28.
41. Dormer HR, Sondheimer JH, Cadnapaphornchai P. Mannitol-induced acute renal failure. Medicine 1990; 69(3):153-159.
42. Mansbach AB, Madden SC, Latta H. Light and electron microscopic changes in proximal tubules of rats after administration of glucose, mannitol, suctose or dextran. Lab Invest 1962; 11:421-432.
43. Dalgard OZ, Pederson KJ. Some observations of the fine structure of human kidneys in acute anuria and osmotic diuresis. In: Renal Biopsy. Wolstenholme GEW, Cameron MP (editors). Little Brown, New York, 1962:
44. Read RC, Johnson JA, Vick JA, Meyre MW. Vascular effects of hypertonic solutions. Circ Research 1960; 8:538-548.
45. Krishnamurty VSR, Adams HR, Smitherman TC, Templeton GH, Willerson JT. Influence of mannitol on contractile responses of isolated perfused arteries. Am J Physiol 1977; 232(1):H59-66.
46. Temes SP, Lilien OM, Chamberlain W. A direct vasoconstrictor effect of mannitol on the renal artery. Surg Gynecol Obstet 1975; 141:223-226.
47. Dzau VJ, Colucci WS, Hollenberg NK, Williams GH. Relation of the rennin-angiotensin-aldosterone system to clinical state in congestive heart failure. Circulation 1981; 63:645-51.
48. Weber KT, Villarreal D. Aldosterone and antialdosterone therapy in congestive heart failure. Am J Cardiol 1993; 71:(suppl)3A-11A.
49. Swedberg K, Eneroth P, Kjekshus J, Wilhelmsen L. Hormones regulating cardiovascular function in patients with servere congestive heart failure and their relation to mortality. Circulation 1990;82:1730-1736.
50. Barr CS, Lang CC, Hanson J, Arnott M, Kennedy N, Struthers AD. Effects of adding spironolactone to an angiotensin-converting enzyme inhibitor in chronic congestive heart failure secondary to coronary artery disease. Am J Cardiol 1995; 76:1259-65.
51. Keidar S, Hayek T, Kaplan M, Povlotsky E, Hamoud S, Coleman R, Aviram M. Effect of eplerenone, a selective aldosterone blocker, on blood pressure, serum and macrophage oxidative stress, and atherosclerosis in apolipoprotein E-deficient mice. J Cardiovasc Pharmacol 2003; 41(6):955-963.
52. Rocha R, Stier CT Jr. Pathophysiological effects of aldosterone in cardiovascular tissues. Trends Endocrinol Metab 2001; 12:308-14.
53. Rocha R, Steir CT Jr, Kifor I, Ochoa-Maya MR, Rennke HG, Williams GH, Adler GK. Aldosterone: a mediator of myocardial necrosis and renal arteriopathy. Endocrinology 2000; 141(10):3871-8.
54. Rossing K, Schjoedt KJ, Smidt UM, Boomsma F, Parving HH. Beneficial effects of adding spironolactone to recommended antihypertensive treatment in diabetic nephropathy. Diabetes Care 2005; 28:2106-2112.
55. Ribstein J, Guilhem DC, Pierre F, Mimran A. Relative glomerular hyperfiltration in primary hyperaldosteronism. J Am Soc Nephrol 2005; 16:1320-1325.
56. Van den Meiracker AH, Baggen RGA, Pauli S, Lindemans A, Vulto AG, Polermans D, Boomsma F. Spironolactone in type 2 diabetic nephropathy: effects on proteinuria, blood pressure and renal function. J Hypertension 2006; 24:2285-2292.

57. Sechi LA, Novello M, Lapenna R, Baroselli S, Nadalini E, Colussi GL, Catena C. Long-term renal outcomes in patients with primary aldosteronism. JAMA 2006; 295:2638-2645.
58. Councilman WM. Acute interstitial nephritis. J Exp Med 1898; 3:393-420.
59. Black-Schaffer B. Pathology of anaphylaxis due to sulfonamide drugs. Arch Path 1943; 39:301-14.
60. Baldwin DS, Levine BB, McClusky RT, Gallo GR. Renal failure and interstitial nephritis due to penicillin and methicillin. N Engl J Med 1968; 279:1245-52.
61. Neilson EG. Pathogenesis and therapy of interstitial nephritis. Kidney Int 1989; 35:1257-1270.
62. Schwartz A, Krause PH, Kunzendorf U, Keller F, Distier A. The outcome of acute interstitial nephritis: risk factors for the transition from acute to chronic interstitial nephritis. Clin Nephrol 2000; 54(3):179-190.
63. Lyons H, Pinn VW, Cortell S, Cohen JJ, Harrington JT. Allergic interstitial nephritis causing reversible renal failure in four patients with idiopathic nephritic syndrome. N Engl J Med 1973; 288(3):124-128.
64. Magil AB, Ballon HS, Cameron EC, Rae A. Acute interstitial nephritis associated with thiazide diuretics. Am J Med 1980; 69:939-943.
65. Bailey RR, Lynn KL, Drennan CJ, Turner GAL. Triamterene-induced acute interstitial nephritis. Lancet 1982; 1:226.
66. Roy LF, Villeneuve J-P, Dumont A, Dufresne LR, Duran MA, Morin C, Jobin J. Irreversible renal failure associated with triamterene. Am J Nephrol 1991; 11(6):486-488.
67. Spence JD, Wong DG, Lindsay RM. Effects of triamterene and amiloride on urinary sediment in hypertensive patients taking hydrochlorothiazide. Lancet 1985;:73-75.
68. Peskoe ST, McMillan JH, Lorch A, Sussman H, Ozawa T. Reversible acute renal failure associated with chlorthalidone therapy: possible drug induced interstitial nephritis. J Med Assoc Ga 1978; 67:17-18.
69. Ooi BS, Jao W, First MR, Mancilla R, Pollak VE. Acute interstitial nephritis. A clinical and pathologic study based on renal biopsies. Am J Med 1975; 59:614-28.
70. Walker RG, Whitworth JA, Kincaid-Smith PS. Acute interstitial nephritis in a patient taking tienilic acid. Brit Med J 1980; 280:1212.
71. Newstead CG, Moore RH, Barnes AJ. Interstitial nephritis associated with indapamide. Brit Med J 1990; 300:1344.
72. Pusey CD, Saltissi D, Bloodworth L, Rainford DJ, Christie JL. Drug associated acute interstitial nephritis: clinical and pathologic features and the response to high dose steroid therapy. Q J Med 1983; 52:194-211.
73. Ten RM, Torres VE, Milliner DW, Schwab TR, Holley KE, Gleich GJ. Acute interstitial nephritis: immunologic and clinical aspects. Mayo Clin Proc 1988; 63:921-930.
74. Kleinknecht D, Vanhille PH, Morel-Moroger L, Kanfer A, Lemaitre V, Mery JP, Laederich J, Callard P. Acute interstitial nephritis due to drug hypersensitivity. An up-to-date review with a report of 19 cases. Adv Nephrol 1983; 12:277-308.
75. Kelly CJ, Neilson EG. Tubulointerstitial diseases. In, The Kidney, seventh edition. Brenner BM (editor). Saunders, Philadelphia 2004; p. 1495.
76. Park CW, You HY, Kim YK, Chang YS, Shin YS, Hong CK, Kim YC, Bang BK. Letter: Chronic tubulointerstitial nephritis and distal renal tubular acidosis in a patient with furosemide abuse. Nephrol Dial Trans 2001; 16:867-869.
77. Larsson GB, Langer L, Nassberger L. Thiazide-induced kidney damage with circulating antibodies against myeloperoxidase and cardiolipin. J Intern Med 1993; 233:493-494.
78. Byornberg A, Gesslen H. Thiazides: a cause of necrotizing vasculitis. Lancet 1965; 2:982.
79. Grunwald MH, Halevy S, Livni E. Allergic vasculitis induces by hydrochlorothiazide: confirmation by mast cell degranulation test. Isr J Med Sci 1989; 25:572-574.
80. Reed BR, Huff JC, Jones SK, Orton PW, Lee LA, Norris PA. Subacute cutaneous lupus erythematosis associated with hydrochlorothiazide treatment. Ann Intern Med 1985 103:49-51.
81. Fitzgerald EW. Fatal glomerulonephritis complicating allergic purpura due to chlorothiazide. Arch Intern Med 1960; 105:305-310.
82. Kjelbo H, Stakeberg H, Mellgren J. Possibly thiazide-induced renal necrotizing vasculitis. Lancet 1965; 2:1035.
83. Cox NH, Hodkin P. Vasculitis due to metolazone. Postgrad Med J 1991; 67:860.
84. DeMartini FE, Wheaton EA, Healey LA, Larugh JH. Effect of chlorothiazide on renal excretion of uric acid. Am J Med 1962; 32:572-577.
85. Puschett JB. Clinical uses of diuretics. In: Handbook of experimental pharmacology. Diuretics. Greger R, Knauf H, Mutschler E (editors). Springer-Verlag, Berlin 1995.
86. Steele TH. Importance and pathogenesis of diuretic-induced hyperuricemia. In: Diuretics IV. Chemistry, pharmacology and clinical applications. Puschett JB, Greenberg A (editors). Elsevier, Amsterdam 1993; p. 231-238.
87. Carlsen JE, Kober L Torp-Pedersen C, Johansen P. Relation between dose of bendrofuazide, anti-hypertensive effect, and adverse biochemical effects. Br Med J 1990; 300:975-978.

88. Berglund G, Andersson O. Low doses of hydrochlorothiazide in hypertension. Antihypertensive and metabolic effects. Eur J Pharmacol 1976; 10:177-182.
89. Liang MH, Fries JF. Asymptomatic hyperuricemia: the case for conservative management. Ann Intern Med 1978; 88:666-670.
90. Hall AP, Barney PE, Dawber TR, McNamara PM. Epidemiology of gout and hyperuricemia. A long-term population study. Am J Med 1967; 42:27-37.
91. Gutman AB, Yü TF. Renal function and gout with a commentary on the renal regulation of urate excretion, and the role of the kidney in the pathogenisis of gout. Am J Med 1957; 23:600-622.
92. Fessel WJ, Siegelaub AB, Johnson ES. Correlation and consequences of asymptomatic hyperuricemia. Arch Intern Med 1973; 132: 44-54.
93. Fessel WJ. Renal outcomes of gout and hyperuricemia. Am J Med 1979; 67:74-82.
94. Klinenberg JR, Gonick HC, Dornfeld L. Renal function abnormalities in patient with asymptomatic hyperuricemia. Arthritis Rheum 1975; 10(supp):725-730.
95. Briney WG, Ogden D, Bartholomew B, Smythe CJ. The influence of allopurinol on renal function in gout. Arthritis Rheum 1975; 18(supp):877-881.
96. Berger L, Yü TF. Renal function in gout IV. Analysis of 524 gouty subjects including long-term follow-up studies. Am J Med 1975; 59:605-613.
97. Rosenfeld JB. Effect of long-term allopurinol administraton on serial GFR in normotensive and hypertensive hyperuricemic subjects. Adv Exp Med Biol 1974; 41:581-596.
98. Steele TH, Manuel MA, Boner G. Diuretics, urate excretion and sodium reabsorption: effect of acetazolamide and urinary alkalinization. Nephron 1975; 14:48-61.
99. Alon US, Scagliotti D, Garola RE. Nephrocalcinosis and nephrolithiasis in infants with congestive heart failure treated with furosemide. J Pediatr 1994; 125:149-151.
100. Downing GJ, Egelhoff JC, Daily DK, Thomas MK, Alon U. Kidney function in very low birth weight infants with furosemide-related renal calcifications at ages 1 to 2 years. J Pediatr 1992; 120:599-604.
101. Hufnagle KG, Khan SN, Penn D, Cacciarelli A, Williams P. Renal calcifications: a complication of long-term furosemide therapy in preterm infants. Pediatrics 1982; 70:360-363.
102. Jacinto JS, Modanlou HD, Crade M, Strauss AA, Bosu SK. Renal calcification incidence in very low birth weight infants. Pediatrics 1988; 81:31-35.
103. Saarela T, Lanning P, Koivisto M, Paavilainen T. Nephrocalcinosis in full-term infants receiving furosemide treatment for congestive heart failure: a study of the incidence and 2-year follow up. Eur J Pediatr 1999; 158:668-672.
104. Saarela T, Lanning P, Koivisto M. Prematurity-associated nephrocalcinosis and kidney function in early childhood. Pediatr Nephrol 1999; 13:886-890.
105. Pope, IV JC, Trusler LA, Klein AM, Walsh WF, Yared A, Brock, III JW. The natural history of nephrocalcinosis in premature infants treated with loop diuretics. J Urol 1996; 156:709-712.
106. Atkinson SA, Shah JK, McGee C, Steele BT. Mineral excretion in premature infants receiving various diuretic therapies. J Pediatr 1988; 113:540-545.
107. Cohanim M, Yendt ER. Reduction of urine oxalate during long-term thiazide therapy in patients with calcium urolithiasis. Invest Urol 1980; 18:170-173.
108. Constanzo LS, Weiner IM. On the hypercalciuric action of chorothiazide. J Clin Invest 1984; 54:628.
109. Campfield T, Braden G, Flynn-Valone P, Powell S. Effect of diuretics on urinary oxalate, calcium, and sodium excretion in very low birth weight infants. Pediatrics 1997; 99:814-818.
110. Puschett JB, O'Donovan R. Renal actions and uses of diuretics. In: Textbook of nephrology. Massry SG, Glassock RJ (editors). Williams & Wilkins, Baltimore.
111. Puschett JB, Rstegar A. Comparative study of the effects of metolazone and other diuretics on potassium excretion. Clin Pharmacol Ther 1973; 15:397-405.
112. Giebisch G. Effect of diuretics on renal transport of potassium. Methods Pharmacol 1976; 4A:121-164.
113. Wright FS, Giebesch G. Regulation of potassium excretion. In: the kidney physiology and pathophysiology. Seldin DW, Giebisch G (editors). Raven Press, New York; 1992:p. 2206-2247.
114. Lawson DH. Allergic reaction to potassium chloride. Q J Med 1974; 43:443-450.
115. Kassirer JP, Harrington JT. Diuretics and potassium metabolism: a reassessment of the need, effectiveness and safety of potassium therapy. Kidney Int 1977; 11:505-515.
116. Cremer W, Bock KD. Symptoms and course of chronic hypokalemic nephropathy in man. Clin Nephrol 1977; 7:112-119.
117. O'Donovan RA, Muhammedi M, Puschett JB. Diuretics in the therapy of hypertension: current status. Am J Med Sci 1992; 304:312-318.

118. Conn JW, Johnson RD. Kaliopenic nephropathy. Am J Clin Nutr 1956; 4:523-528.
119. Relman AS, Schwartz WB. The kidney in potassium depletion. Am J Med 1958; 24:764-773.
120. Cremer W, Blümcke S, Bock KD. Morphologie der kaliopenischen nephropathie beim menschen. Zentrabl Allg Path 1974; 118:481-482.
121. Healy JJ, McKenna TJ, Canning B St J, Brien TG, Duffy GJ, Muldowney FP. Body composition changes in hypertensive subjects on long-term oral diuretic therapy. Brit Med J 1970; 1:716-719.
122. Marples D, Frøkiaer J, Dørup J, Knepper MA, Nielsen S. Hypokalemia-induced downregulation of aquaporin-2 water channel expression in rat kidney medulla and cortex. J Clin Invest 1996; 97(8):1960-1968.
123. Mujais SK, Katz AI. Potassium deficiency. In: The kidney: physiology and pathophysiology. Seldin DW, Giebisch G (editors). Raven Press, New York 1992; p. 2249-2278.
124. Kirk KL, Schaefer JA. Water transport and osmoregulation by antidiuretic hormone in terminal nephron segments. In: The kidney: physiology and pathophysiology. Seldin DW, Giebisch G (editors). Raven Press, New York 1992; p. 1693-1725.
125. Orloff J. Handler JS. The similarity of effects of vasopressin adenosine-3',5'-monophosphate (cyclic AMP) and theophylline on the toad bladder. J Clin Invest 1962; 41:702-709.
126. Zaman F, Pervez A, Abreo K. Isopropyl alcohol intoxication: a diagnostic challenge. Am J Kidney Dis 2002; 40(3):1-4.
127. Ashkar FS, Miller R. Hospital ketosis in the alcoholic diabetic: A syndrome due to isopropyl alcohol intoxication. South Med J 1971; 64:1409-1411.
128. Abramson S, Singh A. Treatment of the alcohol intoxications: Ethylene glycol, methanol and isoproranol. Curr Opin Nephrol Hypertens 2000; 9:695-701.
129. Adelson L. Fatal intoxication with isopropyl alcohol. Am J Clin Pathol 1962; 38:144-151.
130. Hawley PC, Falko JM. "Pseudo" renal failure after isopropyl alcohol intoxication. South Med J 1982; 75:630-631.
131. Winchester JF. Methanol, isopropyl alcohol, higher alcohols, ethylene glycol, cellosolves, acetone and oxalate. In: Clinical Management of Poisoning and Drug Overdose, 3rd edition. Haddad LM, Shannon MW, Winchester JF (editors). WB Saunders Company, Philadelphia 1998; p. 491-504.
132. Janzen IE, Dossetor JF, Seem CP. Model car fuel poisoning. Ann Clin Biochem 2005; 42(Pt 4):308-309.
133. Verhelst D, Moulin P, Haufroid V, Wittebole X, Jadoul M, Hantson P. Acute renal injury following methanol poisoning: analysis of a case series. Int J Toxicol 2004; 23:267-273.
134. Steinhart B. Case report: severe ethylene glycol intoxication with normal osmolal gap—"a chilling thought". J Emerg Med 1990; 8:583.
135. Ammar KA, Heckerling PS. Ethylene glycol poisoning with a normal anion gap caused by concurrent ethanol ingestion: importance of the osmolal gap. Am J Kidney Dis 1996; 27:130.
136. Purssell RA, Lynd LD, Koga Y. The use of the osmole gap as a screening test for the presence of exogenous substances. Toxicol Rev 2004; 23:189.
137. Liu JJ, Daya MR, Carrasquillo O, Kales SN. Prognostic factors in patients with methanol poisoning. J Toxicol Clin Toxicol 1998; 36:175-181.
138. Gosselin RE, Smith RP, Hodge HC (editors). Methyl alcohol. In: Clinical toxicology of commercial products, 5th ed. Williams & Wilkins, Baltimore 1984; p. 111-275.
139. Closs K, Solberg CO. Methanol poisoning. JAMA 1970; 211:497-499.
140. Erlanson PH, Fritz KE, Hagstam B, Liljenberg N, Tryding N, Voigt G. Severe methanol intoxication. Acta Med Scand 1965; 177:393-407.
141. Gufferman SD, Alvarez M, Alvarez J. Methanol poisoning complicated by myoglobinuric renal failure. Am J Emerg Med 1985; 3:24-26.
142. Hoy WE, Scandling JD, Carbonneau RJ. Hemodialysis treatment of methanol intoxication. Artif Organs 1983; 7:479-481.
143. Friedlaender MM, Rosenmann E, Rubinger D, Silver J, Moskovici A, Dranitzki-Elhalel M, Popovtzer MM, Berlatzky Y, Eid A. Successful renal transplantation from two donors with methanol intoxication. Transplantation 1996; 61(10):1549-1552.
144. Davis DP, Bramwell KJ, Hamilton RS, Williams SR. Ethylene glycol poisoning: case report of a record-high level and review. J Emerg Med 1997; 15:653-67.
145. Barceloux DG, Krenzelok EP, Olson K, Watson W. American Academy of Clinical Toxicology practice guidelines on the treatment of ethylene glycol poinsoning. Ad Hoc Committee. J Toxicol Clin Toxicol 1999; 37:537-60.
146. Moreau C, Kerns II W, Tomaszewski CA, McMartin KE, Rose SR, Ford MD, Brent J, and the META study group. Glycolate kinetics and hemodialysis clearance in ethylene glycol poisoning. Clin Toxicol 1998; 36:659-666.
147. Corley RA, Meek ME, Carney EW. Mode of action: oxalate crystal-induced renal tubule degeneration and glycolic acid-induced dysmorphogenesis—renal and developmental effects of ethylene glycol. Crit Rev Toxicol 2005; 35:691-702.
148. Gabow PA, Clay K, Sullivan LB, Lepoff R. Organic acids in ethylene glycol intoxication. Ann Intern Med 1986; 105:16.

149. Guo C, McMartin KE. The cytotoxicity of oxalate, metabolite of ethylene glycol, is due to calcium oxalate monohydrate formation. Toxicology 2005; 208:347-355.
150. Poldelski V, Johnson A, Wright S, Dela Rosa V, Zager RA. Ethylene glycol-mediated tubular injury: identification of critical metabolites and injury pathways. Am J Kid Dis 2001; 38(2):339-348.
151. McMartin KE, Wallace KB. Calcium oxalate monohydrate, a metabolite of ethylene glycol, is toxic for rat renal mitochondrial function. Toxicol Sci 2005; 84:195-200.
152. Hess R, Bartels MJ, Pottenger LH. Ethylene glycol: and estimate of tolerable levels of exposure based on a review of animal and human data. Arch Toxicol 2004; 78:671-680.
153. Petersen CD, Collins AJ, Himes JM, Bullock ML, Keane WF. Ethylene glycol poisoning. N Engl J Med 1981; 304:21-23.
154. Jacobsen D, McMartin KE. Methanol and ethylene glycol poisonings. Mechanism of toxicity, clinical course, diagnosis and treatment. Med Toxicol 1986; 1:309.
155. Jacobsen D, Øvrebø S, Østborg J, Sejersted OM. Glycolate causes acidosis in ethylene glycol poisoning and is effectively removed by hemodialysis. Acta Med Scand 1984; 216:409-16.
156. Jacobsen D, McMartin KE. Antidotes for methanol and ethylene glycol poisoning. J Toxicol Clin Toxicol 1997; 35:127-43.
157. Brent J, McMartin KE, Phillips S, Burkhart KK, Donovan JW, Wells M, Kulig K. Fomepizole for the treatment of ethylene glycol poisoning. Methylpyrazone for the toxic alcohols study group. J Engl J Med 1999; 340(11):832-838.
158. Baud FJ, Galliot M, Astier A, Bien DV, Garnier R, Likforman J, Bismuth C. Treatment of ethylene glycol poisoning with intravenous 4-metylpyrazole. N Engl J Med 1988; 319(2):97-100.
159. Jacobsen D, Hewlett TP, Webb R, Brown ST, Ordinario AT, McMartin KE. Ethylene glycol intoxication: evaluation of kinetics and crystalluria. Am J Med 1988; 84(1):145-52.
160. Sivilotti ML, Burns MJ, McMartin KE, Brent J. Toxicokinetics of ethylene glycol during fomepizole therapy: implications for management. For the Methylpyrazole for Toxic Alcohols Study Group. Ann Emerg Med 2000; 36:114.
161. Borron SW, Mégarbane B, Baud FJ. Fomepizole in treatment of uncomplicated ethylene glycol poisoning. Lancet 1999; 354:831.

22

Anticancer drugs

Corinne ISNARD-BAGNIS, Vincent LAUNAY-VACHER, Svetlana KARIE and Gilbert DERAY

Groupe Hôpitalier Pitié Salpétrière, Paris, France

Introduction

Nephrotoxicity is an inherent adverse effect of certain anticancer drugs. Antineoplastic drugs have a narrow therapeutic index and the amount of drug necessary to produce a significant reduction in tumor burden usually produces significant nephrotoxicity. The dosage used in clinical trials represents often the maximum tolerated doses determined during phase I drug evaluation. Greater toxicity is acceptable during curative therapy than during palliative therapy. But cancer patients often exhibit excretory reduced organ function. Modulation of pharmacokinetics and pharmacodynamics of these drugs in cancer patient is therefore necessary in order to improve tolerance. Patients with malignancies are particularly vulnerable to development of renal abnormalities. Conversely, patients with renal abnormalities who have undergone kidney transplantation are at high risk for malignancy. Clinical syndromes of renal involvement are diverse and sometimes insidious. This chapter focuses on the major anticancer drugs and their renal consequences. Despite the recent physiopathological advances in understanding the mechanism of anticancer drug nephrotoxicity, prevention still relies on drug dosage decrease, and active screening for renal abnormalities as part of the usual biological work up in patients treated with anticancer drugs (Table 1).

Table 1. Potentially nephrotoxic chemotherapeutic agents and options for prevention.

	Type of renal toxicity	Prevention
Alkylating agents		
Cisplatin*	ATN, dose-related (rare if doses <1600 to 2400 mg/m^2), non-oliguric and reversible Hypomagnesemia usually remits when cisplatin is discontinued	Hydration and vigorous diuresis with saline Daily divided doses for 5 days instead of single infusion Cumulative dose <120 mg/m^2 of body surface area
Carboplatin		
Oxazophosphorins		
Cyclophosphamide	Hemorraghic cystitis	Aggressive hydration and Mesna® prevent hemorraghic cystitis induced by both drugs
Ifosfamide	Fanconi syndrome ATN if doses >5 g/m^2	
Nitrosoureas		
Streptozotocin*	Fanconi syndrome (hypophosphatemia + +) Glomerular toxicity and renal failure	
Carmustine*	Late development of renal failure (long treatment or over 6 courses with the conventional dose 200 mg/m^2)	
Antimetabolites		
Methotrexate*	ATN or secondary intrarenal obstructive uropathy (precipitation of methotrexate or methotrexate metabolite in the distal tubules if dose >50 mg/m^2) Fall in glomerular filtration rate in a rapid and dose related fashion if dose >1 g/m^2	Urine alkalinization and hydration Enhanced toxicity if previous treatment with cisplatin, or NSAIDs Charcoal hemoperfusion and sequential hemodialysis if severe renal toxicity (significant clearance of methotrexate can be achieved with high-flux dialyzers
Antitumour antibiotics		
Mitomycin*	HUS (risk 2 to 10%), late onset (6-17 months following the initiation of treatment)	Cumulative dose should be <40 mg/m^2
Immunotherapy		
Interleukin-2* *(Aldesleukin, IL-2)*	Reversible syndrome of hypotension, oliguria, fluid retention, azotemia, and a very low urinary excretion of sodium Capillary leak syndrome Acute interstitial nephritis	Steroids and plasma exchange
Interferon	Proteinuria in up to 5 to 20% patients Rarely nephritic syndrome or/and acute renal failure (acute interstitial nephrotoxicity and minimal change nephropathy	

Abbreviations and notes: **drugs with asterisk are high-risk drugs, other are lower risk; ATN: Acute Tubular Necrosis; NSAIDs: Non-Steroid Anti-Inflammatory Drugs; HUS: Hemolytic and Uremic Syndrome.*

Alkylating agents

Cisplatin

Cis-dichlorodiammine platinum [II], or cisplatin, has emerged as a principal chemotherapeutic agent in the treatment of otherwise resistant solid tumors and is currently among the most widely used agents in the chemotherapy of cancer [1]. The chief limit to its greater efficacy, however, is its nephrotoxicity, which has made it necessary both to lower its dosage and actively hydrate patients to reduce it. These techniques have proven to be only partially successful as acute renal failure occurs even at such low doses and especially after its repeated administration [2, 3]. Use of other means to protect the kidney [4, 5, 6] are only partially successful and of uncertain clinical application [7]. It may not be possible to alter or prevent the renal toxicity of cisplatin, however, until a more basic understanding of that toxicity is obtained.

Pharmacology

The kidney is the principal excretory organ of cisplatin. In the rat, 50% of injected cisplatin is excreted in the urine 24 hours after its administration [8] and most of excreted platinum appears in the urine within the first hour [9]. Platinum is extensively bound to plasma protein. Free cisplatin in the plasma, by virtue of its low molecular weight and uncharged character, is freely filtered at the glomerulus [10]. Rat and human studies suggest that there may be secretion of cisplatin as well [11, 12]. Proximally microinjected radiolabeled cisplatin is almost completely recovered in the urine and is not reabsorbed to any significant degree [13]. Kidney concentration of platinum is several folds above plasma levels and above that in other organs [8]. Almost all of the platinum in the kidney is contained within the cortex and can be found in all subcellular organelles as well as the cytosol [9]. The process by which the kidney accumulates cisplatin is dependent upon normal oxygen utilization [10] and is inhibitable by drugs that compete for the transport of organic bases in a dose dependent manner. Drugs that compete for the organic anion transport system, such as PAH and pyrazinoic acid, do not inhibit uptake. Taken together, these observations suggest that the renal uptake of cisplatin involves some specific interaction of the drug with the kidney, perhaps involving transport or binding to components of the base transport system.

Further evidence that links the kidney's vulnerability to its role in cisplatin transport is provided by autoradiographic studies that show greater uptake of radiolabeled cisplatin in the S3 segments of the proximal nephron [13]. As the S3 segment of the proximal tubule is the principle site of cell toxicity of cisplatin and contains the most platinum, these studies provide further evidence that the particular vulnerability of this cell type depends on its ability to accumulate cisplatin.

Cisplatin is excreted largely unchanged in the urine [10]. Upon entry into the renal cell, however, cisplatin undergoes biotransformation. In addition to binding to cell macromolecules, a large portion [30-50%] of the total cell platinum is in a form whose molecular weight is below 500 Dalton and whose chromatographic behavior is different from cisplatin. Another characteristic of this platinum metabolite is the loss of its biologic activity as a mutagen. Whereas excreted platinum is mutagenic, cell platinum is not [14]. Mutagenic compounds react with or can be converted to compounds that react with DNA to form DNA adducts. The cisplatin DNA adducts cause errors during DNA replication, which lead to mutations, especially G→T transversions [15]. Such mutations may be responsible for second malignancies that arise after cisplatin therapy [16].

Renal tolerance

The clinical use of cisplatin is hampered by nephrotoxicity, expressed by a reduction in glomerular filtration rate in proportion to the repeated cycles of cisplatin chemotherapy. Progressive and partially irreversible declines in glomerular filtration rate and renal blood flow may develop with each successive treatment course [17]. Renal plasma flow, whole kidney glomerular filtration rate, single nephron glomerular filtration rate, and stop-flow pressure are reduced compared to controls [17]. Intratubular hydrostatic pressure is the same as control in euvolemic and volume expanded animals and it is unlikely that intratubular obstruction plays an important role in early cisplatin induced acute renal failure. With the withdrawal of the drug, renal insufficiency stabilizes or remains indefinitely impaired. The cis-platin-induced hypofiltration is usually associated with minimal proteinuria due to tubular injury. Severe salt wasting with orthostatic hypotension has been observed after cisplatin administration in a minority of patient [18].

Polyuria uniformly accompanies cisplatin administration and occurs in two distinct phases. Urine osmolality initially falls over the first 24-48 hrs after it is given but glomerular filtration rate in this phase is normal. This early polyuria usually ameliorates spontaneously. A second phase of increased volume and reduced osmolality occurs between 72 and 96 hrs after cisplatin. This later phase is accompanied by reduced glomerular filtration rate and is persistent.

Hypomagnesemia is a particularly common complication of cisplatin administration in humans [19] and persistent excretion of magnesium in the presence of severe hypomagnesemia suggests that the hypomagnesemia is due to a renal defect in magnesium reabsorption [20]. Recent studies in a rat model of this syndrome suggest that abnormal magnesium excretion may be due to a defect in magnesium transport in juxtamedullary nephrons or collecting ducts [21], much like the situation that exists for defective water transport described above. Secondary hypocalcemia and hypokaliemia may accompany this situation. Cisplatin may also induce and incomplete distal tubular acidosis by altering the cellular respiration leading to changes in tubular handling of hydrogen, magnesium, potassium and calcium ions [22].

The mediators of the fall in glomerular filtration rate and renal blood flow have not been determined although extensively studied but calcium channel blockers [23] and angiotensin converting enzyme inhibitors [24] have been unable to demonstrate a reversal in cisplatin-induced acute renal failure. Several suspected targets of pathogenetic importance in cisplatin nephrotoxicity have been studied extensively, including renal tubule energy production and DNA synthesis. Mitochondrial dysfunction is involved in the pathogenesis of cisplatin-induced renal failure [25, 26]. *In vitro* incubation of normal tubules with cisplatin inhibits basal and stimulated rates of oxygen consumption but at very high concentrations [10^{-3}M] only. Transplatin, which is neither antineoplasic nor nephrotoxic, but also binds to DNA and protein, decreases respiration at lower concentrations [10^{-4}M] and is even a more potent inhibitor of respiration than cisplatin [13]. But in tubules isolated from rats given a nephrotoxic dose of cisplatin, basal and stimulated rates of respiration are entirely normal up to 48 hrs after cisplatin administration [13]. In these studies the concentration of Pt in proximal tubules were several hundred fold less than that of tubules exposed to cisplatin *in vitro* at a dose that inhibited respiration [13]. The results of these studies would seem to indicate that neither the renal cell mitochondria nor the membrane associated Na-K ATPase are important early pathogenetic targets of cisplatin.

There is convincing evidence that the primary biochemical lesion induced by cisplatin in cancer cells is inhibition of DNA synthesis [27, 28]. The inhibition of DNA synthesis is persistent and occurs at much lower doses than that necessary to inhibit RNA and protein synthesis [29]. Cisplatin binds to two sites in DNA [30] inducing DNA inter- and intrastrand as well as DNA-protein crosslinks [30, 31]. What relationship such cisplatin DNA-binding has to renal cytotoxicity is unknown. How such a decline in DNA synthesis throughout the kidney would explain cell-specific necrosis is problematic but at least two explanations might account for such specificity. First, other cells of the kidney repair their DNA lesions while those of the pars recta cannot. Studies in cells whose repair processes are deficient show that cisplatin is especially toxic in them [32] making such a possibility likely. Second, it may be that the levels of the DNA adducts formed in the pars recta cells are lethal while lower levels in other nephron segments are not. Further studies will be necessary to determine the importance of the reduction in DNA synthesis in renal cytotoxicity.

Recovery from nephrotoxic acute renal failure requires replacement of damaged tubule cells with new ones that are actively dividing. Recovery from cisplatin induced acute renal failure is accompanied by increased mitosis in renal epithelial cells, which is preceded by increases in nucleic acid synthesis [33].

Prevention of cisplatin-induced nephrotoxicity

Early in the development of cisplatin, more than 70% of patients developed acute renal failure that appeared to be cisplatin dose-related [34, 35]. Despite aggressive hydration, especially with NaCl solutions, which are routinely applied in the clinical setting to prevent nephrotoxicity [36], renal failure still occurs [37, 38, 39]. Therefore several attempts have been made to reduce nephrotoxicity by either co administration of other compounds, alternate method of administration, or by developing analogues with an improved therapeutic index.

As mannitol and furosemide reduce the concentration of platinum in the urine, it has been suggested that these agents may attenuate cisplatin nephrotoxicity [40, 41]. However, neither platinum content in the plasma or kidney nor the degree of cellular necrosis it produces is modified by these diuretics [41]. Platinum is not reabsorbed to an important degree after its intra tubular microinjection and, therefore, platinum content in the cell should not be dependent on its luminal concentration [13].

Prior hydration with hypertonic salt seems to reduce cisplatin-induced acute renal failure [42]. As previous studies indicated that the degree of azotemia produced by cisplatin was highly dependent on the sodium chloride content of the vehicle used for its administration [42] it has been suggested that the increase in chloride concentration in the urine that occurs after hypertonic salt infusion may reduce the conversion of cisplatin to toxic aquated metabolites, a process known to be sensitive to Cl ion concentration.

While several experimental reports have suggested that diuretics [mannitol and furosemide] decrease cisplatin nephrotoxicity [36, 41] others have shown that they may aggravate it [43]. Further, in humans, there is no convincing evidence than diuretics may attenuate cisplatin nephrotoxicity as shown in a randomized study by Alsarraf *et al.* [44] hydration + cisplatin was compared to hydration + mannitol + cisplatin.

Protection of kidney function by mannitol was observed after the first cycle, but no convincing effect was observed during the subsequent cycles. So far there is thus no reason to advocate for the use of diuretics in prevention of cisplatin induced nephrotoxicity. Hydration well in advance [at least 12 hours] of cisplatin administration will induce a diuresis of at least 100 ml/hr and will not make compensation of electrolytes losses mandatory as it is the case with diuretics.

The use of hypertonic saline was first introduced in the clinic by Schilsky *et al.* [19] who concluded than when 3% saline was used as a vehicle for cisplatin, no renal toxicity was observed as measured by serum creatinine and creatinine clearance in patients treated with a high dose of cisplatin. However, when ^{51}Cr-EDTA was used as a measure of glomerular filtration rate, a significant decrease in the latter was observed despite the use of 3% saline [12, 13]. Thus the interest of hypertonic saline in the prevention of high dose cisplatin nephrotoxicity will have to be further delineated in randomized studies.

As compared to bolus dose, fractionation or continuous infusion of the total dose of cisplatin over 3-5 days is equally effective from the therapeutic standpoint but probably spares renal function [45]. Indeed, for a given total amount of cisplatin, the fall in glomerular filtration rate is dependent on the amount given as single dose.

Infections are a frequent cause of morbidity in the immunocompromised cancer patients and often necessitate antibiotic therapy. The use of certain bread-spectrum antibiotics, which are potentially nephrotoxic by themselves, may add to the renal toxicity of the anticancer agents. Clinically, the incidence of nephrotoxicity has been recognized to be greater in patients receiving cisplatin in combination with aminoglycosides than in patients receiving cisplatin alone [46].

The degree of renal impairment has usually been mild and not clinically significant [46]. However, acute renal insufficiency has been reported following the combined use of cisplatin with gentamicin-cephalotin [47]. Further it has been shown in rats that even a non-nephrotoxic dose of aminoglycosides immediately following a single dose of cisplatin causes a marked potentiation of the impairment to renal function caused by cisplatin alone [48, 49]. The administration of nephrotoxic drugs such as aminoglycosides, non-steroidal anti-inflammatory drugs or iodinated contrast media simultaneously with cisplatin should therefore be avoided.

An impressive list of compounds has been used to decrease cisplatin nephrotoxicity [ANF, glycine, diethyldithiocarbamate, calcium channel blockers, cimetidine, sodium thiosulphate, glutathione, other sulfidryl compounds, ...]. Among them only sodium thiosulphate has received a significant clinical application and has been reported to reduce the renal toxicity of cisplatin administered locally by either the intra-arterial, intra-peritoneal or intrathoracic routes [50, 51]. However, controversies still exists as to the effect of sodium thiosulphate on cisplatin antitumor activity. Thus sodium thiosulphate may be most useful in combination with intraperitoneal cisplatin where it confers renal protection without altering local effects of cisplatin [51].

Hydration with isotonic saline beginning several hours before cisplatin infusion and continuous infusion of saline infusion several days after cisplatin administration are routinely used to prevent cisplatin nephrotoxicity [35, 36, 38, 39]. Even though several days are required for the severe changes in renal function to fully develop, the critical events seem to occur immediately after cisplatin administration. Protective measure should therefore be applied before, during and immediately after cisplatin infusion. We suggest a regimen consisting of prehydration using 100 ml/hr of normal saline solution for the 12 hours prior to the administration of the compound and continuous infusion of saline during and at least 1 day after cisplatin treatment. Efficacious antiemetic drugs should be given concomitantly to avoid dehydration. With the introduction of odansetron it is now the usual clinical practice to stop intravenous hydration very quickly after cisplatin perfusion to shorten the duration of hospitalization. It should be remembered that odansetron is ineffective in avoiding vomiting in more than 10% of patients submitted to chemotherapy [52]. Since antiemetic reaction cannot be predicted in these patients, intravenous hydration should be maintained at least 3 days after stopping cisplatin.

At present, we would strongly urge not to administer platinum compounds to patients before objective evidence of euvolemia is present. Further, the platinum should be administered slowly in conjunction with a saline solution infusion that produces a brisk diuresis. Urine flow should be maintained at 3 to 4 l/24 hrs for the next two to three days.

The vulnerability of the kidney to cisplatin is almost certainly linked to its primary role in the excretion of the drug. The P3 segment of the proximal tubule is particularly vulnerable to it. The cause of renal cell death induced by cisplatin is unknown, but mounting evidence points to its genotoxic effect. In cisplatin nephrotoxicity, as in other forms of nephrotoxic renal damage, reduced renal blood flow and diminished renal conservation of water are common physiologic derangements.

The high incidence of nephrotoxicity of the currently used inorganic platinum compounds stresses the importance of undertaking research to identify platinum complexes that would feature antitumor properties with less nephrotoxicity. Until this goal is achieved, it seems advisable to attempt to explore further the possibility of utilizing platinum in combination with chemotherapy at that are not associated with significant nephrotoxicity and to avoid other concomitant nephrotoxic insults, especially volume depletion.

Carboplatin

Carboplatin is a cytotoxic platinium complex structurally related to cisplatin, which antitumor activity *in vitro* is qualitatively similar to that of cisplatin. Comparative trials with carboplatin alone or in combination with other chemotherapeutic agents suggest comparable efficacy with cisplatin in ovarian cancer. As with cisplatin, nausea and vomiting occur in many patients but symptoms are usually delayed for several hours and mild to moderate in severity. The dose limiting toxicity of carboplatin is myelosuppression enhanced by renal impairment, previous chemotherapy or in older patients.

Pharmacology

Tissue distribution is similar to that seen with cisplatin with the highest concentrations of platinium in the kidney, liver, skin and tumors [53]. Tissue platinium concentrations were generally 0.5 to 3 fold greater than those observed after cisplatin. It has been demonstrated that platin which is bound to plasma protein looses most of its cytotoxicity [54]. In contrast to cisplatin, which is extensively protein bound, carboplatin appears to be less extensively bound [15 to 25%] at least in the initial hours following administration. Renal clearance appears to be the main route of excretion, and urinary excretion of carboplatin is more rapid than that of cisplatin in animals [55] and cancer patients [56]. 50 to 80% of the dose administered is excreted in the urine over the first 24 hours [57, 58, 59]. It has been postulated that repeated administration of cisplatin may cause decreased carboplatin renal clearance and enhanced toxicity [60]. Renal clearance and total body clearances are reduced in patients with reduced renal function [61, 62, 63].

Calculation of dose in renal failure

The dose administered should be adjusted in proportion to the reduction of creatinine clearance for patients with renal impairment since they require lower doses to achieve AUCs comparable with those seen with patients with normal renal function. Calvert *et al.* [64] have proposed the following formula for calculation of dose:

Dose [mg] = AUC x [GFR + 25]

Where the target AUC [area under the plasma concentration x time curve] is in the target range of 5 to 7 mg/ml per min for acceptable toxicity in patients receiving single agent carboplatin.

Renal Tolerance

Carboplatin was developed to avoid the nephrotoxicity of cisplatin and was initially considered as less nephrotoxic [65]. Initial studies in rats demonstrated that carboplatin had minimal renal effects as measured by serum blood urea nitrogen, creatinine, kidney weight and renal histology [66]. Early clinical studies established that, at doses of 400 mg/m^2, carboplatin caused virtually no nephrotoxicity, ototoxicity or peripheral neuropathy [67]. Egorin *et al.* in 1984 [68] found no decrease in creatinine clearance in 22 patients treated with intravenous carboplatin at 400 mg/m^2 and believed that no reduction in dosage was required in patients with diminished renal function. Because the dose-limiting toxicity for carboplatin is myelosuppression, with little renal or neurological toxicity, higher doses [800 mg/m^2 body surface area] were combined with granulocyte-macrophage colony-stimulating factor. In these settings, with no vigorous hydration, a significant decrement in renal function has been described [69, 70]. Out of six patients receiving 1200 mg/m^2 carboplatin, a decrease in glomerular filtration rate of 25% to 50% was observed in 4 [71]. Several studies have also reported the comparative toxicity of carboplatin and cisplatin, all confirming the same general trend.

Oxazaphosphorines / cyclophosphamide and ifosfamide

Cyclophosphamide

Pharmacology

The oxazophosphorine cyclophosphamide is initially oxidized to active and inactive metabolites which are secreted by the kidney [72, 73, 74, 75]. The 24 hour urinary excretion of intact parent compound and alkylating activity is respectively 1-14% and 7-17% [76]. The fraction of cyclophosphamide and metabolites excreted in the urine is high and unchanged in patients with renal failure [77].

Urothelial toxicity

Direct contact of the bladder epithelium with the catabolites acrolein and 4-hydroxy-cyclophosphamide is responsible for the hemorrhagic cystitis that can be a consequence of therapy with cyclophosphamide [78]. Aggressive hydration provides prophylaxis against this toxicity to the efferent urinary tract [79]. The sulfhydryl compound mesna has also demonstrated uroprotective ability during therapy with cyclophosphamide [80]. Although hemorrhagic cystitis is a dose-related toxicity, chronic low doses of orally administered cyclophosphamide are also associated with development of this adverse event [81].

Renal tolerance

Cyclophosphamide can also cause tubular necrosis in experimental animals [82]. No clinical nephrotoxicity has been described, even when carefully assessed in patients receiving high doses of cyclophosphamide [83, 84]. Although there are no detectable alterations of renal function tests, some subtle changes in tubular kidney physiology do occur. Bode and associates [85] studied the mechanism of water retention that occurs from cyclophosphamide. They determined that cyclophosphamide directly affected the tubules, causing increased water resorbtion and sodium loss. This water retention is self-limited and lasts only a day or two. It is not a major clinical problem.

Ifosfamide

Pharmacology

Ifosfamide is used increasingly for the treatment of pediatric malignancies. It is a prodrug that must be biotransformed by the hepatic cytochrome P450 system before it can exert its therapeutic or toxic effects [86, 87]. Ring hydroxylation produces 4-hydroxy-ifosfamide, which is then converted into the active alkylating agent [isophosphoramide mustard] and acroleine [the putative cause of hemorrhagic cystitis and *in vitro* nephrotoxin]. Significant molecular decomposition occurs by dechloroethylation of ifosfamide [88], subsequent chloroethyl side chain breakdown with production of chloroacetaldehyde precipitating neuro and nephrotoxic effects [89, 90, 91].

Urinary excretion of 57 – 80% of the dose as ifosfamide and metabolites is reported and 27-41% of the dose is recovered in the urine as alkylating activity

[92]. Indeed ifosfamide metabolism occurs at a low range in the kidney since ifosfamide metabolites were recovered from urine and renal venous effluent in an isolated perfused rat kidney model after ifosfamide perfusion [93].

Renal Tolerance

Experience with ifosfamide-containing regimens has revealed a consistent clinical pattern of nephrotoxicity. Fanconi syndrome, which is characterized by acid, sodium, potassium, magnesium, and small molecular weight proteins, occurs in 1-5% of the children who have received repeated treatments of ifosfamide [94] [95]. In fact the development of rickets secondary to Fanconi syndrome has been reported following treatment with ifosfamide [96]. Patients who have received therapy with cisplatin or carboplatin in addition to ifosfamide may be at greater risk for development of Fanconi syndrome [97]. Hemorrhagic cystitis is a significant toxicity that occurs with ifosfamide administration [98, 99]. However, appropriate hydration and the sulfhydryl compound mesna are effective in decreasing the urotoxicity of ifosfamide [100, 101]. Less frequently asymptomatic renal functional abnormalities are reported following treatment with ifosfamide when used at a dose below 1.5 gr/m^2 body skin surface [102, 103]. Acute renal failure secondary to tubular necrosis has been described when high-dose therapy [>5 gr/ m2] is administered, especially if patients were treated previously with cisplatin [104, 105]. With escalating doses of a 96 hours infusion of ifosfamide, renal toxicity is dose limiting at 18 gr/ m2 [106].

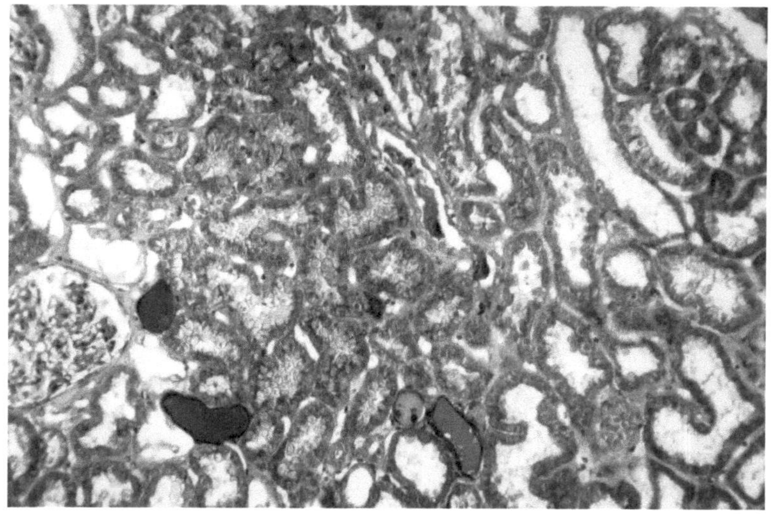

Figure 1. *Focal tubular necrosis with flat epithelial, pauci cellular fibrosis. Patient received cisplatin. Masson's trichrome staining, magn. x125.*

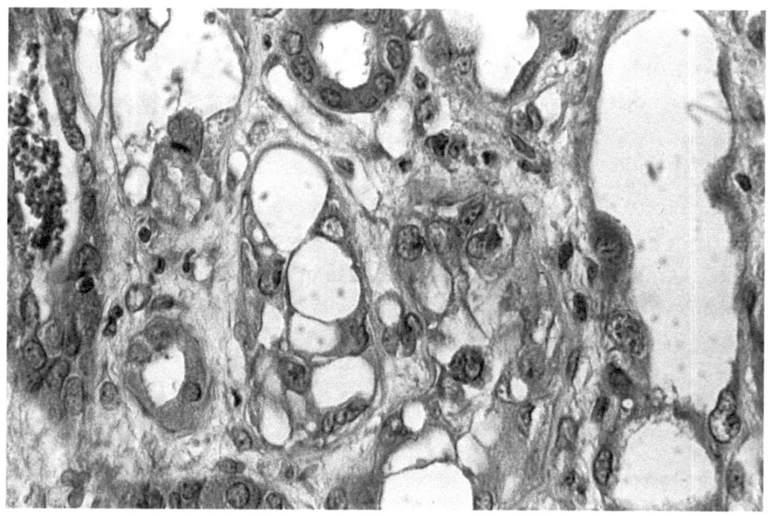

Figure 2. *Tubular necrosis with focal denudation of the basement membrane and pronounced vacuolization, swelling. Some interstitial fibrosis. Patient received ifosfamide. Masson's trichrome staining, magn. x325.*

Nitrosoureas / streptozotocin / carmustine and lomustine

Streptozotocin

Streptozotocin is a naturally occurring nitrosourea useful for the treatment of advanced islet cell carcinomas and carcinoïd tumors [107].

Pharmacology

Animal studies have shown high concentration of streptozotocin in the kidney [108]. Urinary excretion of streptozotocin accounts for 10-20% of the dose [109, 110]. Large concentrations of drug metabolites can also be detected there [109, 110]. Thus, the major excretion pathway of streptozotocin is the kidney.

Renal tolerance

Nephrotoxicity characterized by renal tubular effects, including the Fanconi syndrome, is a documented side effect of streptozotocin therapy. The onset of streptozotocin-induced nephrotoxicity can be insidious with hypophosphatemia as the presenting sign, which is followed by glycosuria, proteinuria and finally increase in creatinine and blood urea nitrogen [111, 112]. In the first phase I trial reported with this drug, all 18 treated patients developed renal dysfunction, and 2 of them became anuric [113]. Schein *et al.* [110] treated 106 patients and noted renal abnormalities in 28%; this was the most common form of toxicity. Nephrotoxicity contributed to the death of 4 patients in this study. Moertel and co-workers [114] saw evidence of nephrotoxicity in two-third of 38 patients treated with streptozotocin. It also occurred in two-thirds of 52 patients in another series, and 5 of these patients died of renal failure.[115]. The incidence of streptozotocin-induced nephrotoxicity seems to increase with prolonged drug administration.

The site of streptozotocin injury is both the glomerulus and the tubule, because histologic changes have been observed in both sites [115, 116, 117]. Although streptozotocin is excreted in the urine, an explanation at the cellular and molecular levels for glomerular and tubular sensitivity to the drug is lacking. Streptozotocin markedly suppresses nicotinamide adenine dinucleotide levels in animal liver and islet cells [which are correlated with the diabetogenic effect of streptozotocin] [118, 119]. This effect could explain why streptozotocin has been reported to induce renal tumors in experimental animals and this effect being modified by nicotinamide administration [120, 121].

Carmustine, lomustine and semustine

Carmustine (BCNU) and Lomustine (CCNU) are antineoplasic drugs widely used in the treatment of brain tumors, multiple myeloma, Hodgkin's disease and non-Hodgkin's lymphoma in combination with other approved drugs [122, 123, 124, 125].

BCNU [1, 3bis[2-chloroethyl]1-nitrosourea] can be administered as a single agent at doses of 50-210 mg/m^2 and in combination chemotherapy regimens at similar or lower doses. BCNU can also be a component of some high-dose chemotherapy regimens with autologous bone marrow reinfusion [126]. BCNU may also be used together with CCNU [1-[2 chloroethyl]-3[cyclohexyl]-1-nitrosourea] or methyl-CCNU [1-[2 chloroethyl]-3[-[4- methyl cyclohexyl]-1-nitrosourea].

Pharmacology

Carmustine is highly lipid soluble, with a rapid metabolism and a bi-phasic half-life [1.4 and 20 minutes]. Carmustine is metabolized to an N-nitroso group, which is secreted into the renal tubule. It has been proposed that this N-nitroso group is pharmacologically active when present in high concentration and capable of spontaneously releasing an active methyl group which may in turn be responsible for its nephrotoxicity [127]. 60 to 70% is excreted in the urine within 96 hours and 6 to 10% is excreted as CO2 by the lungs. No parent compound is excreted in the urine, so nephrotoxicity is most likely due to one of the metabolites. Nitrosoureas have both alkylating and carbamoylating activity, but they vary a great deal in the degree of each [128]. Therefore it is difficult to implicate either chemical action in the mechanism of nephrotoxicity. The toxicity [mainly haematopoietic, hepatic and gastro intestinal] is cumulative therefore the Food and Drug Administration recommends that courses should not be given more frequently than every 6 weeks.

Renal tolerance

Renal toxicity of Carmustine [BCNU] and Lomustine [CCNU] was first noted in the pre clinical studies with these two drugs [129]. In the earliest clinical trial of Carmustine, 10% of the patients had unexplained elevations of BUN, but there were no instances of severe renal problems [130]. Thus, renal problems were believed not to be of major importance with any of these drugs. Reports of Semustine- and Lomustine-induced renal failure later contradicted this impression [131, 132, 133, 134, 135, 136]. Potential renal toxicity seems to be a clinical problem only in patients receiving unusually long treatment. Indeed, 3 single cases have first been reported. These patients received high cumulative doses of Lomustine [2300 to 3360 mg] [137, 132, 136]. Then Schacht *et al.* [138] reported late development of renal functional impairment following at least one year of therapy during which a minimum of 6 courses of these nitrosoureas were administered in conventional dosage [200 mg/m2 at 8 weeks intervals]. 18 patients, having received cumulative doses of 1.5 to 7.4 gr, had developed impaired renal function with elevation of BUN above 20 mg/dl or a decrease in glomerular filtration rate as determined by inulin clearance. 4 patients developed end-stage renal disease 9 to 16 months after following courses of therapy ranging from 28 to 65 months in duration. The clinical records of these patients failed to reveal any history of hypertension or impaired renal function before treatment and no sign of early nephrotoxicity even though each bimonthly dose wad administered under close observation in the hospital. Renal functional impairment developed insidiously, while urinalyses showed no proteinuria or only traces and formed element were absent. 24-hour urinary protein values never exceeded 450 mg. None of the patient had glycosuria. Renal pathology was obtained in 5 patients by percutaneous biopsy and 2 patients post mortem in this study and showed glomerular sclerosis affecting more than 15% of glomeruli, focal thickening and reduplication of the basement membranes in many of the remaining glomeruli. No glomerular abnormality was observed. Focal areas of tubular atrophy, interstitial fibrosis and infiltration with chronic inflammatory cells were observed in all patients but one. In patients with severe damage, there was advanced, widespread sclerosis of glomeruli, varying from contraction of tufts with partial obliteration of lumens to complete obliteration of capillary lumens forming acellular contracted tufts. In these cases, tubular atrophy was extensive and severe. Immunofluorescence studies failed to show any localization of immunoglobulin. The histologic abnormalities were similar to that reported by Harmon *et al.* [133]. The predominance of tubulointerstitial changes in some patients suggested that glomerular sclerosis might have been secondary to a primary interstitial process. However, an independent nephrotoxic effect of the nitrosoureas directed against glomeruli as well as the interstitium could not be ruled out. Despite the histologic and clinical evidence of a chronic progressive parenchymal nephropathy, at no time were there any features of acute nephrotoxicity. Further clinical evidence that no acute renal insult antedates the chronic progressive disease was provided by post mortem renal examination in patients who died from their brain tumors and who received one or two courses of nitrosourea therapy, because no acute renal parenchymal process was on going. Renal function decline is insidious, the initial intimation of renal damage occurring 1 to 6 years after onset of chemotherapy. Once having developed, renal functional impairment may progress rapidly to advanced uremia despite discontinuation of the drug.

The mechanism of BCNU-induced nephrotoxicity is most likely based on a direct nephrotoxic effect but differs from that of streptozotocin manifested by proximal tubular dysfunction and acute renal failure that may abate when the drug is discontinued.

Antimetabolites

Methotrexate

Methotrexate is a folic acid antagonist that inhibits the enzyme dihydrofolate reductase. This agent is mainly used in the treatment of both cancer [trophoblastic neoplasms, leukemias, breast carcinoma, carcinoma of gastric, esophagus, testes, lymphomas] and non-cancer diseases [psoriasis; rheumatoid arthritis]. Recent successful results using high-dose [$>1 g/m^2$] methotrexate followed by leucoverin in the treatment of head and neck carcinomas and osteosarcoma has led to a more widespread use of this therapy in patients with these and other tumors.

Pharmacology

Methotrexate is readily filtered by the kidneys, and renal clearance is influence by both tubular secretion [139, 140, 141, 142] and tubular reabsorption [142]. Intravenous administration of methotrexate 140-350 mg/kg [<6h infusion] results in 70-94% of the dose appearing in the urine over 24 h [143]. In contrast, when methotrexate is administered as a 24-h continuous infusion, 60% of the dose is excreted in the urine during the 24-h infusion [144]. Approximately 10% of the dose is excreted in the urine as 7-hydroxymethotrexate [143, 144]. The 7-hydroxy metabolite is important since it may contribute to the renal toxicity of methotrexate [148] and this moiety becomes a significant metabolite when methotrexate doses are 50 mg/kg or greater [145]. Following oral administration of methotrexate a lesser fraction of the dose is recovered in the urine than following intravenous administration [141]. This may reflect the dose-dependent incomplete absorption of methotrexate [141, 146, 147]. Methotrexate is highly bound to plasma proteins.

Renal tolerance

Nephrotoxicity is a potential adverse effect of treatment with methotrexate, particularly when dosages equal or exceeds 50 mg/$m^{2.}$ The most commonly accepted mechanism for this drug-induced toxicity is precipitation of methotrexate or methotrexate metabolite in the distal tubules with secondary intrarenal obstructive uropathy and tubular necrosis. Particularly during high-doses methotrexate therapy [>1gr/m^2], the urinary concentration of methotrexate and 7-hydroxymethotrexate may exceed the aqueous solubility of these agents at urinary pH [148]. This hypothesis is supported by ability of urinary alkalinization and hydration to decrease the incidence and severity of methotrexate-induced nephrotoxicity [149]. Direct tubular toxicity [148, 150] and decreased tubular filtration [149, 151] may also be components of methotrexate-induced nephrotoxicity. Toxicity is enhanced when patients have been treated previously with cisplatin, or concomitantly with other nephrotoxic drugs [non-steroidal antiinflammatory drugs] [152]. An enhanced toxicity was indeed observed when administered concomitantly with another highly protein bound agent such as ketoprofen [152] but the mechanism of this interaction is unclear. If anything this interaction should actually have resulted in an increased clearance of the drug. It has been suggested that the decrease in renal clearance of methotrexate observed after concomitant nonsteroidal anti-inflammatory drug treatment could be explained by either a competitive inhibition of methotrexate tubular secretion or inhibition of renal prostaglandins secretion inducing altered glomerular filtration rate in the setting of pre renal volume contraction [153].

When high-doses methotrexate are administered, glomerular filtration rate falls in a majority of patients in a rapid and dose related fashion [154, 155]. Patients should be euvolemic prior to receiving treatment with methotrexate. In addition, adjunctive hydration and urinary alkalinization should be included in therapy for patients receiving dosages equal to or exceeding 50 mg/m^2. Due to the significant renal clearance of methotrexate and the risk of increased toxicity associated with increased concentrations of methotrexate over time, dosing of this agent should be done relative to renal function.

It is noteworthy that a significant clearance of methotrexate can be achieved with high-flux dialyzers. Serum methotrexate levels can be successfully lowered in patients with methotrexate-induced acute renal failure by charcoal hemoperfusion and sequential hemodialysis [156, 157].

Gemcitabine

Several therapeutic agents can promote the development of Thrombotic MicroAngiopathy (TMA), which is characterized clinically by microangiopathic hemolytic anemia, thrombocytopenia, and various ischemic end organ manifestations. Pathologically, vessel wall thickening, endothelial cell swelling, intraluminal platelet thrombi, and microvascular occlusion are noted [158]. Some forms of TMA are dominated by renal impairment and are usually referred to as haemolytic uremic syndrome (HUS); others show predominant central nervous system involvement and are referred to as thrombotic thrombocytopenic purpura (TTP).

Gemcitabine is a nucleoside analog that was released in 1996 for the treatment of unresectable pancreatic cancer. Subsequently, it has been employed successfully to treat several malignancies including bladder cancer, non-small cell lung cancer, ovarian cancer, and breast cancer. Initial reports by Flombaum and colleagues of TMA associated with gemcitabine were rare [159] and the manufacturer estimated an incidence of 0.015% according to adverse events reporting through 1997 [160]. Potential underreporting is possible, especially from spontaneous sources, but when compared with the incidence rates ranging from 2.6-13.0% cited in the literature for either malignancy-induced or chemotherapy-induced HUS [160, 161], the incidence of HUS associated with gemcitabine is relatively rare. However, anecdotal experience and review of the literature suggested that TMA occurs more commonly after gemcitabine exposure than initially believed. One retrospective study determined that gemcitabine-associated TMA was more common than previously reported [162]. A cumulative incidence of 0.31% was calculated in this study. Eight of 12 affected patients (67%) required treatment with dialysis. Acute onset or worsening hypertension occurred in 7 (58%) of twelve affected patients. The median duration of treatment with gemcitabine was 5.8 months (range = 3.8 to 13.1 months). Renal dysfunction was universal, while hematuria was present in more than two thirds of patients. Signs and symptoms of HUS developed within 1 to 2 months of the last gemcitabine treatment in all patients. Two of 12 patients (17%) had previously received treatment with a mitomycin-containing regimen [160]. The clinical course of TMA, which developed after chronic therapy was dose-dependent.

More recently, to characterize the clinical presentation of gemcitabine nephrotoxicity, the medical records of 29 patients were reviewed by Flombaum *et al.* [163]. Twenty-eight patients were evaluated for new-onset renal disease and one for microangiopathic hemolytic anemia. Median age was 64 years (50-81). The typical presentation consisted of rising serum urea and creatinine levels occurring over a period of weeks to months, in association with new or worsening hypertension (26 patients). Thrombocytopenia and microangiopathic hemolytic anemia of varying degrees were present in all patients. Twenty-three out of 26 patients have a low or undetectable haptoglobin level. LDH level was elevated in all Pts. Schistocytes were present in 21 of the 24 patients who had their blood smears reviewed. The median cumulative dose of gemcitabine was 22gm/m^2 (4-81) given over 77 months (1.75-34). Prior chemotherapy with mitomycin C (9 patients), especially if given in close proximity (4 patients), may be synergistic and was particularly severe and appeared within a short period after gemcitabine administration. Full or partial recovery of renal function occurred in 19 patients (in 2 patients, after requiring dialysis for 3 and 20 months). Seven patients progressed to end-stage renal disease and 3 patients developed chronic renal failure, but did not need dialysis. Microhematuria and proteinuria was present in 27 patients. Oedema and chronic heart failure was present in 21 and 7 patients respectively. A high index of suspicion is essential and discontinuation of gemcitabine alone often improved the outcome.

Review of literature suggests that cancer-associated HUS usually occurs during widespread metastatic disease or poorly controlled carcinomas, whereas chemotherapy-associated HUS is more common when the patient is in disease remission or has minimal tumor burden [164, 165]. However, the discrimination is not always clear. Murgo [165] attempted to distinguish the characteristics of malignancy-induced and chemotherapy-induced HUS and identified several features to separate the two while Gordon and Kwaan [164] showed that there are more similarities than differences. Some researchers suggest the level of serum factors such as TNF-α, IL-1, and IL-6 as well as von Willebrand factor (vWF) antigen and low molecular weight vWF multimers may be used to distinguish between malignancy-associated HUS and chemotherapy-associated HUS [166, 167]. However, such studies remain experimental and are not readily available in the majority of community settings.

Ancillary treatments or antidotes that effectively prevent or reduce the severity of gemcitabine associated HUS have not be identified. Treatment modalities employed for TMA include immunocomplex removal (plasmapheresis, immunoadsorption, hemodialysis, or exchange transfusion), antiplatelet/anticoagulant therapies (antiplatelet drugs, heparin, prostacyclin, or splenectomy), immunosuppressive therapies (corticosteroids, vincristine, or azathioprine), and fresh frozen plasma transfusion [160, 168, 169]. Most of such modalities of treatment are safe and quite effective, in particular if performed in a specialized setting. Despite the availability of these treatments, the outcome with TMA is poor with a high mortality. Mortality rates rage from 10 to 40% in the majority of series [168, 169] to as high as 60-70% in others [161, 170]. Such a high mortality rate approaching 50% is not surprising because the majority of these patients had advanced disease. Since this adverse effect is frequently associated with a poor outcome, patients should be monitored for signs and symptoms of HUS for 3 months following completion of treatment with gemcitabine.

Upon recognition of gemcitabine-associated TMA, the drug must be discontinued. Depending on the timing of diagnosis, there may be full renal recovery with early recognition. Late diagnosis is associated with chronic kidney disease, development of end stage renal disease requiring dialysis, and death due to progressive disease.

Antitumor antibiotics

Mitomycin

Mitomycin C does not need dosage adjustment in the presence of impaired renal function since less than 20% of the dose appears in the urine [171, 172, 173].

Potentially life-threatening hemolytic uremic syndrome is an adverse event that occurs with Mitomycin C therapy [174.]. Hematological findings include anemia, thrombocytopenia and the presence of schizocytes on peripheral blood smear. Acute renal failure in these settings may be associated with proteinuria and microscopic hematuria [175, 176, 177, 178, 179]. The onset of signs and symptoms associated with renal impairment generally occurs 6-17 months following the initiation of treatment with this agent [180]. Corticoids and plasma exchanges have been associated with drastic improvement of the renal parameters [181]. The mechanism of Mitomycin induced nephrotoxicity is unknown. To prevent the occurrence of this side effect, the maximum cumulative dose should be 40 mg/m2. Severe hemolytic uremic syndrome can also be seen with different other anticancer drugs [5-fluoro-uracile, vincristine, cis-platin, bleomycin, adriamycin] [182].

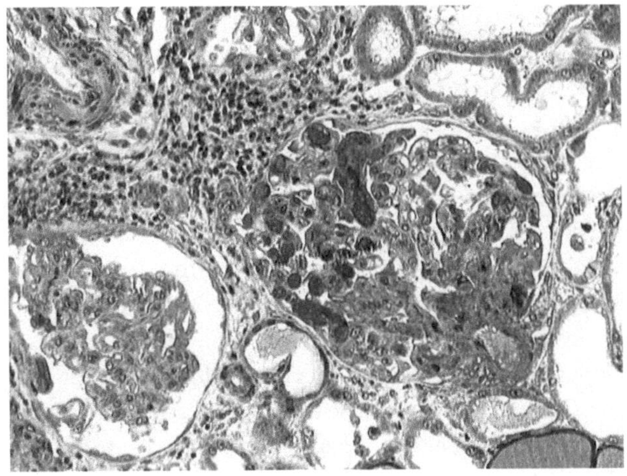

Figure 3. *Mitomycin C induced thrombotic microangiopathy. Glomeruli show swelling and detatchment of endothelial cells and luminal occlusion. The arterioles and arteries show intimal cellular swelling and hyperplasia and fibrin deposition. Masson's trichrome staining, magn. x325.*

Immunotherapy

Interleukin 2

Recombinant Interleukin 2 has opened a new approach in the treatment of renal cell carcinoma [183, 184]. Interleukin 2 alone, or combined with interferon alpha and lymphokine activated killer cells is now used at a high dosage in patients with advanced melanoma or renal cancer to induce regression of solid tumor and metastasis [185, 186, 187]. Renal toxicity is the main limiting side effect of Interleukin 2 administration, more important in aging and subjects with altered renal function and often leads physicians to discontinue or reduce interleukin-2 doses. Clinical studies document a reversible syndrome of hypotension, oliguria, fluid retention, azotemia, and a very low urinary excretion of sodium [188, 189]. It is associated to the so-called vascular leak syndromedescribed in experimental studies as a primary increase in the vascular permeability with consequent shifting of proteinaceous intravascular fluid into the interstitium of many organs, hypoalbuminemia and reduction of the intravascular volume [190]. Therefore, acute renal failure after interleukin-2 administration has initially been considered as secondary to the systemic alterations associated with this treatment. Further studies have suggested that in cancer patients with interleukin-2 continuous infusion, renal failure may occur even in stable hemodynamic conditions [191].

Acute interstitial nephritis characterized by parenchymal infiltration with T lymphocytes was also reported [192] in few patients. It has been suggested that acute tubular nephritis could be the result of a cytotoxic lymphocyte-mediated reaction induced by the interleukin-2 treatment [193].

In human, the pathophysiology of interleukin-2 induced renal dysfunction is still poorly understood. Interleukin-2 may act directly on the vascular tonus and endothelial integrity or may stimulate generation of other cytokines, which in turn would increase vascular permeability. Occurrence of an intrinsic renal lesion has been suggested by Shalmi *et al.* [194] who showed that glomerular filtration rate is altered in 90% of the patients [mean decrease of 43%] whereas renal plasma flow decreases is only slightly altered [mean decrease 5%] in 50% of the patients.

Since interleukin-2 induced rate of response in patients with metastatic melanoma or renal cell cancer is schedule and dose dependent, and because renal toxicity is the main cause of treatment discontinuation, more studies are warranted to elucidate the observed nephrotoxicity.

Alpha-Interferon

Pharmacology

Alpha-interferon, a 165 amino acid glycoprotein, is effective in the treatment of viral hepatitis C and B, and also myeloma, melanoma, and renal carcinoma. Little is known about the renal metabolism of alpha-interferon despite extensive studies in experimental animals. In patients with normal renal function, a serum peak level is obtained 8 hours after a subcutaneous injection of 3 10^6 units of alpha-interferon. Terminal elimination half-life ranges from 4 to 16 hours and after 24 to 48 hours, the interferon molecule is not detected anymore in the serum [195]. Alpha-interferon urinary level is undetectable. Some authors have suggested that, despite the lack of urinary excretion, the kidney could play a role in alpha-interferon metabolism [196]. Indeed, as far as hepatitis C treatment is concerned, dialysis patients often show a better response to therapy than non-dialysis patients do but at the expense of increased side effects. This better efficacy is associated with lower tolerance in this population. This raises the question of pharmacokinetics modifications. Few studies documented that clearance kinetics of interferon alpha in patients with chronic renal failure is about twice as low as in patients with normal renal function [197]. Indeed interferon is filtered by the glomeruli and largely absorbed and catabolized within tubular cells [198].

Main side effects are dose-dependent chills, fatigue and gastrointestinal disturbances. Rarely seizures, encephalopathy and strokes have been reported [199]. Although there has been considerable experience with interferons in clinical trials during the past 20 years, acute renal failure as a side effect of interferon treatment has been rarely reported. In 1976, Gresser *et al.* [200] described experimental lesions induced in the kidney by interferon in mice. Glomerular nephropathy was observed, either hyalynosis or rapidly progressive glomerulonephritis [201]. In human, while proteinuria has been noted in up to 15 to 20% patients treated with interferon [202], acute renal failure syndrome has rarely been observed [203], [204]. Nephrotic syndrome was present in some cases [205] and the histopathology was described as a combination of acute interstitial nephrotoxicity and minimal change nephropathy. This pattern is similar to that seen with renal injury from non-steroidal anti-inflammatory drugs and ampicillin [206]. A pathogenic role for cellular immunity being enhanced by interferon therapy has been therefore suspected. The overall incidence of alpha-interferon acute renal toxicity was recently evaluated as below 5% in patients treated for myeloproliferative syndrome [207].

Acute renal insufficiency as a complication of gamma interferon treatment has been reported anecdotally.

Anti-VEGF agents

Those latter years have seen the emergence of new anticancer molecules with novel pharmacological mechanisms named « targeted therapies ». They differ from conventional chemotherapy and radiotherapy in the way that they demonstrate a high specificity towards their target. Among those new drugs, the inhibitors of angiogenesis are the most developed. Their therapeutic targets include the vascular endothelial growth factor (VEGF), its circulating form or its receptors. Indeed, bevacizumab has been marketed a few years ago. It is a humanized monoclonal antibody targeted to VEGF, or other molecules such as VEGF-Trap. Other classes of anti-angiogenic agents include the inhibitors of tyrosine kinase sunitinib, sorafenib, AG013736, or valatinib, which specifically inhibit the tyrosine kinases from the intracellular domain of VEGF receptor. Most common renal effects of those drugs, which are besides that well-tolerated, were hypertension and proteinuria, witth some differences in their histological presentation.

Bevacizumab

In a Phase III study, Hurwitz *et al.* [208] report an incidence of grade III hypertension of 11% in patients receiving bevacizumab and chemotherapy as compared to 2.3% in patients receiving the same regimen without bevacizumab. The incidence of all grades hypertension was 22.4% in that study and no episode of hypertensive crisis or death secondary to hypertension have been observed. In 2003, Kabbinavar had already reported that 19 out of 104 patients had presented hypertension, 47% of them having a history of hypertension before the introduction of the treatment [209]. The incidence of all grades hypertension was 28% in this study following administration of bevacizumab 10 mg/kg/dose. This incidence was dose-related since it was 11% in the group of patients receiving bevacizumab 5 mg/kg/dose. Similarly, the Summary of Product Characteristics (SmPC) of bevacizumab, Avastin® mentions that an elevated incidence of hypertension has been notes in patients receiving bevacizumab in combination with 5-FU (60 to 67%) as compared to those patients who did not received bevacizumab (43%). The same observation was noted regarding severe hypertension: 7 to 10% in bevacizumab-treated patients versus 2% in non-treated patients [210].

The mechanism of this hypertension is unclear. One hypothesis would be the inhibition of VEGF. Indeed, VEGF stimulates Nitric Oxide production (NO) and thus acts as a vasodilator. Its inhibition could thus lead to vasoconstriction and elevation of blood pressure. In fact, bevacizumab plays a key-role in angiogenesis and hemodynamics through inhibiting VEGF. Some animals and human studies suggest that an appropriate, balanced expression of VEGF is mandatory to maintain the structure and functions of the renal glomerulus. For instance, hyper-expression or under-expression of VEGF may lead to the development of a glomerulopathy. In one study, an elevated concentration of the soluble VEGF receptor R1 is a predictor of pre-eclampsia, associated with proteinuria and hypertension [211]. Animal studies have shown that VEGF is expressed in podocytes and that its receptors are present in endothelial glomerular cells [212] and in another study, the authors demonstrated that under-expression or heterozygous expression of VEGF in podocytes induces endotheliosis with hyaline deposits, clinically accompanied by a nephritic syndrome resembling pre-eclampsia [213]. On the other hand, hyper-expression of VEGF in podocytes may also induce proteinuria, secondary to a collapsing of the glomerulus [214]. Those results demonstrate that an appropriate expression of VEGF is essential in maintaining the function and structure of the renal glomerulus [215].

There are very few histological data from renal biopsies in cancer patients treated with anti-VEGF agents and the precise anatomopathological profile of the proteinuria observed remains unclear. Furthermore, proteinuria may also be due to the elevation of intraglomerular pressure secondary to hypertension, at least partly, or related to other nephrotoxic drugs frequently used in cancer patients. In the article from Miller [216], the incidence of proteinuria was 33.9% in patients receiving bevacizumab and pamidronate alone induced proteinuria in 18.5% of cases. Those two drugs in combination may thus add their nephrotoxic effects, bevacizumab through a proteinuria, sometimes severe, and pamidronate through a collapsing focal and segmental glomerular sclerosis or other glomerulopathies [217]. Bevacizumab-induced renal effects must not favour neglecting other possible causes of renal toxicity. For instance, in two patients with grade 3 proteinuria reported in the literature for whom a renal biopsy was performed, authors show lesions of focal and segmental glomerulo sclerosis due to co-administration of pamidronate for 2 years in one [216] a cryoglobulinemic glomerulonephritis for the second [218].

Among anti-VEGF agents, hypertension and proteinuria have also been reported with sunitib [219], sorafenib [220], AG13736 [221], and VEGF-Trap [222].

Sunitib

The most frequent adverse events encountered under treatment with sunitib are hypertension (18 to 28%) and asthenia (42 to 47%). In two Phase II studies in patients with metastatic renal carcinoma, hypertension has been noted in 48 patients out of 169 (28%), with 6% presenting with a grade 3 hypertension versus 1% of patients receiving placebo. No grade 4 hypertension has been reported and dosage reduction or withdrawal of treatment allowed blood pressure control [219, 223]. The mean time before apparition of hypertension was 131 days [7 – 316] after bevacizumab first dose. Moreover, 12% of those patients from this study had elevation of their serum creatinine.

Sorafenib

Ratain *et al.* report the occurrence of hypertension in 86 patients out of 202 (43%) with 62 (31%) presenting a grade ¾ in a population of metastatic renal carcinoma patients treated with sorafenib for 12 weeks. Forty-six percent of those patients necessitated antihypertensive therapy and none of them died [224]. In another study [220], 75% of 20 metastatic renal carcinoma patients exhibited an increase in their systolic blood pressure of more than 10 mmHg. In 12 patients, this increase was superior to 20 mmHg after 3 weeks under sorafenib therapy. Diastolic blood pressure was also increased, by more than 9.3 mmHg under treatment. In another study in 28 patients presenting solid tumours of different types, hypertension was observed in 5 patients after 3 to 4 weeks of sorafenib treatment [225].

Other anti-VEGF agents

Thirty-three percent of 17 patients treated with AG013736 developed hypertension. In one patient, treatment had to be resumed because of this side effect, and 6 of them (12%) presented a grade ¾ hypertension [221]. Data are even more scanty with VEGF-Trap but it seems that this drug behaves the same way with regard to this issue, as showed in ref [222].

Treatment of anti-VEGF agent-induced renal effects

Optimal treatment of hypertension and proteinuria induced by anti-VEG agents necessitates a clear understanding of their physiopathology. In fact, the association of hypertension with bevacizumab may result from the pharmacological effect of the drug resulting in the blockade of the VEGF pathway. Indeed, the intravenous administration of VEGF in rats induces a dose-dependent hypotension with reflex tachycardia. This manifestation is linked to an interaction with NO [226] and the induction of prostacyclin synthesis [227]. As demonstrated in the VIVA study [228], in rats, hypotension is a limiting and dose-dependent side-effect of VEGF IV infusions.

Angiotensin converting enzyme (ACE) inhibitors or angiotensin II receptor antagonists (ARBs) are usually used to reduce proteinuria which occurs during hypertensive episodes in patients with type 2 diabetes or glomerulopathies. There are no evidence to date that such therapies may be efficient in reducing proteinuria and hypertension secondary to bevacizumab treatment. Furthermore, angiotensin II may increase VEGF secretion in podocytes, as observed in renal cells from mice [229]. As a result, a treatment with either an ACE inhibitors or an ARBs may be tried in such patients, keeping in mind that there are no clinical evidence suggesting their potential efficacy. However, because decreasing blood pressure is a crucial issue to allow maintenance of anti-VEGF therapy, anti-hypertensive therapies may be used with antihypertensive drugs from those classes or calcium inhibitors, beta blockers, or diuretics. None of those classes may be recommended to date. However, in one Phase II study in patients receiving bevacizumab for the treatment of advanced carcinoïd tumours, blood pressure was not in the target in 50% of the patients receiving nifedipine, and in 78% of the patients receiving other antihypertensive therapies [230].

A strict monitoring of blood pressure is thus mandatory in those patients, before treatment is started and every 2 weeks thereafter, and more frequently if hypertension is diagnosed [210]. Proteinuria may be easily monitored with the determination of the protein/creatin ratio on a urine spot, which is an easy and reliable method in this indication [231].

Radiation nephritis

Radiation nephropathy is defined as renal injury caused by ionizing radiation. Number of cases increases steadily and parallels the increase of bone marrow transplant procedures using total body irradiation [232]. Radiation nephritis is dose dependent [233]. Doses traditionally associated with radiation nephropathy are above 2000 cGy. Fractionation, time and chemotherapy may change the time course and severity of radiation-induced nephropathy. Increasing tolerance is observed with increasing fractionation, probably because it allows repair of sublethal damage during the time between fractional doses. Therefore, chronic nephropathy can be prevented by kidney shielding or, alternatively, by fractionating doses. Previous cytotoxic chemotherapy, radiocontrast agents, antibiotics potentiate the effects of ionizing radiation [234].

Radiation nephropathy can present in several forms. An acute form is usually seen within a year after radiation and presents with hypertension, anemia and edema. A more insidious chronic form presents primarily with diminished glomerular filtration, hypertension and occasionally proteinuria. When present, associated accelerated hypertension can promote renal failure. Some patients may develop hypertension within several years after radiation but no azotemia. In a subset of patients, mild proteinuria may be the only feature of chronic renal disease [235].

Interstitial fibrosis is the common pathologic finding in patients with chronic radiation nephritis.

Morphologic studies of radiation nephropathy have documented injury to blood vessels, glomeruli, tubular epithelium and interstitium. Recent ultrastructural studies indicate that glomerular endothelium is an early site of visible injury [236] with endothelial disruption and leukocyte adherence. Later, tubular degeneration and atrophy occur. The second pathophysiologic hypothesis holds vascular injury as the main initial event [237] which helps understand the hypertension occurring in radiation nephritis but does not account for the glomerular lesions.

Even though radiation nephropathy has been known for a long time, first therapeutic attempts were only made recently when it has been documented that ACE inhibitors could attenuate in animals the response to renal irradiation over the short term [238] and slow down the decline in renal function even after the onset of renal injury [239]. Same positive effects were observed with angiotensin II antagonists whereas other antihypertensive agents (hydrochlorothiazide or verapamil) were ineffective. These data point to a role for the renin-angiotensin system in the pathogenesis of radiation nephropathy but clinical data are scarce and no long-term benefit of ACE inhibitors has been yet established.

Acknowledgements

Figures 1-3 by courtesy of Dr. Hélène Beaufils.

References

1. Safirstein RL. Anticancer drugs. In Clinical Nephrotoxins, Debroe ME, Porter GA, Bennett WM, Verpoten GA. [Editors]. Kluwer Academic Publ. Dordrecht, 1998: 261-271.
2. Meijer S, Mulder NH, Sleijfer DT, de Jong PE, Sluiter WJ, Schraffordt Koops H, van der Hem GK. Nephrotoxicity of cis-diamminedichloride platinum [CDDP] during remission-induction and maintenance chemotherapy of the testicular carcinoma. Cancer Chemother Pharmacol 1982; 8: 27-30.
3. Brock PR, Koliouska DE, Baratt TM, Yeomans E, Pritchard J. Partial reversibility of cisplatin nephrotoxicity in children. J Pediatric 1991; 118: 531-4.
4. Yuhas JM, Culo F. Selective inhibition of the nephrotoxicity of cis-dichlorodiamine platinum by WR 272l without altering its antitumor properties. Cancer Treat Rep 1980; 64: 57-64.
5. Borch RF, Pleasants ME. Inhibition of cis-platinum nephrotoxicity by diethyldithiocarbamate rescue in a rat renal model. Proc Natl Acad Sci USA 1979; 76: 6611-4.
6. Berry J-P, Pauwells C, Tlouzeau S, Lespinats G. Effect of Selenium in combination with cis-diamminedichloroplatinum [II] in the treatment of murine fibrosarcoma. Cancer Res 1984; 44: 2864-8.
7. Citkovic E, Hayes DM, Golbey RB, Krakoff IH. Cisplatin-nephrotoxicity: diethyldithiocarbomate, WR2721 or just water. J Clin Oncol 1991; 9: 707-9.
8. Litterst CL, Torres IJ, Guarino AM. Plasma levels and organ distribution of platinum in the rat, dog, and dog fish following intravenous administration of cis-DDP[II]. J Clin Hemat Oncol 1977; 7: 169-78.
9. Safirstein R, Daye M, Miller P, Guttenplan J. Renal disposition and metabolism of liganded platinum: implications to toxicity. Fed Proc 1980; 40: 651A
10. Safirstein R, Miller P, Guttenplan JB. Uptake and metabolism of cisplatin by rat kidney. Kidney Int 1984; 25: 753-8.
11. Jacobs C, Kalman SM, Tretton M, Weiner MW. Renal handling of cis-diammine dichloroplatinum [II]. Cancer Treat Rep 1980; 64: 1223-6.
12. Levi J, Jacobs C, Kalman S, McTigue M, Weiner MWJ. Mechanism of cis-platinum nephrotoxicity I. Effects on sulfhydryl groups in rat kidneys. Pharmacol Exp Ther 1980; 213: 545-50.
13. Safirstein R, Winston J, Moel D, Dikman S, Guttenplan J. Cisplatin nephrotoxicity insights into mechanism. Int J Andrology 1987; 10: 325-46.
14. Safirstein RL, Daye M, Guttenplan JB. Mutagenic activity and identification of excreted platinum in human and rat urine and rat plasma after administration of cisplatin. Cancer Letters 1983; 18: 329-38.
15. Bradley LJN, Yacema KJ, Lippard SJ, Essigmann JM. Mutagenicity and genotoxicity of the major DNA adduct of the antitumor drug cis-diamminedichloroplatinum [II]. Biochemistry 1993; 32: 982-8.
16. Greene MH. Is cisplatin a human carcinogen ? J Natl Cancer Inst 1992; 84: 306-12.
17. Winston JA, Safirstein R. Reduced renal blood flow in early cisplatin-induced acute renal failure in the rat. Am J Physiol. 1985, 249: F490-496.
18. Hutchinson FN, Perez EA, Gandara DR, Lawrence HJ, Kaysen G. Renal salt-wasting in patients treated with cisplatin. Ann Intern Med. 1988, 108:21-5.
19. Schilsky Rl, Anderson T. Hypomagnesemia and renal magnesium wasting in patients receiving cis-diamminedichloroplatinum II. Ann Intern Med 1979; 90: 929-31.
20. Schilsky RL, Barlock A, Ozols RF. Persistent hypomagnesemia following cisplatin chemotherapy for testicular cancer. Cancer Treat Reports 1982; 66: 1767-9.
21. Mavichak v, Wong NLM, Quamme GA, Magil AB, Sutton RAL, Dirks JH. Studies on the pathogenesis of cisplatin-induced hypomagnesemia in rats. Kidney Int 1985; 28: 914-21.
22. Swainson CP, Colls BM, Fitzharris BM. Cisplatinium and distal renal tubule toxicity. N Z Med J, 1985, 98:375-378.

23. Safirstein R, Winston J, Moel D, Dikman S, Guttenplan J. Cisplatin nephrotoxicity insights into mechanism. Int J Andrology 1987; 10: 325-46.
24. Schor N, Ichikawa I, Rennke HG, Troy JL, Brenner BM. Pathophysiology of altered glomerular function in aminoglycoside-treated rats. Kidney Int 1981; 19: 288-92.
25. Gordon JA, Gattone VH. Mitochondrial alterations in cisplatin-induced acute renal failure. Am J Physiol 1986; 250: F991-8.
26. Brady HR, Kone BC, Stroniski ME, Zeidel ML, Giebisch G, Gullans SR. Mitochondrial injury: an early event in cisplatin-toxicity to renal proximal tubules. Am J Physiol 1990; 258: F1181-7.
27. Harder HC, Rosenberg B. Inhibitory effects of anti-tumor platinum compounds on DNA, RNA, and protein synthesis in mammalian cells *in vitro*. Int J Cancer 1970; 6: 207-16.
28. Howle JA, Gale GR. Cis-dichlorodiammine platinum II persistent and selective inhibition of deoxyribonucleic acid synthesis *in vitro*. Biochem Pharmacol 1970; 19: 2757-62.
29. Munchausen LL, Rahn RO. Biological and chemical effects of cis-dichlorodiammineplatinum [II] on DNA. Cancer Chemother Rep 1975; 59: 643-6.
30. Roberts JJ, Prascoe JM. Cross linking of complementary strands of DNA in mammalian cells by antitumor platinum compounds. Nature 1972; 235: 282-4.
31. Zwelling LA, Anderson T, Kohn KW. DNA-protein and DNA interstrand cross-linking by cis- and trans platinum [II] Diamminedichloride in Ll2lO mouse leukemia cells and relation to cytotoxicity. Cancer Res 1979; 39: 365-9.
32. Fraval HNA, Rawlings CJ, Roberts JJ. Increased sensitivity of UV repair deficient human cells to DNA bound platinum products which unlike thymine dimers are not recognized by an endonuclease extracted from Micrococcus leuteus. Mutat Res 1978; 51: 12l-32.
33. Safirstein R, Zelent AZ, Gordon R. Cisplatin-nephrotoxicity: new insights into mechanisms. In: Hacker MP, Lazo JS, Tritton TR, editors. Organ directed toxicities of anticancer drugs. Boston: Martinus Nijhof, 1988: 172-89.
34. Madias NE, Harrington JT. Platinium nephrotoxicity. Am J Med 1978; 65: 307-14.
35. Goldstein RS, Mayor GH. Minireview: the nephrotoxicity of cisplatin. Life Sci 1983; 32: 685-90.
36. Heidemann HTH, Gerkens JF, Jackson EK, Branch RA. Attenuation of cisplatin-induced nephrotoxicity in the rat by high salt diet, furosemide and acetazolamide. Naunyn-Schmiedeberg's Arch Pharmacol 1985; 329: 201-5.
37. Hayes DM, Cvitkovic E, Golbey RB, Scheiner E, Helson L, Krakoff IA. High dose cisplatinium diammine dichloride: amelioration of renal toxicity by mannitol diuresis. Cancer 1977; 39: 1372-81.
38. tark JJ, Howell SB. Nephrotoxicity of cisplatinium [II]-dichlorodiammine. Clin Pharmacol Ther 1978; 23: 461-6.
39. Einhorn LH, Donohue J. Cis diammine dichloroplatinium, uniblastine and gleomycine combination chemotherapy in disseminated testicular cancer. Ann Intern Med. 1977. 87:293.
40. Cvitkovic B, Spaulding J, Bethune V, Martin J, Whitemore WF. Improvement of cis-dichlorodiammineplatinum therapeutic index in an animal model. Cancer 1977; 39: 1357-61.
41. Pera MF Jr, Zook BC, Harder HC. Effects of mannitol or furosemide diuresis on the nephrotoxicity and physiological disposition of cis-dichlorodiammine platinum [II] in rats. Cancer Res 1979; 29: 1269-78.
42. Litterst CL. Alterations in the toxicity of cis- dichlorodiammine platinum II and in tissue localization of platinum as a function of NaCl concentration in the vehicle of administration. Appl Pharmacol 1981; 61: 99-108.
43. Lehane D, Winston A, Gray R, Daskal Y. The effect of diuretic pretreatment on clinical morphological and ultrastructural cis-platinium induced nephrotoxicity. Int J Radiation Oncology Biol Phys 1979; 5: 1393-9.
44. All-Sarraf M, Fletcher W, Oishi N, Pugh R, Hewlett JS, Balducci L, McCracken J, Padilla F. Cisplatin hydration with and without mannitol diuresis in refractory disseminated malignant melanoma: a southwest oncology group study. Cancer Treat Rep 1982; 66: 31-5.
45. Salem P, Khalyl M, Jabboury K, Hashimi L. Cis-diamminedichloroplatinium [II] by a 5-day continuous infusion. Cancer 1984; 53: 837-40.
46. Haas A, Anderson L, Lad T. The influence of aminoglycosides on the nephrotoxicity of cis-diammine-chloroplatinium in cancer patients. J Infect Dis 1983; 147: 363.
47. Gonzales-Vitale JC, Hayes DM, Cvitkovic E, Sternberg SS. Acute renal failure after cis-dichlorodiammine-platinium [II] and gentamicin-cephalotin therapies. Cancer Treat Rep 62: 693
48. Jongejan HTM, Provost AP, Molenar JC. Potentiation of cis-diamminedichloroplatinium nephrotoxicity by amikacin in rats. Cancer Chemother Pharmacol 1988; 22: 178-80.
49. Bregman CL, Williams PD. Comparative nephrotoxicity of carboplatin and cisplatin in combination with actinomycin. Cancer Chemother Pharmacol 1986.
50. Hirosawa A, Niitani H, Hayashibara K, Tsubo IE. Effects of sodium thiosulfate in combination therapy of cis-dichlorodiammine platinium and vindesine. Cancer Chemother Pharmacol 1989; 23: 255-8.

51. Howell S, Pfeifle C, Wung W, Olshen R, Lucas W, Yon J, Green M. Intraperitoneal cisplatin with systemic thiosulfate protection. Ann Intern Med 1982; 97: 845-51.
52. Cubeddu LX, Hoffmann IS, Fuenmayor NT, Finn AL. Efficacity of odansetron and the role of serotonin in cisplatin induced nausea and vomiting. N Engl J Med 1990; 322[12]: 810-5.
53. Boven E, Van der Vijgh WJF, Nauta MM, Schlüper HMM, Pinedo HM. Comparative activity and distribution studies of five platinium analogues in nude mice bearing human ovarian carcinoma xenografts. Cancer Research, 45:86-90, 1985
54. Gormley PE, Bull JM, LeRoy AF, Cysyk R. Kinetics of cis-dichlorodiammineplatinum. Clin Pharmacol Ther. 1979 Mar;25[3]:351-7
55. Siddik ZH, Jones M, Boxall FE, Harrap KR. Comparative distribution and excretion of carboplatin and cisplatin in mice Cancer Chemother Pharmacol. 1988;21[1]:19-24
56. Sharma H, Thatcher N, Baer J, Zaki A, Smith A, McAucliffe CA, Crowther D, Owens S, Fox BW. Blood clearance of radioactively labeled cis-diammine 1, 1-cyclobutane dicarboxylate platinum [II] [CBDCA] in cancer patients. Cancer Chemother Pharmacol. 1983;11[1]:5-7
57. Elferink F, van der Vijgh WJ, Klein I, Pinedo HM. Interaction of cisplatin and carboplatin with sodium thiosulfate: reaction rates and protein binding. Clin Chem. 1986 Apr;32[4]:641-5
58. Harland SJ, Newell DR, Siddik ZH, Chadwick R, Calvert AH, Harrap KR. Pharmacokinetics of cis-diammine-1, 1-cyclobutane dicarboxylate platinum[II] in patients with normal and impaired renal function. Cancer Res. 1984 Apr;44[4]:1693-7
59. Koeller JM, Trump DL, Tutsch KD, Earhart RH, Davis TE, Tormey DC. Phase I clinical trial and pharmacokinetics of carboplatin [NSC 241240] by single monthly 30-minute infusion. Cancer. 1986 Jan 15;57[2]:222-5
60. Trump DL, Elson P, Brodovsky H, Vogl SE. Carboplatin in advanced, refractory germ cell neoplasms: a phase II Eastern Cooperative Oncology Group Study. Cancer Treat Rep. 1987 Oct;71[10]:989-90
61. Egorin MJ, Van Echo DA, Tipping SJ, Olman EA, Whitacre MY, Thompson BW, Aisner J. Pharmacokinetics and dosage reduction of cis-diammine[1, 1-cyclobutanedicarboxylato]platinum in patients with impaired renal function. Cancer Res. 1984 Nov;44[11]:5432-8
62. Gaver RC, George AM, Deeb G. *In vitro* stability, plasma protein binding and blood cell partitioning of 14C-carboplatin. Cancer Chemother Pharmacol. 1987;20[4]:271-6
63. Harland SJ, Newell DR, Siddik ZH, Chadwick R, Calvert AH, Harrap KR. Pharmacokinetics of cis-diammine-1, 1-cyclobutane dicarboxylate platinum[II] in patients with normal and impaired renal function. Cancer Res. 1984 Apr;44[4]:1693-7
64. Calvert AH, Newell DR, Gumbrell LA, O'Reilly S, Burnell M, Boxall FE, Siddik ZH, Judson IR, Gore ME, Wiltshaw E. Carboplatin dosage: prospective evaluation of a simple formula based on renal function. J Clin Oncol. 1989 Nov;7[11]:1748-56
65. Martinez F, Deray G, Dubois M, Beaufils H, Jacquiaud C, Bourbouze R, Benhmida M, Jaudon MC, Jacobs C. Comparative nephrotoxicity of carboplatin and cisplatin in euvolemic and dehydrated rats. Anticancer Drugs 1993; 4: 85-90.
66. Levine BS, Henry MC, Port CD, Richter WR, Urbanek MA. Nephrotoxic potential of cis-diamminedichloroplatinum and four analogs in male Fischer 344 rats. J Natl Cancer Inst. 1981 Jul;67[1]:201-6
67. Canetta R, Rozencweig M, Carter SK. Carboplatin: the clinical spectrum to date. Cancer Treat Rev. 1985 Sep;12 Suppl A:125-36
68. Egorin MJ, Van Echo DA, Tipping SJ, Olman EA, Whitacre MY, Thompson BW, Aisner J. Pharmacokinetics and dosage reduction of cis-diammine[1, 1-cyclobutanedicarboxylato]platinum in patients with impaired renal function. Cancer Res. 1984 Nov;44[11]:5432-8
69. Reed E, Jacob J. Carboplatin and renal dysfunction. Ann Intern Med. 1989 Mar 1;110[5]:409
70. Gore ME, Calvert AH, Smith LE. High dose carboplatin in the treatment of lung cancer and mesothelioma: a phase I dose escalation study. Eur J Cancer Clin Oncol. 1987 Sep;23[9]:1391-7
71. Sleijfer DT, Smit EF, Meijer S, Mulder NH, Postmus PE. Acute and cumulative effects of carboplatin on renal function. Br J Cancer. 1989 Jul;60[1]:116-20
72. Schuler U, Ehninger G and Wagner T. Repeated high_dose cyclophosphamide administration in bone marrow transplantation: exposure to activated metabolites. Cancer Chemother Pharmacol. 20:248-252, 1987
73. Bagley CM, Bostick FW and De Wita. Clinical pharmacology of cyclophosphamide. Cancer Res. 88226-233, 1978
74. Struck RF, Kirk M, C, Mellet LB, el Dareer S and Hill DL. Urinary metabolites of the antitumor agent cyclophosphamide. Mol Pharmacol 7:519-529, 1971
75. Dooley JS, James CA, Rogers HJ and Stuart-Harris. Biliary elimination of cyclophosphamide in man. Cancer Chemother Pharmacol, 9:26-29, 1982
76. Juma FD, Rogers HJ, Trounce JR. Pharmacokinetics of cyclophosphamide and alkylating activity in man after intravenous and oral administration. Br J Clin Pharmacol. 8:209-217, 1979
77. Mouridsen HT, and Jacobsen E. Pharmacokinetics of cyclophosphamide in renal failure. Acta Pharmacol Toxicol 86:409-414, 1975

78. Brock N, Pohl J, and stekarJ. Studies of the urotoxicity of oxazophosphorine cytostatics and its prevention. Eur J Cancer. 17:595-607, 1981
79. Droller MJ, Sral R and Santos G. Prevention of cyclophosphamide-induced hemorrhagic cystitis. Urology, 20:256-258, 1982
80. Link H, Neef V, Niethammer D and Wilms K. Prophylaxis of haemorrhagic cystatis due to cyclophosphamide-conditioning for bone marrow transplantation. Blut, 48:329-330, 1981
81. Ann Intern Med 106:79-94, 1987
82. Philips FS, Sternberg SS, Cronin AP, and Vidal PM. Cyclophosphamide and urinary bladder toxicity. Cancer Res. 21:1577-1589, 1961
83. Bode U, Seif SM, and Levin AS. Studies on the antidiuretic effect of cyclophosphamide: vasopressin release and sodium excretion. Med Pediatr Oncol 8: 295-303, 1980
84. De Fronzo RA, Colvin OM, Braine H, Robertson GL, and Davis PJ. Cyclophosphamide and the kidney. Cancer 33:483-491, 1974
85. Bode U, Seif SM, Levin AS. Studies on the antidiuretic effect of cyclophosphamide: vasopressin release and sodium excretion. Med Pediatr Oncol, 8:295-303, 1980
86. Skinner R, Sharkey IM, Pearson ADJ, et al. Ifosfamide, Mesna and nephrotoxicity in children. J Clin Oncol 11:173-190, 1993.
87. Kaijser G, Bejnen J, Bult A, and Underberg W. Ifosfamide metabolism and pharmacokinetics. Anticancer Res 14:517-532, 1994
88. Boos J, Welslau U, Ritter J, Blaschke G and Schellong G. Urinary excretion of the enantiomers of Ifosfamide and its inactive metabolites in children. Cancer Chemother Pharmacol 28:455-460, 1991
89. Mohrmann M, Pauli A, Ritzer M, Schonfeld B, Seifert B and Brandis M. Inhibition of sodium-dependent transport systems in LLC-PK1 cells by metabolites of ifosfamide. Renal Physiol Biochem 15, 289-301, 1992
90. Mohrmann M, Ansorge S, Schmich U, Schonfeld B, and Brandis M. Toxicity of Ifosfamide, cyclophosphamide and their metabolites in tubular cells in culture. Pediatr Nephrol 8:157-163, 1994
91. Zamlauski-Tucker M, Morris M, and Springate: Ifosfamide metabolite chloroacetaldehyde causes Fanconi syndrome in the perfused rat kidney. Toxicol App Pharmacol 129:170-175, 1994
92. Allen LM, Creaven PJ, and Nelson RL. Studies on the human pharmacokinetics of Ifosfamide [NSC-109724]. Cancer Treat Rep, 60:451-458, 1976
93. Springate J, Zamlauski-Tucker M, Lu H, and ChanKK. Renal Clearance of Ifosfamide. Drug Metab and Dispos, 29, 9:1081-1082, 1997
94. Suarez A, McDowell H, Niaudet P, Comoy E, and Flamant F. Long term follow up of Ifosfamide renal toxicity in children treated for malignant mesenchymal tumors: an international society of pediatric oncology report. J Clin Oncol, 9: 2177-2182, 1991
95. Pratt CB, Meyer WH, Jenkins JJ, Avery L, McKay CP, Wyatt RJ, Hancock ML. Ifosfamide, Fanconi's syndrome and reickets. J Clin Oncol 9:1495-1499, 1991
96. Moncrieff M, and Foot A. Fanconi syndrome after Ifosfamide. Cancer Chemother Pharmacol, 23:121-122, 1989
97. Skinner R, Sharkey IM, Pearson ADJ and Craft AW. Ifosamide, mesna and nephrotoxicity in children. J Clin Oncol. 11:173-190, 1993
98. Brock N, Pohl J and Stekar J. Studies on urotoxicity of oxazophosphorine cytostatics and its prevention. Eur J Cancer 17:595-607, 1981
99. Van Dyck JJ, Falkson HC, Van der Merwe AM, and Falkson G. Unexpected toxicity in patients treated with ifosfamide. Cancer Res 32: 921-924, 1972
100. Falkson G, Van Dick JJ, Stapelberg R and Falkson HC. Mesnum as protector against kidney and bladder toxicity with high-dose ifosfamide treatment. Cancer Chemother Pharmacol 9:81-84, 1982
101. Stuart-Harris R, Harper PG, Kaye SB, and Wiltsaw E. High-dose ifosfamide by infusion with mesna in advanced soft tissue sarcoma. Cancer Treat Rep 10[suppA]:163-164, 1988
102. Newbury-Ecob RA, Noble VW, Barbor PRH. Ifosfamide-induced Fanconi syndrome. Lancet 2, 1328, 1989
103. Patterson WP, Khojasteh A. Ifosfamide-induced renal tubular defects. Cancer 63:649651, 1989
104. Stuart-Harris RC, Harper PJ, Parson CA and coll. High-dose alkylation therapy using Ifosfamide infusion with Mesna in the treatment of adult soft-tissue sarcoma. Cancer Chemother Pharmacol, 11:69-74, 1983
105. Willemse PHB, De Jong PE, Elema JD, Mulder NH. Severe renal failure following high-dose Ifosfamide and Mesna. Cancer Chemother Pharmacol, 23:329-330, 1989
106. Elias AD, Eder JP, Shea T, Begg C, Frei E III, Antman K. High-dose Ifosfamide with mesna uroprotection: a phase I study. J Clin Oncol, 8: 170-178, 1990
107. Rougier P, Mitry E. Digestion; Chemotherapy in the treatment of neuroendocrine malignant tumors, 62 Suppl 1:73-8, 2000
108. Bhuyan BK, Kuentzel SL, Gray LG, Fraser TJ, Wallach D and Neil GL. Tissue distribution of streptozotocin [NCS-85998]. Cancer Chemother Rep. 58:157-165, 1974

109. Adolphe AB, Glasofer ED, Troetel WM, Ziegenfuss J, Stambaugh JE, Weiss AJ, and Manthei RW. Fate of streptozotocin [NSC-85998] in patients with advanced cancer. Cancer Chemother Rep. 59:547-556, 1975
110. Schein PS, O'Connell MJ, Blom J, Hubbard S, Magrath IT, Bergevin P, Wiernik JL, Ziegler PH, and DeVita VT. Clinical antitumor activity and toxicity of streptozotocin [NSC-85998]. Cancer 84:993-1000, 1974
111. Myerowitz RL, Sartiano GP, and Cavallo T. Nephrotoxic and cytoproliferative effects of streptozotocin. Cancer 88:1550-1555, 1976
112. Perry DJ, and Weiss RB. Nephrotoxicity of streptozotocin. Ann Int Med 96:122, 1982
113. Sadoff L. Nephrotoxicity of Streptozotocin [NSC-85998]. Cancer Chemother. Rep 54:457-459, 1970
114. Moertel CG, Reitemeir RJ, Schutt AJ, and Hahn RG. Phase II study of streptozotocin [NSC-85998] in the treatment of advanced gastro-intestinal cancer. Cancer Chemother Rep 55:303-307, 1971
115. Broder LE, and Carter SK. Pancreatic islet cell carcinoma. II Results of therapy with streptozotocin in 52 patients. Ann Intern Med, 79:108-118, 1973
116. Loftus L, Cuppage FE, Hoogstraten B. Clinical and pathological effects of streptozotocin. J Lab Clin Med. 84:407-413, 1974
117. Myerowitz RL, Sartiano GP, and Cavallo T. Nephrotoxic and cytoproliferative effects of streptozotocin. Report of a patient with multiple hormone-secreting islet cell carcinoma. Cancer, 38:1550-1555, 1976
118. Anderson T, Schein PS, McMenamin MG, and Gooney DA. Streptozotocin diabetes. Correlation with extend of depression of pancreatic islet nicotinamide adenine dinucleotide. J Clin Invest 54:672-677, 1974
119. Schein PS and Loftus S. Streptozotocin: depression of mouse liver pyridine nucleotides. Cancer Res 28:1501-1506, 1968
120. Horton L, Fox C, Corrin B and Sönksen PH. Streptozotocin-induced renal tumors in rat.Br J Cancer. 36:692-699, 1977
121. Rakieten N, Gordon BS, Cooney DA, Davis RD and Schein PS. Renal tumorigenesis action of streptozotocin [NSC-85998] in rats. Cancer Chemother Rep. 52:563-567, 1968
122. Dumontet C, Thieblemont C, Espinouse D, Bouafia F, Hequet O, Salles G, Coiffier B. A prospective study of intensive induction therapy with high-dose consolidation in patients with aggressive non-Hodgkin's lymphoma and two or three adverse prognostic factors. Leukemia. 2000 Dec;14[12]:2159-65
123. Dillman RO, Soori G, Wiemann MC, Schulof R, Dobbs TW, Ruben RH, DePriest CB, Church C. Phase II trial of subcutaneous interleukin-2, subcutaneous interferon-alpha, intravenous combination chemotherapy, and oral tamoxifen in the treatment of metastatic melanoma: final results of cancer biotherapy research group 94-11. Cancer Biother Radiopharm. 2000 Oct;15[5]:487-94
124. Nieder C, Grosu AL, Molls M. A comparison of treatment results for recurrent malignant gliomas. Cancer Treat Rev. 2000 Dec;26[6]:397-409
125. Engelhard HH. The role of interstitial BCNU chemotherapy in the treatment of malignant glioma. Surg Neurol. 2000 May;53[5]:458-64
126. Spitzer G, Dickie KA, Litam Y et al. High-dose combination of chemotherapy with autologous bone marrow transplantation in adult solid tumors. Cancer, 45:3075-3085, 1980
127. Olivero VT, Toxicology and pharmacology of the nitrosoureas. Cancer Chemother rep. 4[3]:13-20, 1973
128. Wheeler GP, A review of studies on the mechanism of action of tne nitrosoureas. In [Sartorelli AC ed.] Cancer Chemotherapy, volume 30, Washingtoon, DC:American Chemical Society.pp87-119, 1976
129. Oliverio VT. Toxicology and pharmacology of the nitrosoureas. Cancer Chemother Rep part 3 4:13-20, 1973
130. De Vita VT, Carbone PP, Owens AH, Gold GL, Krant MJ, and Edmonson J. Clinical trials with 1, 3-bis [2-chloroethyl]-1-nitrosourea, NSC 409962. Cancer Res 25:1876-1881, 1965
131. Bagley CM, Bostick FW, DeVita VT. Clinical pharmacology of cyclophosphamide. Cancer Res. 1973 Feb;33[2]:226-33
132. Goupil A, Baglin A, Clavel B, Verger C, Fritel D. Chronic renal failure after CCNU treatment [author's transl]. Nouv Presse Med. 1980 Nov 1;9[41]:3069-70
133. Harmon WE, Cohen HJ, Schneeberger EE, Grupe WE Chronic renal failure in children treated with methyl CCNU. N Engl J Med. 1979 May 24;300[21]:1200-3
134. Nichols WC, Moertel CG. Nephrotoxicity of methyl CCNU. N Engl J Med. 1979 Nov 22;301[21]:1181
135. Schacht RG, Feiner HD, Gallo GR, Lieberman A, Baldwin DS. Nephrotoxicity of nitrosoureas. Cancer. 1981 Sep 15;48[6]:1328-34
136. Silver HKB, and Morton DL. CCNU nephrotoxicity following sustained remission in oat cell carcinoma. Cancer Trea Rep, 63:226-227, 1979
137. Berglund J, Progressive renal insuffisancy after CCNU therapy. Läkartidningen 77:1760, 1980
138. Schacht RG, Feiner HD, Gallo GR, Liebermann A and Baldwin DS. Nephrotoxicity of Nitrosoureas. Cancer 48:1328-1334, 1981
139. Liegler DG, Henderson ES, Hahn MA and Oliverio VT. 1989. The effect of organic acids on renal clearance of methotrexate on man. Clin Pharmacol Ther. 10.849-857.

140. Patel OD, Morgenthaler FR, Khazei AM, Grimaidi R and Watkins E. 1969. Methetrexate excretion patterns and renal toxicity. Arch Surg 98:305-308.
141. Balis FM, Savich JL, and Bleyer WA. 1983. Pharmacokinetics of oral methotrexate in children. Cancer Res. 43:2342-2345.
142. Shen DD and Azarnoff DL. 1978. Clinical pharmacokinetics of methotrexate. Clin Pharmacokinet. 8:1-18.
143. Breithaupt H and Kuenzlen E. 1982. Pharmacokinetics of methotrexate and 7-hydroxymethotrexate following infusions of high-dose methotrexate. Cancer Treat Rep. 66:1733-1741.
144. Winograd B, Lippens RJJ, Oosterbaan MJM, Dirks MJM, Vree TB and van der Kleijn E. 1986. Renal excretion and pharmacokinetics of methotrexate and 7-hyfroxymethotrexate following a 24 hours high dose infusion of methotrexate in children. Eur J Clin Pharmacol. 30:231-238.
145. Jacobs SA, Stoller RG, Chabner BA, and Johns DG. 1977. Dose-dependent metabolism of methotrexate in man and Rhesus monkey. Cancer Treat Rep, 61:651-658.
146. Pearson ADJ. Mills S, Amineddine HA, Long DR, Craft AW and Chessels JM. 1987. Pharmacokinetics of oral and intramuscular methotrexate in children with acute lymphoblastic leukaemia. Cancer Chemother Pharmacol 20:243-247.
147. Sonneveld P, Schultz FW, Nooter K and Hahlen K. 1986. Pharmacokinetics of methotrexate and 7-hydroxymethotrexate in plasma and bone marrow of children receiving, low-doses oral methotrexate. Cancer Chemother Pharmacol 18:111-118.
148. Rieselbach RF and Garnick MB. 1988. Renal diseases indiced by antineoplastic agents. In Schrier RW, Gottschalk CW. [eds], Diseases of the kidney [Fourth edition], Boston, MA Little Brownand Company.pp 1275-1299.
149. Pittman SW, and Frei E. 1977. Weekly methotrexate-calcium leucovorin rescue: effect of alkalinization on nephrotoxicity; pharmacokinetics in the CNS, and use in CNS non Hodgkin's lymphoma. Cancer Treat Rep. 61:695-701.
150. Glode LM, Pitman SW and Ensminger WD. 1979. A phase I study of high dose of aminopterin with leucoverin rescue in patients with advanced metastatic tumors. Cancer Res. 39:3707-3714.
151. Link DA, Fosberg MT and Ingelfinger JR. 1976. Renal toxicity of high-dose methotrexate. Pediatr Res. 10:455 [abstr].
152. Thyss A, Milano G, Kubar J, Namer M, Schneider M. Clinical and pharmacokinetic evidence of a life-threatening interaction between methotrexate and ketoprofen. Lancet, 1986, I:256-258.
153. Kremer JM and Hamilton RA. The effects of nonsteroidal antiinflammatory drugs on methotrexate [MTX]pharmacokinetics: Impairment of renal clearance of MTX at weekly maintenance doses but not at 7.5 mg. J Rheumatol. 1995. 22:2072-2277.
154. Pitman SW, Parker LM, Tattersall MNH, Jaffe N, Frei E. Clinical trial of high-dose methotrexate with citrovorum factor-toxicologic and therapeutic observations. Cancer Chemother Rep. 1975. 6:43-49.
155. Abelson HT, Fosburg MT, Beardsley GP. Methotrexate-induced renal impairment. J Clin Oncol 1983. 1:208-216.
156. Molina R, Fabian C, Cowley B. Use of charcoal hemoperfusion wih sequential hemodialysis to reduce serum methotrexate levels in a patient with acute renal insufficiency. Am J Med. 1987. 82:350-352.
157. Relling MV, Stapelton BF, Ochs J, Jones DB, Meyer W, Wainer IW, Crom WR, McKay CP and Evans WE. Removal of methotrexate, leucoverin and their metabolites by combined hemodialysis and hemoperfusion. Cancer, 62.884-888, 1988.
158. Remuzzi G, Galbusera M, Salvadori M, et al. Bilateral nephrectomy stopped disease progression in plasma-resistant hemolytic uremic syndrome with neurological signs and coma. Kidney Int 49: 282-6, 1996.
159. Flombaum CD, Mouradian JA, Casper ES, et al. Thrombotic microangiopathy as a complication of long-term therapy with gemcitabine. Am J Kidney Dis 33: 555-62, 1999.
160. Fung MC, Storniolo AM, Nguyen B, et al. A review of hemolytic uremic syndrome in patients treated with gemcitabine therapy. Cancer 85: 2023-32, 1999.
161. Sheldon R, Slaughter D. A syndrome of microangiopathic hemolytic anemia, renal impairment, and pulmonary edema in chemotherapy-treated patients with adenocarcinoma. Cancer 58: 1428-36, 1986.
162. Humphreys BD, Soiffer RJ, Magee CC. Renal failure associated with cancer and its treatment: an update. J Am Soc Nephrol 16: 151-61, 2005.
163. Flombaum CD. Gemcitabine Nephrotoxicity and the Hemolytic Uremic Syndrome (HUS): Report of 29 Cases from a Single Institution. J Am Soc Nephrol, 2005, 777°. Poster SA-PO1008.
164. Gordon LI, Kwaan HC. Cancer- and drug-associated thrombotic thrombocytopenic purpura and hemolytic uremic syndrome. Semin Hematol 34: 140-7, 1997.
165. Murgo AJ. Thrombotic microangiopathy in the cancer patient including those induced by chemotherapeutic agents. Semin Hematol 24: 161-77, 1987.
166. Monteagudo J, Pereira A, Roig S, et al. Investigation of plasma von Willebrand factor and circulating platelet aggregating activity in mitomycin C-related hemolytic-uremic syndrome. Am J Hematol 33: 46-9, 1990.
167. Zeigler ZR, Rosenfeld CS, Andrews DF 3rd, et al. Plasma von Willebrand Factor Antigen (vWF:AG) and thrombomodulin (TM) levels in Adult Thrombotic Thrombocytopenic Purpura/Hemolytic Uremic Syndromes (TTP/HUS) and bone marrow transplant-associated thrombotic microangiopathy (BMT-TM). Am J Hematol 53: 213-20, 1996.

168. Hollenbeck M, Kutkuhn B, Aul C, et al. Haemolytic-uraemic syndrome and thrombotic-thrombocytopenic purpura in adults: clinical findings and prognostic factors for death and end-stage renal disease. Nephrol Dial Transplant 13: 76-81, 1998.
169. Sens YA, Miorin LA, Silva HG, et al. Acute renal failure due to hemolytic uremic syndrome in adult patients. Ren Fail 19: 279-82, 1997.
170. Mergenthaler HG, Binsack T, Wilmanns W. Carcinoma-associated hemolytic-uremic syndrome in a patient receiving 5-fluorouracil-adriamycin-mitomycin C combination chemotherapy. Oncology 45: 11-4, 1988.
171. van Hazel GA, Scott M, Rubin J, Moertel CG, Eagan RT, O'Connell MJ and Kovach JS. Pharmacokinetics of mitomycin C in patients receiving the drug alone or in combination. Cancer Treat Rep, 67:805-810, 1982
172. Schilder RB, Young JD, Ratanatharathorn V, Karanes C and Baker LH. Clinical pharmacokinetics of high-dose mitomycin C. Cancer Chemother Pharmacol, 13:186-190, 1984
173. Erlichman C, Rauth AM, Battistella R and Fine S. Mitomycin C pharmacokinetics in patients with recurrent or metastatic colorectal carcinoma. Can J Physiol Pharmacol, 65:407-411, 1987
174. Lelesne JB, Rothschild N, Erickson B, Koreu S, Sisk R, Keller J, Arbus M, Wooley P, Chiazze L, Schein PS, and Neefe JR. Cancer-associated hemolytic-uremic syndrome: analysis of 85 cases from the national registry. J Clin Oncol, 7:781-789, 1989
175. Cantrell JE, Phillips TM, and Schein PS. Carcinoma-associated hemolytic-uremic syndrome: a complication of mitomycin chemotherapy. J Clin Oncol, 3:723-734, 1985
176. Hanna WT, Krauss S, Regester RF and Murphy WM. Renal disease after Mitomycin C therapy. Cancer, 48:2583-2588, 1981
177. Gulati SC, Sordillo P, Kempin S, Reich L, Magill GB, Scheiner E and Clarkson B. Microangiopathic hemolytic anemia observed after treatment of epidermoid carcinoma with mitomycin C and 5-fluorouracil. Cancer, 45:2252-2257, 1980
178. Bayle F, Vialtel P, Bastrenta F, Swiercz P, Dechelette E, Pin I, Carpentier P, Mousseau M, Schaerer R, Couderc P, Cordonnier D. [Thrombotic microangiopathy and chronic renal failure caused by mitomycin C in 4 women treated for breast cancer]. Nouv Presse Med. 1982 Jun 26;11[30]:2300-1
179. Hanna WT, Krauss S, Rolland FR, Murphy WM. Renal disease after mitomycin C therapy. Cancer, 1981, 48:2583-88.
180. LiuK, Mittelmann A, Sproul RR, and Elias EG. Renal toxicity in man treated with mitomycin C Cancer, 28:1314-1320, 1971
181. Lyman NW, Michaelson R, Viscuso RL, Winn R, Mulgaonakar S, Jacobs MG. Mitomycin-induced hemolytic-uremic syndrome. Successful treatment with corticosteroids and intense plasma Arch Intern Med. 1983 Aug;143[8]:1617-8.
182. Jackson AM, Rose BD, Graff LG, Jacobs JB, Schwartz JH, Strauss GM, Yang JP, Rudnick MR, Elfenbein IB, Narins RG. Thrombotic microangiopathy and renal failure associated with antineoplastic chemotherapy. Ann Intern Med. 1984 Jul;101[1]:41-4.
183. Rosenberg SA, Lotze MT, Muul LM, Leitman S, Chang AE, Ettinghause SE, Matory YL, Skibber JM, Shiloni E, Vetto JT, Seipp CA, Simpson CG, Reichert CM: Observations on the systemic administration of autologous lymphokine-activated killer cells and recombinant interleukin-2 to patients with metastatic cancer. N Eng J Med, 1985, 313:1485-1491.
184. Law TM, Motzer RJ, Gluck L et al. Phase III randomized trial of interleukine-2 with or without lymphokine activated killer cells in the treatment of patients with advanced renal cell carcinoma. Cancer, 1995, 76: 824-832.
185. Rozenberg SA, Lotze MT et al. A progress report on the treatment of 157 patients with advanced cancer using lymphokine activated killer cells and interleukine 2 or high dose interleukine 2 alone. N ehg J Med. 1987, 316, 889-897.
186. Thompson JA, Shulman KL, Benyunes MC, Lindgren CG, Collins C, Lange PH, Bush WH Jr, Benz LA, Fefer A. Prolonged continuous intravenous infusion interleukin-2 and lymphokine activated killer cell therapy for metastatic renal cell carcinoma. J Clin Oncol 1992, 10:960-968.
187. Guleria AS, Yang JC, Topalian SL, et al. Renal dysfunction associated with the administration of high-dose interleukin-2 in 199 consecutive patients with metastatic melanoma or renal cell carcinoma. J Clin Oncol. 1994, 12:2714-2722.
188. Webb DE, Austin HA, Belldegrun A, Vaughan E, Linehan WM, Rosenberg SA. Metabolic and renal effects of Interleukin-2 immunotherapy for metastatic cancer. Clin Nephrol. 1988, 30 [3]:141-145.
189. Philip T, Mercatello A, Negrier S, Philip I, Rebattu P, Kaemmerlin P, Gaspard M, Tognier E, Combaret V, Bijman JT, et al. Interleukine-2 with and without LAK cells in renal cell carcinoma: the Lyon first-year experience with 20 patients. Cancer Treat Rev. 1989, 13 [suppA]:91-104.
190. Rosenstein M, Ettinghausen SE, Rosenberg SA: Extravasation of intravascular fluid wediated by the systemic administration of recombinant interleukin-2. J Immunol. 1986, 137:1735-1742.
191. Ponce P, Cruz J, Travassos J, Moreira P, Oliveira J, Melo-Gomes E, Gouveia J. Renal toxicity mediated by continuous infusion of recombinant interleukin-2. Nephron, 1993, 64[1]:114-118.
192. Feinfeld DA, D'Agati Y, Dutcher JP, Werfel SB, Lynn RI, Wiernik PH. Interstitial nephritis in a patient receiving adoptive immunotherapy with recombinant interleukin-2 and lymphokine-activated killer cells. Am J Nephrol. 1991, 11[6], 489-492.
193. Valsveld LT, van de Wiel-van Kamenade E, de Boer AJ, Sein JJ, Galle MP, Krediet RT, Mellief CJ, Rankin EM, Hekman A, Figdor CG. Possible role for cytotoxic lymphocytes in the pathogenesis of acute intertitial nephritis after recombinant interleukin-2 treatment for renal cell cancer. Cancer Immunol Immunother. 1993, 36[3]:210-213.

194. Shalmi CL, Dutcher JP, Feinfeld DA, Chun KJ, Saleemi KR, Freeman LM, Lynn RI, and Wiernik PH. Acute renal dysfunction during interleukin-2 treatment: suggestion of an intrinsic renal lesion. J Clin Oncol, 1990, 8[11]: 1839-1846.
195. Wills RJ, Clinical pharmacokinetics of interferons. Clin Pharmacokinet, 1990, 19:390-399.
196. Grimbert P, Deray G, Lebon P, Faucher C, Malingre P, Raymond F, Petitclerc T, and Jacobs C. Pharmacokinetics of recombinant leukocyte interferon in a patient on continuous ambulatory peritoneal dialysis. Am J Nephrol, 1995, 15:175(2).
197. Rostaing L, Chatelut E, Payen JL, Izopet J, Thalamas C, Ton-That H, Pascal JP, Durand D, and Canal P. Pharmacokinetics of alpha IFN-2b in chronic hepatitis C virus patients undergoing hemodialysis or with normal renal function. Clinical implications. J Am Soc Nephrol. 1998, 9:2344-2348.
198. Bocci V, Pacini A, Muscettola M, Paulesu L, Pessina GP, santiano M, Viano AI. Renal filtration, absorption and catabolism of human alpha interferon. J Interferon Res, 1981, 3: 347-352
199. Bailly F, Mattei A, SiAhmed SN, Trepo C. Uncommon side-effects of interferon. J Viral Hep, 1997, 4 [suppl 1]: 89-94.
200. Gresser I, Maury M, Tovey M, Morel Maroger L, Pontillon F. Progressive glomerulonephritis in mice treated with interferon preparation at birth. Nature. 1976. 263:420-422.
201. Morel-Maroger L, Sloper JC, Vinter J, Woodrow D, Gresser I. An ultrastructural study of the development of nephritis in mice treated with interferon in the neonatal period. Lab Invest. 1978 Nov;39(5):513-22.
202. Quesada J et al. Clinical toxicity of interferons in cancer patients: a review. J Clin Oncol. 1986, 4:234.
203. Quesada JR, Talpaz M, Rios A, Kurzrock R, Gutterman JU. Clinical toxicity of interferons in cancer patients: a review. J Clin Oncol. 1986 4(2):234-43.
204. Miranda-Guardiola F, Fdez-Llama P, Badia J, Botey A, Estruch R, Darnell A, Rozman C and Revert L. Acute renal failure associated with alpha-interferon therapy for chronic hepatitis B. Nephrol. Dial Transplant, 1995, 10:1441-1443.
205. Nair S, Ernstoff M, Bahnson R, Arthur S, Johnston J, Downs M, Neuhart J, and Kirkwood J. Interferon-induced reversible acute renal failure with nephrotic syndrome. Urology, 1992, 39 2), 169-172.
206. Averbuch SD, Austin HA, Sherwin SA, Antonovych T, Bunn PA, Longo DL. Acute interstitial nephritis with the nephrotic syndrome following recombinant leukocyte a interferon therapy for mycosis fungoides. N Engl J Med. 1984 5;310(1):32-5.
207. Kurschel E, Metz-Kurschel U, Niederle N, Aulbert E. Investigations on the subclinical and clinical nephrotoxicity of interferon alpha IIB in patients with myeloproliferative syndromes. Renal Failure, 91:13:87-93.
208. Hurwitz H, Fehrenbacher L, Novotny W, Cartwright T, Hainsworth J, Heim W, Berlin J, Baron A, Griffing S, Holmgren E, Ferrara N, Fyfe G, Rogers B, Ross R, Kabbinavar F.. Bevacizumab plus irinotecan, fluorouracil, and leucovorin for metastatic colorectal cancer. N Engl J Med. 2004; 350: 2335-42
209. Kabbinavar, F, Hurwitz, HI, Fehrenbacher, L. Phase II, randomized trial comparing bevacizumab plus fluorouracil (FU)/leucovorin (LV) with FU/LV alone in patients with metastatic colorectal cancer. J Clin Oncol, 21:60-5, 2003
210. Genentech: Avastin. labeling Text, FDA Approval Date: September 2005
211. Levine, RJ, Maynard, SE, Qian, C. Circulating angiogenic factors and the risk of preeclampsia. N Engl J Med, 350:672-83, 2004
212. Simon, M, Grone, HJ, Johren, O. Expression of vascular endothelial growth factor and its receptors in human renal ontogenesis and in adult kidney. Am J Physiol, 268:F240-50, 1995.
213. Kincaid-Smith P. The renal lesion of preeclampsia revisited. Am J Kidney Dis. 1991 Feb;17(2):144-8.
214. Eremina, V, Sood, M, Haigh, J. Glomerular-specific alterations of VEGF-A expression lead to distinct congenital and acquired renal diseases. J Clin Invest, 111:707-16, 2003.
215. Mathieson, PW: How much VEGF do you need? J Am Soc Nephrol, 17:602-3, 2006.
216. Miller, KD, Chap, LI, Holmes, FA. Randomized phase III trial of capecitabine compared with bevacizumab plus capecitabine in patients with previously treated metastatic breast cancer. J Clin Oncol, 23:792-9, 2005.
217. Markowitz, GS, Appel, GB, Fine, PL. Collapsing focal segmental glomerulosclerosis following treatment with high-dose pamidronate. J Am Soc Nephrol, 12:1164-72, 2001.
218. Johnson, DH, Fehrenbacher, L, Novotny, WF. Randomized phase II trial comparing bevacizumab plus carboplatin and paclitaxel with carboplatin and paclitaxel alone in previously untreated locally advanced or metastatic non-small cell lung cancer. J Clin Oncol, 22:2184-91, 2004.
219. Motzer RJ, Michaelson MD, Redman BG, Hudes GR, Wilding G, Figlin RA, Ginsberg MS, Kim ST, Baum CM, DePrimo SE, Li JZ, Bello CL, Theuer CP, George DJ, Rini BI. Activity of SU11248, a multitargeted inhibitor of vascular endothelial growth factor receptor and platelet-derived growth factor receptor, in patients with metastatic renal cell carcinoma. J Clin Oncol. 2006 Jan 1;24(1):16-24.
220. Veronese ML, Mosenkis A, Flaherty KT, Gallagher M, Stevenson JP, Townsend RR, O'Dwyer PJ. Mechanisms of hypertension associated with BAY 43-9006. J Clin Oncol. 2006 Mar 20;24(9):1363-9.
221. Rini B, Rixe O, Bukowski R, et al. (2005) AG-013736, a multitarget tyrosine kinase receptor inhibitor, demonstrates anti-tumor activity in a phase 2 study of cytokine-refractory, metastatic renal cell cancer (RCC). ASCO Proc (abstract 4509).

222. Nguyen QD, Shah SM, Hafiz G, Quinlan E, Sung J, Chu K, Cedarbaum JM, Campochiaro PA; CLEAR-AMD 1 Study Group. A phase I trial of an IV-administered vascular endothelial growth factor trap for treatment in patients with choroidal neovascularization due to age-related macular degeneration. Ophthalmology. 2006 Sep;113(9):1522.e1-1522.e14.
223. Motzer RJ, Rini BI, Bukowski RM, Curti BD, George DJ, Hudes GR, Redman BG, Margolin KA, Merchan JR, Wilding G, Ginsberg MS, Bacik J, Kim ST, Baum CM, Michaelson MD. Sunitinib in patients with metastatic renal cell carcinoma. JAMA. 2006 Jun 7;295(21):2516-24.
224. Ratain MJ, Eisen T, Stadler WM, Flaherty KT, Kaye SB, Rosner GL, Gore M, Desai AA, Patnaik A, Xiong HQ, Rowinsky E, Abbruzzese JL, Xia C, Simantov R, Schwartz B, O'Dwyer PJ. Phase II placebo-controlled randomized discontinuation trial of sorafenib in patients with metastatic renal cell carcinoma. J Clin Oncol. 2006 Jun 1;24(16):2505-12.
225. Faivre S, Delbaldo C, Vera K, Robert C, Lozahic S, Lassau N, Bello C, Deprimo S, Brega N, Massimini G, Armand JP, Scigalla P, Raymond E. Safety, pharmacokinetic, and antitumor activity of SU11248, a novel oral multitarget tyrosine kinase inhibitor, in patients with cancer. J Clin Oncol. 2006 Jan 1;24(1):25-35.
226. Yang, R, Thomas, GR, Bunting, S. Effects of vascular endothelial growth factor on hemodynamics and cardiac performance. J Cardiovasc Pharmacol, 27:838-44, 1996.
227. Neagoe, PE, Lemieux, C ? Sirois, MG. Vascular endothelial growth factor (VEGF)-A165-induced prostacyclin synthesis requires the activation of VEGF receptor-1 and -2 heterodimer. J Biol Chem, 280:9904-12, 2005.
228. Henry, TD, Annex, BH, McKendall, GR. The VIVA trial. Vascular endothelial growth factor in Ischemia for Vascular Angiogenesis. Circulation, 107:1359-65, 2003.
229. Chen, S, Lee, JS, Iglesias-de la Cruz, MC. Angiotensin II stimulates alpha3 (IV) collagen production in mouse podocytes via TGF-beta and VEGF signalling: implications for diabetic glomerulopathy. Nephrol Dial Transplant, 20:1320-8, 2005.
230. Mares, JE, Worah, S, Mathew, SV. Increased rates of hypertension (HTN) among patients with advanced carcinoid treated with bevacizumab. the 41st Annual Meeting of the American Society of Clinical Oncology (ASCO).Abstract No: 4087, 2005.
231. Ginsberg, JM, Chang, BS, Matarese, RA. Use of single voided urine samples to estimate quantitative proteinuria. N Engl J Med, 309:1543-6, 1983.
232. Cohen E. Radiation nephropathy after bone marrow transplantation. Kidney International, 2000, 58:903-918.
233. Redd BL. Radiation nephritis: review, case report and animal study. Roentgenol. 1960, 83:88.
234. Phillips TL, Wharam MD, Margolis LW. Modification of radiation injury to normal tissues by chemotherapeutic agents. Cancer, 1975, 35:1678-1684.
235. Kelly CJ and Neilson EG. Intertitial diseases. In Brenner & Rector's, Ed by Barry B. Brenner, WB Saunders Company, Phildelphia, 1655-1679, Vth edition, 1996.
236. Jaenke RS, Robbins MEC, Bywaters T, Whitehouse E, Rezvani M, Hopewell JW. Capillary endothelium: target site of renal radiation injury. Lab Invest 1993, 68:396-405.
237. Rubin P, Casarett GW. Clinical Radiation pathology. Philadelphia, Saunders, 1968, pp 293-333.
238. Robbins MEC, Hopewell JW: Physiological factors effecting renal radiation tolerance: A guide to the treatment of late effects. Br J Cancer, 1986, 53:265-267.
239. Cohen EP, Fish BL, Moulder JE: Treatment of radiation nephropathy with captopril. Radiat Res. 1992, 132: 346-350.

23

Anesthetic agents

Per-Olof JARNBERG

Oregon Health & Science University, Portland, Oregon, USA

Introduction

Renal function impairment remains a common event in connection with anesthesia and surgery. Severe perioperative renal dysfunction (SCr > 6 mg/dL, CrCl ≤ 15 ml/min) accounts for one half of all patients requiring acute dialysis [1] and is associated with a mortality in excess of 50% [2]. Mild to moderate renal function impairment is surprisingly common after surgery. In a group of 278 patients undergoing non-emergency general, vascular, or gynecological surgery, 65 of the patients developed an increase in serum creatinine levels ≥ 20% within the first six postoperative days [3]. Thirty-two patients had increases that were sustained for more than 48 hours. For half of these patients, creatinine clearance had not returned to baseline levels by the time of discharge.

In most cases, the perioperative changes in renal function are not due to the anesthetic agent itself, although some volatile anesthetics have nephrotoxic potential due to direct toxicity of their metabolites. Instead, postoperative renal failure is more commonly multifactorial. Risk factors include: 1) preexisting renal or cardiac disease, 2) the type of surgical procedure, 3) occurrence of rhabdomyolysis or hemolysis, 4) adverse hemodynamic events, 5) inappropriate fluid management, and 6) concurrent administration of potentially nephrotoxic substances such as radiographic contrast agents, aminoglycoside antibiotics, and cyclosporine. Such risk factors usually play a more important role than the anesthetic agent in the development of postoperative renal dysfunction [4].

Comparative renal pharmacology of inhaled and injectable anesthetic agents

Inhaled anesthetic agents

Since Pringle et al. described oliguria during ether anesthesia in 1905, many investigators have focused on the effects of anesthesia on renal function [5]. All general anesthetics have significant but reversible effects on renal function. These effects are mediated directly by changes in renal vascular resistance, renal blood flow, glomerular filtration rate, and renal tubular function, or indirectly by changes in cardiovascular function and neuroendocrine activity.

Modern inhaled anesthetic agents - halothane, enflurane, isoflurane, desflurane, and sevoflurane - decrease glomerular filtration rate, sodium excretion, and urine output [6-10]. Studies of the response of renal blood flow to these agents have yielded conflicting results. Initially, investigators using clearance techniques concluded that halothane and enflurane reduce renal blood flow [9, 10]. In later studies, direct measurement techniques indicated that clinical doses of inhaled agents decrease renal vascular resistance thus maintaining renal blood flow when perfusion pressure decreases during anesthesia [11-15]. These changes are transient and usually return to normal in the immediate postoperative period. In one study, even prolonged hypotension to a mean arterial pressure of 60 mm Hg induced with isoflurane was not associated with persistent derangement of renal function postoperatively [16].

Injectable anesthetic agents

Sodium thiopental does not alter renal blood flow although glomerular filtration rate and urine output are moderately affected [17]. The same is true for opioids such as morphine [18] and fentanyl [19, 20] and the more recently introduced I.V. agent propofol [21]. The effects of these drugs on renal function are transient. There is no evidence that injectable anesthetic agents are associated with direct nephrotoxicity.

In addition to the effects of anesthetic agents themselves, other intraoperative interventions may also influence renal function. The initiation of mechanical ventilation, especially with the application of positive end-expiratory pressure, is associated with decreases in sodium excretion and urine output [22-24]. Decreased cardiac output, increased sympathetic outflow and release of renin and decreased release of atrial natriuretic peptide have all been implicated as being responsible for these changes [25, 26].

In summary, virtually all anesthetic agents and techniques are associated with reductions in glomerular filtration rate and urine output. These changes are usually readily reversed in the immediate postoperative period and represent the net effect of complex interactions between direct actions of the anesthetics on the kidney and indirect changes in cardiac output, blood pressure, and neuroendocrine function.

Metabolism of inhaled anesthetic agents

Toxic effects of biodegradation products from anesthetic agents may also directly influence renal function. On rare occasions renal failure will result.

Modern inhalation anesthetics are fluorinated to reduce flammability. Initially, these inhaled agents were believed to be biochemically inert. Over the past 30 years, however, research findings have demonstrated that not only are inhaled anesthetics metabolized *in vivo* [27], but their metabolites are also responsible for both acute and chronic toxicities [28, 29]. Therefore, the use of some anesthetics has been discontinued, including methoxyflurane because of its nephrotoxicity; and other anesthetics are more selectively used, e.g. halothane due to a rare incidence of liver toxicity. Studies have also provided the impetus to develop new agents - isoflurane and desflurane - with properties that lower their toxic potential. The result has been improved safety, but there is room for further improvement as our insight into toxicological mechanisms expands.

Metabolism of inhaled anesthetics usually begins with oxidation and is carried out by cytochrome P-450 enzymes located in the microsomes of the liver and the kidneys [30, 31]. Under certain circumstances, some agents, such as halothane, might also undergo reduction. In addition to their primary metabolism, some anesthetics, sevoflurane for instance, also undergo phase II conjugation reactions prior to excretion.

The cytochrome P-450 enzyme system is comprised of multiple isoenzymes that are inducible to varying degrees [32]. These two characteristics are major determinants of metabolic pathways and rates. Induction can be caused by exposure to one or more of a large variety of compounds, including ethanol, phenobarbital, cimetidine, phenytoin, isoniazid, and some volatile anesthetics. Both transcriptional and translational processes are stimulated by the inducer to produce cytochrome P-450 [33, 34]. Expression of the various isoenzymes depends not only on induction, but also on such factors as sex, obesity, fasting, and diabetes. For example in Streptozotocin- induced diabetes in rats, P-4502E increases several fold, causing an enhanceds enflurane and isoflurane metabolism [35].

Most halogenated anesthetics are similar in composition; however, they vary greatly in their rate and pathway of metabolism. Minor alterations in configuration can be associated with major changes in metabolism. Also, their degree of lipid solubility, which governs the drug's access to and duration at metabolizing enzyme sites, is important in determining metabolic rate and the amount of drug that is biotransformed.

Halothane

Halothane ($CF_3CHBrCl$), the first of the modern halogenated volatile anesthetics, was introduced into clinical practice in 1956. It is normally metabolized in an oxidative pathway forming bromide ions and trifluoroacetic acid, neither of which has potential for tissue toxicity [36, 37]. Reductive metabolism of halothane takes place during low oxygen tension states in the liver [38]. This pathway has been linked to halothane-induced liver necrosis through production of free radicals that bind to cellular macromolecules [39, 40]. Reductive metabolism is also associated with production of fluoride ions [41], although the quantities produced are too small to have nephrotoxic importance.

The extent of halothane metabolism has been reported to be 17-20% of an administered dose [36]. Oxidation to trifluoroacetic acid is the principal pathway of halothane metabolism, and no fluoride ions are released. Therefore, fluoride-induced renal toxicity is not a concern with halothane.

Enflurane

Enflurane (CHF_2OF_2CHClF) has been in clinical use for the last three decades. It is metabolized to a much lesser degree than halothane. Approximately 2-3% of a given dose undergoes biodegradation [42, 43]. Although the chief metabolite is difluoromethoxy-difluoroacetic acid, fluoride ions are also released in sufficient quantity to merit some concern about renal function [44]. Plasma inorganic fluoride concentrations after clinical enflurane anesthesia are usually in the 15-25 µM range [8, 9, 44]. Longer procedures [45] and obesity [46] are associated with higher postanesthetic fluoride levels. A study of surgical patients with pre-anesthetic chronic consumption of enzyme-inducing drugs such as phenobarbital, phenytoin, diazepam, and ethanol did not reveal increased plasma fluoride levels compared to untreated patients [47]. In contrast, about 50% of surgical patients on chronic isoniazid therapy demonstrated significantly elevated plasma fluoride concentrations after enflurane anesthesia [48]. Enflurane is the only modern inhaled anesthetic that may be linked to fluoride-induced renal failure in a very limited number of cases [49, 50], but this has not yet been proven.

Isoflurane

Isoflurane ($CHF_2OCH_2ClCF_3$) is an isomer of enflurane and has been in clinical use for about twenty years. It has a very low degree of defluorination [51]. Approximately 0.2-0.4% of a given dose is metabolized. Fluoride levels in humans after isoflurane anesthesia peak at 4-6 µM, which represents only a modest rise over basal fluoride levels. Although enzyme induction increases defluorination somewhat, it is not associated with plasma fluoride concentrations of clinical significance [52, 53].

Sevoflurane

Sevoflurane [$(CF_3)_2CHOCH_2F$] was first used in Japan and introduced into American clinical practice in 1995. Sevoflurane is defluorinated to approximately the same extent as enflurane. In fact, initial studies reported that plasma levels of fluoride associated with sevoflurane anesthesia are comparable to those seen after enflurane administration [54, 55]. More recent studies, however, report that plasma fluoride concentrations often rise above 50 mM [56, 57]. Due to sevoflurane's low blood/gas solubility, only limited quantities build up during anesthesia; and, as a result, fluoride levels fall very quickly after termination of anesthesia. *In vivo*, defluorination in rats is increased by pretreatment with phenobarbital [58].

Numerous studies have addressed the same issues raised with enflurane regarding fluoride production and nephrotoxic potential including fluoride levels after prolonged exposure [56, 57, 59], urine concentrating ability [57, 59-61], the effect of obesity [57, 60], and the effect of preexisting renal function impairment [62, 63]. The findings demonstrated that sevoflurane has little or no potential for fluoride-induced nephrotoxicity (For further information see section on mechanisms of fluoride toxicity).

Sevoflurane undergoes degradation in the presence of soda lime and barium hydroxide lime, both of which are used in modern anesthesia machines for CO_2 absorption. The chief degradation product is fluoromethyl-2,2-difluoro-1(trifluoromethyl)-vinyl ether, also called compound A [64]. In an anesthesia circle circuit using the above absorbents, compound A concentrations correlate directly with sevoflurane concentrations and absorbent temperature, and inversely with the inflow rate of fresh gas [65]. Increasing inflow rates reduces compound A concentrations by decreasing the rebreathing of gas that has passed through the absorbent, thereby decreasing the amount of CO_2 that reaches the absorbent. The amount of CO_2 absorbed determines the temperature of the absorbent, since CO_2 absorption is an exothermic reaction [65, 66].

Compound A is nephrotoxic in rats at thresholds estimated at 180 ppm/hour [67]. Renal toxicity is characterized histologically by proximal tubular cell degeneration and necrosis in the corticomedullar region of the kidney and biochemically by proteinuria, glucosuria, and enzymuria (NAG and α-GST) with increased serum creatinine and BUN concentrations occurring with severe toxicity [67-70].

In humans, there seems to be a dose-dependent association between compound A exposure and the appearance of urinary biomarkers such as albumin, glucose, and the enzymes NAG or α-GST. These findings appear in studies when the compound A exposure exceeds 160 ppm/hour [71-74], while they are absent in studies with lower compound A exposure [75-77]. In all studies associated with higher exposure of compound A, the urinary markers are transient, lasting 3-5 days with total normalization within one week. There is no correlation between serum creatinine and the urinary markers.

In summary, the available information indicates that sevoflurane anesthesia is nontoxic to the kidney as long as exposure to compound A is kept below 150 ppm/hour. However, there are significant questions regarding the potential for compound A to cause renal injury: Are larger doses than 160 ppm/hour harmful? Do they cause histologically detectable tissue damage? Is there a cumulative effect of repeated exposures? Are particular patients more prone to injury?

The concerns and questions surrounding the degradation of sevoflurane by CO_2 absorbents to toxic compounds would disappear if the use of absorbents that minimally degrade sevoflurane became standard [78-80]. Such absorbents exist, and they do not contain sodium or potassium hydroxide. An example is Amsorb® (Armstong Medica Ltd., Coleraine, Northern Ireland). It is completely inert when brought into contact with sevoflurane [81]. This absorbent is widely used in Europe and is commercially available in the US. Medisorb®, Spherasorb®, Loflosorb®, and Superia® are other examples of CO_2 absorbents which produce little or no sevoflurane degradation. [81a].

Desflurane

Desflurane ($CHF_2OCHFCF_3$) has been in clinical use in the US for more than a decade. It has very low lipid solubility [82] and is highly resistant to metabolism and to degradation in soda lime [83]. Data from studies in rats and humans suggest that desflurane is not toxic to the liver or kidney [84-86]. Serum inorganic fluoride concentrations do not rise above background levels even after prolonged exposure [87, 88]. Since desflurane has a boiling point of 23.5°C, it requires a special vaporizer to ensure a stable output.

Mechanisms of fluoride toxicity

For more than forty years, the potential for nephrotoxicity, particularly when fluoride induced, has influenced every aspect of the development of new inhaled anesthetics. This concern is based on the experience with methoxyflurane, which was introduced in the US in 1960 [89]. The exact mechanism(s) responsible for fluoride nephrotoxicity have not been defined. The fluoride ion interferes with normal cell function on several levels. Fluoride inhibits several cellular enzyme systems and diminishes tissue respiration and anaerobic glycolysis [90]. The lethal dose of sodium fluoride in humans is approximately 5 g [90]. In the kidney, fluoride interferes with the transport of sodium in the proximal convoluted tubule. It also inhibits adenylate cyclase in the collecting tubules and diminishes the action of antidiuretic hormone. Experimental evidence in rats indicates that the chloride-dependent pump in the thick ascending part of Henle's loop is also inhibited [91]. In cultures of human collecting duct cells, exposure to fluoride ions inhibits Na-K-ATPase and causes morphologic changes in mitochondria [92].

In 1966, renal failure was reported in 13 of 41 patients receiving methoxyflurane anesthesia for abdominal surgery [93]. The cause was later associated with methoxyflurane metabolism and increased plasma fluoride levels [94]. Methoxyflurane undergoes oxidative metabolism by cytochrome P450, and inorganic fluoride ions are released [95]. The clinical manifestations of this process consist of vasopressin-resistant polyuria, hypernatremia, hyperosmolality, and azotemia. The degree of nephrotoxicity is positively correlated with plasma fluoride levels. Subclinical toxicity occurs at fluoride levels of 50-80 μM, while fluoride concentrations of 90-120 μM are associated with established renal failure that becomes severe when levels reach 150-175 μM [96]. When animals are injected with inorganic fluoride, the changes in renal function are similar to those seen after the administration of methoxyflurane. The dose of sodium fluoride required to cause nephrotoxicity, however, results in much higher fluoride levels (>400 μM) than those seen after methoxyflurane anesthesia [97, 98]. Despite this observation, the conclusion was drawn that nephrotoxicity from methoxyflurane must be caused by metabolically-released inorganic fluoride ions. This hypothesis was subsequently generalized to include all fluoride-containing volatile anesthetics, and 50 μM of fluoride was considered the nephrotoxic threshold. Plasma fluoride levels exceeding 50 μM or even 100 μM following administration of sevoflurane are not associated with renal damage. This lack of correlation between peak serum fluoride levels and nephrotoxicity led one investigator to suggest that intrarenal production of fluoride is more important in the etiology of nephrotoxicity than the blood levels resulting from hepatic production of fluoride [99]. Indeed, during the last decade, we have learned that hepatic defluorination and blood transport of fluoride to the kidney is not the mechanism responsible for volatile anesthetic nephrotoxicity and that neither plasma fluoride concentrations greater than 50 μM nor the duration of fluoride increase have implications for renal toxicity [99-101].

Based on the seminal work of Evan Kharasch, it now seems clear that nephrotoxicity of inhaled anesthetics is agent-specific (methoxyflurane) and caused by an organic methoxyflurane metabolite in combination with fluoride, rather than by metabolic fluoride generation alone [102, 103]. Methoxyflurane is metabolized by two different pathways [95, 104]. Oxidative dechlorination of the chloromethyl carbon produces 2,2-difluoro-2-methoxyacetic acid (MDFA). Oxidative O-demethylation of the methoxy group results in formation of fluoride and dichloroacetic acid (DCAA). Experiments in rats revealed no functional or histologic signs of nephrotoxicity when either MDFA or DCAA was administered intraperitoneally. Fluoride in combination with DCAA, but not with MDFA, resulted in significant dose-dependent histologic (necrosis) and functional renal injury [103]. Fluoride administered alone in varying doses resulting in a total 4-day urine recovery of fluoride equal or greater than that after methoxyflurane anesthesia caused reduced urine osmolality and significant diuresis at the highest dose [103]. These findings may explain why increased fluoride formation from methoxyflurane, but not other anesthetics, is associated with nephrotoxicity and may have implications for the importance of volatile anesthetic defluorination, future development of inhaled anesthetic agents, and the laboratory methods used to evaluate potential toxicity.

Fluoride elimination

Fluoride is removed from plasma by urinary excretion [105] and uptake into calcified tissues [106]. Normally, each mechanism represents about 50% of the removal [107]. Renal fluoride excretion begins with-glomerular filtration which is followed by variable tubular reabsorption. The tubular reabsorption is influenced by tubular fluid flow rate [108] and urinary pH [109, 110]. Manipulation of urinary pH in patients undergoing a standard enflurane anesthetic resulted in plasma fluoride levels that were 50% lower in patients with alkaline urine than in patients with acidic urine [111].

Bone uptake may also influence plasma fluoride concentrations. Studies in rats have demonstrated that metabolic acidosis increases the rate of bone resorption while metabolic alkalosis increases the rate of osseous accretion [112].

Considerations in pediatric patients

Renal function is markedly diminished in neonates because of low perfusion pressure and immature glomerular and tubular function. Nearly complete maturation of glomerular filtration and tubular function occurs by approximately 20 weeks after birth in term infants but is delayed in premature infants. Complete maturation of renal function occurs by approximately two years of age [113, 114]. The ability to excrete potentially nephrotoxic degradation products associated with anesthesia may, therefore, be impaired in neonates and small children.

Halothane and sevoflurane are commonly used for inhaled induction of anesthesia in children because they do not have a noxious smell. These drugs and isoflurane or desflurane are then used to maintain anesthesia, according to the preference of the anesthesiologist. Enflurane is rarely used today because it irritates the airway [115]. Therefore, of the inhaled agents currently used in pediatric patients, only sevoflurane has nephrotoxic potential.

In two studies of children undergoing sevoflurane anesthesia, mean plasma fluoride levels were 15.8 μM and 21.5 μM in ages 1-12 years and 3 months-7 years, respectively [116, 117]. The latter study also reported on compound A levels in the breathing system. Maximum inspired concentration was 5.4 ± 4.4 ppm (mean ± SD), and maximum expired concentration was 3.7 ± 2.7 ppm. There were no changes in serum creatinine values from samples obtained 24 hours postanesthesia compared with the control. These limited studies give no reason for concern about an increased risk for nephrotoxicity from sevoflurane in the pediatric population.

Clinical implications

Sevoflurane is the only volatile anesthetic that has nephrotoxic potential due to biodegradation by the CO_2 absorbents currently used in anesthesia circuits. Sevoflurane has been used in patients with moderate renal function impairment (average CrCl 30-32 ml/min, CKD3/4) without worsening of renal failure [62, 63]. To minimize the risks with compound A formation from sevoflurane, it seems prudent to follow the Food and Drug Administration's (FDA) recommendations. The FDA warns against administration of sevoflurane at fresh gas flows < 1 L/min. Fresh gas flows at 1-2 L/min are limited to a total of 2 MAC hours after which the recommended flow rate is 2 L or more. However, since its introduction to the US in 1995, sevoflurane has been given to tens of millions of patients without a single report of nephrotoxicity [118].

Isoflurane and desflurane do have no known nephrotoxic properties and are excellent choices for anesthetizing patients with preexisting renal disease.

References

1. Kasiske BL, Kjellstrand CM. Perioperative management of patients with chronic renal failure and postoperative acute renal failure. Urol Clin North Am 1983;10(1):35-50.
2. Metnitz PG, Krenn CG, Steltzer H, Lang T, Ploder J, Lenz K, et al. Effect of acute renal failure requiring renal replacement therapy on outcome in critically ill patients. Crit Care Med 2002;30(9):2051-8.
3. Charlson ME, MacKenzie CR, Gold JP, Shires GT. Postoperative changes in serum creatinine. When do they occur and how much is important? Ann Surg 1989;209(3):328-33.
4. Coggins C, Fang LS-T. Acute renal failure associated with antibiotics, anesthetic agents, and radiographic contrats agents. In: Brenner BM, Lazarus, JM, editor. Acute Renal Failure: Churchill Livingstone; 1988. p. 295-352.
5. Pringle H MR, Pringle S. Clinical effects of ether anaesthesia on renal activity. Brit Med J 1905;2:542-545.
6. Blackmore WP EK, Wiegand OF, Lipsey R. Renal and cardiovascular effects of halothane. Anesthesiology 1960;27:793-803.
7. Mazze RI, Cousins MJ, Barr GA. Renal effects and metabolism of isoflurane in man. Anesthesiology 1974;40(6):536-42.
8. Cousins MJ, Greenstein LR, Hitt BA, Mazze RI. Metabolism and renal effects of enflurane in man. Anesthesiology 1976;44(1):44-53.
9. Jarnberg PO, Ekstrand J, Irestedt L, Santesson J. Renal function and fluoride formation and excretion during enflurane anaesthesia. Acta Anaesthesiol Scand 1979;23(5):444-52.

10. Deutsch S, Goldberg M, Stephen GW, Wu WH. Effects of halothane anesthesia on renal function in normal man. Anesthesiology 1966;27(6):793-804.
11. Bastron RD, Pyne JL, Inagaki M. Halothane-induced renal vasodilation. Anesthesiology 1979;50(2):126-31.
12. Priano LL. Effect of halothane on renal hemodynamics during normovolemia and acute hemorrhagic hypovolemia. Anesthesiology 1985;63(4):357-63.
13. Gelman S, Fowler KC, Smith LR. Regional blood flow during isoflurane and halothane anesthesia. Anesth Analg 1984;63(6):557-65.
14. Jarnberg PO, Marrone, B, Priano, LL. Enflurane preserves renal blood flow. Anesthesiology 1990;73:A572.
15. Hysing ES, Chelly JE, Doursout MF, Merin RG. Comparative effects of halothane, enflurane, and isoflurane at equihypotensive doses on cardiac performance and coronary and renal blood flows in chronically instrumented dogs. Anesthesiology 1992;76(6):979-84.
16. Lessard MR, Trepanier CA. Renal function and hemodynamics during prolonged isoflurane-induced hypotension in humans. Anesthesiology 1991;74(5):860-5.
17. Cho KW KS, Koh GY, Seul KH, Kim HJ, Song HS. Renalm and renin effects of sodium thiopental in rabbits. Ren Physiol 1987;10:261-271.
18. Bidwai AV, Stanley TH, Bloomer HA, Blatnick RA. Effects of anesthetic doses of morphine on renal function in the dog. Anesth Analg 1975;54(3):357-60.
19. Hunter JM, Jones RS, Utting JE. Effect of anaesthesia with nitrous oxide in oxygen and fentanyl on renal function in the artificially ventilated dog. Br J Anaesth 1980;52(3):343-8.
20. Priano LL. Effects of high-dose fentanyl on renal haemodynamics in conscious dogs. Can Anaesth Soc J 1983;30(1):10-8.
21. Jarnberg PO, Leyden P, Woods L. Renal blood flow is maintained during propofol anesthesia in dogs. Anesthesiology 1992;77: A655.
22. Baratz RA, Philbin DM, Patterson RW. Plasma antidiuretic hormone and urinary output during continuous positive-pressure breathing in dogs. Anesthesiology 1971;34(6):510-3.
23. Hall SV, Johnson EE, Hedley-Whyte J. Renal hemodynamics and function with continuous positive-pressure ventilation in dogs. Anesthesiology 1974;41(5):452-61.
24. Jarnberg PO, de Villota ED, Eklund J, Granberg PO. Effects of positive end-expiratory pressure on renal function. Acta Anaesthesiol Scand 1978;22(5):508-14.
25. Kharasch ED, Yeo KT, Kenny MA, Buffington CW. Atrial natriuretic factor may mediate the renal effects of PEEP ventilation. Anesthesiology 1988;69(6):862-9.
26. Andrivet P, Adnot S, Brun-Buisson C, Chabrier PE, Darmon JY, Braquet P, et al. Involvement of ANF in the acute antidiuresis during PEEP ventilation. J Appl Physiol 1988;65(5):1967-74.
27. Van Dyke R CM, Poznak AV. Metabolism of volatile anesthetics: 1. Conversion *in vivo* of several anesthetics to 14 CO2 and chloride. Biochem Pharmacol 1964;13:1239-1248.
28. Subcommittee on the National Halothane Study of the Committee on Anesthesia. National Academy of Sciences-National Research Council. Summary of the national halothane study: possible association halothane anesthesia and postoperative necrosis. JAMA 1966;197:775-83.
29. Mazze RI, Trudell JR, Cousins MJ. Methoxyflurane metabolism and renal dysfunction: clinical correlation in man. Anesthesiology 1971;35(3):247-52.
30. Thummel KE, Kharasch ED, Podoll T, Kunze K. Human liver microsomal enflurane defluorination catalyzed by cytochrome P-450 2E1. Drug Metab Dispos 1993;21(2):350-7.
31. Pacifici GM, Viani A, Franchi M, Gervasi PG, Longo V, Di Simplicio P, et al. Profile of drug-metabolizing enzymes in the cortex and medulla of the human kidney. Pharmacology 1989;39(5):299-308.
32. Nebert DW, Adesnik M, Coon MJ, Estabrook RW, Gonzalez FJ, Guengerich FP, et al. The P450 gene superfamily: recommended nomenclature. DNA 1987;6(1):1-11.
33. Waxman DJ. Interactions of hepatic cytochromes P-450 with steroid hormones. Regioselectivity and stereospecificity of steroid metabolism and hormonal regulation of rat P-450 enzyme expression. Biochem Pharmacol 1988;37(1):71-84.
34. Conney AH. Pharmacological implications of microsomal enzyme induction. Pharmacol Rev 1967;19(3):317-66.
35. Pantuck EJ, Pantuck CB, Conney AH. Effect of streptozotocin-induced diabetes in the rat on the metabolism of fluorinated volatile anesthetics. Anesthesiology 1987;66(1):24-8.
36. Rehder K, Forbes J, Alter H, Hessler O, Stier A. Halothane biotransformation in man: a quantitative study. Anesthesiology 1967;28(4):711-5.
37. Cohen EN, Trudell JR, Edmunds HN, Watson E. Urinary metabolites of halothane in man. Anesthesiology 1975;43(4):392-401.

38. Lind RC, Gandolfi AJ, Sipes IG, Brown BR, Jr., Waters SJ. Oxygen concentrations required for reductive defluorination of halothane by rat hepatic microsomes. Anesth Analg 1986;65(8):835-9.
39. Wood CL, Gandolfi AJ, Van Dyke RA. Lipid binding of a halothane metabolite. Relationship to lipid peroxidation *in vitro*. Drug Metab Dispos 1976;4(4):305-13.
40. Trudell JR, Bosterling B, Trevor AJ. Reductive metabolism of halothane by human and rabbit cytochrome P-450. Binding of 1-chloro-2,2,2-trifluoroethyl radical to phospholipids. Mol Pharmacol 1982;21(3):710-7.
41. Van Dyke RA, Gandolf AJ. Anaerobic release of fluoride from halothane. Relationship to the binding of halothane metabolites to hepatic cellular constituents. Drug Metab Dispos 1976;4(1):40-4.
42. Chase RE, Holaday DA, Fiserova-Bergerova V, Saidman LJ, Mack FE. The biotransformation of ethrane in man. Anesthesiology 1971;35(3):262-7.
43. Burke TR, Jr., Branchflower RV, Lees DE, Pohl LR. Mechanism of defluorination of enflurane. Identification of an organic metabolite in rat and man. Drug Metab Dispos 1981;9(1):19-24.
44. Maduska AL. Serum inorganic fluoride levels in patients receiving enflurane anesthesia. Anesth Analg 1974;53(3):351-3.
45. Mazze RI, Calverley RK, Smith NT. Inorganic fluoride nephrotoxicity: prolonged enflurane and halothane anesthesia in volunteers. Anesthesiology 1977;46(4):265-71.
46. Rice SA, Fish KJ. Anesthetic metabolism and renal function in obese and nonobese Fischer 344 rats following enflurane or isoflurane anesthesia. Anesthesiology 1986;65(1):28-34.
47. Dooley JR, Mazze RI, Rice SA, Borel JD. Is enflurane defluorination inducible in man? Anesthesiology 1979;50(3):213-7.
48. Mazze RI, Woodruff RE, Heerdt ME. Isoniazid-induced enflurane defluorination in humans. Anesthesiology 1982;57(1):5-8.
49. Loehning RW, Mazze RI. Possible nephrotoxicity from enflurane in a patient with severe renal disease. Anesthesiology 1974;40(2):203-5.
50. Eichhorn JH, Hedley-Whyte J, Steinman TI, Kaufmann JM, Laasbert LH. Renal failure following enflurane anesthesia. Anesthesiology 1976;45(5):557-60.
51. Holaday DA, Fiserova-Bergerova V, Latto IP, Zumbiel MA. Resistance of isoflurane to biotransformation in man. Anesthesiology 1975;43(3):325-32.
52. Mazze RI, Hitt BA, Cousins MJ. Effect of enzyme induction with phenobarbital on the *in vivo* and *in vitro* defluorination of isoflurane and methoxyflurane. J Pharmacol Exp Ther 1974;190(3):523-9.
53. Rice SA, Talcott RE. Effects of isoniazid treatment on selected hepatic mixed-function oxidases. Drug Metab Dispos 1979;7(5):260-2.
54. Holaday DA, Smith FR. Clinical characteristics and biotransformation of sevoflurane in healthy human volunteers. Anesthesiology 1981;54(2):100-6.
55. Fujii K, Morio, M, Kikuchi,. Pharmacokinetic study in excretion of inorganic fluoride, a metabolite of sevoflurane. Hiroshima J Med Sci 1987;36:89-94.
56. Kobayashi Y, Ochiai R, Takeda J, Sekiguchi H, Fukushima K. Serum and urinary inorganic fluoride concentrations after prolonged inhalation of sevoflurane in humans. Anesth Analg 1992;74(5):753-7.
57. Frink EJ, Jr., Malan TP, Jr., Isner RJ, Brown EA, Morgan SE, Brown BR, Jr. Renal concentrating function with prolonged sevoflurane or enflurane anesthesia in volunteers. Anesthesiology 1994;80(5):1019-25.
58. Cook TL, Beppu WJ, Hitt BA, Kosek JC, Mazze RI. A comparison of renal effects and metabolism of sevoflurane and methoxyflurane in enzyme-induced rats. Anesth Analg 1975;54(6):829-35.
59. Nishiyama T, Hirasaki A. Effects of sevoflurane anaesthesia on renal function--duration of administration and area under the curve and rate of decrease of serum inorganic fluoride. Eur J Anaesthesiol 1995;12(5):477-82.
60. Frink EJ, Jr., Malan TP, Jr., Brown EA, Morgan S, Brown BR, Jr. Plasma inorganic fluoride levels with sevoflurane anesthesia in morbidly obese and nonobese patients. Anesth Analg 1993;76(6):1333-7.
61. Higuchi H, Arimura S, Sumikura H, Satoh T, Kanno M. Urine concentrating ability after prolonged sevoflurane anaesthesia. Br J Anaesth 1994;73(2):239-40.
62. Conzen PF, Nuscheler M, Melotte A, Verhaegen M, Leupolt T, Van Aken H, et al. Renal function and serum fluoride concentrations in patients with stable renal insufficiency after anesthesia with sevoflurane or enflurane. Anesth Analg 1995;81(3):569-75.
63. Tsukamoto N, Hirabayashi Y, Shimizu R, Mitsuhata H. The effects of sevoflurane and isoflurane anesthesia on renal tubular function in patients with moderately impaired renal function. Anesth Analg 1996;82(5):909-13.
64. Hanaki C, Fujii K, Morio M, Tashima T. Decomposition of sevoflurane by sodalime. Hiroshima J Med Sci 1987;36(1):61-7.
65. Fang ZX, Eger EI, 2nd. Factors affecting the concentration of compound A resulting from the degradation of sevoflurane by soda lime and Baralyme in a standard anesthetic circuit. Anesth Analg 1995;81(3):564-8.
66. Bito H, Ikeda K. Effect of total flow rate on the concentration of degradation products generated by reaction between sevoflurane and soda lime. Br J Anaesth 1995;74(6):667-9.

67. Gonsowski CT, Laster MJ, Eger EI, 2nd, Ferrell LD, Kerschmann RL. Toxicity of compound A in rats. Effect of a 3-hour administration. Anesthesiology 1994;80(3):556-65.
68. Keller KA, Callan C, Prokocimer P, Delgado-Herrera L, Friedman MB, Hoffman GM, et al. Inhalation toxicity study of a haloalkene degradant of sevoflurane, Compound A (PIFE), in Sprague-Dawley rats. Anesthesiology 1995;83(6):1220-32.
69. Morio M, Fujii K, Satoh N, Imai M, Kawakami U, Mizuno T, et al. Reaction of sevoflurane and its degradation products with soda lime. Toxicity of the byproducts. Anesthesiology 1992;77(6):1155-64.
70. Kharasch ED, Thorning D, Garton K, Hankins DC, Kilty CG. Role of renal cysteine conjugate beta-lyase in the mechanism of compound A nephrotoxicity in rats. Anesthesiology 1997;86(1):160-71.
71. Goldberg ME, Cantillo J, Gratz I, Deal E, Vekeman D, McDougall R, et al. Dose of compound A, not sevoflurane, determines changes in the biochemical markers of renal injury in healthy volunteers. Anesth Analg 1999;88(2):437-45.
72. Higuchi H, Sumita S, Wada H, Ura T, Ikemoto T, Nakai T, et al. Effects of sevoflurane and isoflurane on renal function and on possible markers of nephrotoxicity. Anesthesiology 1998;89(2):307-22.
73. Eger EI, 2nd, Koblin DD, Bowland T, Ionescu P, Laster MJ, Fang Z, et al. Nephrotoxicity of sevoflurane versus desflurane anesthesia in volunteers. Anesth Analg 1997;84(1):160-8.
74. Eger EI, 2nd, Gong D, Koblin DD, Bowland T, Ionescu P, Laster MJ, et al. Dose-related biochemical markers of renal injury after sevoflurane versus desflurane anesthesia in volunteers. Anesth Analg 1997;85(5):1154-63.
75. Bito H, Ikeuchi Y, Ikeda K. Effects of low-flow sevoflurane anesthesia on renal function: comparison with high-flow sevoflurane anesthesia and low-flow isoflurane anesthesia. Anesthesiology 1997;86(6):1231-7.
76. Kharasch ED, Frink EJ, Jr., Zager R, Bowdle TA, Artru A, Nogami WM. Assessment of low-flow sevoflurane and isoflurane effects on renal function using sensitive markers of tubular toxicity. Anesthesiology 1997;86(6):1238-53.
77. Ebert TJ, Messana LD, Uhrich TD, Staacke TS. Absence of renal and hepatic toxicity after four hours of 1.25 minimum alveolar anesthetic concentration sevoflurane anesthesia in volunteers. Anesth Analg 1998;86(3):662-7.
78. Forster H, Dudziak R. [Causes for the reaction between dry soda lime and halogenated inhalation anesthetics]. Anaesthesist 1997;46(12):1054-63.
79. Forster H, Warnken UH, Asskali F. [Various reactions of sevoflurane with the individual components of soda lime]. Anaesthesist 1997;46(12):1071-5.
80. Neumann MA, Laster MJ, Weiskopf RB, Gong DH, Dudziak R, Forster H, et al. The elimination of sodium and potassium hydroxides from desiccated soda lime diminishes degradation of desflurane to carbon monoxide and sevoflurane to compound A but does not compromise carbon dioxide absorption. Anesth Analg 1999;89(3):768-73.
81. Murray JM, Renfrew CW, Bedi A, McCrystal CB, Jones DS, Fee JP. Amsorb: a new carbon dioxide absorbent for use in anesthetic breathing systems. Anesthesiology 1999;91(5):1342-8.
81a. Keijzer C, Perez, RSGM, De Lange, JJ. Compound A and carbon monoxide production from sevoflurane and seven different types of carbon dioxide absorbent in a patient model Acta Anaesth Scand 2007;51(1):31-37.
82. Koblin DD, Eger EI, 2nd, Johnson BH, Konopka K, Waskell L. I-653 resists degradation in rats. Anesth Analg 1988;67(6):534-8.
83. Eger EI, 3rd. Stability of I-653 in soda lime. Anesth Analg 1987;66(10):983-5.
84. Eger EI, 2nd, Johnson BH, Strum DP, Ferrell LD. Studies of the toxicity of I-653, halothane, and isoflurane in enzyme-induced, hypoxic rats. Anesth Analg 1987;66(12):1227-9.
85. Eger EI, 2nd, Johnson BH, Ferrell LD. Comparison of the toxicity of I-653 and isoflurane in rats: a test of the effect of repeated anesthesia and use of dry soda lime. Anesth Analg 1987;66(12):1230-3.
86. Jones RM, Koblin DD, Cashman JN, Eger EI, 2nd, Johnson BH, Damask MC. Biotransformation and hepato-renal function in volunteers after exposure to desflurane (I-653). Br J Anaesth 1990;64(4):482-7.
87. Koblin DD, Weiskopf RB, Holmes MA, Konopka K, Rampil IJ, Eger EI, 2nd, et al. Metabolism of I-653 and isoflurane in swine. Anesth Analg 1989;68(2):147-9.
88. Sutton TS, Koblin DD, Gruenke LD, Weiskopf RB, Rampil IJ, Waskell L, et al. Fluoride metabolites after prolonged exposure of volunteers and patients to desflurane. Anesth Analg 1991;73(2):180-5.
89. Artusio JF, Jr., Van Poznak A, Hunt RE, Tiers RM, Alexander M. A clinical evaluation of methoxyflurane in man. Anesthesiology 1960;21:512-7.
90. Haynes RJ. Agents affecting calcification. In: Gilman AF RT, Nies AS, Taylor P, editor. Goodman and Gilman's The Pharmacological Basis of Therapeutics. 8th ed: Pergamon Press; 1990. p. 1518-1522.
91. Roman RJ, Carter JR, North WC, Kauker ML. Renal tubular site of action of fluoride in Fischer 344 rats. Anesthesiology 1977;46(4):260-4.
92. Cittanova ML, Lelongt B, Verpont MC, Geniteau-Legendre M, Wahbe F, Prie D, et al. Fluoride ion toxicity in human kidney collecting duct cells. Anesthesiology 1996;84(2):428-35.

93. Crandell WB, Pappas SG, Macdonald A. Nephrotoxicity associated with methoxyflurane anesthesia. Anesthesiology 1966;27(5):591-607.
94. Mazze RI, Shue GL, Jackson SH. Renal dysfunction associated with methoxyflurane anesthesia. A randomized, prospective clinical evaluation. Jama 1971;216(2):278-88.
95. Holaday DA, Rudofsky S, Treuhaft PS. The metabolic degradation of methoxyflurane in man. Anesthesiology 1970;33(6):589-93.
96. Cousins MJ, Mazze RI. Methoxyflurane nephrotoxicity. A study of dose response in man. Jama 1973;225(13):1611-6.
97. Cousins MJ, Mazze RI, Kosek JC, Hitt BA, Love FV. The etiology of methoxyflurane nephrotoxicity. J Pharmacol Exp Ther 1974;190(3):530-41.
98. Frascino JA. Effect of inorganic fluoride on the renal concentrating mechanism. Possible nephrotoxicity in man. J Lab Clin Med 1972;79(2):192-203.
99. Kharasch ED, Hankins DC, Thummel KE. Human kidney methoxyflurane and sevoflurane metabolism. Intrarenal fluoride production as a possible mechanism of methoxyflurane nephrotoxicity. Anesthesiology 1995;82(3):689-99.
100. Brown BR, Jr. Shibboleths and jigsaw puzzles. The fluoride nephrotoxicity enigma. Anesthesiology 1995;82(3):607-8.
101. Mazze RI, Jamison R. Renal effects of sevoflurane. Anesthesiology 1995;83(3):443-5.
102. Kharasch ED, Schroeder JL, Liggitt HD, Park SB, Whittington D, Sheffels P. New insights into the mechanism of methoxyflurane nephrotoxicity and implications for anesthetic development (part 1): Identification of the nephrotoxic metabolic pathway. Anesthesiology 2006;105(4):726-36.
103. Kharasch ED, Schroeder JL, Liggitt HD, Ensign D, Whittington D. New insights into the mechanism of methoxyflurane nephrotoxicity and implications for anesthetic development (part 2): Identification of nephrotoxic metabolites. Anesthesiology 2006;105(4):737-45.
104. Selinsky BS, Perlman ME, London RE. *In vivo* nuclear magnetic resonance studies of hepatic methoxyflurane metabolism. II. A reevaluation of hepatic metabolic pathways. Mol Pharmacol 1988;33(5):567-73.
105. Chen PS, Jr., Gardner DE, Hodge HC, O'Brien JA, Smith FA. Renal clearance of fluoride. Proc Soc Exp Biol Med 1956;92(4):879-83.
106. Carlson CH, Armstrong WD, Singer L. Distribution and excretion of radiofluoride in the human. Proc Soc Exp Biol Med 1960;104:235-9.
107. Hosking DJ, Chamberlain MJ. Studies in man with 18 F. Clin Sci 1972;42(2):153-61.
108. Ekstrand J, Ehrnebo M, Boreus LO. Fluoride bioavailability after intravenous and oral administration: importance of renal clearance and urine flow. Clin Pharmacol Ther 1978;23(3):329-37.
109. Whitford GM, Pashley DH, Stringer GI. Fluoride renal clearance: a pH-dependent event. Am J Physiol 1976;230(2):527-32.
110. Ekstrand J, Ehrnebo M, Whitford GM, Jarnberg PO. Fluoride pharmacokinetics during acid-base balance changes in man. Eur J Clin Pharmacol 1980;18(2):189-94.
111. Jarnberg PO, Ekstrand J, Irestedt L. Renal fluoride excretion and plasma fluoride levels during and after enflurane anesthesia are dependent on urinary pH. Anesthesiology 1981;54(1):48-52.
112. Barzel US, Jowsey J. The effects of chronic acid and alkali administration on bone turnover in adult rats. Clin Sci 1969;36(3):517-24.
113. Leake RD, Trygstad CW. Glomerular filtration rate during the period of adaptation to extrauterine life. Pediatr Res 1977;11(9 Pt 1):959-62.
114. Jose PA, Fildes RD, Gomez RA, Chevalier RL, Robillard JE. Neonatal renal function and physiology. Curr Opin Pediatr 1994;6(2):172-7.
115. Fisher DM, Robinson S, Brett CM, Perin G, Gregory GA. Comparison of enflurane, halothane, and isoflurane for diagnostic and therapeutic procedures in children with malignancies. Anesthesiology 1985;63(6):647-50.
116. Lerman J, Sikich N, Kleinman S, Yentis S. The pharmacology of sevoflurane in infants and children. Anesthesiology 1994;80(4):814-24.
117. Frink EJ, Jr., Green WB, Jr., Brown EA, Malcomson M, Hammond LC, Valencia FG, et al. Compound A concentrations during sevoflurane anesthesia in children. Anesthesiology 1996;84(3):566-71.
118. Bedford RF, Ives HE. The renal safety of sevoflurane. Anesth Analg 2000;90(3):505-8.

24

Bisphosphonates and the kidney

Jonathan GREEN

Novartis Institutes for BioMedical Research, Basel, Switzerland

Introduction

Bone remodelling is a continuous and dynamic process that normally involves the coordinated interplay among 3 types of cells: the bone resorptive osteoclasts, the bone-forming osteoblasts, and osteocytes, which are thought to act as mechano-transducers in bone [1]. The process becomes unbalanced in the elderly, in patients with benign bone disease [2], and in patients with primary bone lesions from multiple myeloma or bone metastases from solid tumours [3, 4]. Bisphosphonates are synthetic analogues of pyrophosphate—a naturally occurring modulator of mineralisation found in plasma, urine, and bone. They inhibit osteoclast-mediated bone resorption through several mechanisms, including inhibition of osteoclastogenesis, disruption of intracellular vesicular trafficking, and induction of osteoclast apoptosis, as well as indirectly via effects on osteoblasts [5]. Bisphosphonates are transported through the bloodstream and are deposited at sites of active bone remodelling, where they bind avidly to the mineralised bone matrix via the bisphosphonate moiety [5]. During bone resorption, bisphosphonates are internalised by osteoclasts, wherein they mediate their antiresorptive effects [5]. Therefore, bisphosphonates have provided increasing clinical utility in the management of patients with pathologies associated with perturbations in bone metabolism [3, 4, 6].

Several generations of bisphosphonates have been developed for the treatment of bone disease, each with different affinities for their cellular targets and increasing clinical efficacy (Figure 1). First-generation bisphosphonates (e.g., etidronate and clodronate)

are relatively simple pyrophosphate analogues that lack a nitrogen atom and induce apoptosis after they are metabolised by osteoclasts into nonhydrolyzable, cytotoxic analogues of adenosine triphosphate (ATP) [5]. The addition of a nitrogen-containing side chain to the bisphosphonate backbone resulted in a class of compounds that inhibited a key enzyme in the mevalonate pathway, farnesyl pyrophosphate synthase (FPPS), and greatly increased their potency as inhibitors of osteoclast-mediated osteolysis [5, 7]. Early nitrogen-containing bisphosphonates, including pamidronate, alendronate, and ibandronate, contain an aliphatic side chain with a single nitrogen atom. Of the newest-generation bisphosphonates, risedronate contains a heterocyclic side chain with 1 nitrogen atom, and zoledronic acid contains 2 nitrogen atoms in an imidazole ring, giving these molecules increased potency and a higher affinity for the intracellular target enzyme, FPPS [5, 7, 8].

The presence of a nitrogen-containing side chain facilitates interaction with the catalytic site of FPPS, an enzyme in the metabolic pathway that is required for the production of the isoprenoid lipids farnesyl diphosphate and geranylgeranyl diphosphate, essential metabolites for posttranslational protein prenylation [5, 8]. Inhibiting the prenylation of guanosine triphosphate-binding proteins such as Ras, Rho, and Rac disrupts the normal cellular signal transduction that is required for osteoclast function and survival [5].

Bisphosphonates are widely used for the prevention and treatment of osteopenia and osteoporosis and for the reduction of skeletal complications in patients with malignant bone disease. Several oral bisphosphonates, including alendronate, risedronate, and ibandronate, are approved worldwide for the treatment of osteoporosis in postmenopausal women, as are intravenous (i.v.) formulations of ibandronate (3 mg quarterly) and zoledronic acid (5 mg annually). Several i.v. bisphosphonates are available for the treatment of the skeletal complications that frequently occur in malignant disease, such as hypercalcaemia of malignancy (HCM), multiple myeloma, and bone metastases associated with solid tumours. Pamidronate is approved worldwide for the treatment of HCM, multiple myeloma, and breast cancer bone metastases. Although not registered for oncology indications in the United States, i.v. ibandronate is widely available elsewhere for HCM and breast cancer bone metastases, and as an oral formulation for breast cancer bone metastases. Clodronate, which also is not registered in the United States, is approved in many other countries for the treatment of HCM (oral and i.v. formulations) and osteolysis due to malignancy (oral formulation). Zoledronic acid, by contrast, has the broadest label of any i.v. bisphosphonate for use in HCM, multiple myeloma, and bone metastases associated with any solid tumour (e.g. breast, prostate, lung, kidney, thyroid, head and neck).

There are class effects specific to each generation of bisphosphonate. As a result, the therapeutic index is different for each agent. Oral bisphosphonates have been associated with upper gastrointestinal disorders including dysphagia, esophagitis, esophageal ulcers, and gastric ulcers [9]. These effects often limit the long-term compliance with, and therefore the efficacy of, these agents [10]. Patients have reported mild to moderate acute flu-like symptoms after the initial i.v. infusions of nitrogen-containing bisphosphonates [9].

The use of i.v. bisphosphonates is associated with an increased risk of adverse renal events, especially with the intensive dosing regimens used in patients with cancer who, in any case, are more likely to have impaired renal function before the initiation of bisphosphonate therapy and may be receiving other nephrotoxic drugs. The renal tolerability profile of several i.v. bisphosphonates has been investigated in randomised clinical trials, and it appears to be dependent not only on molecular structure but also on the dosing regimen (Table 1) [11-26]. Occasional incidents of renal adverse events with oral alendronate have also been reported but not to the extent of i.v. bisphosphonates [27, 28]. Intravenous bisphosphonates should not be used in patients with renal failure to avoid further impairment of renal function. Therefore, to ensure renal safety, measurement of serum creatinine is recommended before administering i.v. bisphosphonates to patients with mild to moderately impaired renal function, and the dosing regimen should be adjusted appropriately in accordance with the prescribing information for each drug [29-34]. In patients with normal renal function at the initiation of therapy, renal adverse events have typically been infrequent, mild, and transient. Overall, the benefits of i.v. bisphosphonate therapy in the oncology setting far outweigh the risk of adverse events. This chapter provides a detailed review of the pharmacokinetics and renal safety profiles of i.v.

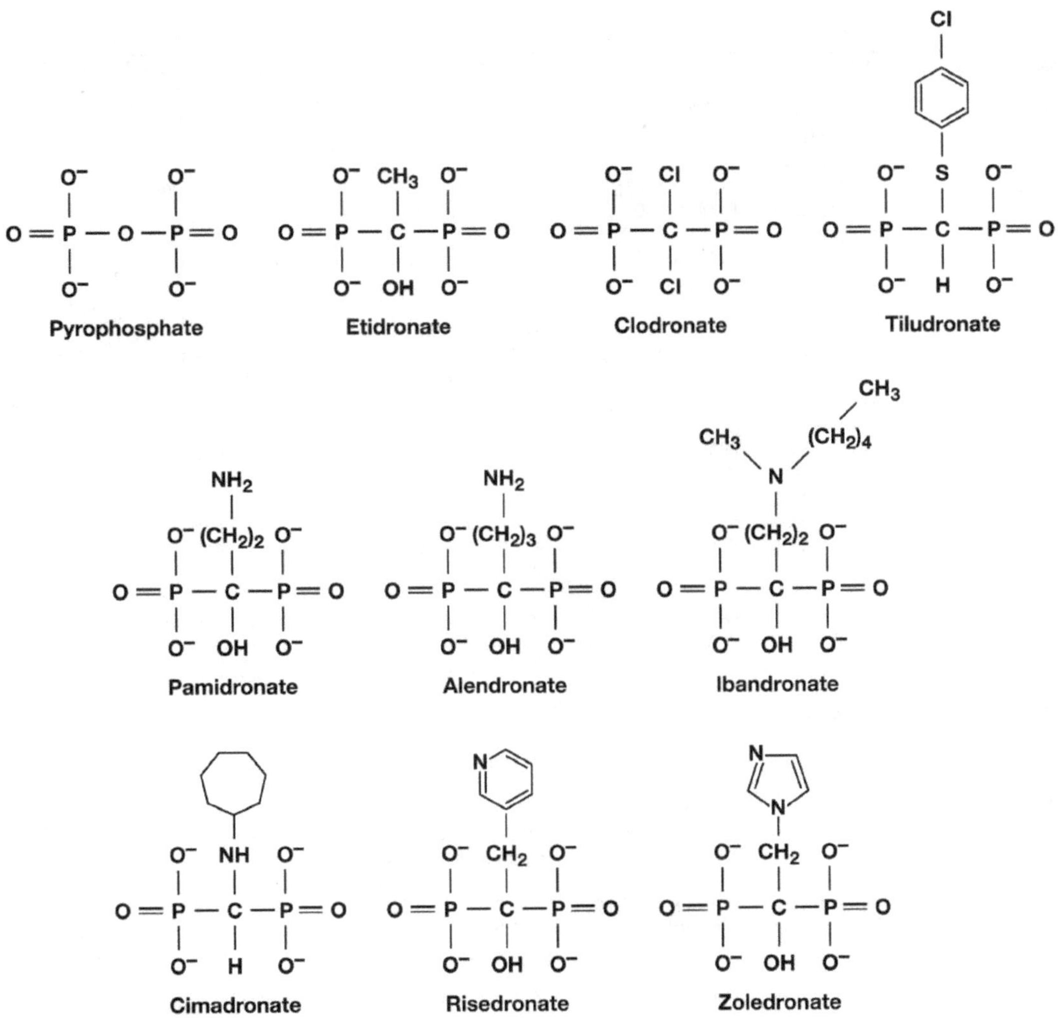

Figure 1. *Chemical structure of bisphosphonates. For consistency all compounds are shown as the dissociated anions. Similarly, zoledronate is used in this figure, although the registered generic name of zoledronic acid is used throughout the text.*

bisphosphonates based on published preclinical and clinical data.

Pharmacokinetics and renal transport of bisphosphonates

Bisphosphonates are transported through the bloodstream bound to plasma proteins; however, the proportion of bound bisphosphonate varies according to agent. For example, the proportions of clodronate, alendronate, and risedronate that bind to human plasma proteins are approximately 40%, 78%, and 24%, respectively [35, 36]. Notable differences exist in the binding of specific bisphosphonates to the plasma proteins of different species: alendronate is highly bound to rat plasma protein (96%) but less so to dog (45%), monkey (62%), or human (78%) plasma [35]. Moreover, binding can vary with experimental conditions, making the direct comparison of the plasma protein binding of different bisphosphonates difficult. In a head-to-head comparison of ibandronate and zoledronic acid, protein binding was investigated in plasma from 3 different species under controlled experimental conditions [37]. No significant differences were observed between the binding of ibandronate and zoledronic acid to human, dog, or rat plasma at

Table 1. Renal tolerability profiles of intravenous bisphosphonates reported in randomised clinical trials.

Publication/ Study drug	Disease	Study design	Patients randomised, N	Regimen	Measure of renal impairment	Renal safety results
Gucalp [11] EHDP PAM	HCM	Randomised, double blind, comparative	EHDP, n = 35; PAM, n = 30	EHDP 7.5mg/kg/day i.v. 2h for 3 days; PAM 60 mg i.v. 24h once	Serum creatinine increase ≥ 0.5 mg/dl	EHDP, 5.7%; PAM, 13.3%
Purohit [12] CLOD PAM	HCM	Randomised, double-blind, comparative	CLOD, n = 21; PAM, n = 20	CLOD 1500 i.v. 4h once; PAM 90 mg i.v. 4h once	Serum creatinine increase	CLOD, 23.8%; PAM, 0%
Atula [13] CLOD PAM	HCM	Randomised, double blind, comparative	CLOD low, n = 10 CLOD high, n = 21; PAM, n = 20	CLOD 900 mg i.v. 4h once; CLOD 1500 mg i.v. 4h once; PAM 90 mg i.v. 4h once	Serum creatinine increase	Slight decrease in both CLOD and PAM groups
Gucalp [14] PAM	HCM	Randomised, double-blind, placebo-controlled	PAM 4h, n = 23; PAM 24h, n = 23; PLA, n = 23	PAM 60 mg i.v. 4h once; PAM 60 mg i.v. 24h once; PLA i.v.	Serum creatinine increase ≥ 0.5 mg/dl	PAM 4h, 13%; PAM 24h, 13%; PLA, 4.3%
Major [15] PAM ZOL	HCM	Randomised, double blind, comparative	PAM, n = 86; ZOL low, n = 90; ZOL high, n = 99	PAM 90 mg i.v. 2h once; ZOL 4mg i.v. 5 min once; ZOL 8 mg i.v. 5 min once	Serum creatinine increase, grade 3/4	PAM, 4.0% ZOL low, 2.3% ZOL high, 5.6%
Berenson [16] PAM	MM	Randomised, double-blind, placebo-controlled	PAM, n = 205; PLA, n = 187	PAM 90 mg i.v. 4h every 4 wks for 21 months	Serum creatinine increase ≥ 1 mg/dl	No difference between PAM and PLA groups
Hortobagyi [17] PAM	BC	Randomised, double-blind, placebo-controlled	PAM, n = 185; PLA, n = 197	PAM 90 mg i.v. 2h every 3-4 wks for 24 months	Serum chemistry, clinical AEs	No evidence of increased renal AEs with PAM*
Theriault [18] PAM	BC	Randomised, double-blind, placebo-controlled	PAM, n = 182; PLA, n = 189	PAM 90 mg i.v. 2h every 4 wks for 24 months	Serum chemistry, clinical AEs in > 10% patients	No evidence of increased renal AEs with PAM
Rosen [19] ZOL	LC, OST	Randomised, double-blind, placebo-controlled	ZOL low, n = 257; ZOL high, n = 266†; PLA, n = 250	ZOL 4 mg i.v. 5-15 min; ZOL 8/4 mg i.v. 5-15 min every 3 wks for 9 months	Notable serum creatinine increase**	ZOL low, 10.9%; ZOL high, 12.7%; PLA 90 mg, 6.7%§
Saad [20] ZOL	PC	Randomised, double-blind, placebo-controlled	ZOL low, n = 214; ZOL high, n = 221†; PLA, n = 208	ZOL 4 mg i.v. 5-15 min; ZOL 8/4 mg i.v. 5-15 min every 3 wks for 15 months	Notable serum creatinine increase‖	ZOL low, 15.2%; ZOL high, 20.7%; PLA, 11.5%¶
Kohno [21] ZOL	BC	Randomised, double-blind, placebo-controlled	ZOL, n = 114; PLA, n = 114	ZOL 4 mg i.v. 15 min every 4 wks for12 months	Notable serum creatinine increase**	No evidence of decreased renal function with ZOL
Rosen [22] ZOL PAM	MM, BC	Randomised, double blind, comparative	ZOL 4 mg, n = 564; ZOL 8/4 mg, n = 526†; PAM 90 mg, n = 558	ZOL or PAM every 3-4 wks for 24 months	Grade 3/4 serum creatinine increases after 25 months	ZOL 4mg, 0.4%; ZOL 8/4 mg, 2.7%; PAM 90 mg, 1.9%‡
Reid [23] ZOL RIS	PDB	Randomised, double-blind, comparative	ZOL, n = 182; RIS, n = 175	ZOL 5 mg i.v. 15 min once; RIS 30 mg/day oral for 60 days	Serum creatinine and urinary protein measured 9-11 days after dosing	No significant difference between ZOL and RIS groups
Black [24] ZOL	PMO	Randomised, double-blind, placebo-controlled	ZOL, n = 3,889; PLA, n = 3,876	ZOL 5 mg i.v. 15 min once a year for 3 years	Serum creatinine increase > 0.5 mg/dl at days 9-11 postinfusion	ZOL, 1.3%; PLA, 0.4%+
Ralston [25] IBN	HCM	Randomised, double-blind, dose escalation	IBN low, n = 45; IBN mid, n = 44; IBN high, n = 42	IBN 2 mg i.v. 2h; IBN 4 mg i.v. 2h; IBN 6 mg i.v. 2h	Serum creatinine	No renal toxicity attributable to IBN
Body [26] IBN	BC	Randomised, double-blind, placebo-controlled	IBN low, n = 154; IBN high, n = 154; PLA, n = 158	IBN 2 mg i.v. bolus; IBN 6 mg i.v. 1-2h every 3-4 wks for 15-24 months	Increased creatinine levels (300 mM)	IBN low, 0.7%; IBN high, 2.6%; PLA, 1.3%

AE = Adverse event; BC = Breast cancer; CLOD = Clodronate; EHDP = Etidronate; HCM = Hypercalcaemia of malignancy; IBN = Ibandronate; i.v. = Intravenous; LC = Lung cancer; MM = Multiple myeloma; OST = Other solid tumours (renal, head and neck, thyroid, other); PDB = Paget's disease of bone; PAM = Pamidronate; PC = Prostate cancer; PLA = Placebo; PMO = Postmenopausal osteoporosis; RIS = Risedronate; ZOL = Zoledronic acid.

**1 patient with preexisting glomerulonephritis developed renal failure, possibly related to study drug.* *(continued on next page)* clinically relevant concentrations (Table 2) [37].

The interaction between bisphosphonates and plasma proteins is not well understood, but it is known to be influenced by both calcium and iron ions [38]. The addition of calcium to human plasma in an *in vitro* study increased the proportion of plasma protein-bound versus free pamidronate, whereas the addition of calcium chelators reduced the proportion of drug bound. Similarly, the addition of ferric ions to plasma increased the proportion of plasma protein-bound versus free pamidronate [38].

It has been reported that 40% to 60% of bisphosphonate that reaches the systemic circulation rapidly binds to bone and remains there for a long time; the terminal half-life of alendronate in the human skeleton has been calculated to be approximately 10.5 years [39]. Bisphosphonates are preferentially deposited on exposed mineral at sites in the bone where turnover is high, especially the growth plates, trabecular bone, and sites of injury, infection, or metastasis. Bisphosphonates are metabolically stable, so the remaining unbound bisphosphonate fraction is rapidly eliminated, unchanged, by the kidneys [29-34, 36]. Pharmacokinetic studies of i.v. clodronate and pamidronate in subjects with different degrees of renal insufficiency have demonstrated that renal clearance of bisphosphonate is markedly compromised with a declining glomerular filtration rate, resulting in an increased area under the serum drug concentration-time curve ($AUC_{0-\infty}$) [40, 41].

Table 2. Bisphosphonate binding to 3 individual human plasma samples at pH 7.4 *in vitro* [37].

Concentration	2 ng/ml	20 ng/ml	200 ng/ml	2,000 ng/ml
Zoledronic acid	40 ± 2	35 ± 2	28 ± 0	23 ± 2
Ibandronate	31 ± 13	26 ± 1	24 ± 1	21 ± 1

Data are expressed as mean percent binding ± standard deviation.

In an open-label pharmacokinetic study of zoledronic acid (4 mg/month for 3 months) in 19 patients with malignant bone disease and varying levels of renal function, renal clearance was consistently lower in patients with impaired renal function [42]. Correspondingly, the 24-hour cumulative urinary excretion of zoledronic acid in patients with renal impairment was lower than in patients with normal renal function. However, in this relatively small study, none of the differences between groups was statistically significant.

Although definitive proof is lacking, there appears to be an active transport mechanism for the elimination of bisphosphonates through the kidney, distinct from the known renal transport systems for organic anions and cations and EDTA [43-45]. In an early study with conscious rats, the clearance of etidronate and clodronate was found to be higher than the glomerular filtration rate by a factor of about 1.5, indicating net tubular secretion of both drugs [43]. Further studies in rats demonstrated that renal excretion of the nitrogen-containing bisphosphonate alendronate is concentration- and dose-dependent and saturable, implying secretion by an active-transport mechanism [44]. Moreover, alendronate clearance could be inhibited by the concomitant addition of the non-nitrogen–containing bisphosphonate etidronate in a dose-dependent manner, suggesting competition between the 2 compounds for an uncharacterised renal transport system. Using a luminal stop-flow tubular microperfusion technique with rat kidney, Ullrich et al. found that only etidronate and clodronate had moderate affinity for the renal sulphate transporter, whereas 5 other nitrogen-containing bisphosphonates had only low or no affinity for any of the contraluminal anion transporters [45].

Although the mechanistic details of bisphosphonate handling by the kidney remain largely unknown, attempts have been made to determine the location

(Footnote Table 1 continued)

***Serum creatinine increase ≥ 0.5 mg/dl from baseline for patients with normal baseline serum creatinine (< 1.4 mg/dl), or increase ≥ 1.0 mg/dl from baseline for patients with baseline serum creatinine above normal (≥ 1.4 mg/dl), or any increase ≥ 2 times the baseline value.*

†To ensure renal safety during the study, the dose was reduced from 8 mg to 4 mg, the infusion volume was increased from 50 ml to 100 ml, and the infusion time from 5 min to 15 min.

‡No significant difference in renal toxicity between ZOL 4 mg/100 ml infused over 15 min and PAM 90 mg/250 ml infused over 2 hours, (risk ratio, 1.057; P = 0.839).

§After protocol amendment, elevated serum creatinine was not statistically significant between the 4-mg ZOL group and the PLA group (hazard ratio = 1.57; P = 0.228).

||Serum creatinine increases of ≥ 0.5 mg/dl (if baseline value was < 1.4 mg/dl) or ≥ 1.0 mg/dl (if baseline value was ≥ 1.4 mg/dl).

¶Compared to patients who received placebo, patients treated with ZOL 4 mg or 8/4 mg had a comparable risk for renal toxicity, relative risk ratio of 1.07 (P = 0.882) and 1.76 (P = 0.165), respectively.

+Transient increase, resolved before the next infusion; no significant difference at 3 years between ZOL and PLA groups for serum creatinine level or creatinine clearance.

of the rate-determining steps. In an *in vivo* rat study with alendronate, Kino et al. determined the influx and efflux at the basolateral membrane, sequestration of the drug at the brush-border membrane, and net secretion via the renal tubules [46]. The data indicated saturable transport from renal tubular cells into the luminal duct, suggesting the presence of a transport system on the renal brush-border membrane. Furthermore, the active transport mechanism appeared to be dependent on bisphosphonate plasma concentration, with the uptake process being the rate-determining step of renal secretion at low plasma concentrations. Increasing plasma concentrations had only a minimal effect on the uptake clearance to renal tubular cells, and secretion from tubular cells into the luminal duct could be saturated. It was concluded that dose-dependent transport mechanisms on both the basolateral and brush-border membranes of renal tubular cells are involved in the renal secretion of alendronate [46]. Clearly, further studies are still required to identify the transporter molecules responsible for the renal clearance of bisphosphonates.

Preclinical renal toxicity

Although the kidney has been identified as a major target organ for all bisphosphonates at the high doses used in preclinical toxicity studies, a clear therapeutic window still exists, enabling bisphosphonates to be safely administered in general clinical use for the inhibition of bone resorption. However, there are differences in the therapeutic indices between individual agents and in their pharmacokinetic and pharmacodynamic profiles in patients with both normal and impaired renal function.

Comparative preclinical studies have provided additional insight into differences in the renal safety profiles of the commonly used bisphosphonates. In a 25-week preclinical rat study [47], renal effects were compared for ibandronate (1 mg/kg) and zoledronic acid (1 mg/kg or 3 mg/kg), with both drugs given either as a single-dose i.v. injection or repeatedly every 3 weeks for 6 months. Both the single and intermittent doses of ibandronate 1 mg/kg resulted in similar incidences of proximal tubular degeneration and single-cell necrosis, without any increase of histopathologic damage (Figure 2) [47]. By contrast, degeneration and single-cell necrosis were observed following intermittent dosing

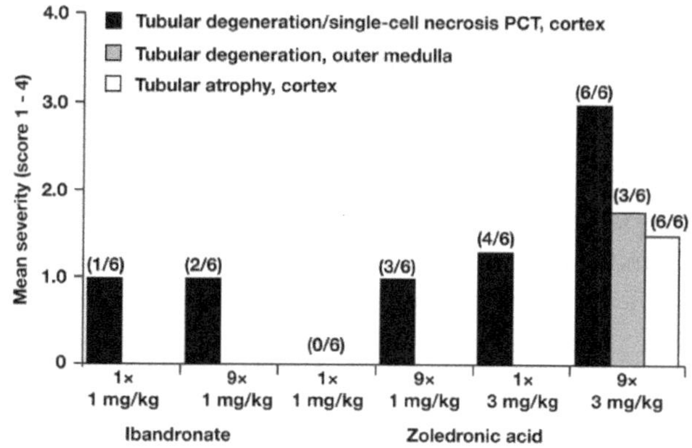

Figure 2. *Histopathologic findings in the kidney of rats after single or intermittent dosing of ibandronate or zoledronic acid. PCT = Proximal convoluted tubules. (Reprinted with permission from [47], Copyright Elsevier 2003)*

of zoledronic acid 1 mg/kg but not after a single i.v. infusion of the same dose. The incidence and severity of damage to the proximal tubules increased with intermittent dosing of zoledronic acid 3 mg/kg. Tubular atrophy and degenerative changes in the outer medulla were associated with this dosing regimen of zoledronic acid but not with the single dose. Hypertrophy and hyperplasia of the collecting ducts and distal tubules were observed following intermittent dosing of both drugs but not after a single dose. These dosing regimens were selected to produce minimally nephrotoxic effects in animals, but they do not reflect the dosing schedules used in the clinical setting [47]. Zoledronic acid is several-fold more potent than ibandronate as an inhibitor of bone resorption [5, 7]; therefore, the doses used in this study were not pharmacologically equivalent. As pointed out by Hirschberg [48], the flaws in the design of this study and in the interpretation of the data make it difficult to draw any clinically relevant conclusions from these experiments.

Another study in rabbits has compared the efficacy and safety of pamidronate (1 mg/kg in 20 ml saline infused over 2 hours) and zoledronic acid (0.1 mg/kg in 20 ml saline infused over 20 minutes). Renal toxicity was identified histologically in 14 of 20 kidneys of pamidronate-treated rabbits but was not detected in the 20 kidneys of rabbits infused with zoledronic acid [49]. Because zoledronic acid is a much more potent inhibitor of bone resorption, this agent could be administered at one tenth of the pamidronate dose and yet still achieve superior therapeutic efficacy without evidence of renal toxicity. In a similar comparative study in rats that were infused with very high doses (1.5-50 mg/kg) of zoledronic acid or pamidronate (~1, 000-fold greater than the therapeutic dose), the dose required to increase serum urea by 100% from baseline was approximately 4 times higher for zoledronic acid than for pamidronate [50]. Furthermore, on subcutaneous injection of 1 mg/kg 9 times over the course of 14 days, zoledronic acid had no effect on the cumulative urinary excretion of a marker enzyme of renal damage, malate dehydrogenase, whereas pamidronate resulted in a 2-fold increase [50]. Again taking into account the different antiresorptive potencies of the 2 compounds, the therapeutic index for zoledronic acid was determined to be 7-fold greater than that of pamidronate. In view of the subsequent clinical data, although these preclinical assays may have some value for early compound screening, they do not appear to be predictive of renal tolerability in humans.

Data from a comparative, preclinical study of single doses of ibandronate (1-20 mg/kg i.v.), zoledronic acid (1-10 mg/kg i.v.), and clodronate (400 mg/kg intraperitoneally), indicated that the proximal tubules were the primary target for renal toxicity as assessed by clinical biochemistry and renal histopathology at 1 and/or 4 days postdosing [51]. Tubular degeneration and single-cell necrosis of the proximal convoluted tubules were observed for all 3 agents at 4 days after dosing, although the severity, type, and location of renal damage differed between compounds. Although high doses of zoledronic acid (10 mg/kg) resulted in granular proteinaceous deposits in the lumen of distal tubules, there was no evidence from X-ray microanalysis of any precipitation of bisphosphonate or formation of aggregates in the kidney. Overall, there were no significant changes in serum biochemical parameters and urinary enzymes in bisphosphonate-treated animals compared with controls [51]. Similarly, in both rats and mice, renal toxicity has been observed with i.v. administration of pamidronate [52]. Renal effects, including renal tubular necrosis and enzymuria, were most prominent when animals received doses of pamidronate (≥10 mg/kg) several-fold greater than those used clinically (~0.5-1.5 mg/kg) [52].

The preclinical toxicity of alendronate has been studied at doses comparable with those used clinically with acute (single-dose) and chronic (repeated-dose) dosing regimens [53]. The most common lethal toxicity observed in mice and rats after oral administration of alendronate was primarily related to gastrointestinal irritation, and no lethality was reported in dogs receiving high oral doses of the drug. Nephrotoxicity was reported in rats and dogs that received high doses of alendronate relative to the clinical doses used in the treatment of osteoporosis (>10 times). Chronic administration of alendronate (at least 0.1 mg/kg/d i.v. for 5 weeks) resulted in microscopic renal damage characterised by very slight to slight focal nephritis in dogs, although no corresponding changes in serum biochemical markers of renal impairment were observed [53]. In further follow-up studies, lower doses of alendronate (0.01 and 0.05 mg/kg/d i.v.) did not cause renal lesions. Similar results were reported in subsequent long-term studies in young dogs receiving oral alendronate at doses of 0.5, 2, or 8 mg/kg/d [53]. No renal lesions were reported at 27 weeks, and only a low incidence of chronic nephritis was seen at 53 weeks with the highest dose. Overall, high doses of alendronate (1 mg/kg/d i.v. or 8 mg/kg/d orally) may cause minimal renal lesions in dogs with no resulting impairment in renal function [53]. These data are consistent with the clinical experience accrued from the extensive use of oral alendronate for the treatment of osteoporosis, which shows minimal risk of renal impairment.

The nephrotoxicity of the experimental bisphosphonate cimadronate (also known as incadronate or YM-175) has also been investigated in dose-escalation studies in rats and dogs. Histopathologic signs of renal toxicity were observed in rats administered i.v. doses of cimadronate ≥0.62 mg/kg/d for 30 days; however, these effects were transient and disappeared after a 30-day recovery period [54]. By contrast, no renal toxicity was observed in rats treated for 26 weeks with weekly i.v. doses of 0.31-1.25 mg/kg/week. In corresponding studies in beagles, 2 dogs were killed in extremis due to renal failure at days 4 and 7 after a single cimadronate dose of 10 mg/kg i.v., whereas there were no drug-related findings at the lower doses of 0.3-3 mg/kg [55]. Animals treated for 30 days with cimadronate at a dose of 1 mg/kg/d i.v. exhibited nephropathy characterised by cortical tubular necrosis or degeneration with tubular dilation and basophilia, as well as slight interstitial nephritis, resulting in the death of 1 animal on day 16. These findings were not observed at lower doses (0.03-0.3 mg/kg/week). No histopathologic changes were observed in the kidney when the compound was administered for 26 weeks at doses of up to 1.25 mg/kg/week [55]. Overall, these findings with cimadronate are consistent with those observed for other bisphosphonates and suggest that renal toxicity, typically proximal tubular degeneration, is most probably a class effect associated with the mechanism of action of these compounds (i.e. inhibition of the enzyme FPPS in the mevalonate pathway). Nevertheless, an acceptable therapeutic window clearly exists for both oral and i.v. bisphosphonates, resulting in the efficacious inhibition of bone resorption with good overall tolerability.

Clinical renal toxicity

Similar to the data from preclinical studies, the tolerability profile of the different bisphosphonates in clinical use is not uniform and is dependent on the dosing regimen as well as the patient population. The extensive use of daily or weekly oral bisphosphonates to treat osteoporosis is primarily associated with gastrointestinal adverse effects including abdominal pain, dyspepsia, nausea, and esophagitis [9]. Renal tolerability has not emerged as an issue in this setting and will not be discussed further [9, 56-58]. For patients with metastatic bone disease, a monthly dosing schedule with i.v. bisphosphonate is established as the standard of care, but some compounds are also available in certain countries as oral formulations for oncology indications. Intravenous bisphosphonates are associated with mild to moderate flu-like symptoms in a significant proportion of patients, predominantly after the initial infusion [9], and adverse effects on renal function may also occur infrequently [9].

Consistent with the preclinical observations, all i.v. bisphosphonates have the potential to affect renal function in clinical use; however, renal adverse effects appear to be dependent on the baseline renal status of the patient and the dosing regimen. Although the incidence of renal adverse events is infrequent when i.v. bisphosphonates are administered at their recommended doses and infusion rates, monitoring of renal function is advisable in all patients receiving i.v. bisphosphonate therapy [29-34]. Attempts to compare the renal safety profiles of different bisphosphonates are confounded by limited head-to-head comparisons between different bisphosphonates. Although limited in number, double-blind, Phase III trials of bisphosphonates in comparison with placebo or active comparator provide the most stringent means to assess the relative effects of specific bisphosphonates on renal tolerability in a controlled setting.

Etidronate, clodronate and tiludronate

Early tolerability studies with the first-generation i.v. bisphosphonates etidronate and clodronate initially identified transient renal effects in patients receiving bisphosphonate therapy for HCM [59-69]. Fatal cases of renal failure were reported after the infusion of high doses of etidronate or clodronate in patients with breast cancer or multiple myeloma [60]. In an early randomised, comparative study of etidronate (3 infusions of 7.5 mg/kg/d for 3 consecutive days), clodronate (600-mg single i.v. infusion), and pamidronate (30-mg single i.v. infusion) in 48 patients with HCM, the latter compound was found to be the most potent at lowering serum calcium and also had the most rapid onset and the longest duration of response [61]. Deterioration of renal function was not observed in patients receiving clodronate or pamidronate; however, significant renal impairment developed in 1 etidronate-treated patient. In further studies with etidronate in patients with HCM, transient increases in serum creatinine were observed in some studies [11, 62, 64, 65]. Overall, in small studies of patients receiving i.v. etidronate for HCM, reports of creatinine elevation ranged from 0% [63] to 13% [64], depending on infusion rate, duration of treatment, and dose [59-65]. Similarly, in trials with a wide range of clodronate i.v. dosing regimens for the treatment of HCM, rates of serum creatinine elevation ranged from 0% to 24% [12, 13, 59, 61, 62, 66-69].

The clinical utility of another first-generation, non-nitrogen–containing bisphosphonate, tiludronate, has been limited because of concern over renal adverse effects observed in early trials. In a dose-finding study for the treatment of HCM, 19 patients received i.v. drug followed by oral maintenance therapy [70]. Three patients had elevated serum creatinine levels after i.v. drug administration of 4.5 or 6.0 mg/kg, 1 of whom developed acute renal insufficiency and subsequently died, most probably due to tiludronate, although renal infection and allopurinol therapy could have played a contributory role.

While receiving oral therapy with either 400 or 800

mg/d, 5 other patients also presented with elevated serum creatinine levels. From the results of this study, it was concluded that, in comparison with the nitrogen-containing bis-phosphonates, tiludronate could not be recommended for the treatment of HCM because of the need for high, potentially nephrotoxic, i.v. doses [70].

Pamidronate

In comparison with the results obtained with earlier bisphosphonates, clinical trials with the nitrogen-containing bisphosphonate pamidronate in more than 1, 300 patients with cancer have reported greater efficacy without a concomitant increase in renal toxicity.

In 3 large, randomised, double-blind, Phase III trials comparing pamidronate 90 mg against placebo in patients with multiple myeloma or breast cancer, renal safety was similar for both treatment groups on the basis of serum chemistry and clinical adverse events (Table 1) [16-18]. In 1 of the studies in patients with malignant bone disease from breast cancer, 1 patient in the pamidronate group discontinued treatment because of renal failure; however, this patient had a history of glomerulonephritis [17]. Similarly, in patients with bone metastases from multiple myeloma, a similar incidence of elevated serum creatinine values (≥1 mg/dl) above baseline was observed in both the pamidronate and placebo treatment groups [16]. However, the administration of pamidronate at doses higher than the recommended 90 mg/month to patients with multiple myeloma has been associated with nephrotic proteinuria, which reversed in the majority of cases after dose reduction or discontinuation [71].

Zoledronic acid

In small Phase I trials, bolus doses of zoledronic acid of up to 16 mg infused over 30 to 60 seconds appeared safe [72], but, subsequently, the infusion time for the 4-mg dose was extended first to 5 and then to 15 minutes, and the infusion volume was increased to 100 ml to ensure renal safety in routine clinical use. Moreover, further investigations with the 8-mg dose were discontinued because there was no evidence of increased efficacy versus 4 mg, and renal tolerability clearly decreased [19, 20, 22].

For the acute treatment of HCM, a single 5-minute infusion of zoledronic acid (4 or 8 mg) was investigated in 2 identical, randomised, double-blind, Phase III trials against a single 2-hour infusion of pamidronate 90 mg [15]. The complete response rates by day 10 were 88.4%, 86.7%, and 69.7% for zoledronic acid 4 mg, zoledronic acid 8 mg, and pamidronate 90 mg, respectively, whereas the corresponding grade 3/4 increases in serum creatinine were 2.3%, 5.2%, and 4%.

The long-term safety and efficacy of zoledronic acid in the oncology setting were investigated in 4 randomised, double-blind clinical trials involving more than 3, 000 patients with multiple myeloma, breast cancer, prostate cancer, and lung cancer or other solid tumours [19-22]. Zoledronic acid has demonstrated an acceptable renal safety profile compared with placebo in 3 long-term, placebo-controlled trials. In patients with prostate cancer who completed the 24-month study (n=122), there was no significant difference in time to first serum creatinine increase between patients who received 4 mg zoledronic acid compared with those who received placebo (P=0.752), and the hazard ratio (HR) of experiencing an elevation in serum creatinine was similar between the 2 groups (HR=1.14) [20, 73]. Similarly, in a randomised, Phase III, double-blind, placebo-controlled trial in 773 patients with lung cancer or other solid tumours, including renal cell carcinoma, there was a slight trend towards increased serum creatinine in patients receiving a 15-minute infusion of 4 mg zoledronic acid compared with those receiving placebo (HR=1.57); however, it was not statistically significant (P=0.228) [19]. Notably, in the subset of patients (n=33) with renal cell carcinoma who were assessed for safety, there was no significant difference in rate of renal adverse events between patients who received zoledronic acid (2/18) and those who received placebo (3/15) [74].

A Japanese study compared the efficacy and safety of zoledronic acid 4 mg, administered as a 15-minute infusion every month for 1 year, versus placebo in 228 women with bone metastases from breast cancer [21]. Zoledronic acid reduced skeletal-related events by 39% and was well tolerated with a safety profile similar to that of placebo. Only 1 patient in the zoledronic acid group had a notable serum creatinine increase (2.0 mg/dl) from a baseline of 1.3 mg/dl compared with 7 patients in the placebo group. Moreover, no patient treated with zoledronic acid developed a grade 3 or 4 serum creatinine increase according to the National Cancer Institute common toxicity criteria, whereas

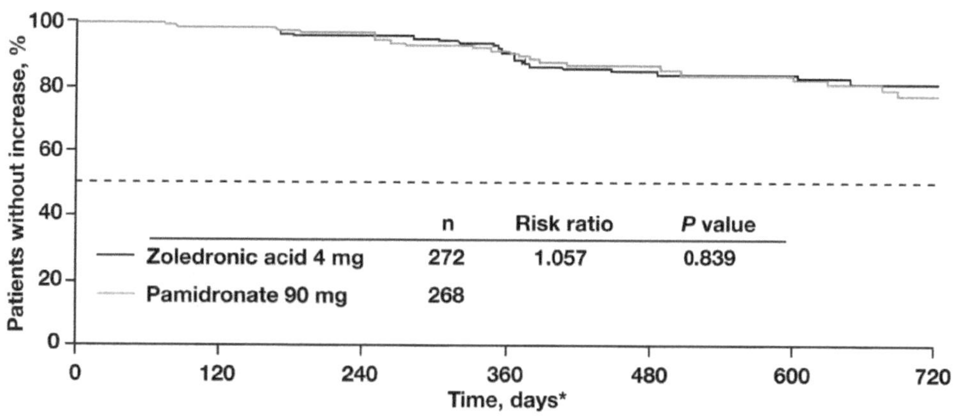

Figure 3. *Kaplan-Meier estimates of time to first notable serum creatinine increase in patients with multiple myeloma or breast cancer with bone metastases receiving 4 mg zoledronic acid or 90 mg pamidronate and Andersen-Gill multiple event analysis of the risk of elevated serum creatinine between treatment groups. *After start of study drug. (Reprinted with permission from [75])*

1 patient in the placebo group had a grade 3 serum creatinine elevation [21].

In the multicentre, Phase III comparative trial in patients with ≥1 bone lesion from breast cancer or multiple myeloma (N=1, 648), there were no significant differences in renal safety profiles between patients given a 15-minute infusion of 4 mg zoledronic acid and those given a 2-hour infusion of 90 mg pamidronate (Table 1) [22]. Kaplan-Meier estimates demonstrated that there were no significant differences in time to first notable serum creatinine increase between treatment groups (HR=1.057; P=0.839; Figure 3) [75].

Zoledronic acid has also been investigated in the prevention of cancer treatment-induced bone loss in 401 premenopausal women receiving adjuvant endocrine therapy for hormone-responsive breast cancer in a randomised, open-label, Phase III clinical trial [76]. In this study, patients received tamoxifen and goserelin with or without zoledronic acid (4 mg i.v. every 6 months) versus anastrozole and goserelin with or without zoledronic acid (4 mg i.v. every 6 months) for 3 years. The combination of zoledronic acid with endocrine therapy was well tolerated and was not associated with changes in renal function in this patient population. Over 3 years, 2, 904 serum creatinine measurements were taken, the mean serum creatinine level was 0.78 ± 0.17 mg/dl, and no patient had serum creatinine levels that exceeded 1.5 times the upper limit of normal [76].

Outside of the controlled clinical trial setting, the renal tolerability of zoledronic acid has also been assessed in routine practice at a single cancer centre. In a retrospective analysis of 446 patients with malignant bone disease who received a total of 3, 115 doses of zoledronic acid (median, 4 doses; range, 1-28 doses) over 2 years, renal deterioration was reported in 9.4% of patients (median rise in creatinine level, 1.0 mg/dl; range, 0.5-4.4 mg/dl) [77]. Eight patients discontinued zoledronic acid therapy because of renal deterioration; however, no patient required dialysis, and no patient died as a result of renal dysfunction [77].

In a retrospective analysis of spontaneous adverse event reports encompassing more than 430, 000 patients who had received zoledronic acid between August 2001 and March 2003, only 72 cases of renal failure were identified by the US Food and Drug Administration [78, 79]. It should be noted, however, that patients with risk factors for renal deterioration, including advanced cancer, previous bisphosphonate exposure, and use of nonsteroidal anti-inflammatory medications, may have contributed to the progression of renal failure [79]. Because of the potentially serious nature of this adverse event, it is recommended to monitor renal function in patients with cancer before each infusion of zoledronic acid, provide adequate hydration, and modify or discontinue treatment if renal complications occur [30, 78, 79].

The renal tolerability of zoledronic acid has also

been investigated in benign bone disease, using a dose of 5 mg infused over 15 minutes, either once for the treatment of Paget's disease or repeated annually for 3 years in postmenopausal osteoporosis. In 2 identical, randomised, double-blind, controlled trials with 357 patients suffering from Paget's disease, patients received either one 15-minute infusion of 5 mg zoledronic acid or 60 days of oral risedronate (30 mg/d) [23]. Zoledronic acid produced a significantly greater and quicker therapeutic response compared with risedronate in this patient population ($P<0.001$). One patient in each group who had pre-existing renal impairment developed moderate, but transient, increases in serum creatinine levels [23]. Similar results were observed in a double-blind, placebo-controlled trial of 7, 765 patients with postmenopausal osteoporosis who were randomly assigned to receive a single infusion of 5 mg zoledronic acid or placebo once a year for 3 years [24]. The annual infusion of zoledronic acid was highly effective at reducing fractures in this patient population. At 9-11 days after infusion, 1.3% of patients in the zoledronic acid group had a transient increase (>0.5 mg/dl) in the serum creatinine level compared with 0.4% in the placebo group ($P=0.001$). However, within 30 days, the levels in greater than 85% of patients returned to within 0.5 mg/dl of preinfusion values, and the remainder reached this level before the next annual infusion. At 3 years, there was no significant difference in either serum creatinine levels or creatinine clearance between the groups, indicating no cumulative effect on renal function [24].

Ibandronate

A Phase III, randomised, clinical trial investigated the efficacy and renal safety of i.v. ibandronate 6 mg (n=154) compared with placebo (n=158) infused over 1-2 hours every 3-4 weeks for up to 2 years in patients with malignant bone disease from breast cancer [26]. Ibandronate 6 mg significantly reduced skeletal events associated with metastatic disease ($P<0.05$) and lowered both pain and analgesic use. There was no evidence of renal toxicity associated with ibandronate treatment, and no patient withdrew from the study as a result of renal adverse events. The percentage of patients with increased creatinine levels (300 mM) was low overall but still 2-fold higher in the ibandronate 6-mg group (2.6%) compared with the placebo group (1.3%) [26]. A post hoc Kaplan-Meier analysis of time to serum creatinine increase revealed that, after 12 treatment months, 4% of patients receiving placebo and 2% of patients receiving ibandronate had increased serum creatinine [80]. At the 24-month time point, the proportion of patients with increased serum creatinine was 12% in the placebo group and 6% in the ibandronate 6-mg group (not significant; $P=0.22$ vs. placebo). Long-term follow-up indicated that the renal safety of ibandronate was maintained in 62 patients who completed an additional 2 years of treatment. The incidence of renal adverse events was comparable between groups (4.0% for ibandronate vs. 4.5% for placebo) [81]. In a small, Phase II, pilot study with a 16 mg loading dose of ibandronate administered as 4 mg over 2 hours for 4 consecutive days, no evidence of a deterioration in renal function was detected [82]. It appears that ibandronate can be safely administered to patients with severe renal impairment (<30 ml/min) at a reduced dose of 2 mg in 500 ml over 1 hour every 3-4 weeks [32, 33, 83]. However, this dose demonstrated only marginal efficacy in Phase III clinical trials in patients with breast cancer and bone metastases [26].

Oral ibandronate has also been investigated in patients with metastatic bone disease. In 2 pooled Phase III studies, 564 patients with metastatic bone disease from breast cancer were randomised to receive 50 mg oral ibandronate or placebo once daily for up to 96 weeks [84]. Oral ibandronate significantly reduced the mean rate of new skeletal complications by almost 20% compared with placebo ($P=0.004$). The incidence of mild treatment-related upper gastrointestinal adverse events was slightly higher for oral ibandronate compared with the placebo group, whereas the renal adverse event rate was comparable between the 2 groups (ibandronate, 5.2%; placebo, 4.7%) with no report of renal failure [84].

Although differences in the incidence of renal adverse events between bisphosphonates have been reported from clinical trials, the reasons for these observations remain unknown but may be specific to a particular drug, dosing regimen, or primary tumour type. Although more common in patients with pre-existing renal impairment, nephrotoxicity is not exclusive to this patient population. Clearly, further comparative clinical trials would be needed to directly compare the renal safety profiles of different i.v. bisphosphonates.

Histopathology

Nephrotoxicity of bisphosphonates is a known complication of this compound class, often exacerbated by diseases that compromise renal function, such as multiple myeloma, and by concomitant use of antineoplastic agents, steroids, and radiation therapy. The first reports of tubulointerstitial damage after treatment with etidronate and clodronate appeared more than 2 decades ago [60]. Subsequently, acute tubular necrosis, focal segmental glomerulosclerosis (FSGS), and granulomatous interstitial nephritis have been reported in renal biopsies from predominantly cancer patients exposed to several bisphosphonates, often at high i.v. doses.

Pamidronate

Not surprisingly, given the drug's widespread use for more than 15 years, the nephrotoxicity associated with pamidronate has been described in the most detail in a series of case reports on more than 20 patients. A prominent feature of the histopathology is often collapsing FSGS, as first reported by Markowitz et al. in biopsies from 6 patients with multiple myeloma (who, in any case, have a higher risk of renal impairment) and 1 patient with breast cancer given pamidronate for 15-48 months at doses ranging from 60-360 mg/month [85]. However, it should be pointed out that the approved pamidronate dose for the oncology indications is 90 mg i.v. every 3-4 weeks for up to 24 months [29]. All 7 biopsies displayed collapsing FSGS characterised by retraction of the glomerular basement membranes and hyperplasia of the overlying podocytes, many of which had numerous small mitochondria and cytoplasmic protein droplets (Figure 4) [85]. Although the proliferating cells were assumed to be hyperplastic podocytes, a subsequent detailed immunohistochemical study concluded that they were probably parietal epithelial cells [86]. Other notable features included diffuse mild to severe tubular atrophy and interstitial fibrosis with focal tubular microcyst formation and extensive degenerative changes in the proximal tubular epithelium. In no biopsy was there any evidence of amyloidosis, myeloma cast nephropathy, or light-chain deposition, indicating the absence of myeloma renal disease. Very similar findings were reported in a further 10 patients in 2 other case series comprising

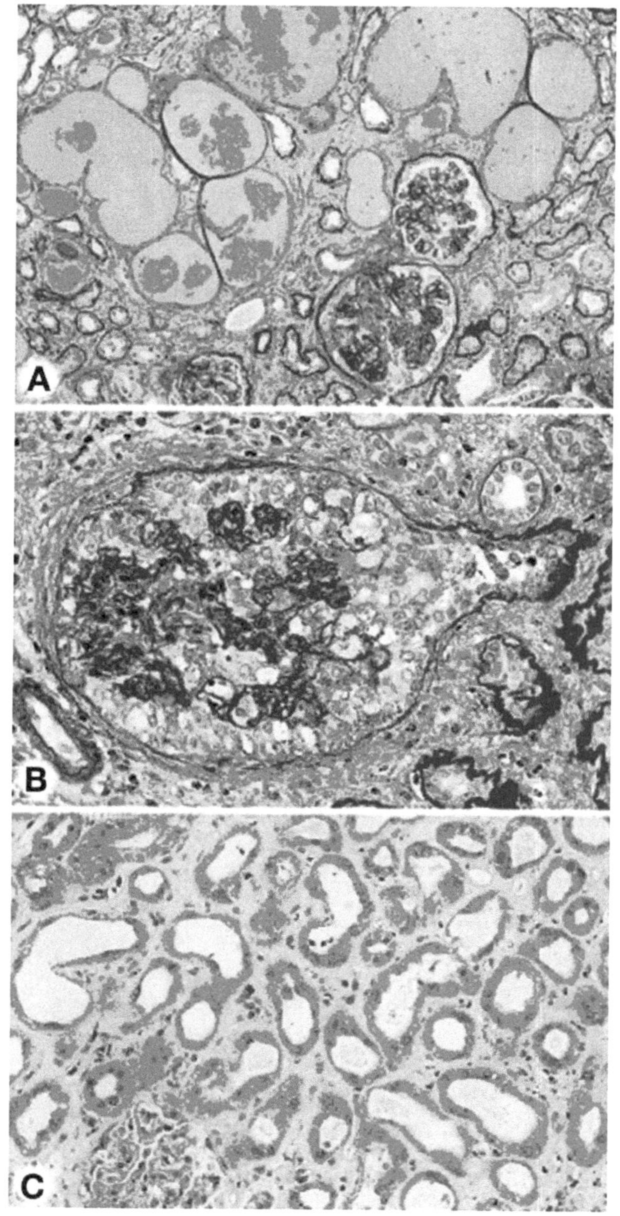

Figure 4. *Examples of renal histopathology from a group of 7 patients receiving pamidronate.* ***A.*** *Low-power view, showing glomeruli with collapsing sclerosis and severe tubulointerstitial damage, including tubular microcyst formation (patient 6). Periodic acid-Schiff stain.* ***B.*** *High-power view of a glomerulus from patient 5, showing global wrinkling and collapse of the glomerular basement membranes and marked hypertrophy and hyperplasia of visceral epithelial cells.* ***C.*** *High-power view showing diffuse tubular injury with interstitial edema, tubular simplification, and regenerative nuclear atypia (patient 1). (Reprinted with permission from [85])*

predominantly myeloma patients with proteinuria [71, 87]. Renal biopsy findings encompassed minimal-change disease, FSGS, collapsing FSGS, global sclerosis, and various degrees of podocyte injury. Again it should be noted that the administered pamidronate doses of up to 180 mg/month [71] or even 700 mg/month [87] greatly exceeded the approved dose.

However, collapsing FSGS may also occur in patients with cancer treated with the standard dose of pamidronate. Kunin et al. reported a myeloma patient with renal failure who had received pamidronate 90 mg/month for more than 3 years [88]. Examination of a renal biopsy by electron microscopy revealed a pathology consistent with collapsing glomerulopathy; namely, glomerular collapse with wrinkling and folding of the basal lamina, foot-process effacement of the glomerular podocytes, and an absence of electron-dense deposits. Similarly, Sauter et al. described a breast cancer patient with proteinuria and renal insufficiency who had been treated with pamidronate 90 mg/month for more than 3 years [89]. Evaluation by light microscopy of 11 glomeruli in a renal biopsy showed focal segmental, and also partly focal global, glomerulosclerosis. Electron microscopy showed disturbed podocyte architecture with foot-process effacement and a pronounced increase in the number of mitochondria that varied considerably in shape and size. At high magnification, focal degenerative changes in mitochondrial ultrastructure with vacuolisation and loss of cristae were observed (Figure 5) [89].

The collapsing FSGS associated with pamidronate therapy is not restricted to the oncology population; it has also been observed in a patient with Langerhans cell histiocytosis who had received a total of 11 doses of pamidronate 90 mg over 1 year and presented with renal failure requiring dialysis [90]. Although collapsing or noncollapsing FSGS appears to be a common feature of the nephrotoxicity associated with pamidronate, other histopathologies have occasionally been described. There is 1 report of renal failure in a patient with breast cancer treated for 11 months with pamidronate, initially at a dose of 60 mg/month for 4 months, rising to 90 mg/month thereafter [91]. The renal biopsy revealed acute tubulointerstitial nephritis with dense interstitial infiltration of lymphocytes, plasmacytes, and neutrophils, but without eosinophils. Renal function improved on withdrawal of pamidronate and initiation of corticosteroid therapy. Other non-oncology case reports have described patients who developed acute tubular necrosis and nephrosclerosis without immunologic or inflammatory tubulointerstitial involvement while receiving i.v. pamidronate therapy for hypercalcaemia of unknown origin [92] or osteoporosis [93]. The former patient had received a dose of 180 mg over 2 weeks; the latter had been infused with 90 mg/month for 20 months after having received oral alendronate 10 mg/day for 2 years. In both cases, renal function recovered after discontinuation of pamidronate treatment; however, the patient with osteoporosis was discovered to have monoclonal gammopathy of uncertain significance with highly elevated serum levels of β_2 microglobulin, which may have contributed to the deterioration of renal function.

Zoledronic acid

The histopathology of biopsies from patients with nephrotoxicity associated with zoledronic acid therapy was first described by Markowitz et al. in a cohort study of 5 patients with multiple myeloma and 1 patient with Paget's disease who all developed renal failure after i.v. administration of zoledronic acid at a dose of 4 mg/month for 3-9 months [94]. (It should be noted that the approved dose of zoledronic acid for Paget's disease is only a single 5-mg infusion [31].) The predominant finding was widespread marked tubular degeneration consistent with toxic, acute tubular necrosis (Figure 6) [94]. Immunohistochemistry revealed a marked increase in proliferating cells (Ki-67 positive) and an altered expression pattern of tubular Na^+/K^+-ATPase. Although all patients had received prior pamidronate treatment at a dose of 90 mg/month for up to 46 months, no biopsy exhibited the collapsing FSGS characteristic of pamidronate nephrotoxicity, but all showed some degree of global glomerulosclerosis. Renal function improved in all 6 patients following discontinuation of zoledronic acid (mean final serum creatinine: 2.3 mg/dl at 1 to 4 months of follow-up). Another case of acute toxic tubular necrosis with a very similar histopathology has been described in a myeloma patient with long-term renal impairment [95]. However, 2 years after discontinuation of zoledronic acid treatment, this patient still required haemodialysis.

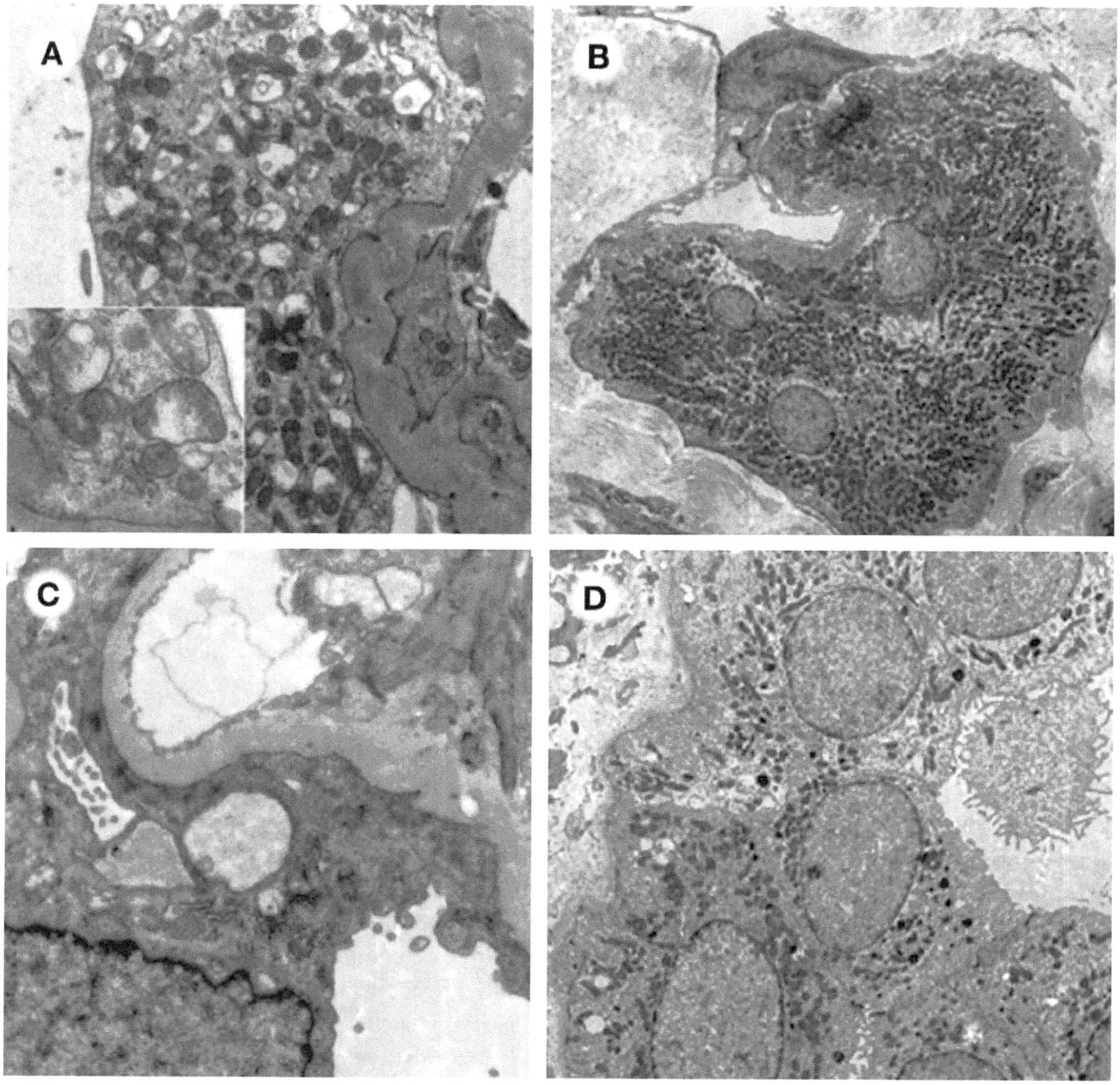

Figure 5. *Histopathology from 1 patient with breast cancer and proteinuria/renal insufficiency who had received pamidronate for 3+ years.* ***A.*** *Glomerulus with thickened and wrinkled basement membrane and a podocyte with prominent proliferation and degeneration of mitochondria (original magnification ×7,000); inlay shows high-power view of podocyte mitochondria with vacuolization and loss of cristae (original magnification ×20,000).* ***B.*** *Collapsed distal tubulus with a widened basement membrane and pronounced proliferation of mitochondria (original magnification ×3,000). In contrast to a biopsy specimen of minimal change disease with nephrotic syndrome, mitochondrial proliferation is absent in (**C**) podocytes (original magnification ×7,000) and (**D**) tubuli (original magnification ×3,000). (Reprinted with permission from [89], Copyright Elsevier 2006)*

Alendronate

Alendronate therapy of a patient with chronic lymphocytic leukaemia has been associated with the onset of acute granulomatous interstitial nephritis, a relatively rare renal pathology primarily caused by adverse drug reactions [27]. In this case, treatment with oral alendronate was initiated 2 weeks before admission for acute renal failure, implicating a causative role of this agent in the absence of any infectious or inflammatory condition. Moreover, the abnormal T-cell function associated with chronic lymphocytic leukaemia and lymphocytic infiltration of the kidney may have predisposed this patient to renal failure. The presence of granuloma distinguishes this case from another report of acute interstitial nephritis associated

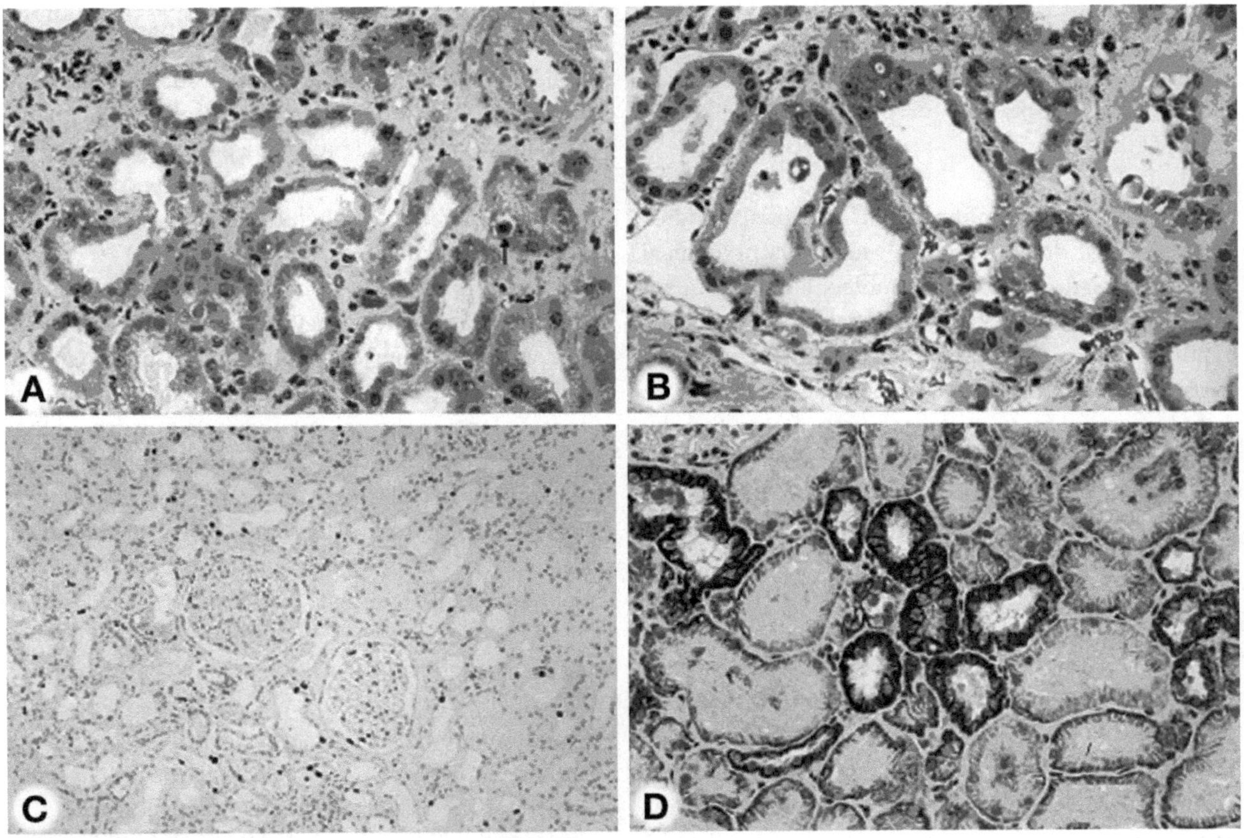

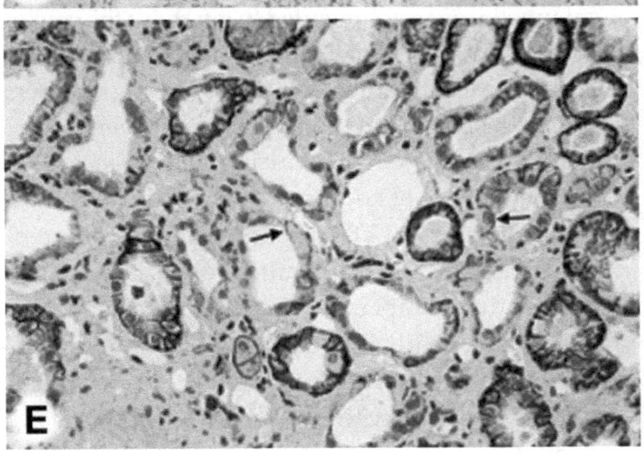

Figure 6. *Light microscopic and immunohistochemical findings in zoledronic acid-associated acute tubular necrosis (ATN). (A) A low power view shows extensive tubular damage including epithelial simplification, loss of brush-border, cytoplasmic hypereosinophilia, enlarged hyperchromatic nuclei, and nucleoli. Some tubular cells are undergoing apoptosis with phagocytosis of apoptotic bodies by neighboring epithelial cells (arrow). There is diffuse interstitial edema and fibrosis with mild mononuclear inflammatory infiltrates, without tubulitis (hematoxylin and eosin, ×160). (B) A high-power view illustrates the tubular cellular detail. The luminal borders are markedly irregular with simplified cells alternating with enlarged, hypereosinophilic cells. There is focal desquamation of apoptotic tubular epithelial cells into the lumen (hematoxylin and eosin, ×250). (C) Immunohistochemical staining for Ki-67 shows greater than 40 positively stained tubular nuclei in this field, indicating numerous cell cycle-engaged epithelial cells (×100). (D) Staining for Na^+,K^+-ATPase shows the normal, diffuse basolateral distribution with greater intensity of staining in distal than proximal tubules (×250). (E) By contrast, staining in zoledronic acid associated ATN shows diffuse reduction in intensity of basolateral staining for Na^+K^+ ATPase with foci of complete loss or apical translocation (arrows) (×250). (Reprinted with permission from [94], Copyright 2003)*

with bisphosphonate treatment in a patient with cancer administered pamidronate, discussed earlier [91]. A case of collapsing FSGS and severe kidney dysfunction has recently been reported in a liver transplant recipient soon after the initiation of oral alendronate therapy (35 mg/week) to prevent steroid-induced osteopenia [96]. In a renal biopsy containing 15 glomeruli, 12 were globally or markedly segmentally sclerosed, and 5 exhibited marked segmental sclerosis with collapsing capillary loops associated with overlying visceral cell hyperplasia. Extensive interstitial lymphocytic infiltrates with increased eosinophils and frequent polymorphonuclear cells associated with interstitial fibrosis were also observed.

Conclusion

The nephrotoxic potential of bisphosphonates has been well documented in numerous preclinical and clinical studies, but the molecular mechanism remains elusive. The observed effects on kidney cells in clinical biopsies are reminiscent of those reported in osteoclasts; namely, the inhibition of FPPS and reduced prenylation of key signalling proteins, thereby impairing normal intracellular metabolism and inducing apoptosis [94]. Moreover, mitochondrial changes revealed by electron microscopy of renal biopsies also resemble those associated with bisphosphonate-induced inhibition of the mevalonate pathway [89, 97]. This hypothesis is supported by the fact that the fraction of a bisphosphonate dose that does not bind bone is exclusively cleared by renal excretion, thus exposing the kidney to high drug levels.

Renal adverse events have been more frequently reported in patients receiving treatment with i.v. pamidronate or zoledronic acid than with other bisphosphonates. Although this may be partly due to the high potency and dosing regimens of these 2 agents, other contributing factors include the widespread use of these compounds in oncology, renal impairment associated with malignant disease, age-related renal insufficiency, and the concomitant administration of nephrotoxic antineoplastic agents. Furthermore, as awareness of the nephrotoxic potential of bisphosphonates increased, renal function was prospectively monitored in the clinical trials with i.v. pamidronate and zoledronic acid, a practice not followed regularly in earlier bisphosphonate studies.

Bisphosphonates have clearly established therapeutic benefits and are widely used to treat both benign and malignant bone disease. Oral bisphosphonates have been prescribed for many years to millions of patients for fracture prevention in the treatment of postmenopausal osteoporosis and have an excellent renal tolerability record. The low incidence of renal complications in patients receiving oral bisphosphonate therapy is most probably related to the minimal systemic exposure associated with the low oral bioavailability of this class of compound. Similarly, the quarterly and annual i.v. dosing regimens of ibandronate and zoledronic acid, respectively, approved for the treatment of postmenopausal osteoporosis are very well tolerated and their use is not associated with progressive renal impairment [9, 98].

In oncology, i.v. bisphosphonates have demonstrated efficacy in delaying the onset and reducing the incidence of skeletal complications in patients with malignant bone disease from a broad range of tumour types. Extensive clinical data have demonstrated that the benefits of bisphosphonate therapy in patients with cancer far outweigh the risks of renal impairment that may occur in a minority of patients. Serious renal side effects are rare in comparison with the large number of patients treated with i.v. bisphosphonates. Postmarketing experience indicates that the approved dosing regimens are well tolerated in most patients with normal renal function as well as in those with mild to moderate renal impairment. Nevertheless, because bisphosphonates are cleared through the kidneys and thus renal exposure to drug is high, monitoring of renal function is recommended throughout the course of treatment. Most renal complications are transient and manageable by adjustment of the dosing regimen; however, bisphosphonates are not recommended for patients with severe renal impairment.

In the absence of additional, head-to-head clinical trials comparing the efficacy and safety of different bisphosphonates, it is difficult to draw conclusions on the relative therapeutic indices of these agents. The available data clearly indicate that an acceptable therapeutic window exists for the currently approved oral and i.v. bisphosphonates. When used appropriately, they offer a large number of patients suffering from a range of benign and malignant bone diseases an efficacious and well-tolerated therapeutic option.

Acknowledgement

The author gratefully acknowledges the editorial assistance of Carol Sledz, PhD, ProEd Communications, Inc.®, in the preparation of this manuscript.

References

1. Seeman E, Delmas PD. Bone quality—the material and structural basis of bone strength and fragility. N Engl J Med 2006; 354: 2250-2261.
2. Raisz LG. Pathogenesis of osteoporosis: concepts, conflicts, and prospects. J Clin Invest 2005; 115: 3318-3325.
3. Lipton A. Pathophysiology of bone metastases: how this knowledge may lead to therapeutic intervention. J Support Oncol 2004; 2: 205-213.
4. Body JJ. Rationale for the use of bisphosphonates in osteoblastic and osteolytic bone lesions. Breast 2003; 12(suppl 2): S37-S44.
5. Rogers MJ. New insights into the molecular mechanisms of action of bisphosphonates. Curr Pharm Des 2003; 9: 2643-2658.
6. Silverman SL, Maricic M. Recent developments in bisphosphonate therapy. Semin Arthritis Rheum 2007; 37: 1-12.
7. Fleisch H. Bisphosphonates: mechanism of action. Endocr Rev 1998; 19: 80-100.
8. Rondeau JM, Bitsch F, Bourgier E, Geiser M, Hemmig R, Kroemer M, Lehmann S, Ramage P, Rieffel S, Strauss A, et al. Structural basis for the exceptional *in vivo* efficacy of bisphosphonate drugs. ChemMedChem 2006; 1: 267-273.
9. Bobba RS, Beattie K, Parkinson B, Kumbhare D, Adachi JD. Tolerability of different dosing regimens of bisphosphonates for the treatment of osteoporosis and malignant bone disease. Drug Saf 2006; 29: 1133-1152.
10. Cramer JA, Amonkar MM, Hebborn A, Altman R. Compliance and persistence with bisphosphonate dosing regimens among women with postmenopausal osteoporosis. Curr Med Res Opin 2005; 21: 1453-1460.
11. Gucalp R, Ritch P, Wiernik PH, Sarma PR, Keller A, Richman SP, Tauer K, Neidhart J, Mallette LE, Siegel R, et al. Comparative study of pamidronate disodium and etidronate disodium in the treatment of cancer-related hypercalcemia. J Clin Oncol 1992; 10: 134-142.
12. Purohit OP, Radstone CR, Anthony C, Kanis JA, Coleman RE. A randomised double-blind comparison of intravenous pamidronate and clodronate in the hypercalcaemia of malignancy. Br J Cancer 1995; 72: 1289-1293.
13. Atula ST, Tahtela RK, Nevalainen JI, Pylkkanen LH. Clodronate as a single-dose intravenous infusion effectively provides short-term correction of malignant hypercalcemia. Acta Oncol 2003; 42: 735-740.
14. Gucalp R, Theriault R, Gill I, Madajewicz S, Chapman R, Navari R, Ahmann F, Zelenakas K, Heffernan M, Knight RD. Treatment of cancer-associated hypercalcemia. Double-blind comparison of rapid and slow intravenous infusion regimens of pamidronate disodium and saline alone. Arch Intern Med 1994; 154: 1935-1944.
15. Major P, Lortholary A, Hon J, Abdi E, Mills G, Menssen HD, Yunus F, Bell R, Body J, Quebe-Fehling E, et al. Zoledronic acid is superior to pamidronate in the treatment of hypercalcemia of malignancy: a pooled analysis of two randomized, controlled clinical trials. J Clin Oncol 2001; 19: 558-567.
16. Berenson JR, Lichtenstein A, Porter L, Dimopoulos MA, Bordoni R, George S, Lipton A, Keller A, Ballester O, Kovacs M, et al. Long-term pamidronate treatment of advanced multiple myeloma patients reduces skeletal events. Myeloma Aredia Study Group. J Clin Oncol 1998; 16: 593-602.
17. Hortobagyi GN, Theriault RL, Lipton A, Porter L, Blayney D, Sinoff C, Wheeler H, Simeone JF, Seaman JJ, Knight RD, et al. Long-term prevention of skeletal complications of metastatic breast cancer with pamidronate. Protocol 19 Aredia Breast Cancer Study Group. J Clin Oncol 1998; 16: 2038-2044.
18. Theriault RL, Lipton A, Hortobagyi GN, Leff R, Gluck S, Stewart JF, Costello S, Kennedy I, Simeone J, Seaman JJ, et al. Pamidronate reduces skeletal morbidity in women with advanced breast cancer and lytic bone lesions: a randomized, placebo-controlled trial. Protocol 18 Aredia Breast Cancer Study Group. J Clin Oncol 1999; 17: 846-854.
19. Rosen LS, Gordon D, Tchekmedyian NS, Yanagihara R, Hirsh V, Krzakowski M, Pawlicki M, De Souza P, Zheng M, Urbanowitz G, et al. Long-term efficacy and safety of zoledronic acid in the treatment of skeletal metastases in patients with nonsmall cell lung carcinoma and other solid tumors: a randomized, phase III, double-blind, placebo-controlled trial. Cancer 2004; 100: 2613-2621.
20. Saad F, Gleason DM, Murray R, Tchekmedyian S, Venner P, Lacombe L, Chin JL, Vinholes JJ, Goas JA, Chen B. A randomized, placebo-controlled trial of zoledronic acid in patients with hormone-refractory metastatic prostate carcinoma. J Natl Cancer Inst 2002; 94: 1458-1468.
21. Kohno N, Aogi K, Minami H, Nakamura S, Asaga T, Iino Y, Watanabe T, Goessl C, Ohashi Y, Takashima S. Zoledronic acid significantly reduces skeletal complications compared with placebo in Japanese women with bone metastases from breast cancer: a randomized, placebo-controlled trial. J Clin Oncol 2005; 23: 3314-3321.
22. Rosen LS, Gordon D, Kaminski M, Howell A, Belch A, Mackey J, Apffelstaedt J, Hussein MA, Coleman RE, Reitsma DJ, et al. Long-term efficacy and safety of zoledronic acid compared with pamidronate disodium in the treatment of skeletal complications in patients with advanced multiple myeloma or breast carcinoma: a randomized, double-blind, multicenter, comparative trial. Cancer 2003; 98: 1735-1744.

23. Reid IR, Miller P, Lyles K, Fraser W, Brown JP, Saidi Y, Mesenbrink P, Su G, Pak J, Zelenakas K, et al. Comparison of a single infusion of zoledronic acid with risedronate for Paget's disease. N Engl J Med 2005; 353: 898-908.
24. Black DM, Delmas PD, Eastell R, Reid IR, Boonen S, Cauley JA, Cosman F, Lakatos P, Leung PC, Man Z, et al. Once-yearly zoledronic acid for treatment of postmenopausal osteoporosis. N Engl J Med 2007; 356: 1809-1822.
25. Ralston SH, Thiebaud D, Herrmann Z, Steinhauer EU, Thurlimann B, Walls J, Lichinitser MR, Rizzoll R, Hagberg H, Huss HJ, et al. Dose-response study of ibandronate in the treatment of cancer-associated hypercalcaemia. Br J Cancer 1997; 75: 295-300.
26. Body JJ, Diel IJ, Lichinitser MR, Kreuser ED, Dornoff W, Gorbunova VA, Budde M, Bergstrom B. Intravenous ibandronate reduces the incidence of skeletal complications in patients with breast cancer and bone metastases. Ann Oncol 2003; 14: 1399-1405.
27. Pena de la Vega L, Fervenza FC, Lager D, Habermann T, Leung N. Acute granulomatous interstitial nephritis secondary to bisphosphonate alendronate sodium. Ren Fail 2005; 27: 485-489.
28. Zazgornik J, Grafinger P, Biesenbach G, Hubmann R, Fridrik M. Acute renal failure and alendronate. Nephrol Dial Transplant 1997; 12: 2797-2798.
29. Aredia® [package insert]. East Hanover, NJ: Novartis Pharmaceuticals Corp; 2005.
30. Zometa® [package insert]. East Hanover, NJ: Novartis Pharmaceuticals Corp; 2005.
31. Reclast® [package insert]. East Hanover, NJ: Novartis Pharmaceuticals Corp; 2007.
32. Boniva® [package insert]. Nutley, NJ: Roche Pharmaceuticals; 2007.
33. Bondronat® [package insert]. Welwyn Garden City, UK: Roche Registration Ltd; 2006.
34. Bonefos® [European SPC]. Schering Health Care Limited, West Sussex, UK; 2006.
35. Lin JH. Bisphosphonates: a review of their pharmacokinetic properties. Bone 1996; 18: 75-85.
36. Actonel® [package insert]. Bridgewater, NJ: Procter & Gamble Pharmaceuticals, Inc; 2006.
37. Cremers S, Weiss M, Moenius T, Fresneau M, Schmid D, Schran H. Plasma protein binding of ibandronate and zoledronic acid. J Bone Miner Res 2006; 21(suppl): S286. Abstract SU319.
38. Daley-Yates PT, Cal JC, Cockshott A, Pongchaidecha M, Gilchrist K. Plasma protein binding of APD: role of calcium and transferrin. Chem Biol Interact 1992; 81: 79-89.
39. Porras AG, Holland SD, Gertz BJ. Pharmacokinetics of alendronate. Clin Pharmacokinet 1999; 36: 315-328.
40. Saha H, Castren-Kortekangas P, Ojanen S, Juhakoski A, Tuominen J, Tokola O, Pasternack A. Pharmacokinetics of clodronate in renal failure. J Bone Miner Res 1994; 9: 1953-1958.
41. Berenson JR, Rosen L, Vescio R, Lau HS, Woo M, Sioufi A, Kowalski MO, Knight RD, Seaman JJ. Pharmacokinetics of pamidronate disodium in patients with cancer with normal or impaired renal function. J Clin Pharmacol 1997; 37: 285-290.
42. Skerjanec A, Berenson J, Hsu C, Major P, Miller WH, Jr., Ravera C, Schran H, Seaman J, Waldmeier F. The pharmacokinetics and pharmacodynamics of zoledronic acid in cancer patients with varying degrees of renal function. J Clin Pharmacol 2003; 43: 154-162.
43. Troehler U, Bonjour JP, Fleisch H. Renal secretion of diphosphonates in rats. Kidney Int 1975; 8: 6-13.
44. Lin JH, Chen IW, Deluna FA, Hichens M. Renal handling of alendronate in rats. An uncharacterized renal transport system. Drug Metab Dispos 1992; 20: 608-613.
45. Ullrich KJ, Rumrich G, Burke TR, Shirazi-Beechey SP, Lang H. Interaction of alkyl/arylphosphonates, phosphonocarboxylates and diphosphonates with different anion transport systems in the proximal renal tubule. J Pharmacol Exp Ther 1997; 283: 1223-1229.
46. Kino I, Kato Y, Lin JH, Sugiyama Y. Renal handling of bisphosphonate alendronate in rats. Biopharm Drug Dispos 1999; 20: 193-198.
47. Pfister T, Atzpodien E, Bauss F. The renal effects of minimally nephrotoxic doses of ibandronate and zoledronate following single and intermittent intravenous administration in rats. Toxicology 2003; 191: 159-167.
48. Hirschberg R. Nephrotoxicity of third-generation, intravenous bisphosphonates. Toxicology 2004; 196: 165-167; author reply 169-170.
49. Williams PR, Smith NC, Cooke-Yarborough C, Little DG. Bisphosphonates and nephrocalcinosis in a rabbit leg lengthening model: a histological and therapeutic comparison. Pharmacol Toxicol 2001; 89: 149-152.
50. Green JR, Seltenmeyer Y, Jaeggi KA, Widler L. Renal tolerability profile of novel, potent bisphosphonates in two short-term rat models. Pharmacol Toxicol 1997; 80: 225-230.
51. Pfister T, Atzpodien E, Bohrmann B, Bauss F. Acute renal effects of intravenous bisphosphonates in the rat. Basic Clin Pharmacol Toxicol 2005; 97: 374-381.
52. Cal JC, Daley-Yates PT. Disposition and nephrotoxicity of 3-amino-1-hydroxypropylidene-1, 1-bisphosphonate (APD), in rats and mice. Toxicology 1990; 65: 179-197.
53. Peter C, Rodan GA. Preclinical safety profile of alendronate. Int J Clin Pract Suppl 1999; 101: 3-8.

54. Okazaki A, Sakai H, Matsuzawa T, Perkin CJ, East PW. Intravenous single and repeated dose toxicity studies of cimadronate (YM175), a novel bisphosphonate, in rats. J Toxicol Sci 1995; 20(suppl 1): 15-26.
55. Okazaki A, Matsuzawa T, Perkin CJ, Barker MH. Intravenous single and repeated dose toxicity studies of cimadronate (YM175), a novel bisphosphonate, in beagle dogs. J Toxicol Sci 1995; 20(suppl 1): 27-36.
56. Miller PD, Roux C, Boonen S, Barton IP, Dunlap LE, Burgio DE. Safety and efficacy of risedronate in patients with age-related reduced renal function as estimated by the Cockcroft and Gault method: a pooled analysis of nine clinical trials. J Bone Miner Res 2005; 20: 2105-2115.
57. Yanik B, Bavbek N, Yanik T, Inegol I, Kanbay M, Turgut FH, Uz E, Akcay A. The effect of alendronate, risedronate, and raloxifene on renal functions, based on the Cockcroft and Gault method, in postmenopausal women. Ren Fail 2007; 29: 471-476.
58. McClung MR, Wasnich RD, Recker R, Cauley JA, Chesnut CH, 3rd, Ensrud KE, Burdeska A, Mills T, Oral Ibandronate Study Group. Oral daily ibandronate prevents bone loss in early postmenopausal women without osteoporosis. J Bone Miner Res 2004; 19: 11-18.
59. Zojer N, Keck AV, Pecherstorfer M. Comparative tolerability of drug therapies for hypercalcaemia of malignancy. Drug Saf 1999; 21: 389-406.
60. Bounameaux HM, Schifferli J, Montani JP, Jung A, Chatelanat F. Renal failure associated with intravenous diphosphonates. Lancet 1983; 1: 471.
61. Ralston SH, Gallacher SJ, Patel U, Dryburgh FJ, Fraser WD, Cowan RA, Boyle IT. Comparison of three intravenous bisphosphonates in cancer-associated hypercalcaemia. Lancet 1989; 2: 1180-1182.
62. Kanis JA, Preston CJ, Yates AJ, Percival RC, Mundy KI, Russell RG. Effects of intravenous diphosphonates on renal function. Lancet 1983; 1: 1328.
63. Flores JF, Singer FR, Rude RK. Effectiveness of a 24-hour infusion of etidronate disodium in the treatment of hypercalcemia of malignant disease. A dose-ranging pilot study. Miner Electrolyte Metab 1991; 17: 390-395.
64. Warrell RP, Jr., Murphy WK, Schulman P, O'Dwyer PJ, Heller G. A randomized double-blind study of gallium nitrate compared with etidronate for acute control of cancer-related hypercalcemia. J Clin Oncol 1991; 9: 1467-1475.
65. Singer FR, Ritch PS, Lad TE, Ringenberg QS, Schiller JH, Recker RR, Ryzen E. Treatment of hypercalcemia of malignancy with intravenous etidronate. A controlled, multicenter study. The Hypercalcemia Study Group. Arch Intern Med 1991; 151: 471-476.
66. Jacobs TP, Siris ES, Bilezikian JP, Baquiran DC, Shane E, Canfield RE. Hypercalcemia of malignancy: treatment with intravenous dichloromethylene diphosphonate. Ann Intern Med 1981; 94: 312-316.
67. Ziegler R, Scharla SH. Treatment of tumor hypercalcemia with clodronate. Recent Results Cancer Res 1989; 116: 46-53.
68. Harjung H, Fritze D. [Monotherapy with clodronate for tumor-induced hypercalcemia]. Dtsch Med Wochenschr 1990; 115: 48-52.
69. O'Rourke NP, McCloskey EV, Vasikaran S, Eyres K, Fern D, Kanis JA. Effective treatment of malignant hypercalcaemia with a single intravenous infusion of clodronate. Br J Cancer 1993; 67: 560-563.
70. Dumon JC, Magritte A, Body JJ. Efficacy and safety of the bisphosphonate tiludronate for the treatment of tumor-associated hypercalcemia. Bone Miner 1991; 15: 257-266.
71. Desikan R, Veksler Y, Raza S, Stokes B, Sabir T, Li ZJ, Jagannath S. Nephrotic proteinuria associated with high-dose pamidronate in multiple myeloma. Br J Haematol 2002; 119: 496-499.
72. Berenson JR, Vescio R, Henick K, Nishikubo C, Rettig M, Swift RA, Conde F, Von Teichert JM. A phase I, open label, dose ranging trial of intravenous bolus zoledronic acid, a novel bisphosphonate, in cancer patients with metastatic bone disease. Cancer 2001; 91: 144-154.
73. Saad F, Gleason D, Murray R, Venner P, Tchekmedyian NS, Lacombe L, Chin J, Vinholes J, Goas JA, Chen B-L, et al. Zoledronic acid is well tolerated for up to 24 months and significantly reduces skeletal complications in patients with advanced prostate cancer metastatic to bone. J Urol 2003; 169(suppl): 394. Abstract 1472.
74. Lipton A, Zheng M, Seaman J. Zoledronic acid delays the onset of skeletal-related events and progression of skeletal disease in patients with advanced renal cell carcinoma. Cancer 2003; 98: 962-969.
75. Conte P, Guarneri V. Safety of intravenous and oral bisphosphonates and compliance with dosing regimens. Oncologist 2004; 9(suppl 4): 28-37.
76. Gnant MF, Mlineritsch B, Luschin-Ebengreuth G, Grampp S, Kaessmann H, Schmid M, Menzel C, Piswanger-Soelkner JC, Galid A, Mittlboeck M, et al. Zoledronic acid effectively prevents cancer treatment-induced bone loss in premenopausal women receiving adjuvant endocrine therapy for hormone-responsive breast cancer: a report from the Austrian Breast and Colorectal Cancer Study Group. J Clin Oncol 2007; 25: 820-828.
77. McDermott RS, Kloth DD, Wang H, Hudes GR, Langer CJ. Impact of zoledronic acid on renal function in patients with cancer: clinical significance and development of a predictive model. J Support Oncol 2006; 4: 524-529.
78. Chang JT, Green L, Beitz J. Renal failure with the use of zoledronic acid. N Engl J Med 2003; 349: 1676-1678.

79. Tarassoff P, Hei Y-J, Maladorno D. Renal failure with the use of zoledronic acid. N Engl J Med 2003; 349: 1678-1679.
80. Body JJ, Diel IJ, Tripathy D, Bergstrom B. Intravenous ibandronate does not affect time to renal function deterioration in patients with skeletal metastases from breast cancer: phase III trial results. Eur J Cancer Care (Engl) 2006; 15: 299-302.
81. Diel I, Body JJ, Bergstrom B. Renal safety of intravenous (i.v.) ibandronate for up to 4 years of treatment in patients with metastatic bone disease [abstract]. Ann Oncol 2004; 15(suppl 3): iii224. Abstract 850P.
82. Mancini I, Dumon JC, Body JJ. Efficacy and safety of ibandronate in the treatment of opioid-resistant bone pain associated with metastatic bone disease: a pilot study. J Clin Oncol 2004; 22: 3587-3592.
83. Pecherstorfer M, Diel IJ. Rapid administration of ibandronate does not affect renal functioning: evidence from clinical studies in metastatic bone disease and hypercalcaemia of malignancy. Support Care Cancer 2004; 12: 877-881.
84. Body JJ, Diel IJ, Lichinitzer M, Lazarev A, Pecherstorfer M, Bell R, Tripathy D, Bergstrom B. Oral ibandronate reduces the risk of skeletal complications in breast cancer patients with metastatic bone disease: results from two randomised, placebo-controlled phase III studies. Br J Cancer 2004; 90: 1133-1137.
85. Markowitz GS, Appel GB, Fine PL, Fenves AZ, Loon NR, Jagannath S, Kuhn JA, Dratch AD, D'Agati VD. Collapsing focal segmental glomerulosclerosis following treatment with high-dose pamidronate. J Am Soc Nephrol 2001; 12: 1164-1172.
86. Dijkman HB, Weening JJ, Smeets B, Verrijp KC, van Kuppevelt TH, Assmann KK, Steenbergen EJ, Wetzels JF. Proliferating cells in HIV and pamidronate-associated collapsing focal segmental glomerulosclerosis are parietal epithelial cells. Kidney Int 2006; 70: 338-344.
87. Barri YM, Munshi NC, Sukumalchantra S, Abulezz SR, Bonsib SM, Wallach J, Walker PD. Podocyte injury associated glomerulopathies induced by pamidronate. Kidney Int 2004; 65: 634-641.
88. Kunin M, Kopolovic J, Avigdor A, Holtzman EJ. Collapsing glomerulopathy induced by long-term treatment with standard-dose pamidronate in a myeloma patient. Nephrol Dial Transplant 2004; 19: 723-726.
89. Sauter M, Julg B, Porubsky S, Cohen C, Fischereder M, Sitter T, Schlondorff D, Grone HJ. Nephrotic-range proteinuria following pamidronate therapy in a patient with metastatic breast cancer: mitochondrial toxicity as a pathogenetic concept? Am J Kidney Dis 2006; 47: 1075-1080.
90. Lockridge L, Papac RJ, Perazella MA. Pamidronate-associated nephrotoxicity in a patient with Langerhans's histiocytosis. Am J Kidney Dis 2002; 40: E2.
91. Janssen van Doorn K, Neyns B, Van der Niepen P, Verbeelen D. Pamidronate-related nephrotoxicity (tubulointerstitial nephritis) in a patient with osteolytic bone metastases. Nephron 2001; 89: 467-468.
92. Banerjee D, Asif A, Striker L, Preston RA, Bourgoignie JJ, Roth D. Short-term, high-dose pamidronate-induced acute tubular necrosis: the postulated mechanisms of bisphosphonate nephrotoxicity. Am J Kidney Dis 2003; 41: E18.
93. Smetana S, Michlin A, Rosenman E, Biro A, Boaz M, Katzir Z. Pamidronate-induced nephrotoxic tubular necrosis—a case report. Clin Nephrol 2004; 61: 63-67.
94. Markowitz GS, Fine PL, Stack JI, Kunis CL, Radhakrishnan J, Palecki W, Park J, Nasr SH, Hoh S, Siegel DS, et al. Toxic acute tubular necrosis following treatment with zoledronate (Zometa). Kidney Int 2003; 64: 281-289.
95. Ramazzina C, Zysset Aschmann Y, Kummer O, Ratz Bravo AE, Bodmer M. [Zoledronate-associated end stage renal failure and hypocalcaemia]. Schweiz Rundsch Med Prax 2007; 96: 673-676; quiz 677-678.
96. Pascual J, Torrealba J, Myers J, Tome S, Samaniego M, Musat A, Djamali A. Collapsing focal segmental glomerulosclerosis in a liver transplant recipient on alendronate. Osteoporos Int 2007; 18: 1435-1438.
97. Cafforio P, Dammacco F, Gernone A, Silvestris F. Statins activate the mitochondrial pathway of apoptosis in human lymphoblasts and myeloma cells. Carcinogenesis 2005; 26: 883-891.
98. Boonen S, Sellmeyer DE, Lippuner K, Orlov-Morozov A, Abrams K, Mesenbrink P, Eriksen EF, Miller PD. Renal safety of zoledronic acid 5 mg annual infusion in osteoporotic postmenopausal women: results of 3 year HORIZON PFT. Kidney Int 2008, in press.

25

Proton pump inhibitors: acute interstitial nephritis and other renal effects

Ursula C. BREWSTER and Mark A. PERAZELLA

Section of Nephrology, Yale University School of Medicine, New Haven, Connecticut, USA

Introduction

Proton pump inhibitors (PPIs) were introduced in 1989 with the development of omeprazole. Since then, they have become one of the most widely prescribed class of drugs on the market today. Over 43 million prescriptions were written for anti-ulcer therapy in the US in 2005 [1]. Currently, there are five PPIs available in the United States and Europe: esomeprazole, lansoprazole, omeprazole, pantoprazole and rabeprazole. Their safety and efficacy profile is excellent, which has been the major factor leading to over 8 billion dollars in sales in 2005; a considerable sum given that omeprazole has been available since 2003 [2]. However, renal complications do occur and it is important that they are recognized. Reported events include rare hyponatremia, drug-drug interactions and acute interstitial nephritis (AIN). There are, as of yet, no data on chronic interstitial disease resulting from these agents. However, it is certainly conceivable that long standing AIN may transition to chronic interstitial nephritis and end-stage renal disease.

Mechanism of action

PPIs decrease acid secretion by binding the H^+/K^+ ATPase at the secretory surface of gastric parietal epithelial cells. The drug is protonated to its active form by the low gastric pH, whereby it then covalently binds the receptor as a non-competitive inhibitor (Figure 1). This decreases both basal and stimulated gastric acid secretion. The drug undergoes hepatic metabolism and inactive metabolites (hydroxy, desmethyl, sulphone) are excreted in the urine. Importantly, although there are H^+/K^+ ATPase on the apical surface of renal tubular cells, omeprazole, when given to healthy male subjects did not disrupt renal electrolyte balance or urinary pH [3]. Thus, there is no *in vivo* effect on renal tubular acid handling, and seemingly no effect on urinary pH.

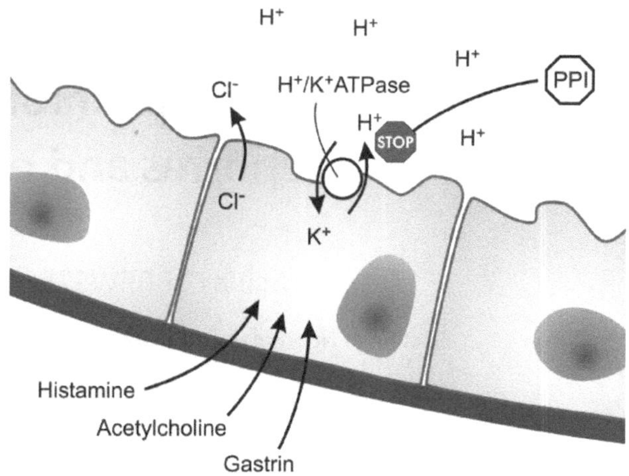

Figure 1. *Gastric parietal epithelial cells possess a H^+/K^+ ATPase that secretes H^+ ions into the gastric lumen in response to stimulation by histamine, acetylcholine or gastrin. Proton pump inhibitors are protonated into their active form by the acidic gastric environment. They covalently bind to the H^+/K^+*

Pharmacokinetics

PPIs are metabolized via the cytochrome P450 (CYP) system. They do, however, have important differences that are briefly noted in Table 1 [4]. Oral bioavailability ranges from 30-90% depending on specific drug, and all are highly protein bound with a small volume of distribution (0.17 L/kg - 0.45 L/kg). Metabolism of active drug occurs primarily via CYP2C19 and CYP3A4 (Figure 2). Lansoprazole is metabolized equally by both enzymes, whereas metabolism of esomeprazole, pantoprazole and omeprazole is predominantly by CYP2C19. This has potentially important implications for interactions with other drugs that are metabolized by these enzymes. For example, drug levels may increase when a PPI is co-administered because they compete for the CYP metabolic pathway. Rabeprazole uses the same cytochrome enzymes, but also has a non-enzymatic metabolic pathway that allows continued metabolism, even in the setting of competing agents.

The PPIs are metabolized to inactive metabolites [5]. Omeprazole's dominant metabolite, 5-hydroxyomeprazole is formed via CYP2C19 metabolism, but there is also a minor component metabolized via CYP3A4 forming an omeprazole sulphone. Both are subsequently metabolized to omeprazole hydroxysulphone,

Table 1. Pharmacology of proton pump inhibitors.

	Lansoprazole	Pantoprazole	Rabeprazole	Omeprazole	Esomeprazole
Dosage (mg/day)	15-30	40	20	20-40	20-40
Volume of Distribution	0.39 L/kg	0.17 L/kg	N/A	0.34-0.37 L/Kg	0.24 L/kg
% Protein Bound	97-99	98	95-98	96	97
Bioavailability	15mg = 81% 30mg = 91%	77%	52%	30-40%	90%
Metabolism by P450 Enzymes in the liver	CYP2C19 = CYP3A4	CYP2C19 > CYP3A4	CYP2C19 = CYP3A4 AND Nonenzymatic	CYP2C19 > CYP3A4	CYP2C19 > CYP3A4
Excretion	14-25% renal inactive metabolites <1% parent drug in urine 67% bile	71-82% renal inactive metabolites No active drug in urine 18-20% fecal	90% renal inactive metabolites No active drug in urine 10% fecal	77% renal inactive metabolites "Minimal" parent drug in urine 19% bile	80% renal inactive metabolites < 1% parent drug in urine

Abbreviations: N/A, not available; CYP, cytochrome P450.

which is the predominant metabolite in plasma. Pantoprazole undergoes O-demethylation via CYP2C19 and this is further metabolized to a pantoprazole sulfate. Pantoprazole is modestly metabolized by CYP3A4 resulting in a pantoprazole sulphone. Esomeprazole is predominantly metabolized to a hydroxy and desmethyl metabolite via the CYP2C19 enzyme, with a small amount of a sulphone metabolite formed via the CYP3A4 enzyme. Lansoprazole is metabolized almost equally by CYP2C19 and CYP3A4 to form a 5-hydroxylansoprazole and lansoprazole sulphone. Rabeprazole has predominantly non-enzymatic pathways for its metabolism, but also uses cytochromes CYP2C19 and CYP3A4, through which it is metabolized to a thioether. The non-enzymatic pathway of metabolism makes it unique in this class of agents and allows it to be used safely with other agents that compete for the CYP pathway, such as cyclosporine (Figure 2). As will be discussed, the CYP450 enzymatic pathway of metabolism of PPIs has broad implications for resulting drug concentrations when these agents are used concurrently with calcineurin inhibitors, which also employ the CYP3A4 pathway for metabolism.

Inactive fragments of metabolized PPI are excreted in the urine, while only 0-1% of active drug are recovered in the urine [4]. Because of this, no dosage adjustments are required in patients with underlying renal impairment, including those with end-stage renal disease (ESRD) on dialysis. Additionally, these drugs are not removed by hemodialysis and do not need special dosing schedules. Dosage adjustment is required, however, in patients with severe liver disease.

Pharmacogenetics

As noted, the major pathway of metabolism for PPIs is the CYP-2C19 (Figure 2). However, gene polymorphisms of this enzyme system do exist that can affect the metabolism of PPIs, and other drugs that utilize this enzyme potentially altering serum drug concentrations. Polymorphisms occur in exon 4 or 5 of the enzyme in 16-25% of Caucasians, 36-47% of Asians and 10% of African-Americans [5]. When these CYP mutations exist, patients are classified as "poor metabolizers". Decreased metabolism in this group of patients is confirmed when the area under the curve (AUC) of the drug is twice that of "normal metabolizers".

Hyponatremia

Hyponatremia is a rare complication of PPI therapy and has occurred in 9 case reports (Table 2) [6-12]. Omeprazole was the causative agent in 8/9 cases, while one case was attributed to esomeprazole. Serum sodium concentrations ranged from 108 -124 mmol/L and in most cases, patients were symptomatic with headache and/or confusion. The causal association between hyponatremia and PPIs is difficult to prove, as three of the published cases had other possible causes, such as volume contraction and concurrent therapy with other suspect drugs [12].

The mechanism of hyponatremia is unclear. Where documented, 4 out of the 6 cases describe a scenario consistent with syndrome of inappropriate antidiuretic hormone (SIADH). In one case, a 66 year old woman

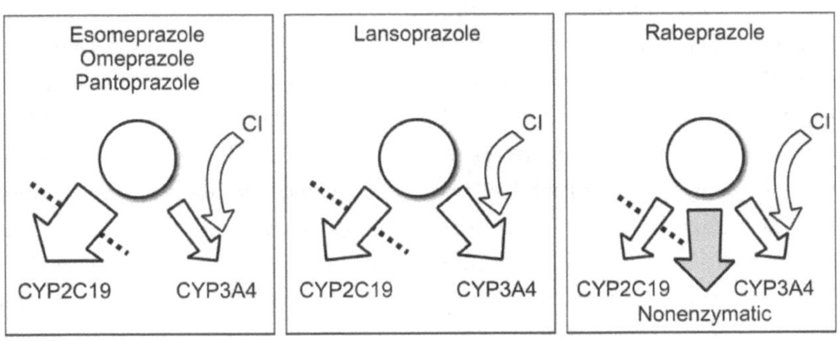

Figure 2. *Relative potency of the various cytochrome P450 enzymes in the metabolism of commonly prescribed proton pump inhibitors (PPI) is noted. Patients with genetic polymorphisms of the CYP2C19 pathway (poor metabolizers) utilize the CYP3A4 pathway (dotted line) for PPI metabolism. Calcineurin inhibitors (CNI) also use the CYP3A4 pathway for their metabolism. As a result, the "poor metabolizers" are at risk to develop elevated CNI levels when concurrently receiving a PPI. In contrast, rabeprazole is safe as it has a "non-enzymatic" pathway for its metabolism, avoiding an interaction with the CNI.*

Table 2. Hyponatremia cases associated with proton pump inhibitors

Patient Age/sex	Drug, Dose and Duration	Serum Na^+ (mEq/L)	Recovery time	Treatment	Cause
70/M (6)	omeprazole 40mg x 4 days	118	5 days	Water restriction, Na supplement	SIADH
84/F (7)	omeprazole 40mg x 11 days	106	8 days	Tetracycline	SIADH
5/M (8)	omeprazole 2mg/kg x 10 days	122	1 day	Na supplement	Renal Na wasting?
66/F (9)	omeprazole 40mg x 5 months	124, 122	? days	Water restriction	SIADH
68/M (10)	omeprazole 20mg x 4 days	111	7 days	Na supplement	Renal Na wasting?
81/F (11)	esomeprazole 20mg x 5 days	122	2 days	Water restriction	SIADH

became profoundly symptomatic with laboratory values consistent with SIADH and a serum sodium concentration of 124mmol/L [9]. Omeprazole with discontinued, she was placed on fluid restriction, and serum sodium concentration improved. Subsequently, she was rechallenged with the drug and re-developed hyponatremia (122 mmol/L). Again, discontinuation of the drug and water restriction normalized the serum sodium concentration.

In two cases thought not to be due to SIADH, renal salt wasting was entertained as a possible mechanism of hyponatremia, but the data are murky [8, 10]. In the first case, a child with Klippel-Feil syndrome received omeprazole therapy and developed hyponatremia and hypokalemia with high urinary sodium and urinary potassium concentrations. The urinary sodium concentration decreased to levels appropriate for underlying volume status with cessation of omeprazole. The authors suggested that hyponatremia was due to volume depletion (from PPI-induced salt wasting) and secondary ADH production while hypokalemia was a result of high distal tubular delivery of sodium from proximal sodium wasting. It is unlikely that these electrolyte disturbances resulted from direct renal tubular effects of the PPIs as the drug metabolites excreted by the kidney are inactive. Further support is garnered by the absence of drug effect on the renal transporters by the study previously noted [3]. Thus, there appears to be a rare association between PPIs and hyponatremia, an effect that is likely found in the entire PPI drug class.

Implications for transplantation

Calcineurin inhibitors are staples of immunotherapy following renal transplantation. Because calcineurin inhibitors are metabolized predominantly by the CYP3A4 enzyme, there is the potential for drug interactions with PPIs that share this enzymatic pathway. In fact, *in vitro* studies in normal subjects note that omeprazole inhibits the metabolism of tacrolimus by liver microsomes by as much as 15% [13]. Specifically, transplant patients treated with PPIs that utilize the CYP3A4 enzyme for metabolism, may develop higher drug levels of calcineurin inhibitors. This effect appears to be largely theoretical, as several studies have looked at dose level: drug dose ratios and found no such interaction. The first of these evaluated 12 transplant patients on pantoprazole and tacrolimus (n=6) or pantoprazole and cyclosporine (n=6) and found no effect on trough levels [14]. A second study examined 51 transplant recipients on tacrolimus who were subsequently placed on omeprazole for 3 months [15]. No change in drug levels was noted. In both studies, CYP gene polymorphisms were not tested.

As most PPIs rely predominantly on the CYP2C19 pathway of metabolism, it is understandable why these drugs are safe in studies examining normal subjects. However, since mutations in the CYP2C19 pathway exist that render the patients "poor metabolizers", a potential interaction between PPIs and calcineurin inhibitors may occur as more PPI metabolism is shifted to the CYP3A4 enzyme.

Case reports have documented this interaction in patients with CYP2C19 mutations. Higher drug level: drug dose ratios of tacrolimus were noted in patients treated with lansoprazole [16]. In contrast, concurrent treatment with tacrolimus and rabeprazole, which has a non-enzymatic pathway of metabolism, did not develop a drug-drug interaction.

Acute interstitial nephritis

The first case of AIN associated with PPIs was published in 1992 [17]. Subsequently, multiple case reports and case series have been noted in the literature [17-32]. PPIs are now considered to be the most common cause of drug-induced acute interstitial nephritis (AIN) worldwide.

AIN is a relatively uncommon cause of kidney disease, accounting for only 2-3% of all renal biopsies [33-35]. However, in patients with acute kidney injury (AKI) who have normal sized kidneys on ultrasound, AIN is much more common, accounting for up to 27% of biopsies [36]. Omeprazole was the first PPI described to cause AIN. In this case, a 74 year old female on omeprazole therapy for 6 months developed fatigue, malaise and was noted to have hematuria, proteinuria and eosinophiluria [17]. Over the next 12 years, 29 cases of AIN associated with omeprazole were published, 23 of which were biopsy proven [18-23]. In 2004 other PPIs were implicated in two large case series that included omeprazole, lansoprazole and pantoprazole [24, 25].

In the first of these case series, all cases of AIN diagnosed at Norwich University Hospital in the United Kingdom were examined over a 4 year period (1995-1999) [24]. Of the 24 cases identified, 14 were drug related, 8 of which (57%) were attributed to PPIs (6 omeprazole, 2 lansoprazole). These patients presented with AKI and non-specific symptoms. Interestingly, although all recovered from AKI, most were left with some level of chronic kidney disease (75%). Subsequently, a large case series from New Zealand in 2005 described 15 cases (12 biopsy proven) of AIN associated with PPIs. Time from initiation of drug to diagnosis (symptoms, renal biopsy) ranged from 10 days to 18 months [25]. Despite improvements in kidney function in all patients, 12 out of 14 patients (86%) were left with chronic kidney disease. The authors also systematically examined data from the Centre for Adverse Reactions Monitoring (CARM) in New Zealand, and found that PPIs were the most common cause of drug-induced AIN in their region (32%), with an incidence of 1:12,500 patient years [25].

The largest report comes from Australia where retrospective data were collected from 2 teaching hospitals from 1993-2003 [27]. Cases were identified and demographics, clinical parameters and histopathology were examined in detail. There were 28 cases of biopsy proven AIN, 18 (64%) of which were due to a PPI (11 omeprazole, 3 pantoprazole, 3 esomeprazole, 1 rabeprazole). Mean time to development of AIN was 11 weeks after initiation of drug. Renal histology revealed classic changes of AIN with interstitial infiltrates and eosinophils present in 83% of biopsy specimens. The authors also queried the Therapeutic Goods Administration (TGA) database from 1991-2004; a governmental organization that records adverse drug events reported by physicians. After extensive review and exclusion of hospital patients in the database (to avoid inclusion of previously noted 18 patients), cases were classified as one of the following based on the quality of data to support causality: "biopsy proven AIN", "suspected interstitial nephritis", "unexplained acute renal failure", and "renal impairment". The TGA database revealed 34 additional cases of "biopsy proven AIN", 10 cases of "suspected interstitial nephritis", 20 cases of "unexplained renal failure" and 26 cases of "renal impairment" that were associated with PPIs. While they do not prove cause and effect, these data are certainly concerning for a higher frequency of AIN from PPIs and support what has been described in case reports and case series.

More recently, additional cases of AIN were reported from the Netherlands (omeprazole, pantoprazole, rabeprazole) [37]. Renal biopsy evidence of AIN was noted in 5 patients, all who had improved symptoms upon drug withdrawal. In this case series, the authors also queried the World Health Organization (WHO) Collaborating Centre for International Drug Monitoring, which is a data bank of over 3.5 million reports of adverse drug reactions (ADR). In this data bank, 150 cases of PPI associated with AIN were noted. Not withstanding the apparent low rate of PPI-induced AIN in this databank study, which is likely explained in part by the lack of awareness of the association of AIN with PPIs, and reliance on spontaneous physician reporting, the association is worth noting.

Mechanism

Drug-induced AIN represents an immune reaction

to the parent drug and/or its metabolites. The fact that AIN is not drug dose dependent, and it occurs in only a small number of patients exposed to any particular drug, makes it unlikely to be purely a nephrotoxic effect of the agent. Also, re-challenge with an agent known to have led to AIN uniformly leads to recurrence of disease. All of these argue for an immune mechanism. Clinically, this is supported by the description of patients with AIN that develop systemic symptoms associated with hypersensitivity reactions, such as rash and fever. In most cases, AIN is a cell mediated immune response as renal histology rarely shows evidence of immune complex deposition. In support of a cell-mediated process, T cells are the predominant cell type in the interstitial infiltrate in kidney biopsy specimens from patients with AIN [38]. Once T-cells are activated in the interstitium, they release a variety of inflammatory cytokines such as IL-4 (Interleukin 4) and IL-5, and chemokines (CXCL8) that act as chemoattractants to cells such as neutrophils, eosinophils and macrophages, that promote local interstitial injury [39].

Drug hypersensitivity is classified into four major categories. Type I reactions include urticaria and anaphylaxis, and are mediated by IgE (Immunoglobulin E). Type II reactions are largely blood cell dyscrasias, and a result of cytotoxic mechanisms of immunoglobulins. Type III reactions are immune complex reactions, such as vasculitis. More important to the discussion of drug-induced AIN are type IV reactions, the so-called delayed-type hypersensitivity reactions, mediated by T cells. This is likely the form of drug hypersensitivity that mediates the development of drug-induced AIN.

T cells recognize antigen via numerous receptors located on the cell surface, which bind major histocompatibility complexes (MHC) on antigen presenting cells (APCs). MHC complexes are characterized as class I or class II and present peptides from differing origins. MHC class I molecules present protein peptides that are synthesized and degraded in the cytosol, and activate CD8+ T cells. Upon activation, CD8+ cells secrete cytokines that kill cells that present cytosolic peptides. One such example of targeted cells are those that present viral particles. MHC class II complexes present peptides that originate from proteins that are first endocytosed, then degraded in vesicles and presented to the surface of the APC. These complexes interact with CD4+ cells, which either kill the APC or activate other immune cells including B cells, macrophages or CD8+ T cells.

Drug-induced AIN is thought to occur when the prescribed drug, or one of its metabolites, acts as a hapten. These small molecules are capable of binding covalently to larger proteins or peptides, and in doing so, confer a conformation change that causes that stable protein or peptide to become immunogenic [40]. These newly immunogenic proteins are either recognized by circulating immunoglobulin, or presented to T cells by MHC complexes. As an example, penicillin G, which covalently binds to lysine groups on cellular proteins, causes a conformational change in the protein that causes it to be recognized as foreign and presented on MHC complexes.

Sometimes, as with sulfamethoxazole, the drug itself does not react with proteins or peptides to induce an immune response. Rather, intracellular metabolism of the parent drug forms the metabolite, sulfamethoxazole-nitroso, which binds covalently to proteins and peptides and induces immunogenicity [41]. This represents a drug that is a pro-hapten, which is immunologically reactive and able to bind to MHC complexes on APCs only after it is metabolized.

More recently, a third mechanism of drug-induced immunogenicity was described. Some drugs are able to bind directly to immune receptors, the so-called pharmacologic-interaction concept, or "p-i concept" [41]. This theory suggests that drugs can directly interact with a T cell receptor without covalent binding or processing by an APC. This "p-i concept", is supported by the following data: 1) T cells are stimulated by drug in the presence of gluaraldehyde-fixed APCs, which are unable to process antigen; 2) drug is not covalently bound to APCs, as the drug can be washed away, unlike covalently bound drugs; and 3) the time course of T cell reactivity in the setting of these drugs occurs much too quickly for either metabolism or processing to occur.

Specific to the kidney, ingested drug or one of its metabolites, can induce AIN by several possible mechanisms [42, 43]. First, the drug (or metabolite) can bind tubular basement membrane and act as a hapten, modifying native renal proteins to induce an immune response. Alternatively, the drug may act as a hapten that mimics an antigen normally present in the tubular basement membrane (TBM) of the kidney, whereby the immune response will be directed against components in the TBM. Experimental models in rats and guinea pigs have shown that extra-renal proteins (like drugs) may be "trapped" in the tubulointerstitium of the kidney, and subsequently induce an immune response by acting like haptens or directly stimulating T cells (p-i concept). This is another proposed mechanism of AIN [42]. Lastly, the drug may form circulating immune complexes that could theoretically be deposited in the kidney and trigger immune-mediated damage. In humans, immune deposits are rarely seen in AIN, suggesting that one of the first two mechanisms is more likely involved.

The exact mechanism of AIN induce by PPI drugs is unknown. It is conceivable that PPIs or their metabolites deposit in the renal tubulointerstitium and behave as either a hapten or directly stimulate T cells to mediate AIN. Further studies in animals on the effect of PPIs on the immune system and induction of AIN are required to allow a clear understanding of the immune processes involved in the kidney injury.

Clinical presentation

The clinical presentation of AIN is somewhat varied. Classically, the presentation of drug-induced AIN is divided into a "methicillin-like" presentation or "non-methicillin-like" presentation. AIN associated with methicillin presents as a classic hypersensitivity reaction consisting of the triad of fever, rash and eosinophilia. This presentation is much less common in patients who develop AIN from PPI's, with symptoms resembling the "non-methicillin-like" pattern. Although data are not available in all reported cases, it appears that less then 10% of patients with PPI-induced AIN have the classic triad of hypersensitivity reactions. Less then half of the patients described manifest fever, less then 10% develop rash and about a third have eosinophilia. Conversely, patients frequently complain of non-specific symptoms including fatigue and nausea in 39% and weakness in 22% [27]. A comparison of the clinical presentation of AIN from methicillin-, non-methicillin- and PPI-associated AIN are shown in Figure 3.

The time interval from initiation of PPI therapy to clinical AIN is quite variable. In all cases published, symptoms are reported to occur anywhere from 1 week to 9 months after initial treatment with the PPI, with a mean time to clinical presentation of 9.9 weeks. Thus, clinicians must be mindful that AIN may occur over a wide time period following drug exposure. AKI that develops without an obvious cause should stimulate the clinician to consider the possibility of PPI-induced AIN if this class of medication is on the drug list. Like many other drugs that cause allergic reactions or AIN, re-challenge with a PPI in a patient previously suspected of PPI-induced AIN causes rapid onset of symptoms of AIN [17, 28-30].

Classic urinalysis findings associated with AIN include pyuria and hematuria. Urine sediment examination classically reveals white blood cells (WBC) alone or with WBC casts. However, these are inconsistent findings and may be absent in biopsy-proven AIN. Thus, PPI-associated AIN (as well as other drugs) should not be excluded solely on the absence of pyuria (Figure 3). Eosinophiluria is also not reliable and, depending on whether a Wright's stain or a Hansel's stain is used, has limited utility in diagnosing AIN. As with other forms of drug-induced AIN, it is likely that sensitivity

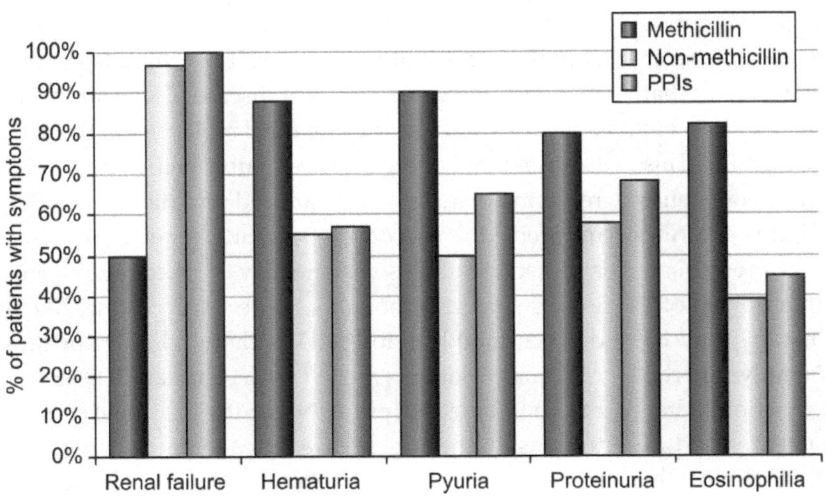

Figure 3. *Clinical features of methicillin-induced AIN, non-methicillin drug-induced AIN and PPI-induced AIN.*

and specificity of eosinophiluria in PPI-induced AIN is suboptimal.

Given the infrequent occurrence of the classic hypersensitivity triad of symptoms, a confirmed diagnosis of PPI-induced AIN can only be definitively made by examination of renal histology. Renal biopsy is diagnostic and typically will demonstrate a cellular interstitial infiltrate with or without tubulitis (Figure 4). Case series that include renal histology describe the presence of eosinophils within the tubulointerstitium in 88% of cases. In general, the glomeruli and vasculature appear to be unaffected [27].

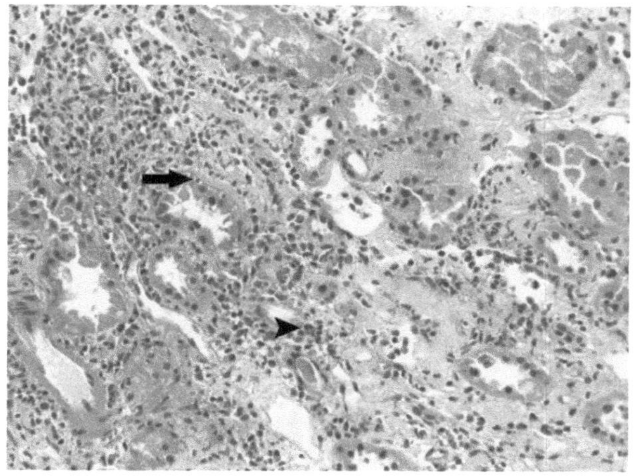

Figure 4. Kidney biopsy demonstrates a diffuse cellular infiltrate within the interstitium with inflammatory cells including eosinophils (arrowhead) and lymphocytes. Tubulitis is present (arrow). Hematoxylin and eosin stain (H&E x 47)

Therapy

Although data are limited, treatment strategies for PPI-induced AIN are similar to those employed in other forms of drug-induced AIN. Critical to preserving kidney function are prompt diagnosis and rapid withdrawal of the offending agent. Many of the published cases of PPI-induced AIN describe treatment with variable courses and doses of corticosteroids. However, it should be noted that treatment of AIN with corticosteroids is a fiercely debated topic in the medical literature. No prospective, controlled trials exist on this topic. A retrospective study of 2,598 patients, of which 67 (2.6%) had AIN, examined the effect of steroids (intravenous pulse followed by oral dosing) in 40 patients as compared with 27 patients not treated with steroids. No statistical difference in the final serum creatinine concentration at 12 months was found between those treated with steroids and controls [34]. Obviously, the retrospective nature of the study is limiting. In particular, "selection for treatment bias" cannot be excluded as those who were given steroids were likely different than untreated patients. However, there are small, uncontrolled studies that suggest that corticosteroid therapy may hasten the time to renal recovery, albeit to a similar level of renal function. This may become important when trying to avoid renal replacement therapy for those with significant AKI from severe forms of AIN [33, 44]. Oral prednisone is the most frequently used agent with a dosage of 1 mg/kg/day commonly employed. Therapy may be continued for 1-2 months and subsequently tapered while concurrently monitoring renal function. Alternatively, high dose intravenous steroids are used in severe cases, but often are not needed. More recently, a few cases of drug-induced AIN that were steroid dependent/resistant derived benefit (as measured by improved kidney function) with oral mycophenylate mofetil (MMF), which allowed discontinuation of steroids [45]. Recurrence of AIN did not occur following discontinuation of MMF. Further study of MMF in the treatment of AIN is required before therapy with this agent can be recommended, but it does hold some promise.

Prognosis

As is the case with all forms of drug-induced AIN, early recognition and intervention lead to a better prognosis. With time, inflammation and damage to the tubulointerstitium leads to interstitial fibrosis and chronic interstitial nephritis (CIN). Ultimately, CIN may result in chronic kidney disease (CKD) and in severe cases, ESRD requiring renal replacement therapy. Upon review of all the cases published to date, AKI requiring dialysis is very rare and no patients with PPI-induced AIN have developed ESRD requiring chronic maintenance dialysis. There may be "recognition bias" in these statistics though, as unrecognized cases likely do occur and lead to ESRD. Although ESRD appears rare, many patients are left with residual CKD as few return to baseline (pre-AIN) serum creatinine concentrations. In the largest case series to date, all patients recovered from AKI, but mean calculated creatinine clearance was 15.9 ml/min and 11.5 ml/min lower then baseline at 3 and 6 months, respectfully [27]. Another series of 15 cases reported an increase in baseline serum creatinine concentration (0.94 mg/dl pre-AIN) to a new baseline serum creatinine concentration (1.57 mg/dl) 3-18 months after PPI discontinuation [25]. Figure 5 demonstrates the change in kidney function in patients with PPI-induced AIN following discontinuation of the drug. Note that patients were left with residual CKD. Other published cases support the development of CKD as noted in these two case series. An average final serum creatinine concentration of 1.3 mg/dl was seen as compared with baseline (pre-AIN) levels of 1.1 mg/dl [31]. Thus, chronic kidney disease, likely due to chronic interstitial scarring and perhaps CIN, is a long-term consequence of PPI-induced AIN.

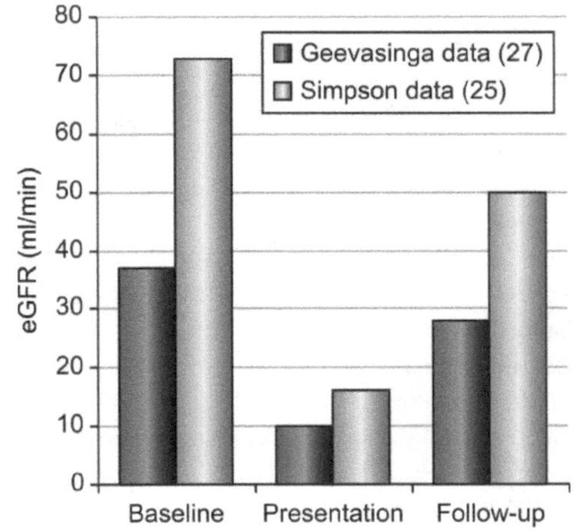

Figure 5. *Bar graph showing estimated GFR (MDRD calculation) of patients presenting with AIN in two large case series. Although GFR does improve from presentation, patients do not return to their previous baseline kidney function and are left with chronic kidney disease. The dark bars represent data from reference 27, the light bars from reference 25.*

Conclusion

Proton pump inhibitors are excellent pharmacologic agents employed in the treatment of acid-related gastrointestinal disease, and are, by in large very safe. They are metabolized by the liver and do not require dosage modification in patients with kidney disease. For nephrologists, an understanding of their pharmacology and metabolism is essential as they are frequently used in combination with calcineurin inhibitors in kidney transplant patients. They have the potential to interact with these immunosuppressive drugs and raise calcineurin blood levels. When calcineurin inhibitor toxicity develops, the patient's medication list should be examined for the recent addition of a PPI. Hyponatremia occurs very rarely, and appears to be the result of a drug-induced SIADH. PPI's are now recognized as the most common cause of drug-induced acute interstitial nephritis, and may often present with "non-methicillin-like" symptoms. Renal biopsy and examination of renal histology is critical to accurate diagnosis. Withdrawal of drug is essential to treatment, and since PPI-induced AIN is a class effect, re-challenge with another PPI is not recommended. There may be some role for corticosteroids in hastening renal recovery, but this is debatable and physicians should use steroids on a case-by-case basis. Finally, patients are frequently left with some degree of CKD from PPI-induced AIN, likely due to chronic interstitial nephritis, and should be monitored routinely following discontinuation of drug for the proper care of CKD.

References

1. Diamanti F. In; 2006:Personal Communication from TAP Pharmaceuticals.
2. New Drugs are not always innovative, just formulas that mirror each other and have been tweaked to gain patient protection and turn big profits. 2005. (Accessed Feb 7, 2007, at http://www.signonsandiego.com/news/business/20051120-9999-lz1b20meds.html#.)
3. Howden CW RJ. Omeprazole, a gastric 'proton pump inhibitor': lack of effect on renal handling of electrolytes and urinary acidification. Eur J Clin Pharmacol 1984;26:639-40.
4. Sanborn K, ed. Physicians Desk Reference. 61 ed. Montvale, NJ: Thompson PDR; 2007.
5. Ishizaki T, Horai Y. Review article: cytochrome P450 and the metabolism of proton pump inhibitors--emphasis on rabeprazole. Aliment Pharmacol Ther 1999;13 Suppl 3:27-36.
6. Kaloustian E, Veyssier P. [Severe hyponatremia: possible role of omeprazole]. Presse Med 1992;21(19):907-8.
7. Gonthier R, Bouchou K, Guy C, Cathebras P, Rousset H. [Severe hyponatremia induced by meprazole]. Presse Med 1993;22(4):176.
8. Melville C, Shah A, Matthew D, Milla P. Electrolyte disturbance with omeprazole therapy. Eur J Pediatr 1994;153(1):49-51.
9. Durst RY, Pipek R, Levy Y. Hyponatremia caused by omeprazole treatment. Am J Med 1994;97(4):400-1.
10. Shiba S, Sugiura K, Ebata A, et al. Hyponatremia with consciousness disturbance caused by omeprazole administration. A case report and literature review. Dig Dis Sci 1996;41(8):1615-7.
11. Mennecier D, Ceppa F, Gidenne S, Vergeau B. Hyponatremia with consciousness disturbance associated with esomeprazole. Ann Pharmacother 2005;39(4):774-5.
12. Castot A, Bidault I, Dahan R, Efthymiou ML. [Evaluation of unexpected and toxic effects of omeprazole (Mopral) reported to the regional centers of pharmacovigilance during the first 22 postmarketing months]. Therapie 1993;48(5):469-74.
13. Christians U, Schmidt G, Bader A, et al. Identification of drugs inhibiting the *in vitro* metabolism of tacrolimus by human liver microsomes. Br J Clin Pharmacol 1996;41(3):187-90.
14. Lorf T, Ramadori G, Ringe B, Schworer H. Pantoprazole does not affect cyclosporin A blood concentration in kidney-transplant patients. Eur J Clin Pharmacol 2000;55(10):733-5.
15. Pascual J, Marcen R, Orea OE, et al. Interaction between omeprazole and tacrolimus in renal allograft recipients: a clinical-analytical study. Transplant Proc 2005;37(9):3752-3.
16. Itagaki F, Homma M, Yuzawa K, Fukao K, Kohda Y. Drug interaction of tacrolimus and proton pump inhibitors in renal transplant recipients with CYP2C19 gene mutation. Transplant Proc 2002;34(7):2777-8.
17. Ruffenach SJ, Siskind MS, Lien YH. Acute interstitial nephritis due to omeprazole. Am J Med 1992;93(4):472-3.
18. Post AT VG, Zanen AL. Reversible renal failure after treatment with omeprazole. Neth J Med 2000;57:58-61.
19. Myers RP, McLaughlin K, Hollomby DJ. Acute interstitial nephritis due to omeprazole. Am J Gastroenterol 2001;96(12):3428-31.
20. Portera-Cailliau C SA. Acute Interstitial Nephritis Due to Omeprazole. Annals of Long-Term Care 1999;7(5):206-7.
21. Wall CA, Gaffney EF, Mellotte GJ. Hypercalcaemia and acute interstitial nephritis associated with omeprazole therapy. Nephrol Dial Transplant 2000;15(9):1450-2.
22. Geetha D. Omeprazole-induced acute interstitial nephritis. Am J Gastroenterol 1999;94(11):3375-6.
23. Torregrosa E, Rovira RE, Calvo C, Hernandez-Jaras J, Maduell F, Garcia H. [Acute interstitial nephritis associated with omeprazole therapy]. Nefrologia 2004;24 Suppl 3:61-3.
24. Torpey N, Barker T, Ross C. Drug-induced tubulo-interstitial nephritis secondary to proton pump inhibitors: experience from a single UK renal unit. Nephrol Dial Transplant 2004;19(6):1441-6.
25. Simpson IJ MM, Pilmore H, Manley P, Williams L, Thein H, Voss D. Proton Pump Inhibitor and acute interstitial nephritis: Report and anlysis of 15 cases. Nephrology 2006;11:381-5.
26. Geevasinga N, Coleman PL, Roger SD. Rabeprazole-induced acute interstitial nephritis. Nephrology (Carlton) 2005;10(1):7-9.
27. Geevasinga N, Coleman PL, Webster AC, Roger SD. Proton pump inhibitors and acute interstitial nephritis. Clin Gastroenterol Hepatol 2006;4(5):597-604.
28. Christensen PB, Albertsen KE, Jensen P. Renal failure after omeprazole. Lancet 1993;341(8836):55.
29. Assouad M, Vicks SL, Pokroy MV, Willcourt RJ. Recurrent acute interstitial nephritis on rechallenge with omeprazole. Lancet 1994;344(8921):549.
30. Gronich JH SE, Stein HD Sirota RA, Yudis M. Omeprazole related acute interstitial nephritis (AIN) with omeprazole (Abstract). JASN 1994;5:394.
31. Brewster UC, Perazella MA. Acute kidney injury following proton pump inhibitor therapy. Kidney Int 2006.
32. Ra A, Tobe SW. Acute interstitial nephritis due to pantoprazole. Ann Pharmacother 2004;38(1):41-5.

33. Buysen JG, Houthoff HJ, Krediet RT, Arisz L. Acute interstitial nephritis: a clinical and morphological study in 27 patients. Nephrol Dial Transplant 1990;5(2):94-9.
34. Clarkson MR, Giblin L, O'Connell FP, et al. Acute interstitial nephritis: clinical features and response to corticosteroid therapy. Nephrol Dial Transplant 2004;19(11):2778-83.
35. Davison AM, Jones CH. Acute interstitial nephritis in the elderly: a report from the UK MRC Glomerulonephritis Register and a review of the literature. Nephrol Dial Transplant 1998;13 Suppl 7:12-6.
36. Farrington K, Levison DA, Greenwood RN, Cattell WR, Baker LR. Renal biopsy in patients with unexplained renal impairment and normal kidney size. Q J Med 1989;70(263):221-33.
37. Harmark L vH, deGroot MC, vanGrootheest AC. Proton pump inhibitor induced acute interstitial nephritis. Br J Clin Pharmacol 2007; 64 (6): 819-823.
38. Spanou Z, Keller M, Britschgi M, et al. Involvement of drug-specific T cells in acute drug-induced interstitial nephritis. J Am Soc Nephrol 2006;17(10):2919-27.
39. Crane IJ, Forrester JV. Th1 and Th2 lymphocytes in autoimmune disease. Crit Rev Immunol 2005;25(2):75-102.
40. Pichler WJ. Delayed drug hypersensitivity reactions. Ann Intern Med 2003;139(8):683-93.
41. Pichler WJ, Beeler A, Keller M, et al. Pharmacological interaction of drugs with immune receptors: the p-i concept. Allergol Int 2006;55(1):17-25.
42. Rossert J. Drug-induced acute interstitial nephritis. Kidney Int 2001;60(2):804-17.
43. Wilson CB. Study of the immunopathogenesis of tubulointerstitial nephritis using model systems. Kidney Int 1989;35(4):938-53.
44. Pusey CD, Saltissi D, Bloodworth L, Rainford DJ, Christie JL. Drug associated acute interstitial nephritis: clinical and pathological features and the response to high dose steroid therapy. Q J Med 1983;52(206):194-211.
45. Preddie DC MG, Radhakrishnan J, Nickolas TL, D'Agati VD, Schwimmer JA, Gardenswartz M, Rosen R, Appel GB. Mycophenolate Mofetil for the Treatment of Interstitial Nephritis. Clin J Am Soc Nephro 2006;11:718-22.

26

Oral sodium phosphate bowel purgatives and acute phosphate nephropathy

Glen S. MARKOWITZ

Department of Pathology, Renal Pathology Laboratory,
Columbia University, New York, NY

Introduction

Phosphorus is a naturally-occurring element with an atomic number of 15 and an atomic mass of 31 g/mol. Within the human body, the majority of phosphorus is bound to 4 oxygen atoms, forming the phosphate anion (PO_4^{3-}). As a result, the terms phosphorus and phosphate are at times used interchangeably. Standard blood chemistries report the serum phosphorus with a normal range of approximately 2.5 – 4.5 mg/dl. This represents a measurement of serum phosphate that has been corrected to reflect the molecular weight of phosphorus alone.

A normal adult has a total body phosphorus content of 700-800 g [1]. The majority of phosphate is present in bone, although approximately 15% is distributed outside of the skeleton where it is present in the form of inorganic phosphate in extra-cellular fluid and organic phosphates within cells, such as adenosine triphosphate (ATP), nucleic acids, and membrane phospholipids. As such, phosphorus plays a vital role in numerous cell processes including cell energetics, cell membrane formation, and DNA & RNA synthesis, to name a few. Within blood, phosphate exists mainly in two forms, HPO_4^{2-} and $H_2PO_4^{1-}$. These two anions are important serum buffers and their relative concentrations are determined by the serum pH.

The average daily dietary intake of phosphorus in the developed world is approximately 1,000 mg, which exceeds the 700 mg adequate daily intake level for adults established by the Food and Nutrition Board of the Institute of Medicine of the National Academy of Sciences (www.IOM.edu). The same group defines the tolerable upper intake level for phosphorus as 4 g for most adults, but 3 g for adults over the age of 70. Phosphorus intake varies with the composition of the diet, and foods that are rich in phosphate include eggs, milk products, meat, and fish.

Within both the kidney and the small intestine, phosphate absorption occurs mainly via sodium-dependent phosphate cotransporter proteins that are members of the SLC34 gene family [2-3]. NaPi-IIa (SLC34A1) and NaPi-IIc (SLC34A3) are expressed in the brush border of the proximal tubule and their expression is down regulated by increases in serum phosphate and parathyroid hormone (PTH). As such, NaPi-IIa knock-out mice have significant hyperphosphaturia and develop early and severe nephrocalcinosis [4]. NaPi-IIb (SLC34A2) has a broader distribution that includes the brush border of the small intestine and levels of this protein increase in response to hypophosphatemia and vitamin D. While expression of NaPi-IIa is acutely controlled over short time periods (i.e. minutes), NaPi-IIb expression in the intestine is slower, requiring days to respond to physiologic changes. Interestingly, recent studies have shown that there is a direct signaling axis by which intestinal phosphate absorption rapidly increases fractional phosphate excretion in the kidney. This effect is apparent within 10 minutes of phosphate ingestion and is independent of serum phosphate concentration or PTH [5].

In the usual state, between 60-80% of ingested phosphate is absorbed in the small intestine. In the kidney, phosphate is freely filtered at the level of the glomerulus. Approximately 80% of phosphate is reabsorbed in the proximal tubule, with smaller amounts reabsorbed in the distal tubule and collecting duct [6-7]. Oral phosphate ingestion has the potential to increase serum levels when the intake is at higher than usual levels or occurs over short periods of time. Similarly hyperphosphatemia may follow phosphate ingestion when it occurs in the setting of impaired gastrointestinal motility leading to increased absorption or with renal dysfunction leading to decreased excretion. Hyperphosphatemia may also result from massive intracellular phosphate release in the setting of tumor lysis syndrome or rhabdomyolysis.

Oral sodium phosphate solution: a common purgative used for colonoscopy preparation

Successful colonoscopy depends upon cleansing of the bowel prior to the procedure in order to have adequate visualization of the mucosal surface. Oral sodium phosphate solution (OSPS), commonly sold under the brand name "Fleet Phospho-soda" (C.B. Fleet Inc.) or as generic equivalents, is a frequently administered over-the-counter purgative used to cleanse the bowel prior to colonoscopy. OSPS is a hyperosmotic laxative that acts by drawing water into the gastrointestinal tract. A commonly recommended regimen consists of two 45-ml doses taken 10-12 hours apart, the evening before and the morning of colonoscopy. Each 45-ml dose contains 21.6 g of monobasic sodium phosphate (NaH_2PO_4) and 8.1 g of dibasic sodium phosphate (Na_2HPO_4), which is equivalent to 5.8 g of elemental phosphorus. Ingestion of 5.8 g of phosphorus diluted into a single 8 ounce glass far exceeds the usual dietary intake of 1 g spread over at least 3 meals in a 24-hour period. Furthermore, it is typically taken twice in a 12-hour period, bringing the total to 11.6 g, an amount that far exceeds the tolerable upper intake level for phosphorus of 4 g, as defined by the Institute of Medicine (www.IOM.edu). Since OSPS is delivered in a relatively small volume and leads to significant fluid loss in the form of diarrhea, ample fluid intake is strongly recommended. A minimum of 36 ounces of clear fluid is recommended with each 45 ml administration.

Oral sodium phosphate solution has been in use as a laxative agent since 1893. In 1990, it began to gain widespread acceptance as a purgative agent prior to colonoscopy. An important paper by Vanner et al. [8] compared OSPS with polyethylene glycol (PEG)-based lavage solution and found that OSPS, with its smaller volume of required oral intake, was associated with better patient compliance, less discomfort, and improved colonic cleansing. Transient hyperphosphatemia was noted, with a mean increase in serum phosphate of 4.1 mg/dl and a peak serum phosphate of 11.6 mg/dl [8]. The changes in serum phosphate resolved within 24 hours and were not associated with hypocalcemia.

Small, statistically-significant, and rapidly reversible increases in serum sodium, serum chloride, hematocrit, and serum osmolality were also noted, along with a 0.5 kg greater decline in body weight in the OSPS group (that did not reach statistical significance). A potential explanation for these findings was a greater degree of hypovolemia in patients who received OSPS.

Subsequent studies similarly have shown that compared to PEG-based purgatives, OSPS is better tolerated and is associated with improved bowel cleansing [9-11]. A recent meta-analysis looked at all 18 randomized, controlled trials comparing OSPS and PEG published from 1990 – 2005 [11]. Among the 16 trials with data that could be analyzed, the efficacy with respect to bowel cleansing was superior for OSPS in 9 studies, inferior in 1 study, and equivalent in 6 [11]. The greater efficacy could be explained in part by the observation that 94.4% of patients completed the OSPS regimen, as opposed to only 70.9% of patients using PEG. The overall adverse event rate was similar between the two groups, although abdominal pain was more common with PEG while dizziness was more common with OSPS. Only 8 of the 18 trials provided details on biochemical changes. Transient hyperphosphatemia and hypokalemia were reported in 7 of 8 studies, but were not associated with clinical symptoms or sequelae. Among the 7 studies, the mean increase in serum phosphate ranged from 1.1 to 4.1 mg/dl. Of note, 3 of the studies also documented a small but statistically significant decline in serum calcium.

Oral sodium phosphate solution is contra-indicated in patients with congestive heart failure, clinically significant impairment in renal function, ascites, gastrointestinal obstruction, or active inflammatory bowel disease. It is not recommended for use in children under the age of 18. OSPS should be used with caution in patients who are elderly, debilitated, pregnant or nursing, have heart disease including myocardial infarction or unstable angina, have increased risk of renal impairment, and have increased risk for or pre-existing electrolyte disturbances (www.phosphosoda.com). Despite these present guidelines, OSPS is frequently used in patients with clear contraindications. A 1997 survey of the Canadian Association of Gastroenterology found that 55% of respondents used OSPS in patients with renal failure, 70% in patients with heart disease, 87% in patients with incomplete bowel obstruction, and 91% in the elderly [12]. Use of OSPS is particularly dangerous in patients with ESRD or significant CKD, where it can produce profound electrolyte abnormalities, loss of consciousness, cardiac arrhythmias, and hypocalcemic tetany [13-14].

Oral sodium phosphate also is available by prescription in a tablet form under the brand names Visicol and more recently OsmoPrep (Salix Pharmaceuticals). Similar to OSPS, Visicol commonly is given in two separate administrations separated by 12 hours. In the evening prior to colonoscopy, patients are instructed to take 3 tablets with at least 8 oz of clear liquids every 15 minutes until reaching a total of 20 tables. This is repeated again in the morning prior to the colonoscopy procedure. The total of 40 tablets has a cumulative sodium phosphate content that is near-identical to the two 45-ml administrations of OSPS. Compared to OSPS, Visicol has the advantages of being tasteless and of mandating greater fluid consumption (when swallowing the pills), thus decreasing the likelihood of underhydration and hypovolumia. Similar to OSPS, Visicol is associated with transient hyperphosphatemia. In one study on 427 patients who received OSP tablets, serum phosphorus levels were elevated by 3.7 mg/dl above baseline at 3-5 hours after the second dose of 20 tablets [15]. These changes spontaneously resolved within 48-72 hours.

Calcium phosphate deposition & the kidney

Renal parenchymal calcium deposition can be associated with significant renal dysfunction. When calcium deposits are encountered on renal biopsy, the calcium salt typically contains either phosphate or oxalate. The two anions are easily differentiated pathologically, as calcium oxalate is identified as refractile crystals under polarized light. In contrast, calcium phosphate is non-polarizable but gives a positive histochemical reaction to the von Kossa stain [16].

The terminology used to describe conditions associated with prominent renal calcium deposits dismisses the importance of the phosphate anion. Renal parenchymal injury with prominent calcium oxalate deposition is referred to as *oxalate nephropathy*. Oxalate nephropathy is seen in the setting of primary hyperoxaluria or enteric hyperoxaluria secondary to fat malabsorption. Renal parenchymal injury with abundant calcium phosphate deposits is referred to as *nephrocalcinosis*, a term that dismisses the importance of the phosphate anion. Nephrocalcinosis is typically attributed to conditions associated with chronic hypercalcemia, including hyperparathyroidism, hypercalcemia related to malignancy, vitamin D intoxication, sarcoidosis, milk alkali syndrome, and distal renal tubular acidosis. Tubulointerstitial calcium phosphate deposits also are commonly encountered in the renal allograft where their presence has been mainly attributed to hyperparathyroidism [17] and chronic calcineurin inhibitor toxicity [18].

Reports of acute kidney injury following the use of oral sodium phosphate bowel purgatives

There have been multiple reports of acute kidney injury following the use of oral sodium phosphate solution [13, 19-33]. Many of these reports are the subject of a recent review [19] and are best divided into 2 categories. In the first group of cases, the clinical course was dominated by immediate and severe electrolyte disorders including hyperphosphatemia, and renal biopsy was not performed [13, 20-28]. In the second group of patients, the clinical course was less acute and the connection between the use of OSPS and renal failure was confirmed by renal biopsy [19, 29-33].

Reports of acute kidney injury immediately following ingestion of OSPS are depicted in Table 1. Review of the literature reveals 12 cases, with a mean age of 69.3 years. Indications for the use of OSPS included preparation for colonoscopy in 7 patients, for abdominal surgery in 2 patients and for abdominal CT scan in 1 patient. One of the two remaining patients used OSPS as a laxative and no indication was provided for the other patient. Detailed clinical information is available for 10 of the 12 cases. Seven of the 10 patients received doses of OSPS far in excess of the quantity typically prescribed for bowel purgation. All ten patients presented with severe hyperphosphatemia and acute kidney injury within 24 hours of exposure. At the time of presentation, the mean serum phosphorus was 31.2 mg/dl (range 13.4 to 59.6 mg/dl). The clinical symptoms were dominated by manifestation of severe hyperphosphatemia and in many cases hypocalcemia, leading to tetany, cardiac arrest, and in five patients, death. Acute management focused on correction of severe electrolyte abnormalities and included hydration, calcium supplementation, phosphate binders, and hemodialysis. All three patients who received acute hemodialysis had excellent outcomes, leading at least one author to recommend this therapeutic approach [23].

The reports in table 1 briefly mention but do not focus on changes in renal function. Among the seven patients who survived the immediate event, six returned to normal or near-normal renal function and the single remaining patient had significant improvement in renal function prior to hospital discharge. Given that electrolyte disorders dominated the clinical presentations and that renal function rapidly improved, none of the patients underwent renal biopsy. Among the 5 patients who expired, one underwent autopsy and no calcium phosphate deposition was identified in the kidney [25]. Of note, an additional, similar case has been reported in which a 48-year-old woman used "huge" doses of oral phosphate on a "daily" basis for chronic constipation. The patient was found at home in a semicomatose state with a blood urea nitrogen of 33 mg/dl and a serum phosphorus of 47 mg/dl *after a five-to-one dilution* [34]. The details of this case are limited and therefore it is not included in table 1. Nonetheless, an interesting finding is that the patient expired within 12 hours and post-mortem evaluation of the kidney was notable for marked hydropic degeneration of the renal tubules, in the absence of calcifications. The cases described in table 1 are part of a larger topic of severe electrolyte abnormalities following the use of OSPS that is reviewed elsewhere [21]. Table 1 focuses only on cases in which acute kidney injury was part of the clinical presentation.

In 2003, Desmeules et al. described a new pattern of renal failure resulting from the use of OSPS [29]. A 71-year-old female with a baseline creatinine of 1.0 mg/dl presented with acute kidney injury and a creatinine of 4.5 mg/dl two weeks following the use of OSPS. Renal biopsy revealed numerous tubular calcium phosphate deposits. Scanning electron microscopy and energy-dispersive x-ray microanalysis revealed that the calcium phosphate deposits formed crystals of hydroxyapatite. The patient's creatinine declined to 1.7 mg/dl at one year of follow-up. The authors described the process as "phosphosoda-induced nephrocalcinosis" and proposed the term "acute phosphate nephropathy".

In 2004, we reported five distinctive cases of ne-

Table 1: Acute kidney injury following the use of OSPS: Cases Without Renal Biopsies

Reference	Age/ Sex	Medical conditions	Indication for OSPS	Dose of OSPS	Interval from OSPS to AKI	Peak serum phosphorus	Baseline sCr	Peak sCr	Final sCr	Duration of follow-up	Treatment
Zipser 1975	41 M	heavy alcohol intake	none	180 ml	< 24 hours	31	na	8.4	1.2	21 days	gastric suction, IV hydration, oral lysine monohydrochloride
Fass 1993	64 M	DM, HTN, CAD, COPD, CHF, pulmonary coccidiosis	ileus	120 ml x 2	< 24 hours	59.6	1	3.4	na	Cardiac arrest & death	phosphorus-binding resin, calcium gluconate
Ahmed 1996	77 F	Parkinson's, Alzheimer's	screening colonoscopy	45 ml (single dose)	< 24 hours	27.8	1	5	2.5	na (prior to discharge)	IV saline, calcium gluconate, aluminum hydroxide
Fine 1997	84 F	HTN, CHF, previous nephrectomy	Purgative prior to abdominal CT	45 ml x 6 (over 4 days)	< 24 hours	35	0.7	2.5	na	Cardiac arrest & death	
Orias 1999	76 M	HTN, colon cancer	Purgative prior to surgery	45 ml x 5	< 24 hours	15.8	1.1	3.7	1.3	1 month	acute HD
Tan 2002 - pt 1	52 F	colon cancer	Purgative prior to surgery	90 ml x 4	< 24 hours	13.4	"normal"	2.9	normal	2 days	
Tan 2002 - pt 2	66 F	benign brain tumor, anemia, pneumonia	colonoscopy; anemia	90 ml x 2 & PEG (1 L)	< 24 hours	57.6	1	1.7	na	central pontine myelinosis, sepsis, death	
Ullah 2002	55 M	DM, HTN, ESRD, renal transplantation	colonoscopy; hematochezia	45 ml x 2	6 hours	17.8	1	3.1	na	Immediate cardiac arrest & death*	
Azzam 2004	79 F	DM, obesity, CKD, cirrhosis	colonoscopy; diarrhea	45 ml x 4 & phos enema x 4	< 24 hours	24	1.3	2	"return to baseline"	5 days	HD, calcium gluconate
Aydogan 2006	82 F	constipation	colonoscopy; constipation	45 ml x 2	8 hours	29.8	"normal"	2.1	na	Immediate cardiac arrest & death	
Ma 2007 - pt 1	75 M	DM, HTN	screening colonoscopy	na	4 days	na	0.9	10.5	1.3	na	continuous renal replacement therapy
Ma 2007 - pt 2	80 F	DM, HTN	screening colonoscopy	na	3 days	na	0.9	7.1	1.1	na	

All creatinine values expressed in mg/dl

Key: M male; F female; DM diabetes mellitus; HTN hypertension; CAD coronary artery disease; COPD chronic obstructive pulmonary disease; CHF congestive heart failure; ESRD end stage renal disease; OSPS oral sodium phosphate solution; PEG polyethylene glycol; AKI acute kidney injury; na not available; HD hemodialysis.

* *Autopsy revealed acute ischemic colitis. No renal calcium phosphate deposits were noted.*

phrocalcinosis that differed from the usual form of disease [35]. The cohort consisted of 2 males and 3 females with a mean age of 69.2 years. All 5 patients had a history of hypertension and 4 were receiving either an angiotensin converting enzyme inhibitor (ACE-I) or an angiotensin receptor blocker (ARB). The cohort was distinctive in that all of the patients had recently undergone colonoscopy, none had a history of hypercalcemia, and the renal failure had an acute onset, unlike the usual insidious presentation of nephrocalcinosis. Patients had a mean baseline creatinine of 0.9 mg/dl at a mean of 4 months prior to colonoscopy. Acute kidney injury with a mean creatinine of 4.9 mg/dl was documented at a mean of 3 weeks post-colonoscopy. In all 5 patients, bowel cleansing with OSPS preceded colonoscopy. Thus, while hypercalcemia was not present, an exogenous source of phosphate was identified. The changes were referred to as "*acute* nephrocalcinosis" to emphasize the rapidity of onset. At a mean of 6 weeks post-colonoscopy, the patients had a mean creatinine of 4.7 mg/dl. We subsequently reported a case in which acute nephrocalcinosis followed the use of visicol [36].

In 2005, we reported a larger series of patients with acute phosphate nephropathy (APhN) [30]. We choose to adopt this more appropriate term because it emphasizes the important pathogenic role of exogenous phosphate administration [29]. The archives of the renal pathology laboratory at Columbia University from 2000 - 2004 were reviewed in an effort to identify additional cases of APhN. Five criteria were required to establish the diagnosis of APhN. Patients had to have: 1) acute kidney injury; 2) recent exposure to OSPS or visicol; 3) renal biopsy findings of acute and chronic tubular injury with abundant calcium phosphate deposits; 4) no evidence of hypercalcemia or conditions associated with hypercalemia; and 5) no other significant pattern of renal injury on renal biopsy. During this 5-year period, 7,349 native renal biopsies were processed, of which 31 met the criteria of acute and chronic tubular injury with abundant calcium phosphate deposits. Among the 31 cases, 10 were excluded for the following reasons. Four patients met criteria for APhN but had a second, significant disease process on renal biopsy, for instance acute post-infectious glomerulonephritis. Two patients were excluded because although they had a history of recent colonoscopy prior to the development of AKI, information was not available on the bowel preparation regimen. Two additional patients were excluded due to a history of hypercalcemia and 2 had no recent history of colonoscopy. Thus, among 31 cases that previously might have been classified as "nephrocalcinosis", a history of hypercalcemia was present in only 2 patients. In contrast, a history of recent colonoscopy preceded by the use of OSPS was present in 25 patients [30].

The remaining 21 patients met all five criteria for the diagnosis of acute phosphate nephropathy and included the 6 cases that had been previous reported [35-36]. The cohort consisted of predominantly women (17 patients; 81.0%) and Caucasians (17 patients; 81.0%) with a mean age of 64.0 years (Table 2). Sixteen patients (76.2%) had a history of hypertension, including 14 who were treated with an ACE-I or ARB. The mean baseline serum creatinine was 1.0 mg/dl and was available within <1 month of colonoscopy in 11 patients and within <4 months of colonoscopy in 19 patients (Table 2). Patients presented with AKI and a mean creatinine of 3.9 mg/dl at a median of <1 month following OSPS use. Specifically, 8 patients presented with AKI <2 weeks after colonoscopy while 18 patients presented within <2 months of OSPS use. The mean 24-hour urine protein was 256 mg, and microscopic evaluation of the urine revealed either a bland sediment or rare RBC's or WBC's. The mean duration of post-colonoscopy follow-up was 16.7 months. During this time, 4 patients progressed to ESRD, requiring dialysis. Sixteen of the remaining 17 patients had a decline in serum creatinine to a mean of 2.4 mg/dl. Only 4 patients reached a creatinine <2.0 mg/dl and no patient returned to baseline.

There have been additional recent reports of acute phosphate nephropathy following the use of OSPS (Table 2) [19, 31-33]. Similar to the majority of cases previously described, these patients appear to have taken OSPS at the correct dose and in the absence of clear contra-indications. Also similar to the previous reports, none of the patients have returned to normal renal function and no patient presented in the initial 24 hours with symptoms of hyperphosphatemia such as tetany or cardiac arrest. One case is of particular interest in that the patient underwent renal biopsy both before and after exposure to OSPS [32]. The patient initially presented with nephrotic syndrome and normal renal function. Renal biopsy revealed membranous nephropathy (MN). In an effort to exclude a secondary form of MN related to malignancy, the patient underwent screening colonoscopy preceded by bowel cleansing with OSPS. The patient had a creatinine of 0.9 mg/dl one month prior to colonoscopy and a creatinine of 4.3 mg/dl one day following colonoscopy. Five days later she had a creatinine of 6.0 when a renal biopsy revealed MN with the additional finding of APhN, which had not been present in the initial renal

Table 2: Biopsy-documented reports of acute phosphate nephropathy.

Cases	Age/ Gender	Baseline creatinine	Interval pre-CSPY	Creatinine upon discovery of AKI	Interval post-CSPY	Creatinine at time of renal biopsy	Interval post-CSPY	Final creatinine	Interval post-CSPY
Desmeules 2003	71 F	1.0	8 weeks	4.5	2 weeks	4.5	2 weeks	1.7	1 year
Markowitz 2005 pt 1	69 M	1.2	2 weeks	6.7	1 month	6.3	7 weeks	ESRD	18 months
Markowitz 2005 pt 2	82 M	0.9	1 day	5.2	1 week	4.9	4 weeks	ESRD	9 months
Markowitz 2005 pt 3	55 F	0.6	3.5 months	4.5	13 days	4.0	4 months	2.7	24 months
Markowitz 2005 pt 4	64 F	0.9	4 months	2.3	2 months	3.0	7 months	ESRD	15 months
Markowitz 2005 pt 5	76 F	0.9	12 months	6.0	3 days	8.0	6 days	1.9	20 months
Markowitz 2005 pt 6	53 M	1.0	1 day	4.8	12 days	2.2	3 months	1.3	55 months
Markowitz 2005 pt 7	81 F	0.9	1 month	3.3	4.5 months	3.3	5 months	2.6	15 months
Markowitz 2005 pt 8	82 F	1.1	3.5 months	4.4	3 weeks	3.3	13 months	3.1	15 months
Markowitz 2005 pt 9	57 F	0.7	1 day	1.8	1 day	3.1	3 weeks	2.7	2 months
Markowitz 2005 pt 10	76 F	0.9	4 months	3.8	2 months	3.6	6 months	2.1	33 months
Markowitz 2005 pt 11	74 F	1.5	2 months	3.9	1 month	3.0	4 months	3.0	5 months
Markowitz 2005 pt 12	57 F	1.0	1 day	3.8	2 days	3.1	14 days	1.5	2 months
Markowitz 2005 pt 13	43 F	0.9	2 weeks	2.2	2 months	2.3	6 months	1.8	13 months
Markowitz 2005 pt 14	39 F	0.7	11 days	4.5	5 days	4.1	17 days	2.7	11 months
Markowitz 2005 pt 15	69 F	1.3	1 month	4.2	5 months	4.6	7 months	ESRD	13 months
Markowitz 2005 pt 16	66 F	1.4	8 years	3.7	19 days	3.9	4 months	3.4	11 months
Markowitz 2005 pt 17	51 F	0.9	2 weeks	3.0	5 weeks	2.7	2 months	2.1	13 months
Markowitz 2005 pt 18	79 F	0.7	3 months	3.4	3 months	3.2	4 months	2.8	6 months
Markowitz 2005 pt 19	44 M	1.7	2 weeks	2.6	2 months	2.3	5 months	2.2	9 months
Markowitz 2005 pt 20	62 F	0.9	7 weeks	5.9	8 days	3.6	17 days	3.4	23 months
Markowitz 2005 pt 21	64 F	0.9	2 months	2.6	2 months	2.3	4 months	1.8	38 months
Gonlusen 2006	56 F	0.8	5 months	3.8	13 days	na	44 days	1.6	10 months
Manley 2006	85 F	1.3	1 month	7.2	6 days	na	na	2.3	na
Aasebo 2006	69 F	0.9	1 month	4.3	1 day	6.0	6 days	1.7	42 months
Beyea 2007	66 F	0.8	na	10.2	1 week	na	na	2.6	na

All creatinine values expressed in mg/dl

Key: F female; M male; na not available; ESRD end stage renal disease; CSPY = colonoscopy; AKI = acute kidney injury.

biopsy performed 4 months prior. This unique case with renal biopsies performed before and after OSPS exposure further strengthens the pathogenic role of OSPS in the development of APhN.

Renal biopsy findings in acute phosphate nephropathy

Renal biopsy findings in acute phosphate nephropathy predominantly involve the tubules and are largely dependent on the time interval between the use of OSPS and renal biopsy. In cases with a short interval from OSPS exposure to renal biopsy, acute tubular degenerative changes predominate and resemble findings seen in acute tubular necrosis [35]. These findings of acute tubular injury involve all tubular segments and include diffuse epithelial simplification, luminal ectasia, loss of proximal tubular brush border, enlarged reparative nuclei with prominent nucleoli, shedding of cellular fragments into tubular lumina, apoptosis, and drop-out of tubular epithelial cells. The tubular degenerative changes are typically diffuse and are accompanied by interstitial edema.

The hallmark of acute phosphate nephropathy is the presence of abundant tubular and interstitial calcifications, commonly involving >40 tubular lumina in a single biopsy [35] (Figure 1A-1C). The calcifications form basophilic rounded concretions and are distributed in the lumina of tubules, within the cytoplasm of tubular epithelia, and, less prominently, within the interstitium. The calcifications often appear clustered in straight segments, suggesting a distribution in medullary rays, and are more prominent in the renal cortex than in the medulla. Importantly, the calcifications do not polarize and have a strong histochemical reaction with the von Kossa stain (Figure 1D), indicating that they are composed of calcium phosphate.

In cases with a longer interval between OSPS exposure and renal biopsy, histologic evaluation reveals a more chronic appearance. Renal biopsies performed more than 3 weeks following OSPS exposure typically exhibit evidence of chronicity in the form of tubular atrophy and interstitial fibrosis. Within a few months of OSPS exposure, the acute tubular degenerative changes begin to become less severe and more localized. This histologic pattern of renal injury may be described as an "acute and chronic tubulointerstitial nephropathy" and resembles changes seen in repeat renal biopsies from patients with non-resolving acute tubular necrosis. In 17 reported cases with this pattern of injury, tubular atrophy and interstitial fibrosis involved a mean of 47.1% of the cortical area sampled [30]. Findings of acute and chronic tubulointerstitial nephropathy have been documented in renal biopsies performed as late as 13 months after OSPS exposure [30]. Importantly, the abundant tubular and interstitial calcium phosphate deposits are a constant requirement to establish the diagnosis of APhN and persist in late biopsies characterized by extensive tubulointerstitial scarring but only mild, localized acute tubular injury.

Acute phosphate nephropathy is commonly accompanied by mild to moderate interstitial inflammation composed of mainly lymphocytes. The interstitial inflammation is not associated with significant tubulitis and likely represents a response to the tubular injury and calcium phosphate deposition. Glomeruli typically appear unremarkable. Vascular disease is commonly encountered but is an expected finding given the mean age and high incidence of hypertension in patients with APhN.

Immunohistochemical and lectin staining have led to insights into the pathogenesis of acute phosphate nephropathy [35]. Tubular calcium phosphate deposits are present in tubular segments that stain positively with Arachis hypogaea, Dolichos biflorus, and epithelial membrane antigen, but not with Tetragonolobus purpureas. These findings indicate that the calcium phosphate deposits are mainly confined to distal tubules and collecting duct. Immunohistochemical staining of tubules also reveals findings commonly encountered in the setting of acute tubular injury including increased staining for Ki-67, a marker of cellular proliferation, and decreased intensity and apical translocation of $Na^{+}K^{+}$-ATPase.

Phosphate administration leading to nephrocalcinosis: human data unrelated to colonoscopy preparation or laxative use

In 1930 and 1932, two separate reports were published, each describing the successful treatment of 2 patients with hypercalcemia secondary to hyperparathyroidism with inorganic phosphate [37-38]. Due to the potential for this treatment to lead to nephrolithiasis or extraskeletal calcifications, it was not widely employed. In 1966, Goldsmith and Ingbar reported the successful treatment of hypercalcemia with inorganic phosphate [39]. This study included 15 patients with hypercalcemia related to malignancy, 4 patients with hyperparathyroidism, and one with vitamin D intoxication. Treatment led to rapid normalization of serum calcium levels in 16 of 20 patients, with hyperphosphatemia documented in only 2 patients. Autopsy was subsequently performed on seven patients and while extraskeletal calcifications were seen, the authors attributed it to the magnitude and duration of hypercalcemia, rather than the administration of phosphate. The authors concluded that there were no deleterious effects of phosphate administration in the acute management of hypercalcemia. As a result largely of this study, and despite the lack of understanding of the mechanism of action, phosphate administration gained acceptance as a treatment option for hypercalcemia.

Not surprisingly, subsequent reports established the danger of utilizing exogenous phosphate to treat hypercalcemia. A 46-year-old woman with multiple myeloma and a calcium of 17.8 mg/dl was treated with oral and intravenous phosphate and developed acute kidney injury with abrupt cessation of calciuria [40]. A 40-year-old male with squamous cell carcinoma

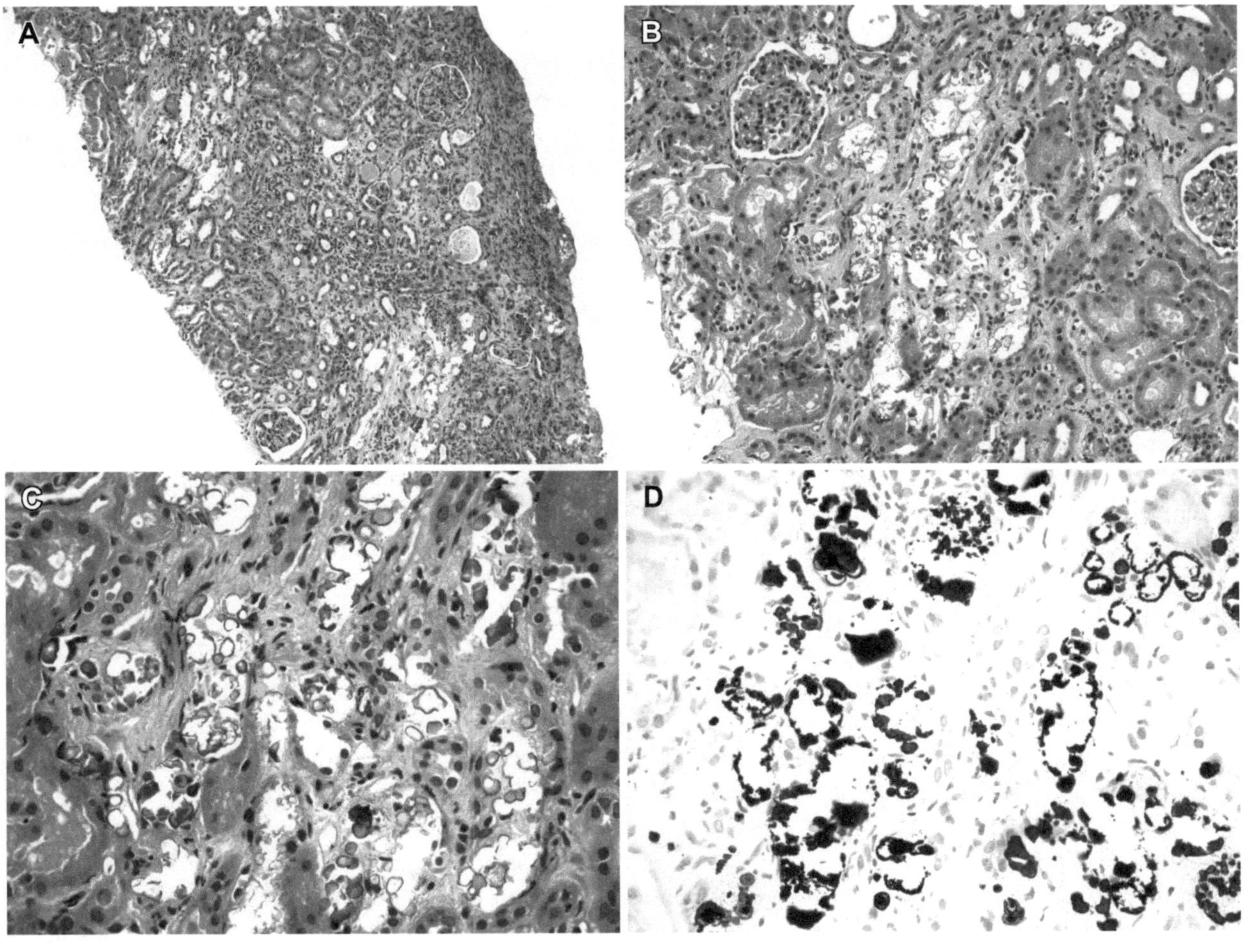

Figure 1.

A. *A low magnification view displays disproportionate tubulointerstitial scarring. There is mild to moderate interstitial chronic inflammation. Prominent tubular calcifications are seen in the upper left and lower right portions of the field. (Hematoxylin & eosin, orig. magn. 100x).*

B. *An intermediate magnification view shows abundant tubular calcifications. The calcifications do not polarize and are mainly confined to distal tubules. (H&E, orig. magn. 200x).*

C. *A high power view shows that the calcifications have an intra-cellular (within tubular epithelia), intra-luminal, and interstitial distribution. (H&E, orig. magn. 400x).*

D. *The tubular calcifications stain intensely with the von Kossa stain, consistent with calcium phosphate. (orig. magn. 400x).*

of the pyriform sinus and a calcium of 12.8 mg/dl was treated with oral and intravenous phosphate and similarly developed acute kidney injury [41]. Post-mortem evaluation of these two patients revealed abundant calcifications in the kidneys, lungs, heart, stomach, spleen, and blood vessels throughout the body. Of note, within the kidney calcifications were seen in tubules, glomeruli, interstitium, and blood vessels. Another report described two patients with hypercalcemia of malignancy who were treated with intravenous phosphate and developed hypocalcemia, hypotension, and acute kidney injury [42]. Acute and subsequent chronic renal failure was described in a patient with primary hyperparathyroidism who received solely oral phosphate [43]. An additional report described calcifications on the conjunctiva, cornea, subcutis, or kidney in 7 of 9 patients treated with oral phosphate for a history of nephrolithiasis or hypercalcemia related to hyperparathyroidism or myeloma [44]. In two patients, a decline in renal function was noted during therapy, including one with extensive renal calcium phosphate deposits noted on post-mortem evaluation. The concept that phosphate infusion leads to calcium phosphate precipitation is supported by experiments showing phosphate infusion produces a concentration-dependent decline in serum calcium that is not explained by a reciprocal degree of calciuria [45].

Oral phosphate administration leading to renal calcium phosphate precipitation has been described in children with X-linked hypophosphatemic rickets. Children with this condition are treated with oral phosphate and vitamin D and frequently developed ultrasonographic evidence of nephrocalcinosis, and the grade of nephrocalcinosis correlates with cumulative phosphate intake [46]. Renal biopsy findings are similar to those seen in acute phosphate nephropathy, with calcifications confined to tubules and the peritubular interstitium [47].

Preterm neonates undergo intensive growth and bone mineralization during the early postnatal period and require calcium and phosphorus supplementation. Not surprisingly, this treatment can lead to nephrocalcinosis. In one study, nephrocalcinosis was documented by ultrasound in 41% of premature infants at full term, and the finding correlated with higher mean intake of calcium or phosphorus [48]. Nephrocalcinosis may resolve in preterm infants following discontinuation of calcium and phosphate supplementation [49].

Phosphate administration leading to nephrocalcinosis: animal data

Studies in rats have shown that exogenous phosphate administration leads to nephrocalcinosis and have provided insight into this process. In one study, female Wistar rats were fed with a 0.4% or 0.6% phosphate diet. The higher level of phosphate intake was associated with increased phosphate retention, increased kidney weight and calcium phosphate deposition, and a greater decline in serum calcium [50]. Renal function in individual rats, as assessed by plasma urea level, correlated with kidney calcium content [50]. The same group went on to show that there is considerable variation in the ability of rat strains to develop nephrocalcinosis and that the differences are reproducible [51]. Susceptible rat strains are characterized by a lower serum phosphorus and higher urine phosphorus concentration after administration of a 0.5% phosphate diet [51]. Exogenous phosphate administration also leads to nephrocalcinosis in mice [47], rabbits [52-53], and dogs [54].

Acute phosphate nephropathy: pathophysiology & risk factors

Calcium phosphorus product (CPP) is generally regarded as an indicator of the likelihood of calcium phosphate precipitation in human tissues and, more specifically, the renal tubules. Based on the normal serum concentration ranges for calcium and phosphorus, the normal range for CPP is 21 to 47.3. Following the use of OSPS, serum phosphorus and CPP transiently increase and the duration and magnitude of this change are likely to be important risk factors for the development of APhN.

Metabolic studies have provided insights into the handling of the small volume of hyperosmotic sodium phosphate that is present in OSPS [55]. A group of 5 normal subjects (age 27-55 years) in a metabolic research unit were administered two 45-ml doses of OSPS at 6 PM and 5 AM the following morning. The patients were instructed to drink liberally and stool and urine were collected for 18 consecutive hours, from 6 PM (when the first OSPS was administered) to 12 PM the following day. The total stool content of phosphorus was 57% of the ingested dose. Thus, despite its osmotic mechanism of action whereby OSPS acts to draw fluid into the bowel lumen, 43% of ingested phosphate is absorbed by the intestine. Urine phosphorus content was 14.7% of the ingest dose. At seven hours following the second OSPS administration, 28.3% of ingested phosphorus was retained [55]. Data was not provided on phosphorus excretion beyond the initial 18 hours.

As previously discussed, phosphate absorption in the small intestine does not appear to be tightly controlled over short periods of time and therefore cannot be physiologically modulated in "real time" following OSPS ingestion [2-3, 5]. In contrast, proximal tubular phosphate reabsorption can be modulated within minutes of OSPS ingestion, leading to decreased proximal tubular reabsorption and a rapid increase in phosphate delivery to the distal tubule. While this physiologic response is beneficial in most situations, it may be detrimental in the setting of the profound volume depletion that can follow OSPS ingestion. Volume depletion leads to avid salt and water reabsorption not only in the proximal tubule but also in the descending limb of the loop of Henle, which is relatively impermeable to calcium and phosphate [56]. The net effect is avid salt and water reabsorption and decreased phosphate reabsorption in proximal segments of the nephron, leading to a marked increase in CPP within the lumen of the distal tubule. This is supported by the observation that calcium phosphate precipitates in APhN occur predominantly in the distal tubule and collecting duct [35]. Hypovolemia leading to tubular injury also may precondition the distal tubular epithelium, leading to surface expression of hyaluronan and osteopontin, which in turn creates a ripe environment for calcium phosphate crystals adherence [57]. Based on these considerations, the critical role of adequate hydration cannot be overstated. OSPS leads to diarrhea and volume depletion. Adequate hydration before, during, and after OSPS exposure diminishes volume depletion, undoubtedly lowering the serum and distal tubular CPP.

Angiotensin converting enzyme inhibitors and angiotensin receptor blockers are likely to exacerbate the pre-renal state caused by the diarrhea and volume depletion that follow the use of OSPS (Table 3). Of the 21 cases of APhN reported in the largest series to date, 14 were receiving one of these two agents [30]. In addition to their effects on volume status, ACE-I and ARB lead to a decline in angiotensin-II dependent bicarbonate reabsorption in the proximal tubule [58]. The resultant bicarbonaturia in the distal tubule has the combined effect of decreasing phosphate absorption [6] and promoting calcium phosphate precipitation [59]. Diuretics and non-steroidal anti-inflammatory agents also exacerbate the effects of volume depletion. A recent study looking at 100 consecutive patients undergoing colonoscopy preceded by bowel cleansing with OSPS found a greater degree of hyperphosphatemia in patients who were taking an ACE-I, ARB, or loop diuretics [60]. Under appropriate conditions, it may be prudent to avoid administering these agents on the day before and the day of the colonoscopy [30, 60].

Age is an important risk factor for the development of acute phosphate nephropathy. Gumurdulu et al. examined electrolyte levels in 70 patients who received two 45-ml doses of OSPS separated by 12 hours and found that the mean increase in serum phosphorus was 3.6 mg/dl in patients between the age of 25-35 years, compared to an increment of 5.5 mg/dl in individuals over the age of 56 [61]. The mean change in phosphate correlated strongly with patient age (Pearson's $r = 0.705$; $p < 0.001$), leading the authors to suggest that this effect was the result of a decline in creatinine clearance with age or increased intestinal transit time leading to increased phosphate absorption. Another study looked at 100 consecutive patients undergoing outpatient colonoscopy and found a correlation between the degree of hyperphosphatemia following the use of OSPS and both patient age and serum creatinine [60]. In a study on 36 hospitalized patients age 65 or older who received OSPS, an inverse relationship between degree of hyperphosphatemia and creatinine clearance was noted [62]. Thus, advanced age is associated with a greater degree of transient hyperphosphatemia following the use of OSPS, and the decline in renal function that occurs with aging is likely to be a component of

Table 3: Risk factors for the development of acute phosphate nephropathy*

I. Probable Risk Factors
A. Inadequate hydration (at the time of OSPS use)
B. Advanced age
C. Hypertension treated with ACE-I, ARB, or loop diuretics
II. Possible Risk Factors
A. Female gender
B. Small body habitus
C. Non-steroidal anti-inflammatory drugs

** Does not include contra-indications listed on the product label*

this process.

Additional risk factors for the development of acute phosphate nephropathy are less well established (Table 3). APhN has been reported more commonly in females than males, including 22 of the 26 cases (84.6%) in Table 2. Similarly, female rats are more susceptible than male rats to developing nephrocalcinosis following exogenous phosphate administration [63]. This effect is likely to be estrogen dependent as it is lost in female rats following oophectomy and gained in male rats following gonadectomy and estrogen therapy [63]. While the findings in rats suggest that the increased incidence in females may be hormone dependent, an alternative or additional factor may be that female subjects are smaller. This raises the possibility that dosing of OSPS should be adjusted for body size. Future studies correlating degree of hyperphosphatemia and both gender and body weight may provide important insights. Studies in rats have also shown reproducible differences between strains in the propensity to develop nephrocalcinosis following phosphate administration [51]. This raises the possibility that genetic factors that influence phosphate handling may also play a role in the development of APhN.

Reducing the incidence of acute phosphate nephropathy

The true incidence of acute phosphate nephropathy is unknown. Unexplained renal failure is not uncommon in elderly patients and until recently, the entity of acute phosphate nephropathy had not been described. Consider the example of a hypothetical 65-year-old female who is being treated with an ACE-I for hypertension and is found to have unexplained renal failure. The patient has minimal proteinuria, bland urine sediment, and negative serologies. The ACE-I is discontinued and the creatinine trends minimally downward over time. The patient may not be referred to a nephrologist. If referred, based on common nephrology practices, it is highly unlikely that she would undergo renal biopsy [64]. In the rare event that the patient undergoes renal biopsy, a diagnosis of nephrocalcinosis would likely be rendered and the nephrologist would investigate for conditions associated with hypercalcemia. It is highly unlikely that a history of recent colonoscopy would be sought.

The role of exogenous phosphate administration (i.e. OSPS) in the development of acute phosphate nephropathy is gaining increased recognition. In May of 2006, the United States Food and Drug Administration issued an alert regarding the potential for OSP products to lead to acute kidney injury and APhN (www.fda.gov/cder/drug/infopage/osp_solution). This warning was subsequently added to a consensus document on bowel preparation jointly issued by the American Society of Colon & Rectal Surgeons, the American Society of Gastrointestinal Endoscopy, and the Society of American Gastrointestinal & Endoscopic Surgeons [65].

Multiple studies have attempted to address the issue of incidence of acute phosphate nephropathy. During calender year 2005, C.B. Fleet, a large producer of OSPS, reported 10 serious adverse events (SAE) for every 1,000,000 doses sold, but did not specify how many of these involved the kidney [66]. Clearly, the overwhelming majority of SAE's are unreported. The relatively small number of enrolled patients significantly flaws prospective studies of APhN, and ethical considerations may limit the ability to perform prospective studies.Retrospective studies may be flawed if they are underpowered, do not take into account biases in selection of bowel preparation, and do not appropriately define renal failure [67, 68].

Among the available retrospective studies on the incidence of APhN, the largest is an observational cohort analysis of 9,799 patients identified through the electronic medical record system of Department of Defense beneficiaries in the U.S. national capital area [69]. This electronic medical record system has the unique feature of tracking over the counter medication use, such as OSPS. The study excluded patients under the age of 50 due to the high incidence of inflammatory bowel disease and applied an appropriately strict definition of acute kidney injury (AKI), requiring a >50% increase in serum creatinine from baseline over 1 year post-colonoscopy. In this study, 114 patients (1.16%) developed AKI, including 1.29% of the 6,432 patients who received OSP and 0.92% of the 3,367 patients who received PEG. The PEG group included patients who were significantly older and had a higher incidence of diabetes mellitus, hypertension, atherosclerotic cardiovascular disease, congestive heart failure, chronic kidney disease, diuretic use, and ACE-I or ARB use (all $p<0.05$). When multiple logistic regression models were applied to adjust for covariates and suspected risk factors, OSPS was found to be the strongest risk factor for the development of AKI following colonoscopy (Odds Ratio 2.35; p<0.001). When AKI was redefined more strictly as doubling of serum creatinine, an even stronger association between OSPS and AKI was found (Odds Ratio 3.52; p=0.03). In attempting to evaluate the risk increase of AKI for OSPS vs. PEG, the authors calculated a "number needed to harm" of only 81. Not surprisingly, the authors concluded that PEG purgatives are preferable in older patients and possibly in patients with comorbidities.

The incidence of acute phosphate nephropathy is likely to significantly decline in the future due to greater awareness of the risk factors for this condition, more careful selection of bowel purgatives for individual patients, and changes in the dosing of OSPS. Increasing the phosphate content of OSPS leads to a greater degree of transient hyperphosphatemia [70]. The converse is true and does not appear to compromise efficacy of bowel cleansing. A randomized, multicenter, endoscopist-blinded study on 98 patients who were prepped with either 32 tablets (48 g sodium phosphate) or 28 tablets (42 g) of Visicol, rather than the full course of 40 tablets, found that colonic cleansing was "good" or "excellent" in 85% of patients and "inadequate" in none [71]. Another study found equal cleansing efficacy when comparing PEG to a combination regimen that included a single 45-ml dose of OSPS, four bisacodyl tablets, and one bisacodyl enema [72]. Only 15.7% of patients who received the combination regimen developed hyperphosphatemia, compared to 81% of patients who received two 45-ml doses of OSPS in a previous study by the same authors [73]. The "next generation of Phospho-soda" is now being marketed and is a kit in which the second dose of OSPS has been reduced from 45-ml to 30-ml (www.fleetez-prep.com/health/health.html). This represents a reduction of phosphate content by 16.7%, which reportedly is associated with equal efficacy and greater tolerability. Similarly Visicol, the tablet form of OSP, is being replaced by OsmoPrep. OsmoPrep has similar phosphate content to Visicol, but current recommendations are for the ingestion of 32 rather than 40 tablets, which represents a 20% reduction in phosphate content that does not appear to impact bowel cleansing efficacy (Osmoprep, Salix Pharmaceuticals).

In addition to decreasing the quantity of OSPS used for bowel preparation, there has also been increased emphasis on the importance of adequate hydration before, during, and after colonoscopy. The current recommendation is for a minimum of 72 ounces of clear liquids to go along with a regimen of 45- & 30-ml of OSPS. Future recommendations may include increasing the interval between OSPS administrations from 12 to 24 hours, as this is likely to produce less significant changes in serum electrolytes [74]. Along the same lines, anesthesia regimens that require no oral intake for 4-6 hours prior to the colonoscopy procedure exacerbate volume depletion, increase the risk of APhN, and should be avoided when possible. Due to the apparent increase in the incidence of APhN in females, future studies may address the potential for altering the dose of OSPS based on gender or body-size. Dose reduction or even complete avoidance of OSPS in elderly patients should also be explored.

Conclusion

The role of oral sodium phosphate bowel purgatives in the development of acute phosphate nephropathy has gained increased recognition. In the United States alone, 14 million colonoscopies are performed each year and over 5 million units of OSPS are sold [75-76]. These numbers underscore the importance of preventing APhN. Further studies are needed to determine the true incidence of APhN, to better understand risk factors for the development of APhN, and to provide guidelines for the most appropriate bowel preparation regimen in different patient populations. Existing data strongly suggest that the mechanism of disease is likely to be dose-dependent. As such, preparations with decreased phosphate content and emphasis on adequate hydration are likely to significantly curtail the incidence of acute phosphate nephropathy.

Disclosure statement
Dr. Glen Markowitz is a consultant to Salix Pharmaceuticals.

References

1. Klemm KM, Klein MJ. Biochemical markers of bone metabolism. In: Henry's Clinical Diagnosis and Management by Laboratory Methods. 21st Edition. McPherson RA, Pincus MR (editors). Saunders Elsevier 2007: p. 170-184.
2. Murer H, Hernando N, Forster L, Biber J. Molecular mechanisms in proximal tubular and small intestinal phosphate reabsorptio. Mol Membr Biol 2001; 18: 3-11.
3. Forster IC, Hernando N, Biber J, Murer H: Proximal tubular handling of phosphate: A molecular perspective. Kidney Int. 2006; 70: 1548-1559.
4. Chau H, El-Maadawy S, McKee MD, Tenenhouse HS: Renal calcification in mice homozygous for the disrupted type IIa Na/Pi cotransporter gene Npt2. J Bone Miner Res. 2003; 18: 644-657.
5. Berndt T, Thomas LF, Craig TA, Sommer S, Li X, Bergstralh EJ, Kumar R: Evidence for a signaling axis by which intestinal phosphate rapidly modulates renal phosphate absorption. Proc Natl Acad Sci USA 2007; 104: 11085-11090.
6. Tenenhouse HS, Gauthier C, Martel J, Gesek FA, Coutermarsh BA, Friedman PA. Na^{+}-phosphate cotransport in mouse distal convoluted tubule cells: Evidence for Glvr-1 and Ram-1 gene expression. J Bone Miner Res 1998; 13: 590-7.
7. Sayer JA, Carr G, Simmons NL. Nephrocalcinosis: Molecular insights into calcium precipitation within the kidney. Clinical Science 2004; 106: 549-561.
8. Vanner SJ, MacDonald PH, Paterson WG, Prentice RS, Da Cost LR, Beck IT. A randomized prospective trial comparing oral sodium phosphate with standard polyethylene glycol-based lavage solution (Golytely) in the preparation of patients for colonoscopy. Am J Gastroenterol 1990; 85: 422-7.
9. Cohen SM, Wexner SD, Binderow SR, Nogueras JJ, Daniel N, Ehrenpreis ED, Jensen J, Bonner GF, Ruderman WB. Prospective, randomized, endoscopic-blinded trial comparing precolonoscopy bowel cleansing methods. Dis Colon Rectum 1994; 37: 689-696.
10. Golub RW, Kerner BA, WiseWE, Meesig DM, Hartmann RF, Khanduja KS, Aguilar PS. Colonoscopic Bowel Preparations – Which One? A Blinded, Prospective, Randomized Trial. Dis Colon Rectum 1995; 38: 594-599.
11. Tan JJ, Tjandra JJ: Which is the optimal bowel preparation for colonoscopy – a meta-analysis. Colorectal Dis 2006; 8: 247-258.
12. Chan A, Depew W, Vanner S. Use of oral sodium phosphate colonic lavage solution by Canadian colonoscopists: pitfalls and complications. Can J Gastroenterol 1997; 11: 334-8.
13. Fine A, Patterson J: Severe Hyperphosphatemia Following Phosphate Administration for Bowel Preparation in Patients With Renal Failure: Two Cases and a Review of the Literature. Am J Kidn Dis 1997; 29: 103-105.
14. Mishra R, Kaufman D, Mattern J 3rd, Dutta SK. Severe hyperphosphatemia and hypocalcemia caused by bowel preparation for colonoscopy using oral sodium phosphate in end-stage renal disease. Endoscopy 2005; 37: 1259-60.
15. Kastenberg D, Chasen R, Cuckoo C, Riff D, Steinberg S, Weiss E, Wruble L: Efficacy and safety of sodium phosphate tablets compared with PEG solution in colon cleansing: two identically designed, randomized, controlled, parallel group multicenter phase III trials. Gastrointestinal Endoscopy 2001; 54: 705-712.
16. Carson FL: Histotechnology: A self-instructional text. Second Edition, Chicago, USA, ASCP Press, 1997.
17. Gwinner W, Suppa S, Mengel M, Hoy L, Kreipe HH, Haller H, Schwarz A. Early calcifications in renal allografts detected by protocol biopsies: Causes and clinical implications. Am J Transplant. 2005; 5:1934-1941.
18. Nankivell BJ, Borrows RJ, Fung CL, O'Connell PJ, Allen RD, Chapman JR. The natural history of chronic allograft nephropathy. N Engl J Med. 2003; 349:2326-2333.
19. Gonlusen G, Akgun H, Ertan A, Olivero J, Truong L. Renal Failure and Nephrocalcinosis Associated with Oral Sodium Phosphate Bowel Cleansing. Arch Patholo Lab Med 2006; 130: 101-6.
20. Zipser RD, Bischel MD, Abrams DE. Hypocalcemic tetany due to sodium phosphate ingestion in acute renal failure. Nephron 1975; 14: 378-381.
21. Fass R, Do S, Hixson LJ: Fatal Hyperphosphatemia following Fleet Phospho-Soda in a Patient with Colonic Ileus. Am J Gastroenterol 1993; 88: 929-932.
22. Ahmed M, Raval P, Buganza G. Oral sodium phosphate catharsis and acute renal failure. Am J Gastroenterol 1996; 6: 1261-2.
23. Orias M, Mahnensmith RL, Perazella MA. Extreme hyperphosphatemia and acute renal failure after a phosphorus-containing bowel regimen. Am J Nephrol 1999; 19: 60-3.
24. Tan HL, Liew QY, Loo S, Hawkins R. Severe hyperphosphatemia and associated electrolyte and metabolic derangement following the administration of sodium phosphate for bowel preparation. Anesthesia 2002; 57: 478-483.
25. Ullah N, Yeh R, Ehrinpreis M. Fatal Hyperphosphatemia From a Phosphosoda Bowel Preparation. J Clin Gastroenterol 2002; 34: 457-458.
26. Azzam I, Kovalev Y, Storch S, Elias N. Life threatening hyperphosphatemia after administration of sodium phosphate in preparation for colonoscopy. Postgrad Med J 2004; 80: 487-488.

27. Aydogan T, Kanbay M, Uz B, Kaya A, Bozalan R, Isik A, Bozalan R, Erkman M, Akcay A. Fatal hyperphosphatemia secondary to phosphosoda bowel preparation in a geriatric patient with normal renal function. J. Clin Gastroenterol 2006; 40: 177.
28. Ma RC, Chow CC, Yeung VT, So WY, Kong AP, Tong PC, Cockram CS, Chan JC. Acute renal failure following oral sodium phosphate bowel preparation in diabetes. Diabetes Care 2007; 30: 182-3.
29. Desmeules S. Gergeron MJ, Isenring P: Acute phosphate nephropathy and renal failure. N Engl J Med 2003; 349: 1006-7.
30. Markowitz GS, Stokes MB, Radhakrishnan J, D'Agati VD. Acute phosphate nephropathy following oral sodium phosphate bowel purgative: An underrecognized cause of chronic renal failure. J Am Soc Nephrol 2005; 16: 3389-3396.
31. Manley P, Somerfield J, Simpson I, Barber A, Zwi J. Bilateral uraemic optic neuritis complicating acute nephrocalcinosis. Nephrol Dial Transplant 2006; 21: 2957-8.
32. Aasebo W, Scott H, Ganss R. Kidney biopsies taken before and after sodium phosphate bowel cleansing. Nephrol Dial Transplant 2006; 22: 920-922.
33. Beyea A, Block C, Schned A. Acute phosphate nephropathy following oral sodium phosphate solution to cleanse the bowel for colonoscopy. Am J Kidn Dis 2007; 50: 151-4, 2007.
34. McConnell TH. Fatal hypocalcemia from phosphate absorption from laxative preparation. JAMA 1971; 216: 147-8.
35. Markowitz GS, Nasr SH, Klein P, Anderson H. Stack JI, Alterman L, Price B, Radhakrishnan J, D'Agati VD. Renal failure and acute nephrocalcinosis following oral sodium phosphate bowel cleansing. Human Pathol 2004; 35: 675-684.
36. Markowitz GS, Whelan, J, D'Agati, VD: Renal failure following bowel cleansing with a sodium phosphate purgative. Nephrol Dial Transplant 2005; 20: 850-851.
37. Bulger HA, Dixon HH, Barr DP, Schregardus O. The functional pathology of hyper-parathyroidism. J Clin Invest 1930; 9:143-190.
38. Albright F, Bauer W, Claflin D, Cockrill JR. Studies in parathyroid physiology III: The effect of phosphate ingestion in clinical hyperparathyroidism. J Clin Invest 1932; 11:411-435.
39. Goldsmith RS, Ingbar SH. Inorganic Phosphate Treatment of Hypercalcemia of Diverse Etiologies. N Eng J Med 1966; 274: 1-7.
40. Breuer I, LeBauer. Caution in the Use of Phosphates in the Treatment of Severe Hypercalcemia. J Clin Endocr 1967; 27: 695-8.
41. Carey RW, Schmitt GW, Kopald HH, Kantrowitz PA. Massive Extraskeletal Calcification During Phosphate Treatment of Hypercalcemia. Arch Intern Med 1968; 122: 150-5.
42. Shackney S, Hasson J. Preciptious Fall In Serum Calcium, Hypotension, and Acute Renal Failure After Intravenous Phosphate Therapy for Hypercalcemia. Ann of Intern Med 1967; 5:906-16.
43. Ayala G, Chertow BS, Shah JH, Williams GA, Kukreja SC. Acute Hyperphosphatemia and Acute Persistent Renal Insufficiency Induced by Oral Phosphate Therapy. Ann of Intern Med 1975; 83: 520-1.
44. Dudley FJ, Blackburn CRB. Extraskeletal Calcification Complicating Oral Neutral- Phosphate Therapy. Lancet 1970; 26: 628-630.
45. Hebert LA, Lemann J, Petersen JR, Lennon EJ. Studies of the mechanism by which phosphate infusion lowers the serum calcium concentration. J Clin Invest 1966; 45: 1886-1894.
46. Verge CF, Lam A, Simpson JM, Cowell CT, Howard NJ, Silink M. Effects of therapy in X-linked hypophosphatemic rickets. N Eng J Med 1991; 325: 1843-8.
47. Alon U, Donaldson DL, Hellerstein S, Warady BA, Harris DJ. Metabolic and histologic investigation of the nature of nephrocalcinosis in children with hypophosphatemic rickets and the Hyp mouse. J Pediatr 1992; 120: 899-905.
48. Schnell-Feith E, Kist-van Holthe J, Conneman N, van Zwietne PHT, Holscher HC, Zonderland HM, Brand R, van der Heijden BJ. Etiology of nephrocalcinosis in preterm neonates: Association of nutritional intake and urinary parameters. Kidney Int 2000; 58: 2102-2110.
49. Pfitzer A, Nelle M, Rohrschneider W, Linderkamp O, Troger J. Incidence of typical nephrocalcinosis ultrasound findings in premature infants during enteral calcium and phosphate administration. Z Geburtshilfe Neonatol 1998; 202: 159-163.
50. Ritkes-Hoitinga J, Lemmens AG, Danse LHJC, Beynen AC. Phosphorous-induced nephrocalcinosis and kidney function in female rats. J Nutr 1989; 119: 1423-1431.
51. Ritkes-Hoitinga J, Mathot JNJJ, Van Zutphen LFM, Beynen AC. Inbred strains of rats have differential sensitivity to dietary phosphorus-induced nephrocalcinosis. J Nutr 1992; 122: 1682-1692.
52. Cramer B, Husa L. Pushpanathan C: Nephrocalcinosis in rabbits – Correlation of ultrasound, computed tomography, pathology and renal function. Pediatr Radiol 1998; 28: 9-13.
53. Cramer B, Husa L. Pushpanathan C: Pattern and permanence of phosphate-induced nephrocalcinosis in rabbits. 1998; 28: 14-19.
54. Schneider P, Ober KM, Ueberberg H. Contribution to the phosphate-induced nephropathy in the dog. Comparative light and electron microscopic investigations on the proximal tubule after oral application of K2HPO4, Na2HPO4, KC1, and NaC1. Exp Patholol 1981; 19: 53-65.

55. Patel VK, Emmett M, Santa Ana C, Fordtran JS. Pathogenesis of nephrocalcinosis after sodium phosphate catharsis to prepare for colonoscopy; Intestinal phosphate absorption and its effect on urine mineral and electrolyte excretion. Human Pathol 2007; 38: 193-4.
56. Asplin JR, Mandel NS, Coe FL. Evidence of calcium phosphate supersaturation in the loop of Henle. Am J Physiol 1996; 270: F604-F613.
57. Verhulst A, Asselman M, De Naeyer S, Vervaet BA, Mengel M, Gwinner W, D'Haese PC, Verkoelen CF, DeBroe ME. Preconditioning of the distal tubular epithelium of the human kidney precedes nephrocalcinosis. Kidney Int. 2005; 68:1643-7.
58. Haithcock D, Jiao H, Cui XL, Hopfer U, Douglas JG. Renal proximal tubular AT2 receptor: Signaling and transport. J Am Soc Nephrol 1999; 10: S69-S74.
59. Hesse A, Heimbach D: Causes of phosphate stone formation and the importance of metaphylaxis by urinary acidification: A review. World J Urol 1999; 17: 308-315.
60. Ainley EJ, Winwood PJ, Begley JP. Measurement of Serum Electrolytes and Phosphate After Sodium Phosphate Colonoscopy Bowel Preparation. Digestive Dis and Sci 2005; 50: 1319-1323.
61. Gumurdulu Y, Serin E, Ozer B, Gokcel A, Boyacioglu S. Age as a predictor of hyperphosphatemia after oral phosphosoda administration for colon preparation. J Gastroenterol Hepatol 2004; 19: 68-72.
62. Beloosesky Y, Grinblat J, Weiss A, Grosman B, Gafter U, Chagnac A: Electrolyte disorders following oral sodium phosphate administration for bowel cleansing in elderly patients. Arch Intern Med 2003; 163: 803-8.
63. Geary CP, Cousins FB. An oestrogen-linked nephrocalcinosis in rats. Br J Exp Pathol 1969; 50:507-515.
64. Fuiano G, Maza G, Comi N, Caglioti A, De Nicola L, Iodice C, Andreucci M, Andreucci VE. Current indications for renal biopsy: A questionnaire-based survey. Am J Kidn Dis 2000; 35: 448-457.
65. Wexner S, Beck D, Baron T, Fanelli, RD, Hyman N, Shen BS, Wasco KE. A consensus document on bowel preparation before colonoscopy: Prepared by Task Force from the American Society of Colon and Rectal Surgeons (ASCRS), the American Society for Gastrointestinal Endoscopy (ASGE), and the Society of American Gastrointestinal and Endoscopic Surgeons (SAGES). Surg Endosc 2006; 20: 1147-1161.
66. Post, S: Changes to Professional Labeling of Fleet Phospho-Soda. 2006. http://www.phosphosoda.com/professionals/pdf/2006DearDrLetter.pdf
67. Abaskharoun R, Depew W, Vanner S. Changes in renal function following administration of oral sodium phosphate or polyethylene glycol cleansing before colonoscopy. Can J Gastroenterol. 2007; 21: 227-231.
68. Brunelli SM, Lewis JD, Gupta M, Latif SM, Weiner MG, Feldman HI. Risk of kidney injury following use of oral phosphosoda bowel preparations. J Am Soc Nephrol. 2007; 18:3199-3205.
69. Hurst FP, Bohen EM, Osgard EM, Oliver DK, Das NP, Gao SW, Abbott KC. Acute kidney injury associated with oral sodium phosphate purgative use: An observational retrospective cohort study. J Am Soc Nephrol. 2007; 18:3192-8.
70. Barclay RL. Safety, efficacy, and patient tolerance of a three-dose regimen of orally administered aqueous sodium phosphate for colonic cleansing before colonoscopy. Gastrointest Endosc 2004; 60: 527-533.
71. Rex DK, Chasen R, Pochapin MB. Safety and efficacy of two reduced dosing regimens of sodium phosphate tablets for preparation following colonoscopy. Aliment Pharmacol Ther. 2002; 16: 937-944.
72. Hookey LC, Depew WT, Vanner SJ. A Prospective Randomized Low-Dose Oral Sodium Phosphate Plus Stimulant Laxatives with Large Volume Polyethylene Glycol Solution for Colon Cleansing. Am J Gastroenterol 2004: 99: 2217-2222.
73. Vanner SJ, MacDonald PH, Paterson WG, Prentice RSA, DaCosta LR, Beck IT: A randomized prospective trial comparing oral sodium phosphate with standard polyethylene glycol-based lavage solution (Golytely) in the preparation of patients for colonoscopy. Am J Gastroenterol 1990; 85: 422-7.
74. Rostom A, JolicoeurE, Dube C, Gregoire S, Patel D, Saloojee N, Lowe C. A randomized prospective trial comparing different regimens of oral sodium phosphate and polyethylene glycol-based lavage solution in the preparation of patients for colonoscopy. Gastrointest Endosc 2006; 64: 544-552.
75. Seeff LC, Richards TB, Shapiro JA, Nadel MR, Manninen DL, Given LS, Dong FB, Winges LD, McKenna MT. How many endoscopies are performed for colorectal cancer screening? Results from the CDC's survey of endoscopic capacity. Gastroenterol 2004; 127: 1670-7.
76. Hookey LC, Vanner S. A review of current issues underlying colon cleansing before colonoscopy. Can J Gastroenterol. 2007; 21: L105-11.

27

Illicit drug abuse and renal disease

Cheryl L. KUNIS, Nidhi AGGARWAL and Gerald B. APPEL

Columbia University College of Physicians and Surgeons, New York, NY, USA

Introduction

The illicit use of drugs involves millions of people worldwide and is associated with a variety of medical complications. In recent years the abuse of both heroin and cocaine have produced major medical problems across the globe. Other illicit agents such as barbiturates, ethyl alcohol, amphetamines, and phencyclidine, as well as drug combinations produce medical complications as well, sometimes with renal manifestations (Table 1). An estimate of 5-6 % of new patients beginning treatment for end stage renal disease in the United States appear to have opiate-related kidney disease [1].

Renal consequences of drug abuse may be related to direct effects of the drug on the kidney, such as cocaine-induced hemodynamic and mesangial effects, while others are caused by the act of drug abuse itself, such as post-infectious or hepatitis-related glomerulonephritis.

Nephrotoxic problems may be relatively specific for abuse of one class of drugs (e.g. cocaine-induced vascular disease) or nonspecific and seen with a variety of abused drugs linked through similar pathogenetic mechanisms (e.g. acute kidney injury due to non-traumatic rhabdomyolysis). Several studies confirm the association between illicit drug abuse and the development of renal failure [2-5]. One well-performed epidemiologic study evaluated all patients 18 to 45 years of age with sclerosing glomerulonephritis who developed end stage renal disease over 4½ years in the Buffalo Standard Metropolitan Statistical Area (SMSA) [3]. The annual incidence of glomerulosclerosis was 41 times greater in addicts than in controls and

Table 1. Nephrotoxicity associated with illicit drug abuse.

Opiate abuse
• heroin nephropathy
• AA amyloidosis
• rhabdomyolysis - acute tubular necrosis
• tubulointerstitial lesions
• glomerulonephritis (membranoproliferative)
• HIV associated nephropathy
Cocaine abuse
• rhabdomyolysis - acute tubular necrosis
• malignant hypertension
• chronic renal failure
Phencyclidine abuse
• rhabdomyolysis - acute tubular necrosis
Amphetamine abuse
• necrotizing angiitis
• rhabdomyolysis - acute tubular necrosis
• acute interstitial nephritis
Other drugs
• ethyl alcohol abuse
- rhabdomyolysis - acute tubular necrosis
- tubular defects
• barbiturates, benzodiazepines, glutethimide
- rhabdomyolysis - acute tubular necrosis
- diazepam - acute interstitial nephritis

29 times greater in Black male addicts than in nonaddicted Black men; end stage renal disease developed 18 times more frequently in addicts than nonaddicts [3]. Another case-controlled study examined the association between drug use and end stage renal disease (ESRD) in 716 patients [4]. They were compared to age matched controls and were examined for lifetime use of heroin, cocaine, and other illicit drugs. After adjustment for age, sex, race, socio-economic status, history of hypertension and diabetes, persons who had ever used heroin or opiates were at increased risk for developing ESRD (odds ratio of 19:1) [4]. Likewise, use of cocaine, crack and psychedelic drugs were associated with ESRD but the effect could not be separated from the effects of heroin [4].

A significant, independent association between illicit drug use and a mild decline in renal function was found in a study of six hundred and forty seven patients followed in the Hypertension Clinic of the VA Medical Center in New Orleans, Louisiana [5]. These patients used a number of illicit substances (heroin, cocaine or crack, psychedelics, amphetamines, marijuana) and were followed for a median of 7 years. They were all hypertensive and the data was adjusted for systolic blood pressure, use of antihypertensive medication, diabetes mellitus, smoking, alcohol consumption, hyperlipidemia, body mass index, age, race, income and education. The decline in renal function was 3 and 3.9 times greater among patients using cocaine and psychedelics, respectively; the risk for renal decline was greater but not statistically significant in patients abusing heroin, amphetamines, marijuana and other illicit substances [5].

This chapter will review the various renal manifestations of illicit drug abuse. It will focus on the clinical and pathologic presentation, the course, the treatment, and the pathogenesis of these lesions. Secondary renal infectious complications will not be discussed, except for the interrelationship of HIV and heroin nephropathy.

Opioids and renal disease

The opioid drugs are responsible for more reported cases of renal damage than any other class of abused drug. While opioids include morphine, codeine, methadone, meperidine, and other agents, most cases of renal damage are related to heroin abuse. Heroin is derived from the acetylation of morphine at two-sites and is rapidly absorbed from all mucous membranes and the lungs.

In the late 1960's and early 1970's intravenous drug addiction became a contributor to renal disease and chronic renal failure in urban centers throughout the USA [6-14]. Almost all patients injected heroin, although it was often mixed with other drugs. Many patients developed albuminuria, the nephrotic syndrome and the glomerular histology described was pleomorphic. Focal segmental and global sclerosis, membranous glomerulopathy, membranoproliferative glomerulonephritis, mesangial proliferative glomerulonephritis, minimal change disease, and amyloidosis were all reported [7-10, 12, 14-20]. Other much less common pathologic diagnoses reported have included chronic interstitial nephritis that may also have granulomatous changes and foreign body giant cells, granulomatous glomerulonephritis, fibrillary glomerulonephritis and hemolytic uremic syndrome [21-24].

The most frequent lesion described has been focal segmental glomerulosclerosis (FSGS) progressing to global sclerosis. This lesion has been classically referred to as "heroin nephropathy" and is the lesion seen in Black heroin addicts in the USA. Ninety percent of all nephrotic black male addicts biopsied in the original report on heroin nephropathy from the Kings County Hospital in Brooklyn, New York were found to have this histologic lesion [12]. One group of investigators found a high incidence of hepatitis C virus infection (HCV) in Black intravenous drug abusers with FSGS and proposed that HCV infection may play a role in the development of FSGS in this predisposed population [25]. Unfortunately HCV testing was not available at the time of the initial reports of heroin nephropathy.

Membranoproliferative glomerulonephritis was initially described in 1972 in 7 heroin addicts and has continued to be the most common pathological finding in Caucasian heroin abusers [9, 20, 26]. A study of renal specimens from 179 autopsies of European intravenous drug abusers in Germany (almost all Caucasian) over a ten year period (1987-1997) demonstrated membranoproliferative glomerulonephritis and no cases of FSGS; there was only a weak association between the glomerular disease and hepatitis B or C infection [20]. In another European study, membranoproliferative glomerulonephritis was seen in 13 of 19 biopsies (68.4%) in Caucasian heroin abusers, all of whom were hepatitis C positive; one of these 19 patients was also hepatitis B positive and 3 were HIV positive [26]. The remaining 6 patients in this series had chronic interstitial nephritis, acute proliferative glomerulonephritis, amyloidosis and granulomatous glomerulonephritis with interstitial inflammation [26]. Hepatitis as the most common causative agent for renal disease in drug abusers remains controversial.

The different pathologies seen in Caucasian and Black heroin abusers along with the incidence of hepatitis furthers the debate as to whether heroin nephropathy is a unique lesion and what the role of genetics, infection and/or the drug itself plays in producing renal disease. Since Black patients have a greater tendency to develop idiopathic FSGS, the use of intravenous drugs might merely potentiate this predisposition. A genetic basis for this predisposition has been suggested by the increased incidence of HLA-Bw53 genotype among Black drug addicts with heroin nephropathy as well as recent data on mutations in podocyte-associated proteins implicated in the development of FSGS [27-32]. A recent critical review suggests that there is no convincing data that the entity "heroin nephropathy" truly exists [33]. These authors believe that the heterogeneity of the pathology, the lack of any good laboratory model for the disease and the almost disappearance of heroin nephropathy despite an increase in intravenous heroin abuse confirms their belief that heroin itself does not produce renal disease [33].

Addicts typically use street heroin mixed with a number of adulterants, such as quinine or lactose, and they often inject combinations of illicit drugs. Three patients who developed the clinical and morphologic picture of heroin nephropathy claimed to have used only intravenous pentazocine and tripelennamine [41]. It has been suggested that the contaminants rather than the narcotic itself might be the inciting factor through the mechanism of mesangial overload [34].

An abnormal immune response may play a role in the development of FSGS in intravenous drug abusers since abnormalities in humoral and cellular immunity have been described in addicts [35, 36]. The repeated injection of heroin could induce an immunologic response to the narcotic as a tissue haptene. Morphine binding activity in the serum of rabbits has been demonstrated with repeated injections of opiates [37]. While some researchers have found that the alpha 2 globulin fraction of serum from heroin addicts also has morphine binding activity [38], this has not been a uniform finding [39]. An increased incidence of antinuclear and anticardiolipin antibodies in ten heroin addicts suggests that these immune responses may play a role in heroin-related systemic complications, including renal disease [40]. Chronic administration of morphine to rats has produced both biochemical abnormalities as well as electron microscopic findings of microprojections on the podocytes [41,42]. Thus, morphine itself may directly affect the kidney, perhaps via altered intracellular cyclic AMP levels [42].

The effects of morphine on cultured mesangial cell proliferation and matrix formation suggest that the drug itself may induce cell proliferation and mesangial sclerosis [43]. Morphine intensifies the accumulation of macromolecules in the mesangium and stimulates TNF-alpha production by lipopolysaccharide activated mesangial cells in culture, which in turn, amplifies mesangial cell nitrite production [44, 45]. The latter effect appears to be morphine receptor mediated since opiate receptor antagonists abolish this effect; in addition, anti-TNF-alpha antibody diminishes morphine-induced nitrite generation [45].

In vitro laboratory studies have suggested that morphine may also have direct effects on renal interstitial fibrosis. Morphine enhances proliferation of cultured rat medullary interstitial cells as well as their mRNA expression for c-jun and c-myc [46]. Morphine increased the accumulation of types 1 and 3 collagen in the renal interstitium and enhanced the proliferation of kidney fibroblasts, inducing apoptosis as well as synthesis of p53 by the kidney fibroblasts at higher doses [46,47]. Thus, opiates may play a role in the development of "heroin nephropathy" via an effect on the renal interstitium as well as the glomerulus.

The use of narcotics in cancer patients may be a useful model to study the role of opioids in producing renal abnormalities. Although renal dysfunction in cancer patients is most likely multifactorial, the significant doses of narcotics which these patients receive may shed light on a direct renal effect. Chronic opioid administration in a murine cancer model recently demonstrated renovasodilatation with a decrease in mean arterial pressure (MAP), an increase in kidney weight, proteinuria and an elevated BUN [48]. Glomerular enlargement with hypercellularity and peritubular congestion occurred with upregulation of iNOS, eNOS, HO-1 and COX-2; L-NAME, an inhibitor of NOS, prevented this opioid-induced increase in renal perfusion and weight [48]. This laboratory model suggests that narcotics may stimulate vasoregulatory mechanisms, inducing histological and functional renal abnormalities.

Heroin nephropathy/clinical course

There are over three hundred cases of classic FSGS associated with intravenous drug abuse described in the literature, including 30 cases from the Columbia Presbyterian Medical Center and Harlem Hospital in New York City [3,6,10,12,16,18,49-57]. The preponderance of patients are young Black males (95% Black, 92% male, mean age 29 years). In three of the larger series, including our own study, all patients were Black [3, 12, 50]. Duration of drug abuse varied from 6 months to 30 years prior to the onset of renal disease with a mean duration of 6 years. Two thirds of patients presented with the nephrotic syndrome with an average 24 hour urinary protein excretion of 9-10 g. Over 40% of patients had greater than 10 g of proteinuria daily with a mean serum albumin of 2.6 g/dl. Despite the presence of substantial proteinuria, the mean serum cholesterol concentrations were not very elevated, probably due to chronic illness and/or malnutrition in this population. Urinalyses demonstrated pyuria in 50% of cases and microhematuria in over 30%. Occasionally patients presented with gross hematuria.

At initial presentation 3/4 of the patients had renal insufficiency with an average serum creatinine concentration of 3.6 mg/dl. Ten percent of patients presented with serum creatinine concentrations greater than 9 mg/dl. Hypertension correlated best with the presence of renal insufficiency [3,50,57]. In one large series serum creatinine averaged 4.7 mg/dl in hypertensive patients and only 1.4 mg/dl in normotensive patients [57].

Our own study compared 30 patients with FSGS due to heroin nephropathy to patients with the idiopathic form of FSGS [50]. The mean serum creatinine at presentation was 4.5 mg/dl in those patients with heroin nephropathy versus 1.2 mg/dl in those with idiopathic FSGS, despite similar degrees of proteinuria, hypoalbuminemia and glomerulosclerosis. Hypertension and hypercholesterolemia were more prevalent in the idiopathic form of FSGS despite greater renal dysfunction in the drug abusers.

The pathologic lesions of heroin nephropathy can be either focal or diffuse with sclerosis involving glomeruli segmentally or globally depending on the serum creatinine at biopsy. The glomeruli show collapse, thickening, and wrinkling of the glomerular basement membrane, sometimes with an increase in mesangial matrix (Figure 1). In early stages, there is often swelling and proliferation of visceral epithelial cells with foam cells in the capillary lumina. Hyalinosis develops similar to the hyaline deposits in other sclerosing glomerulopathies. The immunofluorescent findings of granular IgM and C3 deposition in the areas of sclerosis are thought to represent nonspecific trapping, similar to that seen in other sclerotic processes [12, 50]. Linear staining for IgG along the glomerular basement membrane without evidence for anti-glomerular basement membrane antibodies has been described and probably also represents nonspecific trapping of plasma proteins [3,10, 57]. The electron microscopic findings are similar to those seen in idiopathic focal segmental glomerulosclerosis with glomerular basement membrane thickening and new basement membrane formation without electron dense deposits. Occasionally deposits have been described which do not represent immune complexes.

More severe interstitial mononuclear cell infil-

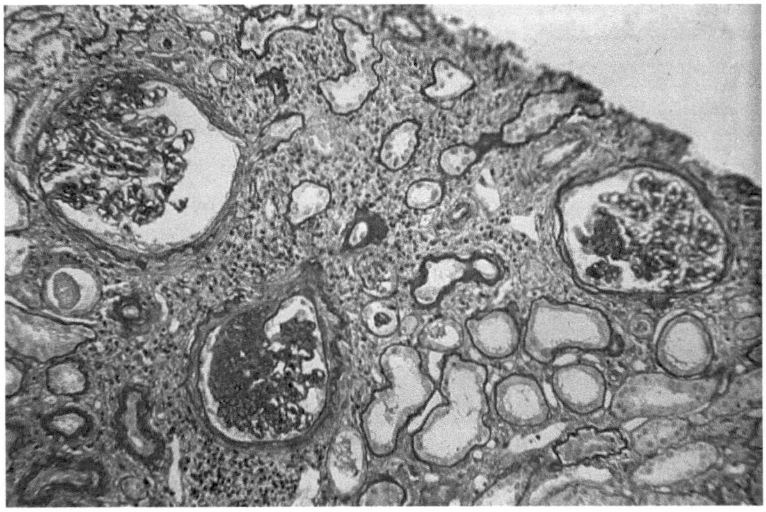

Figure 1. *Renal biopsy of patient with heroin nephropathy showing focal glomerulosclerosis plus severe tubulointerstitial damage. H&E staining, orig. magn. x300.*

trates, greater tubular atrophy, and more interstitial fibrosis have been described in heroin nephropathy as compared to idiopathic FSGS in most reported series [10, 50-52, 58]. Although several investigators believe that the severity of the tubulointerstitial changes are consistent with the degree of glomerular damage, other workers have found the degree of interstitial inflammation to be out of proportion to the degree of glomerular disease and most likely explains the more severe renal dysfunction and more rapid progression to end stage renal disease [3, 10, 50, 55, 57].

Most patients with heroin nephropathy develop end stage renal disease from several months to five years following diagnosis. There appears to be a spectrum in terms of rapidity of progression from the idiopathic form of FSGS to heroin nephropathy and then to the collapsing form seen in HIV nephropathy. Idiopathic FSGS typically progresses to end stage renal disease over a 5 to 10 year period, collapsing FSGS and HIV nephropathy progress over several weeks to months to end stage, and heroin nephropathy appears to be in between these two extremes.

One study demonstrated that the mean time to end stage renal disease for heroin addicts with an initial glomerular filtration rate (GFR) greater than 60cc/min was 43 months compared to 3.6 months for patients with HIV nephropathy who had a similar GFR [59]. By stratifying the patients with heroin nephropathy, those with a GFR from 20-60 cc/min took a mean of 20 months to reach uremia, while those with an initial clearance less than 20 cc/min progressed to uremia in a mean of 7 months [59]. Isolated reports have suggested that abstinence from substance abuse may allow for improvement and/or stabilization of renal function [16, 50, 56], but this data has not been confirmed by any systematic study. As opposed to HIV nephropathy, the use of immunosuppressive therapy has not been successfully used in heroin nephropathy, but in those few patients who have remained drug free after renal transplantation, results have been favorable without recurrence [60, 61].

Amyloidosis associated with intravenous drug abuse

In the late 1970's and early 1980's there was a change in the spectrum of heroin nephropathy [49, 62-67]. FSGS was replaced by secondary amyloidosis as the most common biopsy finding in intravenous drug abusers with the nephrotic syndrome. After prolonged intravenous drug abuse, addicts had exhausted their venous accesses and resorted to subcutaneous injection of drugs, so-called "skin-popping". The persistent subcutaneous injections led to chronic ulcerations and suppurative skin infections which appeared to be the stimulus for the development of secondary amyloidosis [63, 64, 50, 68].

Between 1978 and 1992, almost seventy cases of heroin-related renal amyloidosis were reported [49, 50, 57, 62-65, 69-71]. Most patients were Black males with a mean age almost ten years greater than those patients with the classic heroin nephropathy and a significantly longer course of drug abuse. Since 1992 there have only been isolated case reports of renal amyloidosis in addicts, including one in an HIV+ patient [72], until a group in London recently reported on 20 cases, 13 occurring between 2000-2005 [73]. Interestingly, these 20 patients were all Caucasian but the rest of their clinical parameters were similar to the earlier reports with a high mortality and rapid progression to ESRD.

Table 2 compares the clinical data in our patients with heroin related amyloidosis (n=24) and heroin related FSGS (n=30) [50]. Most patients with renal amyloidosis had exhausted their intravenous access for drug abuse and resorted to subcutaneous "skin-popping". Almost all patients used heroin, some mixed with cocaine, and two patients reportedly abused only pentazocine and tripelennamine [64]. All patients had chronic dermal ulcerations and suppurative skin infections.

Most patients have nephrotic range proteinuria with an average daily urinary protein excretion of 13 g, marked hypoalbuminemia (mean serum albumin 2.1 g/dl), and an elevated serum cholesterol (mean 247 mg/dl). Hypertension has been variable, occurring in less than 20% of most reported series, but it was as high as 40% in one series [49, 50, 57]. Most patients present with renal insufficiency, the average serum creatinine concentration being 2.5 mg/dl. In our patients the initial serum creatinine concentration was significantly higher (6.2 mg/dl) [50].

The amyloid is of the secondary type, amyloid A protein. Serum amyloid A, an acute phase reactant produced by hepatocytes, circulates complexes to high density lipoprotein and is cleaved into smaller fragments which subsequently polymerize into the alpha pleated sheet configuration of amyloid [57, 68]. The renal amyloid is heavily distributed in the tubular basement membranes, vessel walls and interstitium as well as the glomeruli. There is greater tubular basement membrane and interstitial amyloid deposition in drug related renal amyloid than in other forms of secondary renal amyloid [53]. Amyloid was not found in the skin biopsies of several of our patients with heroin related secondary amyloidosis, although interestingly, multiple pulmonary nodules due to AA amyloid have been described in an HIV positive intravenous drug abuser [40].

Similar to FSGS in drug abusers, the interstitial cell inflammation is more prominent in the biopsies of patients with substance abuse amyloidosis than in other forms of secondary amyloidosis [50]. Accompanying the tubulointerstitial involvement are a number of physiologic and clinical tubular abnormalities including renal tubular acidosis, glycosuria, phosphaturia, and symptoms of nephrogenic diabetes insipidus [74].

Our patients with illicit drug-related secondary amyloidosis progressed to end stage renal disease more rapidly than patients with other forms of secondary renal amyloidosis [50]. This more rapid progression correlated with the presence of marked interstitial inflammation. In contrast, the control patients with amyloidosis often died of their underlying disease before developing end stage renal disease. Both groups experienced a high mortality rate by two years following the diagnosis (64 and 66%) [50]. Four patients with heroin related renal amyloidosis who subsequently abstained from subcutaneous drug abuse experienced remissions of proteinuria and improvement or stabilization of renal function [69, 70, 73]. However, most

Table 2. Heroin nephropathy – clinical features.

	FGS	Amyloid	
Number of patients	30	24	
Age (years)	35 (range 23-51)	40 (range 27-56)	$p < 0.05$
Drug abuse (years)	14.5 (range 4-30)	18.6 (range 5-33)	NS
Proteinuria (g/24 hrs)	7.7 ± 1.18*	6.1 ± 1.37*	NS
Nephrotic syndrome (%)	85%	66%	NS
Plasma albumin (g/dl)	2.3 ± 0.18*	2.0 ± 0.18*	NS
Plasma cholesterol (mg/dl)	234 ± 31.8*	199 ± 33.6*	NS
Plasma creatinine (mg/dl)	4.5 ± 0.97*	6.2 ± 1.45*	NS
Hypertension (%)	27%	15%	NS
Skin ulcers/abcessess (%)	13%	100%	$p < 0.01$

** Mean ± S.E.*

patients developed progressive renal failure despite abstinence from drug abuse and/or improvement in their suppurative skin infections. Colchicine was reported to markedly lower proteinuria to near normal levels and improve renal function in one patient with drug-related renal amyloidosis despite no demonstrable change in a repeat renal biopsy [75]. Transplantation has generally not been recommended for these patients because of the severe chronic skin infections, aside from the risk of their continuing and/or returning to substance abuse post transplantation.

HIV nephropathy and its relationship to heroin nephropathy

The association between HIV and renal disease was first reported in 1984, shortly after the discovery of HIV [76]. While infection with this virus has been associated with a number of patterns of renal disease, the most frequent pattern has been designated HIV-associated nephropathy (HIVAN), an aggressive form of collapsing FSGS [58, 59, 77-88]. In some cities in the USA, such as New York, there is a 60-85% carriage rate for HIV among intravenous drug abusers [79]. In the initial ten years of the AIDS epidemic, HIVAN surpassed any other cause for ESRD among intravenous drug abusers.

This collapsing variant of FSGS, HIVAN, appears clinically and pathologically distinct from the lesion formerly described as heroin nephropathy [58, 77, 78]. As HIVAN emerged as the major glomerulopathy among intravenous drug abusers, the lesion of classic "heroin nephropathy" essentially disappeared [89]. Perhaps the speed with which HIV nephropathy develops among addicts may not allow for the longer time interval required to express the lesion of heroin nephropathy. Moreover, the lesion of heroin nephropathy may be underdiagnosed in the HIV infected population since, by definition, heroin nephropathy must exclude the presence of the HIV virus. Regardless, the reported incidence of both heroin nephropathy and amyloidosis has decreased in the addict population as HIV seropositivity and HIV nephropathy has increased [89]. The incidence of HIVAN has plateaued at approximately 800 to 900 new cases per year in the USA since the introduction of highly active antiretroviral therapy.

HIV nephropathy is characterized by heavy proteinuria, large echogenic kidneys on ultrasonography and rapid progression to renal failure with characteristic renal biopsy findings [80-88]. HIV-associated nephropathy is a better term than AIDS nephropathy since this lesion may occur in patients with early manifestations of HIV infection, and asymptomatic HIV carriers as well as patients with overt AIDS [81]. While HIVAN has an incidence of only 3-7% of unselected autopsy series in HIV infected patients, it is by far the most common lesion found in HIV patients undergoing renal biopsy. Of 104 biopsies in HIV positive patients with glomerular disease at the Columbia Presbyterian Medical Center, 73 had classic HIVAN [58]. In both intravenous drug abusers and non-drug users who are HIV positive, the incidence of HIVAN has been far greater in African Americans. In San Francisco where most AIDS patients are Caucasian and homosexual men, HIVAN has been extremely uncommon [84-86]. Akin to the predilection for idiopathic FSGS and heroin nephropathy in African Americans, the Black race is probably the single most important predisposing epidemiologic risk factor for the development of HIVAN in HIV infected individuals. In addition, patients with ESRD secondary to HIVAN are more likely to have a family history of ERSD. These observations have lead to studies in mouse models which demonstrate that murine genetic background affects the development of kidney disease in HIV in addition to the expression of viral genes; the genetic susceptibility locus for HIVAN has been identified on mouse chromosome 3 [90]. In a cohort of Black and Caucasian HIV positive individuals followed for a mean duration of 4.5 years, there was more than a 6-fold greater decline in glomerular filtration rate, a higher prevalence of aggressive disease features and a 20 fold more rapid progression to ESRD in Black than Caucasian people with chronic kidney disease [91].

The typical patient with HIVAN presents with renal insufficiency and signs of the nephrotic syndrome. Hypertension is uncommon and urinalysis often shows a bland sediment with varying numbers of proteinaceous casts and renal tubular epithelial cells. In our patients with HIVAN the initial serum creatinine was markedly elevated (mean 5.4 mg/dl], the serum albumin low (mean 2.2 g/dl] and edema frequent (62%) [81]. Ultrasonography demonstrates large echogenic kidneys (mean size 12.3 cm); the echogenicity correlates with dilated cystic renal tubules rather than with glomerular changes.

The pathology of HIVAN has several distinct features which differ from classic idiopathic FSGS and heroin nephropathy [58, 78, 84-89, 92]. Light microscopy demonstrates a diffuse global collapsing glomerulosclerosis with striking visceral epithelial cell hypertrophy accompanied by large cytoplasmic vacuoles and resorption droplets. There are also severe tubulointerstitial changes with interstitial inflammation, edema, microcystic dilatation of tubules (Figure 2) and severe tubular degenerative changes. Tubulo-reticular inclusions are prevalent in the glomerular endothelium on electron microscopy. While these tubulo-reticular inclusions may only be markers for the presence of severe viral infection, their presence in a patient with classic light microscopic findings of HIVAN confirms the diagnosis. Children with AIDS often have other glomerular lesions such as minimal change disease.

HIVAN usually progresses quite rapidly to renal failure. An early study by Rao et al.found that the average time from diagnosis to uremia was 3-4 months when the GFR was greater than 60cc/min [59]. By contrast the time course for heroin nephropathy to progress to ESRD with a similar GFR is almost 44 months; even with a GFR < 20cc/min at the time of diagnosis, the time course to uremia for heroin nephropathy was 7 months. In a subsequent study, Rao et al. followed 55 patients with HIVAN in which 43 progressed rapidly to uremia, 2 died without uremia and ten were lost to follow-up [80]. In our study of 26 patients with HIVAN, life table analysis confirmed the rapid progression to end stage renal disease [81]. Patient survival most closely correlated with the stage of HIV infection. Patients with AIDS and end stage renal disease had a mean survival of only 1.9 months; patients with early symptoms of HIV infection survived a mean of 3.6 months, while patients with asymptomatic HIV infection survived a mean of 9.7 months [81]. Since these early reports, HAART therapy has clearly changed these statistics. In our experience all patients with classic HIV nephropathy eventually developed AIDS.

Data suggests that HIV nephropathy is a late consequence of HIV infection associated with a high viral load [88], although the nephrotic syndrome and renal failure can be the initial presentation of HIV infection. The kidney appears to be an important long-term reservoir for the HIV-1 virus [93]. The presence of viral transcripts in renal epithelial cells has been documented even in the presence of effective therapy [93]. In addition to ACE inhibition, the use of antiretroviral therapy, especially when begun early in the course of HIVAN, has markedly improved the prognosis for progression to end stage renal disease and discontinuing such therapy can lead to rapid viral replication [93-95]. Some patients with asymptomatic HIV infection can survive many years on dialysis and recent statistics demonstrate a much improved prognosis for HIV-infected patients maintained on hemodialysis [96].

Interestingly, a recent study of 61 Black patients diagnosed with HIVAN from 1998 though 2004 in the United Kingdom did not demonstrate any additional renal benefit from early initiation of highly active antiretroviral therapy [97]. This was of course in contrast to the improved overall patient survival from

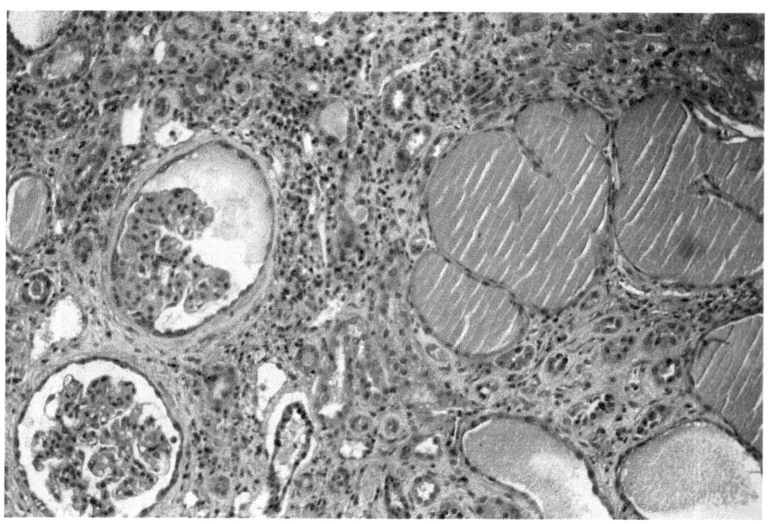

Figure 2. *Renal biopsy of patient with HIV nephropathy showing pronounced tubular dilatation. H&E staining, orig. magn. x300.*

early initiation of antiretroviral therapy. These patients were followed for a median of 4.2 years at which time 56% or 34 patients had developed ESRD. There was no difference in the rate of HIV RNA suppression, renal function or HIV parameters at baseline between those patients with stable renal function and those who went on to ESRD [97]. The patients who developed ESRD had a greater chronicity index on renal biopsy and thus, the severity of sclerosis on biopsy was the strongest predictor of renal outcome [97].

Recent studies have shown that the pathogenesis of HIVAN results from direct infection of renal tubular and glomerular epithelial cells by HIV-1. The HIV genome is commonly found in renal tissue in HIV seropositive patients by the DNA polymerase chain reaction. HIV core protein (p-24) and pro-viral HIV DNA have been localized to the tubular cells and visceral epithelial cells, but their role in the pathogenesis of HIV nephropathy is unclear [92, 98]. One group of investigators found that the HIV virus was readily able to infect 90% of cultured human glomerular endothelial cells and 5% of mesangial cells, but glomerular epithelial cells could not be infected [99]. More recent studies have detected HIV-1 in tubular cells as well as glomerular visceral and parietal epithelial cells by PCR amplification and RNA *in situ* hybridization [100].

Experiments with mice made transgenic for HIV-1 proviral DNA show a characteristic course of proteinuria and progressive azotemia [101]. Histology reveals focal segmental sclerosing lesions and microcyst formation with interstitial infiltrates similar to the histologic pattern seen in human HIVAN. These findings implicate HIV gene constructs directly in the pathogenesis of HIVAN. Specific HIV viral genes, nef and vpr, appear to be involved in the pathogenesis of HIVAN. Ongoing studies show that when expressed exclusively in podocytes, Nef induces a dedifferentiated state and initiates changes in the cell cycle. However, Nef alone is unable to stimulate the massive proliferation seen in HIVAN; thus, the human disease may require additional factors to generate the appearance of a collapsing glomerulopathy [102]. Laboratory data has demonstrated a role for the HIV-1 gp120 envelope protein on tubular cell interaction products in promoting renal fibroblast proliferation and apoptosis; in addition, this response was enhanced by morphine [103]. Thus, this effect may play a role in the renal interstitial disease which is so prominent in HIVAN.

HIVAN is clearly a different entity from the previously described heroin nephropathy, both clinically and histologically. While heroin nephropathy by definition occurs only in heroin addicts, the classical clinical and histologic picture of HIVAN has been seen in patients who acquired the virus through homosexual contact, blood transfusions and maternal transmission as well as intravenous drug abuse. The progression to ESRD as described above is much more rapid in patients with HIVAN. The pathology of HIVAN has unique features of the collapsing form of glomerulosclerosis, marked tubular microcyst formation and electron microscopic tubulo-reticular inclusions. Moreover, the transgenic animal models with features typical of HIVAN also suggest a unique pathogenesis for this form of collapsing FSGS. Since dysregulation of VEGF (vascular endothelial growth factor) expression within the glomerulus has been demonstrated in a variety of renal diseases, recent animal data has shown that podocyte-specific overexpression of the VEGF-164 isoform can produce a collapsing glomerulopathy, similar to that seen in HIVAN [104]. HIV-1 induces expression of VEGF and its cell surface receptor VEGFR2 in podocytes and this may be a critical step in the pathogenesis of HIVAN [105]. Recent studies of chemokines have demonstrated higher levels of MCP-1, RANTES, and IL-8 interstitial and glomerular tissue levels in HIV infected patients, regardless of renal disease, but MHC Class II, interferon alpha and beta receptor protein expression was greater in HIV patients with nephropathy [106]. This suggests that upregulation of these proteins may also be important in the pathogenesis of HIVAN [106].

Acute kidney injury due to drug-induced rhabdomyolysis

In addition to chronic renal failure, illicit drug abuse is associated with a characteristic pattern of acute kidney injury. Overdoses can cause traumatic or non-traumatic rhabdomyolysis associated with myoglobinuric acute kidney injury [107-113]. Rhabdomyolysis has been reported with various illicit drugs including heroin and other opiates, methadone, cocaine and drug combinations [107, 108, 114]. In a number of centers rhabdomyolysis is responsible for 5-7% of all cases of acute kidney injury [107, 109, 115]. While drug-related cases comprised only 11 of 157 cases of rhabdomyolysis in one large series, drug ingestion has a very high likelihood of being complicated by acute kidney injury.

The typical patient is a young male addict who presents with coma or stupor after the intravenous use of heroin. Decreased levels of consciousness can develop rapidly since such patients are soemtimes found comatose with the injection needle still inserted in their veins [114]. This occurs commonly in inexperienced addicts who misjudge the dose of drug administered or when there is a sudden change in the potency of available street heroin. Most of the patients with acute kidney injury have had a prolonged period of coma prior to presentation [114]. Less frequently an addict will present with rhabdomyolysis and acute kidney injury and deny prior coma or stupor. In some of these cases seizures, trauma or excessive exertion prior to the use of the drug may explain the rhabdomyolysis. At presentation many patients will be hypotensive, hypoxic, acidotic, and dehydrated [107,108]. Patients may or may not have clinical evidence of muscle damage with myalgias and tender swollen muscle groups. Evidence for muscle damage, however, is readily documented by very elevated levels of muscle enzymes (CPK and aldolase) and myoglobinuria.

The acute kidney injury is typical for acute tubular necrosis and is characterized by a urine sediment with granular pigmented casts and benzidine positive urine often in the absence of significant hematuria. Acute tubular necrosis from rhabdomyolysis does not always have an elevated urinary sodium concentration and fractional excretion of sodium as in classic acute tubular necrosis [116]. One half to two-thirds of patients have oliguria which may last from hours to many weeks. During this phase of acute kidney injury, there is a very rapid rise in the serum creatinine (often > 2.0 mg/dl/day) and profound increases in the serum levels of a variety of solutes normally found in muscle or produced from muscle derived precursors. Thus, the levels of potassium, phosphate, and uric acid all rise dramatically. Associated with the oliguria many patients develop severe hypocalcemia [107, 109, 114]. This may be due to deposition of calcium salts in the damaged muscle, tissue deposition of calcium salts elsewhere due to the high circulating levels of phosphate, decreased parathyroid hormone levels, or altered vitamin D metabolism [117, 118]. During the polyuric recovery phase of the acute kidney injury, a rebound hypercalcemia occurs in many patients due to reversal of the processes that led to hypocalcemia [107, 109, 117, 118].

Almost half of the reported patients with acute kidney injury due to rhabdomyolysis have required dialytic support. Nevertheless, the majority of patients regain significant renal function. The mortality from drug-induced rhabdomyolysis and ATN has been low despite the common occurrence of intercurrent infection. This may be related to the patients being young and without prior multisystem disease.

The mechanism of muscle damage with opiates is most likely related to profound and prolonged compression of muscle with compromise of the regional vascular supply [107, 109, 113, 118-120]. The presence of hypovolemia and hypotension may further contribute to the ischemic damage. There is a direct correlation between the duration of altered consciousness and the severity of the rhabdomyolysis. Moreover, there is no evidence for any major direct toxic effect of narcotics on muscle in the vast majority of addicts who present without coma or stupor. Trauma, exertion and seizures may contribute to the muscle damage in some patients.

The mechanism of the acute kidney injury is thought to be multifactorial and similar to other cases of myoglobinuric renal failure [118, 121-126]. These factors include obstruction of tubules, toxic effects of the pigment or iron on renal tubular cells and altered hemodynamics in association with inhibition of the vasodilator nitric oxide by myoglobin. Experimental animals exposed to heme pigment have increases in the renal synthesis of both heme oxidase and ferritin [125]. This allows for more rapid heme degradation and greater sequestration of potentially toxic iron by the tubular cells [125]. Whether narcotics or the hypotensive, hypoxic environment associated with rhabdomyolysis interfere with these protective effects of the kidney is unknown.

Initial treatment of the acute kidney injury consists of intravascular volume repletion and restoration of the blood pressure. Treatment with mannitol, alkalinization of the urine and diuretics have all been tried with variable success [110, 111, 122, 127]. Clearly, supportive care and dialytic intervention when necessary are crucial to allow for adequate recovery. Hemodialysis may be more effective than peritoneal dialysis in highly catabolic patients with rhabdomyolysis-induced renal failure.

Cocaine-induced renal disease

Cocaine has been used by the Indians of South America for at least 2500 years. Its central nervous system effects have been long known and ironically in 1884 Freud wrote one of the first reports on the mental effects of cocaine. In the mid 1980's widespread abuse of various forms of cocaine led to major medical and social problems [128]. This coincided with a decrease in the price of the drug "on the street" and more widespread availability. The use of cocaine has changed from that of "social and recreational" use by the wealthy to a common addiction and affliction that affects all segments of the population, as many millions of Americans use cocaine.

Cocaine HCl is an alkaloid derived from the leaves of the South American coca plant. The free base alkaloid, made by extraction from cocaine HCl, is relatively insoluble in water, but dissolves in a variety of organic solvents. There has been a dramatic increase in the use of cocaine free base, which is most commonly known by its street name "crack". Since free base is not destroyed by heating, but rather vaporizes, it can be smoked and inhaled [129]. This provides speedy absorption from the respiratory tract inducing a short-lived but rapid euphoria. The free base is also well absorbed by nasal, vaginal, gastrointestinal and sublingual mucous membranes. Cocaine can be injected intravenously, intramuscularly or subcutaneously. Crack is often combined with heroin or other drugs of abuse and taken intravenously [128]. Cocaine is detoxified by cholinesterases and cocaine or its metabolites may be present in the urine for one to two days after use.

Cocaine is a central nervous system stimulant that inhibits the peripheral reuptake of catecholamines, leading to increased sympathomimetic activity [129]. Its abuse is associated with a variety of medical problems. These include acute myocardial infarction, cardiac arrhythmias, cerebrovascular accidents, hyperpyrexia and stimulated sympathetic activity, seizures and coma, obstetrical complications, intestinal ischemia and a variety of psychiatric complications [128-131]. A number of reports in the mid to late 1980's described patients who developed rhabdomyolysis while using cocaine [132-134]. Some of these patients experienced acute kidney injury [135-139]. While the exact incidence of acute kidney injury secondary to cocaine rhabdomyolysis is unknown, in one reported series it occurred in only three of 211 admissions for cocaine related complications [128]. In a series of nearly 40 patients the incidence of cocaine related acute rhabdomyolysis increased over the period of enrollment from 2 patients in 1985 to 22 patients in 1987 [140]. Several reports of patients with cocaine-induced rhabdomyolysis have clearly defined both the clinical syndrome and the risk factors for the development of acute kidney injury and an adverse outcome [137, 140, 141]. Most patients have been previously healthy young males (mean age 30-35 years old, 80-85% male). The cocaine has been smoked, snorted, used intravenously, or taken orally, implying that the route of administration was not relevant [136, 137, 140, 141]. In contrast to narcotic related rhabdomyolysis, a history of prolonged coma or stupor is absent. The majority of patients are combative and agitated on presentation. Only one-half of the patients have evidence of muscle tenderness or myalgias. The creatinine phosphokinase was more than 10 times normal in all patients developing acute kidney injury. Between 30 and 50% of patients with cocaine associated rhabdomyolysis develop acute kidney injury.

Several features identify patients at risk for developing acute kidney injury [140]. While hypertension (blood pressure greater than 140/90 mmHg) was present in about 20 to 30% of the patients, severe hypotension (blood pressure less than 100 mmHg) on presentation occurred in 46% of those patients who developed acute kidney injury compared to only 4% of those who maintained renal function [140]. In this same series patients developing acute kidney injury were also more likely to have severe hyperpyrexia (70% versus 15%) and documented seizure activity (30% versus 8%). Patients with acute kidney injury have also had higher creatinine phosphokinase levels than those without renal failure [140, 141]. The mean creatinine phosphokinase level for patients developing renal failure has been greater than 20,000 U/L. As might be expected, serum uric acid levels have been higher and serum calcium levels lower in patients with acute kidney injury. The mean hematocrit has also been higher on admission in the renal failure group, implying more severe volume depletion. Admission serum creatinine ranged from 1.9 mg/dl to greater than 12 mg/dl with peaks as high as 24 mg/dl [140, 141]. About 50% of the patients with acute kidney injury were oliguric with 70% having a positive urinalysis for heme pigment.

A bleeding tendency was reported in many of the patients and 7 of 9 patients with acute kidney injury in one series had abnormal coagulation tests with increased fibrin degradation products, decreased fibrinogen levels, prolonged prothrombin times and thrombocytopenia [140]. These 7 patients were felt to have disseminated intravascular coagulation and six of them died despite treatment with plasma infusion and heparin. The associated disseminated intravascular coagulation has been noted by other authors [141]. In one large study, 85% of the acute kidney injury patients had evidence of severe liver function abnormalities with markedly elevated levels of serum aspartate aminotransferase (at least 40 times above normal for the laboratory) as opposed to only 8% of the patients without acute kidney injury [140].

Almost all patients with cocaine induced rhabdomyolysis without renal failure survive and are discharged after an average hospital stay of 5 days. The patients with acute kidney injury who require hemodialysis have a prolonged hospitalization and a lower survival rate. Of patients with acute kidney injury who died, most did so between 2 to 15 days after admission with associated disseminated intravascular coagulation and severe liver dysfunction. Autopsies on these patients showed no evidence of pre-existing renal disease or underlying glomerulopathy.

The exact pathogenesis of cocaine associated rhabdomyolysis remains to be defined [135, 138, 140]. The route of cocaine administration does not predispose to rhabdomyolysis. Moreover, hypotension, hyperpyrexia, coma, muscle crush injury and associated nephrotoxins do not appear to be crucial to the muscle toxicity. Whether there is any direct role of cocaine induced muscle necrosis or a role in combination with sympathetic discharge causing severe arterial vasoconstriction and subsequent ischemia remains to be clarified [128]. The factors predisposing to acute kidney injury are similar to other forms of non-traumatic rhabdomyolysis and include volume depletion, hypotension and increased severity of muscle damage [140, 141]. Rhabdomyolysis may release tissue thromboplastin and other factors inciting disseminated intravascular coagulation and the resulting thrombotic process might accentuate the renal ischemia. The mechanism(s) by which cocaine rhabdomyolysis and myohemoglobinuria produce acute kidney injury are probably similar to other forms of myohemoglobinuric acute kidney injury.

While acute kidney injury due to rhabdomyolysis is by far the most common form of renal damage associated with cocaine, acute kidney injury secondary to malignant hypertension has also been described [142]. Theses patients can regain renal function with treatment of the malignant hypertension, even if they require dialysis. This form of renal failure is thought to be due to drug-induced acute vasoconstriction resembling the hypertensive crises seen in patients with scleroderma. Scleroderma with a scleroderma renal crisis has actually been reported as a complication of cocaine abuse [143]. Kidney biopsies in 2 reported cases of cocaine associated malignant hypertension with acute kidney injury revealed evidence of thrombotic microangiopathy with fibrinoid necrosis of arterioles and glomerular tufts [144]. Cocaine-mediated endothelial injury and platelet activation may play an important pathogenic role in cocaine abusers who develop malignant hypertension and renal failure.

Several patients have presented with angiographic evidence of renal infarction in the setting of active intravenous cocaine use [145,146]. The hypertension abated and the patients were left with no long-term sequelae. There has been a recent case report of renal vein thrombosis associated with cocaine use in the absence of other possible causes [147]. Potential mechanisms might involve vascular injury caused by cocaine induced vasoconstriction, direct endothelial injury and/or alteration in endothelial cytokine expression. A number of other case reports of renal disease associated with cocaine abuse include acute interstitial nephritis [148], anti-GBM antibody-mediated glomerulonephritis [149, 150], Henoch-Schonlein purpura with necrotizing vasculitis [151] and a syndrome resembling thrombotic thrombocytopenic purpura [152, 153]. Cocaine during pregnancy may lead to acute kidney injury due to pre-eclampsia and abruption placentae. There has been a report of urinary tract infections in infants exposed to cocaine in utero, possibly due to ischemia/hypoxia producing renal scar formation [154]. HIVAN is also occurring more frequently in cocaine abusers [155].

The association of cocaine abuse with progressive chronic renal failure has received increased attention in recent years [156-158]. Ward and co-workers have reported on the possibility of a progressive nephropathy with features of hypertension, azotemia and proteinuria in 50 African American cocaine abusers [159]. The renal presentation is often nonspecific with low-grade proteinuria and lack of specific findings on urinalysis although some patients displayed nephrotic range proteinuria. A renal biopsy was obtained in 20 of these patients and revealed the presence of a variety of glomerular and vascular abnormalities including focal glomerulosclerosis, collapsing FSGS, immune complex glomerulonephritis and ischemic arteriolitis. On average, the patients were predominantly African American with one to ten years of using cocaine at least once weekly. However, an earlier study by the same group noted that Caucasian cocaine users also displayed an increased risk for renal disease [156]. A discharge diagnosis of hypertensive renal disease was associated with cocaine use in over one third of cases in that study. Cocaine use is associated with hypertensive renal changes in HIV-infected patients in the absence of hypertension and/or diabetes [160]. Renal biopsies performed over 11 years in 193 HIV positive patients were retrospectively reviewed. Of 53 patients without a history of hypertension or diabetes mellitus, 29 were found to have hypertensive renal changes [160]. Cocaine was used in 16 of these 29 patients (55%) and in only 6 of the remaining 24 patients (25%) without any hypertensive renal changes [OR 3.7 (CI 1.2-11.7)].

Finally, cocaine has been implicated as a risk factor for the development of ESRD in young dialysis patients with a shorter duration of hypertension by history [158]. The relative risk of developing ESRD with cocaine abuse was nearly 10 times higher than that of race and blood pressure matched controls. In summary, evidence for a progressive nephropathy associated with cocaine abuse is accumulating and could contribute to the increasing incidence of ESRD in the United States.

Phencyclidine

Phencyclidine is an anesthetic, analgesic, hallucinogenic drug which was widely abused in the 1970's. As a street drug it was known as "peace pill", "crystal", "hog" and most commonly "PCP" or "angel dust" [161]. It is often used in combination with other illicit drugs and may be smoked, inhaled, snorted, or taken by injection. The abuse of phencyclidine has been associated with respiratory depression, convulsions, hyperpyrexia, hypertensive crisis and schizoid psychoses. It has also produced rhabdomyolysis in many reported cases, often with acute kidney injury [161-166]. In one group of 1000 patients admitted with a diagnosis of phencyclidine abuse, 25 patients (2.5%) experienced rhabdomyolysis and 10 developed acute kidney injury [162]. Thus, 40% of the patients with phencyclidine-associated rhabdomyolysis develop acute kidney injury, while others may develop mild, rapidly reversible renal insufficiency probably related to volume depletion. As with cocaine and heroin induced acute kidney injury most patients have been young males [162, 165]. About 50% are comatose on admission while others display a variety of organic brain syndromes and mental dysfunctions. Hyperpyrexia, tachycardia, hypertension, myalgias with exaggerated muscle activity and acute dystonic motor reactions are all commonly seen on admission [161, 162, 165]. Patients often display a leukocytosis and markedly elevated levels of serum creatinine phosphokinase. The serum creatinine is usually elevated in the patients presenting with acute kidney injury (range 1.2 mg/dl to 12.7 mg/dl with a mean of 4.1 mg/dl in one large series). The urine is typically orthotoluidine positive in the absence of significant hematuria; granular casts and a positive test for myoglobin are common. The serum creatinine rapidly peaks and then returns toward normal. Even though some patients will require dialytic support, the majority recover significant renal function. Fifty percent of patients in acute kidney injury are oliguric but most have hyperuricemia, hyperphosphatemia and hypocalcemia. Rebound hypercalcemia may occur during the recovery phase of acute kidney injury.

The etiology of the acute kidney injury may be related to isometric tension in restrained limbs or to ischemic damage to muscle in the presence of hyperthermia and/or limb compression [161, 166]. While it is possible that the drug itself may possess direct myopathic toxicity when abused in certain settings, it does not induce rhabdomyolysis in unrestrained animals [167]. Animals restrained in immobilizing cages, however, develop rhabdomyolysis, which correlates with isometric muscle tension during the restrained period which can be prevented by prior denervation [167].

Avoiding restraints, intravascular volume repletion and perhaps muscle paralyzing drugs have been advocated. Although urinary acidification has been recommended to promote phencyclidine excretion, this may be deleterious in patients with rhabdomyolysis, hyperuricemia and myoglobinuria and should thus be avoided [166].

Amphetamines and renal disease

Amphetamines are sympathomimeticamines with central nervous system stimulatory activity. They may induce a number of patterns of renal damage including rhabdomyolysis related acute kidney injury, acute interstitial nephritis and an angiitis resembling polyarteritis nodosa.

Methamphetamine alone or in combination with heroin or d-lysergic acid diethylamide has been associated with a necrotizing angiitis similar to that seen in idiopathic polyarteritis nodosa [168]. Although most of these patients have been intravenous abusers of multiple drugs, the common denominator in most cases and the sole drug in others has been methamphetamine [168, 169]. One study described 14 patients with drug (and presumably methamphetamine) related vasculitis seen in a short time period [169]. While others cite the rarity of this lesion with no case in over 1000 consecutive autopsies in addicts, the diligence with which the lesions were sought in this population has been questioned [170, 171]. The lesions have occurred in both male and female intravenous drug abusers who usually present with a prodromal illness of fever, weight loss, malaise and weakness. The angiitis may involve any body organ and patients may experience central nervous system symptoms, abdominal pain, arthralgias, myalgias and other systemic findings akin to idiopathic polyarteritis [169]. Renal involvement is characterized by mild proteinuria, hematuria, hypertension and often progressive renal failure. The lesions in the kidneys on arteriography and at autopsy are similar to those found in classic polyarteritis with involvement of middle size vessels, especially at bifurcations, aneurysms, luminal irregularities and sacculations [168]. The lesions are noted to be in different stages of development with some showing active inflammation of the vessel wall, neighboring lesions showing more chronic healing lesions, and others demonstrating occluded vessels with evidence of distal infarction [168].

The relationship between amphetamine abuse, the presence of hepatitis B antigenemia and immune complex vasculitis remains unclear [172-174]. While similar lesions have been described in non-drug abusing patients who are hepatitis B antigen positive, only 30% of amphetamine abusers were hepatitis B antigen positive in the largest series [171]. Nevertheless, the method and sensitivity of these earlier screening tests for hepatitis B have been questioned. The situation may be even less clear now that hepatitis C has been shown to be associated with a polyarteritis like syndrome and vasculitis [175]. It is also possible that the direct effects of amphetamines or the immune complexes formed by drug-induced release of tissue antigens can produce a vasculitis similar to polyarteritis nodosa [168].

Interestingly, two patients who each received a kidney transplant from the same donor who had used methamphetamine prior to death lost their allografts within one week of the transplant [176]. The transplant renal biopsies revealed a necrotizing vasculopathy which was attributed to the donor's methamphetamine use. In addition, the level of methamphetamine was much higher than other cases where amphetamine abusers were donors with favorable recipient outcomes. Thus, a high level of methamphetamine in a renal donor may produce a vasculopathy that can lead to early renal allograft loss [176].

Amphetamines have also been associated with a syndrome of acute kidney injury and rhabdomyolysis. Several series have described patients following intravenous injection of methamphetamine or phenmetrazine who presented with hyperactivity, fever, chills, sweats, abdominal cramps, diarrhea, and hypotension [177, 178]. The patients have developed acute kidney injury which is usually oliguric and associated with classic rhabdomyolysis, similar to cases of cocaine-induced rhabdomyolysis. Several patients have had disseminated intravascular coagulation and liver function abnormalities as well. Methamphetamine abuse has also been associated with accelerated hypertension, unexplained chronic renal failure, acute lead poisoning (a common reagent used in its production utilizes lead acetate) and at least one case of biopsy proven interstitial nephritis; the latter patient responded to intravenous corticosteroids but whether the nephritis was truly due to amphetamines remains unproven [179].

Ecstacy (MDMA; methylenedioxymethamphetamine) use has been a fast growing new form of drug abuse in the USA and has been implicated as a cause of rhabdomyolysis and acute kidney injury [2]. Ironically, efforts to pre-empt overheating and dehydration by drinking large fluid volumes ("chill out" rooms at "rave" parties) have led to cases of life-threatening hyponatremic encephalopathy [180]. The postulated mechanism may be SIADH exacerbated by polydipsia. Methamphetamine is an indirect serotonin agonist and augments antidiuretic hormone release from the neurohypophysis [181]. In addition, the acute stress and excessive visual and auditory stimuli contribute to the exaggerated antidiuretic hormone secretion. The mechanism for polydipsia due to methamphetamine abuse is still unclear [182].

Marijuana, ethyl alcohol and other drugs

Marijuana has not been known to produce renal disease, although a recent report suggested that de novo membranous glomerulonephritis in the renal transplant may have been associated with heavy marijuana abuse [183]. Since de novo membranous glomerulonephritis is the most common de novo glomerular lesion in the renal transplant and occurs in up to 9% of allografts, it seems unlikely that marijuana was the causative agent in this case report. Although a recent article described lead intoxication due to marijuana use in a number of patients, renal disease was not noted [184]. In this report, lead was being used to increase the weight of the marijuana and investigation into the neurological disorders it produced led to the discovery of lead in the marijuana.

A variety of illicit drugs and other abused substances, most commonly ethyl alcohol, have been associated with acute kidney injury due to rhabdomyolysis [107-109, 120]. There are many potential etiologies for rhabdomyolysis in these patients including trauma to muscles, alcohol related hypokalemia and metabolic disturbances, sustained seizure activity and a direct toxic effect of the alcohol [119, 120]. Alcohol has been shown to produce a rise in muscle enzymes and electron microscopic morphologic changes in muscles even without trauma, seizures or ischemia to a limb. Nevertheless, the vast majority of patients present with coma or stupor, limb compression and a picture similar to that seen with other drugs. Indeed, many patients have a combined overdose of alcohol and a second drug as the etiology of their altered mental state [107, 120].

While alcohol abuse may be associated with a variety of electrolyte and acid-base disorders, the role of the kidneys in this process has only recently been fully defined [185]. Renal functional abnormalities have now been related to chronic alcoholism in patients without liver disease and these defects have reverted to normal with abstinence from alcohol. These abnormalities include decreases in the maximal reabsorptive ability and threshold for glucose, a decrease in the threshold for phosphate excretion and increases in the fractional excretion of beta -2 microglobulin, uric acid, calcium, magnesium and amino acids [185]. Defective tubular acidification and impaired concentrating ability are also commonly found. Thus, defects at multiple sites along the nephron are common in patients with chronic alcohol abuse.

Acute kidney injury has also been associated with a variety of sedatives and hypnotics including barbiturates, benzodiazepines, glutethimide and chlorpromazine [107, 108, 119]. The acute kidney injury is usually related to rhabdomyolysis but the classical clinical picture of acute interstitial nephritis has been reported in one patient with the use of diazepam, although no renal biopsy was performed [186]. In those patients with rhabdomyolysis, multiple seizures often develop prior to the rhabdomyolysis and others are febrile at the time. However, the most common presentation is that of a young person without a prior medical history who presents with coma-stupor of one to several days duration, variable signs of volume depletion, limb compression and follows the typical course of acute tubular necrosis with a high likelihood of renal recovery [107-109].

Summary

The use of illicit drugs has become a worldwide health problem and has been associated with various forms of renal disease, often requiring renal replacement therapy. Renal disease may be due to a direct effect of the drug itself on the kidney or a complication from the act of drug abuse itself. Treatment is clearly costing millions of dollars yearly to treat this self-inflicted disorder. Whether heroin produces FSGS or is just a stimulus for glomerular disease in a population with a genetic predisposition is still a debatable issue. The role of hepatitis C as the causative agent for the development of renal disease in drug abusers is also not fully defined. There has been an evolution in the types of renal diseases which some drug abusers develop. As heroin addicts resorted to subcutaneous injections because of the lack of intravenous access, suppurative skin infections predisposed these patients to the development of secondary renal amyloidosis. With the advent of the HIV virus into the addict population, a new entity of collapsing FSGS appeared as HIV infects the glomerular epithelial and renal tubular cells. Cocaine-induced vasoconstriction with vascular endothelial damage and malignant hypertension can produce renal vascular disease as well as rhabdomyolysis with ATN. Traumatic rhabdomyolysis producing ATN has also been well described with intravenous narcotic and amphetamine abuse. Other illicit substances have been reported to be associated with varying renal diseases such as vasculitis and interstitial nephritis, but these cases are not common and therefore their association with the illicit substances is not well defined. Laboratory investigation has demonstrated upregulation of certain growth factors, such as VEGF, and mutations in podocyte proteins in certain renal diseases. These findings will hopefully better define the true mechanisms by which certain substances and various diseases induce proteinuria and renal failure.

References

1. Orth SR. Adverse renal effects of legal and illicit drugs. Ther Umsch 2002; 59(3):122-130.
2. Crowe AV, Howse M, Bell GM, Henry JA. Substance abuse and the kidney. Quart J Med 2000; 93: 147-152.
3. Cunningham EE, Brentjens JR, Zielezny MA, Andres GA, Venuto RC. Heroin nephropathy - a clinicopathologic and epidemiologic study. Am J Med 1980; 68: 47-53.
4. Perneger TV, Klag MJ, Whelton PK. Recreational drug use: a neglected risk factor for end-stage renal disease. Am J Kidney Dis 2001; 38 (1): 49-56.
5. Vupputuri S, Batuman V, Muntner P, Bazzano LA, Lefante JJ, Whelton PK, He J. The risk for mild kidney function decline associated with illicit drug use among hypertensive men. Am J Kidney Dis 2004; 43:629-635.
6. Avram MM, Iancu M, Weiss S. Heroin usage nephropathy - subclinical to end stage nephrotic syndrome. J Am Soc Nephrol 1971; 5A.
7. Eknoyan G, Gyorkey F, Dichoso C, Hyde SE, Gyorkey P, Suki WN, Matinez-Maldonado M. Renal involvement in drug abuse. Arch Intern Med 1973; 132: 801-806.
8. Friedman EA, Rao TKS, Nicastri AD. Heroin-associated nephropathy. Nephron 1974; 13: 421-426.
9. Kilcoyne MM, Gocke DJ, Meltzer JI, Daly JJ, Thomason GE, Hsu KC, Tannenbaum M. Nephrotic syndrome in heroin addicts. Lancet 1972; 1: 17-20.
10. Matalon R, Katz L, Gallo G. Glomerular sclerosis in adults with nephrotic syndrome. Ann Int Med 1974; 80: 488-495.
11. McGinn JT, McGinn TG, Cherubin CE, Hoffman RS. Nephrotic syndrome in drug addicts. NY State J Med 1974; 74: 92-95.
12. Rao TKS, Nicastri AD, Friedman EA. A natural history of heroin associated nephropathy. N Engl J Med 1974; 290: 19-23.
13. Sapira JD, Ball JC, Penn H. Causes of death among institutional narcotic addicts. J Chronic Dis 1970; 22: 733-742.
14. Salomon MI, Poon TP, Goldblatt M, Tchertkoff V. Renal lesions in heroin addicts: a study based on kidney biopsies. Nephron 1972; 9: 356-363.
15. Arruda JAL, Kurtzman NA, Pillay VKG. Prevalence of renal disease in asymptomatic heroin addicts. Arch Intern Med 1975; 135: 535-537.
16. Llach F, Descoeudres C, Massry SG. Heroin associated nephropathy: clinical and histological studies in 19 patients. Clin Nephrol 1979; 11: 7-12.
17. Thompson AM, Anthonovych T, Lin R. Focal membranoproliferative glomerulonephritis in heroin users. J Am Soc Nephrol 1973; 105A.
18. Treser G, Cherubin C, Lonergan ET, Yoshizawa N, Viswanathan V, Tannenberg AM, Pompa D, Lange K. Renal lesions in narcotic addicts. Am J Med 1974; 57: 687-694.
19. Gallo G, Neugarten J, Buxbaum J, Katz L. Renal amyloidosis in subcutaneous heroin abusers. ASN (New Orleans) 1985; 38A.
20. Dettmeyer R, Wessling B, Madea B. Heroin-associated nephropathy – a post-mortem study. Forensic Sci Int 1998; 95: 109-116.
21. Steinmuller DR, Bolton WK, Stillman MM, Couser WG. Chronic interstitial nephritis and mixed cryoglobulin associated with drug abuse. Arch Pathol Lab Med 1979; 103: 63-66.
22. McAllister CJ, Horn R, Havron A, Abramson JH. Granulomatous interstitial nephritis: a complication of heroin abuse. S Med J 1979; 72: 162-165.
23. Hill P, Dwyer K, Kay T, Murphy B. Severe chronic renal failure in association with oxycodone addiction: a new form of fibrillary glomerulopathy. Hum Pathol 2002; 33(8): 783-787.

24. Peces R, Diaz-Corte C, Baltar J, Seco M, Alvarez-Grande J. Haemolytic-uraemic syndrome in a heroin addict. Nephrol Dial Transplant. 1998; 13: 3197-3199.
25. Stehman-Breen C, Alpers CE, Fleet WP, Johnson RJ. Focal segmental glomerular sclerosis among patients infected with hepatitis C virus. Nephron 1999; 81: 37-40.
26. Do Sameiro Faria M, Sampaio S, Faria V, Carvalho E. Nephropathy associated with heroin abuse in Caucasian patients. Nephrol Dial Transplant 2003;18:2308-2313.
27. Glicklich D, Haskell L, Senitzer D, Weiss RA. Possible genetic predisposition to idiopathic focal segmental glomerulosclerosis. Am J Kidney Dis 1988; 12: 26-30.
28. Haskell LP, Glicklich D, Senitzer D. HLA associations in heroin-associated nephropathy. Am J Kidney Dis 1988; 12: 45-50.
29. Kaplan JM, Kim SH, North KN, Rennke H, Correia LA, Tong HQ, Mathis BJ, Rodriguez-Perez JC, Allen PG, Beggs AH, Pollak MR. Mutations in ACTN4, encoding alpha-actin-4, cause familial focal segmental glomeruloscerosis. Nat Genet 2000; 24:251-256.
30. Boute N, Gribouval O, Roselli S, Benessy F;, Attie T, Gubler MC, Niaudet P, Antignac C. NPHS2, encoding the glomerular podocin, is mutated in autosomal recessive steroid-resistant nephrotic syndrome. Nat Genet 2000; 24: 349-354.
31. Niranjan T, Bielesz B, Gruenwald A, Ponda MP, Kopp JB, Thomas DB, Susztak K. The Notch pathway in podocytes plays a role in the development of glomerular disease. Nat Med. 2008; 14 (3):290-298
32. Mukerji N, Damodaran TV, Winn MP. TRPC6 and FSGS: the latest TRP channelopathy. Biochim Biophys Acta 2007;1772 (8):859-868.
33. Jaffe JA, Kimmel PL. Chronic nephropathies of cocaine and heroin abuse: a critical review. Clin J Am Soc Nephrol 2006;1:655-667.
34. Moody C, Kaufman R, McGuire D, Grossman S. The role of adulterants in heroin nephropathy. NKF (New Orleans) 1985; 32.
35. Brown SM, Stimmel B, Taub RN, Kochwa S, Rosenfield RE. Immunologic dysfunction in heroin addicts. Arch Intern Med 1974; 134: 1001-1006.
36. Nikolova M., Liubomirova M, Iliev A, Krasteva R, Andreev E, Radenkova J, Minkova V, Djerassi R, Kiperova B, Vlahov ID. Clinical significance of antinuclear antibodies, anti-neutrophil cytoplasmic antibodies and anticardiolipin antibodies in heroin abusers. Isr Med Assoc J 2002 ;4 (11 Suppl):908-910.
37. Ringle DA, Herndon BL. In-vitro morphine binding by sera from morphine-treated rabbits. J Immunol 1972; 109: 174-175.
38. Ryan JJ, Parker CW, Williams RC. Gamma-globulin binding of morphine in heroin addicts. J Lab Clin Med 1972; 80: 155-164.
39. Weksler ME, Cherubin C, Kilcoyne M, Koppel G, Yoel M. Absence of morphine-binding activity in serum from heroin addicts. Clin Exp Immunol 1973; 13: 613-617.
40. Shah SP, Khine M, Anigbogu J, Miller A. Nodular amyloidosis of the lung from intravenous drug abuse: an uncommon cause of multiple pulmonary nodules. South Med J 1998 ;91 (4):402-404.
41. Marchand C, Cantin M, Cote M. Evidence for the nephrotoxicity of morphine sulfate in rats. Can J Physiol Pharmacol 1969; 47: 649-655.
42. Johnson JE, White JJ, Walovitch RC, London ED. Effects of morphine on rat kidney glomerular podocytes. A scanning electron microscope study. Drug Alcohol Depend 1987; 19: 249-257.
43. Singhal PC, Gibbons N, Abromovici M. Long term effects of morphine on mesangial cell proliferation and matrix synthesis. Kidney Int 1992; 41: 1560-1570.
44. Singhal PC, Pan CQ, Sagar S, Valderrama E, Stahl RA. Morphine modulates mesangial immunoglobulin G uptake in rats with antithymocyte serum-induced mesangial cell injury. Nephron 1996; 74: 197-203.
45. Kapasi AA, Gibbons N, Mattana J, Singhal PC. Morphine stimulates mesangial cell TNF-a and nitrite production. Inflammation 2000; 24: 463-476.
46. Singhal PC, Sharma P, Gibbons N, Franki N, Kapasi A, Wagner JD. Effect of morphine on renomedullary interstitial cell proliferation and matrix accumulation. Nephron 1997; 77: 225-234.
47. Singhal PC, Sharma P, Sanwal V, Prasad A, Kapasi A, Ranjan R, Franki N, Reddy K, Gibbons N. Morphine modulates proliferation of kidney fibroblasts. Kidney Int 1998; 53: 350-357.
48. Arerangaiah R, Chalasani N, Udager AM, Weber ML, Manivel JC, Griffin RJ, Song CW, Gupta K. Opioids induce renal abnormalities in tumor-bearing mice. Nephron Exp Nephrol 2007; 105(3): e80-89
49. Dubrow A, Mittman N, Ghali V, Ghali V, Flamenbaum W. The changing spectrum of heroin-associated nephropathy. Am J Kidney Dis 1985; 5: 36-41.
50. Kunis C, Olesnicky M, Nurse H. Heroin nephropathy-clinical pathologic correlations. Proc 9th Int Congr Nephrol 1984; 102A.
51. Cunningham EE, Zielezny MA, Venuto RC. Heroin-associated nephropathy - a nationwide problem. JAMA 1983; 250: 2935-2936.
52. Davis JS, Lie JT. Extracellular glomerular microparticles in nephrotic syndrome of heroin users. Arch Pathol 1975; 99: 278-282.
53. Gardiner H, Mahajan S, Briggs W. Renal disease in heroin addicts. J Am Soc Nephrol 1977; 15A.

54. Grishman E, Churg J. Focal glomerular sclerosis in nephrotic patients. An electron microscope study of glomerular podocytes. Kidney Int 1975; 7: 111-122.
55. Grishman E, Churg J, Porush JG. Glomerular morphology in nephrotic heroin addicts. Lab Invest 1976; 35: 415-424.
56. Rao TKS, Nicastri AD, Friedman EA. Renal consequences of narcotic abuse. Adv Nephrol 1979; 7: 261-290.
57. Baldwin DS, Gallo GR, Neugarten J. Drug abuse with narcotics and other agents in diseases of the kidney. In: Diseases of the kidney, 5th ed. Schrier RW, Gottschalk CW (editors). Little Brown and Co, Boston 1992; p 1219-1236.
58. D'Agati V, Appel GB. HIV infection and the kidney. J Am Soc Nephrol 1997; 8: 138-152.
59. Rao TK, Filippone EJ, Nicastri AD, Landesman SH, Frank E, Chen CK, Friedman EA. Associated focal and segmental glomerulosclerosis in the acquired immunodeficiency syndrome. N Engl J Med 1984; 310: 669-673.
60. Ross G, Weinstein S, Dutton S, Whittier FC. Renal transplantation in end stage renal disease of drug abuse. J Urol 1983; 129: 14-15.
61. Gordon MJ, White R, Matas A, Tellis VA, Glicklich D, Quinn T, Soberman R, Veith FJ. Renal transplantation in patients with history of heroin abuse. Transplantation 1986; 42: 556-557.
62. Brus I, Steiner G, Maceda A, Lejano R. Amyloid fibrils in urinary sediment. Heroin addiction with renal amyloidosis. NY State J Med 1979; 79: 768-771.
63. Jacob H, Charytan C, Rascoff JH, Golden R, Janis R. Amyloidosis secondary to drug abuse and chronic skin suppuration. Arch Intern Med 1978; 138: 1150-1151.
64. Meador KH, Sharon Z, Lewis EJ. Renal amyloidosis and subcutaneous drug abuse. Ann Intern Med 1979; 91: 565-567.
65. Novick DM, Yancovitz SR, Weinberg PG. Amyloidosis in parenteral drug abusers. Mt Sinai J Med 1979; 46: 163-167.
66. Scholes JV, Derosena R, Appel GB. Amyloidosis and the nephrotic syndrome in chronic heroin addicts. Proc 7th Int Congr Nephrol 1978; L9.
67. Scholes J, Derosena R, Appel GB, Ao W, Boyd MT, Pirani CL. Amyloidosis in chronic heroin addicts with the nephrotic syndrome. Ann Intern Med 1979; 91: 26-29.
68. Menchel S, Cohen D, Gross E, Frangione B, Gallo G. AA protein-related renal amyloidosis in drug addicts. Am J Pathol 1983; 112: 195-199.
69. Amigo JS, Orriols J, Modol J. Resolution of nephrotic syndrome secondary to heroin-associated renal amyloidosis. Nephrol Dial Transplant 1990; 158.
70. Crowley S, Feinfeld DA, Janis R. Resolution of nephrotic syndrome and lack of progression of heroin associated renal amyloidosis. Am J Kidney Dis 1989; 13: 333-335.
71. Derosena R, Koss MN, Pirani CL. Demonstration of amyloid fibrils in urinary sediment. N Engl J Med 1975; 293: 1131-1133.
72. Chan-Tack KM, Ahuja N, Weiman EJ Wali RK, Uche A, Greisman LA, Drachenberg C, Hawkins PN, Redfield RR. Acute renal failure and nephrotic range proteinuria due to amyloidodsis in an HIV-infected patient. Am J Med Sci 2006; 332 (6):364-367
73. Connolly JO, Gillmore JD, Lachmann HJ, Davenport A, Hawkins PN, Woolfson RG. Renal amyloidosis in intravenous drug abusers. QJMed 2006; 99:737-742.
74. Neugarten J, Gallo GR, Buxbaum J, Katz LA, Rubenstein J, Baldwin DS. Amyloidosis in subcutaneous heroin abusers. Am J Med 1986; 81: 635-640.
75. Tan AU Jr, Cohen AH, Levine BS. Renal amyloidosis in a drug abuser. J Am Soc Nephrol 1995; 5: 1653-1658.
76. Ray PE, Xu L, Rakusan T, Liu XH. A 20-year history of childhood HIV-associated nephropathy. Pediatr Nephrol. 2004;19(10):1075-1092
77. D'Agati V, Cheng JI, Carbone L, Cheng JT, Appel G. The pathology of HIV-nephropathy: a detailed morphologic and comparative study. Kidney Int 1989; 35: 1358-1370.
78. D'Agati V, Appel GB. Renal pathology of human immunodeficiency virus infection. Sem Nephrol 1998; 18: 406-421.
79. Appel GB, Nicolaides M. HIV-AIDS nephropathy in the inner city. New York State J Med 1991; 91: 207-210.
80. Rao TK, Friedman EA, Nicastri AD. The types of renal disease in the acquired immunodeficiency syndrome. N Engl J Med 1987; 316: 1062-1068.
81. Carbone L, D'Agati V, Cheng J-T, Appel GB. Course and prognosis of human immunodeficiency virus-associated nephropathy. Am J Med 1989; 87: 389-395.
82. Pardo V, Aldana M, Colton RM, Fischl MA, Jaffe D, Moskowitz L, Hensley GT, Bourgoignie JJ. Glomerular lesions in the acquired immunodeficiency syndrome. Ann Intern Med 1984; 101: 429-434.
83. Strauss J, Abibol C, Zilleruelo G, Scott G, Paredes A, Malaga S, Montane B, Mitchell C. Renal disease in children with the acquired immunodeficiency syndrome. N Engl J Med 1989; 321: 625-630.
84. Bourgoigne JJ. Renal complications of human immuodeficiency virus type I. Kidney Int 1990; 37: 1571-1584.
85. Seney FD, Burns DK, Silva FG. Acquired immunodeficiency syndrome and the kidney. Am J Kidney Dis 1990; 16: 1-13.

86. Glassock RJ, Cohen AH, Danovitch G, Parsa P. Human immunodeficiency virus infection and the kidney. Ann Int Med 1990; 112: 35-49.
87. Pardo V, Meneses R, Ossa L, Jaffe DJ, Strauss J, Roth D, Bourgoignie JJ. AIDS-related glomerulopathy: occurrence in specific risk groups. Kidney Int 1987; 31: 1167-1173.
88. Winston JA, Burns GC, Klotman PE. The human immunodeficiency virus epidemic and HIV associated nephropathy. Sem Nephol 1998; 18: 373-377.
89. Friedman EA, Tao TK. Disappearance of uremia due to heroin-associated nephropathy. Am J Kidney Dis 1995: 5: 689-693.
90. Gharavi AG, Ahmad T, Wong RD, et al. Mapping a locus for susceptibility to HIV-1-associated nephropathy to mouse chromosome 3. Proc Natl Acad Sci U S A. 2004;101(8):2488-2493.
91. Lucas GM, Lau B, Atta MG, Fine DM, Keruly J, Moore RD. Chronic Kidney Disease Incidence, and Progression to End-Stage Renal Disease, in HIV-Infected Individuals: A Tale of Two Races. J Infect Dis. Apr 18 2008.
92. Cohen AH, Sun NCJ, Shapshak P, Imagawa DT. Demonstration of HIV in renal epithelium in HIV associated nephropathy. Modern Path 1989; 2: 125-128.
93. Winston JA, Bruggeman LA, Ross MD, Jacobson J, Ross L, D'Agati V, Klotman PE, Klotman ME. Nephropathy and establishment of a renal reservoir of HIV type 1 during primary infection. N Engl J Med 2001; 344: 1979-1984.
94. Wali RK, Drachenberg CI, Papadimitriou JC, Keay S, Ramos E. HIV-1-associated nephropathy and respose to highly-active antiretroviral therapy. Lancet 1998; 352: 783-784.
95. Ho DD, Zhang L. HIV-1 rebound after abti-retroviral therapy. Nat Med 2000; 6: 736-737.
96. Monahan M, Tanji N, Klotman PE. HIV-associated nephropathy: An urban epidemic. Semin Nephrol 2001; 21: 394-402.
97. Post FA, Campbell LJ, Hamzah L, Collins L, Jones R, Siwani R Johnson L, Fisher M, Holt SG, Bhaagani S, Frankel AH, et al. Predictors of renal outcome in HIV-associated nephropathy. CID 2008; 46:1282-1289.
98. Kimmel PL, Ferreira-Centeno A, Farkas-Szallasi T, Abraham AA, Garrett CT. Viral DNA in microdissected renal biopsy material from HIV infected patients with the nephrotic syndrome. Kidney Int 1993; 43: 1347-1352.
99. Green DF, Resnick L, Bourgoignie J. HIV infects glomerular endothelial and mesangial cells but not epithelial cells *in vitro*. Kidney Int 1992; 41: 956-960.
100. Bruggeman LA, Ross MD, Tanji N, et al. Renal epithelium is a previously unrecognized site of HIV-1 infection. J Am Soc Nephrol 2000;11(11):2079-2087
101. Kopp JB, Klotman ME, Adler SH, Bruggeman LA, Dickie P, Marinos NJ, Eckhaus M, Bryant JL, Notkins AL, Klotman PE. Progressive glomerulosclerosis and enhanced renal accumulation of basement membrane components in mice transgenic for HIV type 1 genes. Proc Nat Acad Sci 1992; 89: 1577-1581.
102. Husain M, D'Agati VD, He JC, Klotman ME, Klotman PE. HIV-1 Nef induces dedifferentiation of podocytes *in vivo*: a characteristic feature of HIVAN. AIDS. 2005;19(17):1975-1980
103. Singhal PC, Sagar S, Reddy K, Sharma P, Ranjan R, Franki N. HIV-1 gp120 envelope protein and morphine-tubular cell interaction products modulate kidney fibroblast proliferation. J Invest Med 1998; 46: 243-248.
104. Eremina V, Sood M, Haigh J, Nagy A, Lajoie G, Ferrara N, Gerber HP, Kikkawa Y, Miner JH, Quaggin SE. Glomerular-specific alterations of VEGF-A expression lead to distinct congenital and acquired renal diseases. J Clin Invest 2003; 111 (5):707-716.
105. Korgaonkar SN, Feng X, Ross MD, et al. HIV-1 upregulates VEGF in podocytes. J Am Soc Nephrol. 2008;19(5):877-883.
106. Kimmel PL, Cohen DJ, Abraham AA, Bodi I, Schwartz AM, Philips TM. Upregulation of MHC class II, interferon-a and interferon-g receptor protein expression in HIV-associated nephropathy. Nephrol Dial Transplant 2003; 18 (2):285-292.
107. Koffler A, Friedler RM, Massry SG. Acute renal failure due to nontraumatic rhabdomyolysis. Ann Intern Med 1976; 85: 23-28.
108. Penn AS, Rowland LP, Fraser DW. Drugs, coma, and myoglobinuria. Arch Neurology 1972; 26: 336-344.
109. Grossman RA, Hamilton RW, Morse BM, Penn AS, Goldberg M. Nontraumatic rhabdomyolysis and acute renal failure. N Engl J Med 1974; 291: 807-811.
110. Ward MM. Factors predictive of acute renal failure in rhabdomyolysis. Arch Intern Med 1988; 148: 1553-1557.
111. Eneas JF, Schoenfeld PY, Humphreys MH. The effect of infusion of mannitol-sodium bicarbonate on the clinical course of myoglobinuria. Arch Intern Med 1979; 139: 801-805.
112. Robinson SF, Woods AH. Heroin induced rhabdomyolysis and acute renal failure: a case report. Arizona Med 1974; 31: 246-251.
113. Richter RW, Challenor YB, Pearson J, Kagen LJ, Hamilton LL, Ramsey WH. Acute myoglobinuria associated with heroin addiction. JAMA 1971; 216: 1172-1176.
114. Rao TK, Nicastri AD, Friedman EA. Natural history of heroin associated nephropathy. In: Nephrology. Hamburger J, Crosnier J, Maxwell MH (editors). Wiley, New York 1979; p 843-856.
115. Rice EK, Isbel NM, Becker GJ, Atkins RC, McMahon LP. Heroin overdose and myoglobinuric acute renal failure. Clin Nephol 2000; 54:449-454.

116. Corwin HL, Schreiber MJ, Fang LS. Low fractional excretion of sodium. Occurrence with hemoglobinuric and myoglobinuric-induced acute renal failure. Arch Intern Med 1984; 144: 981-982.
117. Llach F, Felsenfeld AJ, Haussler MR. The pathophysiology of altered calcium metabolism in rhabdomyolysis-induced acute renal failure. N Engl J Med 1981; 305: 117-123.
118. Gabow PA, Kaehny WD, Kelleher SP. The spectrum of rhabdomyolysis. Medicine 1982; 61: 141-152.
119. Penn AS. Myoglobin and myoglobinuria. In: The handbook of clinical neurology - disease of muscle. Vinken PJ, Bruyn GW (editors). North-Holland Publishing Co, Amsterdam, New York, Oxford 1979; 41: 259-285.
120. Rowland LP, Penn AS. Myoglobinuria. Med Clin N Am 1972; 56: 1233-1256.
121. Zager RA. Studies of mechanisms and protective maneuvers in myoglobinuric acute renal failure. Lab Invest 1989; 60: 619-629.
122. Better OS. Early management of shock and prophylaxis of acute renal failure in traumatic rhabdomyolysis. N Engl J Med 1990; 322: 825-828.
123. Venuto RC. Pigment-associated acute renal failure: is the water clearer 50 years later ? J Lab Clin Med 1992; 119: 452-454.
124. Odeh M. The role of reperfusion-induced injury in the pathogenesis of the crush syndrome. N Engl J Med 1991; 324: 1417-1422.
125. Nath KA, Balla G, Vercellotti GM, Balla J, Jacob HS, Levitt, Rosenberg ME. Induction of heme oxidase is a rapid protective response in rhabdomyolysis in the rat. J Clin Invest 1992; 90: 267-270.
126. Zager RA. Combined mannitol and desferoxamine therapy for myohemoglobinuric renal injury and oxidant tubular stress. Mechanistic and therapeutic implications. J Clin Invest 1992; 90: 711-719.
127. Ron D, Taitelman U, Michaelson M, Bar-Joseph G, Bursztein S, Better OS. Prevention of acute renal failure in traumatic rhabdomyolysis. Arch Intern Med 1984; 144: 277-280.
128. Rubin RB, Neugarten J. Medical complications of cocaine: changes in pattern of use and spectrum of complications. Clin Toxicology 1992; 30: 1-12.
129. Adverse effects of cocaine abuse. Med Letter 1984; 26: 51-52.
130. Cregler LI, Mark H. Medical complications of cocaine abuse. N Engl J Med 1986; 315: 1495-1500.
131. Isner JM, Estes NA, Thompson PD, Costanzo-Nordin MR, Subramanian R, Miller G, Katsas G, Sweeney K, Sturner WQ. Acute cardiac events temporally related to cocaine abuse. N Engl J Med 1986; 315: 1438-1443.
132. Zamoa-Quezada JC, Dinerman H, Stadecker MJ, Kelly JJ. Muscle and skin infarction after free-basing cocaine (Crack). Ann Intern Med 1988; 108: 564-566.
133. Krohn KD, Slowman-Kovacs S, Leapman SB. Cocaine and rhabdomyolysis. Ann Intern Med 1988; 108: 639-640.
134. Rubin RB, Neugarten J. Cocaine-induced rhabdomyolysis masquerading as myocardial ischemia. Am J Med 1989; 86: 551-553.
135. Lombard J, Wong B, Young JH. Acute renal failure due to rhabdomyolysis associated with cocaine toxicity. West J Med 1988; 148: 466-468.
136. Herzlich BC, Arsura EL, Pagala M, Grob D. Rhabdomyolysis related to cocaine abuse. Ann Intern Med 1988; 109: 335-336.
137. Pogue VA, Nurse HM. Cocaine-associated acute myoglobinuric renal failure. Am J Med 1989; 86: 183-186.
138. Merigian KS, Roberts JR. Cocaine intoxication: hyperpyrexia, rhabdomyolysis and acute renal failure. Clin Toxicol 1987; 25: 135-148.
139. Faulkner M, Singhal P, Peters A. Rhabdomyolysis and acute renal failure following cocaine abuse. Kidney Int 1989; 35: 225A.
140. Roth D, Alarcon FJ, Fernandez JA, Preston RA, Bourgoignie JJ. Acute rhabdomyolysis associated with cocaine intoxication. N Engl J Med 1988; 319: 673-677.
141. Singhal PC, Rubin RB, Peters A, Santiago A, Neugarten J. Rhabdomyolysis and acute renal failure associated with cocaine abuse. Clin Toxicology 1990; 28: 321-330.
142. Barrido DT, Joseph AJ, Rao TK, Friedman EA. Renal disease associated with acute and chronic "Crack" abuse. Kidney Int 1988; 33: 181A.
143. Attoussi S, Faulkner ML, Oso A, Umoru B. Cocaine-induced scleroderma and scleroderma renal crisis. South Med J 1998; 91: 961-963.
144. Gu X, Herrera GA. Thrombotic microangiopathy in cocaine abuse-associated malignant hypertension: report of 2 cases with review of the literature. Arch Pathol Lab Med. 2007;131(12):1817-1820.
145. Sharff JA. Renal infarction associated with intravenous cocaine use. Ann Emerg Med 1984; 13: 1145-1147.
146. Goodman PE, Rennie WP. Renal infarction secondary to nasal insufflation of cocaine. Am. J Emerg Med 1995; 13: 421-423.
147. Zoghby Z, Sekhon IS, Miller DV, Sethi S. Cocaine, loin pain, and renal vein thrombosis. Am J Kidney Dis. 2007;49(6):859-861.
148. Alvarez D, Nzerue CM, Daniel JF, Faruque S, Hewan-Lowe K. Acute interstitial nephritis induced by crack cocaine binge. Nephrol Dial Transplant 1999; 14: 1260-1262.

149. Peces R, Navascues RA, Baltar J, Seco M, Alvarez J. Antiglomerular basement membrane antibody-mediated glomerulonephritis after intranasal cocaine use. Nephron 1999; 81: 434-438.
150. Garcia-Rostan GM, Garcia-Bragado F, Puras-Gil AM. Pulmonary hemorrhage and antiglomerular membrane antibody-mediated glomerulonephritis after exposure to smoked (crack) cocaine: A case report and review of the literature. Pathol Int 1997: 47: 692-697.
151. Chevalier X, Rostoker G, Larget-Piet B, Gherardi R. Schoenlein-Henoch pupura with necrotizing vasculitis after cocaine snorting. Clin Nephrol 1995; 43: 348-349.
152. Volcy J, Nzerue CM, Oderinde A, Hewan-Lowe K. Cocaine-induced acute renal failure, hemolysis, and thrombocytopenia mimicking thrombotic thrombocytopenic purpura. Am J Kidney Dis 2000; 35: E3.
153. Tumlin JA, Sands JM, Someren A. Hemolytic uremic syndrome following "crack" cocaine inhalation. Am J Med Sci 1990; 299: 366-371.
154. Gottbrath-Flaherty EK, Agrawal R, Thaker V, Patel D, Ghai K. Urinary tract infections in cocaine-exposed infants. J Perinatol 1995; 15: 203-207.
155. Klotman PE. HIV-associated nephropathy. Kidney Int 1999; 56: 1161-1176.
156. Ward HJ, San Diego R, Pan DK. Substance abuse as a risk factor for hypertensive renal disease. J Am Soc Nephrol 1998; 162 A (abstract).
157. Norris K, Thornhill-Joynes M, Robinson C, Strickland T, Alperson B, Witana S, Ward HJ. Cocaine use, hypertension and end stage renal disease. Am J Kidney Dis 2001; 38: 523-528.
158. Dunea G, Arruda JL, Bakin-Share DS, Smith C. Role of cocaine in end-stage renal disease in some hypertensive African-Americans. Am J Nephrol 1995; 15: 5-9.
159. Ward HJ, Pickett R, Tovar L. Cocaine associated nephropathy: a new clinicopathologic entity. J Am Soc Nephrol 2000; 11; 79A (abstract).
160. Fine DM, Garg N, Haas M, Hafizur Rahman M, Lucas GM, Scheel PJ, Atta MG. Cocaine use and hypertensive renal changes in HIV-infected individuals. Clin J Am Soc Nephrol. 2007;2(6):1125-1130.
161. Cogen FC, Rigg G, Simmons JL, Domino EF. Phencyclidine-associated acute rhabdomyolysis. Ann Intern Med 1978; 88: 210-212.
162. Akmal M, Valdin JR, McCarron MM, Massry SG. Rhabdomyolysis with and without acute renal failure in patients with phencyclidine intoxication. Am J Nephrol 1981; 1: 91-96.
163. Hoogwerf B, Kern J, Bullock M, Comty CM. Phencyclidine-induced rhabdomyolysis and acute renal failure. Clin Toxicol 1979; 14: 47-53.
164. Patel R, Ansari A, Hughes JL. Myoglobinuric acute renal failure associated with phencyclidine abuse. West J Med 1979; 131: 244-247.
165. Patel R, Das M, Patazzolo M, Ansari A, Balasubramaniam J. Myoglobinuric acute renal failure in phencyclidine overdose. Report of observations in eight cases. Ann Emerg Med 1980; 9: 549-553.
166. Barton CH, Sterling ML, Vaziri ND. Rhabdomyolysis and acute renal failure associated with phencyclidine intoxication. Arch Intern Med 1980; 140: 568-569.
167. Kuncl RW, Meltzer HY. Pathologic effect of phencyclidine and restraint on rat skeletal muscle: prevention by prior denervation. Exp Neurology 1974; 45: 3887-3402.
168. Appel GB, Radhakrishnan J, D'Agati V, Secondary glomerular disease. In: The Kidney (chapter 30), 6th edition. BH Brenner (editor). WB Saunders Company, Philadelphia 2000; p 1350-1449.
169. Citron BP, Halpern M, McCarron M, Lundberg GD, McCormick R, Pincus IJ, Tatter D, Haverback BJ. Necrotizing angiitis associated with drug abuse. N Engl J Med 1970; 283: 1003-1011.
170. Baden MM. Angiitis in drug abuse. N Engl J Med 1971; 284: 111-112.
171. Citron BP, Peters RL. Angiitis in drug abuse. N Engl J Med 1971; 284: 112.
172. Gocke DJ, Hsu K, Morgan C, Bombardieri S, Lockshin M, Christian CL. Association between polyarteritis and Australia antigen. Lancet 1970; 2: 1149-1153.
173. Koff RS, Widrich WC, Robbins AH. Necrotizing angiitis in a methamphetamine user with hepatitis B. N Engl J Med 1973; 288: 946-947.
174. Lignelli GJ, Buchheit WA. Angiitis in drug abuse. N Engl J Med 1971; 284: 112-123.
175. Cacoub P, Lunel-Fabiani F, Huong Dup LT. Polyarteritis nodosa and hepatitis C virus infection. Ann Intern Med 1992; 116: 605-606.
176. Hurault de Ligny B, El Haggan W, Comoz F, et al. Early loss of two renal grafts obtained from the same donor: role of ecstasy? Transplantation. 2005;80(1):153-156.

177. Ginsberg MD, Hetrzman M, Schmidt-Nowara WW. Amphetamine intoxication with coagulopathy, hyperthermia, and reversible renal failure. Ann Intern Med 1970; 73: 81-85.
178. Kendrick WC, Hull AR, Knochel JP. Rhabdomyolysis and shock after intravenous amphetamine administration. Ann Intern Med 1977; 86: 381-387.
179. Foley RJ, Kapatkin K, Verani R, Weinman E. Amphetamine-induced acute renal failure. Southern Med J 1984; 77: 258-260.
180. Verebey K, Alraze J, Depace A. The complications of "Ecstacy" (MDMA). JAMA 1988; 259: 1649-1658.
181. Hartung TK, Schofield E, Short AI, Parr MJ, Henry JA. Hyponatraemic states following 3,4-methylenedioxymethamphetamine (MDMA, 'ecstasy') ingestion. Quart J Med. 2002;95(7):431-437.
182. Brvar M, Kozelj G, Osredkar J, Mozina M, Gricar M, Bunc M. Polydipsia as another mechanism of hyponatremia after 'ecstasy' (3,4 methyldioxymethamphetamine) ingestion. Eur J Emerg Med. 2004;11(5):302-304.
183. Bohatyrewicz M, Urasinska E, Rozanski J, Ciecharowski K. Membranous glomerulonephritis may be associated with heavy marijuana abuse. Transplant Proc. 2007; 39(10):3054-3056.
184. Busse F, Omidi L, Leichtle A, Windgassen M, Kluge E, Stumvoll M. Lead Poisoning due to adulterated marijuana. N Engl J Med 2008;358 (15):1641-1642.
185. De Marchi S, Cecchin E, Basile A. Renal tubular dysfunction in chronic alcohol abuse - effects of abstinence. N Engl J Med 1993; 329: 1927-1934.
186. Sadjadi SA, McLaughlin K, Shah RM. Allergic interstitial nephritis due to Diazepam. Arch Intern Med 1987; 141: 579-580.

28

Nephrotoxicity of calcineurin and mTOR inhibitors

Emmanuel A. Burdmann[1] and William M. Bennett[2]

[1]Division of Nephrology, São José do Rio Preto Medical School, São José do Rio Preto, São Paulo, Brazil
[2]Northwest Renal Clinic, Transplant Services, Legacy Good Samaritan Hospital, Portland, Oregon, USA

Introduction

Cyclosporine A (CSA) was introduced into clinical practice in the early 80s resulting in a large decrease in the incidence of acute rejection in renal transplantation and increasing solid organ transplant graft and patient survival to unparalleled levels. Subsequently, its use was extended to bone marrow transplant immunosuppression and to the treatment of a variety of autoimmune diseases refractory to conventional therapy, again with noteworthy efficacy [1-6]. The subsequent development of CSA self-emulsifying formulations improved bioavailability, decreased inter- and intra-patient variability and allowed more precise drug dose-tailoring [3, 7]. More recently, generic CSA brands have become available, decreasing treatment costs substantially. The combination of efficacy, accumulated experience and decreasing cost makes CSA still widely used in the clinical practice, and large numbers of patients are currently exposed to this drug.

In 1989 tacrolimus (TAC), a second calcineurin inhibitor was approved for clinical use [8]. Tacrolimus has an immunosuppressive effect approximately 100 times more potent than CSA and early clinical trials demonstrated that TAC was effective in reversing refractory acute rejection in renal, liver and heart transplantation. Subsequently, this drug was shown to be at least as effective as CSA in the primary immunosuppression schedules for solid organ and bone marrow transplantation and, similar to CSA, has proven to be a valuable alternative in the treatment of autoimmune diseases [3, 9-11]. Because the facility of drug monitoring by trough levels, less cosmetic side effects and a putative better profile in preventing acute rejection, TAC use has increased significantly and in fact, it has become the calcineurin inhibitor of choice for the prevention of rejection in solid organ transplantation in the majority of centers.

Both drugs inhibit interleukin-2 gene transcription and the transition of T lymphocytes from the G0 to G1 phase of the cell cycle. They bind to cytoplasmic immunophilins, cyclophilin for CSA and FK-binding protein (FKBP12) for TAC. The immunosuppressive drug-immunophilin complex reduces calcium signaling, blocking a calcium dependent enzyme, calcineurin phosphatase, responsible for the nuclear translocation and dephosphorylation of the cytosolic nuclear factor of activating T lymphocytes (NF-AT-c). NF-AT-c regulates the transcription of genes responsible for several cytokines, including interleukin 2 [3].

The most important side effects for both drugs are kidney-related: acute and chronic renal dysfunction, hemolytic-uremic syndrome, hypertension, electrolyte disturbances (hyperkalemia, hypomagnesemia and hypocalcemia), renal tubular acidosis and defects in urinary concentrating ability. Among them, nephrotoxicity is considered the most significant and limiting adverse effect. Interestingly, sirolimus which reduces interleukin 2 production without blocking calcineurin has a different pattern of nephrotoxicity [12]. When calcineurin is inhibited, the interleukin 2 gene is not the only gene which has its transcription impaired. Actually, the list includes genes for other interleukins, interleukin 2 receptor, nitric oxide synthase, transforming growth factor β (TGF-β), endothelin, collagen I and IV and bcl-2, responsible for protein Bcl-2, which is likely implicated in cellular protection against apoptosis [13]. It is possible that calcineurin inhibition at the same time that it blocks immune cell-mediated reaction against the transplanted tissue triggers a sequence of undesirable events that will eventually lead to renal injury [13]. The development of selective calcineurin inhibitors that disrupt genes transcription of particular genes without affecting the others may clarify this important issue [14].

Calcineurin inhibitor nephrotoxicity presents as two distinct forms of renal injury. Acute nephrotoxicity is a dose-dependent, hemodynamically mediated disorder, not accompanied by particular or permanent structural changes which is reversible with decrease or discontinuation of the offending drug. On the other hand, calcineurin inhibitor-induced chronic nephrotoxicity is an insidious lesion, characterized by an irreversible and progressive renal interstitial fibrosis, which may cause important impairment in renal function and even stage 5 chronic kidney disease.

Cyclosporine A nephrotoxicity

Acute nephrotoxicity

Acute CSA-induced nephrotoxicity is a functional abnormality caused by a disproportion of the balance of vasoconstrictor and vasodilator mediators. The main characteristic of this form of nephrotoxicity is an intense intra-renal vasoconstriction , causing RBF decrease and RVR increase, accompanied by variable degree of GFR impairment. The main site for this vasoconstriction is the afferent arteriole but it also occurs in adjacent small arteries, including the glomerular tuft [13, 15, 16].

CSA administration causes acute changes in renal hemodynamics and function in patients and in healthy human volunteers [17]. The phenomenon is reversible with drug dosage decrease or withdrawal. These changes were also demonstrated after different doses and route of administration in animals and indeed, acute CSA-induced nephrotoxicity models are consistent. Renal structural abnormalities seem in experimental studies or in patients' biopsies are minimal to absent and non-specific, even when renal dysfunction is severe [15, 18].

The list of possible mediators for acute CSA nephrotoxicity is extensive (see Table 1). Most of the studies assessing the mechanisms involved in acute CSA nephrotoxicity have been done through pharmacological blockade of the candidate system using experimental models. Individual blockade of a particular system resulted in improvement but not total prevention of impairment in renal hemodynamics, indicating that CSA-induced vasoconstriction is likely a complex phenomenon caused by the interaction of different mechanisms [19, 20].

Table 1. Mediators and mechanisms possibly involved in the pathogenesis of acute CSA nephrotoxicity.

Angiotensin II
Endothelin
Nitric oxide
Prostaglandins
Leukotrienes
Sympathetic system
Free radicals
Adenosine
Vasopressin
Platelet activation factor
Atrial natriuretic factor
Kallikrein-kinin system
Cholesterol
Hypomagnesemia
Extracellular volume depletion
Cremophor
Direct contraction – mesangial and smooth vascular cells
Direct tubular epithelial cell toxicity

Mechanisms of vascular/hemodynamic injury

Renin-angiotensin aldosterone system

The interaction of cyclosporine with the plasma and tissue renin-angiotensin-aldosterone systems (RAS) has been extensively studied [21, 22]. Sodium depletion, a condition that stimulates renin release, enhances acute CSA nephrotoxicity [23, 24]. In rats, CSA treatment enhanced plasma renin activity (PRA) [21, 25, 26], increased renal renin content [21], promoted juxtaglomerular hypertrophy and hyperplasia [27, 28], increased renin staining cells in juxtaglomerular apparatus (JGA) and renin containing cells in the afferent arterioles [29] and increased the number of renal angiotensin II AT_1 receptors [30]. *In vitro*, CSA induced renin release in renal cortical slices and culture of juxtaglomerular cells of rats, stimulated renin synthesis in juxtaglomerular cells and up-regulated angiotensin II receptors in cultured human smooth muscle cells [31-33]. In humans, CSA shows no effect or even decreases PRA [34]. Conversely, it increases levels of pro-renin and total renin and promotes JGA hyperplasia in heart and liver transplant recipients [35]. Gardiner et al showed that conversion from CSA to azathioprine decreased the number of renin-containing cells in renal allograft biopsies, suggesting a CSA-induced intra-renal RAS activation [36]. If there is little doubt that CSA has an important effect on the RAS, the actual role of this system in CSA-induced renal vascular changes is less clear. In fact, blocking of the RAS in experimental acute CSA nephrotoxicity produced conflicting results. Saralasin prevented renal blood flow decrease and intra-renal vasoconstriction in a model of isolated hydronephrotic rat kidney [37], losartan attenuated the increase in RVR [19], angiotensin converting enzyme inhibitor minimized GFR and RBF decreases [38, 39] and aldosterone blockade by spironolactone completely prevented GFR and RBF reductions caused by CSA [40]. On the other hand, multiple authors did not find preservation of renal function and/or hemodynamics when angiotensin converting enzyme inhibitors were given concomitantly with CSA [41-44]. In humans, attempts of prevention or attenuation of CSA-induced acute nephrotoxicity by pharmacological blockade of RAS have been mostly disappointing, with some studies finding improvement in RBF and RVR but not in GFR when angiotensin converting enzyme inhibitors or angiotensin II receptor blockers were administered to CSA-treated patients [45-47].

Endothelin

In 1987 O'Brien et al reported that cultured endothelial cells produced a potent vasoconstrictor substance [48]. In 1988, Yanagisawa et al identified this substance as endothelin (ET), a 21-amino acid peptide [49]. Then, three distinct genes for endothelin were discovered, each encoding a particular peptide, named ET-1, ET-2 and ET-3 [50]. Different renal resident and infiltrating cells can produce ET-1, such as vascular smooth muscle, endothelial, epithelial, mesangial and tubular cells, macrophages and monocytes. Moreover, endothelin-converting enzyme-1 (ECE-1), the enzyme responsible for ET-1 production, has a ubiquitous intra-renal distribution and ECE-1 mRNA can be found in glomeruli and in different tubular segments. The hemodynamics effects of ET include mesangial cells contraction, intra-renal vessels and afferent and efferent arterioles vasoconstriction, RVR increasing and RBF and GFR decreasing [51, 52]. The first evidence linking endothelin to acute CSA nephrotoxicity came out from the demonstration that CSA stimulated endothelin release from cultured renal epithelial cells (LLC-PK1) and that renal ET receptors were up-regulated in rats with CSA-induced nephrotoxicity [53, 54]. At that time, it was found that CSA administration to rats increased circulating ET-1, that anti-endothelin antibodies partially prevented CSA-induced renal hemodynamics changes and that an endothelin-1 receptor antagonist blunted *in vitro* mesangial cells contraction caused by CSA [55-57]. Subsequently, several authors reported increased urinary and/or plasma levels of ET after CSA treatment in animals and solid organ transplant recipients [58-63]. Additionally, molecular biologic studies disclosed up-regulation of arterial ET_A receptor mRNA, and increased pre-pro-ET1 mRNA expression and up-regulation of endothelin-converting enzyme 1 mRNA expression in renal cortex of CSA-treated rats [64, 65]. Nakayama et al, showed that a single IV injection of CSA in rats caused a rapid increase in glomerular pre-pro ET-1 mRNA and plasma ET-1 followed by a late glomerular and tubular decrease of ECE-1, ET_A and ET_B mRNA and protein levels, suggesting that CSA-induced ET1 synthesis induced down-regulation of ECE-1 expression [66]. Marsen et al demonstrated that CSA induces a calcium-dependent pre-pro endothelin gene transcription and ET-1 mRNA production in human endothelial cells in culture [67]. Experimental use of ET_A or ET_A/ET_B receptors antagonists attenuated CSA-induced hemodynamic changes [68], vasoconstriction of large pre-glomerular arteries and reduction in glomerular blood flow [69], afferent arteriole vasoconstriction [70], myosin light chain phosphorylation in glomerular mesangial cells [57] and calcium rise in smooth muscle cells [71]. When ET_A and ET_A/ET_B receptors antagonists were compared in the same study, additional ET_B blockade did not provide further protection against CSA effects [69]. Actually, blockade of ET receptors provided some conflicting results. Fogo et al found that an ET_A antagonist attenuated CSA-induced fall in GFR and RBF only when infused in the renal artery before CSA administration. When the ET_A antagonist was infused systemically or after CSA there was no protection [68]. Davis et al showed that the use of a selective ET_A antagonist or a combination of an ET_A and ET_B receptor antagonists did not prevent CSA-induced renal vasoconstriction in rats [72]. Binet et al reported that bosentan, a non-peptide mixed ET_A and ET_B receptor antagonist, attenuated RBF decrease, but not GFR fall caused by CSA in healthy human volunteers [73].

Nitric oxide

There are several lines of evidence demonstrating that CSA causes endothelial cell injury. CSA has a direct cytotoxic effect on cultured endothelial cells and inhibits human umbilical endothelial cell proliferation [74, 75]. CSA increases the plasma level of endothelial damage markers, such as Von Willebrand factor, endothelin tissue factor pathway inhibitor, P-selectin and thrombin-antithrombin complexes in renal and heart transplant patients [76-79]. Similarly, the release of Von

Willebrand factor, endothelin tissue factor pathway inhibitor and thrombomodulin was enhanced by CSA in the supernatant of endothelial cells in culture [79, 80]. The vascular endothelium produces nitric oxide (NO), which modulates relaxation of adjacent smooth muscle cells by a cyclic GMP-dependent mechanism. NO is produced from L-arginine by the action of NO synthase (NOS) family. Three NOS isoforms have been identified: neuronal NOS (nNOS), markedly expressed in brain, inducible NOS (iNOS) expressed in macrophages and endothelial NOS (eNOS) mainly expressed in endothelial cells. The three isoforms are present in different renal structures and have a major function in the regulation of glomerular and vascular tone and tubular function [81, 82]. There is a robust body of data linking acute CSA nephrotoxicity to disturbances in L-arginine-NO pathway. CSA impairs NO-mediated endothelium-dependent vasodilatation of human subcutaneous vessels and forearm vessels of heart transplant recipients [83, 84]. In the same way, studies in rodents, evaluating different aortic or arterial preparations, found CSA-induced impairment of NO dependent vasodilatation [85-91]. On the other hand, evaluations of CSA influence on tissue, plasma and urinary levels of NO and on tissue expression of NOS isoforms have provided contradictory results. *In vivo* experiments in rats showed CSA not changing, increasing or decreasing urinary NO metabolites [92-95]. Experiments using murine macrophage cell line, thoracic aorta or VSMC of rats found CSA-induced decrease in tissue NO metabolites [88] or NO production [96]. Studies performed in healthy volunteers showed that CSA increases NOS activity [97], whereas studies in renal transplant recipients found CSA-induced impairment of basal and stimulated NO production [98] and a biphasic pattern of decrease and then increase in plasma NO accompanied by a non significant decrease in urinary excretion of NO metabolites after the CSA first dose [99]. The evaluation of CSA effects on NOS genes showed increase of eNOS mRNA in renal cortex and increased induction of eNOS gene in bovine aortic endothelial cells [81, 100, 101] and no change in vascular eNOS [88]. CSA-promoted decreases in iNOS and nNOS mRNA and iNOS protein in renal tissue, aorta, macrophages and VSMC [81, 88, 95, 96, 101]. Enhancement of NO production by administration of L-arginine improved and blockade of NO by L-NAME administration worsened CSA-induced changes in endothelium-dependent vasodilation and in renal and glomerular hemodynamics in animals [81, 86, 88, 93, 94, 102-106]. Nifedipine prevented the changes induced by CSA in renal NOS mRNA [101] and in tissue and urinary NO levels in rats [101, 107]. Enalapril and and valsartan restored acetylcholine-dependent relaxation in the renal arteries of CSA-treated spontaneously hypertensive rats [108]. Interestingly, Asberg et al found better long-term microvascular function in CSA-treated renal transplant recipients receiving lisinopril as compared to patients receiving nifedipine [109]. Recently, Chander et al showed that resveratrol, a polyphenolic phytoalexin, protected rats against cyclosporine-induced nephrotoxicity through nitric oxide dependent mechanisms [110]. Clinical trials assessing the effects of L-arginine supplementation in CSA-treated renal or heart transplant patients were mostly negative, without improvement of renal function and/or hemodynamics [111-113], with the exception of Andrés et al who found increases in RPF, GFR and natriuresis after administration of L-arginine to stable renal transplant recipients [114].

Prostaglandins

Eicosanoids (arachidonic acid metabolites) have an important role in the local control of renal blood flow, mainly in the setting of systemic or intra-renal hemodynamic disorders. They are produced by renal resident cells (endothelial, mesangial, tubular and interstitial cells) as well as by infiltrating cells (macrophages, lymphocytes platelets and neutrophils). The cyclooxygenase pathway produces the vasodilators prostaglandins PGI_2 or prostacyclin (that undergoes spontaneous hydrolysis to 6-keto-$PGF_{1\alpha}$) and PGE_2 and the vasoconstrictor thromboxane A_2 (TXA_2) whereas the lipoxygenase pathway produces the vasoconstrictor leukotrienes. CSA-induced imbalance in the vasodilator/vasoconstrictor rate of these metabolites favors vasoconstriction and is implicated in the development of the functional changes seem in acute CSA nephrotoxicity [3, 115]. CSA administration to rodents consistently resulted in increased urinary excretion of TXA_2 metabolites: thromboxane B_2 (TXB_2), 2, 3 dinor-TXB_2 and 11-dehydro-TXB_2, reflecting enhancement of renal and systemic thromboxane production [116-124]. Many authors disclosed that this activation of thromboxane synthesis was paralleled by GFR and RBF decreases and RVR increase [117-119, 121, 122-127].

In fact, a strong and significant negative correlation between GFR decrease and urinary TXB_2 levels was found in rats receiving CSA [122, 124]. Experimental CSA administration increased *ex-vivo* renal production of TXB_2 [111, 112], renal tissue thromboxane levels [125, 127, 128] and production of TXB_2 by isolated glomeruli and peritoneal macrophage [116, 128]. Supporting these experimental findings, clinical studies have also showed CSA-related urinary TXB_2 and 11-dehydro-TXB_2 increases in renal and liver transplant recipients and healthy volunteers [76, 129-131]. The enhancement of thromboxane production by CSA has been related to activated infiltrating platelets and macrophage in renal tissue, increased renal lipid peroxidation and reactive oxygen species production, endothelial injury and systemic platelet activation [76, 116, 124]. Administration of thromboxane synthase inhibitors, thromboxane receptor antagonists, fish or seal oil (both reduce the production of thromboxane) to animals resulted in decrease or normalization of urinary thromboxane metabolites and variable degrees of improvement in renal function and hemodynamics [119, 121-123, 125-128, 132-134]. Contrasting with the animal studies, the clinical use of selective thromboxane synthase inhibitors did not prevent CSA-induced renal dysfunction, even decreasing urinary and blood levels of thromboxane metabolites [129, 135, 136]. In the same way, the use of fish oil in CSA-treated patients resulted in contradictory results, with some authors finding improvement in renal function and decrease in urinary TXB_2, and others no effect at all [130, 137-139]. A role for the 5-lipoxygenase pathway in acute CSA nephrotoxicity has also been suggested by the demonstration that a leukotriene receptor antagonist partially prevented the decrease in GFR and RPF after intravenous CSA administration. The same authors showed that the simultaneous administration of a leukotriene receptor antagonist and a thromboxane receptor antagonist completely abolished CSA-induced changes in renal function [133]. Butterly et al reported a CSA-related increase in urinary excretion of leukotriene metabolites in a rat model of renal transplantation. In this study, the use of a leukotriene receptor antagonist totally prevented the GFR impairment caused by CSA [140]. The precise role of vasodilative prostaglandins in CSA-induced acute nephrotoxicity is elusive. CSA has been shown to increase, decrease or did not change the levels of 6-keto-$PGF_{1\alpha}$ and PGE_2 in urine, blood, renal venous effluent of *ex-vivo* preparations, renal tissue and supernatant of cultured mesangial cells and isolated glomeruli of rodents and humans [63, 99, 117-119, 122, 126-129, 131, 136, 141, 142]. CSA decreased COX-2 expression and PGE_2 production in cultured mouse medullary thick ascending limb cells [143]. Manipulation of vasodilative prostaglandins by prostacyclin analogues or PGE precursors afforded protection against the renal functional abnormalities caused by CSA in animals [144, 145]. However, data derived from clinical studies or human tissue is conflicting. Misoprostol, a synthetic PGE_2 analogue, improved renal function in CSA-treated renal recipients [146] and iloprost, a prostacyclin analogue, prevented CSA-induced glomerular constriction in human isolated glomeruli [147]. In contrast, several authors failed to demonstrate any beneficial effect after the administration of PGE_2 or prostacyclin analogues to patients receiving CSA [148-152].

Sympathetic system

CSA-stimulated activation of the sympathetic system was demonstrated in animals and humans and linked to development of hypertension and systemic and renal hemodynamic abnormalities [153-155]. Some of the mechanisms which have been implicated in this adrenergic stimulation are augmented norepinephrine release from terminal nerves, blockade of neuronal calcineurin, activation of excitatory neural reflexes in the subdiaphragmatic area and elevation of plasma and platelets catecholamines [156-159]. Zhang et al showed that knockout mice lacking synapsin (synaptic vesicle proteins that regulated neurotransmitter release at synapses) were protected against efferent sympathetic nerve activation and blood pressure increase after CSA administration [160]. Adrenergic pharmacological blockade, renal denervation, chemical sympathectomy, administration of glycine (an inhibitory neurotransmitter) and depletion of catecholamine stores by reserpine prevented or significantly reduced CSA-induced hemodynamic changes and hypertension in animal studies [161-165]. However, other authors did not find protection against CSA-induced renal functional impairment after renal denervation in transplanted or native kidneys in animals [166-169] and several clinical studies were unable to correlate the changes in renal and systemic hemodynamics found in CSA-treated patients to increased sympathetic activity [170-174].

Oxidative stress

There is extensive evidence favoring the participation of reactive oxygen species (ROS) in acute CSA nephrotoxicity. Experimental *in vivo* and *in vitro* studies found increased renal tissue content of malondialdehyde, lipid hydroperoxides and conjugated dienes, increased glomerular synthesis of hydrogen peroxide, superoxide anion and malondialdehyde accompanying functional derangements caused by CSA. Cyclosporine also increased production of malondialdehyde by cultured human endothelial cells, formation of malondialdehyde and hydrogen peroxide by renal mitochondria, urinary excretion of free radicals and levels of plasma malondialdehyde [165, 175-182]. Results regarding CSA effect on glutathione renal content showed decreased glutathione levels or increased tissue concentrations of oxidized and reduced glutathione [178, 183]. If we consider the pivotal role of glutathione in cellular protection against free radicals damage, these results can be reconciled. It is possible that the increase in oxidized and reduced glutathione was caused by accelerated glutathione peroxidase activity and adaption of glutathione pathway in order to counterbalance excessive free radicals production and that reduced glutathione levels ultimately indicate an exhaustion of the system. This excessive ROS production might be attributed to renal ischemia, hypoxia-reoxygenation injury or direct cellular membrane injury caused by CSA [165]. CSA-induced ROS generation was related to increased thromboxane production, increased mRNA production for cyclooxygenase I and decreased mRNA production for cyclooxygenase II, up-regulation of Bcl-2 protein expression and increased expression of eNOS mRNA, indicating an important cross-talk between these systems [176, 177, 184, 185]. Inhibition of ROS production by antioxidants such as lazaroid, vitamin E, melatonin, taurine, L-propionyl carnitine, lipoic acid and N-acetylcysteine, by administration of the xanthine oxidase inhibitor allopurinol, by blockade of renal sympathetic system by glycine or renal denervation and by viral delivery of superoxide dismutase genes consistently resulted in renal function improvement in animals models of acute CSA nephrotoxicity [93, 165, 177-182, 184, 186-191]. More recently, it has been demonstrated that several natural-derived anti-oxidants such as plants polyphenol, epigallocatechin gallate, green tea extract, curcumin, garlic extract, provinol (a red wine polyphenol), spirulina, sulphated polysaccharides, black grape extract, lycopene (a carotenoid), quercetin (a flavanoid), and Nigella sativa oil attenuated experimental CSA-induced functional injury [192-203]. Conversely, administration of vitamin E and selenium deficient diet to rats enhanced acute CSA nephrotoxicity [180]. Among the few clinical studies that addressed the role of free radicals in acute CSA nephrotoxicity two found negative results [204, 205]. The remaining tested the effects of garlic ingestion on 50 renal transplant recipients with stable renal function. The use of 1g of garlic by day for two months induced small but significant decreases in blood pressure, serum creatinine and malondialdehyde [206].

Other mediators

Other mediators have been related to CSA-induced functional nephrotoxicity. Increased plasma level of adenosine was observed in CSA-treated renal transplant recipients [207, 208]. In the same way, rats receiving CSA showed increased concentration of adenosine in renal artery paralleled by a decrease in mRNA expression for A_1 and A_{2a} renal adenosine receptors [209]. Experimental use of selective A_1 adenosine receptors antagonists or theophylline provided contradictory results with some authors finding renal hemodynamic protection whereas other did not [39, 210-213]. Moderate increases in plasma vasopressin were observed in CSA-treated renal transplant recipients [214] and CSA enhanced vasopressin-induced rise in intracellular calcium in cultured glomerular mesangial cells, human coronary myocytes and vascular smooth muscle cells [215-217]. In addition, incubation of vascular smooth muscle cells with CSA increased the expression of AVP receptors and vasopressin V1A receptor mRNA [217, 218]. Use of platelet activating factor (PAF) antagonists improved CSA-induced changes in GFR, RBF and glomerular hemodynamics as well as CSA toxicity in cultured tubular LLC-PKI cells [219-222]. Cyclosporine impaired atrial natriuretic factor-induced glomerular guanylyl cyclase activation in rats. Indeed, experimental or clinical administration of atrial natriuretic factor (ANF), use of neutral endopeptidase (ANF degrading enzyme) inhibitors or simultaneous utilization of both maneuvers prevented the adverse effects of CSA on renal function and hemodynamics, smooth muscle cells, cultured proximal renal tubular epithelial cells and blood vessels [223-228]. Reduced kallikrein urinary excretion was found in CSA-treated patients [229-231]. Studies in rats showed that 3 days of CSA administration decreased cortical mRNA expression for kallikrein and bradykinin 2 receptors [232] whereas CSA administration for 28 days increased renal tissue kallikrein mRNA and kallikrein content, increased urinary excretion of kallikrein, increased hepatic expression of kininogen mRNA and increased renal bradykinin B_2 receptor mRNA, suggesting an enhancement in the activity of the kallikrein-kinin system trying to compensate for CSA nephrotoxicity [233]. A potential role for cholesterol, a known vasoconstrictor substance, in CSA-acute nephrotoxicity is suggested by the finding of renal dysfunction aggravation in hereditary hypertriglyceridemic rats receiving CSA or when dietary cholesterol supplementation was provided to CSA-treated rats [234, 235]. CSA-induced hypomagnesemia has been proposed as a possible factor in the pathogenesis of the functional changes induced by the drug. Effects of human magnesium dietary supplementation on CSA nephrotoxicity are conflicting, with lack of functional protection in normotensive rats on low salt diet versus improvement of renal function in SHR rats on high sodium diet [236, 237]. Extracellular fluid volume depletion due to increased vascular permeability and loss of renal auto-regulatory capacity have also been linked to acute CSA nephrotoxicity [238-240]. Systemic administration of insulin-like growth factor-I, human recombinant human relaxin and methoxyethyl-modified intercellular adhesion molecule-1 antisense phosphorothiateoligonucleotides ameliorated acute CSA nephrotoxicity in rats [241-243].

Action on mesangial cells

CSA have an intrinsic capacity to stimulate direct contraction of animal and human mesangial cells, smooth vascular cells and resistance vessels with obvious consequence for renal function and hemodynamics. These effects are associated to augmented intracellular influx of calcium, impaired relaxation response of vascular wall to vasodilatory stimuli and endothelin-1 [16, 20, 91, 223, 244-249]. CSA-induced cultured mesangial cell contraction was prevented by mycophenolic acid [250].

Cremophor

Cyclosporine is a very lipophilic and hydrophobic compound, making mandatory the use of lipid vehicles in order to obtain stable preparations for experimental or clinical use. The commercial intravenous formulation of CSA uses as vehicle Cremophor-EL, a polyethylated castor oil, which possess important hemodynamics effects already demonstrated in animals and humans [251-253]. This intravenous formulation has been incriminated in episodes of AKI in transplant recipients and patients with autoimmune diseases and caused abrupt GFR decrease after a single dose in healthy volunteers [254-257]. Substitution of Cremophor by a soybean lipid used for parenteral nutrition in an experimental model of CSA-induced AKI resulted in preservation of GFR with maintenance of CSA immunosuppressive activity measured by decrease in interleukin 2 production and inhibition of lymphocyte activation. This favorable profile was related to increased CSA clearance and lower trough level but similar tissue amount of CSA [258]. In a similar way, Aliabadi et al demonstrated that the IV administration of CSA polymeric micellar formulation to rats prevented CSA/Cremophor-induced decrease in creatinine clearance. However, differently from the previous study, this micellar formulation reduced CSA kidney uptake and increased CSA blood levels [259].

Mechanisms of tubular injury

The seminal study by English et al clearly showed that major proximal tubular functions were preserved in acute CSA nephrotoxicity [15] and in fact, documented ATN is rarely seen in CSA-treated patients. On the other hand, experimental and clinical studies provided evidences of subtile CSA-induced tubular cell injury such as increased urinary excretion of tubular enzymes, increased fractional excretion of magnesium in the presence of hypomagnesemia, impaired urinary concentrating ability and hyperkalemia consequent to impaired tubular excretion of potassium [236, 260, 261]. Experiments using cultured LLC-PK1 and MDCK renal tubular cell lines showed direct, dose-dependent, CSA-induced cell toxicity [262]. This cytotoxicity is manifested in tubular cells as reduction of cell proliferation, interference with membrane transporters activity (such as Na-K-ATPase, Na-K-2Cl and Ca^{2+} pump), impairment of membrane tonicity-enhancer binding protein, tubular cell apoptosis and necrosis, increased LDH release, DNA damage, cell cycle arrest and decreased cell viability [236-270]. CSA cytotoxicity was related to lipid peroxidation, increase in p53b protein expression, increase in intracellular calcium and reduction in NO production [265, 267, 271-273]. More indirect evidence for CSA-induced tubular cell damage is the induction of heat shock proteins in renal tubular cells after CSA addition to cultured cells or CSA administration to rats [274, 275] and CSA-induced inhibition of potassium channels in cortical collecting tubules cells of rabbits [276]. Using fresh isolated proximal tubules from rats, da Costa et al showed that only very high concentrations of CSA caused direct tubular injury, which was prevented by low calcium or high magnesium concentrations in the medium [277].

Clinical aspects of acute CSA nephrotoxicity

There are four potential clinical presentations for acute CSA nephrotoxicity: asymptomatic increases in serum creatinine (SCr) without overt renal dysfunction, acute kidney injury, delayed graft function after renal transplantation and recurrent or *de novo* hemolytic uremic syndrome (Table 2).

Table 2. Clinical presentations of acute cyclosporine A nephrotoxicity.

Asymptomatic increases in serum creatinine
Acute renal failure
Delayed recovery of renal graft function
Hemolytic-uremic syndrome

The most frequent presentation of acute CSA nephrotoxicity is a dose-related, clinically asymptomatic increase in SCr, which can occur even when drug whole blood trough levels are in the so-called "therapeutic range" [3, 278]. This situation may be difficult to distinguish from kidney rejection in renal transplant recipients or from primary renal disease progression in patients with glomerulonephritis treated with the drug. Moreover, CSA nephrotoxicity and allograft rejection or worsening of primary renal disease can co-exist. Otherwise, in extra-renal organ transplantation and non-renal autoimmune disease patients, these SCr elevations are very likely caused by acute CSA nephrotoxicity. Actually, this form of renal impairment is relatively frequent after cardiac, hepatic and pulmonary transplantation [279-281]. The renal histology of these patients is usually normal or shows non-specific changes like vacuolization or presence of giant mitochondria in tubular cells [18, 282, 283]. The defining parameter for diagnosis will be improvement in SCr in about one week after dosage manipulation or drug discontinuation [3]. There are clinical studies which found that even CSA-treated patients who are apparently doing well in terms of renal function suffer a significant renal hemodynamic impact from this immunosuppressive drug. Curtis el al showed that CSA withdrawal for economic reasons in renal transplant recipients with stable and normal SCr was followed by a 30% increase in renal blood flow with a parallel drop in renal vascular resistance and blood pressure [284]. A particularly important aspect of this paper was that this improvement in renal function occurred after a long period of CSA treatment. More recently, Hilbrands et al studied patients without clinical evidence of acute nephrotoxicity who discontinued CSA at 3 months after renal transplantation. One week after the withdrawal there was a significant increase in GFR and decrease in SCr [285]. A single daily dose of CSA in stable renal transplant patients chronically treated with CSA caused a significant and transitory decrease in GFR [62], which was prevented by the use of a calcium channel blocker [286]. Various studies showed enhancement in renal function when transplant patients on "classic" dosages of CSA had their immunosuppressive regimes changed to low dosage CSA plus mofetil mycophenolate (MMF) or when CSA was withdrawn and replaced by other immunosuppressive drugs. It is very likely that the price to be paid for effective immunosuppression with full doses of CSA is some degree of renal hemodynamic impairment [287].

Clinically important acute kidney injury (AKI) associated with CSA can occur in a significant number (ranging from 10 to more than 50%) of patients in the post-operative period of heart, liver and bone marrow transplantation [255, 278-280, 288-292]. AKI in these patients is generally multifactorial and seldom related exclusively to CSA. More than 40% of heart transplant recipients are re-hospitalized in the first year post-transplantation and roughly 30% of them require intensive care unit admission. Moreover, cardiac transplant patients may have impaired pre-transplant renal function due to chronic heart failure, suffer the insult of cardiopulmonary bypass during surgery, require CSA doses 30% higher than the doses used for other solid organs transplantation and may have activated renin-angiotensin-aldosterone system due to chronic renal ischemia [280, 293-295]. Liver transplant recipients usually don't have previous renal impairment, but liver transplantation is major surgery, which induces significant cytokine activation, and not infrequently is associated to intravascular volume depletion, hypotension and coagulopathy. Additionally, the early liver transplant post-operative period, when usually CSA administration is initiated, may be complicated by sepsis, liver graft dysfunction, use of other nephrotoxic drugs and multi-organ failure syndrome [278, 279]. In the same way, the early period after bone marrow transplantation might be affected by graft-versus-host-disease, veno-occlusive liver disease, infection, hemodynamic instability, volume depletion and use of nephrotoxic antibiotics, [289, 296-298]. When AKI occurs in these situations, CSA withdrawal or substitution should always be considered [299]. The development of AKI in CSA-treated patients is also likely to occur when this immunosuppressive agent is administered in combination with other nephrotoxic drugs such as aminoglycoside, amphotericin B, foscarnet or iodinated contrast media or with drugs with important action on intrarenal vascular tonus regulation, like non steroidal anti-inflammatory drugs or angiotensin converting enzyme inhibitors [300-309]. In rare occasions, CSA can induce acute kidney injury in patients with autoimmune diseases [254, 310] or extremely high CSA dosages can cause acute tubular necrosis [311, 312].

Delayed graft function recovery (DGFR) after renal transplant was seen more often in the past, when elevated doses of cyclosporine were used, principally with the concomitant occurrence of prolonged ischemic times. This event has been modified by the delay of CSA administration until adequate renal graft function is present or by the use of alternative schedules with induction immunosuppression that spare calcineurin blockers [2, 3]. In fact, anti-lymphocyte antibodies were used in kidney transplant patients with high risk for acute tubular necrosis with encouraging results [313]. Withdrawal of CSA in renal transplant patients with delayed graft function has been associated with less severe and shorter renal dysfunction [314]. Patients with DGFR on a CSA-sparing regimen had faster renal function recovery, less occult rejections throughout the anuria period, earlier hospital discharge and significantly lower treatment costs than patients on a CSA-based regimen [315].

CSA can rarely cause fulminant AKI due to an immune-mediated phenomenon involving the ADAMTS13 metalloprotease or due to direct endothelial cell injury, clinically manifested as an entity similar to the hemolytic-uremic syndrome (HUS) [316]. This serious problem occurs more frequently in bone marrow transplantation (BMT) but has also been reported in kidney transplantation, where it may be very difficult to distinguish from acute vascular rejection, and in other solid organs transplant. CSA-related HUS is usually considered as associated with renal allograft poor prognosis, but recent publications disclosed a more benign scenario [317]. The clinical presentation of CSA-related HUS can be fulminant with severe anemia, low platelet count, increased numbers of schistocytes and increased serum levels of lactic dehydrogenase or be more subtle, with inconsistent laboratory findings. In the same way, renal biopsy may show the typical findings of thrombotic microangiopathy, eventually associated to afferent arteriolar thrombosis, or be misleading in the early phases of the disease [3, 287, 318-322]. CSA should be halted and replaced by alternative immunosuppressive drugs in these cases. However, it is important to stress that HUS has also been described with both tacrolimus and sirolimus use. Plasmapheresis and intravenous immunoglobulin has been employed with some success for rescue of these patients [323, 324]. A case-control study found that early therapy with isradipine, aspirin and pentoxifylline resulted in increased transplant survival as compared to previous reports [318].

Management of acute CSA nephrotoxicity

Regular monitoring of CSA blood levels in order to keep drug concentration within its narrow therapeutic window would be in theory a rational way to prevent CSA nephrotoxicity [238, 278, 290]. Nevertheless, the clinical reality is quite different, since many patients develop renal toxicity with CSA trough blood levels in the "therapeutic" range [238, 325, 326]. In reality, area under the curve (AUC) but not trough levels represents real exposure and may predict CSA efficacy and nephrotoxicity. Lower AUC is associated with acute rejection and higher AUC with acute nephrotoxicity. Unfortunately, the correlation between CSA trough levels and AUC is very poor, even with the new microemulsion formulation [327, 328]. Furthermore, a prospective study, which tried to adjust CSA daily intake by optimized AUC, found that was very difficult to control CSA exposure by examining AUC and modifying CSA dose in accord [327]. Administration of CSA once a day, instead half dose twice a day, was associated with less acute nephrotoxicity in heart transplant recipients [329]. Since hepatic metabolism and biliary excretion are the major route for elimination of CSA and its metabolites, downstream adjustments in CSA dosage are required in patients with liver disease in order to avoid episodes of acute nephrotoxicity [3, 287].

Special attention is needed when new medications are prescribed to CSA-treated patients. CSA is extensively metabolized by the cytochrome P450 liver microsomal enzyme system [2, 3], and consequently drugs that interfere with this pathway can cause important changes in CSA blood levels (Table 3). Compounds inhibiting P450 enzymes, such as ketoconazole, erythromycin, verapamil, and diltiazem increase concentration of parent CSA and may cause acute nephrotoxicity. On the other hand, drugs that increase P450 enzyme activity, such as phenobarbital, carbamazepine and rifampicin, can lower CSA blood levels and impair immunosuppression [287]. As mentioned before, potentially nephrotoxic drugs ((aminoglycosides, amphotericin B, foscarnet, vancomycin, , contrast media, NSAID, anesthetics, etc) or drugs that induce efferent arteriole vasodilatation (angiotensin converting enzyme inhibitors and angiotensin II AT_1 receptors antagonists) should be used with extreme discretion in CSA-treated patients, since they can act synergistically with CSA-induced preglomerular vasoconstriction to promote renal injury.

Table 3. Some drugs that change CSA blood concentration.

INCREASE LEVEL	DECREASE LEVEL
Verapamil	Rifampicin
Diltiazem	Isoniazid
Nicardipine	Phenytoin
Amlodipine	Carbamazepine
Erythromycin	Barbiturates
Clarithromycin	Octreotide
Ketoconazole	Ticlopidine
Fluconazole	Orlistat
Itraconazole	Nafcillin
Lansoprazole	St. John's Wort
Rabeprazole	
Cimetidine	
Methylprednisolone	
Allopurinol	
Bromocriptine	
Metoclopramide	
Colchicine	
Amiodarone	
Danazole	
Grapefruit juice	

The ability of calcium cannel antagonists to induce afferent arteriole vasodilation makes this class of drugs a potential pharmacological antidote against acute CSA vascular effects [278]. In fact, several studies showed improvement in renal hemodynamics and/or function when different calcium antagonists like verapamil, diltiazem, nifedipine, lacidipine, isradipine and amlodipine were given for CSA-treated patients [46, 286, 330-336]. Some studies also suggest that perioperative administration of calcium antagonists to donors or recipients may prevent or diminish the time and intensity of delayed graft function and improve long-term kidney outcome [238, 337, 338]. The use of lacidipine in a two-year randomized placebo-controlled study was associated to better late renal allograft function, independent of blood pressure reduction [339]. A further potential advantage of adding these drugs to CSA therapy is an adjunctive immunosuppressive effect, since calcium antagonists may have some intrinsic immunomodulatory activity [340, 341].

The antiinflammatory, antithrombotic, hypolipidemic, vasodilatory and immunomodulatory properties of fish oil (omega-3 fatty acids) make then an attractive potential treatment for CSA nephrotoxicity [115, 342]. Omega-3 fatty acids decrease the formation of prostaglandin E_2 metabolites, inhibit the production of thromboxane A_2, reduce production of biologically active leukotrienes and enhance prostacyclin release. In result, they inhibit platelet aggregation, promote vasodilation, low blood pressure and are antiatherogenic [342]. Daily dietary supplementation of 6 to 18 g of fish oil to CSA-treated patients has been performed in different clinical trials with inconsistent results. . Psoriatic patients receiving CSA plus 6 g of fish oil/day for 3 months did not change their RBF and RVR and had less GFR impairment than the control group, which received only CSA [343]. In a series of placebo-controlled, randomized, prospective studies, Homan van der Heide et al showed that supplementation of 6g of fish oil to CSA-treated renal transplant recipients increased GFR, improved RPF, and decreased blood pressure and RVR. Fish oil also influenced favorably the recovery of renal function after early acute rejection and, at one year pos-transplant, was associated with higher GFR, lower blood pressure, fewer rejection episodes and a non statistically significant trend to better graft survival [139, 344, 345]. In contrast, other three placebo-controlled, randomized, double-blind, prospective studies did not find any renal function improvement after omega-3 fatty acid supplementation in CSA-treated renal transplant recipients [346-348]. Liver transplant recipients using CSA and supplemented with 12g of fish oil for two months significantly improved renal hemodynamics and had a marginally statistically significant increase in GFR, whereas corn-oil treated controls did not change any of these parameters [130]. Finally, a study in hypertensive heart transplant patients showed that one year of omega-3 fatty acids supplementation resulted in stable blood pressure, systemic vascular resistance, and GFR, in opposite to the findings of the placebo group, where a significant increase in blood pressure and systemic vascular resistance and a significant decrease in GFR were observed [349].

There are some other pharmacological interventions for treatment of acute CSA nephrotoxicity already tried clinically with positive results. Atrial natriuretic factor has opposite effects on renal hemodynamics as compared to CSA. Candoxatrilat inhibits neutral endopeptidase, an enzyme found most abundantly in the kidney, which degrades atrial natriuretic factor. Intravenous infusion of candoxatrilat in stable renal transplant recipients increased significantly GFR, RBF, diuresis, fractional excretion of sodium, plasma atrial natriuretic factor and decreased RVR [227]. Dehydropeptidase-I is a glutathione-processing enzyme, found on both the brush border and the basolateral membranes of proximal tubular cells. Administration of cilastatin, an inhibitor of dehydropeptidase, prevented elevations of serum creatinine in the early post-operative phase of CSA-treated heart transplant patients, decreased the frequency of AKI after allogeneic bone marrow transplantation (BMT) and reduced serum creatinine levels in the first 2 weeks after kidney transplantation [350-353]. A recent systematic review reported that cilastatin significantly reduced serum creatinine and odds ratio for AKI in CSA-treated patients [354]. The mechanisms of cilastatin prevention of CSA acute nephrotoxicity are still unclear, but might be related to preservation of tubular cell membrane fluidity and inhibition of CSA transport across membranes, causing lower intracellular accumulation of the drug [355]. Activation of the endothelin (ET) system has been consistently correlated to the adverse renal vascular effects of CSA. Administration of bosentan, an ET_A and ET_B receptor antagonist, blunted CSA-induced fall in RPF but not GFR decrease in healthy human volunteers [73].

CSA has more than 700 analogues, but few have immunosuppressive capacity. The finding of an analogue with similar immunosuppressive effect but with lesser nephrotoxicity than CSA has been an obvious target for the pharmaceutical industry. Cyclosporine G (CSG), a natural occurring analogue of CSA with potent immunosuppressive activity, disclosed significantly less acute and chronic nephrotoxicity when administered to rats [356]. Clinical phase II and III studies in renal transplant and patients with uveitis showed comparable efficacy and less functional nephrotoxicity when CSG was compared to CSA [357, 358]. However, the short-term differences between CSA and CSG in renal function were not dramatic which hampered the introduction of this drug to the market. Likewise, SDZ IMM 125, a derivative of cyclosporine, showed substantial immunosuppressive activity and less renal toxicity than CSA in animal studies. The limited clinical information about this drug did not demonstrate significant differences in renal effects but more hepatotoxicity when it was compared to CSA [359, 360].

CSA standard oral formulation in olive oil has an erratic and unpredictable gastrointestinal absorption, causing marked inter- and intra-patient variability. To overcome this problem a microemulsion pre-concentrate was developed. When used in healthy volunteers and transplant recipients this new galenic formulation had faster time to peak concentration, reached higher peak concentration, greater AUC and was not affected by the physiological state of the gastrointestinal tract [3, 361, 362]. Undoubtedly, the microemulsion formulation provides a more regular and reliable pharmacokinetic profile and improves bioavailability, allowing reduction in the daily dosage of CSA [7, 363-365]. The new microemulsion formula was also used as an alternative for the intravenous CSA formulation in the induction of immunosuppression in liver transplantation, resulting in a not statistically significant reduction in nephrotoxicity episodes from 45 to 25% [366]. The microemulsion formulation showed similar immunosuppressive efficacy when compared to the standard presentation, although some studies have suggested a reduction in the rate of acute rejection with the new formula [7, 364, 366-368]. However, the high peak levels reached by the microemulsion administration might be associated with an increase in acute nephrotoxicity [369]. Like the standard formulation, the microemulsion reduced GFR and RBF after a single daily dose in healthy subjects [204] or in animal models of CSA nephrotoxicity [370]. The nadir of RBF impairment occurs 5 hours after drug ingestion [73]. Conversion from the standard formula to microemulsion apparently did not cause long-term nephrotoxicity when dosages were adjusted for the same blood level, but some studies showed transitory impairment of renal function in the early phase of microemulsion treatment [363, 365, 367]. When standard to microemulsion switch was done in a 1:0.8 ratio instead of a 1:1 ratio there was an alleviation of this short-term nephrotoxicity, indicating that conversion should be done in an individualized manner [371].

A simple way to prevent or reverse functional CSA nephrotoxicity is to reduce its dosage or to halt the drug. The rationale for this maneuver is that the most noteworthy benefit of CSA use in transplantation is a remarkable decrease in early acute rejection, and thus the drug might be decreased or even withdrawn after the initial immunosuppression phase [278, 372]. However, this approach is controversial, particularly in the field of transplantation, where inadequate immunosuppression could result in morbidity and mortality. [373-376]. Reduced doses of CSA at one year post-transplant have been associated with major risk of acute and chronic rejection, whereas higher CSA doses correlated with better long-term graft survival in some studies [377, 378]. Accordingly, many authors found high rates of acute rejection when cyclosporine was electively discontinued in stable renal transplant recipients [379-381], or development of rejection in heart or liver transplant patients who had CSA withdrawn due to impaired renal function [382, 383]. On the other hand, several studies, including a large meta-analysis by Kasiske et al [372], reported that CSA withdrawal, 3 to 12 months after renal transplantation, did not result in worst graft or patient survival, independent of increased rate of acute rejection, as compared to controls that continued on CSA therapy [374, 384, 385]. Some authors found better long-term renal function in the groups where CSA was withdrawn [384, 386, 387]. Recently, two studies reported the results of an extended follow-up of 15 years after CSA withdrawal in renal transplantation. In the first one, Bakker et al randomly assigned the patients, three months after transplant, to continue on CSA or to be converted to azathioprine treatment. Patients on the azathioprine arm had better graft survival, higher GFR and less incidence of chronic allograft nephropathy [388]. In the second study, Gallagher et al randomized patients in three groups: azathioprine, long term CSA and short term CSA followed by azathioprine. Patients treated with short term CSA followed by azathioprine presented better graft survival and function, whereas long term CSA treatment reduced long term graft survival [389]. So, the available data suggests that long-term CSA treatment is not obligatory in a significant number of renal transplant patients, and that CSA withdrawal is potentially a useful maneuver to control functional nephrotoxicity in selected sub-groups.

The advent of the new potent immunosuppressors mofetil mycophenolate (MMF) and sirolimus made the replacement of CSA or its decrease in immunosuppressive protocols more feasible [390].

MMF is a non-competitive, reversible, inhibitor of inosine monophosphate dehydrogenase, which inhibits lymphocyte proliferation. The use of MMF allowed concomitant CSA dose reduction or withdrawal, with significant improvement in renal function and hemodynamics in renal, liver and heart transplant recipients with stable or impaired renal function [391-400]. David-Neto et al analyzed a group of children with renal transplants and with biopsy-confirmed chronic transplant nephropathy in whom CSA dose was reduced or withdrawn and azathioprine switched to MMF. Six months after the introduction of MMF serum creatinine decreased and no acute rejection occurred [401]. In another group of children with nephrotic syndrome, CSA treatment had to be discontinued and switched to MMF due to significant GFR decrease. Interruption of CSA lead to rapid GFR increase, whereas MMF maintained nephrotic syndrome remission [402]. Gregoor et al randomized 64 stable renal transplant recipients for conversion of CSA to azathioprine or MMF. Both groups had a significant decrease in serum creatinine, but the azathioprine group presented significantly more acute rejections than the MMF group [403]. MMF use may be extremely useful in patients receiving grafts from marginal donors, such as advanced age donors, since these kidneys are more vulnerable to acute CSA nephrotoxicity [394, 404]. MMF has also shown to be a safe and effective therapeutic option when CSA has to be discontinued due to CSA-associated HUS [405]. Stepwise replacement of CSA by MMF induced a dose-related decrease in von Willebrand Factor and sP-selectin in renal transplant recipients, indicating that the endothelial dysfunction is reversible [78]. Although the vast majority of the studies analyzing MMF as a sparing regime for CSA showed positive outcomes, there have also been some unfavorable results. A switch from cyclosporine A to MMF in eight patients with severe psoriasis resulted in renal function improvement in 90% of then, but all subjects had disease re-activation [406]. In a multicenter French study, 20 cadaveric kidney recipients had CSA gradually discontinued and azathioprine switched to MMF. All patients had a baseline renal biopsy in the previous 12 months. Worsening of the histological injury was observed in 50% of the patients after a mean follow-up of 9 months after MMF conversion and 5.4 months after CSA withdrawal. These patients did not change their serum creatinine or GFR, in contrast with the nine patients without structural deterioration, who had a significant improvement in renal function. Although the histological worsening might already be present when patients switched to MMF and started CSA withdrawal (some of the baseline biopsies were done up to 6 months before study initiation) the trial was discontinued [407]. In a recent study, stable renal transplant recipients were randomized to either CSA and MMF or MMF and CSA-free regimen. After five years of follow-up, the CSA-free group presented higher creatinine clearance but had more acute rejection episodes and more graft loss due to chronic rejection [408].

Sirolimus (rapamycin) is a macrolide compound related to erythromycin and tacrolimus. It binds to the same immunophilin as tacrolimus, but it does not inhibit calcineurin. Sirolimus blocks T-cell activation at a late stage, interfering with the signal from IL2 receptors and receptors for other cytokines and growth factors, and so blocking the cytokine or growth factor-induced activation of the proliferation cell cycle response [409]. This powerful immunosuppressive drug has demonstrated excellent efficacy in the prevention of acute rejection and did not caused renal hemodynamic impairment in animal or clinical studies [12, 410-412]. However, when used together CSA, sirolimus may intensify CSA-induced functional nephrotoxicity [413-415], probably due to pharmacokinetic interaction between the two drugs, increasing CSA concentrations in whole blood and renal tissue [416]. These results, and the already known synergistic immunosuppressive interaction between CSA and sirolimus, indicate that if the two drugs are used simultaneously, CSA dosages should be reduced [327, 415, 417]. Conversion from cyclosporine to sirolimus in renal, heart and liver transplant patients with chronic or acute CSA nephrotoxicity resulted in significant renal function improvement [327, 418-422]. Early CSA withdrawal in kidney recipients receiving sirolimus was followed by renal function improvement [423].

Chronic nephrotoxicity

Chronic CSA-induced nephropathy is best defined as "a clinicopathologic entity produced by exposure of the patient to cyclosporine, characterized by tubulointerstitial fibrosis in a striped pattern beginning in the medulla and progressing to the medullary rays of the cortex. Usually, but not inevitably, this pathologic finding is associated with some degree of renal dysfunction" [424]. Unfortunately, several authors use inadequately the term "chronic CSA nephrotoxicity" when describing renal functional changes without histological evaluation after variable times of CSA administration to humans or animals. This expression must be reserved for the description of CSA-induced nephrotoxicity associated with irreversible interstitial fibrosis. This injury has been classically coupled to degenerative hyaline changes in the afferent arteriole walls, consisting of endothelial swelling, nodular hyaline protein deposition and areas of smooth muscle cell lesions and necrosis [18, 425]. In kidney transplant recipients, this arteriolar hyaline thickening is considered the key for the discrimination between chronic CSA nephropathy from rejection [282, 425]. Clinical and experimental studies have shown that this arteriopathy, which was considered irreversible, can remit after CSA discontinuation, in distinction to the tubulointerstitial fibrosis, which is irreversible [18, 425-428]. CSA-induced chronic nephrotoxicity has been described in renal and non-renal transplant recipients and in patients with autoimmune diseases receiving the drug for periods of 6 months or more [429, 430].

The lack of a suitable animal model hampered the study of the mechanisms leading to chronic CSA nephrotoxicity for some years after CSA introduction. Using the observation that sodium depletion exacerbates CSA nephrotoxicity [431, 432], Rosen et al. and Elzinga et al. developed a reproducible animal model of chronic CSA nephrotoxicity [433, 434]. In this model, CSA administration to rats on low salt diet produced a profound decrease in GFR and histological changes similar to those described in patients with chronic CSA nephrotoxicity [433-435]. When the drug was discontinued, GFR improved, returning to baseline values, but the tubulointerstitial injury was progressive, even in the absence of CSA [433].

Mechanism of injury

CSA effects on afferent arterioles led to the hypothesis that afferent arteriolopathy would ultimately result in downstream renal tissue ischemia with consequent fibrosis, nephron dropout and tubular atrophy in the affected areas [425, 436, 437]. In fact, experimental renal ischemia induced by unilateral clamping of renal artery for 28 days can induce significant chronic interstitial fibrosis [438]. On the other hand, several experimental studies found dissociation between the mechanisms promoting the interstitial scarring and the hemodynamics changes in CSA nephropathy [433, 439]. Felodipine prevented functional changes but did not avoid interstitial damage induced by CSA [440]. Increased collagen mRNA was demonstrated in a murine model of CSA nephrotoxicity, while SCr was still normal [441]. Endothelin receptor blockade normalized renal hemodynamics but had no effect on structural injury in the low salt model of chronic CSA nephrotoxicity [442, 443]. Conversely, pharmacological RAS blockade strikingly reduced the progression of CSA-induced tubulointerstitial fibrosis despite failure to normalize GFR [444]. Vieira Jr et al reported that salt-depleted rats receiving low and clinically relevant dosages of CSA (5 mg/kg) for 8 weeks developed significant interstitial fibrosis without any decrease in RBF or afferent arteriole structural injury, clearly demonstrating that the interstitial injury can occur independently from pre-glomerular vasoconstriction [445].

Angiotensin II plays a major role in CSA-induced chronic nephrotoxicity. As already pointed, there are several lines of evidence showing intra-renal RAS activation by CSA [36, 446]. Salt depletion used in the chronic CSA nephrotoxicity model enhances systemic and intra-renal RAS, and consequently angiotensin II generation [447, 448]. Angiotensin II can act as a potent growth factor inducing fibroblast activation, extracellular matrix deposition and tissue scarring [449-451]. Chronic infusion of angiotensin II in rats induced tubulointerstitial injury similar to that following CSA chronic nephropathy [452]. A high concentration of angiotensin II AT_1 receptors is present in the inner zone of the outer medulla, particularly in longitudinal bands paralleling the vasa recta bundles, which is the most affected area in CSA damage [453, 454]. Likewise, renal outer medulla type 1 interstitial cells have a high density of angiotensin II receptors. These interstitial cells have extensive cytoplasmic processes, which are intimally related to the vasa recta basement membrane [455]. When taken together this evidence strongly suggests that the regional regulation of medullary blood flow is mediated by angiotensin II. Therefore, it is possible that CSA-induced activation of intra-renal RAS promotes an interstitial ischemia via vasa recta constriction.

Attenuation of chronic CSA-induced nephrotoxicity independently of hemodynamic changes has been consistently shown with RAS blockade. Lafayette et al compared the effects of enalapril and the combination of minoxidil/ hydrochlorothiazide/reserpine in rats on normal salt diet treated with CSA for 12 months. Enalapril and the three drugs combination reduced blood pressure similarly, but whereas the ACE inhibitor reduced interstitial fibrosis, the combination therapy worsened it [456]. In a different model of CSA nephrotoxicity, using spontaneously hypertensive rats on high salt diet, enalapril and valsartan co-treatment prevented CSA-induced renal dysfunction and interstitial fibrosis [457]. In an interesting study, Johnson et al showed that enalaprilat, the active metabolite of enalapril, completely reversed the stimulatory effect of CSA on collagen synthesis by cultured renal cortical fibroblasts, stressing that RAS blockade can prevent CSA chronic nephrotoxicity independently of hemodynamic or systemic angiotensin II effects [458]. RAS blockade by enalapril and/or an AT_1 angiotensin II receptor antagonist (losartan) in salt-depleted CSA-treated rats reduced blood pressure, promoted afferent arteriole vasodilation and significantly attenuated interstitial fibrosis development without improving renal hemodynamics. Losartan and losartan plus enalapril, but not enalapril alone decreased renal cortical α1 (I) procollagen mRNA. Treatment with hydralazine plus furosemide reduced blood pressure in the same extent as enalapril and/or losartan but did not prevent tubulointerstitial injury [444]. Losartan protection in the chronic CSA nephrotoxicity model has been related to prevention of changes in epidermal and vascular endothelial growth factor and TGF-β1 inducible gene-h3 expression [459-461]. The coadministration of losartan with MMF or pravastatin was synergic to protect against the effects of CSA in the chronic nephrotoxicity model [462, 463]. Other AT_1 angiotensin II receptor antagonists, such as irbesartan and telmisartan, also attenuated the renal structural injury seem in animal models of chronic CSA nephrotoxicity [464, 465]. In an elegant series of consecutive papers, Bobadilla et al disclosed an important role for aldosterone in the development of chronic CSA nephrotoxicity [466]. Spironolactone administration reduced arteriolopathy and interstitial fibrosis, prevented renal functional impairment and up-regulation of TGF-β, collagen I and fibronectin mRNA expression in the salt-depleted rat model of chronic CSA nephrotoxicity [467]. This protection was related to reduction of ET_B endothelin receptors and to prevention of up-regulation of pro-renin [40]. Finally, spironolactone reduced the progression of renal dysfunction and tubulointerstitial fibrosis even in pre-existing chronic CSA nephrotoxicity. This protection was associated with TGF- β, procaspase-3 and KIM-1 mRNA level reduction [468].

CSA stimulates renal and systemic production of TGF-β [445, 469-473]. The potential sources for renal TGF-β include interstitial macrophages and fibroblasts and tubular epithelial cells. Using a double immunolabeling technique, Pichler et al suggested that the majority cells expressing TGF-β in CSA-treated rats were fibroblasts [471]. TGF-β plays a major role in the generation of renal fibrosis by directly stimulating the production of extracellular matrix components and reducing collagenase production, ultimately leading to renal scarring [474]. Recent data also suggest that CSA-induced increase in osteopontin, a glycoprotein involved in the genesis of chronic CSA nephrotoxicity, might be mediated by TGF-β. In fact, mice injected with recombinant TGF-β presented a significant increase in osteopontin mRNA and anti-TGF-β antibody injection inhibited osteopontin mRNA expression in CSA-treated mice [475]. Animal and clinical studies data indicate that TGF-β over expression is an important factor in the development of chronic CSA nephrotoxicity. Indeed, CSA induced a progressive increase in mRNA TGF-beta 1 expression preceding the later development of tubulointerstitial fibrosis in the salt-depleted rat model [476]. Vieira Jr et al, showed an early and progressive TGF-β immunostaining in renal tissue of CSA-treated rats on low salt diet, which was more prominent at the juxtaglomerular arterioles [445]. It has also been shown that CSA administration increased c-fos, c-jun and TGF-β renal mRNA expression before the development of fibrosis [477]. Calcineurin alpha-isoform is apparently the key component for modulation of TGF-β and fibrosis. Mice lacking this isoform developed histological lesions resembling calcineurin inhibitors-induced chronic nephrotoxicity and showed increased renal expression of TGF-β. These data open the possibility that targeted inhibition of calcineurin beta-isoform may be immunosuppressive without nephrotoxicity [478]. Cuhaci et al found that 72% of the renal biopsies from CSA-treated transplant patients with chronic allograft fibrosis expressed high levels of TGF-β. These patients had a rate of renal function decline approximately 3 times higher than patients with minimal or no TGF-β renal expression [479]. In heart transplant recipients, the presence of TGF-β 1 codon 10-gene polymorphism was associated to a higher prevalence of renal dysfunction seven years after transplantation [480]. There is a well-defined link between RAS and TGF- β, traduced by angiotensin II-induced stimulation of TGF-β expression in the kidney [481]. In fact, renal mRNA TGF-β expression was enhanced only in salt depleted rats in contrast to normal salt diet rats treated with CSA [482]. Enalaprilat prevented the CSA-induced TGF-β secretion by cultured human proximal tubular cells and losartan and enalapril decreased mRNA TGF-β and extracellular matrix proteins expression and reduced interstitial fibrosis in the salt-depleted rat model [458, 483]. Similarly, losartan decreased plasma levels of TGF-β in CSA-treated renal transplant recipients [46]. Use of anti-TGF-β antibodies in salt-depleted rats receiving CSA reduced renal TGF-β expression, normalized alfa-1 (I) collagen mRNA expression, partially prevented the decrease in renal tissue levels of metalloproteinase-9 and tissue increase of metalloproteinase-1 inhibitor, prevented GFR impairment and attenuated arteriolar hyalinosis but surprisingly did not change the extent of tubulointerstitial fibrosis [469]. These results were confirmed by Khanna et al, who also showed that anti TGF-β anti-body decreased CSA-induced renal expression of fibrinogenic molecules in rodents. However, in this paper the authors did not describe the presence of interstitial fibrosis [484].

Experimental data point for the involvement of renal infiltrating and resident cells in the induction of chronic CSA nephrotoxicity. The presence of infiltrating mononuclear cells has been shown in the interstitial area of the cortex and outer medulla of salt-depleted rats treated with CSA [432, 485]. Significant renal macrophage infiltration occurs very early in the salt-depletion model of chronic CSA nephropathy, preceding GFR decrease and development of interstitial fibrosis [445, 486]. This infiltration was accompanied by an impressive interstitial and tubular cell proliferation, which started in the medullary area and progressed to the areas of cortical fibrosis [432, 486]. An up-regulation of the macrophage chemoattractant osteopontin was observed in proximal tubular cells of CSA-treated rats, and was closely correlated to the degree of macrophage infiltration and fibrosis development [471, 486]. Indeed, CSA-treated osteopontin null mice on low salt diet developed less renal macrophage infiltration and interstitial fibrosis than their wild type counterparts [487]. Likewise, Benigni et al found an intense staining for monocyte chemoattractant protein 1 (MCP-1) in renal biopsies with CSA nephrotoxicity from kidney transplant recipients [488]. Recently, Hudkins el al confirmed the presence of osteopontin in human biopsies with CSA nephrotoxicity, but there was no significant inflammatory cells infiltration, suggesting that this molecule might be important in the early but not in the established phase of chronic CSA nephrotoxicity [489]. Macrophages are known sources of cytokines and other mediators of inflammation and play a key factor in several processes that lead to progressive renal fibrosis [490, 491]. Activated infiltrating macrophages amplify and retro-activate the inflammatory and pro-fibrogenic response by recruiting immunocompetent cells, stimulating fibroblast proliferation and migration and increasing of collagen synthesis [492]. Thus, there is an intense and close relationship between angiotensin II and macrophage function. Angiotensin II stimulates the production of monocyte chemoattractant protein 1 (MCP-1) and osteopontin and induces the expression of adhesion molecules, responsible for the rolling, adhesion and penetration of monocytes into the interstitial spaces [491]. Additionally, rat and human macrophage express functional components of the RAS [493, 494]. Angiotensin not only recruits but also activates macrophages [491], and in fact human cells show RAS activation during human monocyte/macrophage differentiation [494]. There is no doubt about the relevance of macrophage as an important participant in chronic CSA nephrotoxicity, but a crucial question remains unanswered: what is (or are) the stimulus for renal macrophage infiltration and activation? Clearly, preglomerular ischemia has a role, but as already pointed CSA can cause significant interstitial fibrosis with normal renal blood flow. Conceivable candidates are post-glomerular ischemia due to vasa recta constriction, sublethal tubular epithelial cell injury, and endothelial cell lesions allowing plasma leakage into renal interstitial area or activation of resident renal interstitial cells.

There are a number of studies showing that CSA could act directly on resident renal cells inducing pro-fibrotic changes. CSA stimulated procollagen production by cultured murine tubulointerstitial fibroblasts and proximal tubule cells [495]. Even very low concentrations of CSA induced collagen synthesis in a variety of cultured human and rat renal fibroblasts, mesangial and tubular epithelial cells [496]. Addition of CSA to primary culture of human renal cortical fibroblasts and proximal tubule cells resulted in direct toxicity, release of pro-fibrotic cytokines and increased collagen synthesis. CSA stimulated insulin-like growth factor secretion and inhibited secretion of IGF-I binding protein by fibroblasts. In tubular cells CSA enhanced the secretion of TGF-beta and platelet-derived growth factor [497]. CSA may have different effects on diverse types of cells, namely cultured human epithelial and endothelial cells and fibroblasts. Collagen production was enhanced in endothelial and epithelial cells, whereas mRNA for tissue inhibitors of metalloproteinase was up regulated in fibroblasts. Toxicity occurred only in endothelial and epithelial cells and was associated with apoptosis. It should be noted that only the epithelial cells had a renal origin, since the fibroblasts and endothelial cells came from human skin, what may limit the generalization of these findings [498]. Impairment of the proteolytic system responsible for renal matrix degradation is also an important element in chronic CSA nephrotoxicity. CSA significantly increased *in vivo* expression of tissue inhibitor of matrix metalloproteinase type 1 by renal interstitial and epithelial cells and promoted intense staining for plasminogen activator inhibitor type 1 in atrophic cortical proximal tubules [499], up-regulated mRNA for tissue inhibitors of metalloproteinase in human skin fibroblasts [498] and inhibited metalloproteinase production by cultured human renal fibroblasts [497]. It was shown that only mesangial cells from mice susceptible to glomerulosclerosis increased collagen content and inhibited matrix metalloproteinase activity and mRNA after exposure to low CSA doses in contrast with mesangial cells from a strain of glomerulosclerosis resistant mice, suggesting that the genetic background may influence CSA-induced pro-fibrotic cellular response [500].

Sub-lethal injury of tubular epithelial cells may be another trigger for CSA-induced fibrosis. In the salt depletion model of chronic CSA nephrotoxicity there was an early activation of pro-apoptotic genes, preceding cells apoptosis and fibrosis [501]. Once again, angiotensin II is likely related to this phenomenon, since co-treatment with losartan significantly reduced the number of tubular and interstitial apoptotic cells in CSA-treated animals [502]. There is also evidence of NO participation in apoptosis induced by CSA. L-arginine administration decreased significantly the magnitude of tubulointerstitial apoptosis in CSA-treated salt-depleted rats [502]. CSA-stimulated apoptosis in various renal cell lines, including human tubular cells, was related to increased inducible NO synthase mRNA via activated p53 proteins [503]. A possible mechanism for CSA-induced tubular injury is an impairment of the P-glycoprotein system (P-GP). This transporter expels hydrophobic substances from the cell, acting as a detoxification system. CSA inhibits P-GP, and so it can potentially promote intracytoplasmic accumulation of its own metabolites and toxic cell catabolism metabolites. Moreover, other P-GP inhibitors, such as verapamil and quinine, enhanced CSA toxicity to cultured epithelial cells [504]. Sustaining this premise, tubular cells expression of P-GP in salt depleted rats receiving CSA was inversely related to interstitial fibrosis and intra-renal angiotensin II deposits [505]. When three different renal cells lines were exposed to CSA *in vitro*, the cells expressing the higher amount of P-GP were the more resistant and the line without P-GP was the more sensitive to CSA toxicity [506]. In renal transplant recipients, increased P-GP expression was found in infiltrating and resident cells of biopsies showing ATN, acute rejection and chronic rejection but not in chronic CSA nephrotoxicity, suggesting that failure to up-regulate P-GP is associated with CSA-induced apoptosis and fibrosis [507]. In the same way, when renal biopsies from solid organ transplant recipients with and without calcineurin inhibitor-induced nephrotoxicity were compared, p-glycoprotein expression was significantly less marked in the biopsies with nephrotoxicity [508]. Recently, Hauser el al performed a case-control study assessing the role of the multi drug resistance (ABCB) 1 gene, which encodes P-GP, in CSA-induced chronic nephrotoxicity and found that the donor's ABCB1 3435TT polymorphism, associated with decreased renal expression of P-GP, was strongly associated to CSA-nephrotoxicity [509].

NO pathway manipulation affects CSA chronic nephrotoxicity. Supplementation of the NO substrate, -L-arginine, ameliorated whereas use of -L-NAME, a NO synthase inhibitor, aggravated tubulointerstitial fibrosis [102]. Likewise, CSA-induced up-regulation of TGF-β1, plasminogen activator inhibitor-1 and deposition of extracellular matrix components were aggravated by NO blockade and ameliorated by NO enhancement [510].

As previously stated, there is abundant evidence that CSA markedly increases endothelin production and endothelin up-regulates TGF-β expression, which in its turn is clearly involved in CSA chronic nephrotoxicity. Therefore, the existence of an endothelin-TGF- β pathway in CSA-induced fibrosis was proposed [511]. Supporting this hypothesis, increased tubular cells endothelin mRNA expression was found in human biopsies with chronic CSA nephrotoxicity; [488] and Ramirez et al found dramatic elevations in endothelin system components in CSA-treated rats that strongly correlate with renal structural lesions [446]. In contrast, experimental use of an endothelin receptor antagonist did not prevent interstitial fibrosis in the salt-depleted chronic CSA nephrotoxicity model [442, 443].

Vascular endothelial growth factor (VEGF) has been considered as a possible factor for CSA chronic nephrotoxicity development. VEGF is a potent endothelial cell mitogen that mediates endothelial cell proliferation and survival, induces angiogenesis, participates in vascular remodeling and repair and causes vasodilation and increased vascular permeability through increase in NO production. Shihab et al. found an increased VEGF expression in salt-depleted CSA-treated rats, which was prevented by angiotensin II blockade via losartan and NO enhancement via L-arginine [460, 512, 513]. In an interesting study, Kang et al. found that VEGF administration to rats with established chronic CSA nephropathy resulted in improvement of interstitial fibrosis, decrease in osteopontin expression, macrophage infiltration and collagen III deposition and caused blood pressure reduction [514].

Hypomagnesemia has been associated to chronic CSA nephrotoxicity. Miura et al supplemented magnesium to rats receiving CSA on low salt diet. The improvement of CSA-induced hypomagnesemia was followed by an impressive prevention of interstitial fibrosis, abrogation of the up-regulation of pro-fibrotic molecule genes (TGF-β, plasminogen activator inhibitor-1, tissue inhibitor of matrix metalloproteinase) and GFR enhancement [515]. The protective effects of magnesium supplementation were independent from RAS-associated mechanisms but linked to prevention of the activation of the transcription factors activator protein-1 and nuclear factor -kappa B and to adjusting of nitric oxide synthase activity and NO production [516-518]. Confirming these experimental data, Holzmacher et al studied a population of renal transplant recipients with biopsy proven CSA nephrotoxicity divided in low and normal serum magnesium groups. Low magnesium levels were significantly associated to faster rate of kidney function decline and increased rates of graft loss in long term follow-up [519].

Other mechanisms and mediators have been implicated in the genesis and prevention of chronic CSA nephrotoxicity. Reactive oxygen species, besides their functional effects on renal function, are also mediators of tissue injury favoring fibrosis. Use of the antioxidant vitamin E inhibited increases in TGF-beta and osteopontin mRNA and development of renal fibrosis in CSA-treated rats [184]. Mazzali et al showed that hyperuricemia exacerbates experimental chronic CSA nephrotoxicity, apparently due to activation of the RAS and inhibition of renal NO production [520]. The complement system was studied in a mouse model of chronic CSA nephrotoxicity, and the authors found an increased expression of C3, C4d and membrane attack complex (C9) associated with upregulation of complement regulatory proteins CD46 and CD55. These changes were mostly confined to the injured tubules and interstitium, suggesting a role for the complement system in chronic CSA nephrotoxicity [521]. Use of a TXA_2 receptor antagonist in a CSA-treated renal isograft model strikingly prevented the development of interstitial fibrosis [522]. Preliminary evidence showed that prednisone altered the structural changes induced by CSA in salt-depleted rats, enhancing tubular hypertrophy in medullary area and favoring less tubulointerstitial fibrosis [523]. Colchicine administration to CSA-treated rats attenuated renal interstitial fibrosis, reduced apoptosis, osteopontin expression and macrophage interstitial influx [524-526]. Johnson el al demonstrated that simvastatin, a 3-hydroxy-3-methylglutaryl CoA reductase inhibitor, completely prevented CSA-stimulated collagen synthesis and IGF-I secretion in cultured human renal fibroblasts [527]. Confirming the protective effects of statins, pravastatin abrogated transforming growth factor β1-inducible gene h3 and TGF-β mRNA expression and attenuated interstitial inflammation and fibrosis in the low-salt model of chronic CSA nephrotoxicity [528, 529]. Pioglitazone, a thiazolidinedione antidiabetic drug, limited the increase in plasminogen activator inhibitor-1 (a pro-fibrotic cytokine) and TGF-β, attenuated afferent arteriopathy and improved renal function in rats receiving CSA, although the authors did not mention renal fibrosis [530]. The new anti-fibrotic drug pirfenidone was used in the salt-depleted chronic CSA nephrotoxicity model, limiting interstitial fibrosis and strikingly decreasing TGF-β and matrix components levels. In addition, pirfenidone decreased the expression of the pro-apoptotic genes p53 and Fas-ligand, increased the expression the anti-apoptotic gene Bcl-xL and consequently, reduced the number of CSA-induced apoptotic cells [531, 532]. Electroporation-mediated hepatocyte growth factor gene transfer to rats receiving CSA reduced interstitial fibrosis and actin expression, tubular cells apoptosis, macrophage infiltration, and TGF-β and type-I collagen cortical expression [533, 534]. Heme oxygenase (HO), the rate-limiting enzyme in heme catabolism, has been related to prevention of ischemic and inflammatory renal injury. CSA decreased renal tissue HO-1 isoenzyme to undetectable levels in rats and the use of cobalt protoporphyrin, an HO inducer, restored HO-1 expression to normal levels and afforded impressive protection against CSA-induced renal fibrosis [535, 536].

A working hypothesis for chronic CSA nephrotoxicity

Chronic CSA nephrotoxicity can be caused by preglomerular vasoconstriction-dependent and independent mechanisms. In the clinical setting and in most of the animal models used it is likely that interstitial fibrosis occurs through a combination of both processes. Mechanisms dissociated from preglomerular ischemia seem to be closely dependent on CSA-induced intra-renal angiotensin II enhancement, macrophage infiltration and fibroblasts/interstitial cell activation. The signals causing macrophage migration may come from interstitial ischemia due to vasa recta constriction, activation of interstitial resident cells, leakage of plasma into interstitial area due to endothelial cells damage or inflammatory stimulus originated from injured or apoptotic tubular cells. Obviously, more than one factor may be occurring at the same time. The final pathway is an inflammatory interstitial microenvironment where cross-talk among angiotensin II, macrophages, fibroblasts and resident cells will result in over expression of pro-fibrotic substances (cytokines, growth factors, ROS) inhibition of antifibrotic components (metalloproteinase etc) in a self-perpetuating cycle of RAS system activation, macrophage recruitment and activation and enhancement of extracellular matrix deposition (Figure 1).

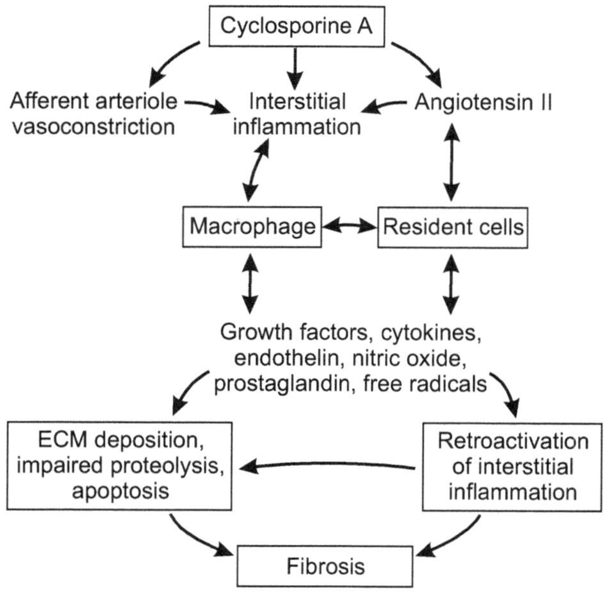

Figure 1. *A working hypothesis for chronic CSA nephrotoxicity.*

Clinical aspects

Renal transplantation

It is almost impossible to individualize the exact role of CSA-induced chronic nephrotoxicity in renal allograft outcomes. From the moment of implantation, the transplanted kidney will suffer from mechanical manipulation, ischemic injury and immunologic attack. Later on acute rejection, recurrent or *de novo* renal disease, hypertension, chronic viral infection, metabolic derangements (dyslipidemia, diabetes, and hyperuricemia), chronic rejection and aging may work in various combinations causing progressive structural damage and functional impairment.

In this complex situation, the histological diagnosis of chronic CSA nephrotoxicity usually relies in the finding of the typical afferent arteriolar lesion with nodular focal or circular protein deposits in the *tunica media* [278, 537]. However, when renal biopsies are performed late, after months or years of continuous renal injury, the morphological picture may be difficult to characterize. In addition, as previously pointed, CSA-induced fibrosis can occur without afferent arteriolar injury and CSA-induced afferent arteriole hyalinosis can remit without parallel improvement in renal fibrosis, strongly suggesting that the vascular lesion and renal fibrosis may occur in independent ways [426, 428, 445]. Moreover, vascular or chronic rejection may co-exist with chronic CSA nephrotoxicity. Potential clues for the differentiation of these two entities came from a study by Abrass el al. These authors showed that extracellular matrix composition of renal fibrosis found in human renal allograft biopsies was different depending on the pathological diagnosis made. Fibrosis associated with chronic CSA nephrotoxicity had a widespread interstitial accumulation of collagens I and III, whereas biopsies with rejection showed an increased expression of proximal tubular basement membrane collagen IV alpha chain 3 and laminin-β2, suggesting that interstitial fibrosis in these patients can result from different pathogenic mechanisms [538]. Subsequently, Bakker et al, found dissimilar results comparing renal allograft biopsies with chronic CSA nephrotoxicity, chronic rejection and chronic allograft nephropathy. Chronic CSA nephrotoxicity was associated with collagen III and IV interstitial accumulation, whereas early deposition of collagen I, associated to collagen III and IV was more specific for chronic rejection [539]. The same group found that mRNA levels for laminin beta 2 and TGF-β were significantly increased only in renal biopsies from patients with chronic CSA nephrotoxicity when compared to chronic rejection patients [540].

Unfortunately, few prospective studies concomitantly assessed functional and histological changes in kidney transplant recipients. Studies claiming the absence of negative chronic effects for CSA on renal allografts are largely based on retrospective analysis of functional data, which frequently are only serum creatinine measurements [541, 542]. On the other hand, when renal histology was obtained, most of the evidences indicating a role for CSA-induced fibrosis in the chronic kidney disease of transplanted kidneys were indirect. As stated before, CSA-treated patients with significant interstitial fibrosis may maintain "normal" serum creatinine for long periods. For instance, Abbas et al found 5.8% of chronic CSA nephrotoxicity among 120 elective biopsies realized one year or more after renal transplant in stable patients with well-functioning grafts and no history of rejection [543]. Other authors found significant development of interstitial fibrosis occurring after 6 months or more of CSA treatment [544, 545]. When CSA-treated and azathioprine-treated renal recipients were compared, the first had significantly more intense interstitial fibrosis [546, 547]. An important additional aspect to be considered is that the contribution of CSA-induced interstitial fibrosis to progressive renal dysfunction in kidney transplant recipient is probably related to individual patients' susceptibility. Genetic background, concomitant diseases and many other factors may modulate different degrees of interstitial fibrosis, inducing individual and unequal patients' response [548].

While CSA remarkably improved short-term graft and patient survival as compared to azathioprine-based immunosuppression, the same outcome has not been consistently demonstrated on long-term survival. One of the factors possibly related to this paradox is the role of chronic CSA nephrotoxicity in chronic allograft nephropathy. Marcén et al compared 128 CSA-treated and 185 azathioprine-treated cadaveric first renal transplant recipients followed for at least 10 years. In the first three years, post-transplant actuarial graft survival was significantly higher in CSA-treated patients. Afterward, this difference disappeared and azathioprine-treated patients showed a non-statistically significant tendency to better graft survival at 5 and 10 years. The leading cause of graft failure in CSA-treated patients was chronic allograft nephropathy [549]. In fact, chronic allograft nephropathy, an entity with obscure pathogenesis, is considered the most important cause of progressive renal failure in renal transplant patients. Potential CSA participation in chronic allograft nephropathy was supported by the finding of a significant reduction in the rate of the loss of renal function in patients with histologically confirmed disease when CSA dosage was reduced or suspended [550]. Strong evidence favoring the importance of CSA in chronic allograft nephropathy came from the paper of Nankivell et al. Ninety-eight recipients of combined kidney-pancreas transplant and one kidney transplant alone, using CSA as the primary immunosuppressive drug, composed the study population. Protocol biopsies were performed at defined intervals for 10 years, with a final total of 888 specimens. Chronic CSA nephrotoxicity (striped fibrosis, progressive arteriolar hyalinosis and ischemic glomerulosclerosis) occurred with a point prevalence of 67.3% by 5 years and was almost universal by 10 years after transplantation. GFR was significantly reduced in patients with chronic CSA nephrotoxicity as compared with those with early acute CSA nephrotoxicity or no nephrotoxicity [551]. The same group found that CSA immunosuppressive therapy was a factor independently associated to the progression of chronic interstitial fibrosis in 839 pairs of renal biopsies taken up to 10 years after renal transplantation [552].

Other solid organ transplantation

CSA use in patients with healthy native kidneys is clearly associated with the potential of renal injury, which ultimately may lead to severe chronic kidney disease (CKD), dialysis or renal transplantation [271, 280, 424, 553, 554]. In fact, recent data indicate an 11-fold increase in the referral for renal transplant evaluation among non-solid organ transplant recipients [555].

Myers et al were the first to describe that CSA use in heart transplantation was associated with development of CKD. They showed that CSA treatment for more than 12 months caused a progressive GFR and

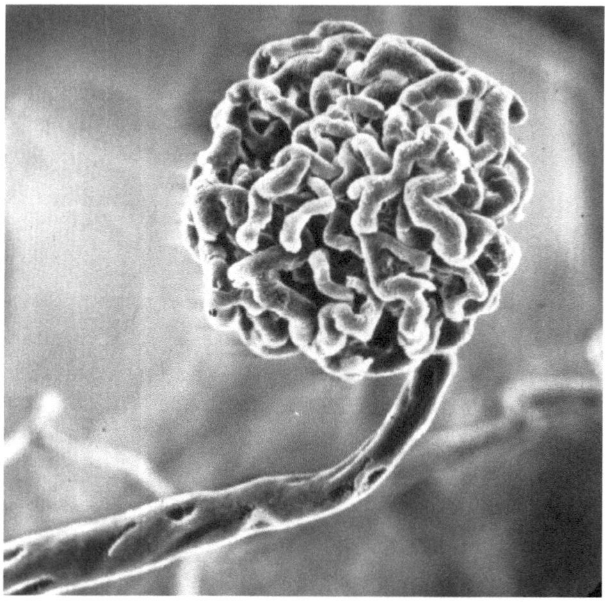

Figure 2. *Striking afferent arteriole vasoconstriction in a Sprague-Dawley rat on low salt-diet treated for 28 days with CSA 15 mg/kg/day. The narrowest point of the arteriole measured 11.02 mm, whereas control animals presented a mean diameter of 12.67 mm. Vascular cast, scanning electron micrograph, orig. magn. x450.*
From [444], with permission.

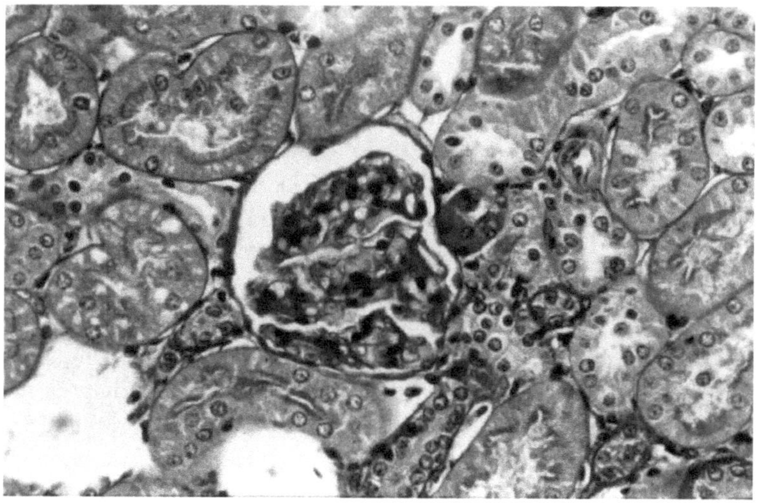

Figure 3. *Afferent arteriole hyalinosis in a Munich-Wistar rat on low salt diet treated with CSA 15 mg/kg for 4 weeks.*
H&E staining, orig. magn. x400.

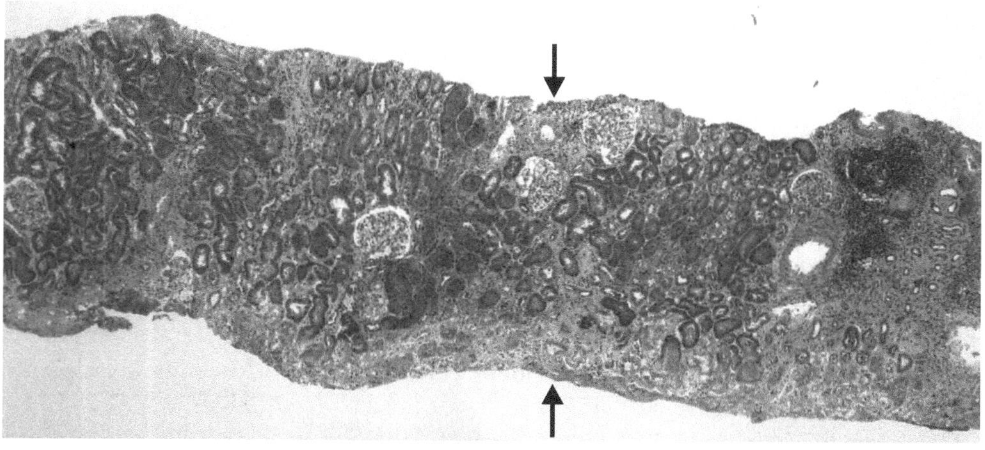

Figure 4. *Striped interstitial fibrosis (arrows) in a CSA treated recipient. Masson's trichrome staining, orig. magn. x40.*
By courtesy of Dr. JL Bosmans.

RBF decline, RVR increase, obliterative arteriolopathy, striped interstitial fibrosis, tubular atrophy and glomerulosclerosis [429]. In a subset of patients followed over 48 m, CSA was reduced or withdrawn, but GFR did not improve and repeated biopsies disclosed further histological deterioration [437]. The starting doses of CSA (17 mg/kg) and target trough levels used in the first studies were substantially higher than dosages currently used. However, when patients on "old high-doses" were compared to patients on "modern low-doses" by the same group of investigators, the intensity and progression of renal injury were the same [436]. In the last paper of this seminal series, the authors reported a 10% cumulative incidence of CKD stage 5 in a 10-year period of observation [556]. A number of subsequent studies substantiated these findings, confirming that prolonged CSA administration to heart transplant recipients causes a progressive renal impairment, with a sharp functional decline in the first year followed by a slower rate of deterioration thereafter, and a prominent structural injury represented by afferent arteriole arteriolopathy, tubulointerstitial fibrosis and glomerulosclerosis [288, 557, 558]. Variable frequencies of severe CKD were reported by different groups, ranging from 1 to 10% [288, 554, 556, 559-565], with an apparent trend for increased frequency with longer follow-up time (Table 4). The mean time elapsed from cardiac transplantation to initiation of dialysis was around 6 to 7 years [559, 561, 562, 564] and development of CKD requiring renal replacement was associated with higher mortality in these patients [280, 559, 564, 566]. Attempts to identify risk factors for CKD development produced conflicting results. Some studies suggested that early decrease in GFR, CSA dose, length of time exposure to CSA, previous renal dysfunction, older age and hypertriglyceridemia were associated to CKD. However, several studies did not find any significant correlation among CSA dosages, CSA trough blood levels, patients' age, presence of hypertension or use of antihypertensive drugs and CSA-induced CKD [280, 554]. These data suggest that heart transplant recipients have different susceptibility to CSA-induced injury, which results in large inter-individual variability for development of renal fibrosis and progression to CKD.

Table 4. The frequency of severe chronic kidney disease after heart transplantation increased in conjunction with longer follow-ups, with few exceptions.

Authors	Number of patients	Follow-up time (years)	CKD frequency (%)
Lewis et al [563]	100	4	1.0
Gonwa et al [575]	69	4	1.3
Zietse et al [565]	187	5	3.2
Goral et al [561]	39	6	4.0
Greenberg et al [288]	228	7	2.2
Herlitz and Lindelöw [554]	151	9	4.0
Goldstein et al [559]	293	9	6.5
van Gelder [564]	304	10	8.0
Myers and Newton [556]	200	10	10.0
Kuo et al [562]	430	13	3.3

CKD: chronic kidney disease

The picture observed in lung and lung/heart transplantation is quite similar to that found after heart transplantation. There is a long-term impairment of GFR, structural arteriolar, interstitial and glomerular damage and development of severe CKD in up to 6.7% of the patients [553, 567-569]. Need for dialysis seems to be progressive over time, reaching the rate of 19%, nine years after transplantation [570].

Information about chronic CSA nephrotoxicity in liver transplantation is scanty, with few papers analyzing renal histology. In a similar way to what was described for heart transplantation, different authors reported an early and marked GFR decrease with a tendency to subsequent renal function stabilization. Liver transplant recipients with ACE gene D/D genotype were reported as having higher risk for developing CSA-induced renal dysfunction [571]. Dagöö et al followed 25 liver transplant patients maintained on low CSA dosages for 5 years. There was a sharp decrease of GFR in the first year and after 5 years, all recipients presented an average GFR loss of 50% (or a reduction of 3 ml/year). However, the authors did not perform renal biopsies or change immunosuppression, making impossible to differentiate how much of this lesion was functional and reversible or chronic and irreversible [572]. When renal histology was available in liver transplant recipients, the usual CSA-induced structural changes were found: preglomerular arteriolopathy, interstitial fibrosis, tubular atrophy and signs of glomerular ischemia [558, 573, 574]. Lately, there have been reports of severe CKD in CSA-treated liver transplant recipients. Gonwa et al reported prevalences of 8.6% for severe CKD and 9.5% for stage 5 CKD, 13 years after liver transplantation. Development of CKD stage 5 was associated with poor prognosis (28.2% survival compared with 54.6% in the control group). Patients developing CKD had a higher preoperative and 1-year serum creatinine and a higher prevalence of hepatorenal syndrome [575]. Coopersmith reported renal transplantation in seven liver-transplant recipients who developed CSA-induced CKD [553]. Fisher et al analyzed 883 consecutive liver transplants, mostly treated with CSA. Severe CKD developed in 25 patients (4.4%) surviving one year or more. Twenty-four out these 25 were on CSA therapy. Among these 25 patients 48% required dialysis, despite CSA dose reduction or withdrawal. The median time for developing severe CKD was three years, and for development of CKD stage 5 was five years. Development of severe CKD was associated with higher mortality. Renal biopsies obtained from 13 out 25 patients were consistent with chronic CSA nephrotoxicity in 10. The risk factors analysis found two sub-groups with different characteristics. One consisted of patients with early renal dysfunction preceding later CKD. These patients presented older age, perioperative dialysis, cytomegalovirus infection, infection and re-grafting as risk factors for later development of CKD stage 5. The second group included patients with late onset renal failure without early renal dysfunction. Trough CSA blood level at month 1 and cumulative CSA dosage at 5 years were predictors of CKD stage 5 development in this group [574]. The better recent prognosis and longer survival time of liver transplantation recipients will probably be associated with a higher frequency of development of CSA-induced CKD in this setting.

Native kidneys of insulin-dependent diabetes mellitus (IDDM) patients submitted to pancreas transplantation can also develop chronic CSA nephrotoxicity. Fiorettto et al studied 13 IDDM pancreas transplantation recipients, using as control group IDDM patients not transplanted or who had early failure of pancreas allograft. Baseline renal function and histology were assessed and repeated up to 5 years of follow-up. They found a 34% GFR decrease in the transplant group with subsequent renal function stabilization versus no GFR change in the control group. Renal histology was preserved or slightly impaired in the first 2 years post-transplant, but 5-year biopsies revealed a remarkable increase in interstitial fibrosis, interstitial cortical volume, tubular atrophy and frequency of sclerosed glomeruli. There were no significant histological changes in the control group. Stepwise multiple regression analysis identified intensity of GFR decline in the first year, CSA blood levels and CSA daily dose as good predictors of structural injury at 5 years [576]. When compared to kidney-alone transplant, simultaneous pancreas-kidney transplant recipients presented higher frequency of calcineurin-inhibitor nephrotoxicity in intermediate and late biopsies [577].

Bone marrow transplantation

CSA therapy is used in bone marrow transplantation (BMT) for prevention of graft versus host disease for limited periods, normally from six to 18 months. Dosages are high, around 10 to 12 mg/kg, with target trough blood levels up to 400 ng/ml. Few studies have explored the issue of chronic nephrotoxicity in this setting. Nizze et al studied autopsy material from 112 BMT recipients treated with either CSA or CSA-free immunosuppression. They found higher prevalence of interstitial fibrosis, tubular atrophy, arteriolopathy, glomerular and/or arteriolar thrombi and glomerular collapse in the CSA group. When these data were compared with autopsies of heart transplant recipients, the frequency of structural injury was clearly more elevated in BMT (54 versus 19.5%) [578]. Diertele et al found structural renal lesions indicative of chronic CSA nephrotoxicity in 67% of 49 BMT recipients. The risk factors for structural injury were longer duration of CSA therapy, severe renal dysfunction in the first 3 months post-transplant and use of total body irradiation [579]. Indeed, Miralbell et al found that total body irradiation and graft versus host disease were associated with increased serum creatinine levels in BMT patients [580].

Autoimmune diseases

The situation where the CSA impact on native kidneys is most evident is the treatment of autoimmune diseases. In these patients rejection is not an issue, and the native kidneys are usually healthy and not submitted to other potential insults, making it easier to establish a direct cause-effect correlation. In fact, Feutren and Mihatsch, on behalf of the International Kidney Biopsy Registry of Cyclosporine in Autoimmune Diseases, found interstitial fibrosis and tubular atrophy and/or arteriolar alterations in 21% of 192 patients with insulin-dependent diabetes mellitus of recent onset, uveitis, psoriasis, Sjögren's syndrome or polychondritis that had been treated with CSA for 4 to 39 months (median 13 m). Use of multivariate logistic-regression analysis found risk factors for CSA nephropathy to be older age, larger initial CSA dose and larger maximal increase in SCr [581]. In a meta-analysis, Vercauteren et al. selected 18 papers (among 423) for systematic review of renal function changes in CSA-treated patients with autoimmune diseases. Patients receiving CSA had a risk difference of 20.9% for developing nephrotoxicity as compared to other therapies. In seven studies, CSA withdrawal induced only a partial reversion of renal dysfunction. Renal histology analysis was reported in 19 papers and 10 of them were selected for review. These studies included 163 patients with uveitis, psoriasis, and rheumatoid arthritis. Time of biopsy was always over 12 months. All papers reported mild to moderate interstitial fibrosis and/or tubular atrophy and/or arteriolar hyalinosis. Three studies performed baseline and post-treatment biopsies and found *de novo* interstitial fibrosis or worsening of pre-treatment injury [582].

Autoimmune uveitis was one of the first autoimmune diseases treated with CSA. In 1986 Palestine et al compared renal biopsies from 17 young patients with normal baseline SCr, treated for an average time of two years, to renal biopsies from patients with idiopathic hematuria not receiving CSA. Interstitial fibrosis and/or tubular atrophy were present in all patients treated with CSA, independently of having impaired or normal renal function at the time of the biopsy, and interstitial infiltrate was found in 14 patients. At the time of the biopsy, mean inulin clearance for CSA-treated group was 69±6 ml/min/1.73 m^2 BSA, SCr was 1.5±0.1 mg/dl and mean CSA dose was 10±0.7 mg/kg [430]. In a subsequent study, the same authors performed sequential renal function and histological evaluation in these patients after two to four years of therapy. Despite CSA dose reductions inulin clearance did not improve in 12 patients and actually, decreased significantly in three. All patients had arteriolar injury, including hyaline changes. CSA-induced chronic histological damage progressed in three of the six follow-up biopsies. It is noteworthy that renal function was stable in two out three patients with progressive interstitial injury [583]. In a recent study irreversible GFR loss was associated with cumulated CSA exposure in uveitis patients on low CSA doses after two and half years of therapy [584]. Another study assessing renal histology in CSA-treated patients with autoimmune uveitis found a lymphocytic infiltrate (predominantly T lymphocytes) and arteriolar changes in 80% of the studied population. Patients were treated for three years, with an initial CSA dose of 10 mg/kg that was tapered to 5 mg/kg [585]. Bagnis et al studied eleven patients on low dose CSA treatment for uveitis, performing renal biopsies before and after two years of therapy. They found significant interstitial fibrosis and tubular atrophy, high prevalence of hypertension and significant decrease in isotopic GFR. All renal changes were CSA dose-dependent [586].

Due to its effectiveness, CSA has been largely used in the treatment of psoriasis. The fact that this autoimmune disease does not cause intrinsic renal abnormalities provides a unique opportunity to assess CSA direct impact on the development of chronic structural injury in healthy kidneys. Indeed, most of the papers that evaluated CSA-induced changes in renal histology of autoimmune diseases are about psoriasis. These studies showed that low CSA doses (initial 5 mg/kg, tapered to 1 to 2 mg/kg) consistently induced mild to moderate renal scarring (interstitial fibrosis and tubular atrophy) and frequently caused arteriolopathy associated with variable degrees of renal dysfunction [587-592]. Sequential biopsies found progression of renal scarring and arteriolopathy accompanied by a concomitant GFR decrease, although development and progression of interstitial fibrosis with stable SCr was also demonstrated [587, 591, 592]. Two studies are particularly relevant because they performed pre and post-treatment biopsies. Svarstad et al studied 10 psoriatic patients treated with an average CSA dose of 3.2 mg/kg for 12 m. At baseline biopsies, just one patient had moderate fibrosis. After one year of therapy, renal scarring worsened in this patient and four patients had *de novo* interstitial fibrosis [590]. Zachariae reported up to eight years of functional and histological follow-up in 30 psoriatics treated with low CSA doses (2.5 to 6 mg/kg). Pre-treatment biopsies were done in 25 of them and 17 had completely normal renal tissue. After two years of treatment all patients presented histological changes compatible with chronic CSA nephrotoxicity. Renal injury, consisting of focal tubulointerstitial fibrosis, arteriolopathy and glomerulosclerosis was progressive over time. After four years, all biopsied patients had moderate to severe striped fibrosis, with a mean injury score two times higher than that found after one year. All patients except one developed significant hyalinosis and the percent of sclerotic glomeruli increased from 1% to 8%. These changes were paralleled by GFR decrease and GFR values correlated negatively with the degree of fibrosis [592]. So far, there is no clear definition of risk factors related to development of structural renal lesions in CSA-treated psoriatic patients. Correlations with dose or trough levels were negative. One study found that late fibrosis correlated with older age and presence of hypertension [587], but others did not [592]. Powles et al reported lack of improvement in renal function after one month of CSA discontinuation as a good predictor for the finding of chronic injury at biopsy [589].

The use of low doses of CSA in rheumatoid arthritis (RA) has also been associated with functional impairment, occasional development of CKD and chronic structural nephropathy [593-598]. Interpretation of renal biopsies in these patients is complicated by the possibility of RA-induced renal changes, such as tubulointerstitial injury, glomerulosclerosis, amyloidosis or NSAIDS and analgesic-induced tubulointerstitial lesions. Landewe et al compared renal biopsies from eleven RA patients treated with low CSA dose (< 5mg/kg) for a mean of 26 m with renal tissue from autopsy of 22 RA patients who did not receive CSA. The two groups were matched for age, disease duration, sex and previous use of gold and/or D-penicillamine. Although GFR decreased 26% from baseline in the CSA group, structural injury (glomeruli obsolescence, arteriolopathy, tubular atrophy and interstitial fibrosis) was minimal and similar in both groups [599]. A possible methodological flaw in this study is the lack of report of the cause of death in the control group, and the fact that kidney biopsies were not performed in patients withdrawn from CSA treatment due to decreased renal function [582]. Another study biopsied fourteen RA patients treated with low dosages of CSA (<5 mg/kg) for 6 months. Mean SCr at biopsy time was 0.84 mg/dl, thirteen patients showed non-specific renal injury and only one had moderate striped interstitial fibrosis attributable to CSA nephrotoxicity. However, there was no baseline, control or consecutive biopsies in this study [595]. Reports of the International Kidney Biopsy Registry of Cyclosporin in Autoimmune diseases showed a more meaningful figure for CSA nephrotoxicity in RA [593, 596]. The initial paper compared 41 patients treated with CSA at a maximum dose of 4.6±1.2 mg/kg for 16±7 m with 11 RA patients not treated with CSA and 41 sex and age matched normal controls (kidney donors). The CSA-treated group showed interstitial fibrosis and tubular atrophy score higher than values for normal controls and RA patients not treated with CSA, although statistical significance was only seen between normal controls and CSA-treated RA. Typical CSA arteriolopathy was not found. Moderate focal interstitial fibrosis with tubular atrophy and/or arteriolopathy affecting more than 30% of the biopsy area were found in four patients of the CSA-treated group and interpreted as CSA nephropathy. CSA structural injury seemed to correlate with initial SCr level and CSA dose, but not with treatment length [593]. Subsequently, the same group reported data originated from first (60) and second (14) biopsies in RA patients treated with CSA for up to 87 m. At first biopsy, they found changes consistent wit CSA nephropathy in five patients, and a further patient presented these changes at second biopsy. None individual developed CSA nephrotoxicity among 22 patients who started treatment with doses below 4 mg/kg and subsequently did not receive doses higher than 5 mg/kg [596]. Sund et al compared pre and post treatment renal biopsies in RA patients given CSA. They studied 10 patients, with mean age of 58 y, without known renal disease, who received a low dose of CSA (< 5mg/kg) for up to 46 months. The second biopsy was performed after a mean of 17.8 months and a third biopsy after a mean of 38.6 months of treatment. A semiquantitative chronicity index (CI) was used for evaluation of renal tissue. GFR was depressed at the time of both post-treatment biopsies. In the baseline biopsy glomeruli were normal or showed slight changes and there was no fibrosis or just a slight increase in interstitial area. In the two subsequent post-treatment biopsies, the frequency of sclerotic glomeruli increased in two and four patients, respectively. Slight to moderate focal interstitial fibrosis and tubular atrophy developed in about half of the patients. In the seven patients that had three biopsies, CI increased from 2.3 to 3.9 in the second biopsy and remained stable in the third. Just one patient presented progressive CI in the three biopsies. Arteriolar changes were non-specific and similar between the baseline and later biopsies. There was no correlation between structural injury, cumulative CSA dose, and duration of treatment or decrease in GFR. This study showed that low doses of CSA can cause chronic nephropathy in RA patients, but also showed that the injury did not occur equally in all of them and is not inevitably progressive, suggesting an important role for individual susceptibility in the development of CSA-induced structural lesions [597]. The number of months with elevated SCr was shown to be an independent predictor for development of irreversible CSA-induced renal dysfunction. Van der Borne et al studying CSA-treated RA patients found higher percent of irreversible SCr increase among patients that remained with SCr ≥ 30% from baseline values for more than two months [598].

CSA has also been used in the early phases of insulin-dependent diabetes mellitus (IDDM), and was associated to variable degrees of structural and functional impairment in these patients [600-602]. Mihatsch et al. reported that 25% of 40 individuals with recent onset IDDM treated with CSA 7 to 9 mg/kg for at least one year had renal interstitial fibrosis and tubular atrophy, and to a lesser extent, arteriolopathy. Serum creatinine at the time of biopsy was 43% higher than baseline values. There was a significant correlation between tubular atrophy intensity and CSA trough blood level [601]. Another study analyzed renal function and histology of 125 IDDM patients (74 adults and 51 children) treated with CSA 7.5 to 10 mg/kg for an average of 13 months. All patients were in remission from insulin dependency and without other possible causes of renal dysfunction at the time of the biopsy. Slight interstitial fibrosis and tubular atrophy were found in 26% of the patients. Moderate injury was observed in additional 16% and considered definitely related to CSA. A non-significant trend towards GFR decrease was observed in the group with moderate structural lesion, but functional changes reversed with CSA dose reduction. Age, excessive CSA dose and trough blood level were considered risk factors for chronic injury. The magnitude of SCr increase was the best predictor of chronic nephropathy presence at biopsy [600].

Although CSA has been used for treatment of other autoimmune diseases such as atopic dermatitis, myasthenia gravis, systemic sclerosis and primary biliary cirrhosis, data about chronic structural injury in these situations are scarce. There are occasional reports of end stage renal failure or development of interstitial fibrosis in kidney biopsies in demyelinating polyradiculoneuropathy, Sjögren's syndrome, , polychondritis, Behçet's and Alport's syndromes [581, 603-605].

In conclusion, there is no doubt that even low doses of CSA can induce chronic irreversible structural injury and sometimes CKD stage 5 in patients with autoimmune diseases. The most usual histological lesions found are interstitial fibrosis and tubular atrophy. The typical CSA-related arteriolopathy has rarely been demonstrated, with a rather more usual finding of non-specific arteriolar hyalinosis. The available data strongly suggest that the development of chronic injury and its severity depend on different individual susceptibilities to CSA. The best predictors for the presence of fibrosis in renal tissue are the length of time in which renal function remained depressed and the lack of reversibility of functional impairment after CSA discontinuation. Whereas in solid organs or bone marrow transplantation CSA use is necessary and justified by obvious reasons, its use in patients with non-fatal autoimmune diseases should be carefully balanced against the risk of causing progressive renal fibrosis, chronic renal failure or even CKD stage 5.

Primary renal disease

CSA is a valid option for treatment of steroid-resistant or relapsing nephrotic syndrome and for some types of glomerulopathies. The clinical and histological differentiation of underlying disease progression from chronic CSA nephrotoxicity in these patients is particularly hard to discern. A baseline biopsy is mandatory for reliable renal tissue evaluation in this setting, but studies analyzing pre and post-treatment biopsies have shown conflicting results. Clasen et al did not find significant vascular or interstitial changes in post-treatment renal biopsies from five patients with minimal-change nephrotic syndrome treated with CSA for 10 months [606]. The same group studied 21 patients with severe steroid-resistant or steroid-dependent nephrotic syndrome treated with CSA for 6 to 71 months. At this time possible CSA nephrotoxicity was diagnosed in three and definite CSA-induced nephropathy in two patients. The mean GFR value remained stable over time [607]. Kranz et al followed 20 CSA-treated children with minimal change nephrotic syndrome for up to 10 years and did not find CSA toxicity in renal biopsies [608]. On the other hand, Meyrier et al found different patterns of response for

CSA treatment in 36 patients with minimal change disease and focal segmental glomerulosclerosis who had baseline and sequential renal biopsies performed. Those with minimal change disease had stable normal function and less severe tubulointerstitial injury on follow-up biopsies. In contrast, the group with focal segmental glomerulosclerosis increased their SCr as compared to minimal change disease patients and presented a further deterioration of renal histology, i.e. an increased number of sclerotic glomeruli and worsening of interstitial fibrosis. CSA doses higher than 5.5 mg/kg were associated with more severe structural injury [609]. On the other hand, Waldo et al did not find progression of interstitial fibrosis in four follow-up biopsies done after at least two years of CSA therapy in children with steroid-resistant nephrotic syndrome due to focal and segmental glomerulosclerosis [610]. Habib and Niaudet performed baseline and sequential biopsies in 42 CSA-treated children with idiopathic nephrotic syndrome. The pre-treatment biopsy showed only one patient with moderate tubulointerstitial lesions, but nine patients presented severe interstitial injury in the first follow-up biopsy (13±4 months of therapy). A second follow-up biopsy was done (29±6 months of therapy) and showed progressive tubulointerstitial injury in 13 out 23 children. There was no correlation between the histological changes and length of treatment, CSA blood or trough levels and no impairment of renal function [611]. Other studies found renal structural injury compatible with CSA-induced nephropathy in 4 to 18% of children and adults with nephrotic syndrome due to minimal change disease or focal segmental glomerulosclerosis after long term CSA treatment [612-615]. Seikaly et al found mild, but progressive tubular atrophy and interstitial fibrosis in 75% of children with minimal change disease treated with CSA for more than three years, while only 25% of children with primary nephrotic syndrome not receiving CSA had similar interstitial injury. Cortical interstitial fibrosis and tubular atrophy areas were significantly wider in kidneys from the CSA-treated group [616]. Few studies have assessed markers or factors which may influence the characteristic of this lesion. Increased renal osteopontin expression and higher cumulative CSA dose were related to development of irreversible interstitial fibrosis, whereas children treated with a single daily dose of CSA did not develop chronic CSA nephrotoxicity at follow-up biopsies [617-619].

Clinical management of chronic nephrotoxicity

The first challenge for prevention and treatment of chronic CSA nephrotoxicity is to recognize it early. Since the diagnosis of chronic nephrotoxicity relies on the presence of irreversible structural injury, a renal biopsy is clearly the diagnostic gold standard. However, renal biopsies are time consuming, relatively expensive and not free of risks. Moreover, due the focal characteristics of the process and a limited sample, early or mild lesions may go undiscovered. Changes in renal function or irreversible renal functional impairment are other possible diagnostic tools. However, renal function is most often monitored by SCr levels, a method with notoriously poor sensitivity. GFR measurement by creatinine, radioisotope or inulin clearance can also underestimate actual structural injury due to the kidney's functional reserve capacity. Urinary enzymes such as alanine aminopeptidase or N-acetyl Beta-D-glucosaminidase have high sensitivity but lack specificity. There is an absolute necessity for an accurate and non-invasive process for early detection of chronic nephrotoxicity, in order to prevent or minimize CSA effects on renal tissue. Some potential diagnostic markers have been recently described. Urinary collagen III, and to a lesser extent serum collagen III were shown to be good markers for the amount of renal fibrosis in biopsies from patients with subacute and chronic nephropathies [620]. Haas et al tested the presence of smooth muscle-specific isoform of α-actin (SMA) in the urine of renal transplant patients submitted to renal biopsy. Patients with CSA or TAC chronic nephrotoxicity had increased SMA in urine samples when compared to patients without toxicity or healthy controls. SMA correlated well with arteriolopathy severity at biopsy. Nevertheless, there was an overlapping of values among the three groups, making SMA an unreliable marker for clinical diagnosis of chronic CSA nephrotoxicity [621]. Câmara et al used the rationale that CSA-induced interstitial fibrosis may be associated to subtle proximal tubule dysfunction to test the role of urinary retinol-binding protein as an early marker for development of chronic CSA nephropathy. Retinol-binding protein is a small protein filtered by the glomeruli and almost totally reabsorbed by the proximal tubule, and thus increases in its urinary concentration indicate proximal tubule dysfunction. They studied 36 stable CSA-treated heart transplant recipients and identified two sub-sets of patients, one with high (13 patients) and other with normal (23 patients) urinary concentrations of retinol binding protein. During a five year follow-up period, 46% of the patients in the high urinary retinol binding protein group doubled SCr and 38% of them required dialysis versus 13% doubling SCr and none developing CKD stage 5 in the normal retinol binding protein urinary group [622]. Recently, urinary transforming growth factor-beta-induced gene-h3 (betaig-h3) was found to be higher in patients with histological diagnostic of chronic CSA nephrotoxicity. In addition, betaig-h3 levels correlated positively with the extent of tubulointerstitial fibrosis and decreased in response to CSA discontinuation [623].

At the present time, the availability of preventive measures or treatment for chronic CSA nephrotoxicity is limited. A simple way to avoid CSA-induced renal interstitial fibrosis would be to reduce its dosage or completely withdraw the drug. Different authors have questioned the need for long-term CSA therapy in transplant recipients. This perspective is supported by the point that the most noteworthy benefit of CSA use is a remarkable decrease in early acute rejection rate, and so the drug might have this dose decreased or be discontinued after the initial months of immunosuppression phase, without compromising long term graft survival [278, 372]. As already discussed in the acute CSA nephrotoxicity section this strategy is a matter of debate. Mourad et al. reported that conversion to a sparing or CSA-free immunosuppressive schedule in long-term therapy of renal transplant recipients with histologically demonstrated chronic CSA nephropathy resulted in significant renal function improvement. Unfortunately, renal biopsies after immunosuppressive regime changes were done only in few patients, who demonstrated improvement of the structural injury [624]. Bakker et al randomized patients, three months after renal transplantation, to continue on CSA or to be converted to azathioprine treatment. Patients on the azathioprine arm had 6.4% incidence of chronic allograft nephropathy, while in the CSA group the incidence was 23.5% [388].

A number of authors report a beneficial effect of CSA dose reduction or discontinuation in conjunction with maintenance or introduction of mycophenolate mofetil (MMF) in patients with histologically proved or clinically suspected chronic CSA nephropathy. Improvement in renal function was the rule and decrease in serum TGF-β after MMF introduction has been described. Nearly all studies did not perform sequential or follow-up biopsies after the immunosuppressive schedule change [401, 408, 551, 625-629]. One of the few papers with histological data available showed that MMF immunosuppressive therapy was associated with less renal fibrosis and delayed expression of CSA nephrotoxicity, in a retrospectively evaluation of protocol kidney biopsies from renal transplant recipients [630]. The number of papers showing that MMF arrests renal injury in experimental models of progressive nephropathy [631-633] raised the question if the beneficial effects of MMF in CSA-treated patients is just the result of CSA dose change/withdrawal or a specific consequence of MMF therapy. In our laboratory, we did not find a specific MMF effect on the prevention of chronic CSA nephrotoxicity in the salt-depleted rat model, suggesting that the renal function improvement seen in the clinical studies was probably due to CSA reduction or discontinuation [634]. Consistent with our results, co-treatment of CSA and MMF in salt-depleted rats did not prevent chronic CSA nephrotoxicity, but MMF treatment after CSA withdrawal promoted a further improvement in renal function and histology when compared to CSA withdrawal-only group [635].

Another alternative for CSA reduction or withdrawal is the introduction of sirolimus in the immunosuppressive schedule. At the moment, there is already some information on the effects of this maneuver on the renal histology changes caused by CSA. In prospective renal transplant trials, the early discontinuation of CSA with sirolimus maintenance was associated with better renal function, reduction in the progression of chronic histologic damage and lower incidence of new cases and severity of chronic allograft nephropathy [636, 637]. When renal transplant recipients were switched from CSA to sirolimus for biopsy-proved chronic allograft nephropathy or calcineurin inhibitor nephrotoxicity, a significant improvement in renal function has been observed in the majority of the patients. However, kidney biopsies performed two years after conversion, did not show renal histology improvement [421]. The concomitant use of CSA and sirolimus should be considered with caution. In the salt-depleted rat chronic CSA nephrotoxicity model, sirolimus given together CSA potentiated the functional and structural toxic effects of CSA on the kidney, and the increases in renal

TGF-β and extracellular matrix proteins [638].

There are few data about pharmacological management of chronic CSA nephrotoxicity in the clinical setting. McCulloch et al studied the effects of nifedipine in CSA-induced interstitial fibrosis in renal transplantation. The authors compared three groups of patients (conventional CSA dose versus conventional CSA dose plus nifedipine versus low CSA dose plus azathioprine) measuring baseline cortical interstitial volume fraction after one, six and 12 months of therapy. After six and 12 months interstitial volume was lower in patients treated with CSA plus nifedipine as compared with the two other groups, but the results only reached statistical significance at 6 months. GFR was significantly lower in CSA-treated patients as compared to CSA plus nifedipine and CSA plus azathioprine. There was a negative correlation between GFR and interstitial volume fraction [639]. Use of losartan in renal transplant recipients with chronic allograft nephropathy decreased systemic TGF-beta levels, indirectly suggesting a possible reduction in the renal fibrogenic process [640].

Tacrolimus nephrotoxicity

The nephrotoxic profile of tacrolimus is usually considered similar to that of CSA, although some authors attribute less functional nephrotoxicity to TAC [641-643]. In fact, when these drugs were administrated to healthy individuals, only the individuals receiving CSA showed decreases in GFR and RBF and blood pressure increase [644].

Tacrolimus can induce acute and reversible renal dysfunction, chronic and irreversible renal structural injury, electrolyte disturbances, renal tubular acidosis and hemolytic-uremic syndrome [278, 645-651]. On the other hand, TAC induces less hypertension and more impairment of glucose metabolism than CSA [278, 646, 647, 651-653]. Similar to CSA, concomitant TAC administration with drugs interfering with the cytochrome P450 system or nephrotoxic drugs, can precipitate acute kidney dysfunction [654-659]. Acute tacrolimus nephrotoxicity was also reported with the co-administration of TAC and metoclopramide. This association caused high TAC blood levels, probably due to increased drug bioavailability caused by improved gastric motility [660].

Acute nephrotoxicity

Tacrolimus acute nephrotoxicity can be manifested as asymptomatic changes in GFR, clinically significant AKI and HUS [290, 661-675]. Paradoxically, TAC has been used as an alternative treatment for patients with CSA-induced HUS [676, 677]. However, cases of HUS recurrence after conversion from CSA to TAC have been reported, indicating that this approach is not completely safe [678].

Tacrolimus causes acute reversible renal dysfunction in renal [661-663, 667], liver [290, 664-666, 679, 680], heart [681-683] and pulmonary [684, 685] transplant recipients and in patients with immunologically mediated diseases [686]. Tacrolimus-induced GFR and RBF decrease is associated with an important increase in renal vascular resistance, both in humans and rodents [63, 679, 687-692]. Calcium channel blockers improved renal function in TAC-treated liver transplant recipients [693] and in animal models of TAC nephrotoxicity [689, 694-696]. Tacrolimus acute nephrotoxicity, similar to CSA, shows normal renal histology or non-specific changes such as isometric cytoplasmic vacuolation in tubular epithelial cells, microcalcification, giant mitochondria and lysosomes, and necrosis and early hyalinosis of individual smooth muscle cells in the afferent arterioles, which revert with drug reduction or discontinuation [697-699].

Tacrolimus dose does not correlate with renal dysfunction, but TAC trough levels have a strong correlation with drug exposure and high trough levels have been associated with episodes of nephrotoxicity [327, 660, 662, 700]. Tacrolimus trough levels < 5 ng/ml are associated with a 5% risk of nephrotoxicity but a 50% risk of rejection. At trough levels of 25 ng/ml there was no rejection but the nephrotoxicity frequency rose to 90%. Therefore, a good compromise for efficient immunosuppression with less nephrotoxicity is to keep TAC blood levels between 10 to 15 ng/ml [327].

Clinical and animal studies suggest that TAC and CSA may have distinct effects on renal vascular resistance. Some authors did not find changes in RVR after high single IV injection of TAC *in vivo* or when the drug was used in the isolated auto perfused rat kidney model [701, 702]. Two weeks of CSA but not TAC administration to healthy individuals reduced GFR and RBF and increased blood pressure [644]. In an interesting study, intra-renal transplant hemodynamics were assessed immediately after CSA or TAC dosing and only CSA caused renal hypoperfusion [703]. Conversely, Hadad et al found glomerular hemodynamic changes in rats treated with TAC similar to that previously described for CSA. Tacrolimus caused a significant decrease in single nephron GFR, glomerular plasma flow rate and glomerular ultrafiltration coefficient and a significant increase in total arteriolar resistance. The addition of this drug to cultured mesangial cells significantly reduced cell cross sectional area and increased intracellular calcium concentration [688].

Most of the mechanisms associated to CSA-induced acute nephrotoxicity are also evoked for TAC functional nephrotoxicity. Evidence favoring a role for RAS came from studies showing juxtaglomerular apparatus (JGA) hyperplasia, increase of renin-containing JGA, increased extent of renin immunostaining along afferent arterioles, enhancement of TAC nephrotoxicity by salt-depletion, increased PRA and cortical renin mRNA in TAC-treated rats [687, 704-708]. Stillman et al showed that JGA granularity did not correlate with systemic PRA levels in TAC-treated rats, which suggests a local activation of the RAS [705]. Administration of captopril did not prevent TAC-induced GFR fall in rats [709].

A possible role for prostaglandins in TAC acute nephrotoxicity has been explored with conflicting results. Textor et al reported a TAC-induced decrease in urinary 6-keto-PG-F1-α and thromboxane B_2 in liver transplant recipients [679]. In SHR rats, acute TAC nephrotoxicity was associated with increased urinary TXB_2 and decreased 6-keto-PG-F1-α [695]. Benigni et al did not find changes in the release of TxB_2 and 6-keto-PG-F1-α by bovine endothelial cells, even after 24-hr incubation with increasing concentrations of TAC [701]. In contrast, McCauley et al showed a TAC-induced decrease in TXB_2 and increase in PGE_2 production by mesangial cells [710]. Juniper oil supplementation in TAC-treated rats elevated significantly urinary PGF2-alpha, and incorporated vasodilatory prostanoids in the renal cell membrane while completely preventing the GFR fall caused by TAC [711].

Data about TAC effects on endothelin system and its association with acute nephrotoxicity are conflicting. Tacrolimus caused urinary endothelin increase in denervated isolated perfused rat kidney and in liver transplant recipients [63, 689]. Elevated serum levels of endothelin were found in kidney and simultaneous kidney/pancreas transplant recipients suffering from TAC-induced microangiopathy [669]. Tacrolimus stimulated the secretion of ET-1 by cultured tubular cells and increased serum endothelin levels in rats [712]. Tacrolimus enhanced ET release by rat mesangial cells and rabbit proximal tubule cells [713, 714] but not by LLC-PK1 epithelial cells or cultured bovine endothelial cells [701, 715]. In human endothelial cells, TAC only increased ET-1 secretion and ET-1 mRNA when extremely high doses were used, but not when clinically relevant doses were added to the medium [716]. In a comparative study, TAC showed a weaker effect than CSA on stimulation of pre-pro ET-1 mRNA [717]. Use of ET receptor antagonists for prevention of acute TAC nephrotoxicity was disappointing. Although TAC augmented ET-1 mRNA levels in SHR, use of an ET_A/ET_B receptor antagonist did not reverse GFR fall and only partially attenuated RVR increase [718]. In the same way, use of an ET_A receptor antagonist, in a dose previously demonstrated as effective for blocking renal effects of exogenous ET infusion, did not prevent GFR decrease in TAC-treated rats [719]. Likewise, an ET_A receptor antagonist only provided partial prevention against TAC-induced GFR decrease but did not alleviate perfusate flow rate fall and perfusion resistance increase in an isolated perfused rat kidney model [689]. Taken together these data show that, as opposed to what was demonstrated for CSA, the role of endothelin in acute TAC nephrotoxicity remains to be unproven.

Tacrolimus capacity to blockade NO pathway is well demonstrated. NO plays a major role in the pathogenesis of cerebral hypoxia-ischemia injury mediated by glutamate/N-methyl-D-aspartate (NDMA). This injury depends on intracellular calcium influx through NDMA receptor channels, which activate calcineurin with consequent dephosphorylation of constitutive NO synthase (cNOS). Tacrolimus addition to cultured neuronal cells reduced NDMA-mediated toxicity, through the inhibition of calcineurin activation, inhibition of cNOS dephosphorylation and consequent decrease in

NO production [720]. Tacrolimus reduced NO activity and NO production in cultured mice macrophage and rat vascular smooth muscle cells. In these studies TAC showed a weaker inhibitory effect than CSA, suggesting that suppression of NO synthase by both drugs occurred through distinct mechanisms [96, 721, 722]. Dusting et al found that only CSA but not TAC suppressed NO production when clinically relevant doses of these drugs were added to a murine macrophage cell line and rat vascular smooth muscle cells in culture, raising doubts if NO blockade is really implicated in TAC nephrotoxicity [96]. Strestikova et al using cultured rat peritoneal macrophages, showed that TAC and CSA blocked inducible NO synthase by different mechanisms, at the transcriptional level for TAC and post-transcriptionally for CSA. However, in this study the inhibitory effect elicited by TAC was clearly more potent than the one obtained with CSA [723]. The evaluation of the interplay between TAC and NO has also provided some divergent results, which do not fit the concept of TAC-induced NO blockade as a key mechanism in TAC nephrotoxicity. For instance, TAC has been shown to up regulate endothelial NO synthase mRNA expression in cultured bovine aortic cells [185]. Tacrolimus-treated rats presented an increase in urinary nitric oxide excretion [724] and nitric oxide enhanced TAC-induced proximal tubular epithelial cell apoptosis [725]. Incubation with L-arginine caused a significant reduction in acetylcholine-induced sensitivity in arteries isolated from rats treated with TAC [726] and CSA, but not TAC inhibited mRNA expression of inducible NO synthase in murine macrophage cells [727]. Manipulation of the system has also provided contradictory results. L-NAME administration to TAC treated rats resulted in decreased NO urinary excretion and enhancement of renal dysfunction [724]. Wataray et al only found RBF reduction and RVR increase when rats were treated concomitantly with TAC and L-NAME, but not with TAC alone [728]. Administration of L-arginine simultaneously to renal arteries clamping in a rat model of ischemic AKI in TAC-treated animals induced partial protection on renal function and hemodynamics [729]. In contrast, administration of L-arginine in a rat model of TAC acute nephrotoxicity was unable to prevent functional renal injury, although L-arginine-treated rats presented significantly higher amounts of urinary NO [730].

Other mediators and mechanisms have been related to TAC acute nephrotoxicity, such as decreased serum fibrinolytic activity [731], sympathetic overactivity [156, 732], increased renal glutathione levels [733], increased serotonin production [690], adenosine [734] and dose timing of TAC administration [735].

Tacrolimus may induce tubular dysfunction characterized as an increased excretion of urinary enzymes, decreased urinary concentrating ability, increased fractional excretion of magnesium in the presence of hypomagnesemia, hyperkalemia, hyperuricemia and tubular acidosis [12, 260, 645, 647, 705, 736, 737]. *In vitro* studies showed that TAC inhibit Na/K – ATPase in rat microdissected cortical collecting duct and medullary thick ascending limb [738], and that high TAC doses added to primary human proximal tubules cultures decreased cell proliferation after 72 hours of incubation [739]. In the same way, only elevated concentrations of TAC had a direct cytotoxic effect on LLC-PK1 tubular cell line [712]. In accordance with these results, Cuvello Neto et al found that TAC was toxic to oxygenated isolated proximal tubules only in high concentrations [740]. Tacrolimus cytotoxicity seems to be mediated by a transient increase in intracellular calcium and by oxygen free radicals [740-742]. In fact, tea polyphenols, substances with anti-oxidant properties, protected LLC-PK1 cells against TAC induced-apoptosis [743].

When analyzed as a whole, the data about acute TAC nephrotoxicity suggest that although the net effect of this drug on vascular reactivity, tubular cells and renal function is similar to that caused by CSA, the mechanisms of TAC-induced functional renal injury are probably distinct from those implicated in CSA-induced acute nephrotoxicity.

Attempts to minimize TAC-induced renal dysfunction by TAC switch to sirolimus [419, 744, 745] or use of low-dose maintenance TAC therapy associated with lymphocyte depleting agents, mycophenolate mofetil or sirolimus have been successfully achieved [746-750]. However, the association of TAC and sirolimus does not seem to be problem-free. Severe acute kidney injury in renal transplant recipients and thrombotic microangiopathy in intestinal transplant have been associated to combined use of TAC and sirolimus [751, 752], renal function improved in renal transplant recipients after conversion from TAC/sirolimus to TAC/MMF therapy [753] and TAC/sirolimus combination was associated to worst renal allograft survival than TAC/MMF immunosuppression [754].

Chronic nephrotoxicity

After the launching of TAC for clinical use, it rapidly became apparent that the new immunosuppressive drug could induce chronic kidney structural injury identical to that seen in CSA-treated patients. In a blinded analysis of renal biopsies from renal transplant recipients randomized to receive either CSA or TAC, Randhawa et al documented for the first time that chronic renal histological injury caused by the two drugs was indistinguishable, qualitatively and quantitatively. Both groups showed a similar prevalence and severity of striped fibrosis, arteriolar hyalinosis and peritubular calcification [755]. Subsequently, several authors confirmed these findings, describing TAC-related chronic structural changes absolutely similar to that caused by CSA in transplant recipients and in patients with immunologically mediated disease [697, 756-761]. Moreover, Solez et al reported that CSA and TAC caused a similar prevalence of chronic allograft nephropathy in 144 cadaveric kidney recipients (62% in TAC and 72.3% in CSA). The authors did not find any histological difference when comparing TAC and CSA biopsies. A multivariate analysis disclosed nephrotoxicity and acute rejection as the most significant predictors for chronic allograft nephropathy in this group of patients [762]. Permanent functional impairment and CKD stage 5 have been described in in liver and heart transplant recipients treated with TAC [664, 681].

Andoh et al developed an experimental model of TAC-induced chronic nephrotoxicity using salt-depletion in rats [687, 704]. A particular characteristic of this model is that renal functional changes and structural injury occur with TAC blood levels equivalent to those found in treated patients, in a striking contrast with the CSA chronic nephrotoxicity model, where extremely high CSA blood levels are necessary to produce injury. In this TAC model, there is an early and dose-dependent decrease in GFR and RBF with a parallel RVR increase followed by a late development of renal interstitial fibrosis involving the inner strip and medullary rays, arteriolar hyalinosis, tubular atrophy and hypertrophy and medullary thick ascending limb size variance. Structural injury showed a significant positive correlation with decreased renal function [687, 704, 705].

Using this model, Shihab et al explored some of the possible mechanisms of TAC-induced chronic nephrotoxicity. They found that TAC induced a progressive increase in renal vessels and tubulointerstitial expression of mRNA for TGF-β, matrix proteins and the protease inhibitor, plasminogen activator inhibitor 1. Therefore, TAC at the same time it induces a TGF-β-related increase in extracellular matrix proteins blocked its degradation. There was an early and sustained increase in systemic PRA and renal tissue renin mRNA, suggesting a participation of this system in the genesis of interstitial fibrosis [763]. Additional evidence pointing for a role of RAS in chronic TAC nephrotoxicity came from the study of Stillman et al, which demonstrated increased juxtaglomerular apparatus granularity in sal-depleted rats given TAC. Juxtaglomerular apparatus granularity did not correlate with systemic renin, suggesting local RAS activation, but strongly correlate with the degree of structural injury [705]. Andoh et al provided supplementary support for RAS role in TAC-induced chronic nephrotoxicity, showing that concomitant treatment with losartan partially prevented the development of TAC-induced interstitial fibrosis in salt-depleted rats [764]. Pharmacological inhibition of the RAS by quinapril or valsartan also attenuated renal fibrosis and decreased fibrogenic cytokine expression in TAC-treated rats [765].

Another mechanism that may contribute to TAC-induced renal fibrosis is increased IL-6 production through NF-Kappa B activation of non-lymphoid cells. Tacrolimus stimulates this inducible transcription factor, which enhances IL-6 production in fibroblasts and mesangial cells. IL-6 in turn triggers mesangial cell proliferation and extracellular matrix production [651, 766]. Inhibition of NF-Kappa B suppressed monocyte/macrophage renal infiltration and attenuated interstitial fibrosis and tubular atrophy in TAC treated rats [767, 768].

Functional and histological protection was also provided in rat models of chronic TAC nephrotoxicity by the anti-fibrotic agent pirfenidone, by plant polyphenols and by anti-TGF-β antibodies [769-771].

There are few data on clinical strategies to avoid or minimize TAC-induced chronic nephrotoxicity. Patients with biopsy proved chronic allograft nephropathy or TAC chronic nephrotoxicity showed renal function improvement after switch from TAC to sirolimus or reduction of TAC dosage and introduction of MMF [421, 772, 773]. Early calcineurin inhibitor withdrawal, before significant renal structural damage occurs, may be the best option for improve chronic calcineurin inhibitors nephrotoxicity [774].

Clinical and experimental studies suggest that TAC might have less renal pro-fibrogenic potential than CSA. Using a rat model of renal ischemia-reperfusion associated with pro fibrotic genes up-regulation, Jain et al found that TAC-treated animals developed less proteinuria and lower SCr than CSA-treated rats. The authors also found that TAC-treated rats had decreased expression of TGF-β and tissue inhibitor of metalloproteinase 1 mRNA. CSA did not change TGF-β or tissue inhibitor of metalloproteinase 1 mRNA, but increased collagen III expression and reduced matrix degrading proteins expression (MMP-2 and MMP-9), although those changes did not reach statistical significance [775]. One possible explanation for the discrepancy in TGF-β expression results between this and the previous study that showed enhancement of TGF-β is that Jain et al used 0.2 mg/kg of TAC while Shihab et al used 1 mg/kg of the drug [763, 775]. When TGF-β and its receptors type I and type II were measured in rats treated with CSA or TAC, the expression of mRNA and protein for TGF-β and both receptors was lower in TAC-treated animals as compared to the CSA group [776]. Differences between the fibrogenic potential of CSA and TAC were also suggested by the analysis of fibrosis-associated genes in isolated glomeruli obtained from renal biopsies of TAC and CSA-treated transplant recipients. Expression of collagen III and tissue inhibitor of metalloproteinase 1 were significantly higher in CSA-treated individuals. Interestingly, mRNA expression for TGF-β was similar in both groups [777]. The improvement in renal function seem in patients with biopsy proved chronic allograft nephropathy after switch from CSA to TAC might be related to this putatively less pro-fibrogenic effect of TAC [778-781].

In summary, TAC produces tubulointerstitial fibrosis indistinguishable from that seen with CSA. The pathogenic mechanisms for this structural injury are apparently similar to those described for CSA. The premise that TAC has less fibrogenic effect on renal tissue than CSA remains to be conclusively determined.

mTOR inhibitors - Sirolimus and Everolimus nephrotoxicity

The molecular targets of rapamycin inhibitors (mTOR), sirolimus and everolimus, have a distinct mechanism of immunosuppressive action different from the calcineurin inhibitors cyclosporine and TAC. As such, they are expected to be minimally nephrotoxic per se.

Renal tubular dysfunction is described in animals but human expression in unclear [12]. Most use of mTOR inhibitors is in conjunction with lowered doses of calcineurin inhibitors since it is known that these two drug classes have a potent drug-drug interaction leading to enhanced renal dysfunction compared to the calcineurin inhibitor alone [782]. This may be explained by inhibition of drug efflux pump P-glycoprotein since both sirolimus and the calcineurin inhibitors are competitive substrates [783, 784].

Other manifestations of mTOR inhibitor renal effects are delayed recovery from ischemic renal injury. In rats not on cyclosporine, sirolimus impairs recovery from acute renal ischemia [785]. Human series describe delayed recovery from post-transplant ischemic injury, and worsening function in glomerulonephritis in the presence of sirolimus [786-787]. Few studies have tested TAC and everolimus for similar changes [788].

Proteinuria usually reversible on drug withdrawal is a recently described adverse effect associated with sirolimus [789-791]. The renal pathological picture is focal glomerulosclerosis and the pathogenesis is obscure, although podocyte dysregulation is suggested [792]. "Release" from vasoconstriction imposed by prior calcineurin inhibitors also has been proposed but direct evidence for this is lacking [793]. mTOR inhibitors may have differential effects producing no renal dysfunction in uninjured kidneys while structural and functional effects may occur in kidneys undergoing ischemic or inflammatory stress [788].

References

1. Cohen DJ, Loertscher R, Rubin MF, Tilney NL, Carpenter CB, Strom TB. Cyclosporine: a new immunosuppressive agent for organ transplantation. Ann Intern Med 1984; 101: 667-682.
2. Kahan BD. Cyclosporine. N Engl J Med 1989; 321: 1725-1738.
3. de Mattos AM, Olyaei AJ, Bennett WM. Pharmacology of immunosuppressive medications used in renal diseases and transplantation. Am J Kidney Dis 1996; 28: 631-667.
4. Langford CA, Klippel JH, Balow JE, James SP, Sneller MC. Use of cytotoxic agents and cyclosporine in the treatment of autoimmune disease. Part 1: rheumatologic and renal diseases. Ann Intern Med 1998; 128: 1021-1028.
5. Langford CA, Klippel JH, Balow JE, James SP, Sneller MC. Use of cytotoxic agents and cyclosporine in the treatment of autoimmune disease. Part 2: Inflammatory bowel disease, systemic vasculitis, and therapeutic toxicity. Ann Intern Med 1998; 129: 49-58.
6. Ponticelli C. Calcineurin-inhibitors in renal transplantation. Too precious to be abandoned. Nephrol Dial Transplant 2000; 15: 1307-1309.
7. Keown P, Niese D. Cyclosporine microemulsion increases drug exposure and reduces acute rejection without incremental toxicity in de novo renal transplantation. International Sandimmun Neoral Study Group. Kidney Int 1998; 54: 938-944.
8. Starzl TE, Todo S, Fung J, Demetris AJ, Venkataramman R, Jain A. FK 506 for liver, kidney, and pancreas transplantation. Lancet 1989; 2: 1000-1004.
9. A comparison of tacrolimus (FK 506) and cyclosporine for immunosuppression in liver transplantation. The U.S. Multicenter FK506 Liver Study Group. N Engl J Med 1994; 331: 1110-1115.
10. Spencer CM, Goa KL, Gillis JC. Tacrolimus. An update of its pharmacology and clinical efficacy in the management of organ transplantation. Drugs 1997; 54: 925-975.
11. Opelz G. Immunosuppression with FK 506 does not improve kidney graft survival. Collaborative Transplant Study. Transplant Proc 1999; 31: 1147-1148.
12. Andoh TF, Burdmann EA, Fransechini N, Houghton DC, Bennett WM. Comparison of acute rapamycin nephrotoxicity with cyclosporine and FK506. Kidney Int 1996; 50: 1110-1117.
13. Campistol JM, Sacks SH. Mechanisms of nephrotoxicity. Transplantation 2000; 69: SS5-SS10.
14. Aramburu J, Yaffe MB, Lopez-Rodriguez C, Cantley LC, Hogan PG, Rao A. Affinity-driven peptide selection of an NFAT inhibitor more selective than cyclosporin A. Science 1999; 285: 2129-2133.
15. English J, Evan A, Houghton DC, Bennett WM. Cyclosporine-induced acute renal dysfunction in the rat. Evidence of arteriolar vasoconstriction with preservation of tubular function. Transplantation 1987; 44: 135-141.
16. Potier M, Wolf A, Cambar J. Comparative study of cyclosporin A, cyclosporin G, and the novel cyclosporin derivative IMM 125 in isolated glomeruli and cultured rat mesangial cells: a morphometric analysis. Nephrol Dial Transplant 1998; 13: 1406-1411.
17. Klein IH, Abrahams A, van Ede T, Hené RJ, Koomans HA, Ligtenberg G. Different effects of tacrolimus and cyclosporine on renal hemodynamics and blood pressure in healthy subjects. Transplantation 2002; 73: 732-736.
18. Mihatsch MJ, Thiel G, Ryffel B. Histopathology of cyclosporine nephrotoxicity. Transplant Proc 1988; 20: 759-771.
19. Conger JD, Kim GE, Robinette JB. Effects of ANG II, ETA, and TxA2 receptor antagonists on cyclosporin A renal vasoconstriction. Am J Physiol 1994; 267: F443-F449.
20. L'Azou B, Medina J, Frieauff W, Cordier A, Cambar J, Wolf A. *In vitro* models to study mechanisms involved in cyclosporine A-mediated glomerular contraction. Arch Toxicol 1999; 73: 337-345.
21. Mason J, Muller-Schweinitzer E, Dupont M, Casellas D, Mihatsch M, Moore L, Kaskel F. Cyclosporine and the renin-angiotensin system. Kidney Int Suppl 1991; 32: S28-S32.
22. Lee DB. Cyclosporine and the renin-angiotensin axis. Kidney Int 1997; 52: 248-260.
23. Whiting PH, Cunningham C, Thomson AW, Simpson JG. Enhancement of high dose cyclosporin A toxicity by frusemide. Biochem Pharmacol 1984; 33: 1075-1079.
24. Swan SK, Bennett WM. Role of the sodium ion in acute renal failure. Miner Electrolyte Metab 1991; 17: 89-99.
25. Lustig S, Stern N, Eggena P, Tuck ML, Lee DB. Effect of cyclosporin on blood pressure and renin-aldosterone axis in rats. Am J Physiol 1987; 253: H1596-H1600.
26. Perico N, Zoja C, Benigni A, Ghilardi F, Gualandris L, Remuzzi G. Effect of short-term cyclosporine administration in rats on renin-angiotensin and thromboxane A2: possible relevance to the reduction in glomerular filtration rate. J Pharmacol Exp Ther 1986; 239: 229-235.
27. Shehata M, el Nahas M, Barkworth E, Cope GH, Raftery AT. Localization of PDGF-BB in the juxtaglomerular cells of cyclosporin-treated rats. Exp Nephrol 1995; 3: 173-179.
28. Verpooten GA, Wybo I, Pattyn VM, Hendrix PG, Giuliano RA, Nouwen EJ, Roels F, De Broe ME. Cyclosporine nephrotoxicity: comparative cytochemical study of rat kidney and human allograft biopsies. Clin Nephrol 1986; 25 Suppl 1: S18-S22.

29. Tufro-McReddie A, Gomez RA, Norling LL, Omar AA, Moore LC, Kaskel FJ. Effect of CsA on the expression of renin and angiotensin type 1 receptor genes in the rat kidney. Kidney Int 1993; 43: 615-622.
30. Regitz-Zagrosek V, Auch-Schwelk W, Hess B, Klein U, Duske E, Steffen C, Hildebrandt AG, Fleck E. Tissue- and subtype-specific modulation of angiotensin II receptors by chronic treatment with cyclosporin A, angiotensin-converting enzyme inhibitors and AT1 antagonists. J Cardiovasc Pharmacol 1995; 26: 66-72.
31. Avdonin PV, Cottet-Maire F, Afanasjeva GV, Loktionova SA, Lhote P, Ruegg UT. Cyclosporine A up-regulates angiotensin II receptors and calcium responses in human vascular smooth muscle cells. Kidney Int 1999; 55: 2407-2414.
32. Baxter CR, Duggin GG, Hall BM, Horvath JS, Tiller DJ. Stimulation of renin release from rat renal cortical slices by cyclosporin A. Res Commun Chem Pathol Pharmacol 1984; 43: 417-423.
33. Kurtz A, Della BR, Kuhn K. Cyclosporine A enhances renin secretion and production in isolated juxtaglomerular cells. Kidney Int 1988; 33: 947-953.
34. Hestin D, Mertes PM, Hubert J, Claudon M, Mejat E, Renoult E, Pertek JP, Frimat L, Burlet C, Kessler M. Relationship between blood pressure and renin, angiotensin II and atrial natriuretic factor after renal transplantation. Clin Nephrol 1997; 48: 98-103.
35. Julien J, Farge D, Kreft-Jais C, Guyene TT, Plouin PF, Houssin D, Carpentier A, Corvol P. Cyclosporine-induced stimulation of the renin-angiotensin system after liver and heart transplantation. Transplantation 1993; 56: 885-891.
36. Gardiner DS, Watson MA, Junor BJ, Briggs JD, More IA, Lindop GB. The effect of conversion from cyclosporin to azathioprine on renin- containing cells in renal allograft biopsies. Nephrol Dial Transplant 1991; 6: 363-367.
37. Abraham JS, Bentley FR, Garrison RN. The role of intrarenal prostaglandins and angiotensin II in acute cyclosporine-induced vasoconstriction. Surgery 1991; 110: 343-349.
38. Barros EJ, Boim MA, Ajzen H, Ramos OL, Schor N. Glomerular hemodynamics and hormonal participation on cyclosporine nephrotoxicity. Kidney Int 1987; 32: 19-25.
39. Prevot A, Semama DS, Tendron A, Justrabo E, Guignard JP, Gouyon JB. Endothelin, angiotensin II and adenosine in acute cyclosporine A nephrotoxicity. Pediatr Nephrol 2000; 14: 927-934.
40. Pérez-Rojas JM, Derive S, Blanco JA, Cruz C, Martínez de la Maza L, Gamba G, Bobadilla NA. Renocortical mRNA expression of vasoactive factors during spironolactone protective effect in chronic cyclosporine nephrotoxicity. Am J Physiol Renal Physiol 2005; 289: F1020-1030.
41. Gerkens JF, Smith AJ. Effect of captopril and theophylline treatment on cyclosporine-induced nephrotoxicity in rats. Transplantation 1985; 40: 213-214.
42. Gillum DM, Truong L. Effects of chronic volume expansion and enalapril on chronic cyclosporine nephropathy. Am J Physiol 1990; 258: F934-F939.
43. Grieve EM, Hawksworth GM, Simpson JG, Whiting PH. Effect of thromboxane synthetase inhibition and angiotensin converting enzyme inhibition on acute cyclosporin A nephrotoxicity. Biochem Pharmacol 1990; 40: 2323-2329.
44. Kaskel FJ, Devarajan P, Arbeit LA, Partin JS, Moore LC. Cyclosporine nephrotoxicity: sodium excretion, autoregulation, and angiotensin II. Am J Physiol 1987; 252: F733-F742.
45. Bantle JP, Paller MS, Boudreau RJ, Olivari MT, Ferris TF. Long-term effects of cyclosporine on renal function in organ transplant recipients. J Lab Clin Med 1990; 115: 233-240.
46. Inigo P, Campistol JM, Lario S, Piera C, Campos B, Bescos M, Oppenheimer F, Rivera F. Effects of losartan and amlodipine on intrarenal hemodynamics and TGF- beta(1) plasma levels in a crossover trial in renal transplant recipients. J Am Soc Nephrol 2001; 12: 822-827.
47. Rondeau E, Paillard F, Peraldi MN, Violet I, Tasse S, Dussaule JC, Ardaillou R, Sraer JD. Role of the renin-angiotensin system on the renal functional reserve in renal transplant recipients. Kidney Int 1993; 44: 165-172.
48. O'Brien RF, Robbins RJ, McMurtry IF. Endothelial cells in culture produce a vasoconstrictor substance. J Cell Physiol 1987; 132: 263-270.
49. Yanagisawa M, Kurihara H, Kimura S, Tomobe Y, Kobayashi M, Mitsui Y, Yazaki Y, Goto K, Masaki T. A novel potent vasoconstrictor peptide produced by vascular endothelial cells. Nature 1988; 332: 411-415.
50. Inoue A, Yanagisawa M, Kimura S, Kasuya Y, Miyauchi T, Goto K, Masaki T. The human endothelin family: three structurally and pharmacologically distinct isopeptides predicted by three separate genes. Proc Natl Acad Sci U S A 1989; 86: 2863-2867.
51. Kohan DE. Endothelins in the normal and diseased kidney. Am J Kidney Dis 1997; 29: 2-26.
52. Watschinger B, Sayegh MH. Endothelin in organ transplantation. Am J Kidney Dis 1996; 27: 151-161.
53. Nakahama H. Stimulatory effect of cyclosporine A on endothelin secretion by a cultured renal epithelial cell line, LLC-PK1 cells. Eur J Pharmacol 1990; 180: 191-192.
54. Nambi P, Pullen M, Contino LC, Brooks DP. Upregulation of renal endothelin receptors in rats with cyclosporine A- induced nephrotoxicity. Eur J Pharmacol 1990; 187: 113-116.

55. Kon V, Sugiura M, Inagami T, Harvie BR, Ichikawa I, Hoover RL. Role of endothelin in cyclosporine-induced glomerular dysfunction. Kidney Int 1990; 37: 1487-1491.
56. Perico N, Dadan J, Remuzzi G. Endothelin mediates the renal vasoconstriction induced by cyclosporine in the rat. J Am Soc Nephrol 1990; 1: 76-83.
57. Takeda M, Breyer MD, Noland TD, Homma T, Hoover RL, Inagami T, Kon V. Endothelin-1 receptor antagonist: effects on endothelin- and cyclosporine-treated mesangial cells. Kidney Int 1992; 41: 1713-1719.
58. Abassi ZA, Pieruzzi F, Nakhoul F, Keiser HR. Effects of cyclosporin A on the synthesis, excretion, and metabolism of endothelin in the rat. Hypertension 1996; 27: 1140-1148.
59. Grekas D, Bamichas G, Karamouzis M, Bacharaki D, Savidis N, Tourkantonis A. Plasma endothelin in cyclosporine A-treated renal transplant patients. Transplant Proc 1999; 31: 1703-1705.
60. Grieff M, Loertscher R, Shohaib SA, Stewart DJ. Cyclosporine-induced elevation in circulating endothelin-1 in patients with solid-organ transplants. Transplantation 1993; 56: 880-884.
61. Kon V, Awazu M. Endothelin and cyclosporine nephrotoxicity. Ren Fail 1992; 14: 345-350.
62. Perico N, Ruggenenti P, Gaspari F, Mosconi L, Benigni A, Amuchastegui CS, Gasparini F, Remuzzi G. Daily renal hypoperfusion induced by cyclosporine in patients with renal transplantation. Transplantation 1992; 54: 56-60.
63. Textor SC, Burnett JC, Jr., Romero JC, Canzanello VJ, Taler SJ, Wiesner R, Porayko M, Krom R, Gores G, Hay E. Urinary endothelin and renal vasoconstriction with cyclosporine or FK506 after liver transplantation. Kidney Int 1995; 47: 1426-1433.
64. Gonzalez-Santiago L, Lopez-Ongil S, Lamas S, Quereda C, Rodriguez-Puyol M, Rodriguez-Puyol D. Imbalance in endothelial vasoactive factors as a possible cause of cyclosporin toxicity: a role for endothelin-converting enzyme. J Lab Clin Med 2000; 136: 395-401.
65. Takeda Y, Miyamori I, Wu P, Yoneda T, Furukawa K, Takeda R. Effects of an endothelin receptor antagonist in rats with cyclosporine-induced hypertension. Hypertension 1995; 26: 932-936.
66. Nakayama Y, Nonoguchi H, Kiyama S, Ikebe M, Tashima Y, Shimada K, Tanzawa K, Tomita K. Intranephron distribution and regulation of endothelin-converting enzyme-1 in cyclosporin A-induced acute renal failure in rats. J Am Soc Nephrol 1999; 10: 562-571.
67. Marsen TA, Weber F, Egink G, Suckau G, Baldamus CA. Cyclosporin A induces prepro endothelin-1 gene transcription in human endothelial cells. Eur J Pharmacol 1999; 379: 97-106.
68. Fogo A, Hellings SE, Inagami T, Kon V. Endothelin receptor antagonism is protective in *in vivo* acute cyclosporine toxicity. Kidney Int 1992; 42: 770-774.
69. Cavarape A, Endlich K, Feletto F, Parekh N, Bartoli E, Steinhausen M. Contribution of endothelin receptors in renal microvessels in acute cyclosporine-mediated vasoconstriction in rats. Kidney Int 1998; 53: 963-969.
70. Lanese DM, Conger JD. Effects of endothelin receptor antagonist on cyclosporine-induced vasoconstriction in isolated rat renal arterioles. J Clin Invest 1993; 91: 2144-2149.
71. Meyer-Lehnert H, Bokemeyer D, Friedrichs U, Backer A, Kramer HJ. Cellular mechanisms of cyclosporine A-associated side-effects: role of endothelin. Kidney Int Suppl 1997; 61: S27-S31.
72. Davis LS, Haleen SJ, Doherty AM, Cody WL, Keiser JA. Effects of selective endothelin antagonists on the hemodynamic response to cyclosporin A. J Am Soc Nephrol 1994; 4: 1448-1454.
73. Binet I, Wallnofer A, Weber C, Jones R, Thiel G. Renal hemodynamics and pharmacokinetics of bosentan with and without cyclosporine A. Kidney Int 2000; 57: 224-231.
74. Storogenko M, Pech-Amsellem MA, Kerdine S, Rousselet F, Pallardy M. Cyclosporin-A inhibits human endothelial cells proliferation through interleukin-6-dependent mechanisms. Life Sci 1997; 60: 1487-1496.
75. Zoja C, Furci L, Ghilardi F, Zilio P, Benigni A, Remuzzi G. Cyclosporin-induced endothelial cell injury. Lab Invest 1986; 55: 455-462.
76. Averna M, Barbagallo CM, Ganci A, Giammarresi C, Cefalu AB, Sparacino V, Caputo F, Basili S, Notarbartolo A, Davi G. Determinants of enhanced thromboxane biosynthesis in renal transplantation. Kidney Int 2001; 59: 1574-1579.
77. Malyszko J, Malyszko JS, Pawlak K, Mysliwiec M. The coagulo-lytic system and endothelial function in cyclosporine- treated kidney allograft recipients. Transplantation 1996; 62: 828-830.
78. Schrama YC, van Dam T, Fijnheer R, Hene RJ, de Groot P, Rabelink TJ. Cyclosporine is associated with endothelial dysfunction but not with platelet activation in renal transplantation. Neth J Med 2001; 59: 6-15.
79. Tiemann C, Prohaska W, Korfer R, Korner M, Brinkmann T, Kleesiek K. Effect of cyclosporine A on the release of tissue factor pathway inhibitor from endothelial cells in heart transplant patients and cell culture. Eur J Clin Chem Clin Biochem 1997; 35: 661-667.
80. Evans SM, Giddings JC, Muraki T, Yamamoto J. Expression of von Willebrand factor, P-selectin (CD62P) and thrombomodulin in human endothelial cells in culture modulated by cyclosporin A. Clin Lab Haematol 1997; 19: 115-122.

81. Bobadilla NA, Gamba G, Tapia E, Garcia-Torres R, Bolio A, Lopez-Zetina P, Herrera-Acosta J. Role of NO in cyclosporin nephrotoxicity: effects of chronic NO inhibition and NO synthases gene expression. Am J Physiol 1998; 274: F791-F798.
82. Kone BC, Baylis C. Biosynthesis and homeostatic roles of nitric oxide in the normal kidney. Am J Physiol 1997; 272: F561-F578.
83. Bracht C, Yan XW, LaRocca HP, Sutsch G, Kiowski W. Cyclosporine A and control of vascular tone in the human forearm: influence of post-transplant hypertension. J Hypertens 1999; 17: 357-363.
84. Richards NT, Poston L, Hilton PJ. Cyclosporine A inhibits relaxation but does not induce vasoconstriction in human subcutaneous resistance vessels. J Hypertens 1989; 7: 1-3.
85. Diederich D, Yang Z, Luscher TF. Chronic cyclosporine therapy impairs endothelium-dependent relaxation in the renal artery of the rat. J Am Soc Nephrol 1992; 2: 1291-1297.
86. Gallego MJ, Lopez FA, Riesco A, Monton M, Grandes SM, Barat A, Hernando L, Casado S, Caramelo CA. Blockade of endothelium-dependent responses in conscious rats by cyclosporin A: effect of L-arginine. Am J Physiol 1993; 264: H708-H714.
87. Gallego MJ, Garcia Villalon AL, Lopez Farre AJ, Garcia JL, Garron MP, Casado S, Hernando L, Caramelo CA. Mechanisms of the endothelial toxicity of cyclosporin A. Role of nitric oxide, cGMP, and Ca2+. Circ Res 1994; 74: 477-484.
88. Lee J, Kim SW, Kook H, Kang DG, Kim NH, Choi KC. Effects of L-arginine on cyclosporin-induced alterations of vascular NO/cGMP generation. Nephrol Dial Transplant 1999; 14: 2634-2638.
89. Rego A, Vargas R, Wroblewska B, Foegh ML, Ramwell PW. Attenuation of vascular relaxation and cyclic GMP responses by cyclosporin A. J Pharmacol Exp Ther 1990; 252: 165-170.
90. Roullet JB, Xue H, McCarron DA, Holcomb S, Bennett WM. Vascular mechanisms of cyclosporin-induced hypertension in the rat. J Clin Invest 1994; 93: 2244-2250.
91. Takenaka T, Hashimoto Y, Epstein M. Diminished acetylcholine-induced vasodilation in renal microvessels of cyclosporine-treated rats. J Am Soc Nephrol 1992; 3: 42-50.
92. Assis SM, Monteiro JL, Seguro AC. L-Arginine and allopurinol protect against cyclosporine nephrotoxicity. Transplantation 1997; 63: 1070-1073.
93. Bobadilla NA, Tapia E, Franco M, Lopez P, Mendoza S, Garcia-Torres R, Alvarado JA, Herrera-Acosta J. Role of nitric oxide in renal hemodynamic abnormalities of cyclosporin nephrotoxicity. Kidney Int 1994; 46: 773-779.
94. Vaziri ND, Ni Z, Zhang YP, Ruzics EP, Maleki P, Ding Y. Depressed renal and vascular nitric oxide synthase expression in cyclosporine-induced hypertension. Kidney Int 1998; 54: 482-491.
95. Blanton A, Nsaif R, Hercule H, Oyekan A. Nitric oxide/cytochrome P450 interactions in cyclosporin A-induced effects in the rat. J Hypertens 2006; 24: 1865-1872.
96. Lessio C, de Assunção Silva F, Glória MA, Di Tommaso AB, Gori Mouro M, Di Marco GS, Schor N, Higa EM. Cyclosporine A and NAC on the inducible nitric oxide synthase expression and nitric oxide synthesis in rat renal artery cultured cells. Kidney Int 2005; 68: 2508-2516.
97. Stroes ES, Luscher TF, de Groot FG, Koomans HA, Rabelink TJ. Cyclosporin A increases nitric oxide activity *in vivo*. Hypertension 1997; 29: 570-575.
98. Morris ST, McMurray JJ, Rodger RS, Farmer R, Jardine AG. Endothelial dysfunction in renal transplant recipients maintained on cyclosporine. Kidney Int 2000; 57: 1100-1106.
99. Gossmann J, Radounikli A, Bernemann A, Schellinski O, Raab HP, Bickeboller R, Scheuermann EH. Pathophysiology of cyclosporine-induced nephrotoxicity in humans: a role for nitric oxide? Kidney Blood Press Res 2001; 24: 111-115.
100. Navarro-Antolin J, Rey-Campos J, Lamas S. Transcriptional induction of endothelial nitric oxide gene by cyclosporine A. J Biol Chem 2000; 275: 3075-3080.
101. Sanchez-Lozada LG, Gamba G, Bolio A, Jimenez F, Herrera-Acosta J, Bobadilla NA. Nifedipine prevents changes in nitric oxide synthase mRNA levels induced by cyclosporine. Hypertension 2000; 36: 642-647.
102. Andoh TF, Gardner MP, Bennett WM. Protective effects of dietary L-arginine supplementation on chronic cyclosporine nephrotoxicity. Transplantation 1997; 64: 1236-1240.
103. de Nicola L, Thomsom SC, Wead LM, Brown MR, Gabbai FB. Arginine feeding modifies cyclosporine nephrotoxicity in rats. J Clin Invest 1993; 92: 1859-1865.
104. Chander V, Chopra K. Effect of molsidomine and L-arginine in cyclosporine nephrotoxicity: role of nitric oxide. Toxicology 2005; 207: 463-474.
105. Gardner MP, Houghton DC, Andoh TF, Lindsley J, Bennett WM. Clinically relevant doses and blood levels produce experimental cyclosporine nephrotoxicity when combined with nitric oxide inhibition. Transplantation 1996; 61: 1506-1512.
106. Kuruş M, Eşrefoğlu M, Bay A, Oztürk F. Protective effect of oral L-arginine supplementation on cyclosporine induced nephropathy in rats. Int Urol Nephrol 2005; 37: 587-594.
107. Chander V, Chopra K. Nifedipine attenuates changes in nitric oxide levels, renal oxidative stress, and nephrotoxicity induced by cyclosporine. Ren Fail 2005; 27: 441-450.

108. Lassila M, Finckenberg P, Pere AK, Vapaatalo H, Nurminen ML. Enalapril and valsartan improve cyclosporine A-induced vascular dysfunction in spontaneously hypertensive rats. Eur J Pharmacol 2000; 398: 99-106.
109. Åsberg A, Karsten M, Vassbotn, Hartmann A. Better microvascular function on long-term treatment with lisinopril than nifedipine in renal transplant recipients. Nephrol Dial Transplant 2001; 16: 1465-1470.
110. Chander V, Tirkey N, Chopra K. Resveratrol, a polyphenolic phytoalexin protects against cyclosporine-induced nephrotoxicity through nitric oxide dependent mechanism. Toxicology 2005; 210: 55-64.
111. Gaston RS, Schlessinger SD, Sanders PW, Barker CV, Curtis JJ, Warnock DG. Cyclosporine inhibits the renal response to L-arginine in human kidney transplant recipients. J Am Soc Nephrol 1995; 5: 1426-1433.
112. Koller-Strametz J, Wolzt M, Fuchs C, Putz D, Wisser W, Mensik C, Eichler H, Laufer G, Schmetterer L. Renal hemodynamic effects of L-arginine and sodium nitroprusside in heart transplant recipients. Kidney Int 1999; 55: 1871-1877.
113. Viganò E, Badalamenti G, Paone G, Como G, Finazzi S, Tarantino A, Galmarini D, Ponticelli C. Renal effects of L-arginine infusion in cyclosporine-treated transplant recipients. Transplant Proc 1994; 26: 2622-2623.
114. Andrés A, Morales JM, Praga M, Campo V, Lahera R, García-Robles R, Rodicio JL, Ruilope LM. L-arginine reverses the antinatriuretic effect of cyclosporin in renal transplant patients. Nephrol Dial Transplant 1997; 12: 1437-1440.
115. Bennett WM. Therapeutic implications of arachidonic acid metabolism in transplant-associated acute renal failure. Ren Fail 1992; 14: 261-265.
116. Benigni A, Chiabrando C, Piccinelli A, Perico N, Gavinelli M, Furci L, Patino O, Abbate M, Bertani T, Remuzzi G. Increased urinary excretion of thromboxane B_2 and 2, 3-dinor-TxB_2 in cyclosporin A nephrotoxicity. Kidney Int 1988; 34: 164-174.
117. Coffman TM, Carr DR, Yarger WE, Klotman PE. Evidence that renal prostaglandin and thromboxane production is stimulated in chronic cyclosporine nephrotoxicity. Transplantation 1987; 43: 282-285.
118. Darlametsos IE, Papanikolaou EN, Varonos DD. Effect of nifedipine in cyclosporine-induced nephrotoxicity in rats: roles of the thromboxane and endothelin systems. Prostaglandins Leukot Essent Fatty Acids 2000; 63: 263-269.
119. Grieve EM, Hawksworth GM, Simpson JG, Whiting PH. The reversal of experimental cyclosporin A nephrotoxicity by thromboxane synthetase inhibition. Biochem Pharmacol 1993; 45: 1351-1354.
120. Kawaguchi A, Goldman MH, Shapiro R, Foegh ML, Ramwell PW, Lower R.D. Increase in urinary thromboxane B_2 in rats caused by cyclosporine. Transplantation 1985; 40: 214-216.
121. Kim Y.J., Park Y.H., Moon H.K. Reduction of chronic ciclosporin nephrotoxicity by thromboxane synthase inhibition with OKY-046. Kidney Blood Press Res 1997; 20: 38-43.
122. Perico N, Benigni A, Zoja C, Delaini F, Remuzzi G. Functional significance of exaggerated renal thromboxane A2 synthesis induced by cyclosporin A. Am J Physiol 1986; 251: F581-F587.
123. Spurney RF, Mayros S.D., Collins D, Ruiz P, Klotman P.E., Coffman T. Thromboxane receptor blockade improves cyclosporine nephrotoxicity in rats. Prostaglandins 1990; 39: 135-146.
124. Parra T, de Arriba G, Conejo JR, Cantero M, Arribas I, Rodriguez-Puyol D, Rodriguez-Puyol M, Carballo F. Cyclosporine increases local glomerular synthesis of reactive oxygen species in rats: effect of vitamin E on cyclosporine nephrotoxicity. Transplantation 1998; 66: 1325-1329.
125. Elzinga L, Kelley VE, Houghton DC, Bennett WM. Modification of experimental nephrotoxicity with fish oil as the vehicle for cyclosporine. Transplantation 1987; 43: 271-274.
126. Smeesters C, Chaland P, Giroux L, Moutquin JM, Etienne P, Douglas F, Corman J, St Louis G, Daloze P. Prevention of acute cyclosporine A nephrotoxicity by a thromboxane synthetase inhibitor. Transplant Proc 1988; 20: 658-664.
127. Torras J, Valles J, Sanchez J, Sabate I, Seron D, Carrera M, Castelao AM, Herrero I, Puig-Parellada P, Alsina J, Grino JM. Prevention of experimental cyclosporine nephrotoxicity by dietary supplementation with LSL 90202, a lysine salt of eicosapentaenoic acid. Role of thromboxane and prostacyclin in renal tissue. Nephron 1994; 67: 66-72.
128. Rogers TS, Elzinga L, Bennett WM, Kelley VE. Selective enhancement of thromboxane in macrophages and kidneys in cyclosporine-induced nephrotoxicity. Dietary protection by fish oil. Transplantation 1988; 45: 153-156.
129. Smith SR, Kubacki VB, Rakhit A, Martin LL, Schaffer AV, Jasani MK, Hefty DJ, Johnston T, Cannon C, Bennett WM, Coffman TM. Chronic thromboxane synthase inhibition with CGS 12970 in human cyclosporine nephrotoxicity. Transplantation 1993; 56: 1422-1426.
130. Badalamenti S, Salerno F, Lorenzano E, Paone G, Como G, Finazzi S, Sacchetta AC, Rimola A, Graziani G, Galmarini D, Ponticelli C. Renal effects of dietary supplementation with fish oil in cyclosporine- treated liver transplant recipients. Hepatology 1995; 22: 1695-71.
131. Hansen JM, Johansen NJ, Mollerup HM, Fogh-Andersen N, Strandgaard S. Effects of nitric oxide blockade and cyclosporin A on cardiovascular and renal function in normal man. J Hypertens 1999; 17: 1707-1713.
132. Gladue RP, Newborg MF. The protective effects of the thromboxane synthetase inhibitor Dazmegrel on nephrotoxicity in cyclosporine-treated rats. Transplantation 1991; 52: 837-841.

133. Perico N, Pasini M, Gaspari F, Abbate M, Remuzzi G. Co-participation of thromboxane A2 and leukotriene C4 and D4 in mediating cyclosporine-induced acute renal failure. Transplantation 1991; 52: 873-878.
134. Yang W, Herzberg GR, Kang Z, Wang L, Robb D, Randell E, Smeda J, Xiong J, Kara M, Liu H. Attenuation of ciclosporin-induced nephrotoxicity by dietary supplementation of seal oil in Sprague-Dawley rats. J Pharm Pharmacol 2005; 57: 1485-1492.
135. Chouinard ML, Martin LL, Coffman T, Hamilton BH, Linberg LF, Pamidi A, Simke JP, Rakhit A. Pharmacokinetics and biochemical efficacy of pirmagrel, a thromboxane synthase inhibitor, in renal allograft recipients. Clin Pharmacol Ther 1992; 52: 597-604.
136. Weir MR, Klassen DK, Burdick JF. A pilot study to assess the ability of an orally available selective thromboxane synthase inhibitor to improve renal function in cyclosporine-treated renal transplant recipients. J Am Soc Nephrol 1992; 2: 1285-1290.
137. Berthoux FC, Guerin C, Burgard G, Berthoux P, Alamartine E. One-year randomized controlled trial with omega-3 fatty acid-fish oil in clinical renal transplantation. Transplant Proc 1992; 24: 2578-2582.
138. Hansen JM, Hoy CE, Strandgaard S. Fish oil and cyclosporin A-induced renal hypoperfusion in kidney- transplanted patients. Nephrol Dial Transplant 1995; 10: 1745-1750.
139. Homan van der Heide JJ, Bilo HJ, Donker AJ, Wilmink JM, Sluiter WJ, Tegzess AM. The effects of dietary supplementation with fish oil on renal function and the course of early postoperative rejection episodes in cyclosporine-treated renal transplant recipients. Transplantation 1992; 54: 257-263.
140. Butterly DW, Spurney RF, Ruiz P, Griffiths R, Albrightson C, Coffman TM. A role for leukotrienes in cyclosporine nephrotoxicity. Kidney Int 2000; 57: 2586-2593.
141. Bunke M, Wilder L, Martin A. The effect of cyclosporine on agonist-stimulated glomerular and mesangial cell vasodilatory prostaglandin production. Transplantation 1991; 52: 718-722.
142. Copeland KR, Yatscoff RW. Comparison of the effects of cyclosporine and its metabolites on the release of prostacyclin and endothelin from mesangial cells. Transplantation 1992; 53: 640-645.
143. Chang CT, Hung CC, Yang CW, Vandewalle A, Wu MS. Cyclosporine decreases prostaglandin E2 production in mouse medullary thick ascending limb cultured cells. Transpl Int 2005; 18: 871-878.
144. Dumble LJ, Gibbons S, Tejpal N, Chou TC, Redgrave NG, Boyle MJ, Kahan BD. 15 AU81, a prostacyclin analog, potentiates immunosuppression and mitigates renal injury due to cyclosporine. Transplantation 1993; 55: 1124-1128.
145. Scholey JW, Mills DE. Dietary fatty acids and the glomerular hemodynamic response to cyclosporine in borderline hypertensive rats. Kidney Int 1995; 47: 611-617.
146. Moran M, Mozes MF, Maddux MS, Veremis S, Bartkus C, Ketel B, Pollak R, Wallemark C, Jonasson O. Prevention of acute graft rejection by the prostaglandin E1 analogue misoprostol in renal-transplant recipients treated with cyclosporine and prednisone. N Engl J Med 1990; 322: 1183-1188.
147. Le Guen E, Morel D, L'Azou B, Cambar J, Potaux L. Effect of cyclosporin and the prostacyclin analogue iloprost on human glomerular vasoreactivity. Nephrol Dial Transplant 1994; 9: 413-415.
148. Adams MB. Enisoprost in renal transplantation. The Enisoprost Renal Transplant Study Group. Transplantation 1992; 53: 338-345.
149. Manasia AR, Leibowitz AB, Miller CM, Silverstein JH, Schwartz M, Delgiudice R, Vallabhajosula S, Oropello JM, Benjamin E. Postoperative intravenous infusion of alprostadil (PGE1) does not improve renal function in hepatic transplant recipients. J Am Coll Surg 1996; 182: 347-352.
150. Pouteil-Noble C, Chapuis F, Berra N, Hadj-Aissa A, Lacavalerie B, Lefrancois N, Martin X, Touraine JL. Misoprostol in renal transplant recipients: a prospective, randomized, controlled study on the prevention of acute rejection episodes and cyclosporin A nephrotoxicity. Nephrol Dial Transplant 1994; 9: 552-555.
151. Ray JG. Prostaglandin E1 analogs do not improve renal function among either transplant or nontransplant patients: no further trials required. Transplantation 1998; 66: 476-483.
152. Weinblatt ME, Germain BF, Kremer JM, Wall BA, Weisman MH, Maier AL, Coblyn JS. Lack of a renal-protective effect of misoprostol in rheumatoid arthritis patients receiving cyclosporin A. Results of a randomized, placebo-controlled trial. Arthritis Rheum 1994; 37: 1321-1325.
153. Morgan BJ, Lyson T, Scherrer U, Victor RG. Cyclosporine causes sympathetically mediated elevations in arterial pressure in rats. Hypertension 1991; 18: 458-466.
154. Moss NG, Powell SL, Falk RJ. Intravenous cyclosporine activates afferent and efferent renal nerves and causes sodium retention in innervated kidneys in rats. Proc Natl Acad Sci U S A 1985; 82: 8222-8226.
155. Scherrer U, Vissing SF, Morgan BJ, Rollins JA, Tindall RS, Ring S, Hanson P, Mohanty PK, Victor RG. Cyclosporine-induced sympathetic activation and hypertension after heart transplantation. N Engl J Med 1990; 323: 693-699.
156. Lyson T, Ermel LD, Belshaw PJ, Alberg DG, Schreiber SL, Victor RG. Cyclosporine- and FK506-induced sympathetic activation correlates with calcineurin-mediated inhibition of T-cell signaling. Circ Res 1993; 73: 596-602.

157. Lyson T, McMullan DM, Ermel LD, Morgan BJ, Victor RG. Mechanism of cyclosporine-induced sympathetic activation and acute hypertension in rats. Hypertension 1994; 23: 667-675.
158. Reis F, Tavares P, Teixeira F. The distribution of catecholamines between plasma and platelets in cyclosporin A-induced hypertensive rats. Pharmacol Res 2000; 41: 129-135.
159. Rossi NF, Churchill PC, McDonald FD, Ellis VR. Mechanism of cyclosporine A-induced renal vasoconstriction in the rat. J Pharmacol Exp Ther 1989; 250: 896-901.
160. Zhang W, Li JL, Hosaka M, Janz R, Shelton JM, Albright GM, Richardson JA, Sudhof TC, Victor RG. Cyclosporine A-induced hypertension involves synapsin in renal sensory nerve endings. Proc Natl Acad Sci U S A 2000; 97: 9765-9770.
161. Grobecker HF, Riebel K, Wellenhofer T. Cyclosporine A-induced hypertension in SHR and WKY: role of the sympatho-adrenal system. Clin Exp Pharmacol Physiol 1995; 22 Suppl 1: S94-S95.
162. Ishikawa A, Suzuki K, Fujita K. Prevention of cyclosporine-induced nephrotoxicity by prazosin hydrochloride, an alpha-1-adrenoreceptor blocker. Transplant Proc 1996; 28: 1360-1361.
163. Murray BM, Paller MS, Ferris TF. Effect of cyclosporine administration on renal hemodynamics in conscious rats. Kidney Int 1985; 28: 767-774.
164. Murray BM, Paller MS. Beneficial effects of renal denervation and prazosin on GFR and renal blood flow after cyclosporine in rats. Clin Nephrol 1986; 25 Suppl 1: S37-S39.
165. Zhong Z, Connor HD, Yin M, Moss N, Mason RP, Bunzendahl H, Forman DT, Thurman RG. Dietary glycine and renal denervation prevents cyclosporin A-induced hydroxyl radical production in rat kidney. Mol Pharmacol 1999; 56: 455-463.
166. Carrier M, Tronc F, Stewart D, Pelletier LC. Dose-dependent effect of cyclosporin on renal arterial resistance in dogs. Am J Physiol 1991; 261: H1791-H1796.
167. Churchill MC, Churchill PC, Bidani AK. The effects of cyclosporine in Lewis rats with native and transplanted kidneys. Transplantation 1993; 55: 1256-1260.
168. Elzinga LW, Rosen S, Burdmann EA, Hatton DC, Lindsley J, Bennett WM. The role of renal sympathetic nerves in experimental chronic cyclosporine nephropathy. Transplantation 2000; 69: 2149-2153.
169. Wyss JM, Mozaffari MS, St John PL, Abrahamson DR. Cyclosporine-induced nephrotoxicity in deoxycorticosterone-NaCl treated rats. Int J Exp Pathol 1993; 74: 615-626.
170. Carvalho MJ, van den Meiracker AH, Boomsma F, Freitas J, Man in 't Veld AJ, Costa O, de Freitas AF. Role of sympathetic nervous system in cyclosporine-induced rise in blood pressure. Hypertension 1999; 34: 102-106.
171. Kaye D, Thompson J, Jennings G, Esler M. Cyclosporine therapy after cardiac transplantation causes hypertension and renal vasoconstriction without sympathetic activation. Circulation 1993; 88: 1101-1109.
172. Lucini D, Milani RV, Ventura HO, Mehra MR, Messerli FH, Murgo JP, Regenstein F, Copley B, Malliani A, Pagani M. Cyclosporine-induced hypertension: evidence for maintained baroreflex circulatory control. J Heart Lung Transplant 1997; 16: 615-620.
173. Lucini D, Milani RV, Ventura HO, Mehra MR, Messerli F, Pagani M. Study of arterial and autonomic effects of cyclosporine in humans. Hypertension 2000; 35: 1258-1263.
174. Stein CM, He H, Pincus T, Wood AJ. Cyclosporine impairs vasodilation without increased sympathetic activity in humans. Hypertension 1995; 26: 705-710.
175. Lee SH, Yoon YC, Jang YY, Song JH, Han ES, Lee CS. Effect of iron and ascorbate on cyclosporine-induced oxidative damage of kidney mitochondria and microsomes. Pharmacol Res 2001; 43: 161-171.
176. Longoni B, Boschi E, Demontis GC, Ratto GM, Mosca F. Apoptosis and adaptive responses to oxidative stress in human endothelial cells exposed to cyclosporin A correlate with BCL-2 expression levels. FASEB J 2001; 15: 731-740.
177. Parra T, de Arriba G, Arribas I, Perez dL, Rodriguez-Puyol D, Rodriguez-Puyol M. Cyclosporine A nephrotoxicity: role of thromboxane and reactive oxygen species. J Lab Clin Med 1998; 131: 63-70.
178. Tariq M, Morais C, Sobki S, Al Sulaiman M, Al Khader A. N-acetylcysteine attenuates cyclosporin-induced nephrotoxicity in rats. Nephrol Dial Transplant 1999; 14: 923-929.
179. Wang C, Salahudeen AK. Cyclosporine nephrotoxicity: attenuation by an antioxidant-inhibitor of lipid peroxidation *in vitro* and *in vivo*. Transplantation 1994; 58: 940-946.
180. Wang C, Salahudeen AK. Lipid peroxidation accompanies cyclosporine nephrotoxicity: effects of vitamin E. Kidney Int 1995; 47: 927-934.
181. Zhong Z, Arteel GE, Connor HD, Yin M, Frankenberg MV, Stachlewitz RF, Raleigh JA, Mason RP, Thurman RG. Cyclosporin A increases hypoxia and free radical production in rat kidneys: prevention by dietary glycine. Am J Physiol 1998; 275: F595-F604.
182. Zhong Z, Connor HD, Yin M, Wheeler MD, Mason RP, Thurman RG. Viral delivery of superoxide dismutase gene reduces cyclosporine A-induced nephrotoxicity. Kidney Int 2001; 59: 1397-1404.
183. Haberland A, Henke W, Grune T, Siems W, Jung K, Schimke I. Differential response of oxygen radical metabolism in rat heart, liver and kidney to cyclosporine A treatment. Inflamm Res 1997; 46: 452-454.

184. Jenkins JK, Huang H, Ndebele K, Salahudeen AK. Vitamin E inhibits renal mRNA expression of COX II, HO I, TGFbeta, and osteopontin in the rat model of cyclosporine nephrotoxicity. Transplantation 2001; 71: 331-334.
185. Navarro-Antolin J, Hernandez-Perera O, Lopez-Ongil S, Rodriguez-Puyol M, Rodriguez-Puyol D, Lamas S. CsA and FK506 up-regulate eNOS expression: role of reactive oxygen species and AP-1. Kidney Int Suppl 1998; 68: S20-S24.
186. Krysztopik RJ, Bentley FR, Spain DA, Wilson MA, Garrison RN. Lazaroids prevent acute cyclosporine-induced renal vasoconstriction. Transplantation 1997; 63: 1215-1220.
187. Kumar KV, Naidu MU, Shifow AA, Prayag A, Ratnakar KS. Melatonin: an antioxidant protects against cyclosporine-induced nephrotoxicity. Transplantation 1999; 67: 1065-1068.
188. Hagar HH, El Etter E, Arafa M. Taurine attenuates hypertension and renal dysfunction induced by cyclosporine A in rats. Clin Exp Pharmacol Physiol 2006; 33: 189-196.
189. Lexis LA, Fassett RG, Coombes JS. Alpha-tocopherol and alpha-lipoic acid enhance the erythrocyte antioxidant defence in cyclosporine A-treated rats. Basic Clin Pharmacol Toxicol 2006; 98: 68-73.
190. Origlia N, Migliori M, Panichi V, Filippi C, Bertelli A, Carpi A, Giovannini L. Protective effect of L-propionylcarnitine in chronic cyclosporine-a induced nephrotoxicity. Biomed Pharmacother 2006; 60: 77-81.
191. Louhelainen M, Merasto S, Finckenberg P, Lapatto R, Cheng ZJ, Mervaala EM. Lipoic acid supplementation prevents cyclosporine-induced hypertension and nephrotoxicity in spontaneously hypertensive rats. J Hypertens 2006; 24: 947-956.
192. Chang EJ, Mun KC. Effect of epigallocatechin gallate on renal function in cyclosporine-induced nephrotoxicity. Transplant Proc 2004; 36: 2133-2134.
193. Mohamadin AM, El-Beshbishy HA, El-Mahdy MA. Green tea extract attenuates cyclosporine A-induced oxidative stress in rats. Pharmacol Res 2005; 51: 51-57.
194. Tirkey N, Kaur G, Vij G, Chopra K. Curcumin, a diferuloylmethane, attenuates cyclosporine-induced renal dysfunction and oxidative stress in rat kidneys. BMC Pharmacol 2005; 5:15.
195. Wongmekiat O, Thamprasert K. Investigating the protective effects of aged garlic extract on cyclosporin-induced nephrotoxicity in rats. Fundam Clin Pharmacol 2005; 19: 555-562.
196. Buffoli B, Pechánová O, Kojsová S, Andriantsitohaina R, Giugno L, Bianchi R, Rezzani R. Provinol prevents CsA-induced nephrotoxicity by reducing reactive oxygen species, iNOS, and NF-kB expression. J Histochem Cytochem 2005; 53: 1459-1468.
197. Khan M, Shobha JC, Mohan IK, Rao Naidu MU, Prayag A, Kutala VK. Spirulina attenuates cyclosporine-induced nephrotoxicity in rats. J Appl Toxicol 2006; 26: 444-451.
198. Josephine A, Veena CK, Amudha G, Preetha SP, Varalakshmi P. Evaluating the effect of sulphated polysaccharides on cyclosporine a induced oxidative renal injury. Mol Cell Biochem 2006; 287: 101-108.
199. Durak I, Cetin R, Candir O, Devrim E, Kiliçoğlu B, Avci A. Black grape and garlic extracts protect against cyclosporine a nephrotoxicity. Immunol Invest 2007; 36: 105-114
200. Ateşşahin A, Ceribaşi AO, Yilmaz S. Lycopene, a carotenoid, attenuates cyclosporine-induced renal dysfunction and oxidative stress in rats. Basic Clin Pharmacol Toxicol 2007; 100: 372-376.
201. Zal F, Mostafavi-Pour Z, Vessal M. Comparison of the effects of vitamin E and/or quercetin in attenuating chronic cyclosporine A-induced nephrotoxicity in male rats. Clin Exp Pharmacol Physiol 2007; 34:720-724. (Erratum in: Clin Exp Pharmacol Physiol 2007;34: 953.
202. Uz E, Bayrak O, Uz E, Kaya A, Bayrak R, Uz B, Turgut FH, Bavbek N, Kanbay M, Akcay A. Nigella sativa Oil for Prevention of Chronic Cyclosporine Nephrotoxicity: An Experimental Model. Am J Nephrol. 2008; 28: 517-522.
203. Wongmekiat O, Leelarugrayub N, Thamprasert K. Beneficial effect of shallot (Allium ascalonicum L.) extract on cyclosporine nephrotoxicity in rats. Food Chem Toxicol 2008 (in press).
204. Barany P, Stenvinkel P, Ottosson-Seeberger A, Alvestrand A, Morrow J, Roberts JJ, Salahudeen AK. Effect of 6 weeks of vitamin E administration on renal haemodynamic alterations following a single dose of neoral in healthy volunteers. Nephrol Dial Transplant 2001; 16: 580-584.
205. McGrath LT, Treacy R, McClean E, Brown JH. Oxidative stress in cyclosporin and azathioprine treated renal transplant patients. Clin Chim Acta 1997; 264: 1-12.
206. Jabbari A, Argani H, Ghorbanihaghjo A, Mahdavi R. Comparison between swallowing and chewing of garlic on levels of serum lipids, cyclosporine, creatinine and lipid peroxidation in Renal Transplant Recipients. Lipids Health Dis 2005; 4: 11.
207. Guieu R, Dussol B, Devaux C, Sampol J, Brunet P, Rochat H, Bechis G, Berland YF. Interactions between cyclosporine A and adenosine in kidney transplant recipients. Kidney Int 1998; 53: 200-204.
208. Capecchi PL, Rechichi S, Lazzerini PE, Collini A, Guideri F, Ruggieri G, Carmellini M, Laghi-Pasini F. Cyclosporin and tacrolimus increase plasma levels of adenosine in kidney transplanted patients. Transpl Int 2005; 18: 289-295.
209. Halimi G, Sampol J, Clot-Faybesse O, Mercier L, Devaux C, Berland Y, Dussol B, Rochat H, Guieu R. Cyclosporine A and purinergic receptors in rat kidney. Life Sci 1999; 65: 2801-2813.

210. Balakrishnan VS, von Ruhland CJ, Griffiths DF, Coles GA, Williams JD. Effects of a selective adenosine A1 receptor antagonist on the development of cyclosporin nephrotoxicity. Br J Pharmacol 1996; 117: 879-884.
211. Churchill PC, Rossi NF, Churchill MC, Bidani AK, McDonald FD. Acute cyclosporine-induced renal vasoconstriction: lack of effect of theophylline. Am J Physiol 1990; 258: F41-F45.
212. Heyne N, Wolf S, Petersen P, Merten S, Schober W, Erley CM, Risler T, Osswald H. Adenosine receptor antagonism in the prevention of acute cyclosporine A- nephrotoxicity in normal, diabetic and hypertensive rats. Nephrol Dial Transplant 1999; 14 Suppl 4: 23-24.
213. Prévot A, Liet JM, Semama DS, Justrabo E, Guignard JP, Gouyon JB. Disparate effects of chronic and acute theophylline on cyclosporine A nephrotoxicity. Pediatr Nephrol 2002; 17: 418-424.
214. Stanek B, Kovarik J, Rasoul-Rockenschaub S, Silberbauer K. Renin-angiotensin-aldosterone system and vasopressin in cyclosporine-treated renal allograft recipients. Clin Nephrol 1987; 28: 186-189.
215. Frapier JM, Choby C, Mangoni ME, Nargeot J, Albat B, Richard S. Cyclosporin A increases basal intracellular calcium and calcium responses to endothelin and vasopressin in human coronary myocytes. FEBS Lett 2001; 493: 57-62.
216. Kremer S, Margolis B, Harper P, Skorecki K. Cyclosporine induced alterations in vasopressin signalling in the glomerular mesangial cell. Clin Invest Med 1989; 12: 201-206.
217. Lo RA, Passaquin AC, Ruegg UT. Mechanism of enhanced vasoconstrictor hormone action in vascular smooth muscle cells by cyclosporin A. Br J Pharmacol 1997; 121: 248-252.
218. Cottet-Maire F, Avdonin PV, Roulet E, Buetler TM, Mermod N, Ruegg UT. Upregulation of vasopressin V1A receptor mRNA and protein in vascular smooth muscle cells following cyclosporin A treatment. Br J Pharmacol 2001; 132: 909-917.
219. Bagnis C, Deray G, Dubois M, Pirotzky E, Jacquiaud C, Baghos W, Aupetit B, Braquet P, Jacobs C. Prevention of cyclosporin nephrotoxicity with a platelet-activating factor (PAF) antagonist. Nephrol Dial Transplant 1996; 11: 507-513.
220. dos Santos OF, Boim MA, Bregman R, Draibe SA, Barros EJ, Pirotzky E, Schor N, Braquet P. Effect of platelet-activating factor antagonist on cyclosporine nephrotoxicity. Glomerular hemodynamics evaluation. Transplantation 1989; 47: 592-595.
221. Kawaguchi A, Sugimoto K, Fujimura A. Preventive effect of platelet-activating factor antagonist, Y-24180, against cyclosporine-induced acute nephrotoxicity. Life Sci 2001; 68: 1181-1190.
222. Massicot F, Lamouri A, Martin C, Pham-Huy C, Heymans F, Warnet JM, Godfroid JJ, Claude JR. Preventive effects of two PAF-antagonists, PMS 536 and PMS 549, on cyclosporin-induced LLC-PK1 oxidative injury. J Lipid Mediat Cell Signal 1997; 15: 203-214.
223. Bokemeyer D, Kramer HJ, Meyer-Lehnert H. Atrial natriuretic peptide blunts the cellular effects of cyclosporine in smooth muscle. Hypertension 1993; 21: 166-172.
224. Capasso G, Rosati C, Ciani F, Giordano DR, Russo F, De Santo NG. The beneficial effect of atrial natriuretic peptide on cyclosporine nephrotoxicity. Am J Hypertens 1990; 3: 204-210.
225. Capasso G, Unwin R, Ciani F, Rizzo A, Russo F, Pica A, De Santo NG. Inhibition of neutral endopeptidase potentiates the effects of atrial natriuretic peptide on acute cyclosporin-induced nephrotoxicity. Nephron 2000; 86: 298-305.
226. Lang CC, Henderson IS, Mactier R, Stewart WK, Struthers AD. Atrial natriuretic factor improves renal function and lowers systolic blood pressure in renal allograft recipients treated with cyclosporin A. J Hypertens 1992; 10: 483-488.
227. Lipkin GW, Thuraisingham R, Dawnay AB, Harwood SM, Raine AE. Acute reversal of cyclosporine nephrotoxicity by neutral endopeptidase inhibition in stable renal transplant recipients. Transplantation 1997; 64: 1007-1017.
228. Polte T, Hemmerle A, Berndt G, Grosser N, Abate A, Schröder H. Atrial natriuretic peptide reduces cyclosporin toxicity in renal cells: role of cGMP and heme oxygenase-1. Free Radic Biol Med 2002; 32: 56-63.
229. Martinez L, Vio CP, Valdes G, Kychenthal W, Mendoza S. Decreased kallikrein excretion in renal transplant treated with cyclosporine A. Transplant Proc 1990; 22: 294-296.
230. Rodier M, Ribstein J, Parer-Richard C, Mimran A. Renal changes associated with cyclosporine in recent type I diabetes mellitus. Hypertension 1991; 18: 334-340.
231. Spragg J, Coblyn JS, Fraser PA, Austen KF, Weinblatt ME. The effect of cyclosporine on urinary kallikrein excretion in patients with rheumatoid arthritis. Adv Exp Med Biol 1989; 247A: 389-392.
232. Bompart G, Tack I, Castano EM, Pesquero JB, Girolami JP, Bascands JL. Cyclosporine A decreases kallikrein and BK2 mRNA expression in the rat renal cortex. Immunopharmacology 1996; 32: 99-101.
233. Wang C, Ford P, Chao C, Chao L, Chao J. Effect of cyclosporin A on the expression of tissue kallikrein, kininogen, and bradykinin receptor in rat. Am J Physiol 1997; 273: F783-F789.
234. Bohdanecka M, Schuck O, Chadimova M, Sedivy J, Glagolicova A, Skibova J, Kunes J, Dobesova Z, Stuchlik M, Vesela J, Kazdova L. Nephrotoxicity of cyclosporin A in hereditary hypertriglyceridemic rats. Physiol Res 1999; 48: 437-443.
235. Duymelinck C, Dauwe SE, Nouwen EJ, De Broe ME, Verpooten GA. Cholesterol feeding accentuates the cyclosporine-induced elevation of renal plasminogen activator inhibitor type 1. Kidney Int 1997; 51: 1818-1830.

236. Burdmann EA, Andoh TF, Lindsley J, Houghton DC, Bennett WM. Effects of oral magnesium supplementation on acute experimental cyclosporin nephrotoxicity. Nephrol Dial Transplant 1994; 9: 16-21.
237. Pere AK, Lindgren L, Tuomainen P, Krogerus L, Rauhala P, Laakso J, Karppanen H, Vapaatalo H, Ahonen J, Mervaala EM. Dietary potassium and magnesium supplementation in cyclosporine-induced hypertension and nephrotoxicity. Kidney Int 2000; 58: 2462-2472.
238. Bennett WM. Mechanisms of acute and chronic nephrotoxicity from immunosuppressive drugs. Ren Fail 1996; 18: 453-460.
239. Devarajan P, Kaskel FJ, Arbeit LA, Moore LC. Cyclosporine nephrotoxicity: blood volume, sodium conservation, and renal hemodynamics. Am J Physiol 1989; 256: F71-F78.
240. Moore LC, Mason J, Feld L, Van Liew JB, Kaskel FJ. Effect of cyclosporine on endothelial albumin leakage in rats. J Am Soc Nephrol 1992; 3: 51-57.
241. Huang X, Cheng Z, Sunga J, Unemori E, Zsebo K. Systemic administration of recombinant human relaxin (RHRLX) ameliorates the acute cyclosporine nephrotoxicity in rats. J Heart Lung Transplant 2001; 20: 253-
242. Maestri M, Dafoe DC, Adams GA, Gaspari A, Luzzana F, Innocente F, Rademacher J, Dionigi P, Barbieri A, Zonta F, Zonta A, Rabkin R. Insulin-like growth factor-I ameliorates delayed kidney graft function and the acute nephrotoxic effects of cyclosporine. Transplantation 1997; 64: 185-190.
243. Chen W, Langer RM, Janczewska S, Furian L, Geary R, Qu X, Wang M, Verani R, Condon T, Stecker K, Bennett CF, Stepkowski SM. Methoxyethyl-modified intercellular adhesion molecule-1 antisense phosphorothiateoligonucleotides inhibit allograft rejection, ischemic-reperfusion injury, and cyclosporine-induced nephrotoxicity. Transplantation 2005; 79: 401-408.
244. Beall A, Epstein A, Woodrum D, Brophy CM. Cyclosporine-induced renal artery smooth muscle contraction is associated with increases in the phosphorylation of specific contractile regulatory proteins. Biochim Biophys Acta 1999; 1449: 41-49.
245. Lo RA, Passaquin AC, Cox C, Ruegg UT. Cyclosporin A potentiates receptor-activated [Ca2+]c increase. J Recept Signal Transduct Res 1997; 17: 149-161.
246. Medina J, Cordier A, Wolf A. Cyclosporine A-induced contraction of isolated rat aortic smooth muscle cells. Life Sci 1997; 61: L-32.
247. Meyer-Lehnert H, Schrier RW. Cyclosporine A enhances vasopressin-induced Ca2+ mobilization and contraction in mesangial cells. Kidney Int 1988; 34: 89-97.
248. Ressureicao FA, Ballejo G, Salgado MC, Ferraz AS. Effect of cyclosporine administration on vascular reactivity of the isolated mesenteric bed. Transplant Proc 1995; 27: 1806-1808.
249. Xue H, Bukoski RD, McCarron DA, Bennett WM. Induction of contraction in isolated rat aorta by cyclosporine. Transplantation 1987; 43: 715-718.
250. Dubus I, Sena S, Labouyrie JP, Bonnet J, Combe C. *In vitro* prevention of cyclosporin-induced cell contraction by mycophenolic acid. Life Sci 2005; 77: 3366-3374.
251. Abraham JS, Bentley FR, Garrison RN, Cryer HM. The influence of the cyclosporine vehicle, cremophor EL, on renal microvascular blood flow in the rat. Transplantation 1991; 52: 101-105.
252. Hardy G, Stanke-Labesque F, Deveaux G, Devillier P, Sessa C, Bessard G. Cyclosporine A and cremophor EL induce contractions of human saphenous vein: involvement of thromboxane A2 receptor-dependent pathway. J Cardiovasc Pharmacol 2000; 36: 693-698.
253. Thiel G, Hermle M, Brunner FP. Acutely impaired renal function during intravenous administration of cyclosporine A: a cremophore side-effect. Clin Nephrol 1986; 25 Suppl 1: S40-S42.
254. Hermida-Rodriguez C, Cantero PJ, Garcia-Valriberas R, Pajares Garcia JM, Mate-Jimenez J. High-dose intravenous cyclosporine in steroid refractory attacks of inflammatory bowel disease. Hepatogastroenterology 1999; 46: 2265-2268.
255. Macris MP, Ford EG, Van Buren CT, Frazier OH. Predictors of severe renal dysfunction after heart transplantation and intravenous cyclosporine therapy. J Heart Transplant 1989; 8: 444-448.
256. Powell-Jackson PR, Young B, Calne RY, Williams R. Nephrotoxicity of parenterally administered cyclosporine after orthotopic liver transplantation. Transplantation 1983; 36: 505-508.
257. Weir MR, Klassen DK, Shen SY, Sullivan D, Buddemeyer EU, Handwerger BS. Acute effects of intravenous cyclosporine on blood pressure, renal hemodynamics, and urine prostaglandin production of healthy humans. Transplantation 1990; 49: 41-47.
258. Burdmann EA, Andoh TF, Prado EAB, Franceschini N, Fujihara C, Zatz R, Bennett WM. Renal, immunosuppressive and pharmacokinetic effects of the substitution of intralipid (LIP) for cremophor (CRE) as vehicle for parenteral cyclosporine (CSA) administration. J Am Soc Nephrol 1995; 6: 995.
259. Aliabadi HM, Elhasi S, Brocks DR, Lavasanifar A. Polymeric micellar delivery reduces kidney distribution and nephrotoxic effects of Cyclosporine A after multiple dosing. J Pharm Sci. 2008, in press.
260. Burdmann EA, Andoh TF, Lindsley J, Russell J, Bennett WM, Porter G. Urinary enzymes as biomarkers of renal injury in experimental nephrotoxicity of immunosuppressive drugs. Ren Fail 1994; 16: 161-168.

261. Laine J, Holmberg C. Renal and adrenal mechanisms in cyclosporine-induced hyperkalaemia after renal transplantation. Eur J Clin Invest 1995; 25: 670-676.
262. Rezzani R, Angoscini P, Borsani E, Rodella L, Bianchi R. Cyclosporine A-induced toxicity in two renal cell culture models (LLC-PK1 and MDCK). Histochem J 2002; 34: 27-33.
263. Deppe CE, Heering PJ, Tinel H, Kinne-Saffran E, Grabensee B, Kinne RK. Effect of cyclosporine A on Na+/K(+)-ATPase, Na+/K+/2Cl-cotransporter, and H+/K(+)-ATPase in MDCK cells and two subtypes, C7 and C11. Exp Nephrol 1997; 5: 471-480.
264. Healy E, Dempsey M, Lally C, Ryan MP. Apoptosis and necrosis: mechanisms of cell death induced by cyclosporine A in a renal proximal tubular cell line. Kidney Int 1998; 54: 1955-1966.
265. Lally C, Healy E, Ryan MP. Cyclosporine A-induced cell cycle arrest and cell death in renal epithelial cells. Kidney Int 1999; 56: 1254-1257.
266. Lima R, Serone AP, Schor N, Higa EM. Effect of cyclosporin a on nitric oxide production in cultured LLC-PK1 cells. Ren Fail 2001; 23: 43-52.
267. Yang JJ, Finn WF. Effect of oxypurinol on cyclosporine toxicity in cultured EA, LLC-PK1 and MDCK cells. Ren Fail 1998; 20: 85-101.
268. Younes-Ibrahim M, Barnese M, Burth P, Castro-Faria MV. Inhibition of purified human kidney Na+, K+-ATPase by cyclosporine A: a possible mechanism for drug human nephrotoxicity. Ann N Y Acad Sci 2003; 986: 633-635.
269. Calderaro V, Boccellino M, Cirillo G, Quagliuolo L, Cirillo D, Giovane A. Cyclosporine A amplifies Ca2+ signaling pathway in LLC-PK1 cells through the inhibition of plasma membrane Ca2+ pump. J Am Soc Nephrol 2003; 14: 1435-1442.
270. Lim SW, Ahn KO, Sheen MR, Jeon US, Kim J, Yang CW, Kwon HM. Downregulation of renal sodium transporters and tonicity-responsive enhancer binding protein by long-term treatment with cyclosporin A. J Am Soc Nephrol 2007; 18: 421-429.
271. Gordjani N, Epting T, Fischer-Riepe P, Greger RF, Brandis M, Leipziger J, Nitschke R. Cyclosporin-A-induced effects on the free Ca2+ concentration in LLC-PK1-cells and their mechanisms. Pflugers Arch 2000; 439: 627-633.
272. Galletti P, Di Gennaro CI, Migliardi V, Indaco S, Della Ragione F, Manna C, Chiodini P, Capasso G, Zappia V. Diverse effects of natural antioxidants on cyclosporin cytotoxicity in rat renal tubular cells. Nephrol Dial Transplant 2005; 20: 1551-1558.
273. Jeon SH, Piao YJ, Choi KJ, Hong F, Baek HW, Kang I, Ha J, Kim SS, Chang SG. Prednisolone suppresses cyclosporin A-induced apoptosis but not cell cycle arrest in MDCK cells. Arch Biochem Biophys 2005; 435: 382-392.
274. Paslaru L, Rallu M, Manuel M, Davidson S, Morange M. Cyclosporin A induces an atypical heat shock response. Biochem Biophys Res Commun 2000; 269: 464-469.
275. Stacchiotti A, Rezzani R, Angoscini P, Corsetti G, Bianchi R. Distribution of heat shock proteins in kidneys of rats after immunosuppressive treatment with cyclosporine A. Acta Histochem 2001; 103: 167-177.
276. Ling BN, Eaton DC. Cyclosporin A inhibits apical secretory K+ channels in rabbit cortical collecting tubule principal cells. Kidney Int 1993; 44: 974-984.
277. Carvalho da Costa M, de Castro I, Neto AL, Ferreira AT, Burdmann EA, Yu L. Cyclosporin A tubular effects contribute to nephrotoxicity: role for Ca2+ and Mg2+ ions. Nephrol Dial Transplant 2003; 18:2262-2268.
278. de Mattos AM, Olyaei AJ, Bennett WM. Nephrotoxicity of immunosuppressive drugs: long-term consequences and challenges for the future. Am J Kidney Dis 2000; 35: 333-346.
279. Fisher NC, Malag M, Gonzlez-Pinto I. The clinical impact of nephrotoxicity in liver transplantation. Transplantation 2000; 69: SS18-SS22.
280. Parry G, Meiser B, Rabago G. The clinical impact of cyclosporine nephrotoxicity in heart transplantation. Transplantation 2000; 69: SS23-SS26.
281. Tsimaratos M, Viard L, Kreitmann B, Remediani C, Picon G, Camboulives J, Sarles J, Metras D. Kidney function in cyclosporine-treated paediatric pulmonary transplant recipients. Transplantation 2000; 69: 2055-2059.
282. Davies DR, Bittmann I, Pardo J. Histopathology of calcineurin inhibitor-induced nephrotoxicity. Transplantation 2000; 69: SS11-SS13.
283. Solez K. International standardization of criteria for histologic diagnosis of chronic rejection in renal allografts. Clin Transplant 1994; 8: 345-350.
284. Curtis JJ, Luke RG, Dubovsky E, Diethelm AG, Whelchel JD, Jones P. Cyclosporin in therapeutic doses increases renal allograft vascular resistance. Lancet 1986; 2: 477-479.
285. Hilbrands LB, Hoitsma AG, Wetzels JF, Koene RA. Detailed study of changes in renal function after conversion from cyclosporine to azathioprine. Clin Nephrol 1996; 45: 230-235.
286. Ruggenenti P, Perico N, Mosconi L, Gaspari F, Benigni A, Amuchastegui CS, Bruzzi I, Remuzzi G. Calcium channel blockers protect transplant patients from cyclosporine- induced daily renal hypoperfusion. Kidney Int 1993; 43: 706-711.
287. Bennett WM, Burdmann EA, Andoh TF, Houghton DC, Lindsley J, Elzinga LW. Nephrotoxicity of immunosuppressive drugs. Nephrol Dial Transplant 1994; 9 Suppl 4: 141-145.

288. Greenberg A, Egel JW, Thompson ME, Hardesty RL, Griffith BP, Bahnson HT, Bernstein RL, Hastillo A, Hess ML, Puschett JB. Early and late forms of cyclosporine nephrotoxicity: studies in cardiac transplant recipients. Am J Kidney Dis 1987; 9: 12-22.
289. Noel C, Hazzan M, Noel-Walter MP, Jouet JP. Renal failure and bone marrow transplantation. Nephrol Dial Transplant 1998; 13: 2464-2466.
290. Platz KP, Mueller AR, Blumhardt G, Bachmann S, Bechstein WO, Kahl A, Neuhaus P. Nephrotoxicity following orthotopic liver transplantation. A comparison between cyclosporine and FK506. Transplantation 1994; 58: 170-178.
291. Lima EQ, Zanetta DM, Castro I, Massarollo PC, Mies S, Machado MM, Yu L. Risk factors for development of acute renal failure after liver transplantation. Ren Fail 2003; 25: 553-560.
292. Hingorani SR, Guthrie K, Batchelder A, Schoch G, Aboulhosn N, Manchion J, McDonald GB. Acute renal failure after myeloablative hematopoietic cell transplant: incidence and risk factors. Kidney Int 2005; 67: 272-277.
293. Brann WM, Bennett LE, Keck BM, Hosenpud JD. Morbidity, functional status, and immunosuppressive therapy after heart transplantation: an analysis of the joint International Society for Heart and Lung Transplantation/United Network for Organ Sharing Thoracic Registry. J Heart Lung Transplant 1998; 17: 374-382.
294. Hosenpud JD, Bennett LE, Keck BM, Fiol B, Boucek MM, Novick RJ. The Registry of the International Society for Heart and Lung Transplantation: sixteenth official report--1999. J Heart Lung Transplant 1999; 18: 611-626.
295. Woolfson RG, Neild GH. Cyclosporin nephrotoxicity following cardiac transplantation. Nephrol Dial Transplant 1997; 12: 2054-2056.
296. Zager RA, O'Quigley J, Zager BK, Alpers CE, Shulman HM, Gamelin LM, Stewart P, Thomas ED. Acute renal failure following bone marrow transplantation: a retrospective study of 272 patients. Am J Kidney Dis 1989; 13: 210-216.
297. Zager RA. Acute renal failure in the setting of bone marrow transplantation. Kidney Int 1994; 46: 1443-1458.
298. Zager RA. Acute renal failure syndromes after bone marrow transplantation. Adv Nephrol Necker Hosp 1997; 27: 263-280.
299. Bestetti RB, Theodoropoulos TA, Burdmann EA, Santos MA, Abbud-Filho M. Switch from cyclosporine to sirolimus as a treatment of acute renal failure complicating cardiogenic shock in a heart transplant recipient. Int J Cardiol 2006; 112: e83-84.
300. Ahuja TS, Niaz N, Agraharkar M. Contrast-induced nephrotoxicity in renal allograft recipients. Clin Nephrol 2000; 54: 11-14.
301. Altman RD, Perez GO, Sfakianakis GN. Interaction of cyclosporine A and nonsteroidal anti-inflammatory drugs on renal function in patients with rheumatoid arthritis. Am J Med 1992; 93: 396-402.
302. Deray G, Le Hoang P, Aupetit B, Achour A, Rottembourg J, Baumelou A. Enhancement of cyclosporine A nephrotoxicity by diclofenac. Clin Nephrol 1987; 27: 213-214.
303. Garcia TM, da Costa JA, Costa RS, Ferraz AS. Acute tubular necrosis in kidney transplant patients treated with enalapril. Ren Fail 1994; 16: 419-423.
304. Luber AD, Maa L, Lam M, Guglielmo BJ. Risk factors for amphotericin B-induced nephrotoxicity. J Antimicrob Chemother 1999; 43: 267-271.
305. Morales JM, Andres A, Prieto C, Diaz Rolon JA, Rodicio JL. Reversible acute renal toxicity by toxic sinergic effect between gentamicin and cyclosporine. Clin Nephrol 1988; 29: 272.
306. Morales JM, Munoz MA, Fernandez ZG, Garcia CC, Garcia Rubiales MA, Andres A, Aguado JM, Gonzalez Pinto I. Reversible acute renal failure caused by the combined use of foscarnet and cyclosporin in organ transplanted patients. Nephrol Dial Transplant 1995; 10: 882-883.
307. Murray BM, Venuto RC, Kohli R, Cunningham EE. Enalapril-associated acute renal failure in renal transplants: possible role of cyclosporine. Am J Kidney Dis 1990; 16: 66-69.
308. Schiff MH, Whelton A. Renal toxicity associated with disease-modifying antirheumatic drugs used for the treatment of rheumatoid arthritis. Semin Arthritis Rheum 2000; 30: 196-208.
309. Termeer A, Hoitsma AJ, Koene RA. Severe nephrotoxicity caused by the combined use of gentamicin and cyclosporine in renal allograft recipients. Transplantation 1986; 42: 220-221.
310. Denton CP, Sweny P, Abdulla A, Black CM. Acute renal failure occurring in scleroderma treated with cyclosporin A: a report of three cases. Br J Rheumatol 1994; 33: 90-92.
311. Dussol B, Reynaud-Gaubert M, Saingra Y, Daniel L, Berland Y. Acute tubular necrosis induced by high level of cyclosporine A in a lung transplant. Transplantation 2000; 70: 1234-1236.
312. Shechter P. Acute tubular necrosis following high-dose cyclosporine A therapy. Eur J Clin Pharmacol 1996; 49: 521-523.
313. Rivera CF, Hernández AA, Verdejo PV, García JO, Rego SC, Cañedo FV. Basiliximab (Simulect) in acute tubular necrosis high-risk kidney transplantation. Transplant Proc 2005; 37: 3733-3735.
314. Kahn D, Botha JF, Pascoe MD, Pontin AR, Halkett J, Tandon V. Withdrawal of cyclosporine in renal transplant recipients with acute tubular necrosis improves renal function. Transpl Int 2000; 13 Suppl 1: S82-S83.
315. Cravedi P, Codreanu I, Satta A, Turturro M, Sghirlanzoni M, Remuzzi G, Ruggenenti P. Cyclosporine prolongs delayed graft function in kidney transplantation: are rabbit anti-human thymocyte globulins the answer? Nephron Clin Pract 2005; 101: c65-71.

316. Zakarija A, Bennett C. Drug-induced thrombotic microangiopathy. Semin Thromb Hemost 2005; 31: 681-90.
317. Bren A, Pajek J, Grego K, Buturovic J, Ponikvar R, Lindic J, Knap B, Vizjak A, Ferluga D, Kandus A. Follow-up of kidney graft recipients with cyclosporine-associated hemolytic-uremic syndrome and thrombotic microangiopathy. Transplant Proc 2005; 37: 1889-1891.
318. Young BA, Marsh CL, Alpers CE, Davis CL. Cyclosporine-associated thrombotic microangiopathy/hemolytic uremic syndrome following kidney and kidney-pancreas transplantation. Am J Kidney Dis 1996; 28: 561-571.
319. Mazzali M, Dias EP, Ribeiro-Alves MA, Homsi E, Alves-Filho G. Nonrecurrent hemolytic uremic syndrome (HUS de novo) as cause of acute renal failure after renal transplant. Ren Fail 1997; 19: 271-277.
320. Shulman H, Striker G, Deeg HJ, Kennedy M, Storb R, Thomas ED. Nephrotoxicity of cyclosporin A after allogeneic marrow transplantation: glomerular thromboses and tubular injury. N Engl J Med 1981; 305: 1392-1395.
321. Zarifian A, Meleg-Smith S, O'donovan R, Tesi RJ, Batuman V. Cyclosporine-associated thrombotic microangiopathy in renal allografts. Kidney Int 1999; 55: 2457-2466.
322. Hale GA, Bowman LC, Rochester RJ, Benaim E, Heslop HE, Krance RA, Horwitz EM, Cunningham JM, Tong X, Srivastava DK, Handgretinger R, Jones DP. Hemolytic uremic syndrome after bone marrow transplantation: clinical characteristics and outcome in children. Biol Blood Marrow Transplant. 2005; 11: 912-920.
323. Gatti S, Arru M, Reggiani P, Como G, Rossi F, Fassati LR, Ponticelli C. Successful treatment of hemolytic uremic syndrome after liver-kidney transplantation. J Nephrol 2003; 16: 586-590.
324. 329. Wen YK, Chen ML. Rescue treatment for cyclosporine-associated hemolytic-uremic syndrome with intravenous immunoglobulin. Clin Nephrol. 2006; 66: 58-62.
325. Bennett WM, Burdmann E, Andoh T, Elzinga L, Franceschini N. Nephrotoxicity of immunosuppressive drugs. Miner Electrolyte Metab 1994; 20: 214-220.
326. Mahalati K, Belitsky P, West K, Kiberd B, Fraser A, Sketris I, Macdonald AS, McAlister V, Lawen J. Approaching the therapeutic window for cyclosporine in kidney transplantation: a prospective study. J Am Soc Nephrol 2001; 12: 828-833.
327. Macdonald AS. Management strategies for nephrotoxicity. Transplantation 2000; 69: SS31-SS36.
328. Mahalati K, Belitsky P, Sketris I, West K, Panek R. Neoral monitoring by simplified sparse sampling area under the concentration-time curve: its relationship to acute rejection and cyclosporine nephrotoxicity early after kidney transplantation. Transplantation 1999; 68: 55-62.
329. Bunke M, Sloan R, Brier M, Ganzel B. An improved glomerular filtration rate in cardiac transplant recipients with once-a-day cyclosporine dosing. Transplantation 1995; 59: 537-540.
330. Chan C, Maurer J, Cardella C, Cattran D, Pei Y. A randomized controlled trial of verapamil on cyclosporine nephrotoxicity in heart and lung transplant recipients. Transplantation 1997; 63: 1435-1440.
331. Madsen JK, Sorensen SS, Hansen HE, Pedersen EB. The effect of felodipine on renal function and blood pressure in cyclosporin-treated renal transplant recipients during the first three months after transplantation. Nephrol Dial Transplant 1998; 13: 2327-2334.
332. Rahn KH, Barenbrock M, Fritschka E, Heinecke A, Lippert J, Schroeder K, Hauser I, Wagner K, Neumayer HH. Effect of nitrendipine on renal function in renal-transplant patients treated with cyclosporin: a randomised trial. Lancet 1999; 354: 1415-1420.
333. Rodicio JL. Calcium antagonists and renal protection from cyclosporine nephrotoxicity: long-term trial in renal transplantation patients. J Cardiovasc Pharmacol 2000; 35: S7-S11.
334. Shin GT, Cheigh JS, Riggio RR, Suthanthiran M, Stubenbord WT, Serur D, Wang JC, Rubin AL, Stenzel KH. Effect of nifedipine on renal allograft function and survival beyond one year. Clin Nephrol 1997; 47: 33-36.
335. van Riemsdijk IC, Mulder PG, de Fijter JW, Bruijn JA, van Hooff JP, Hoitsma AJ, Tegzess AM, Weimar W. Addition of isradipine (Lomir) results in a better renal function after kidney transplantation: a double-blind, randomized, placebo-controlled, multi-center study. Transplantation 2000; 70: 122-126.
336. Wilkie ME, Beer JC, Evans SJ, Raftery MJ, Lord RH, Moore R, Marsh FP. A double-blind, randomized, placebo-controlled study of nifedipine on early renal allograft function. Nephrol Dial Transplant 1994; 9: 800-804.
337. Neumayer HH, Kunzendorf U, Schreiber M. Protective effects of calcium antagonists in human renal transplantation. Kidney Int Suppl 1992; 36: S87-S93.
338. Harper SJ, Moorhouse J, Abrams K, Jurewicz A, Nicholson M, Horsburgh T, Harris K, Combe C, Bell PR, Walls J, Donnelly PK, Veitch PS, Feehally J. The beneficial effects of oral nifedipine on cyclosporin-treated renal transplant recipients--a randomised prospective study. Transpl Int 1996; 9: 115-125.
339. Kuypers DR, Neumayer HH, Fritsche L, Budde K, Rodicio JL, Vanrenterghem Y; Lacidipine Study Group. Calcium channel blockade and preservation of renal graft function in cyclosporine-treated recipients: a prospective randomized placebo-controlled 2-year study. Transplantation 2004; 78: 1204-1211.

340. Lapointe N, Chen H, Qi S, Xu D, Daloze P, Dumont L. Immunomodulating effects of second-generation calcium channel blockers on experimental heart transplantation. Eur Surg Res 1999; 31: 259-266.
341. Blaheta RA, Hailer NP, Brude N, Wittig B, Leckel K, Oppermann E, Bachmann M, Harder S, Cinatl J, Scholz M, Bereiter-Hahn J, Weber S, Encke A, Markus BH. *In vitro* analysis of verapamil-induced immunosuppression: potent inhibition of T cell motility and lymphocytic transmigration through allogeneic endothelial cells. Transplantation 2000; 69: 588-597.
342. Simopoulos AP. Essential fatty acids in health and chronic disease. Am J Clin Nutr 1999; 70: 560S-569S.
343. Stoof TJ, Korstanje MJ, Bilo HJ, Starink TM, Hulsmans RF, Donker AJ. Does fish oil protect renal function in cyclosporin-treated psoriasis patients? J Intern Med 1989; 226: 437-441.
344. Homan van der Heide JJ, Bilo HJ, Tegzess AM, Donker AJ. The effects of dietary supplementation with fish oil on renal function in cyclosporine-treated renal transplant recipients. Transplantation 1990; 49: 523-527.
345. van der Heide JJ, Bilo HJ, Donker JM, Wilmink JM, Tegzess AM. Effect of dietary fish oil on renal function and rejection in cyclosporine-treated recipients of renal transplants. N Engl J Med 1993; 329: 769-773.
346. Bennett WM, Carpenter CB, Shapiro ME, Strom TB, Hefty D, Tillman M, Abrams J, Ryan D, Kelley VR. Delayed omega-3 fatty acid supplements in renal transplantation. A double-blind, placebo-controlled study. Transplantation 1995; 59: 352-356.
347. Kooijmans-Coutinho MF, Rischen-Vos J, Hermans J, Arndt JW, van der Woude FJ. Dietary fish oil in renal transplant recipients treated with cyclosporin-A: no beneficial effects shown. J Am Soc Nephrol 1996; 7: 513-518.
348. Schut NH, Bilo HJ, Popp-Snijders C, Goedhart PT, Wilmink JM. Erythrocyte deformability, endothelin levels, and renal function in cyclosporin-treated renal transplant recipients: effects of intervention with fish oil and corn oil. Scand J Clin Lab Invest 1993; 53: 499-506.
349. Holm T, Andreassen AK, Aukrust P, Andersen K, Geiran OR, Kjekshus J, Simonsen S, Gullestad L. Omega-3 fatty acids improve blood pressure control and preserve renal function in hypertensive heart transplant recipients. Eur Heart J 2001; 22: 428-436.
350. Carmellini M, Frosini F, Filipponi F, Boggi U, Mosca F. Effect of cilastatin on cyclosporine-induced acute nephrotoxicity in kidney transplant recipients. Transplantation 1997; 64: 164-166.
351. Carmellini M, Matteucci E, Boggi U, Cecconi S, Giampietro O, Mosca F. Imipenem/cilastatin reduces cyclosporin-induced tubular damage in kidney transplant recipients. Transplant Proc 1998; 30: 2034-2035.
352. Gruss E, Tomas JF, Bernis C, Rodriguez F, Traver JA, Fernandez-Ranada JM. Nephroprotective effect of cilastatin in allogeneic bone marrow transplantation. Results from a retrospective analysis. Bone Marrow Transplant 1996; 18: 761-765.
353. Markewitz A, Hammer C, Pfeiffer M, Zahn S, Drechsel J, Reichenspurner H, Reichart B. Reduction of cyclosporine-induced nephrotoxicity by cilastatin following clinical heart transplantation. Transplantation 1994; 57: 865-870.
354. Tejedor A, Torres AM, Castilla M, Lazaro JA, de Lucas C, Caramelo C. Cilastatin protection against cyclosporin A-induced nephrotoxicity: clinical evidence. Curr Med Res Opin 2007; 23: 505-513.
355. Pérez M, Castilla M, Torres AM, Lázaro JA, Sarmiento E, Tejedor A. Inhibition of brush border dipeptidase with cilastatin reduces toxic accumulation of cyclosporin A in kidney proximal tubule epithelial cells. Nephrol Dial Transplant 2004; 19: 2445-2455.
356. Burdmann EA, Andoh TF, Rosen S, Lindsley J, Munar MY, Elzinga LW, Bennett WM. Experimental nephrotoxicity, hepatotoxicity and pharmacokinetics of cyclosporin G versus cyclosporin A. Kidney Int 1994; 45: 684-691.
357. Gruber SA, Gallichio M, Rosano TG, Kaplan SS, Hughes SE, Urbauer DL, Singh TP, Lempert N, Conti DJ, Stein DS, Drusano G. Comparative pharmacokinetics and renal effects of cyclosporin A and cyclosporin G in renal allograft recipients. J Clin Pharmacol 1997; 37: 575-586.
358. Nussenblatt RB, de Smet MD, Rubin B, Freidlin V, Whitcup SM, Davis J, Herman D, Bloom JN, Sran PK, Whitcher S, et al. A masked, randomized, dose-response study between cyclosporine A and G in the treatment of sight-threatening uveitis of noninfectious origin. Am J Ophthalmol 1993; 115: 583-591.
359. Hiestand PC, Graber M, Hurtenbach U, Herrmann P, Cammisuli S, Richardson BP, Eberle MK, Donatsch P, Ryffel B, Borel JF. New cyclosporine derivative SDZ IMM 125: *in vitro* and *in vivo* pharmacologic effects and toxicologic evaluation. Transplant Proc 1993; 25: 691-692.
360. Witkamp L, Zonneveld IM, Jung EG, Schopf RE, Christophers E, Grossman R, Meffert H, Belaich S, Mahrle G, van Joost T, et al. Efficacy and tolerability of multiple-dose SDZ IMM 125 in patients with severe psoriasis. Br J Dermatol 1995; 133: 95-103.
361. Bennett WM. The nephrotoxicity of new and old immunosuppressive drugs. Ren Fail 1998; 20: 687-690.
362. Noble S, Markham A. Cyclosporin. A review of the pharmacokinetic properties, clinical efficacy and tolerability of a microemulsion-based formulation (Neoral). Drugs 1995; 50: 924-941.
363. Bartucci M, Koshla B, Fleming-Brooks S, Weigel K, Donley V, Schulak JA, Knauss TC, Hricik DE. Renal function following conversion from Sandimmune to Neoral in stable renal transplant recipients. J Transpl Coord 1997; 7: 78-81.
364. Gennery AR, O'Sullivan JJ, Hasan A, Hamilton JR, Dark JH. Changing cyclosporin A formulation: an analysis in paediatric cardiac transplant recipients. Pediatr Transplant 1999; 3: 215-218.

365. Neumayer HH, Budde K, Farber L, Haller P, Kohnen R, Maibucher A, Schuster A, Vollmar J, Waiser J, Luft FC. Conversion to microemulsion cyclosporine in stable renal transplant patients: results after one year. Clin Nephrol 1996; 45: 326-331.
366. Hemming AW, Greig PD, Cattral MS, Chung SW, Lilly LB, Aljumah AA, Levy GA. A microemulsion of cyclosporine without intravenous cyclosporine in liver transplantation. Transplantation 1996; 62: 1798-1802.
367. Cole E, Keown P, Landsberg D, Halloran P, Shoker A, Rush D, Jeffrey J, Russell D, Stiller C, Muirhead N, Paul L, Zaltzman J, Loertscher R, Daloze P, Dandavino R, Boucher A, Handa P, Lawen J, Belitsky P, Parfrey P, Tan A, Hendricks L. Safety and tolerability of cyclosporine and cyclosporine microemulsion during 18 months of follow-up in stable renal transplant recipients: a report of the Canadian Neoral Renal Study Group. Transplantation 1998; 65: 505-510.
368. Pollard SG, Lear PA, Ready AR, Moore RH, Johnson RW. Comparison of microemulsion and conventional formulations of cyclosporine A in preventing acute rejection in de novo kidney transplant patients. The U.K. Neoral Renal Study Group. Transplantation 1999; 68: 1325-1331.
369. Olyaei AJ, deMattos AM, Bennett WM. Switching between cyclosporin formulations. What are the risks? Drug Saf 1997; 16: 366-373.
370. Cibulskyte D, Pedersen M, Hjelm-Poulsen J, Hansen HE, Madsen M, Mortensen J. The pharmacokinetics and acute renal effects of oral microemulsion ciclosporin A in normal pigs. Int Immunopharmacol. 2006; 6: 627-634.
371. Hricik DE, Dixit A, Knauss TC, Donley V, Bartucci MR, Schulak JA. Benefits of pre-emptive dose reduction for Sandimmune to Neoral conversion in stable renal transplant recipients. Clin Transplant 1998; 12: 575-578.
372. Kasiske BL, Chakkera HA, Louis TA, Ma JZ. A meta-analysis of immunosuppression withdrawal trials in renal transplantation. J Am Soc Nephrol 2000; 11: 1910-1917.
373. Helderman JH, Goral S. Cyclosporin withdrawal: to be or not to be! Nephrol Dial Transplant 1998; 13: 31-33.
374. Newstead CG, Johnston PA, Will EJ, Davison AM. The case for withdrawal of cyclosporin after renal transplantation. Nephrol Dial Transplant 1998; 13: 28-31.
375. Thervet E, Martinez F, Legendre C. Benefit-risk assessment of ciclosporin withdrawal in renal transplant recipients. Drug Saf 2004; 27: 457-476.
376. Srinivas TR, Meier-Kriesche HU. Minimizing immunosuppression, an alternative approach to reducing side effects: objectives and interim result. Clin J Am Soc Nephrol 2008; 3 (Suppl 2): S101-116.
377. Almond PS, Matas A, Gillingham K, Dunn DL, Payne WD, Gores P, Gruessner R, Najarian JS. Risk factors for chronic rejection in renal allograft recipients. Transplantation 1993; 55: 752-756.
378. Opelz G. Effect of the maintenance immunosuppressive drug regimen on kidney transplant outcome. Transplantation 1994; 58: 443-446.
379. Jha V, Muthukumar T, Kohli HS, Sud K, Gupta KL, Sakhuja V. Impact of cyclosporine withdrawal on living related renal transplants: a single-center experience. Am J Kidney Dis 2001; 37: 119-124.
380. Kasiske BL, Heim-Duthoy K, Ma JZ. Elective cyclosporine withdrawal after renal transplantation. A meta- analysis. JAMA 1993; 269: 395-400.
381. Rocher LL, Milford EL, Kirkman RL, Carpenter CB, Strom TB, Tilney NL. Conversion from cyclosporine to azathioprine in renal allograft recipients. Transplantation 1984; 38: 669-674.
382. Hunt SA, Stinson EB, Oyer PE, Billingham ME, Gamberg P, Miller J, Schroeder JS, Baldwin JC, Shumway NE. Results of "immunoconversion" from cyclosporine to azathioprine in heart transplant recipients with progressive nephrotoxicity. Transplant Proc 1987; 19: 2522-2524.
383. Sandborn WJ, Hay JE, Porayko MK, Gores GJ, Steers JL, Krom RA, Wiesner RH. Cyclosporine withdrawal for nephrotoxicity in liver transplant recipients does not result in sustained improvement in kidney function and causes cellular and ductopenic rejection. Hepatology 1994; 19: 925-932.
384. Dubey D, Kumar A, Srivastava A, Mandhani A, Sharma AP, Gupta A, Sharma RK. Cyclosporin A withdrawal in live related renal transplantation: long-term results. Clin Transplant 2001; 15: 136-141.
385. Heim-Duthoy KL, Chitwood KK, Tortorice KL, Massy ZA, Kasiske BL. Elective cyclosporine withdrawal 1 year after renal transplantation. Am J Kidney Dis 1994; 24: 846-853.
386. Hollander AA, van Saase JL, Kootte AM, van Dorp WT, van Bockel HJ, van Es LA, van der Woude FJ. Beneficial effects of conversion from cyclosporin to azathioprine after kidney transplantation. Lancet 1995; 345: 610-614.
387. MacPhee IA, Bradley JA, Briggs JD, Junor BJ, MacPherson SG, McMillan MA, Rodger RS, Watson MA. Long-term outcome of a prospective randomized trial of conversion from cyclosporine to azathioprine treatment one year after renal transplantation. Transplantation 1998; 66: 1186-1192.
388. Bakker RC, Hollander AA, Mallat MJ, Bruijn JA, Paul LC, de Fijter JW. Conversion from cyclosporine to azathioprine at three months reduces the incidence of chronic allograft nephropathy. Kidney Int 2003; 64: 1027-1034.

389. Gallagher MP, Hall B, Craig J, Berry G, Tiller DJ, Eris J; Australian Multicenter Trial of Cyclosporine Withdrawal Study Group and the ANZ Dialysis and Transplantation Registry. A randomized controlled trial of cyclosporine withdrawal in renal-transplant recipients: 15-year results. Transplantation 2004; 78: 1653-1660.
390. Pescovitz MD, Govani M. Sirolimus and mycophenolate mofetil for calcineurin-free immunosuppression in renal transplant recipients. Am J Kidney Dis 2001; 38: S16-S21.
391. de Sevaux RG, Gregoor PJ, Hene RJ, Hoitsma AJ, Vos P, Weimar W, Van Gelder T, Hilbrands LB. A controlled trial comparing two doses of cyclosporine in conjunction with mycophenolate mofetil and corticosteroids. J Am Soc Nephrol 2001; 12: 1750-1757.
392. Schrama YC, Joles JA, van Tol A, Boer P, Koomans HA, Hene RJ. Conversion to mycophenolate mofetil in conjunction with stepwise withdrawal of cyclosporine in stable renal transplant recipients. Transplantation 2000; 69: 376-383.
393. Weir MR, Anderson L, Fink JC, Gabregiorgish K, Schweitzer EJ, Hoehn-Saric E, Klassen DK, Cangro CB, Johnson LB, Kuo PC, Lim JY, Bartlett ST. A novel approach to the treatment of chronic allograft nephropathy. Transplantation 1997; 64: 1706-1710.
394. Zanker B, Schneeberger H, Rothenpieler U, Hillebrand G, Illner WD, Theodorakis I, Stangl M, Land W. Mycophenolate mofetil-based, cyclosporine-free induction and maintenance immunosuppression: first-3-months analysis of efficacy and safety in two cohorts of renal allograft recipients. Transplantation 1998; 66: 44-49.
395. Aleksic I, Baryalei M, Busch T, Pieske B, Schorn B, Strauch J, Sirbu H, Dalichau H. Improvement of impaired renal function in heart transplant recipients treated with mycophenolate mofetil and low-dose cyclosporine. Transplantation 2000; 69: 1586-1590.
396. Herrero JI, Quiroga J, Sangro B, Girala M, Gomez-Manero N, Pardo F, Alvarez-Cienfuegos J, Prieto J. Conversion of liver transplant recipients on cyclosporine with renal impairment to mycophenolate mofetil. Liver Transpl Surg 1999; 5: 414-420.
397. Schlitt HJ, Barkmann A, Boker KH, Schmidt HH, Emmanouilidis N, Rosenau J, Bahr MJ, Tusch G, Manns MP, Nashan B, Klempnauer J. Replacement of calcineurin inhibitors with mycophenolate mofetil in liver-transplant patients with renal dysfunction: a randomised controlled study. Lancet 2001; 357: 587-591.
398. Koch RO, Graziadei IW, Schulz F, Nachbaur K, Königsrainer A, Margreiter R, Vogel W. Long-term efficacy and safety of mycophenolate mofetil in liver transplant recipients with calcineurin inhibitor-induced renal dysfunction. Transpl Int 2004; 17: 518-524.
399. Al-Aly Z, Sachdeva A, Philoctete Ashley JM, Bastani B. Preliminary experience with mycophenolate mofetil for preservation of renal function in cardiac transplant patients with documented cyclosporine nephrotoxicity. Nephrology (Carlton) 2006; 11: 151-155.
400. Hamour IM, Lyster HS, Burke MM, Rose ML, Banner NR. Mycophenolate mofetil may allow cyclosporine and steroid sparing in de novo heart transplant patients. Transplantation 2007; 83: 570-576.
401. David-Neto E, Araujo LM, Lemos FC, David DS, Mazzucchi E, Nahas WC, Arap S, Ianhez LE. Introduction of mycophenolate mofetil and cyclosporin reduction in children with chronic transplant nephropathy. Pediatr Transplant 2001; 5: 302-309.
402. Ulinski T, Dubourg L, Saïd MH, Parchoux B, Ranchin B, Cochat P. Switch from cyclosporine A to mycophenolate mofetil in nephrotic children. Pediatr Nephrol 2005; 20: 482-485.
403. Smak Gregoor PJ, Van Gelder T, van Besouw NM, van der Mast BJ, Ijzermans JN, Weimar W. Randomized study on the conversion of treatment with cyclosporine to azathioprine or mycophenolate mofetil followed by dose reduction. Transplantation 2000; 70: 143-148.
404. Theodorakis J, Schneeberger H, Illner WD, Stangl M, Zanker B, Land W. Nephrotoxicity-free, mycophenolate mofetil based induction/maintenance immunosuppression in elderly recipients of renal allografts from elderly cadaveric donors. Transplant Proc 2000; 32(1A Suppl): 9S-11S.
405. Lecornu-Heuze L, Ducloux D, Rebibou JM, Martin L, Billerey C, Chalopin JM. Mycophenolate mofetil in cyclosporin-associated thrombotic microangiopathy. Nephrol Dial Transplant 1998; 13: 3212-3213.
406. Davison SC, Morris-Jones R, Powles AV, Fry L. Change of treatment from cyclosporin to mycophenolate mofetil in severe psoriasis. Br J Dermatol 2000; 143: 405-407.
407. Thervet E, Morelon E, Ducloux D, Bererhi L, Noel LH, Janin A, Bedrossian J, Puget S, Chalopin JM, Mihatsch M, Legendre C, Kreis H. Cyclosporine withdrawal in stable renal transplant recipients after azathioprine-mycophenolate mofetil conversion. Clin Transplant 2000; 14: 561-566.
408. Abramowicz D, Del Carmen Rial M, Vitko S, del Castillo D, Manas D, Lao M, Gafner N, Wijngaard P; Cyclosporine Withdrawal Study Group. Cyclosporine withdrawal from a mycophenolate mofetil-containing immunosuppressive regimen: results of a five-year, prospective, randomized study. J Am Soc Nephrol 2005; 16: 2234-2240.
409. Sehgal SN. Rapamune (RAPA, rapamycin, sirolimus): mechanism of action immunosuppressive effect results from blockade of signal transduction and inhibition of cell cycle progression. Clin Biochem 1998; 31: 335-340.
410. Groth CG, Backman L, Morales JM, Calne R, Kreis H, Lang P, Touraine JL, Claesson K, Campistol JM, Durand D, Wramner L, Brattstrom C, Charpentier B. Sirolimus (rapamycin)-based therapy in human renal transplantation: similar efficacy and different toxicity compared with cyclosporine. Sirolimus European Renal Transplant Study Group. Transplantation 1999; 67: 1036-1042.

411. Kreis H, Cisterne JM, Land W, Wramner L, Squifflet JP, Abramowicz D, Campistol JM, Morales JM, Grinyo JM, Mourad G, Berthoux FC, Brattstrom C, Lebranchu Y, Vialtel P. Sirolimus in association with mycophenolate mofetil induction for the prevention of acute graft rejection in renal allograft recipients. Transplantation 2000; 69: 1252-1260.
412. Morelon E, Mamzer-Bruneel MF, Peraldi MN, Kreis H. Sirolimus: a new promising immunosuppressive drug. Towards a rationale for its use in renal transplantation. Nephrol Dial Transplant 2001; 16: 18-20.
413. Andoh TF, Lindsley J, Franceschini N, Bennett WM. Synergistic effects of cyclosporine and rapamycin in a chronic nephrotoxicity model. Transplantation 1996; 62: 311-316.
414. Kahan BD. Efficacy of sirolimus compared with azathioprine for reduction of acute renal allograft rejection: a randomised multicentre study. The Rapamune US Study Group. Lancet 2000; 356: 194-202.
415. Macdonald AS. A worldwide, phase III, randomized, controlled, safety and efficacy study of a sirolimus/cyclosporine regimen for prevention of acute rejection in recipients of primary mismatched renal allografts. Transplantation 2001; 71: 271-280.
416. Podder H, Stepkowski SM, Napoli KL, Clark J, Verani RR, Chou TC, Kahan BD. Pharmacokinetic interactions augment toxicities of sirolimus/cyclosporine combinations. J Am Soc Nephrol 2001; 12: 1059-1071.
417. Kahan BD, Kramer WG. Median effect analysis of efficacy versus adverse effects of immunosuppressants. Clin Pharmacol Ther 2001; 70: 74-81.
418. Dominguez J, Mahalati K, Kiberd B, McAlister VC, Macdonald AS. Conversion to rapamycin immunosuppression in renal transplant recipients: report of an initial experience. Transplantation 2000; 70: 1244-1247.
419. Fairbanks KD, Eustace JA, Fine D, Thuluvath PJ. Renal function improves in liver transplant recipients when switched from a calcineurin inhibitor to sirolimus.Liver Transpl 2003; 9: 1079-1085.
420. Lyster H, Panicker G, Leaver N, Banner NR. Initial experience with sirolimus and mycophenolate mofetil for renal rescue from cyclosporine nephrotoxicity after heart transplantation. Transplant Proc 2004; 36: 3167-3170.
421. Bumbea V, Kamar N, Ribes D, Esposito L, Modesto A, Guitard J, Nasou G, Durand D, Rostaing L. Long-term results in renal transplant patients with allograft dysfunction after switching from calcineurin inhibitors to sirolimus. Nephrol Dial Transplant 2005; 20: 2517-2523.
422. Bestetti R, Theodoropoulos TAD, Burdmann EA, AbbudFilho M, Cordeiro JÁ, Villafanha D. Switch from calcineurin inhibitors to sirolimus induced renal recovery in heart transplant recipients in the midterm follow-up. Transplantation 2006; 81: 692-696.
423. Ruiz JC, Campistol JM, Grinyó JM, Mota A, Prats D, Gutiérrez JA, Henriques AC, Pinto JR, García J, Morales JM, Gómez JM, Arias M. Early cyclosporine a withdrawal in kidney-transplant recipients receiving sirolimus prevents progression of chronic pathologic allograft lesions. Transplantation. 2004; 78: 1312-1318.
424. Bennett WM, DeMattos A, Meyer MM, Andoh T, Barry JM. Chronic cyclosporine nephropathy: the Achilles' heel of immunosuppressive therapy. Kidney Int 1996; 50: 1089-1100.
425. Mihatsch MJ, Ryffel B, Gudat F. The differential diagnosis between rejection and cyclosporine toxicity. Kidney Int Suppl 1995; 52: S63-S69.
426. Franceschini N, Alpers CE, Bennett WM, Andoh TF. Cyclosporine arteriolopathy: effects of drug withdrawal. Am J Kidney Dis 1998; 32: 247-253.
427. Hamahira K, Iijima K, Tanaka R, Nakamura H, Yoshikawa N. Recovery from cyclosporine-associated arteriolopathy in childhood nephrotic syndrome. Pediatr Nephrol 2001; 16: 723-727.
428. Iijima K, Hamahira K, Kobayashi A, Nakamura H, Yoshikawa N. Immunohistochemical analysis of renin activity in chronic cyclosporine nephropathy in childhood nephrotic syndrome. J Am Soc Nephrol 2000; 11: 2265-2271.
429. Myers BD, Ross J, Newton L, Luetscher J, Perlroth M. Cyclosporine-associated chronic nephropathy. N Engl J Med 1984; 311: 699-705.
430. Palestine AG, Austin HA, III, Balow JE, Antonovych TT, Sabnis SG, Preuss HG, Nussenblatt RB. Renal histopathologic alterations in patients treated with cyclosporine for uveitis. N Engl J Med 1986; 314: 1293-1298.
431. Gerkens JF, Bhagwandeen SB, Dosen PJ, Smith AJ. The effect of salt intake on cyclosporine-induced impairment of renal function in rats. Transplantation 1984; 38: 412-417.
432. Jackson NM, Hsu CH, Visscher GE, Venkatachalam MA, Humes HD. Alterations in renal structure and function in a rat model of cyclosporine nephrotoxicity. J Pharmacol Exp Ther 1987; 242: 749-756.
433. Elzinga LW, Rosen S, Bennett WM. Dissociation of glomerular filtration rate from tubulointerstitial fibrosis in experimental chronic cyclosporine nephropathy: role of sodium intake. J Am Soc Nephrol 1993; 4: 214-221.
434. Rosen S, Greenfeld Z, Brezis M. Chronic cyclosporine-induced nephropathy in the rat. A medullary ray and inner stripe injury. Transplantation 1990; 49: 445-452.
435. Young BA, Burdmann EA, Johnson RJ, Andoh T, Bennett WM, Couser WG, Alpers CE. Cyclosporine A induced arteriolopathy in a rat model of chronic cyclosporine nephropathy. Kidney Int 1995; 48: 431-438.

436. Myers BD, Newton L, Boshkos C, Macoviak JA, Frist WH, Derby GC, Perlroth MG, Sibley RK. Chronic injury of human renal microvessels with low-dose cyclosporine therapy. Transplantation 1988; 46: 694-703.
437. Myers BD, Sibley R, Newton L, Tomlanovich SJ, Boshkos C, Stinson E, Luetscher JA, Whitney DJ, Krasny D, Coplon NS, Perlroth MG. The long-term course of cyclosporine-associated chronic nephropathy. Kidney Int 1988; 33: 590-600.
438. Truong LD, Farhood A, Tasby J, Gillum D. Experimental chronic renal ischemia: morphologic and immunologic studies. Kidney Int 1992; 41: 1676-1689.
439. Burdmann EA, Young B, Andoh TF, Evans A, Alpers CE, Lindsley J, Johnson RJ, Couser W, Bennett WM. Mechanisms of cyclosporine-induced interstitial fibrosis. Transplant Proc 1994; 26: 2588-2589.
440. Dieperink H, Hansen HV, Kemp M, Leyssac PP, Starklint H, Kemp E. Antagonist capacity of felodipine on cyclosporin A nephrotoxicity in the rat. Nephrol Dial Transplant 1992; 7: 1124-1129.
441. Wolf G, Neilson EG. Increases in levels of collagen types I and IV messenger ribonucleic acid in murine kidneys after treatment with ciclosporin. Nephron 1992; 60: 87-91.
442. Hunley TE, Fogo A, Iwasaki S, Kon V. Endothelin A receptor mediates functional but not structural damage in chronic cyclosporine nephrotoxicity. J Am Soc Nephrol 1995; 5: 1718-1723.
443. Kon V, Hunley TE, Fogo A. Combined antagonism of endothelin A/B receptors links endothelin to vasoconstriction whereas angiotensin II effects fibrosis. Studies in chronic cyclosporine nephrotoxicity in rats. Transplantation 1995; 60: 89-95.
444. Burdmann EA, Andoh TF, Nast CC, Evan A, Connors BA, Coffman TM, Lindsley J, Bennett WM. Prevention of experimental cyclosporin-induced interstitial fibrosis by losartan and enalapril. Am J Physiol 1995; 269: F491-F499.
445. Vieira JM, Jr., Noronha IL, Malheiros DM, Burdmann EA. Cyclosporine-induced interstitial fibrosis and arteriolar TGF-beta expression with preserved renal blood flow. Transplantation 1999; 68: 1746-1753.
446. Ramirez C, Olmo A, O'Valle F, Masseroli M, Aguilar M, Gomez-Morales M, Revelles F, Garcia-Chicano MJ, Arrebola F, Reguero ME, del Moral RG. Role of intrarenal endothelin 1, endothelin 3, and angiotensin II expression in chronic cyclosporin A nephrotoxicity in rats. Exp Nephrol 2000; 8: 161-172.
447. Fox J, Guan S, Hymel AA, Navar LG. Dietary Na and ACE inhibition effects on renal tissue angiotensin I and II and ACE activity in rats. Am J Physiol 1992; 262: F902-F909.
448. Holmer S, Eckardt KU, LeHir M, Schricker K, Riegger G, Kurtz A. Influence of dietary NaCl intake on renin gene expression in the kidneys and adrenal glands of rats. Pflugers Arch 1993; 425: 62-67.
449. Ruiz-Ortega M, Egido J. Angiotensin II modulates cell growth-related events and synthesis of matrix proteins in renal interstitial fibroblasts. Kidney Int 1997; 52: 1497-1510.
450. Wolf G, Neilson EG. Angiotensin II as a renal growth factor. J Am Soc Nephrol 1993; 3: 1531-1540.
451. Wolf G, Kalluri R, Ziyadeh FN, Neilson EG, Stahl RA. Angiotensin II induces alpha3(IV) collagen expression in cultured murine proximal tubular cells. Proc Assoc Am Physicians 1999; 111: 357-364.
452. Johnson RJ, Alpers CE, Yoshimura A, Lombardi D, Pritzl P, Floege J, Schwartz SM. Renal injury from angiotensin II-mediated hypertension. Hypertension 1992; 19: 464-474.
453. Meister B, Lippoldt A, Bunnemann B, Inagami T, Ganten D, Fuxe K. Cellular expression of angiotensin type-1 receptor mRNA in the kidney. Kidney Int 1993; 44: 331-336.
454. Sechi LA, Grady EF, Griffin CA, Kalinyak JE, Schambelan M. Distribution of angiotensin II receptor subtypes in rat and human kidney. Am J Physiol 1992; 262: F236-F240.
455. Zhuo J, Alcorn D, Allen AM, Mendelsohn FA. High resolution localization of angiotensin II receptors in rat renal medulla. Kidney Int 1992; 42: 1372-1380.
456. Lafayette RA, Mayer G, Meyer TW. The effects of blood pressure reduction on cyclosporine nephrotoxicity in the rat. J Am Soc Nephrol 1993; 3: 1892-1899.
457. Lassila M, Finckenberg P, Pere AK, Krogerus L, Ahonen J, Vapaatalo H, Nurminen ML. Comparison of enalapril and valsartan in cyclosporine A-induced hypertension and nephrotoxicity in spontaneously hypertensive rats on high-sodium diet. Br J Pharmacol 2000; 130: 1339-1347.
458. Johnson DW, Saunders HJ, Vesey DA, Qi W, Field MJ, Pollock CA. Enalaprilat directly ameliorates *in vitro* cyclosporin nephrotoxicity in human tubulo-interstitial cells. Nephron 2000; 86: 473-481.
459. Yang CW, Ahn HJ, Kim WY, Shin MJ, Kim SK, Park JH, Kim YO, Kim YS, Kim J, Bang BK. Influence of the renin-angiotensin system on epidermal growth factor expression in normal and cyclosporine-treated rat kidney. Kidney Int 2001; 60: 847-857.
460. Shihab FS, Bennett WM, Isaac J, Yi H, Andoh TF. Angiotensin II regulation of vascular endothelial growth factor and receptors Flt-1 and KDR/Flk-1 in cyclosporine nephrotoxicity. Kidney Int 2002; 62: 422-433.
461. Sun BK, Li C, Lim SW, Choi BS, Lee SH, Kim IS, Kim YS, Bang BK, Yang CW. Blockade of angiotensin II with losartan attenuates transforming growth factor-beta1 inducible gene-h3 (betaig-h3) expression in a model of chronic cyclosporine nephrotoxicity. Nephron Exp Nephrol 2005; 99: e9-16.

462. Yang CW, Ahn HJ, Kim WY, Li C, Jung JY, Yoon SA, Kim YS, Cha JH, Kim J, Bang BK. Synergistic effects of mycophenolate mofetil and losartan in a model of chronic cyclosporine nephropathy. Transplantation 2003; 75: 309-315.

463. Li C, Lim SW, Choi BS, Lee SH, Cha JH, Kim IS, Kim J, Yang CW. Inhibitory effect of pravastatin on transforming growth factor beta1-inducible gene h3 expression in a rat model of chronic cyclosporine nephropathy. Am J Nephrol 2005; 25: 611-620.

464. Chander V, Singh D, Tirkey N, Chander H, Chopra K. Amelioration of cyclosporine nephrotoxicity by irbesartan, A selective AT1 receptor antagonist. Ren Fail 2004; 26: 467-477.

465. Cibulskyte D, Pedersen M, Hørlyck A, Marcussen N, Hansen HE, Frøkiaer J, Madsen M, Mortensen J. Telmisartan attenuates chronic ciclosporin A nephrotoxicity in a pig model. Nephrol Dial Transplant 2007; 22: 369-375.

466. Bobadilla NA, Gamba G. New insights into the pathophysiology of cyclosporine nephrotoxicity: a role of aldosterone. Am J Physiol Renal Physiol 2007; 293: F2-9.

467. Feria I, Pichardo I, Juárez P, Ramírez V, González MA, Uribe N, García-Torres R, López-Casillas F, Gamba G, Bobadilla NA. Therapeutic benefit of spironolactone in experimental chronic cyclosporine A nephrotoxicity. Kidney Int 2003; 63: 43-

468. Pérez-Rojas J, Blanco JA, Cruz C, Trujillo J, Vaidya VS, Uribe N, Bonventre JV, Gamba G, Bobadilla NA. Mineralocorticoid receptor blockade confers renoprotection in preexisting chronic cyclosporine nephrotoxicity. Am J Physiol Renal Physiol 2007; 292: F131-139.

469. Islam M, Burke JF, Jr., McGowan TA, Zhu Y, Dunn SR, McCue P, Kanalas J, Sharma K. Effect of anti-transforming growth factor-beta antibodies in cyclosporine-induced renal dysfunction. Kidney Int 2001; 59: 498-506.

470. Khanna A, Kapur S, Sharma V, Li B, Suthanthiran M. *In vivo* hyperexpression of transforming growth factor-beta1 in mice: stimulation by cyclosporine. Transplantation 1997; 63: 1037-1039.

471. Pichler RH, Franceschini N, Young BA, Hugo C, Andoh TF, Burdmann EA, Shankland SJ, Alpers CE, Bennett WM, Couser WG. Pathogenesis of cyclosporine nephropathy: roles of angiotensin II and osteopontin. J Am Soc Nephrol 1995; 6: 1186-1196.

472. Shin GT, Khanna A, Ding R, Sharma VK, Lagman M, Li B, Suthanthiran M. *In vivo* expression of transforming growth factor-beta1 in humans: stimulation by cyclosporine. Transplantation 1998; 65: 313-318.

473. Wolf G, Thaiss F, Stahl RA. Cyclosporine stimulates expression of transforming growth factor-beta in renal cells. Possible mechanism of cyclosporines antiproliferative effects. Transplantation 1995; 60: 237-241.

474. Campistol JM, Inigo P, Larios S, Bescos M, Oppenheimer F. Role of transforming growth factor-beta1 in the progression of chronic allograft nephropathy. Nephrol Dial Transplant 2001; 16 Suppl 1: 114-116.

475. Khanna A. Tacrolimus and cyclosporine *in vitro* and *in vivo* induce osteopontin mRNA and protein expression in renal tissues. Nephron Exp Nephrol 2005; 101: e119-126.

476. Shihab FS, Andoh TF, Tanner AM, Noble NA, Border WA, Franceschini N, Bennett WM. Role of transforming growth factor-beta 1 in experimental chronic cyclosporine nephropathy. Kidney Int 1996; 49: 1141-1151.

477. Saggi SJ, Andoh TF, Safirstein R, Bennett WM. Cyclosporin induces renal proto-oncogene RNA message and increased transforming growth factor-beta prior to renal fibrosis: Modification by calcium channel blockade in the salt replete rat. Nephrology (Carlton). 2004; 9: 58-64.

478. Gooch JL, Roberts BR, Cobbs SL, Tumlin JA. Loss of the alpha-isoform of calcineurin is sufficient to induce nephrotoxicity and altered expression of transforming growth factor-beta. Transplantation 2007; 83: 439-447.

479. Cuhaci B, Kumar MS, Bloom RD, Pratt B, Haussman G, Laskow DA, Alidoost M, Grotkowski C, Cahill K, Butani L, Sturgill BC, Pankewycz OG. Transforming growth factor-beta levels in human allograft chronic fibrosis correlate with rate of decline in renal function. Transplantation 1999; 68: 785-790.

480. Baan CC, Balk AH, Holweg CT, van Riemsdijk IC, Maat LP, Vantrimpont PJ, Niesters HG, Weimar W. Renal failure after clinical heart transplantation is associated with the TGF-beta 1 codon 10 gene polymorphism. J Heart Lung Transplant 2000; 19: 866-872.

481. Wolf G. Link between angiotensin II and TGF-beta in the kidney. Miner Electrolyte Metab 1998; 24: 174-180.

482. Shihab FS, Andoh TF, Tanner AM, Bennett WM. Sodium depletion enhances fibrosis and the expression of TGF-beta1 and matrix proteins in experimental chronic cyclosporine nephropathy. Am J Kidney Dis 1997; 30: 71-81.

483. Shihab FS, Bennett WM, Tanner AM, Andoh TF. Angiotensin II blockade decreases TGF-beta1 and matrix proteins in cyclosporine nephropathy. Kidney Int 1997; 52: 660-673.

484. Khanna AK, Plummer MS, Hilton G, Pieper GM, Ledbetter S. Anti-transforming growth factor antibody at low but not high doses limits cyclosporine-mediated nephrotoxicity without altering rat cardiac allograft survival: potential of therapeutic applications. Circulation 2004; 110: 3822-3829.

485. Gillum DM, Truong L, Tasby J. Characterization of the interstitial cellular infiltrate in experimental chronic cyclosporine nephropathy. Transplantation 1990; 49: 793-797.

486. Young BA, Burdmann EA, Johnson RJ, Alpers CE, Giachelli CM, Eng E, Andoh T, Bennett WM, Couser WG. Cellular proliferation and macrophage influx precede interstitial fibrosis in cyclosporine nephrotoxicity. Kidney Int 1995; 48: 439-448.

487. Mazzali M, Hughes J, Dantas M, Liaw L, Steitz S, Alpers CE, Pichler RH, Lan HY, Giachelli CM, Shankland SJ, Couser WG, Johnson RJ. Effects of cyclosporine in osteopontin null mice. Kidney Int 2002; 62: 78-85.
488. Benigni A, Bruzzi I, Mister M, Azzollini N, Gaspari F, Perico N, Gotti E, Bertani T, Remuzzi G. Nature and mediators of renal lesions in kidney transplant patients given cyclosporine for more than one year. Kidney Int 1999; 55: 674-685.
489. Hudkins KL, Le QC, Segerer S, Johnson RJ, Davis CL, Giachelli CM, Alpers CE. Osteopontin expression in human cyclosporine toxicity. Kidney Int 2001; 60: 635-640.
490. Ghielli M, Verstrepen WA, Nouwen EJ, De Broe ME. Inflammatory cells in renal regeneration. Ren Fail 1996; 18: 355-375.
491. Rodriguez-Iturbe B, Pons H, Herrera-Acosta J, Johnson RJ. Role of immunocompetent cells in nonimmune renal diseases. Kidney Int 2001; 59: 1626-1640.
492. Becker GJ, Hewitson TD. The role of tubulointerstitial injury in chronic renal failure. Curr Opin Nephrol Hypertens 2000; 9: 133-138.
493. Iwai N, Inagami T, Ohmichi N, Kinoshita M. Renin is expressed in rat macrophage/monocyte cells. Hypertension 1996; 27: 399-403.
494. Okamura A, Rakugi H, Ohishi M, Yanagitani Y, Takiuchi S, Moriguchi K, Fennessy PA, Higaki J, Ogihara T. Upregulation of renin-angiotensin system during differentiation of monocytes to macrophages. J Hypertens 1999; 17: 537-545.
495. Wolf G, Killen PD, Neilson EG. Cyclosporin A stimulates transcription and procollagen secretion in tubulointerstitial fibroblasts and proximal tubular cells. J Am Soc Nephrol 1990; 1: 918-922.
496. Ghiggeri GM, Altieri P, Oleggini R, Valenti F, Ginevri F, Perfumo F, Gusmano R. Cyclosporine enhances the synthesis of selected extracellular matrix proteins by renal cells "in culture". Different cell responses and phenotype characterization. Transplantation 1994; 57: 1382-1388.
497. Johnson DW, Saunders HJ, Johnson FJ, Huq SO, Field MJ, Pollock CA. Cyclosporin exerts a direct fibrogenic effect on human tubulointerstitial cells: roles of insulin-like growth factor I, transforming growth factor beta1, and platelet-derived growth factor. J Pharmacol Exp Ther 1999; 289: 535-542.
498. Esposito C, Fornoni A, Cornacchia F, Bellotti N, Fasoli G, Foschi A, Mazzucchelli I, Mazzullo T, Semeraro L, Dal Canton A. Cyclosporine induces different responses in human epithelial, endothelial and fibroblast cell cultures. Kidney Int 2000; 58: 123-130.
499. Duymelinck C, Deng JT, Dauwe SE, De Broe ME, Verpooten GA. Inhibition of the matrix metalloproteinase system in a rat model of chronic cyclosporine nephropathy. Kidney Int 1998; 54: 804-818.
500. Fornoni A, Lenz O, Tack I, Potier M, Elliot SJ, Striker LJ, Striker GE. Matrix accumulation in mesangial cells exposed to cyclosporine A requires a permissive genetic background. Transplantation 2000; 70: 587-593.
501. Shihab FS, Andoh TF, Tanner AM, Yi H, Bennett WM. Expression of apoptosis regulatory genes in chronic cyclosporine nephrotoxicity favors apoptosis. Kidney Int 1999; 56: 2147-2159.
502. Thomas SE, Andoh TF, Pichler RH, Shankland SJ, Couser WG, Bennett WM, Johnson RJ. Accelerated apoptosis characterizes cyclosporine-associated interstitial fibrosis. Kidney Int 1998; 53: 897-908.
503. Amore A, Emancipator SN, Cirina P, Conti G, Ricotti E, Bagheri N, Coppo R. Nitric oxide mediates cyclosporine-induced apoptosis in cultured renal cells. Kidney Int 2000; 57: 1549-1559.
504. Anglicheau D, Pallet N, Rabant M, Marquet P, Cassinat B, Méria P, Beaune P, Legendre C, Thervet E. Role of P-glycoprotein in cyclosporine cytotoxicity in the cyclosporine-sirolimus interaction. Kidney Int 2006; 70: 1019-1025.
505. del Moral RG, Andujar M, Ramirez C, Gomez-Morales M, Masseroli M, Aguilar M, Olmo A, Arrebola F, Guillen M, Garcia-Chicano MJ, Nogales FF, O'Valle F. Chronic cyclosporin A nephrotoxicity, P-glycoprotein overexpression, and relationships with intrarenal angiotensin II deposits. Am J Pathol 1997; 151: 1705-1714.
506. Nascimento CR, Braga F, Capella LS, Santos OR, Lopes AG, Capella MA. Comparative study on the effects of cyclosporin A in renal cells in culture. Nephron Exp Nephrol 2005; 99: e77-86.
507. Koziolek MJ, Riess R, Geiger H, Thevenod F, Hauser IA. Expression of multidrug resistance P-glycoprotein in kidney allografts from cyclosporine A-treated patients. Kidney Int 2001; 60: 156-166.
508. 508. Joy MS, Nickeleit V, Hogan SL, Thompson BD, Finn WF Calcineurin inhibitor-induced nephrotoxicity and renal expression of P-glycoprotein. Pharmacotherapy 2005; 25:779-789.
509. Hauser IA, Schaeffeler E, Gauer S, Scheuermann EH, Wegner B, Gossmann J, Ackermann H, Seidl C, Hocher B, Zanger UM, Geiger H, Eichelbaum M, Schwab M. BCB1 genotype of the donor but not of the recipient is a major risk factor for cyclosporine-related nephrotoxicity after renal transplantation. J Am Soc Nephrol 2005; 16: 1501-1511.
510. Shihab FS, Yi H, Bennett WM, Andoh TF. Effect of nitric oxide modulation on TGF-beta1 and matrix proteins in chronic cyclosporine nephrotoxicity. Kidney Int 2000; 58: 1174-1185.
511. Hutchinson IV. An endothelin-transforming growth factor beta pathway in the nephrotoxicity of immunosuppressive drugs. Curr Opin Nephrol Hypertens 1998; 7: 665-671.

512. Shihab FS, Bennett WM, Yi H, Andoh TF. Expression of vascular endothelial growth factor and its receptors Flt-1 and KDR/Flk-1 in chronic cyclosporine nephrotoxicity. Transplantation 2001; 72: 164-168.
513. Shihab FS, Bennett WM, Yi H, Andoh TF. Nitric oxide modulates vascular endothelial growth factor and receptors in chronic cyclosporine nephrotoxicity. Kidney Int 2003; 63: 522-533.
514. Kang DH, Kim YG, Andoh TF, Gordon KL, Suga S, Mazzali M, Jefferson JA, Hughes J, Bennett W, Schreiner GF, Johnson RJ. Post-cyclosporine-mediated hypertension and nephropathy: amelioration by vascular endothelial growth factor. Am J Physiol Renal Physiol 2001; 280: F727-F736.
515. Miura K, Nakatani T, Asai T, Yamanaka S, Tamada S, Tashiro K, Kim S, Okamura M, Iwao H. Role of hypomagnesemia in chronic cyclosporine nephropathy. Transplantation 2002; 73: 340-347.
516. Asai T, Nakatani T, Yamanaka S, Tamada S, Kishimoto T, Tashiro K, Nakao T, Okamura M, Kim S, Iwao H, Miura K. Magnesium supplementation prevents experimental chronic cyclosporine a nephrotoxicity via renin-angiotensin system independent mechanism. Transplantation 2002; 74: 784-791.
517. Asai T, Nakatani T, Tamada S, Kuwabara N, Yamanaka S, Tashiro K, Nakao T, Komiya T, Okamura M, Kim S, Iwao H, Miura K. Activation of transcription factors AP-1 and NF-kappaB in chronic cyclosporine A nephrotoxicity: role in beneficial effects of magnesium supplementation. Transplantation 2003; 75: 1040-1044.
518. Yuan J, Zhou J, Chen BC, Zhang X, Zhou HM, Du DF, Chang S, Chen ZK. Magnesium supplementation prevents chronic cyclosporine nephrotoxicity via adjusting nitric oxide synthase activity. Transplant Proc 2005; 37: 1892-1895.
519. Holzmacher R, Kendziorski C, Michael Hofman R, Jaffery J, Becker B, Djamali A. Low serum magnesium is associated with decreased graft survival in patients with chronic cyclosporin nephrotoxicity. Nephrol Dial Transplant 2005; 20: 1456-1462.
520. Mazzali M, Kim YG, Suga S, Gordon KL, Kang DH, Jefferson JA, Hughes J, Kivlighn SD, Lan HY, Johnson RJ. Hyperuricemia exacerbates chronic cyclosporine nephropathy. Transplantation 2001; 71: 900-905.
521. Kim YO, Lim SW, Li C, Kang HJ, Ahn KO, Yang HJ, Ghee JY, Kim SH, Kim JY, Choi BS, Kim J, Yang CW. Activation of intrarenal complement system in mouse model for chronic cyclosporine nephrotoxicity. Yonsei Med J 2007; 48: 517-525.
522. Perico N, Rossini M, Imberti O, Malanchini B, Cornejo RP, Gaspari F, Bertani T, Remuzzi G. Thromboxane receptor blockade attenuates chronic cyclosporine nephrotoxicity and improves survival in rats with renal isograft. J Am Soc Nephrol 1992; 2: 1398-1404.
523. Stillman IE, English J, Burdmann EA, Andoh TF, Franschini N, Bennett WM, Rosen S. Prednisone alters the histopathology of chronic cyclosporine nephropathy. Exp Nephrol 1997; 5: 61-68.
524. Sobh M, Sabry A, Moustafa F, Foda MA, Sally S, Ghoneim M. Effect of colchicine on chronic ciclosporin nephrotoxicity in Sprague-Dawley rats. Nephron 1998; 79: 452-457.
525. Li C, Yang CW, Ahn HJ, Kim WY, Park CW, Park JH, Lee MJ, Yang JH, Kim YS, Bang BK. Colchicine decreases apoptotic cell death in chronic cyclosporine nephrotoxicity. J Lab Clin Med 2002; 139: 364-371.
526. Li C, Yang CW, Ahn HJ, Kim WY, Park CW, Park JH, Cha JH, Kim J, Kim YS, Bang BK. Colchicine suppresses osteopontin expression and inflammatory cell infiltration in chronic cyclosporine nephrotoxicity. Nephron 2002; 92: 422-430.
527. Johnson DW, Saunders HJ, Field MJ, Pollock CA. *In vitro* effects of simvastatin on tubulointerstitial cells in a human model of cyclosporin nephrotoxicity. Am J Physiol 1999; 276: F467-F475.
528. Li C, Yang CW, Park JH, Lim SW, Sun BK, Jung JY, Kim SB, Kim YS, Kim J, Bang BK. Pravastatin treatment attenuates interstitial inflammation and fibrosis in a rat model of chronic cyclosporine-induced nephropathy. Am J Physiol Renal Physiol 2004; 286: F46-57.
529. Li C, Lim SW, Choi BS, Lee SH, Cha JH, Kim IS, Kim J, Yang CW. Inhibitory effect of pravastatin on transforming growth factor beta1-inducible gene h3 expression in a rat model of chronic cyclosporine nephropathy. Am J Nephrol 2005; 25: 611-620.
530. Pereira MG, Câmara NO, Campaholle G, Cenedeze MA, de Paula Antunes Teixeira V, dos Reis MA, Pacheco-Silva A. Pioglitazone limits cyclosporine nephrotoxicity in rats. Int Immunopharmacol 2006; 6: 1943-1951.
531. Shihab FS, Bennett WM, Yi H, Andoh TF. Pirfenidone treatment decreases transforming growth factor-beta1 and matrix proteins and ameliorates fibrosis in chronic cyclosporine nephrotoxicity. Am J Transplant 2002; 2: 111-119.
532. Shihab FS, Bennett WM, Yi H, Andoh TF. Effect of pirfenidone on apoptosis-regulatory genes in chronic cyclosporine nephrotoxicity. Transplantation 2005; 79: 419-426.
533. Yazawa K, Isaka Y, Takahara S, Imai E, Ichimaru N, Shi Y, Namba Y, Okuyama A. Direct transfer of hepatocyte growth factor gene into kidney suppresses cyclosporin A nephrotoxicity in rats. Nephrol Dial Transplant 2004; 19: 812-826.
534. Mizui M, Isaka Y, Takabatake Y, Mizuno S, Nakamura T, Ito T, Imai E, Hori M. Electroporation-mediated HGF gene transfer ameliorated cyclosporine nephrotoxicity. Kidney Int 2004; 65: 2041-2453.
535. Rezzani R, Rodella L, Bianchi R, Goodman AI, Lianos EA. Protective effects of heme-oxygenase expression in cyclosporine A-induced injury. Curr Neurovasc Res 2005; 2: 157-1561.
536. Rezzani R, Rodella L, Buffoli B, Goodman AA, Abraham NG, Lianos EA, Bianchi R. Change in renal heme oxygenase expression in cyclosporine A-induced injury. J Histochem Cytochem 2005; 53: 105-112.

537. Sis B, Dadras F, Khoshjou F, Cockfield S, Mihatsch MJ, Solez K. Reproducibility studies on arteriolar hyaline thickening scoring in calcineurin inhibitor-treated renal allograft recipients. Am J Transplant. 2006 Jun;6(6):1444-50.

538. Abrass CK, Berfield AK, Stehman-Breen C, Alpers CE, Davis CL. Unique changes in interstitial extracellular matrix composition are associated with rejection and cyclosporine toxicity in human renal allograft biopsies. Am J Kidney Dis 1999; 33: 11-20.

539. Bakker RC, Koop K, Sijpkens YW, Eikmans M, Bajema IM, De Heer E, Bruijn JA, Paul LC. Early interstitial accumulation of collagen type I discriminates chronic rejection from chronic cyclosporine nephrotoxicity. J Am Soc Nephrol 2003; 14: 2142-2149.

540. Koop K, Bakker RC, Eikmans M, Baelde HJ, de Heer E, Paul LC, Bruijn JA. Differentiation between chronic rejection and chronic cyclosporine toxicity by analysis of renal cortical mRNA. Kidney Int 2004; 66: 2038-2046.

541. Burke JF, Jr., Pirsch JD, Ramos EL, Salomon DR, Stablein DM, Van Buren DH, West JC. Long-term efficacy and safety of cyclosporine in renal-transplant recipients. N Engl J Med 1994; 331: 358-363.

542. Lewis RM. Long-term use of cyclosporine A does not adversely impact on clinical outcomes following renal transplantation. Kidney Int Suppl 1995; 52: S75-S78.

543. Abbas TM, Wafa EW, Bakr MA, Refaie AF, Sheashaa HA, Elagroudy AE, El-Baz MA, Mohsen TA, Shehab El Dein AB, Sobh MA, Ghoneim MA. Histologic and clinical findings in living donor allografts with long-term stable function. Am J Nephrol 2006; 26: 491-496.

544. Jacobson SH, Jaremko G, Duraj FF, Wilczek HE. Renal fibrosis in cyclosporin A-treated renal allograft recipients: morphological findings in relation to renal hemodynamics. Transpl Int 1996; 9: 492-498.

545. Kon SP, Templar J, Dodd SM, Rudge CJ, Raftery MJ. Diagnostic contribution of renal allograft biopsies at various intervals after transplantation. Transplantation 1997; 63: 547-550.

546. Klintmalm G, Bohman SO, Sundelin B, Wilczek H. Interstitial fibrosis in renal allografts after 12 to 46 months of cyclosporin treatment: beneficial effect of low doses in early post- transplantation period. Lancet 1984; 2: 950-954.

547. Ruiz P, Kolbeck PC, Scroggs MW, Sanfilippo F. Associations between cyclosporine therapy and interstitial fibrosis in renal allograft biopsies. Transplantation 1988; 45: 91-95.

548. Dudley J, Truman C, McGraw M, Tizard J, Haque G, Bradley B. Estimation of individual sensitivity to cyclosporin in children awaiting renal transplantation. Nephrol Dial Transplant. 2003; 18: 403-410.

549. Marcen R, Pascual J, Teruel JL, Villafruela JJ, Rivera ME, Mampaso F, Burgos FJ, Ortuno J. Outcome of cadaveric renal transplant patients treated for 10 years with cyclosporine: is chronic allograft nephropathy the major cause of late graft loss? Transplantation 2001; 72: 57-62.

550. Weir MR, Ward MT, Blahut SA, Klassen DK, Cangro CB, Bartlett ST, Fink JC. Long-term impact of discontinued or reduced calcineurin inhibitor in patients with chronic allograft nephropathy. Kidney Int 2001; 59: 1567-1573.

551. Nankivell BJ, Borrows RJ, Fung CL, O'Connell PJ, Chapman JR, Allen RD. Calcineurin inhibitor nephrotoxicity: longitudinal assessment by protocol histology. Transplantation 2004; 78:557-565.

552. Nankivell BJ, Borrows RJ, Fung CL, O'Connell PJ, Chapman JR, Allen RD. Delta analysis of posttransplantation tubulointerstitial damage. Transplantation 2004; 78: 434-441.

553. Coopersmith CM, Brennan DC, Miller B, Wang C, Hmiel P, Shenoy S, Ramachandran V, Jendrisak MD, Ceriotti CS, Mohanakumar T, Lowell JA. Renal transplantation following previous heart, liver, and lung transplantation: an 8-year single-center experience. Surgery 2001; 130: 457-462.

554. Herlitz H, Lindelow B. Renal failure following cardiac transplantation. Nephrol Dial Transplant 2000; 15: 311-314.

555. Chandrakantan A, de Mattos AM, Naftel D, Crosswy A, Kirklin J, Curtis JJ. Increasing referral for renal transplant evaluation in recipients of nonrenal solid-organ transplants: a single-center experience. Clin J Am Soc Nephrol. 2006; 1: 832-836.450.

556. Myers BD, Newton L. Cyclosporine-induced chronic nephropathy: an obliterative microvascular renal injury. J Am Soc Nephrol 1991; 2: S45-S52.

557. Bertani T, Ferrazzi P, Schieppati A, Ruggenenti P, Gamba A, Parenzan L, Mecca G, Perico N, Imberti O, Remuzzi A, Remuzzi G. Nature and extent of glomerular injury induced by cyclosporine in heart transplant patients. Kidney Int 1991; 40: 243-250.

558. Falkenhain ME, Cosio FG, Sedmak DD. Progressive histologic injury in kidneys from heart and liver transplant recipients receiving cyclosporine. Transplantation 1996; 62: 364-370.

559. Goldstein DJ, Zuech N, Sehgal V, Weinberg AD, Drusin R, Cohen D. Cyclosporine-associated end-stage nephropathy after cardiac transplantation: incidence and progression. Transplantation 1997; 63: 664-668.

560. Gonwa TA, Mai ML, Pilcher J, Johnson C, Pierson S, Capehart JE, Alivizatos PA. Stability of long-term renal function in heart transplant patients treated with induction therapy and low-dose cyclosporine. J Heart Lung Transplant 1992; 11: 926-928.

561. Goral S, Ynares C, Shyr Y, Yeoh TK, Johnson HK. Long-term renal function in heart transplant recipients receiving cyclosporine therapy. J Heart Lung Transplant 1997; 16: 1106-1112.

562. Kuo PC, Luikart H, Busse-Henry S, Hunt SA, Valantine HA, Stinson EB, Oyer PE, Scandling JD, Alfrey EJ, Dafoe DC. Clinical outcome of interval cadaveric renal transplantation in cardiac allograft recipients. Clin Transplant 1995; 9: 92-97.

563. Lewis RM, Van Buren CT, Radovancevic B, Frazier OH, Janney RP, Powers PL, Golden DL, Giannakis JG, Macris MP, Kerman RH, et al. Impact of long-term cyclosporine immunosuppressive therapy on native kidneys versus renal allografts: serial renal function in heart and kidney transplant recipients. J Heart Lung Transplant 1991; 10: 63-70.
564. Van Gelder T, Balk AH, Zietse R, Hesse C, Mochtar B, Weimar W. Renal insufficiency after heart transplantation: a case-control study. Nephrol Dial Transplant 1998; 13: 2322-2326.
565. Zietse R, Balk AH, vd Dorpel MA, Meeter K, Bos E, Weimar W. Time course of the decline in renal function in cyclosporine-treated heart transplant recipients. Am J Nephrol 1994; 14: 1-5.
566. Sénéchal M, Dorent R, du Montcel ST, Ghossou JJ, Pavie A, Petitclerc T, Dubois M, Isnard R, Gandjbakhch I. End-stage renal failure and cardiac mortality after heart transplantation. Clin Transplant 2004; 18: 1-6.
567. Griffiths MH, Crowe AV, Papadaki L, Banner NR, Yacoub MH, Thompson FD, Neild GH. Cyclosporin nephrotoxicity in heart and lung transplant patients. QJM 1996; 89: 751-763.
568. Pattison JM, Petersen J, Kuo P, Valantine V, Robbins RC, Theodore J. The incidence of renal failure in one hundred consecutive heart-lung transplant recipients. Am J Kidney Dis 1995; 26: 643-648.
569. Zaltzman JS, Pei Y, Maurer J, Patterson A, Cattran DC. Cyclosporine nephrotoxicity in lung transplant recipients. Transplantation 1992; 54: 875-878.
570. Mason DP, Solovera-Rozas M, Feng J, Rajeswaran J, Thuita L, Murthy SC, Budev MM, Mehta AC, Haug M 3rd, McNeill AM, Pettersson GB, Blackstone EH. Dialysis after lung transplantation: prevalence, risk factors and outcome. J Heart Lung Transplant 2007; 26: 1155-1162.
571. Gallon L, Akalin E, Lynch P, Rothberg L, Parker M, Schiano T, Abecassis M, Murphy B. ACE gene D/D genotype as a risk factor for chronic nephrotoxicity from calcineurin inhibitors in liver transplant recipients. Transplantation 2006; 81: 463-468.
572. Dagoo T, Backman L, Mjornstedt L, Olausson M, Friman S. Progressive renal impairment in liver transplant recipients on a cyclosporine-based protocol: 5 year follow-up with glomerular filtration rate measurements. Transplant Proc 1997; 29: 3116-3118.
573. Dische FE, Neuberger J, Keating J, Parsons V, Calne RY, Williams R. Kidney pathology in liver allograft recipients after long-term treatment with cyclosporin A. Lab Invest 1988; 58: 395-402.
574. Fisher NC, Nightingale PG, Gunson BK, Lipkin GW, Neuberger JM. Chronic renal failure following liver transplantation: a retrospective analysis. Transplantation 1998; 66: 59-66.
575. Gonwa TA, Mai ML, Melton LB, Hays SR, Goldstein RM, Levy MF, Klintmalm GB. End-stage renal disease (ESRD) after orthotopic liver transplantation (OLTX) using calcineurin-based immunotherapy: risk of development and treatment. Transplantation 2001; 72: 1934-1939.
576. Fioretto P, Steffes MW, Mihatsch MJ, Strom EH, Sutherland DE, Mauer M. Cyclosporine associated lesions in native kidneys of diabetic pancreas transplant recipients. Kidney Int 1995; 48: 489-495.
577. Rerolle JP, Thervet E, Anglicheau D, Desgrandchamps F, Nochy D, Janin A, Fornairon S, Passa P, Bedrossian J, Legendre C. Long-term renal allograft outcome after simultaneous kidney and pancreas transplantation. Nephrol Dial Transplant 2002; 17: 905-909.
578. Nizze H, Mihatsch MJ, Zollinger HU, Brocheriou C, Gokel JM, Henry K, Sloane JP, Stovin PG. Cyclosporine-associated nephropathy in patients with heart and bone marrow transplants. Clin Nephrol 1988; 30: 248-260.
579. Dieterle A, Gratwohl A, Nizze H, Huser B, Mihatsch MJ, Thiel G, Tichelli A, Signer E, Nissen C, Speck B. Chronic cyclosporine-associated nephrotoxicity in bone marrow transplant patients. Transplantation 1990; 49: 1093-1100.
580. Miralbell R, Bieri S, Mermillod B, Helg C, Sancho G, Pastoors B, Keller A, Kurtz JM, Chapuis B. Renal toxicity after allogeneic bone marrow transplantation: the combined effects of total-body irradiation and graft-versus-host disease. J Clin Oncol 1996; 14: 579-585.
581. Feutren G, Mihatsch MJ. Risk factors for cyclosporine-induced nephropathy in patients with autoimmune diseases. International Kidney Biopsy Registry of Cyclosporine in Autoimmune Diseases. N Engl J Med 1992; 326: 1654-1660.
582. Vercauteren SB, Bosmans JL, Elseviers MM, Verpooten GA, De Broe ME. A meta-analysis and morphological review of cyclosporine-induced nephrotoxicity in auto-immune diseases. Kidney Int 1998; 54: 536-545.
583. Austin HA, III, Palestine AG, Sabnis SG, Balow JE, Preuss HG, Nussenblatt RB, Antonovych TT. Evolution of ciclosporin nephrotoxicity in patients treated for autoimmune uveitis. Am J Nephrol 1989; 9: 392-402.
584. Tostivint I, du Montcel ST, Jaudon MC, Mallet A, Le Hoang P, Bodaghi B, Deray G, Bagnis CI. Renal outcome after ciclosporin-induced nephrotoxicity. Nephrol Dial Transplant 2007; 22: 880-885.
585. Andersen CB, Larsen S, Elmgreen J, Tvede N, Andersen V. Cyclosporine-induced renal morphologic and immunohistologic changes in patients with chronic uveitis. APMIS 1991; 99: 576-582.
586. Isnard Bagnis C, Tezenas du Montcel S, Beaufils H, Jouanneau C, Jaudon MC, Maksud P, Mallet A, LeHoang P, Deray G. Long-term renal effects of low-dose cyclosporine in uveitis-treated patients: follow-up study. J Am Soc Nephrol. 2002; 13: 2962-2968.

587. Lowe NJ, Wieder JM, Rosenbach A, Johnson K, Kunkel R, Bainbridge C, Bourget T, Dimov I, Simpson K, Glass E, Grabie MT. Long-term low-dose cyclosporine therapy for severe psoriasis: effects on renal function and structure. J Am Acad Dermatol 1996; 35: 710-719.
588. Messana JM, Johnson KJ, Mihatsch MJ. Renal structure and function effects after low dose cyclosporine in psoriasis patients: a preliminary report. Clin Nephrol 1995; 43: 150-153.
589. Powles AV, Cook T, Hulme B, Baker BS, Lewis HM, Thomas E, Valdimarsson H, Fry L. Renal function and biopsy findings after 5 years' treatment with low- dose cyclosporin for psoriasis. Br J Dermatol 1993; 128: 159-165.
590. Svarstad E, Helland S, Morken T, Bostad L, Myking A, Iversen BM, Ofstad J. Renal effects of maintenance low-dose cyclosporin A treatment in psoriasis. Nephrol Dial Transplant 1994; 9: 1462-1467.
591. Young EW, Ellis CN, Messana JM, Johnson KJ, Leichtman AB, Mihatsch MJ, Hamilton TA, Groisser DS, Fradin MS, Voorhees JJ. A prospective study of renal structure and function in psoriasis patients treated with cyclosporin. Kidney Int 1994; 46: 1216-1222.
592. Zachariae H, Kragballe K, Hansen HE, Marcussen N, Olsen S. Renal biopsy findings in long-term cyclosporin treatment of psoriasis. Br J Dermatol 1997; 136: 531-535.
593. Renal morphology after cyclosporin A therapy in rheumatoid arthritis patients. International Kidney Biopsy Registry of Cyclosporin (Sandimmun) in Autoimmune Diseases. Br J Rheumatol 1993; 32 Suppl 1: 65-71.
594. Berg KJ, Forre O, Bjerkhoel F, Amundsen E, Djoseland O, Rugstad HE, Westre B. Side effects of cyclosporin A treatment in patients with rheumatoid arthritis. Kidney Int 1986; 29: 1180-1187.
595. Ludwin D, Alexopoulou I, Esdaile JM, Tugwell P. Renal biopsy specimens from patients with rheumatoid arthritis and apparently normal renal function after therapy with cyclosporine. Canadian Multicentre Rheumatology Group. Am J Kidney Dis 1994; 23: 260-265.
596. Rodriguez F, Krayenbuhl JC, Harrison WB, Forre O, Dijkmans BA, Tugwell P, Miescher PA, Mihatsch MJ. Renal biopsy findings and followup of renal function in rheumatoid arthritis patients treated with cyclosporin A. An update from the International Kidney Biopsy Registry. Arthritis Rheum 1996; 39: 1491-1498.
597. Sund S, Forre O, Berg KJ, Kvien TK, Hovig T. Morphological and functional renal effects of long-term low-dose cyclosporin A treatment in patients with rheumatoid arthritis. Clin Nephrol 1994; 41: 33-40.
598. van den Borne BE, Landewe RB, Goei The HS, Breedveld FC, Dijkmans BA. Cyclosporin A therapy in rheumatoid arthritis: only strict application of the guidelines for safe use can prevent irreversible renal function loss. Rheumatology (Oxford) 1999; 38: 254-259.
599. Landewe RB, Dijkmans BA, van der Woude FJ, Breedveld FC, Mihatsch MJ, Bruijn JA. Longterm low dose cyclosporine in patients with rheumatoid arthritis: renal function loss without structural nephropathy. J Rheumatol 1996; 23: 61-64.
600. Assan R, Timsit J, Feutren G, Bougneres P, Czernichow P, Hannedouche T, Boitard C, Noel LH, Mihatsch MJ, Bach JF. The kidney in cyclosporin A-treated diabetic patients: a long-term clinicopathological study. Clin Nephrol 1994; 41: 41-49.
601. Mihatsch MJ, Helmchen U, Casanova P, Habib R, Larsen S, Magil A, Noel LH, Rapola J, Ulrich J, Wallace AC. Kidney biopsy findings in cyclosporine-treated patients with insulin- dependent diabetes mellitus. Klin Wochenschr 1991; 69: 354-359.
602. Parving HH, Tarnow L, Nielsen FS, Rossing P, Mandrup-Poulsen T, Osterby R, Nerup J. Cyclosporine nephrotoxicity in type 1 diabetic patients. A 7-year follow-up study. Diabetes Care 1999; 22: 478-483.
603. Kolkin S, Nahman NS, Jr., Mendell JR. Chronic nephrotoxicity complicating cyclosporine treatment of chronic inflammatory demyelinating polyradiculoneuropathy. Neurology 1987; 37: 147-149.
604. Svenson K, Bohman SO, Hallgren R. Renal interstitial fibrosis and vascular changes. Occurrence in patients with autoimmune diseases treated with cyclosporine. Arch Intern Med 1986; 146: 2007-2010.
605. Charbit M, Gubler MC, Dechaux M, Gagnadoux MF, Grünfeld JP, Niaudet P. Cyclosporin therapy in patients with Alport syndrome. Pediatr Nephrol 2007; 22: 57-63.
606. Clasen W, Kindler J, Mihatsch MJ, Sieberth HG. Long-term treatment of minimal-change nephrotic syndrome with cyclosporin: a control biopsy study. Nephrol Dial Transplant 1988; 3: 733-737.
607. Sieberth HG, Clasen W, Fuhs M, Ittel T, Kindler J, Mihatsch MJ. Serial kidney biopsies in patients with nephrotic syndrome treated with cyclosporin. J Autoimmun 1992; 5 Suppl A: 355-361.
608. Kranz B, Vester U, Büscher R, Wingen AM, Hoyer PF. Cyclosporine-A-induced nephrotoxicity in children with minimal-change nephrotic syndrome: long-term treatment up to 10 years. Pediatr Nephrol 2008; 23: 581-586.
609. Meyrier A, Noel LH, Auriche P, Callard P. Long-term renal tolerance of cyclosporin A treatment in adult idiopathic nephrotic syndrome. Collaborative Group of the Societe de Nephrologie. Kidney Int 1994; 45: 1446-1456.
610. Waldo FB, Benfield MR, Kohaut EC. Therapy of focal and segmental glomerulosclerosis with methylprednisolone, cyclosporine A, and prednisone. Pediatr Nephrol 1998; 12: 397-400.
611. Habib R, Niaudet P. Comparison between pre- and posttreatment renal biopsies in children receiving ciclosporine for idiopathic nephrosis. Clin Nephrol 1994; 42: 141-146.

612. Hino S, Takemura T, Okada M, Murakami K, Yagi K, Fukushima K, Yoshioka K. Follow-up study of children with nephrotic syndrome treated with a long- term moderate dose of cyclosporine. Am J Kidney Dis 1998; 31: 932-939.
613. Ittel TH, Clasen W, Fuhs M, Kindler J, Mihatsch MJ, Sieberth HG. Long-term ciclosporine A treatment in adults with minimal change nephrotic syndrome or focal segmental glomerulosclerosis. Clin Nephrol 1995; 44: 156-162.
614. Kano K, Kyo K, Yamada Y, Ito S, Ando T, Arisaka O. Comparison between pre- and posttreatment clinical and renal biopsies in children receiving low dose ciclosporine-A for 2 years for steroid- dependent nephrotic syndrome. Clin Nephrol 1999; 52: 19-24.
615. El-Husseini A, El-Basuony F, Mahmoud I, Sheashaa H, Sabry A, Hassan R, Taha N, Hassan N, Sayed-Ahmad N, Sobh M. Long-term effects of cyclosporine in children with idiopathic nephrotic syndrome: a single-centre experience. Nephrol Dial Transplant 2005;20: 2433-2438.
616. Seikaly MG, Prashner H, Nolde-Hurlbert B, Browne R. Long-term clinical and pathological effects of cyclosporin in children with nephrosis. Pediatr Nephrol 2000; 14: 214-217.
617. Lim BJ, Kim PK, Hong SW, Jeong HJ. Osteopontin expression and microvascular injury in cyclosporine nephrotoxicity. Pediatr Nephrol 2004; 19: 288-294.
618. Nakamura T, Nozu K, Iijima K, Yoshikawa N, Moriya Y, Yamamori M, Kako A, Matsuo M, Sakurai A, Okamura N, Ishikawa T, Okumura K, Sakaeda T. Association of cumulative cyclosporine dose with its irreversible nephrotoxicity in Japanese patients with pediatric-onset autoimmune diseases. Biol Pharm Bull 2007; 30: 2371-2375.
619. Kranz B, Vester U, Büscher R, Wingen AM, Hoyer PF. Cyclosporine-A-induced nephrotoxicity in children with minimal-change nephrotic syndrome: long-term treatment up to 10 years. Pediatr Nephrol 2008; 23: 581-586.
620. Soylemezoglu O, Wild G, Dalley AJ, MacNeil S, Milford-Ward A, Brown CB, el Nahas AM. Urinary and serum type III collagen: markers of renal fibrosis. Nephrol Dial Transplant 1997; 12: 1883-1889.
621. Haas M, Meehan SM, Josephson MA, Wit EJ, Woodle ES, Thistlethwaite JR. Smooth muscle-specific actin levels in the urine of renal transplant recipients: correlation with cyclosporine or tacrolimus nephrotoxicity. Am J Kidney Dis 1999; 34: 69-84.
622. Camara NO, Matos AC, Rodrigues DA, Pereira AB, Pacheco-Silva A. Early detection of heart transplant patients with increased risk of ciclosporin nephrotoxicity. Lancet 2001; 357: 856-857.
623. Kim CD, Cho YJ, Park SH, Ha SW, Lee EG, Kim YJ, Kwon TH, Kim IS, Kim YL. Urinary transforming growth factor-beta-induced gene-h3 (betaig-h3) as a sensitive predictor in chronic cyclosporine nephrotoxicity. Transplant Proc 2006; 38: 1314-1319.
624. Mourad G, Vela C, Ribstein J, Mimran A. Long-term improvement in renal function after cyclosporine reduction in renal transplant recipients with histologically proven chronic cyclosporine nephropathy. Transplantation 1998; 65: 661-667.
625. Ducloux D, Fournier V, Bresson-Vautrin C, Rebibou JM, Billerey C, Saint-Hillier Y, Chalopin JM. Mycophenolate mofetil in renal transplant recipients with cyclosporine- associated nephrotoxicity: a preliminary report. Transplantation 1998; 65: 1504-1506.
626. Filler G, Gellermann J, Zimmering M, Mai I. Effect of adding Mycophenolate mofetil in paediatric renal transplant recipients with chronical cyclosporine nephrotoxicity. Transpl Int 2000; 13: 201-206.
627. Houde I, Isenring P, Boucher D, Noel R, Lachanche JG. Mycophenolate mofetil, an alternative to cyclosporine A for long-term immunosuppression in kidney transplantation? Transplantation 2000; 70: 1251-1253.
628. Hueso M, Bover J, Seron D, Gil-Vernet S, Sabate I, Fulladosa X, Ramos R, Coll O, Alsina J, Grinyo JM. Low-dose cyclosporine and mycophenolate mofetil in renal allograft recipients with suboptimal renal function. Transplantation 1998; 66: 1727-1731.
629. Al-Aly Z, Sachdeva A, Philoctete Ashley JM, Bastani B. Preliminary experience with mycophenolate mofetil for preservation of renal function in cardiac transplant patients with documented cyclosporine nephrotoxicity. Nephrology (Carlton) 2006; 11: 151-155.
630. Nankivell BJ, Wavamunno MD, Borrows RJ, Vitalone M, Fung CL, Allen RD, Chapman JR, O'Connell PJ. Mycophenolate mofetil is associated with altered expression of chronic renal transplant histology. Am J Transplant 2007; 7: 366-376.
631. Badid C, Vincent M, McGregor B, Melin M, Hadj-Aissa A, Veysseyre C, Hartmann DJ, Desmouliere A, Laville M. Mycophenolate mofetil reduces myofibroblast infiltration and collagen III deposition in rat remnant kidney. Kidney Int 2000; 58: 51-61.
632. Fujihara CK, De LN, I, Malheiros, Antunes GR, de Oliveira IB, Zatz R. Combined mycophenolate mofetil and losartan therapy arrests established injury in the remnant kidney. J Am Soc Nephrol 2000; 11: 283-290.
633. Remuzzi G, Zoja C, Gagliardini E, Corna D, Abbate M, Benigni A. Combining an antiproteinuric approach with mycophenolate mofetil fully suppresses progressive nephropathy of experimental animals. J Am Soc Nephrol 1999; 10: 1542-1549.
634. Araujo IM, Mendes GEF, Baptista MAF, Burdmann EA. Effects of mycophenolate mofetil (MMF) on chronic cyclosporine (CSA) nephrotoxicity. J Am Soc Nephrol 2001; 12: 797A.
635. Yang CW, Ahn HJ, Kim WY, Li C, Kim HW, Choi BS, Cha JH, Kim YS, Kim J, Bang BK. Cyclosporine withdrawal and mycophenolate mofetil treatment effects on the progression of chronic cyclosporine nephrotoxicity. Kidney Int 2002; 62: 20-30.
636. Stallone G, Di Paolo S, Schena A, Infante B, Grandaliano G, Battaglia M, Gesualdo L, Schena FP. Early withdrawal of cyclosporine A improves 1-year kidney graft structure and function in sirolimus-treated patients. Transplantation 2003; 75: 998-1003.

637. Ruiz JC, Campistol JM, Grinyó JM, Mota A, Prats D, Gutiérrez JA, Henriques AC, Pinto JR, García J, Morales JM, Gómez JM, Arias M. Early cyclosporine a withdrawal in kidney-transplant recipients receiving sirolimus prevents progression of chronic pathologic allograft lesions. Transplantation 2004;7 8: 1312-1318.
638. Shihab FS, Bennett WM, Yi H, Choi SO, Andoh TF. Sirolimus increases transforming growth factor-beta1 expression and potentiates chronic cyclosporine nephrotoxicity. Kidney Int 2004; 65: 1262-1271.
639. McCulloch TA, Harper SJ, Donnelly PK, Moorhouse J, Bell PR, Walls J, Feehally J, Furness PN. Influence of nifedipine on interstitial fibrosis in renal transplant allografts treated with cyclosporin A. J Clin Pathol 1994; 47: 839-842.
640. Campistol JM, Inigo P, Jimenez W, Lario S, Clesca PH, Oppenheimer F, Rivera F. Losartan decreases plasma levels of TGF-beta1 in transplant patients with chronic allograft nephropathy. Kidney Int 1999; 56: 714-719.
641. Martins L, Ventura A, Branco A, Carvalho MJ, Henriques AC, Dias L, Sarmento AM, Amil M. Cyclosporine versus tacrolimus in kidney transplantation: are there differences in nephrotoxicity? 1: Transplant Proc 2004; 36: 877-879.
642. Krämer BK, Montagnino G, Del Castillo D, Margreiter R, Sperschneider H, Olbricht CJ, Krüger B, Ortuño J, Köhler H, Kunzendorf U, Stummvoll HK, Tabernero JM, Mühlbacher F, Rivero M, Arias M; European Tacrolimus vs Cyclosporin Microemulsion Renal Transplantation Study Group. Efficacy and safety of tacrolimus compared with cyclosporin A microemulsion in renal transplantation: 2 year follow-up results. Nephrol Dial Transplant 2005; 20: 968-973.
643. Lucey MR, Abdelmalek MF, Gagliardi R, Granger D, Holt C, Kam I, Klintmalm G, Langnas A, Shetty K, Tzakis A, Woodle ES. Comparison of tacrolimus and cyclosporine in liver transplantation: effects on renal function and cardiovascular risk status. Am J Transplant 2005; 5:1111-1119.
644. Klein IH, Abrahams A, van Ede T, Hené RJ, Koomans HA, Ligtenberg G. Different effects of tacrolimus and cyclosporine on renal hemodynamics and blood pressure in healthy subjects. Transplantation. 2002; 73: 732-736.
645. Schwarz C, Benesch T, Kodras K, Oberbauer R, Haas M. Complete renal tubular acidosis late after kidney transplantation. Nephrol Dial Transplant 2006; 21: 2615-2620.
646. McCauley J. The nephrotoxicity of FK506 as compared with cyclosporine. Curr Opin Nephrol Hypertens 1993; 2: 662-669.
647. Morales JM, Andres A, Rengel M, Rodicio JL. Influence of cyclosporin, tacrolimus and rapamycin on renal function and arterial hypertension after renal transplantation. Nephrol Dial Transplant 2001; 16 Suppl 1: 121-124.
648. Ogita K, Takada N, Taguchi T, Suita S, Soejima Y, Suehiro T, Shimada M, Maehara Y. Renal tubular acidosis secondary to FK506 in living donor liver transplantation: a case report. Asian J Surg 2003; 26: 218-220.
649. Plosker GL, Foster RH. Tacrolimus: a further update of its pharmacology and therapeutic use in the management of organ transplantation. Drugs 2000; 59: 323-389.
650. Sakamoto K, Yamada K, Arita S, Hamaguchi K, Kashiwabara H, Yokoyama T. Sodium-losing nephropathy and distal tubular damage of transplant kidneys with FK506 administration. Transplant Proc 1995; 27: 826-828.
651. Finn WF. FK506 nephrotoxicity. Ren Fail 1999; 21: 319-329.
652. Webster A, Woodroffe RC, Taylor RS, Chapman JR, Craig JC. Tacrolimus versus cyclosporin as primary immunosuppression for kidney transplant recipients. Cochrane Database Syst Rev 2005; 4:CD003961.
653. Haddad EM, McAlister VC, Renouf E, Malthaner R, Kjaer MS, Gluud LL. Cyclosporin versus tacrolimus for liver transplanted patients. Cochrane Database Syst Rev 2006; 4:CD005161.
654. Chenhsu RY, Loong CC, Chou MH, Lin MF, Yang WC. Renal allograft dysfunction associated with rifampin-tacrolimus interaction. Ann Pharmacother 2000; 34: 27-31.
655. Gomez G, Alvarez ML, Errasti P, Lavilla FJ, Garcia N, Ballester B, Garcia I, Purroy A. Acute tacrolimus nephrotoxicity in renal transplant patients treated with clarithromycin. Transplant Proc 1999; 31: 2250-2251.
656. Ocran KW, Plauth M, Mai I, Lochs H. Tacrolimus toxicity due to drug interaction with mibefradil in a patient after liver transplantation. Z Gastroenterol 1999; 37: 1025-1028.
657. Olyaei AJ, deMattos AM, Norman DJ, Bennett WM. Interaction between tacrolimus and nefazodone in a stable renal transplant recipient. Pharmacotherapy 1998; 18: 1356-1359.
658. Sheiner PA, Mor E, Chodoff L, Glabman S, Emre S, Schwartz ME, Miller CM. Acute renal failure associated with the use of ibuprofen in two liver transplant recipients on FK506. Transplantation 1994; 57: 1132-1133.
659. Soubhia RM, Mendes GE, Mendonça FZ, Baptista MA, Cipullo JP, Burdmann EA. Tacrolimus and nonsteroidal anti-inflammatory drugs: an association to be avoided. Am J Nephrol 2005; 25:327-334.
660. Prescott WA Jr, Callahan BL, Park JM. Tacrolimus toxicity associated with concomitant metoclopramide therapy. Pharmacotherapy 2004; 24: 532-537.
661. Ahsan N, Johnson C, Gonwa T, Halloran P, Stegall M, Hardy M, Metzger R, Shield C, III, Rocher L, Scandling J, Sorensen J, Mulloy L, Light J, Corwin C, Danovitch G, Wachs M, VanVeldhuisen P, Salm K, Tolzman D, Fitzsimmons WE. Randomized trial of tacrolimus plus mycophenolate mofetil or azathioprine versus cyclosporine oral solution (modified) plus mycophenolate mofetil after cadaveric kidney transplantation: results at 2 years. Transplantation 2001; 72: 245-250.

662. Katari SR, Magnone M, Shapiro R, Jordan M, Scantlebury V, Vivas C, Gritsch A, McCauley J, Starzl T, Demetris AJ, Randhawa PS. Clinical features of acute reversible tacrolimus (FK 506) nephrotoxicity in kidney transplant recipients. Clin Transplant 1997; 11: 237-242.
663. Mayer AD, Dmitrewski J, Squifflet JP, Besse T, Grabensee B, Klein B, Eigler FW, Heemann U, Pichlmayr R, Behrend M, Vanrenterghem Y, Donck J, van Hooff J, Christiaans M, Morales JM, Andres A, Johnson RW, Short C, Buchholz B, Rehmert N, Land W, Schleibner S, Forsythe JL, Talbot D, Neumayer H-H, Hauser I, Ericzon B-G, Brattstrom C, Claesson K, Muhlbacher F, Pohanka E. Multicenter randomized trial comparing tacrolimus (FK506) and cyclosporine in the prevention of renal allograft rejection: a report of the European Tacrolimus Multicenter Renal Study Group. Transplantation 1997; 64: 436-443.
664. Mor E, Patel T, Glabman S, Sheiner P, Emre S, Guy S, Schwartz M, Miller C. Comparison of short and long-term renal function in liver transplant patients receiving cyclosporin or FK 506. Transpl Int 1994; 7 Suppl 1: S77-S80.
665. Porayko MK, Textor SC, Krom RA, Hay JE, Gores GJ, Richards TM, Crotty PH, Beaver SJ, Steers JL, Wiesner RH. Nephrotoxic effects of primary immunosuppression with FK-506 and cyclosporine regimens after liver transplantation. Mayo Clin Proc 1994; 69: 105-111.
666. Porayko MK, Gonwa TA, Klintmalm GB, Wiesner RH. Comparing nephrotoxicity of FK 506 and cyclosporine regimens after liver transplantation: preliminary results from US Multicenter trial. U.S. Multicenter Liver Study Group. Transplant Proc 1995; 27: 1114-1116.
667. Vincenti F, Laskow DA, Neylan JF, Mendez R, Matas AJ. One-year follow-up of an open-label trial of FK506 for primary kidney transplantation. A report of the U.S. Multicenter FK506 Kidney Transplant Group. Transplantation 1996; 61: 1576-1581.
668. McLaughlin GE, Abitbol CL. Reversal of oliguric tacrolimus nephrotoxicity in children. Nephrol Dial Transplant 2005; 20: 1471-1415.
669. Burke GW, Ciancio G, Cirocco R, Markou M, Olson L, Contreras N, Roth D, Esquenazi V, Tzakis A, Miller J. Microangiopathy in kidney and simultaneous pancreas/kidney recipients treated with tacrolimus: evidence of endothelin and cytokine involvement. Transplantation 1999; 68: 1336-1342.
670. Gharpure VS, Devine SM, Holland HK, Geller RB, O'Toole K, Wingard JR. Thrombotic thrombocytopenic purpura associated with FK506 following bone marrow transplantation. Bone Marrow Transplant 1995; 16: 715-716.
671. Schmidt RH, Lenz T, Grone HJ, Geiger H, Scheuermann EH. Haemolytic-uraemic syndrome after tacrolimus rescue therapy for cortisone-resistant rejection. Nephrol Dial Transplant 1999; 14: 979-983.
672. Schmidt RJ, Venkat KK, Dumler F. Hemolytic-uremic syndrome in a renal transplant recipient on FK 506 immunosuppression. Transplant Proc 1991; 23: 3156-3157.
673. Pham PT, Peng A, Wilkinson AH, Gritsch HA, Lassman C, Pham PC, Danovitch GM. Cyclosporine and tacrolimus-associated thrombotic microangiopathy. Am J Kidney Dis 2000; 36: 844-850.
674. Pandirikkal VB, Jain M, Gulati S. Tacrolimus-induced HUS: an unusual cause of acute renal failure in nephrotic syndrome. Pediatr Nephrol 2007; 22: 298-300.
675. Saito M, Satoh S, Kagaya H, Tsuruta H, Obara T, Kumazawa T, Inoue T, Inoue K, Miura M, Yuasa T, Komatsuda A, Tsuchiya N, Habuchi T. Thrombotic microangiopathy developing in early stage after renal transplantation with a high trough level of tacrolimus. Clin Exp Nephrol. 2008 (in presss).
676. Abdalla AH, al Sulaiman MH, al Khader AA. FK 506 as an alternative in cyclosporin-induced hemolytic uremic syndrome in a kidney transplant recipient. Transpl Int 1994; 7: 382-384.
677. McCauley J, Bronsther O, Fung J, Todo S, Starzl TE. Treatment of cyclosporin-induced haemolytic uraemic syndrome with FK506. Lancet 1989; 2: 1516.
678. Abraham KA, Little MA, Dorman AM, Walshe JJ. Hemolytic-uremic syndrome in association with both cyclosporine and tacrolimus. Transpl Int 2000; 13: 443-447.
679. Textor SC, Wiesner R, Wilson DJ, Porayko M, Romero JC, Burnett JC, Jr., Gores G, Hay E, Dickson ER, Krom RA. Systemic and renal hemodynamic differences between FK506 and cyclosporine in liver transplant recipients. Transplantation 1993; 55: 1332-1339.
680. McDiarmid SV, Colonna JO, Shaked A, Ament ME, Busuttil RW. A comparison of renal function in cyclosporine- and FK-506-treated patients after primary orthotopic liver transplantation. Transplantation 1993; 56: 847-853.
681. Asante-Korang A, Boyle GJ, Webber SA, Miller SA, Fricker FJ. Experience of FK506 immune suppression in pediatric heart transplantation: a study of long-term adverse effects. J Heart Lung Transplant 1996; 15: 415-422.
682. Reichart B, Meiser B, Vigano M, Rinaldi M, Martinelli L, Yacoub M, Banner NR, Gandjbakhch I, Dorent R, Hetzer R, Hummel M. European Multicenter Tacrolimus (FK506) Heart Pilot Study: one-year results--European Tacrolimus Multicenter Heart Study Group. J Heart Lung Transplant 1998; 17: 775-781.
683. Taylor DO, Barr ML, Radovancevic B, Renlund DG, Mentzer RM, Jr., Smart FW, Tolman DE, Frazier OH, Young JB, VanVeldhuisen P. A randomized, multicenter comparison of tacrolimus and cyclosporine immunosuppressive regimens in cardiac transplantation: decreased hyperlipidemia and hypertension with tacrolimus. J Heart Lung Transplant 1999; 18: 336-345.

684. Griffith BP, Bando K, Hardesty RL, Armitage JM, Keenan RJ, Pham SM, Paradis IL, Yousem SA, Komatsu K, Konishi H, Fung JJ, Starzl TE. A prospective randomized trial of FK506 versus cyclosporine after human pulmonary transplantation. Transplantation 1994; 57: 848-851.
685. Kur F, Reichenspurner H, Meiser BM, Welz A, Furst H, Muller C, Vogelmeier C, Schwaiblmaier M, Briegel J, Reichart B. Tacrolimus (FK506) as primary immunosuppressant after lung transplantation. Thorac Cardiovasc Surg 1999; 47: 174-178.
686. Segarra A, Vila J, Pou L, Majó J, Arbós A, Quiles T, Piera LL. Combined therapy of tacrolimus and corticosteroids in cyclosporin-resistant or -dependent idiopathic focal glomerulosclerosis: a preliminary uncontrolled study with prospective follow-up. Nephrol Dial Transplant 2002; 17: 655-662.
687. Andoh TF, Burdmann EA, Lindsley J, Houghton DC, Bennett WM. Functional and structural characteristics of experimental FK 506 nephrotoxicity. Clin Exp Pharmacol Physiol 1995; 22: 646-654.
688. Hadad SJ, Souza ER, Ferreira AT, Oshiro ME, Boim MA, Razvickas CV, Moura LA, Schor N. FK 506: effects on glomerular hemodynamics and on mesangial cells in culture. Kidney Int 1995; 48: 56-64.
689. Kumano K, Chen J, He M, Endo T, Masaki Y. Role of endothelin in FK 506-induced renal hypoperfusion in rats. Transplant Proc 1995; 27: 550-553.
690. Mugiya S, Fujita K, Malyszko J, Takada Y, Takada A. Renal blood flow and serotonin metabolism in tacrolimus treated rats. Int J Urol 1996; 3: 187-190.
691. Nielsen FT, Leyssac PP, Kemp E, Starklint H, Dieperink H. Nephrotoxicity of FK-506 in the rat. Studies on glomerular and tubular function, and on the relationship between efficacy and toxicity. Nephrol Dial Transplant 1995; 10: 334-340.
692. Ueda D, Suzuki K, Kawabe K. Influence of FK 506 on renal blood flow. Transplant Proc 1993; 25: 2722-2723.
693. Seifeldin R, Marcos-Alvarez A, Lewis WD, Gordon FD, Jenkins RL. Effect of nifedipine on renal function in liver transplant recipients receiving tacrolimus. Clin Ther 1996; 18: 491-496.
694. Andoh TF, Burdmann EA, Houghton DC, Lindsley J, Bennett WM. Protective effects of nilvadipine on experimental acute FK 506 nephrotoxicity. J Am Soc Nephrol 1993; 4: 760.
695. Mitamura T, Yamada A, Ishida H, Fujihira S, Ohara K, Noguchi H, Mine Y. Tacrolimus (FK506)-induced nephrotoxicity in spontaneous hypertensive rats. J Toxicol Sci 1994; 19: 219-226.
696. Tada H, Yanagiwara S, Ito K, Suzuki T. Role of diltiazem on tacrolimus pharmacokinetics in tacrolimus-induced nephrotoxic rats. Pharmacol Toxicol 1999; 84: 241-246.
697. Mihatsch MJ, Kyo M, Morozumi K, Yamaguchi Y, Nickeleit V, Ryffel B. The side-effects of ciclosporine-A and tacrolimus. Clin Nephrol 1998; 49: 356-363.
698. Ninova D, Covarrubias M, Rea DJ, Park WD, Grande JP, Stegall MD. Acute nephrotoxicity of tacrolimus and sirolimus in renal isografts: differential intragraft expression of transforming growth factor-beta1 and alpha-smooth muscle actin. Transplantation 2004; 78: 338-44.
699. Liptak P, Ivanyi B. Primer: Histopathology of calcineurin-inhibitor toxicity in renal allografts. Nat Clin Pract Nephrol 2006; 2: 398-404;
700. Shimizu T, Tanabe K, Tokumoto T, Ishikawa N, Shinmura H, Oshima T, Toma H, Yamaguchi Y. Clinical and histological analysis of acute tacrolimus (TAC) nephrotoxicity in renal allografts. Clin Transplant 1999; 13 Suppl 1: 48-53.
701. Benigni A, Morigi M, Perico N, Zoja C, Amuchastegui CS, Piccinelli A, Donadelli R, Remuzzi G. The acute effect of FK506 and cyclosporine on endothelial cell function and renal vascular resistance. Transplantation 1992; 54: 775-780.
702. Bagnis C, Deray G, Dubois M, Adabra Y, Jacquiaud C, Jaudon MC, Jacobs C. Comparative acute nephrotoxicity of FK-506 and ciclosporin in an isolated *in situ* autoperfused rat kidney model. Am J Nephrol 1997; 17: 17-24.
703. Nankivell BJ, Chapman JR, Bonovas G, Gruenewald SM. Oral cyclosporine but not tacrolimus reduces renal transplant blood flow. Transplantation 2004; 77: 1457-1459.
704. Andoh TF, Burdmann EA, Lindsley J, Houghton DC, Bennett WM. Enhancement of FK506 nephrotoxicity by sodium depletion in an experimental rat model. Transplantation 1994; 57: 483-489.
705. Stillman IE, Andoh TF, Burdmann EA, Bennett WM, Rosen S. FK506 nephrotoxicity: morphologic and physiologic characterization of a rat model. Lab Invest 1995; 73: 794-803.
706. Su Q, Weber L, Le Hir M, Zenke G, Ryffel B. Nephrotoxicity of cyclosporin A and FK506: inhibition of calcineurin phosphatase. Ren Physiol Biochem 1995; 18: 128-139.
707. Yamada K, Sugisaki Y, Akimoto M, Yamanaka N. FK 506-induced juxtaglomerular apparatus hyperplasia and tubular damage in rat kidney--morphologic and biologic analysis. Transplant Proc 1992; 24: 1396-1398.
708. Nakatani T, Uchida J, Iwai T, Matsumura K, Naganuma T, Kuratsukuri K, Sugimura K. Renin mRNA expression and renal dysfunction in tacrolimus-induced acute nephrotoxicity. Int J Mol Med 2003; 11: 75-78.
709. Kumano K, Wang G, Endo T, Kuwao S. FK 506-induced nephrotoxicity in rats. Transplant Proc 1991; 23: 512-515.

710. McCauley J, Studer R, Craven P, Murray S. The effects of cyclosporine A, cyclosporine G, and FK 506 upon prostaglandin production in renal mesangial cells in culture. Transplant Proc 1991; 23: 3141-3142.
711. Butani L, Afshinnik A, Johnson J, Javaheri D, Peck S, German JB, Perez RV. Amelioration of tacrolimus-induced nephrotoxicity in rats using juniper oil. Transplantation 2003; 76: 306-11.
712. Moutabarrik A, Ishibashi M, Fukunaga M, Kameoka H, Kawaguchi N, Takano Y, Kokado Y, Sonoda T, Onishi S, Takahara S, Okuyama A. FK506-induced kidney tubular cell injury. Transplantation 1992; 54: 1041-1047.
713. Goodall T, Kind CN, Hammond TG. FK506-induced endothelin release by cultured rat mesangial cells. J Cardiovasc Pharmacol 1995; 26 Suppl 3: S482-S485.
714. Haug C, Grill C, Schmid-Kotsas A, Gruenert A, Jehle PM. Endothelin release by rabbit proximal tubule cells: modulatory effects of cyclosporine A, tacrolimus, HGF and EGF. Kidney Int 1998; 54: 1626-1636.
715. Nakahama H, Fukunaga M, Kakihara M, Horio M, Fujiwara Y, Fukuhara Y, Ueda N, Orita Y, Kamada T. Comparative effects of cyclosporine A and FK-506 on endothelin secretion by a cultured renal cell line, LLC-PK1. J Cardiovasc Pharmacol 1991; 17 Suppl 7: S172-S173.
716. Takeda Y, Yoneda T, Ito Y, Miyamori I, Takeda R. Stimulation of endothelin mRNA and secretion in human endothelial cells by FK 506. J Cardiovasc Pharmacol 1993; 22 Suppl 8: S310-S312.
717. Marsen TA, Weber F, Egink G, Suckau G, Baldamus CA. Differential transcriptional regulation of endothelin-1 by immunosuppressants FK506 and cyclosporin A. Fundam Clin Pharmacol 2000; 14: 401-408.
718. Uchida J, Miura K, Yamanaka S, Kim S, Iwao H, Nakatani T, Kishimoto T. Renal endothelin in FK506-induced nephrotoxicity in spontaneously hypertensive rats. Jpn J Pharmacol 1998; 76: 39-49.
719. Burdmann EA, Mattar AL, Fujihara C, Andoh TF, Zatz R, Bennett WM. Effects of an endothelin Et_A receptor antagonist on experimental FK 506-induced acute renal dysfunction. J Am Soc Nephrol 1994; 5: 918.
720. Dawson TM, Steiner JP, Dawson VL, Dinerman JL, Uhl GR, Snyder SH. Immunosuppressant FK506 enhances phosphorylation of nitric oxide synthase and protects against glutamate neurotoxicity. Proc Natl Acad Sci U S A 1993; 90: 9808-9812.
721. Akita K, Dusting GJ, Hickey H. Suppression of nitric oxide production by cyclosporin A and FK506A in rat vascular smooth muscle cells. Clin Exp Pharmacol Physiol 1994; 21: 231-233.
722. Conde M, Andrade J, Bedoya FJ, Santa MC, Sobrino F. Inhibitory effect of cyclosporin A and FK506 on nitric oxide production by cultured macrophages. Evidence of a direct effect on nitric oxide synthase activity. Immunology 1995; 84: 476-481.
723. Strestikova P, Otova B, Filipec M, Masek K, Farghali H. Different mechanisms in inhibition of rat macrophage nitric oxide synthase expression by FK 506 and cyclosporin A. Immunopharmacol Immunotoxicol 2001; 23: 67-74.
724. Wang L, Kubodera S, Ueno A, Takeda M. Effects of nitric oxide synthesis inhibition on FK506-induced nephrotoxicity in rats. Ren Fail 2001; 23: 11-19.
725. Hortelano S, Castilla M, Torres AM, Tejedor A, Bosca L. Potentiation by nitric oxide of cyclosporin A and FK506-induced apoptosis in renal proximal tubule cells. J Am Soc Nephrol 2000; 11: 2315-2323.
726. De Lima JJ, Xue H, Coburn L, Andoh TF, McCarron DA, Bennett WM, Roullet JB. Effects of FK506 in rat and human resistance arteries. Kidney Int 1999; 55: 1518-1527.
727. Attur MG, Patel R, Thakker G, Vyas P, Levartovsky D, Patel P, Naqvi S, Raza R, Patel K, Abramson D, Bruno G, Abramson SB, Amin AR. Differential anti-inflammatory effects of immunosuppressive drugs: cyclosporin, rapamycin and FK-506 on inducible nitric oxide synthase, nitric oxide, cyclooxygenase-2 and PGE2 production. Inflamm Res 2000; 49: 20-26.
728. Watarai Y, Morita K, Shimoda N, Miura M, Yoshioka M, Togashi H, Nonomura K, Koyanagi T. Effect of tacrolimus and cyclosporine on renal microcirculation and nitric oxide production. Transplant Proc 2004; 36: 2130-2132.
729. Lopau K, Kleinert D, Erler J, Schramm L, Heidbreder E, Wanner C. Tacrolimus in acute renal failure: does L-arginine-infusion prevent changes in renal hemodynamics? Transpl Int 2000; 13: 436-442.
730. Tome LA, Castro I, Yu L, Andoh TF, Seguro AC, Burdmann EA. Role of nitric oxide (NO) on FK506-induced acute nephrotoxicity - *in vivo* and *in vitro* studies. J Am Soc Nephrol 1996; 7: 1897.
731. Mugiya S, Suzuki K, Ueda D, Ohtawara Y, Fujita K, Malyszko J, Urano T, Knofler R, Takada Y, Takada A. Renal blood flow, fibrinolysis, and platelet aggregation following tacrolimus (FK 506) treatment in rats. Thromb Res 1995; 79: 337-341.
732. Zhang W, Victor RG. Calcineurin inhibitors cause renal afferent activation in rats: a novel mechanism of cyclosporine-induced hypertension. Am J Hypertens 2000; 13: 999-1004.
733. Edkins RD, Rybak LP, Hoffman DW. Comparison of cyclosporine and FK506 effects on glutathione levels in rat cochlea, brain, liver and kidney. Biochem Pharmacol 1992; 43: 911-913.
734. McLaughlin GE, Schober M, Perez M, Ruiz P, Steele BW, Abitbol C. Benefit of theophylline administration in tacrolimus-induced nephrotoxicity in rats. Pediatr Nephrol 2003; 18: 860-864.
735. Yamauchi A, Oishi R, Kataoka Y. Tacrolimus-induced neurotoxicity and nephrotoxicity is ameliorated by administration in the dark phase in rats. Cell Mol Neurobiol 2004; 24: 695-704.

736. Jain A, Reyes J, Kashyap R, Rohal S, Abu-Elmagd K, Starzl T, Fung J. What have we learned about primary liver transplantation under tacrolimus immunosuppression? Long-term follow-up of the first 1000 patients. Ann Surg 1999; 230: 441-448.

737. Ryffel B, Weber E, Mihatsch MJ. Nephrotoxicity of immunosuppressants in rats: comparison of macrolides with cyclosporin. Exp Nephrol 1994; 2: 324-333.

738. Lea JP, Sands JM, McMahon SJ, Tumlin JA. Evidence that the inhibition of Na+/K(+)-ATPase activity by FK506 involves calcineurin. Kidney Int 1994; 46: 647-652.

739. Blaehr H, Andersen CB, Ladefoged J. Acute effects of FK506 and cyclosporine A on cultured human proximal tubular cells. Eur J Pharmacol 1993; 228: 283-288.

740. Cuvello Neto AL, Castro I, Costa MC, Ferreira AT, Burdmann EA, Yu L. Tacrolimus (FK-506)-induced tubular toxicity: role of intracellular calcium, nitric oxide (NO) and hydroperoxides. J Am Soc Nephrol 2001; 12: 799A.

741. Han SY, Mun KC, Choi HJ, Kwak CS, Bae JH, Suh SI, Park SB, Kim HC, Chang EJ. Effects of cyclosporine and tacrolimus on the oxidative stress in cultured mesangial cells. Transplant Proc 2006; 38:2 240-241.

742. Zhou X, Yang G, Davis CA, Doi SQ, Hirszel P, Wingo CS, Agarwal A. Hydrogen peroxide mediates FK506-induced cytotoxicity in renal cells. Kidney Int 2004; 65: 139-147.

743. Hisamura F, Kojima-Yuasa A, Kennedy DO, Matsui-Yuasa I. Protective effect of green tea extract and tea polyphenols against FK506-induced cytotoxicity in renal cells. Basic Clin Pharmacol Toxicol 2006; 98: 192-196.

744. Neff GW, Montalbano M, Slapak-Green G, Meyer D, Berney T, Safdar K, Schiff ER, Tzakis AG. Sirolimus therapy in orthotopic liver transplant recipients with calcineurin inhibitor related chronic renal insufficiency. Transplant Proc 2003; 35: 3029-3031.

745. Watson CJ, Firth J, Williams PF, Bradley JR, Pritchard N, Chaudhry A, Smith JC, Palmer CR, Bradley JA. A randomized controlled trial of late conversion from CNI-based to sirolimus-base immunosuppression following renal transplantation. Am J Transplant 2005; 5: 2496-2503.

746. Ellis D, Shapiro R, Moritz M, Vats A, Basu A, Tan H, Kayler L, Janosky J, Starzl TE. Renal transplantation in children managed with lymphocyte depleting agents and low-dose maintenace tacrolimus monotherapy. Transplantation 2007; 83: 1563-1570.

747. Jain A, Mohanka R, Orloff M, Abt P, Kashyap R, Kelley M, Burlee K, Bozorgzadeh A. Intravenous mycophenolate mofetil with low-dose oral tacrolimus and steroid induction for live donor liver transplantation. Exp Clin Transplant 2005; 3: 361-365.

748. Jain A, Vekatramanan R, Eghtesad B, Gadomski M, Mohanka R, Marcos A, Fung J. Long-term outcome of adding mycophenolate mofetil to tacrolimus for nephrotoxicity following liver transplanatation. Transplantation 2005; 80; 859-864.

749. Casas-Melley AT, Falkenstein KP, Flynn LM, Ziegler VL, Dunn SP. Improvement in renal function and rejection control in pediatric liver transplant recipients with the introduction of sirolimus. Pediatr Transplant 2004; 8: 362-366.

750. Meiser B, Kaczmarek I, Mueller M, Groetzner J, Weis M, Knez A, Stempfle HU, Klauss V, Schmoeckel M, Reichart B, Ueberfuhr P. Low-dose tacrolimus/sirolimus and steroid withdrawal in heart recipients is highly efficacious. J Heart Lung Transplant 2007; 26: 598-603.

751. Lawsin L, Light JA. Severe acute renal failure after exposure to sirolimus-tacrolimus in two living donor kidney recipients. Transplantation 2003; 75: 157-160.

752. Paramesh AS, Grosskreutz C, Florman SS, Gondolesi GE, Sharma S, Kaufman SS, Fishbein TM. Thrombotic microangiopathy associated with combined sirolimus and tacrolimus immunosuppression after intestinal transplantation. Transplantation 2004; 77: 129-131.

753. Augustine JJ, Chang PC, Knauss TC, Aeder MI, Bodziak KA, Schulak JA, Hricik DE. Improved renal function after conversion from tacrolimus/sirolimus to tacrolimus/mycophenolate mofetil in kidney transplant recipients. Transplantation 2006; 81: 1004-1009.

754. Meier-Kriesche HU, Schold JD, Srinivas TR, Howard RJ, Fujita S, Kaplan B. Sirolimus in combination with tacrolimus is associated with worse renal allograft survival compared to mycophenolate mofetil combined with tacrolimus. Am J Transplant 2005; 5: 2273-2280.

755. Randhawa PS, Shapiro R, Jordan ML, Starzl TE, Demetris AJ. The histopathological changes associated with allograft rejection and drug toxicity in renal transplant recipients maintained on FK506. Clinical significance and comparison with cyclosporine. Am J Surg Pathol 1993; 17: 60-68.

756. Hatori M, Takahara S, Kyo M, Kokado Y, Nagano S, Okuyama A. Clinical and histopathologic examination of renal allografts treated with tacrolimus (FK506) for at least one year. Int J Urol 1998; 5: 526-533.

757. Kyo M, Hatori M, Takahara S, Kyakuno M, Nakamura T, Okada M, Kokado Y, Toki K, Ding XQ, Miki T, Miyamoto M, Okuyama A. Morphological findings in non-episode biopsies of kidney transplant allografts treated with FK506 or cyclosporine. Transpl Int 1998; 11 Suppl 1: S100-S103.

758. Sugito K, Morozumi K, Oikawa T. A comparative study of clinicopathologic characteristics of renal allografts under cyclosporine and FK506 immunosuppression. Transplant Proc 1996; 28: 1335-1337.

759. Pillebout E, Nochy D, Hill G, Conti F, Antoine C, Calmus Y, Glotz D. Renal histopathological lesions after orthotopic liver transplantation (OLT). Am J Transplant 2005; 5: 1120-1129.

760. Sinha MD, MacLeod R, Rigby E, Clark AG. Treatment of severe steroid-dependent nephrotic syndrome (SDNS) in children with tacrolimus. Nephrol Dial Transplant 2006; 21: 1848-1854.

761. Tse KC, Lam MF, Tang SC, Tang CS, Chan TM. A pilot study on tacrolimus treatment in membranous or quiescent lupus nephritis with proteinuria resistant to angiotensin inhibition or blockade. Lupus 2007; 16: 46-51.

762. Solez K, Vincenti F, Filo RS. Histopathologic findings from 2-year protocol biopsies from a U.S. multicenter kidney transplant trial comparing tacrolimus versus cyclosporine: a report of the FK506 Kidney Transplant Study Group. Transplantation 1998; 66: 1736-1740.

763. Shihab FS, Bennett WM, Tanner AM, Andoh TF. Mechanism of fibrosis in experimental tacrolimus nephrotoxicity. Transplantation 1997; 64: 1829-1837.

764. Andoh TF, Burdmann EA, Houghton DC, Lindsley J, Franceschini N, Bennett WM. Calcium antagonist (CA) versus angiotensin II antagonist (ATA) in a rat model of chronic FK506 nephrotoxicity. J Am Soc Nephrol 1994; 5: 915.

765. Deniz H, Oğütmen B, Cakalağaoğlu F, Tuğlular S, Ozener C, Akoğlu E. Inhibition of the renin angiotensin system decreases fibrogenic cytokine expression in tacrolimus nephrotoxicity in rats. Transplant Proc 2006; 38: 483-486.

766. Muraoka K, Fujimoto K, Sun X, Yoshioka K, Shimizu K, Yagi M, Bose H, Jr., Miyazaki I, Yamamoto K. Immunosuppressant FK506 induces interleukin-6 production through the activation of transcription factor nuclear factor (NF)-kappa(B). Implications for FK506 nephropathy. J Clin Invest 1996; 97: 2433-2439.

767. Tamada S, Nakatani T, Asai T, Tashiro K, Komiya T, Sumi T, Okamura M, Kim S, Iwao H, Kishimoto T, Yamanaka S, Miura K. Inhibition of nuclear factor-kappaB activation by pyrrolidine dithiocarbamate prevents chronic FK506 nephropathy. Kidney Int 2003; 63: 306-314.

768. Tamada S, Asai T, Kuwabara N, Iwai T, Uchida J, Teramoto K, Kaneda N, Yukimura T, Komiya T, Nakatani T, Miura K. Molecular mechanisms and therapeutic strategies of chronic renal injury: the role of nuclear factor kappaB activation in the development of renal fibrosis. J Pharmacol Sci 2006; 100: 17-21.

769. Brook NR, Waller JR, Bicknell GR, Nicholson ML. The experimental agent pirfenidone reduces pro-fibrotic gene expression in a model of tacrolimus-induced nephrotoxicity. J Surg Res 2005; 125:137-143.

770. Zhong Z, Connor HD, Li X, Mason RP, Forman DT, Lemasters JJ, Thurman RG. Reduction of ciclosporin and tacrolimus nephrotoxicity by plant polyphenols. J Pharm Pharmacol 2006; 58: 1533-1543.

771. Khanna AK, Pieper GM. NADPH oxidase subunits (NOX-1, p22phox, Rac-1) and tacrolimus-induced nephrotoxicity in a rat renal transplant model. Nephrol Dial Transplant 2007; 22: 376-385.

772. Boyer O, Le Bidois J, Dechaux M, Gubler MC, Niaudet P. Improvement of renal function in pediatric heart transplant recipients treated with low-dose calcineurin inhibitor and mycophenolate mofetil. Transplantation 2005; 79: 1405-1410.

773. Wu MS, Chang CT, Hung CC. Rapamycin in patients with chronic renal allograft dysfunction. Clin Transplant 2005; 19: 236-242.

774. Flechner SM, Kobashigawa J, Klintmalm G. Calcineurin inhibitor-sparing regimens in solid organ transplantation: focus on improving renal function and nephrotoxicity. Clin Transplant 2008; 22: 1-15.

775. Jain S, Bicknell GR, Nicholson ML. Tacrolimus has less fibrogenic potential than cyclosporin A in a model of renal ischaemia-reperfusion injury. Br J Surg 2000; 87: 1563-1568.

776. Bing P, Maode L, Li F, Sheng H. Comparison of expression of TGF-beta1, its receptors TGFbeta1R-I and TGFbeta1R-II in rat kidneys during chronic nephropathy induced by cyclosporine and tacrolimus. Transplant Proc 2006; 38: 2180-2182

777. Bicknell GR, Williams ST, Shaw JA, Pringle JH, Furness PN, Nicholson ML. Differential effects of cyclosporin and tacrolimus on the expression of fibrosis-associated genes in isolated glomeruli from renal transplants. Br J Surg 2000; 87: 1569-1575.

778. Morris-Stiff G, Baboolal K, Singh J, Balaji V, Ostrowski K, Moore R, Lord R, Jurewicz A. Conversion from cyclosporine to tacrolimus in renal allograft recipients with chronic graft nephropathy: preliminary report. Transplant Proc 1998; 30: 1245-1246.

779. Duncan N, Dhaygude A, Owen J, Cairns TD, Griffith M, McLean AG, Palmer A, Taube D. Treatment of focal and segmental glomerulosclerosis in adults with tracrolimus monotherapy. Nephrol Dial Transplant 2004; 19: 3062-3067.

780. Lee WC, Lian JD, Wu MJ, Cheng CH, Chen CH, Shu KH. Long-term beneficial effect of tacrolimus conversion on renal transplant recipients. Ren Fail 2005; 27: 501-506.

781. Cantarovich D, Renou M, Megnigheto A, Giral-Class M, Hourmant M, Dantal J, Blancho G, Karam G, Soulillou JP. Switching from cyclosporine to tacrolimus in patients with chronic transplant dysfunction or cyclosporine-induced adverse effects. Transplantation 2005; 79: 72-78.

782. Schwarz C, Oberbauer R. Calcineurin inhibitor sparing in renal transplantation. Curr Opin Organ Transplant 2006; 11: 632-636.

783. Anglicheau D, Pallet N, Rabant M, Marquet P, Cassinat B, Meria P, Beaune P, Legendre C, Thervet E. Role of P-glycoprotein in cyclosporine cytotoxicity in the cyclosporine-sirolimus interaction. Kidney Int 2006; 70: 1019-1025.

784. Knight RJ, Kahan BD. The place of sirolimus in kidney transplantation: Can we reduce calcineurin inhibitor renal toxicity? Kidney Int 2006; 70: 994-999.

785. Lieberthal W, Fuhro R, Andry CC, Rennke H, Abernathy VE, Koh JS, Valeri R, Levine JS. Rapamycin impairs recovery from acute renal failure: Role of cell-cycle arrest and apoptosis of tubular cells. Am J Physiol Renal Physiol 2001; 281: F693-F706.

786. McTaggart RA, Gottlieb D, Brooks J, Bacchetti P, Roberts JP, Tomlanovich S, Feng S. Sirolimus prolongs recovery from delayed graft function after cadaveric renal transplantation. Am J Transplant 2003; 3: 416-423.

787. Fervenza FC, Fitzpatrick PM, Mertz J, Erickson SB, Liggett S, Popham S, Wochos DN, Synhavsky A, Hippler S, Larson TS, Bagniewski SM, Velosa JA, Mayo Nephrology Collaborative Committee. Acute rapamycin nephrotoxicity in native kidneys of patients with chronic glomerulopathies. Nephrol Dial Transplant 2004; 19: 1288-1292.

788. Dunn C, Croom KF. Everolimus: A review of its use in renal and cardiac transplantation. Drugs 2006; 66: 547-570.

789. Senior PA, Paty BW, Cockfield SM, Ryan EA, Shapiro AM. Proteinuria developing after clinical islet transplantation resolves with sirolimus withdrawal and increased tacrolimus dosing. Am J Transplant 2005; 5: 2318-2323.

790. van den Akkar JM, Wetzels JFM, Hoitsma AJ. Proteinuria following conversion from azathioprine to sirolimus in renal transplant recipients. Kidney Int 2006; 70: 1355-1357.

791. Stephany BR, Augustine JJ, Krishnamurthi V, Goldfarb DA, Flechner SM, Braun WE, Hricik DE, Dennis VW, Poggio ED. Differences in proteinuria and graft function in de novo sirolimus-based vs. calcineurin inhibitor-based immunosuppression in live donor kidney transplantation. Transplantation 2006; 82: 368-374.

792. Tomlanovich SJ, Vincenti F. Sirolimus: Defining nephrotoxicity in the renal transplant recipient. Clin J Am Soc Nephrol 2007; 2: 198-199.

793. Mulay AV, Cockfield S, Stryker R, Fergusson D, Knoll GA. Conversion from calcineurin inhibitors to sirolimus for chronic renal allograft dysfunction: A systematic review of the evidence. Transplantation 2006; 82: 1153-1162.

29

Immunomodulators: interleukins, interferons, and IV immunoglobulin

Joris J. ROELOFS[1], Daniel ABRAMOWICZ[2] and Sandrine FLORQUIN[1]

[1]Department of Pathology, Academic Medical Center, Amsterdam, The Netherlands
[2]Department of Nephrology, Hopital Erasme, Brussels, Belgium

Introduction

The outstanding progress in immunology and the development of new technologies have resulted in the introduction of new immunotherapies, the so-called "immunomodulators", for autoimmune diseases, inflammatory disorders, allograft rejection, and cancer. These immunomodulators comprise recombinant cytokines and specific blocking or depleting antibodies. Many of these therapies achieve their effect by stimulating the release of cytokines. The term cytokines includes interleukins (IL-), chemokines, growth factors, interferons (IFN), colony stimulating factors (CSF), and tumor necrosis factors (TNF). These molecules are involved in inflammation, cell proliferation and apoptosis, tissue injury and repair.

These new therapeutic tools can be associated with side effects among which nephrotoxicity. The most common immunomodulators associated with nephrotoxicity are described in Table 1. The nephrotoxic side effects of immunomodulators can be roughly divided into (ischemic) tubular necrosis, thrombotic microangiopathy, serum sickness, and autoimmune disorders.

This chapter aims to address the nephrotoxic potential of the cytokines or monoclonal antibodies at the doses being used in the treatment of cancer, auto-immune diseases, and transplantation.

Table 1. The most common immunomodulators associated with nephrotoxicity.

Agent	Pharmacological substance	Indications	Renal toxicity	References
Aldesleukine	Recombinant **IL-2**	- Metastatic renal cell carcinoma - Melanoma	- Acute renal failure	9, 15-18
Interferon-α	Recombinant **IFN-α**	- Viral hepatitis - Non-Hodgkin lymphoma - Several other malignancies	- Acute renal failure - Proteinuria - Lupus-like disease - Pauci-immune GN - RPGN - FSGS - Minimal change nephrotic syndrome - Allograft rejection	27, 31, 32, 33-35, 38-40, 42-48, 51, 52, 54, 58, 59
Peginterferon-α	Pegylated **IFN-α**	- Hepatitis C	- Acute renal failure - Exacerbation of vasculitis	60, 61
Interferon-β	Recombinant **IFN-β**	- Multiple sclerosis	- None reported	62, 63
Interferon-γ	**IFN-γ**-1b	- Chronic granulomatous disease	- Proteinuria - Acute renal failure	64, 66, 67
Muromonab (OKT3)	Anti-**CD3** Ab	- Allograft rejection	- Acute renal failure - Thrombotic microangiopathy	76, 78-82
Rituximab	Anti-**CD20** Ab	- Rheumatoid arthritis - Non-Hodgkin lymphoma	- Acute renal failure - Serum sickness	86-89
Infliximab	Anti-**TNFα** Ab	- Rheumatoid arthritis - Crohn's disease - Ankylosing spondylitis	- Serum sickness - Lupus-like disease - Extracapillary glomerulonephritis	90-93
Alemtuzumab (Campath)	Anti-**CD52** Ab	- B-cell chronic lymphocytic leukemia - Preconditioning regimen for bone marrow and renal transplantation	- HUS - Acute renal failure - Acute humoral rejection	98, 99, 101
Intravenous immune globulin (**IVIG**)	Human IgG	- Primary immunodeficiency syndromes - Kawasaki disease	- Acute renal failure	103, 106-108
Thymoglobulin (**ATG**)	Anti-thymocyte globulin	- Acute kidney and liver allograft rejection	- Acute renal failure	110, 111

Pathogenesis

Tubular necrosis

Cytokine associated renal dysfunction is regularly observed in the setting of sepsis syndrome or systemic inflammatory response syndrome. The cytokine release syndrome associated for example with OKT3 administration is similar to systemic inflammatory response syndrome. During systemic inflammatory response syndrome, it has been observed that even in the absence of systemic hypotension, acute tubular necrosis (ATN) can occur. Certain cytokines released during systemic inflammatory response syndrome mediate peripheral vasodilation in the absence of systemic hypotension. The renal response to peripheral vasodilation is vasoconstriction of the renal vasculature and reduced renal blood flow. TNF-α is a pro-inflammatory cytokine which plays a central role in the pathogenesis of systemic inflammatory response syndrome. TNF-α stimulates the secretion of IL-1β and regulates genes coding for other inflammatory mediators such as IL-1, IL-6, IL-8, and macrophage inflammatory protein (MIP-2). The major cellular sources of TNF-α are monocytes and T cells but upon injury, renal tubular cells start also to produce TNF-α as well as other pro-inflammatory cytokines [1-3] leading to an amplification of the inflammatory responses. TNF-α and IL-1 have also been shown to induce glomerular endothelial and mesangial cell production of vasoconstricting mediators like platelet activating factor (PAF), endothelin-1 (ET-1) and adenosine, but also of the vasodilators nitric oxide and prostaglandin E2. Local release of TNF-α reduces glomerular blood flow and glomerular filtration rate, induces the synthesis of other proinflammatory mediators, and, along with reactive oxygen species, increases glomerular albumin permeability. Pro-inflammatory cytokines recruit neutrophils and monocytes to the kidney and enhance their adhesion to endothelial cells.

Thrombotic microangiopathy

Thrombotic microangiopathy results from a massive activation of the clotting cascade. The major initiating factors are the release or expression of tissue factor, usually involving entry of tissue thromboplastins into the circulation, extensive injury to vascular endothelium exposing tissue factor, or enhanced expression of tissue factor by monocytes in response to endotoxin and various cytokines. Very high doses of systemic TNF can cause thrombotic microangiopahy as observed by Bertani in an experimental rabbit model. He showed that an intravenous TNF infusion did induce glomerular endothelial damage, neutrophil accumulation, and fibrin deposition within capillary lumens [4]. TNF-α induces production of reactive oxygen species by mesangial cells and tissue factor production by mesangial and endothelial cells, leading to fibrin deposition [5].

Serum sickness

The originators of the term 'serum sickness' are von Pirquet and Schick, who published a book with that title (Das Serumkrankheit) in 1905 [6]. The authors described an illness that developed in some patients after administration of horse serum that had been given as an antitoxin for the treatment of diphtheria and scarlet fever. Serum sickness is characterized by fever, rash, arthralgias, and eventually glomerulonephritis. Serum sickness is the prototypic example of the Coombs 'type III' or immune complex mediated hypersensitivity disease. The disease requires the presence of the antigen coincident with antibodies directed against the antigen, leading to the formation of antigen-antibody or immune complexes. These should normally be cleared by the mononuclear phagocyte system. If this system is not functioning well or is saturated by the immune complex load, then excess immune complexes may form in the circulation and deposit in tissues, or form directly in the involved tissues. The deposition of antigen-antibody (immune) complexes in tissues triggers the activation of the complement cascade, recruitment of leukocytes, and release of inflammatory mediators, such as histamine. Classic serum sickness can occur after injections of chimeric monoclonal antibodies but a variety of drugs can also cause reactions that clinically resemble classical serum sickness, but are believed to be caused by different mechanisms. In most cases, the specific mechanism is not known.

Auto-immune disorders

Drug-induced lupus is a syndrome which shares symptoms and laboratory characteristics with idiopathic systemic lupus erythematosus (SLE). Similarly to idiopathic lupus, drug-induced lupus can be divided into systemic, sub-acute cutaneous and chronic cutaneous lupus. The syndrome is characterized by arthralgia, myalgia, pleurisy, rash and fever in association with antinuclear antibodies in the serum. The clinical and laboratory manifestations of drug-induced SLE are similar to those of idiopathic SLE, but central nervous system and renal involvement are rare in drug-induced lupus [7]. Blockade of TNF in human rheumatoid arthritis or Crohn's disease led to the development of autoantibodies, lupus-like syndrome, and glomerulonephritis in some patients. These data raise concern about using TNF-blocking therapies in renal disease because the kidney may be especially vulnerable to the manifestation of autoimmune processes. Interestingly, recent experimental evidence suggests distinct roles for the 2 TNF receptors in mediating local inflammatory injury in the kidney and systemic immune-regulatory functions [8].

Recombinant cytokines

Interleukin-2

IL-2 is a 15 kilodalton glycoprotein which is normally produced by antigen or mitogen activated circulating T lymphocytes. It induces natural killer cell activity, enhances the allogeneic response, and activates cytotoxic T lymphocytes [9].

IL-2 has been used in the treatment of solid tumors such as metastatic melanoma, metastatic renal cell carcinoma, and colorectal carcinoma. Interleukin-2 infusions are associated with significant dose-dependent toxicity characterized by fevers, malaise, nausea, vomiting, diarrhea, hepatic dysfunction, pulmonary edema, somnolence, confusion, dysrhythmias, myocardial infarction, hematopoietic suppression, and renal insufficiency [10]. IL-2 has a short serum half-life of 6-10 min and a clearance of 30-60 min after bolus intravenously infusion [11]. Resultant toxicity is generally transient and reversible. It is possible that IL-2 induced renal failure only occurs in the setting of profound hypotension, prior volume depletion, concurrent administration of potentially nephrotoxic drugs, or the presence of underlying renal disease.

Morroquin *et al.* [12] studied the effect of high-dose IL-2 therapy in the treatment of patients with metastatic melanoma and renal cell cancer. They found that there was a subset of patients who could not tolerate high doses or retreatment due to renal toxicity. Pre-treatment factors that were significantly associated with renal toxicity were male sex, diagnosis of renal cancer, previous nephrectomy, and older age. These patients also had higher baseline creatinine.

Kozeny [13] evaluated IL-2 associated fluid and electrolyte disorders in 8 patients with metastatic cancer. All patients developed capillary leak syndrome, pre-renal azotemia, hypophosphatemia, hypocalcemia, hypomagnesemia, and respiratory alkalosis. As noted in other studies, albumin fell precipitously with an associated fall in serum calcium. However, measurement of ionized calcium and urinary calcium demonstrated true hypocalcemia and hypocalciuria. There was an associated hypomagnesemia and hypomagnesurea, hypophosphatemia, hypophosphaturea. Primary hyperventilation and respiratory alkalosis were thought to have caused an increased binding to albumin and intracellular shifts of these ions. Likewise, severe hypophosphatemia can be seen in gram negative sepsis in association with respiratory alkalosis. All patients developed a compensatory metabolic acidosis due to chronic hyperventilation. Respiratory alkalosis was thought to have developed because of capillary leak into the lungs producing borderline or frank pulmonary edema. After several days a superimposed normal anion gap acidosis developed from dilution by large volumes of saline fluid resuscitation. The authors found no defects in renal handling of calcium, phosphorous, or magnesium. There was no evidence of a renal acidification defect or renal tubular acidosis.

Shalmi *et al.* [14] suggested that an intrinsic renal defect may contribute to the renal dysfunction since the creatinine appeared to increase out of proportion to the blood urea nitrogen. If the predominant lesions were pre-renal azotemia, one would expect relative preservation of glomerular filtration rate in the face of renal hypoperfusion, thereby increasing the filtration fraction. The urinalysis did not show an active sediment as one might see in acute tubular necrosis. The authors suggested that the generalized capillary leak syndrome associated with the administration of IL-2 might have contributed to intra-renal edema and congestion leading to increased back-pressure and a decrease in ultrafiltration pressure and glomerular filtration rate.

Vlasveld [15] obtained biopsy material from a patient with renal cell cancer who developed acute renal failure in the sixth week of a continuous rIL-2 infusion. Acute tubulo-interstitial nephritis was present on pathology. Further studies on cryopreserved peripheral blood lymphocytes revealed specific cytotoxic activity against an autologous renal cell line cultured from the biopsy specimen.

In the past indomethacin was commonly given as prophylaxis against the chills, fever, arthralgias, myalgia's, and malaise associated with IL-2 administration. Non-steroidal anti-inflammatory drugs (NSAIDs) block prostaglandin-mediated glomerular afferent arteriolar vasodilation that is part of the auto-regulatory response to hypotension and renal hypo-perfusion. Co-administration of an NSAID with IL-2 sometimes precipitated acute renal failure.

Belldegrun [9] studied 99 patients with various types of metastatic cancer who had no identified renal disease, had a serum creatinine <1.9 mg/dl (despite unilateral nephrectomy in some) and had no autoimmune disorders and no exposure to immunosuppressive drugs. A confounding factor in the study was the prophylactic administration of indomethacin. The mean percentage of increase in creatinine was 219±15%. Mean peak serum creatinine level correlated with dose of IL-2 administered. Patients with baseline elevation of serum creatinine greater than 1.4mg/dl, renal cell carcinoma and radical nephrectomy represented a high risk group who were more sensitive to the IL-2 regimen and had a prolonged recovery of renal function. Weight gain and edema were observed in conjugation with the renal dysfunction. Textor *et al.* [16] noted progressive hypotension, sodium avidity, weight gain and edema, diminished glomerular filtration rate and evidence of ongoing tubular injury after administration of recombinant interleukin-2 to 12 patients. All patients received indomethacin which may have contributed to the development of acute renal failure. Serum creatinine returned to normal one week following discontinuation of therapy. The above 2 studies were seriously flawed because of the co-administration of NSAIDs.

Administration of cytokine combinations may be synergistic in their toxicity. Dutcher *et al.* reported a phase II trial of outpatient subcutaneous IL-2 plus IFNα [17]. They noted higher grade toxicity of fatigue, nausea, vomiting diarrhea, anorexia, fluid overload, rash, aseptic meningitis, chest pain, atrial fibrillation, and hypotension. One patient developed irreversible, dialysis dependent renal failure with crescentic glomerulonephritis.

Negrier *et al.* have compared the toxic effects of IL-2 and IFN-α in a cohort of 425 patients with metastatic renal cell carcinoma [18]. They found that the response rate of IL-2 and IFN-α were comparable, whereas the response rate of combined IL-2 and IFN-α therapy was significantly higher than during monotherapy. Nephrotoxicity however, was more common in patients receiving IL-2 than in those receiving IFN-α. Interestingly, Schomburg [19] demonstrated that palliative low to intermediate-dose of IL-2 in combination with IFN-α therapy was less nephrotoxic and less vasculo-toxic, especially if given subcutaneously rather than intravenously. Although there was a significant increase in serum creatinine and blood urea nitrogen (mean peak of 115.1±21.4 mmol/l, 6.5±2.5 mmol/l), there was no clinical evidence of renal dysfunction.

IL-2 appears to cause a generalized increase in capillary permeability, reduced systemic vascular resistance, fluid shifts and low effective circulating blood volume. It is not known if the vascular effects are a direct effect of IL-2 or due to IL-2 induced release of other mediators such as IFN, IL-1, TNF, and lymphotoxin [11, 20].

Rosentein *et al.* [21] injected high dose IL-2 into mice followed by intravenous I^{125} bovine serum albumin as a marker of capillary leak. The severity of the vascular leak syndrome was dependent upon the number of days of treatment and the dose given. Severity could be reduced by immune suppression with cyclophosphamide, corticosteriods, or whole body irradiation implying that lymphokines released by lymphocytes placed a role in the induction of the vascular leak phenomenon.

Renal toxicity has been attributed to sequelae from the development of the capillary leak syndrome. Vascular leak resulted in significant extravascular fluid accumulation (ascites, pleural effusions, peripheral edema) and weight gains of as much as 17 kg in 3 weeks [11]. As in sepsis syndrome, hypotension, oliguria and reduced fractional excretion of sodium accompanied the capillary leak.

Ponce treated 5 patients who had metastatic colorectal carcinoma with continuous intravenous infusions of IL-2 for 5 days and 9 cycles. They attempted to maintain a stable blood pressure with aggressive fluid replacement. However systemic vascular resistance declined from 1304 to 871 dyn/s/cm-5 and mean arterial blood pressure still dropped from 105 to 86 mm/Hg. Urine output dropped significantly and serum creatinine rose significantly. Urine sediment was normal on day 1 but contained multiple epithelial cells and brown casts by day 5 [22].

Others have shown that oliguria accompanying IL-2 infusions, responds to low-dose dopamine infusions, fluid resuscitation, and alpha agonists such as phenylephrine [20, 23, 24].

Rafi-Janajreh et al [25] examined the mechanism of IL-2 induced vascular leak syndrome in a mouse model. The vascular leak was especially significant in the lung and liver of wild-type mice but was markedly reduced in the lungs and liver of CD44 knockout mice. Both groups had similar levels of perivascular infiltration with lymphocytes but the CD44 knockout mice did not have endothelial cell damage and also exhibited a marked decrease in IL-2-induced lymphokine-activated killer cell activity. These investigators also showed that the vascular leak syndrome was dependent on the expression of CD44 on immune cells and not on the endothelial cells.

The above-mentioned studies have suggested or proposed a direct renal injury by IL-2, but none of them have been able to conclusively distinguish a direct IL-2 renal effect from simple renal under-perfusion severe enough to cause ischemia and ATN. The toxicity of IL-2 has been clearly associated with widespread endothelial cell damage and capillary leak [25]. This is consistent with a generalized, systemic effect of IL-2 rather than proof of a specific direct effect on the kidney.

Hall *et al.* [26] examined the nephrotoxic effects of IL-2 and its putative mediator, TNFα, in a pig kidney cell line. Levels of IL-2 comparable to those used in human studies, caused vacuolization, cell shrinkage and growth inhibition. Dexamethasone, which is used clinically to inhibit TNFα, failed to protect the cultured cells from the effects of IL-2. TNFα when given alone had no apparent effect on morphology or cell growth, suggesting that the nephrotoxic effect of IL-2 was direct.

Interferons

IFNα and IFNβ share 29% amino acid homology. Type I IFN (α and β) differ from Type II IFN (γ) in biochemical properties, biological function, and receptor specificity. Side effects common to both classes of IFN include chills, fever, rigors, headache, myalgia's, hypotension, nausea, vomiting, anorexia, constipation, fatigue, neutropenia, and elevated transaminases. This constellation of symptoms frequently results in mild to moderate hypotension and volume depletion and could potentially contribute to pre-renal azotemia or ATN.

Interferon-α

IFNα has anti-viral and anti-proliferative effects which have proven useful in the treatment of hepatitis B and C, cryoglobulinemia, and various tumors including rectal cancer, lymphoma, breast cancer, ovarian malignancies, cutaneous T-cell leukemia (mycosis fungoides), bladder cancer, cervical dysplasia, melanoma, and chronic lymphocytic lymphoma. Side effects include fever, chills, malaise, headache, myalgia's, neuropathy, somnolence, confusion, and fatigue. Leukopenia and elevation of serum transaminases are the most common dose limiting side effects. Nephrotoxicity is uncommon and usually noted in individual case reports as an association with administration of IFNα. Often there are other factors contributing to acute renal failure such as concomitant renal disease (nephrectomy, hepatitis C infection, or nephrotoxic drugs). Phillips reviewed this topic in 1996 [27]. Gutterman [28] reported no effects of treatment on serum creatinine and blood urea nitrogen, although transient pyuria was noted in 5 of 16 patients. Abdullhay [29] noted mild elevations of blood urea nitrogen and creatinine in 10 patients and more severe dysfunction in 2 of 36 patients with ovarian malignancies. The latter 2 patients had prior renal impairment.

Reports of isolated proteinuria associated with IFNα therapy have cropped up in the literature. Sherwin [30] observed 2 patients with transient proteinuria of less than 2 g/day which recurred with rechallenge with IFNα. Quesada [31] initially reported proteinuria of less than 2 g/day which recurred with rechallenge with IFNα. In a later publication, Quesada [32] cited an overall incidence of non-dose related proteinuria in 15-20% of patients. Quantitation rarely exceeded 1 gram and was not associated with a decline in glomerular filtration rate. Ferri [33] also noted proteinuria in patients being treated for mixed cryoglobulinemia but admitted that subclinical glomerular involvement with cryoglobulins could have been present. A few cases of acute renal failure and nephrotic syndrome have also been reported [34, 35].

As far back as 1976 IFNα was shown to be able to induce glomerulonephritis in animal models. Gresser [36] was able to develop an animal model of acute glomerulonephritis (GN) by injecting high dose IFNα into mice. Experimental evidence supports an immunologic effect of IFNα the kidney. Morel-Maroger [37] injected partially purified mouse interferon into newborn mice and found marked thickening of the glomerular basement membrane preceding the deposition of immunoglobin and complement.

Since then there have been a number of case reports of IFNα associated GN in humans. A variety of lesions have been reported including minimal change disease, pauci-immune GN, rapidly progressive GN, and focal segmental glomerulosclerosis [38, 39]. Two studies reported the onset of a nephrotic syndrome during treatment with IFNα. The nephrotic syndrome reversed after treatment was withdrawn [34, 40]. Herman [41] published a report of a patient with hairy cell leukemia who developed mesangio-capillary GN during treatment with IFNα. He developed hematuria, pyuria, and depressed complements. Colovic reported a patient with Philadelphia chromosome positive CML and nephrotic syndrome in whom renal insufficiency developed after the onset of IFNα treatment [42]. A renal biopsy showed the characteristics of mesangio-capillary glomerulonephritis. In spite of the discontinuation of treatment, renal function deteriorated and the patient died six months after the onset of the symptoms. Averbuch [43] reported a patient with Mycosis Fungoides who developed a minimal change nephropathy and acute interstitial nephritis after 6 doses of IFNα. After IFNα was discontinued, renal function returned to normal, but low grade proteinuria persisted for 2 months. Rechallenge with IFNα again produced azotemia and nephrotic range proteinuria. The authors suggested that activated cytotoxic T cells were responsible for a cell mediated delayed hypersensitivity mechanism of injury. Similar cases of minimal change disease associated with IFNα were reported by Traynor et al [44] and Rettmar et al [45]. Shah et al reported 2 cases of renal failure associated with IFNα treatment of chronic myeloid leukemia. Both patients had proteinuria and focal segmental glomerulosclerosis on biopsy [46]. Recently, two case reports were issued that concerned the occurrence of acute renal failure in patients that were treated with IFNα for metastatic carcinoid tumors [47, 48]. In both cases, renal function recovered after cessation of therapy.

Unusual immune side-effects have also been reported in association with IFNα therapy. Chronic hemolytic uremic syndrome was observed in a patient with multiple myeloma treated with IFNα (De Broe ME, personal communication). The post bone marrow transplantation course was complicated and he received several nephrotoxic antibiotics. Three months later a treatment with IFNα was started. Towards the end of the treatment renal function deteriorated. There was partial renal recovery after cessation of therapy. Renal biopsy showed focal mesangio-capillary lesions, mesangiolysis and intracapillary thrombosis consistent with a chronic form of hemolytic uremic syndrome. Ravandi-Kashani et al. [49] and Harvey et al. [50] reported 3 other cases of HUS/TTP. Two patients developed renal failure requiring dialysis. E. coli OH157.H7 was grown from the stool of one patient.

Acute renal failure or deterioration has frequently been cited in association with IFNα treatment of hepatitis C and even hepatitis B. It is well known that hepatitis C virus infection can cause GN. Mesangio-capillary GN is the most common manifestation and biopsy specimens have shown deposition of immune complexes composed of hepatitis C virus-related antigen and cryoglobulin. The difficulty lies in distinguishing glomerulonephritis caused by hepatitis C from glomerulonephritis seen in association with IFNα therapy or from occult underlying renal disease that is exacerbated by IFNα. There have been reports of nephrotic range proteinuria and focal segmental glomerulosclerosis on biopsy in patients who are being treated with IFNα for hepatitis C [51, 52]. Gordon *et al.* [53] reported a case of IFNα induced exacerbation of vasculitis (rash and renal impairment) in a patient with hepatitis C-associated cryoglobinulemia. Ohta *et al.* [54] examined 24 patients who manifested the appearance of or exacerbation of proteinuria after IFN therapy for chronic hepatitis C infection. One patient had known hepatitis C-related glomerulopathy and cryoglobulinemia and showed a good response to therapy including improved renal function and remission of proteinuria. Yamabe *et al.* and also Sarac *et al.* confirmed good responses to IFN therapy without renal deterioration in patients with hepatitis C-related glomerulonephritis [55, 56]. In Ohta's study only 3 subjects were treated with IFNα, the remainder were treated with IFNβ. As was shown by Johnson [57] improvement in mesangiocapilarry GN with IFNα correlated with clearance of viremia but did not correlate with remission of proteinuria. Other results were quite variable. The authors felt that absence (or minimal presence) of Hepatitis C core antigens or cryoglobulin deposits in the glomeruli indicated non-hepatitis C virus related or primary GN and that these patients might be at higher risk for exacerbation or direct injury from IFN. There was no clear explanation for which patients would benefit from or fail to respond to IFN and which patients might develop irreversible renal injury.

Renal transplant patients with hepatitis C seem to be especially susceptible to injury from IFNα. IFNα triggers renal graft rejection in a substantial number of patients, and is now considered contra-indicated in this setting [58, 59].

In recent years, pegylated IFN (peginterferon) in combination with ribavirin has shown to attain higher virological response rates in chronic hepatitis C than standard interferon. Therefore, Peginterferon-α is rapidly becoming the standard of care for chronic hepatitis C infections. Peginterferon is produced by the addition of a polyethylene glycol molecule to standard interferon alfa-2 and results in important changes in drug metabolism, with marked prolongation of its half-life. Peginterferon-α causes virtually no toxic side effects and hitherto only two case reports on renal adverse effects of this medicine have been published. Gordon described the case of a 54-year-old patient, who developed acute renal failure nine days after commencing treatment [60]. A renal biopsy showed ATN, and exacerbation of (probably pre-existent) IgA-nephropathy. After cessation of therapy, renal function was restored. In addition, Batisse described exacerbation of cryoglobulinemia-related vasculitis in one patient, following treatment of hepatitis C with peginterferon-α [61]. Symptoms included a purpuric rash, peripheral neuropathy and acute renal failure, which resolved slowly after discontinuation of peginterferon-α therapy.

In summary, other symptoms of IFNα toxicity are far more common than nephrotoxicity (fevers, chills, malaise, arthralgias, fatigue anorexia, weight loss, depression, impaired cognitive function, diminished libido, abnormal thyroid function). Nevertheless, IFNα has a complicated and important relationship to the kidney but there are many confounding factors that tend to obscure the molecular dynamics of that relationship.

Interferon-β

IFNβ has been used in the treatment of multiple sclerosis. IFNβ has been also used in combination with IFNγ because of synergistic anti-tumor effects. The combinations of IFN appear to potentiate systemic effects and cumulative toxicity compared to administration of either interferon alone. Synergistic toxicity limits the tolerated dose maximum and may also limit efficacy. Low doses of IFN-β and -γ given in combination, either by intravenous bolus or continuous infusion, do not appear to cause renal damage or dysfunction [62, 63].

The particular renal effects of IFN-β have not been specifically evaluated. Increased insensible losses via skin or the gastrointestinal tract or fluid sequestration from capillary leak and hypoalbuminemia can contribute to the development of pre-renal azotemia. Volume depletion and hypotension stimulate Angiotensin II and renal sympathetic nerves to try to maintain filtration fraction. Angiotensin II is a potent vasoconstrictor and also up-regulates the expression of growth factors and cytokines such as TGFβ, TNFα, vascular cell adhesion molecule-1 (VCAM-1), platelet derived growth factor (PDGF), basic fibroblast growth factor (bFGF) and insulin-like growth factor that are involved in renal injury and repair.

Interferon-γ

There are several subspecies of IFNγ determined by differential glycosylation. IFNγ is the most potent immunomodulator of all IFN. IFNγ is cidal to human tumor cell lines, activates monocyte/macrophages, upregulates Class II MHC expression and increases natural killer cell activity [64]. In the kidney, IFNγ regulates Class I and II MHC expression in the basal state, in response to inflammatory stimuli, and after ischemia or ischemia-reperfusion renal injury [65].

Systemic side effects are similar to those of other IFN, namely fever, chills, rigors, hypotension, confusion, disorientation, anorexia, lethargy, nausea, vomiting, diarrhea, myalgia, leukopenia, hepatotoxicity. Side effects are reversible and limited to the time of administration of the drug. Mild changes in liver function have been observed at higher dose levels and include hypoalbuminemia. There have been no significant changes noted in blood urea nitrogen and creatinine, although a small degree of proteinuria has occasionally been observed [64, 66].

Ault [67] reported a case of acute renal failure in a 12 year old child which required temporary hemodialysis after 19 days of therapy with IFNγ. The urinary sediment contained numerous white cells, red cells, and waxy and granular casts. Open renal biopsy revealed focal segmental glomerosclerosis in 3 of 43 glomeruli and irregular wrinkling of the capillary walls in others. A tuft adhesion to Bowman's capsule was seen in one glomerulus. There was also diffuse tubular damage and interstitial edema consistent with acute tubular necrosis. Electron microscopy demonstrated foot process effacement. Direct immunofluoroscence was negative for IgG, IgA, IgM, kappa and lambda light chains, C3, Clq, properdin, and fibrin reactive products. Renal function returned to normal after withdrawal of the drug. The authors suggested that structural distortion of the basement membrane and absence of immune complexes was evidence for direct glomerular injury by the cytokine. However the authors could not exclude prior sub-clinical focal and segmental glomerulosclerosis in the child. To support their hypothesis, the authors cited studies in newborn Swiss mice exposed to mouse interferon in which there was diffuse glomerular basement membrane wrinkling and capillary IgG and C3 deposition which progressed to focal segmental glomerulosclerosis.

Monoclonal antibodies

Monoclonal antibodies can vary tremendously in terms of isotype, construction (animal derived, chimeric, humanized, bound to toxin), ability to activate complement, binding avidity, target specificity, and whether it binds and blocks or binds and activates the receptor. Monoclonal antibodies may be directed toward soluble or membrane bound receptors or receptor ligands, tumor antigens, growth factor or their receptors. Therefore toxicity and side effects are equally variable [68].

In general, complement-binding monoclonal antibodies are more likely to cause a first dose response and cytokine release and potentially renal failure.

Monoclonal antibodies that are associated with systemic response consistent with cytokine release include:

Anti-CD3 antibodies

OKT3 is a murine monoclonal antibody recognizing the CD3 complex closely associated with the T cell receptor (TCR). The immunosuppressive properties of OKT3 are related to its ability to deplete CD3+ T cells, to induce the internalization of the CD3-TCR complexes, and to sterically inhibit residual CD3-TCR complexes [69]. The ability of OKT3 to induce multivalent cross-linking of both the TCR-CD3 complexes and the monocyte Fc receptor results in T cell and monocyte activation [70]. This is accompanied by the systemic release of pro-inflammatory cytokines including TNF-α, IFN-γ, IL-2 and IL-6 [71-75]. This leads to a cytokine release syndrome similar to systemic inflammatory response syndrome. This is associated with the development of a transient renal dysfunction [76]. In some cases renal biopsies were obtained at the time of renal dysfunction that showed only mild interstitial edema [77]. Beside the transient kidney dysfunction described above, OKT3 exerts pro-coagulant effects which can precipitate intragraft thromboses [78-82].

Anti-CD4

Anti-CD4 monoclonal antibodies have been used in the treatment of rheumatoid arthritis, psoriasis, systemic lupus erythematosus, and multiple sclerosis. First dose reactions were observed consisting of dyspnea, chills and hypotension [83].

Anti-CD20 antibodies

Rituximab, a B cell-depleting chimeric anti-CD20 monoclonal antibody, has been used with increasing frequency in the treatment of rheumatologic diseases. First dose effect was noted with rituximab (fever, rigors, hypotension) suggesting cytokine release. Some patients have experienced severe hypotension with the first two infusions [84, 85]. Recent publications reported the occurrence of serum sickness in patients with autoimmune diseases and marked hypergammaglobulinemia [86]. Also in patients suffering from hematological malignancies such as mantle cell lymphoma [87] and marginal zone B-cell lymphoma [88] rituximab-induced serum sickness has been described. Usually, there are no, or only mild renal side effects. Recently however, Ramamoorthy presented an unusual case of a 56-year-old man, who developed intravascular hemolysis, rhabdomyolysis and acute renal failure upon treatment with rituximab for high-grade non-Hodgkin lymphoma [89].

Anti-TNF antibodies

Despite a good overall safety profile, anti-TNF antibodies can induce a number of adverse effects, including autoimmunity and infections. A trial in the treatment of Crohn's disease noted infusion reactions, transient increased of anti-dsDNA antibodies, and serum sickness-like delayed hypersensitivity with retreatment. Induction of human-antichimeric-antibodies was suggested as the cause of some of the infusion reactions [90]. A prospective study in 35 patients with Crohn's disease showed induction of ANA and anti-dsDNA autoantibodies in 53% and 35% of infliximab-treated patients [91]. A single patient showed clinical features consistent with drug-induced lupus, including the presence of ANA and anti-dsDNA autoantibodies, which quickly resolved after discontinuation of infliximab. Reports on renal adverse effects of anti-TNF antibodies are very rare. Saint Marcoux described the occurrence of crescentic GN in as few as 2 patients out of a cohort of 39 patients, treated with an anti-TNF antibody for rheumatoid arthritis [92]. A case report by Chin *et al.* [93] described the case of a 29-year-old Australia-born Vietnamese who presented with nephrotic syndrome. A renal biopsy showed membranous nephropathy. Symptoms attenuated after discontinuation of infliximab therapy.

Etanercept is a recombinant dimeric fusion protein consisting of a TNF-α receptor ligand-binding region linked to the Fc portion of human IgG, used in the treatment of rheumatoid arthritis, ankylosing spondylitis, juvenile rheumatoid arthritis and psoriasis. Since 1998, there have been reports of vasculitic adverse events, including necrotizing vasculitis and leukocytoclastic vasculitis [92]. Etanercept has relatively little renal toxicity [94]. Recently, a case report was published that described the occurrence of Henoch-Schönlein Purpura, 11 months after starting etanercept therapy for psoriasis in a 57-yr old man [95]. Purpura was accompanied by renal failure, proteinuria and hematuria with red blood cell casts. Symptoms disappeared after discontinuation of etanercept. A second case study by Stokes described onset of renal failure, 4 months after initiation of etanercept therapy for rheumatoid arthritis [96]. On renal biopsy, the diagnosis of pauci-immune crescentic GN was established.

Anti-IL-2 Receptor

Of note, the *anti-IL-2 Receptor* (alpha chain) antibodies daclizumab and basiliximab, widely studied in renal transplant recipients, did not induce cytokine release or first dose reactions [97].

Anti-CD52-antibody

Campath-1H is a humanized CD52-specific depleting complement-fixing cytotoxic IgG1 monoclonal antibody. CD52 antigen is located on the surface of T and B lymphocytes, natural killer (NK) cells, and less densely on monocytes. Campath-1H depletes T lymphocytes from the peripheral blood for several months. Anti-CD52-Ab is used in the treatment of chronic lymphocytic leukemia, as induction therapy in renal transplantation and as a conditioning agent for bone marrow transplantation. Recently, a limited number of studies have been published that demonstrate possible renal adverse effects of anti-CD52-Ab. Bonatti reported the occurrence of hemolytic uremic syndrome in a renal transplant patient treated with Campath-1H [98]. In addition, Osborne described the case of a 37 year old woman who developed acute renal failure and disseminated intravascular coagulation following one dose of Campath-1H and Fludarabine, in preparation for bone marrow transplantation [99]. Campath-1H was thought to be the most likely causal agent although Fludarabine alone or in combination with Campath cannot be excluded. Renal function did not recover, requiring dialysis treatment up to 9 months after onset of symptoms. Recently, in a retrospective study in 443 renal transplant patients with biopsy-proven glomerular disease, the recurrence of glomerular disease under treatment with Campath-1H was studied [100]. In this study, the recurrence of biopsy-proven glomerular disease was similar in patients induced with Campath-1H or IL-2 receptor antagonists, while patients receiving antithymocyte antibody had a borderline lower recurrence rate than patients treated with other induction agents (P=0.047). Hill presented the rare case of a 38-yr-old renal transplant patient, who developed severe early acute humoral rejection, resulting in allograft loss after Campath-1H induction therapy [101].

Intravenous immune globulin

Intravenous immune globulin (IVIG) is purified, sterile IgG derived from pooled human plasma. Stabilizing agents such as glucose, maltose or sucrose are added in high concentrations in order to prevent or reduce immunoglobulin aggregation. IVIG modulates cytokine production and down-regulates IL-1, IL-2, IL-3, IL-4, IL-5, IL-10, TNFα, and granulocyte-macrophage colony-stimulating factor (GM-CSF). However, flushing, myalgia, headache, fever, chills, wheezing, hypotension and tachycardia have been noted after the start of the infusion and have been attributed to activation of complement and the complement cascade. Reversible rises in serum creatinine occurred in 4/17 patients treated for ANCA-associated vasculitis [102].

Acute renal failure is a well-recognized but infrequent finding after IVIG treatment and is thought to be at least partly related to the high solute load-induced injury to the proximal tubule [103]. Indeed, renal biopsies from patients with IVIG-induced acute renal failure show swelling and vacuolization of proximal tubular epithelial cells, leading to obstruction of the tubular lumen [104]. Other studies have shown that intravenous immunoglobulin infusions are more likely to result in acute renal failure in the presence of underlying renal disease or with simultaneous use of certain other drugs such as non-steroidals and angiotensin-converting-enzyme inhibitors.

IVIG is increasingly used in the treatment of auto-immune nephropathies, mainly lupus-nephritis and ANCA-associated glomerulonephritis [105]. In these diseases, IVIG is reported to reduce proteinuria and improve renal function (comprehensively reviewed by Orbach *et al.* [105]). However, the occurrence rate of acute renal failure in patients with lupus-nephritis and ANCA-associated glomerulonephritis, treated with IVIG), seems higher than in patients with other auto-immune diseases, although prospective studies are still lacking. Generally, the injury is reversible [106, 107]. More severe acute renal failure was noted in a patient who had underlying mixed cryoglobulinemia [108].

Although acute renal failure is an infrequent complication of IVIG therapy, clinicians should monitor renal function and sucrose-containing products should be avoided, especially in older patients with preexisting renal disease, dysfunction of other organs or volume depletion.

Anti-thymocyte globulin

Anti-thymocyte globulin (ATG, thymoglobulin) is a polyclonal rabbit antithymocyte globulin that has been used as an immunosuppressive agent in kidney and liver transplant patients. Despite a fairly high safety profile, reported side effects of ATG include hypertension, leucopenia and ARDS [109]. Renal adverse effects are extremely rare; only two case reports describe the occurrence of acute renal failure in patients treated with ATG [110, 111]. Cessation of ATG therapy in both cases and plasmapheresis in one case resulted in full recovery.

References

1. Giroir BP, Johnson JH, Brown T, Allen GL, Beutler B: The tissue distribution of tumor necrosis factor biosynthesis during endotoxemia, J Clin Invest 1992, 90:693-698
2. Ramesh G, Reeves WB: TNF-alpha mediates chemokine and cytokine expression and renal injury in cisplatin nephrotoxicity, J Clin Invest 2002, 110:835-842
3. Leemans JC, Stokman G, Claessen N, Rouschop KM, Teske GJ, Kirschning CJ, Akira S, van der Poll T, Weening JJ, Florquin S: Renal-associated TLR2 mediates ischemia/reperfusion injury in the kidney, J Clin Invest 2005, 115:2894-2903
4. Bertani T, Abbate M, Zoja C, Corna D, Perico N, Ghezzi P, Remuzzi G: Tumor necrosis factor induces glomerular damage in the rabbit, Am J Pathol 1989, 134:419-430
5. Wang J, Dunn MJ: Platelet-activating factor mediates endotoxin-induced acute renal insufficiency in rats, Am J Physiol 1987, 253: F1283-1289
6. von Pirquet C, Schick B: Das Serumkrankheit. Edited by Leipzig, Deuticke, 1905, p
7. Sarzi-Puttini P, Atzeni F, Capsoni F, Lubrano E, Doria A: Drug-induced lupus erythematosus, Autoimmunity 2005, 38:507-518
8. Vielhauer V, Mayadas TN: Functions of TNF and its receptors in renal disease: distinct roles in inflammatory tissue injury and immune regulation, Semin Nephrol 2007, 27:286-308
9. Belldegrun A, Webb DE, Austin HA, 3rd, Steinberg SM, White DE, Linehan WM, Rosenberg SA: Effects of interleukin-2 on renal function in patients receiving immunotherapy for advanced cancer, Ann Intern Med 1987, 106:817-822
10. Rosenberg SA, Lotze MT, Muul LM, Chang AE, Avis FP, Leitman S, Linehan WM, Robertson CN, Lee RE, Rubin JT, et al.: A progress report on the treatment of 157 patients with advanced cancer using lymphokine-activated killer cells and interleukin-2 or high-dose interleukin-2 alone, N Engl J Med 1987, 316:889-897
11. Lotze MT, Matory YL, Rayner AA, Ettinghausen SE, Vetto JT, Seipp CA, Rosenberg SA: Clinical effects and toxicity of interleukin-2 in patients with cancer, Cancer 1986, 58:2764-2772
12. Marroquin CE, White DE, Steinberg SM, Rosenberg SA, Schwartzentruber DJ: Decreased tolerance to interleukin-2 with repeated courses of therapy in patients with metastatic melanoma or renal cell cancer, J Immunother (1997) 2000, 23:387-392
13. Kozeny GA, Nicolas JD, Creekmore S, Sticklin L, Hano JE, Fisher RI: Effects of interleukin-2 immunotherapy on renal function, J Clin Oncol 1988, 6:1170-1176
14. Shalmi CL, Dutcher JP, Feinfeld DA, Chun KJ, Saleemi KR, Freeman LM, Lynn RI, Wiernik PH: Acute renal dysfunction during interleukin-2 treatment: suggestion of an intrinsic renal lesion, J Clin Oncol 1990, 8:1839-1846
15. Vlasveld LT, van de Wiel-van Kemenade E, de Boer AJ, Sein JJ, Gallee MP, Krediet RT, Mellief CJ, Rankin EM, Hekman A, Figdor CG: Possible role for cytotoxic lymphocytes in the pathogenesis of acute interstitial nephritis after recombinant interleukin-2 treatment for renal cell cancer, Cancer Immunol Immunother 1993, 36:210-213
16. Textor SC, Margolin K, Blayney D, Carlson J, Doroshow J: Renal, volume, and hormonal changes during therapeutic administration of recombinant interleukin-2 in man, Am J Med 1987, 83:1055-1061
17. Dutcher JP, Fisher RI, Weiss G, Aronson F, Margolin K, Louie A, Mier J, Caliendo G, Sosman JA, Eckardt JR, Ernest ML, Doroshow J, Atkins M: Outpatient subcutaneous interleukin-2 and interferon-alpha for metastatic renal cell cancer: five-year follow-up of the Cytokine Working Group Study, Cancer J Sci Am 1997, 3:157-162
18. Negrier S, Escudier B, Lasset C, Douillard JY, Savary J, Chevreau C, Ravaud A, Mercatello A, Peny J, Mousseau M, Philip T, Tursz T: Recombinant human interleukin-2, recombinant human interferon alfa-2a, or both in metastatic renal-cell carcinoma. Groupe Francais d'Immunotherapie, N Engl J Med 1998, 338:1272-1278
19. Schomburg A, Kirchner H, Atzpodien J: Renal, metabolic, and hemodynamic side-effects of interleukin-2 and/or interferon alpha: evidence of a risk/benefit advantage of subcutaneous therapy, J Cancer Res Clin Oncol 1993, 119:745-755
20. Margolin KA, Rayner AA, Hawkins MJ, Atkins MB, Dutcher JP, Fisher RI, Weiss GR, Doroshow JH, Jaffe HS, Roper M, et al.: Interleukin-2 and lymphokine-activated killer cell therapy of solid tumors: analysis of toxicity and management guidelines, J Clin Oncol 1989, 7:486-498
21. Rosenstein M, Ettinghausen SE, Rosenberg SA: Extravasation of intravascular fluid mediated by the systemic administration of recombinant interleukin 2, J Immunol 1986, 137:1735-1742
22. Ponce P, Cruz J, Travassos J, Moreira P, Oliveira J, Melo-Gomes E, Gouveia J: Renal toxicity mediated by continuous infusion of recombinant interleukin-2, Nephron 1993, 64:114-118
23. Memoli B, De Nicola L, Libetta C, Scialo A, Pacchiano G, Romano P, Palmieri G, Morabito A, Lauria R, Conte G, et al.: Interleukin-2-induced renal dysfunction in cancer patients is reversed by low-dose dopamine infusion, Am J Kidney Dis 1995, 26:27-33
24. Palmieri G, Morabito A, Lauria R, Montesarchio V, Matano E, Memoli B, Libetta C, Rea A, Merola C, Correale P, et al.: Low-dose dopamine induces early recovery of recombinant interleukin-2--impaired renal function, Eur J Cancer 1993, 29A:1119-1122

25. Rafi-Janajreh AQ, Chen D, Schmits R, Mak TW, Grayson RL, Sponenberg DP, Nagarkatti M, Nagarkatti PS: Evidence for the involvement of CD44 in endothelial cell injury and induction of vascular leak syndrome by IL-2, J Immunol 1999, 163:1619-1627
26. Hall TJ, James PR, Cambridge G: Interleukin-2 nephrotoxicity assessed *in vitro*, Res Commun Chem Pathol Pharmacol 1991, 73:375-378
27. Phillips TM: Interferon-alpha induces renal dysfunction and injury, Curr Opin Nephrol Hypertens 1996, 5:380-383
28. Gutterman JU, Fine S, Quesada J, Horning SJ, Levine JF, Alexanian R, Bernhardt L, Kramer M, Spiegel H, Colburn W, Trown P, Merigan T, Dziewanowski Z: Recombinant leukocyte A interferon: pharmacokinetics, single-dose tolerance, and biologic effects in cancer patients, Ann Intern Med 1982, 96:549-556
29. Abdulhay G, DiSaia PJ, Blessing JA, Creasman WT: Human lymphoblastoid interferon in the treatment of advanced epithelial ovarian malignancies: a Gynecologic Oncology Group Study, Am J Obstet Gynecol 1985, 152:418-423
30. Sherwin SA, Knost JA, Fein S, Abrams PG, Foon KA, Ochs JJ, Schoenberger C, Maluish AE, Oldham RK: A multiple-dose phase I trial of recombinant leukocyte A interferon in cancer patients, Jama 1982, 248:2461-2466
31. Quesada JR, Hawkins M, Horning S, Alexanian R, Borden E, Merigan T, Adams F, Gutterman JU: Collaborative phase I-II study of recombinant DNA-produced leukocyte interferon (clone A) in metastatic breast cancer, malignant lymphoma, and multiple myeloma, Am J Med 1984, 77:427-432
32. Quesada JR, Talpaz M, Rios A, Kurzrock R, Gutterman JU: Clinical toxicity of interferons in cancer patients: a review, J Clin Oncol 1986, 4:234-243
33. Ferri C, Marzo E, Longombardo G, Lombardini F, La Civita L, Vanacore R, Liberati AM, Gerli R, Greco F, Moretti A, et al.: Interferon-alpha in mixed cryoglobulinemia patients: a randomized, crossover-controlled trial, Blood 1993, 81:1132-1136
34. Dimitrov Y, Heibel F, Marcellin L, Chantrel F, Moulin B, Hannedouche T: Acute renal failure and nephrotic syndrome with alpha interferon therapy, Nephrol Dial Transplant 1997, 12:200-203
35. Dhib M, Bakhache E, Postec E, Vanrenterghem B, Le Roy F, Azar R, Francois A, Boldron A, Amaria R, Ozenne G, Hermelin A: [Nephrotic syndrome complicating treatment with interferon alpha], Presse Med 1996, 25:1066-1068
36. Gresser I, Maury C, Tovey M, Morel-Maroger L, Pontillon F: Progressive glomerulonephritis in mice treated with interferon preparations at birth, Nature 1976, 263:420-422
37. Morel-Maroger L, Sloper JC, Vinter J, Woodrow D, Gresser I: An ultrastructural study of the development of nephritis in mice treated with interferon in the neonatal period, Lab Invest 1978, 39:513-522
38. Lederer E, Truong L: Unusual glomerular lesion in a patient receiving long-term interferon alpha, Am J Kidney Dis 1992, 20:516-518
39. Parker MG, Atkins MB, Ucci AA, Levey AS: Rapidly progressive glomerulonephritis after immunotherapy for cancer, J Am Soc Nephrol 1995, 5:1740-1744
40. Selby P, Kohn J, Raymond J, Judson I, McElwain T: Nephrotic syndrome during treatment with interferon, Br Med J (Clin Res Ed) 1985, 290:1180
41. Herrman J, Gabriel F: Membranoproliferative glomerulonephritis in a patient with hairy-cell leukemia treated with alpha-II interferon, N Engl J Med 1987, 316:112-113
42. Colovic M, Jurisic V, Jankovic G, Jovanovic D, Nikolic LJ, Dimitrijevic J: Interferon alpha sensitisation induced fatal renal insufficiency in a patient with chronic myeloid leukaemia: case report and review of literature, J Clin Pathol 2006, 59:879-881
43. Averbuch SD, Austin HA, 3rd, Sherwin SA, Antonovych T, Bunn PA, Jr., Longo DL: Acute interstitial nephritis with the nephrotic syndrome following recombinant leukocyte a interferon therapy for mycosis fungoides, N Engl J Med 1984, 310:32-35
44. Traynor A, Kuzel T, Samuelson E, Kanwar Y: Minimal-change glomerulopathy and glomerular visceral epithelial hyperplasia associated with alpha-interferon therapy for cutaneous T-cell lymphoma, Nephron 1994, 67:94-100
45. Rettmar K, Kienast J, van de Loo J: Minimal change glomerulonephritis with reversible proteinuria during interferon alpha 2a therapy for chronic myeloid leukemia, Am J Hematol 1995, 49:355-356
46. Shah M, Jenis EH, Mookerjee BK, Schriber JR, Baer MR, Herzig GP, Wetzler M: Interferon-alpha-associated focal segmental glomerulosclerosis with massive proteinuria in patients with chronic myeloid leukemia following high dose chemotherapy, Cancer 1998, 83:1938-1946
47. Roeloffzen WW, Hospers GA, De Vries EG, Navis GJ: Renal failure after treatment with interferon alpha 2b, Anticancer Res 2002, 22:1929-1931
48. Laboudi A, Makdassi R, Choukroun G, Fournier A: [Acute renal insufficiency secondary to interferon], Nephrologie 2003, 24:181-185
49. Ravandi-Kashani F, Cortes J, Talpaz M, Kantarjian HM: Thrombotic microangiopathy associated with interferon therapy for patients with chronic myelogenous leukemia: coincidence or true side effect?, Cancer 1999, 85:2583-2588
50. Harvey M, Rosenfeld D, Davies D, Hall BM: Recombinant interferon alpha and hemolytic uremic syndrome: cause or coincidence?, Am J Hematol 1994, 46:152-153

51. Coroneos E, Petrusevska G, Varghese F, Truong LD: Focal segmental glomerulosclerosis with acute renal failure associated with alpha-interferon therapy, Am J Kidney Dis 1996, 28:888-892
52. Bellaiche G, Guettier C, Duboust A, Ley G, Slama JL: [Nephrotic syndrome with acute renal failure due to focal segmental glomerulosclerosis in a patient treated with alpha-interferon for chronic hepatitis C], Gastroenterol Clin Biol 2000, 24:465
53. Gordon AC, Edgar JD, Finch RG: Acute exacerbation of vasculitis during interferon-alpha therapy for hepatitis C-associated cryoglobulinaemia, J Infect 1998, 36:229-230
54. Ohta S, Yokoyama H, Wada T, Sakai N, Shimizu M, Kato T, Furuichi K, Segawa C, Hisada Y, Kobayashi K: Exacerbation of glomerulonephritis in subjects with chronic hepatitis C virus infection after interferon therapy, Am J Kidney Dis 1999, 33:1040-1048
55. Yamabe H, Johnson RJ, Gretch DR, Osawa H, Inuma H, Sasaki T, Kaizuka M, Tamura N, Tsunoda S, Fujita Y, et al.: Membranoproliferative glomerulonephritis associated with hepatitis C virus infection responsive to interferon-alpha, Am J Kidney Dis 1995, 25:67-69
56. Sarac E, Bastacky S, Johnson JP: Response to high-dose interferon-alpha after failure of standard therapy in MPGN associated with hepatitis C virus infection, Am J Kidney Dis 1997, 30:113-115
57. Johnson RJ, Gretch DR, Couser WG, Alpers CE, Wilson J, Chung M, Hart J, Willson R: Hepatitis C virus-associated glomerulonephritis. Effect of alpha-interferon therapy, Kidney Int 1994, 46:1700-1704
58. Rostaing L, Izopet J, Baron E, Duffaut M, Puel J, Durand D, Suc JM: Preliminary results of treatment of chronic hepatitis C with recombinant interferon alpha in renal transplant patients, Nephrol Dial Transplant 1995, 10 Suppl 6:93-96
59. Rostaing L, Modesto A, Baron E, Cisterne JM, Chabannier MH, Durand D: Acute renal failure in kidney transplant patients treated with interferon alpha 2b for chronic hepatitis C, Nephron 1996, 74:512-516
60. Gordon A, Menahem S, Mitchell J, Jenkins P, Dowling J, Roberts SK: Combination pegylated interferon and ribavirin therapy precipitating acute renal failure and exacerbating IgA nephropathy, Nephrol Dial Transplant 2004, 19:2155
61. Batisse D, Karmochkine M, Jacquot C, Kazatchkine MD, Weiss L: Sustained exacerbation of cryoglobulinaemia-related vasculitis following treatment of hepatitis C with peginterferon alfa, Eur J Gastroenterol Hepatol 2004, 16:701-703
62. Schiller JH, Storer B, Willson JK, Borden EC: Phase I trial of combinations of recombinant interferons beta(ser) and gamma in patients with advanced malignancy, Cancer Treat Rep 1987, 71:945-952
63. Schiller JH, Storer B, Witt PL, Nelson B, Brown RR, Horisberger M, Grossberg S, Borden EC: Biological and clinical effects of the combination of beta- and gamma-interferons administered as a 5-day continuous infusion, Cancer Res 1990, 50:4588-4594
64. Thompson JA, Cox WW, Lindgren CG, Collins C, Neraas KA, Bonnem EM, Fefer A: Subcutaneous recombinant gamma interferon in cancer patients: toxicity, pharmacokinetics, and immunomodulatory effects, Cancer Immunol Immunother 1987, 25:47-53
65. Takei Y, Sims TN, Urmson J, Halloran PF: Central role for interferon-gamma receptor in the regulation of renal MHC expression, J Am Soc Nephrol 2000, 11:250-261
66. Sriskandan K, Garner P, Watkinson J, Pettingale KW, Brinkley D, Calman FM, Tee DE: A toxicity study of recombinant interferon-gamma given by intravenous infusion to patients with advanced cancer, Cancer Chemother Pharmacol 1986, 18:63-68
67. Ault BH, Stapleton FB, Gaber L, Martin A, Roy S, 3rd, Murphy SB: Acute renal failure during therapy with recombinant human gamma interferon, N Engl J Med 1988, 319:1397-1400
68. Green MC, Murray JL, Hortobagyi GN: Monoclonal antibody therapy for solid tumors, Cancer Treat Rev 2000, 26:269-286
69. Goldstein G: Overview of the development of Orthoclone OKT3: monoclonal antibody for therapeutic use in transplantation, Transplant Proc 1987, 19:1-6
70. Van Wauwe JP, De Mey JR, Goossens JG: OKT3: a monoclonal anti-human T lymphocyte antibody with potent mitogenic properties, J Immunol 1980, 124:2708-2713
71. Abramowicz D, Schandene L, Goldman M, Crusiaux A, Vereerstraeten P, De Pauw L, Wybran J, Kinnaert P, Dupont E, Toussaint C: Release of tumor necrosis factor, interleukin-2, and gamma-interferon in serum after injection of OKT3 monoclonal antibody in kidney transplant recipients, Transplantation 1989, 47:606-608
72. Chatenoud L, Ferran C, Reuter A, Legendre C, Gevaert Y, Kreis H, Franchimont P, Bach JF: Systemic reaction to the anti-T-cell monoclonal antibody OKT3 in relation to serum levels of tumor necrosis factor and interferon-gamma [corrected], N Engl J Med 1989, 320:1420-1421
73. Chatenoud L, Ferran C, Legendre C, Thouard I, Merite S, Reuter A, Gevaert Y, Kreis H, Franchimont P, Bach JF: *In vivo* cell activation following OKT3 administration. Systemic cytokine release and modulation by corticosteroids, Transplantation 1990, 49:697-702
74. Bloemena E, ten Berge IJ, Surachno J, Wilmink JM: Kinetics of interleukin 6 during OKT3 treatment in renal allograft recipients, Transplantation 1990, 50:330-331
75. Gaston RS, Deierhoi MH, Patterson T, Prasthofer E, Julian BA, Barber WH, Laskow DA, Diethelm AG, Curtis JJ: OKT3 first-dose reaction: association with T cell subsets and cytokine release, Kidney Int 1991, 39:141-148

76. Toussaint C, De Pauw L, Vereerstraeten P, Kinnaert P, Abramowics D, Goldman M: Possible nephrotoxicity of the prophylactic use of OKT3 monoclonal antibody after cadaveric renal transplantation, Transplantation 1989, 48:524-526
77. Batiuk TD, Bennett WM, Norman DJ: Cytokine nephropathy during antilymphocyte therapy, Transplant Proc 1993, 25:27-30
78. Abramowicz D, Pradier O, Marchant A, Florquin S, De Pauw L, Vereerstraeten P, Kinnaert P, Vanherweghem JL, Goldman M: Induction of thromboses within renal grafts by high-dose prophylactic OKT3, Lancet 1992, 339:777-778
79. Abramowicz D, Pradier O, De Pauw L, Kinnaert P, Mat O, Surquin M, Doutrelepont JM, Vanherweghem JL, Capel P, Vereerstraeten P, et al.: High-dose glucocorticosteroids increase the procoagulant effects of OKT3, Kidney Int 1994, 46:1596-1602
80. Gomez E, Aguado S, Gago E, Escalada P, Alvarez-Grande J: Main graft vessels thromboses due to conventional-dose OKT3 in renal transplantation, Lancet 1992, 339:1612-1613
81. Noel C, Hazzan M, Coppin MC, Pruvot FR, Bridoux F, Lelievre G: Renal transplant artery thrombosis following treatment of allograft rejection with monoclonal anti-CD3 antibodies (OKT3), Transplant Proc 1995, 27:2438-2439
82. Shankar R, Bastani B, Salinas-Madrigal L, Sudarshan B: Acute thrombosis of the renal transplant artery after a single dose of OKT3, Am J Nephrol 2001, 21:141-144
83. Isaacs JD, Burrows N, Wing M, Keogan MT, Rebello PR, Watts RA, Pye RJ, Norris P, Hazelman BL, Hale G, Waldmann H: Humanized anti-CD4 monoclonal antibody therapy of autoimmune and inflammatory disease, Clin Exp Immunol 1997, 110:158-166
84. Gopal AK, Press OW: Clinical applications of anti-CD20 antibodies, J Lab Clin Med 1999, 134:445-450
85. Nguyen DT, Amess JA, Doughty H, Hendry L, Diamond LW: IDEC-C2B8 anti-CD20 (rituximab) immunotherapy in patients with low-grade non-Hodgkin's lymphoma and lymphoproliferative disorders: evaluation of response on 48 patients, Eur J Haematol 1999, 62:76-82
86. Finger E, Scheinberg M: Development of serum sickness-like symptoms after rituximab infusion in two patients with severe hypergammaglobulinemia, J Clin Rheumatol 2007, 13:94-95
87. Todd DJ, Helfgott SM: Serum sickness following treatment with rituximab, J Rheumatol 2007, 34:430-433
88. Schutgens RE: Rituximab-induced serum sickness, Br J Haematol 2006, 135:147
89. Ramamoorthy SK, Marangolo M, Durrant E, Akima S, Gottlieb DJ: Unusual reaction to Rituximab with intra-vascular hemolysis, rhabdomyolysis, renal failure and bone marrow necrosis, Leuk Lymphoma 2006, 47:747-750
90. Van Deventer SJ: Immunotherapy of Crohn's disease, Scand J Immunol 2000, 51:18-22
91. Nancey S, Blanvillain E, Parmentier B, Flourie B, Bayet C, Bienvenu J, Fabien N: Infliximab treatment does not induce organ-specific or nonorgan-specific autoantibodies other than antinuclear and anti-double-stranded DNA autoantibodies in Crohn's disease, Inflamm Bowel Dis 2005, 11:986-991
92. Saint Marcoux B, De Bandt M: Vasculitides induced by TNFalpha antagonists: a study in 39 patients in France, Joint Bone Spine 2006, 73:710-713
93. Chin G, Luxton G, Harvey JM: Infliximab and nephrotic syndrome, Nephrol Dial Transplant 2005, 20:2824-2826
94. Schiff MH, Whelton A: Renal toxicity associated with disease-modifying antirheumatic drugs used for the treatment of rheumatoid arthritis, Semin Arthritis Rheum 2000, 30:196-208
95. Lee A, Kasama R, Evangelisto A, Elfenbein B, Falasca G: Henoch-Schonlein purpura after etanercept therapy for psoriasis, J Clin Rheumatol 2006, 12:249-251
96. Stokes MB, Foster K, Markowitz GS, Ebrahimi F, Hines W, Kaufman D, Moore B, Wolde D, D'Agati VD: Development of glomerulonephritis during anti-TNF-alpha therapy for rheumatoid arthritis, Nephrol Dial Transplant 2005, 20:1400-1406
97. Berard JL, Velez RL, Freeman RB, Tsunoda SM: A review of interleukin-2 receptor antagonists in solid organ transplantation, Pharmacotherapy 1999, 19:1127-1137
98. Bonatti H, Brandacher G, Boesmueller C, Cont M, Hengster P, Rosenkranz AR, Krugmann J, Margreiter R: Hemolytic uremic syndrome following Campath-1H induction, Transpl Int 2007, 20:386-389
99. Osborne WL, Lennard AL: Acute renal failure and disseminated intravascular coagulation following an idiosyncratic reaction to Alemtuzumab (Campath 1H) or fludarabine, Haematologica 2005, 90:ECR05
100. Pascual J, Mezrich JD, Djamali A, Leverson G, Chin LT, Torrealba J, Bloom D, Voss B, Becker BN, Knechtle SJ, Sollinger HW, Pirsch JD, Samaniego MD: Alemtuzumab induction and recurrence of glomerular disease after kidney transplantation, Transplantation 2007, 83:1429-1434
101. Hill P, Gagliardini E, Ruggenenti P, Remuzzi G: Severe early acute humoral rejection resulting in allograft loss in a renal transplant recipient with Campath-1H induction therapy, Nephrol Dial Transplant 2005, 20:1741-1744
102. Jayne DR, Chapel H, Adu D, Misbah S, O'Donoghue D, Scott D, Lockwood CM: Intravenous immunoglobulin for ANCA-associated systemic vasculitis with persistent disease activity, Qjm 2000, 93:433-439
103. Gupta N, Ahmed I, Nissel-Horowitz S, Patel D, Mehrotra B: Intravenous gammglobulin-associated acute renal failure, Am J Hematol 2001, 66:151-152

104. Cantu TG, Hoehn-Saric EW, Burgess KM, Racusen L, Scheel PJ: Acute renal failure associated with immunoglobulin therapy, Am J Kidney Dis 1995, 25:228-234

105. Orbach H, Tishler M, Shoenfeld Y: Intravenous immunoglobulin and the kidney--a two-edged sword, Semin Arthritis Rheum 2004, 34:593-601

106. Tan E, Hajinazarian M, Bay W, Neff J, Mendell JR: Acute renal failure resulting from intravenous immunoglobulin therapy, Arch Neurol 1993, 50:137-139

107. Kobosko J, Nicol P: Renal toxicity of intravenous immunoglobulin, Clin Nephrol 1992, 37:216-217

108. Barton JC, Herrera GA, Galla JH, Bertoli LF, Work J, Koopman WJ: Acute cryoglobulinemic renal failure after intravenous infusion of gamma globulin, Am J Med 1987, 82:624-629

109. Walton GD, Gualtieri RJ: Antithymocyte globulin-induced adult respiratory distress syndrome, Arch Intern Med 1998, 158:1380

110. Busani S, Rinaldi L, Begliomini B, Pasetto A, Girardis M: Thymoglobulin-induced severe cardiovascular reaction and acute renal failure in a patient scheduled for orthotopic liver transplantation, Minerva Anestesiol 2006, 72:243-248

111. Levine JM, Lien YH: Antithymocyte globulin-induced acute renal failure, Am J Kidney Dis 1999, 34:1155

30

Imaging agents

Christiane M. ERLEY[1], Ihab M. WAHBA[2] and George A. PORTER[2]

[1]St. Joseph Krankenhaus Berlin, Germany
[2]Oregon Health Sciences University, Portland, Oregon, USA

1. Radiocontrast agents

Introduction

The use of iodinated contrast media (CM) continues to be a common cause of hospital-acquired acute renal failure (ARF) and its development increases the in-hospital mortality significantly [1, 2, 3, 4] as well as increasing the length of hospital stay [5]. Contrast media-induced nephropathy (CMIN) is defined as an otherwise unexplained acute deterioration of renal function after intravascular administration of iodinated CM. Although the clinical features and the histopathological findings of CMIN have been well described [6-9], its pathogenesis, prevention and best treatment modality remain uncertain.

Definition

Most authors define CMIN by an increase of serum creatinine of more than 1 mg/dl 2-3 days after CM exposure. Other reasons for an acute deterioration of renal function have to be excluded. Some investigators even believe that a lower increase of serum creatinine (0.5 mg/dl 2-4 days after CM) also should be classified as CMIN. It would also be prudent to look for a fall of GFR (general > 25% from baseline) with more sensitive methods (i.e. inulin clearance, iothalmate clearance, iohexol clearance [10]. Next to changes in GFR or serum creatinine levels an increase in urinary enzyme excretion seems to also be a sensitive marker of tubular damage after CM exposure [10, 11]. However, no conclusive relationship has been demonstrated between the detection of enzymes in urine and the fall in GFR [11-14]. Newer developments of early biomarkers i.e. the neutrophil gelatinase-associated lipocalin (NGAL), one of the most strikingly upregulated genes (HUGO approved gene name *LCN2*) and overexpressed proteins in the kidney after ischaemia, has been successful evaluated in the detection of renal impairement after CM, especially in children [15, 16). Further studies with this new markers are needed to verify the benefit CMIN.

Clinical findings and histopathology

In most cases, the increase in serum creatinine starts 24 to 48 hours after CM exposure, will peak after 3-5 days and return to baseline 7-10 days after exposure. Except for patients with a profound degree of renal function impairment, CMIN presents as a non-oliguric form of ARF. Temporary or continuous dialysis is rarely required. Although the majority of patients will show only minor and transient effects on renal function after CM exposure, a recent study showed that an increase of serum creatinine that did not require dialysis was associated with a higher in-hospital mortality rate compared to patients without CMIN [1, 2]. For post-angiographic patients who develop CMIN, 10% will require long-term dialysis [17]. A recent study demonstrate that, regardless of the presence of CKD, baseline characteristics and periprocedural hemodynamic parameters predict CMIN, the development of CMIN is associated with worse in-hospital and 1-year outcomes[18].

Morphological changes have been observed mainly as vacuolar changes in the proximal convoluted tubular cells [9, 19, 20]. These morphological changes parallel the increases in urinary enzyme excretion [9, 21], but a strong relationship to renal function impairment after CM has not been demonstrated [22]. It is more likely that these morphologic changes are consistent with CM exposure rather than evidence of tubular toxicity [22A]. Further evidence against traditional proximal tubular toxicity in patients with CMIN is the observation by Han et al that kidney ischemia molecule-1 (KIM-1) could not be detected in the urine of patients with CMIN [22B].

Incidence

The incidence of CMIN in the literature ranges from less than 1% to over 70% [23-27]. This discrepancy results from the lack of a single reliable definition, different methods of investigation, different types of radiological procedures, use of high or low osmolar contrast media and the presence or absence of risk factors. In patients without any risk factor the incidence is less than 1% despite the use of up to 800 ml of contrast media [28]. In patients at high risk the frequency of CMIN has been reported to increase in the last few years, which seems to be related to the wider use of diagnostic and therapeutic interventions in elderly and critically ill patients [29]. Multivariate analysis revealed in-hospital dialysis and an increase in baseline serum creatinine levels as the most important predictors of in-hospital and long-term mortality. Thus, acute kidney injury that requires dialysis after percutaneous coronary interventions is associated with very high in-hospital and 1-year mortality rates and a dramatic increase in hospital resource utilization [29A].

Risk Factors

A preexistent impairment of renal function is commonly regarded as the most important risk factor [32-36]. Consistent with multivariate regression analyses, diabetes mellitus is frequently citied next to renal insufficiency as an independent risk factor for CMIN [2, 6, 7, 32, 35-37]. However, in controlled studies diabetic patients without renal function impairment have not been shown to be at higher risk for developing CMIN [38, 39]. Because diabetic patients suffer from multiple vascular abnormalities, especially endothelial dysfunction, which contribute to renal damage, the vascular contribution still has to be clarified. After having developed renal insufficiency, diabetics are at significantly higher risk for CMIN compared to patients with other forms of renal failure [40]. In distinction to other patients given contrast media, diabetic often develop an oliguric form of CMIN and subsequently require dialysis. Contrary to previous reports [37, 41, 42], the volume of CM is only a risk factor in azotemic, diabetic patients [26, 43, 45]. Patients with server congestive heart failure [33, 36, 44] are at greater risk of developing CMIN, as are patients with hypertension [46,47] and anemia [48]. Female gender seems also to be an independent predictor of CIN development after PCI and a marker of worse 1-year mortality after CIN in patients without baseline CRF [46].

Based on a laboratory demonstration that CM addition caused intratubular precipitations of Bence-Jones protein, multiple myeloma has long been held out as an independent risk factor; however, a recent retrospective analysis [49] concluded that patients with multiple myeloma where not at increased risk for developing CMIN (Table 1).

Pathogenesis

In general, CM attenuates both renal hemodynamics and renal tubular function [50]. Mainly demonstrated in animal models injection of CM resulted in a transient increase, followed by a more prolonged decrease in renal blood flow (RBF) [51-53].

Recently, data has been published measuring the effect of CM on renal blood flow velocity (RBFV) directly. The authors used a 0.014 inch Doppler guide wire which was inserted through a separate contralateral femoral sheath via a 5 F Cobra diagnostic catheter into therenal artery during a PTCA maneuver showed that the administration of non-ionic low-osmolal contrast media has no immediate effect on renal perfusion in patients with CKD [54]. However, during the course of coronary angiography a gradual decline in renal blood flow may occur, the extent of which varies, presumably depending on individual pre-disposition as well as the amount and possibly the type of contrast medium.

A variety of vasoactive substances may modulate the CM-induced vasoconstriction, including prostaglandins, ANF, adenosine, endothelin, vasopressin, noradrenaline and angiotensin [53A, 55]. Of particular interest has been the possible role of superoxide radicals in the pathogenesis of CMIN. Not only do they induce renal vasoconstriction, but, as noted above, they also cause direct renal cell injury. Superoxide dismutase prevents the fall in GFR associated with CM, while in a dehydrated animal model, renal levels of superoxide dismutase is diminished which may account for the demonstrated increased susceptibility to

Table 1. Risk factors for contrast media-induced nephropathy.

Confirmed	Suspected	Disproved
Age	Anemia	Myeloma
Chronic renal failure	Urgent procedures	Diabetes without nephropathy
Diabetic nephropathy	Hypertension	
Severe congestive heart failure	Generalized atherosclerosis	
Amount and frequency of contrast media	Abnormal liver function tests	
Volume depletion/hypotension	Hyperuricemia	

CMIN [2]. By sequentially measuring these substances before and after CM exposure and by using antagonists of these vasoactive substances (misoprostol, bosentan, ace-inhibitors, α-blockers, etc.) [53, 56-60] the degree of involvement for each of these potential mediators in the process of developing CMIN has been investigated. To date, only endothelin and adenosine have been shown to play a role as important mediators in CMIN [58, 59, 61].

CM-induces intrarenal hypoxia, possibly related to the hemodynamic changes and/or increased tubular energy expenditure in response to osmotic stress [50]. Heyman et al have summarized the data supporting hypoxic medullary injury as being central to CMIN [62]. Because this region of the kidney functions in a relative low ambient pO_2, small reductions in O_2 delivery can have profound effects of cellular function. Confirmation of the reduction in medullary oxygenation following CM injection was provided by Heyman el al [71]. This observation was subsequently confirmed by Liss and co-workers [63]. The fall in medullary oxygenation is paralleled by a fall in medullary blood flow [64]. A key role for intact NO or prostaglandin synthesis was found by Agmon et al [75] who noted that outer medullary blood flow increased following CM injection provided that NO or prostaglandin synthesis was not inhibited. In conclusion, Heyman et al [53A] conclude that "CM-induced accentuation of inner medullary hypoxia is medidated to large extent by a decline in regional blood flow and oxygen supply. In contrast, intensification of outer medullary hypoxia predominately represents enhanced oxygen consumption, not fully compensated by increasedregional oxygen delivery." The final pathway for tubular necrosis may well be the formation of reactive oxygen species which activate energy consuming cellular reparative processes.

It has been proposed that increased renal adenosine levels arising from enhanced ATP hydrolysis may be a major contributor to development of acute kidney injury after CM application (Figure 1). This is corroborated by the finding that application of CM increases urinary adenosine excretion [65, 66] and the observation that dipyridamol, a nucleoside uptake blocker, magnifies the renal hemodynamic effects of CM [65, 66]. In addition, there are many similarities between CM-induced nephrotoxicity and the renal hemodynamic changes induced by adenosine. Sodium depletion potentate both adenosine action in the kidney [67, 68], and augments the nephrotoxicity of CM [52, 57]. Blockade of the production of vasodilatory prostaglandins by indomethacin potentates both the adenosine effect in the kidney [69], as well as the vasoconstriction induced by CM [22, 70, 71]. Pre-existing

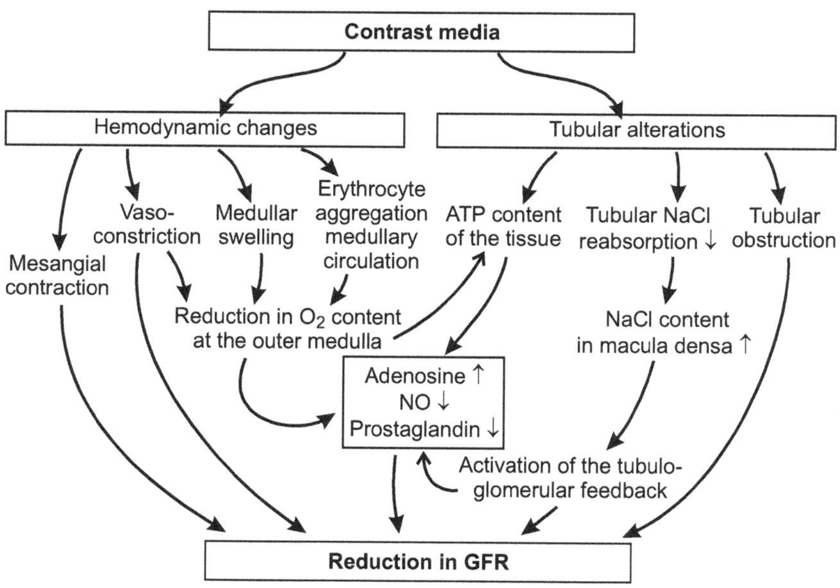

***Figure 1.** Pathogenesis of CMIN.*

renal ischemia prior to application of CM increases the severity of toxicity [51] and renal ischemia is associated with enhanced adenosine generation inducing renal vasoconstriction [67, 73, 74]. CM and adenosine both showed disparate effects regarding regional blood flow of the kidney with cortical vasoconstriction and medullary vasodilation [71, 75]. An additional role for adenosine comes from evidence that the diabetic kidney, due to attenuation of nitric oxide mediated renal vasodilation, has increased sensitivity to adenosine-induced vasoconstriction possible through up-regulation of adenosine A1 receptors [76].

Experimental studies in a variety of animal models of acute kidney injury reveal a consistent nephroprotective effect of adenosine antagonism [78-85]. Theophylline, for instance, acts as a non-specific adenosine receptor antagonist. Studies in both dogs and rats show a nephroprotective effect of theophylline after application of CM [65]. Our own group showed that rats subjected to chronic NO-blockade are highly sensitive to CM damage and when given adenosine antagonists (theophylline and DPCPX) demonstrate favorable effects concerning the prevention of a decline in GFR and RBF (Figure 2) in this animal model of CMIN [86].

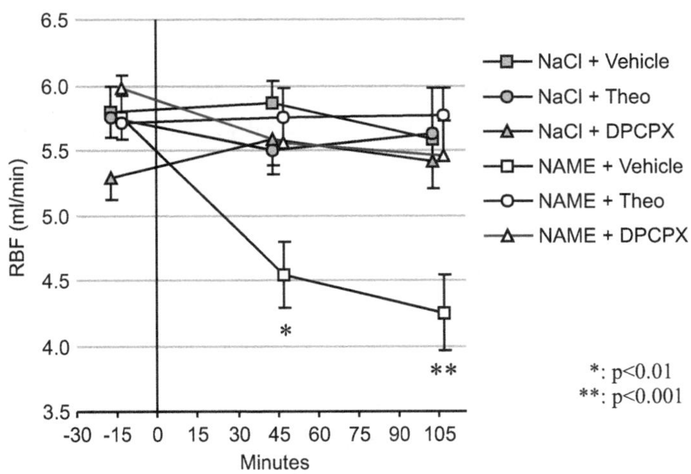

***Figure 2.** Decline in renal blood flow (RBF) in rats with hypertension and renal vasoconstriction due to chronic NO-inhibition by L-NAME compared to controls after CM-application. Data obtained after the administration of adenosine antagonists (theophylline and DPCPX) are also shown.*

Prevention/treatment

Choice of contrast media

Studies performed after the introduction of new low osmolar (nonionic) contrast media have failed to consistently demonstrate that these more costly substances reduce the incidence of CMIN when compared to high osmolar (ionic) CM [7, 87-90]. The largest trial involving a substantial number of azotemic patients (509 out of a total of 1, 196 patients), including 213 diabetics, also found a negligible incidence of CMIN with either low osmolar or high osmolar CM [37]. Patients suffering from renal function impairment due to diabetic nephropathy had a twofold incidence of CMIN when high osmolar CM was used as compared to low osmolar CM [37]. A recent published meta-analysis concluded that low osmolar CM may be beneficial for patients with azotemia [91], although the difference was very small and the higher price of low osmolar CM must be taken into consideration when choosing contrast agents. One has to keep in mind that the definition of "low osmolar" still involves CM's with an osmolarity of around 600 mOsmol/kg (compared to high osmolar CM with an osmolarity of around 1, 400 mOsmol/kg).

The development of new iso-osmolar CM (i.e. iodixanol) seems to promise a lesser toxicity compared to "low" osmolar CM [55, 92, 93], but a number of prospective randomized comparison trials conducted in patients with normal renal function, who underwent cardiac, abdominal, and peripheral arteriography, failed to show any superiority of iso-osmolality CM over LOCM [94, 95, 97]. Data from the Swedish Coronary Angiography and Angioplasty Registry based on Swedish Hospital Discharge Register, revealed that iso-osmolar CM iodixanol (iso-osmolar) was used in 45 485 patients, ioxaglate (low osmolar) in 12 440 subjects [96]. The incidence of CMIN was higher when patients received iodixanol than ioxaglate or iohexol. The authors mentioned that these effect may be due to the higher viscosity of the iso-osmolar CM, which has been shown in animal models to play a significant role in contrast-induced nephropathy.

Recently, a number of studies reported magnetic resonance CM as alternative CM in hopes of preventing CMIN in azotemic patients undergoing CT-scanning or angiography [98-100]. However, the only proven benefit of these substances in conventional radiology (despite magnetic resonance) is the lack of iodine exposure in highly allergic patients. Disadvantages of the magnetic resonance CM are their high viscosity and osmolarity. This physical characteristic theoretically also limits their use for CMIN prevention (especially because the volume of contrast agents needed for computed tomography or angiography is much higher than for a magnetic resonance examination, 100 ml versus 15 ml). Controlled studies in azotemic patients treated with either iso-osmolar CM or with magnetic resonance CM are not available, especially because in 2006, it was demonstrated that some gadolinium based contrast agents may trigger the development of nephrogenic systemic fibrosis, a generalized fibrotic disorder, in renal failure patients. Accordingly, the use of gadodiamide and gadopentate dimeglumine for renal failure patients was banned in Europe in spring 2007 (except for the use of gadoterate meglumine (Dotarem®), where no case of nephrogenic fibrosis was described so far). The same two compounds should only be used cautiously in patients with moderate renal dysfunction.(see next section on gadolinium).

Another promising imaging agent alternative to conventional X-ray CM is carbon dioxide, which is used to provide a negative contrast. Studies performed so far showed less nephrotoxicity [101, 102], but an image that lasts a short time. However, this agent induces ischemia of the infused organs. This effect on vascular perfusion prevents carbon dioxide from being used for the investigation of cerebral vessels or for detecting smaller vessels. Although not available at the present time, future development of alternative contrast media or alternative investigations could supplant imaging investigations using iodinated CM.

Hydration/mannitol/diuretics

From a theoretical point of view, pre-hydrating patients prior to contrast imaging studies would have the following beneficial effects on the kidney:

- decreased activity of the renin-angiotensin-system;
- down-regulation of the tubulo-glomerular feed back;
- augmentation of diuresis and sodium excretion;
- dilution of the contrast media and thus minimizing renal cortical vasoconstriction;
- reduced pre-constriction of the vessels;
- avoidance of tubular obstruction;
- reduction of endothelin and other intrarenal vasoconstrictive mediators (e.g. vasopressin).

Most studies involve either saline hydration in the role of mannitol or the value of vasodilators such as dopamine, atrial natriuretic peptide, Ca-antagonists or ACE-inhibitors with regard to protecting the kidney from contrast media damage [104-106]. The authors found that hydration alone was as equal to or more effective than the additional administration of hypertonic mannitol or the administration of one of the vasodilative agents. Other investigators compared results in patients submitted to special hydration protocols with historical control groups [107, 108] or data reported in the literature [109-111]. Pre-study hydration was the only preventative maneuver consistently associated with a lower incidence of acute kidney injury. So far, only one controlled, randomized study compared saline administration alone (0.45% saline over 24 hours, starting 12 hours before administration of radiocontrast dye) with mannitol (25 g of mannitol given 60 minutes before administration of radiocontrast dye) or furosemide (80 mg i.v.) [103]. In this study administration of saline alone was the most successful strategy.

Which fluid and when to start ?

Most investigators administer 0.45% saline in combination with 5% dextrose intravenously in various amounts (around 1000-1500 ml starting 12 hours before administration of radiocontrast agents). There is no controlled study that assessed oral hydration in these patients. Until now, there has been no investigation as to how long hydration should be continued. From a theoretical point of view the use of hyperosmolar fluids (such as 15% mannitol) in addition to the administration of the hyperosmolar contrast media may have adverse effects. Therefore, it is not surprising that most studies failed to observe a beneficial effect of mannitol in this setting [40, 103, 107]. In accordance with the reported investigational data, humans have been significantly protected against the development of CMIN when hydrated prior to and up to 12 hours after contrast media exposure [103, 107, 110]. Only a minor protective effect could be demonstrated when fluid was administered during the procedure [108, 111] or shortly before the CM administration [112].

The hypothesis that intravenous fluid that contains sodium bicarbonate might decrease the incidence of CIN compared with NaCl was recently tested in some randomized trials [113-116]. The hypothesis for a potential benefit of bicarbonate is based on the concept that alkalinizing tubular fluid reduces the generation of injurious hydroxyl radicals. Within a retrospective Cohort Study of 7977 Patients at Mayo Clinic N-acetylcysteine alone and in combination with sodium bicarbonate was not associated with any significant difference in the incidence of contrast nephropathy. The use of intravenous sodium bicarbonate was associated with increased incidence of contrast nephropathy [117]. As with any retrospective study confounding by indication is always exists since patients at preceived high risk often receive the treatment that is suspected of being superior even when unproven.

There remains a clear need for well-powered studies with large numbers of high-risk patients to help answer the outstanding questions of composition, route of administration, rate, and duration of volume expansion toprevent CIN.

Use of diuretics?

No conclusive evidence is available to support a protective role of loop-active diuretics with regard to the prevention of CMIN. It has been claimed that a reduction of the workload of the tubular cells of the thick ascending limb of Henle, by decreasing the rate of sodium reabsorption, might be tubuloprotective. Additionally, there might be a dilution effect by an increment of diuresis after furosemide. Most studies that have investigated this application showed either no beneficial effect or sometimes even worse results in case of furosemide application [103, 118, 119]. The negative effect of furosemide could be due to the reduction of cortical resistance inducing a redistribution of renal perfusion with reduced perfusion of the medulla. In combination with the contrast media-induced vasoconstriction, the oxygen content could be reduced to a critical point and thereby contributing to further deterioration of renal ischemia. Furosemide should be used with caution because there is always the fear of dehydration, which would enhance the nephrotoxicity of contrast agents.

Use of vasoactive substances as prophylaxis

Many of the therapeutic approaches to the prevention of CMIN involve the use of vasodilator agents. The lack of efficacy of such approaches may be contained in a recent concept articulated by a group from Mayo Clinic [76]. Starting with the evidence that the diabetic kidney has a diminished vasodilatory capacity, they reason that CM released vasoconstrictor, such as endothelin, would inhibit the production and release of nitric oxide and further compromise an already diminished endothelial mediated vasodilation. Thus, they suggest that administration of vasoconstrictor antagonist may be more effective in preventing or minimizing the vasoconstriction induced by CM, rather than applying a direct vasodilator to vessels with dysfunctional capacity. While the concept is most applicable to diabetics, there is evidence that hypertensive patients share a diminished capacity for generation of nitric oxide in response to renal vasoconstriction [77].

Calcium channel blockers

Due to their vasodilating effect and the hope to prevent calcium overload in the tubular cells [52], calcium channel blockers have been used in both experimental [80] and clinical studies [65, 120, 121]. Despite early promising results large prospective trials failed to observe a beneficial effect regarding the decline in GFR after CM exposure [122-124]. Taken together a prophylactic value of calcium channel blockers (either short or long acting) has not been proven.

Dopamine

Dopamine, given in the so-called "renal doses" of around 2 μg/kg/min is widely used to prevent and to treat an acute kidney injury induced under various circumstances. So far, most prospective studies have failed to demonstrate any real benefit of dopamine in the setting of CMIN [105, 125]. An interesting point seems to be the observation, that a prophylactic treatment with dopamine in 497 patients with ARF increased the mortality rate, which could be due to the pro-arrhythmic effect of this substance [126]. Fenoldopam, a selective dopamine type 1 receptor agonist has shown promise in the prevention of CMIN. In a retrospective evaluation of CRF patients given CM and fenoldopam, Madyoon et al [127] reported a CMIN incidence of only 13% that was significantly less that the 38% derived from historic controls. In a prospective trial of CRF patients undergoing coronary angiography, Kini et al [128] found significantly fewer patients had elevated serum creatinine values post procedure than would have been predicted from previously reported incidences. Obviously, in order to confirm a beneficial effect of fenoldopam, a prospective, randomized control trial will be required.

Atrial natriuretic factor (ANF)

Because of its natriuretic and vasodilative activity, in addition to its effect on the intracellular ATP-concentration [129], ANF seems to be a good candidate for the prevention of CMIN. To date no conclusive beneficial results have been obtained in clinical studies [40, 104, 130]. This may be due to the route of application (i.v. versus i.a. in experimental studies) and to intrarenal hemodynamic changes caused by ANF with induction of an arterial-steal phenomenon.

Adenosine Antagonists

In preliminary studies in both animals and humans a nephroprotective effect of theophylline (an unspecific adenosine antagonist) indicated a modification of the reduction of GFR after application of CM [66, 131]. However, a large, double blind, placebo-controlled study performed in patients with chronic renal failure failed to show a benefit of theophylline when given to otherwise stable and well hydrated mildly azotemic patients [12]. Thus, it can be argued that the prolonged tubular exposure to CM because of low tubular flow rates in dehydrated patients in combination with a stimulation of the renin-angiotensin system is the main reason for a fall in GFR after CM and that adenosine role in developing CMIN involving vasoconstriction [61]. Patients with heart failure or inability to be tolerate hydrated due to other conditions and a higher degree of renal insufficiency have been excluded from prospective trials, which investigated the effects of theophylline. Clinical trials involving patients with contraindications for hydration should be carried out in order to clearly evaluate the value of theophylline in the prevention of CM-induced nephropathy. Preliminary results obtained through a retrospective study showed that theophylline administration on an intensive care unit showed good results regarding the incidence of CMIN in patients with cardiac insufficiency (incidence of acute kidney injury without theophylline: 15%, with theophylline: 7%) [132].

Antioxidant agents

Reactive oxygen species may have a role in renal damage caused by contrast agents. Acetylcysteine, a thiol-containing antioxidant has been used to treat a variety of pulmonary diseases and to treat acute acetaminophen poisoning. Recently, however, it has been used successfully to ameliorate the toxic effects of a variety of experimentally or clinically induced ischemia-reperfusion syndromes of the heart, kidney, lung, and liver. In each of these syndromes, it is thought that the activity of acetylcysteine is related to its action as a free-radical scavenger, or as a reactive sulphydryl compound that increases the reductive capacity of the cell. Tepel et al. [133] recently published the first clinical trial using acetylcysteine (1200 mg of acetylcysteine per day, given orally in divided doses on the day before and on the day of the administration of the radiocontrast agent) in order to prevent the decline in renal function in patients with moderate renal insufficiency, who were undergoing computed tomography [133]. On closer evaluation of the data they do not really show a conclusive benefit of acetylcysteine since the placebo comparison group did not show a significant decline in renal function after contrast media exposure and the significant difference between the groups resulted from an unexplained decline in creatinine levels in the acetylcysteine group compared to stable creatinine levels in the placebo group.

Since that time there have been many published studies with great heterogeneity in results some finding substantial benefit for NAC [134-136], others reporting no effect [137]. Most of the studies included patient populations at relatively increased risk for CIN, generally defined by an increased baseline SCr. ARF developing after contrast exposure has generally been defined as an increase in SCr of ≥0.5 mg/dl or ≥25% above the baseline value. There are > 20 published studies investigating NAC for the prevention of CIN, with 30 to 487 subjects enrolled in each study [138]. Studies with negative results outnumber those with positive results by a 2-to-1 margin. However, the magnitude of benefit in some of the positive studies was substantial [134]. Most published studies have been underpowered to adequately test efficacy end points. In the largest published study, by Webb *et al.*, [139] 487 patients with renal dysfunction were randomized to receive either placebo or NAC 500 mg intravenously before undergoing cardiac catheterization. The study was terminated prematurely by the Data Safety Monitoring Committee because of futility and the lack of any trend toward benefit with NAC treatment [139]. Because of the larger sample size of this study compared with other NAC studies, the negative findings carry particular weight. In contrast to Webb's findings is the recent publication of Marenzi *et al.*, which reports on 354 patients with myocardial infarction undergoing coronary angiography with primary angioplasty [140]. Patients were randomized to treatment with placebo, a standard dose of NAC (600 mg by intravenous bolus before primary angioplasty and 600 mg orally twice daily for 48 h after angioplasty), or a double dose of NAC (1200 mg by intravenous bolus and 1200 mg orally twice daily for 48 h after intervention). ARF was defined as a 25% increase in SCr level. The risk for CIN was reduced by 54.5% in the standard-dose NAC group and by 75.8% in the high-dose NAC group. This gradient of effect was particularly impressive and not found in prior studies. More remarkable, the risk for death was also reduced by the use of NAC at both dosage strengths. The most likely explanation for this find is that NAC may have had a cardioprotective effect, as has been recently suggested. However, this result would be strengthened by confirmation by other investigators. It should be noted that intravenous NAC is associated with a small risk for anaphylactoid reactions. The findings of Marenzi *et al* [140] stand in stark contrast to the other large study, that of Webb *et al* [139], and further add to the murkiness of the literature on NAC for prevention of CIN. Within a retrospective (real-world) cohort study of 7977 Patients at Mayo Clinic N-acetylcysteine alone and in combination with sodium bicarbonate was not associated with any significant difference in the incidence of contrast nephropathy [117].

It has to be claimed that *N*-Acetylcysteine artifactually lower plasma creatinine concentration [98H]. Although these hypothesis was not confirmed by others who showed that although NAC may have a small effect on measurement of SCr, it is probably not large enough to diminish the value of SCr as a study end point [138].

Endothelin antagonists

Endothelin as a potent vasoconstrictor has been implicated in the pathogenesis of CMIN. Although animal studies showed promising results by application of endothelin antagonists [143] the first clinical study using an endothelin receptor antagonist showed a negative result with an exacerbation [144].

Hemodialysis after exposure to contrast media

Some nephrologists have used hemodialysis in azotemic patients to enhance the elimination rate of CM from the body. From a pathophysiological point of view hemodialysis, which was normally initiated around 30-120 minutes after CM application, cannot prevent the effects on the renal hemodynamic situation. The only prospective study done so far by Lehnert et al. [145] showed no benefit regarding the development of ARF in dialyzed patients compared to controls. In our own institute we performed a controlled study with azotemic patients. Fifteen patients with an impaired renal function (mean serum creatinine concentration 2.7 ± 0.2 mg/dl) were randomly assigned to receive either a hemodialysis procedure for 2-3 hours, started as early as possible after administration of CM (106 ± 25 minutes), or a conservative treatment. The course and absolute changes in serum creatinine over the entire observation period was not different in either groups. The percentage increase of serum creatinine the day after CM application was higher in the group that underwent hemodialysis [146]. The rate of CMIN (defined as serum creatinine increase of greater than or equal to 0.5 mg/dl within 48 h after administration of CM) was significantly higher in the dialyzed group (43% in the hemodialysis group and 13% in the group with conservative treatment, respectively). The serum iodine concentration declined earlier in the dialyzed group. A randomized controlled trial comparing hydration therapy to additional hemodialysis or N-acetylcysteine for the prevention of contrast medium-induced nephropathy: the Dialysis-versus-Diuresis (DVD) Trial did not find a benefit for hemodyialysis [147].

One study in 114 patients showed that in patients with severe chronic renal impairment (serum creatinine ≥2 mg/dL [≥176.8 μmol/L]), continuous venovenous hemofiltration (1,000 mL/hr without weight loss) was more effective than intravenous volume expansion in reducing the risk for CIN (normal saline 1 mL/kg per hr). Hemofiltration and intravenous volume expansion were both started 4–8 hours before percutaneous coronary intervention (PCI) and continued for 18–24 hours afterward. It is important to note that CIN was defined in this study as a ≥25% increase in serum creatinine; this occurred less frequently in the group receiving hemofiltration than in the group treated with volume expansion (5% vs 50%; p <0.001). However, because the intervention of hemofiltration itself affected the serum creatinine level, it cannot be determined whether there was a beneficial effect of hemofiltration. Although the inhospital and 1-year mortality were significantly lower in the patients who underwent hemofiltration, the flawed nature of the trial design does not allow for definitive conclusions regarding this technique [148].

The CIN Consensus Working Panel considered that hemofiltration deserves further investigation using end points unaffected by the experimental intervention, but the high cost and need for intensive care unit admission will also limit the utility of this prophylactic approach. [149].

In summary, dialysis has no proven benefit in regard to a prevention of CMIN in azotemic patients.

Conclusions

Table 2 summarizes the clinical maneuvers that, based on current evidence, can be implemented to reduce the chance of CMIN. Before undertaking an imaging study, a risk/benefit analysis is needed. Will the information obtained lead to a change in treatment or is it simply to confirm a clinical suspicion? If the latter, then a compelling need for such confirmation must exist. By following the six recommendations on Table 2, the risk for CMIN can be significantly reduced. A more detailed algorithm for managing CM injections in patients with risk factors as outlined on Table 1 can be found in the report by Pannu et al [150].

2. Gadolinium use in the setting of renal dysfunction

Introduction

As noted in the preceding section, the use of IV iodinated imaging contrast agents in patients with renal dysfunction is associated with the risk of contrast nephropathy [151]. The consequences of the latter not only include acute kidney injury (AKI) and the need for dialysis, but also an increased mortality risk [1]. Therefore, IV iodinated contrast agents are often avoided in the setting of renal dysfunction, especially when the risk of contrast nephropathy is high, such as in patients with diabetic nephropathy and/or a creatinine greater than 1.5 mg/dL [1]. The use of gadolinium-containing contrast agents (GCCA) has traditionally been considered a safe alternative in the setting of renal dysfunction, because of the low risk of gadolinium-induced AKI. Gadolinium is a rare-earth lanthanide metallic element used in magnetic resonance imaging (MRI) and magnetic resonance angiography (MRA) because of its paramagnetic properties that enhance imaging quality. Occasionally, GCCA are used in lieu of iodinated contrast agents for traditional angiography in patients allergic to iodinated contrast or in the setting of reduced glomerular filtration rate (GFR).

Despite the widely accepted myth that GCCA are safe to use in the setting of reduced GFR, this may not be true. Several reports have associated the administration of IV gadolinium with AKI, similar to iodinated contrast-induced nephropathy. This association, although not definitively proven, is concerning. More concerning, is the recently reported association between gadolinium and an emerging serious disorder in patients with reduced GFR, especially those

Table 2. Clinical maneuvers that may prove beneficial in reducing the risk of CMIN.

1.	Hydrate patients with intravenous saline and sustain in the immediate post-procedure interval.
2.	Minimize the amount of CM used, sufficient to insure a interpretable study.
3.	Perform diagnostic angiographic studies on separate days.
4.	Discontinue any drugs with nephrotoxic potential.
5.	Use low-osmolar CM in patients with renal insufficiency, especially diabetics.
6.	Consider the use of bicarbonate infusion in patients with renal insufficiency.

undergoing dialysis therapy, namely nephrogenic systemic fibrosis (NSF). In addition, GCCA administration may result in transient laboratory abnormalities that could be misinterpreted. This section will address the potential toxicity and pitfalls associated with the administration of GCCA to patients with chronic kidney disease (CKD).

Gadolinium and the risk of acute kidney injury

The use of GCCA is generally thought of as a "renally-safe" alternative to iodinated contrast agents in patients with reduced GFR. However, no well designed studies have rigorously examined the effect of IV GCCA on renal function as compared to IV iodinated contrast. Earlier reports suggested that the risk of AKI is low with GCCA [1, 152-155]. However, most of these reports represent retrospective studies of small number of patients and are uncontrolled. More recently, several reports with a lager number of patients suggested that the use of GCCA may be followed by AKI in a substantial percentage of patients with CKD (up to 50%) [155-161]. In addition, diabetes mellitus and low GFR, two well known risk factors for iodinated contrast media-induced AKI, have also been shown to be independent predictors of AKI in patients with stages 3 and 4 CKD exposed to IV gadolinium [158]. Gadolinium-induced AKI may be the result of acute tubular necrosis, as has been documented in one case [10], but the exact mechanisms by which GCCA may cause AKI are not fully elucidated. Animal data support the nephrotoxicity potential of GCCA [161]. On the basis of the possible nephrotoxicity of gadolinium, the Contrast Media Safety Committee of the European Society of Urogenital Radiology recommended, in a position paper, against the use of GCCA in patients with CKD [162]. Given the lack of evidence that GCCA are safer than IV iodinated contrast agents in patients with stages 3 CKD or higher, including those at high risk for contrast nephropathy, we recommend against their use as an alternative.

Gadolinium and NSF

History of NSF

NSF was first reported in 2000 when Cowper et al published a series of patients with a newly diagnosed skin condition that resembled scleromyxedema and systemic sclerosis [163]. The first case was recognized in 1997. Since most cases were receiving dialysis, it was first thought to be exclusively associated with dialysis [163]. It was later termed "nephrogenic fibrosing dermopathy" (NFD) since it was found to occur not only in dialysis recipients, but also in patients with reduced renal function not receiving dialysis. It has been reported in the setting of both AKI and CKD [164, 165]. Kidney dysfunction appears to be required for the development of NSF, and with the exception of one case report [166], all reported cases had a significantly reduced GFR (GFR< 30 ml/min/1.73 m^2). In 2004, several case series indicated that NFD may not be limited to the skin, and may cause fibrotic changes in several tissues and organs, including the skeletal muscle, diaphragm, pericardium, myocardium, pleura, lungs, kidneys, testes, and other organs [167-170]. Therefore, the nomenclature was changed to NSF. It remains unclear, however, if the fibrotic changes in some organs are specifically related to NSF or simply coincidental findings.

Clinical presentation and prognosis

NSF presents with skin induration and tethering, most commonly affecting the extremities in a symmetric distribution [164, 170]. Usually, the distal lower and/or upper extremities are affected first, followed by other areas becoming involved, including the proximal limbs, trunk and neck, usually sparing the face [170]. Occasionally, a fulminant presentation occurs, with all areas being affected simultaneously. Skin induration is usually preceded by edema, induration, and skin rash in the affected areas [164, 165]. It is unclear if the edema is caused by the triggering events causing NSF or if it is due to unrelated preexisting conditions and simply facilitates the development of NSF. The skin rash is typically pink to violaceous or brownish, maculopapular, often with a raised ameboid advancing edge (Figure 3A). Intense pruritus induration and pain in affected areas may occur and may last for weeks [164, 165]. Over the ensuing several weeks or months, a peau d'orange appearance and skin induration and tethering occur. Severe fibrosis of the skin and underlying tissues may result in flexion deformities and joint contractures (Figure 3B), loss of function, and falls [171-173]. Yel-

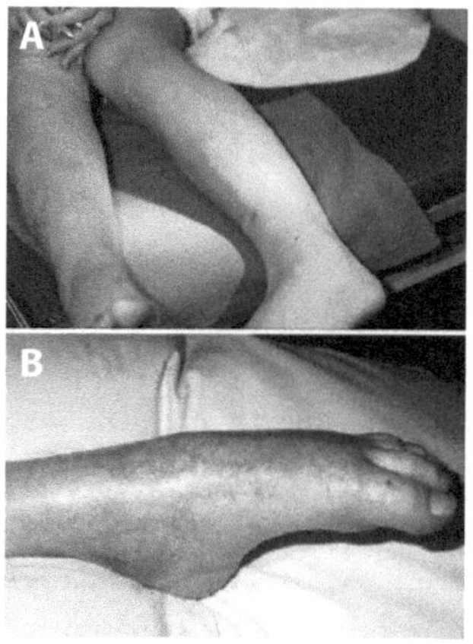

Figure 3. **A.** *Raised erythematous plaques with an "ameboid" edge and a bosselated peau d'orange appearance on the legs of a patient with NSF.* **B.** *Contracture of the ankle and flexion deformity of the foot in a patient with advanced NSF (Reproduced with permission from ref 23).*

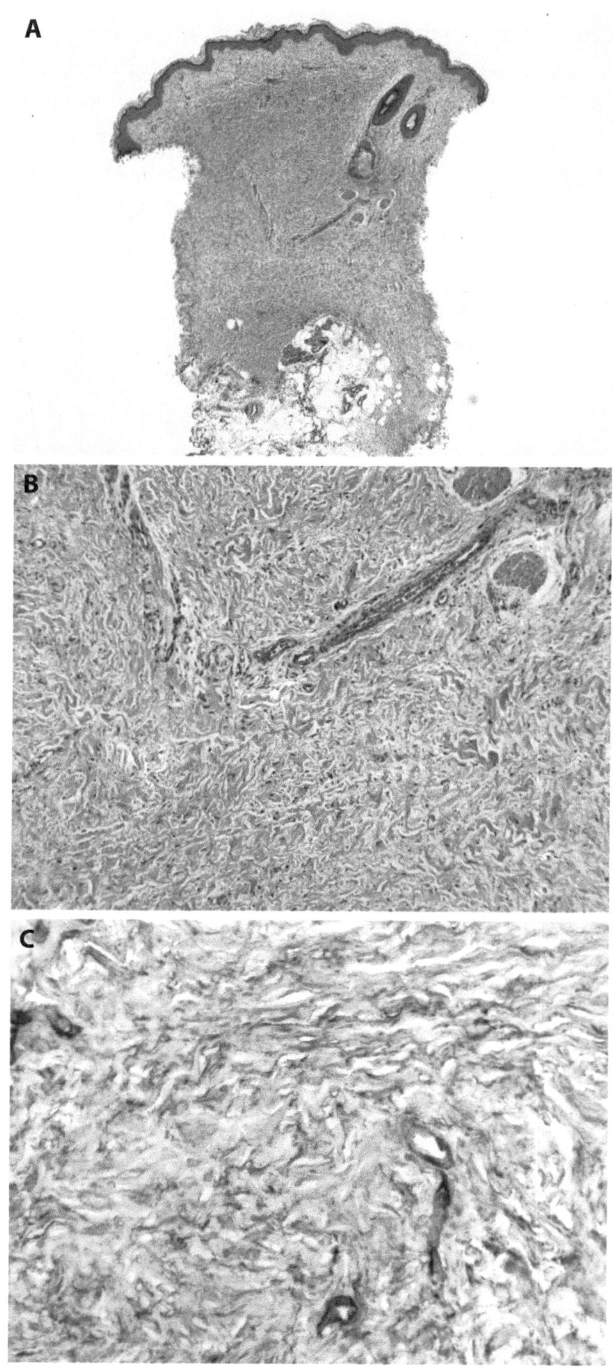

Figure 4. ***A.*** *Hematoxylin and eosin-stained skin biopsy showing increased spindled fibrocytes between thickened collagen bundles in a patient with NSF (x25).* ***B.*** *A higher magnification showing the spindle cells between broad collagen bundles (x100).* ***C.*** *Immunohistochemical stain for CD34-positive dendritic cells between collagen bundles, a characteristic feature of NSF.*

low scleral patches have also been described in some patients [164, 174].

In addition to being a disabling disease, NSF may result in other morbidities and has been associated with a high mortality rate. For instance, in later stages of the disease, edema resulting from fluid retention may be masked by skin fibrosis and induration, which may lead to underestimation of fluid gains for patients on dialysis. This may mislead clinicians in estimating the dialysis patient's dry weight and may result in lack of adequate fluid removal and subsequent fluid overload.

NSF has been associated with high mortality. In a small series of NSF patients, mortality was found to be 65%, and in another 48% within 2 years of diagnosis [175, 176]. Most of the mortalities in the latter study were related to cardiovascular causes, which is the most common cause of death in CKD. Therefore, it is unclear if this high mortality is directly related to NSF or simply to CKD. In addition, given some inherent problems with these studies, including a small sample size and a probable underdiagnosis of NSF in one study [39], and many histologically unconfirmed diagnoses in the other [176], it is still too early to determine if these high mortality rates are disease-related. What is clear, however, is that NSF may result in a disabling poor quality of life leading some patients to withdraw from dialysis [169, 175].

Histopathology

A deep skin biopsy is usually needed to make a diagnosis of NSF. Increased dermal infiltration by fibrocyte-like spindle cells intermingled with broad collagen bundles, is the hallmark of the histopathology (Figure 4 A&B) [163, 164]. These cells may extend into the subcutaneous fat septae and underlying muscles [168, 177]. Immunohistochemical staining is usually positive for cell surface markers CD34 (Figure 4C), CD45RO, CD68 and procollagen I, features of circulating fibrocytes [169, 177, 178]. These cells are usually found in wounds during healing and repair, and are thought to originate from the bone marrow and migrate to sites of injury [178, 179]. The stimuli for such translocation remain to be determined.

Differential diagnosis

In its early stages, NSF may be missed altogether, or may mimic inflammatory skin conditions such as cellulitis. In the later stages, NSF resembles other fibrotic skin disorders, such as scleromyxedema, morphea and systemic sclerosis, eosinophilic fasciitis, eosinophilia mayalgia syndrome, Spanish toxic oil syndrome and others [165, 171, 173, 180]. A detailed review of the differential diagnosis is beyond the scope of this chapter, but a few hints may help distinguish NSF from the other entities (Table 3). NSF is characterized by increased dermal fibrocytes, little or no mucin deposits, and absence of inflammatory cell infiltration, contrary to most other sclerosing skin conditions. Paraproteinemia, which is almost always present in scleromyxedema, is absent in NSF. Therefore, given the appropriate clinical setting, a skin biopsy is usually diagnostic of NSF, and there is little room for confusing it with the above skin disorders. The case can also be made to diagnosing the condition on clinical grounds alone without a biopsy [176], since the latter may miss the typical dermal changes in some cases owing to sampling error, or when a biopsy is deemed unsafe. However, obtaining a biopsy to confirm the diagnosis is the preferred approach.

Gadolinium is a likely trigger for NSF

For years, a possible trigger for NSF was not discovered, until Grobner reported 9 patients on dialysis who had received IV GCCA, 5 of whom developed NSF shortly thereafter [181]. He suggested that gadolinium may be an NSF trigger. Following this report, several similar case series and observational studies were published, strengthening the gadolinium-NSF link [175, 182-186]. Case-control studies have shown that gadolinium exposure in the preceding 6 months is a strong risk factor for NSF in patients with reduced GFR [183, 187]. In fact, NSF occurred within 12 weeks of exposure in most reported cases. Over 400 cases of NSF preceded by gadolinium exposure have been reported to the Federal Drug Administration (FDA)

Table 3. Most common cutaneous fibrosing disorders mimicking Nephrogenic Systemic Fibrosis (NSF).

Disease	NSF	Scleroderma/ systemic sclerosis	Scleromyxedema	Eosinophilic fasciitis	Eosinophilia-myalgia syndrome
Skin distribution	Extremities, hand and feet> trunk, face usually spared	Face usually affected, hands and feet	Face and neck usually affected	Extremities	Extremities, erythematous rash
Systemic features	Possible visceral fibrosis	CREST, pulmonary hypertension, major organ dysfunction	CNS and cardiac involvement	Hematologic abnormalities, hypergamma-globulinemia	Myalgia, neuropathy, ingestion of L-tryptophan
Paraproteinemia	Absent	Absent	Present	Absent	Absent
Eosinophilia	Absent	Absent	Absent	Present	Present
Fibroblastic proliferation	Prominent	Usually absent	Present	Usually absent	Usually absent
Inflammatory infiltration	Absent or mild	Present, mixed infiltrate	Present, lymphocytes and plasma cells	Present, mixed, eosinophils	Present, mixed infiltrate, eosinophils
Mucin deposits	Mild or absent	Large	Usually not increased	Large	Variable

Abbreviations: NSF, nephrogenic systemic fibrosis; CREST, calcinosis, Raynaud's phenomenon, esophageal dysmotility, sclerodactyly and telangiectasia.

to date [188].

The gadolinium-NSF link is plausible, since most GCCA are renally excreted, and thus expected to be retained for prolonged periods in patients with reduced GFR. In subjects with normal renal function, GCCA half-life is about 1.5 hours, whereas it reaches up to 60 hours in patients with renal failure [189]. Thus the prolonged retention of gadolinium in patients with moderate to severe reduction in GFR can predispose to tissue injury by gadolinium. Gadolinium deposits have recently been found in fibrotic skin lesions of patients with NSF, further strengthening the gadolinium-NSF link [190-194]. Automated scanning electron microscopy and X-Ray spectroscopy were used in these studies for in-situ quantification of gadolinium deposits in the skin. It was found that gadolinium deposits were likely located intracellularly in lysosomes, and co-localized with other elements such as calcium, phosphorus, sodium, iron, cupper and zinc. Furthermore, exposure of rats with normal renal function to very high doses of gadolinium over a prolonged period of time has been shown to cause skin redness, loss of hair and a skin histolopathologic appearance reminiscent of NSF, further strengthening the gadolinium-NSF causality link [195].

The prevalence of NSF has been estimated at 4.3 cases per 1000 patient-years in one study, with a 2.4% risk per gadolinium exposure [175]. However, it is clear that NSF is underdiagnosed and frequently missed by clinicians, and that these percentages may be underestimates. A higher prevalence was observed in more recent studies ranging from 13-18% in patients with stage 5 CKD, particularly among those on dialysis [176, 196]. These percentages are probably more reflective of the true prevalence of NSF. It still remains unclear why only a few patients with advanced CKD develop NSF after gadolinium exposure. Furthermore, not all studies have clearly shown a relationship between the dose or the number of GCCA exposures and the risk of NSF [182]. The risk may thus vary, depending on the presence of other facilitating co-factors. Interestingly, a few NSF cases have recently been reported without a clear history of preceding GCCA exposure [197, 198]. These cases may represent a different phenotype and may follow solid organ transplantation [197].

Other risk factors for NSF

Other factors that may increase the risk of NSF in the setting of gadolinium exposure include a markedly reduced renal function, edema [187], a high dose of erythropoietin (a pro-fibrotic agent) [187, 199], systemic inflammation [183], recent vascular procedures or surgery [164], a high calcium-phosphorus product [200], a hypercoagulable state and/or history of deep venous thrombosis [164), liver disease [164, 201], acidosis [181], and possibly hypothyroidism [187). Several reported cohorts have an unusually higher prevalence of immunosuppressed patients or solid organ transplant recipients than one would typically expect in a CKD population, indicating that immunologic factors may facilitate the development of NSF [163, 168, 170, 183, 185, 186, 197]. The role any of those co-factors may be playing in NSF, singly or in combination, remains unclear and definitely not proven.

Do all gadolinium-based contrast agents confer a similar risk of NSF?

Free gadolinium ions (Gd^{+++}) are highly toxic and can be splenic and hepatotoxic in animals [202, 203]. Therefore, GCCA contain a chelate (ligand) that binds free gadolinium and renders it non-toxic when infused in humans. Gd^{+++} is present at the core of the chelate molecule, and is valently bonded via 9 coordination sites to the ligand [204]. Table 4 lists the most commonly used gadolinium chelates world-wide: The first 5 are FDA-approved for use in the U.S.A. [204, 205]. They differ in ionic and structural composition. The chelate's molecule may be ionic or non-ionic, linear or cyclic (Figure 5 A&B) [204, 206]. Ionic molecules, which generally have a greater number of carboxyl groups, bind Gd^{+++} more avidly than non-ionic molecules. Cyclic molecules, which completely surround the Gd^{+++} core, offer better protection and binding to Gd^{+++} than linear molecules. The molecular configuration and ionic composition therefore affect the stability of the molecule, which in turns, determines the likelihood that Gd^{+++} will dissociate from its chelate *in vivo*. Ionic cyclic chelates are more stable than non-ionic or linear chelates, and are less likely to release free Gd^{+++} in the tissues. The stability of the molecule is assessed by the thermodynamic stability constant and kinetic stability (dissociation half-life), both of which are greater with

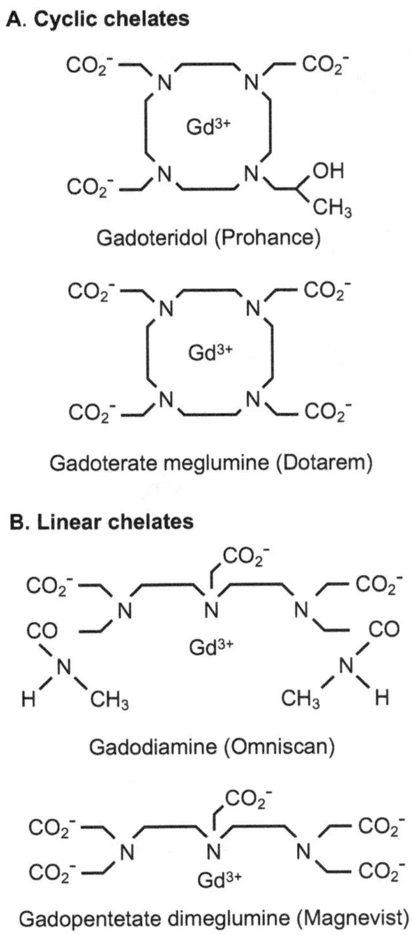

Figure 5. *Molecular configuration of gadolinium contrast agents. Gadolinium ions are valently bonded to carboxy and other groups within the molecule (bonds not shown for simplification).* ***A.*** *Examples of cyclic agents: Gadoteridol (non-ionic) and Gadoterate (ionic).* ***B.*** *Examples of linear agents: Gadodiamide (non-ionic) and Gadopentetate dimeglumine (ionic).*

more stable agents (Table 4). A greater amount of excess chelate is usually added to less stable GCCA to reduce the toxicity of free Gd^{+++} (Table 4) [204, 206].

It is plausible that the less stable GCCA are more liable to induce NSF than the more stable agents. In support of this hypothesis, most cases of NSF that have been reported in the literature and to the FDA followed exposure to gadodiamide or gadopentetate, two linear molecules with lower kinetic stability than cyclic more stable molecules. Interestingly, only 2 cases of NSF have been reported with gadoteridol, a more stable cyclic chelate, and only one of those cases was exclusively exposed to gadoteridol before NSF developed. In a large US cohort of dialysis patients exposed to gadoteridol, no cases of NSF were found [207]. Similarly, no cases of NSF have been reported following the administration of gadoterate, a highly stable GCCA used in France [208]. Although the stability of the chelate is likely an important factor determining the safety of GCCA use in the setting of renal failure, the data may be confounded by the market share of these agents. Gadodiamide, for instance, is one of the most commonly used agents in the U.S.A. Since NSF has been reported with all GCCA except gadoterate, we recommend that GCCA of any kind be avoided all together if the GFR is less than 30 ml/min/1.73 m^2, as the FDA has recently warned [188]. Some authorities, including the FDA, recommended immediate hemodialysis and for 3 consecutive days following GCCA exposure in patients receiving chronic hemodialysis This is based on data that one hemodialysis session clears over 65% of gadolinium, and 3 sessions more than 95%, whereas peritoneal dialysis does not effectively remove

Table 4. Molecular structure and characteristics of the most commonly used gadolinium-containing chelates. (Adapted with permission from ref 55)

Gadolinium-containing chelate	**Structure**	**Charge**	**Thermodynamic stability**	**Kinetic stability** (Dissociation half-life at pH 1.0)	**Amount of excess chelate (mg/ml)**
Gadodiamide (Omniscan)	Linear	Non-ionic	16.9	35 seconds	12
Gadoversetamide (OptiMark)	Linear	Non-ionic	16.6	Not available	28.4
Gadopentetate dimeglumine (Magnavist)	Linear	Ionic	22.1	10 minutes	0.4
Gadobenate meglumine (MultiHance)	Linear	Ionic	22.6	Not available	Not available
Gadoteridol (ProHance)	Cyclic	Non-ionic	23.8	3 hours	0.23
Gadoterate (Dotarem)	Cyclic	Ionic	25.8	> 1 month	Not available
Gadobutrol (Gadovist)	Cyclic	Non-ionic	21.8	5 minutes	Not available

gadolinium [188, 189, 209, 210]. Whether this practice is protective and whether it is effective in removing gadolinium sequestered in extravascular spaces such as the subcutaneous tissues, remain unclear and not supported by any data.

Pathogenesis of NSF

The pathogenesis of NSF remains unclear. The most plausible explanation is that following the administration of GCCA in a patient with low GFR, gadolinium is not promptly excreted and is retained. In patients with increased vascular permeability, extravasation of GCCA to subcutaneous tissues and other organs is facilitated [211]. This may explain why edema has been shown to be a strong risk factor for NSF in the best designed case-control study to date [187], and perhaps also explains why edema precedes the development of NSF in many cases. In the presence of favorable risk factors, Gd^{+++} is released from its chelate, replaced by other ions, such as iron, zinc or copper, a process called transmetallation, and induces tissue injury [190-192, 204, 205)] Gd^{+++} is likely phagocytosed by macrophages which produce profibrotic cytokines and promote fibrosis [211]. Circulating fibrocytes may also be recruited to the sites of injury, causing fibrosis.

The role other co-factors may be playing, such as calcium, phosphorus, erythropoietin, acidosis, or other metals, remains unclear. A higher calcium-phosphorus product was found in one study to be a risk factor for NSF in GCCA-exposed patients [200]. The role of iron in the transmetallation hypothesis was specifically explored. Following GCCA administration, a transient rise of serum iron, ferritin and transferritin saturation and a decrease in iron binding capacity, were observed by some investigators, hinting to mobilization of iron from its stores [212]. The authors postulated that Gd^{+++} may then be replaced by iron in the process of transmetallation, which may cause oxidative stress and trigger fibrosis in the tissues [212, 213]. However, the changes observed in iron saturation may simply be due to the interference of GCCA during in-vitro measurement of serum iron markers [202, 214], and these observations have not been convincingly reproduced. Therefore, the evidence that iron or any other metals is playing a significant role in the pathogenesis of NSF is still not supported by rigorous data. Figure 6 summarizes the potential triggers and probable pathogenesis of NSF based on published data.

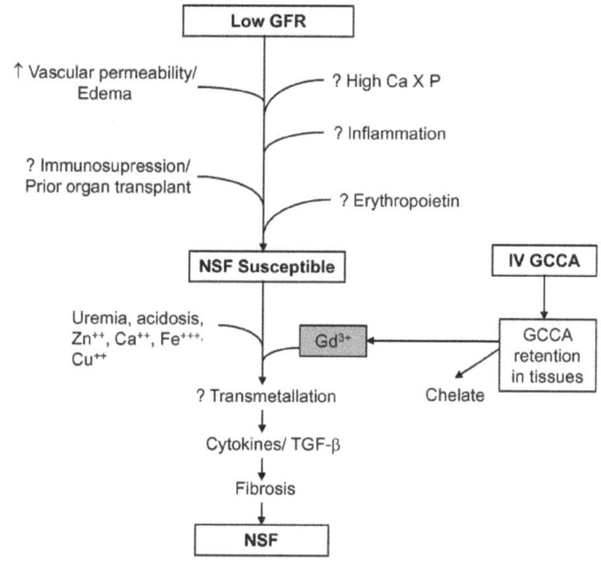

Figure 6. *Postulated pathogenesis of NSF (Explanation in the text). Abbreviations: GFR, glomerular filtration rate; Ca x P, calcium-phosphorus product; NSF, nephrogenic systemic fibrosis; IV, intravenous; GCCA, gadolinium-containing contrast agents.*

Treatment of NSF

Unfortunately, there is not an effective treatment modality at present, and once severe skin fibrosis has occurred, it is unlikely to significantly regress. Several therapeutic modalities have been tried, but they remain anecdotal. The most successful palliative therapies include aggressive physical therapy and ultraviolet light therapy, especially photopheresis, which can result in skin softening in some patients [166, 215-217]. Improvement following renal transplantation and worsening following deterioration of renal function has been reported, but it is unclear if gadolinium re-exposure occurred or played any role before NSF recurrence [218]. Other reported therapeutic modalities include plasmapheresis [219-221], thalidomide therapy [164, 171], and sodium thiosulfate [222], however, there is no convincing evidence that any of these modalities is effective.

Prevention of NSF

Given the high morbidity and mortality associated with NSF and the lack of controlled trials for therapy, we recommend avoiding GCCA in patients with GFR< 30 ml/min/1.73 m^2, and especially for those undergoing dialysis. Risk stratification should probably be implemented in the future when more studies on risk factors are available, to determine which patients are more prone to NSF than others. Alternative imaging modalities, including non-contrast MRI or iodinated contrast agents should be substituted if deemed safe to use. If GCCA use is indispensably needed for a life-threatening emergency, we recommend the use of a cyclic GCCA with a high kinetic stability, and only after appropriate informed discussion with the patient or surrogate. Potential risks and benefits must be explained, and preferably an informed consent obtained. Hemodialysis immediately following GCCA administration and for 3 consecutive days is probably prudent for patients already receiving hemodialysis, although there are no data to support the prophylactic outcome of such a practice.

Gadolinium and associated laboratory abnormalities

Several laboratory abnormalities can occur after the administration of GCCA, the most common being pseudohypocalcemia [202]. Other abnormalities include reduction of angiotensin converting enzyme levels, alteration of serum iron (a rise or a reduction), increased total iron-binding capacity, and reduction of serum zinc levels [202, 214]. These abnormalities particularly occur with the use of specific measurement assays, indicating that they may be artifacts, but their exact mechanisms are unclear.

Reduction of serum calcium levels can be detected shortly after IV administration of GCCA if a calorimetric assay is used [223-227]. This phenomenon does not occur if atomic emission spectroscopy or ion-selective electrodes are used to measure serum calcium concentration, indicating an artifactual and not a true reduction [228]. The mechanism of pseudohypocalcemia is not clear, but is thought to be related to binding of calcium by excess chelate present in GCCA, or alternatively, to the interaction between gadolinium and orthocrescolphthalein, the agent used in calorimetric assays. The former hypothesis is more likely, since some and not all GCCA, particularly those with excess chelates (e.g. gadodiamide and gadoversetamide) have been found to cause pseudohypocalcemia [217, 227, 228]. Pseudohypocalcemia may last 4-6 hours post GCCA administration in patients with normal renal function, and is prolonged for several days in patients with CKD [224]. Therefore, the concentrations of serum calcium measured too soon after GCCA administration should be interpreted with caution.

Summary

The administration of GCCA in the setting of renal dysfunction may be associated with serious adverse effects in patients with CKD, particularly in those with moderate to severe reduction of GFR. The most serious complication is NSF. AKI, similar to contrast nephropathy seems to be also a potential adverse effect. Pseudohypocalcemia, although benign, can last for several days post GCCA administration in patients with CKD and serum calcium levels should be interpreted with caution in this setting. The administration of GCCA in patients with GFR< 30 ml/min/1.73 m^2 should be discouraged and limited to life-threatening indications and only when no alternative imaging agents can be used. Appropriate informed consent outlining the risks and benefits of GCCA administration in patients with CKD should be obtained.

References

1. Levy EM, Viscoli CM, Horwitz RI. The effect of acute renal failure on mortality: a cohort analysis. JAMA 1996; 275: 1489-1494.
2. Porter GA. Contrast-associated nephropathy: presentation, pathophysiology and management. Mineral&Electrolyte Metabolism 1994; 20: 232-243.
3. Kurnik BR, AllgrenRI, GenterFC, Solomon RJ, Bates ER, Weisberg LS: Prospective study of atrial natriuretic peptide for the prevention of radiocontrast-induced nephropathy. Am J Kid Dis. 1998;31:674-80 .
4. Gruberg L., Mintz GS, Mehran R, Gangas G, Lansky AJ, Kent KM, Pichard AD, Satler LF, Leon MB: The prognostic implications of further renal function deterioration within 48 h of interventional coronaryprocedures in patients with pre-existing chronic renal insufficiency. J Am Coll Cardiol. 2000;36:1542-8.
5. Abizaid AS, Clark CE, Mintz GS, Dosa S, Popma JJ, Pichard AD, Satler LF, Harvey M, Kent KM, Leon MB: Effects of dopamine and aminophylline on contrast-induced acute renal failure after coronary antioplasty in patients with preexisiting renal insufficiency. Am J. Cardiol. 1999; 83;260-3.
6. Berns AS. Nephrotoxicity of contrast media (clinical conference). Kidney Int 1989; 36: 730-740.
7. Barrett BJ, Parfrey PS, Vavasour HM, McDonald J, Kent G, Hefferton D, O'Dea F, Stone E, Reddy R, McManamon PJ. Contrast nephropathy in patients with impaired renal function: high versus low osmolar media. Kidney Int 1992; 41: 1274-1279.
8. Rudnick MR, Berns JS, Cohen RM, Goldfarb S. Contrast media-associated nephrotoxicity. Curr Opin Nephrol Hypert 1996; 5: 127-133.
9. Moreau JF, Droz D, Sabto J, Jungers P, Kleinknecht D, Hinglais N, Michel JR. Osmotic nephrosis induced by water soluble triiodinated contrast media in man. Radiology 1975; 115: 329-336.
10. Bettmann MA. The evaluation of contrast-related renal failure (comment). AJR Am J Roentgenol 1991; 157: 66-68.
11. Hunter JV, Kind PRN. Nonionic iodinated contrast media: potential renal damage assessed with enzymuria. Radiology 1992; 183: 101-104.
12. Erley CM, Duda SH, Rehfuss D, Scholtes B, Bock J, Müller C, Osswald H. Prevention of radiocontrast-media-induced nephropathy in patients with preexisting renal insufficiency by hydration in combination with the adenosine antagonist theophylline. Nephrol Dial Transplant 1999; 14: 1146-1149.
13. Donadio C, Tramonti G, Giordani R, Lucchetti A, Calderazzi A, Sbragia P, Bianchi C. Glomerular and tubular effects of ionic and nonionic contrast media (diatrizoate and iopamidol). Contrib Nephrol 1988; 68: 212-219.
14. Porter GA. Urinary biomarkers and nephrotoxicity. Mineral&Electrolyte Metabolism 1994; 20: 181-186.
15. NGAL may represent a sensitive early biomarkers of renal impairment after PCI. Int J Cardiol. 2007 Jun 11,.
16. NGAL is an early predictive biomarker of contrast-induced nephropathy in children.Pediatr Nephrol. 2007.
17. Scanlon PJ, Faxon DP, Audet AM, Carabello, B, Dehmer GJ, Eagle KA, Legako RD, Leon DF, Murray JD, Nissen SE, Pepine CJ, Watson, RM, Ritchie JL, Gibbons RJ, Cheitlin MD, Gardner TJ, Garson A, Russell RO, Ryan TJ, Smith SC: ACC/AHA guidelines for coronary angiography: a report of the American College of Cardiology/American Heart Associateion Task force on Practic Guidelines (Committee on Coronary Angiography). J Am Coll Cardiol. 1999;33:1756-824.
18. Dangas,G., Iakovou,I., Nikolsky,E., Aymong,E.D., Mintz,G.S., Kipshidze,N.N., Lansky,A.J., Moussa,I., Stone,G.W., Moses,J.W., Leon,M. B., and Mehran,R. (2005): Contrast-induced nephropathy after percutaneous coronary interventions in relation to chronic kidney disease and hemodynamic variables. *Am J Cardiol.*, 95:13-19.
19. Tervahartiala P, Kivisaari L, Kivisaari R, Vehmas T, Virtanen I. Structural changes in the renal proximal tubular cells induced by iodinated contrast media. Nephron 1997; 76: 96-102.
20. Dobrota M, Powell CJ, Holtz E, Wallin A, Vik H. Biochemical and morphological effects of contrast media on the kidney. Acta Radiol (Suppl) 1995; 399: 196-203.
21. Battenfeld R, Khater AE, Drommer W, Guenzel P, Kaup FJ. Ioxaglate-induced light and electron microscopic alterations in the renal proximal tubular epithelium of rats (see comments). Invest Radiol 1991; 26: 35-39.
22. Heyman SN, Brezis M, Reubinoff CA, Greenfeld Z, Lechene C, Epstein FH, Rosen S. Acute renal failure with selective medullary injury in the rat. J Clin Invest 1988; 82: 401-412.

22A. Heyman SN, Brezis M, Epstein FH, Spokes K, Silva P, Rosen S. Early medullary hypoxic injury from radio-contrast and indomethacin. Kidney Int 1991; 40: 632-642

22B. Han Wkj, Vaily V, Abischandani, R, Thadlhani R, Bonventre JV. Kidney injury molecule-1 (KIM-1): A novel biomarker for human renal proximal tubule injury. Kidney Int. 2002; 62: 237-244.

23. Rich MW, Crecelius CA. Incidence, risk factors, and clinical course of acute renal insufficiency after cardiac catheterization in patients 70 years of age or older. A prospective study. Arch Intern Med 1990; 150: 1237-1242.
24. Davidson CJ, Hlatky M, Morris KG, Pieper K, Skelton TN, Schwab SJ, Bashore TM. Cardiovascular and renal toxicity of a nonionic radiographic contrast agent after cardiac catheterization. A prospective trial. Ann Intern Med 1989; 110: 119-124.

25. D'Elia JA, Gleason RE, Alday M, Malarick C, Godley K, Warram J, Kaldany A, Weinrauch LA. Nephrotoxicity from angiographic contrast material. A prospective study. Am J Med 1982; 72: 719-725.
26. Manske CL, Sprafka JM, Strony JT, Wang Y. Contrast nephropathy in azotemic diabetic patients undergoing coronary angiography. Am J Med 1990; 89: 615-620.
27. Agrawal M, Stouffer GA: Contrast induced nephropathy after angiography. Am J Med Sci. 2002;323:252-58.
28. Rosovsky MA, Rusinek H, Berenstein A, Basak S, Setton A, Nelson PK. High-dose administration of nonionic contrast media: a retrospective review. Radiology 1996; 200: 119-122.
29. Rudnick M, Berns JS, Cohen RM, Goldfarb S. Contrast media-associated nephrotoxicity. Curr Opin Nephrol Hypertens 1996; 5: 127-133.
29A. Gruberg L, Mehran R, Dangas G, Mintz GS, Waksman R, Kent KM, Pichard AD, Satler LF , Wu H, and Leon MB. Acute renal failure requiring dialysis after percutaneous coronary interventions. Catheter Cardiovasc Interv 2001; 52: 409-416.
31. Vanzee BE, Hoy WE, Talley TE, Jaenike JR. Renal injury associated with intravenous pyelography in nondiabetic and diabetic patients. Ann Intern Med 1978; 89: 51-54.
32. Moore RD, Steinberg EP, Powe NR, Brinker JA, Fishman EK, Graziano S, Gopalan R. Nephrotoxicity of high-osmolality versus low-osmolality contrast media: randomized clinical trial. Radiology 1992; 182: 649-655.
33. Freeman RV, O'donnell M, Share D. Nephropathy requiring dialysis after percutanheous coro ary intervention and the critical role of an adjusted contrast dose. Am J, Cardiol. 2002;90:1068-1073.
34. Ashby DT, Mehran R, Aymong EA . Comparison of outcomes in men versus woment having percutaneous coronary interventions in small coronay artieries. Am. J.l Cardiol 2003;91:979-981. .
35. Bartholomew BA, Harjal KJ, Dukkipati S. Impact of nephropathy aftr percutaneous coronary intervention a method for risk stratification Am J Cardiol. 2004;93;1515-1519.
36. Mehran R, Aymong ED, Nikolsky E. A simple risk scorfe for prediction of contrast-induced nephropathy after percutaneous coronary intervention. Development and initial validation. J Am Coll Cardiol. 2004;44:1393-1399. .
37. Rudnick MR, Goldfarb S, Wexler L, Ludbrook PA, Murphy MJ, Halpern EF, Hill JA, Winneford M, Cohen MB, Vanfossen DB. Nephrotoxicity of ionic and nonionic contrast media in 1196 patients: a randomized trial. Kidney Int 1995; 47: 254-261.
38. Parfrey PS, Griffiths SM, Barrett BJ, Paul MD, Genge M, Withers J, Farid N, McManamon PJ. Contrast material-induced renal failure in patients with diabetes mellitus, renal insufficiency, or both. A prospective controlled study. N Engl J Med 1989; 320: 143-149.
39. Lautin EM, Freeman NJ, Schoenfeld AH, Bakal CW, Haramati N, Friedman AC, Lautin JL, Braha S, Kadish EG, Sprayregen S. Radiocontrast-associated renal dysfunction: incidence and risk factors (see comments). AJR Am J Roentgenol 1991; 157: 49-58.
40. Weisberg LS, Kurnik PB, Kurnik BR. Risk of radiocontrast nephroathy in patients with and without diabetes mellitus. Kidney Int 1994; 45: 259-265.
41. Gomes AS, Baker JD, Martin-Paredero V, Dixon SM, Takiff H, Machleder HI, Moore WS. Acute renal dysfunction after major arteriography. AJR Am J Roentgenol 1985; 145(6): 1249-1253.
42. Taliercio CP, McCallister SH, Holmes DR, Ilstrup DM, Vlietstra RE. Nephrotoxicity of nonionic contrast media after cardiac angiography. Am J Cardiol 1989; 64: 815-816.
43. Rudnick MR, Berns JS, Cohen RM, Goldfarb S. Contrast media-associated nephrotoxicity. Sem Nephrol 1997; 17: 15-26.
44. Gruberg L, Mehran R, Dangas G. Acute renal failure reuiring dialysis after percutaneous coronary intervention. Catheter Cardiovas. Interv. 2001;52:409-416.
45. Cigarroa RG, Lange RA, Williams RH, Hillis LD. Dosing of contrast material to prevent contrast nephropathy in patients with renal disease. Am J Med 1989; 86: 649-652.
46. Lakovou,I., Dangas,G., Mehran,R., Lansky,A.J., Ashby,D.T., Fahy,M., Mintz,G.S., Kent,K.M., Pichard,A.D., Satler,L.F., Stone,G.W., and Leon,M.B. (2003): Impact of gender on the incidence and outcome of contrast-induced nephropathy after percutaneous coronary intervention. *J Invasive.Cardiol.*, 15:18-22.
47. Nikolsky E, Aymong ED, Dangas G, Mehran R. Radiocontrast nephropathy identifying the high-risk pataient and the implications of exacerbating renal function. Rev Cardiovasc. Med 2003;4(S1):s7-s14.
48. Nikolsky E, Mehran R, Lasic Z . Low hematocrit predicts contrast-induced nephropathy after percutaneous coronary interventions. Kidney Int. 2005;67:706-713. .
49. McCarthy CS, Becker JA. Multiple myeloma and contrast media. Radiology 1992; 183: 519-521.
50. Heyman SN, Rosen S, Brezis M. Radiocontrast nephropathy: a paradigm for the synergism between toxic and hypoxic insults in the kidney. Exp Nephrol 1994; 2: 153-157.
51. Katzberg RW, Morris TW, Burgener FA, Kamm DE, Fischer HW. Renal renin and hemodynamic responses to selective renal artery catheterization and angiography. Invest Radiol 1977; 12: 381-388.
52. Bakris GL, Burnett JCJ. A role for calcium in radiocontrast-induced reductions in renal hemodynamics. Kidney Int 1985; 27: 465-468.

53. Caldicott WJ, Hollenberg NK, Abrams HL. Characteristics of response of renal vascular bed to contrast media. Evidence for vasoconstriction induced 53 renin-angiotensin system. Invest Radiol 1970; 5: 539-547.
53A. Heyman SN, Rosenberger C, Rosen S. Regional alterations in renal haemodynamics and oxygentation: a role in contrast medium-induced nephropathy. Nephrol Dial Transplant 2005; 20(S1): i6-i11.
54. Mockel,M., Radovic,M., Kuhnle,Y., Combe,V., Waigand,J., Schroder,S., Dietz,R., Frei,U., and Eckardt,K.U. (2008): Acute renal haemodynamic effects of radiocontrast media in patients undergoing left ventricular and coronary angiography. *Nephrol Dial Transplant.*
55. Katzberg RW. Urography into the 21st century: new contrast media, renal handling, imaging characteristics, and nephrotoxicity. Radiology 1997; 204: 297-312.
56. Workman RJ, Shaff MI, Jackson RV, Diggs J, Frazer MG, Briscoe C. Relationship of renal hemodynamic and functional changes following intravascular contrast to the renin-angiotensin system and renal prostacyclin in the dog. Invest Radiol 1983; 18: 160-166.
57. Larson TS, Hudson K, Mertz JI, Romero JC, Knox FG. Renal vasoconstrictive response to contrast medium. The role of sodium balance and the renin-angiotensin system. J Lab Clin Med 1983; 101: 385-391.
58. Heyman SN, Clark BA, Kaiser N, Spokes K, Rosen S, Brezis M, Epstein FH. Radiocontrast agents induce endothelin release *in vivo* and *in vitro*. J Am Soc Nephrol 1992; 3: 58-65.
59. Oldroyd SD, Haylor JL, Morcos SK. Bosentan, an orally active endothelin antagonist: effect on the renal response to contrast media. Radiology 1995; 196: 661-665.
60. Russo D, Minutolo R, Cianciaruso B, Memoli B, Conte G, De Nicola L. Early effects of contrast media on renal hemodynamics and tubular function in chronic renal failure. J Am Soc Nephrol 1995; 6: 1451-1458.
61. Erley CM, Osswald H. Prevention of contrast media-induced renal impairment by adenosine antagonists in humans. Drug Dev Res 1998; 45: 172-175.
62. Heyman SN, Rosenberger C, Rosen S. regional alterations in renal heamodynamics and oxygenation: a role in contrast medium-induced nephropathy. Nephrol Dial Transpl. 2005;20(S1): i6-i11..
63. Liss P, Nygren A, Erikson U, Ulfendahl HR. Injection of low and iso-osmolar contrast medium decreases oxygen tension in the renal medlulla. Kidney Int. 1998;53:698-702.
64. Liss P, Nygren A, Olsson U, Ulfendahl HR. Effects of contrast media and mannitol on renal medullary blood flow and red cell aggregation in the rat kidney. Kidney Int. 1996;49:1268-1275..
65. Arend LJ, Bakris GL, Burnett JCJ, Megerian C, Spielman WS. Role for intrarenal adenosine in the renal hemodynamic response to contrast media. J Lab Clin Med 1987; 110: 406-411.
66. Katholi RE, Taylor GJ, McCann WP, Woods WT, Womack KA, McCoy CD, Katholi CR, Moses HW, Mishkel GJ, Lucore CL, Holloway RM, Miller BD, Woodruff RC, Dove JT, Mikell FL, Schneider JA. Nephrotoxicity from contrast media: attenuation with theophylline. Radiology 1995; 195:17-22.
67. Osswald H, Schmitz HJ, Heidenreich O. Adenosine response of the rat kidney after saline loading, sodium restriction and hemorrhagia. Pflugers Arch 1975; 357: 323-333.
68. Hall JE, Granger JP. Adenosine alters glomerular filtration control by angiotensin II. Am J Physiol 1986; 250: F917-F923.
69. Haas JA, Osswald H. Adenosine induced fall in glomerular capillary pressure: effect of ureteral obstruction and aortic constriction in the Munich- Wistar rat kidney. Naunyn Schmiedebergs Arch Pharmacol 1981; 317: 86-89.
70. Cantley LG, Spokes K, Clark B, McMahon EG, Carter J, Epstein FH. Role of endothelin and prostaglandins in radiocontrast-induced renal artery constriction. Kidney Int 1993; 44: 1217-1223.
71. Heyman SN, Brezis M, Epstein FH, Spokes K, Silva P, Rosen S. Early renal medullary hypoxic injury from radiocontrast and indomethacin. Kidney Int 1991; 40: 632-642.
72. Cederholm C, Almen T, Bergqvist D, Golman K, Takolander R. Acute renal failure in rats. Interaction between contrast media and temporary renal arterial occlusion. Acta Radiol 1989; 30: 321-326.
73. Deray G, Dubois M, Martinez F, Baumelou B, Beaufils H, Bourbouze R, Baumelou A, Jacobs C. Renal effects of radiocontrast agents in rats: a new model of acute renal failure. Am J Nephrol 1990; 10: 507-513.
74. Osswald H, Schmidt HJ, Kemper R. Tissue content of adenosine, inosine and hypoxanthine in the rat kidney after ischemia and postischemic recirculation. Pflügers Arch 1977; 371: 45-49.
75. Agmon Y, Peleg H, Greenfeld Z, Rosen S, Brezis M. Nitric oxide and prostanoids protect the renal outer medulla from radiocontrast toxicity in the rat. J Clin Invest 1994; 94: 1069-1075.
76. Pflueger A, Larson, TS, Nath KA, King BF, Gross JM, Knox, FG: Role of adenosine in constrast media-induced acute renal failure in diabetes mellitus. Mayo Clin Proc. 2000; 75:1275-83..
77. Taddei S, Virdis A, Ghiadoni L, Magagna A, Salvetti A: Cyclooxygenase inhibition restores nitric oxide activity in essential hypertension. Hyperten. 1997;29(1Pt2):274-9.

78. Osswald H, Helminger I, Jendralski A, Abrar B. Improvement of renal function by theophylline in the acute renal failure of the rat. Naunyn-Schmiedeberg´s Arch Pharmacol 1979; 307: R47 (abstract).
79. Gouyon JB, Guignard JP. Theophylline prevents the hypoxemia-induced renal hemodynamic changes in rabbits. Kidney Int 1988; 33: 1078-1083.
80. Deray G, Martinez F, Cacoub P, Baumelou B, Baumelou A, Jacobs C. A role for adenosine calcium and ischemia in radiocontrast-induced intrarenal vasoconstriction. Am J Nephrol 1990; 10: 316-322.
81. Rossi N, Ellis V, Kontry T, Gunther S, Churchill P, Bidani A. The role of adenosine in HgCl2-induced acute renal failure in rats. Am J Physiol 1990; 258: F1554-F1560.
82. Lin JJ, Churchill PC, Bidani AK. Theophylline in rats during maintenance phase of post-ischemic acute renal failure. Kidney Int 1988; 33: 24-28.
83. Lin JJ, Churchill PC, Bidani AK. Effect of theophylline on the initiation phase of postischemic acute renal failure in rats. J Lab Clin Med 1986; 108: 150-154.
84. Bidani AK, Churchill PC. Aminophylline ameliorates glycerol-induced acute renal failure in rats. Can J Physiol Pharmacol 1983; 61: 567-571.
85. Bidani AK, Churchill PC, Packer W. Theophylline-induced protection in myoglobinuric acute renal failure: Further chracterization. Can J Physiol Pharmacol 1987 ; 65: 42-45.
86. Erley CM, Heyne N, Burgert K, Langanke J, Risler T, Osswald H. Prevention of radiocontrast induced nephropathy by adenosine antagonists in rats with chronic nitric oxide deficiency. J Am Soc Nephrol 1997; 8: 1125-1132.
87. Barrett BJ, Parfrey PS, McDonald JR, Hefferton DM, Reddy ER, McManamon PJ. Nonionic low-osmolality versus ionic high-osmolality contrast material for intravenous use in patients perceived to be at high risk: randomized trial (see comments). Radiology 1992; 183: 105-110.
88. Deray G, Jacobs C. Radiocontrast nephrotoxicity. A review. Invest Radiol 1995; 30: 221-225.
89. Katholi RE, Taylor GJ, Woods WT, Womack KA, Katholi CR, McCann WP, Moses HW, Dove JT, Mikell FL, Woodruff RC. Nephrotoxicity of nonionic low-osmolality versus ionic high- osmolality contrast media: a prospective double-blind randomized comparison in human beings. Radiology 1993; 186: 183-187.
90. Schwab SJ, Hlatky MA, Pieper KS, Davidson CJ, Morris KG, Skelton TN, Bashore TM. Contrast nephrotoxicity: a randomized controlled trial of a nonionic and an ionic radiographic contrast agent. N Engl J Med 1989; 320: 149-153.
91. Barrett BJ, Carlisle EJ. Metaanalysis of the relative nephrotoxicity of high- and low-osmolality iodinated contrast media. Radiology 1993; 188: 171-178.
92. Jakobsen JA. Renal effects of iodixanol in healthy volunteers and patients with severe renal failure. Acta Radiol (Suppl) 1995; 399: 191-195.
93. Jakobsen JA. Renal experience with Visipaque. Eur Radiol 1996; 6 (Suppl 2): S16-S19.
94. Solomon,R., The role of osmolality in the incidence of contrst-induced nephyropathy: a syhstematic review of angiographic contrast mediain high risk patients. Kid. Elnternat. 2005;68:2256-2263.
95. Liss,P., Persson,P.B., Hansell,P., and Lagerqvist,B. (2006): Renal failure in 57 925 patients undergoing coronary procedures using iso-osmolar or low-osmolar contrast media. *Kidney Int*, 70:1811-1817.
96. Seeliger E, Flemming B, Wronski T, Ladwig M, Arakelyan K, Godes M, Mockel M, Persson PB. Viscosity of contrast media perturbs renal hemodynamics. J Am Soc Nephrol 2007; 18: 2912-2920.
97. Sharma SK, Kini A . Effect of non-ionic radiocontrast agents on the occurrence of contgrast-induced in patients with mild-moderate chrnic renal insufficiency: pooled analysis of the randomized trials. Catherter Cardiovascular Interv. 2005;65:386-393.
98. Weissleder R. Can gadolinium be safely nephropathy in patients given in renal failure? AJR Am J Roentgenol 1996; 167: 278-279.
99. Kaufman JA, Geller SC, Waltman AC. Renal insufficiency: gadopentetate dimeglumine as a radiographic contrast agent during peripheral vascular interventional procedures. Radiology 1996; 198: 579-581.
100. Hatrick AG, Jarosz JM, Irvine AT. Gadopentate dimeglumine as an alternative contrast agent for use in interventional procedures. Clin Radiology 1997; 52: 948-952.
101. Seeger JM, Self S, Harward TR, Flynn TC, Hawkins IF Jr. Carbon dioxide gas as an arterial contrast agent. Ann Surgery 1993; 217: 688-697.
102. Hawkins IF Jr, Wilcox CS, Kerns SR, Sabatelli FW. CO_2 digital angiography: a safer contrast agent for renal vascular imaging ? Am J Kidney Dis 1994; 24: 685-694.
103. Solomon R, Werner C, Mann D, D'Elia J, Silva P. Effects of saline, mannitol, and furosemide on acute decreases in renal function induced by radiocontrast agents. N Engl J Med 1994; 331: 1416-1420.
104. Kurnik BR, Weisberg LS, Cuttler IM, Kurnik PB. Effects of atrial natriuretic peptide versus mannitol on renal blood flow during radiocontrast infusion in chronic renal failure. J Lab Clin Med 1990; 116: 27-36.

105. Weisberg LS, Kurnik PB, Kurnik BR. Dopamine and renal blood flow in radiocontrast-induced nephropathy in humans. Renal Failure 1993; 15: 61-68.
106. Weisberg LS, Kurnik PB, Kurnik BR. Radiocontrast-induced nephropathy in humans: role of renal vasoconstriction. Kidney Int 1992; 41: 1408-1415.
107. Anto HR, Chou SY, Porush JG, Shapiro WB. Infusion intravenous pyelography and renal function. Effect of hypertonic mannitol in patients with chronic renal insufficiency. Arch Intern Med 1981; 141: 1652-1656.
108. Eisenberg RL, Bank WO, Hedgock MW. Renal failure after major angiography can be avoided with hydration. Am J Radiol 1981; 136: 859-861.
109. Carraro M, Stacul F, Collari P, Toson D, Zucconi F, Torre R, Faccini L, Dalla Palma L. Contrast media nephrotoxicity: urinary protein and enzyme pattern in patients with or without saline infusion during digital subtracting angiography. Contrib Nephrol 1993; 101: 251-254.
110. Kerstein MD, Puyau FA. Value of periangiography hydration. Surgery 1984; 96: 919-922.
111. Louis BM, Hoch BS, Hernandez C, Namboodiri N, Neiderman G, Nissenbaum A, Foti FP, Magno A, Banayat G, Fata F, Manohar NL, Lipner HI. Protection from the nephrotoxicity of contrast dye. Renal Failure 1996; 18: 639-646.
112. Krasuski RA, Beard BM, Geoghagan JD, Thompson CM, Guidera SA: Optimal timing of hydration to erase contrastassociated nephropathy: The OTHER CAN study. *J Invasive Cardiol* 15: 699–702, 2003.
113. Merten GJ, Burgess WP, Gray LV, Holleman JH, Roush TS, Kowalchuk GJ, Bersin RM, Van Moore A, Simonton CA 3rd, Rittase RA, Norton HJ, Kennedy TP: Prevention of contrast-induced nephropathy with sodium bicarbonate: A randomized controlled trial. *JAMA* 291: 2328–2334, 2004.
114. Briguori C, Airoldi F, D'Andrea D, Bonizzoni E, Morici N, Focaccio A, Michev I, Montorfano M, Carlino M, Cosgrave J, Ricciardelli B, Colombo A: Renal Insufficiency Following Contrast Media Administration Trial (REMEDIAL): A randomized comparison of 3 preventive strategies. *Circulation*115: 1211–1217, 2007.
115. ecio-Mayoral A, Chaparro M, Prado B, Cozar R, Mendez I, Banerjee D, Kaski JC, Cubero J, Cruz JM: The Reno-Protective Effect of Hydration with Sodium Bicarbonate Plus N-Acetylcysteine in Patients Undergoing Emergency Percutaneous Coronary Intervention: The RENO Study*J Am Coll Cardiol* 49: 1283–1288, 2007.
116. Schmidt P, Pang D, Nykamp D, Knowlton G, Jia H: N-acetylcysteine and sodium bicarbonate versus N-acetylcysteine and standard hydration for the prevention of radiocontrast-induced nephropathy following coronary angiography. *Ann Pharmacother* 41: 46–50, 2007.
117. From AM, Bartholmai BJ, Williaws AW, Cha SS, PfluegerA, McDonald S. Sodium bicarbonate is associated with a increased incidence of contrast nephropathy: a retrospective cohort study of 7977 patients at the mayo clinicl *Clin J Am Soc Nephrol* 3: 10–18, 2008. doi: 10.2215/CJN.03100707.
118. Weinstein JM, Heyman S, Brezis M. Potential deleterious effect of furosemide in radiocontrast nephropathy. Nephron 1992; 62: 413-415.
119. Golman K, Cederholm C. Contrast medium-induced acute renal failure. Can it be prevented ? Invest. Radiol. 1990; 25(Suppl 1): S127-S128.
120. Neumayer HH, Gellert J, Luft FC. Calcium antagonists and renal protection. Renal Failure 1993; 15: 353-358.
121. Russo D, Testa A, Volpe LD, Sansone G. Randomised propspective study on renal effects of two different contrast media in humans: protective role of a calcium channel blocker. Nephron 1990; 55: 254-257.
122. Carraro M, Mancini W, Artero M, Stacul F, Grotto M, Cova M, Faccini L. Dose effect of nitrendipine on urinary enzymes and microproteins following non-ionic radiocontrast administration. Nephrol Dial Transplant 1996; 11: 444-448.
123. Spangberg Viklund B, Berglund J, NikonoffT, Nyberg P, Skau T, Larsson R. Does prophylactic treatment with felodipine, a calcium antagonist, prevent low-osmolar contrast-induced renal dysfunction in hydrated diabetic and nondiabetic patients with normal or moderately reduced renal function? Scand J Urol Nephrol 1996; 30: 63-68.
124. Khoury Z, Schlicht JR, Como J, Karschner JK, Shapiro AP, Mook WJ, Weber RJ. The effect of prophylactic nifedipine on renal function in patients administered contrast media. Pharmacother 1995; 15: 59-65.
125. Hall KA, Wong RW, Hunter GC, Camazine BM, Rappaport WA, Smyth SH, Bull DA, McIntyre KE, Bernhard VM, Misiorowski RL. Contrast-induced nephrotoxicity: the effects of vasodilator therapy. J Surg Res 1992; 53: 317-320.
126. Chertow GM, Sayegh MH, Allgren RL, Lazarus JM. Is the administration of dopamine associated with adverse or favorable outcomes in acute renal failure? Auriculin Anaritide Acute Renal Failure Study Group. Am J Med 1996; 101: 49-53.
127. Madyoon H, Croushore L, Weaver D, Mathur V: Use of fenoldopam to prevent radiocontrast nephropathy in high-risk patients. Cather Cardiovasc. Intervent 2001;53;341-5.
128. Kini A, Sharma S: Managing the high-risk patients: Experience with fenoldopam, a selective dopamine receptor agonist, in prevention of radiocontrast nephropathy during percutaneous coronary intervention. Rev Cardiovas Med. 2001;2(s1):S19-25.

129. Wambach G, Winkert T. Nierenfunktionsstörungen nach Röntgenkontrastmittelgabe: Prophylaxe durch das atriale natriuretische Peptid? Nieren- und Hochdruckkrankheiten 1990; 19: 312-317.
130. Kurnik BR, Allgren RL, Genter FC, Solomon RJ, Bates ER, Weisberg LS. Prospective study of atrial natriuretic peptide for the prevention of radiocontrast-induced nephropathy. Am J Kidney Dis 1998; 31: 674-680.
131. Erley CM, Duda SH, Schlepckow S, Koehler J, Huppert PE, Strohmaier WL, Bohle A, Risler T, Osswald H. Adenosine antagonist theophylline prevents the reduction of glomerular filtration rate after contrast media application. Kidney Int 1994; 45: 1425-1431.
132. Erley CM. Prävention des kontrastmittelbedingten Nierenversagens. Intensivmed 1997; 34: 769-777.
133. Tepel M, van der Giet M, Schwarzfeld C, Laufer U, Liermann D, Zidek W. Prevention of radiographic-contrast-agent-induced reductions in renal function by acetylcysteine. New Engl J MED 2000; 343: 180-184.
134. Diaz-Sandoval LJ, Kosowsky BD, Losordo DW: Acetylcysteine to prevent angiography-related renal tissue injury (The APART Trial). Am J Cardiol. 2002;89:356-8.
135. Mehran R, Ashby DT. Radiocontrast-induced acute renal failure: allocations and outcomes. Rev Cardiovas Med 2001;2(suppl1): S9-S13.
136. Tadros GM, Mouhayar EN, Akinwande AO, Campbell B, Wood C, Blankenship JA. Prevention of radiocontrast-induced nephropathy with n-acetylcysteine in patients undergoing coronary angiography. J Invas Cardiol 2003; 15: 311-314.
137. Briguori C, Manganelli F, Scarpato P, Elia PP, Golia B, Riviezzo G, Lepore S, Librera M, Villari B, Colombo A, Ricciardelli B. Acetylcysteine and contrast agent-associated nephrotoxicity. J Am Coll Cardiol. 2002; 40: 298-303.
138. Fishbane S. N-acetylcysteine in the prevention of contrast-induced nephropathy. Clin J Am Soc Nephrol 2008; 3: 281-287.
139. Webb JG, Pate GE, Humphries KH, Buller CE, Shalansky S, Al Shamari A, Sutander A, Williams T, Fox RS, Levin A: A randomized controlled trial of intravenous N-acetylcysteine for the prevention of contrast-induced nephropathy after cardiac catheterization: Lack of effect. *Am Heart J* 148: 422–429, 2004.
140. Marenzi G, Assanelli E, Marana I, Lauri G, Campodonico J, Grazi M, De Metrio M, Galli S, Fabbiocchi F, Montorsi P, Veglia F, Bartorelli AL: N-acetylcysteine and contrast-induced nephropathy in primary angioplasty. *N Engl J Med*354: 2773–2782, 2006.
141. Hoffmann U, Fischereder M, Kruger B *et al.* The value of *N*-acetylcysteine in the prevention of radiocontrast agent-induced nephropathy seems questionable. *J Am Soc Nephrol* 2004; 15: 407–410,) .
143. Oldroyd S, Slee SJ, Haylor J, Morcos SK, Wilson C. Role for endothelin in the renal responses to radiocontrast media in the rat. Clin Sci Colch 1994; 87: 427-434.
144. Wang A, Holcslaw T, Bashore TM, Freed MI, Miller D, Rudnick MR, Szerlip H, Thames MD, Davidson CJ, Shusterman N, Schwab SJ. Exacerbation of radiocontrast nephrotoxicity by endothelin receptor antagonism. Kidney Int 2000; 57: 1675-1680.
145. Lehnert T, Keller E, Gondolf K, Schaffner T, Pavenstandt H, Schollmeyer P. Effect of haemodialysis after contrast medium administration in patients with renal insufficiency. Nephrol Dial Transplant 1998; 13: 358-362.
146. Berger ED, Bader BD, Bosker J, Risler T, Erley CM. Kontrastmittelinduziertes Nierenversagen läßt sich durch Hämodialyse nicht verhindern. (Contrast media-induced kidney failure cannot be prevented by hemodialysis). Dtsch Med Wochenschr 2001; 16; 126(7): 162-166 (German).
147. Clin Res Cardiol. 2007 Mar;96(3):130-9. Epub 2006 Dec 22.
148. Marenzi G, Marana I, Lauri G, Assanelli E, Grazi M, CampodonicoJ, Trabattoni D, Fabbiocchi F, Montorsi P, Bartorelli AL. The prevention of radiocontrast-agent-induced nephropathy by hemofiltration. *N Engl J Med* 2003;349:1333–1340.
149. Stacul F, Adam A, Becdker CR, Davidson C, Lameire N, McCullough PA, Tumlin J. Strategies to reduce the risk of contrast-induced nephropathy. Am J Cardiol 2006;98[suppl]:59K–77K.
150. Pannu N, Wiebe N, Tonelli M. Prophylaxis strategiesfor contrast-induced nephropathy. JAMA. 2006;295:2765-2779..
151. Barrett BJ, & Parfrey PS: Clinical practice. Preventing nephropathy induced by contrast medium. *N Engl J Med* 354: 379-386, 2006.
152. Hammer FD, Goffette PP, Malaise J, Mathurin P: Gadolinium dimeglumine: An alternative contrast agent for digital subtraction angiography. *Eur Radiol* 9: 128-136, 1999.
153. Hammer FD, Malaise J, Goffette PP, Mathurin P: Gadolinium dimeglumine: An alternative contrast agent for digital subtraction angiography in patients with renal failure. *Transplant Proc* 32: 432-433, 2000.
154. Kaufman JA, Geller SC, Bazari H, Waltman AC: Gadolinium-based contrast agents as an alternative at vena cavography in patients with renal insufficiency--early experience. *Radiology* 212: 280-284, 1999.
155. Rieger J, Sitter T, Toepfer M, Linsenmaier U, Pfeifer KJ, Schiffl H: Gadolinium as an alternative contrast agent for diagnostic and interventional angiographic procedures in patients with impaired renal function. *Nephrol Dial Transplant* 17: 824-828, 2002.
156. Akgun H, Gonlusen G, Cartwright J,Jr, Suki WN, Truong LD: Are gadolinium-based contrast media nephrotoxic? A renal biopsy study. *Arch Pathol Lab Med* 130: 1354-1357, 2006.

157. Briguori C, Colombo A, Airoldi F, Melzi G, Michev I, Carlino M, Montorfano M, Chieffo A, Bellanca R, Ricciardelli B: Gadolinium-based contrast agents and nephrotoxicity in patients undergoing coronary artery procedures. *Catheter Cardiovasc Interv* 67: 175-180, 2006.
158. Ergun I, Keven K, Uruc I, Ekmekci Y, Canbakan B, Erden I, Karatan O: The safety of gadolinium in patients with stage 3 and 4 renal failure. *Nephrol Dial Transplant* 21: 697-700, 2006.
159. Erley CM, Bader BD, Berger ED, Tuncel N, Winkler S, Tepe G, Risler T, Duda S: Gadolinium-based contrast media compared with iodinated media for digital subtraction angiography in azotaemic patients. *Nephrol Dial Transplant* 19: 2526-2531, 2004.
160. Sam AD,2nd, Morasch MD, Collins J, Song G, Chen R, Pereles FS: Safety of gadolinium contrast angiography in patients with chronic renal insufficiency. *J Vasc Surg* 38: 313-318, 2003.
161. Kwak HS, Lee YH, Han YM, Jin GY, Kim W, Chung GH: Comparison of renal damage by iodinated contrast or gadolinium in an acute renal failure rat model based on serum creatinine levels and apoptosis degree. *J Korean Med Sci* 20: 841-847, 2005.
162. Thomsen HS, Almen T, Morcos SK, Contrast Media Safety Committee Of The European Society Of Urogenital Radiology (ESUR): Gadolinium-containing contrast media for radiographic examinations: A position paper. *Eur Radiol* 12: 2600-2605, 2002.
163. Cowper SE, Robin HS, Steinberg SM, Su LD, Gupta S, LeBoit PE: Scleromyxoedema-like cutaneous diseases in renal-dialysis patients. *Lancet* 356: 1000-1001, 2000.
164. Cowper SE: Nephrogenic fibrosing dermopathy: The first 6 years. *Curr Opin Rheumatol* 15: 785-790, 2003.
165. Perazella MA, Ishibe S, Perazella MA, Reilly RF: Nephrogenic fibrosing dermopathy: An unusual skin condition associated with kidney disease. *Semin Dial* 16: 276-280, 2003.
166. Wahba IM, White K, Meyer M, Simpson EL: The case for ultraviolet light therapy in nephrogenic fibrosing dermopathy--report of two cases and review of the literature. *Nephrol Dial Transplant* 22: 631-636, 2007.
167. Ting WW, Stone MS, Madison KC, Kurtz K: Nephrogenic fibrosing dermopathy with systemic involvement. *Arch Dermatol* 139: 903-906, 2003.
168. Jimenez SA, Artlett CM, Sandorfi N, Derk C, Latinis K, Sawaya H, Haddad R, Shanahan JC: Dialysis-associated systemic fibrosis (nephrogenic fibrosing dermopathy): Study of inflammatory cells and transforming growth factor beta1 expression in affected skin. *Arthritis Rheum* 50: 2660-2666, 2004.
169. Daram SR, Cortese CM, Bastani B: Nephrogenic fibrosing dermopathy/nephrogenic systemic fibrosis: Report of a new case with literature review. *Am J Kidney Dis* 46: 754-759, 2005.
170. Mendoza FA, Artlett CM, Sandorfi N, Latinis K, Piera-Velazquez S, Jimenez SA: Description of 12 cases of nephrogenic fibrosing dermopathy and review of the literature. *Semin Arthritis Rheum* 35: 238-249, 2006.
171. Moschella SL, Kay J, Mackool BT, Liu V: Case records of the Massachusetts General Hospital. Weekly clinicopathological exercises. Case 35-2004. A 68-year-old man with end-stage renal disease and thickening of the skin. *N Engl J Med* 351: 2219-2227, 2004.
172. Mackay-Wiggan JM, Cohen DJ, Hardy MA, Knobler EH, Grossman ME: Nephrogenic fibrosing dermopathy (scleromyxedema-like illness of renal disease). *J Am Acad Dermatol* 48: 55-60, 2003.
173. Evenepoel P, Zeegers M, Segaert S, Claes K, Kuypers D, Maes B, Flamen P, Fransis S, Vanrenterghem Y: Nephrogenic fibrosing dermopathy: A novel, disabling disorder in patients with renal failure. *Nephrol Dial Transplant* 19: 469-473, 2004.
174. Streams BN, Liu V, Liegeois N, Moschella SM: Clinical and pathologic features of nephrogenic fibrosing dermopathy: A report of two cases. *J Am Acad Dermatol* 48: 42-47, 2003.
175. Deo A, Fogel M, Cowper SE: Nehprogenic systemic fibrosis: A population study examining the relationship of disease development to gadolinium exposure. *Clin J Am Soc Nephrol* 2: 264-267, 2007.
176. Todd DJ, Kagan A, Chibnik LB, Kay J: Cutaneous changes of nephrogenic systemic fibrosis: Predictor of early mortality and association with gadolinium exposure. *Arthritis Rheum* 56: 3433-3441, 2007.
177. Cowper SE, Su LD, Bhawan J, Robin HS, LeBoit PE: Nephrogenic fibrosing dermopathy. *Am J Dermatopathol* 23: 383-393, 2001.
178. Ortonne N, Lipsker D, Chantrel F, Boehm N, Grosshans E, Cribier B: Presence of CD45RO+ CD34+ cells with collagen synthesis activity in nephrogenic fibrosing dermopathy: A new pathogenic hypothesis. *Br J Dermatol* 150: 1050-1052, 2004.
179. Quan TE, Cowper S, Wu SP, Bockenstedt LK, Bucala R: Circulating fibrocytes: Collagen-secreting cells of the peripheral blood. *Int J Biochem Cell Biol* 36: 598-606, 2004.
180. Swartz RD, Crofford LJ, Phan SH, Ike RW, Su LD: Nephrogenic fibrosing dermopathy: A novel cutaneous fibrosing disorder in patients with renal failure. *Am J Med* 114: 563-572, 2003.
181. Grobner T: Gadolinium--a specific trigger for the development of nephrogenic fibrosing dermopathy and nephrogenic systemic fibrosis? *Nephrol Dial Transplant* 21: 1104-1108, 2006.
182. Marckmann P, Skov L, Rossen K, Dupont A, Damholt MB, Heaf JG, Thomsen HS: Nephrogenic systemic fibrosis: Suspected causative role of gadodiamide used for contrast-enhanced magnetic resonance imaging. *J Am Soc Nephrol* 17: 2359-2362, 2006.
183. Sadowski EA, Bennett LK, Chan MR, Wentland AL, Garrett AL, Garrett RW, Djamali A: Nephrogenic systemic fibrosis: Risk factors and incidence estimation. *Radiology* 24: 148-157, 2007.

184. Khurana A, Runge VM, Narayanan M, Greene JF,Jr, Nickel AE: Nephrogenic systemic fibrosis: A review of 6 cases temporally related to gadodiamide injection (omniscan). *Invest Radiol* 42: 139-145, 2007.
185. Pryor JG, Poggioli G, Galaria N, Gust A, Robison J, Samie F, Hanjani NM, Scott GA: Nephrogenic systemic fibrosis: A clinicopathologic study of six cases. *J Am Acad Dermatol* 57: 105-111, 2007.
186. Broome DR, Girguis MS, Baron PW, Cottrell AC, Kjellin I, Kirk GA: Gadodiamide-associated nephrogenic systemic fibrosis: Why radiologists should be concerned. *AJR Am J Roentgenol* 188: 586-592, 2007.
187. Centers for Disease Control and Prevention (CDC): Nephrogenic fibrosing dermopathy associated with exposure to gadolinium-containing contrast agents--st. louis, missouri, 2002-2006. *MMWR Morb Mortal Wkly Rep* 56: 137-141, 2007.
188. US Food and Drug Administration: Information for healthcare professionals: Gadolinium-based contrast agents for magnetic resonance imaging (marketed as magnevist, MultiHance, omniscan, OptiMARK, ProHance). Food and Drug administration web site. Published June 2006. Updated May 23, 2007. Accessed February 12, 2008. *Http://www.Fda.gov/cder/drug/InfoSheets/HCP/gcca_200705HCP.Pdf.* 2006.
189. Joffe P, Thomsen HS, Meusel M: Pharmacokinetics of gadodiamide injection in patients with severe renal insufficiency and patients undergoing hemodialysis or continuous ambulatory peritoneal dialysis. *Acad Radiol* 5: 491-502, 1998.
190. Boyd AS, Zic JA, Abraham JL: Gadolinium deposition in nephrogenic fibrosing dermopathy. *J Am Acad Dermatol* 56: 27-30, 2007.
191. High WA, Ayers RA, Chandler J, Zito G, Cowper SE: Gadolinium is detectable within the tissue of patients with nephrogenic systemic fibrosis. *J Am Acad Dermatol* 56: 21-26, 2007.
192. High WA, Ayers RA, Cowper SE: Gadolinium is quantifiable within the tissue of patients with nephrogenic systemic fibrosis. *J Am Acad Dermatol* 56: 710-712, 2007.
193. Thakral C, & Abraham JL: Automated scanning electron microscopy and X-ray microanalysis for *in situ* quantification of gadolinium deposits in skin. *J Electron Microsc (Tokyo)* 56: 181-187, 2007.
194. Abraham JL, Thakral C, Skov L, Rossen K, Marckmann P: Dermal inorganic gadolinium concentrations: Evidence for *in vivo* transmetallation and long-term persistence in nephrogenic systemic fibrosis. *Br J Dermatol* 158: 273-280, 2008.
195. Sieber MA, Pietsch H, Walter J, Haider W, Frenzel T, Weinmann HJ: A preclinical study to investigate the development of nephrogenic systemic fibrosis: A possible role for gadolinium-based contrast media. *Invest Radiol* 43: 65-75, 2008.
196. Rydahl C, Thomsen HS, Marckmann P: High prevalence of nephrogenic systemic fibrosis in chronic renal failure patients exposed to gadodiamide, a gadolinium-containing magnetic resonance contrast agent. *Invest Radiol* 43: 141-144, 2008.
197. Wahba IM, Simpson EL, White K: Gadolinium is not the only trigger for nephrogenic systemic fibrosis: Insights from two cases and review of the recent literature. *Am J Transplant* 7: 2425-2432, 2007.
198. Anavekar NS, Chong AH, Norris R, Dowling J, Goodman D: Nephrogenic systemic fibrosis in a gadolinium-naive renal transplant recipient. *Australas J Dermatol* 49: 44-47, 2008.
199. Swaminathan S, Ahmed I, McCarthy JT, Albright RC, Pittelkow MR, Caplice NM, Griffin MD, Leung N: Nephrogenic fibrosing dermopathy and high-dose erythropoietin therapy. *Ann Intern Med* 145: 234-235, 2006.
200. Marckmann P, Skov L, Rossen K, Heaf JG, Thomsen HS: Case-control study of gadodiamide-related nephrogenic systemic fibrosis. *Nephrol Dial Transplant* 22: 3174-3178, 2007.
201. Chiu H, Wells G, Carag H, Canova E, Firpi RJ: Nephrogenic fibrosing dermopathy: A rare entity in patients awaiting liver transplantation. *Liver Transpl* 10: 465-466, 2004.
202. Penfield JG, & Reilly RF,Jr: What nephrologists need to know about gadolinium. *Nat Clin Pract Nephrol* 3: 654-668, 2007.
203. Spencer AJ, Wilson SA, Batchelor J, Reid A, Rees J, Harpur E: Gadolinium chloride toxicity in the rat. *Toxicol Pathol* 25: 245-255, 1997.
204. Morcos SK: Nephrogenic systemic fibrosis following the administration of extracellular gadolinium based contrast agents: Is the stability of the contrast agent molecule an important factor in the pathogenesis of this condition? *Br J Radiol* 80: 73-76, 2007.
205. Thomsen HS, Marckmann P, Logager VB: Nephrogenic systemic fibrosis (NSF): A late adverse reaction to some of the gadolinium based contrast agents. *Cancer Imaging* 7: 130-137, 2007.
206. Thomsen HS, Morcos SK, Dawson P: Is there a causal relation between the administration of gadolinium based contrast media and the development of nephrogenic systemic fibrosis (NSF)? *Clin Radiol* 61: 905-906, 2006.
207. Reilly RF: Risk of nephrogenic systemic fibrosis (NSF) with gadoteridol (ProHance) [Abstract]. *J Am Soc Nephrol,* 18: 716A, 2007.
208. Launay-Vacher V, Karie S, Janus N, Choukroun G, Clement O, Frances C, Deray G: Prevalence of nephrogenic systemic fibrosis in renal insufficiency patients. results of the FINEST study. [Abstract]. *J Am Soc Nephrol,* 18: 775A, 2007.
209. Okada S, Katagiri K, Kumazaki T, Yokoyama H: Safety of gadolinium contrast agent in hemodialysis patients. *Acta Radiol* 42: 339-341, 2001.
210. Morcos SK, Thomsen HS, Webb JA, Contrast Media Safety Committee of the European Society of Urogenital Radiology (ESUR): Dialysis and contrast media. *Eur Radiol* 12: 3026-3030, 2002.

211. Perazella MA: Nephrogenic systemic fibrosis, kidney disease, and gadolinium: Is there a link? *Clin J Am Soc Nephrol* 2: 200-202, 2007.

212. Swaminathan S, Horn TD, Pellowski D, Abul-Ezz S, Bornhorst JA, Viswamitra S, Shah SV: Nephrogenic systemic fibrosis, gadolinium, and iron mobilization. *N Engl J Med* 357: 720-722, 2007.

213. Swaminathan S, & Shah SV: New insights into nephrogenic systemic fibrosis. *J Am Soc Nephrol* 18: 2636-2643, 2007.

214. Proctor KA, Rao LV, Roberts WL: Gadolinium magnetic resonance contrast agents produce analytic interference in multiple serum assays. *Am J Clin Pathol* 121: 282-292, 2004.

215. Lauchli S, Zortea-Caflisch C, Nestle FO, Burg G, Kempf W: Nephrogenic fibrosing dermopathy treated with extracorporeal photopheresis. *Dermatology* 208: 278-280, 2004.

216. Gilliet M, Cozzio A, Burg G, Nestle FO: Successful treatment of three cases of nephrogenic fibrosing dermopathy with extracorporeal photopheresis. *Br J Dermatol* 152: 531-536, 2005.

217. Richmond H, Zwerner J, Kim Y, Fiorentino D: Nephrogenic systemic fibrosis: Relationship to gadolinium and response to photopheresis. *Arch Dermatol* 143: 1025-1030, 2007.

218. Goddard DS, Magee CC, Lazar AJ, Miller DM: Nephrogenic fibrosing dermopathy with recurrence after allograft failure. *J Am Acad Dermatol* 56: S109-111, 2007.

219. Baron PW, Cantos K, Hillebrand DJ, Hu KQ, Ojogho ON, Nehlsen-Cannarella S, Concepcion W: Nephrogenic fibrosing dermopathy after liver transplantation successfully treated with plasmapheresis. *Am J Dermatopathol* 25: 204-209, 2003.

220. Gremmels JM, & Kirk GA: Two patients with abnormal skeletal muscle uptake of tc-99m hydroxymethylene diphosphonate following liver transplant: Nephrogenic fibrosing dermopathy and graft vs host disease. *Clin Nucl Med* 29: 694-697, 2004.

221. Hubbard V, Davenport A, Jarmulowicz M, Rustin M: Scleromyxoedema-like changes in four renal dialysis patients. *Br J Dermatol* 148: 563-568, 2003.

222. Yerram P, Saab G, Karuparthi PR, Hayden MR, Khanna R: Nephrogenic systemic fibrosis: A mysterious disease in patients with renal failure--role of gadolinium-based contrast media in causation and the beneficial effect of intravenous sodium thiosulfate. *Clin J Am Soc Nephrol* 2: 258-263, 2007.

223. Lin J, Idee JM, Port M, Diai A, Berthommier C, Robert M, Raynal I, Devoldere L, Corot C: Interference of magnetic resonance imaging contrast agents with the serum calcium measurement technique using colorimetric reagents. *J Pharm Biomed Anal* 21: 931-943, 1999.

224. Prince MR, Erel HE, Lent RW, Blumenfeld J, Kent KC, Bush HL, Wang Y: Gadodiamide administration causes spurious hypocalcemia. *Radiology* 227: 639-646, 2003.

225. Kang HP, Scott MG, Joe BN, Narra V, Heiken J, Parvin CA: Model for predicting the impact of gadolinium on plasma calcium measured by the o-cresolphthalein method. *Clin Chem* 50: 741-746, 2004.

226. Emerson J, & Kost G: Spurious hypocalcemia after omniscan- or OptiMARK-enhanced magnetic resonance imaging: An algorithm for minimizing a false-positive laboratory value. *Arch Pathol Lab Med* 128: 1151-1156, 2004.

227. Lowe A, Balzer T, Hirt U: Interference of gadolinium-containing contrast-enhancing agents with colorimetric calcium laboratory testing. *Invest Radiol* 40: 521-525, 2005.

228. Brown JJ, Hynes MR, Wible JH,Jr: Measurement of serum calcium concentration after administration of four gadolinium-based contrast agents to human volunteers. *AJR Am J Roentgenol* 189: 1539-1544, 2007.

31

Lithium-associated kidney effects

Daniel BATLLE, Edgar V. LERMA, Parveen NAAZ and Santosh HAKKAPAKKI

Northwestern University, Feinberg School of Medicine, Chicago, IL, USA

Introduction

Since its introduction several decades ago for the occasional treatment of "psychotic excitement", lithium is still a mainstay in the treatment and prophylaxis of manic-depressive disorders [1]. The biologic basis for the clinical efficacy of lithium is not completely known. Interestingly, the agent relieves both mania and depression, states which appear to be opposites. Its therapeutic range, however, is narrow, and even at the lowest effective dosage, some unwanted side effects may occur [2]. Serum levels above 1.5 mEq/L often result in acute intoxication, which may be severe. The therapeutic range varies, depending on methodology, but it is advisable to target a level of about 0.5 mEq/L, with an upper range at 1.0 mEq/L. Values above this level signify a warning range of impending toxicity.

An equation to predict daily lithium dose has been suggested:

Daily lithium carbonate dose (mg) =
100.5
+ 752.7 x desired lithium concentration (mEq/L)
- 3.6 x age (years)
+ 7.2 x weight (kg)
- 13.7 x blood urea nitrogen [BUN] (mg/dl) [3].

Lithium is one of the smallest elements, between H and Na in the Periodic Table of elements, and is always ionized (Li^+) in watery solutions [1]. In living organisms it has strong pharmacologic and toxic activity. Lithium occurs in two isotopic forms of mass number 6 and 7, with natural abundances of 7.4 and 92.6% respectively [4]. Pharmaceutical lithium is prepared from the isotope mixture [4]. The smaller ^{6}Li has higher charge to mass and radius ratio. This can produce differences in the isotopes' electrostatic interactions with water molecules and negatively charged membranes. An increase in the rate of ^{6}Li transport, compared to ^{7}Li transport, across membranes is expected [4]. Accordingly, elimination or reduction of ^{6}Li from pharmaceutical preparations may merit further evaluation as a way to develop potentially less nephrotoxic form of lithium [4].

The red blood cell, which is a convenient model, shows a cell-to-plasma lithium ratio of 0.3-0.6, whereas the Nernst equation would predict a 1.6 ratio. When red blood cells are loaded with lithium *in vitro* its extrusion is accomplished by a Na^+/Li^+ countertransporter (SLC), the physiological role of which is unclear, but some believe it represents a mode of operation of the Na^+/H^+ exchanger. Interestingly, a recent paper suggested that red cell SLC may be a marker of the activity of Na^+/H^+ exchanger-3 the isoform expressed in the kidney proximal tubule rather than the ubiquitous Na^+/H^+ exchanger-1 isoform [5].

Because lithium is cleared from the body by the kidneys, its blood level at a given dosage depends critically on renal excretion, which is subject to various physiological and pathological influences. An insight into renal "lithium handling" is a prerequisite for effective prevention of complications and treatment of lithium intoxication when it occurs. Another reason why lithium is of interest to nephrologists is that its clearance has been used as a tool to investigate segmental tubular function [6-9].

With the widespread use of lithium in the treatment of affective disorders, many questions have centered on its long-term effect on the kidneys. Of particular interest is the action of lithium at distal nephron sites where it inhibits water transport, hydrogen secretion, and possibly potassium secretion as well [10, 11]. The most common side effect of chronic lithium therapy is an impairment of renal concentrating ability [11]. Lithium therapy is also associated with side effects related to hormonal alterations and changes in calcium metabolism.

Lithium transport along the nephron

Lithium is freely filtered by the glomeruli, whereas excretion into the urine is 20-30% of that amount [2]. Thus, at least 70% of the filtered load undergoes tubular reabsorption. Lithium clearance closely parallels changes in natrium delivery from the proximal tubule (Figure 1).

a. Proximal tubule. Early micropuncture studies reported Lithium concentration at the end of the convoluted proximal tubule to be close to unity [12]. Subsequent recent studies [13-19] using lower lithium plasma concentrations and more sensitive methods all found filtrate-to-plasma ratios to be definitely higher, the average value being 1.14. This value was not influenced by various manipulations such as natrium depletion, osmotic diuresis, prostaglandin inhibition, or infusion of acetazolamide, furosemide, or angiotensin [13, 14, 16]. Lithium can enter the cells via the

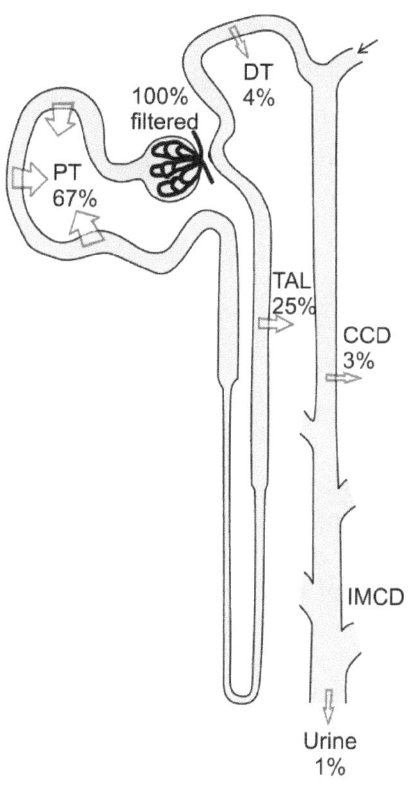

Figure 1. *Scheme of Li^+ transport along different nephron segments.*

Na^+/H^+ exchanger (Na^+/H^+ exchanger-1 isoform) but it is not clear how it may leave these cells. Although some possibilities in this regard have been suggested, the transcellular transport of lithium if it occurs at all is likely to be much less than that of natrium. Importantly, the remarkable constant fluid to blood ratio for lithium, despite large changes in proximal fluid reabsorption, suggests that lithium delivery from this part of the nephron, while systematically overestimating natrium delivery, can be considered a marker of proximal natrium reabsorption [13, 18]. It is generally believed that this also is true for the straight part of the proximal tubule, because paracellular transport in this part is even more important than in the convoluted tubules. However, because of their inaccessibility to micropuncture no direct evidence exists.

b. Henle's loop. Earlier investigations suggested that the amount of lithium arriving at the early distal tubule was the same as the amount calculated to enter the loop of Henle [12]. Recent studies, however, showed that the difference between the amounts of lithium reaching the late proximal and early distal tubule is about 25% of the filtered load [13-17]. This does not necessarily indicate that lithium is actively transported by the thick ascending limb. In the thick ascending limb of Henle's loop, a $Na^+/K^+/2Cl^-$ cotransporter is responsible for NaCl reabsorption. Lithium may substitute for natrium in isolated cell models including rabbit thick ascending limb cells. It has been shown that lithium can be reabsorbed through a paracellular pathway with an affinity 1.5 that of Cl^- and 65% that of Na^+ [20]. Moreover, some lithium might be reabsorbed through $Na^+/K^+/2Cl^-$ cotransporter and extruded at the basolateral site through a K^+/Cl^- cotransporter [20]. It is likely that transport also occurs in the highly lithium permeable thin descending limb along the osmotic gradient to the hyperosmolar inner medulla [21]. Indeed, studies using loop diuretics suggest that lithium is concentrated in the medulla to the same extent as natrium and this accumulation is largely abolished by such diuretics.

About 5% of the filtered lithium may be actively reabsorbed in the thick ascending limb [19]. This active "reabsorption" can increase to about 15% after prostaglandin inhibition [9, 17]. These observations suggest that lithium clearance cannot be used as a precise marker of proximal fluid reabsorption.

c. Distal tubule. Micropuncture studies have shown that urinary excretion of lithium is almost equal to the amount reaching the early distal tubule, indicating no further reabsorption beyond this point [12]. The permeability and transport characteristics of this "tight" epithelium also suggest no active or passive lithium transport. Thiazide diuretics whose action is confined to the distal tubule did not affect lithium clearance in a recent micropuncture study since identical amounts of lithium were found at the beginning and at the end of this segment [19].

d. Collecting duct. Although this is also a "tight" epithelium with high electrical resistance and low natrium permeability, there is evidence that lithium can be transported under certain conditions. In rats and dogs lithium clearance drops markedly on severe salt restriction (a reflection of enhanced proximal reabsorption) and increases after the diuretic amiloride, which acts in the cortical collecting tubule. This drug, though, does not affect lithium clearance on a normal diet [22, 23]. The limitation in reabsorption of Li^+ during Na^+-replete conditions may be either the cellular influx across the apical membrane or extrusion through the basolateral membrane making the rate of distal tubular Na^+ delivery a crucial determinant for reabsorption of Li^+. Under Na^+-depleted conditions, the apical membrane becomes hyperpolarized due to a low-Na^+ influx, and distal Li^+ reabsorption can occur [23]. However, an acute decrease in urine volume induced by antidiuretic hormone administration causes a definite but limited fall in lithium excretion particularly during a low sodium diet.

This effect likely results from enhanced reabsorption in the cortical collecting tubule.

In normal humans, values for fractional excretion of lithium varying from 19 to 38% have been reported [9]. These marked discrepancies are probably due mainly to variable experimental conditions such as natrium intake and urine flow rate. Of note also are the marked inter-individual differences in lithium clearance documented by Boer et al. [18, 24]. Fortunately, intra-individual variability is small. Thus, lithium clearance is still a sensitive tool to detect changes in tubular sodium handling for a given individual studied on different occasions. The limitations and advantages of this method have been discussed elsewhere [6-8, 14, 18]. The use of lithium clearance as a research tool to analyze segmental tubular sodium reabsorption has been controversial. Recent investigations, while refuting the claim that it is an absolute measure of fluid delivery from the proximal tubule, have confirmed its value as a directional, non-quantitative marker of proximal fluid and sodium reabsorption [13, 18]. Indeed, in clinical practice it provides information which cannot be obtained by any other non-invasive method [13].

Effect of lithium on water transport

Overview of experimental studies

Polyuria is a common side effect associated with lithium use, and is often found in patients whose levels are within the therapeutic range [10, 11]. The mechanism whereby lithium causes polyuria has been studied extensively in humans, experimental animals, and epithelial analogs of the mammalian collecting tubule [26, 49-59]. In the aggregate, these studies have provided compelling evidence for a direct inhibitory effect of lithium on arginine vasopressin-mediated water reabsorption by renal tubules.

In the toad urinary bladder, an experimental model of the mammalian collecting tubule, addition of lithium to the mucosal surface (but not to the serosal surface) markedly inhibited both basal and arginine vasopressin-stimulated water flow [50]. The concentration of mucosal lithium used in these studies (10 mEq/L) was comparable to or even lower than that usually found in the urine of patients on well-controlled lithium therapy (that is, 10 to 40 mEq/L) [63] Fernandez et al. [53] confirmed the inhibitory effect of lithium on water flow in toad urinary bladders exposed only submaximal concentrations of arginine vasopressin. Inhibition of cyclic adenosine monophosphate-stimulated water flow when lithium (2 mEq/L) was applied to the serosal surface of the toad bladder was reported in one study. Such an effect of lithium, when applied to the serosal surface has, to our knowledge, not been found by any other investigators. As herein discussed, the bulk of evidence supports the notion that the action of lithium on water transport is the result of its cell uptake from the luminal (apical) surface of the collecting tubule.

The mechanism of the action of lithium on H_2O transport lies at some point along the arginine vasopressin-mediated transport process, either before or beyond the formation of cyclic adenosine monophosphate. Forrest et al. [51] suggested that lithium interference with the cellular action of arginine vasopressin occurs, in part, at a step beyond the formation of cyclic adenosine monophosphate. This was deduced from their findings that infusions of dibutyryl cyclic adenosine monophosphate to lithium-treated rats had only a marginal effect on urine osmolality. Another study in rats treated with intraperitoneal lithium injections suggested that lithium impairs the action of arginine vasopressin on water transport at steps both proximal and distal to the intracellular formation of cyclic adenosine monophosphate [52].

Cogan and Abramow [55] addressed this issue more directly. These authors showed that addition of lithium to the luminal perfusion solution of isolated cortical collecting tubules reduces the hydro-osmotic action of arginine vasopressin. This effect persisted after removal of lithium from the luminal fluid, which strongly suggests that its inhibitory effect on H_2O transport is exerted only after cell uptake from the luminal site. To determine whether the lithium-arginine vasopressin interaction affected the generation of cyclic adenosine monophosphate or the effect of this second messenger in the cell, these authors investigated the effect of lithium on the hydro-osmotic action of 8-Br-cyclic adenosine monophosphate, a derivative of cyclic adenosine monophosphate resistant to the action of phosphodiesterase. The hydro-osmotic action of 8-Br-cyclic adenosine monophosphate was not diminished by the presence of lithium in the lumen of cortical collecting tubules perfused *in vitro*. This finding strongly suggests that the inhibitory effect of lithium on the hydro-osmotic action of arginine vasopressin occurs at a step preceding the formation of cyclic adenosine monophosphate [55].

These *in vitro* findings were expanded by Christien-sen et al. [56] using an experimental model that closely resembles the clinical setting of chronic lithium therapy. In this model, lithium was administered to rats for several weeks in conjunction with a NaCl drinking solution to prevent sodium depletion. At serum lithium levels within the accepted therapeutic range (0.7 to 1.5 mEq/L), marked polyuria and polydipsia developed after four weeks of lithium administration. Cortical collecting tubules isolated from lithium-treated rats displayed decreased ability to generate cyclic adenosine monophosphate *in vitro* in response to arginine vasopressin stimulation. In contrast, tubules from polyuric rats with hypothalamic diabetes insipidus

(Brattleboro homozygotes) had intact arginine vasopressin-dependent cyclic adenosine monophosphate generation. The activity of cyclic adenosine monophosphate phosphodiesterase was not affected in lithium-treated rats. Hence, it seems that the main cellular effect of lithium involves impairment of arginine vasopressin-sensitive adenylate cyclase and that this results in impairment of intracellular cyclic adenosine monophosphate formation.

Other studies also support lithium's primary effect at the level of cyclic adenosine monophosphate generation [57, 58]. Though the greatest effect of arginine vasopressin is in the cortical collecting tubule, an arginine vasopressin-mediated cyclic adenosine monophosphate response has been demonstrated throughout the distal nephron. Jackson, Edwards and Dousa [58] evaluated the effects of lithium on the medullary thick ascending limb and medullary collecting tubule. Isolated tubules perfused in a hyper-osmotic medium (800 mOsm) displayed a significant rise in arginine vasopressin-dependent cyclic adenosine monophosphate generation. In contrast, in tubules exposed to lithium there was a significant decrease in arginine vasopressin-dependent cyclic adenosine monophosphate formation in both the medullary ascending limb and medullary collecting tubule segments when compared to controls [58]. This study also showed a dose-dependent decrease in cyclic adenosine monophosphate levels with increasing lithium concentrations [58]. Thus, reduced arginine vasopressin-sensitive adenyl cyclase activity in the medullary collecting tubule of lithium-treated polyuric rats may contribute to the observed reduction in concentrating ability. In other work, micro-dissected medullary collecting tubules from rats chronically treated with lithium responded to pertussis toxin, an inhibitor of inhibitory GTP binding protein, with an increase in arginine vasopressin dependent cyclic adenosine monophosphate production similar to that seen in control rats [59]. This finding suggests that lithium may inhibit arginine vasopressin dependent cyclic adenosine monophosphate formation by activation of inhibitory GTP binding protein [59]. The notion that lithium acts via cAMP, however, has been challenged. In a recent study [138] using a mouse cortical collecting duct mpkCCDc14 cells, the effect of lithium was found to be cAMP independent. Lithium did not alter AVP-stimulated cAMP production or PKA-dependent phosphorylation of AQP2 or cAMP responsive element binding protein [138]. In addition, lithium exposure decreased AQP2 mRNA expression [138]. Most of the previous studies have used LLP-PK-cells which are derived from pig proximal tubule cells, whereas the greatest effect of arginine vasopressin mediated AQP2 expression is in the cortical collecting tubule. The mouse cortical collecting duct cell line used in this study retains many of the hallmarks of principal cells from native epithelium, including the expression of endogenous AQP2. These findings suggest that the lithium-induced down regulation of AQP2 and development of NDI occur independent of adenyl cyclase activity *in vitro* and *in vivo*. Hensen and Gross [139] in an earlier study showed that lithium significantly reduces vasopressin receptor density in rats developing NDI. Thus, despite considerable investigative efforts, the mechanism of lithium induced impairment of concentrating ability in not fully understood. What is most striking, in our opinion, is the marked suppression of AQP2 expression observed *in vitro* and *in vivo* (Figure 2).

Renal urinary concentration is associated with enhanced expression of rBSC1, a rat sodium cotransporter, in the thick ascending limb of Henle. In two recent studies by Kwon et al [60] and Michimata et al [62] dehydration or high plasma AVP resulted in an enhanced expression of rBSC1 in rats with lithium induced nephrogenic diabetes insipidus. rBSC1 expression was closely associated with the adverse effects of Li ions on collecting duct function [60, 62].

Role of aquaporin-2

In recent years our understanding of the mechanism of H_2O transport and concentrating ability has widened with the discovery of aquaporin-2. The gene for aquaporin-2 [AQP2], a member of the aquaporin family of water channels, has been identified and sequenced [63-65]. Several studies have shown that AQP2 is the predominant vasopressin-sensitive water channel of the renal collecting duct [63-65]. AQP2 is selectively localized in the collecting duct principal cells, mainly in the apical plasma membrane and intracellular vesicles. Vasopressin acutely increases the water permeability of the collecting ducts by stimulating insertion of AQP2 water channels from intracellular vesicles into the apical plasma membrane [66]. Normally, the expression of AQP2 was increased by dehydration or

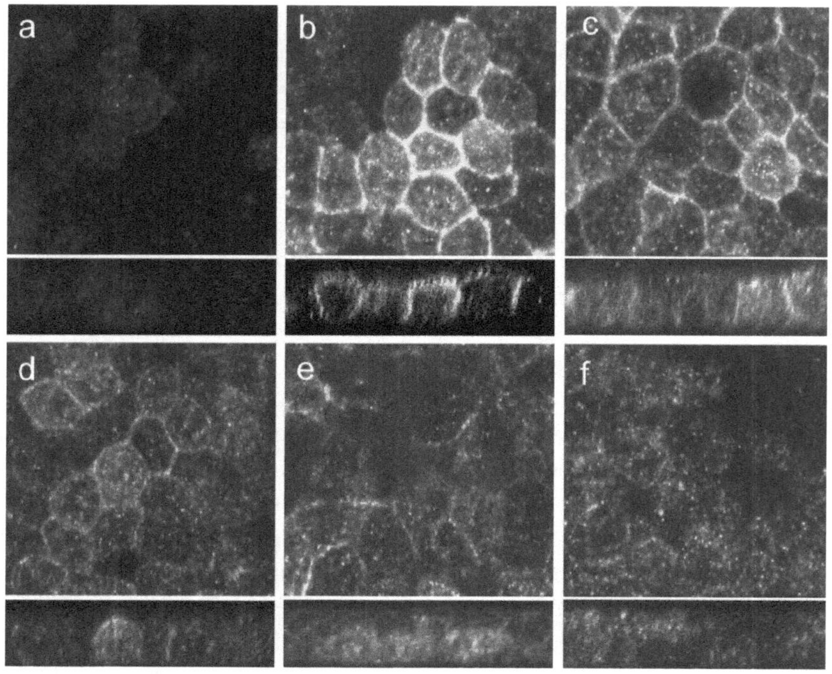

Figure 2. *Effects of lithium on the cellular distribution of AQP2 in mpkCCD cells. Confluent mpkCCD monolayers were left untreated (**a**), treated with 1nM dDAVP for 96 h (**b**), or treated with both dDAVP for 96 h and either 1 mM lithium for 24h (**c**) or 48h (**d**) or 10 mM lithium for 24h(**e**) or 48h (**f**). (Reproduced with permission from Yeudan et al [138]).*

chronic vasopressin administration, providing a long-term regulatory mechanism in antidiuresis. Mutations of AQP2 can result in severe nephrogenic diabetes insipidus, thus demonstrating that AQP2 is necessary for urinary concentrating ability [66].

Inner medullary collecting ducts (IMCD) isolated from rats treated with lithium for either 1 or 2 weeks were subjected to differential 2D gel electrophoresis combined with mass spectrometry and bioinformatic analysis to identify signaling pathways affected by lithium indicated that proteins involved in cell death, apoptosis, cell proliferation, and morphology are highly affected by lithium. Lithium treatment increased the intracellular accumulation of β-catenin in association with increased levels of phosphorylated glycogen synthase kinase type 3β (GSK3β) [61].

Chronic lithium administration to rats results in marked down regulation of AQP2 expression in medullary collecting ducts, parallel with the development of severe polyuria [66]. This effect of lithium therapy on AQP2 expression is only partially reversed by thirsting, intravenous 1-desamino-8-D-arginine-vasopressin [dDAVP], or return to a lithium-free diet [66]. After a one-week cessation of lithium administration, AQP2 was only partly reversed, consistent with the clinical findings of slow recovery of concentrating ability after lithium therapy [66].

In contrast to the process of spontaneous recovery after downregulation of AQP2 expression, which appears to be a slow process, up regulation in response to a stimulus such as thirsting occurs within 1-2 days despite continued lithium treatment [66]. The level of AQP2 expression was still below control levels, presumably reflecting a continued effect of lithium. It is to be noted that thirsting induces a considerably greater increase in expression of AQP2 than with dDAVP, but fails to induce significant redistribution of AQP2. This raises the possibility of a differing mechanism involved in water channel delivery to the plasma membrane during thirsting and dDAVP administration [64, 66] .

In rats treated with lithium, dDAVP, a specific V2 agonist, produced an increase in urine osmolality associated with increased apical plasma membrane AQP2 labeling. The action of dDAVP was likely due, at least in part, to its ability to overcome the block of adenylate cyclase caused by lithium. This may cause relocation of AQP2 to the apical part of the cell, and presumably induction of water channel insertion into the plasma membrane may be restored [63, 66]. The stimulatory effect of dDVAP in the presence of lithium, to our knowledge, has not been shown to be clinically useful for treating the polyuria associated with long-term lithium therapy.

Renal histological findings

Kidney biopsy findings consistent with chronic interstitial nephritis were first described by Hestbech et al. [98] in 14 patients who were selected on the basis of impaired concentrating ability or previous episodes of lithium intoxication. Renal function as judged by plasma creatinine was normal in all but one patient. The abnormalities described in this study included tubular atrophy, cortical and medullary fibrosis, sclerotic glomeruli, tubular dilatation, and cyst formation. Similar lesions were subsequently described by the same investigators in patients selected for biopsy on the basis of either impaired concentrating ability or reduced glomerular filtration rate [99] and confirmed by other investigators [67,68, 100,101]. A significant positive correlation between the duration of lithium therapy and the extent of tubular atrophy and interstitial fibrosis has been noted by other investigators [94, 97]. One of the most consistent findings observed in biopsies from lithium-treated patients is microcyst formation and distal tubular dilation [67, 99-103].

An important issue is whether this type of tubulointerstitial lesions develop in individuals not selected on the basis of abnormal clinical findings. In a group of 23 nonselected lithium-treated patients reported by Jorgensen et al. [80], focal interstitial fibrosis and glomerular sclerosis were found. These changes were more pronounced than those found in a "control" group of patients who had been biopsied for either acute oliguria or proteinuria. However, tubular atrophy and total fibrosis did not differ between the two groups. Rafaelson et al. [103] performed biopsies in 37 randomly chosen lithium-treated patients. Analysis of their data reveals that in nine of 12 patients who had polyuria (>3 L/d), kidney biopsies disclosed either borderline or advanced tubulointerstitial changes. Renal biopsies were normal in most patients who were not polyuric (18 of the remaining 25 patients). These observations suggest that the impairment of concentrating ability has, at least in part, a structural basis. The impairment in concentrating ability, which is evident shortly after initiation of lithium therapy, is usually mild and probably reversible. Over the course of long-term therapy, the impairment in concentrating ability may be progressive and related to structural tubulointerstitial alterations as discussed below.

In a study of 24 biopsies performed on bipolar disorder patients with lithium-associated chronic tubulo-interstitial nephropathy was characterized by tubular atrophy and interstitial fibrosis, typically out of proportion to the extent of glomerular or vascular disease with tubular cysts in 62.5% and lesser degrees of tubular dilatation in additional 33% of biopsies [101]. All these patients had serum creatinine of >2.5 at time of biopsy. Another important but unexplained finding was that lesions of FSGS were present in 50% of their biopsies, with a strong correlation between the FSGS lesions and presence of proteinuria >1.0 g/d [101]. This could indicate a potential direct glomerular toxicity of lithium. The presence of significant foot process fusion in some cases and recurrence of FSGS in the single transplant patient in whom lithium was not withdrawn lend further support to the above hypothesis. By cox regression analysis, it was found that a serum creatinine > 2.5 at the time of biopsy was a reliable predictor of progression to end-stage renal disease, even on discontinuation of lithium in 42% of patients [101]. Immunohistochemical and lectin staining revealed tubular cysts of predominantly distal tubular and collecting duct origin and rare cysts of proximal propagation of the distal portions of the cysts of the nephron [101].

The specificity of the chronic tubulointerstitial changes ascribed to lithium administration has been rightfully questioned because similar lesions have been described in psychiatric patients not receiving lithium [67, 105-107]. Walker et al. [67] compared biopsies from 47 patients treated with lithium for an average duration of 5 years to 32 patients with affective disorders who had never been treated with lithium. Using a semiquantitative analysis, they found no difference in interstitial fibrosis between the two groups even though the lithium group had a significantly lower glomerular filtration rate. Therefore, psychiatric patients, with or without the use of lithium, may develop chronic tubulointerstitial changes as compared to healthy controls. This may explain the reduced concentrating ability demonstrated in many psychiatric patients not receiving lithium therapy [73, 74, 108, 109].

Of interest is the finding of a lesion confined to the distal nephron that has been described in patients taking lithium but not in psychiatric controls [67, 103-106]. Several studies from Australia have reported this lesion, which appears to involve the distal convoluted tubules and collecting ducts of lithium-treated patients

[103-107]. Their findings include cytoplasmic swelling with the accumulation of glycogen deposits, dilated tubules, and microcyst formation. The lesion appears to be specific for lithium in that a similarly localized accumulation of glycogen has not been found in kidney biopsy material obtained from either psychiatric patients who have never taken lithium or from normal subjects donating a kidney for transplant [106]. Walker et al. [102] described a similar lesion in rabbits and speculated that the accumulation of glycogen in the distal nephron might be related to decreased intracellular formation of cyclic adenosine monophosphate by lithium. If this hypothesis were true, one could anticipate that the lesion should be reversible once cyclic adenosine monophosphate formation normalized after removal of lithium from distal tubular cells. Various studies have shown that the distinctive distal tubular lesion ascribed to lithium therapy appears very early after therapy is started and is reversible [106-108]. Burrows et al. [108] observed this lesion in two patients who had been on lithium for less than a year. Renal biopsies from patients who had discontinued lithium for 2 months to 5 years prior to biopsy did not show this type of distal tubular lesion [107].

In a study using rabbits, renal biopsies were performed at 1, 3, 6 and 12 months of lithium administration [102]. Cytoplasmic vacuolization and glycogen accumulation in cells lining distal convoluted tubules and collecting ducts was found. Thus, lithium induces a tubular lesion in rabbits which resembles the lesion described in humans. McAuliffe et al. [108] examined kidney specimens from rats given lithium for 7 weeks whose lithium levels were within the therapeutic range. They found glycogen deposits, cellular edema, and cellular detachment from type I basement membrane in cells lining the collecting tubule. The aggregate of these observations suggests that this specific lesion associated with lithium is manifested functionally by inhibition of H_2O transport in the collecting tubule, appears very early in therapy, and is likely to be reversible.

In a recent study using male Wistar rats fed lithium containing diet for 16 weeks postnatally, a marked decrease in glomerular volume was found [110]. This was not associated with detectable changes in structural parameters. Moreover, no effect of ACE inhibitor treatment could be demonstrated on glomerular volume [110].

Clinical studies on lithium-induced polyuria

An early study by Forrest et al. [51] demonstrated a significant decline in maximal urinary osmolality (from 1,110 to 854 mOsm/kg H_2O) in ten patients studied before and after only eight weeks of lithium therapy. Since urine osmolalities around 800 mOsm/kg H_2O after fluid deprivation are in the low range of normal, this investigation also demonstrated the importance of having information on urinary osmolality prior to lithium use. A subtle but significant decrement in concentrating ability caused by lithium could otherwise go unnoticed. This early and mild impairment in concentrating ability appears to be, at least in part, a functional defect caused by the temporal exposure of distal tubular cells to lithium [10].

The prevalence of polyuria among unselected lithium-treated patients has been difficult to ascertain [11]. Polyuria, as defined by a 24-hour urine output exceeding 3 L, varies considerably among patients on chronic lithium therapy [67-80]. In a review of a total of 841 unselected patients evaluated for 24-hour urine volume, we found that 160 (or 19%) had polyuria as defined by these criteria [11]. It was found that 85% of lithium treated patients have a normal glomerular filtration rate and that the remaining 15% have only mild reductions in renal function [11]. After fluid deprivation of approximately 24-hours duration, normal individuals should be able to raise urinary osmolality above 800 mOsm/kg H_2O. In a survey of a total of 1,105 lithium-treated patients [69-74], we found that at least 602 (or 54%) had a subnormal concentrating ability defined by this criterion [11].

The impairment of concentrating ability was reported to be mild or moderate in many studies [72, 74-77]. However, maximal urine osmolalities below 400 mOsm/kg H_2O were not infrequent [72]. Difficulties in completing 24-hour urine collections may also explain the relatively low prevalence of urine outputs exceeding 3 L/24-hours in relation to the high prevalence of reduced concentrating ability disclosed by urine osmolality measurements. Nocturia, an indirect but useful marker of polyuria, is a frequent complaint among lithium-treated patients [11]. For instance, of 153 lithium-treated patients, 105 (or 68%) reported at least one urination per night. Of these 105 subjects, 50 reported one urination, 35 reported two urinations, and the remaining 20 reported more than two urinations per night [70]. Several studies have shown that impairment of concentrating ability directly correlates with the duration of lithium therapy [67, 68, 72-75].

Persistence of a concentrating defect despite the discontinuation of lithium therapy is common [81-86]. In a study including 87 patients, maximal urine osmolality measured 8 weeks after discontinuation of lithium increased only slightly (from 517 ± 197 to 658 ± 203 mOsm/kg H_2O) [87]. These investigators also described a persistent defect in concentrating ability (urinary osmolality 800 mOsm/kg H_2O) in 17 of 27 patients who were studied one year after discontinuation of lithium. Although concentrating ability improved significantly during the first two months after lithium was stopped, there was no further improvement thereafter [87]. Persistence of nephrogenic diabetes insipidus following the discontinuation of lithium has been associated with renal biopsy findings consistent with chronic interstitial nephritis. The impairment in concentrating ability which is evident shortly after initiation of lithium therapy is usually mild and reversible [11]. Over the course of long-term therapy, the impairment in concentrating ability may be progressive and non-reversible as it is caused by structural tubulo-interstitial damage [11].

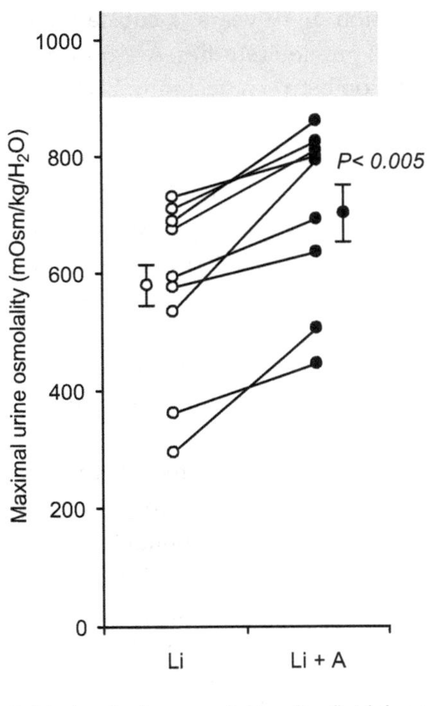

Figure 3. *Maximal urine osmolality after fluid deprivation and vasopressin administration during (closed circles) and before (open circles) amiloride administration. The shaded area shows the range of urine osmolality in normal subjects tested after fluid deprivation and vasopressin administration in our laboratory. Li denotes lithium and Li + A lithium plus amiloride (reproduced from Batlle et al [26]).*

Treatment of lithium-induced polyuria

The management of lithium-induced polyuria includes the use of thiazide diuretics alone, amiloride alone, or a combination of both. The use of thiazide diuretics to treat the polyuria induced by lithium therapy has had the problems of potentiating overt lithium toxicity by contracting the extracellular space, thereby causing compensatory proximal reabsorption of sodium and lithium. In the toad urinary bladder, an epithelium that transports water in a manner analogous to that of the mammalian collecting duct, amiloride blocks the entry of lithium across the apical surface, much as it does that of sodium [50]. Importantly, the addition of this agent to the mucosal side of this membrane markedly diminishes the inhibitory effect of lithium on arginine vasopressin-mediated water transport.

We utilized the above principle to treat lithium-induced polyuria [26]. This reduction in urine output could not be ascribed to increased proximal fluid reabsorption and decreased delivery of fluid to the distal nephron as a result of the volume contraction caused by amiloride. Fractional lithium excretion, a marker of proximal sodium reabsorption, did not fall during amiloride treatment, arguing against volume contraction induced by amiloride as possible mechanism [26]. In lithium treated patients, urinary osmolality increased when treated with amiloride. Amiloride attenuates the inhibitory effect of lithium on vasopressin-mediated water reabsorption [26](Figure 3).

In cases where sufficient tubulointerstitial damage causing impaired concentrating ability has occurred, amiloride is less effective; still, it can be used in combination with a thiazide diuretic to reduce polyuria [2]. Moreover, hypokalemia, a common side effect of thiazides, is not observed with amiloride [26]. Amiloride obviates the need for potassium supplementation, which is required when thiazide diuretics are used to treat polyuria and, in addition, is less likely to cause lithium intoxication. Although both lithium and amiloride interfere with distal urinary acidification, the development of metabolic acidosis is uncommon with therapeutic dosages of either drug. Further, no significant change in plasma bicarbonate levels was noted when given in combination [26]. This suggests that the suppressive effect of these two agents on distal acidification is not additive.

Other complications of lithium administration

Renal failure

In rats with lithium-induced tubulo-interstitial damage, a rise in plasma urea levels after 16 weeks of treatment has been demonstrated even though plasma lithium levels were in the accepted therapeutic range for humans with mood disorders [111]. In contrast to this finding in rats, progression of the chronic tubulo-interstitial lesion towards renal insufficiency is unusual in humans.

In our analysis of glomerular filtration rate data available from reports published up to 1986 we found only minor changes in glomerular filtration rate despite prolonged lithium therapy [11]. The majority of studies used endogenous creatinine clearance as a marker of glomerular filtration rate. Of 491 patients investigated using this method, 78 (or 15%) had a somewhat reduced glomerular filtration rate [72, 76, 79, 112-113]. In one study, glomerular filtration rate measured by the EDTA clearance method was found to be reduced in 39 of 179 patients (or 22%) [74]. A study involving 153 patients revealed that 31 patients (20%) had an EDTA clearance below the 95th percentile confidence limits corrected for age and sex [70]. Combined analysis of data from six studies using EDTA clearance showed that glomerular filtration rate was reduced in 92 of 538 patients (17%) [69, 70, 74, 80, 114, 115]. Of a total of 1,172 patients in whom glomerular filtration rate was measured by different methods we found it to be reduced in only 15% [11].

The overall prevalence (15%) of reduced glomerular filtration rate among unselected lithium-treated patients probably overestimates the proportion of patients in whom such reduction can be ascribed to lithium [11]. First, a sizeable number of patients had prior episodes of lithium intoxication [76, 80, 113-115]. A reduced glomerular filtration rate could be related to factors other than lithium, such as the common use of other psychotropic drugs. The latter possibility is suggested from studies that found tubulo-interstitial damage in psychiatric patients taking drugs other than lithium [96].

Of particular importance is the level of glomerular filtration rate among the patients in whom it was felt to be reduced. The distribution of glomerular filtration rates in the large series of patients studied by Wallin et al. [73] and Lokkegaard et al. [70] revealed that the reduction of glomerular filtration rate in lithium populations, when present, is very moderate. If lithium therapy were to result in lowering of glomerular filtration rate, it would be expected that there would be a progressive decline with the continuation of lithium therapy. A significant correlation between reduced glomerular filtration rate and the duration of therapy has not been found in the majority of studies that addressed this issue [67, 69, 75, 78, 109, 114, 116]. A significant but weak correlation (r= 0.29) between glomerular filtration rate and time on lithium was found among 231 patients on lithium for an average of 6.5 years [74]. Lokkegaard et al. [70] studied 153 patients treated for a mean duration of 10 years, a substantially longer period than all previous studies. A significant but also weak correlation between declining EDTA clearances and the duration of treatment was also found by these authors (r= 0.29).

Recent studies have shown that Lithium induced nephropathy develops slowly over several decades [142]. This is well demonstrated in the two multi centric studies performed by the same group in Sweden 12 years apart. Only 4% of the patients receiving lithium for a mean duration of 6.5 years had elevated serum creatinine levels where as this was found in 12% of the patients after 19 years of Lithium administration [69,146, 148] . Presne et al in a recent study involving 74 patients treated with lithium for a mean period of 20 years have shown that the annual loss of creatinine clearance in patients with lithium induced nephropathy is 2.29 ml/min [142] (Figure 4). The study results also suggested that the duration of lithium therapy and the cumulative dose of lithium are major determinants of nephrotoxicity .From the survey performed in France the prevalence of lithium induced ESRD among dialysis patients is estimated to be 3 per 1000 [142]. Maskowitz et al in his study of 24 patients with lithium induced nephrotoxicity noticed high prevalence of CKD [100]. He also found that serum creatinine at the time of biopsy was the only reliable predictor of progression to

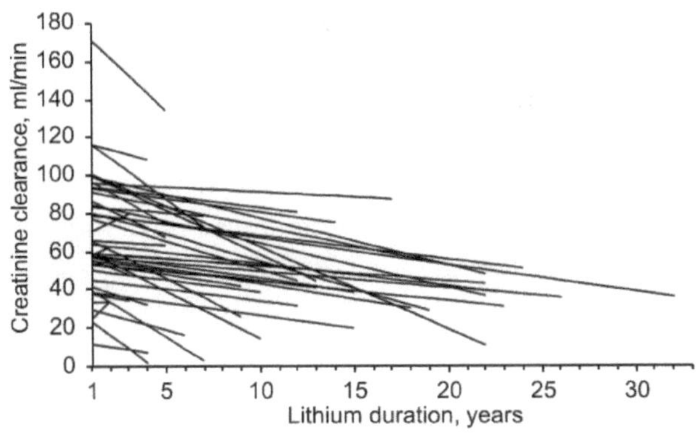

***Figure 4.** Evolution of estimated creatinine clearance over time in 35 patients on lithium therapy. Each line denotes the evolution in one patient up for more than 1 year. (Reproduced with permission from Presne et al [142]).*

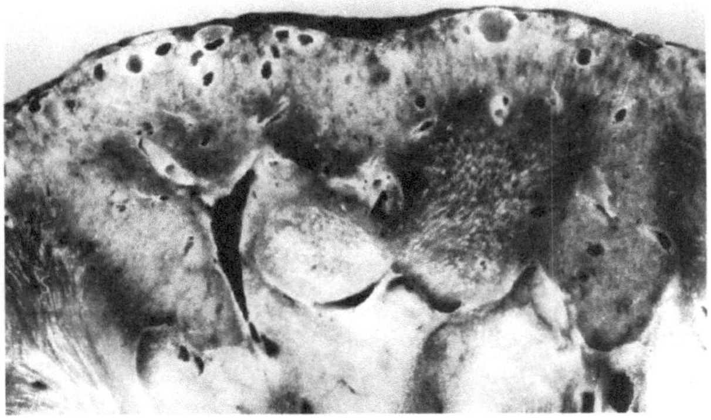

***Figure 5**. The cut surface of kidney from a patient, obtained at autopsy, showing granular scarring and a multitude of small cysts. (Reproduced with permission from Hestbech et al. [141]).*

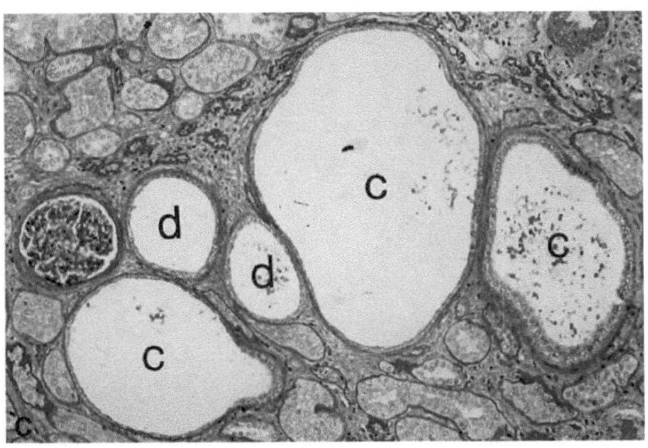

***Figure 6.** High power view of tubular cysts lined by simple cuboidal epithelium (labeled c). Adjacent tubules show tubular dilatation (labeled d). PAS stain, orig. magn. x 100. (Reproduced with permission from Markowitz et al [100]).*

ESRD. In this study progression to ESRD was noted in 8 of 9 patients with serum creatinine > 2.5 mg/dl at the time of biopsy compared to 1 of 10 patients with serum creatinine < 2.5 mg/dl [100]. A recently published Dutch article mentions that some decrease in renal function occurs in approximately 20% of the patients on long term lithium therapy [147]. So it seems likely that at least in some susceptible individuals prolonged lithium administration results in chronic renal failure, although this is relatively rare.

Renal cysts

The predominant form of chronic renal disease associated with lithium therapy is chronic tubulointerstitial nephropathy (CTIN). Biopsy findings in patients with lithium induced CTIN include tubular atrophy and interstitial fibrosis interspread with tubular cysts and dilatations [99-103]. Infact, tubular dilatations and micro cysts are characteristic specific findings in lithium nephropathy [100]. In a study involving New Zealand white rabbits when treated with lithium developed a pattern of CTIN with tubular cysts that is virtually identical to human disease [101]. Various studies have shown that cysts are seen in 33-62.5% of the patients undergoing lithium therapy (100-103, 141,142](Figure 5). Cysts are found to be in both cortex and medulla particularly in the regions with extensive atrophy and fibrosis. They tend to be spare and do not normally exceed 1-2 mm diameter. Immunohistochemical and lectin staining revealed tubular cysts of predominantly distal tubular and collecting duct origin [100](Figure 6). In another study in France involving 74 patients with lithium nephropathy treated for 20 years, renal biopsy showed tubular cysts in 28% and tubular dilatation in 66% of the patients [142]. Tubular dilatation and cysts were more frequent in patients with longer duration of lithium therapy [142]. Various imaging modalities have been studied in the diagnosis of renal cysts. Studies have shown that MR imaging is highly capable of defining renal morphological features and has been demonstrated to be superior to US and CT scan for the visualization of small renal cysts [143]. One study involving 16 patients with renal insufficiency and clinical and biochemical evidence of lithium nephropathy concluded that these patients have normal sized kidney with very abundant uniformly and symmetrically distributed renal micro cysts [144]. This MR imaging pattern is very characteristic of lithium nephropathy and may aid in diagnosis in a patient with long standing lithium therapy [144]. (Figure 7,8).

Renal tubular acidosis

The administration of large doses of lithium to experimental animals consistently results in hyperchloremic metabolic acidosis and inability to normally lower urine pH, features that are characteristic of the distal form of renal tubular acidosis [88,89]. In humans on well-controlled lithium therapy, however, metabolic acidosis usually does not ensue. None of the 14 patients studied by us had metabolic acidosis, and they were all able to lower urine pH below 5.5 after the administration of ammonium chloride for three consecutive days [90]. The capacity of the collecting tubule to secrete hydrogen ions was examined further using the urine PCO_2 in highly alkaline urine as an index of urinary acidification. Urine PCO_2 examined as a function of urine bicarbonate concentration was found to be reduced in lithium-treated individuals. This defect was apparent in patients with near normal and in those with frankly reduced urine osmolality [25]. The findings of reduced urine PCO_2 was taken as evidence that lithium administration, at therapeutic doses, causes a mild distal acidification detect. Since metabolic acidosis did not spontaneously develop in these patients, it was proposed that lithium therapy results in a variant of incomplete distal renal tubular acidosis [90].In the turtle bladder, mucosal lithium inhibits hydrogen ion secretion by reducing the transepithelial electrical potential [92]. Laski and Kurtzman [92] investigated the effect of lithium on bicarbonate transport and transepithelial voltage in both the cortical collecting tubule and medullary collecting tubule. Acidification in the cortical collecting tubule is facilitated by the active reabsorption of sodium, which results in the formation of a transtubular voltage (lumen negative). When sodium reabsorption is inhibited acidification declines, and vice versa. If, however, sodium reabsorption is inhibited while the lumen is kept at a constant negative potential, acidification proceeds. This effect is seen in the cortical collecting tubule but not in the medullary collecting tubule where acidification occurs without active sodium absorption [93]. When lithium is substituted for sodium in the bath of isolated rabbit cortical collecting tubules, the potential difference decreases. This effect is associated with a reduction in the rate of bicarbonate (TCO_2) transport. In contrast, neither an effect on potential difference nor TCO_2 transport is seen in medullary collecting tubules exposed to lithium. Thus, this study demonstrated a nephron segment-specific site of action for lithium within the collecting tubule [93]. In a more recent study, Kurtzman's group has shown that lithium administration to rats also inhibits H^+/K^+ ATPase activity in the cortical but not in the medullary collecting tubule [93].

Hyperkalemia

The effects of lithium on potassium balance have

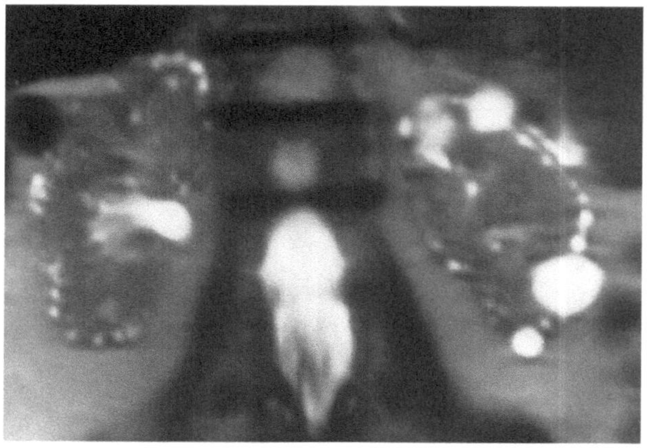

Figure 7. *Coronal half-Fourier single-shot turbo spin-echo MR image (10.9/87; flip angle, 180°) in a 73-year-old woman shows the predominance of the high-signal-intensity microcysts in the cortical regions.*
(Reproduced with permission from Farres et al [144]).

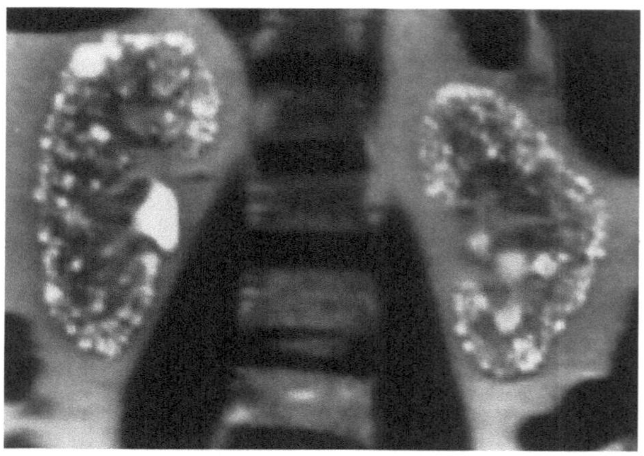

Figure 8. *Coronal half-Fourier single-shot turbo spin-echo MR image (10.9/87; flip angle, 180°) in a 68-year-old man shows very abundant microcysts in the cortical and medullary regions.*
(Reproduced with permission from Farres et al [144]).

not been well characterized. Galla et al. [94] suggested that distal potassium secretion is impaired in rats given lithium to produce high serum levels (2 to 5 mEq/L). We found similar results under acute potassium loading conditions [95]. Prior to potassium loading, however, potassium excretion was higher in lithium-treated rats than in controls. These two findings can be explained by postulating that potassium reabsorption in the proximal tubule is inhibited by lithium, while potassium secretion in the distal nephron is impaired. These two effects may offset each other so that plasma potassium does not need to change under ordinary conditions.

The inhibitory effect of lithium on distal potassium secretion is likely to occur in the cortical collecting tubule where it decreases Na^+ uptake and the transepithelial voltage (lumen-negative) that normally favors potassium secretion.

Usually neither hyperkalemia nor hypokalemia pose a problem for the management of lithium treated patients. However, in lithium-treated subjects given thiazide diuretic, hypokalemia often develops [97]. This is due to the diuretic-induced increase in sodium delivery to the collecting tubule combined with the lithium-induced increase in urine flow.

Hypothyroidism

It has been long recognized that prolonged lithium therapy can cause hypothyroidism. In fact, determination of serum thyroid-stimulating hormone once a year is recommended in all subjects on prolonged lithium therapy [32, 33]. Lithium perturbs receptor-mediated signaling events such as cyclic adenosine monophosphate and inositol phosphate accumulation [34]. These effects likely explain many hormonal side effects of lithium.

Hypercalcemia

Lithium can increase the Ca^{2+} set-point for inhibition of parathyroid hormone secretion during both *in vitro* and *in vivo* studies [35]. The calcium receptor plays a central role in calcium sensing by the parathyroid gland and other organs, including the brain. Chronic lithium therapy causes a significant alteration in calcium-sensing by the calcium receptor-expressing parathyroid chief cells through an unknown mechanism. As a result of this the parathyroid hormone set-point (the level of calcium that half-maximally suppresses parathyroid hormone secretion) is shifted to the right [35] (Figure 9). In other words, it takes a higher serum calcium concentration to inhibit parathyroid hormone secretion, a phenomenon known as a reset of the "set-point" [35, 36].

Hyperparathyroidism

A causal relationship between lithium treatment and hyperparathyroidism has been suggested [37]. Lithium seems to induce morphological changes in the parathyroid glands with an increase in parathyroid volume, and an increase in cellular DNA synthesis [37-39], which may explain why its effects may not be completely reversible. It is not rare to find patients with hypercalcemia, usually mild, after discontinuation of prolonged lithium therapy. A number of cases have been reported where hypercalcemia and hypocalciuria persisted even after discontinuation. We also have seen persistence of hypercalcemia and hyperparathyroidism several years after discontinuation of lithium therapy [Batlle et al unpublished, 2000].

However, the exact mechanism by which lithium induces such morphologic changes in the parathyroid tissues remain a mystery. Some studies suggest that a similar process occurs in those with familial hypercalcemic hypocalciuria (FHH), such that it is presumed that lithium interferes with the calcium-mediated

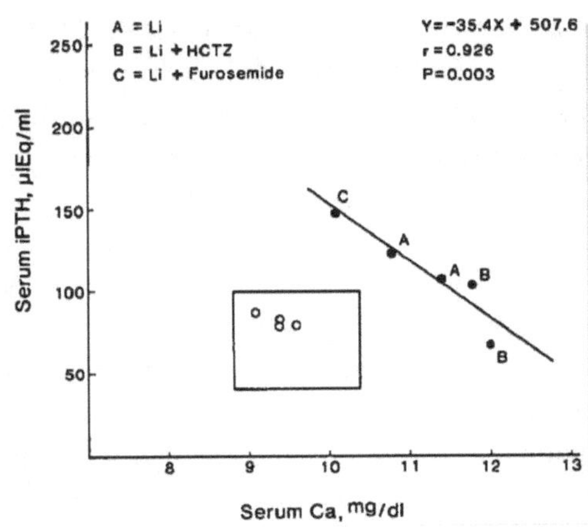

Figure 9. *Inverse correlation between serum calcium concentration and serum immunoreactive parathyroid hormone (iPTH) level when patient was on lithium (Li) treatment (solid line). The square denotes the normal range for serum calcium and iPTH. Solid circles denote when patient was taking lithium and open circles when lithium had been withdrawn. HCTZ = hydrochlorothiazide.*

transmembrane signal transduction by the calcium sensing receptor (CaSR), thereby increasing the set-point for inhibition of PTH release [40]. Furthermore, it is suggested that lithium occupies, but does not stimulate, the CaSR, thereby competitively inhibiting calcium from doing so. This leads to continued PTH secretion, which promotes bone resorption and release of calcium into the bloodstream. This competitive inhibition of the CaSR (in the ascending limb of the loop of Henle) can also interfere with the inhibitory effects of the potassium channels, thereby preventing further calcium reabsorption. On the otherhand, lithium could also directly stimulate PTH production by yet unknown mechanisms, e.g., interference with other parathyroid cell-surface receptors involved in the regulation of intracellular calcium levels [41]. Haven et al [42] suggested that perhaps, loss of tumor suppressor genes is behind such expression of parathyroid gland mutations and adenoma formations. Cinacalcet HCl. A calcimimetic agent and a known allosteric activator of the CaSR may play a role in the treatment of lithium associated renal disease. It is believed, that such allosteric activation of the CaSR, may either offset the receptor's affinity for lithium or magnify calcium mediated effects that can potentially override the effects induced by lithium. Much needs to be learned regarding the intricate interaction between lithium, cinacalcet HCl, and CaSR. To date, there are no known drug-drug interactions between lithium and cinacalcet HCl.

Most cases of lithium-induced hyperparathyroidism are mild [43]. Both pre-existing parathyroid abnormalities which may have been unmasked by lithium therapy and *de novo* hypercalcemia and hyperparathyroidism have been documented [44]. Parathyroid hyperplasia [33%] and adenomas [67%] were reported in one series of hypercalcemic patients treated with lithium [45]. Bilateral neck exploration has been proposed as an appropriate management approach because of a relatively high frequency of multi-gland involvement. However, parathyroid resection should be limited to those with overt disease [46].

Features of lithium-induced hyperparathyroidism include: a) a low urinary calcium excretion and the absence of nephrolithiasis; b) normal urinary cyclic adenosine monophosphate excretion; and c) normal plasma inorganic phosphate [32]. In lithium-induced hypercalcemia, a higher frequency of conduction defects has been noted [47]. Lithium also inhibits parathyroid hormone-mediated renal reabsorption of Ca^{2+} and Mg^{2+} and blunts parathyroid hormone–mediated phosphaturia [48]. Lithium interferes with the formation of renal cyclic adenosine monophosphate, which is regulated by parathyroid hormone. Levels of urinary cyclic adenosine monophosphate are typically normal in patients with elevated levels of parathyroid hormone related to lithium maintenance, rather than high, as in cases of primary hyperparathyroidism [32].

In lithium treated subjects, there is no evidence of reduced bone mass at any of the measured sites in relation to that of control subjects. The mechanism responsible for the maintenance of bone mass despite biochemical evidence of hyperparathyroidism is not clear [45]. We suspect that it is due to renal calcium retention. Indeed, in dogs lithium administration for only 3 days causes a striking decrease in urinary calcium excretion which is independent of the presence of parathyroid hormone and occurs despite the concurrent development of metabolic acidosis [Batlle D, Arruda J, and Kurtzman NA 1981 unpublished observations].

Nephrotic syndrome

Several case reports [129-136] have been published regarding the association of lithium with nephrotic syndrome in both adult and pediatric patients. Majority of the cases are due to minimal change disease, although there are some reports of focal segmental glomerulosclerosis as well. The mechanism by which lithium causes glomerular injury is not clearly understood. In general, in those with minimal change disease, the degree of proteinuria either resolves completely or partially within 1 to 4 weeks of discontinuation of lithium. Later re-institution of lithium led to recurrence of nephrosis. In some cases, requirement of subsequent corticosteroid therapy (aside from discontinuation of lithium) to achieve remission led to suggestions that perhaps lithium was not the underlying etiology.

The relationship to focal segmental glomerulosclerosis (FSGS) on the otherhand, has led to some questions. In majority of cases, cessation of lithium therapy did not translate into any improvement. It was therefore suggested, that either such cases were not due to lithium or were secondary forms of FSGS secondary to tubular injury brought about by chronic lithium therapy [136].

Edema

Demers, et al [137] described the observation of pretibial edema and sodium retention in lithium treated patients, in the absence of clear evidence of renal, hepatic or cardiac disease. The mechanism for such fluid retention remains unclear, but two plausible mechanisms have been suggested: an excessive sodium intake, perhaps related to the manic phase; and a lithium-induced reduction in maximum sodium excretory capacity which tends to be negligible when sodium intake is normal. Such patients manifested varying degrees of edema, combined with significantly increased urinary sodium > 200 mEqs/ day. Furthermore, due to increased urinary excretion of lithium, actual serum lithium levels may fall below therapeutic ranges, thereby leading to precipitation of manic crises. As volume expands, there is decreased reabsorption of sodium in the proximal tubules; similarly, since lithium is reabsorbed via the same channels and transporters as sodium, lithium reabsorption also decreases [11].

Perinatal/neonatal complications

Maternal lithium therapy may also endanger the fetus. Neonatal diabetes insipidus, hypothyroidism, cardiac dysfunction, respiratory difficulties, low muscle tone and lethargy have all been reported. Lithium has been shown to equilibrate completely across the placenta, with higher lithium concentrations at delivery associated with more perinatal complications [149].

Drug interactions

As can be expected, many drugs that interfere with renal function also influence lithium excretion. This and other drug interactions are listed in Table 1.

a. Diuretics. All diuretics cause a negative natrium balance and various degrees of contraction of the extracellular volume. The extent to which this occurs is dependent on the dose of the drug and the level of sodium intake. Extracellular volume contraction caused by thiazide diuretics predictably decreases lithium clearance by increasing proximal reabsorption. For clinical purposes, there is an important risk of causing lithium intoxication when diuretics are administered to patients on maintenance lithium therapy, and they should be given under close control of serum lithium levels or avoided altogether. Loop diuretics (furosemide, ethacrynic acid, torsemide and bumetanide) all have a powerful enhancing effect on lithium excretion. At their usual dosage they double lithium clearance when given acutely [8, 25]. This has been ascribed to the combined effect of increasing glomerular filtration rate and decreasing proximal reabsorption. Their marked effect, however, clearly suggests inhibition of lithium reabsorption in the loop of Henle as well. Recent micropuncture studies [14, 16] indicate that they inhibit 10-12% of filtered lithium reabsorption in this region. If lost salt and water are replaced concurrently these drugs have a role for treating lithium intoxication. Because of their short duration of action, this will be followed by a period of lithium retention which is dependent on the frequency of the dosage. The net effect may be no change in 24-hour lithium excretion.

Acetazolamide, and probably other diuretics which inhibit carbonic anhydrase, cause a strong inhibition of proximal $NaHCO_3$ reabsorption and lithium reabsorption. However, unlike loop diuretics, acetazolamide does not interfere with tubuloglomerular feedback and causes a 20% decrease in glomerular filtration rate. The increase in absolute lithium excretion is somewhat lower than that caused by loop diuretics [22]. Colussi et al. [25] reported the effect of furosemide and acetazolamide to be additive, indicating a dual site of action (i.e., inhibition of lithium reabsorption in both the proximal tubule and the loop of Henle).

Table 1. Drug interactions with lithium.

Drug	Effect on serum lithium concentration
Thiazide diuretics	Increase
Acetazolamide and other carbonic anhydrase inhibitors	Decrease*
Osmotic diuretics	Decrease
K^+ Sparing	Minimal decrease or no effect
Methyl xanthine inhibitors	Decrease
Loop diuretics	Decrease*
ACE inhibitors	Increase
NSAIDs:	
Indomethacin	Increase
Ibuprofen	Increase
Mefenamic acid	Increase
Naproxen	Increase
Sulindac	No effect
Aspirin	No effect

** When given acutely for lithium intoxication.*

Thiazide diuretics predictably increase serum lithium levels. However, they differ among themselves in that they may or may not have a carbonic anhydrase inhibitory action. Those which have such an activity, e.g. chlorothiazide, inhibit proximal reabsorption and thus may increase lithium excretion, at least when given acutely. Those devoid of such an effect (such as bendroflumethiazide) may not change lithium clearance [22]. Potassium-sparing drugs (spironolactone, triamterene and amiloride) have no obvious action on lithium excretion in humans. Amiloride enhances lithium excretion in rats and dogs only during sodium restriction under conditions, where natrium uptake by distal tubule is more abbit. In humans, however, no effect has been reported even when natrium retention was severe [12]. However, small changes in distal and cortical collecting tubule lithium reabsorption could easily be missed by clearance studies. Amiloride seems to prevent lithium uptake in the cortical collecting tubule [26].

b. Antihypertensives. Angiotensin II and noradrenaline infusions reduce lithium excretion [27]. Although no systematic experimental studies or controlled clinical observations are available, lithium is known to activate the renin-angiotensin system through several mechanisms. This effect can be reversed by angiotensin converting enzyme inhibitors (ACE-I). When given alone, however, converting enzyme inhibitors have little influence on lithium excretion. Anecdotal observations suggest that renal dysfunction may occur when unadjusted doses of angiotensin converting enzyme inhibitors are administered to patients on long-term lithium treatment [27]. Potential mechanisms involved in this are: a) Lithium causing volume loss and activation of RAS by interfering with H_2O reabsorption and to a lesser extent Na^+; b) Effects of lithium on cellular events including reduced specific angiotensin II binding, inhibition of sympathetic transmission and phosphatidylinositol signaling [27]. In addition, direct interactions between lithium and angiotensin II may take place at a cellular level.

Renal function should be closely monitored when patients on lithium treatment are given ACE-I. Doses of both drugs should be chosen with caution to avoid serious drug interaction [27].

c. NSAIDs. These drugs, in particular indomethacin, have a depressing effect on lithium clearance which is enhanced by salt restriction [28]. Micropuncture studies showed that an additional 13% reabsorption of filtered lithium is caused by these drugs, probably half of it in the thick ascending limb, the rest in the thin limb of Henle [17]. Therefore, when drugs of this group are given to patients on lithium treatment, close control of blood levels is recommended.

d. Cyclosporine. Of some practical importance is the finding that cyclosporine decreases lithium clearance. This likely reflects enhanced proximal fluid reabsorption secondary to vasoconstriction caused by this drug.

e. Ethylene glycol. A protective effect of lithium carbonate has been suggested in patients who were treated for ethylene glycol toxicity. Leon [29] reported a case of severe ethylene glycol poisoning who did not manifest with severe acidosis, contrary to what was expected. It was postulated that concomitant ingestion of 80 tablets of lithium carbonate, amounting to 320 mEqs of bicarbonate load, had a serendipitous protective effect.

f. N-Acetylcysteine. Efrati et al [30] showed that co-administration of N-acetylcysteine (NAC) during lithium chloride therapy had a significant renoprotective effect in a rat model of lithium-induced renal failure. Those rats treated with lithium and NAC had normal appearing glomeruli and basement membrane without signs of cellular proliferation. Although tubular damage was demonstrated in both treated and non-treated groups, the authors noted significantly fewer tubular dilatations, and less swelling of tubular cells; and also less tubular luminal obstructions in the NAC group. It remains to be seen whether such positive findings would also be demonstrated in human subjects.

Clinical conditions that affect lithium metabolism

a. Volume status. Salt intake is an important determinant of lithium excretion. Acute as well as chronic NaCl loading increases absolute as well as fractional lithium clearance, while salt restriction causes a marked decrease. Upright posture and tilt also cause a decrease in absolute as well as fractional lithium excretion, while head-out water immersion increases it.

These investigations of lithium handling by the kidneys have provided information which is useful for prevention and treatment of lithium intoxication. In general, all conditions associated with salt depletion strongly impair renal capacity to eliminate lithium.

Abnormal values of fractional lithium excretion have been reported in a variety of conditions. In hyperthyroidism and Bartter's syndrome fractional lithium clearance is increased. After unilateral nephrectomy, lithium clearance by the remaining kidney increases. After two weeks, fractional lithium clearance returns to normal. Rombola et al. [8] reported markedly increased fractional lithium clearance values in patients with Fanconi syndrome, renal glycosuria, and hypercalciuria.

b. Pregnancy. After investigations in animals suggested the potential of lithium to disrupt embryonic development, questions arose regarding the safety of lithium in human pregnancy [31]. These concerns emerged as data from anecdotal case descriptions and a registry of infants born to women treated with lithium during pregnancy indicated that such treatment might pose a substantial risk of cardiovascular anomalies. More recent controlled epidemiologic investigations demonstrate that most women who are treated with lithium during pregnancy have normal infants and that the risk to the fetus is less than previously believed. This more modest risk estimate may have a dramatic effect on clinical management of women with bipolar disorder, given the morbidity associated with discontinuation of lithium therapy [31].

c. Lithium intoxication

Symptoms of lithium toxicity can be expected when serum lithium level increases above 1.5 mEq/L. Most patients receiving lithium have side effects, reflecting the drug's narrow therapeutic index [1]. Many symptoms and signs of toxicity correlate with serum lithium concentrations (Table 2). The amount of lithium inside the cells, however, may be more predictable for lithium toxicity. Equilibration between intra- and extracellular lithium occurs rather slowly. Therefore intoxication develops more easily during chronic therapy, while after an acute high intake symptoms may be less despite higher serum levels.

Typical symptoms of lithium intoxication are summarized in Table 2 [122-127]. The clinical picture of lithium intoxication is dominated by neuromuscular and cerebral symptoms: in mild cases apathy, muscle weakness, tremor, and unsteady gait are seen. In more severe cases speech disturbances, myoclonic twitching, coma and convulsion can occur. Pulse irregularities and circulatory collapse may supervene. Lithium often causes T-wave flattening or inversion on the electrocardiogram, but clinically important cardiovascular effects are rare, with sinus-node dysfunction reported most often [123]. Residual neurological sequelae consisting of cerebellar dysfunction with ataxia, neuropathy and supra-bulbar symptoms are not unusual.

As discussed above, lithium inhibits the synthesis of thyroid hormone and its release from the thyroid, and stimulates the formation of antithyroid antibodies in susceptible subjects [122]. Lithium-induced hypothyroidism responds to thyroxine therapy. Lithium

Table 2. Clinical symptomatology associated with lithium poisoning.

Organ system	Acute poisoning	Chronic poisoning
Endocrine	None	Hypothyroidism, hyperparathyroidism
Gastrointestinal	Nausea, vomiting	Minimal
Heart	Prolonged QT interval ST and T wave changes	Myocarditis
Hematological	Leukocytosis	Aplastic anemia
Neurological		
a. Mild	Fine tremors, lightheadedness, weakness	Same
b. Moderate	Apathy, drowsiness, hyper-reflexia, muscle twitching, slurred speech, tinnitus	Same
c. Severe	Choroathetoid movements, clonus, coma, confusion, muscle irritability, seizures	Memory deficits, Parkinson's disease, pseudo-tumor cerebri, psychosis
Neuromuscular	Myopathy, peripheral neuropathy	Same
Renal	Urine concentrating defect	Chronic interstitial nephritis, nephrogenic diabetes insipidus, ESRD (rare)
Skin	None	Dermatitis, localized edema, ulcers

can increase the secretion of parathyroid hormone and therefore can increase serum calcium concentrations, but symptomatic hypercalcemia is rare.

Acute renal insufficiency with or without oliguria can occur, usually in association with severe volume depletion in, which case renal function is rapidly restored with appropriate fluid therapy. The picture may resemble that of acute tubular necrosis but prerenal failure seems more likely. Histological biopsy findings show remarkably few abnormalities.

Lithium poisoning can be categorized into two groups:

(1) Acute poisoning, in patients who are not actually being treated for lithium, but have obtained the medication either voluntarily (e.g. suicide attempts) or involuntarily (e.g. accidental childhood mishaps). Usually, these patients have an excellent prognosis as a result of normal baseline renal functioning, hence not interfering with the renal elimination of lithium.

(2) Acute on top of chronic poisoning occurs in individuals who have been on a chronic lithium prescription, and who in one way or another ingest an overdose of the lithium, or are given medications that increase lithium levels. Conditions where sodium conservation is stimulated, such as low salt intake, loss of body fluid by way of vomiting, diarrhea, or use of diuretics which decrease lithium clearance (thiazides) are usually the precipitating factors.

The polyuria which often accompanies lithium treatment is normally compensated for by drinking water, but when consciousness is impaired severe hypernatremia may develop. When any acute illness (particularly if associated with gastrointestinal symptoms) occurs or when new medication is given, lithium blood levels should be closely monitored, and the lithium dose adjusted.

Management of lithium intoxication

Regardless of the manner of presentation, the initial management is the same. If the patient presents with mental status changes (e.g. decreased consciousness), an oral airway must be secured in the immediate instance. Volume status should be assessed and isotonic saline administered for volume repletion. A serum lithium level and a serum chemistry panel (serum sodium, potassium, chloride, CO_2, BUN and creatinine, and calcium) should be drawn immediately to assess the degree or level of intoxication, as well as underlying renal function.

Volume resuscitation is the cornerstone of management of lithium toxicity (Table 3) [124, 125]. Patients with underlying lithium-induced diabetes insipidus may initially present with volume depletion. It must be borne in mind, however, that hypernatremia [125] is a potential complication, especially in those with underlying diabetes insipidus. Forced saline diuresis is expected to increase lithium clearance by decreasing proximal tubular reabsorption. With normal renal function, lithium can be cleared at a rate of 10-40 mL/min [125]. The excretion of lithium can be further increased acutely by using acetazolamide and/or loop diuretics [124,125].

Peritoneal dialysis clears only 9-15 mL/min of lithium, and is therefore not recommended for the treatment of acute lithium toxicity [125,126]. Conventional hemodialysis, on the other hand, decreases serum lithium levels at a rate of 1 mEq/L with every 4 hours of treatment [126]. Several treatment sessions of hemodialysis may be required, and serum lithium levels need to be checked frequently even after hemodialysis, because of the shifting of lithium from inside the cells (lithium rebound phenomenon). In those patients who may have ingested the sustained-release form of lithium, continued absorption from the GI tract may cause a rise in serum lithium levels between hemodialysis sessions [128].

Continuous arteriovenous hemodialysis and continu-

Table 3. Management of lithium intoxication.

1. Protect oral airway if consciousness is impaired
2. Volume resuscitation
3. Gastric lavage, whole bowel irrigation with polythene glycol to prevent continued absorption of lithium
4. Lithium removal: • Serum lithium level>3.5-4 mEq/L: most patients require hemodialysis. • Serum lithium level 2-4 mEq/L: unstable patients and patients with severe nephrogenic signs of renal insufficiency require hemodialysis. • Serum lithium levels 1.5-2.5 mEq/L: hemodialysis indicated for patients with renal failure or if patient fails to reach a lithium level below 1 mEq/L. Fluid therapy or forced diuresis treatment should be recommended in patients with early signs of lithium intoxication and normal renal function, and when it is known that lithium levels have been elevated for only a few days.

ous venovenous hemodialysis can clear 60-85 L per day of lithium [129]. The main advantage of this treatment is that it decreases chances of lithium rebound. The disadvantages pertain to the fact that such continuous therapies do not reduce levels as quickly as hemodialysis and are often limited by the need for anticoagulation.

References

1. Price LH, Heininger GR. Lithium in the treatment of mood disorders. N Engl J Med 1994; 331: 591-598.
2. Batlle D, Dorhout-Mees EJ. Lithium and the kidney. In: Clinical Nephrotoxins - renal injury from drugs and chemicals. De Broe ME, Porter GA, Bennett WM, Verpooten GA (editors). Kluwer Academic Publ, Dordrecht 1998; p. 383-395.
3. Terao T, Okuno K, Okuno T, Nakano H, Shinkai T, Ohmori O, Yoshimura R, Suzuki T, Abe K. A simpler and more accurate equation to predict daily lithium dose. J Clin Psychopharmacol 1999; 19(4): 336-340.
4. Stoll PM, Stokes PE, Okamoto M. Lithium isotopes: differential effects on renal function and histology. Bipolar Disorders 2001; 3: 174-180.
5. Ng LL, Quinn PA, Paulene A, Baker F, Carr SJ. Red cell Na/Li countertransport and Na/H exchanger isoforms in human proximal tubules. Kidney Int 2000; 58(1): 229-235.
6. Thomsen K, Schou M, Steiness I, Hansen E. Lithium as an indicator of proximal tubular reabsorption. Pflugers Arch 1969; 308: 180-184.
7. Navar LG, Schafer JA. Comments on lithium clearance: a new research area. News Physiol Sci 1987; 2: 34-35.
8. Rombola G, DeFerrari Colussi G ME, Surian M, Malberti F, Minetti L. Clinical evaluation of segmental tubular reabsorption of sodium and fluid in man: lithium vs free water clearance. Nephrol Dial Transplant 1987; 2: 212-218.
9. Boer WH, Koomans HA, Dorhout Mees EJ. Lithium clearance in healthy humans suggesting lithium reabsorption beyond the proximal tubules. Kidney Int 1990; 37 (suppl 28): 39-44.
10. Godinich MJ, Batlle DC. Renal tubular effects of lithium. Kidney Int 1990; 37 (suppl 28): S52-S57.
11. Boron R, Gaviria M, Batlle DC. Prevalence, pathogenesis, and treatment of renal dysfunction associated with chronic lithium therapy. Am J Kidney Dis 1987; 10(5): 329-345.
12. Hayslett IP, Kashgarian M. A micropuncture study of the renal handling of lithium. Plugers Arch 1979; 380: 159-163.
13. Leyssac PP, Holstein-Rathlou NH, Skott P, Alfrey AC. A micropuncture study of proximal tubular transport of lithium during osmotic diuresis. Am J Physiol 1990; 258: F1090-F1095.
14. Shirley DG, Walter SJ, Sampson B. A micropuncture study of renal lithium reabsorption; effects of amiloride and furosemide. Am J Physiol 1992; 263: F1128-F1133.
15. Fransen R, Boer WH, Boer P, Koomans HA. Amiloride sensitive lithium reabsorption in rats; a micropuncture study. J Pharmacol Exp Therapy 1992; 263: 646-650.
16. Fransen R, Boer WH, Boer P, Dorhout Mees EJ, Koomans HA. Effects of furosemide or acetazolamide infusion on renal handling of lithium; a micropuncture study in rats. Am J Physiol 1993; 264: 129-34.
17. Boer WH, Fransen R, Boer P, Roos R de, Koomans HA. Prostaglandin synthesis inhibition stimulates lithium reabsorption in Henle's loop in rats. Kidney Int 1993; 43: 301-306.
18. Koomans HA, Boer WH, Dorhout Mees EJ. Evaluation of lithium clearance as a marker of proximal tubule sodium handling. Kidney Int 1989; 36: 2-12.
19. Kirchner KA. Lithium as a marker for proximal tubular delivery during low salt uptake and diuretic infusion. Am J Physiol 1987; 253: F188-F196.
20. Greger R. Possible sites of lithium transport in the nephron. Kidney Int. 1990; 37 (suppl 28): S26-S30.
21. Imai M, Isozaki T, Yasoshima K, Yoshitomi K. Permeability characteristics and probability of lithium transport in the thin limbs of Henle's loop. Kidney Int 1990; 37 (suppl 28): S31-S35.
22. Atherton JC, Green R, Higgins A. Large A, McNicholas C, Parker D. Pempkowiak L, Rajani K, Smith J. Lithium clearance in healthy humans: effects of sodium intake and diuretics. Kidney Int. 1990; 37 (suppl 28): 36-38.
23. Shalmi M, Jonassen T, Thomsen K, Kibble JD, Bie P, Christensen S. Am J Physiol 1998; 274 (Renal Physiol 43): F445-F452.
24. Boer WH, Koomans HA, Beutler JJ. Gaillard CA, Rabelink AJ, Dorhout Mees EJ. Small intra- and large inter-individual variability in lithium clearance in humans. Kidney Int 1989; 35: 1183-1188.
25. Colussi G, Rombola G, Surian M, DeFerrari ME, Airaghi C. Benazzi E, Malberti F, Minetti L. Lithium clearances in humans: effects of acute administration of acetazolamide and furosemide. Kidney Int 1990; 39 (suppl 28): S63-S66.
26. Batlle DC, Von Riotte AB, Gaviari M, Grupp M. Amelioration of polyuria by amiloride in patients receiving long-term lithium therapy. N Engl J Med 1985; 312: 409-414.

27. Lehmann K, Ritz E. Angiotensin-converting enzyme inhibitors may cause renal dysfunction in patients on long-term lithium treatment. Am J Kidney Dis. 1995; 25: 82-87.
28. Ragheb M. The clinical significance of lithium non-steroidal anti-inflammatory drug interactions. J Clin Psychopharmacol 1990; 10: 350-354.
29. Leon M, Graeber C. Absence of high anion gap metabolic acidosis in severe ethylene glycol poisoning: A potential effect of simultaneous lithium carbonate ingestion. Am J Kidney Dis 1994; 23: 313-316.
30. Efrati S, Averbukh M, Berman S, et al. N-Acetylcysteine ameliorates lithium-induced renal failure in rats. Nephrol Dial Transplant 2004. 20; 1: 65-70.
31. Cohen LS, Friedman JM, Jefferson JW, Johnson EM, Weiner ML. A re-evaluation of risk of in utero exposure to lithium. JAMA 1994; 271: 146-150.
32. Stancer HC, Forbath N. Hyperparathyroidism, hypothyroidism, and impaired renal function after 10 to 20 years of lithium treatment. Arch Intern Med 1989; 149: 1042-1045.
33. Schou M, Dr. H C Mull. Forty years of lithium treatment. Arch Gen Psychol 1997; 54(1): 9-13.
34. Racke F, McHenry C, Wentworth D. Lithium-induced alterations in parathyroid cell function: insight into the pathogenesis of lithium-associated hyperparathyroidism. Am J Surg 1994; 168(5): 462-465.
35. Shen F-H, Sherrad DJ. Lithium-induced hyperparathyroidism: an alteration of the "set-point". Ann Int Med 1982; 96(1): 63-65.
36. Haden ST, Brown EM, Stoll AL, Scott J, El-Hajj F, Ghada. The effect of lithium on calcium-induced changes in adrenocorticotrophin levels. J Clin Endocrin Met 1999; 84(1): 198-200.
37. Bendz H, Sjodin I, Toss G, Berglund K. Hyperparathyroidism and long term effects of lithium therapy - a cross-sectional study and the effect of lithium withdrawal. J Int Med 1996; 240: 357-365.
38. Saxe AW, Gibson G. Lithium increase tritiated thymidine by abnormal human parathyroid tissue. Surgery 1991; 110: 1067-1077.
39. Saxe AW, Gibson G, Silvera E. Effects of long-term lithium infusion on normal parathyroid. Surgery 1995; 117: 577-580.
40. McHenry CR, Lee K: Lithium therapy and disorders of the parathyroid glands. Endocr Pract 2: 103-109, 1996.
41. Hershfinkel M, Moran A, Grossman N, Sekler I: A zinc-sensing receptors triggers the release of intracellular calcium and regulated ion transport. Proc Natl Acad Sci 98: 11749-11754, 2001.
42. Haven CJ, Howell VM, Eilers PH, et al: A mouase model of human familial hypocalciuric hypercalcemia and neonatal severe hyperparathyroidism. Nat Genet 11: 389-394, 1995.
43. Wolff ME, Moffat M, Dempsey S. Lithium therapy, hypercalcemia, and hyperparathyroidism. Am J Therap 1997; 4: 323-325.
44. McHenry C, Stenger D, Racke F. Investigation of calcium-induced hydrolysis of Phosphoinositedes in normal and lithium treated parathyroid cells. Am J Surgery 1995; 170 (5): 484-487.
45. Nordenstrom J, Elvius M., Zhao B, Torring O. Biochemical hyperparathyroidism and bone mineral status in patients treated long-term with lithium. Metabolism 1994; 43(12): 1563-1567.
46. Abdullah H, Bliss R, Guinea AI, Delbridge L. Pathology and outcome of surgical treatment for lithium-associated hyperparathyroidism. Brit J Surgery 1999; 86(1): 91-93.
47. Wolf EM, Ranade V, Molnar J, Somberg J, Mosnaim A. Hypercalcemia, arrhythmia and mood stabilizers. J Clin Psychopharmacol 2000; 20(2): 260-264.
48. Carney S, Jackson P. Acute effect of lithium administration on renal Ca, Mg, and PO_4 transport in the rat. Kidney Int 1996; 50(4): 1406.
49. Singer I, Rottenberg D, Puschett IB. Lithium-induced nephrogenic diabetes insipidus: *in vivo* and *in vitro* studies. J Clin Invest 1972; 51: 1081-1091.
50. Singer I, Franko EA. Lithium-induced ADH resistance in toad bladders. Kidney Int 1973; 3: 151-159.
51. Forrest J Jr, Cohen AD, Torretti J, Himmelhoch JM, Epstein FH. On the mechanism of lithium-induced diabetes insipidus in man and the rat. J Clin Invest 1974; 53: 115-123.
52. Martinez-Maldonado M, Stravroulaki-Tsapar A, Tsaparas N. Renal effects of lithium administration in rats: alterations in water and electrolyte metabolism and the response to vasopressin and cyclic adenosine monophosphate during prolonged administration. J Lab Clin Med 1975; 86: 445-461.
53. Fernandez-Repollet E, LeFurgey A, Hardy MA, Tisher CC. Structural and functional response of toad urinary bladder of LiCi. Kidney Int 1983; 24: 719-730.
54. Harris CA, Jenner FA. Some aspects of the inhibition of the action of antidiuretic hormone by lithium ions in the rat kidney and bladder of the toad *Bufo marinus*. Brit J Pharmacol 1972; 44: 223-232.
55. Cogan E, Abramow M. Inhibition by lithium of the hydro-osmotic action of vasopressin in the isolated perfused conical collecting tubule of the rabbit. J Clin Invest 1986; 77: 1507-1514.

56. Christiensen S, Kusano E, Yusufi ANK. Pathogenesis of nephrogenic diabetes insipidus due to chronic administration of lithium in rats. J Clin Invest 1985; 75: 1869-1879.
57. Dousa TP, Barnes LD. Lithium-induced diuretic effect of antidiuretic hormone in rats. Am J Physiol 1976; 231: 1754-1759.
58. Jackson BA, Edwards RM, Dousa TR. Lithium-induced polyuria: effect of lithium on adenylate cyclate and adenosine 3'5' monophosphate phosphodisterase in medullary ascending limb of Henle's loop and in medullary collecting tubules. Endocrinol 1980; 107(6): 1693-1698.
59. Yamaki M, Kusano E, Homma S. Cellular mechanisms of lithium induced nephrogenic diabetes insipidus. Am Soc Nephrol 1989; 404A.
60. Kwon TH, Laursen UH, Marples D. Altered expression of renal AQP2s and Na^+ transporters in rats with lithium induced NDI. Am J Physiol 2000; 279:F552-F564.
61. Nielsen J, Hoffert JD, Knepper MA, Agre P, Nielsen S, Fenton RA . Proteomic analysis of lithium-induced nephrogenic diabetes insipidus:mechanisms for aquaporin 2 down-regulation and cellular proliferation.Proc Natl Acad Sci U S A.2008 Mar 4;105(9):3634-9.
62. Michimata M, Fujita S, Araki T, Mizukami K, Kazama I, Muramatsu Y, Suzuki M, kimura T, Sasaki Ss, Imai Y, Matsubara M. Reverse pharmacological effect of loop diuretics and altered rBSC1 expression in rats with lithium nephropathy. Kidney Int 2003;63(1):165-171.
63. Agre P, Preston GM, Smith BL, Neilsen S. Aquaporin CHIP: the archetypal molecular water channel. Am J Physiol 1993; 265: F463-F476.
64. Nielsen S, Marples D, Knepper M, Agre P. The Aquaporin family of water channels in the kidney: An update on physiology and pathophysiology of Aquaporin-2. Kidney Int 1996; 49: 1718-1723.
65. Fushimik Fushimi K, Uchida S, Hara Y, Hirata Y, Marumo F, Sasaki S. Cloning and expression of apical membrane water channel of rat kidney collecting tubule. Nature 1993; 361(6412): 549-552.
66. Marples D, Christensen S, Oltosen P, Nielsen S. Lithium-induced Down-regulation of Aquaporin -2 water channel experession in the rat kidney medulla. J Clin Invest 1995; 95 (4): 1838-1845.
67. Walker RG, Bennett WM, Davies BM. Structural and functional aspects of long-term lithium therapy. Kidney Int 1982; 21: 513-519.
68. Albrecht J, Kampf D, Muller-Oerlinghausen B. Renal function and biopsy in patients on lithium therapy. Pharmako-psychiatne 1980; 13: 228-234.
69. Bendz H, Andersch S, Aurell M. Kidney function in an unselected lithium population. A cross-sectional study. Acta Psychiatry Scand 1983; 68: 325-334.
70. Lokkegaard H, Anderson HF, Henriksen E, Bartels PD, Brahm M, Baastrup PC, Jorgensen HE, Larsen M. Munck O, Rasmussen K. Renal function in 153 manic depressive patients treated with lithium for more than five years. Acta Psychiatry Scand 1985; 71: 347-355.
71. Baylis PH, Heath DA. Water disturbances in patients treated with oral lithium carbonate. Ann Intern Med 1978; 88: 607-609.
72. Uldall PR, Awad AG, McCormick WO, Caner LB, Gonsick T, Grass CL, Kugelmass ML. Renal function in patients receiving long-term lithium therapy. Can Med Assoc J 1981; 124(11): 1471-1474.
73. Wahlin A, Bucht G, Von Knorring L, Smigan L. Kidney function in patients with affective disorders with and without lithium therapy. Pharmacopsych 1980; 15: 253-259.
74. Wallin L, Aling C, Aurell M. Impairment of renal function in patients on long-term lithium treatment. Clin Nephrol 1982; 18: 23-28.
75. Donker AJM, Prins E, Meijer S, Sluiter W, Van Berkestijn JW, Dols LC. A renal function study in 30 patients on long-term lithium therapy. Clin Nephrol 1979; 12: 254-262.
76. Vestergaard R, Amdisen A, Hansen AE, Schou M. Lithium treatment and kidney function. Acta Psychiatry Scan 1979; 60: 504-520.
77. Johnson GF, Hunt G, Duggin GG, Horvath JJ, Tiller DJ. Renal function and lithium treatment: initial and follow up tests in manic-depressive patients. J Affective Disord 1984; 6: 249-263.
78. Coppen A, Bishop ME, Bailey JE, Cattell WR, Price RG. Renal function in lithium and non-lithium treated patients with affective disorders. Acta Psychiatry Scand 1980; 62: 343-355.
79. Grof P, MacCrimmon DJ, Smith EKM, Daigle L, Saxena B, Varma R, Grof E, Keitner G, Kenny J. Long-term lithium treatment and the kidney. Can J Psychiatry 1980; 25: 535-544.
80. Jorgensen F, Larsen S, Spanager E, Clausen E, Tango M, Brinch E, Brun C. Kidney function and quantitative histological changes in patients on long-term lithium therapy. Acta Psychiatry Scand 1984; 70: 455-462.
81. Rabin EZ, Garston RG, Weir RV, Posen GA. Persistent nephrogenic diabetes insipidus associated with long term lithium carbonate treatment. Can Med Assoc J 1979; 121(2): 194-198.

82. Lee R, Jampol L, Brown W. Nephrogenic diabetes insipidus and lithium intoxication: complications of lithium carbonate therapy. N Engl J Med 1971; 284: 93-94.
83. Simon NM, Garber E, Arieff AJ. Persistent nephrogenic diabetes insipidus after lithium carbonate. Ann Intern Med 1977; 86: 446-447.
84. Hansen HE, Hestbech J, Olsen S, Amdisen A. Renal function and renal pathology in patients with lithium induced impairment of renal concentrating ability. Proc EDTA 1977; 14: 518-527.
85. Price TRP, Beisswenger PJ. Lithium and diabetes insipidus. Ann Int Med 1989; 88: 576-577.
86. Forrest J Jr. Lithium-induced polyuria: cellular mechanisms and response to diuretics. In: Lithium - controversies and unresolved issues. Cooper TB, Gershon S, Kline NS (editors). Excerpta Medica, Amsterdam 1979; p. 632-641.
87. Bucht G, Wahlin A. Renal concentration capacity in long-term lithium treatment and after withdrawal of lithium. Acta Med Scand 1980; 207: 309-314.
88. Nascimento L, Rademacher D, Hamburger R, Arruda JA, Kurtzman A. On the mechanism of lithium-induced renal tubular acidosis. J Lab Clin Med 1977; 89: 455-462.
89. Mehta PK. Sodhi B, Arruda JAL, Kunzman NA. Interaction of amiloride and lithium on distal urinary acidificalion. J Lab Clin Med 1979; 93: 93-94.
90. Batlle DC, Gaviria M, Grupp M. Distal nephron function in patients receiving chronic lithium therapy. Kidney Int 1982; 21: 477-485.
91. Arruda JAL, Dytko G, Mola R. Kurtzman NA. On the mechanism of lithium-induced renal tubular acidosis; studies in the turtle bladder. Kidney Int 1980; 17: 196-204.
92. Laski ME, Kurtzman NA. Characterization of acidification in the cortical and medullary collecting tubule of the rabbit. J Clin Invest 1983; 72: 2050-2059.
93. Eiam-Ong B, Dafnis E, Spohn M, Kurtzman NA, Sabatini S. H/K/ATpase in distal renal tubular acidosis: urinary tract obstraction, lithium, and amiloride. Am J Physiol 1993; 265 (6Pt2): F675-F680.
94. Galla JN, Forrest JN, Hecht B, Kashgarian M, Hayslett JP. Effect of lithium on water and electrolyte metabolism. Yale J Biol Med 1975; 48: 305-314.
95. Batlle DC, Tarka J, Kurtzman NA. Renal handling of potassium after chronic lithium administration. Clin Res 1983; 31: 424A.
96. Jefferson JW. Potassium supplementation in lithium patients: a timely intervention or premature speculation ? J Clin Psychiatry 1992; 53: 370.
97. Hestbech J, Hansen H, Amdisen A, Olsen S. Chronic renal lesions following long-term treatment with lithium. Kidney Int 1977; 12: 205-213.
98. Hansen HE, Hestbech J, Sorenson JL, Norgaard K, Heilskov J, Amdisen A. Chronic interstitial nephropathy in patients with long term treatment. Q J Med 1979; 192: 577-591.
99. Aurell M, Svalander C, Wallin L, Alling G. Renal function and biopsy finding in patients on long-term lithium treatment. Kidney Int. 1981; 20: 663-670.
100. Markowitz GS, Radhakrishnan J, Kambhaam N, Valer AM, Hines WH, D'Agati VD. J Am Soc Nephrol 2000; 11: 1439-1448.
101. Walker RG, Escott M, Birchall J, Dowling JP, Kincaid-Smith P. Chronic progressive renal lesions induced by lithium. Kidney Int 1986; 29: 875-881.
102. Walker RG, Davies BM, Holwill BJ. A chronic pathological study of lithium nephrotoxicity. J Chro Dis 1982; 35: 655-695.
103. Rafaelson OJ, Bolwig TG, Ladefoged J. Kidney function and morphology in long-term lithium treatment. In: Lithium. Cooper TB, Gershon S, Kline NS (editors). pta Medica 1979; p. 578-583.
104. Davies B, Kincaid-Smith P. Renal biopsy studies of lithium and pre-lithium patients and comparison with cadaver transplant kidneys. Neuropharmacol 1979; 18: 1001-1002.
105. Walker RG, Dowling JF, Alcorn D, Ryan GB, Kincaid-Smith P. Renal pathology associated with lithium therapy. Pathology 1983; 15: 403-11.
106. Kincaid-Smith P, Burrows GD, Davies BM. Renal biopsy findings in lithium and pre-lithium patients. Lancet 1979; 2: 700-701.
107. Burrows GD, David B, Kincaid-Smith P. Unique tubular lesion after lithium. Lancet 1978; 1: 1210.
108. McAuliffe WG, Olesen OV. Effects of lithium on the structure of the rat kidney. Nephron 1983; 34: 114-124.
109. Ottosen PD, Sign B, Kristensen J, Olsen S, Christensen S. Lithium-induced interstitial nephropathy associated with chronic renal failure. Reversibility and correlation between functional and structural changes. Acta Pathol Microbiol Immunol Scand 1984; 92: 447-454.
110. Min G, Christensen S, Marcussen N, Osterby R. Glomerular structure in lithium-induced chronic renal failure in rats. APMIS 2000; 108: 652-62.
111. Gerner RH, Psarras J, Kirschenbaum MA. Results of the clinical renal function tests in lithium patients. Am J Psychiatry 1980; 137: 834-837.

112. Hullin RP, Coley VP, Birch NJ, Thomas TH, Morgan DB. Renal function after long-term treatment with lithium. Brit Med J 1979; 1: 1457-1459.
113. Thysell H, Brante G, Sjostedt L, Lindergard B, Lindholm T, Franzen G, Rorsman B. Glomerular filtration rate and calcium metabolism in long-term lithium treatment. Neuropsychobiol 1981; 7: 105-111.
114. Depaulo JR Jr, Correa EJ, Sapir DG. Renal glomerular function and long-term lithium therapy. Am J Psychiatry 1981; 138: 324-327.
115. Halgren R, Alm PO, Hellsing K. Renal function in patients on lithium treatment. Brit J Psychiatry 1979; 135: 22-27.
116. Hestbech J, Aurell M. Lithium-induced uremia. Lancet 1979; 1: 212-213.
117. Nue C, Manschreck TC, Flockx JM. Renal damage associated with long-term use of lithium carbonate. J Clin Invest 1979; 40: 460-463.
118. Vestergaard P. Lithium-induced uremia ? Lancet 1979; 1: 491.
119. Chugh S, Yager H. End stage renal diseases after treatment with lithium. J Clin. Psychopharmacol 1997; 17 (6): 495-497.
120. Von Knorring K, Wahlin A, Nystrom K, Bohman SO. Urema induced by long term lithium treatment. Lithium 1990; 1: 251-253.
121. Lazarus JH. Endocrine and metabolic effects of lithium. New York: Plenum Medical, 1986.
122. Mitchell JE, Mackenzie TB. Cardiac effects of lithium therapy in man: a review. J Clin Psychiatry 1982; 43: 47-51.
123. Timmer RT, Sands JM. Disease of the month: lithium intoxication. J Am Soc Nephrol 1999; 10: 666-674.
124. Okusa MD, Crystal LJT. Clinical manifestations and management of acute lithium intoxication. Am J Med 1994; 97: 383-389.
125. Ellenhorn MJ, Schonwald S, Ordog G, Wasserberger J. Lithium. In: Medical toxicology - diagnosis and treatment of human poisoning. Ellenhorn MJ, Schonwald S, Ordog G, Wasserberger J (editors). Williams and Wilkins, Baltimore 1997; p. 1579.
126. Henry GC. Lithium. In: Toxicologic emergencies. Goldfrank LR, Flomenbaum NE, Lewin NA, Weisman RS, Howland MA, Hoffman RS (editors). Appleton and Lange, Stampford CT 1998; p. 969.
127. Dupuis RE, Cooper AA, Rosamund LJ, Campbell-Bright S. Multiple delayed peak lithium concentrations following acute intoxication with an extended release product. Ann Pharmacother 1996; 30: 356-360.
128. Leblanc M, Raymond M, Bonnardeaux A, Isenring P, Pichette V, Geadah D, Quimet D, Ethier J, Cardinal J. Lithium poisoning treated by high-performance continuous arteriovenous and venovenous hemodiafiltration. Am J Kidney Dis 1996; 27: 365-372.
129. Sakarcan A, Thomas DB, O'Reilly KP, Richards RW: Lithium-induced nephritic syndrome in a young pediatric patient. Pediatr Nephrol. 2002; 17: 290-2.
130. Schreiner A, Waldherr R, Rohmeiss P, Hewer W: Focal segmental glomerulosclerosis and lithium treatment. Am J Psychiatry. 2000; 157: 834.
131. Bosquet S, Descombes E, Gauthier T, Fellay G, Regamey C: Nephrotic syndrome during lithium therapy. Nephrol Dial Transplant. 1997;12: 2728-31.
132. Gills DS, Chhetri M, Milne JR: Nephrotic syndrome associated with lithium therapy. Am J Psychiatry. 1997; 154: 1318-9.
133. Tam VK, Green J, Schwieger J, Cohen AH: Nephrotic syndrome and renal insufficiency associated with lithium therapy. Am J Kidney Dis. 1996;27: 715-20.
134. Wood IK, Parmelee DX, Foreman JW: Lithium-induced nephritic syndrome. Am J Psychiatry 1989; 146: 84
135. Alexander F, Martin J: Nephrotic syndrome associated with lithium therapy. Clin Nephrol 1981; 15: 267.
136. Santella RN, Rimmer JM, MacPherson BR: Focal segmental glomerulosclerosis in patients receiving lithium carbonate. Am J Med 1988; 84: 951.
137. Demers R, Heninger G: Pretibial edema and sodium retention during lithium carbonate treatment. JAMA 1970; 214: 1845.
138. Yeudan Li, Stephen Shaw, Peter MT Deen: Development of lithium –induced NDI is dissociated from adenel cyclase activity. J AM Soc Nephrol 2006; 17: 1063-1072.
139. Hensen and Gross : Lithium induced polyuria and renal vasopressin receptor density: Nephrol Dial Transplant 1996 11: 622-627.
140. Chronic progressive renal lesions induced by lithium Kidn Int 1986; 29: 875-881.
141. Hestbech J, Hansen HE, Amdisen A, Olsen S. Chronic renal lesions following long-term treatment with lithium. Kidney Int 1977; 12: 205-213.
142. Presne C, Fakhouri F, Noël LH, Stengel B, Even C, Kreis H, Mignon F, Grünfeld JP. Lithium induced nephropathy: Rate of progression and prognostic factors. Kidney Int 2003; 64: 585-592.
143. Krestin GP, Genitourinary MR : kidneys and adrenal gland. Eur Radiology 1999: 9: 1705-1714
144. Farres MT, Ronco : Chronic Lithium Nephropathy: MRI imaging for diagnosis. Radiology 2003; 229: 570-574.
145. Aurell M, Brun C, Clemmensen L, Ladefoged J: Renal function and biopsy finding findings on long term lithium treatment. Kidney Int 20: 663-670, 1981.
146. Bendz H, Aurell M, Balldin J et al : kidney damage in long term lithium patients; a cross sectional study of patients with 15 years or more on lithium Nephrol Dial Transpl 9,1250-1254: 1994.

147. van Gerven HA, Boer, WH: Ned Tijdschr Geneeskunde Chronic renal function disorders during lithium use : 2006; 150: 1715-8. Review in Dutch.
148. Gitlin M: Lithium and kidney: an updated review: Drug Saf 20: 231-243, 1999
149. Newport DJ, Viguera AC, Beach AJ, Ritchie JC, Cohen LS and Stowe ZN, Lithium placental passage and obstetrical outcome: implications for clinical management during late pregnancy, Am J Psychiatry 2005; 162: 2162–2170.

32

Oxalate

Anja VERHULST and Marc E. DE BROE

Laboratory of Pathophysiology, University of Antwerp, Belgium

Oxalate, oxalic acid and calcium oxalate

Oxalic acid (chemical formula of this dicarboxylate HOOC-COOH) is a strong organic acid, widely spread in both plants and animals. The name comes from the *Oxalis* plant (wood sorrel) from which it was first isolated.

Oxalic acid has the ability to form strong bonds with various minerals, such as sodium, potassium, magnesium, and calcium. When this occurs, the compounds formed are usually referred to as oxalate salts. Thus, "*oxalate*" usually refers to the salt forming ion of oxalic acid. Although both sodium and potassium oxalate salts are water soluble, calcium oxalate is practically insoluble (8.76×10^{-8} mol/L at 37°C in a urine like solution [1]) which is why calcium oxalate, when present in high enough levels, has the propensity to precipitate (or solidify) in the kidneys or in the urinary tract to form calcium oxalate crystals. Calcium oxalate crystals, in turn, contribute to the formation of kidney stones of which approximately 75% are composed predominantly of calcium oxalate.

Oxalates in plants, animals and humans

Oxalate is found in plants, animals, and in humans. Oxalate content of plants is, compared to that of animals and humans, much higher. The calcium oxalate found in plants can even account for a large amount of their total calcium. Plant oxalate is the main regulator of calcium concentrations in plant tissues, an important factor in plants defense (against herbivores), and in heavy metal tolerance [2]. In contrast to these important roles that have been dedicated to oxalate in plants, in animals it is an almost useless end-product of metabolism. The human metabolism routinely converts other substances into oxalates (for example glycine and vitamin C). In addition to oxalate that is made inside of our body, dietary oxalate is an important oxalate source. The primary sources of dietary oxalate are plants and their products. It has been proposed that an increased oxalate delivery to the kidney is nephrotoxic. It is therefore worthwhile to describe the metabolism and particularly renal handling and toxicity of oxalate.

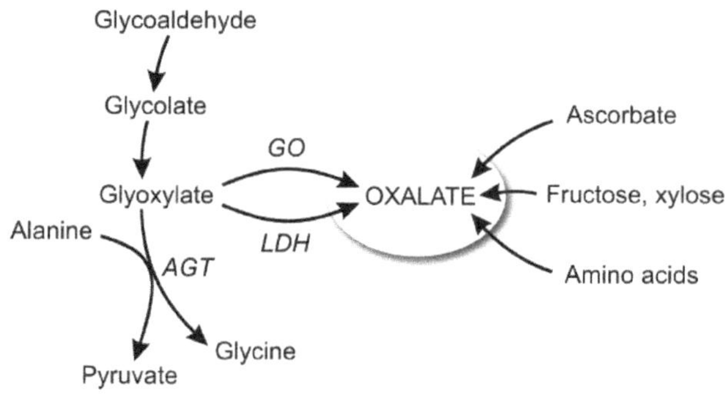

Figure 1. *Schematic overview of cellular oxalate production pathways.*

(Abbreviations: GO = glyoxylate oxidase, LDH = lactate dehydrogenase, AGT = alanine glyoxylate aminotransferase)

Intestinal uptake, endogenous production and renal excretion

Dietary oxalate is absorbed throughout the length of the intestine, but mainly in the small intestine [3]. Oxalate absorption from the gut is dependent on the amount of free oxalate present in the intestinal lumen, often referred to as bioavailable oxalate. When calcium is plentiful in the gut, a greater proportion of oxalate will be complexed to the cations leaving less free for absorption. Hence patients with hyperoxaluria should be advised to consume a calcium rich diet.

Glyoxylate is the major precursor for hepatic production of oxalic acid (oxalate). Glyoxylate is metabolized to either glycine or oxalate. The metabolism of glyoxylate to glycine, however, limits the amount of glyoxylate that can be converted to oxalate. Glyoxylate can be converted to oxalate by lactate dehydrogenase or glycolate oxidase. Oxalate is also produced from metabolic breakdown of ascorbic acid. By far less important precursors are the carbohydrates fructose and xylose and finally a number of amino acids may also be metabolic precursors of oxalate. Figure 1 summarizes oxalate production pathways.

Oxalate is excreted primarily by the kidney. Oxalate is freely filtered at the glomerulus, where its concentration is normally1~5 μM. One of the few physiologic functions of oxalate occurs in the proximal tubule where it plays a role in transcellular reabsorption of chloride (mainly present as sodium chloride). Cl^- entry across the apical membrane is mediated by Cl^-/oxalate exchange (oxalate is recycled from the tubular lumen to the cell by oxalate/sulfate exchange, in parallel with Na^+/sulfate cotransport) [4]. Early studies of renal oxalate clearance using radio-labeled oxalate showed secretion in almost all subjects studied. More recent studies using direct measurement of serum and urine oxalate demonstrated that net tubular reabsorption can occur as well. Nevertheless tubular oxalate concentrations rise in response to fluid reabsorption, resulting in cortical collecting duct oxalate concentrations of ≥ 300-500 μM. Depending on dietary intake, daily oxalate excretion in healthy volunteers varies from 0.1 to 0.45 mmol. Renal excretion has been thought to be the sole route for oxalate excretion. It has been shown however that the gut is able to secrete oxalate as well. Intestinal secretion seems to be an important route of oxalate excretion in end stage renal disease or other states with elevated serum oxalate levels [5, 6]. The role of intestinal oxalate secretion in normal physiology is not clear [7].

States of hyperoxaluria

Dietary oxalate load

Urinary oxalate is derived from three sources: (i) hepatic synthesis, (ii) breakdown of ascorbic acid and (iii) diet. Because of an overestimation of the ascorbic acid fraction, it has long been thought that the dietary fraction was responsible for only 10 to 20% [8]. A more recent study identified a dietary fraction of around 50%, making it an important determining factor in the urinary oxalate concentration [9]. Another study demonstrated that a dietary oxalate load resulted in transiently increasing plasma and urine oxalate levels peaking in the 2 to 4 hour post-load period [10], implying that an oxalate rich meal is able to induce a temporally state of hyperoxaluria. The fact that oxalate is an unavoidable component of the human diet since it is a ubiquitous component of plants, further highlights the role of diatary oxalate load in final urinary oxalate concentrations. Table 1 gives an overview of oxalate rich foods.

Table 1. Moderate and high oxalate containing foods.

High oxalate content (>0.9%)	Moderate oxalate content (0.2-0.9%)
beet greens	beans, green or wax
chocolate, cocoa	blackberries
figs	carrots
lamb's quarters	celery
pepper, black	coffee
poppy seeds	currants
purslane	endive
rhubarb	gooseberries
sorrel	grapes, Concord
spinach	green pepper
Swiss chard	lemon peel
tea (black)	okra
	onions, green
	oranges, orange peel
	raspberries
	strawberries
	sweet potatoes
	tomatoes
	wheat

(Adapted from Yarnell E. Naturopathic Urology and Men's Health. Wenatchee, WA, Healing Mountain Publishing, 2001.http://dryarnell.com/Files/Oxalate_foods_Yarnell.pdf)

Renal transplantation following chronic renal failure

When glomerular filtration rate declines, the clearance of oxalate becomes compromised. Therefore in chronic renal failure oxalate accumulates causing hyperoxalemia and crystals of calcium oxalate occur in the tissues of uremic patients. Renal replacement therapy is not able to remove the already accumulated oxalate from the body. Hence, following renal transplantation oxalate is released from the body resulting in an increased oxaluria (419±191 in transplanted patients versus 311±79 μmol/day in control patients; P<0.001) [11, 12].

Primary hyperoxaluria

Primary hyperoxaluria type 1 (PH1) is an autosomal-recessive disorder caused by a deficiency of the peroxysomal liver enzyme pyridoxal-phosphate-dependent enzyme alanine:glyoxylate aminotransferase (AGT) [13]. AGT catalyses the transamination of the intermediary metabolite glyoxylate to glycine, but its deficiency in PH1 allows glyoxylate to be reduced to glycolate and oxidized to oxalate instead (see figure 1). Primary hyperoxaluria type 2 (PH2) results from the deficiency of a cytosolic liver enzyme with glycolate reductase activities [13]. Both PH1 and 2 show an increased liver oxalate production. Since renal excretion is the major excretion route for oxalate, this results in hyperoxaluria. In patients suffering from primary hyperoxaluria the excretion can attain 1 to 3.5 mmol/day (up to ten times normal).

Enteric hyperoxaluria

Enteric hyperoxaluria refers to a state in which oxalate is over-absorbed in the bowel because of a defect in absorption of fat and bile acids. In those patients, suffering from Crohn's disease or patients with jejunoileal bypass [14, 15], Ca is complexated to fatty (bile) acids by which Ca-oxalate is no longer formed making oxalate available for intestinal absorption. Daily oxalate excretion is in between that of healthy volunteers and primary hyperoxaluria patients.

In a recent publication Sikora et al. found that increased intestinal oxalate absorption is an important risk factor for idiopathic calcium oxalate nephrolithiasis [16]. This observation may have important implications for the prevention of this disease.

Ethylene glycol poisoning

Ethylene glycol (EG) can be found in many agents, such as antifreeze. Ingestion of EG may cause serous poisoning [17, 18]. Adults are typically exposed when EG is ingested as a cheap substitute for ethanol or in suicide-attempts. Children may be exposed by accidental ingestion. EG itself has a low toxicity, but is in *vivo* metabolized to four organic acids: glycoaldehyde, glycolic acid, glyoxylic acid and ultimately oxalic acid (oxalate). Hence, 4 to 8 hours after the ingestion this results in hyperoxaluria and calcium oxalate precipitation in the kidney. The other metabolites induce metabolic acidosis, central nervous system depression, and cardio-pulmonary failure. As oxalate precursor, ethylene glycol is often used in rats to induce hyperoxaluria as an experimental animal-model for nephrocalcinosis/nephrolithiasis [19-24].

Oxalate and calcium oxalate as toxic agent for renal cells

Evidence for renal oxalate toxicity was found from studies describing urinary enzyme excretion suggesting renal (tubular) damage in patients with stones [25]. Rat models of stone disease have been used to study such damage in greater detail and revealed brush border loss, release of cellular enzymes, and epithelial erosion [19, 26, 27]. However, all these arguments are indirect and cannot distinguish oxalate (or oxalic acid) mediated effects from calcium oxalate crystal induced effects.

In order to investigate the direct effect of oxalate onto renal tubular cells, renal tubular cell cultures were exposed to elevated oxalate concentrations. Those studies elicited similar toxic effects *in vitro* as were seen *in vivo*: loss of cell integrity, release of cellular enzymes and cell (necrotic and apoptotic) death (reviewed in [28, 29].

A broad range of toxic responses that possibly induce these severe cellular effects have been reported:

(1) Redistribution of phosphatidylserine to the surface of renal cells

Redistribution of phosphatidylserine (PS) to the surface of renal epithelial cells as a consequence of oxalate exposure was first seen by Wiessner et al. [30] and later confirmed by Cao et al. [31]. When cells were exposed to various levels of oxalate, a dose-dependent PS externalization occurred. PS is a phospolipid molecule normally present in the inner leaflet of the plasma membrane. Externalization of PS to the outer leaflet of the plasma membrane may play a role in induction of apoptosis and may serve as signal molecule to engulf these cells [32].

(2) Activation of phospholipase A2

Oxalate is able to activate cytosolic phospholipase A2 ($cPLA_2$) in Madin Darby Canine Kidney (MDCK) cells and thereby mediates arachidonic acid release [33]. Using a selective inhibitor of $cPLA_2$, cytotoxic effects of oxalate could be attenuated.

(3) Free radical production [34]

Oxalate imposes an oxidant stress on renal cells by stimulating the generation of reactive oxygen species (ROS) [31]. ROS are produced as a byproduct of electron transport in mitochondria. Recent evidence suggests that mitochondria are a significant source of the ROS that are produced in renal cells following exposure to oxalate [34].

An excess of oxalate ions is also thought to stimulate the production of pro-inflammatory molecules by renal epithelial cells, directing the kidney towards inflammation. Oxalate stimulates production of monocyte chemoattractive protein-1 (MCP-1) [35], osteopontin, matrix gla protein, bikunin, fibronectin and prothrombin (reviewed in [28, 36]).

Some of these molecules may also limit urinary crystal growth and thereby inhibit nephrolithiasis (see below).

A manuscript published in 2005 by Schepers et al.[37] is questioning all the above described studies in which oxalate is identified as a nephrotoxic agent. Both *in vivo* and *in vitro*, high oxalate concentrations cannot exist without crystal formation since oxalate rapidly forms crystals in calcium-containing urine and growth media. According to these authors, the toxicological response induced by oxalate should be the result of calcium oxalate crystals and not of oxalate (oxalic acid) itself. Another point of their concern was that renal tubular cells are grown on plastic dishes, receiving calcium and oxalate in the same compartment. Especially in the high oxalate range this leads to calcium depletion and its deleterious effects. Finally, they state that most oxalate toxicity studies in cell culture are performed with renal proximal tubular cells, while high oxalate concentrations occurs at the distal part of the nephron. Therefore the possible toxic effect of oxalate to cells of both renal proximal and more distal tubular segments were studied using a two compartment system in which calcium depletion could be avoided. It was found that oxalate is only toxic to renal tubular cells at supraphysiologic concentrations (5 to 10mM). Lack of oxalate toxicity to mouse proximal tubular cells is also described by Podelski et al [38]. They investigated the toxicity of ethylene glycol metabolites and found glyoxylate and glycoaldehyde to be highly toxic, in contrast to ethylene glycol, glycolate and oxalate which did not show any toxicity to renal tubular cells.

Oxalate as component and/or inducer of renal calcifications (nephrocalcinosis) and stones (nephrolithiasis)

Calcifications of the renal tissue can be found either in the tubules (tubular nephrocalcinosis) or in the interstitium (interstitial nephrocalcinosis). Interstitial nephrocalcinosis starts in the interstitium beneath the basement membrane around the thin limbs of Henle and is thought to give rise to subepithelial calcifications on the level of the renal papillae, which are better known as Randall's plaques [15, 39]. In comparision to nephrocalcinosis, nephrolithiasis (kidney stones) occurs further on in the urological tract, i.e. the renal calyces and pelvis. Both intratubular [40] and interstitial nephrocalcinosis [41] have been proposed to play a role in the development of (particular) kidney stones. Nephrolithiasis is a major health problem in the western world where it affects 12% of men and 6% of women during their lives. Kidney stones are responsible for about 10% of urological hospital admissions per year and account for a significant number of visits to the hospital emergency departments [42].

Although nephrolithiasis is associated with much pain and suffering, kidney stones seldom lead to loss of kidney function. Although less painfull, intratubular nephrocalcinosis may constitute a much greater health risk. The incidence of tubular nephrocalcinosis is often under-estimated because of the low sensitivity of radiological imaging techniques and because most crystals (~90%) are lost from the renal tubules during tissue processing for routine histology [43]. Apart from the possibility that tubular nephrocalcinosis may lead to nephrolithiasis, tubular nephrocalcinosis can lead to a (obstruction-induced) tubulopathy. Massive tubular nephrocalcinois ultimately leads to end-stage renal failure in primary hyperoxaluria [13]. Furthermore, there is accumulating evidence that also milder forms of tubular nephrocalcinosis may induce tubular dysfunction to some degree: following kidney transplantation a 12 year allograft survival rate of 75% is observed in the absence of nephrocalcinosis, whilst in the presence of nephrocalcinosis allograft survival decreased to 48% [44, 45].

Renal stones (nephrolithiasis) consist of an organic and an anorganic phase. The organic phase, also called the stone matrix, is rich in proteins and carbohydrates. Depending on the composition of the anorganic- or crystal-phase, renal stones are subdivided in different categories: calcium stones (calcium oxalate or calcium phosphate crystals), uric acid stones and cysteine stones [46]. In industrialized countries, calcium and in particular calcium oxalate stones are most abundant: more than 75% of all detected stones contain calcium oxalate in their anorganic phase [46-48]. The composition of renal calcifications (nephrocalcinosis) depends on its origin. Interstitial nephrocalcinosis are found to be build up out of calcium phosphate [39] but when evolving to Randall plaques may become adhesion points for calcium oxalate crystals/stones that passed through the tubules [41]. Tubular nephrocalcinosis often is build up out of calcium oxalate crystals as in primary hyperoxaluria, intestinal bypass and inflammatory bowel disease patients [13-15].

The high prevalence of oxalate containing renal (tubular) and urinary tract calcifications is related to the low solubility of the oxalate-calcium salt. High urine oxalate excretion increases urine calcium oxalate supersaturation and, therefore the risk of crystal formation in tubular fluid and urine. In human urine, calcium concentration is about ten fold higher than oxalate on molar base. Relatively modest increases in urine oxalate excretion will have significant effects on urine supersaturation [49], especially in patients with hypercalciuria where calcium is even in greater excess of oxalate. Nevertheless, most people do not suffer from renal calcifications [50-54], suggesting that renal protection mechanisms exist.

A *first* defence mechanism is that a high urinary calcium concentration is able to reduce ADH-stimulated water permeability of the collecting duct via the calcium sensing receptor at the luminal site of the thick ascending loop of Henle, leading to an increased urinary volume and a reduced risk of supersaturation.

Secondly, urine contains molecules that inhibit crystallization *in vitro*. These molecules can be divided into two major classes: (1) small molecules such as citrate and pyrophosphate, and (2) macromolecular, organic molecules such as Tamm-Horsfall protein, nephrocalcin, osteopontin[55] and glycosaminoglycans [56]. These protective molecules have the collective property of being poly-anionic. They inhibit crystal formation by (1) complexation of Ca^{2+} ions by small molecules like citrate, and (2) coating the surface of nascent crystals by the macromolecules, thereby preventing further deposition of lattice ions. Furthermore, crystal formation alone is not enough to cause nephrolithiasis/calcinosis, which depends as well on the retention of crystals in the kidney. Retention can occur when crystals aggregate and/or grow big enough to obstruct the renal tubules but also when crystals adhere to the tubular cells [57]. However, Finlayson and Reid [40] calculated based on the velocity of crystal growth and tubular flow that crystalline particles, during normal transit times through the kidney, can never become large enough to be retained in the nephron solely by their size. Although, these findings were a matter of dispute in a later study [58], there is currently no doubt that crystal-cell interactions are an important event in the process of nephrolithiasis. Providing epithelial cells of the tubular epithelium, collecting ducts, ureters, bladder and the urethra with a non-adherent surface might be a *third* natural defense mechanism against tubular nephrocalcinosis/nephrolithiasis [59]. This defense mechanism is hampered when the anti-adherence properties are compromised. For example, damage to epithelial cells lining the renal tubules may play a crucial role in the disturbance of this defense mechanism. This is argumented by several studies of us and others. In rats, the deposition of crystals in the kidneys is higher when their crystal-inducing diet is combined with nephrotoxic agents [26;27]. Likewise, crystals adhere to the damaged bladder urothelium, but not to the healthy tissue [59]. The urine of recurrent stone formers contains enhanced levels of renal tubular cell-derived enzymes [25;26] and cytokines [60], indicating that the renal tissue is injured in these patients. Both *in vivo* and *in vitro* studies performed in our laboratory furthermore proved that proliferating, dedifferentiated cells [61-63], showed increased crystal binding when compared to normal epithelium. Molecules present on the luminal membrane (membrane that is exposed to the crystals) of proliferating/dedifferentiated cells that may be responsible for the crystal retention are osteopontin (OPN), hyaluronic acid (HA), nucleolin related protein and annexin [19, 62, 64-67]. Observations in preterm- and transplanted human kidneys with nephrocalcinosis demonstrated that the retention-prone epithelial phenotype (characterized by the expression of crystal binding molecules) precedes crystal adhesion leading to tubular nephrocalcinosis [68]. The underlying etiology, responsible for changes in the composition of the cell surface, is often not known and can be different for the diverse forms of nephrolithiasis and -calcinosis. It is important to remark that although oxalate (oxalic acid) might not be toxic to renal cells [37], calcium oxalate (crystals) might cause injury to these cells and in this way they can promote their own retention in the kidney [69-71].

Our latest research concerning renal defense against calcifications [72] identified a new and *fourth* defense mechanism of the kidney. It comprises an active crystal clearing mechanism of already retained crystals involving epithelial crystal overgrowth and interstitial degradation of the crystals.

In conclusion, the kidney protects itself against calcium oxalate nephrocalcinosis/lithiasis at different levels. Failure or saturation of these protection mechanisms, might explain why patients develop renal and/or urinary tract calcifications.

References

1. Streit J, Tran-Ho LC, Königsberger E. Solubility of the three calcium oxalate hydrates in sodium chloride solutions and urine-like liquors. Monatshefte Für Chemie 2008;129:1225-36.
2. Franceschi VR, Nakata PA. Calcium oxalate in plants: formation and function. Ann.Rev.Plant Biol. 2005;56:41-71.
3. Holmes RP, Goodman HO, Assimos DG. Dietary oxalate and its intesitnal absorption. Scanning Micr. 1995;9(4):1109-18.
4. Aronson PS. Ion exchangers mediating NaCl transport in the renal proximal tubule. Cell Biochem.Biophys. 2002;36:147-53.
5. Hatch M, Freel RW, Vaziri ND. Intestinal excretion of oxalate in chronic renal failure. J.Am.Soc.Nephrol. 1994;5:1339-43.
6. Hatch M, Cornelius JG, Allison M, Sidhu H, Peck AB and Freel RW. Oxalobacter sp. reduces urinary oxalate excretion by promoting enteric oxalate secretion. Kidney Int. 69, 691-698. 2006. Ref Type: Generic
7. Hatch M, Freel RW. Renal and intestinal handling of oxalate following oxalate loading in rats. Am.J.Nephrol 2003;23:18-26.
8. Mazzachi BC, Teubner JK, Ryall RL. Factors affecting measurement of urinary oxalate. Clin.Chem. 1984;30:1339-43.
9. Holmes RP, Goodman HO, Assimos DG. Contribution of dietary oxalate to urinary oxalate secretion. Kidney Int. 2001;59:270-6.
10. Holmes RP, Ambrosius WT. Dietary oxalate loads and renal oxalate handling. J.Urol. 2005;174(3):943-7.
11. Dumoulin G, Hory B, Nguyen NU, Henriet MT, Bresson C, Bittard H et al. Lack of increased urinary calcium-oxalate supersaturation in long-term kidney transplant recipients. Kidney Int. 1997;51:804-10.
12. Worcester EM, Fellner SK, Nakagawa Y, Coe FL. Effect of renal transplantation on serum oxalate and urinary oxalate excretion. Nephron 1994;67:414-8.
13. Milliner DS, Wilson RD, Smith LH. Phenotypic expression of primary hyperoxaluria: comparative features of type I and II. Kidney Int. 2001;59:31-6.

14. Worcester EM. Stones from bowel disease. Endocrinol.Metab.Clin.North.Am. 2002;31(4979):4999.
15. Evan AP, Coe FL, Lingeman JE, Worcester EM. Insights on the pathology of kidney stone formation. Urol Res 2005;33:383-9.
16. Sikora P, von Unruh G, Beck B, Feldkotter M, Zajaczdowska M, Hesse A et al. [13C2] Oxalate absorption in children with idiopathic calcium oxalate urolithiasis or primary hyperoxaluria . Kidney Int. 2008;73:1181-6.
17. Davis DP, Bramwell KJ, Hamilton RS, Williams SR. Ethylene glycol poisoning: case report of a record-high level and a review. J.Emergency.Med. 1997;15(5):653-67.
18. Leth PM, Gregersen M. Ethylene glycol poisoning. Forensic Sci.Int. 2005;155:179-84.
19. Asselman M, Verhulst A, De Broe ME, Verkoelen CF. Calcium oxalate crystal adherence to hyaluronan-, osteopontin- and CD44-expressing injured/regenerating tubular epithelial cells in rat kidneys. J.Am.Soc.Nephrol. 2003;13:3155-266.
20. Khan SR, Johnson JM, Peck AB, Cornelius JG, Glenton PA. Expression of osteopontin in rat kidneys: induction during ethylene glycol induced calcium oxalate nephrolithiasis. J.Urol. 2002;168:1173-81.
21. Lyon ES, Borden TA, Vermeulen CW. Experimental oxalate lithiasis produced with ethylene glycol. Invest.Urol. 1966;4(2):143-51.
22. Thamiselvan S, Hackett RL, Khan SR. Lipid peroxidaition in ethylene glycol induced hyperoxaluria and calcium oxalate nephrolithiasis. J.Urol. 1997;157:1059-63.
23. Yasui T, Sato M, Fujita K, Tozawa K, Nomura S, Kohri K. Effects of citrate on renal stone formation and osteopontin expression in a rat urolithiasis model. Urol Res 2001;29:50-6.
24. Marengo SR, Chen DH, Kaung HL, Resnick MI, Yang L. Decreased renal expression of the putative calcium oxalate inhibitor Tamm-Horsfall protein in the ethylene glycol rat model of calcium oxalte urolithiasis. J.Urol. 2002;167:2192-7.
25. Baggio B, Gambaro G, Ossi E, Favaro S, Borsatti A. Increased urinary excretion of renal enzymes in idiopathic calcium oxalate nephrolithiasis. J.Urol. 1983;129(6):1161-2.
26. Khan SR, Shevok PN, Hackett RL. Acute hyperoxaluria, renal injury and calcium oxalate urolithiasis. J.Urol. 1992;147:226-30.
27. Kumar S, Sigmon D, Miller T, Carpenter B, Khan SR, Malhotra R et al. A new model of nephrolithiasis involving tubular dysfunction/injury. J.Urol. 1991;147:1384-9.
28. Khan SR, Thamiselvan S. Nephrolithiasis: a consequence of renal epithelial cell exposure to oxalate and calcium oxalate. Mol. Urol. 2000;4(4):305-11.
29. Jonassen Ja, Cao LC, Honeyman T, Scheid C. Mechanisms mediating oxalate-induced alterations in renal cell functions. Crit.Rev. Eukaryotic Gene Expr. 2003;13(1):55-72.
30. Wiessner JH, Hasegawa AT, Hung LY, Mandel GS. Oxalate-induced exposure of phophatidylserine on the surface of renal epithelial cells in culture. J.Am.Soc.Nephrol. 1999;10:S441-5.
31. Cao LC, Jonassen Ja, Honeyman T, Scheid C. Oxalate-induced redistribution of phosphatidylserine in renal epithelial cells: implications for kidney stone disease. Am.J.Nephrol 2001;21(69):77.
32. Fadok VA, Voelker DR, Campbell PA, Cohen JJ, Bratton DL, Henson PM. Exposure of phosphatidylserine on the surface of apoptotic lymphocytes triggers specific recognition and removal by macrophages. J.Immunol. 1992;148:2207-16.
33. Kohjimoto Y, Kennington L, Scheid C, Honeyman T. Role of phosphlipase A2 in the cytotoxic effects of oxalate in cultured renal epithelial cells. Kidney Int. 1999;56:1432-41.
34. Thamiselvan S, Khan SR. Oxalate and calcium oxalate are injurious to renal epithelium cells: results of *in vivo* and *in vitro* studies. J.Pathol. 1998;Suppl 1:66-9.
35. Umekawa T, Chegini N, Khan SR. Oxalate ions and calcium oxalate crystals stimulate MCP-1 expression by renal epithelium cells. Kidney Int. 2002;61:105-12.
36. Scheid C, Cao LC, Honeyman T, Jonassen Ja. How elevated oxalate can promote kidney stone disease: changes at the surface and in the cytosol of renal cells that promote crystal adherence and growth. Frontiers in Bioscience 2004;1(9):797-808.
37. Schepers MS, Van Ballegooijen E, Bangma CH, Verkoelen CF. Oxalate is toxic to renal tubular cells only at supraphysiological concentrations. Kidney Int. 2005;68:1660-9.
38. Podelski V, Johnson A, Wright S, Rosa VD, Zager RA. Ethyleneglycol-mediated tubular injury: identification of critical metabolites and pathways. Am.J.Kidney Dis. 2001;38:339-48.
39. Evan AP, Lingeman JE, Coe FL, Parks JH, Bledsoe SB, Shao Y et al. Randall's plaque of patients with nephrolithiasis begins in basement membranes of thin loops of Henle. J.Clin.Invest. 2003;111:607-16.
40. Finlayson B, Reid F. The expectation of free and fixed particles in urinary stone diseaese. Invest.Urol. 1979;15:442-8.
41. Evan AP, Lingeman JE, Coe FL, Worcester EM. Randall's plaque: pathogenesis and role in calcium oxalate nephrolithiasis. Kidney Int. 2006;69:1313-8.
42. Taylor EN, Curhan GC. Diet and fluid prescription in stone disease. Kidney Int. 2006;70(70):-835.
43. Kummeling MT, de Jong BW, Laffeber C, Kok DJ, Verhagen PC, Leenders GJ et al. Tubular and interstitial nephrocalcinosis. J.Urol. 2007;178:in press.

44. Pinheiro H, Camara N, Osaki K, De Moura L, Pacheco-Silva A. Early presence of calcium oxalate deposition in kidney graft biopsies is associated with poor long-term graft survival. Am.J.Transplantation 2005;5:323-9.
45. Nankivell BJ, Borrows RJ, Fung CL, O'Connel PJ, Allen DM, Chapman JR. The natural history of chronic allograft nephropathy. N.Eng.J.Med 2003;349:2326-33.
46. Mandel NS, Mandel GS. Urinary tract stone disease in the United States veteran population. II. Geographical analysis of variations in composition. J.Urol. 1989;142:1516-21.
47. Serio A, Fraioli A. Epidemiology of nephrolithiasis. Nephron 1999;81:26-30.
48. Coe FL, Parks JH, Asplin JR. The pathogenesis and treatment of kidney stones. J.Clin.Invest. 1992;327(16):1141-52.
49. Robertson WG. The effect of high animal protein uptake on the risk of calcium stone formation in the urinary tract. Clin.Sci. 1979;57(3):285-8.
50. Worcester EM, Blumenthal SS, Behensky AM, Lewand DL. The calcium oxalate crystal growth inhibitor protein produced by mouse kidney cortical cells in culture is osteopontin. J.Bone.Min.Res. 1992;7(9):1029-36.
51. Worcester EM, Nakagawa Y, Wabner CL, Kumar S, Coe FL. Crystal adsorption and growth slowing by nephrocalcin, albumin, and Tamm-Horsfall protein. Am.J.Physiol. 1888;255:F1179-F1205.
52. Hess B, Nakagawa Y, Coe FL. Inhibition of calcium oxalate monohydrate crystal aggregation by urine proteins. Am.J.Physiol. 1989;257:F99-F106.
53. Hess B, Nakagawa Y, Parks JH, Coe FL. Molecular abnormality of Tamm-Horsfall glycoprotein in calcium oxalate nephrolithiasis. Am.J.Physiol. 1991;260:569-78.
54. Asplin JR, Deganello S, Nakagawa Y, Coe FL. Evidence that nephrocalcin and urine inhibit nucleation of calcium oxalate monohydrate crystals. Am.J.Physiol. 1991;261:F824-F830.
55. Asplin JR, Arsenault D, Parks JH, Coe FL, Hoyer JR. Contribution of human uropontin to inhibition of calcium oxalate crystallization. Kidney Int. 1998;53:194-9.
56. Worcester EM. Inhibitors of stone formation. Sem.Nephrol. 1996;16(5):474-86.
57. Verkoelen CF. The involvement of renal tubule epithelial cells in the pathophysiology of calcium oxalate nephrolithiasis. PhD thesis 1996.
58. Kok DJ, Khan SR. Calcium oxalate nephrolithiasis, a free or fixed particle diseaese. Kidney Int. 1994;46:847-54.
59. Khan SR, Cockrell CA, Finlayson B, Hackett RL. Crystal retention by injured urothelium of the rat urinary bladder. J.Urol. 1984;132:153-7.
60. Rhee E, Santiago L, Park E, Lad P, Bellman GC. Urinary IL-6 is elevated in patients with urolithiasis. J.Urol. 1998;160:2284-8.
61. Verkoelen CF, Romijn HC, de Bruijn WC, Boeve ER, Cao LC, Schroder FH. Association of calcium oxalate monohydrate crystals with MDCK cells. Kidney Int. 1995;48:129-38.
62. Verhulst A, Asselman M, Persy VP, Schepers MS, Helbert MF, Verkoelen CF et al. Crystal retention capacity of cells in the human nephron: involvement of CD44 and its ligands hyaluronic acid and osteopontin in the transition from a crystal binding- into a non-adherent epithelium. J.Am.Soc.Nephrol. 2002;14:107-15.
63. Verkoelen CF, van der Boom BG, Houtsmuller AB, Schroder FH, Romijn HC. Increased calcium oxalate monohydrate crystal binding to injured renal tubular epithelial cells in culture. Am.J.Physiol. 1998;274:F958-F965.
64. Verkoelen CF, van der Boom BG, Romijn JC. Identification of hyaluronan as a crystal-binding molecule at the surface of migrating and proliferating MDCK cells. Kidney Int. 2000;58:1045-54.
65. Sorokina EJ, Kleinman JG. Cloning and preliminary characterization of a calcium-binding protein closely related to nucleolin on the apical surface of inner medullary collecting duct cells. J.Biol.Chem. 1999;274(39):27491-6.
66. Sorokina EJ, Wesson JA, Kleinman JG. An acidic peptide sequence of nucleolin-related protein mediate the attachement of calcium oxalate to renal tubule cells. J.Am.Soc.Nephrol. 2004;15:2057-65.
67. Kumar S, Farell G, Deganello S, Lieske JC. Annexin II is present on renal epithelial cells and binds oxalate monohydrate crystals. J.Am.Soc.Nephrol. 2003;14:289-97.
68. Verhulst A, Asselman M, De Naeyer S, Vervaet B, Mengel M, Gwinner W et al. Preconditioning of the distal tubular epithelium of the human kidney precedes nephrocalcinosis. Kidney Int. 2005;68:1643-7.
69. Hackett RL, Shevok PN, Khan SR. Cell injury associated calcium oxalate crystalluria. J.Urol. 1990;144:1535-8.
70. Hackett RL, Shevok PN, Khan SR. Alterations in MDCK and LLC-PK1 cells exposed to oxalate and calcium oxalate monohydrate crystals. Scanning Micr. 1995;9(2):587-96.
71. Hackett RL, Shevok PN, Khan SR. Madin-Darby canine kidney cells are injured by exposure to oxalate and to calcium oxalate crystals. Urol Res 1994;22(4):197-203.
72. Vervaet B, Verhulst A, Dauwe SE, Verberckmoes SC, De Broe M, D'Haese P. An active renal crystal clearing mechnism in rat and man. Kidney Int. 2008;in press.

33

Herbal remedies containing aristolochic acid and mushroom nephrotoxicity

Frédéric DEBELLE, Marie-Carmen MUNIZ-MARTINEZ, Jean-Louis VANHERWEGHEM and Joëlle NORTIER

Hôpital Erasme, Université Libre de Bruxelles, Brussels, Belgium

Aristolochic acid nephropathy

Introduction

Numerous myths have grown around medicinal herbs and their healing powers [1]. The myth of beneficent nature is resistant to the accumulated evidence of health problems resulting from unknown or underestimated toxicity as well as from adulteration and misidentification of medicinal herbs [2]. Many plants contain substances toxic to humans and therefore, not surprisingly, to the human kidney. In early 1993, a rapidly progressive kidney failure leading to end-stage renal disease was reported in a number of women who had ingested slimming pills that contained powdered Chinese herbs [3]. Further investigations showed that this so called "Chinese herb nephropathy" was, in fact, secondary to the replacement of one of the prescribed Chinese herb, *Stephania tetrandra*, by other mixtures of Chinese herbs containing *Aristolochia Fang chi* [4]. The term "Aristolochia nephropathy" was thus proposed to be used instead of "Chinese herb nephropathy (CHN)" [5]. Finally, due to the presence of aristolochic acids (AA) in *Aristolochia spp.* and to their further demonstrated nephrotoxicity (see below), the term of "Aristolochic acid nephropathy" (AAN) is now commonly used.

History

In early 1992, two women presented to our nephrology department in Brussels (Belgium) with an extensive interstitial fibrosis of the kidney that rapidly progressed to terminal renal failure [3]. These two women who had no previous history of renal disease had followed, just before the onset of the renal disease, the same weight loss regimen in the same medical clinic in Brussels. This clinic specialized in weight loss regimens for more than 15 years and no renal problems had been previously encountered. Interestingly, the diet regimen was changed in mid 1990 by introducing powdered extracts of Chinese herbs, nominally *Stephania tetrandra* and *Magnolia officinalis* in the slimming pills [3]. A 1992 – epidemiological survey of the nephrology centers of Brussels showed that seven other women with "interstitial nephritis of unknown origin" were admitted for dialysis in 1991 and 1992. They had all followed the same slimming regimen including the Chinese herbs in the same medical clinic [3]. *Stephania tetrandra* and *Magnolia officinalis* were withdrawn from the Belgian market at the end of 1992. However, the outbreak of renal failure after absorption of these Chinese herbs eventually resulted in the accumulation of about 100 cases by 1998, 70 % of them being in end stage renal disease [6].

Phytochemical analyses of 12 different samples of *Stephania tetrandra* delivered in Belgium from 1990 to 1992 showed that only one sample corresponded to uncontaminated *Stephania* while the others were most probably *Aristolochia* sp [4], confirming the results of the analyses performed in Hong Kong on a sample sent by the Belgian importers [7].

After the publication of the index cases [3], similar cases were reported all around the world: four cases in France secondary to the intake of Arkomedika n°28 slimming pills containing *Stephania tetrandra* which was, in fact, *Aristolochia Fangchi* [8,9], one case in Spain after the chronic intake of an infusion made with a mixture of herbs containing *Aristolochia pistolochia* [10], four cases in United Kingdom consisting of two cases after the local treatment of eczema with AA containing *Aristolochia manshuriensis* (Mu-tong) [11], and in two other cases following a 5-year period of ingesting a Chinese herbal preparation to treat hepatitis B for the first one [12] and the Chinese herb *Longdan Xieganwan* for "liver enhancement" for the second one [13], and one case in USA after the intake of AA containing Chinese herbal remedies for pain relief [14]. Two series, one of 12 [15] and the other of 20 cases [16] were also reported in Taiwan related to the use of various unidentified herbal medications. In Japan, four cases presenting with a Fanconi syndrome were related to the use of different Chinese herb remedies (Boui and Mokutsu) containing AA [17,18]. A reversible Fanconi syndrome after the intake of a Chinese herbal remedy (*Akebia*) containing aristolochic acids was also reported in Germany [19]. In two CHN cases, paralysis secondary to profound hypokaliemia was the initial manifestation of the Fanconi syndrome [20,21]. Acute kidney injury due to tubular necrosis was also reported in one patient after the ingestion of Chinese herbal medicine as "tonic herbal remedies" containing Mu-tong (*A. manshuriensis*) and Fangchi (*A. fangchi*), and in 8 patients after the intake of Guan Mu-tong (*A. manshuriensis Kom*) [22,23].

Clinical features and functional aspects

Renal failure was rarely suspected and, in most of the cases, was discovered by routine blood testing. Dipstick analysis for proteinuria was negative and urinary sediment was unremarkable. Blood pressure was initially normal in half of the patients. Anemia was present and usually more severe that might be anticipated from the degree of renal failure [24]. Further investigations of renal functions indicated that proximal tubular cells were a primary target in Aristolochia nephropathy. First, some cases presented with a Fanconi syndrome [17-19]. Second, urinary excretion of five low molecular weight proteins (β2-microglobulin, cystatin C, Clara cell protein, retinol binding protein and α1-microglobulin) was markedly increased in five patients with CHN and the urinary low molecular weight protein/albumin ratio was higher than in control patient with glomerular diseases [25]. Third, levels of urinary neutral endopeptidase, an ectoenzyme of the proximal tubule brush border were significantly decreased in patients with renal failure secondary to CHN as compared to patients with glomerular diseases. Moreover, neutral endopeptidase enzymuria correlated positively with creatinine clearance and negatively with urinary low molecular weight protein levels [26]. Finally, the pattern of aminoaciduria in four cases of CHN with Fanconi syndrome (increased excretion of proline, hydroxyproline and citrulline with an almost normal excretion of glycine) suggested that aristolochic acids was predominantly affect the low affinity transport system of proline in the brush border membrane of proximal tubule [17].

Despite cessation of the exposure to Chinese herbs, progression of renal failure is usually relentless over a period of few months to several years. Six year after the withdrawal of the incriminated herbs from the Belgian market, more than 100 patients with CHN were confirmed in Belgium, 30 % of them having a moderate renal failure and 70 % being treated by maintenance dialysis or renal grafting [6].

A pilot study involving 35 CHN patients demonstrated that a steroid therapy could slow the progression of the renal failure: after one year, only two of the 12 CHN patients treated with steroids required dialysis as compared with 16 of the 23 CHN control patients [27]. The beneficial effect of steroid therapy was confirmed 8 years later in a larger group of patients [28]. Curiously, asymptomatic aortic insufficiency was observed in one third of the patients with CHN [24,29]. This cardiac complication was thought to be a result of extrarenal toxicity of Chinese herbs [30]. However, an alternate possibility was the role of appetite suppressants in the development of valvular heart diseases [31]. Since most of the CHN patients we have seen have been given appetite suppressants (fenfluramine, dexfenfluramine, phentermine alone or in combination) besides the Chinese herbs, the puzzling association of aortic insufficiency with CHN is more likely linked to the concomitant use of (dex)-fenfluramine rather than an extrarenal effect of the Chinese herbs [29]. In fact, the presence of aortic regurgitation was detected in 21 out of 40 CHN patients and was significantly correlated in a dose-response relationship with the cumulative dose of fenfluramine [32].

Pathology

Macroscopically, the kidneys were shrunk, asymmetric in about half of the cases with irregular outlines in one third [30].

Microscopically, the description of the pathologic aspects were derived from the analysis of 4 pieces of native nephroureterectomies obtained at the time of transplantation [33] and of 33 renal biopsies performed at different degrees of renal failure [34].

As shown on Figure 1, extensive interstitial fibrosis with atrophy and loss of the tubules was the major lesion. It was predominantly located in superficial cortex. The glomeruli were relatively spared. They nevertheless showed a mild collapse of the capillaries and a wrinkling of the basement membrane. Thickening of Bowman's capsule was the rule.

Interlobular and afferent arterioles showed thickening of their walls due to a swelling of the endothelial cells. These aspects suggest that the primary lesions could be located in the vessel walls leading to ischemia and interstitial fibrosis [34]. In one case, an extension of the fibrotic process to the pelvis and the ureter was observed [33], what may explain the unusual presentation of this case with a bilateral hydronephrosis [35].

Association with urinary tract carcinomas

Moderate atypia and atypical hyperplasia of the urothelium were first described in 4 pieces of nephroureterectomies performed in 3 CHN patients prior or at the time of transplantation [33]. Then, four cases of cancers of the urinary tract were reported: the first

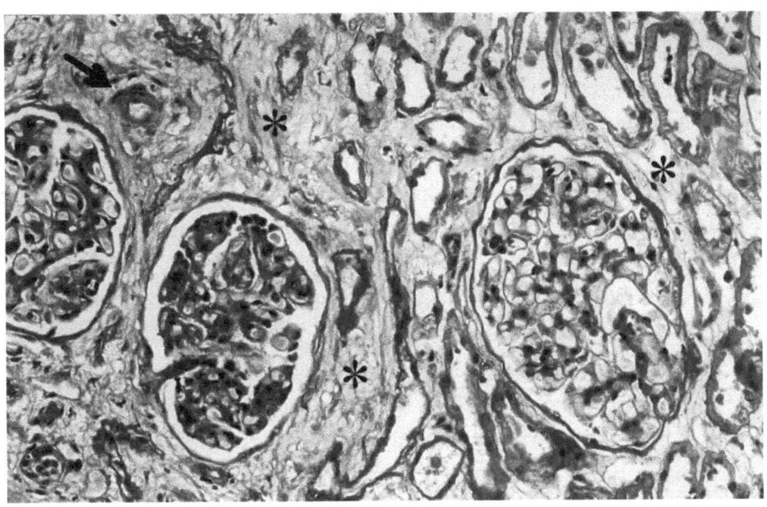

Figure 1. *Pathological aspect of Chinese herb nephropathy. Paucicellular interstitial fibrosis around atrophic tubules (*). Fibrous thickening of the arteriolar walls (arrow). No glomerular lesion. H&E staining, original magnification 300x. By courtesy of Dr. M. Depierreux.*

case, a 28 year old woman with CHN, developed two papillary transitional cell carcinomas in the posterior bladder wall 12 months after a renal transplantation [36] the second case, a 42 year old woman with CHN, presented with hematuria secondary to a papillary transitional cell carcinoma of the right pelvis [37]. The third case was a 49 year old woman previously published as a CHN case in UK [11]. She developed a hydronephrosis of the left native kidney after a successful renal transplantation. The piece of nephroureterectomy showed a multifocal transitional cell carcinoma of the ureter [38]. The fourth case was a 30-year-old Chinese man in whom the diagnosis of multifocal transitional cell carcinoma of the bladder was made following the assessment of macroscopic hematuria. He admitted having ingested for at least 5 years the Chinese herb *Longdan Xieganwan* which contains *Caulis Aristolochia manshuriensis* to "enhance" his liver [13]. Patients with end-stage CHN treated by dialysis or renal transplantation were therefore systematically offered bilateral removal of their native kidneys and ureters. Doing that, multifocal high grade transitional cell carcinomas, mainly in the upper urinary tract, were observed in four patients among 10 in one series [39] and in 18 among 39 in an other series [40]. The cumulative ingested dose of *Stephania* (in fact, *Aristolochia*) was shown to be a significant risk factor for the development of urothelial carcinomas [40].

A further bladder follow-up of these kidney recipients (cystoscopy and biopsies per 6 months) resulted in the diagnosis of 8 urothelial carcinoma *in situ*, 4 non-invasive low-grade papillary urothelial carcinoma and 3 infiltrating urothelial cancer, 68 to 169 months after cessation of AA exposure (cumulative incidence of 39.5%). Despite local and/or systemic chemotherapy, 3 patients died and 2 radical cystectomies had to be performed [41].

Urothelial cancer seemed to be a late complication of CHN since all the cases had been detected in patients with ESRD. However, the observation of a generalized urinary tract cancer in a 69 year old woman after intake of Chinese herbal medicine containing aristolochic acids but without a significant renal failure suggests that a dissociation between carcinogenicity and nephrotoxicity of aristolochic acids is possible [42].

Pathogenesis: The role of aristolochic acids

The time between the introduction of Chinese herbs in weight loss regimens and the outbreak of renal diseases in Brussels (Belgium) circumscribed the search for the culprit to the Chinese herbs [3]. Further epidemiological survey demonstrated that only the so-called *Stephania* was associated with all the cases of renal interstitial fibrosis [34].

Replacement of *Stephania* by *Aristolochia* was suspected [3] because : 1) *Stephania tetrandra* (Han Fang-ji) belongs to the family of Fang-ji besides *Aristolochia Fang chi* (Guang Fang ji); 2) pathological aspect of CHN is very similar to that of Balkan endemic nephropathy [3,33,34], the cause of which is still under controversies but some suggested causes included fungal and plant toxins such as ochratoxin A from *Penicillium* and aristolochic acids from *Aristolochia clematitis* [43].

Actually, the replacement of *Stephania* by *Aristolochia* species was confirmed using different batches of powders delivered in Belgium under the name of *Stephania tetrandra*. Most of these batches did not contain tetrandrine but aristolochic acids (0.65 ± 0.56 mg/g) [4].

Aristolochic acids (AA) were thus considered as the offending substance because AA induced nephrotoxic effects in experimental animals [44] as well as in human beings [45]. They also induced carcinomas in rodents [46].

However, some controversies were raised against the AA hypothesis. First, promoters of Chinese herbs claimed that the renal disease originated, in fact, from the injection of a "hidden" serotonin-like substance, with the mesotherapy which was a part of the slimming regimen [47,48]. Serotonin was indeed shown to induce ischemic renal lesions progressing in a short time to renal fibrosis [48]. Moreover the Belgian patients were also given (dex)fenfluramine which is a serotonin agonist [50]. Second, Chinese herbs originated from batches imported in Belgium at the same time were used without apparent untoward effects [50]. Third, similarities with Balkan endemic nephropathy suggested that ochratoxin A could be an alternative hypothesis.

However, further evidences support the AA hypothesis. The presence of 7(desoxyadenosin-N^6-yl) aristolactam I DNA adducts (dA-AAI) was demonstrated in renal tissue samples obtained from five patients with

CHN while dA-AAI was absent in the renal tissue of six patients with other renal diseases [51]. That was also the case for 7(deoxyguanosine-N^2-yl) aristolactam I DNA adducts (dG-AAI) and 7(deoxy-adenosin-N^6-yl) aristolactam II DNA adducts (dA-AAII) [52]. A larger series of kidney samples from 38 patients with CHN confirmed the presence of DNA adducts six year after the exposure to Chinese herbs; the levels ranging from 1.2 to 165 per 10^9 normal nucleotides for dA-AAI, from 0.6 to 6.8 per 10^9 normal nucleotides for dA AAII and from 0.4 to 8.2 per 10^9 normal nucleotides for dG AAI. These adducts were absent in kidney samples obtained in eight patients with renal diseases of other origin [40]. The renal tissue samples of 25 among these 38 patients with CHN were also analyzed for ochratoxin A related adducts. Levels of these adducts were low and close to the background level of the assay [40]. On the other hand, for 71 patients with CHN followed in our department, a comprehensive analysis of the medical charts and of the prescriptions filled between 1990 and 1992 directly obtained from the pharmacists was conducted. This survey showed that eleven patients with Chinese herbs - related end-stage renal disease did not receive mesotherapy. Moreover, using a multiple regression analysis, the cumulative dose of *Stephania* (in fact, *Aristolochia*) appeared as the only significant factor predicting the slope of the time course of the inverse of plasma creatinine levels [53]. Although these observations can not rule out a possible potentiating effect of anorexigens [49], the description of similar renal diseases after the intake of *Stephania* without slimming pills [54,55] as well as in different clinical settings all around the world [8-19] indicates that (dex)fenfluramine is not necessary to induce renal disease. Moreover, dexfenfluramine did not enhance the nephrotoxicity of AA in a rat model of CHN [56].

On the other hand, AA are activated by nitroreduction in aristolactams which form DNA adducts with adenosine and guanosine. The formation of AA-DNA adducts was studied *in vitro*: cytochrome P450 1A1 and 1A2 [57] as well as prostaglandin H synthetase [58] were shown to be involved in the metabolic activation of AA. These observations could explain variations between individuals in the susceptibility to aristolochic acid toxicity as well as the preferential localization in the kidney and the urinary tract. Carcinogenicity of AA DNA adducts has been related to the mutation in the codon 61 of the protooncogen Ha-ras [59] as well as in a mutation of p53 [39]. Finally, the effects of AA on proximal tubules were investigated on the opossum kidney (OK) cell line. Aristolochic acids impaired the process of receptor-mediated endocytosis of albumin and β2-microglobulin, decreased megalin expression and formed specific DNA adducts in OK cells. These data support the involvement of AA in the proximal tubule dysfunction found in CHN patients [60].

Experimental aristolochic acid nephropathy

First attempts to experimentally reproduce CHN failed: two groups of seven Wistar rats were orally administered either pure aristolochic acids (10 mg/kg for 5 days a week during 3 months) or herbs powders (containing AA) mixed with fenfluramine. At sacrifice animals in both groups had developed the expected tumors but not fibrosis of the renal interstitium [61]. However, when 12 female New Zeeland white rabbits were injected intraperitoneally with 0.1 mg aristolochic acids per kg, 5 days a week, for 17 to 21 months, they developed a severe hypocellular interstitial fibrosis, urothelial atypias and, in 3 of them, tumors of the urinary tract [62].

In the Wistar rat model, the daily administration of 10 mg per kg body weight of AA induced, after 35 days, renal failure with interstitial fibrosis (Figure 2) as well as a papillary urothelial carcinoma of the pelvis in some animals [63,64]. Nephrotoxicity of different components of AA was also studied in three strains of inbred male mice. The C3H/He mice intraperitoneally injected with 2.5 mg/Kg of AA, five days a week, for 2 weeks, developed on day 14 foci of proximal tubule injury surrounded by mononuclear cell infiltration. Two weeks later, signs of proximal tubule cell proliferation were observed whereas the inflammatory cells infiltration became more severe and interstitial fibrosis occurred [65]. In this mice model, AAI exhibited a higher nephrotoxicity than AAII [65], which was also confirmed in *in vitro* studies on proximal tubular LLC-PK1 cells line [66].

Despite these findings, the pathophysiological mechanisms by which AA induce renal interstitial fibrosis remain hypothetic. In the Wistar rat model, pathways leading to interstitial fibrosis seem to be independent of the renin-angiotensin system (RAS), as suggested by experiments where functional and structural renal impairments were not modified either

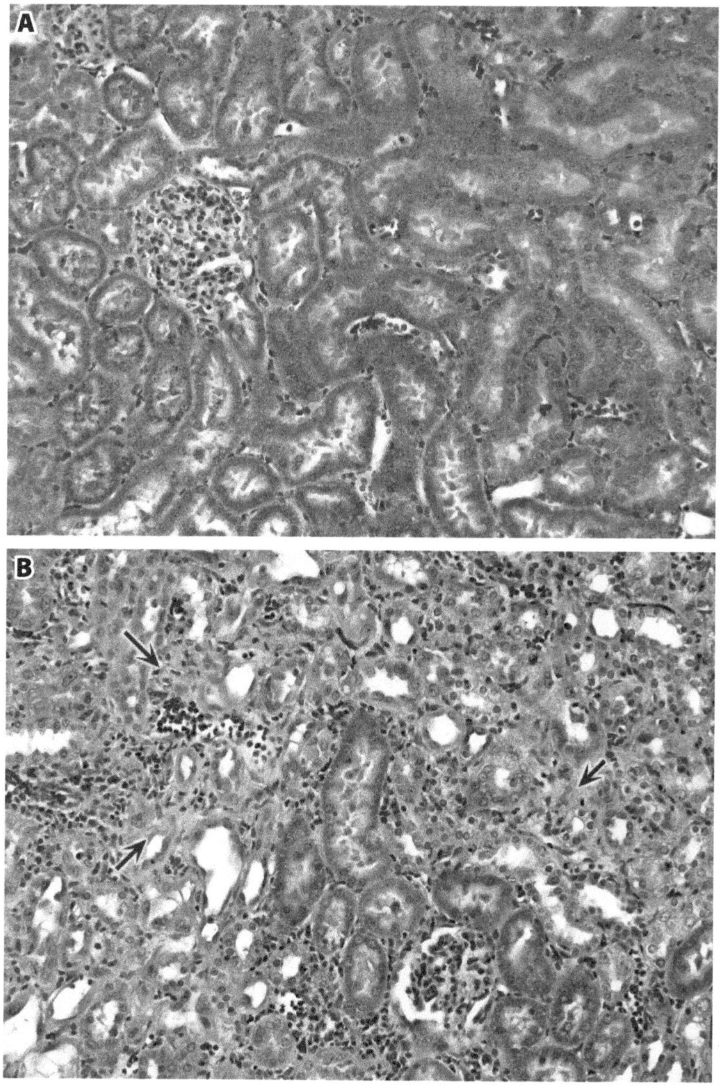

Figure 2. *Photomicrographs of renal cortex.* ***A.*** *For a control rat on day 35, no abnormalities were noted.* ***B.*** *For an aristolochic acid-treated (10 mg/Kg bw) rat on day 35, severe tubular atrophy and interstitial fibrosis (arrows) were observed. Goldner's trichrome staining, original magnification 100x.*

by enhancing (via salt-depletion) or blocking (via angiotensin converting enzyme inhibitor ± angiotensin II receptor blocker) the RAS [64]. On the other hand, an activation defect of antioxidant enzymes was observed and could be involved in an early dedifferentiation process of proximal tubular epithelial cells. The development of interstitial fibrosis was preceded by an influx of inflammatory cells (lymphocytes and mononuclear cells) and by an increased urinary excretion of the active form of transforming growth factor beta (TGB-β), which is a key profibrosing cytokine [67].

Several experimental studies revealed an early phase of acute tubular necrosis preceding the development of tubular atrophy and interstitial fibrosis [65,68,69]. By using a transgenic mice model, Okada et al demonstrated that hepatocyte growth factor (HGF) did not interfere with the acute phase but reduced the severity of interstitial fibrosis during the tubular regeneration phase, partially through a decreased expression of tissue inhibitor of metalloproteinase-1 and increased matrix metalloproteinase-9 activity [68].

Additionally, apoptosis probably also plays a role in the AA-induced proximal tubular atrophy according to several *in vivo* and *in vitro* studies [66,68,70]. In an *in vitro* study conducted by Hsin et al [71], LLC-PK1 cells exposed to AA showed a rapid increase in their intracellular calcium content leading to endoplasmic reticulum and mitochondrial stress which in turn causes activation of the caspase pathway and finally apoptosis.

Conclusion

From an outbreak of end stage renal disease occurring around a slimming clinic in Brussels [3] a new cause of renal interstitial fibrosis [3,33,34] complicated by urinary tract carcinomas [39,40] was identified. Finally, the disease was related to the intake of Chinese herbs containing aristolochic acids (see above). After the publication of the Belgian cases, similar cases were reported all around the world [8-19,22,23,72-74]. The existence of more cases should be suspected. Indeed, Fang ji, a commonly used traditional Chinese medicine, purchased from herbs shops in Hong Kong contained aristolochic acids [75] as well as *Akebia* used in traditional Sino Japanese prescriptions ("Kampo") [76]. Indian traditional medicine used more than 7500 plant species which include *Aristolochia bracteata, Aristolochia tagala* and *Aristolochia indica* and chronic interstitial nephritis of unknown origin is a frequent cause of terminal renal disease in Indians [77]. Moreover, AA is proposed as the environmental causal factor for the Balkan endemic nephropathy, a familial chronic tubulointerstitial disease frequently associated with urothelial malignancies, which affect thousands of people living in the Danube basin [78,79].

Nephrotoxins are usually easy to identify when deriving from well known therapeutic agents. However, their identification requires a detective work when causes involve the unregulated use of herbs ingredients in home remedies or folk medicine. The difficulty is compounded by the fact that patients do not mention their regular use of herbal powders or infusions because they consider these natural products to be harmless [1].

Faced with a case of interstitial renal nephritis of unknown origin, all nephrologist should be encouraged to examine with the utmost care whether herbal remedies containing aristolochic acids as summarized by the US Food and Drug Administration [80] (Table 1) can genuinely be ruled out. Moreover, taking into account that herbal remedies containing plant species of the genus *Aristolochia* are carcinogenic to humans [81], this alert should be extended to the diagnosis of urinary tract carcinoma.

Table 1. Botanicals known or suspected to contain or to be adultered with aristolochic acids.

Botanical names
Aristolochia sp (n=30), *Asarum sp* (n=6), *Akebia sp* (n=3), *Bragantia sp* (n=1), *Clematis sp* (n=6), *Cocculus sp* (n=17), *Sinomenium sp* (n=1), *Stephania sp* (n=1)
Common names
• Aristolochia, Akebia, Clematis, Clematidis, Cocculus, Serpentaria, Stephania
• Dutchman's pipe, Birthwort, Snakeroot, wild (Indian) Ginger, False Coltsfoot, Colic root, Chocolate vine, Virgin bower, Indian cockle, Colombo, Columba, Ukulwe, Orient vine
• Fang-ji 1, Mu-tong 1, Boui, Mokutsu, Saishin, Mokku, Ma dou ling, Tian Xian teng, Mokuboi, Kwang banggi, Moktong, Yu Zhi zi, Bei Xi Xin, Xin Xin, Ireisen, Wojoksum, Weiling Xian, Fengteng, Kanboi.

[1] Fang-ji and Mu-tong are ingredients in the following products : Ba Zheng Wan, Chan Yang Zheng Ji Wan, Da Huang Quing Wei Wan, Dang Gui Si Ni Wan, Dao Chi Wan, Dieda Wan, Fu Ke Fen Quing Wan, Guan Xin Su He Wan, Ji Sheng Ju He Wan, Kat Kit Wan, Long Dan Xie Gan Wan, Quell Fire, Shi Xiang Fan Shen Wan, Xin Yi Wan (From ref. [79] in which more details can be found).

Mushroom nephrotoxicity

Introduction

Mushroom poisoning is another example of the identification of hazardous natural substances leading to accidental exposure and occasionally to renal damage. The failure to recognize mushrooms and the likeness between some edible and poisonous species are usual sources of mushroom intoxication. Although infrequent, the incidence of mushroom poisoning could be rising since the use of wild mushrooms in cooking preparations is becoming more popular. Among the poisonous species, *Amanita phalloides* ("Deathcap") which causes a life-threatening illness with liver and renal failure is the most widely recognized. However, less known species such as *Amanita proxima* and *smithiana*, *Cortinarius orellanus* and *C. speciosissimus*, and *Tricholoma equestre* were also reported to induce renal injury (Table 2).

Amanita phalloides and amatoxin-containing mushrooms

Amatoxins which are thermostable toxins interfering with the RNA enzyme polymerase II [82] are retrieved in high concentration levels in *Amanita phalloides* but also, to a lesser extent, in other *Amanita* species (*A. virosa, A. verna., A. ocreata, A. bisporigera, A. suballiacea, A. tenuifolia* and *A. hygroscopica*) as well as *Lepiota* and *Galerina species* mushrooms [83]. Ingestion of *Amanita phalloides* rapidly provokes severe digestive disturbance and liver injury 36 to 48 hours later, whereas acute kidney injury generally develops 3 to 5 days after ingestion. Renal impairment may be related to profound hypovolemia, hepatorenal syndrome or direct toxic renal injury [83]. Diagnosis is based on the history of recent absorption of mushrooms and can be confirmed by the detection of amatoxins in fluids and tissue samples [84]. The treatment mainly consists in supportive care. Considering the enterohepatic cycle of amatoxins [85], activated charcoal may be given during the first days of poisoning to reduce the re-absorption of toxins. On the other hand, the efficacy of hemodialysis, hemoperfusion, and plasmapheresis in reducing amatoxins levels has not been proven [86]. Different pharmaceutical agents either interfering with liver uptake of toxins (silibinin, benzylpenicillin) or protecting against the liver oxidative stress (*N*-acetylcystein) were tried in amatoxins poisoning [87]. However, their efficacy remains unclear due to difficulties obtaining solid scientific documentations for such poisoning.

Cortinarius orellanus, C. speciosissimus, C. rainierensis

Cortinarius species usually grow in semimountainous and deciduous forests at the end of the summer or in autumn, and may be easily mistaken for the *Psylocybe* genus, the so-called "magic mushrooms" appreciated by drug-abuser people for its hallucinogenic properties. The toxicity of *Cortinarius* is related to the orellanine toxin, a hydroxypyridine with structural analogy to paraquat, which blocks protein synthesis and induces oxidative stress [88,89]. Numerous cases of orellanine-induced nephrotoxicity have been reported in Europe (*C. orellanus* and *C. speciosissimus*) [90-92], North America and Canada [88] and suspected in 3 patients in Australia [93].

Intoxication by *Cortinarius* induces nonspecific digestive symptoms which precede the worsening of the patient's general condition. In most cases, liver is spared and renal damage is delayed by a mean period of 8.5 days, which makes the diagnosis of mushroom poisoning quite difficult [88]. Although hard to perform and not routinely available, different analytical methods can detect orellanine in serum, urine and renal tissue, confirming the diagnosis of poisoning [88].

Renal manifestations are characterized by loin pains, oliguria or less frequently polyuria, as well as leukocyturia, hematuria and proteinuria in 50 %, 45 % and 30 % of the cases, respectively [88]. Renal failure is generally reversible. However, about 30 % of the cases are reported to progress to chronic renal failure and for some to end-stage renal disease [88,90]. The histopathology reveals acute tubular necrosis with marked interstitial edema, signs of interstitial nephritis, and in more advanced stages, areas of atrophic tubules surrounded by interstitial fibrosis [94-96]. The glomeruli may show a mild increase in mesangial matrix, but no deposit of immunoglobulins or complement component has been detected by immunofluorescence [96].

Just like for amatoxin intoxication, the treatment is mainly supportive care. Orellanine seems to be rapidly concentrated in renal tissue [97], making toxins extraction techniques such as hemoperfusion, hemodialysis or plasma exchange, probably ineffective [90,94]. Antioxydant therapy with *N*-acetylcysteine [98] and selenium [99] as well as corticosteroids treatment [90,98] were also proposed but the data are limited to case reports.

Amanita proxima, A. smithiana and Tricholoma equestre

Contrary to *Amanita* phalloides, both *A. proxima* and *smithiana* do not contain amatoxins. Cases of poisoning with *Amanita proxima*, mistaken for the edible *Amanita ovoidae*, were reported in 36 patients in France [100,101]. These patients developed mild gastrointestinal symptoms, renal impairment requiring hemodialysis in about 25 % of cases and hepatic insufficiency in 10 patients with a complete recovery within one month [100,101]. The toxin is still unknown.

The renal toxins of *A. smithiana* are identified as allenic norleucine and chlorocrotylglycine [102]. Poisoning with *A. smithiana* which were mistaken for the edible *Tricholoma magnivelare* (edible pine mushroom or matsutake) was reported in three Asian patients in the Pacific Northwest and two patients in Taiwan [103,104]. Nausea, vomiting, water diarrhea and abdominal discomfort without liver injury developed 4 - 11 hours post ingestion. Renal failure occurred 2 to 4 days later and temporary required hemodialysis. After several weeks, renal function recovered to the baseline level [104].

In southwestern France, twelve cases of delayed rhabodmyolysis and acute kidney injury in 3 cases, were reported after repeated ingestion of *Tricholoma equestre* containing meals [105]. The responsible toxin was not identified.

Conclusion

Mushroom-induced nephrotoxicity is mainly related to amatoxins containing *Amanita* and orellanine containing *Cortinerius*. It commonly occurs in harvesters who are mistaken by look-alikes edible wild mushrooms. Its incidence is hopefully limited to case series (mostly in parts of the world where mushroom harvesting is common). However, its consequences may be dramatic. In the absence of specific "antidote", the treatment is largely based on vigorous supportive care.

Faced with renal failure of uncertain etiology, especially in association with digestive disturbance and liver damage, the nephrologist must consider mushroom poisoning as a putative cause and question the patient about recent dietary history.

Table 2. Mushrooms-induced nephrotoxicity.

Botanical names	Mistaken for	Toxins	Renal manifestations	Ref.
Amanita phalloides ("Deathcap") A. virosa, A. verna., A. ocreata, A. bisporigera, A. suballiacea, A. tenuifolia and A. hygroscopica Lepiota and Galerina species	Volvariella gloiocephale, V. volvacea	Amatoxins	Early onset of acute renal failure (3 – 5 days) Related to severe hypovolemia, hepatorenal syndrome or direct tubular toxicity High mortality rate	[82]
Cortinarius orellanus, C. orellanoides, C. speciosissimus, C. splendens	Psilocybe semilanceata ("Magic mushrooms")	Orellanine	Late onset of acute renal failure (3 – 17 days), dialysis may be required Chronic renal failure in 30 – 45% of cases	[87]
Amanita proxima	Amanita ovoidea	Unknown	Acute renal failure requiring in 25 % of cases hemodialysis Recovery without sequellae	[99]
Amanita smithiana	Tricholoma nauseosum or matsutake ("Matsutake" or "Songi"), Tricholoma magnivelare ("Penderosa" or pine mushroom or American Matsutake)	Allenic norleucine (aminohexadienoic acid) and chlorocrotylglycine	Early onset of renal dysfunction: 2 – 4 days Dialysis support required No chronic renal impairment	[103]
Tricholoma equestre (Tricholoma flavovirens) "Yellow trich", "shimokoshi", "man on horseback" or "yellow-knight fungus"	None	Unkown	Repeated ingestion may lead to severe rhabdomyolysis and renal impairment	[104]

References

1. Vanherweghem JL. Nephropathy and herbal medicine. Am J Kidney Dis 2000; 35: 330-332
2. Huxtable RJ. The myth of beneficent nature: the risks of herbal preparations. Ann Intern Med 1992; 117: 165-166
3. Vanherweghem JL, Depierreux M, Tielemans C, Abramowicz D, Dratwa M, Jadoul M, Richard C, Vandervelde D, Verbeelen D, Vanhaelen-Fastre R. Rapidly progressive interstitial renal fibrosis in young women: association with slimming regimen including Chinese herbs. Lancet 1993; 341: 387-391
4. Vanhaelen M, Vanhaelen-Fastre R, But P, Vanherweghem JL. Identification of aristolochic acid in Chinese herbs. Lancet 1994; 343: 174 (letter)
5. Vanherweghem JL. Aristolochia nephropathy in humans: an outbreak in Belgium. J Am Soc Nephrol 1993; 4: 327 (abstract)
6. Vanherweghem JL. Misuse of herbal remedies: the case of an outbreak of terminal renal failure in Belgium (Chinese herbs nephropathy). J Altern Complement Med 1998; 4: 9-13
7. But PP. Need for correct identification of herbs in herbal poisoning. Lancet 1993; 341: 637 (letter)
8. Pourrat J, Montastruc JL, Lacombe JL, Cisterne JM, Rascol O, Dumazer P. Néphropathie associée à des herbes chinoises - 2 cas. Presse Med 1994; 23: 1669 (letter)
9. Stengel B, Jones E. Insuffisance rénale terminale associée à la consommation d'herbes chinoises en France. Néphrologie 1998; 19: 15-20
10. Pena JM, Borras M, Ramos J, Montoliu J. Rapidly progressive interstitial renal fibrosis due to a chronic intake of a herb (Aristolochia pistolochia) infusion. Nephrol Dial Transplant 1996; 11: 1359-1360
11. Lord GM, Tagore R, Cook T, Gower P, Pusey CD. Nephropathy caused by Chinese herbs in the UK. Lancet 1999; 354: 481-482

12. Cronin AJ, Maidment G, Cook T, Kite GC, Simmonds MS, Pusey CD, Lord GM. Aristolochic acid as a causative factor in a case of Chinese herbal nephropathy. Nephrol Dial Transplant 2002; 17: 524-525
13. Laing C, Hamour S, Sheaff M, Miller R, Woolfson R. Chinese herbal uropathy and nephropathy. Lancet 2006; 368: 338
14. Meyer MM, Chen TP, Bennett WM. Chinese herb nephropathy. Proc (Bayl Univ Med Cent) 2000; 13: 334-337
15. Yang CS, Lin CH, Chang SH, Hsu HC. Rapidly progressive fibrosing interstitial nephritis associated with Chinese herbal drugs. Am J Kidney Dis 2000; 35: 313-318
16. Chang CH, Wang YM, Yang AH, Chiang SS. Rapidly progressive interstitial renal fibrosis associated with Chinese herbal medications. Am J Nephrol 2001; 21: 441-448
17. Tanaka A, Nishida R, Yokoi H, Kuwahara T. The characteristic pattern of aminoaciduria in patients with aristolochic acid-induced Fanconi syndrome: could iminoaciduria be the hallmark of this syndrome? Clin Nephrol 2000; 54: 198-202
18. Tanaka A, Nishida R, Maeda K, Sugawara A, Kuwahara T. Chinese herb nephropathy in Japan presents adult-onset Fanconi syndrome: could different components of aristolochic acids cause a different type of Chinese herb nephropathy? Clin Nephrol 2000; 53: 301-306
19. Krumme B, Endmeir R, Vanhaelen M, Walb D. Reversible Fanconi syndrome after ingestion of a Chinese herbal 'remedy' containing aristolochic acid. Nephrol Dial Transplant 2001; 16: 400-402
20. Yang SS, Chu P, Lin YF, Chen A, Lin SH. Aristolochic acid-induced Fanconi's syndrome and nephropathy presenting as hypokalemic paralysis. Am J Kidney Dis 2002; 39: E14
21. Tsai CS, Chen YC, Chen HH, Cheng CJ, Lin SH. An unusual cause of hypokalemic paralysis: aristolochic acid nephropathy with Fanconi syndrome. Am J Med Sci 2005; 330: 153-155
22. Lo SH, Mo KL, Wong KS, Poon SP, Chan CK, Lai CK, Chan A. Aristolochic acid nephropathy complicating a patient with focal segmental glomerulosclerosis. Nephrol Dial Transplant 2004; 19: 1913-1915
23. Yang L, Li X, Wang H. Possible mechanisms explaining the tendency towards interstitial fibrosis in aristolochic acid-induced acute tubular necrosis. Nephrol Dial Transplant 2007; 22: 445-456
24. van Ypersele de Strihou C, Vanherweghem JL. The tragic paradigm of Chinese herbs nephropathy. Nephrol Dial Transplant 1995; 10: 157-160
25. Kabanda A, Jadoul M, Lauwerys R, Bernard A, van Ypersele de Strihou C. Low molecular weight proteinuria in Chinese herbs nephropathy. Kidney Int 1995; 48: 1571-1576
26. Nortier JL, Deschodt-Lanckman MM, Simon S, Thielemans NO, de Prez EG, Depierreux MF, Tielemans CL, Richard C, Lauwerys RR, Bernard AM, Vanherweghem JL. Proximal tubular injury in Chinese herbs nephropathy: monitoring by neutral endopeptidase enzymuria. Kidney Int 1997; 51: 288-293
27. Vanherweghem JL, Abramowicz D, Tielemans C, Depierreux M. Effects of steroids on the progression of renal failure in chronic interstitial renal fibrosis: a pilot study in Chinese herbs nephropathy. Am J Kidney Dis 1996; 27: 209-215
28. Muniz Martinez MC, Nortier J, Vereerstraeten P, Vanherweghem JL. Steroid therapy in chronic interstitial renal fibrosis: the case of Chinese-herb nephropathy. Nephrol Dial Transplant 2002; 17: 2033-2034
29. Vanherweghem JL. Association of valvular heart disease with Chinese-herb nephropathy. Lancet 1997; 350: 1858 (letter)
30. Reginster F, Jadoul M, van Ypersele de Strihou C. Chinese herbs nephropathy presentation, natural history and fate after transplantation. Nephrol Dial Transplant 1997; 12: 81-86
31. Connolly HM, Crary JL, McGoon MD, Hensrud DD, Edwards BS, Edwards WD, Schaff HV. Valvular heart disease associated with fenfluramine-phentermine. N Engl J Med 1997; 337: 581-588
32. Unger P, Nortier J, Muniz Martinez MC, Plein D, Vandenbossche JL, Vereerstraeten P, Vanherweghem JL. High prevalence of fenfluramine-related aortic regurgitation in women with end-stage renal disease secondary to Chinese herb nephropathy. Nephrol Dial Transplant 2003; 18: 906-910
33. Cosyns JP, Jadoul M, Squifflet JP, de Plaen JF, Ferluga D, van Ypersele de Strihou C. Chinese herbs nephropathy: a clue to Balkan endemic nephropathy? Kidney Int 1994; 45: 1680-1688
34. Depierreux M, Van Damme B, Vanden Houte K, Vanherweghem JL. Pathologic aspects of a newly described nephropathy related to the prolonged use of Chinese herbs. Am J Kidney Dis 1994; 24: 172-180
35. Jadoul M, de Plaen JF, Cosyns JP, van Ypersele de Strihou C. Adverse effects from traditional Chinese medicine. Lancet 1993; 341: 892-893
36. Cosyns JP, Jadoul M, Squifflet JP, Van Cangh PJ, van Ypersele de Strihou C. Urothelial malignancy in nephropathy due to Chinese herbs. Lancet 1994; 344: 188 (letter)
37. Vanherweghem JL, Tielemans C, Simon J, Depierreux M. Chinese herbs nephropathy and renal pelvic carcinoma. Nephrol Dial Transplant 1995; 10: 270-273
38. Lord GM, Cook T, Arlt VM, Schmeiser HH, Williams G, Pusey CD. Urothelial malignant disease and Chinese herbal nephropathy. Lancet 2001; 358: 1515-1516

39. Cosyns JP, Jadoul M, Squifflet JP, Wese FX, van Ypersele de Strihou C. Urothelial lesions in Chinese-herb nephropathy. Am J Kidney Dis 1999; 33: 1011-1017
40. Nortier JL, Muniz Martinez MC, Schmeiser HH, Arlt VM, Bieler CA, Petein M, Depierreux MF, De Pauw L, Abramowicz D, Vereerstraeten P, Vanherweghem JL. Urothelial carcinoma associated with the use of a Chinese herb (Aristolochia fangchi). N Engl J Med 2000; 342: 1686-1692
41. Lemy A, Wissing KM, Rorive S, Zlotta A, Roumeguere T, Muniz Martinez MC, Decaestecker C, Salmon I, Abramowicz D, Vanherweghem JL, Nortier J. Late onset of bladder urothelial carcinoma after kidney transplantation for end-stage aristolochic acid nephropathy: a case series with 15-year follow-up. Am J Kidney Dis 2008; 51: 471-477
42. Nortier JL, Schmeiser HH, Muniz Martinez MC, Arlt VM, Vervaet C, Garbar CH, Daelemans P, Vanherweghem JL. Invasive urothelial carcinoma after exposure to Chinese herbal medicine containing aristolochic acid may occur without severe renal failure. Nephrol Dial Transplant 2003; 18: 426-428
43. Stefanovic V, Polenakovic MH. Balkan nephropathy. Kidney disease beyond the Balkans? Am J Nephrol 1991; 11: 1-11
44. Mengs U. Acute toxicity of aristolochic acid in rodents. Arch Toxicol 1987; 59: 328-331
45. Jackson L, Kofman S, Weiss A, Brodovsky H. Aristolochic Acid (NSC-50413): Phase I Clinical Study. Cancer Chemotherapy Reports 1964; 35-37
46. Mengs U, Lang W, Poch J-A. The carcinogenic action of aristolochic acid in rats. Arch Toxicol 1982; 57: 107-119
47. Malak J. Chinese herb nephropathy is not a (dex)fenfluramine nephropathy but a serotonin nephropathy. J Altern Complement Med 1998; 4: 131-132
48. McIntyre M. Chinese herbs: risk, side effects, and poisoning: the case for objective reporting and analysis reveals serious misrepresentation. J Altern Complement Med 1998; 4: 15-16
49. Colson CR, De Greef KE, Duymelinck C, Simoens PJ, Verpooten GA, De Broe ME. Role of serotonin in the development of Chinese herbs nephropathy? Nephrol Dial Transplant 1999; 14 Suppl 4: 16 (abstract)
50. De Broe ME. On a nephrotoxic and carcinogenic slimming regimen. Am J Kidney Dis 1999; 33: 1171-1173
51. Schmeiser HH, Bieler CA, Wiessler M, van Ypersele de Strihou C, Cosyns JP. Detection of DNA adducts formed by aristolochic acid in renal tissue from patients with Chinese herbs nephropathy. Cancer Res 1996; 56: 2025-2028
52. Bieler CA, Stiborova M, Wiessler M, Cosyns JP, van Ypersele de Strihou C, Schmeiser HH. 32P-post-labelling analysis of DNA adducts formed by aristolochic acid in tissues from patients with Chinese herbs nephropathy. Carcinogenesis 1997; 18: 1063-1067
53. Muniz Martinez MC, Nortier J, Vereerstraeten P, Vanherweghem JL. Progression rate of Chinese herb nephropathy: impact of Aristolochia fangchi ingested dose. Nephrol Dial Transplant 2002; 17: 408-412
54. Gillerot G, Jadoul M, Arlt VM, van Ypersele de Strihou C, Schmeiser HH, But PP, Bieler CA, Cosyns JP. Aristolochic acid nephropathy in a Chinese patient: time to abandon the term "Chinese herbs nephropathy"? Am J Kidney Dis 2001; 38: E26
55. Vanherweghem JL, Cuykens JJ, Vandenbergh P, Bouman KP, Hagers Y. Valvular heart disease and Chinese-herb nephropathy. Lancet 1998; 351: 991
56. Debelle F, Nortier J, Arlt VM, De Prez E, Vienne A, Salmon I, Phillips DH, Deschodt-Lanckman M, Vanherweghem JL. Effects of dexfenfluramine on aristolochic acid nephrotoxicity in a rat model for Chinese-herb nephropathy. Arch Toxicol 2003; 77: 218-226
57. Stiborova M, Frei E, Wiessler M, Schmeiser HH. Human enzymes involved in the metabolic activation of carcinogenic aristolochic acids: evidence for reductive activation by cytochromes P450 1A1 and 1A2. Chem Res Toxicol 2001; 14: 1128-1137
58. Stiborova M, Frei E, Breuer A, Wiessler M, Schmeiser HH. Evidence for reductive activation of carcinogenic aristolochic acids by prostaglandin H synthase -- (32)P-postlabeling analysis of DNA adduct formation. Mutat Res 2001; 493: 149-160
59. Schmeiser HH, Scherf HR, Wiessler M. Activating mutations at codon 61 of the c-Ha-ras gene in thin-tissue sections of tumors induced by aristolochic acid in rats and mice. Cancer Lett 1991; 59: 139-143
60. Lebeau C, Arlt VM, Schmeiser HH, Boom A, Verroust PJ, Devuyst O, Beauwens R. Aristolochic acid impedes endocytosis and induces DNA adducts in proximal tubule cells. Kidney Int 2001; 60: 1332-1342
61. Cosyns JP, Goebbels RM, Liberton V, Schmeiser HH, Bieler CA, Bernard AM. Chinese herbs nephropathy-associated slimming regimen induces tumours in the forestomach but no interstitial nephropathy in rats. Arch Toxicol 1998; 72: 738-743
62. Cosyns JP, Dehoux JP, Guiot Y, Goebbels RM, Robert A, Bernard AM, van Ypersele de Strihou C. Chronic aristolochic acid toxicity in rabbits: A model of Chinese herbs nephropathy? Kidney Int 2001; 59: 2164-2173
63. Debelle FD, Nortier JL, de Prez EG, Garbar CH, Vienne AR, Salmon IJ, Deschodt-Lanckman MM, Vanherweghem JL. Aristolochic acids induce chronic renal failure with interstitial fibrosis in salt-depleted rats. J Am Soc Nephrol 2002; 13: 431-436
64. Debelle FD, Nortier JL, Husson CP, de Prez EG, Vienne AR, Rombaut K, Salmon IJ, Deschodt-Lanckman M, Vanherweghem JL. The renin-angiotensin system blockade does not prevent renal interstitial fibrosis induced by aristolochic acids. Kidney Int 2004; 66: 1815-1825

65. Sato N, Takahashi D, Chen SM, Tsuchiya R, Mukoyama T, Yamagata S, Ogawa M, Yoshida M, Kondo S, Satoh N, Ueda S. Acute nephrotoxicity of aristolochic acids in mice. J Pharm Pharmacol 2004; 56: 221-229
66. Balachandran P, Wei F, Lin RC, Khan IA, Pasco DS. Structure activity relationships of aristolochic acid analogues: toxicity in cultured renal epithelial cells. Kidney Int 2005; 67: 1797-1805
67. Pozdzik AA, Salmon IJ, Debelle FD, Decaestecker C, Van den Branden C, Verbeelen D, Deschodt-Lanckman MM, Vanherweghem JL, Nortier JL. Aristolochic acid induces proximal tubule apoptosis and epithelial to mesenchymal transformation. Kidney Int 2008; 73: 595-607
68. Okada H, Watanabe Y, Inoue T, Kobayashi T, Kanno Y, Shiota G, Nakamura T, Sugaya T, Fukamizu A, Suzuki H. Transgene-derived hepatocyte growth factor attenuates reactive renal fibrosis in aristolochic acid nephrotoxicity. Nephrol Dial Transplant 2003; 18: 2515-2523
69. Lebeau C, Debelle FD, Arlt VM, Pozdzik A, de Prez EG, Phillips DH, Deschodt-Lanckman MM, Vanherweghem JL, Nortier JL. Early proximal tubule injury in experimental aristolochic acid nephropathy: functional and histological studies. Nephrol Dial Transplant 2005; 20: 2321-2332
70. Liu MC, Maruyama S, Mizuno M, Morita Y, Hanaki S, Yuzawa Y, Matsuo S. The nephrotoxicity of Aristolochia manshuriensis in rats is attributable to its aristolochic acids. Clin Exp Nephrol 2003; 7: 186-194
71. Hsin YH, Cheng CH, Tzen JT, Wu MJ, Shu KH, Chen HC. Effect of aristolochic acid on intracellular calcium concentration and its links with apoptosis in renal tubular cells. Apoptosis 2006; 11: 2167-2177
72. Lee S, Lee T, Lee B, Choi H, Yang M, Ihm CG, Kim M. Fanconi's syndrome and subsequent progressive renal failure caused by a Chinese herb containing aristolochic acid. Nephrology (Carlton) 2004; 9: 126-129
73. Arlt VM, Stiborova M, Schmeiser HH. Aristolochic acid as a probable human cancer hazard in herbal remedies: a review. Mutagenesis 2002; 17: 265-277
74. Vanherweghem JL. Urémie chronique et cancer des voies urinaires secondaires à la prise d'extraits végétaux utilisés en phytothérapie chinoise. Med Sciences 2003; 18: 1095-1101
75. Zhu M, Phillipson JD. Hong Kong samples of the traditional Chinese Medicine "Fang ji" contain aristolochic acid toxins. Int J Pharmacognosy 1996; 34: 283-289
76. Hashimoto K, Higuchi M, Makino B, Sakakibara I, Kubo M, Komatsu Y, Maruno M, Okada M. Quantitative analysis of aristolochic acids, toxic compounds, contained in some medicinal plants. J Ethnopharmacol 1999; 64: 185-189
77. Vanherweghem JL. Aristolochia sp and chronic interstitial nephropathies in Indians. Lancet 1997; 349: 1399
78. Grollman AP, Shibutani S, Moriya M, Miller F, Wu L, Moll U, Suzuki N, Fernandes A, Rosenquist T, Medverec Z, Jakovina K, Brdar B, Slade N, Turesky RJ, Goodenough AK, Rieger R, Vukelić M, Jelaković B. Aristolochic acid and the etiology of endemic (Balkan) nephropathy. Proc Natl Acad Sci 2007;104:12129-12134
79. Debelle FD, Vanherweghem JL, Nortier JL. Aristolochic acid nephropathy: a worldwide problem. Kidney Int 2008; *in press*
80. Lewis CJ, Alpert S. Letter to health Care Professionals on FDA concerned about botanical products, including dietary supplements containing aristolochic acid. Us Food and Drug Administration – Center for Food Safety and Applied Nutrition – Office of Natritional Products. Labeling and Dietary supplements 2000; May 31
81. World Health Organization - International Agency for research on cancer: IARC monographs on the evaluation of carcinogenic risks to humans: some traditional herbal medicines, some mycotoxins, naphtalene and styrene. IARC Press, Lyon, France 2002; 82: 118
82. Wieland T. The toxic peptides from Amanita mushrooms. Int J Pept Protein Res 1983; 22: 257-276
83. Karlson-Stiber C, Persson H. Cytotoxic fungi--an overview. Toxicon 2003; 42: 339-349
84. Jehl F, Gallion C, Birckel P, Jaeger A, Flesch F, Minck R. Determination of alpha-amanitin and beta-amanitin in human biological fluids by high-performance liquid chromatography. Anal Biochem 1985; 149: 35-42
85. Jaeger A, Jehl F, Flesch F, Sauder P, Kopferschmitt J. Kinetics of amatoxins in human poisoning: therapeutic implications. J Toxicol Clin Toxicol 1993; 31: 63-80
86. Mullins ME, Horowitz BZ. The futility of hemoperfusion and hemodialysis in Amanita phalloides poisoning. Vet Hum Toxicol 2000; 42: 90-91
87. Enjalbert F, Rapior S, Nouguier-Soule J, Guillon S, Amouroux N, Cabot C. Treatment of amatoxin poisoning: 20-year retrospective analysis. J Toxicol Clin Toxicol 2002; 40: 715-757
88. Danel VC, Saviuc PF, Garon D. Main features of Cortinarius spp. poisoning: a literature review. Toxicon 2001; 39: 1053-1060
89. Prast H, Werner ER, Pfaller W, Moser M. Toxic properties of the mushroom Cortinarius orellanus. I. Chemical characterization of the main toxin of Cortinarius orellanus (Fries) and Cortinarius speciosissimus (Kuhn & Romagn) and acute toxicity in mice. Arch Toxicol 1988; 62: 81-88
90. Bouget J, Bousser J, Pats B, Ramee MP, Chevet D, Rifle G, Giudicelli CP, Thomas R. Acute renal failure following collective intoxication by Cortinarius orellanus. Intensive Care Med 1990; 16: 506-510

91. Short AI, Watling R, MacDonald MK, Robson JS. Poisoning by Cortinarius speciosissimus. Lancet 1980; 2: 942-944

92. Gryzmala S. Massenvergiftungen durch den orangefuchsigen Hautkopf. Z Pilzkd 1957; 23: 139-142

93. Mount P, Harris G, Sinclair R, Finlay M, Becker GJ. Acute renal failure following ingestion of wild mushrooms. Intern Med J 2002; 32: 187-190

94. Montoli A, Confalonieri R, Colombo V. Lack of efficacy of early plasma exchange in renal toxicity from Cortinarius orellanus. Nephron 1999; 81: 248

95. Calvino J, Romero R, Pintos E, Novoa D, Guimil D, Cordal T, Mardaras J, Arcocha V, Lens XM, Sanchez-Guisande D. Voluntary ingestion of Cortinarius mushrooms leading to chronic interstitial nephritis. Am J Nephrol 1998; 18: 565-569

96. O'Donnell M, Fleming S. The renal pathology of mushroom poisoning. Histopathology 1997; 30: 280-282

97. Rapior S, Delpech N, Andary C, Huchard G. Intoxication by Cortinarius orellanus: detection and assay of orellanine in biological fluids and renal biopsies. Mycopathologia 1989; 108: 155-161

98. Kilner RG, D'Souza RJ, Oliveira DB, MacPhee IA, Turner DR, Eastwood JB. Acute renal failure from intoxication by Cortinarius orellanus: recovery using anti-oxidant therapy and steroids. Nephrol Dial Transplant 1999; 14: 2779-2780

99. Wornle M, Angstwurm MW, Sitter T. Treatment of intoxication with Cortinarius speciosissimus using an antioxidant therapy. Am J Kidney Dis 2004; 43: e3-e6

100. de Haro L, Jouglard J, Arditti J, David JM. Insuffisance rénale aiguë lors d'intoxications par Amanita proxima: expérience du Centre anti-poisons de Marseille. Néphrologie 1998; 19: 21-24

101. Leray H, Canaud B, Andary C, Klouche K, Beraud JJ, Mion C. Intoxication par Amanita proxima; une nouvelle cause d'insuffisance rénale aiguë. Néphrologie 1994; 15: 197-199

102. Pelizarri V, Feifel E, Rohrmoser MM, Gstraunthaler G, Moser M. Partial purification and characterization of a toxic component of Amanita smithiana. Mycologia 1994; 86: 555-560

103. Yang WS, Lin CH, Huang JW, Fang CC. Acute renal failure caused by mushroom poisoning. J Formos Med Assoc 2006; 105: 263-267

104. Leathem AM, Purssell RA, Chan VR, Kroeger PD. Renal failure caused by mushroom poisoning. J Toxicol Clin Toxicol 1997; 35: 67-75

105. Bedry R, Baudrimont I, Deffieux G, Creppy EE, Pomies JP, Ragnaud JM, Dupon M, Neau D, Gabinski C, De WS, Chapalain JC, Godeau P, Beylot J. Wild-mushroom intoxication as a cause of rhabdomyolysis. N Engl J Med 2001; 345: 798-802

C

Environmental and Occupational Nephrotoxins

34

Lead nephropathy

Richard P. WEDEEN

Department of Veterans Affairs, New Jersey Health Care System,
East Orange, New Jersey, USA

Introduction

Occupational exposure to lead originated over 10,000 years ago in the region of the Aegean sea. The earliest description of lead poisoning is a poem dating from about 200 BC by the Greek philosopher Nikander of Colophon [1]. Although possible recognition of renal effects of lead can be traced to the 17th century, Lancereaux provided the first description of lead nephrotoxicity in modern terms in 1862. Lancereaux's patient had saturnine (lead-induced) gout; his kidneys showed interstitial nephritis at postmortem examination [2]. Controversy concerning the renal effects of lead stems from this 19th century description compounded by the recurrent difficulty in recognizing the late sequelae of chronic absorption of relatively low levels of lead. Early reports failed to distinguish glomerular from extraglomerular renal disease. Additional confusion has been created by the failure to distinguish the transient Fanconi syndrome of acute symptomatic lead poisoning from the insidious chronic interstitial nephritis characteristic of lead nephropathy in adults.

In addition to the difficulty in assigning cause when the effect is delayed in time, identification of the renal effects of lead was further obscured because the late complications of excessive lead absorption, namely, gout and hypertension, can themselves produce renal damage unrelated to lead. The kidney has permissive control of blood pressure by modulating fluid volume and more direct control by intrarenal hormones which effect vascular tone. Hypertension and kidney disease are therefore inextricably interrelated.

In the past, lead nephropathy was identified in individuals who had repeated episodes of symptomatic lead intoxication [1]. The classic symptoms of inorganic lead poisoning (abdominal colic, extensor muscle weakness due to peripheral neuropathy, encephalopathy, and pallor) in patients known to have excessive lead absorption made the diagnosis straightforward. In the early twentieth century, the diagnosis was confirmed in the clinical laboratory by finding anemia in association with excessive urinary excretion of lead, and coproporphyrins, or δ-aminolevulinic acid (compounds accumulated in the blood because of lead inhibition of hemoglobin synthesis). Following the extensive studies of lead metabolism by Robert Kehoe as medical director of the Ethyl Corporation beginning in the 1930s [1], the mainstay of laboratory diagnosis has been the blood lead concentration. Robert Kehoe considered blood lead levels up to 80 µg/dL safe for lead workers. He was reluctant to acknowledge that the more subtle, non-specific symptoms of lead poisoning such as headache, constipation, arthralgia, and loss of libido seen at blood lead levels below 80 µg/dL were attributable to lead. Kehoe did not recognize the effects of lead on cognitive function, blood pressure or the kidneys in individuals not exhibiting classical symptoms.

While the acceptable blood lead level set by the US Occupational Safety and Health Agency (OSHA) remained 50 µg/dL in 2007, that for children had been progressively lowered by the Center for Disease Control and Prevention (CDC) to 10 µg/dL by 1991. The disparity between acceptable blood lead levels in adults and children can be explained in part by the paucity of studies of lead toxicity in adults, and the increased sensitivity of the developing brain in children to toxins. The efforts of the lead industry to thwart public health regulation in the workplace contributed to the disparity in standards for children and adults. OSHA is reluctant to revise the occupational lead standard because of the risk of litigation. The mounting evidence of the impact of lower and lower lead levels on blood pressure and the kidneys in industry and the general public is reviewed in this chapter.

Biomarkers of lead absorption

Cumulative absorption of lead over time is a more reliable predictor of adverse effects of lead than a single blood lead measurement. The blood concentration tends to fall markedly within weeks of removal from exposure. The biologic half-life of lead in blood approximates four weeks. However, up to 95% of the body lead stores are retained in bone with a half-life approximating two decades in cortical bone and about four years in trabecular bone. [3]. Consequently, a number of approaches to assess cumulative lead absorption have been explored: 1) the calcium disodium ethylenediamine tetraacetic acid ($CaNa_2EDTA$) lead-mobilization test, 2) *in vivo* bone x-ray induced x-ray fluorescence (XRF), and 3) the blood lead index (area under the time-concentration curve for multiple blood lead measurements).

The $CaNa_2EDTA$ mobilization test is performed by parenteral administration of 1 to 3 g of $CaNa_2EDTA$ over 4 to 12 hours with subsequent collection of 24-hour urine samples over 1 to 4 days. A dosage of 20 to 30 mg of EDTA per kg is used in children. In the presence of renal failure (serum creatinine >1.5 mg/dL) urine collections are extended to at least 3 days. [4]. The $CaNa_2EDTA$ lead mobilization test has proved useful in detecting excessive lead absorption. It permitted an unbiased assessment of the consequences of lead absorption at a time when blood leads up to 80 µg/dL were deemed acceptable. The validity of arbitrary standards for the $CaNa_2EDTA$ lead mobilization test is, however, unclear since recent epidemiologic studies demonstrate an adverse impact of levels of blood lead far lower than previously considered dangerous. Setting an "acceptable" level of urinary lead excretion during the $CaNa_2EDTA$ test is, therefore, problematic. The same caveat applies to the lead mobilization test performed with the oral chelating agent, succimer. Despite these considerations the blood lead concentration remains the "gold standard" for assessing lead exposure. Adverse effects of lead on blood pressure and kidney function have been found at blood lead levels as low as 2 µg/dL [5]. There thus appears to be no threshold below which adverse effects of lead are not found. From the point of view of protecting health, there is no safe level for blood lead, chelatable lead, or bone lead.

Bone lead measured by non-invasive K-XRF is particularly useful for assessing cumulative lead absorption in population studies. However, the relationship of XRF to the $CaNa_2EDTA$ mobilization test or the blood lead index over the full range of possible exposure situations is unknown. The fraction of urinary lead coming from bone following the administration of chelators presumably varies with the time, duration and level of recent and past exposure as well as with physiologic factors modulating bone remodeling and renal function. Under steady-state conditions (absent ongoing heavy exposure) the $CaNa_2EDTA$ mobilization test correlates well with direct chemical measurement of lead in transiliac bone biopsies [6, 7]. Because lead in bone has a biologic half-life of years, compared to a biologic half-life of lead in blood of weeks [3], bone more closely reflects cumulative lead stores. In groups heavily exposed to lead over many years, blood lead correlates well with bone lead [7, 8].

Although the blood lead concentration reflects absorption of both organic and inorganic lead, the clinical symptoms of organic lead absorption (e.g. tetraethyl lead gasoline additive) are of rapid onset and primarily cerebral. Colic, peripheral neuropathy, and anemia, characteristic symptoms of inorganic lead poisoning, are absent. Chelation therapy, highly effective for inorganic lead poisoning, is ineffective in organic lead poisoning [9]. The distinctive hallucinogenic effects induced by massive absorption of tetraethyl lead was dramatized when DuPont's Chambers Works in Deepwater, New Jersey, became known as the "House of Butterflies" shortly after manufacture of the antiknock gasoline additive began in 1923 [10]. Differentiating the residual cognitive defects induced by lead from those induced by organic compounds is challenging [11]. Neither the acute Fanconi syndrome (aminoaciduria, phosphaturia, and glycosuria without hyperglycemia) nor chronic interstitial nephritis have been described as a consequence of tetraethyl lead exposure [9]. A longitudinal study of tetraethyl lead workers, however, showed a positive correlation between blood pressure and both blood and tibial lead [12].

Acute lead nephropathy

In children with lead encephalopathy, proximal tubule reabsorptive defects characterized by the Fanconi syndrome have been observed [13]. The Fanconi syndrome appears when blood lead levels approach 150 μg/dL. It is rapidly reversed by chelation therapy designed to treat the far more dangerous lead encephalopathy. The proximal tubule reabsorptive defect can regularly be induced experimentally in rats fed dietary lead [14]. In both children and experimental animals, acute lead nephropathy is consistently associated with acid-fast intranuclear inclusions in proximal tubule epithelial cells [14]. The intranuclear inclusion bodies consist of a lead–protein complex and may be seen in tubular epithelial cells in the urinary sediment during acute poisoning [15]. Lead-containing intranuclear inclusions have also been observed in liver, neural tissue, and osteoclasts. Acute poisoning is associated with morphologic and functional defects in tubular epithelial cell mitochondria.

Chronic lead nephropathy

The phrase *chronic lead nephropathy* refers to the slowly progressive interstitial nephritis occurring infrequently in adults following prolonged exposure to lead and manifested by a reduced glomerular filtration rate (GFR), and meager proteinuria. It is frequently associated with hypertension, and gout. Interstitial nephritis following symptomatic lead poisoning was described in the nineteen century and was widely identified among symptomatic lead workers, and consumers of contaminated illegal whiskey ("moonshiners") in the twentieth century [1]. Recognition of the adverse effects of lead in asymptomatic individuals depended on the development of chemical methods for measuring lead in blood in the twentieth century. Identifying the effects of lead when blood levels are below 20 μg/dL had to await large epidemiologic studies in community populations as opposed to clinically or occupationally defined groups. Epidemiologic studies demonstrated the statistical significance of small alterations in blood pressure and renal function due to low-level lead, alterations that have major public health implications. Lead may contribute to the finding that almost four million Americans have both elevated creatinines and hypertension [16].

Occupational lead nephropathy has developed after as little as 3 years of intense occupational exposure [4] Analysis of death certificates of 601 men employed at the Bunker Hill Lead Mine and Smelter in Kellogg, Idaho, up to 1977 indicated a twofold-increased risk of dying from chronic renal disease [17]. The increased risk approached fourfold after 20 years of occupational exposure. Although most frequently recognized in lead workers after decades of occupational exposure, chronic lead nephropathy was originally described among young adults in Australia who sustained acute childhood lead poisoning [18]. Sporadic case reports of lead nephropathy arising from unusual accidental exposure such as geophagia [19] or Asian folk remedies and cosmetics continue to appear in the medical literature [1].

Lead-induced chronic interstitial nephritis in the absence of symptomatic lead poisoning was first described among American workers [4, 20], and in U.S. Armed Service veterans suffering from renal failure that had been initially attributed to gout or essential hypertension [21, 22]. The contribution of excessive lead absorption to hypertension and interstitial nephritis was indicated by urinary excretion of more than 600 μg of lead during the $CaNa_2EDTA$ lead-mobilization test performed after renal failure was apparent. Medical histories obtained from these men were misleading with respect to prior lead exposure; patient recall frequently contradicted the objective evidence of the chelation test. In the 1960s and 1970s the arbitrary cut off of 600 μg/3days for lead excretion during the $CaNa_2EDTA$ test proved useful for identifying excessive lead exposure groups in Australia, the United States, Spain and Italy [4, 6, 18, 23]. Studies using this cut off identified the relatively frequent appearance of renal insufficiency with hypertension and/or gout at high exposure levels ($CaNa_2EDTA$ lead mobilization test > 600μg/3d). Detecting the lower prevalence of adverse effects at low body lead burdens required studies of asymptomatic populations with lower exposure [24, 25].

"Queensland nephritis" appears to represent the transition from the proximal tubule reabsorptive defects of acute lead poisoning in children, to the chronic interstitial nephritis of adults [18]. Lead-induced interstitial nephritis was first recognized among young adults in Queensland, Australia, who were lead poisoned as children in the 1890s through the 1920s. The evolution of acute lead nephropathy to chronic interstitial nephritis has been produced in experimental animals but was only recently reported in follow-up studies of Americans adults exposed in childhood. In an early follow-up study of untreated childhood lead poisoning, diagnostic criteria for both lead poisoning and renal disease were unacceptably vague [26]. A 50-year follow-up of untreated lead-poisoned children in the United States found evidence of an increased prevalence of renal disease [27].

Chronic lead nephropathy from moonshine came to medical attention because of the dramatic symptoms of acute lead poisoning. Lead colic and anemia were associated with reduced GFR, which often improved following chelation therapy. Transient renal failure, apparently the result of renal vasoconstriction [28], was superimposed on structural renal damage that appeared to be less responsive to chelating agents. This therapeutic response in pre-azotemic lead nephropathy may reflect reversal of functional impairment rather than reversal of established interstitial nephritis.

Acute reductions in GFR and acute elevations of blood pressure may be mediated by the blood lead concentration whereas long-term effects such as interstitial nephritis and sustained hypertension may be determined by cumulative lead absorption [12, 29]. This difference in the short-term (days) effects of lead on GFR and blood pressure compared to the effects of long-term (years) exposure corresponds to the difference between Fanconi syndrome following brief acute exposure and the delayed development of chronic interstitial nephritis following prolonged exposure. The acute and chronic effects of lead on the kidney may have different pathogenetic mechanisms. Epidemiologic evidence suggests that modest azotemia is significantly more prevalent among lead-exposed workers than among nonexposed counterparts, presumably owing to both morphologic changes mediated by cumulative exposure and functional changes mediated by current blood lead levels [30].

Chronic lead nephropathy in moonshiners, more often than not, is accompanied by gout and hypertension, in accord with 19th century descriptions of plumbism and reports from Australia [1]. A statistically significant odds ratio of 2.4 has been reported for moonshine consumption and end-stage renal disease, suggesting a causal association with lead in the absence of symptomatic lead poisoning [31].

Renal biopsies in chronic lead nephropathy show nonspecific tubular atrophy and interstitial fibrosis with minimal inflammatory response as well as mitochondrial swelling, loss of cristae, and increased lysosomal dense bodies within proximal tubule cells [4, 18]. (Figure 1)

Intra-renal arteriolar changes indistinguishable from nephrosclerosis are found, often in the absence of clinical hypertension [4]. The appearance of arteriolar nephrosclerosis before hypertension develops and the relatively short duration of hypertension before renal failure supervenes suggest that the initial renal injury from lead may be in the microvascular endothelium

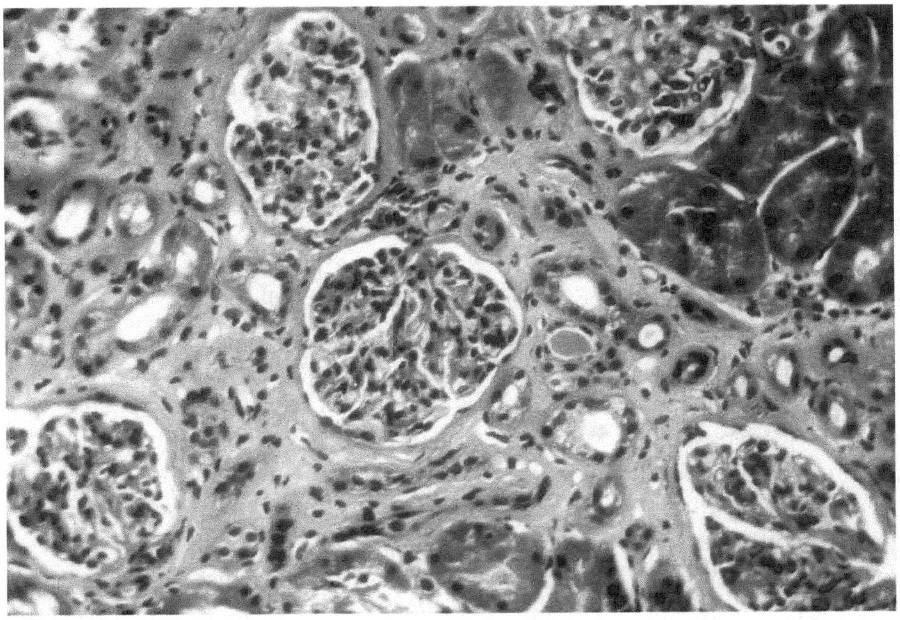

Figure 1. *Tubular atrophy and interstitial fibrosis in a case of chronic lead nephropathy. H&E staining, orig. magn. x300.*

[30, 32]. This view is consistent with the possibility that the acute effects of lead on blood pressure are mediated by the current blood lead concentration whereas the long-term effects are mediated by endothelial injury resulting from cumulative lead absorption. Intranuclear inclusion bodies are often absent when the renal disease is long-standing and advanced or following the administration of chelating agents. Clumped chromatin and nuclear invaginations of cytoplasmic contents may be found even in the absence of intranuclear inclusions. Morphologic alterations are minimal in glomeruli until the reduction in GFR is advanced

The functional changes in chronic lead nephropathy appear to be less specific than those observed in acute poisoning. As in other forms of interstitial nephritis, proteinuria and glycosuria are initially absent. In contrast to cadmium nephropathy, the excretion of a large array of urinary marker proteins such as retinal binding protein, lysozyme, and β_2-microglobulin [33, 34] is not increased in the absence of a reduced GFR.

The increase in urinary *N*-acetyl-ß-D-glucosaminidase (NAG) with increasing blood lead concentrations reflects the proximal tubule dysfunction seen in acute lead nephropathy rather than the chronic interstitial nephritis associated with occupational lead exposure [35, 36]. NAG excretion correlates positively with the blood lead concentration but not with the bone lead concentration [37]. Eicosanoid excretion in lead workers is similar to that in patients with essential hypertension [33, 36].

In contrast to the reabsorptive defect of acute lead nephropathy, saturnine gout is characterized by renal retention of uric acid [18]. The clearance (C_{PAH}) and maximal secretion rate (Tm_{PAH}) for *p*-aminohippurate (PAH) have been found to be variable in patients with occupational lead nephropathy.

Saturnine gout

Hyperuricemia and gout are common among individuals with excessive exposure to lead, apparently the result of decreased excretion and increased production of uric acid. Although hyperuricemia invariably accompanies azotemia, gout is uncommon in patients with renal failure except in those with lead nephropathy. Half of uremic patients with lead nephropathy have clinical gout [18] but in the absence of renal failure, gout cannot usually be attributed to lead despite coexisting hypertension [23, 37].

There is substantial evidence that renal failure in gout is often secondary to overt or unsuspected lead poisoning. In Queensland, Australia, as many as 80% of gout patients with renal failure had elevated EDTA lead-mobilization tests [18]. In New Jersey, chelatable lead was found to be significantly greater among gout patients with renal failure than among gout patients with normal renal function [21]. Because patients with comparable renal failure owing to known causes other than lead show no increase in chelatable lead, the excessive mobilizable lead in these gout patients appears to be the cause rather than consequence of their renal failure. Measurement of lead levels in transiliac bone biopsy specimens from patients with end-stage renal disease confirms the finding that renal failure per se does not cause increased mobilizable lead or bone lead [6, 7]. The conclusion that lead absorption causes renal damage rather than the reverse is supported by longitudinal studies [4, 6]. Unrecognized lead poisoning, therefore, may explain the occurrence of renal failure in some gout patients who have neither urinary calculi nor intratubular uric acid deposition disease. Similarly, overt lead poisoning may explain the protean manifestations of gout in past centuries, *irregular gout,* as well as the almost forgotten association of gout with (lead-laden) wine [1]. Sporadic contamination of alcoholic drinks with lead throughout history may have been responsible for irregular gout that terminated in cerebral disease (e.g., uremia, stroke, lead encephalopathy).

Lead-induced hyperuricemia may contribute to chronic lead nephropathy. Uric acid *per se* induces endothelial cell injury, renal microvascular disease, and hypertension, at least in part mediated by oxidative stress [38]. Independent of uric acid, reactive oxygen species induced by lead have been implicated in endothelial cell injury, increased vascular reactivity, and the production of hypertension in humans and experimental animals [39].

Hypertension

The association between lead and hypertension has been a subject of controversy since the first use of the sphygmomanometer. The early view that renal injury induced by lead causes hypertension has gained increasing support. The duration of hypertension in patients with lead nephropathy tends to be shorter than that in hypertensives without renal failure, suggesting that lead-induced renal vascular damage precedes, and therefore causes the hypertension. This view is consistent with the finding that creatinine clearance decreases with increasing blood lead in the general population, an effect that is independent of blood pressure [40]. Mortality data show that death from hypertensive cardiovascular disease is more frequent among lead workers than the general population [17]

Lead nephropathy does not account for renal failure in all hypertensives with kidney disease any more than it accounts for renal failure in all gout patients with kidney disease. The heavy metal may, however, contribute to the association of gout with hypertension, as well as to the variable incidence of renal failure in each of these conditions.

An etiologic role for lead in hypertension is supported by epidemiologic studies in populations with mean blood leads > 10 μg/dL, but with exposure too low to produce symptomatic lead poisoning. The Second National Health and Nutrition Examination Survey (NHANES II) performed between 1976 and 1980 included blood lead and blood pressure measurements in almost 10,000 non-institutionalized Americans aged 6 months to 74 years [41] Correlation between blood lead and blood pressure was robust even when both measurements were within the (at the time) accepted "normal" range [42, 43]. Similar observations have been made in studies performed throughout the world, although non-statistically significant findings in small studies have also been reported.

Low-level exposure

Epidemiologic evidence that low-level lead absorption (blood leads < 10 μg/dL) increases blood pressure and decreases renal function has been obtained from studies undertaken after lead was removed from gasoline as blood lead levels were falling in the United States population as a whole. Analysis of data on over 15,000 Americans from 1988 to 1994 in NHANES III showed that hypertensives had significantly higher blood leads (4.21 vs 3.30 μg/dL) and a higher frequency of elevated creatinines (11.5 vs 1.8%) than non-hypertensives [44]. Cross-sectional studies showed a significant positive association between low-level lead exposure and serum creatinine [40, 45]. Major adverse consequences of hypertension, mortality from cardiovascular disease, myocardial infarction, and stroke, have been found to correlate positively with blood lead levels above [45] and below 10 μg/dL [5]. Even as the mean blood lead in the US population fell below 2 μg/dL, those in the highest lead quartile were 2.72 time more likely to have chronic kidney disease than those in the lowest blood lead quartile [47].

The adverse effect of low-level lead exposure on renal function is supported by longitudinal observations in non-occupationally exposed populations. Among 509 randomly selected men in the Department of Veterans Affairs Normative Aging Study who had a mean blood lead of 9.9 μg/dL, Kim et al. found that blood lead correlated positively and significantly with serum creatinine [48]. In 1171 of these veterans (mean blood lead of 6.3 μg/dL), tibia, patella and blood lead levels were significantly higher in those who developed hypertension than in those who did not [49]. In another subset of the Normative Aging Study, Thais et al. reported that the rate of progression of renal failure was 17.6- and 12.8-fold greater in diabetics in the highest tibial and blood lead quartiles, respectively, than in non-diabetics indicating high vulnerability to the adverse effects of low-level lead in diabetics [50]. Similarly, increased sensitivity to the additional adverse effects of low-level lead exposure on kidney function was observed among hypertensives [49]. Among 964 subjects (mean blood lead 3.5 μg/dL) blood (but not tibial) lead was significantly correlated with systolic and diastolic blood pressure but not with hypertension [29]. Tibia lead correlated with hypertension suggesting that current blood lead levels influence blood pressure but cumulative absorption influences the development of sustained hypertension.

Cross-sectional studies of normal populations also show adverse effects of exposure to lead at blood lead levels < 10μg/dL. Tibial lead (but not blood or patella lead) was a significant predictor of hypertension and systolic pressure in the normotensive range in the Normative Aging Study (mean blood lead 6.09 μg/dL) [51]. In contrast, patella lead, but not tibia lead, was found to be a significant predictor of hypertension in nurses [52]. In one study, the impact of low level lead exposure assessed by blood lead on blood pressure was statistically significant in blacks but not in whites [53]. The impact of cumulative lead absorption on blood pressure may be ameliorated by high dietary calcium intake (> 800 mg/day), and further modulated by polymorphisms in the vitamin D receptor gene [54, 55].

A study in pregnant women with a geometric mean blood lead of 1.9 μg/dL found increased bone leads were associated with an increased risk of hypertension [56]. Diastolic and systolic blood pressure were significantly and positively associated with blood lead concentration. The major portion of the effect was found with blood leads < 5 μg/dL. Blood lead < 10 μg/dL also was a risk factor for postpartum hypertension among women in Tehran [57]. A compelling case is therefore emerging indicating adverse effects on blood pressure and the kidneys at blood lead levels < 5 μg/dL in diverse populations [58].

Causality and environmental exposure

The variability of the positive correlations found between blood pressure or GFR with biomarkers of lead absorption (see above) has been used as an argument to deter preventive action. Such hesitancy may in part derive from a fundamental misunderstanding of the scientific rationale (i.e.Bradford Hill's considerations) for determining causality in environmental disease [59] By convention, statistical analysis favors accepting the null hypothesis; finding no significant difference between groups. The methodology results in finding false negatives more readily than false positives. Measurement error and human variability tend to support the null hypothesis.

Because control of renal function and blood pressure is multifactorial, the causal contribution of lead is difficult to isolate. A number of biomarkers (blood, tibial, and patella lead), and a variety of populations differing by age, gender, race, and level of exposure are examined. Systolic and diastolic pressures are assessed separately and may be analyzed both as continuous or dichotomous variables. Kidney function is assessed by the serum creatinine concentration or empirical adjustments of the creatinine to estimate GFR. Large populations are required to achieve statistical significance amidst the noise of the multifactorial causality and the imprecision of outcome measures. Inconsistent results and weak correlations are, therefore, expected as smaller and smaller outcome effects are evaluated.

Consequently, the finding of statistical significance for some but not all of the biomarkers of lead absorption does not nullify the importance of the positive associations. On the contrary, statistical inference is stacked against finding false positives and therefore may underestimate real associations. The failure to find statistical significance does not have weight equal to the finding of significance. Despite the inevitable persistence of uncertainty, the obligation to recognize the importance of statistically significant findings, and to undertake preventive action, remains.

Although some controversy exists about the magnitude of the dose-response relationship, there is a growing consensus that lead contributes to hypertension in the general population, particularly in the presence of renal dysfunction. Lead may also contribute to the disproportionate representation of black men with hypertensive nephrosclerosis and diabetic nephropathy in end-stage renal disease programs in the United States [60].

The observation reported from Ja-Liang Lin's laboratory in Taiwan that chelation therapy improves renal function in renal failure patients with low body lead stores ($CaNa_2EDTA$ lead mobilization tests < 80 μg/3d) reinforces the conclusion that unrecognized low-level lead absorption contributes to renal failure due to other causes [25]. Lin's laboratory reported that blood lead levels correlate with the rate of fall of GFR in patients with diabetic nephropathy (serum creatinine range 1.7-3.9 mg/dl) such that an increase in blood lead of 1 μg/dL predicted a reduction in GFR of 0.56 ml/min/1.73 m^2 over 1 year of observation before chelation therapy (mean low blood lead group 5.9 μg/dL, N=15; mean high blood lead 7.5 μg/dL, N=15) [61]. These data reinforce the observation that low-level lead absorption accelerates the reduction in GFR in diabetic nephropathy made in Boston [50]. Following 2 years of chelation therapy (averaging a total of 7.0 g $CaNa_2EDTA$) the GFR increased an average of 6 ml/min/1.73 m^2 compared to a *decrease* of 1.4 ml/min/1.73 m^2 in the untreated group [61].

Additional observations from Lin's laboratory raise the possibility that $CaNa_2EDTA$ may improve GFR in all patients with reduced GFR. They treated 32 non-diabetic patients (mean creatinine 2.1 mg/dL; mean blood lead 5.3 μg/dL) with $CaNa_2EDTA$, 4-13 g IV, over two years. The treated group had an increase in GFR averaging 3.4 ml/min while untreated controls (N=32) had a *decrease* in GFR of 1.0 ml/min [62]. The effect of comparable chelation on an important control group of renal failure patients with virtually no lead absorption was, unfortunately, not studied. Although these findings from Taiwan need to be confirmed in other laboratories, they raise the possibility that the beneficial effect of $CaNa_2EDTA$ may be unrelated to urinary lead excretion. The salutary results might, for example, be due to a non-specific antioxidant effect of $CaNa_2EDTA$ that increases GFR.

Treatment

Lead nephropathy is important because it is one of the few renal diseases that is preventable. Moreover, lead-induced acute renal dysfunction can sometimes be reversed by chelation therapy [19, 28, 63]. The salutary effect of chelation therapy appears to be on the acute reduction in GFR and the acute elevation of blood pressure associated with elevated blood lead concentration rather than on the long-term effects of cumulative exposure associated with endothelial dysfunction, hypertension, and interstitial nephritis. There is no evidence that such therapy reverses established interstitial nephritis. The partial remission achieved among moonshiners and lead workers appears to represent reversal of the physiologic effects of acute poisoning superimposed on chronic lead nephropathy. No improvement in renal function has been observed once advanced interstitial nephritis is present and the steady-state serum creatinine concentration exceeds about 3 mg/dL [64].

Despite the effectiveness of chelation therapy in increasing the rate of lead excretion, the most appropriate treatment for asymptomatic excessive lead absorption is preventing further exposure. Elderly males store about 500 mg of lead in their bones in the absence of unusual exposure while occupational exposure may result in several grams stored in bones. Chelation therapy briefly increases the rate of removal of lead from the body, but, in the long run, the negative balance established by preventing further exposure is far more effective in reducing the body burden. The unstimulated daily excretion of lead ranges from a few micrograms in those without unusual exposure to hundreds of micrograms per day in those with heavy exposure. Chelation therapy increases lead excretion 10 or 20 fold for a few days, but in total cannot match the negative balance due to unstimulated daily excretion occurring over decades when intake of lead approaches zero. Prevention of lead intake is therefore far more effective than chelation therapy in asymptomatic individuals. However, chelation therapy is justified in the face of symptomatic lead poisoning or when blood levels exceed about 80 μg/dL because of the danger of lead encephalopathy.

In summary, chelation therapy is justified in cases of symptomatic lead poisoning or when the blood lead exceeds about 80 μg/ dL. When no symptom end-point is clearly defined, chelation for blood lead < 80 μg/ dL is not usually justified.

References

1. Wedeen RP. Poison in the Pot: the Legacy of Lead. Carbondale, Ill: Southern Illinois University Press, 1984.
2. Lancereaux E. Saturnisme chronique avec acces de goutte et Arthritis uratiques. Compt Rend Soc de Biol (Paris) 1872; 2: 99-106.
3. Rabinowitz MB. Kinetic analysis of lead metabolism in healthy humans. J Clin Invest 1976; 58: 260-270.
4. Wedeen RP, Maesaka JK, Weiner B, Lipat GA, Lyons MM, Vitale LF. Joselow MM. Occupational lead nephropathy. Am J Med 1975; 59: 630 641.
5. Menke A, Munter P, Batuman V, Silbergeld EK, Guallar E. Blood lead below 0.48 βmol/L (10 ug/dL) and mortality among US adults. Circulation 2006; 114: 1388-1394.
6. Sanchez-Fructuoso AI, Torralbo A, Arroyo M, Luque,\ M, Ruilope LM, Santos JL, Cruycyera A, Barrientes A. Occult lead intoxication as a cause of hypertension and renal failure. Nephrol Dial Transplant 1996; 11:1775-178.
7. Van de Vyver FL, D'Haese PC, Visier WJ, Elseviers MM, Knippenberg LI, Lamberts LW, Wedeen, RP, De Broe ME. Bone lead in dialysis patients. Kidney Int 1988; 33: 601-607.
8. Inglis JA, Henderson DA, Emmerson BT. The pathology and pathogenesis of chronic lead nephropathy occurring in Queensland. J Path 1978; 124: 65-76.
9. Grandjean P. Biological effects of organolead compounds. Boca Raton, FL: CRC Press, 1984.
10. Wedeen RP. The politics of lead. In: Sheehan HE, Wedeen RP, eds. Toxic circles: environmental hazards from the workplace into community. New Brunswick: Rutgers University, 1993:168-200.
11. Fiedler, N., Weisel, C., Lynch, R., Kelly-McNeil, K., Wedeen, R., Jones, K., Udasin, I., Ohman-Strickland, P., and Gochfeld, M. Cognitive effects of chronic exposure to lead and solvents. Am. J. Indust. Med. 2003; 4: 413-423.
12. Glenn BS, Stewart WF, Links JM, Todd AC, Schwartz BS. The longitudinal association of lead and blood pressure. Epidemiology 2003; 14: 30-36.
13. Chisolm JJ, Harrison HC, Eberlern WR, Harrison HE. Aminoaciduria, hypophosphatemia and rickets in lead poisoning. Am J Dis Child 1955; 89: 159-68.
14. Goyer RA, Wilson MH. Lead-induced inclusion bodies. Results of ethylenediaminetetraacetic acid treatment. Lab Invest 1975; 32: 149-56.
15. Schumann GB, Lerner SI, Weiss MA, Gawronski L, Lohiya GK. Inclusion-bearing cells in industrial workers exposed to lead. Am J Clin Pathol 1980; 74: 192-6.
16. Coresh J, Wei GL, McQuillan G, Brancati FL, Levey AS, Jones C, Klag MJ. Prevelence of high blood pressure and elevated serum creatinine level in the United States. 2001; 161; 1206-1216.
17. Selevan SG, Landrigan PJ, Stern FB, Jones JH. Mortality of lead smelter workers. Am J Epidemiol 1985; 122: 673-83.
18. Emmerson BT. Chronic lead nephropathy. The diagnostic use of calcium EDTA and the association with gout. Aust Med J 1963; 12: 310-324.
19. Wedeen RP, Mallik DK, Batuman V, Bogden JD. Geophagic lead nephropathy: A case report. Environ Res 1978; 17: 409-415.
20. Wedeen RP, Mallik DK, Batuman V. Detection and treatment of occupational lead nephropathy. Arch Intern Med 1979; 139: 53-57.
21. Batuman, V., Maesaka, J.K., Haddad, B., Tepper, E., Landy, E. and Wedeen, R.P. The role of lead in gout nephropathy. N. Engl. J. Med. 1981; 304: 520 523.
22. Batuman V, Landy E, Maesaka JK, Wedeen RP. Contribution of lead to hypertension with renal failure. N Engl J Med 1983; 309: 17-21.
23. Colleoni N, D'Aminco G. Chronic lead accumulation as a possible cause of renal failure in gouty patients. Nephron 1986: 44; 32-35.
24. Behringer D, Craswell P., Mohl C. Stoeppler M, Tritz E. Urinary lead excretion in uremic patients. Nephron 1986: 42 323-329.
25. Lin J-A, Ho H-H, Yu C-C. Chelation therapy for patients with elevated body lead burden and progressive renal insufficiency. A randomized controlled trial. Ann Intern Med 1999; 130:7-13.
26. Tepper L. Renal function subsequent to childhood plumbism. Arch Environ Health 1963; 7: 76-85.

27. Hu H. A 50-year follow-up of childhood plumbism: hypertension, renal function, and hemoglobin levels among survivors. Am J Dis Child 1991; 145:681-687.
28. Lilis R, Garvrilescu N, Nestroescu R, Dumitriu C, Roventa A. Nephropathy in chronic lead poisoning. Br J Ind Med 1968;25:196-202.
29. Martin D, Glass TA, Bandeen-Roche K, Todd AC, Shi W, Schwartz BS. Association of blood lead and tibia lead with blood pressure and hypertension in a community sample of older adults. Am J Epidemiol 2006; 163: 467-478.
30. Chai S S, Webb RC. Effects of lead on vascular reactivity. Environ Health Perspect 1988; 78: 85-91.
31. Steenland NK, Thun Mj, Furguson W, Port FK. Occupational and other exposures associated with male end stage renal disease: a case/control study. Am J Public Health 1990; 80: 153-159.
32. Kopp SJ, Barron JT, Tow JP. Cardiovascular actions of lead and relationship to hypertension: a review. Scand J Work Environ Health 1985; 11: 15-23.
33. Cardenas A, Roels H, Bernard AM, Barbon R, Buchet JP, Lauwerys RR, Rosello J, Ramis I, Mutti A, Franchini I, Fels LM, Stolte H, De Broe ME, Nuyts GD, Taylor SA, Price RG. Markers of early renal changes induced by industrial pollutants. II. Application to workers exposed to lead. Brit J Ind Med 1993; 50: 28-36.
34. Mueller PW, Paschal PC, Hammel RR, Klincewitz SL, McNeil ML, Speirto B, Steinberg KK. Chronic effects in three studies of men and women occupationally exposed to cadmium. Arch Environ Contam Toxicol 1992; 23: 125-136.
35. Endo G, Horiguchi S, Kiyota I. Urinary N-acetyl-ß-D-glucosaminidase activity in lead-exposed workers. J Appl Toxicol 1990; 10: 235-238.
36. Wedeen RP, Udasin I., Fiedler N, D'Haese P, De Broe ME, Gelpi E, Jones KW, Gochfeld M. Urinary biomarkers as indicators of renal disease. Renal Failure. 1999; 21: 241-249.
37. Peitzman SJ, Bodison W, Ellis I. Moonshine drinking among hypertensive veterans in Philadelphia. Arch Intern Med 1985; 145: 632-634.
38. Nakagawa t, Kang D-H, Sanchez-Lozada LG, Srinivas TR, Sautin Y, Ejaz AA, Segal M, Johnson RJ. Unearthing uric acid: An ancient factor with recently found significance in renal cardiovascular disease. Kidney International 2006; 69:1722-1735.
39. Vaziri ND, Sica DA. Lead-induced hypertension: Role of oxidative stress. Curreent Hypertension Reports 2004; 6: 314-320.
40. Staessen J, Lauwerys RR, Buchet J-P, Bulpitt CJ, Rondia D, Vanenterghem Y, Amery A. Impairment of renal function with increasing blood lead concentration in the general population. The Cadmibel study group. N Engl J Med 1994; 327: 151-156.
41. Mahaffey KR, Annest JL, Roberts J, Murphy RS. National estimates of blood lead levels: United States, 1976–1980. Association with selected demographic and socioeconomic factors. N Engl J Med 1982; 307: 573-579.
42. Harlan WR. The relationship of blood lead levels to blood pressure in the U.S. population. Environ Health Perspect 1988; 78: 9-13.
43. Pirkle JL, Schwartz J, Landia JR, Harlan WR. The relationship between blood lead levels and blood pressure and its cardiovascular risk implications. Am J Epidemiol 1985; 121: 246-258.
44. Munter P, He J, Vupputuri S, Coresh J, Batuman V. Blood lead and chronic kidney disease in the general United States population: Results from NHANES III. Kidney Int 2003; 63: 1044-1050.
45. Payton M, Hu H, Sparrow D, Young JB, Landsberg L, Weiss S. Relation between blood lead and urinary biogenic amines in community-exposed men. Am J Epidemiology. 1993; 138(10): 815-825.
46. Lustberg M, Silbergeld E. Blood lead levels and mortality. Arch Intern Med 2002; 162: 2443-2449.
47. Munter P, Menke A, DeSalvo KB, Rabito FA, Batuman V. Continued decline in blood lead levels among adults in the United States. Arch Intern Med 2006; 165: 2155-2161.
48. Kim R, Rotnitski A, Parrow D, Weiss ST, Wager C, Hu H. A longitudinal study of low-level lead exposure and impairment of renal function. The Normative Aging Study. JAMA 1996; 275: 1177-1176.
49. Hu H, Aro A, Payton M, Korrick S, Sparrow D, Weiss ST. The relationship of bone and blood lead to hypertension. The Normative Aging Study. JAMA 1996; 275: 1171-1176.
50. Thais S-W, Korrick S, Schwartz J, Amasirlwardena C, Aro A, Sparrow D, Hu H. Lead diabetes, hypertension, and renal function: Normative Aging Study. Environ Health Perspect 2004; 112: 1178-1182.
51. Cheng Y, Schwartz J, Sparrow D, Aro A, Weiss, ST, Hu H. Bone lead and bone lead levels in relation to baseline blood pressure and the prospective development of hypertension: The Normative Aging Study. Am J Epidemiology. 2001; 153(2): 164-171.
52. Korrick SA, Hunter DJ, Rotnitzky A, Hu H, Speizer FE. Lead and hypertension in a sample of middle-aged women. Am J Public Health. 1999; 89(3): 330-335.
53. Vupputuri S, He J, Munter P, Bazzano LA, Whelton PK, Batuman V. Blood lead level is associated with elevated blood pressure in blacks. Hypertension 2003; 41: 463-468.

54. Byung-Kook L, Lee G-S, Stewert WF, Kyu-Dong A, Simon D, Kelsey KT, Todd AC, Schwartz BS. Associations of blood pressure and hypertension with lead dose measures and polymorphisms in the vitamin D receptor and β-aminolevulinic acid dehydratase genes. Environ Health Perspectives 2001; 109: 383-389.
55. Elmarsafawy SF, Nitin J, Schwartz J, Sparrow D, Nie H, Hu H. Dietary calcium as a potential modifier of the relationship between lead burden to blood pressure. Epidemiology 2006; 17(5): 531-7.
56. Rothenberg S, Khondrashov V, Manalo M, Jiang J, Cuellar R, Garcia M, et al. Increases in hypertension and blood pressure during pregnancy with increased bone lead levels. Am J Epidemiology 2002; 156(12):1079-1087
57. Vigeh M, Ghazizadeh S, Yokayama K, Sakai T, Mazaheri M, Morita Y, Beheshti S, Kitamura F, Araki S. Relationship between increased blood lead and preganacy hypertension in women without occupational lead exposure in Tehran, Iran. Arch Environ Health 2004; 59: 70-75.
58. Ekong EB, Jaar BJ, Weaver VM. Lead-related nephrotoxicity: A review of the epidemiologic evidence. Kidney Int 2006; 70: 2074-2084.
59. Legator MS, Morris DL. What did Sir Bradford Hill really say? Arch Environ Health 2003; 58: 718-720.
60. Wedeen RP. Blood lead levels, dietary calcium, and hypertension. Ann Intern Med 1985; 102:403.
61. Lin J-L, Lin-Tan D-T, Yu C-C, Li Y-J, Huang Y-Y, li K-L. Environmental exposure to lead and progressive diabetic nephropathy in patients with type II diabetes. Kidney International 2006; 69: 2049-2056.
62. Lin J-L, Lin-Tan D-T, Hsu K-H, Yu C-C. Environmental lead exposure and progression of chronic renal diseases in patients without diabetes. N Eng J Med 2003; 348: 277-286.
63. Sehnert KW, Claque AF, Cheraskin E. The improvement in renal function following EDTA chelation and multi-vitamin-trace mineral therapy: a study in creatinine clearance. Med Hypoth 1984; 15: 301-304.
64. Germain MJ, Braden GL, Fitzgibbons JP. Failure of chelation therapy in lead nephropathy. Arch Intern Med 1984; 144: 2419-2420.

35

Cadmium-induced renal effects

Gunnar F. NORDBERG[1], Teruhiko KIDO[2] and Harry A. ROELS[3]

[1]Umea University, Umea, Sweden,
[2]Kanazawa University, Kodatsuno, Kanazawa, Japan
[3]Université catholique de Louvain, Brussels, Belgium

Introduction

The first observations on adverse renal effects of cadmium (Cd) exposure in humans were made by Friberg in the late 1940s [1]. He reported a high prevalence of proteinuria (65% using the nitric acid test and 81% using the trichloroacetic acid test) in Cd-exposed workers.

In Japan, an unusual disease named "itai-itai byo" or "ouch-ouch disease" was reported in 1955 [2]. This disease is characterized clinically by bone and kidney damage. In 1968, the Japanese Ministry of Health and Welfare concluded that itai-itai disease was caused by chronic Cd poisoning [3].

The kidneys are particularly affected by Cd following long-term exposure [4, 5]. Studies of workers chronically exposed to air borne Cd report renal effects as well as respiratory effects though less frequently. Therefore, the kidneys are considered the critical target organ for Cd in the general population as well as occupationally exposed population.

Exposure

Low concentrations of the element Cd occur naturally in the environment. Human exposure in the general environment occurs mainly from ingested foods. Concentrations of Cd in food items from areas without industrial contamination are summarized in Table 1.

For basic food items such as rice, potatoes and wheat, Cd concentrations usually are lower than 0.1 mg/kg, while higher concentrations occur naturally in certain meats or shellfish. The daily dietary intake of Cd has been estimated to be 10-20 μg in several countries of the European Union and in several studies from the USA [3, 5]. In areas contaminated by emissions from industrial activities much higher daily oral intakes have occurred with amounts up to 200-1800 μg in people living in such areas in Japan and China [3, 6, 7].

Cadmium can also occur as an aerosol in air. While inhalation of ambient air usually does not contribute significantly to the daily intake of Cd, cigarette smoking does. The content of Cd often is 1-2 μg per cigarette. Based on data concerning the Cd content of cigarettes, it has been estimated that smoking of 20 cigarettes per day results in a daily inhalation of 2-4 μg [3]. Since approximately 50% may be absorbed, this can result in an uptake of 1-2 μg of Cd per day.

Occupational exposure in the Cd-related industries can be associated with the inhalation of considerable amounts of Cd. In the 1950s, before the health hazards of Cd were recognized, Cd concentrations in the air of the working environment were sometimes high, i.e. in the order of milligrams per m^3. In recent years, concentrations in industrial air have been reduced to 2-50 $\mu g/m^3$, with higher values being reported in some exceptional cases. Examples of Cd-related industrial activities include: manufacturing of alkaline (nickel-Cd) batteries, smelting operations involving copper/zinc-Cd ores or alloys, production of Cd-based pigments, soldering with silver-Cd containing solder and welding in Cd-containing materials. In several EU countries (e.g. Sweden) certain uses of Cd such as its use in pigments, in electroplating and in soldering have been banned.

Toxicokinetics

Uptake

Inhalation of airborne Cd leads to variable uptake depending on size and solubility of particles. The systemic uptake of aerosolized Cd with a particle size of 10 μm has been estimated to be about 7%, while the uptake following inhalation of a particle size of 0.1 μm may be as high as 50% [8].

Table 1. Concentrations of cadmium in different foodstuffs*.

Food	Mean mg/kg wet weight
Beef meat	0.005-0.02
Beef kidney	0.2-1.3
Fish meat (other than crab)	0.004-0.1
Oysters	0.1-4.7
Wheat grains	0.005-0.08
Rice (non-contaminated areas)	0.008-0.13
Milk	0.00017-0.002
Potatoes	0.01-0.06

From Nordberg et al. [5].

After oral ingestion, systemic uptake has been reported to be 1-6% in animal experiments. Factors that have been shown to influence oral uptake are dose and composition of the diet. In humans, the systemic uptake usually varies between 3 and 10% of the oral intake. In individuals with depleted body iron stores, uptake may be as high as 20% or even higher [5, 8].

Transport and distribution

Figure 1 represents the uptake and transfer of Cd to the kidney. Following uptake, Cd is primarily bound in serum to albumin, the form in which it is transported to the various body pools. Cadmium bound to albumin (which is the dominating form in plasma shortly after uptake) is taken up primarily by the liver where it accumulates, and is dissociated. Released Cd-ions induce the synthesis of metallothionein which results in an increasing proportion of liver Cd being bound to metallothionein. The uptake of albumin-bound Cd by liver cells may be mediated by albumin receptors on the sinusoidal surfaces of hepatocytes [9]. In long-term chronic exposure a slow release of Cd-metallothionein from liver to blood occurs. During the phase when plasma Cd is bound to albumin, there is only limited uptake of Cd in the kidney. A long time after a single exposure or in a long-term chronic exposure situation, a considerable proportion of plasma Cd is bound to metallothionein. The Cd-metallothionein complex, because of its small molecular size, is filtered by the glomerular membrane and is efficiently taken up by renal tubular cells. Moreover, metallothionein-bound Cd is taken up more efficiently by renal cells of Cd-exposed animals than by cells from non-exposed animals [10]. After entering renal tubule cells via

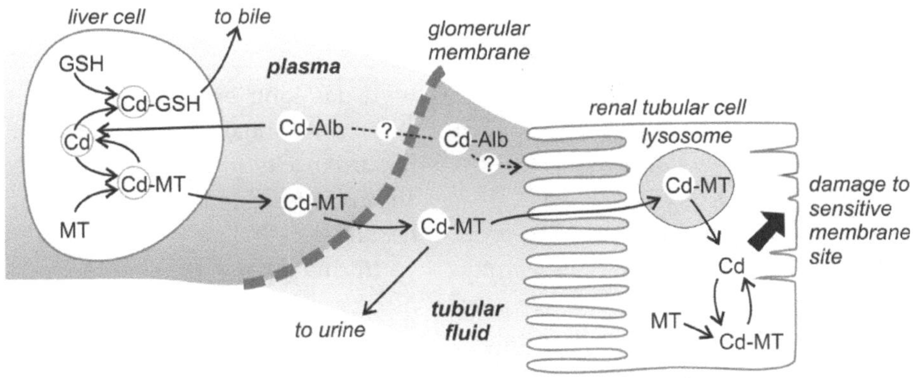

Figure 1. *Pathways of cadmium uptake and interaction with target sites in the kidney.*

pinocytosis [11] or, as shown by Bernard et al. [12], by adsorptive endocytosis the Cd-metallothionein complex is catabolized in lysosomes releasing toxic Cd ions [13]. The balance between metallothionein-bound and non-metallothionein-bound Cd in the cell is considered of importance for the expression of toxicity. Non-metallothionein Cd in renal cells induces *de novo* synthesis (Figure 1). This process may account for the long biological half-life of Cd in the kidney where the element may be retained 10-20 years [5, 8]. Such a long biological half-life explains why Cd continues to accumulate in humans up to 50 years of age, reflecting the historical intake from the environment.

Cadmium does not readily pass the blood-brain barrier, the blood-testis barrier or the placental barrier, but it accumulates in the placenta of animals and humans [14]. In humans, placental transfer of Cd seems to be very low and Cd is found to accumulate in the placenta [15, 16].

Excretion of cadmium

The daily elimination of Cd (0.01-0.02 % of the body burden per day) via urine and feces is small as would be expected from the element's long biological half-life [5, 8]. This implies that there is an age-related accumulation of Cd in the body and the increased urinary excretion of Cd with age is due to the increasing body burden. While this interrelationship has been documented in humans on a group basis, there exists a large variation among individuals. Cadmium is also excreted in the feces, but the majority of fecal Cd consists of the unabsorbed fraction of the metal passing through the gastrointestinal tract. The fecal content is, often a good indicator of dietary Cd intake since 90% or more of the ingested amount is unabsorbed and eliminated via feces. True fecal elimination of the body burden of Cd is difficult to study in humans due to the preponderance of unabsorbed Cd. Data from animal experiments indicate that fecal elimination is dependent both on dose and body burden. Thus, in long-term low-level exposures, the fecal excretion may be largely related to body burden [5, 13]. The daily fecal content of Cd in persons whose exposure is limited to the general environment, is approximately 50 times higher than the urinary excretion.

Mathematical models of cadmium toxicokinetics

A mathematical model of long-term toxicokinetics in humans has been developed [17, 18]. Subsequently, a more detailed description of Cd toxicokinetics was formulated considering additional events that modify the behaviour of Cd in humans and includes relationships between levels in urine, blood and major organs [19, 20]. The kidney and particularly the cortex, is considered the critical target tissue for Cd and its accumulation is of decisive importance for risk assessment. In long-term exposures (life-long) either a simple one-compartment model or a multi-compartment model predicts that 1/3 to 1/2 of the total body burden accumulates in the kidney and that the concentration of Cd in the kidney cortex is 1.25 times higher than the average concentration in the whole kidney [5, 8].

Toxic effects of cadmium

Acute toxicity

Acute effects of excess Cd in the diets or drinking water of humans (more than 15 mg Cd/kg) involve vomiting and diarrhoea [21]. Acute inhalation of high concentrations of Cd (about 5 mg/m^3 or higher) causes effects on the lungs in the form of pneumonitis and may be lethal [3, 5].

Long-term exposure

Pulmonary toxicity may occur after long-term exposure to inhaled Cd. In such situations emphysema and other chronic pulmonary effects have been observed both in animals and in humans. Respiratory effects of Cd have not been recorded in the general population [3, 5].

Reproductive toxicity

It is well known that the injection of Cd in experimental animals induces testicular necrosis in males and placental necrosis in pregnant females. Whether such effects may also occur after long-term dietary or environmental exposure in animals or humans is still a matter of discussion [5, 22, 23]. In humans placental transfer of Cd is limited (see above). A protective role of metallothionein in both human placenta and pregnant rats exposed to Cd may explain the lack of an effect on birth weights of children from Cd-exposed female Cd battery workers [23, 24].

Carcinogenicity

Cadmium has been reported to induce cancer in animals at the site of injection. Respiratory cancers may occur after inhalation of Cd compounds [25]. There is also epidemiological evidence of an association between Cd exposure and cancer in occupational groups such as smelter and battery workers [26]. Both prostate and lung cancers have been reported to occur in increased frequency. The International Agency for Research on Cancer (IARC) [25] concluded that there was sufficient evidence supporting the carcinogenicity of Cd, although methodological problems in the interpretation of the studies have been recognized [26, 27]. The overall standardized mortality and incidence ratios of all malignant neoplasms among persons in Japan previously exposed to environmental Cd, were not significantly increased [28].

Some studies performed after the IARC assessment, have not given support for carcinogenicity of Cd [29] while other studies have given such support [30, 31].

Nephrotoxicity

It has long been recognized that Cd exposure either after inhalation or ingestion, can give rise to nephrotoxicity in humans and that this effect is usually considered to be the earliest and most important health effect [32].

In this regard, the dominating effect was recognized early and consisted primarily of injury to the renal tubules inducing a proteinuria characterized by the excretion of low molecular weight (LMW) plasma proteins. As noted previously, in long-term exposures to Cd, both in experimental animals and in humans there is continuous accumulation of Cd in liver and kidneys. Nephrotoxicity in animal experiments usually does not develop until the concentration of Cd in the renal cortex is in the range of 100-400 μg/g wet weight. Increased concentrations of urinary LMW proteins were found in ±10% of a study population of industrial workers, having a Cd concentration in the kidney cortex of about 200 μg/g as assessed by *in vivo* neutron activation analysis [33-35]. Reports from Belgium indicate that, in workers with a urinary Cd excretion lower than 10 μg/g creatinine, renal effects may occur [36, 37], whilst concentrations of urinary Cd as low as 2 to 4 μg/g creatinine have been associated with an increased prevalence of various indicators of renal tubular dysfunction in the general population [38]. This concentration in urine corresponds to a renal cortical concentration varying between 50-100 μg/g wet weight [29].

Although renal cortical concentrations greater than 50 μg/g wet weight may be accompanied with mild effects on the renal tubules in humans who have been exposed to Cd for a long time, it has been demonstrated in animal models that renal tubular injury can occur following injection of Cd-metallothionein at concentrations in renal cortex as low as 10-20 μg/g wet weight [39, 40], whereas in animals with long-term exposure concentrations of 100 μg/g wet weight or higher are required [3]. The explanation for this discrepancy is most likely due to differences in metallothionein induction that may occur in these two situations. Indeed, in the long-term exposure situation, ample time will be available for the induction of a protective level of metallothionein synthesis, whereas this will not be the case of acute exposure after Cd-metallothionein injection. The acute injection delivers a bolus dose of this complex to the renal tubule where it is metabolized in the lysosomes and toxic Cd ions are released [11]. This non-metallothionein bound Cd interacts with sensitive sites in the renal cells like enzymes and high molecular weight membrane proteins, particularly in the basolateral membrane and causes cellular damage with related changes in cellular calcium balance (Figure 1) [41-43]. In addition to the protective effect of metallothionein, stress proteins may also participate in this protection [42, 44]. Cadmium is the most potent inducer of metallothionein synthesis. The detailed mechanisms underlying the induction, regulation and toxicological role in various tissues of metallothionein remain to be elucidated, but the metallothionein genes have been identified [45] and the toxicological role has been reviewed [46].

Biomarkers of exposure and internal dose in humans

Cadmium levels in blood are generally recognised as a biomarker of recent exposure to cadmium. It can also be used as biomarker of cumulative internal dose and accumulation of cadmium, but only when there is long-term (decade long) continuous exposure, for example in subsistence farmers consuming their own crops. Cadmium levels in urine are a widely recognised biomarker of cumulative internal dose, kidney and body burden of Cd. Dose-response relationships between urinary Cd and occurrence of kidney effects are described in the subsequent sections of this chapter "Sweden", "Japan", "Belgium", and "Other countries".

Reports concerning metallothionein in plasma and urine of Cd-exposed persons are limited [47-49]. This is at least in part due to the fact that the accurate measurement of Cd and metallothionein levels in plasma appears to be difficult [50]. The concentration of metallothionein in urine and blood has to be measured using the Onosaka saturation method, radio-immunoassay (RIA) or enzyme-linked immunosorbent assay (ELISA). The detection limits in human serum and urine for metallothionein by RIA is 1 pg [50]. For ELISA the detection limits are higher. Normal values range between 0.01-1 ng/ml for serum and between 1-10 ng/ml for urine. Metallothionein concentrations in Cd-exposed workers are reported to vary between 2-11 ng/ml in plasma and 2-155 ng/ml in urine [47].

Human nephrotoxicity by cadmium exposure

Sweden

As mentioned in the introduction to this chapter, chronic Cd poisoning with proteinuria resulting from occupational exposure was identified in Sweden in the late 1940s by Friberg [1]. Subsequently, it was shown that the proteinuria is of the tubular type and that the LMW proteins that were plasma proteins were not reabsorbed because of tubular damage [51, 52]. As a result of the discovery of the role of metallothionein in the toxicology of Cd [47, 53, 54] and the recognition of metallothionein binding as an explanation of the long biological half-life of Cd, interest was focused on the long-term intake of Cd via food. Kjellström et al. [55] assessed the temporal evolution of Cd in Swedish wheat, sampled from 1880 to 1970, and found a statistically significant time-dependent increase. The possibility of a risk for renal dysfunction and disease as a result of long-term dietary Cd intake was recognized and the relationship between occupational Cd exposure, renal accumulation of the element and tubular proteinuria was established [56]. Based on animal and human studies investigating long-term exposure to Cd from food and inhalation, a critical concentration of Cd in renal cortex was related to the risk of developing renal effects. These estimates were published in extensive reviews and evaluation volumes [13, 17, 56-58]. They were confirmed and/or partly revised according to epidemiological data from Japan, Belgium, and China (see the respective separate sections) and later on summarized in reviews by Järup et al. [29] and Nordberg et al. [5]. It was concluded that a small increase (less than one percent above background) in the prevalence of tubular dysfunction is expected to occur at renal cortical Cd concentrations exceeding 50 μg/g wet weight. The corresponding level of urinary Cd was estimated at 2.5 μg/g creatinine. These levels distinguishing apparent thresholds in renal cortex and urine are valid for persons not simultaneously exposed to other toxic substances and not suffering diabetes [5] or other conditions with increased risks of renal disease (see following text "Other countries"). In an epidemiological study reporting data from subjects previously exposed to higher levels of Cd in Sweden [59] a relationship between current urinary Cd levels and increased excretion of tubular proteins was demonstrated. Relationships between urinary Cd and occurrence of osteoporosis have also been established [60]. Since the slightly increased urinary Cd levels observed in these studies resulted from past exposures whilst recent exposure to Cd most probably was considerably lower, it is difficult to estimate from these data at what levels of cumulative exposures and urinary Cd, one might expect increased proteinuria and osteoporosis. Studies in another Swedish area (Skane) reported a statistically significant increase of age-adjusted urinary β_2-microglobulin clearance in relation to urinary Cd at urinary Cd levels below 1 µg/g creatinine, but there were no statistically significant increases in other indicators of renal dysfunction [61]. Another study among women in the same area [62], however reported statistically significant increases in urinary NAG (N-acetyl-β-D-glucosaminidase) and protein HC (α_1-microglobulin) in those women having urinary Cd of 0.8 µg/g creatinine compared to those having 0.48 µg/g creatinine. Interactions with diabetes were indicated. These studies give support to the notion that tubular proteinuria/enzymuria might already be induced at lower cumulative exposures than those giving rise to 2.5 µg/g creatinine, particularly among diabetics (see also section "Other countries").

Japan

Clinical features of itai-itai disease

The main features of itai-itai disease are osteomalacia and osteoporosis [2]. The patients usually have several fractures that are caused by events as trivial as coughing. They suffer from severe pain when sleeping or even breathing. Compression fractures in the spine resulting in skeletal deformity and eventually shortening of the stature may occur. Patients also develop a duck-like gait and progressive difficulties in walking. While most of the itai-itai patients are postmenopausal women with several pregnancies no hereditary factors have been identified. X-ray findings include marked decalcification and the presence of "Looser's zones" localized at areas where pressure causes pain. In severe cases, multiple pathological fractures are found. Skeletal deformities are frequently observed in pelvic bones, costae, and thoracic and lumbar vertebrae. Blood chemistry showed an increase in serum alkaline phosphatase and decreases in serum inorganic phosphorus and calcium, while urinalysis revealed proteinuria, glucosuria, and aminoaciduria. The urinary protein excretion is characterized by the so-called 'tubular protein pattern' consisting of mainly LMW proteins such as β_2-microglobulin, retinol-binding protein, and lysosomal enzymes. The aminoaciduria of the patient is of the "generalized aminoaciduria" type. The Cd content in urine is remarkably high. Increased excretion of calcium is also noticed. The principal pathological changes in bones are similar to the combined findings of osteomalacia and osteoporosis. Nearly 60% of 75 autopsied itai-itai disease patients had some degree of osteomalacia. All of them had severe to extreme osteoporosis [63]. Although the kidney is contracted, there is no obvious change in the glomeruli. The tubuli however, show a marked atrophy and degeneration. By the end of March, 2006, 188 inhabitants living in the Jinzu River basin had been diagnosed with itai-itai disease and 2 were still alive [64].

Renal effects by cadmium exposure

The typical Cd-induced proteinuria reported by Butler and Flynn resembles that of acquired Fanconi syndrome [65] and mainly consists of LMW proteins derived from the plasma [66].

β2-microglobulin excretion is considered as one of the best indicators of early Cd-induced nephropathy since serum concentrations are stable and analysis of β2-microglobulin using radio-, latex-, or ELISA-assays is sensitive and accurate [67].

Unlike β2-microglobulin, urinary α1-microglobulin is stable at pH down to 4.5 [17]. It can be analyzed using commercially available ELISA assays. A significant correlation has been reported between α1-microglobulin and β2-microglobulin in the urine of Cd-exposed subjects [17, 68].

The urinary excretion of metallothionein parallels urinary Cd and evidences early renal dysfunction as indicated by increased excretion of either β2-microglobulin or α1-microglobulin. Based on these results, the urinary excretion of metallothionein reflects not only the level of Cd exposure but also any renal dysfunction caused by long-term Cd exposure [18, 29].

Enzymes of higher molecular weight, which preclude filtration, enter the urine from renal proximal tubuli. They are also indicators of Cd-induced renal damage, which confirm renal tubular damage even in clinical states where the overproduction of LMW proteins in blood occurs.

Of all the urinary enzymes, N-acetyl-β-D-glucosaminidase is the most widely studied and used indicator of renal tubular damage. An increased urinary N-acetyl-β-D-glucosaminidase activity has been documented in Cd-exposed subjects [69]. However, the N-acetyl-β-D-glucosaminidase activity in urine of itai-itai patients was less than twice that of the controls, while β2-microglobulin levels were more than 100-fold those of the controls [70, 71]. This suggests that urinary N-acetyl-β-D-glucosaminidase activity decreases when renal tubular epithelia destruction becomes so severe that the cells can no longer excrete the enzyme into the urine. N-acetyl-β-D-glucosaminidase is probably a better marker for the acute effects or initial stage of chronic effects.

Urinary trehalase activity in inhabitants of Cd-polluted areas was significantly higher than in the reference area [72].

Intestinal-type alkaline phosphatase is specifically located in the S3-segment of the proximal tubuli [73]. Urinary intestinal-type alkaline phosphatase activity is significantly higher in the Cd-exposed subjects than in the non-exposed subjects [74]. The relationship between β2-microglobulin and intestinal-type alkaline phosphatase can be fit to a fourth-order mathematical function. The β2-microglobulin level corresponding to the inflexion point of intestinal-type alkaline phosphatase activity is smaller than that for N-acetyl-β-D-glucosaminidase. This result supports the contention that intestinal-type alkaline phosphatase is more useful for detecting renal tubular damage in the early stage of Cd exposure.

Higher molecular weight (HMW) proteins such as albumin or mucoproteins are also excreted by the Cd-exposed subjects [75].

Urinary levels of various indicators of Cd exposure assessed in subjects living near the Kakehashi River basin (one of the Cd-polluted areas in Japan) and non-exposed subjects are compared in Table 2.

Some causal relations among various urinary indices were identified using path analysis method. Cadmium-induced renal dysfunction develops in the following order: Cd exposure → increased β2-microglobulin and/or metallothionein → increased excretion of amino-nitrogen and/or total protein → increased excretion of glucose [76].

A decline of the creatinine clearance was also evident during the early stage of renal dysfunction and a significant correlation between tubular reabsorption of phosphate and glomerular filtration rate was reported in subjects exposed to Cd [77, 78]. These results provide evidence of Cd-induced glomerular dysfunction. However, histopathological examination revealed that while the glomeruli were relatively well maintained in number and size, renal tubuli were markedly damaged, resulting in obstruction of the lumen [79]. The mechanism responsible for the changes in glomerular

Table 2. Proteinuria and urinary cadmium in cadmium-exposed and non-exposed subjects.

		Cadmium-exposed subjects			Non-exposed subjects		
	Sex	N	Mean	S.D.	N	mean	S.D.
β2-microglobulin (μg/g creatinine)	M	67	7116	6.38**	26	141	387
	F	102	10934	5.11**	55	174	3.47
α1–microglobulin (μg/g creatinine)	M/F	27	18880	5.5**	10	352	4.2
N-acetyl-β-D-glucosaminidase (U/g creatinine)	M	39	51.1	2.45**	22	25.3	1.60
	F	36	43.9	2.21*	26	27.2	1.88
Human intestinal alkaline phosphatase (IU/g creatinine)	M	18	4.62	2.07**	18	1.26	1.75
	F	22	4.74	2.99**	22	1.82	2.28
Mucoprotein (mg/g creatinine)	M	67	228.6	1.82**	26	75.9	1.75
	F	102	309.2	1.84**	55	81.5	1.90
Albumin (mg/g creatinine)	M	67	93.6	4.79**	26	29.3	2.47
	F	102	140.0	3.60**	55	31.7	2.80
Total protein (mg/g creatinine)	M	67	185.6	3.62**	26	68.3	1.81
	F	102	251.7	2.73**	55	73.4	2.01
Cadmium (μg/g creatinine)	M	67	7.5	1.82**	26	2.5	1.58
	F	102	10.1	1.74**	55	4.0	1.45

*Mean S.D.: Geometric mean and geometric standard deviation. **: Significant difference from control (p <0.05). **: Significant difference from control (p <0.01).*

function following Cd exposure is still uncertain. It has been proposed that Cd exerts a direct effect on the glomeruli [80]. It has also been suggested that Cd-induced tubular damage leads to a certain degree of interstitial nephritis, which in turn results in a decreased glomerular filtration rate [66].

As renal tubular damage progresses the concentration of serum creatinine increases. One of the most severe cases in the Cd-polluted Kakehashi River basin had a serum creatinine value of 4.4 mg/100 ml. Progression to renal failure was evidenced by high blood nitrogen, severe anemia, acidosis, hyponatremia, hyperphosphatemia and hypocalcemia [81]. It was reported that four out of six itai-itai disease patients died of uremia [82].

Epidemiological studies

In 1967 and 1968, data of an extensive epidemiological investigation involving 13,183 inhabitants (6,155 men and 7,028 women) aged 30 years and older living in the district where itai-itai disease occurred and adjacent districts were reported [83]. The prevalence of proteinuria and glucosuria in the endemic area was found to be markedly higher than that in the non-endemic district.

Using the Cd concentration in rice as an index of exposure and the prevalence of proteinuria with glucosuria as an index of health effect, a significant dose-response relationship was demonstrated between the two indices. The allowable values of Cd concentration in rice were estimated to be in the range of 0.05-0.20 mg/kg, representing values lower than the 0.4 mg/kg provisionally adopted by the Japanese government [84].

A large number of epidemiological studies were subsequently performed in 10 Cd-polluted areas using urinary protein and glucose levels as indicators of renal damage [85]. However, statistically significant differences in the prevalence of proteinuria and glucosuria could not be demonstrated in any of the studies suggesting that these indicators are rather insensitive to detect early renal effects. It should be noted that the level of Cd exposure in these areas was generally lower than that in the itai-itai disease endemic district.

The LMW protein, β2-microglobulin, which is considered to be a more sensitive indicator of Cd-induced renal tubular dysfunction, was measured in an epidemiological study in 3,178 inhabitants over 50 years of age and living in the Kakehashi River basin [86]. The prevalence of β2-microglobulinuria (β2-microglobulin >1000 μg/g creatinine) was significantly higher in Cd-exposed subjects than in the non-exposed subjects although no significant difference was noted in the concurrent prevalence of proteinuria and glucosuria, as shown in Table 3.

Ten years after cessation of Cd exposure, urinary Cd concentrations in men >40 years and in women >30 years old were significantly higher than those of younger ages, whilst levels of subjects >50 years were significantly lower than those of subjects aged >60 years [87].

The epidemiological study reported by the Japan Environment Agency in 1989 failed to detect any renal tubular dysfunction among 7,196 persons in the Cd non-polluted areas, while in 202 persons among 13,570 (1.5%) of the Cd-polluted areas, proximal renal tubular dysfunction was seen [88].

A follow-up survey on 2,101 inhabitants (1,566 men and 535 women), who participated in a 1967-health survey and had resided in their actual rural community since birth, was conducted to determine the influence of environmental Cd exposure on the mortality of the general population in the Jinzu River basin. The Cox hazard ratios for males and females exposed to Cd concentration in rice >0.30 mg/kg were 1.42 and 1.10, respectively. Especially, this value is statistically significant in men. Since the mean Cd concentration in rice was closely related to the development of renal injury, the Cd-induced renal injury is believed to be the factor underlying the increased mortality observed [89].

Relationship between cadmium-induced renal and bone effects

Itai-itai disease is considered the most advanced stage of chronic Cd intoxication. Cadmium-induced bone effects are also suggested to occur in the more advanced stage. Originally, attention was focused on osteomalacia in the diagnosis of this disease. Recent studies, however, showed that osteopenia, a main characteristic of osteoporosis, can be detected in the early stage of chronic Cd intoxication.

Bone density was analyzed in 28 women with itai-itai disease, 92 men and 114 women with Cd-induced renal dysfunction and 44 men and 66 women living in non-polluted areas using a microdensitometer [90]. To assess the degree of bone density by microdensitometry, an X-ray of the hands along with an aluminum step-wedge was obtained and the bone density was measured at the middle site of the metacarpal bone 11 [91]. The values of indices for both cortical width and bone mineral content were significantly lower in itai-itai disease patients than the Cd-exposed subjects. The Cd-exposed women also showed a decrease in bone density compared with the non-exposed subjects. A significant decrease in bone density was also observed between Cd-exposed men and the non-exposed subjects, although the difference was not as distinct as in women. In other Cd-polluted areas such as the Jinzu River basin or Tsushima Island, a decrease in bone density in Cd-exposed subjects has also been reported using the same method [92, 93].

The relationship between the bone density and renal dysfunction was studied in 85 female inhabitants of the Cd-polluted Jinzu River basin aged 55 to 71 years who had various concentrations of β2-microglobulin in urine [92]. A significant negative correlation between the urinary β2-microglobulin level and indicators of microdensitometry was found.

In a study involving 203 Cd-exposed subjects with renal dysfunction and 80 non-exposed subjects an association was observed between Cd-induced renal dysfunction and osteopenia [94]. The relationship between biological parameters such as urinary β2-microglobulin and serum creatinine, calcium and phosphorus, and microdensitometric indices were analyzed using multivariate analysis. Age, urinary β2-microglobulin, and serum creatinine were significantly associated with indices of osteopenia in Cd-exposed men. In contrast, age showed the most significant association with the microdensitometric parameters in women of both groups. However, only in Cd-exposed women did urinary β2-microglobulin levels significantly correlate with indices of microdensitometry.

Using ultrasonic equipment, bone density was measured in 35 Cd-exposed and 68 non-exposed subjects [95]. The bone density was significantly decreased in Cd-exposed subjects as compared to the non-exposed subjects. Values obtained with this method (which is considered to be safer since it lacks radiation exposure) showed a significant correlation with those measured by microdensitometry.

Bone-G1a protein ((osteocalcin) is rapidly emerging as a clinically important diagnostic parameter of bone pathology since bone-G1a protein appears to be a highly specific marker of osteoblast function and is expressed during bone formation. Serum levels of bone-G1a protein were evaluated in 76 Cd-exposed subjects with renal tubular dysfunction and 133 non-exposed subjects [96]. Serum bone-G1a protein levels were higher in Cd-exposed subjects than in the non-exposed subjects. In 29 Cd-exposed men, bone-G1a protein, % tubular reabsorption of phosphorus (TRP) and base excess were found to show significant associations with the microdensitometry indicators. In 42 Cd-exposed women, parathyroid hormone, age, blood Cd and bone-G1a protein significantly correlated with the microdensitometric indicators. Only serum bone-G1a protein showed a significant correlation in both

Table 3. Prevalence (%) of abnormal urinary findings in cadmium-exposed and non-exposed subjects.

	Cadmium-exposed subjects					Non-exposed subjects				
Age:	50-59	60-69	70-79	80-	Total	50-59	60-69	70-79	80-	Total
Male										
N	600	494	265	65	1424	62	38	26	7	133
Glucose ≥20 mg/dl with protein ≥5 mg/dl	1.3	2.6	4.2	7.7	2.6	4.8	0	0	0	2.3
Amino acids ≥300 mg/g creatinine	0.0	1.6	3.0	9.2	1.8	1.6	2.6	0	0	1.5
β2-microglobulin ≥1000 μg/g creatinine	4.8	13.0**	28.7	52.3	14.3**	0	0	26.9	14.3	6.0
Metallothionein ≥638 μg/g creatinine	1.5	6.5	7.5	6.2	4.6	4.9	0	0	0	2.3
Female										
N	713	591	340	110	1754	64	49	34	14	161
Glucose ≥20 mg/dl with protein ≥5mg/dl	0.6	1.9	7.1	20.0	3.5	0	4.1	0	7.1	1.9
Amino acids ≥300 mg/g creatinine	5.9	7.8	10.6	23.6*	8.6**	1.6	2.0	2.9	0	1.9
β2-microglobulin ≥1000 μg/g creatinine	4.9*	17.1*	36.5**	61.8*	18.7**	0	6.1	5.9	21.4	5.0
Metallothionein ≥693 μg/g creatinine	4.5	10.2	10.9	16.5	8.4*	0	10.2	0	0	3.1

**: Significant difference from control (p<0.05).*
***: Significant difference from control (p<0.01).*

sexes of the Cd-exposed subjects, and a sex difference was found in the relationship between bone metabolic markers and osteopenia.

Urinary type-1 collagen cross-linked N-telopeptides (NTx) are related to bone resorption activity. Urinary NTx concentrations of Cd-exposed women aged more than 65 years were significantly higher than those in corresponding non-exposed women although no significant difference was shown in men. Urinary aminoN and Cd showed significant association with NTx only in women using stepwise multiple regression analysis [97].

Out of these results, one may deduce that itai-itai disease only represents the tip of the iceberg. Indeed, in the earlier stage of chronic Cd exposure, the presence of Cd-induced bone effects such as osteopenia may be reflected by both microdensitometry and biochemical indices of bone turn-over. The degree of bone damage closely parallels the degree of renal damage.

To investigate the mechanism of bone disease caused by exposure to Cd, 1α,25-dihydroxyvitamin D, parathyroid hormone, β2-microglobulin, calcium and inorganic phosphorus were assessed in serum samples of 5 itai-itai disease patients, 36 Cd-exposed residents with renal tubular damage and 17 non-exposed individuals [98]. Measurements of %TRP were performed only on the Cd-exposed subjects. Serum 1α,25-dihydroxyvitamin D levels were lower in the itai-itai disease patients and Cd-exposed subjects with renal damage than in non-exposed subjects. Parathyroid hormone and serum β2-microglobulin concentrations were higher in the Cd-exposed subjects [98, 99]. Decreases in serum lα,25-dihydroxyvitamin D levels were closely related to serum concentrations of parathyroid hormone, β2-microglobulin and %TRP. This study suggests that Cd-induced bone effects were mainly due to a disturbance in vitamin D and parathyroid hormone metabolism, which most probably resulted from the Cd-induced kidney damage.

In a further study, serum concentrations of 25-hydroxyvitamin D, 24,25-dihydroxyvitamin D and 1α,25-dihydroxyvitamin D were measured in 10 Cd-exposed subjects and 5 non-exposed subjects [100]. The Cd-exposed subjects were divided into two groups according to serum 1α,25-dihydroxyvitamin D levels. No significant differences for 25-hydroxyvitamin D were found between the Cd-exposed group with low or normal serum 1α,25-dihydroxyvitamin D and the non-exposed group. The concentrations of 24,25-dihydroxyvitamin D were lowest in the Cd-exposed group with low serum 1α,25-dihydroxyvitamin D, highest in the non-exposed group, and significantly lower in the Cd-exposed group with normal serum 1α,25-dihydroxyvitamin D than in the non-exposed group. Renal function was substantially worse in the Cd-exposed group with low serum 1α,25-dihydroxyvitamin D than in the group with normal serum 1α,25-dihydroxyvitamin D. These findings suggest that Cd initially disturbs the hydroxylation of 25-hydroxyvitamin D into 24,25-dihydroxyvitamin D and then disturbs the hydroxylation of 25-hydroxyvitamin D into 1α,25-dihydroxyvitamin D. The decrease of serum 24,25-dihydroxyvitamin D and 1α,25-dihydroxyvitamin D in Cd-exposed subjects most probably is not due to a decrease of the serum 25-hydroxyvitamin D level.

Based on the current knowledge obtained from both experimental and human studies, three different mechanisms might be active in development of Cd-induced bone effects.

Firstly, Cd causes renal damage with effects principally on renal tubular cells, i.e. the site of 1α,25-dihydroxyvitamin D synthesis resulting in an intrinsic vitamin D deficiency. This will impair the gastrointestinal absorption of calcium, reduce the calcium incorporation in bone and ultimately result in the development of osteomalacia. It is well known that 1α,25-dihydroxyvitamin D is the biologically active metabolite of vitamin D. As there is a sequential relationship between the synthesis of 1α,25-dihydroxyvitamin D in the kidney and cyclic-adenosine monophosphate, adenylcyclase, parathyroid hormone, a direct interference of Cd with any of these steps cannot be excluded.

Secondly, Cd directly interferes with the gastrointestinal calcium absorption leading to the bone decalcification found in osteoporosis.

Finally, Cd may directly affect bone collagen formation as indicated by a reduction in lysyl-oxidase activity.

To date, however, no clear-cut data are available that inevitably present evidence for a particular mechanism underlying the development of Cd-induced bone effects in human subjects.

Dose-response relationship between cadmium exposure and renal effects

It is assumed that urinary Cd reflects the body burden of Cd at low exposure (environmental pollution), whilst it might be a valuable index of current exposure when exposure is high (industrial situation with high level exposure) [101].

In an epidemiological study involving 1,815 Cd-exposed and 240 non-exposed inhabitants of the Kakehashi River basin, the significance of the urinary Cd concentration as an indicator of the internal dose for subjects living in a Cd-polluted environment was investigated [102]. The mean urinary Cd concentration increased in a dose-related manner as assessed by classifying subjects according to the average Cd concentration in their rice and to their residence period in the polluted area. A strong direct correlation was found (r=0.93 in men and r=0.88 in women) between the total Cd intake and urinary Cd excretion. This made the authors conclude that, on a group basis, urinary Cd is a useful indicator of the internal dose resulting from environmental Cd exposure.

In another study investigating the dose-effect and dose-response relationship between the Cd concentration in rice and urinary concentrations/prevalence of abnormal levels of markers of renal dysfunction, significant correlations between Cd concentration in rice and concentrations as well as prevalence rates of abnormal urinary β2-microglobulin, metallothionein, glucose and amino-nitrogen levels were found. The highest maximum allowable concentration of Cd in rice calculated for these indicators was 0.34 mg/kg when the uncorrected urinary value was used and 0.29 mg/kg when the creatinine corrected value was used. Both values are lower than 0.4 mg/kg, the tentative limit prescribed by the Japanese government [103].

A benchmark dose low (BMDL) was used as a replacement for the no-observed adverse effect level (NOAEL). The threshold levels of urinary Cd as BMDL were estimated using the former epidemiological data [86]. Using cut-off values for β_2-microglobulinuria, the BMDL at which the excess risk is 0.05 was determined to be 2.9-4.0 µg/g creatinine (men) and 1.5-3.6 µg/g creatinine (women) [104]. These values correspond to those calculated from previous studies.

Reversibility of renal effects

The reversibility of β2-microglobulinuria, glucosuria and aminoaciduria was evaluated in 74 inhabitants over the age of 50 who lived in the Cd-polluted Kakehashi River basin [105]. The initiation of the examinations coincided with the cessation of Cd exposure after which patients were followed-up during 5 years. The geometric mean concentrations of β2-microglobulinuria, glucosuria and aminoaciduria indicated significant increases in excretion during the 5-year follow-up period. In cases where the initial level of β2-microglobulin in urine exceeded 1000 µg/g creatinine, almost all individuals showed a further increase of β2-microglobulinuria, whereas in the cases in which the urinary excretion of β2-microglobulin was less than 1000 µg/g creatinine, no progression was observed. A 15-year follow-up study in the Jinzu River basin and a 10-year follow-up study in Nagasaki also confirmed the irreversibility of β2-microglobulinuria when the initial urinary level of β2-microglobulin was over 1000 µg/g creatinine.

In 21 Cd-exposed subjects who had renal tubular dysfunction, serum creatinine and arterial blood pH were measured annually during 9-14 years [81]. During this time period, mean serum creatinine increased significantly from 1.19±1.28 mg/100 ml to 1.68±1.56 mg/100 ml. Even after cessation of Cd exposure, a progressive deterioration of glomerular filtration was seen. The mean arterial blood pH values decreased significantly in all subjects (from 7.40±0.02 to 7.36±0.03), which, in the absence of respiratory disease, was ascribed to metabolic acidosis resulting from the severe renal tubular dysfunction. In Nagasaki, serum creatinine levels were followed in 15 inhabitants living in the Cd-polluted area for 15 years [106]. Although most of the serum creatinine levels were below 2 mg/100 ml, a gradual increase was noted.

Prognosis of cadmium-induced renal effects

Despite the fact that a number of studies on the influence of environmental Cd exposure on the mortality of inhabitants of Cd-polluted areas have been conducted, to date no consensus has been achieved. Shigematsu et al. investigated the outcome of residents of Cd-polluted areas in Akita, Miyagi, Nagasaki, and Toyama Prefectures and reported lower standardized mortality rates in these polluted areas as compared to non-polluted areas with even greater decreases in the standardized mortality ratios in the most severely polluted areas [107].

However, in contrast, in a 20-year follow-up study in which (i) patients diagnosed as having itai-itai disease, (ii) subjects who were suspected of having the disease, and (iii) controls (95 subjects per category matched for age, sex, and residential area) were included [108], the cumulative survival rate of the patients who had a definite diagnosis of itai-itai disease was significantly lower than that of the control group as from a >3year follow-up period on. Moreover, the cumulative survival rate of the subjects who were suspected of having itai-itai disease with evidence of severe renal dysfunction due to Cd pollution was significantly lower than that of the control group.

In another 9-year follow-up study of 3,178 persons living in a Cd-polluted area, the standardized mortality rates of the urinary β2-microglobulin positive subjects (>1000 μg/g creatinine) of both sexes were higher than those of the general Japanese population, whereas the cumulative survival curves were lower than those of the urinary β2-microglobulin negative group [109]. A significant association was also found between urinary β2-microglobulin and mortality, using a Cox's proportional hazards model.

In multiple comparisons using four indices of renal dysfunction (i.e. urinary β2-microglobulin, protein, glucose and amino acid), urinary protein and β2-microglobulin in women and urinary protein in men were the most contributory factors to the mortality rates [110].

Data from a 7-year follow-up study in another Cd-polluted area (Nagasaki) showed that, in both men and women, serum β2-microglobulin and creatinine, as well as urinary total protein and β2-microglobulin were significantly related to mortality independent of age as assessed by the Cox's proportional hazards model [111]. In advanced cases, the excess mortality of subjects with Cd-induced renal tubular dysfunction might, to some extent, be ascribed to a reduction in GFR.

In conclusion, these results suggest that the prognosis of subjects with Cd-induced renal dysfunction is unfavourable. The mortality rate tended to become higher as the severity of renal dysfunction progressed. Moreover, an isolated increase in urinary β2-microglobulin is an important factor in assessing the prognosis of a person's mild proximal tubular dysfunction.

Belgium

Cadmium is an important occupational and environmental pollutant in Belgium. This is mainly due to the long-standing commercial production of this metal as a "by-product" of the mining and refining of zinc ores, which contain minor quantities of Cd (0.1–0.3 %). Because of the presence of zinc/lead ores, non-ferrous metallurgy workshops developed in the Meuse–Vesdre Valley near Liège as early as the 18th century. After Canon Jean-Jacques Dony discovered in Liège a coal-based thermic process to extract zinc from zinc blende (ZnS), an industrial revolution occurred in the zinc metallurgy from the 1850s on. This industry expanded rapidly in the Liège area concomitantly with coal mining and iron and steel works. After the 1st world war, increasing amounts of imported zinc ores were refined using the DONY-process, which in 1972 was replaced by electrolytic zinc refinery. Dust and waste from the primary zinc industry constituted the bulk of the basic material for the production of Cd using thermic refinery processes. After the 2nd world war, however, the heavy industrial activity in the Meuse Valley basin declined which resulted in a progressive shut down of non-ferrous industries of which all activity ceased in the early 1980s.

In 1888, a similar non-ferrous metallurgic activity developed in the northeast of Belgium, a rural region near the Dutch border (Noorderkempen), where during the 20th century several primary zinc smelters and Cd refineries were in operation. Thermic processes, such as the horizontal retort zinc furnace for reduction of zinc calcine with coal at 1100-1300°C (DONY-process), were widely used in zinc refineries. As the boiling point of Cd (765°C) is much lower and the technology to recover Cd fume/dust from zinc furnaces was not very efficient, thermic processes were one of the main causes of the large scale dispersion of Cd in this rural area comprising about 300 km^2. For instance, the Lommel-Overpelt smelters refined 250 metric tonnes of Cd in 1950 whereby 340 kg Cd/day were emitted in the air. Technological improvements raised the Cd production to 300 metric tonnes in 1970 while the atmospheric Cd losses, though still high, had dropped to 200 kg Cd/day. By 1974, the ore-roasting/electrolysis-based zinc refining process had replaced the zinc furnaces and in the 1980s the electrolytic Cd refinery process, used since 1935 in the Balen smelter, was generalized and the re-melting and casting ovens modernized. Hence, for 600 metric tonnes of Cd produced in 1989 only 0.35 kg Cd/day was lost in the air. In 1992, the two remaining smelters in the Noorderkempen produced 1000 metric tonnes of Cd whereby barely 0.04 kg Cd/day escaped in the atmosphere [112]. Belgium has always been a major Cd producer in Europe and by 1997 its share of the Cd production in the European Union was 20%. To date, one high-performing big zinc smelter remains in the Noorderkempen, however, its Cd refinery facility shut down in the spring of 2002.

Although cases of acute Cd intoxication were first recorded in 1858 in Belgium (domestic servants polishing silverware with Cd carbonate) [113], it should be pointed out that before 1970 systematic epidemiological studies had never been conducted in Belgium to assess health risks of Cd exposure in the industrial setting or the general population. For historical reasons, however, it is interesting to mention the 1953-report of the occupational physician of the Balen plant (Vieille Montagne at that time) dealing with clinical observations made in a group of 30 workers who were exposed to fume and dust of Cd in the Cd production facility of this plant [114]. In 10 workers with less than 2 years of exposure, a slight reticulocytosis was seen and the urinary Cd concentrations ranged 10-20 μg Cd/L as assessed by the dithizon method. In 8 workers with 2-8 years of exposure, the characteristic yellow dental Cd line was noticed together with a reticulocytosis exceeding 2%, a mild hyperchromic anemia, and a urinary Cd varying from 20 to 90 μg Cd/L. The same observations were made in twelve workers with 8 to 30 years of exposure and urinary Cd levels usually of 60 μg Cd/L, but interestingly in seven of them a proteinuria was found which displayed the same LMW protein characteristics as the Cd proteinuria already described by Friberg in 1948 [115].

Occupational exposure to cadmium in Belgium

Critical cadmium concentration in kidney and urine

In the early 1970s, Lauwerys et al. conducted the first cross-sectional epidemiological survey ever in Belgian factories. The workers (31 women, 49 men) were exposed to Cd dust and fume and were recruited from an electronic workshop, a nickel-Cd storage battery factory, and a Cd producing plant [116]. At the time of the study, the average airborne Cd ranged from 31 to 134 μg Cd/m^3 (total dust), which was below the American Conference of Governmental Industrial Hygienists' (ACGIH) threshold limit value (TLV) being 200 μg Cd/m^3 in 1972. The kidney was found more sensitive to Cd exposure than the lung. Proteinuria showed abnormal electrophoretic patterns of LMW and/or HMW proteins in 4/27 male workers with less than 20 years of exposure and in 15/22 with more than 20 years of exposure. Moreover, on the basis of the correlation between total proteinuria and cadmium concentration in urine (CdU), it was suggested that the risk of renal damage would be low when CdU is kept below 15 μg Cd/g creatinine [116]. In addition, blood Cd was found to reflect current exposure to Cd, whereas Cd in urine would reflect body burden of Cd when industrial exposure is low to moderate, but it would reflect current exposure when industrial exposure is high [116].

Subsequent studies in male workers of two Cd refineries confirmed previous findings of other investigators [117-119], in that prolonged Cd exposure is usually characterized by microproteinuria due to impairment of the tubular reabsorption of plasma-derived LMW proteins, e.g. β_2-microglobulin and retinol-binding protein [120]. An isolated glomerular effect with increased permeability of HMW proteins, e.g. albumin and transferrin, was less commonly found [120, 121]. To obtain a reliable and direct estimate of the critical body burden of Cd in relation to Cd nephropathy, the Cd concentrations of liver and left kidney were determined in 1978 in about 300 male workers from two Cd refineries using *in vivo* neutron activation analysis, and the urinary β_2-microglobulin concentration was measured as well. A dose-response relation between liver Cd and prevalence of increased β_2-microglobulinuria was found, indicating an increased prevalence (>5%) of abnormal β_2-microglobulinuria when hepatic Cd was exceeding 30 μg Cd/g wet weight (Table 4). Unlike liver Cd, renal Cd was found to drop in workers with abnormal urinary β_2-microglobuline concentrations and a concomitant steep rise in urinary Cd excretion may be seen. This study established that abnormal β_2-microglobulinuria is likely to occur when Cd in the renal cortex or in the urine exceeds the critical concentrations of 216 μg Cd/g wet weight and 10.8 μg Cd/g creatinine respectively [34, 35].

Predictive significance of tubular proteinuria

Further research on occupational Cd nephropathy aimed at a better understanding of the predictive value of Cd-induced microproteinuria and explored underlying features of early glomerular impairment seen in a few Cd-exposed workers. A retrospective examination

Table 4. Dose-response relation between cadmium concentration in liver and abnormal β2-microglobulinuria in a group of 148 workers from two zinc/cadmium smelters in Belgium.

Cadmium in liver[a]	Number of workers	Prevalence of abnormal β2-microglobulinuria[b]		Mean β2-microglobulinuria in workers with abnormal values
(μg/g)		n	%	(mg/g creatinine)
10-19	54	0	0	
20-29	27	1	4	7.30
30-39	28	3	11	0.28
40-49	18	3	17	1.42
50-59	8	2	25	7.00
60-69	5	2	40	4.89
70-160	8	8	100	6.45

Adapted from Roels et al. [34].
[a]Cadmium concentration measured in vivo by neutron activation analysis.
[b]β2-microglobulinuria was considered abnormal when exceeding 0.20 mg/g creatinine.

of serum creatinine, total proteinuria, aminoaciduria, albuminuria, and microproteinuria (retinol-binding protein and β_2-microglobulin) was carried out in a group of nineteen workers (40 to 60 years old) with 16 to 42 years of occupational Cd exposure. These renal markers were measured on average 1.2 years before and 4.2 years after removal from exposure and showed in this group of workers that the Cd-induced nephropathy was not reversible when exposure ceased, that in particular the microproteinuria exacerbated, and that serum creatinine tended to increase [122]. A few workers turned into end-stage renal insufficiency (unpublished data). To better assess the health significance of Cd-induced microproteinuria in male Cd workers three studies were carried out.

The first study was a 5-year prospective study conducted in 23 Cd workers removed from exposure because of the discovery of microproteinuria [123]. They were exposed for 25 years on average and at the time of the first examination the mean age of the group was 59 (46-68 years). The mean±SEM CdU in the subjects amounted to 22.2±2.9 μg Cd/L, the geometric means of urinary retinol-binding protein and β_2-microglobulin were 1.57 and 1.77 mg/L respectively, whilst serum creatinine was normal (<1.4 mg/100 ml) in all subjects, except in two (2.0 and 2.2 mg/100 ml). This longitudinal study corroborated not only the irreversibility of Cd-induced microproteinuria (about 30 and 50% increase in urinary retinol-binding protein and β_2-microglobulin respectively at the end), but unequivocally showed that creatinine and β_2-microglobulin in serum significantly increased with time indicating a progressive reduction of the GFR. The estimated GFR was found to decrease five times more rapidly than what could be expected due to aging alone. Elevated microproteinuria predicts thus an exacerbation of the age-related decline of GFR and, hence, it should be regarded as an early adverse health effect in occupational exposure to Cd. This finding raised the question whether a CdU threshold value of 10 μg Cd/g creatinine would not only prevent the occurrence of microproteinuria, but also the loss of nephron mass. In other words, does an increased CdU not yet sufficient to modify the urinary excretion of plasma-derived proteins, impair the renal filtration reserve capacity?

The second study addressed this point by investigating the GFR in Cd workers without (n=31) or with (n=12) increased microproteinuria, i.e. urinary β_2-microglobulin or retinol-binding protein >0.30 mg/g creatinine, and whose geometric mean (range) of CdU was 4.7 (2.1-8.8) and 11.1 (5.8-21.7) μg Cd/g creatinine respectively. The subjects in both groups aged on average 55 years (50 to 64 years) and all had a normal serum creatinine (<1.4 mg/100 ml) [124]. GFR was estimated as the creatinine clearance under baseline conditions and after an acute oral protein load to assess the hyperfiltration capacity of the kidney. The baseline creatinine clearance was normal in both groups (mean 116 ml/min). The creatinine clearance after protein load, however, failed to rise in the group with microproteinuria (mean 114 ml/min) and remained significantly lower than that in the group without microproteinuria (mean 124 ml/min). The mean creatinine clearance after protein load in the latter group was similar to that of an age-matched control group (n=35; CdU <2 μg Cd/g creatinine).

This study showed that the filtration reserve capacity of the kidney is lost when elevated microproteinuria is present, but that there was no functional impairment at a renal Cd burden not yet causing microproteinuria. Implicitly, it validated the proposal of a CdU of 10 μg Cd/g creatinine as biological exposure limit to prevent microproteinuria in male Cd workers.

The third study was prospective (observation periods 1980-84 and 1990-92) and aimed at an evaluation of Cd-induced microproteinuria by assessing its evolution in 32 Cd workers as a function of CdU and severity of the microproteinuria at the time exposure was substantially reduced or had ceased [125]. The finding that 15/24 workers with historical CdU >10 μg Cd/g creatinine had an elevated β_2-microglobulinuria (>0.30 mg/g creatinine) corroborated our earlier finding, namely that the risk of abnormal microproteinuria may dramatically increase when CdU regularly exceeds 10 μg Cd/g creatinine. However, when reduction of Cd exposure took place at the time β_2-microglobulinuria did not exceed 0.30 mg/g creatinine, the risk of developing tubular dysfunction at a later stage was low, even in cases with historical CdU values occasionally >10 but always <20 μg Cd/g creatinine. There was also indication that the tubulotoxic effect of Cd may be reversible, provided that the historical CdU values never exceeded 20 μg Cd/g creatinine and the β_2-microglobulinuria was mild (<1.5 mg/g creatinine) at the time the Cd exposure was reduced. When a β_2-microglobulinuria >1.5 mg/g creatinine was found in combination with historical CdU values above 20 μg Cd/g creatinine, Cd-induced tubular dysfunction exacerbated in spite of reduction or cessation of Cd exposure. The latter condition was present in 10 of the 15 above-mentioned workers who compared well with the Cd-exposed workers of our previous studies [122, 123, 126]. Their past Cd exposure was characterized by a mean CdU_{max} of 35 μg Cd/g creatinine (range: 19-83) and in 1980-84 a frank microproteinuria was diagnosed which in the observation period 1990-92 exacerbated for β_2-microglobulin from 8.96 to 18.1 mg/g creatinine (mean values) and for retinol-binding protein from 4.28 to 6.81 mg/g creatinine. The severe microproteinuria was thus irreversible and still progressive 15 years after removal from exposure. That only 5 workers were identified with a reversible microproteinuria was after all not surprising, because in the 1980s technological improvements, industrial hygiene controls, and systematic health surveillance were implemented in the Cd-producing plants to reduce overexposure and to prevent health risks. It should also be noted, that the exact point in time at which the first sign of a Cd-induced microproteinuria would appear in a subject is yet unpredictable and that the accumulation of Cd in the kidney and the ability to develop a concomitant tubulopathy are time-dependent processes likely to display inter-individual variability [34]. Hence, in ongoing Cd exposure variable time windows would exist within which abnormal microproteinuria would show up and remain "reversible" before it would turn into a progressive exacerbation. Interestingly, the five Cd workers with reversible microproteinuria had a mean historical CdU_{max} = 16.6 μg Cd/g creatinine (range: 14-19) which was half that of the workers with irreversible and more severe microproteinuria. Mean age (57 vs 61) and mean duration of exposure (26 vs 28 years) did not differ significantly between both subgroups. Thus, age and the years of exposure did not seem to play a role, but it would rather be the cumulative exposure of the past (body burden of Cd) in combination with the severity of the tubulopathy at the time exposure was reduced or ceased that were the determining factors. The past Cd exposure of the 5 workers with reversible microproteinuria apparently did not result in a renal cortex Cd level sufficient to induce progressive tubulopathy 7-12 years after cessation of exposure.

Target-segment nephrotoxicity of cadmium

One of the characteristics of the kidney is its ability to compensate for renal damage and for this reason classical function tests, for example serum creatinine clearance, are insensitive since they only deviate late in the cascade of damage events when there is a large reduction in nephron mass. The last decade has seen a lot of effort in developing diagnostic tests that are sensitive enough to assess changes in renal integrity at an early stage, that is, before clinical manifestations. In the frame of a large collaborative network-project, involving laboratories of 5 countries of the European Union, the diagnostic potential of more than 25 urine or serum markers of kidney function/integrity was evaluated in a cohort of male Cd workers (n=37; CdU=2-16 μg Cd/g creatinine) and an age-matched control group (n=43; CdU <2 μg Cd/g creatinine). The aim was to assess whether one or more of the anatomical regions of the nephron segments (glomerulus, proximal or distal tubule, loop of Henle, and interstitium) may be targets of Cd toxicity. The tests comprised functional markers (e.g., creatinine and β_2-microglobulin in serum; LMW and HMW proteins in urine), cytotoxicity markers (e.g., tubular antigens or enzymes in urine), and biochemical markers (e.g., glycosaminoglycans, kallikrein, sialic acids, and eicosanoids in urine) [37]. The results demonstrated a target-segment nephrotoxicity and the first Cd-induced alterations were at the proximal tubule as evidenced by increased urinary excretion of brush-border antigens and lysosomal as well as brush-border enzymes such as N-acetyl-β-D-glucosaminidase and intestinal-type alkaline phosphatase, a specific and sensitive marker of the S3 segment of the proximal tubule [73]. Cadmium exposure was found to have an early effect on the urinary excretion of 6-keto-prostaglandin $F_{1\alpha}$ of which the glomerulus is the principal site of synthesis. Nearly half of the subjects had abnormally increased urinary values of this eicosanoid. As long as the biological significance and implication(s) of this marker in Cd nephropathy is not elucidated, it would be premature to propose a biological exposure threshold based on this highly sensitive marker. An increased urinary excretion of HMW proteins (transferrin and albumin) occurring at a Cd body burden where the protein reabsorption capacity of tubular cells does not yet seem to be impaired was shown as well, which would indicate a slight loss of the glomerular barrier function. This glomerular-type proteinuria may be ascribed to a depletion of the glomerular polyanion charge [127, 128] and suggests that in some subjects subtle alterations of the glomerular filter may precede the onset of tubular-type proteinuria. Traditional markers indicative of tubular damage, i.e. a rise in urinary excretion of plasma-derived LMW proteins like β_2-microglobulin and retinol-binding protein, are likely to be affected at a higher Cd body burden. As a cumulative nephrotoxicant, Cd can thus produce a broad spectrum of site-specific dose-related effects on the nephron over a wide range of Cd body burden, as estimated on the basis of CdU. Logistic regressions showed significant dose-response rate (CdU - %) curves for renal marker values (cut-off: 95th centile of values observed in control group) and allowed to determine marker-specific CdU threshold values which were arbitrarily set at a response rate twice the background of elevated values (Table 5). Three main groups of CdU thresholds could be identified: one around 2 µg Cd/g creatinine associated with biochemical alterations (6-keto-PGF$_{1\alpha}$ and sialic acids in urine), a second around 4 µg Cd/g creatinine associated with cytotoxic effects (renal brush-border antigen, intestinal-type alkaline phosphatase, and N-acetyl-β-D-glucosaminidase in urine) or glomerular barrier dysfunction (albumin

Table 5. Thresholds of urinary cadmium concentration for abnormal values of urinary markers of renal effects found in male workers with chronic occupational cadmium exposure.

Urinary markers	Cut-off values[a]	Threshold effect concentration of urinary cadmium (µg Cd/g creatinine)
Biochemical alterations		
6-keto-prostaglandin $F_{1\alpha}$	280 ng/L	2.3
Sialic acid	501 mg/L	2.4
Cytotoxic effects/enzymuria		
Brush border antigen BBA	6.70 U/L	3.7
N-acetyl-β-*D*-glucosaminidase	2.19 U/L	4.0
Intestinal-type alkaline phosphatase	2.72 U/L	4.1
Renal function changes		
Glomerulus		
Transferrin	0.90 mg/L	3.6
Albumin	19 mg/L	4.1
Proximal tubule		
Retinol binding protein	0.19 mg/L	10.4
β_2-microglobulin	0.32 mg/L	11.5

Adapted from Roels et al. [37].
[a]Upper limit of normal, defined as the 95th centile of the values in control workers with a urinary cadmium concentration < 1 µg Cd/g creatinine.
BBA: Brush border antigen

and transferrin in urine), and a third around 10 μg Cd/g creatinine associated with tubular reabsorption dysfunction (microproteinuria), or changes in other markers (e.g. glycosaminoglycans in urine). In this study, a few other renal markers were tested as well, including the structural protein fibronectin in urine as a marker of the integrity of the extracellular matrix of the glomerulus, the renal kallikrein activity in urine as a structure/function marker of the distal tubule, and anti-glomerular basement membrane antibodies in serum as a marker of dysfunction of the glomerular basement membrane. None of these last three markers was disturbed in the present group who got a rather moderate Cd exposure and whose current CdU averaged 5.4 μg Cd/g creatinine (range: 2.1-16.4). Previous studies in male workers with much higher Cd exposure, however, showed a significantly decreased urinary kallikrein activity [129] in a group with a mean CdU of 10.4 μg Cd/g creatinine and in another group a significantly increased prevalence of circulating anti-laminin antibodies [130] was found at CdU >20 μg Cd/g creatinine.

Conclusions from studies of occupational exposures in Belgium

The studies in the occupational setting of Cd-exposed male workers in Belgium carried out in the period 1970-2000 validated that on average the critical Cd concentration in the renal cortex lies around 200 μg/g wet weight which is associated with an increased risk of microproteinuria and a CdU threshold of 10 μg Cd/g creatinine. So far, Cd-induced LMW proteinuria is the only renal effect of Cd with documented health risk significance. Indeed, ongoing overexposure to Cd may lead to irreversible tubular damage predictive of a severe exacerbation of the age-related decline in GFR and a decrease in the filtration reserve capacity. However, for several reasons like the long biological half-life of Cd, the safety margin, the occurrence of other renal effects of which the health significance is still unknown, and the fact that no efficient treatment to remove Cd from its storage sites is presently available, several investigators proposed to revise the health-based limit for CdU of 10 μg Cd/g creatinine recommended by the World Health Organization [131] for occupational exposure to Cd. The adoption by the ACGIH of 5 μg Cd/g creatinine as biological exposure index for Cd seems for the time-being justified [132]. Studies on the predictive value of renal changes other than microproteinuria are needed to assess the validity of this biological exposure index. It is interesting to note that suggestive evidence of excess of neurotoxic complaints has been shown in Cd smelter workers from the Balen plant before signs of Cd-induced microproteinuria occurred [133].

Environmental exposure to cadmium in Belgium

First, it should be pointed out that the severe renal and skeletal outcomes of the endemic Cd exposure in Japanese people [88] had never been reported in the Belgian general population. Nevertheless, at the end of the 1970s a few pilot surveys were conducted in the Liège area, the first epidemiological studies ever done in groups of the Belgian general population environmentally exposed to Cd. In the wake of the experience with exposure to Cd in Belgian industries a crucial question emerged whether the health conservation strategies, as applied to 20-55 year-old men in the industry to avoid nephrotoxic effects of Cd exposure, could be extrapolated to the general population with long-term low-level exposure to historical Cd contamination of their environment? In other words, are more stringent exposure guidelines justified for the general population, for example as to the urinary Cd excretion, and which are the critical adverse effects to be taken into account?

Pilot studies in the Liège area

Aged women who had lived in the contaminated Liège area (n=60) were compared with a group from a 'control' industrial area (Charleroi, n=70) who were matched for age and socioeconomic characteristics. Only women of Belgian nationality were recruited. They were non-smokers, not bedridden, more than 60 years old (mean about 80), and resided in the respective areas more than 25 years (mean about 70). They were not suffering from diabetes mellitus or clinically confirmed renal disease and had not been treated in the past for renal diseases (e.g. glomerulonephritis, pyelonephritis, ...) [134, 135]. The median values for the estimated urinary excretion of Cd were 2.02 μg/24h (range: 0.36-8.76) in the Liège group against 0.79 μg/24h (range 0.05-3.74) in the Charleroi group, and for the urinary excretion of β_2-microglobulin it was 0.18 against 0.12 mg/24h respectively. The prevalence of women with a β_2-microglobulinuria exceeding 1.2 mg/24h was 18% in Liège and 7% in Charleroi. This study suggested that living in the Liège area may significantly increase the body burden of Cd, though the CdU values were much lower than in Japan. The higher β_2-microglobulinuria in Liège suggested further that the critical level of urinary Cd (thus also in the renal cortex) might be much lower in groups of the general population than in middle-aged male workers. A retrospective mortality study in the same two areas showed that in both males and females the standardized mortality ratios from nephritis and nephrosis (ICD 580 and 584) for the years 1969-1976 were twice as high in Liège compared to Charleroi [136]. This finding, which did not seem to be confounded by a difference in analgesic consumption between the two areas [137], supported the hypothesis that Cd may be a contributing environmental factor of renal insufficiency. Post-mortem analysis of Cd in liver and kidney cortex of Belgian citizens corroborated that people who had lived in the industrial area of Liège had accumulated significantly more Cd in their tissues than those who resided in Brussels or the southern provinces of Belgium. In the age group 40-49 years, the Cd concentration in the renal cortex of nonsmoker women was about 40 μg Cd/g wet weight in the Liège area against 14 μg Cd/g wet weight in the other areas [138].

Cadmibel study

The outcomes of these three pilot studies provided the incentive to carry out a large scale cross-sectional population-based investigation in Belgium. Hence, from 1985 to 1989 the Cadmibel study was conducted in about 2,300 subjects to assess the extent of exposure and health effects associated with low-level environmental Cd pollution. Citizens of Belgian nationality were randomly recruited from four areas: Liège (urban) and Noorderkempen (rural), two areas documented with records of environmental Cd pollution due to the activities of various zinc/Cd smelters in the past, and Charleroi (urban) and Hechtel-Eksel (rural), two areas without such industries [139]. Some selection criteria were applied so that the statistical analysis pertaining to renal effects was carried out on about 1,700 adults (males and females aged 20-80 years) who had never been occupationally exposed to heavy metals and who resided the last 8 years in the respective areas. After allowing for major covariates like age and smoking habits, the 24-hour urinary Cd excretion averaged 25% higher in women than in men and was found 20 to 60% higher in both genders living in the polluted areas Liège or Noorderkempen [140]. Stepwise multiple regression analysis showed that only markers of tubulotoxicity (e.g. 24-hour urinary excretion of calcium, N-acetyl-β-D-glucosaminidase, retinol-binding protein, β_2-microglobulin, and amino acids) were significantly and positively associated with CdU. In logistic regression, the likelihood of 10% abnormal values for these tubular effect markers (cut-off: 95th centile of values observed in an "internal control group") would occur at urinary Cd excretion values different from those seen in male Cd workers (Table 6) [38]. For example, the threshold effect level of urinary Cd approximates 3 μg Cd/g creatinine for microproteinuria (retinol-binding protein and β_2-microglobulin) in the general population, whereas it is 10 μg Cd/g creatinine in adult male Cd workers. Järup et al. [59] also reported that renal tubular damage due to exposure to Cd develops at lower levels of Cd body burden than previously anticipated. A 5-year follow-up of a subcohort from the Cadmibel study (about 1,100 subjects from the rural area) suggested that the subclinical renal effects seen at baseline were not progressive and that tubular effects were not necessarily associated with a subsequent deterioration in glomerular function [141].

A striking and unexpected outcome of the Cadmibel study was the clear-cut interference of the low-level Cd exposure with calcium metabolism. For example, when urinary Cd excretion increased twofold, serum alkaline phosphatase activity and urinary calcium excretion rose by 3-4% and 0.25 mmol/24h respectively [142]. The dose (CdU)-response rate of increased calciuria (>9.8 mmol/24h) suggested a 10% prevalence of hypercalciuria when CdU exceeded 1.9 μg Cd/24h [38]. Hypercalciuria should be considered an early adverse tubulotoxic effect, because it may exacerbate the development of osteoporosis, especially in the elderly. A prospective study from 1992-1995 (median follow-up of 6.6 years) in the above-mentioned Cadmibel subcohort from the rural area showed for a two-fold increase in urinary Cd a significant ($p<0.02$) decrease of 0.01 g/cm^2 in forearm bone density in post-menopausal women. In addition, the relative risks associated with doubled urinary Cd were 1.73 (95% CI: 1.16-2.57; p=0.007) for fractures in women and 1.60 (0.94-2.72; p=0.08) for height loss in men. Cadmium excretion in the four districts near the smelters was 22.8% higher (p=0.001) than in the six other districts, with fracture rates of 16.0 and 10.3 cases per 1000 person-year, respectively, and a population-attributable risk of 35% [143]. In Belgium, low-level environmental exposure to Cd may thus promote skeletal demineralization, which may lead to increased bone fragility and raised risk of fractures. Therefore it has been proposed that a CdU value of 2 μg Cd/g creatinine should be regarded as the maximum tolerable internal Cd dose for individuals from the general population. Hence, one may assume that in the early 1990s about 10% of the general population in Belgium exceeded this threshold value and that it amounted to 20% in the rural area with historical pollution by Cd from non-ferrous smelters. In this area, a clear-cut impact of a preventive action to decrease the Cd transfer from the environment to the inhabitants was observed, because the Cd concentration had decreased by about 30% in blood and 15% in urine; the decrease was, however, less pronounced in subjects living closer to the smelters and in pre-menopausal women [144].

General conclusion from studies in Belgium

The results of the various epidemiological investigations performed since the 1970s in Belgium indicate that the efforts made by industries and the health authorities to reduce occupational and environmental exposure to Cd are fully justified. As practical guidelines to control kidney effects at an early stage in occupational or environmental exposure to Cd, the urinary Cd concentration should not exceed 5 μg Cd/g creatinine in male workers and 2 μg Cd/g creatinine in the general population. However, recent findings in groups of Belgian subjects (Cd workers, adolescents, rural Cadmibel cohort) are likely to question whether Cd-associated neuropsychological deficits [133, 145] and increased lung cancer incidence [31] could be adequately prevented on the basis of guidelines derived to avoid early renal effects.

Other countries

A relationship between urine Cd levels and increased excretion of tubular proteins in long-term occupationally exposed workers has been reported from USA [146]. In Germany, Jung et al. [147] reported increased prevalence of elevated urinary excretion of N-acetyl-β-D-glucosaminidase and retinol-binding protein both in occupationally and non-occupationally Cd-exposed groups. In occupationally Cd-exposed workers in Singapore [148] elevated urinary levels of β2-microglobulin, N-acetyl-β-D-glucosaminidase, and α1-microglobulin were reported. The latter two indicators were positive at urine Cd levels of only a few μg per gram creatinine.

In China, increased occurrence of tubular proteinuria has been reported in Cd-contaminated areas [6, 7, 149, 150]. In an area in southeast China, there was high dietary exposure via the intake of cadmium containing rice. Mean levels of cadmium in rice in the most polluted area was 3.7 mg/kg [7]. Contamination occurred by effluents of a non-ferrous smelter. Increased excretion of tubular proteinuria was reported among the inhabitants of this area. Urinary β2-microglobulin and albumin correlated in a dose-related pattern with the urinary Cd excretion [7]. Urinary β2-microglobulin and N-acetyl-β-D-glucosaminidase excretion was evident also at relatively low urinary Cd concentrations [151]. Consumption of cadmium-contaminated rice was stopped in 1996 in this area, but because of the long biological half-life of cadmium in the human body, relatively high levels of cadmium in urine remained when this population was again investigated in 1998 [152]. Statistically significant dose-response relationships were found between biomarkers of internal dose (Cd in blood or urine) and the prevalence of increased retinol-binding protein in urine as well as decreased bone mineral density [152] and an increased prevalence of fractures [153]. The connection between renal dysfunction and osteoporosis in this population group was illustrated by statistical analyses [154]. A Symposium summarizing the studies in China was held in 2003 and published in 2004 [155]. Nutritional interactions on intestinal uptake of Cd were reviewed and data was presented on interactions related to combined exposures of Cd and As in China. Renal and bone effects as well as male reproductive effects including potential precursors of cancer were reported. Low benchmark dose-05 values for increased urinary NAG-B was reported at urinary Cd of 3.99 μg/g creatinine and higher values for other indicators of renal dysfunction [156]. Critical Cd exposure levels for elevated urinary metallothionein have been reported among occupationally cadmium-exposed persons in China [157].

In some Chinese areas there are combined exposures to cadmium and inorganic arsenic. It was shown that there is a strong interaction between these two toxicants for induction of adverse renal effects in terms of tubular markers like increased β2-microglobulin and glomerular marker urinary albumin [158].

In Chinese Cd-exposed workers it was demonstrated that those with a high ability to induce metallothionein suffered less tubular damage than those with a low ability to induce metallothionein in peripheral blood lymphocytes [159]. Similar observations were reported from a population group in China environmentally exposed to cadmium [160]. These observations give support for an important role of metallothionein induction in humans and that such induction in peripheral blood lymphocytes can be used as a biomarker of individual sensitivity to development of renal damage.

Auto-antibodies against metallothionein can be determined in plasma by enzyme-linked immunosorbent assay. It was shown in an occupationally Cd-exposed group in China, that persons with elevated levels of antibodies against metallothionein in plasma displayed a greater sensitivity to developing renal tubular dysfunction – odds ratio 4.2 (95% CI: 1.2-14.5) [161]. In a group of Chinese type-2 diabetics with urinary cadmium levels (geometric mean) of 0.43 μg/g creatinine in women and 0.32 μg/g creatinine in men, the odds ratio for tubular dysfunction after adjustment for confounding covariates was 5.6 (95% CI: 2.3–13.7) when subgroups with low and high levels of plasma metallothionein antibodies were compared [162].

Conclusions from studies in other countries

The observations of dose-response relationships between cumulative absorbed dose of Cd, reflected by urinary Cd levels, and occurrence of tubular proteinuria in other countries support the relationships observed in Sweden, Japan, and Belgium. Recent observations in China indicate that the presence of diabetes, increased levels of tissue antibodies against metallothionein, poor ability of the individual to synthesize metallothionein and/or concomitant exposure to inorganic arsenic may give rise to the occurrence of renal tubular and glomerular dysfunction at cadmium levels as low as those occurring in the general population in China (and many other countries). For persons with such constitution, disease, or exposure there may not exist a threshold level for cadmium-related renal dysfunction above background cadmium exposure. These findings in China need be confirmed in population groups residing in other countries.

References

1. Friberg L. Health hazards in the manufacture of alkaline accumulators with special reference to chronic cadmium poisoning. Act Med Scand 1950; 138 (suppl. 240): 1-124.
2. Nogawa K. Itai-itai disease and follow-up studies. In: Nriagu JO (editor). Cadmium in the environment. Part II: Health effects. John Wiley & Sons, New York 1981; p. 1-37.
3. World Health Organization. Cadmium (environment health criteria; 134). World Health Organization, Geneva 1992; p. 174-188.
4. Kjellström T. Critical organs, critical concentrations, and whole body dose-response relationships. In: Cadmium and health: a toxicological and epidemiological appraisal. Volume II: effects and response. Friberg L, Elinder C-G, Kjellström T, Nordberg GF (editors). CRC Press, Boca Raton, Florida 1986; p. 231-246.
5. Nordberg GF, Nogawa K, Nordberg M, Friberg L. Cadmium. In: Nordberg GF, Fowler BA, Nordberg M, Friberg LT (editors). Handbook on the Toxicology of Metals, 3rd edition. Elsevier, Amsterdam, 2007.
6. Cai SW, Yue L, Hu ZN, Zhong XZ, Y ZL, Xu HD, Liu YR, Ji RD, Zhang WH, Zhang FY. Cadmium exposure and health effects among residents in an irrigation area with ore dressing wastewater. Sci Total Environ 1990; 90: 67-73.
7. Nordberg GF, Jin T, Kong Q, Ye T, Cai S, Wang Z, Zuang F, Wu X. Biological monitoring of cadmium exposure and renal effects in a population group residing in a polluted area in China. Sci Total Environ 1997; 119: 111-114.
8. Nordberg GF, Kjellström T, Nordberg M. Kinetics and metabolism. In: Friberg L, Elinder C-G, Kjellström T, Nordberg GF (editors). Cadmium and health: a toxicological and epidemiological appraisal, Volume I. CRC Press, Boca Raton, Florida 1985; p. 103-178.
9. Berk PD, Stremmel W. Hepatocellular uptake of organic anions. Prog Liver Dis 1986; 8: 125-144.
10. Jin T, Nordberg GF, Nordberg M. Uptake of cadmium in isolated kidney cells - influence of binding forms and *in vivo* pretreatment. J Appl Toxicol 1986; 6: 397-400.

11. Fowler BA, Nordberg GF. Renal toxicity of cadmium metallothionein: morphometric and X-ray microanalytical studies. Toxicol Appl Pharmacol 1978; 46: 609-623.
12. Bernard AM, Ouled AA, Lauwerys RR. The effects of low doses of cadmium-metallothionein on the renal uptake of β_2-microglobulin in rats. Toxicol Appl Pharmacol 1987; 87: 440-445.
13. Nordberg GF. Metabolism of cadmium. In: Nephrotoxic mechanisms of drugs and environmental toxins. Porter G (editor). Plenum Publishing Co, New York, London, Paris 1982; p. 285-303.
14. Lagerkvist BJson, Sandberg S, Frech W, Jin T, Nordberg GF. Is placenta a good indicator of cadmium and lead exposure? Arch Environ Health 1996; 112: 151-156.
15. Roels H, Hubermont G, Buchet JP, Lauwerys R. Placental transfer of lead, mercury, cadmium, and carbon monoxide in women. III. Factors influencing the accumulation of heavy metals in the placenta and the relationship between metal concentration in the placenta and in maternal and cord blood. Environ Res 1978; 16: 236-247.
16. Lagerkvist BJson, Soderberg H-A, Nordberg GF, Ekesrydh S, EnglystV. Biological monitoring of arsenic, lead and cadmium in occupationally and environmentally exposed pregnant women. Scand J Work Environ Health 1993; 19 (suppl 1): 39-44.
17. Friberg L, Piscator M, Nordberg GF (editors). Cadmium in the environment. CRC Press, Boca Raton, Florida 1971.
18. Friberg L, Piscator M, Nordberg GF, Kjellström T (editors). Cadmium in the environment, 2nd edition. CRC Press, Boca Raton, Florida 1974.
19. Kjellström T, Nordberg GF. A kinetic model of cadmium metabolism in the human being. Environ Res 1978; 16: 248-269.
20. Kjellström T, Nordberg GF. Kinetic model of cadmium metabolism. In: Cadmium and health: a toxicological and epidemiological appraisal. Friberg L, Elinder C-G, Kjellström T, Nordberg GF (editors). CRC Press, Boca Raton, Florida 1985; p. 179-197.
21. Nordberg GF, Slorach S, Stenström T. Kadmium-forgiftning orsakad av kalldrycksautomat. Lakartidningen 1973; 70: 601-604.
22. Clarkson TW, Nordberg GF, Sager PR. Reproductive and developmental toxicity of metals. Scand J Work Environ Health 1985; 11: 145-154.
23. Goyer RA, Cherian MG. Role of metallothionein in human placenta and rats with cadmium exposure. In: Cadmium in the human environment: toxicity and carcinogenicity. Nordberg G, Herber R, Alessio L (editors). International Agency for Research on Cancer (IARC) Scientific Publications, Vol 118, Lyon 1992; p. 239-247.
24. Berlin M, Blanks R, Catton M, Kazantzis G, Mottet N, Samiullah Y. Birth weight of children and calcium accumulation in placentas of female nickel-cadmium (long-life) battery workers. In: Cadmium in the human environment: toxicity and carcinogenicity. Nordberg G, Herber R, Alessio L (editors). International Agency for Research on Cancer (IARC) Scientific Publications, Vol 118, Lyon 1992; p. 257-262.
25. IARC. Beryllium, cadmium, mercury and exposure in the glass manufacturing industry. International Agency for Research on Cancer (IARC) Monographs on the evaluation of carcinogenic risks to humans, Vol 58, Lyon 1993.
26. Verougstraete V, Lison D, Hotz P. Cadmium, lung and prostate cancer: a systematic review of recent epidemiological data. J Toxicol Environ Health 2003; 6: 227-255.
27. Doll R. Cadmium in the human environment: closing remarks. In: Cadmium in the human environment: toxicity and carcinogenicity. Nordberg G, Herber R, Alessio L (editors). International Agency for Research on Cancer (IARC) Scientific Publications, Vol 118, Lyon 1992; p. 459-464.
28. Arisawa K, Nakano A, Saito H, Liu XJ, Yokoo M, Soda M, Koba T, Takahashi T, Kinoshita K. Mortality and cancer incidence among a population previously exposed to environmental cadmium. Int Arch Occup Environ Health 2001; 74: 255-262.
29. Järup L, Berglund M, Elinder C-G, Nordberg GF, Vahter M. Health effects of cadmium exposure - a review of the literature and a risk estimate. Scand J Work Environ Health 1998; 24 (suppl 1): 1-51.
30. Nordberg G. Lung cancer and exposure to environmental cadmium. Lancet Oncology 2006; 7: 99-101.
31. Nawrot T, Plusquin M, Hogervorst J, Roels HA, Celis H, Thijs L, Vangronsveld J, Van Hecke E, Staessen JA. Environmental exposure to cadmium and risk of cancer: a prospective population-based study. Lancet Oncology 2006; 7: 119-126.
32. Nordberg G. Effects of dose-response relationships of toxic metals. Elsevier Publishing Co, Amsterdam 1976; p. 111.
33. Ellis KJ, Yuen K, Yasumura S, Cohn SH. Dose-response analysis of cadmium in man: body burden versus dysfunction. Environ Res 1984; 33: 216-229.
34. Roels HA, Lauwerys RR, Buchet JP, Bernard A, Chettle DR, Harvey TC, Al-Haddad IK. *In vivo* measurement of liver and kidney cadmium in workers exposed to this metal: its significance with respect to cadmium in blood and urine. Environ Res 1981; 26: 217-240.
35. Roels H, Lauwerys R, Dardenne AN. The critical level of cadmium in human renal cortex: a re-evaluation. Toxicol Lett 1983; 15: 357-360.
36. Bernard A, Roels H, Buchet JP, Cardenas A, Lauwerys R. Cadmium and health: the Belgian experience. In: Cadmium in the human environment: toxicity and carcinogenicity. Nordberg G, Herber R, Alessio L (editors). International Agency for Research on Cancer (IARC) Scientific Publications, Vol 118, Lyon 1992; p. 15-33.

37. Roels H, Bernard AM, Cardenas A, Buchet JP, Lauwerys RR, Hotter G, Ramis I, Mutti A, Franchini I, Bundschuh I, Stolte H, De Broe ME, Nuyts GD, Taylor SA, Price RG. Markers of early renal changes induced by industrial pollutants. III. Application to workers exposed to cadmium. Br J Ind Med 1993; 50: 37-48.
38. Buchet JP, Lauwerys R, Roels H, Bernard A, Bruaux P, Claeys F, Ducoffre G, De Plaen P, Staessen J, Amery A, Lijnen P, Thijs L, Rondia D, Sator F, Saint-Remy A, Nick L. Renal effects of cadmium body burden of the general population. Lancet 1990; 336: 699-702.
39. Nordberg GF, Goyer RA, Nordberg M. Comparative toxicity of cadmium metallothionein and cadmium chloride on mouse kidney. Arch Pathol 1975; 99: 192-197.
40. Squibb KS, Pritchard JB, Fowler BA. Cadmium metallothionein nephrotoxicity: ultrastructural/biochemical alterations and intracellular cadmium-binding. J Pharmacol Exp Ther 1984; 229: 311-321.
41. Nordberg GF, Jin T, Nordberg M. Subcellular targets of cadmium nephrotoxicity: cadmium binding to renal membrane proteins in animals with or without protective metallothionein synthesis. Environ Health Perspect 1994; 102 (suppl 3): 191-194.
42. Fowler BA, Akkerman M. The role of Ca^{++} in cadmium-induced renal tubular cell injury. In: Cadmium in the human environment: toxicity and carcinogenicity. Nordberg G, Herber R, Alessio L (editors). International Agency for Research on Cancer (IARC) Scientific Publications, Vol 118, Lyon 1992; p. 271-277.
43. Leffler PE, Jin T, Nordberg GF. Differential calcium transport disturbances in renal membrane vesicles after cadmium-metallothionein injection in rats. Toxicology 2000; 143: 227-234.
44. Liu X, Squibb KS, Akkerman M, Nordberg GF, Lipsky M, Fowler BA. Cytotoxicity, zinc protection and stress protein induction in rat proximal tubule cells exposed to cadmium chloride in primary cell culture. Renal Failure 1996; 8: 867-882.
45. Karin M, Richards RJ. The human metallothionein gene family. Structure and expression. Environ Health Perspect 1984; 54: 111-115.
46. Nordberg M, Nordberg G. Toxicological aspects of metallothionein. Cellul Mol Biol 2000; 46: 451-463.
47. Nordberg GF, Garvey JS, Chang CC. Metallothionein in plasma and urine of cadmium workers. Environ Res 1982; 28: 179-182.
48. Roels HA, Lauwerys R, Buchet JP, Bernard A, Garvey JS, Linton HJ. Significance of urinary metallothionein in workers exposed to cadmium. Int Arch Occup Environ Health 1983; 52: 159-166.
49. Tohyama C, Shaikh ZA, Nogawa K, Kobayashi E, Honda R. Elevated urinary excretion of metallothionein to environmental cadmium. Toxicology 1981; 20: 289-297.
50. Garvey JS. Metallothionein: structure/antigenicity and detection/quantification in normal physiological fluids. Environ Health Perspect 1984; 54: 117-127.
51. Piscator M. Proteinuria in chronic cadmium poisoning. I. An electrophoretic and chemical study of urinary and serum proteins from workers with chronic cadmium poisoning. Arch Environ Health 1962; 4: 607-621.
52. Piscator M. Proteinuria in chronic cadmium poisoning. II. The applicability of quantitative methods of protein determination for the demonstration of cadmium proteinuria. Arch Environ Health 1962; 5: 325-332.
53. Nordberg GF. Cadmium metabolism and toxicity. Environ Physiol Biochem 1972; 2: 7-36.
54. Nordberg M. Studies on metallothionein and cadmium. Environ Res 1978; 15: 381-404.
55. Kjellström T, Linnman L, Elinder C-G. Variation of cadmium concentration in Swedish wheat and barley. An indicator of changes in daily cadmium intake during the 20th century. Arch. Environ Health 1975; 30: 321-328.
56. Kjellström T, Evrin P-E, Rahnster B. Dose-response analysis of cadmium induced tubular proteinuria. A study of urinary β_2-microglobulin excretion among workers in a battery factory. Environ Res 1977; 13: 303-317.
57. Nordberg GF. Health hazards of environmental cadmium pollution. Ambio 1974; 3: 55-66.
58. Friberg L, Elinder C-G, Kjellström T, Nordberg GF (editors). Cadmium and health: a toxicological and epidemiological appraisal. CRC Press, Boca Raton, Florida 1986.
59. Järup L, Hellström L, Alfvén T, Carlsson MD, Grubb A, Persson B, Petterson C, Spång G, Schultz A, Elinder C-G. Low level cadmium exposure and early kidney damage – the OSCAR study. Occup Environ Med 2000; 57: 668-672.
60. Alfvén T, Elinder C-G, Carlsson MD, Grubb A, Hellström L, Persson B. Low level cadmium exposure and osteoporosis. J Bone Mineral Res 2000; 15: 1579-1586.
61. Olsson IM, Bensryd I, Lundh T, Ottosson H, Skerfving S, Oskarsson A. Cadmium in blood and urine--impact of sex, age, dietary intake, iron status, and former smoking-association of renal effects. Environ Health Perspect 2002; 210: 1185–1190.
62. Akesson A, Lundh T, Vahter M, Bjellerup P, Lidfeldt J, Nerbrand C, Samsioe G, Stromberg U, Skerfving S. Tubular and glomerular kidney effects in Swedish women with low environmental cadmium exposure. Environ Health Perspect 2005; 113: 1627–1631.
63. Kitagawa M, Yamashita H. Studies on histopathological findings of osteomalacia of itai-itai disease. Kankyo Hoken Report (in Japanese) 1993; 60: 172-174.
64. Health and Welfare Statistics Association. Trend of Environmental Health. J Health and Welfare Statistics 2006: 53; 309-312.
65. Butler EA, Flynn FV. The proteinuria of renal tubular disorders. Lancet 1958; 2: 978-980.

66. Piscator M. The nephropathy of chronic cadmium poisoning. In: Cadmium. Foulkes EC (editor). Springer-Verlag, Berlin 1986; p. 179-194.
67. Piscator M. Markers of tubular dysfunction. Toxicol Lett 1989; 46: 197-204.
68. Kido T, Honda R, Yamada Y, Tsuritani I, Ishizaki M, Nogawa K. α_1-microglobulin determination in urine for the early detection of renal tubular dysfunctions caused by exposure to cadmium. Toxicol Lett 1985; 24: 195-201.
69. Sugihira N, Saito H. Urinary excretion of N-acetyl-β-D-glucosaminidase and β_2-microglobulin in people living in a cadmium-polluted area. Jpn J Hyg 1986; 41: 665-671.
70. Nogawa K, Yamada Y, Honda R, Tsuritani I, Ishizaki M, Sakamoto M. Urinary N-acetyl-β-D-glucosaminidase and β_2-microglobulin in 'itai-itai' disease. Toxicol Lett 1983; 16: 317-322.
71. Nogawa K, Yamada Y, Kido T, Honda R, Ishizaki M, Tsuritani I, Kobayashi E. Significance of elevated urinary N-acetyl-β-D-glucosaminidase activity in chronic cadmium poisoning. Sci Total Environ 1986; 53: 173-178.
72. Nakano M, Aoshima K, Katoh T, Teranishi H, Kasuya M. Urinary trehalase activity and renal brush-border damage in inhabitants of a cadmium-polluted area (Jinzu River basin). Toxicol Lett 1986; 34: 159-166.
73. Verpooten GF, Nouwen EJ, Hoylaerts MF, Hendrix PG, De Broe ME. Segment-specific localization of intestinal-type alkaline phosphatase in human kidney. Kidney Int 1989; 36: 617-625.
74. Kido T, Hayano M, Kobayashi E, Nogawa K, Nishijo M, Tabata M, Nakagawa H, Tsuritani I. Significance of elevated urinary human intestinal alkaline phosphatase in Japanese people exposed to environmental cadmium. Toxicol Lett 1995; 80: 49-54.
75. Kido T, Honda R, Tsuritani I, Ishizaki M, Yamada Y, Nakagawa H, Nogawa K. Significant increase of urinary mucoprotein in environmental cadmium-exposed Japanese subjects. Toxicol Lett 1991; 55: 303-309.
76. Abe T, Kobayashi E, Okubo Y, Suwazono Y, Kido T, Shaikh ZA, Nogawa K. Application of path analysis to urinary findings of cadmium-induced renal dysfunction. J Environ Sci Health Part A Tox Hazard Subst Environ Eng 2001; 36: 75-87.
77. Nogawa K, Kobayashi E, Honda R, Ishizaki A, Kawano S, Matsuda H. Renal dysfunction of inhabitants in a cadmium-polluted area. Environ Res 1980; 23: 1323-1330.
78. Nogawa K. Biologic indicators of cadmium nephrotoxicity in persons with low-level cadmium exposure. Environ Health Perspect 1984; 54: 163-169.
79. Takebayashi S. First autopsy case, suspicious of cadmium intoxication, from the cadmium-polluted area in Tsushima, Nagasaki Prefecture. In: Cadmium-induced osteopathy. Shigematsu I, Nomiyama K (editors). Japan Public Health Association, Tokyo 1980; p. 124-138.
80. Bernard A, Lauwerys R. Effects of cadmium exposure in humans. In: Cadmium. Foulkes EC (editor). Springer-Verlag, Berlin 1986; p. 150-159.
81. Kido T, Nogawa K, Ishizaki M, Honda R, Tsuritani I, Yamada Y, Nakagawa H, Nishi M. Long-term observation of serum creatinine and arterial blood pH in persons with cadmium-induced renal dysfunction. Arch Environ Health 1990; 45: 35-41.
82. Kajikawa K, Kitagawa M, Nakanishi I, Ueshima H, Katsuda S, Kuroda K. A pathological study of "itai-itai disease". J Juzen Med Soc (in Japanese) 1974; 83: 309-347.
83. Fukushima M. Environmental pollution by cadmium and its health effects: an epidemiological approach to the "itai-itai" disease. In: New methods in environmental chemistry and toxicology. Coulston F, Koprte F, Goto M (editors). International Academic Printing Co, Tokyo 1973; p. 231-252.
84. Osawa K, Kobayashi E, Okubo Y, Suwazono Y, Kido T, Nogawa K. A retrospective study on the relation between renal dysfunction and cadmium concentration in rice in individual hamlets in the Jinzu River basin, Toyama Prefecture, Japan. Environ Res 2001; 86: 51-59.
85. Tsuchiya K. Environmental pollution and health effects. In: Cadmium studies in Japan: a review. Tsuchiya K (editor). Kodansya Ltd, Tokyo 1978; p. 144-253.
86. Kido T, Honda R, Tsuritani I, Yamaya H, Ishizaki M, Yamada Y, Nogawa K. An epidemiological study on renal dysfunction of inhabitants in cadmium-exposed areas in the Kakehashi River basin in Ishikawa Prefecture. Jpn J Hyg (in Japanese) 1987; 42: 964-972.
87. Kido T, Nishijo M, Nakagawa H, Kobayashi E, Nogawa K, Tsuritani I, Honda R, Kito H. Urinary findings of inhabitants in a cadmium-polluted area ten years after cessation of cadmium exposure. Hokuriku J Public Health 2001; 27: 81-84.
88. Japan public health association cadmium research committee. Summary report on studies of health effects of cadmium. Japan Public Health Association, Tokyo 1989; p. 53-67.
89. Ishihara T, Kobayashi E, Okubo Y, Suwazono Y, Kido T, Nishijo M, Nakagawa H, Nogawa K. Association between cadmium concentration in rice and mortality in the Jinzu River basin, Japan. Toxicology 2001; 163: 23-28.
90. Kido T, Nogawa K, Yamada Y, Honda R, Tsuritani I, Ishizaki M, Yamaya H. Osteopenia in inhabitants with renal dysfunction induced by exposure to environmental cadmium. Int Arch Occup Environ Health 1989; 61: 271-276.
91. Inoue T, Kusida K, Miyamoto S, Sumi Y. Quantitative assessment of bone density on X-ray picture. J Jpn Orthop Ass 1983; 57: 1923-1936.

92. Aoshima K, Iwata K, Kasuya M. Environmental exposure to cadmium and effects on human health. Part 2. Bone and mineral metabolism in inhabitants of the cadmium-polluted Jinzu River basin in Toyama Prefecture. Jpn J Hyg (in Japanese) 1988; 43: 864-871.
93. Harada T, Matsuo S, Hara K, Yoshimura S. The association between proximal renal tubular dysfunction and osteopenia using microdensitometry in subjects required observation in cadmium-polluted areas. Kankyo-Hoken Report (in Japanese) 1986; 52: 109-113.
94. Kido T, Nogawa K, Honda R, Tsuritani I, Ishizaki M, Yamada Y, Nakagawa H. The association between renal dysfunction and osteopenia in environmental cadmium-exposed subjects. Environ Res 1990; 51: 71-82.
95. Tsuritani I, Honda R, Ishizaki M, Yamada Y, Nishijo M, Nakagawa H. Bone mineral measurement in inhabitants in a cadmium polluted area by ultrasound bone densitometer. Jpn J Hyg (in Japanese) 1994; 49: 125.
96. Kido T, Honda R, Tsuritani I, Ishizaki M, Yamada Y, Nakagawa H, Nogawa K, Dohi Y. Serum levels of bone G1a-protein in inhabitants exposed to environmental cadmium. Arch Environ Health 1991; 46: 43-49.
97. Omote S, Kido T, Nishijo M, Nakagawa H, Suwazono E, Kobayashi E, Nogawa K. Urinary type 1 collagen cross-linked N-telopeptides in inhabitants 18 years after cessation of exposure to cadmium in Japan. Bull Environ Contam Toxicol 2006; 76: 187-194.
98. Nogawa K, Tsuritani I, Kido T, Honda R, Yamada Y, Ishizaki M. Mechanism for bone disease found in inhabitants environmentally exposed to cadmium; decreased serum 1α,25-dihydroxyvitamin D level. Int Arch Occup Environ Health 1987; 59: 21-30.
99. Nogawa K, Kobayashi E, Yamada Y, Honda R, Kido T, Tsuritani I, Ishizaki M. Parathyroid hormone concentration in the serum of people with cadmium-induced renal damage. Int Arch Occup Environ Health 1984; 54: 187-193.
100. Nogawa K, Tsuritani I, Kido T, Honda R, Ishizaki M, Yamada Y. Serum vitamin D metabolites in cadmium-exposed persons with renal damage. Int Arch Occup Environ Health 1990; 62: 189-193.
101. Lauwerys RR, Buchet JP, Roels H. The relationship between cadmium exposure or body burden and the concentration of cadmium in blood and urine in man. Int Arch Occup Environ Health 1976; 36: 275-285.
102. Kido T, Nogawa K, Ohmichi M, Honda R, Tsuritani I, Ishizaki M, Yamada Y. Significance of urinary cadmium concentration in a Japanese population environmentally exposed to cadmium. Arch Environ Health 1992; 47: 196-202.
103. Nakashima K, Kobayashi E, Nogawa K, Kido T, Honda R. Concentration of cadmium in rice and urinary indicators of renal dysfunction. Occup Environ Med 1997; 54: 750-755.
104. Shimizu A, Kobayashi E, Suwazono Y, Uetani M, Oishi M, Inaba T, Kido T, Nogawa K. Estimation of benchmark doses for urinary cadmium based on β_2-micoroglobulin excretion in cadmium-polluted regions of the Kakehashi River basin, Japan. Int J Environ Health Res 2006; 16: 329-337.
105. Kido T, Honda R, Tsuritani I, Yamaya H, Ishizaki M, Yamada Y, Nogawa K. Progress of renal dysfunction in inhabitants environmentally exposed to cadmium. Arch Environ Health 1988; 43: 213-217.
106. Harada T, Hara K, Ogata T, Nishimura K, Shigeno N, Shichijo T, Kuwazuka M, Sato S. Changes of main biochemical findings of subjects required observation in cadmium-polluted areas in Tsushima, Nagasaki Prefecture. Kankyo Hoken Report (in Japanese) 1991; 58: 205-211.
107. Shigematsu I, Takeuchi J, Minowa M, Nagai M, Usui T, Fukushima M. A retrospective mortality study on cadmium-exposed population in Japan. Kankyo Hoken Report (in Japanese) 1980; 46 (part 2): 1-71.
108. Nakagawa H, Tabata M, Morikawa Y, Senma M, Kitagawa Y, Kawano S, Kido T. High mortality and shortened life-span in patients with itai-itai disease and subjects with suspected disease. Arch Environ Health 1990; 45: 283-287.
109. Nakagawa H. Nishijo M, Morikawa Y, Tabata M, Senma M, Kitagawa Y, Kawano S. Ishizaki M, Sugita N, Nishi M, Kido T, Nogawa K. Urinary β_2-microglobulin concentration and mortality in a cadmium-polluted area. Arch Environ Health 1993; 48: 428-434.
110. Nishijo M, Nakagawa H, Morikawa Y, Tabata M, Senma M. Kitagawa Y, Kawano S. Ishizaki M, Sugita N, Nishi M, Kido T, Nogawa K. Prognostic factors of renal dysfunction induced by environmental cadmium pollution. Environ Res 1994; 64: 112-121.
111. Iwata K, Saito H, Nakano A. Association between cadmium-induced renal dysfunction and mortality: further evidence. Tohoku J Exp Med 1991; 164: 319-330.
112. Staessen JA, Roels H, Vangronsveld J, Clijsters, H, De Schrijver K, De Temmerman L, Dondeyne F, Van Hulle S, Wildemeersch D, Wilms L. Preventiemaatregelen voor bodemverontreiniging met cadmium. Tijdschr Geneesk 1995; 51: 1387-1395.
113. Sovet. Empoisonnement par une poudre servant à écurer l'argenterie; symptômes graves; gastro-entérite suraigue; accidents dyssentériques; antidote; antiphlogistiques; ipécacuana; analyse chimique. Press Méd Belge 1858; 10: 69-70.
114. Leduc V. Pathologie du cadmium. Report to the Vieille Montagne plant management, September 10, 1953.
115. Friberg L. Proteinuria and kidney injury among workmen exposed to cadmium and nickel dust. J Ind Hyg Toxicol 1948; 30: 32-36.
116. Lauwerys RR, Buchet JP, Roels HA, Brouwers J, Stanescu D. Epidemiological survey of workers exposed to cadmium. - Effects on lung, kidney, and several biological indices. Arch Environ Health 1974; 28: 145-148.

117. Butler EA, Flynn FV, Harris H, Robson EB. A study of urine proteins by two dimensional electrophoresis with special reference to the proteinuria of renal tubular disorders. Clin Chim Acta 1962; 7: 172-178.
118. Kazantzis G, Flynn FV, Spowage JS, Trott DG. Renal tOubular malfunction and emphysema in cadmium pigment workers. Quart J Med 1963; 32: 165-192.
119. Piscator M. Proteinuria in chronic cadmium poisoning. III. Electrophoretic and immuno-electrophoretic studies on urinary proteins from cadmium workers, with special reference to the excretion of low molecular weight proteins. Arch Environ Health 1966; 12: 335-344.
120. Lauwerys RR, Roels HA, Buchet JP, Bernard A, Stanescu D. Investigations on lung and kidney function in workers exposed to cadmium. Environ Health Perspect 1979; 28: 137-145.
121. Bernard A, Buchet JP, Roels H, Masson P, Lauwerys R. Renal excretion of proteins and enzymes in workers exposed to cadmium. Eur J Clin Invest 1979; 9: 11-22.
122. Roels H, Djubgang J, Buchet JP, Bernard A, Lauwerys R. Evolution of cadmium-induced renal dysfunction in workers removed from exposure. Scand J Work Environ Health 1982; 8: 191-200.
123. Roels HA, Lauwerys RR, Buchet JP, Bernard AM, Vos A, Oversteyns M. Health significance of cadmium induced renal dysfunction: a five year follow up. Br J Ind Med 1989; 46: 755-764.
124. Roels HA, Lauwerys RR, Bernard AM, Buchet JP, Vos A, Oversteyns M. Assessment of the filtration reserve capacity of the kidney in workers exposed to cadmium. Br J Ind Med 1991; 48: 365-374.
125. Roels HA, Van Assche FJ, Oversteyns M, De Groof M, Lauwerys RR, Lison D. Reversibility of microproteinuria in cadmium workers with incipient tubular dysfunction after reduction of exposure. Am J Ind Med 1997; 31: 645-652.
126. Buchet JP, Roels H, Bernard A, Lauwerys R. Assessment of renal function of workers exposed to inorganic lead, cadmium or mercury vapor. J Occup Med 1980; 22: 741-750.
127. Bernard AM, Ouled Amor A, Lauwerys RR. Decrease of erythrocyte and glomerular membrane negative charges in chronic cadmium poisoning. Br J Ind Med 1988; 45: 112-115.
128. Cardenas A, Bernard AM, Lauwerys R. Disturbance of sialic acid metabolism by chronic cadmium exposure and its relation to proteinuria. Toxicol Appl Pharmacol 1991; 108: 547-558.
129. Roels HA, Lauwerys RR, Buchet JP, Bernard AM, Lijnen P, Van Houte G. Urinary kallikrein activity in workers exposed to cadmium, lead, or mercury vapour. Br J Ind Med 1990; 47: 331-337.
130. Bernard AM, Roels HA, Foidart JM, Lauwerys RR. Search for anti-laminin antibodies in the serum of workers exposed to cadmium, mercury vapour or lead. Int Arch Occup Environ Health 1987; 59: 303-309.
131. World Health Organization (WHO). Recommended health-based limits in occupational exposure to heavy metals. Report of a study group. WHO Technical Report Series No. 647. Geneva, 1980.
132. American Conference of Governmental Industrial Hygienists (ACGIH). Supplement: Cadmium and inorganic compounds. Biological Exposure Indices. Cincinnati, Ohio 1996.
133. Viaene MK, Masschelein R, Leenders J, De Groof M, Swerts LJVC, Roels HA. Neurobehavioral effects of occupational exposure to cadmium: a cross sectional epidemiological study. Occup Environ Med 2000; 57: 19-27.
134. Lauwerys R, Roels H, Bernard A, Buchet JP. Renal response to cadmium in a population living in a nonferrous smelter area in Belgium. Int Arch Occup Environ Health 1980; 45: 271-274.
135. Roels HA, Lauwerys RR, Buchet JP, Bernard A. Environmental exposure to cadmium and renal function of aged women in three areas of Belgium. Environ Res 1981; 24: 117-130.
136. Lauwerys R, de Wals Ph. Environmental pollution by cadmium and mortality from renal diseases. Lancet 1981; 1: 383.
137. Vanherweghem JL, Even-Adin D. Epidemiology of analgesic nephropathy in Belgium. Clin Nephrol 1982; 17: 129-133.
138. Lauwerys R, Hardy R, Job M, Buchet JP, Roels H, Bruaux P, Rondia D. Environmental pollution by cadmium and cadmium body burden: an autopsy study. Toxicol Lett 1984; 23: 287-289.
139. Lauwerys R, Amery A, Bernard A, Bruaux P, Buchet JP, Claeys F, De Plaen P, Ducoffre G, Fagard R, Lijnen P, Nick L, Roels H, Rondia D, Saint-Remy A, Sartor F, Staessen J. Health effects of environmental exposure to cadmium: objectives, design and organization of the Cadmibel study: a cross-sectional morbidity study carried out in Belgium from 1985 to 1989. Environ Health Perspect 1990; 87: 283-289.
140. Sartor FA, Rondia DJ, Claeys FD, Staessen JA, Lauwerys RR, Bernard AM, Buchet JP, Roels HA, Bruaux PJ, Ducoffre GM, Lijnen PJ, Thijs LB, Amery AK. Impact of environmental cadmium pollution on cadmium exposure and body burden. Arch Environ Health 1992; 47: 347-353.
141. Hotz Ph, Buchet JP, Bernard A, Lison D, Lauwerys R. Renal effects of low-level environmental cadmium exposure: 5-year follow-up of a subcohort from the Cadmibel study. Lancet 1999; 354: 1508-1513.

142. Staessen J, Amery A, Bernard A, Bruaux P, Buchet JP, Claeys F, De Plaen P, Ducoffre G, Fagard R, Lauwerys RR, Lijnen P, Nick L, Saint-Remy A, Roels H, Rondia D, Sartor F, Thijs L. Effects of exposure to cadmium on calcium metabolism: a population study. Br J Ind Med 1991; 45: 710-714.
143. Staessen JA, Roels HA, Emelianov D, Kuznetsova T, Thijs L, Vangronsveld J, Fagard R. Environmental exposure to cadmium, forearm bone density, and risk of fractures: a prospective population study. Lancet 1999; 353: 1140-1144.
144. Staessen JA, Kuznetsova T, Roels HA, Emelianov D, Fagard R. Exposure to cadmium and conventional and ambulatory blood pressures in a prospective population study. Am J Hypertens 2000; 13: 146-156.
145. Vermeir G, Viaene M, Staessen J, Den Hond E, Roels HA. Neurobehavioural investigations in adolescents exposed to environmental pollutants. Env Toxicol Pharmacol 2005; 19: 707-713.
146. Mueller PW, Smith SJ, Steinberg KK, Thun MJ. Chronic renal tubular effects in relation to urine cadmium levels. Nephron 1989; 52: 45-54.
147. Jung K, Pergande M, Graubaum H C, Fels LM, Endl U, Stolte H. Urinary proteins and enzymes as early indicator of renal dysfunction in chronic exposure to cadmium. Clin Chem 1993; 39: 757-765.
148. Chia KS, Tan AL, Chia SE, Ong CN Jeyaratnam J. Renal tubular function of cadmium exposed workers. Ann Acad Med Singapore 1992; 21: 756-759.
149. Cai S, Yue L, Shang Q, Nordberg G. Cadmium exposure among residents in an area contaminated by irrigation water. Bull WHO 1995; 73: 359-367.
150. Cai,S, Yue L, Jin T, Nordberg G. Renal dysfunction from cadmium contamination of irrigation water: dose-response analysis in a Chinese population. Bull WHO 1998; 76: 153-159.
151. Jin T, Nordberg GF, Wu X, Ye T, Kong Q, Wang Z, Zhuang F, Cai S. Urinary N-acetyl-β-D-glucosaminidase isoenzymes as biomarker of renal dysfunction caused by cadmium in a general population. Environ Res Sect A 1999; 81: 167-173.
152. Nordberg G, Jin T, Bernard A, Fierens S, Buchet JP, Ye T, Kong Q, Wang H. Low bone density and renal dysfunction following environmental cadmium exposure in China. Ambio 2002; 31: 478-481.
153. Wang H, Zhu G, Shi Y, Weng S, Jin T, Kong Q, Nordberg GF. Influence of environmental cadmium exposure on forearm bone density. J Bone Miner Res 2003; 18: 553-560.
154. Jin T, Nordberg G, Ye T, Bo M, Wang H, Zuh G, Kong Q, Bernard A. Osteoporosis and renal dysfunction in a general population exposed to cadmium in China. Environ Res 2004; 96: 353-359.
155. Nordberg GF, Jin T, Nordberg M. International Symposium on Health Impacts of Cadmium Exposure and its Prevention in China. BioMetals 2004; 17: 483-597.
156. Jin T, Wu X, Tang Y, Nordberg M, Bernard A, Ye T, Kong Q, Lundstrom N-G, Nordberg G. Environmental epidemiological study and estimation of benchmark dose for renal dysfunction in a cadmium-polluted area in China. BioMetals 2004; 17: 525-530.
157. Chen L, Jin T, Huang B, Nordberg G, Nordberg M. Critical exposure level of cadmium for elevated urinary metallothionein – an occupational population study in China. Toxicol Appl Pharmacol 2006; 215: 93-99.
158. Nordberg GF, Jin T, Hong F, Zhang A, Buchet JP, Bernard A. Biomarkers of cadmium and arsenic interactions. Toxicol Appl Pharmacol 2005; 206: 191-197.
159. Lu J, Jin T, Nordberg GF, Nordberg M. Metallothionein gene expression in peripheral lymphocytes from cadmium exposed workers. Cell Stress Chaperones 2001; 6: 97-104.
160. Lu J, Jin T, Nordberg G, Nordberg M. Metallothionein gene expression in peripheral lymphocytes and renal dysfunction in a population environmentally exposed to cadmium. Toxicol Appl Pharmacol 2005; 206: 150-156.
161. Chen L, Jin T, Huang B, Chang X, Lei L, Nordberg GF, Nordberg M. Plasma metallothionein antibody and cadmium-induced renal dysfunction in an occupational population in China. Toxicol Sci 2006; 91: 104-112.
162. Chen L, Lei L, Jin T, Nordberg M, Nordberg GF. Plasma metallothionein antibody, urinary cadmium and renal dysfunction in a Chinese type 2 diabetic population. Diabetes Care 2006; 29: 2682-2687.

36

Mercury-induced renal effects

Bruce A. FOWLER[1], Margaret H. WHITTAKER[2] and Carl-Gustaf ELINDER[3]

[1]ATSDR, Atlanta, Georgia, USA, [2]Toxservices, LLC, Washington DC, USA,
[3]Department of Renal Medicine, Karolinska University Hospital, Solna and Huddinge, Sweden

Physical and chemical properties of mercury

Mercury (Hg, CAS Number 7439-97-6) is a naturally-occurring metal that has an atomic number of 80 and an atomic weight of 200.6. Many different organic and inorganic mercury compounds are found in nature because of mercury's ability to form covalent and ionic bonds with other chemicals. Mercury exists in three forms in three oxidation states (0, +1, +2): elemental mercury (Hg^0), organic mercury (e.g., methyl mercury), and inorganic mercury (e.g., Hg^{1+}, Hg^{2+}). Elemental mercury is a silvery, white liquid at room temperature, and because of this, Aristotle named mercury "quicksilver."

History of human use of mercury

Mercury has been used by humans since antiquity. More than 10,000 years ago, prehistoric humans used the bright red stone of mercury ore (cinnabar, mercury sulphide, HgS) to color cave drawings. Theofrastos, the disciple of Aristotle, described the production of metallic mercury from cinnabar. Egyptians and Romans identified several of the occupational hazards in mercury mines. During the Roman period, slaves, convicts, and political enemies were sent to the mercury mines in Almadén in Spain where they succumbed to the toxic effects of mercury. In 1700, the Italian physician Ramazzini, regarded as the founder of occupational medicine, in his classical book 'De Morbis Artificum' (Diseases of Workers) described several signs of mercury poisoning, which he observed not only among miners but also gilders, mirror makers, and syphilis patients given treatment with mercury ointments. It was not uncommon for the doctor who administered mercury ointment to also suffer from mercury poisoning.

The use of mercury in the treatment of diseases such as syphilis, psoriasis, and congestive heart failure began more than two centuries ago. Although mercury's medicinal use has tapered off in recent years, mercury compounds such as thimerosal and phenylmercuric nitrate still have a limited use in human and veterinary medicines to prevent bacterial growth in injection solutions (e.g. vaccines), antiseptics, and skin ointments. The United States Food and Drug Administration [1] estimates that approximately 200 human and veterinary drug products marketed in the U.S. contain mercury as an active or inactive ingredient.

The unique physical properties of metallic mercury led to its widespread industrial use during the 19th century. Because of this, epidemics of occupational poisonings were documented in the mirror and felt hat industries. Symptoms and signs of severe poisoning included pneumonitis, tremor, inflammation of the gums with excessive salivation, and psychiatric symptoms such as excitability, insomnia, irritation, and shyness.

Worldwide production of mercury has declined in recent years. Total world production of mercury was 1, 400 tons in 2001, compared to 2, 750 tons in 1997 [2, 3]. Mercury recovered from primary sources accounts for about 60% of world consumption, with the remainder being supplied from recycled sources [4]. Spain, Kyrgyzstan, and Algeria accounted for approximately 70% of the world's mined mercury in 2001 [2].

Mercury compounds continue to have numerous commercial uses. Besides its use as a preservative, mercury is used in the manufacture of many technical and medical instruments including blood pressure measurement devices, manometers, thermometers, and barometers. Mercury is also used in production of certain types of fluorescent lamps and in the chloralkali industry, where chlorine and caustic soda are produced using brine electrolysis in mercury cells. Metallic mercury is used in the production of precious metals such as gold and silver. As part of the production process, metallic mercury can be used to concentrate gold from crushed ore or sediments. This method, also known as the amalgamation method, results in occupational and environmental exposures to vaporized mercury, posing an immediate health threat. Such a health hazard was a common occurrence in the in the 1850s during the California gold rush. Although phased out by most gold producing countries, the amalgamation method is still used in several countries. It has been estimated that some 500, 000 gold miners in Brazil are exposed to liquid mercury during the concentration of gold from sediments [5, 6].

Mercury has been used for more than 150 years in dental silver amalgams. Dental silver amalgams in tooth fillings are composed of a mixture of 50% metallic mercury and metal powder, usually silver, tin, copper and zinc.

Exposure

Humans can be exposed to mercury compounds via the oral, inhalation, and dermal routes. The primary sources of mercury exposure among the general population are dental amalgams and the diet, with amalgam fillings being the most important source of inorganic mercury, and fish and other seafood (marine mammals, crustaceans) the principle sources of methylated or organic mercury.

The release of mercury from amalgam fillings is proportional to both the number of fillings and the total amalgam surface area. It has been challenging to accurately estimate the release from amalgam fillings, but according to the National Research Council, estimates of average daily mercury intake from dental amalgams range from 3.8-21 μg/day [7]. Measurements of urinary excretion of mercury have revealed that individuals with a habit of tooth grinding or 'Bruxism' release considerably more mercury from their dental fillings compared to persons who do not grind their teeth [8]. Most of the exposure from amalgam fillings probably comes from release of mercury vapor (Hg^0) but uptake from amalgam particles in the gastrointestinal tract, at least after dental treatment, may contribute [9].

The concentration of mercury in most foodstuffs is generally below the reported limit of detection, which is usually 20 μg/kg fresh weight [10]. Fish and other seafood products are the primary dietary sources of mercury, and scientists have determined that mercury concentrations in fish and shellfish are approximately 10 to 100 times greater than in other foods, including cereals, potatoes, vegetables, fruits, meats, poultry, eggs, and milk [11]. It only takes a small amount of mercury to pollute aquatic organisms, and render them unfit for consumption. Mercury in fish and seafood is almost completely in the form of methyl mercury, which is a particular health threat to infants and the developing fetus [12]. Certain marine fish, (e.g. shark, swordfish, king mackerel, and tuna), as well as certain freshwater fish (e.g. pike, walleye and bass) may contain high concentrations of mercury. Levels of mercury among these marine fish species range from 0.05-4.54 mg methyl mercury/kg fish (wet weight), while mercury levels in these freshwater fish species range from 0.5 to 2 mg methyl mercury/kg fish (wet weight) [11, 13]. Daily consumption of 100 g of fish possessing an average mercury concentration of 1 mg methyl mercury/kg results in an intake of 100 μg methyl mercury, which exceeds the tolerable limits recommended by the World Health Organization, the United States Environmental Protection Agency, and the United States Food and Drug Administration [14, 15].

Besides dietary and dental amalgam exposure to mercury compounds, accidental exposure to mercury vapors may occur among the general population (e.g., from breakage of a mercury-containing thermometer), or from use of metallic mercury or mercury containing ointments, creams, and drugs.

Occupational exposure to inorganic mercury is quite common, and occurs in the dental and chloralkali industries, as well as in thermometer factories, and in mercury mines. Approximately 70,000 workers in the United States are regularly exposed to mercury [16]. Measurements of mercury in blood and urine are useful in quantifying the magnitude of exposure (see section about biological monitoring below). In most instances there is a linear relationship between ambient air and urine concentration of mercury, where the urine concentration (μg/L) corresponds to air concentration (μg/m^3) multiplied by 1-2 [17]. In dentistry, ambient mercury vapor concentrations during the1960s-1970s were often around 25 μg/m^3. Due to improved ventilation and handling of amalgam, most dental offices have reduced levels below 5 μg/m^3.

Ambient mercury vapor concentrations of 100 μg/m^3 or higher have been measured during chloralkali production and mercury mining [18]. Adverse health effects were common sequelae from such exposures. During recent years, most countries have reduced mercury's occupational threshold limit value to 50 μg/m^3 or less.

Toxicokinetics

The toxicokinetics (i.e., absorption, distribution, metabolism, and excretion) of mercury is highly dependent on the form of mercury to which an individual has been exposed [15]. This difference in toxicokinetics is illustrated in Figures 1 and 2, where intravenous administration of 10 ml (135 grams) of elemental mercury distributed in the lung, while oral ingestion of 236 ml (3212 grams) of elemental mercury distributed in the large intestine. The subject in Figure 1 attempted suicide by injecting elemental mercury intravenously because elemental mercury is poorly absorbed via other routes, such as the gastrointestinal route, as illustrated in Figure 2.

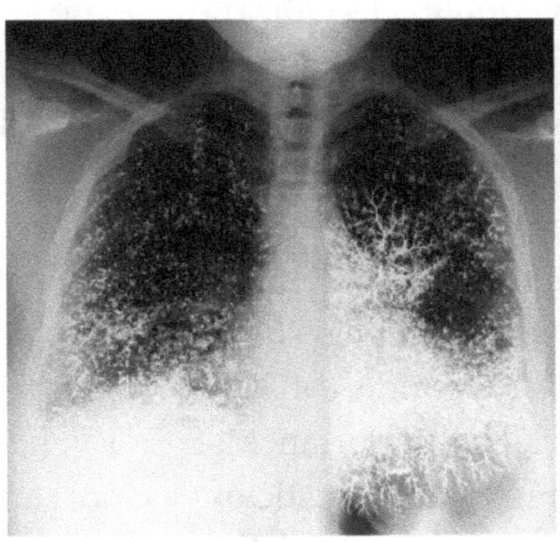

Figure 1. *Elemental mercury embolism to the lung. (reproduced from Gutiérrez and Leon [19], with permission)*

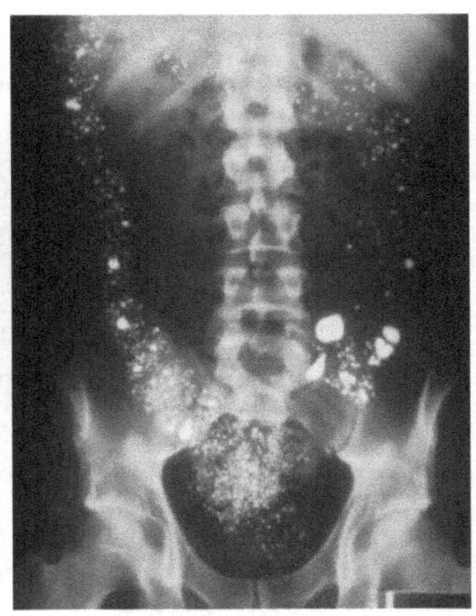

Figure 2. *Elemental mercury distribution in the intestine. (reproduced from Diner and Brenner [20], with permission)*

Mercury vapor (Hg°)

While pulmonary absorption of mercury vapor is high (75-85%) [21], this particular chemical form of mercury is poorly absorbed from either the gastrointestinal tract or across the skin. The gastrointestinal absorption of mercury from amalgam powder in humans has been estimated as 0.04% [9]. The kidney is the major site of mercury deposition following mercury vapor exposure [15]. The half-life of mercury in kidneys following inhalation has been calculated [22] to be approximately 64 days in humans. The half-life of mercury in blood of workers following an acute high dose exposure was reported [23] to be biphasic with a fast phase (3.1 days) and a slow phase (18 days). A significant fraction of the inhaled mercury vapor is eliminated during exhalation with a majority of the absorbed remainder eliminated in the feces.

Ionized inorganic mercury (Hg^{1+}, Hg^{2+})

As with other metals, the pulmonary absorption of Hg^{1+} and Hg^{2+} varies with particle size [24]. Clarkson [25] reports a 40% pulmonary absorption of mercuric chloride in dogs. The gastrointestinal absorption of Hg^{1+} or Hg^{2+} is approximately 15%. The kidney is the major site of deposition following inorganic mercury exposure. Inorganic mercury has a relatively long half-life in the body, and has been estimated to be 40 days [26] and 67 days with a range of 49-96 days [26]. Urinary and fecal elimination are the major routes of removal from the body. Concomitant exposure to selenium results in the formation of Hg-Se intranuclear inclusion bodies in renal proximal tubule cells [28]. The formation of these complexes may temporarily prevent mercury-induced tissue damage as well as delay excretion [15]. Recent studies [29, 30, 31] have demonstrated that the human organic anion transporter -1 (OAT1) and other anion transporters plays a major role in the uptake of mercuric thiol conjugates (N-acetylcysteine, cysteine, glutathione) by Madin-Darby canine (MDCK) and rat kidney cells respectively. The importance of these findings rests with providing a mechanistic explanation for the high degree of mercury accumulation renal tubule cells and subsequent nephrotoxicity.

Organomercurials

Organomercurials can be found in three forms: aryl compounds (aromatics containing mercury atoms, such as phenyl mercury), and short- and long-chain alkyl compounds (aliphatic compounds containing carbon, hydrogen, and mercury atoms, such as methyl mercury). The absorption of organomercurials from the gastrointestinal tract and skin varies with the nature of the organic moiety and stability of the organomercurial bond. Alkyl mercurials such as methyl mercury are highly absorbed. Humans absorb approximately 95% of methyl mercury contained in contaminated fish [32, 33]. Alkyl mercurials are dealkylated [34]. This dealkylation process is extremely slow, as evidenced by continued inorganic mercury excretion among Macaca fascicularis monkeys administered oral doses of methyl mercury [35] (the inorganic mercury was thought to have been demethylated in the brains of monkeys). Methyl mercury has a relatively long half-life of 70-80 days in the human body [33]. While the kidney is a major site of deposition, the hair and central nervous system are other important sites of deposition. There also exist sex-related differences in the handling of organomercurials by rodents [36, 37]. Methyl mercury is primarily excreted in the feces but dealkylation reactions result in sex-related differences in urinary excretion of Hg^{2+} [38]. The OAT1 transporter plays a central role in the cysteine-S-conjugates of methylmercury in MDCK cells and rat NRK52E cells expressing human the OAT1 transporter [31]. These data also provide a mechanistic explanation for the known extensive accumulation and observed tubular effects following methyl mercury exposure in renal tubule cells as described below.

Biological monitoring of mercury

Analytical methods are available to measure mercury in blood, urine, tissue, hair, and breast milk [11]. Biological monitoring of mercury is very useful for assessing exposure as well as risk for health effects [17], but complicated by the fact that both organic and inorganic forms of mercury occur in the body and can be identified in blood and urine. Mercury concentration in individuals who are not occupationally exposed, and whose fish intake is moderate or low, varies between 0.1 and 7 μg/L. The lower values are found in urine and the higher in blood. Urinary mercury is thought to indicate most closely the mercury levels present in the kidneys [39]. The concentration of mercury in urine relates primarily to an exposure to metallic mercury vapor or inorganic mercury compounds. There is a relationship between the number of amalgam fillings and the excretion of mercury in urine. However, for people who are not occupationally exposed, the urinary levels are seldom higher than 10 μg/L. In the case of occupational exposure, there is a linear relationship between air and urine concentrations of mercury. Urine concentrations (μg/L) correspond to air concentrations (μg Hg/m^3) multiplied by 1–2. If mercury concentrations in urine exceed 100 μg Hg/g creatinine, the risk of adverse effects in the nervous system becomes significant. Tremor, nervousness, irritation and kidney damage with proteinuria may be observed. At exposure levels between 50 and 100 μg Hg/g creatinine in urine, these symptoms are less pronounced. Some studies indicate that early signs of adverse effects relating to the nervous system or kidneys can be observed even at urinary levels between 25 and 35 μg Hg/g creatinine [40]. There is a general consensus that if 24-hour urine levels of mercury are greater than 50 μg Hg/g creatinine, nephrotoxicity is probable, comprising cytotoxic effects at the proximal tubule (e.g. enzymuria and increase in tubular antigens) and functional changes (e.g. proteinuria, increase in serum β2-microglobulin) [41, 42].

Because methyl mercury freely distributes throughout the body, monitoring of mercury in the *blood* is usually carried out to identify exposure to methyl mercury. The concentration of total mercury in blood among people who are not occupationally exposed is influenced by their consumption of fish. Heavy consumers of lake fish have higher blood mercury levels than those who eat fish only rarely. People who never eat fish have blood levels of around 2 μg Hg/L, while the mercury concentrations of those who eat fish three times a week may reach close to 10 μg Hg/L.

During long-term constant exposure (several months) to methyl mercury in food, there is a linear relationship between daily intake of methyl mercury and the concentration of mercury in blood. The mercury concentration in blood (μg/L) corresponds to the daily intake of methyl mercury (μg/day) multiplied by 0.5–1. When exposure is continuous, the blood mercury concentration is proportional to the concentration in the brain, the critical organ for methyl mercury toxicity. Because of mercury's short half-life in the blood (2-4 days), evaluation of blood mercury is of limited clinical value if a substantial amount of time has passed since time of exposure [43].

Analyses of methyl mercury in scalp *hair* can be used to make a retrospective estimation of maternal exposure during pregnancy. It has been found that children born to mothers, whose hair mercury concentrations ranged between 70 and 640 μg Hg/g, show a considerably higher prevalence of developmental changes than controls. Scalp hair levels exceeding 6 μg/g are considered elevated and should be confirmed by a 24-hour urine collection.

Studies from New Zealand and the Faroe Island indicate that adverse effects in children can be correlated with maternal hair levels as low as 10–20 μg/g [44]. Mercury analyses conducted on a single human hair can be used to monitor daily variations in methyl mercury exposure among fish eaters [45, 46], and have been utilized to track maternal fish consumption and risk of preterm delivery [47]. Other investigators [48] have utilized measurements of total mercury in hair, toenails and urine to assess exposures in a group of non-occupationally exposed women in relation to renal tubular effects.

As identified in Table 1, the most common methods used to determine mercury levels in blood, urine, and hair of humans and animals include atomic absorp-

Table 1. Analytical methods for the detection of mercury in biological samples.

Method	Able to distinguish methyl mercury?	Detection limit (ppm)	Reference
NAA	No	0.1	Byrne and Kosta [49]; WHO [50]
AAS	No	2 ppb range	Hatch and Ott [51]
	No[a]		Magos and Clarkson [52]
GC-Electron Capture	Yes	0.1	Von Burg et al [53]; Cappon and Smith [54]
XRF	No	"Low ppm"	Marsh et al [55]

[a]*The Magos and Clarkson method estimates methyl mercury by subtracting the inorganic mercury content from the total mercury content. Adapted from U.S. EPA [15]*

tion spectrometry (AAS), neutron activation analysis (NAA), x-ray fluorescence (XRF), and gas chromatography (GC).

Roels et al. [42] points out that the analytical techniques identified in Table 1 are not easily available and are not well-suited for routine biomonitoring of occupational or environmental exposures. Instead, indirect biomarkers such as urinary enzymes are often used with success to evaluate mercury exposure and injury. Zalups [39] identifies numerous methods used to detect renal tubular injury induced by mercury. These methods monitor the urinary excretion of enzymes that leak from injured and necrotic proximal tubules, including lactate dehydrogenase (LDH), aspartate aminotransferase (AST), alanine aminotransferase (ALT), and N-acetyl-β-D-glucosaminidase (NAG). Although advocated by Zalups [39] to detect renal tubular injury, Mason et al [56] questions the practical utility of such biomarkers in occupational surveillance. According to Mason et al., small increases in NAG, leucine aminopeptidase (LAP), and other markers of renal tubular cell function are of unclear significance in the prediction of clinical renal disease among occupationally-exposed workers.

General human toxicity

In the assessment of patients with possible mercury exposure, the three key determinants of clinical toxicity are the form of mercury, the route of exposure, and the dose [57]. Diagnosis of mercury poisoning is usually made by obtaining a patient's complete history and performing a physical examination. In addition, laboratory tests may demonstrate increased mercury levels [58]. In 1998, there were 3, 861 documented cases of mercury-related poisonings in the United States [59]. Among these cases, 1 death was reported, while 6 and 52 cases of major and minor illnesses were reported, respectively. Toxic effects from mercury exposure can result from mercury inhalation, injection, ingestion, or dermal absorption. Because of the importance of the chemical form of mercury, toxicity is discussed separately for mercury vapor, inorganic, and organic mercury compounds. Adverse renal effects from all forms of mercury are presented in detail in the next section.

Mercury vapor

The inhalation of mercury vapor at concentrations exceeding 1 mg/m^3 produces a severe and sometimes fatal interstitial pneumonitis. At air concentrations between 100 to 1000 μg/m^3, a variety of signs and symptoms occur after mercury vapor exposure. Typically the mercury-poisoned subject displays severe intention tremor involving the fingers and hands, which make handwriting difficult. In the mouth, gums become tender and inflamed. Salivation is excessive and the salivary glands often are swollen. The third hallmark in mercury poisoning comprises personality changes and psychiatric symptoms that include: anxiety, erethism, irritability, excitability, fearfulness, shyness, memory loss, depression, fatigue, weakness, and drowsiness [6, 21, 60].

Recent occupational health studies have focused on detecting early effects from mercury on the central nervous system. A dose-response relationship between subjective symptoms and/or impaired performance on psychological tests has been reported [61-64]. It is now conceded that an increased prevalence of neurotic symptoms may occur following long-term exposure to mercury vapor at concentrations exceeding 25 μg/m^3 [21]. An air concentration of 25 μg/m^3 roughly corresponds to a urinary excretion of 50 μg Hg/L.

Small children who are accidentally exposed to high concentrations of mercury vapor may develop acrodynia, or Pink disease. This is a syndrome characterized by a body rash, swelling and irritation of palms and feet followed by skin desquamation, irritability, photophobia, fever, insomnia, and perfusesweating [60, 65]. Curtis et al. [66] describes a typical case. A healthy 18-month old boy moved with his family to a different house. After one month, he became irritable and anorexic. He developed a cough and dribbled saliva. His hands and feet were swollen. On examination his hands and feet were bright pink with peeling skin. He could not sit up because of profound proximal muscle weakness. Pink disease was suspected and confirmed by measuring mercury in urine and detecting a concentration of 70 μg Hg/L. Subsequent analysis of mercury at the boy's home revealed high air levels, in particular near the floor level (up to 300 μg/m^3). Lifting the carpet displayed droplets of mercury underneath. The former occupant of the house had used metallic mercury when building silver telescopic mirrors.

Although it has been suspected and claimed by some there are no hard scientific evidence that mercury released from amalgam fillings may cause significant health effects. In a thorough examination of more than 400 individuals with suspected adverse health effects from release of mercury from amalgam fillings not a single case of toxicity from mercury could be confirmed [67]. Likewise extensive recent reviews from the US uncovered no evidence for any adverse health effects of mecury released from dental amalgam, besides local hypersensitivity in some individuals [68, 69].

Inorganic mercury compounds

Mercuric mercury compounds are inorganic salts with mercuric ions (Hg^{2+}), e.g. mercuric chloride and mercuric iodide. *Mercurous* mercury compounds are salts with Hg^{2+} ions having an apparent valence of +1, e.g. calomel (mercurous chloride, Hg_2Cl_2).

Previously, inorganic mercury compounds were used as medicines. For example, calomel was used as a teething powder in small children, and in the treatment of severe congestive heart failure, but today its use is rare. Accidental and suicidal intoxications have occurred. Generally, the ingestion of inorganic mercury compounds is associated with acute toxicity characterized by erosive damage in the gastrointestinal tract, accompanied by severe abdominal pain, gastrointestinal bleeding, and in severe cases circulatory collapse. Also, kidney lesions with tubular necrosis and oliguria may develop following ingestion of high doses of soluble inorganic mercury [21, 60].

Acrodynia, or Pink disease, discussed above, was common among infants in the UK and USA until the late 1940s when it became evident that the condition was caused by exposure to calomel in teething powders and in antihelmintic preparations. An allergic reaction towards mercury with variable susceptibility is considered to be involved in the pathogenesis of Pink disease because the syndrome develops in only a small proportion of all exposed (less than 1%) [65]. Furthermore, only infants and small children are affected.

Organic mercury compounds

For organic mercury compounds, the mercury is covalently bound to carbon in compounds of the R-Hg^+ and R-Hg-R type where R represents the organic moiety. With regard to human exposure and health effects, methyl mercury is most important. Consumption of methyl mercury-contaminated seafood and grain products (e.g., bread) has been associated with severe epidemics of poisonings in both Japan and Iraq, respectively [14, 60]. Such epidemics were caused by industrial discharge of methyl mercury in Minimata Bay, Japan, and the accidental ingestion of bread baked from methyl mercury-treated grain in Iraq. As is the case with mercury vapor, the central nervous system is affected, albeit the symptoms slightly different. Symptoms of poisoning include paraesthesia, notably around the mouth, malaise, constriction of the visual field, deafness, and ataxia. The fetus is particularly vulnerable to methyl mercury, and may succumb to the neurotoxic effects of methyl mercury even if the pregnant mother shows no signs of toxicity [44].

Although there is experimental evidence of nephrotoxicity from methyl mercury in animals, no reports of human renal toxicity from methyl mercury exposure have been identified [14].

Certain organic mercury compounds, such as phenyl mercury and methoxyalkyl mercury, are metabolized relatively fast in the human body and are excreted in urine. In contrast to methyl mercury, these compounds do not accumulate in the body nor do they cause toxicity in the central nervous system. On the other hand they affect renal function, and mercury-containing diuretics have been used in the management of congestive cardiac failure. Membranous glomerulonephritis with nephrotic syndrome and severe tubular damage complicating the nephrotic syndrome have been reported as side effects during the treatment of heart failure with organic mercurials [70, 71].

Immunotoxicity

Over the past decade there has, as result of experimental studies, been a growing appreciation that mercury may exert an effect on the immune system. As summarized by Silbergeld and Devine [72], mercury has at least two types of effects on the immune system. First, mercury induces autoimmunity to renal basement membrane proteins, causing mercury-induced glomerulonephritis in certain strains of mice and rats. Secondly, mercury exposure impairs cell-mediated and humoral immunity by affecting Th1 and Th2 responses, which in turn impairs the body's ability to effectively respond to antigens or pathogens.

However, most studies on humans occupationally exposed to mercury identify no effects on immunological markers such as serum immunoglobulins and autoantibodies [73, 74], albeit Ellingsen et al. [75] noted subtle elevations in plasma antibodies against myeloid peroxidase (anti-MPO) and proteinase 3 (anti-PR3).

Adverse renal effects

Bioaccumulation of mercuric ions occurs preferentially in the kidney after exposure to inorganic or elemental mercury. At sufficiently high concentrations, profound nephrotoxicity can occur after exposure to inorganic or elemental mercury. Organic mercurials, such as methyl mercury are much less nephrotoxic, although they do have the potential to cause adverse effects, secondary to other effects such as neurotoxicity. As illustrated in Figure 3, the pars recta of the proximal tubule (the S3 segment) is most vulnerable to the toxic effects of mercury, particularly at the junction of the cortex and the outer medulla [39]. This can be explained in part because tubular transport of heavy metals (and subsequent accumulation) is localized primarily in the proximal tubule. The S3 segment of the proximal tubule comprises proteins that contain sulfhydryl groups, which bind readily to heavy metals such as mercury. It is hypothesized that interaction between protein sulfhydryl groups and mercury may result in cellular dysfunction and death.

Experimental studies

Mercury vapor (Hg°)

Prolonged exposure to Hg° is known to result in renal damage characterized by proteinuria and edema. This effect involves both tubular and immunological mechanisms [77].

Ionized inorganic mercury (Hg^{1+}, Hg^{2+})

For many years, acute administration of either Hg^{1+} or Hg^{2+} has been known to produce necrosis of the third segment of the proximal tubule [78-84]. The mechanisms that lead to these effects appear to involve alterations in intracellular calcium concentrations secondary to membrane damage. The mechanisms of Hg^{2+} toxicity to renal tubule cells has been studied at the molecular level. Tarabova et al [85] reported that Hg^{2+}

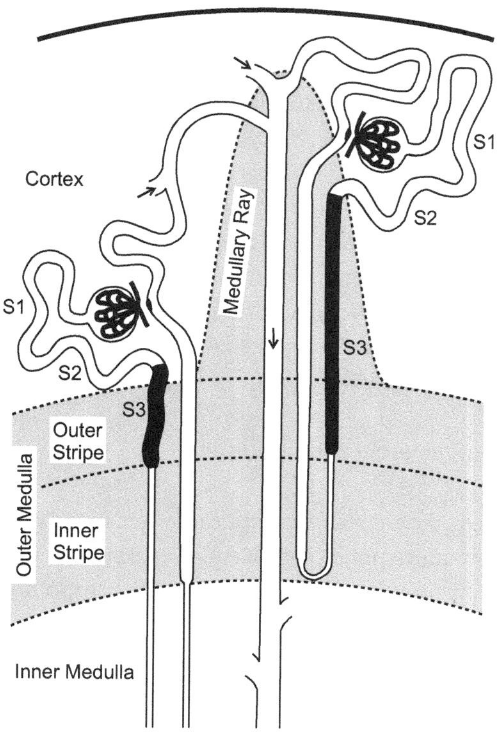

***Figure 3.** Illustration of the kidney. (reproduced from De Broe [76], with permission)*

and methyl mercury both altered the Cav3.1 calcium channel in human embryonic kidney 293 cells without decreasing cell viability. Wang et al [86] reported a number of metabolic alterations, as measured by high resolution NMR, in kidneys of rats injected with $HgCl_2$ and sacrificed 48 hours post treatment. Brandao et al [87] reported inhibition of renal ALA-dehydratase and increased concentrations of metllothionein and non-protein thiol groups in mice injected with $HgCl_2$ for 3 consecutive days. They examined the potential therapeutic effects of a number of anti-oxidants and reported that only DMPS was effective in preventing inhibition of ALA-dehydratase. Brkljacic et al [88] studied alterations in chaperoning of the glucocorticoid receptor by Hsp90 and the constitutive and inducible forms of Hsp 70 in rats treated with $Hg2^{+}$ at 3 different dose levels. They found that mercury treatment increased the association of the GR complex with both Hsp groups. Hsp90 concentrations were increased in the cytosol while the Hsp 70s were unaltered. In addition, exposure to Hg^{2+} also produces immunological effects in rodents [89-95, 96] with glomerular lesions since proteinuria is composed mainly of albumin. The inducibility of such immune lesions appears to be highly strain dependent.

Organomercurials

A number of animal studies confirm that high concentrations of mercury accumulate in the kidneys following acute [81] or chronic exposure to methyl mercury [36, 38, 98] and produce renal tubular toxicity. Similar results have been reported using aryl mercury [99]. At present, it is unclear whether these effects are the result of the inorganic mercury yielded by demethylation of methyl mercury in the kidney or the combined action of both organic and inorganic mercurials in renal proximal tubule cells. There are data suggesting that pretreatment with agents that stimulate microsomal drug metabolizing enzyme systems reduce the nephrotoxicity of methyl mercury by increasing urinary excretion of Hg^{2+} [34, 36]. There is also evidence of marked differences in gender sensitivity between male and female animals to methyl mercury nephrotoxicity [36, 37]. Alterations in renal heme biosynthesis following prolonged exposure to methyl mercury cause a relatively specific porphyrinuria pattern [89, 100].

Kidney toxicity – the human experience

Mercury gives rise to different types of renal effects in humans, including acute kidney injury, and tubular and glomerular damage with a nephrotic syndrome. In 1818, Blackall documented that mercury caused proteinuria in humans (cited in [71]). A nephrotic syndrome characterized by edema, marked proteinuria and a pronounced decrease in plasma albumin, may develop from mercury exposure and result in a combination of either predominantly tubular or glomerular lesions. The tubular lesions appear early and are dose-related, whereas the glomerular ones may have an immunologic basis. The risk for glomerular damage giving rise to a nephrotic syndrome increases with dose.

Ingestion of large doses of soluble mercuric salts causes acute kidney injury with *tubular necrosis* and possibly coexisting renal vasospasm [60]. In the 1950's, when acute treatment with dialysis was not available, the lethal dose of mercuric bichloride, was estimated to range from 2 to 3.5 g [101]. Long-term ingestion of a laxative containing mercurous chloride by two demented patients resulted in renal impairment with elevated serum urea and creatinine [102]. Microscopic examination of renal biopsy tissue revealed *chronic tubular lesions*. Analysis of mercury in tissues confirmed the diagnosis of mercury poisoning with high concentrations of mercury in the kidney. One of the patients also had moderate proteinuria.

In addition to tubular lesions, a classic *nephrotic syndrome* may develop following mercury exposure [70, 103-105]. Preddy and Russel [106], describe a 54-year old woman who developed severe tubular damage with excessive urinary losses of sodium and a nephrotic syndrome, but with trivial morphological glomerular damage (i.e., minimal change nephropathy) after 68 weeks of treatment with an intravenous mercurial diuretic. Six similar cases of nephrotic syndrome and tubular damage following mercurial diuretics are presented by Burston et al. [104] and Riddle et al. [70]. Williams and Bridge [107] present a 52-year old man with nephrotic syndrome after prolonged use of a mercury containing ointment in the treatment of psoriasis. Diagnosis was confirmed by a urinary mercury excretion of 240 µg Hg/24h. After treatment with a chelating agent, dimercaprol, and withdrawal of the mercury skin ointment, the nephrotic syndrome resolved. Five cases of mercury-induced nephrosis in infants were reported by Wilson et al. [108]. The children had been given mercury containing teething powders or drugs for at least three months, with cumulative mercury doses in the order of several grams. Urinary excretion of mercury was excessive in all cases, in the order of 1000 µg/L. Four of the infants recovered completely, three of them after treatment with dimercaprol.

Nephrotic syndrome with specific histopathological signs of a primarily glomerular damage has also been seen after mercury exposure. Becker et al. [105] report on five cases of biopsy proven membranous glomerulonephritis after exposure to ammoniated mercury ointments (3 cases), mercury paint additive (1 case), and mercury diuretics (1 case). The tubular lesions were not prominent and the authors suggested that mercury induced an autoimmune response that in turn caused the glomerular lesions. Cameron and Trounce [71] present a 64-year old man with heart failure who developed a full blown nephrotic syndrome with urinary excretion of up to 44 g protein daily after receiving injections of organic mercury (chlormerodrin Mersalyl®). The glomerular filtration rate, estimated by creatinine clearance, was 40 ml/min. Postmortem examination of renal tissue revealed a typical membranous glomerulonephritis with no signs of tubular damage. From Nairobi, nephrotic syndrome has been reported in young females who used mercury containing *skin lightning creams*. Most of those affected had minimal changes in the kidney (50%) at renal biopsy examination. Urinary excretion of mercury was excessive in most of the nephrotic patients, and it was suspected that the mercury containing cream was involved in the pathogenesis of the nephrotic syndrome [110]. Another case of nephrotic syndrome possibly attributable to the use of a skin lightning cream was reported by Olivera et al. [111]. A 46-year old female developed a membranous glomerulonephritis after using a cream containing 1% mercury. The urinary excretion of mercury was markedly elevated. Although no kidney toxicity was reported, Weldon et al. [112] reported elevated urine mercury concentrations among a predominantly female, Hispanic population living in the Southwestern portion of the United States who used a Mexican mercury chloride-containing creme called "Crema de Belleza-Manning." Median urinary mercury levels were 79 μg/L, with individual values as large as 1,170 μg/L, providing clear evidence that systemic absorption mercury can occur via topical application of a cosmetic containing mercury. From Hong Kong two cases of nephrotic syndrome from minimal change glomerulonephritis was reported after use of a skin lightning cream containing 3% mercury [113]. Initially blood and urine concentrations of mercury were in the order of 30-60 μg/L, but decreased to normal levels after cessation of usage the cream and treatment with D-penicillamine.

Pink disease in children may be accompanied by a nephrotic syndrome [114]. Two sisters developed severe proteinuria four days apart a few weeks after that their parents had spilled metallic mercury in the bedroom. The younger girl had typical red-colored palms.

Albuminuria and nephrosis may also follow *occupational exposure*. Friberg et al. [115] found two such cases in a group of 50 workers exposed to metallic mercury. Both men recovered after the exposure was eliminated. Likewise, Kazantzis et al. [116] describe four cases from two factories where 72 men were exposed to mercury compounds. The urinary excretion of mercury was excessive in most of the workers, ranging from not detectable to more than 1000 μg Hg/L. Recovery from the nephrotic syndrome was complete after removal from exposure. Two cases of membranous nephropathy and a nephrotic syndrome were recently reported from a fluorescent-tube recycling industry in Germany [117]. Heavy occupational exposure to mercury was evident from markedly elevated urinary excretion of mercury; 118 and 158 μg Hg/L respectively. After withdrawal from exposure and treatment with 2,3 dimercaptopropane-1 sulphonate (DMPS) urinary excretion of mercury and protein in one patient was almost normalized after two years whereas the second patient was also treated but lost for follow.

There are also data showing more subtle effects of mercury on the kidneys after occupational exposure.

Roels et al. [63] and Buchet et al. [118] observed a slightly higher prevalence of elevated urinary excretion of albumin, transferrin, retinol binding protein and the tubular enzyme β-galactosidase in chloralkali workers with a urinary excretion of mercury exceeding 50 μg/g creatinine.

Analysis of the tubular enzyme N-acetyl-β-D-glucosaminidase appears to be particularly effective in detecting early evidence of adverse renal effects from mercury [119, 120]. In an extensive cross sectional examination of chloralkali workers exposed to mercury at air concentrations around 25 μg/m^3, Langworth et al. [121] noted a significant correlation and dose-response relationship between urinary excretion of mercury and

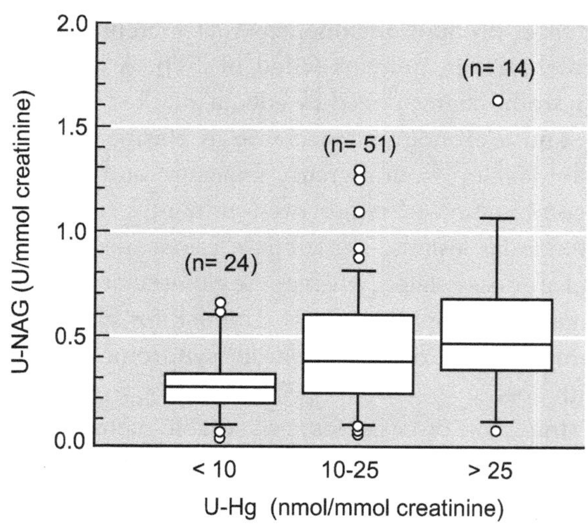

Figure 4. *Box-plots showing the relation between U-Hg and U-NAG in the exposed group (10th, 25th, 50th, 75th, 90th percentiles, and outliers indicated).*
(reproduced from Langworth [121], with permission)

N-acetyl-β-D-glucosaminidase (Figure 4). No significant correlation was evident for other renal parameters: U-albumin, U-orosomucoid, U-β2-microglobulin, U-copper, S-creatinine, and S-β2-microglobulin. Studies on chlor-alkali workers in Scandinavia [122-124] have reported minimal and apparently reversible renal effects from mercury exposures in this occupational group as evaluated by urinary excretion of NAG, albumin and titers of autoantibodies. These investigators noted that a small number of susceptible individuals may exist and that selenium status appears to have a major effect on urinary NAG excretion [124].

There are no reports of human nephrotoxicity caused by release of mercury from amalgam fillings. This is supported by experimental data from ten humans where standard measurements of renal function (glomerular filtrate rate, urinary albumin excretion, β2-microglobulin, N-acetyl-β-D-glucosaminidase) were monitored before and 60 days after the removal of mercury amalgam fillings [125]. Bellinger et al [126] conducted a proper randomized controlled clinical trial in 534 children aged 6 to 10 years to find out if mercury released from amalgam fillings could give rise to any neuropsychological or renal (glomerular) effects. The number of amalgam resorted surfaces over five years was 14.6 in the amalgam group (n=267) and none in the composite group (n=267). Urinary excretion of mercury was slightly higher in the amalgam group; 0.9 μg and 0.6 Hg/g creatinine in amalgam and composite respectively but there was no difference in the urinary albumin excretion, and likewise no difference in a battery of neuropsychological tests.

In an environmental epidemiological study from the UK [127] calculated airborne exposure to mercury and mortality in 'Nephritis, nephritic syndrome and nephrosis' have been significantly associated. However, as most individuals in the UK and other developed countries have access to Renal Replacement Therapy (RRT) nowadays and die from mostly other causes than nephritis and nephritic syndrome, the associations seen between modeled air levels of mercury and mortality in kidney disease should be regarded as 'suggestive' at the most.

Treatment

Treatments currently available for mercurial poisoning in humans involve the use of thiol-based chelating agents such as British Anti-Lewisite (BAL), penicillamine [60] and more recently, agents such as 2, 3 dimercaptopropane-1 sulphonate (DMPS) [128] or 2, 3 dimercaptosuccinic acid (DMSA). Chelation is the formation of a metal ion complex in which the metal ion is association with a charged or uncharged electron donor. Studies by Bluhm et al. [129] compared the efficacy of D-penicillamine with dimercaptosuccinic acid (DMSA), and demonstrated that DMSA was able to increase the excretion of mercury to a greater extent than D-penicillamine. Studies in humans demonstrate that chelation therapy successfully lowers body burden of mercury and increases urinary mercury levels [130, 131]. However, the impact of chelation on long-term outcome of parenteral mercury exposure remains uncharacterized [132]. Standard dose regimens for the above chelators are as follows: penicillamine given with paradoxen at doses of 500 mg P.O., every 6 hours for 5 days; DMPS given at total a dose of 250 mg I.M. or I.V./4 hours on day 1, 6 hours on day 2, and on 6 to 8 hours on day 3 for the remaining course; DMSA given at 10 mg/kg P.O. every 8 hours for 5 days [133]. DMPS given IV at a dose of 50 mg/day to a 22-year-old man who had injected about 8 g of elemental mercury dramatically increased the urinary excretion of mercury but was - due to the relative small amount of mercury chelated and excreted daily - unable to eliminate the total load of mercury efficiently and it was not until residual mercury droplets were surgically extirpated, after three years, that the blood levels of mercury went down and the remaining symptoms of mercury poisoning (mainly tremor) disappeared [134]. Although DMPS has been used in Europe for the past 25 years (under the names Unithiol and Dimaval), it is not widely used in the United States because it is not approved as a drug.

References

1. United States Food and Drug Administration. Mercury compounds in drugs and foods. Center for Biologics Evaluation and Research (CBER). 2001.
2. United States Geological Service (U.S.G.S.). U.S. Geological Survey, Mineral Commodity Summaries (Mercury). 2002.
3. United States Geological Service (U.S.G.S.). U.S. Geological Survey, Mineral Commodity Summaries (Mercury). 1999.
4. Chevalier, P. Mercury. Canadian Minerals Yearbook 1999. Natural Resources Canada. 2000.
5. Byrne L. Brazil's mercury poisoning disaster. Brit Med J 1992; 304: 1397.
6. Schutte NP, Knight AL, Jahn O. Mercury and its compounds. In: Dickerson OB, Horovath EP, Zenz C, editors. Occupational medicine, 3rd ed. St Louis: Mosby-Year Book Inc, 1994: 549-57.
7. National Research Council (NRC). Toxicological effects of methylmercury. 2000.
8. Sällsten G, Barregård L, Österberg T. Tandgnissling hos amalgambärare – en orsak till hög kvicksilverutsöndring ? (Tooth grinding among wearers of amalgam fillings – a cause of high mercury release ?). Läkartidningen (Sweden) 1991; 88: 232-3.
9. Geijersstam E, Sandborgh-Englund G, Jonsson F, Ekstrand J. Mercury uptake and kinetics after ingestion of dental amalgam. J Dent Res 2001; 80:1793-6.
10. International Agency for Research on Cancer (IARC). IARC monograph on Beryllium, Cadmium, Mercury, and Exposures in the Glass Manufacturing Industry. Volume 58. Lyon, France. 1994: 239-345.
11. United States Environmental Protection Agency (U.S. EPA). Mercury update: impact on fish advisories. 2001. Office of Water.
12. Grandjean P, Weihe P, White RF, Debes F, Araki S, Yokoyama K, Murata K, Sorensen N, Dahl R, Jorgensen PJ. Cognitive deficit in 7-year old children with prenatal exposure to methylmercury. Neurotoxicol. Teratol. 1997; 19: 417-28.
13. United States Food and Drug Administration (U.S. FDA). Methyl mercury levels in commercial seafood species. 2000. Center for Food Safety and Applied Nutrition. Office of Seafood.
14. World Health Organization. Methylmercury. Environmental Health Criteria 101. World Health Organization, Geneva 1990.
15. United States Environmental Protection Agency (U.S. EPA). Mercury study report to Congress. 1997. Office of Air Quality Planning and Standards and Office of Research and Development.
16. Campbell D, Gonzales M, Sullivan JB. 1992. Mercury. In, Sullivan, J.B. & Krieger, G.R., eds, Hazardous Materials Toxicology. 824-33. Clinical Principles of Environmental Health, Baltimore:Williams and Wilkins.
17. Elinder C-G, Friberg L, Nordberg GF, Kjellström T, Oberdoerster G. Biological monitoring of metals. Chemical safety monographs. International Programme on Chemical Safety. WHO/EHG/94.2 1994: 1-80.
18. Sällsten G, Barregård L, Järvholm B. Mercury in the Swedish chloralkali industri - an evaluation of the exposure and preventive measures over 40 years. Ann Occup Hyg 1990; 34: 205-14.
19. Gutiérrez F, Leon L. Elemental mercury embolism to the lung. New England Journal of Medicine 2000; 342(24): 1791.
20. Diner B, Brenner B. Toxicity, mercury. eMed J. 2001; 2:1-13. Available at: www.emedicine.com/EMERG/topic813.htm.
21. World Health Organization. Inorganic mercury. Environmental Health Criteria 118. World Health Organization, Geneva 1991.
22. Hursh JB, Clarkson TW, Cherian MG, Vostal J, Mallie RV. Clearance of mercury (Hg-197 and Hg-203) vapor inhaled by human subjects. Arch Env Health 1976; 31: 302-9.
23. Barregård L, Ställsten G, Schutz A, Attwell R, Skerfving S, Jarvholm B. Kinetics of mercury in blood and urine after brief occupational exposure. Arch Env Health 1992; 47: 176-84.
24. Morrow PE, Gibb FR, Johnson L. Clearance of insoluble dust from the lower respiratory tract. Health Phys 1964; 10: 543-55.
25. Clarkson TW. Human toxicity of mercury. The Journal of Trace Elements in Experimental Medicine 1998; 11: 303-17.
26. Rahola T, Hattula T, Korolainen A, Miettinen JK. Elimination of free and protein-bound ionic mercury in man. Ann Clin Res 1973; 5: 214-19.
27. Hall LL, Allen PV, Fisher HL, et al. 1994. The kinetics of intravenously-administered inorganic mercury in humans. In: Kinetic Models of Trace Elements and Mineral Metabolism During Development, K.M.S. Subramanian and M.E. Wastney, Ed. CRC Press, Boca Raton, FL. p. 1-21.
28. Carmichael NG, Fowler BA. Effects of separate and combined chronic mercuric chloride and sodium selenite administration in rats: histologic, ultrastructural and x-ray microanalytical studies of liver and kidney. J Env Pathol Toxicol 1979; 3: 399-412.
29. Aslamkhan AG, Han YH, Yang XP, et al.Human renal anion transporter 1 dependent uptake and toxicity of mercuric thiol conjugates in Madin-Darby canine kidney cells. Mol Pharmacol 2003; 63(3):590-6.
30. Lash LH, Hueni SE, Putt DA, et al. Role of organic anion and amino acid carriers in transport of inorganic mercury in rat renal basolateral membrane vesicles: influence of compensatory renal growth. Toxicol Sci 2005; 88(2):630-44.
31. Zalups RK, Ahmad S. Handling of cysteine S-conjugates of methylmercury in MDCK cells expressing human OAT1. Kidney Int 2005; 68(4):1684-99

32. Aberg B, Ekman L, Falk R, Greitz U, Persson G, Snihs J. Metabolism of methyl mercury (Hg) compounds in man: Excretion and distribution. Arch Environ. Health 1969; 19: 478-84.
33. Miettinen JK. 1973. Absorption and elimination of dietary (Hg^{++}) and methyl mercury in man. In: Mercury, Mercurial, and Mercaptans, M.W. Miller and T.W. Clarkson, Ed. Springfield, IL. p. 233-43.
34. Fowler BA, Lucier GW, Mushak P. Phenobarbital protection against methylmercury nephrotoxicity. Proc Soc Exp Biol Med 1975; 149: 75-9.
35. Vahter M, Mottet NK, Friberg L, Lind B, Shen DD, Burbacher T. Speciation of mercury in the primate blood and brain following long-term exposure to methyl mercury. Toxicol Appl Pharmacol 1994; 124(2): 221-29.
36. Fowler BA. The morphologic effects of dieldrin and methyl mercuric chloride on pars recta segments of rat kidney proximal tubules. Am J Pathol 1972; 69: 163-74.
37. Yasutake A, Hirayama K, Inouye M. Sex difference in acute renal dysfunction induced by methyl mercury in mice. Renal Failure 1990; 12: 233-40.
38. Fowler BA, Brown HW, Lucier GW, Krigman MR. The effect of chronic oral methylmercury exposure on the lysosome system of rat kidney. Morphometric and biochemical studies. Lab Invest 1975; 32: 313-22.
39. Zalups RK. Molecular interactions with mercury in the kidney. Pharmacological Reviews. 2000; 52(1):113-143.
40. Clarkson TW. Mercury. J. Am. Coll. Toxicol. 1989; 8(7): 1291-96.
41. Hu H. Exposure to metals. Occupational and Environmental Medicine 2000; 27(4):983-96.
42. Roels HA, Hoet P, Lison D. Usefulness of biomarkers of exposure to inorganic mercury, lead, or cadmium in controlling occupational and environmental risks of nephrotoxicity. Renal Failure 1999; 21(3 & 4): 251-62.
43. Satoh H. Occupational and environmental toxicology of mercury and its compounds. Industrial Health 2000; 38: 153-64.
44. Grandjean P, Weihe P, White RF, Debes F: Cognitive performance of children prenatally exposed to "safe" levels of methylmercury. Environ Res 1998; 77(2): 165-72.
45. Legrand M, Passos CJ, Mergler D, et al. Biomonitoring of mercury exposure with single human hair strand. Environ Sci Technol 2005; 39(12):4594-8.
46. Legrand M, Lam R, Passos CJ, et al. Analysis of mercury in sequential micrometer segments of single hair strands of fish-eaters 2007; 41(2):593-8.
47. Xue F, Holzman C, Rahbar MH, et al. Maternal fish consumption, mercury levels, and risk of preterm delivery. Environ Health Perspect 2007; 115(1):42-7.
48. Ohno T, Sakamoto M, Kurosawa T, et al. Total mercury levels in hair, toenail, and urine among women free from occupational exposure and their relations to renal tubular function. Environ Res 2007; 103(2):191-7.
49. Byrne AR, Kosta L. Simultaneous neutron-activation determination of selenium and mercury in biological samples by volatilization. Talanta. 1974; 21: 1083-90.
50. WHO (World Health Organization). 1976. Environmental Health Criteria: Mercury. World Health Organization, Geneva, Switzerland, 121.
51. Hatch WR, Ott WL. Determination of sub-microgram quantities of mercury by atomic absorption spectrophotometry. Anal Chem 1968; 40(14): 2085-87.
52. Magos L, Clarkson TW. Atomic absorption and determination of total, inorganic, and organic mercury in blood. J AOAC 1972; 55(5): 966-71.
53. Von Burg R, Rustam H. Electrophysiological investigations of methyl mercury intoxication in humans: Evaluation of peripheral nerve by conduction velocity and electromyography. Electroenceph Clin Neurophysiol 1974; 37: 381-92.
54. Cappon CJ, Smith JC. A simple and rapid procedure for the gas-chromatographic determination of methylmercury in biological samples. Bull Environ Contam. Toxicol 1978; 19(5): 600-7.
55. Marsh, DO, Clarkson TW, Cox C, Amin-Zaki L, Al-Tikriti S. Fetal methyl mercury poisoning: Relationship between concentration in single strands of maternal hair and child effects. Arch Neurol 1987; 44: 1017-22.
56. Mason HJ, Hindell P, Williams NR. Biological monitoring and exposure to mercury. Occup Med 2001; 51(1): 2-11.
57. Kulig, K. A tragic reminder about organic mercury. The New England Journal of Medicine. 1998; 338(23): 1692-94.
58. Goldman L, Shannon MW, The Committee on Environmental Health. Technical Report: Mercury in the Environment: Implications for Pediatricians. Pediatrics 2001; 108(1): 197-205.
59. Litovitz TL, Klein-Schwartz W, White S, Cobaugh DJ, Youniss J, Drab A., Benson BE. The 1999 annual report of the American Association of Poison Control Centers Toxic Exposure Surveillance Systems. The American Journal of Emergency Medicine 1999; 18(5): 517-74.
60. Berlin M. Mercury. In: Friberg L, Nordberg GF, Vouk VB, editors. Handbook on the toxicology of metals, Vol II. Amsterdam: Elsevier, 1986: 387-445.

61. Smith RG, Vorwald AJ, Patil LS, Mooney TF. Effects of exposure to mercury in the manufacture of chlorine. Am Ind Hyg Ass J 1970; 31: 687-700.
62. Smith PJ, Langolf GD, Goldberg J. Effects of occupational exposure to elemental mercury on short term memory. Brit J Ind Med 1983; 40: 413-9.
63. Roels H, Gennart JP, Lauwerys R, Buchet JP, Malchaire J, Bernard A. Surveillance of workers exposed to mercury vapour: validation of a previously proposed biological threshold limit value for mercury concentration in urine. Am J Ind Med 1985; 7: 45-71.
64. Langworth S, Almkvist O, Söderman E, Wikström BO. Effects of occupational exposure to mercury vapour on the central nervous system. Brit J Ind Med 1992; 49: 545-55.
65. Clarkson TW. Mercury - an element of mystery. New Eng J Med 1990; 323: 1137-9.
66. Curtis HA, Ferguson SD, Kell RL, Samuel AH. Mercury as a health hazard. Arch Dis Childhood 1987; 62: 293-5.
67. Langworth S, Bjorkman L, Elinder CG, Jarup L, Savlin P. Multidisciplinary examination of patients with illness attributed to dental fillings. J Oral Rehabil 2002; 29:705-13.
68. Brownawell AM, Berent S, et al. "The potential adverse health effects of dental amalgam." Toxicol Rev 2005; 24: 1-10.
69. Bates MN. "Mercury amalgam dental fillings: an epidemiologic assessment." Int J Hyg Environ Health 2006; 209: 309-16
70. Riddle M, Gardner F, Beswick I, Filshie I. The nephrotic syndrome complicating mercurial diuretic therapy. Brit Med J 1958; 1: 1274-7.
71. Cameron JS, Trounce R. Membranous glomerulonephritis and the nephrotic syndrome appearing during mersalyl therapy. Guy's Hosp Report 1965; 114: 101-7.
72. Silbergeld E, Devine PJ. Mercury- are we studying the right endpoints and mechanisms. Fuel Processing Technology 2000; 65-66: 35-42.
73. Langworth S, Elinder CG, Sundqvist KG: Minor effects of low exposure to inorganic mercury on the human immune system. Scand J Work Environ Health 1993; 19(6): 405-13.
74. Langworth S, Elinder CG, Sundquist KG, Vesterberg O: Renal and immunological effects of occupational exposure to inorganic mercury. Br J Ind Med 1992; 49(6): 394-401.
75. Ellingsen DG, Efskind J, Berg KJ, Gaarder PI, Thomassen Y. Renal and immunologic markers for chloralkali workers with low exposure to mercury vapor. Scand J Work Environ Health 2000; 26(5): 427-35.
76. De Broe M. Renal toxicity from environmental toxins, drugs, and contrast agents. In: Essential Atlas of Nephrology. Lippincott, Williams & Wilkins, 2001.
77. Hua J, Pelletier L, Berlin M, Druet P. Autoimmune glomerulonephritis induced by mercury vapour exposure in the Brown Norway rat. Toxicology 1993; 79: 119-29.
78. Gritzka TL, Trump BF. Renal tubular lesions caused by mercuric chloride: electron microscopic observations. Am J Pathol 1968; 52: 1225-78.
79. Ganote CE, Reimer KA, Jennings RB. Acute mercuric chloride nephrotoxicity: an electron microscopic and metabolic study. Lab Invest 1975; 31: 633-47.
80. Kempson SA, Ellis BG, Price RG. Changes in rat renal cortex, isolated plasma membranes, and urinary enzymes following the injection of mercuric chloride. Chem Biol Interact 1977; 18: 217-34.
81. Trump BF, Berezesky IK, Sato T, Laiho KU, Phelps PC, DeClaris N. Cell calcium, cell injury and cell death. Environ Health Perspect 1984; 54: 281-7.
82. Trump BF, Berezesky IK, Smith MW, Phelps PC, Eliget KA. The relationship between cellular ion deregulation and acute and chronic toxicity. Toxicol Appl Pharmacol 1989; 97: 6-22.
83. Smith MW, Ambudkar IS, Phelps PC, Regec AL, Trump BF. $HgCl_2$-induced changes in cytosolic Ca^{2+} of cultured rabbit renal tubular cells. Biochim Biophys Acta 1987; 931: 130-42.
84. Nielsen JB, Andersen HR, Andersen O, Starklint H. Mercuric chloride-induced kidney damage in mice: time course and effect of dose. J Toxicol Environ Health 1991; 34: 469-83.
85. Tarabova B, Kurejova M, Sulova Z, et al. Inorganic mercury and methylmercury inhibit the Cav3.1 channel expressed in human embryonic kidney 293 cells by different mechanisms. J Pharmacol Exp Ther 2006; 317(1):418-27.
86. Wang Y, Bollard ME, Nicholson JK, et al. Exploration of the direct metabolic effects of mercury II chloride on the kidney of Sprague-Dawley rats using high-resolution magic angle spinning 1H NMR spectroscopy of intact tissue and pattern recognition. J Pharm Biomed Anal 2006; 40(2):375-81.
87. Brandao R, Santos FW, Farina M, et al. Antioxidants and metallothionein levels in mercury-treated mice. Cell Biol Toxicol 2006; 22(6):429-38.
88. Brkljacic J, Perisic T, Dundjerski J, et al. Interaction of rat renal glucocorticoid receptor with Hsp90 and Hsp70 upon stress provoked by mercury 2007; 27(1):43-50.
89. Woods JS, Fowler BA. Renal porphyrinuria during chronic methyl mercury exposure. J Lab Clin Med 1977; 90: 266-72.

90. Hultman P, Bell LJ, Eneström S, Pollard KM. Murine susceptibility to mercury. I. Autoantibody profiles and systemic immune deposits in inbred, congenic, and intra-H-2 recombinant strains. Clin Immunol Immunopathol 1992; 65: 98-109.
91. Hultman P, Eneström S. Mercury induced antinuclear antibodies in mice: characterization and correlation with renal immune complex deposits. Clin Exp Immunol 1988; 71: 269-74.
92. Hultman P, Eneström S. Mercury induced b-cell activation and antinuclear antibodies in mice. J Clin Lab Immunol 1989; 28: 143-50.
93. Bernard AM, Collette C, Lauwerys R. Renal effects of in utero exposure to mercuric chloride in rats. Arch Toxicol 1992; 66: 508-13.
94. Bellon B, Capron M, Druet E, Verroust M-CV, Sapin C, Girard JF, Foidart JM, Mathieu P, Druet P. Mercuric chloride induced autoimmune disease in Brown-Norway rats: sequential search for anti-basement membrane antibodies and circulating immune complexes. Eur J Clin Invest 1982; 12: 127-33.
95. Esnault VLM, Mathieson PW, Thiru S, Olveira DBG, Lockwood M. Autoantibodies to myeloperoxidase in Brown Norway rats treated with mercuric chloride. Lab Invest 1992; 67: 114-20.
96. Havarinasab, S, Bjorn, E, Ekstrand, J, et al. Dose and Hg species determine the T-helper cell activation in murine autoimmunity. Toxicology 2007; 229(1-2):23-32.
97. Klein R, Herman SP, Bullock BC, Talley FA. Early functional and pathological changes in rat kidney during methyl mercury intoxication. Arch Pathol 1976; 96: 83-90.
98. Fowler BA. Ultrastructural evidence for nephropathy induced by long-term exposure to small amounts of methylmercury. Science 1972; 175: 780-1.
99. Gage JC. The toxicity of alkyl- and arylmercury salts. Biochem Pharmacol 1961; 8: 77.
100. dos Santos AP, Mateus ML, Carvalho CM, et al. Biomarkers of exposure and effect as indicators of the interference of selenomethionine on methylmercury toxicity. Toxicol Lett 2007; 169(2):121-8.
101. Troen P, Seymour A, Kaufman SA, Katz KH. Mercuric bichloride poisoning. N Engl J Med 1951; 244: 459-63.
102. Wands JR, Weiss SW, Yardley JH, Maddrey WC. Chronic inorganic mercury poisoning due to laxative abuse. Am J Med 1987; 57: 92-101.
103. Munck O, Nissen NI. Development of nephrotic syndrome during treatment with mercurial diuretics. Acta Med Scand 1956; 153: 397-413.
104. Burston J, Darmady EM, Stranack F. Nephrosis due to mercurial diuretics. Brit Med J 1958; 1: 1277-8.
105. Becker CG, Becker EL, Maher JF, Schreiner GE. Nephrotic syndrome after contact with mercury. Arch Intern Med 1962; 83: 178-86.
106. Preedy LRK, Russel DS. Acute salt depletion associated with the nephrotic syndrome. Development during the treatment with a mercurial diuretic. Lancet 1953; 2: 1181-4.
107. Williams NE, Bridge HG. Nephrotic syndrome after the application of mercury ointment. Lancet 1958; 2: 602.
108. Wilson VK, Thomson ML, Holzel A. Mercury nephrosis in young children. Brit Med J 1952; 1: 358-60.
109. Langworth S, Bjorkman L, Elinder CG, Jarup L, Savlin P. Multidisciplinary examination of patients with illness attributed to dental fillings. J Oral Rehabil 2002; 29:705-13.
110. Barr RD, Rees PH, Cordy PE, Kungu A, Woodger BA, Cameron HM. Nephrotic syndrome in adult African in Nairobi. Brit Med J 1972; 2:131-4.
111. Oliviera DBG, Foster G, Savill J, Syme PD, Taylor A. Membranous nephropathy caused by mercury-containing skin lightning cream. Postgr Med J 1987; 63: 303-4.
112. Weldon MM, Smolinski MS, Maroufi A, Hasty BW, Gilliss DL, Boulanger LL, Balluz LS, Dutton RJ. Mercury poisoning associated with a Mexican beauty cream. West J Med 2000; 173:15-18.
113. Tang HL, Chu KH, et al. "Minimal change disease following exposure to mercury-containing skin lightening cream." Hong Kong Med J 2006; 12(4): 316-8.
114. Agner E, Jans H. Mercury poisoning and nephrotic syndrome in two siblings. Lancet 1978; 2: 951.
115. Friberg L, Hammarström S, Nyström A. Kidney injury after chronic exposure to inorganic mercury. Arch Ind Hyg Occup Med 1953; 8: 149-53.
116. Kazantzis G, Schiller KFR, Asscher AW, Drew RG. Albuminuria and the nephrotic syndrome following exposure to mercury and its compounds. Quart J Med 1962; 31: 403-19.
117. Aymaz S, Gross O, et al. "Membranous nephropathy from exposure to mercury in the fluorescent-tube-recycling industry." Nephrol Dial Transplant 2001; 16(11): 2253-5.
118. Buchet JP, Roels H, Bernard A, Lauwerys R. Assessment of renal function of workers exposed to inorganic lead, cadmium or mercury vapor. J Occup Med 1980; 22: 741-50.

119. Stonard MD, Chater BV, Duffield DP, Nevitt AL, O'Sullivan JJ, Steel GT. An evaluation of renal function in workers occupationally exposed to mercury vapor. Int Arch Environ Health 1983; 52: 177-89.
120. Langworth S, Elinder CG, Sundquist KG, Vesterberg O. Renal and immunological effects of occupational exposure to inorganic mercury. Br J Ind Med 1992; 49: 394-401.
121. Langworth S. Early effects of occupational and environmental exposure to inorganic mercury (dissertation). Karolinska Institute Stockholm, Sweden 1992.
122. Ellingsen DG, Barregard L, Gaarder PI, et al. Assessment of renal dysfunction in workers previously exposed to mercury vapour at a chloralkali plant. Br J Ind Med 1993; 50(10):881-7.
123. Barregard L, Enestrom S, Ljunghuse O, et al. A study of autoantibodies and circulating immune complexes in mercury-exposed chloralkali workers. Int Arch Occup Environ Health 1997; 70(2):101-6.
124. Efskind J, Ellingsen DG, Hartman A, et al. Renal function of chloralkali workers after the cessation of exposure to mercury vapor. Scan J Work Environ Health 2006; 32(3):241-9.
125. Sandborgh-Englund G, Nygren, AT, Ekstrand J, Elinder CG. 1996. No evidence of renal toxicity from amalgam fillings. Am J Physiol 271(4 Pt 2):R941-945.
126. Bellinger DC, Trachtenberg F, et al. "Neuropsychological and renal effects of dental amalgam in children: a randomized clinical trial." JAMA 2006; 295(15): 1775-83.
127. Hodgson S, Nieuwenhuijsen MJ, et al. "Kidney disease mortality and environmental exposure to mercury." Am J Epidemiol 2007; 165(1): 72-7.
128. Sällsten G, Barregård L, Schutz A. Clearance half-life of mercury in urine after the cessation of long term occupational exposure: influence of a chelating agent (DMPS) on excretion of mercury in urine. Brit J Occupational Environ Med 1994; 51: 337-42.
129. Bluhm RE, Bobbit RG, Welch LW, Wood AJ. Elemental mercury vapour toxicity, treatment and prognosis after acute, intensive exposure in chloralkali plant workers. Part I: History, neuropsychological findings and chelator effects. Human Exp Toxicol 1992; 11: 201-10.
130. Gonzalez-Ramirez D, Zuniga-Charles M, Narro-Juarez A, Molina-Recio Y, Hurlbut KM, Dart RC, Aposhian HV. DMPS (2, 3-dimercaptopropane-1-sulfonate, dimaval) decreases the body burden of mercury in humans exposed to mercurous chloride. J Pharmacol Exp Ther 1998; 287(1):8-12.
131. Garza-Ocanas L, Torres-Alanis O, Pineyro-Lopez A. Urinary mercury in twelve cases of cutaneous mercurous chloride (calomel) exposure: effect of sodium 2, 3-dimercaptopropane-1-sulfonate (DMPS) therapy. J Toxicol Clin Toxicol 1997; 35(6): 653-5.
132. McFee RB, Caraccio TR. Intravenous mercury injection and ingestion: clinical manifestations and management. J Toxicol Clin Toxicol 2001; 39(7): 733-8.
133. McFee RB. and Caraccio TR. "Intravenous mercury injection and ingestion: clinical manifestations and management." J Toxicol Clin Toxicol 2001; 39(7): 733-8.
134. Winker R., Schaffer AW, et al. „Health consequences of an intravenous injection of metallic mercury." Int Arch Occup Environ Health 2002; 75(8): 581-6.

37

Organic solvents, silicon-containing compounds and pesticides

Patrick C. D'HAESE[1], Monique M. ELSEVIERS[1], Muhammed YAQOOB[2] and Marc E. DE BROE[1]

[1]University of Antwerp, Belgium
[2]The Royal London Hospital, London, UK

Summary

Environmental/industrial exposure to heavy metals, light hydrocarbons, pesticides and silicon-containing compounds all have been associated with the development and/or progression of renal failure. Exposure to heavy metals, more particularly lead, cadmium and mercury has been linked with the development of acute or chronic renal failure. The current literature also contains a growing body of information linking solvent exposure with renal injury. To what extent exposure to environmental/occupational contaminants such as pesticides play either a causal or contributive role in the development of chronic renal failure is less clear. Reported observations suggest either a primary or secondary role of silicon-containing compounds in the development of anti-neutrophil cytoplasmic antibody-positive rapidly progressive glomerulonephritis and Wegener's granulomatosis. Such observations deserve further confirmation as do studies suggesting a particular sensitivity of the diabetic kidney for the damaging effects of certain occupational exposures.

Introduction

Despite the overwhelming amount of information dealing with the nephrotoxic effects of particular environmental/occupational exposures that have appeared in the literature, to date no data have been reported on the incidence of renal diseases resulting from exposure to particular toxins and chemicals. In view of this it is worth noting that recent data (year 2006) from the Belgian Society of Nephrology indicate that the cause of the disease is not known in up to 11% of cases of end-stage renal disease. This allows us to suggest that the impact of exposure to environmental and occupational toxins on the development of renal disease probably is more important than generally assumed. Hence, better information as to the impact of such exposure is of paramount importance because it can lead to both primary and secondary prevention, a rather exceptional privilege in nephrology. With the exception of lead [1], the failure to demonstrate an etiological role for other potential "environmental/occupational nephrotoxins" in the development or progression of renal disease is due, in fact, to the lack of well elaborated clinical or epidemiological studies.

In the search for a role for such exposure, the following questions need to be answered: (i) does occupational/environmental exposure to a potential nephrotoxic substance play a direct etiological role in the induction of a particular renal disease, (ii) does the exposure correlate with an increased risk for the progression of renal damage already present in patients with glomerulonephritis, diabetic nephropathy, hypertensive renal disease etc. (iii) do both possibilities have to be considered concomitantly or separately?

Some interesting observations have been published recently. While some authors confirm the role of previously identified risk factors others have, based on some experimental evidence, put forward an additional number of potential occupational/environmental nephrotoxins. Also a contributive role for specific occupational exposures, such as organic solvents, on the progression of diabetic nephropathy been suggested. Finally, studies reporting a striking association between exposure to silicon containing compounds and the occurrence of Wegener's granulomatosis may contribute to a better insight in the pathogenesis of that disease.

Organic solvents

Hydrocarbons: *what's in a name?*

The term "hydrocarbon" refers to any aliphatic, alicyclic, aromatic, halogenated and oxygenated hydrocarbons, glycols and organic solvents. Exposure may occur either via abuse or in during various industrial processes or household activities. *Halogenated* hydrocarbons (carbon tetrachloride, chloroform) are contained in cleaning agents, insecticides, plastics, degreasers, paint removers, household cleaners. *Aromatic* hydrocarbons are additives in glues and plastics while the *aliphatic* compounds occur in fuels. The *oxygenated* hydrocarbons include alcohols, ketones and ethers and are mostly contained in paint removers, varnishes and glues. Glycols (e.g. ethylene glycol, diethylene glycol, dioxane, glycerol) are used in household and industry. Solvents of abuse are e.g. toluene and xylene.

As can be appreciated, solvents possess a wide variety of chemical and physical properties. Because of this diversity there are many different health effects associated with excessive exposure to solvents. While acute renal failure has been documented following exposure to halogenated hydrocarbons [2], glycols [3] and aromatic hydrocarbons, those attributed to light petroleum hydrocarbon exposure are restricted to isolated clinical case reports [4]. More important, but less well proven, is the role of organic solvents in the development or progression of glomerulonephritis or other types of renal diseases.

Exposure to organic solvents

Exposure to organic solvents can occur either through inhalation, skin and/or mouth contact. For most solvents, inhalation is considered the most important route of exposure. Once inhaled, the solvent vapors directly irritate the upper respiratory tract (nose, throat and bronchial tubes) and the lungs. Solvent vapors are easily absorbed from the lungs into the bloodstream and are distributed to other parts of the body to produce additional toxic effects. Solvents can also be absorbed through the skin and thus be distributed to various organs. Although not a common route of entry, mouth contact with contaminated hands, food and cigarettes may provide solvents entry into the body and the bloodstream via the digestive system.

The route of entry of any solvent depends, to a certain extent, on the chemical group involved. Thus, alcohols enter the body through inhalation, skin absorption, and ingestion. Aromatic hydrocarbons are readily absorbed through the skin, whilst chlorinated hydrocarbons vaporize, presenting an inhalation hazard. Glycols are water-soluble and glycol ethers and several ketones are absorbed through the skin; an exposure route which can be more serious than inhalation.

Nephrotoxicity of organic solvents

Epidemiological studies

Sprecace [5] was the first to suggest an association between gasoline exposure and the pulmonary renal presentation of "idiopathic pulmonary hemosiderosis", more commonly known as Goodpasture's syndrome. Following this observation several *cross-sectional* [6, 7-14] and *case-control* [15-29] studies investigating the relation between renal impairment and occupational hydrocarbon exposure have been published.

Cross-sectional studies [6, 7-14] mainly involve the determination of a few up to 23 urinary markers of early tubular or glomerular changes/dysfunction in individuals chronically exposed to organic solvents with various compositions. In these studies renal effects were defined as early subclinical effects. Overt clinical problems have not been reported. In a critical literature review on cross-sectional epidemiological studies of gasoline associated glomerulonephritis Churchill et al. [30] concluded that based upon study design and execution only the study by Ravnskov et al. [18] made a compelling case for a causal association. Furthermore they judged that neither a cohort analytical study nor randomized clinical trial hold a feasible approach to confirm a suspected association. Hence, additional case-control studies are recommended [30].

From 1975 on, several *case-control* studies [15-29] investigating possible nephrotoxic effects of occupational exposure to solvents have been reported. Although in general the reported findings are highly suggestive of a relation between hydrocarbon exposure and glomerulonephritis, the applied methodology and statistical power have been criticized. These shortcomings are summarized in two excellent reviews by Churchill et al. [30] and Angell [31] who identify four areas of methodological weaknesses: (i) inappropriate control groups, (ii) use of unblinded interviewers, (iii) no consideration of recall bias and (iv) failure to define a credible measure of the degree and duration of solvent exposure. Moreover most of these studies suffer from small sample size, equivocal case definition and lack of information on important covariates. [32]. In addition, epidemiological studies should consider the magnitude of the observed effect and weigh it against the "biological plausibility". It must be noted that experimental models are not available which possess the genetic and/or environmental factors that make specific individuals susceptible to solvent nephropathy.

Based on epidemiological studies the relation between hydrocarbon exposure and glomerulonephritis seems to be well established by both case-control and cross-sectional studies. However, at present it is unclear which solvents are associated with which type of glomerulonephritis. The studies by Stengel et al. [29] and Porro et al. [25] suggest that the risk is highest for IgA nephropathy and that the possible role of oxygenated solvents in the development of this particular renal disease should be further investigated. Yaqoob et al. [26] found risk factors of 15.5, 5.3, 2.0 for respectively aliphatic, halogenated (greasing/degreasing agents) and aromatic and oxygenated (glue/paints) compounds. Furthermore, they demonstrated a direct correlation between the intensity of hydrocarbon exposure and the appearance of (early) markers of renal dysfunction such as serum creatinine, proteinuria, urinary N-acetyl-β-D-glucosaminidase, leucine aminopeptidase, and γ-glutamyl transferase [6].

An accelerated progression of glomerulonephritis has been reported in patients with intense and continued solvent exposure [33, 34]. A cohort study has investigated the contributive role of solvent exposure in the progression of primary glomerulonephritis [6]. Yaqoob et al. found that progressive renal failure was associated with a greater exposure to organic solvents when compared to individuals presenting with stable or improving renal function. Moreover patients whose occupational solvent exposure continued following the diagnosis of glomerulonephritis, presented with heavy proteinuria and more severe hypertension. In two recent reviews, Ravnskov [35, 36] considered both the hypothesis of a direct casual effect of solvent exposure and the hypothesis that the exposure worsens renal function separately. Results from 14 cross-sectional, 18 case-control studies, 2 cohort studies and 15 experiments on laboratory animals and 2 on humans, together with many case reports satisfied all but one (lack of specificity) of Hill's criteria for both hypotheses prompting the author to conclude that early elimination of the exposure may prevent the progress of renal failure in many patients.

Aside from glomerulonephritis, the impact of solvent exposure in other renal diagnoses needs to be explored. Indeed, it is of particular note that all these studies are limited to the former type of renal disease while the role of hydrocarbons in the other renal diagnoses such as diabetic nephropathy should be considered [27, 28]. Interestingly in this context is the recent observation by Nuyts et al. [28] in a group of patients with diabetic nephropathy where hydrocarbon exposure was found in 39% of the patients with that particular type of renal disease. This corroborates the results of Yaqoob et al. [27] who found higher exposure scores to hydrocarbons in patients with incipient (odds ratio 4.0) and overt (odds ratio 5.8) diabetic nephropathy as compared to diabetic individuals without clinical evidence of nephropathy.

In contrast to the above, data from a recent large nation-wide case-control study by Fored et al. [32] in which 926 incident cases in a pre-uremic stage (serum creatinine: men >3.4 mg/dl; women >2.8 mg/dl) and 998 control subjects were included the overall risk for chronic renal failure among subjects ever exposed to organic solvents was virtually identical to that among never-exposed individuals (odds ratio 1.01; 95% CI: 0.81 to 1.25). Also there were no dose-response relationships observed for lifetime cumulative solvent exposure, average dose, or exposure frequency or duration. Moreover, the absence of association pertained to all subgroups of chronic renal failure: glomerulonephritis (odds ratio 0.96; 95% CI 0.68 to 1.34), diabetic nephropathy (odds ratio 1.02; 95% CI 0.74 to 1.41), renal vascular disease (odds ratio 1.16; 95% CI 0.76 to 1.75), and other types of chronic renal failure (OR 0.92; 95% CI 0.66 to 1.27).

Pathology and mechanism(s) of solvent induced nephrotoxicity

Whereas acute renal failure has been documented following exposure to halogenated hydrocarbons [2], glycols [3] and aromatic hydrocarbons, episodes attributed to exposure to light hydrocarbons are restricted to isolated clinical case reports [4]. More important, and less well proven is the role of organic solvents in the development or progression of glomerulonephritis or other types of renal diseases.

One of the portals for entry of volatile hydrocarbons is the lung. Lipophilic hydrocarbons rapidly penetrate the lipid membranes thus gaining intracellular access. The link between pulmonary and renal lesions is believed to result from the antigenic similarity shared by the basement membranes of the alveolus and the glomerulus. The immunodominant or epitope is located within the glomerular non-collagenous domain of type IV collagen. It has been proposed that organic solvents or other environmental agents may expose the otherwise cryptic Goodpasture antigen (type IV collagen α 3 chain) to the immune response system in susceptible individuals [37, 38].

The major pathologic presentation of solvent associated nephropathy is that of anti-glomerular basement membrane disease [39] but epimembraneous and subacute proliferative glomerulonephritis have also been demonstrated. In addition, Narvarte et al. [40] reported on a patient with ulcerative colitis in which chronic interstitial nephritis developed that later was attributed to long-term exposure to organic solvents.

The histological severity of tubulointerstitial damage in primary glomerular disorders appears to correlate with severity of renal impairment and can predict the future outcome of renal disease [41]. Recent data correlating solvent exposure with morphological parameters of tubulointerstitial damage in 59 patients with biopsy-proven primary glomerulonephritis showed that solvent exposure correlated significantly with relative interstitial volume and serum creatinine. Solvent exposure, relative interstitial volume, degree of interstitial fibrosis and magnitude of chronic inflammatory cellular infiltrate in the renal cortex at the time of renal biopsy were higher in these glomerulonephritic patients developing progressive renal failure as compared to those presenting a stable or improving renal function [6].

Since, in solvent associated nephropathy, the renal injury is insidious its accurate detection/diagnosis remains an intriguing challenge. Indeed, to be of clinical value methods of detection must be sensitive, quantitative, and correlate with the usual parameters of renal impairment. Measurements of enzymuria, proteinuria and specific tubular antigens have all been proposed. However, until now there is no consensus on their diagnostic sensitivity, specificity and predictive value [12, 42-45]. At present albuminuria, compatible with altered membrane permeability [45], turns out to be the most consistent renal abnormality in solvent-associated nephropathy. Indeed, in a recent analysis of the available literature evaluating relevant cross-sectional studies were evaluated and a series of markers were analyzed with respect to their suitability as biomarker for renal damage, an increased albumin excretion was observed more frequently in groups of workers exposed to various solvents (like toluene, styrene, aliphatic/aromatic hydrocarbon mixtures, tetrachloroethene, mixtures of chlorinated hydrocarbons) as compared to controls whilst no clear pattern emerged for the other markers [46].

The issue of coexisting solvent-associated tubular damage is more controversial. While a urinary increase in tubular derived enzymes has been reported by some authors [12, 43, 44], others have failed to detect any change using either β2-microglobulin or retinol binding protein excretion [13, 43, 45].

The mechanism underlying solvent-induced glomerulopathy remains speculative. Possible pathways have been proposed by Roy et al. [4] (Figure 1). Conceptually it is proposed that when a genetically sensitive individual is exposed to environmental hydrocarbons, any or all three of the pathways could induce a hypersensitive reaction leading to glomerulonephritis. Glomerulonephritis appears to be mainly an immune-mediated disease and some solvents are found to act as immunosuppressants [47-48]. Experimentally, solvent exposure results in glomerular and tubulointerstitial injury [50] which can be explained since membranous glomerulonephritis can be induced by administration of proximal tubular brush border antigens [51], thus suggesting that solvent exposure may induce a low-grade tubular injury. This tubular injury could provoke local autoimmunity by releasing tubular or basement membrane antigens (antibodies to proximal tubular changes, laminin, Goodpasture's antigens) with activation or damage of the underlying endothelium resulting in the induction of glomerulonephritis. Alternatively potential glomerulotoxic immune factors may arise independently of solvent exposure. Also, the immunosuppressant action of solvents may facilitate the deposition of these mediators of immune damage in renal tissue.

Experimental studies

Several animal models have been used for studying the nephrotoxic effects of solvent exposure. Using rats exposed to petroleum vapors Klavis and Drommer [52] demonstrated renal lesions similar to those noted in Goodpasture's syndrome. In another study 60% of rats fed N,N'-diacetylbenzidine [53] had an increased blood urea nitrogen level. The N,N'-diacetylbenzidine induced glomerulonephritis was characterized by rapid crescent formation, fragmentation of the capsular basement membrane and early obliterative glomerulosclerosis. The site of action of N,N'-diacetylbenzidine appeared to be localized at Bowman's capsule and was not dependent on either deposition of fibrin or coagulative mechanisms [54]. Zimmerman and Norbach [55] demonstrated mesangial proliferative glomerulonephritis with focal glomerulosclerosis after long-term administration of carbon tetrachloride to rats. Although the pathogenesis of the glomerular lesion was not clear, glomerular deposits of antigen-antibody complexes were not observed. In addition to the glomerular lesions the same workers also noted tubulointerstitial damage in a similar experiment [55]. Exposing LLC-PK1 cells to either toluene or p-xylene resulted in reduced cell viability and increased DNA fragmentations which might indicate that long-term

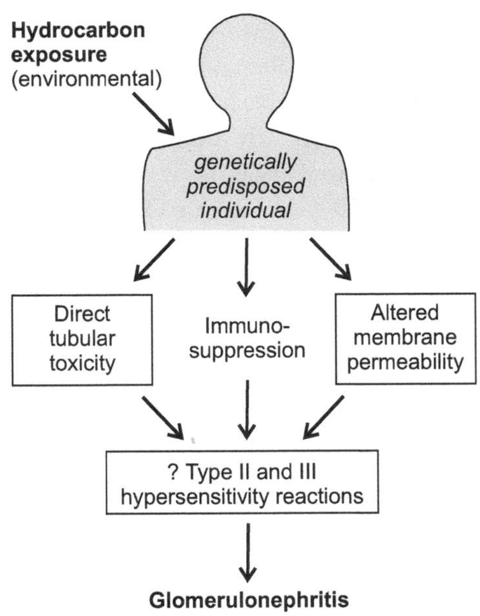

***Figure 1.** Possible mechanism of hydrocarbon associated glomerulonephritis (adapted with permission from Roy et al. [4]). See also Chapter 7 by Pelletier et al.*

exposure to organic solvents may be associated with proximal tubule cell apoptosis [56].

Silicon containing compounds

Silicon: occurrence, uses and essential chemistry

Silicon (Si) is the second most abundant element in the earth's crust, contributing around 28%. Silicon acts as a nonmetal in its chemical behavior but its electrical and physical properties are those of a semimetal. Crystalline silicon is a gray, lustrous solid. The chemistry of silicon is dominated by compounds that contain the silicon-oxygen (Si-O) linkage.

The element is used in ceramic industries and for the fabrication of semiconductors. Silicon-based polymers (*silicones*: polymeric chains containing alternately linked silicon and oxygen atoms) have wide application in industry as well as for clinical and pharmaceutical purposes.

In the literature the nomenclature used to describe the various silicon containing compounds is confusing. In nature silicon does not occur as the free element; rather it is either found as silicon dioxide (SiO_2), the so-called *silica,* in an enormous variety of *silicates* or in its carbide form i.e. carborundum (SiC). The soil water or the so-called 'soil solution' [57] contains silicon as silicic acid (H_4SiO_4). In the form of silicic acid silicon is readily absorbed by plants and all soil grown plants contain it as an appreciable but variable fraction of the dry matter [57]. Particularly the hulls of grains and the macrohairs of a number of grasses may contain high concentrations of the element (up to 10% of the plant's dry weight).

Exposure to silicon containing compounds

Due to the element's abundance in nature, human beings are exposed to relatively large but variable amounts of silicon through food, drinking water and dust. In the human body, however, the element is only present in trace amounts. The prolonged inhalation of crystalline silica dust is associated with silicosis. Amorphous silica is considered much less pathogenic than crystalline forms. In occupational settings, the main concern regarding exposure to silicon containing compounds with inhalation of silica and silicate-containing mineral dust. Since silica is such an abundant mineral, there are multiple industries in which exposure may occur. However, in modern, industrialized societies, due to the extensive enforcement of occupational health standards, exposure from well recognized sources such as mining and quarrying activities, sandblasting, stonecutting, ceramics, glass, abrasives etc. ... is well controlled, while other sources such as cosmetics, electrical and electronic machinery, grain dust and cotton or wool textiles are less well recognized.

Nephrotoxicity of silicon containing compounds

Epidemiology

Silicon toxicity is virtually limited to occupational exposure to silicon compounds e.g. miners, sandblasters, bricklayers, pottery workers in which inhalation of the compounds has been associated with the diseases of the lung. The later being evidenced by nodule formation and acute silicosis, mixed dust fibrosis and diatomite pneumoconiosis.

Knowledge regarding renal injury and the development of anti-neutrophil cytoplasmic antibody (ANCA) positivity associated with silica exposure is rudimentary being limited to epidemiological observations. Moreover, information about the health significance of the occupational exposure to other silicon containing compounds apart from silica and crystalline silicates is lacking.

During the past decade a number of case reports have described the occurrence of different forms of renal disease in patients exposed to silica [58-66]. However, only a few reports concerned subjects exposed to silica but without silicosis. Most of the cases demonstrated renal lesions compatible with rapidly progressive glomerulonephritis with a necrotizing component present in most cases. Crescent formation was described in a patient with proliferative glomerulonephritis [59] and three individuals with IgA nephropathy [60].

Renal lesions observed after silica exposure have been associated with ANCA positivity suggesting a pathogenetic role of ANCA [64-67]. Other autoimmune manifestations have been reported in a cohort of 50 workers after occupational exposure to a scouring powder mainly containing silica [68]. Systemic symptoms were present in 32 of these subjects including Sjögren's syndrome (n=6), systemic lupus erythematosus (n=3), "overlap" syndrome (n=5) and with undifferentiated findings (n=13) not meeting the criteria for a defined disease (Table 1). In most patients renal disease occurred after a long latency period. In the reports where the information is available, renal symptoms occurred 3 to 27 years after silica exposure. Data of a retrospective cohort study including 2412 white male gold miners which had been working underground for at least 1 year between 1940 and 1965 showed an elevated relative risk for non-systemic end-stage renal disease (i.e. glomerulonephritis or interstitial nephritis) of 4.22 (95% CI: 1.54-9.19) increasing to 7.70 (95% CI: 1.59-22.48) among workers with 10 or more years of employment [69] when compared to the incidence of end-stage renal disease in the US population. These data could be confirmed in a more recent cohort study in which 2670 men employed before 1980 for 3 years or more in North-American sand-producing plants. Although evaluation of death from renal disease was not the primary objective of their study the total number of deaths from nephritis or nephrosis was 16 against 7.6 (SMR 212, P = 0.002) from state/provincial rates, with the excess present only in workers employed for 10 years or more [70].

Increased levels of early markers of renal dysfunction have been demonstrated even in currently exposed workers [71, 72]. The cross-sectional observations in workers exposed to silica confirmed signs of renal impairment in patients with silicosis [71, 73] as well as in workers exposed to silica dust for less than 2 years and without lung injury [74].

In a cross-sectional study by Boujemaa et al. [72], who evaluated early indicators of renal dysfunction in silicotic workers (n=116), recorded a delay after cessation of exposure up to 30 years (mean 23 years). The

Table 1. Observations in silica exposed workers.

Cross sectional studies				
Reference	**Exposed workers**	**Non-exposed workers**	**Lung**	**Early markers of renal dysfunction: increased compared to controls**
Ng et al. 1992 [71]	33 drillers/crushers in granite quarries current exposure	19 age-matched non-exposed workers	Silicosis (7)	Albumin α-1-microglobulin ß-N-acetyl-glucosaminidase
Boujemaa et al. 1994 [72]	116 underground miners past exposure	61 age-matched general population	Silicosis	Albumin Retinol-binding protein ß-N-acetyl-glucosaminidase
Hotz et al. 1995 [74]	86 workers in quartzite rock quarry current exposure	86 age-matched non-exposed workers	No silicosis	Albumin Transferrin Retinol-binding protein ß-N-acetyl-glucosaminidase
Mortality studies				
Reference	**Exposed workers**	**Non-exposed workers**	**Disease**	**Standardized mortality ratio**
Marsh et al. 1985 [75]	16661 man-made mineral fiber workers	/	Malignant neoplasms Respiratory cancer	108.3 112.1
Goldsmith 1993 [76]	Man-made mineral fiber workers	/	Renal disease	/
Steenland et al. 2001 [77]	4626 workers in sand industry	US population	Renal disease	161.0
Cohort studies				
Reference	**Exposed workers**	**Non-exposed workers**	**Disease**	
Prospective Sanchez-Roman 1993 [68]	50 scouring powder producing factory	/	Systemic illness (32) - Sjörgen (6) - Systemic sclerosis (5) - Overlap syndrome (5) - Systemic lupus erythematosis (3) - Undifferentiated findings (13)	
Retrospective Calvert et al. 1997 [69]	2412 silica exposed gold miners	US population	Non-systemic end-stage renal disease - Glomerulonephritis or interstitial nephritis Standard incidence ratio 4.22 (1.54-9.19)	

(continued on next page)

Table 1 (continued)

Case control studies				
Reference	**Cases**	**Controls**	**Occupational exposure**	**OR (95% CI)**
Steenland et al. 1990 [78]	325 end-stage renal failure patients	325 age-matched general population	Silica Brick and foundry	1.67 (1.02-2.74) 1.92 (1.06-3.46)
Gregorini et al. 1993 [79]	16 patients with ANCA-positive rapidly progressive glomerulonephritis	32 age-matched other renal failure patients	Silica dust	14.0 (1.7-113.8)
Nuyts et al. 1995 [28]	272 renal failure patients	272 age-matched general population	Silicon containing compounds Grain dust	2.51 (1.37-4.60) 2.96 (1.24-7.04)
Nuyts et al. 1995 [80]	16 patients with Wegener's granulomatosis	32 age-matched general population	Silica Silicon containing compounds	5.0 (1.4-11.6) 6.5 (1.3-13.5)
Duna et al. 1998 [84]	101 patients with Wegener's granulomatosis	54 'Healthy' gender-matched patients from medical clinics	Construction & farm workers	OR not reported Construction 31% cases versus 19% controls Farm 36% versus 22% controls
Stratta et al. 2001 [81]	31 cases of biopsy proven vasculitis*	58 age/sex residence-matched controls	Silica	2.4 (p=0.04)
Hogan et al. 2001 [82]	65 ANCA-SVV patients with pauci-immune necrotizing GN	65 other renal patients matched for age, gender and race	Silica dust	4.4 (1.4-14.4)
Flores-Suarez et al. 2003 [86]	76 ANCA-positive primary systemic vasculitis	159 healthy, age-matched patients	Dusty areas Silica	3.1 (1.5-6.8) 3.2 (1.1-9.2)
Lane et al., 2003 [83]	75 patienst with primary systemic vasculitis	220 age-matched hospital patients	Silica Agricultural silica	3.0 (1.0-8.4) 4.4 (1.1-18.1)
Beaudreuil et al., 2005 [67]	60 ANCA-positive patients	120 age and gender-matched hospital patients	High Silica Medium silica Low silica	6.9 (1.3-35.1) 2.3 (0.6-8.2) 0.8 (0.1-3.9)
Rihova et al., 2005 [87]	31 ANCA-positive vasculitis with renal and lung involvement	30 age, gender and residence-matched office workers	Silica & asbestos	22% (13% silica and 9% asbestos) versus 0% in controls ($P < 0.05$)
Hogan et al., 2007 [85]	129 ANCA-SVV with renal biopsy proven glomerular involvement	109 healthy age, gender, state-matched controls	Silica Crop harvesting	1.9 (1.0-3.5) 2.5 (1.1-5.4)

OR = Odds ratio; ANCA = anti-neutrophil cytoplasmic antibody ; CI = Confidence interval; SVV = small vessel vasculitis; GN = glomerulonephritis

**18 pauci-immune crescentic glomerulonephritis, 9 microscopic polyangitis, 4 Wegener's granulomatosis*

(Adapted with permission from De Broe et al. [117])

silicotic subjects excreted, on average, slightly higher amounts of albumin, retinol binding protein and N-acetyl-β-D-glucosaminidase [71, 72, 74].

A survey of the literature [28, 58-65, 71, 72, 74-80] indicates that the most frequent exposure to silicon involves exposure to silica and silicates mainly in their crystalline forms. Health risks associated with the exposure to other silicon containing compounds were reported in the mortality study of 16.661 man-made mineral fiber workers employed during 1945 to 1963 at one of 17 U.S. manufacturing plants [75]. Fiber exposure in the plants producing fibrous glass or mineral wool, or both, was associated with increased standardized mortality ratios for overall mortality as well as for mortality from nephritis and nephrosis. Further evidence of the nephrotoxic role of these and other kinds of silicon containing compounds was reported by Goldsmith and Goldsmith [76]. They argued that in California an increased mortality from diseases of the urinary system was observed for farmers and farm workers. More recently, Steenland et al. [77] examined renal disease morbidity and mortality as well as arthritis mortality in a cohort of 4.626 silica-exposed workers in the industrial sand industry (an industry previously unstudied). Comparison of the cohort with the US population revealed an excess mortality ratio from chronic renal disease of 1.61 [95% CI = 1.13-2.22]. Linking of the cohort with the US registry of end-stage renal disease for the years 1977-1996 demonstrated an excess of end-stage renal disease incidence (standardized incidence ratio: 1.97, 95% CI: 1.25-2.96), which was highest for glomerulonephritis (3.85, 95% CI: 1.55-7.93) and increased with increasing cumulative exposure.

The most firmly based epidemiological observations are derived from recently published case-control studies [78-80]. Two studies, based on a large sample size, retrospectively examined occupational exposures of renal failure patients. Amongst others, an increased odds ratio's for silicon-containing compounds was also observed [28, 78]. Nuyts et al. [28] were the first to demonstrate an increased risk for the exposure to grain dust that potentially may contain high amounts of silicon, an observation that later on has been confirmed by others [80-82]. Other studies only [79, 80] focused on a small sample of patients with rapidly progressive glomerulonephritis and the specific exposure to silicon containing compounds. Gregorini et al. [79] selected only ANCA positive patients and Nuyts et al. [80] investigated patients with Wegener granulomatosis, 80% of who were ANCA positive. Studying a group of 31 cases of biopsy proven vasculitis (18 pauci-immune crescentic glomerulonephritis, 9 microscopic polyangitis, 4 Wegener granulomatosis) Stratta et al. [81] also found an increased odds ratio (2.4) for exposure to silica whilst no other significant association with a series of other exposures could be found. Hogan et al. [82] studying 65 patients with ANCA-associated small-vessel vasculitis (all of them having biopsy-proven pauci-immune crescentic glomerulonephritis) also demonstrated the odd's ratio of silica dust exposure in the development of the disease to be 4.4 times greater as compared to control subjects. In contrast to an increased risk for the development of ANCA-associated small-vessel vasculitis, exposure to silica could not be associated with systemic lupus erythematosus [82]. In a more recent studies these and other groups confirmed the association between silica exposure and onset of biopsy-proven glomerulonephritis resulting from ANCA-associated small vessel vasculitis (Table 1) [67, 83-87].

Pathology and mechanism(s) of silicon-induced nephrotoxicity

Data presented above are highly indicative for an association between silica and renal disease. The underlying pathophysiological mechanisms, however, are far from clear. At least two mechanisms have been proposed. A direct nephrotoxic effect of silicon has been suggested by Hauglustaine et al. [88]. Recently, Hotz et al. [74] reported on subclinical renal effects as indicated by an increased excretion of albumin, transferrin, retinol binding protein and N-acetyl-β-D-glucosaminidase following short time (less then 2 years) exposure to silica in non-silicotic workers. In a recent review on the association between renal disease and silica exposure Kallenberg [89] suggested that the tubular dysfunction observed in silica workers resulted from a direct nephrotoxic effect of the silicon compound. Experimentally, the nephrotoxic potential of silica has been demonstrated in the dog [90].

The exact mechanism responsible for the nephrotoxic effect of silicon remains to be elucidated although membrane damage possibly related to oxidant generation [89] or inhibition of superoxide dismutase activity [91] might be rational explanations. Based on reports on lung toxicity related to the chemical, morphological and surface characteristics of the various silicon compounds, it is not known yet to which extent these exhibit direct toxic effects at the level of the kidney [90, 92].

A second possible mechanism consists in the interaction of the inhaled silicon compounds with the cell membrane particularly that of macrophages. Once engulfed a series of events may ensue resulting in an important inflammatory reaction at the alveolar level. In addition silica particles have been shown to induce rupture of phagosomes of macrophages [93] with the release of lysosomal enzymes such as proteinase 3 or myeloperoxidase the antigens of ANCA into the microenvironment that in turn may be followed by the genration of the autoantibodies. Recently, increasing interest has been raised in the role of apoptosis in the induction of autoimmunity [94]. There is growing evidence that apoptotic antigens are the natural targets for many autoantibodies [95]. The possibility that silica, *in vitro*, may induce apoptosis of monocytes or macrophages and possibly neutrophils may represent an alternative mechanism that is operative in the induction of ANCA-associated vasculitis [95, 96]. Surface expression of ANCA antigens proteinase 3 and myeloperoxidase have been demonstrated during apoptosis of neutrophils [95, 97]. Therefore, ANCA's may bind to their target antigen on apoptotic cells and via an Fc-dependent bridging, the antibodies may amplify the release of cytokines, oxygen radicals, and lysosomal enzymes.

To which extent the generated ANCA's are responsible for initiating vasculitis, or may increase or even perpetuate vasculitis remains to be determined. Since ANCA (i) may directly activate neutrophils *in vitro*, (ii) may damage endothelial cells expressing the proteinase-3 antigen, (iii) are capable of inducing *in vitro* adherence of neutrophils to endothelial cells, (iv) block (c-ANCA) the inactivation of proteinase-3 by α-1 antitrypsin, a pathophysiological role may be suggested.

Based on experimental studies it has been suggested that silicates may stimulate lymphocytes via a T-cell receptor Vβ-specific T-cell activation pathway resulting in the production of autoantibodies or autoimmune diseases [94, 98, 99]. In this context it must be noted that not only ANCA's but also other autoantibodies such as antinuclear antibodies and rheumatoid factors frequently occur in workers heavily exposed to silicon-containing compounds [68, 77].

An intriguing observation made from case-control studies remains the controversy that exists between silica exposure and the development of a particular renal disease. Indeed, in a recent case-control study on occupational risk factors for chronic renal failure, Nuyts et al. [28] demonstrated exposure to silicon containing compounds to be related to the development of virtually all diagnostic groups of chronic renal failure. On the other hand, in two other studies [79, 80] silicon exposure was linked to a significantly higher relative risk for the development of ANCA-associated rapidly progressive glomerulonephritis or Wegener disease. These observations might indicate that silicon-containing compounds may act as a contributive as well as a causative factor in the development of renal disease. A similar observation has also been made in subjects taking analgesics. Here, besides the development of the so-called analgesic nephropathy identifiable with high accuracy by the visualization of renal papillary necrosis [100], analgesic abuse also seems to accelerate the development and evolution of the other types of renal diseases [101]. In a recent study it was demonstrated that acetaminophen and aspirin exhibit exacerbating effects on the development of all types of chronic renal failure [102].

Pesticides

The information linking environmental/occupational exposure to pesticides (including herbicides/fungicides/insecticides) is confined to some case reports and an occasional retrospective review on occupational exposure and acute renal failure [103]. Serious exposure to pesticides is usually accidental although suicidal ingestion's have occurred [103, 104]. Since many of these compounds have both commercially and domestic application exposures usually occur when proper protective precautions are ignored. Usually the acute renal failure following pesticide poisoning turns out to be multifactorial. For example, poisoning by the now banned pesticide Lindane® caused both acute volume depletion [105] and rhabdomyolysis [106], either of which could account for the subsequent acute renal failure. Other examples of multifactorial causes of acute renal failure due to pesticide exposure are reviewed by Abuelo [103].

Due to the increased litigation based on premise of product liability a renewed interest in the renal effects of herbicides, fungicides, pesticides, and insecticides has been noted during the last years. However, because of the lack of a valuable experimental animal model the current knowledge of the pathophysiologic mechanisms of the pesticide-induced renal injury is highly limited. The possibility that these pesticides act similar to that of light hydrocarbons is worthwhile to be considered, however, at the present is at is still highly speculative.

Little is also known of the long term renal effects of chronic low dose exposure to pesticides. Chronic exposure to the now banned dichlorodiphenyltrichloroethane (DDT), a lipophilic compound with prolonged body fat retention, has been associated with renal injury [105].

Insights in the renal handling of 2,4-dichlorophenoxyacetic acid have contributed to a better knowledge of the extent of occupational exposure to this widely used herbicide [107-111]. Recently, Kancir et al. [112] reported on a case of oliguric acute renal failure complicated by profound and recurrent hypocalcemia, severe hyperphosphatemia, and inappropriately high urinary sodium concentrations following exposure to this compound. In the studies of Manninen et al. [111] the peak herbicide concentration which was noted during the first 12 hours post exposure turned out to be associated with an increased excretion of both sodium and potassium. In *in-vitro* experiments the uptake of either 2,4-dichlorophenoxyacetic acid or 2,4,5-trichlorophenoxyacetic acid via a proximal tubule organic acid transport system was demonstrated in both rat and rabbit renal cortical slices [113]. Based on these experiments it was suggested that once 2,4-dichlorophenoxyacetic acid is secreted into the proximal tubule, it is probably non-reabsorbable an acts to bind intraluminal sodium and potassium. This, in turn, induces electrolyte depletion which could cause the rhabdomyolysis and severe hypocalcemia and hyperphosphatemia observed by Kancir et al. in the above mentioned study [112]. Lindane® [106], diquat® [104], copper sulphate [114] and paraphenylene diamine [115, see also Chapter 40] all have been reported to induce rhabdomyolysis and acute renal failure. Recently, Talbot et al. [116] reported the poisoning of 93 patients with the glyphosphate-surfactant herbicide (Round-up®). In ten patients (14%) manifest renal abnormalities were noted which was accompanied by a nearly uniform increase in serum creatinine (>180 µM/L) and oliguria in 3 patients. Based on their own investigations and those of Japanese workers, the authors concluded [116] that in 50% of the cases in which exposure to glyphosphate-surfactant herbicide was reported renal failure resulted.

Conclusion

Recent literature clearly points to a role for exposure to solvents in the development or progression, or both, of chronic renal failure. With regard to long-term exposure to pesticides no clear-cut evidence for a linkage with renal disease has been presented to date. Furthermore, a number of observations of the past two years supports the prveviously suggested primary or secondary role of substances such as silicon-containing compounds in the development of ANCA-associated rapidly progressive glomerulonephritis or Wegener's granulomatosis as well as an increased susceptibility of the diabetic kidney to the toxic effects of particular occupational pollutants. Further experimental and clinical studies are required to gain insight in the underlying mechanisms by which the environmental/occupational contaminants exert their toxic action at the level of the kidney.

References

1. Croll DG. The incidence of chronic nephritis amongst young people in Queensland. Med J Aust 1929; 2: 144-145.
2. Pederen LM. Biological studies in human exposure to and poisoning with organic solvents. Pharmacol Toxicol 1987; 3: 1-38.
3. Porter GA. The treatment of ethylene glycol poisoning simplified. N Eng J Med 1988; 319(2): 109-110.
4. Roy AT, Brautbar N, Lee DBN. Hydrocarbons and renal failure. Nephron 1991; 58: 385-392.
5. Sprecace GA. Idiopathic pulmonary hemosiderosis. Am Rev Resp Dis 1963; 8: 330-337.
6. Yaqoob M, Bell GM, Stevenson A, Mason H, Percy DF. Renal impairment with hydrocarbon exposure. Quart J Med 1993; 86: 165-174.
7. Krusell L, Nielsen HK, Baelum J, Lundqvist G, Omland O, Vaeth M, Husted SE, Mogensen CE, Geday E. Renal effects of chronic exposure to organic solvents: a clinically controlled trial. Acta Med Scand 1985; 218: 323-327.
8. Enarson DA, Chan-Yeung M, Embree V, Wang R, Schulzer M. Occupational exposure to chlorophenates. Scand J Work Environ Health 1986; 12: 144-148.
9. Ng TP, Ong SG, Lam WK, Jones MG, Cheung CK, Ond CN. Urinary levels of proteins and metabolites in workers exposed to toluene. Int Arch Occup Environ Health 1990; 62: 43-46.
10. Hotz P, Pilliod J, Bernard A, Berode M, Rey F, Mazzocato C, Guillemin M, Boillat MA. Hydrocarbon exposure, hypertension and kidney function tests. Int Arch Occup Environ Health 1990; 62: 501-508.
11. Lauwerys R, Herbrand J, Buchet JP, Bernard A, Gaussin J. Health surveillance of workers exposed to tetrachloroethylene in dry-cleaning shops. Int Arch Occup Environ Health 1983; 52: 69-77.
12. Mutti A, Lucertini S, Falzoi M, Cavatorta A, Franchini I. Organic solvents and chronic glomerulonephritis: a cross-sectional study with negative findings for aliphatic and alicyclic C5-C7 hydrocarbons. J Appl Toxicol 1981; 1(4): 224-226.
13. Viau C, Bernard A, Lauwerys R, Buchet JP, Quaeghebeur L, Cornu L, Cornu M, Phillips SC, Mutti A, Lucertini S, Francini I. A cross-sectional survey of kidney function in refinery employees. Am J Ind Med 1987; 11: 177-187.

14. Mutti A, Alinovi R, Bergamaschi E, Giagini C, Cavazinni S, Franchini I, Lauwerys RR, Bernard AM, Roels H, Gelpi E, Rosello J, Ramis I, Price RG, Taylor SA, De Broe ME, Nuyts GD, Stolte H, Fels LM, Herbort C. Nephropathies and exposure to perchloroethylene in dry cleaners. Lancet 1992; 340: 189-193.
15. Zimmerman SW, Groehler K, Beirne GJ. Hydrocarbon exposure and chronic glomerulonephritis. Lancet 1975; 2: 199-201.
16. Lagrue G, Kamalodine T, Hirbec G et al. Rôle de l'inhalation de substances toxiques dans la genèse des glomérulonéphritis. Nouv Press Med 1977; 6: 3609-3613.
17. Ravnskov U. Exposure to organic solvents - a missing link in poststreptococcal glomerulonephritis ? Acta Med Scand 1978; 203: 351-356.
18. Ravnskov U, Forsberg B, Skerfving S. Glomerulonephritis and exposure to organic solvents: a case control study. Acta Med Scan 1979; 205: 575-579.
19. Finn R, Fennerty AG, Ahmad R. Hydrocarbon exposure and glomerulonephritis. Clin Nephrol 1980; 14(4): 173-175.
20. Van der Laan G. Chronic glomerulonephritis and organic solvents: a case control study. Int Arch Occup Environ Health 1980; 47: 1-8.
21. Ravnskov U, Lundström S, Nordén A. Hydrocarbon exposure and glomerulonephritis evidence from patients' occupations. Lancet 1983; 2: 1214-1216.
22. Bell GM, Gordon ACH, Lee P, Doig A, MacDonald MK, Thomson D, Anderton JL, Robson JS. Proliferative glomerulonephritis and exposure to organic solvents. Nephron 1985; 40: 161-165.
23. Harrison DJ, Thomson D, MacDonald MK. Membranous glomerulonephritis. J Clin Pathol 1986; 39: 167-171.
24. Harrington JM, Whitby H, Gray CN, Reid FJ, Aw TC, Waterhouse JA. Renal disease and occupational exposure to organic solvents: a case referent approach. Brit J Ind Med 1989; 46: 643-650.
25. Porro A, Lomonte C, Coratelli P, Passavanti G, Maria Ferri G, Assennato G. Chronic glomerulonephritis and exposure to solvents: a case referent study. Brit J Ind Med 1992; 49: 738-742.
26. Yaqoob M, Bell GM, Percy D, Finn R. Primary glomerulonephritis and hydrocarbon exposure: a case control study and literature review. Quart J Med 1992; 301: 409-418.
27. Yaqoob M, Patrick AW, McClelland P, Stevenson A, Mason H, Percy DF, White MC, Bell GM. Occupational hydrocarbon exposure in diabetic nephropathy. Diabetic Med 1994; 11(8): 789-793.
28. Nuyts GD, Van Vlem E, Thys J, De Leersnijder D, D'Haese PC, Elseviers MM, De Broe ME. New occupational risk factors for chronic renal failure. Lancet 1995; 346: 7-11.
29. Stengel B, Cénée S, Limasset JC, Protois JC, Marcelli A, Brochard P, Hémon D. Organic solvent exposure may increase the risk of glomerular nephropathies with chronic renal failure. Int J Epidem 1995; 24: 427-434.
30. Churchill DN, Fine A, Gault MH. Association between hydrocarbon exposure and glomerulonephritis. An appraisal of the evidence. Nephron 1983; 33: 169-172.
31. Angell M. The interpretation of epidemiologic studies. N Engl J Med 1990; 323: 823-825.
32. Fored CM, Nise G, Ejerblad E, Fryzek JP, Lindblad P, McLaughlin JK, Elinder C-G, Nyrén O. Absence of Association between Organic Solvent Exposure and Risk of Chronic Renal Failure: A Nationwide Population-Based Case-Control Study. J Am Soc Nephrol 2004; 15:180-186.
33. Bell GM, Doig D, Thompson D, Anderton JL, Robson JS. End-stage renal disease associated with occupational exposure into organic solvents. Proc EDTA-ERA 1985; 22: 725-729.
34. Ravnskov U. Influence of hydrocarbon exposure on the course of glomerulonephritis. Nephron 1986; 42: 156-160.
35. Ravnskov U. Hydrocarbon exposure may cause glomerulonephritis and worsen renal function: evidence based on Hill's criteria for causality. Q J Med 2000; 93: 551-556.
36. Ravnskov U. Hydrocarbons may worsen renal function in glomerulonephritis: A meta-analysis of the case-control studies. Am J Ind Med 2000; 37: 599-506.
37. Salant DJ. Immunopathogenesis of crescentic glomerulonephritis and lung purpura. Kidney Int 1987; 32: 408-425.
38. Kalluri R, Gattone VH 2nd, Noelken ME, Hudson BG. The α 3 chain of type IV collagen induces autoimmune Goodpasture syndrome. Proc Natl Acad Sci USA 1994; 91(13): 6201-6205.
39. Daniell WE, Couser WG, Rosenstock L. Occupational solvent exposure and glomerulonephritis. A case report and review of the literature. JAMA 1988; 259: 2280-2283.
40. Narvarte J, Sabe SR, Ramirez G. Occupational exposure to organic solvents causing chronic tubulointerstitial nephritis. Arch Intern Med 1989; 149: 154-158.
41. Cameron JS. Tubular and interstitial factors in the progression of glomerulonephritis. Pediatr Nephrol 1992; 6: 292-303.
42. Meyer BR, Fischbein A, Rosenman K, Lerman Y, Drayer DE, Reidenberg MM. Increased urinary enzyme excretion in workers exposed to nephrotoxic chemicals. Am J Med 1984; 76: 989-998.

43. Askergen A. Studies in kidney function in subjects exposed to organic solvents. III. Excretion of cells in the urine. Acta Med Scand 1981; 210: 103-108.
44. Francini I, Cavatorta A, Folzoi M Lucertini S, Mutti A. Early indicators of renal damage in workers exposed to organic solvents. Int Arch Occup Environ Health 1983; 52: 1-9.
45. Lauwerys R, Bernard A, Viau C, Buchet JP. Kidney disorders and hemotoxicity from organic solvent exposure. Scan J Work Environ Health 1985; II (suppl 1): 84-90.
46. Voss JU, Roller M, Brinkmann E, Mangelsdorf I. Nephrotoxicity of organic solvents: biomarkers for early detection. Int Arch Occup Environm Health 2005; 78: 475-485.
47. Ravnskov U. Possible mechanism of hydrocarbon-associated glomerulonephritis. Clin Nephrol 1985; 23: 294-298.
48. Bekesi JG, Holland JF, Anderson HA, Fischbein AS, Rom W, Wolff MS, Selikoff IJ. Lymphocyte function of Michigan dairy farmers exposed to polybrominated biphenyls. Science 1978; 199: 1207-1209.
49. Peters DK, Lachmann PJ. Immunity deficiency in the pathogenesis of glomerulonephritis. Lancet 1974; 1: 58-61.
50. Shibita S, Yokoyama M. Nephritogenic glycoproteins. Nephron 1990; 55: 152-158.
51. Glassock RJ, Lachmann PJ, Watson JI, Dixon FJ. Autologous immune complex nephritis induced by renal tubular antigens. J Exp Med 1986; 127: 573-587.
52. Klavis G, Drommer W. Goodpasture's syndrome and the effects of benzene. Arch Toxicol 1970; 26: 40-55.
53. Harman JW, Miller EC, Miller JA. Chronic glomerulonephritis and nephrotic syndrome induced in rats by N, N'-diacetylbenzidine. Am J Pathol 1952; 28: 529.
54. Harman JW. Chronic glomerulonephritis and nephrotic syndrome induced in rats with N, N'-diacetylbenzidine. J Pathol 1970; 104: 119-128.
55. Zimmerman SW, Norbach DH. Nephrotoxic effects of long term carbon tetrachloride administration in rats. Arch Pathol Lab Med 1980; 104: 94-99.
56. Al-Ghamdi SS, Raftery MJ, YAqoob MM. Toluene and p-xylene induced LLC-PK1 apoptosis. Drug Chem Toxicol 2004; 27(4): 425-432.
57. Epstein E. The anomaly of silicon in plant biology. Proc Natl Acad Sci 1994; 91: 11-17.
58. Slavin RE, Swedo JL, Brandes D, Gonzalez-Vitale JC, Osornio-Vargas A. Extrapulmonary silicosis: a clinical, morphologic, and ultrastructural study. Hum Pathol 1985; 16: 393-412.
59. Osorio AM, Thun MJ, Novak RF, Van Cura EJ, Avner ED. Silica and glomerulonephritis: case report and review of the literature. Am J Kidney Dis 1987; 9(3): 224-230.
60. Bonnin A, Mousson C, Justrabo E, Tanter Y, Chalopin JM, Rifle G. Silicosis associated with crescentic IgA mesangial nephropathy. Nephron 1987; 47: 229-230.
61. Sherson D, Jorgensen F. Rapidly progressive crescenteric glomerulonephritis in a sandblaster with silicosis. Brit J Ind Med 1989; 46: 675-676.
62. Arnalich F, Lahoz C, Picazo ML, Monerero A, Arribas JR, Martinez Ara J, Vazques JJ. Polyarteritis nodosa and necrotizing glomerulonephritis assciated with long-standing silicosis. Nephron 1989; 51: 544-547.
63. Dracon M, Noel C, Wallaert B, Dequiedt P, Lelievre G, Tacquet A. Glomérulonéphrites rapidement progressives chez les mineurs de charbon pneumoconiotiques. Néphrologie 1990; 11: 61-65.
64. Gregorini G, Tira P, Lancini L, Bozzola G, Maiorca R. Silica exposure as a risk factor in the development of necrotising and crescentic glomerulonephritis with anti-mieloperoxidase antibodies. Nephrol Dial Transplant 1991; 6: 773 (abstract).
65. Neyer U, Wöss E, Neuweiler J. Wegener's granulomatosis associated with silicosis. Nephrol Dial Transplant 1994; 9: 559-561.
66. Nakajima H, Miyazaki M, Imai N, Yokokawa T, Yamamoto S. A case of silicosis with MPO-ANCA-associated glomerulonephritis and alveolar hemorrhage. Nippon Jinzo Gakkai Shi 2001; 43: 351-356.
67. Beaudreuil, S, Lasfargues G, Lauériere, Ghoul ZE, Fourquet F, Longuet C, Halimi J-M, Nivet H, Büchler M. Occupatiopal exposure in ANCA-positive patients: A case-control study. Kidney Int 2005; 67: 1961-1966.
68. Sanchez-Roman J, Wichmann I, Salaberri J, Varela JM, Nunez-Roldan A. Multiple clinical and biological autoimmune manifestations in 50 workers after occupational exposure to silica. Ann Rheum Dis 1993; 52: 534-538.
69. Calvert GM, Steenland K, Palu S. End-stage renal disease among silica-exposed gold miners. A new method for assessing incidence among epidemiologic cohorts. JAMA 1997; 277: 1219-1223.
70. McDonald AD, McDonald DC, Rando RJ, Hughes JM, Well H. Cohort mortality study of North American industrial sand workers. I. Mortality from lung cancer, silicosis and other causes. Ann Occup Hyg 2001; 45: 193-199.
71. Ng TP, Ng YL, Lee HS, Chia KS, Ong HY. A study of silica nephrotoxicity in exposed silicotic and non-silicotic workers. Brit J Ind Med 1992, 49: 35-37.
72. Boujemaa W, Lauwerys R, Bernard A. Early indicators of renal dysfunction in silicotic workers. Scand J Work Environ Health 1994; 20: 188-191.

73. Rosenman KD, Moore-Fuller M, Reilly MJ. Kidney disease and silicosis. Nephron 2000; 85: 14-19.
74. Hotz P, Gonzalez-Lorenzo J, Siles E, Trujillano G, Lauwerys R, Bernard A. Subclinical signs of kidney dysfunction following short exposure to silica in the absence of silicosis. Nephron 1995; 70: 438-442.
75. Marsh GM, Enterline PE, Stone RA, Henderson VL. Mortality among a cohort of U.S. manmade mineral fiber workers: 1985 follow-up. J Occup Med 1985; 32: 594-604.
76. Goldsmith JR, Goldsmith DF. Fiberglass or silica exposure and increased nephritis or end-stage renal disease. Am J Ind Med 1993; 23: 873-881.
77. Steenland K, Sanderson W, Calvert GM. Kidney disease and arthritis in a cohort study of workers exposed to silica. Epidemiology 2001; 12: 405-412
78. Steenland NK, Thun MJ, Ferguson CW, Port FK. Occupational and other exposures associated with male end-stage renal disease: a case/control study. Am J Public Health 1990; 80: 153-159.
79. Gregorini G, Ferioli A, Donato F, Tira P, Morassi L, Tardanico R, Lancini L, Maiorca R. Association between silica exposure and necrotizing crescentic glomerulonephritis with P-ANCA and anti-MPO antibodies: a hospital-based case-control study. Adv Exp Med Biol 1993; 336: 435-439.
80. Nuyts GD, Van Vlem E, De Vos A, Daelemans RA, Rorive G, Elseviers MM, Schurgers M, Segaert M, D'Haese PC, De Broe ME. Wegener granulomatosis is associated to exposure to silicon compounds: a case-control study. Nephrol Dial Transplant 1995; 10: 1162-1165.
81. Stratta P, Messuerotti A, Canavese C, Coen M, Luccoli L, Bussolati B, Giordia L, Malavenda P, Cacciabu M, Bugiani M, Bo M, Ventura M, Camussi G, Fubini B. The role of metals in autoimmune vasculitis: epidemiological and pathogenic study. Sci Total Environ 2001; 270: 179-190.
82. Hogan SL, Satterly KK, Dooley MA, Nachman PH, Jennette JC, Falk RJ. Silica exposure in anti-neutrophil cytoplasmic autoantibody-associated glomerulonephritis and lupus nephritis. J Am Soc Nephrol 2001; 12: 134-142.
83. Lane SE, Watts RA, Bentham G, Innes NJ, Scott DG. Are environmental factors important in primary systemic vasculitis? A case-control study. Arthritis Rheum 2003; 48: 814-823.
84. Duna GF, Cotch MF, Galperin C, Hoffman DB, Hoffman GS. Wegener's granulomatosis: role of environmental exposures. Clin Exp Rheumatol 998; 16(6): 669-674.
85. Hogan SL, Cooper GS, Savitz DA, Nylander-French LA, Parks CG, Chin H, Jennette CE, Lionakin S, Jennette JC, Falk RJ. Association of silica exposure with anti-neutrophil cytoplasmic autoantibody small-vessel vasculitis: a population-based, case-control study. Clin J Am Soc Nephrol 2007; 2(2): 290-299.
86. Flores-Suarez LF, Contreras I, Brise CA, Tilde N, Villa AR. Environmental risk factors important in primary systemic vasculitides. Kidney Blood Press Res 2003; 26: 249-302.
87. Rihova Z, Maixnerova, D, Jancova E, Pelclova D, Bartukova J, Fenclova Z, Vankova Z, Reiterova J, Merta M, Rysava R, Tesar V. Silica and asbestos exposure in ANCA-associated vasculitis with pulmonary involvement. Ren Fail 2005; 27(5): 605-8.
88. Hauglustaine, Van Damme B, Daenens P, Michielsen P. Silicon nephropathy: a possible occupational hazard. Nephron 1980; 26: 219-224.
89. Kallenberg CGM. Renal disease-another effect of silica exposure. Nephrol Dial Transplant 1995; 10: 1117-1119 (Editorial Comment).
90. Warheit DB, Driscoll KE, Oberdoerster G, Walker C, Kuschner M, Hesterberg TW. Symposium overview. Contemporary issues in fiber toxicology. Fund Appl Toxicol 1995; 25: 171-183.
91. Schainkin-Kerstenbaum R, Adler AJ, Berlyne GM. Inhibition of superoxide dismutase activity by silicon. J Trace Elem Electrolytes Health Dis 1990; 4: 97-99.
92. Fubini B, Bolis V, Giamell E, Volante M. Chemical functionalities at the broken fiber surface relatable to free radical production. In: Mechanisms in fibre carcinogenisis. Brown RC, editor. Plenum Press, New York 1991, p. -.
93. Fubini B. The possible role of surface chemistry in the toxicity of inhaled fibres. In: Fiber toxicology. Warheit DB (editor). Academic Press, San Diego 1993; p. 229-257.
94. Tervaert JWC, Stegeman CA, Kallenberg CGM. Silicon exposure and vasculitis. Current Opinion Rheumatol 1998; 10: 12-17.
95. Gilligan HM, Bredy B, Brady HR, Hebert MJ, Slayter HS, Xu Y, Rauch J, Shia MA, Koh JS, Levine JS. Antineutrophil cytoplasmatic autoantibodies interact with primary granule constituents on the surface of apoptotic neutrophils in the absence of neutrophil priming. J Exp Med 1996; 184: 2231-2241.
96. Iyer R, Hamilton RF, Li L, Holian A. Silica-induced apoptosis mediated via scavenger receptor in human alveolar macrophages. Toxicol Appl Pharmacol 1996; 141: 84-92.
97. Yang JJ, Tuttle R, Taylor JG, Jennette JC, Falk RJ. ANCA target antigens are not on the surface of normal neutrophils but are present on both primed and apoptotic neutrophils. J Am Soc Nephrol 1997; 8; 546 (abstract).

98. Ueki A, Yamaguchi M, Ueki H, Watanabe Y, Ohsawa G, Kinuguwa K, Kawakami Y, Hyodoh F. Polyclonal human T-cell activation by silicate *in vitro*. Immunology 1994; 82: 332-335.
99. Shiffenbauer J, Johnson H, Soos J. Superantigens in autoimmunity: their role as etiologic and therapeutic agents. In: Superantigens: Molecular biology, immunology, and relevance to human disease. Leung DYM, Huber BT, Schlievert PM (editors). Marcel Dekker, New York 1997; p. 525-549.
100. Elseviers MM, De Schepper A, Corthouts R, Bosmans JL, Cosyn L, Lins RL, Lornoy W, Matthys E, Roose R, Van Caesbroeck D, Waller I, Horackova M, Schwarz A, Svrcek P, Bonucchi D, Franek E, Morlans M, De Broe ME. High diagnostic performance of CT scan for analgesic nephropathy in patients with incipient to severe renal failure. Kidney Int 1995; 48: 1316-1323.
101. Perneger TV, Whelton PK, Klag MJ. Risk of kidney failure associated with the use of acetaminophen, aspirin and nonsteroidal antiinlammatory drugs. New Engl J Med 1994; 331: 1675-1679.
102. Fored CM, Ejerblad E, Lindblad P, Fryzek JP, Dickman PN, Signorello LB, Lipworth L, Elinder CG, Blot WJ, McLaughlin JK, Zack MM, Nyrén O. N Engl J Med 2001; 345: 1801-1808.
103. Abuelo JG. Renal failure caused by chemicals, foods, plants, animal venoms, and misuse of drugs. Arch Intern Med 1990; 150: 505-510.
104. Vanholder R, Colardyn F, De Reuck J, Praet M, Lameire N, Ringoir S. Diquat intoxication: report of two cases and review of the literature. Am J Med 1981; 70: 1267-1271.
105. Poisoning: toxicology, symptoms, treatments. Arena JM, Drew RH, editors. Charles C Thomas Publ, Springfield Ill 1983; p. 177-179.
106. Munk ZM, Nantel A. Acute lindane poisoning with development of muscle necrosis. Can Med Assoc J 1977; 117: 1050-1052.
107. Nash RG, Kearney PC, Maitlen JC, Sell CR, Fertig SN. Agricultural applicators exposure to 2, 4-Dichlorophenoxyacetic acid. In: Pesticide residues and exposure. Plimmer JR, editor. ACS symposium series #182, 1982, Chap 10: 119-132.
108. Kolmodin-Hedman B, Hoglund S, Akerblom M. Studies on phenoxy acid herbicides. I. Field study. Occupational exposure to phenoxy acid herbicides (MCPA, dichlorprop, mecoprop and 2, 4-D) in agriculture. Arch Toxicol 1983; 54(4): 257-265.
109. Kolmodin-Hedman B, Hoglund S, Swensson A, Akerblom M. Studies on phenoxy acid herbicides. II. Oral and dermal uptake and elimination in urine of MCPA in humans. Arch Toxicol 1983; 54(4): 267-273.
110. Libich S, To JC, Frank R, Sirons GJ. Occupational exposure of herbicide applicators to herbicides used along electric power transmission line right-of-way. Am Ind Hyg Assoc J 1984; 45: 56-62.
111. Manninen A, Kangas J, Klen T, Savolainen H. Exposure of finnish farm workers to phenoxy acid herbicides. Arch Envir Contam Toxicol 1986; 15: 107-111.
112. Kancir CB, Andersen C, Olesen AS. Marked hypocalcemia in a fatal poisoning with chlorinated phenoxy acid derivatives. Clin Toxicol 1988; 26: 257-264.
113. Berndt WO, Koschier F. *In vitro* uptake of 2, 4-dichlorophenoxyacetic acid (2, 4-D) and 2, 4, 5-trichlorophenoxyacetic acid (2, 4, 5-T) by renal cortical tissue of rabbits and rats. Toxicol Appl Pharmacol 1973; 26: 559-570.
114. Chugh KS, Singhal PC, Nath IVS, Pareek SK, Ubroi HS, Sarkar AK. Acute renal failure due to non-traumatic rhabdomyolysis. Postgrad Med J 1979; 55: 386-392.
115. Averbukh Z, Modai D, Leonov V, Weissgarten J. Rhabdomyolysis and acute renal failure induced by paraphenylenediamine. Hum Toxicol 1989; 8: 345-348.
116. Talbot AR, Shiaw MH, Huang JS, Yang SF, Goo TS, Wang SH, Chen CL, Sanford TR. Acute poisoning with a glyphosate-surfactant herbicide ('Round-up'): a review of 93 cases. Hum Exper Toxicol 1991; 10: 1-8.
117. De Broe ME, D'Haese PC, Nuyts GD, Elseviers MM. Occupational renal diseases. Current Opinion Nephrol Hypert 1996; 5: 114-121.

38

Balkan nephropathy

Ljubica DJUKANOVIĆ[1] and Zoran RADOVANOVIĆ[2]

[1]Clinical Centre of Serbia, Beograd, Serbia
[2]Faculty of Medicine, Kuwait University, Kuwait

Introduction

Balkan (or endemic) nephropathy is a chronic tubulointerstitial disease of unknown, presumably exotoxic etiology. It has been shown to exist only in some parts of the southeastern Europe.

While there have been many meetings and papers [1, 2] concerning both cause and treatment of Balkan nephropathy, sociopolitical turmoil, including wars, and economical hardship prevented any meaningful research on the problem during the 1990's. Thus, despite numerous proceedings and a large number of publications on the subject, many features of Balkan nephropathy, its etiology and natural history in particular, remained nearly as mysterious as when described in the mid-fifties.

Meetings organized by international organizations [3-7] had a key role in informing the international scientific community on the disease. A recent source of information is a bilingual (in English and Serbian) monograph published in 2000 [8].

Epidemiological features

Distribution and frequency

Though exclusive geographical restriction of the agent(s) of Balkan nephropathy is not very likely, the disease has been diagnosed only among people living (or those who used to live) in more or less well defined areas of the Balkans. Along with Bulgaria and Romania, three republics of the former Yugoslavia have been affected: Bosnia, Croatia and Serbia, including Kosovo (Figure 1).

As recently summarized [9], the affected territory has a shape of a rhomboid. Its longer diameter spreads over 500 km (from the Vratza municipality in Bulgaria to villages west of Slavonski Brod in Croatia), while its transversal diameter has about 300 km (from endemic foci in eastern Romania to Vitina municipality in Kosovo). The disease affects individuals who live (or used to live) in rural environment. There are spared households even in the most affected areas, leading

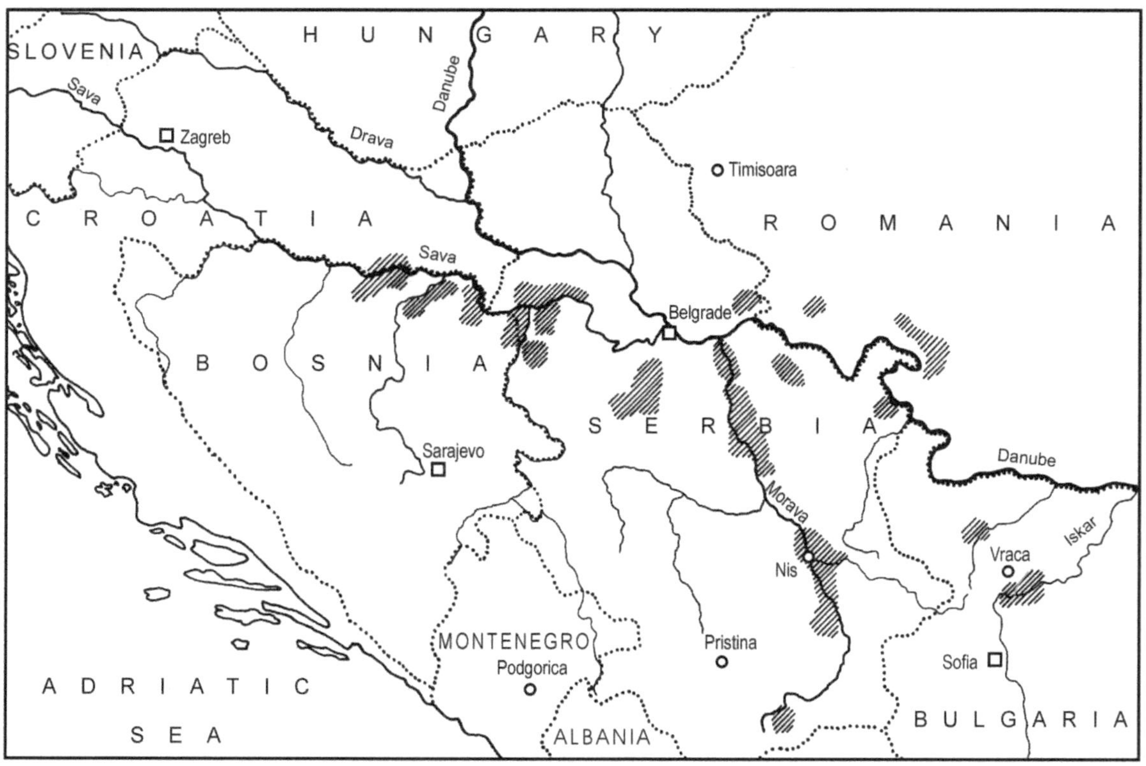

Figure 1. *Medical geography of Balkan nephropathy.*

to frequently cited remarks on mosaic distribution of the disease.

Topography of the terrain differs between endemic regions. All 14 endemic villages in Croatia are located in a single lowland municipality, at an altitude of about 100 m, while Bosnian foci are found up to 130 m. About 90% of all endemic settlements in Serbia are also situated at a low altitude, below 200 m. [10], either in large plains, river valleys or, much more seldom, in hilly regions. There have been no studies of medical geography of Balkan nephropathy in Romania for the last 40 years and endemic localities are yet to be determined [11], but the original findings pointed out to hilly areas, with endemic villages laying at the bottom of valleys eroded by flooding, at an altitude of 200-300 m. The endemic region in Bulgaria was described as mountainous or semi-mountainous, without any relationship between endemicity and altitude. Hydrogeological features [12] and lack of floods differentiate (at least some) Bulgarian foci from other typical endemic regions.

Controversial data on the frequency of Balkan nephropathy were mainly result of methodological shortcomings [9]. A main obstacle was the operational definition of the disease, leading to huge differences in estimated prevalence rates. The highest ever recorded average annual incidence rate was 16.6 per 1000 in Cakonica, Bulgaria. The average cause-specific mortality rate from Balkan nephropathy over 15 years in one of the most affected Serbian foci was 3.3 per 1000 [13].

Demographic data

During initial Balkan nephropathy research, patients were frequently in their thirties [14], and it was widely accepted that azotemia usually affects the age group 30-50 [3]. Later an apparent shift towards the older ages occurred, with most identified patients being above the age of 60 [9]. The diagnosis of clinical forms before the age of 20 was rare and never independently confirmed. Despite occasional statements on laboratory and bioptic abnormalities in the first decade of life among clinically healthy children from endemic areas, no follow up study ever showed that these children developed subsequently kidney disorder.

Both genders are similarly affected, especially considering mortality. As explained in details elsewhere [9], higher prevalence rates among women reported by some authors appears to be a consequence of unreliable diagnostic criteria.

A vast majority of experts believe that a link exist between agricultural activity and exposure to the agent(s) of Balkan nephropathy. There is also near consensus on the absence of ethnic and/or religious differences as a risk of developing the disease. The most convincing data come from Croatia, where the large group of Ukrainians who settled a century ago had the same odds of being affected as the indigenous population. The first generation immigrants developed Balkan nephropathy usually a couple of decades after moving into an endemic region.

Initial studies of affected households showed a low standard of living, poor hygienic level, and insufficient nutrition. However, socio-economic factors, including living conditions and well water quality, did not differ between contiguous affected and non-affected households or between endemic and neighboring non-endemic villages.

Chronological characteristics

The initial description of Balkan nephropathy emanated from Bulgaria [15, 16] and Serbia [17-19]. By 1957, the disease was recognized in Bosnia and Croatia and by 1958 in Romania [20].

On retrospect, it was not a newly emerging condition but rather recognition of an already existing endemic process, a previous epidemic wave seems having occurred in the early forties. Unfortunately, attempts to trace the disease prior to World War 2 are speculative, due to the absence of reliable data and a high frequency of the competing causes of morbidity, notably tuberculosis and malaria.

As for the secular trend, two facts, common to all endemic areas, are crucial in assessing any future dynamics of the disease. These are, an apparent shift of the age distribution of the incidence towards the older age groups, and a much longer natural history of the condition compared to previous data. Consequently, it suggests that the intensity of exposure diminished (if still present at all).

Other epidemiological characteristics

Clustering of cases within a household is one of the most conspicuous features of the disease. It is generally agreed that the disease affects both blood related and non-blood related family members. The "phenomenon of simultaneous deaths" (dying of parents and their children within a short interval) was also observed.

Between 1/3 and 1/2 of patients with Balkan nephropathy develop urothelial tumors [21]. An exceptionally high frequency of these tumors was also observed in the general population of endemic regions [22]. When initially studied, the attributive risk of developing upper urothelial tumors in inhabitants of endemic foci amounted to several dozen or even to as much as 100-200.

There is no evidence that domestic and/or wild animals in endemic regions develop a similar condition.

Overview of the descriptive epidemiological research

There is general agreement on the following descriptive-epidemiological characteristics of Balkan nephropathy [9]: The disease is known to exist only in some parts of the southeastern Europe, with Central Serbia as the most affected region. Balkan nephropathy does not spread beyond its already defined foci; the disease is distributed mosaically: non-endemic villages exist in the most affected regions, and there are spared families and households in the most affected settlements. Clustering of cases in families and households has been described. Children and adolescents are spared of clinical disease. Incidence is proportional to age, except for the oldest age groups. There are no major sex differences in the cause-specific mortality rates. The excess risk of developing transitional cell urothelial tumors was expressed by two- or even three-digit numbers.

The large majority of researchers support the following statements [9]: autochthonous urban population is spared; rural way of life, i.e., agricultural activity is needed for exposure to the agent(s). Separation from an endemic focus early may prevent the disease, while immigration to an endemic area provides risk of disease development, providing that the exposure was sufficient. Prevalence of the disease has been stable over many years, but now appears to decline in most affected settlements. Incidence rates are shifting towards the older age groups, and the clinical course is much more protracted suggesting a less intensive contact with the agent(s) and, consequently, possible future spontaneous disappearance of Balkan nephropathy.

Etiology

Genetic factors

The most elaborate and, seemingly consistent, hypotheses regarding etiology initially came from proponents of heredity as an explanation of the disease occurrence. These authors assumed that the risk of developing the disease was restricted only to specific, ethnically distinct, population groups, irrespectively of their place of birth and residence history. Wider acceptance of these hypotheses was hampered by the different perception of descriptive epidemiology of Balkan nephropathy by a majority of researchers on the topic.

A specific chromosome marker (3q25) in Balkan nephropathy patients from Bulgaria was identified, and this isolated finding was used to support arguments in favor of a crucial role of genetic factors [24-26]. More recently, the same authors acknowledged that environment is also important [27]. Some aberrations of the X chromosome have been reported, but they resembled changes occurring after exposure to ochratoxin A [28].

Major anomalies of urinary organs allegedly occurred in a high percentage of otherwise healthy children from affected households. However, such a finding has never been replicated.

Genetic epidemiological approach suggest two possibilities, either polygenic type of inheritance with an insufficient expression of the main gene [29], or monofactorial model with a crucial role of a single gene of incomplete penetrance [30]. In both cases, contributing environmental factor is needed.

There is no evidence supporting an immunological mechanism in Balkan nephropathy.

Biological agents and their products

Unspecified viral particles [31], an unidentified cythopathogenic agent, serially propagated slow viruses [32], and an unknown virus associated with foci of natural infection [33] have been mentioned in the context of Balkan nephropathy etiology. Several specific viruses, notably West Nile [34], coronavirus [35], and papova virus [36], were also suggested as a causative agent. A common feature of all these hypotheses was unimpressive supporting evidence and ignorance of basic epidemiological features of the disease, in particular its absence of spreading [37].

Bacteria received particular attention in initial stages of the Balkan nephropathy research but their possible etiological importance has been unanimously considered as ruled out [2]. Protozoa have never attracted any attention.

Toxic fungal products were until recently the principle and prime potential culprits. Most efforts have concentrated on ochratoxin A, a mycotoxin responsible for porcine (swine) nephropathy [38]. The substance is found in endemic foci but it is also present in neighboring non-endemic areas, and the differences are not statistically significant [39, 40]. Still, the consistent isolating of ochratoxin A in greater frequency and higher concentrations from food and sera samples obtained from endemic, compared to control villages, offered some arguments in favor of this hypothesis.

Association of ochratoxin A with chronic interstitial nephropathy in Tunisia [41] and its relation to renal tumors [42] provides additional support for the idea of the etiological role of this mycotoxin. Other fungal toxins, as zerealenone, citrinin [43] and aflatoxin were also isolated in endemic foci. Experimental models suggested that a combination of mycotoxins, rather than a single one, might be involved in the etiology of Balkan nephropathy [44].

Aristolochic acid and its salts, originated from a weed, *Aristolochia clematitis*, have toxic and carcinogenic effects to the kidneys and urothelium [45], respectively. Ivic [46] postulated that this plant may be a cause of Balkan nephropathy, but failed to provide convincing evidence from field surveys. Evidence that *A. clematitis* played a central role in the etiology of Chinese herb nephropathy [47-49], a condition similar to Balkan nephropathy, initiated a second look at this previously abandoned hypothesis and it gained a lot of weight by recent data on the association between DNA adduct formation derived from AA, mutation pattern and tumour development in BEN [50] (see also chapter 33).

No local practice in terms of the use of teas or folk medicine could have been implicated. No one has ever studied flora of the local wells.

Agents from the inanimate environment

Chronologically, lead poisoning was first offered as an explanation for the occurrence of Balkan nephropathy [17-19]. The idea on lead-contaminated flour led to abandonment of water mills in a part of Central Serbia. This energetic public health action had no impact on the disease frequency.

Effects of non-occupational exposure to cadmium [51], itai-itai disease in particular [52, 53], were occasionally compared with kidney damage seen in Balkan nephropathy patients. In spite of some resembling features, the idea of a common etiology between cadmium nephropathy (including itai-itai disease) and Balkan nephropathy was refuted [52, 54].

Many other metals, including radioactive ones such as uranium [55], were also suggested as possible causative agents of the disease. Results were non-convincing and non-reproducible. Inability to identify a single toxic effect of any metal or metalloid as a cause of Balkan nephropathy led researchers to two alternative approaches. First, deficiency, rather than abundance of such a chemical element was proposed [56], with selenium as the most likely candidate [57]. Second, attention was paid to a combined adverse effect of several elements. Synergism of uranium and some other elements, none of which exceeding maximal allowed levels, was proposed [58]. It was also noted that criteria used in occupational medicine (exposure only during working hours) have been applied to an ecological problem (constant exposure) and that concentrations of lead or cadmium within formally acceptable level, combined with other factors, such as selenium deficiency, might lead to the disease [58]. All these suggestions remained speculative.

As for non-metals, there were attempts to relate Balkan nephropathy to silicon [59-62]. However, when affected and non-affected households were compared, there was even an inverse relationship between the silica content and endemicity. On one occasion, small differences in silica content happened to reach the level of statistical significance but the association was explained as a result of confounding variables [63].

Common hydrogeological characteristics of endemic foci [12] and inverse relationship between altitude of wells and disease frequency in a longitudinal (cohort) study [63], pointed to potable water as a vehicle of the agent(s). However, none of the already mentioned or several dozen other non-organic substances were associated with the disease [64].

Organics in water have been investigated and provided some interesting data [65]. Except for nitrites [66], chemically unstable substances have not been studied. Wells associated with the disease were reported as situated on alkali soil [67], but the finding was restricted to a single endemic area and never reproduced.

Based on chronological data, it is clear that no pesticides, fertilizers or chemicals introduced during the last few decades may be blamed for the occurrence of Balkan nephropathy. Except for exposure to agricultural activities, no occupation, habit (e.g., smoking, alcohol consumption), or hobby (e.g., hunting, fishing) might have been shown to precede the disease onset.

Overview of the etiological research

Genetic factors may play a role in different individual risk of developing Balkan nephropathy, upper urothelial tumors, both diseases or none of them [68]. However, epidemiological data indicate that one or more external, environmental factors are crucial for the occurrence of both Balkan nephropathy and excessive frequency of these tumors in endemic areas.

Among biological agents and their products, the candidates for etiological agents are mycotoxins and, much more probably, toxic plants, notably *Aristolochia clematitis*. The possible role of viruses is very unlikely, indeed.

As for inanimate environment, there is no chemical element that has been consistently detected in higher concentrations in biological material of Balkan nephropathy patients and/or their environment, as compared to the controls. However, though unlikely, insufficiency of an essential element has not been completely ruled out. Speculations on a combination of vaguely defined environmental factors have never been substantiated by facts.

Pathomorphological Changes

Balkan nephropathy is non-destructive and non-inflammatory tubulointerstitial renal disease [69]. The changes are non-specific and in the chronic, sclerotic phase they may be quite similar to changes observed in other chronic interstitial diseases such as analgesic nephropathy [70], vascular nephrosclerosis [69] cyclosporine-induced nephropathy [71], radiation nephritis [72, 73] and aging [72], intoxication with silicate, cadmium, lead, uranium [74], mycotoxin ochratoxin A [75], Aristolochia clematitis [46], and recently with Chinese herbs [47, 49].

Macroscopic features

Before introduction of hemodialysis in the treatment of chronic renal patients, the kidneys of patients who died of Balkan nephropathy used to be the smallest seen at post mortem examinations, weighing 14.8-80 g each (Figure 2A) the difference between the left and right kidneys being small (5-20 g) [74, 76-78]. Surface of the kidneys is smooth, occasionally wavy but never granulated or roughly nodular. The section shows markedly narrowed cortex, pyramid and Bertin's columns are fairly well preserved, and corticomedular border is well differentiated. Papillary necrosis of the pyramids has not been found.

Small, papillary, usually multiple tumors of the renal pelvis and ureters are also one of the characteristic findings (Figure 2B]. In post-mortem studies tumors were reported in 8-50% of cases [74, 79].

Morphological studies of renal changes in post mortem material

Diffuse fibrosis of cortical interstitium and tubular atrophy may be observed along in the absence of sig-

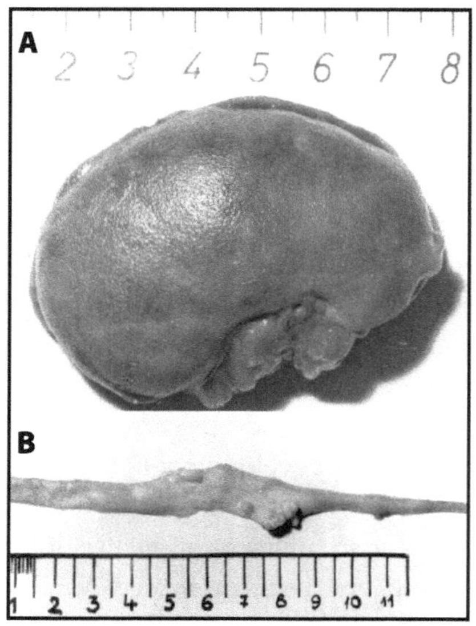

Figure 2. A. *Macroscopic appearance of the right kidney weighing 35 g in a case of BN, surface if smooth, occasionally mildly wrinkled (Autopsy, a man aged 48).*
B. *Multifocal papillary tumor of the right ureter (autopsy).*

nificant cellular interstitial infiltration. In contrast to the cortex, Bertin's columns are less markedly affected. Even in severe tubulointerstitial cortical changes, glomeruli are well preserved, partially collapsed, and subsequently subjected to focal or generalized sclerosis mainly collapsing. Glomeruli in Bertin's column are occasionally compensatorily enlarged. Pyramids are preserved or less markedly affected [74, 76, 79].

Blood vessels, arcuate or interlobular arteries, and arterioles are affected in the form of intimal sclerosis and thickening of lamina elastica interna. In addition, the blood vessels are compressed and torsioned [79].

In cases of tumors of the renal pelvis and ureters morphological signs of pyelonephritis are often found [74].

Optic microscopic, immunofluorescent and electron microscopic studies of renal biopsies

In oligosymptomatic clinical cases, rare disseminated foci of interstitial fibrosis and tubular atrophy with preserved glomeruli are seen. These changes have no special predilection of distribution and are not inflammatory. They tend to be triangular, with the base oriented toward the renal surface [69, 79]. In cases with initial renal failure, the fields of acellular interstitial fibrosis are larger and even diffuse.

The striking atrophic process observed in Balkan nephropathy suggests that apoptosis may play a role in this disease. In this context it is of interest that Savin et al. observed an increased apoptosis to proliferation ratio at the level of the tubuli [80].

The glomeruli are usually affected by generalized [80%] or segmental sclerosis [10%]/ and only in 8% hyalinosis is recorded. Double contour glomerular basement membrane was recorded in 22% of the cases. In 2.7-6% of cases fetal-like glomeruli can be seen in the kidneys, while glomerular hypercellularity was recorded in 4% [72, 79, 81].

The most interesting changes are recognized in pre- and postglomerular blood vessels. In about 50% of cases PAS positive proteins are deposited in vas afferens walls in a focal segmental or circumferent manner in the form of droplets, bands or granules [72, 79, 81].

Interlobular capillaries are filled with thick proteinaceous substances that are also deposited below the capillary endothelium and may even be found free in the interstitium. These changes are described as capillary sclerosis [70]. Although renal vascular changes in Balkan nephropathy have been pointed out as very important, they are not specific and can be encountered in other renal diseases. Ferluga et al. [72] and Sindjić [79] commented on their similarities with cyclosporine induced nephrotoxic changes.

Immunofluorescence revealed irregular and scarce deposits of C3, fibrin and IgM, and occasionally IgA, C1q and C4, mainly on the vascular walls, Bowman's capsule and some sclerotic glomeruli [69, 82, 83].

Electron microscopic findings are either normal or correspond to degenerative and sclerotic changes. While some authors describe virus-like particles [35, 84, 85], others point out that such particles were not found [72, 73].

Despite these findings, some authors described Balkan nephropathy as a form of glomerulonephritis [81, 86]. However, the lack of reliable evidence supporting glomerulonephritis has lead to it being discarded [73, 77] and abandoned even by its advocates [87].

Optic microscopic, immunofluorescent and electron microscopic studies of renal biopsies in children aged 5-15 from affected families in endemic regions failed to detect any Balkan nephropathy related changes [79].

Overview of morphological studies

It is generally agreed that the morphological changes of Balkan nephropathy are not specific and correspond to non-destructive, non-inflammatory kidney disease accompanied by marked changes on the blood vessels in both early and late stages of the disease, interstitial, multifocal fibrous expansion and severe tubular atrophy mainly in the upper cortex [69, 72, 73, 79, 81].

Changes on kidneys arterioles have been described suggesting that the changes in early stage of the disease may be responsible for the development of multifocal, ischemic, vascular nephrosclerosis encountered in chronic stages of the disease [69, 72]. On the other hand, close similarity of Balkan nephropathy with analgesic and cyclosporin-induced nephropathy has been recognized [71, 72, 79]. All this leads to a suggestion that Balkan nephropathy develops following a model of toxic nephropathy, targeting primarily the vascular endothelium where the tubular epithelium is affected either directly or indirectly due to accompanying ischemia.

Clinical features, diagnostics and treatment

Clinical picture and course

Balkan nephropathy is a chronic tubulointerstitial disease with occult, insidious onset, usually progressing slowly with no apparent signs of symptoms. After a long asymptomatic period, the disease is manifested as chronic renal failure. Less commonly blunt lumbar pain or renal colic may develop or, occasionally, dysuric symptoms induced by urinary tract infection. If hematuria exists, urothelial tumor should be suspected. In an advanced case polyuria and nocturia are present due to impaired concentrating ability of the kidneys. The disease is tolerated well and the patients preserve their working ability until advanced stages of renal failure [18, 76, 88, 89].

Objective examination reveals characteristic skin tan of Balkan nephropathy patients: a pale yellow with copperish glow on the cheeks has been recognized since the augural reports on the disease [18, 88]. Besides, xantochromia of the palms and soles is also frequently observed. In the advanced phase of the disease physical examination detects signs of chronic renal failure [19].

Patients with Balkan nephropathy do not suffer from edema, and their blood pressure is usually described as normal [18, 88-90]. Recently, several studies reported a higher prevalence of hypertension even in offspring of Balkan nephropathy families [91, 92, 93].

As Balkan nephropathy is characterized with slow asymptomatic course, most authors identify two main stages of the disease: the first, asymptomatic (latent, subclinical) and second, manifest (symptomatic). The latter is usually subdivided into the stage without renal failure (early, compensated Balkan nephropathy, with no azotemia) and chronic renal failure (decompensated Balkan nephropathy, uremia) [19, 88, 89].

An important feature of Balkan nephropathy is its association with a high incidence of tumors of the renal pelvis and ureters, but not urinary bladder tumors [22, 94, 95]. However, the difference between the incidence of upper urothelial tumors in endemic and non-endemic regions diminished in the last decades. In the sixties and seventies the incidence of these tumors was reported to be several dozen times higher in endemic than in non-endemic regions, while in the last decades this difference almost disappeared [21, 22, 94, 96, 97]. Upper urothelial tumors of patients originating from the region with Balkan nephropathy differ from tumors identified in patients from other regions in their similar incidence in both sexes, bilateral occurrence, and more common association with chronic renal failure [95].

Laboratory findings

Appearance and urine color are unchanged in most patients with Balkan nephropathy. Urine sediment is usually scarce, while microhematuria or leukocyturia are usually associated with the occurrence of tumors or urinary tract infection [88, 89].

Bacteriological studies usually reveal sterile urine, but in 8.3-31.8% significant bacteriuria was confirmed and considered as superimposed urinary tract infection [88, 89].

Proteinuria is a common finding in patients with Balkan nephropathy [18, 88]. It is usually intermittent, less than 1 g per day and it becomes permanent in advanced renal failure [98]. Although proteinuria is one of the criteria for diagnosis of Balkan nephropathy, it has been reported in healthy members of endemic families [30, 98, 99]. Tubular proteinuria is the most common and increased excretion of low-molecular weight proteins such as β_2-microglobulins, lysozyme, ribonuclease, light chains of immunoglobulin, retinol-binding protein has been reported [100-105]. Beside tubular proteinuria, smaller numbers of patients manifest mixed proteinuria, while in patients with renal failure, glomerular proteinuria may be encountered [103, 105].

Anemia has been noted in patients with Balkan nephropathy in early studies [18] and described as normocytic and normochromic or mildly hypochromic [88]. It has been suggested that anemia occurs earlier in the course of the disease progression than is the case in other renal diseases and that it precedes azotemia [88, 106]. However, recent studies have failed to substantiate this claim [98, 107]. Also, there is no evidence that anemia in Balkan nephropathy differs from anemia accompanying other renal diseases in either features [107] or rate of deterioration in the progression of renal failure [108]. Nevertheless, anemia in Balkan nephropathy patients treated with hemodialysis is more severe than in patients with other renal diseases [108].

The leukocyte count in the peripheral blood of patients with Balkan nephropathy is normal and without

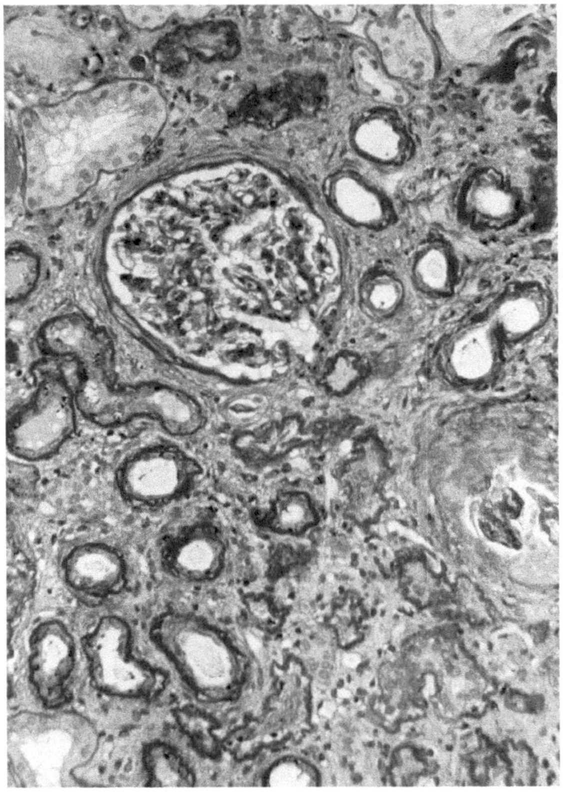

Figure 3. *Interstitial fibrosis and tubular atrophy; glomerulus with mild mesangial hypercellularity and another with incomplete hyalinosis. PAS, x120.*

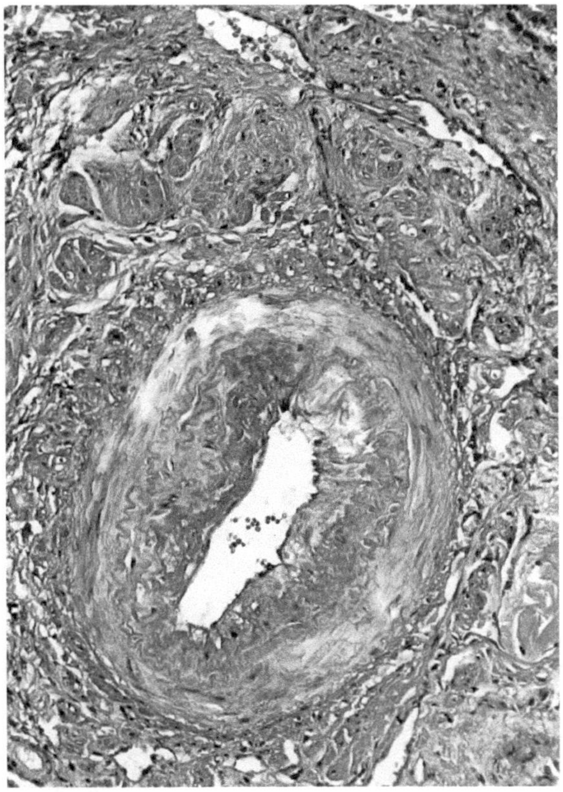

Figure 4. *Interlobar artery showing intimal fibrosis. PAS, x240.*

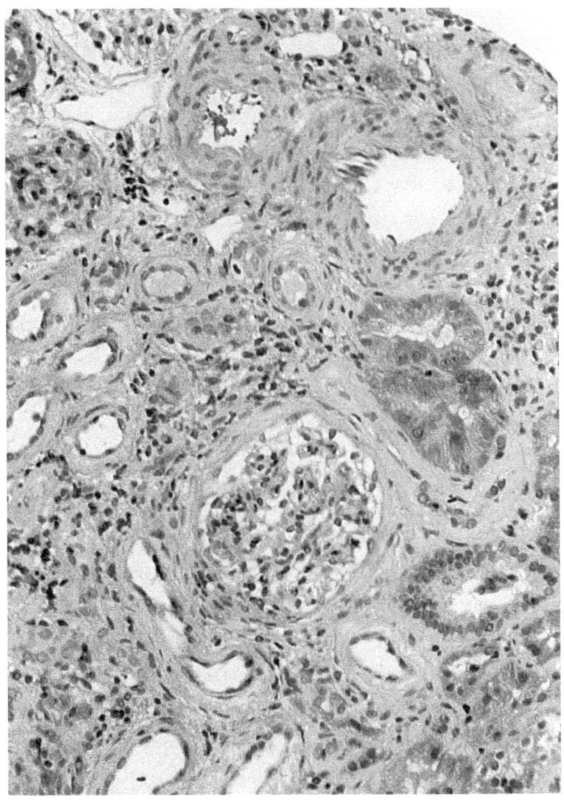

Figure 5. *Reduced number of tubules; fibrotic interstitium; few infiltrating cells. Masson's trichrome, x120.*

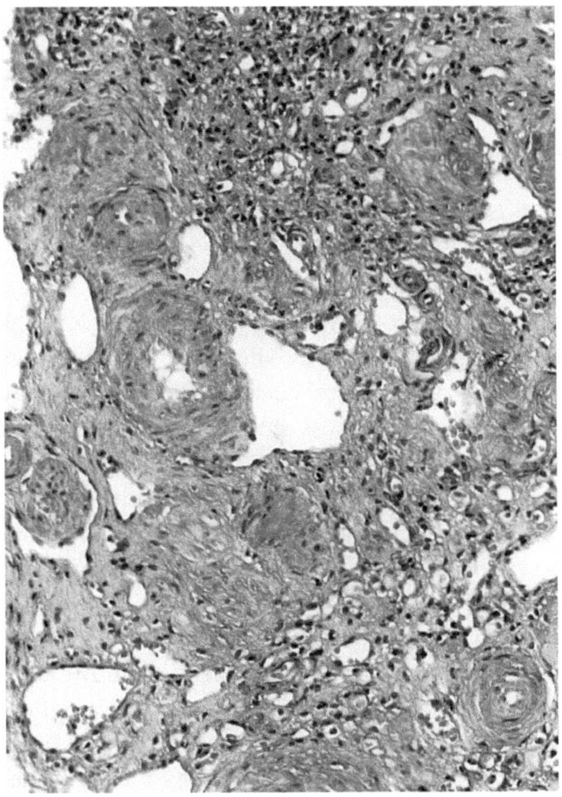

Figure 6. *Extensive interstitial scarring associated with severe arterio and arteriolosclerosis. PAS, x120.*

pathological changes in the differential count and bone marrow [19, 88].

Investigation of renal function in patients with endemic nephropathy has revealed tubular dysfunctions in the earliest stage of the disease: renal glycosuria, increased uric acid and amino acid excretion [101], as well as increased excretion of low molecular weight proteins [104]. Significantly higher activity of cellular enzymes in the urine and increased urinary excretion of Tamm-Horsfall protein was described in patients with Balkan nephropathy, as well as in healthy members of endemic families [109]. Findings of a distal tubular disorders (impaired urinary acidification, impaired urine concentrating ability) were described in earlier studies [88, 89] but could not be confirmed in studies conducted in larger groups of patients with normal or mildly impaired glomerular filtration rate [98, 110]. The occurrence of certain disorders of the tubular function recorded in the course of chronic renal failure (increased natriuria, phosphaturia) can be considered as the result of kidney adaptation to the lost nephron mass, instead of Balkan nephropathy properties [110].

The immunological studies have failed to indicate that immune disorders participate in the pathogenesis of Balkan nephropathy, with some of detected changes having been attributed to advanced renal failure [111].

Imaging methods

Different methods of kidney imaging have shown that Balkan nephropathy patients with chronic renal failure have symmetrically shrunken kidneys with smooth surface and no calcifications [90]. The time at which the shrinking occurs remains to be determined. While some authors suggest that the size of the kidneys remains normal in patients in the latent phase of the disease and with normal renal function, others report cases of shrunken kidneys in patients in an early phase with normal glomerular filtration rate, and it was even proposed that the disease was characterized with primarily small kidneys [98, 110, 112]. As ultrasound became a standard imaging method in the evaluation of kidney dimensions, several recent studies that used this method showed diminished kidney length and cortex width in members of Balkan nephropathy families with normal kidney function [113, 114]. Besides, significantly shorter kidney length, as well as higher protein, albumin and b2-microglobulin excretion was found among offspring with a maternal history of Balkan endemic nephropathy (BEN), not a paternal one [113] .

Excretory urography does not reveal changes in the pyelocaliceal system, except in cases with secondary infection or urothelial tumors.

Radionuclide methods have shown that renal plasma flow impairment is the first sign of the early phase. Glomerular and tubular functions correspond to the severity of the disease.

Diagnosis

The most commonly used criteria for the diagnosis of Balkan nephropathy are still those proposed by Danilović [106]. They include: 1) farmers living in the endemic villages, (2) familial history positive for Balkan nephropathy, (3) mild proteinuria, (4) low specific gravity of the urine, (5) anemia, (6) retention of nitrogen compounds in the blood (urea > 50 mg/dl, creatinine > 1.5 mg/dl) and (7) symmetrically shrunken kidneys. Using these criteria, Danilović suggested classification of patients in field studies into the following groups:

1. *potential,* a group with intermittent proteinuria, those that fulfill at least the first three criteria,
2. *suspected patients,* that in addition to the first three fulfill at least one of the remaining three criteria,
3. *affected patients,* that fulfill at least 5 out of 6 criteria,
4. *decompensated* patients that fulfill at least 5 out of 6 criteria and have urea values >150 mg% and manifested signs of uremia.

Analysis of these criteria leads to the conclusion that they enable detection only of patients with overt disease, and the criteria are not sufficiently specific to enable a reliable diagnosis. Therefore, numerous studies have been focused on developing sufficiently sensitive and specific criteria to enable diagnosis in the early phase. Although markers of tubular disorders, particularly tubular proteinuria, may be used as sufficiently specific diagnostic criteria, so far not a single clinical or laboratory finding is considered pathognomonic for Balkan nephropathy when differentiate it from other, specially, tubulointerstitial diseases.

The diagnosis of Balkan nephropathy is now established according to the first two criteria (residence in endemic village and positive family history) suggested by Danilović [106], presence of tubular proteinuria and ruling out other renal diseases.

Histopathological analysis makes the diagnosis of Balkan nephropathy significantly easier [72, 79], and it is considered indispensable in classifying the following groups of patients with urinary abnormalities suggestive of endemic nephropathy:

1. Patients from families that were not previously been affected with endemic nephropathy, but live in an endemic village,
2. In cases of nephropathy of unknown etiology in villages close to endemic foci,
3. In immigrants to endemic regions and in emigrants from these regions [111].

Differential diagnosis of Balkan nephropathy should include all chronic, slowly progressive renal diseases, primarily chronic tubulointerstitial diseases. Although no specific indicators of Balkan nephropathy have been recognized, epidemiological data, familial history as well as clinical characteristics of the disease enable differential diagnosis. Thus, shrunken kidneys with smooth surface are characteristic of Balkan nephropathy and they differentiate it from analgesic nephropathy, pyelonephritis or reflux nephropathy that are characterized by shrunken kidneys with uneven surface. Pyelocaliceal system of the kidneys remains unaffected in patients with Balkan nephropathy, unlike the characteristic changes observed in pyelonephritis or obstructive nephropathy. Absence of papillary necrosis/calcifications also enables differentiation of Balkan nephropathy from analgesic, obstructive, reflux nephropathy [110, 115].

Recently similarity of Balkan nephropathy and nephropathy induced by Chinese herbs used in slimming diets have been suggested [48]. Nevertheless, Chinese herb nephropathy is rapid progressive tubulointerstitial diseases with pronounced fibrosis and progression towards end-stage renal disease within few years, clearly different from the protracted clinical course of Balkan nephropathy.

Prevention and treatment

Balkan nephropathy is a disease of unknown etiopathogenesis, so that recommendations regarding effective prevention are not possible. Efforts have been made to improve the living conditions, bring high quality drinking water to endemic villages and undertake other hygienic measures. Treatment is planned according to the stage of the disease. In principle, the treatment involves the measures for slowing down deterioration of renal function and those applied in chronic renal failure [116].

End-stage renal disease is treated with dialysis and kidney transplantation. Hypertension and cardiovascular diseases affect the Balkan nephropathy patients less frequently, so they tolerate hemodialysis rather well compared to patients with other renal diseases. The Balkan nephropathy patients on long-term hemodialysis frequently develop upper urothelial or urinary bladder carcinoma.

Although the number of reported cases with kidney transplant is small, neither specific post-transplantation problems nor disease recurrency on the transplanted kidney have been described.

However, recent studies indicated that patients with Balkan nephropathy are at increased risk for the development of upper urothelial tumors in both native and transplanted kidneys [117].

Overview of clinical and laboratory studies

Balkan nephropathy is a chronic tubulointerstitial disease with insidious occult onset progressing without symptoms. Agreement as to how to define the early asymptomatic phase of the disease is lacking, since no specific indicators for the diagnosis have been recognized. The diagnosis is established according to epidemiological criteria (farmers in endemic villages, familial history positive for endemic nephropathy), presence of tubular proteinuria, findings of symmetrically shrunk kidneys with smooth surface, without calcifications and ruling out of other renal disease. Renal biopsy may make the diagnosis easier, although the changes are non-specific. One of the important features of Balkan nephropathy is its association to high incidence of tumors of the renal pelvic and ureters, comparable to analgesic nephropathy (se chapter 17) and aristolochic acid nephropathy (see chapter 33).

So far, laboratory studies have failed to detect any disorder as a specific marker for early detection of the disease or a reliable indicator for differential diagnosis. Laboratory studies have confirmed that Balkan nephropathy is a tubulointerstitial disease so that tubular disorders precede impairment of glomerular filtration. Although anemia is one of the criteria for the diagnosis of the disease, it has not been evidenced that pathogenesis and features of this anemia differ from that observed in other chronic renal diseases. It is only more severe in end-stage Balkan nephropathy patients than in patients with other kidney diseases.

Acknowledgement

Photos of all tissue specimens were provided by Professor Jovan Dimitrijević.

References

1. Astrug A (editor). Endemic Nephropathy – Bibliography 1956-1970, Sofia: Ministry of Public Health; 1971.
2. Radovanović Z. Aetiology of Balkan nephropathy: A reappraisal after 30 years. Eur J Epidemiol 1989; 5:372-7.
3. World Health Organization. The "Endemic Nephropathy" of South-Eastern Europe. Bull Wld Hlth Org 1965; 32(3):431-448.
4. Wolstenholme GEW, Knight J (editors). The Balkan Nephropathy. Ciba Foundation Study Group No. 30. London: Churchill; 1967.
5. World Health Organization. WHO Meeting of Investigators on Endemic Nephropathy, Belgrade and Lazarevac, November 1974, NCD/WP/74.
6. Castegnaro M, Plestina R, Dirheimer G, Chernozemsky IN, Bartsch H (editors). Mycotoxins, Endemic Nephropathy and Urinary Tract Tumours. IARC Scientific Publications No. 115. Lyon: International Agency for Research on Cancer; 1991.
7. Hall P, Batuman V (guest editors). Kidney Int 1991; 40: Suppl 34 (Proceedings of the IUPAB meetings, Belgrade, 1989 and 1990).
8. Radovanović Z, Sinđić M, Polenaković M, Djukanović Lj, Petronić V. Endemic Nephropathy. Belgrade: Office for Textbooks and Teaching Aids, 2000.
9. Radovanović Z. Epidemiology and aetiology of endemic nephropathy. In: Radovanović Z, Sinđić M, Polenaković M, Djukanović Lj, Petronić V. Endemic Nephropathy. Belgrade: Office for Textbooks and Teaching Aids, 2000.
10. Radovanović Z. Topographical distribution of the Balkan endemic nephropathy in Serbia (Yugoslavia). Trop geogr Med 1979; 31:185-189.
11. Gluhovschi G, Stefanovic V, Dimitrov Tz et al. Endemic Balkan Nephropathy. Helicon, Timisoara, 1994.
12. Radovanović Z, Perić J. Hydrogeological characteristics of endemic nephropathy foci. Public Health (Lond.) 1979; 93:76-81.
13. Radovanović Z, Danilović V, Velimirović D et al. Beta2-microglobulinuria as a predictor of death in a population exposed to Balkan endemic nephropathy. Kidney Int 1991; 40(S34):32-34.
14. Danilović V. Effet des recherches des néphrites endemiques en Yougoslavie. Arch. Union Méd. Balkan. 1964; 2(1): 31-40.
15. Tančev I, Evstatijev P, Dorosiev D, Penceva Z, Cvetkov G. Proučvanija na nefritite v'v Vracanska okolija. S'vr. med. 1956; 7(9): 14-29.
16. Ivanov L. Proučvanija v'rhu etiologijata na b'brežnite zaboljavanija v'v Vracanska okolija. S'vr. med. 1956; 7(9): 30-34.
17. Danilović V, Djurišić M, Mokranjac M, Stojimirović B, Živojinović J, Stojaković P. Porodična oboljenja bubrega u selu Šopic izazvana hroničnom intoksikacijom olovom. Srp. arh. celok. lek. 1957; 85(10): 1115-25.
18. Danilović V, Djurišić M, Mokranjac M, Stojimirović B, Živojinović J, Stojaković P. Néphrites chroniques provoquées par l'intoxication au plomb par voie digestive (farine). Presse méd. 1957; 65(90): 2039-40.
19. Danilović V. Chronic nephritis due to ingestion of lead-contaminated flour. Brit. Med. J. 1958; 1: 27-8.
20. Milojčić B. Epidemic of chronic nephritis of unknown aetiology. Brit. Med. J. 1960; i:244-5.
21. Radovanović Z, Janković S, Jevremović I. Incidence of tumors of urinary organs in a focus of Balkan endemic nephropathy. Kidney Int 1991; 40(S34): 75-76.
22. Petković S, Mutavdžić M, Petronić V, Marković V. Les tumeurs du bassinet et de l'uretere. Recherches cliniques et étiologique. J. Urol. Néphrol. 1971; 77(6): 429-39.
23. Radovanović Z, Krajinović S, Petković S, Hall PW. Papillary transitional cell tumours, Balkan nephropathy, and beta2-microglobulin. The Lancet 1981; 2:689.
24. Toncheva D, Dimitrov Ts, Tzoneva M. Cytogenetic studies in Balkan endemic nephropathy. Nephron 1988; 48:18-21.
25. Toncheva D, Gergov T, Tzoneva M, Bouchakliev Z. Spontaneous and induced chromosome aberrations in Balkan endemic nephropathy. Kidney Int. 1991; 40 (Suppl. 34): 97-101.
26. Toncheva D, Dimitrov T. Genetic predisposition to Balkan endemic nephropathy. Nephron 1996; 72(4):564-9.
27. Toncheva D, Dimitrov T, Stojanova S. Etiology of Balkan endemic nephropathy: a multifactorial disease? Eur J Epidemiol. 1998 Jun;14(4):389-94.

28. Manolova Y, Manolov G, Parvanova L, Petkova-Bocharova T, Castegnaro M, Chernozemsky IN. Induction of characteristic chromosomal aberrations, particularly X-trisomy, in cultured human lymphocytes treated by ochratoxin A, a mycotoxin implicated in Balkan endemic nephropathy. Mutat. Res. 1990; 231(2):143-9.
29. Tucić N, Marinković D. The inheritance of liability of Balkan nephropathy. Genetika 1979; 11(3): 213-20.
30. Banjević D, Tucić N. The monofactorial model for inheritance of liability to disease and its implications for relatives at risk. Genetika 1979;11(3): 221-30.
31. Georgescu L, Litvac B, Manescu N, Petrovici A, Schnjartzkopf A, Zosin C. Particules virales dans le rein de la nephropathie endemique Balcanique. Sem. Hôp. Paris 1970; 46:3526.
32. Draganescu N, Antipa C, Girjabu E, Melencu M. Endemic Balkan nephropathy, a slow virus disease? Rev. Roum. Med.-Virol. 1983; 34(1): 3-6.
33. Birtašević B, Vuković B, Drndarević D et al. Endemska (Balkanska) nefropatija kao prirodno-žarišna infekcija? Vojnosanit pregl 1983; 40: 319-24.
34. Kraus N. Studien über die endemische Nephrozirrhose der Balkanhalbinsel. Zeitschrift für ärztliche Fortbildung 1966; 60:829-34.
35. Apostolov K, Spasić P, Bojanić N. Evidence of a viral etiology in endemic (Balkan) nephropathy. Lancet 1975; ii: 1271-3.
36. Nastac E, Stoian M, Hozoc M, Iosipenco M, Melencu M. Further data on the prevalence of serum antibodies to papova viruses (BK and SV40) in subjects from the Romanian area with Balkan endemic nephropathy. Rev. Roum. Med.-Virol. 1984; 35(1):65-7.
37. Radovanović Z. Epidemiological evidence on Balkan nephropathy as a viral disease. Medical Hypotheses 1987; 22:171-5.
38. Krogh P. Causal association of mycotoxic nephropathy. Acta Path Microbiol Scand Sect A (Suppl) 1978; 269:1-28.
39. Petkova-Bocharova T, Castegnaro M. Ochratoxin A contamination of cereals in an area of high incidence of Balkan endemic nephropathy in Bulgaria. Food Addit Contam 1985; 2: 267-70.
40. Cvetnić Z, Pepeljnjak S. Ochratoxinogenicity of Aspergillus ochraceus strains from nephropathic and non-nephropathic areas in Yugoslavia. Mycopathologia 1990; 110(2): 93-9.
41. Maaroufi K, Achour A, Betbeder AM et al. Foodstuffs and human blood contamination by the mycotoxin ochratoxin A: correlation with chronic interstitial nephropathy in Tunisia. Arch. Toxicol. 1995; 69:552-8.
42. Maaroufi K, Pfohl-Leszkowicz A, Achour A et al. Ochratoxin A genotoxicity, relation to renal tumors. Arch Inst Pasteur Tunis 1994; 71(1-2):21-31.
43. Yeulet SE, Mantle PG, Rudge MS, Greig JB. Nephrotoxicity of Penicillium aurantiogriseum, a possible factor in the aetiology of Balkan endemic nephropathy. Mycopathologia 1988; 102: 21-30.
44. Bach PH, Gregg NJ, Delacruz L. Relevance of a rat model of papillary necrosis and upper urothelial carcinoma in understanding the role of ochratoxin A in Balkan endemic nephropathy and its associated carcinoma. Food Chem Toxicol. 1992; 30(3): 205-11.
45. Mengs U, Lang W, Poch JA. The carcinogenic action of aristolochic acid in rats. Arch. Toxicol. 1982; 51:107-19.
46. Ivić M. Problem etiologije endemske nefropatije. Acta Fac Med Naiss 1970; 1:29-38.
47. Vanherweghem JL, Depierreux M, Tielemans C, Abramowicz D, Dratwa M, Jadoul M, Richard C, Vandervelde D, Verbeelen D, Vanhaelen-Fastre R, et al.Rapidly progressive interstitial renal fibrosis in young women: association with slimming regimen including Chinese herbs. Lancet. 1993;341(8842):387-91.
48. Cosyns JP, Jadoul M, Squifflet JP et al. Chinese herbs nephropathy: a clue to Balkan endemic nephropathy? Kidny Int. 1994; 45(6):1680-8.
49. Cosyns JP, Dehoux JP, Guiot Y, Goebbels RM, Robert A, Bernard AM, van Ypersele de Strihou C. Chronic aristolochic acid toxicity in rabbits: a model of Chinese herbs nephropathy? Kidney Int. 2001; 59(6):2164-73
50. Grollman AP, Shibutani S, Moriya M, Miller F, Wu L, Moll U, Suzuki N, Fernandes A, Rosenquist T, Medverec Z, Jakovina K, Brdar B, Slade N, Turesky RJ, Goodenough AK, Rieger R, Vukelić M, Jelaković B. (2007) Aristolochic acid and the etiology of endemic (Balkan) nephropathy. PNAS 2007; 104: 12129-12134.
51. Nogawa K, Kobayashi E, Honda R, Ishizaki A, Kawano S, Matsuda H. Renal dysfunctions of inhabitants in a cadmium-polluted area. Environ Res 1980; 23(1): 13-23.
52. Danilović V (editor). Bulletin, T. LXIX, Classe des sciences medicales No. 12. Beograd: Academie Serbe des Sciences et des Arts, 1980.
53. Frieberg L, Elinder C-G, Kjellstrom T, Nordberg GF (editors). Cadmium and Health: A Toxicological and Epidemiological Appraisal. Boca Raton, CRC Press, 1986.
54. Piscator M, Kostial K, Plestina R. Urinary excretion of cadmium and zink among women with Balkan endemic nephropathy. Trace Elements Med. 1984; 1:134-8.
55. Ignjatović B. Prilog proučavanju etiologije hroničnog nefrita. Narodno zdravlje 1962; 18: 329-34.

56. Maksimović Z, Radovanović Z. Balkan endemic nephropathy in Yugoslavia and geochemical studies. In: Hemphill DD, ed. Trace Substances in Environmental Health (18). Univ. Missouri, 1984; p. 230-6.
57. Maksimović Z. Selenium deficiency and Balkan endemic nephropathy. Kidney Int 1991; 40 (suppl. 34):S12-14.
58. Wedeen RP. Environmental renal disease: Lead, cadmium and Balkan endemic nephropathy. Kidney Int 1991; 40 (suppl. 34): S4-8.
59. Duančić V. Essai d'explication de la manifestation de l'affection rénale de masse å Slavonski Kobas. Biol. glasnik 1960; 3:43-50.
60. Marković B, Lebedev S. Role étiopathogénique des silicates érosifs dans la néphrite endémique. Presse méd. 1965; 73(8):401-4.
61. Marković B, Arambašić M. Experimental chronic interstitial nephritis compared with endemic human nephropathy. J. Pathol. 1971; 103: 35-40.
62. Goldsmith JR, Goldsmith DF. Fiberglass or silica exposure and increased nephritis or ESRD (end-stage renal disease). Am J Ind Med 1993; 23:873-81.
63. Radovanović Z, Marković-Denić Lj, Marinković J, Jevremović I, Janković S. Well water characteristics and the Balkan nephropathy. Nephron 1991; 57:52-54.
64. Radovanović Z, Edmunds WM. Groundwater chemistry and the incidence of Balkan endemic nephropathy. Environ Geochem Health 1991; 13(2):43-9.
65. Finkelman RB, Feder GL, Orem WH, Radovanovic Z. Relationship between low-rank coal deposits and Balkan endemic nephropathy. AGID News, 1991; 65: 23.
66. Radovanović Z, Stevanović D. Different forms of mineral nitrogen in drinking water and the Balkan nephropathy. Arch Environm Contam Toxicol 1988; 17: 813-5.
67. Filipović A, Abinun A, Nijemčević S, Leković G, Popović N. Ispitivanje ovisnosti pojave endemske nefropatije i sastava zemljišta iz kojeg stanovništvo uzima vodu za piće u opštini Modriča. Med arhiv 1977; 31(5): 277-84.
68. Radovanović Z, Velimirović D, Naumović T. Upper urothelial tumours and the Balkan nephropathy - Inference from the study of a family pedigree. Eur J Cancer 1990; 26:391-2.
69. Sindjić M. Pathomorphology of the kidneys in endemic nephropathy. Academie Serbe des Scientes et des Arts Bulletin 1980; 69: 127-140.
70. Zollinger H U, Mihatsch M J, Torhost J. Nephropathy due to analgesics. Morphological aspects. XIII Inter. Congr. of Inter. Acad. of Pathology, Paris, Abstracts, 1980; 17.
71. Mihatsch MJ, Thuel G, Ryffel N. Morphology of cyclosporin nephropathy. Prog Allergy 1986; 38: 447-465.
72. Ferluga D, Hvala A, Vizjak A, Trnavcevic S, Halibasic A. Renal function, protein excretion and pathology of Balkan endemic nephropathy. III Light and electron micorscopy studies. Kidney Int 1991; 40 (Suppl 34): S54 - S67.
73. Hall PW III, Dammin GJ Balkan nephropathy. In: Renal pathology with clinical and functional correlations. Fisher G, Brenner BM (editors). J.B. Lippincott Co., Philadelphia, 1989; 913-924.
74. Sindjić M. Resultats des recheches patho-anatomiques, faites jusqu'a present, concernant la nephropathie endemique.In: I Symposium sur la nephropathie endemique. 1973 Beograd. Danilovic V (redacteur). Academie Serbe des Scientces et des Arts, Beograd 1973; 187-202.
75. Krogh P, Hald B, Pleština R, Čeović S. Enviromental Ochratoxin A and Balkan (endemic) nephropathy: Evidence for support of a casual relationship. In: Endemic (Balkan) Nephropathy, Proc. 4th Symp., Nis 1979. Eds. S. Strahinjic & V. Stefanovic. Inst. Nephr. Haemod., Nis 1981, 35-43.
76. Radonić M, Radošević Z, Županić V. Endemic nephropathy in Yugoslavia. In: The Kidney. Mostby S, David E (editors). Wiliams & Wilkins Co., Baltimore, 1966; 503-522.
77. Zosin L et al. Aspects anatomo-cliniques de la néphropathie endémique balkanique. Sém Hôp, 1966; 42(3/1):194-201.
78. Hall PW et al. Investigation of chronic endemic nephropathy in Yugoslavia. II Renal Pathology. Am J Med 1965; 39(2): 210-217.
79. Sindjić M. Morphological changes in kidneys affected by endemic nephropathy. In: Radovanović Z, Sindjić M, Polenaković M, Djukanović Lj, Petronić V. Endemic nephropathy. Belgrade: Office for Textbooks and Teaching Aids, 2000.
80. Savin M, Bumbaširević V, Djukanović Lj, Petronić V. The significance of apoptosis for early diagnosis of Balkan nephropathy. Nephrol Dial Transplant 2001; 16(Suppl 6): 30-32.
81. Doichinov D, Todorov D, Dinev I, Milev B. Biopsy specimen examination during the early stage of endemic nephropathy. In: Endemic Nephropathy. Proc. 2nd Int. Symp. on End. Nephr., Sofia 1972, Bulg. Acad. Sc. Press, Sofia 1974, 189-194.
82. Polenaković M, Hrizoho D. Endemska nefropatija – imunofluorescentna mikroskopska ispitivanja. In: II Simpozijum o endemskoj nefropatiji, Beograd-Lazarevac 1977. Ur. V. Danilovic, SANU, Beograd 1979, 137-150.
83. Vizjak A., Trnačević S., Ferluga D., Halilbašić A. Renal function, protein excretion and pathology of Balkan endemic nephropathy. IV-Immunohistology. Kidney Int 1991; 40 (Suppl 34) 68-74.
84. Georgescu L, Litvac B, Diosi P, Plavosin L, Herzog G. Viruses in endemic (Balkan) nephropathy. Lancet 1976; i: 1086.

85. Uzelac-Keserovic B, Vasic D, Ikonomovski J, Bojanic N, Apostolov K. Isolation of a coronavirus from urinary tract tumours of endemic Balkannephropathy patients. Nephron 200;86:93-4
86. Pantić VR, Suša S. Ultrastructure of nephrons in kidney of endemic nephropathy patients. In: Endemic (Balkan) Nephropathy, Proc. 4th Symp., Nis 1979. Strahinjic S & Stefanovic V (editors). Inst Nephr Haemod, Nis 1981; 123-132.
87. Doitchinov D. Immunohistochemical studies in Balkan endemic nephropathy. In: Endemic (Balkan) Nephropathy, Proc. 4th Symp., Nis 1979. Strahinjic S & Stefanovic V (editors). Inst. Nephr. Haemod., Nis 1981, 265.
88. Puchlev A, Popov N, Astrug A, Dotchev D. Clinical studies on endemic nephropathy in Bulgaria. In: Int. Symp. on End. Nephr., Sofia, 1963, Bulg. Acad. Sc. Press, Sofia 1965; 17-24.
89. Bruckner I., Zosin C ., Lazarescu R, et al. A clinical study of nephropathy of an endemic character in the people's Republic of Rumania. In: Int. Symp. on Endemic Nephropathy, Sofia 1963. Bulg. Acad. Sc. Press, Sofia 1965; p. 25-35.
90. Djukanović Lj, Velimirović D, Sindjić M. Balkan Nephropathy. In: Clinical Nephrotoxins. Renal Injury from Drugs and Chemicals. De Broe ME, Porter GA, Bennett WM, Verpoolen GA (editors) Kluwer Academic Publishers. Dordrecht 1988; 426-436.
91. Arsenovic A, Bukvic D, Trbojevic S, Maric I, Djukanovic L. Detection of renal dysfunctions in family members of patients with Balkan Endemic Nephropathy. Am J Nephrol 2005; 25: 50–54.
92. Dimitrov P, Tsolova S, Georgieva R, Bozhilova D, V Simeonov V, Bonev A, Karmaus W. Clinical markers in adult offspring of families with and without Balkan endemic nephropathy. Kidney Int 2006; 69: 723–729.
93. Bukvić D, Marić I, Arsenović A, Janković S, Djukanović Lj. The prevalence of Balkan endemic nephropathy has not changed since 1971 in the Kolubara region in Serbia. Kidney Blood Press Res 2007;30:117-123
94. Petković S. Epidemiology and treatment of renal pelvic and ureeral tumours. J Urol 1971; 114: 858.
95. Petronić V. Tumors of the upper urothelium and endemic nephropathy. In: Endemic nephropathy. Radovanović Z, Sindjić M, Polenaković M, Djukanović Lj, Petronić V. Office for Textbooks and Teaching Aids, Beograd, 2000.
96. Markovic N, Ignjatovic I, Cukuranovic R, Petrovic B, Kocic B, Stefanovic V. Decreasing incidence of urothelial cancer in a Balkan endemic nephropathy region in Serbia. A surgery based study from 1969 to 1998. Pathol Biol (Paris). 2005;53: 26-9.
97. Dragicevic D, Djokic M, Pekmezovic T, Micic S, Hadzi-Djokic J, Vuksanovic A, Simic T. Survival of patients with transitional cell carcinoma of the ureter and renal pelvis in Balkan endemic nephropathy and non-endemic areas of Serbia. BJU Int. 2007;
98. Trnačević S, Halilbšić A, Ferluga D et al. Renal function, protein excretion and pathology of Balkan endemic nephropathy. I. Renal function. Kidney Int 1991; 40 (Suppl 34): S49-S51.
99. Čvorišćec D, Radonić M, Čeović S, Aleraj B. Characteristics of proteinuria in endemic nephropathy. J Clin Chem Clin Biochem 1983; 21: 569-571.
100. Bruckner I, Stoica G, Serban M. Studies on urinary proteins. In: The Balkan Nephropathy. Wolstenholme GEW & Knight J (editors). Ciba Foundation Study Group No. 30. Churchill, London 1967; p. 15-20.
101. Hall PW, III, Piscator M, Vasiljević M, Popović N. Renal function studies inindividuals with the tubular proteinuria of endemic Balkan nephropathy. Q J Med 1972; 41: 385 - 393.
102. Radošević Z, Traeger J, Radonić M, Manuel Y, Revillard J P. Etude elctrophoretique de la proteinurie de 31 sujet crates vivant en pays de nephropathie endemique. J Urol Nephrol 1968; 74: 703-10.
103. Bruckner I, Stoica Gh. Urinary proteins in renal diseases. II. Alpha2-microglobulins in tubular protienuria with special reference to endemic nephropathy. Rev Roum Med Med Int 1978; 16: 2-8.
104. Hall PW, Vasiljević M. Beta2-microglobulin excretion as an index of renal tubular disorders with special reference to endemic Balkan nephropathy. J Lab Clin Med 1973; 81: 897-904.
105. Raičević S, Trnačević S, Hranisavljević J, Vučelić D. Renal function, protein excretion, and pathology of Balkan endemic nephropathy. II. Protein excretion. Kidney Int 1991; 40(Suppl. 34): S-52-56.
106. Danilović V. Endemic nephropathy in Yugoslavia. In: Endemic (Balkan) Nephropathy, Proc. of the 4th Symp., Ni{ 1979. Strahinji} S & Stefanovi} V (editors). Inst. Nephr. Haemod., Nis 1981; 1-5.
107. Pavlović -Kentera V, Djukanović Lj, Clemons G K, Trbojević S, Dimković N, Slavković A. Anaemia in Balkan endemic nephropathy. Kidney Int 1991; 40 (Suppl. 34): S46-S48.
108. Pavlovic-Kentera V, Clemons G K, Trbojevic S, Dimkovic N, Djukanovic Lj. Erythropoietin and anemia in the progression of Balkan endemic nephropathy and other renal diseases. Nephron 1990; 54: 139-143.
109. Čvorišćec D, Stavljenić A, Radonić M. Relationship between tubular and Tamm-Horsfall proteinuria in Balkan endemic nephropathy. Nephron 1998; 42: 152-155.
110. Djukanović Lj. Laboratory studies. In: Endemic nephropathy. Radovanović Z, Sindjić M, Polenaković M, Djukanović Lj, Petronić V (editors). Office for Textbooks and Teaching Aids, Beograd 2000.
111. Polenakovic M, Stefanovic V. Balkan Nephropathy. In: Oxford Textbook of Clinical Nephrology, Oxford medical Publications, Sec. ed. Davison A., Cameron JS, Grunfeld JP, Kerr DNS, Ritz E and Winearls Ch (editors). Oxford, Oxford University Press, 1998; 1202-1210.

112. Hrisoho DT. Balkan Endemic Nephropathy. Study of pathogenesis based on genetic factors. In: Endemic (Balkan) Nephropathy, Proc. 4th Symp., Nis 1979. Eds. S. Strahinjic & V. Stefanovic. Inst. Nephr. Haemod., Nis 1979; 1981; p. 147-154.
113. Dimitrov P, Tsolova S, Georgieva R, Bozhilova D, V Simeonov V, Bonev A, Karmaus W: Clinical markers in adult offspring of families with and without Balkan endemic nephropathy. Kidney Int 69: 723–729, 2006.
114. Djukanovic L, Bukvic D, Maric I. Creatinine clearance and kidney size in Balkan endemic nephropathy patients. Clin Nephrol 61:384-6, 2004.
115. Elseviers MM, De Schepper A, Corthouts R et al. High diagnostic performance of CT scan for analgesic nephropathy in patients with incipient to severe renal failure. Kidney Int 1995; 48: 1316-1323.
116. Polenaković M, Djukanović Lj. Clinical picture, diagnostics and treatment of endemic nephropathy. In: Endemic nephropathy. Radovanović Z, Sindjić M, Polenaković M, Djukanović Lj, Petronić V (editors). Belgrade: Office for Textbooks and Teaching Aids, 2000.
117. Basic-Jukic N, Hrsak-Puljic I, Kes P et al. Renal transplantation in patients with Balkan endemic nephropathy. Transplant Proc 2007; 39:1432-5.

39

Nephrotoxins in Africa

Charles SWANEPOEL[1], Marc BLOCKMAN[2] and Joe TALMUD[2]

Divisions of [1]Nephrology and [2]Pharmacology,
University of Cape Town and Groote Schuur Hospital, Cape Town, South Africa

Introduction

Toxin-induced acute kidney injury (AKI) is a common cause of morbidity and mortality in Africa. However reports in the medical literature are limited because in the majority of cases, identification of the precise toxin is missing [1].

A majority of the toxin induced acute kidney injury in South Africa follows a visit to the traditional diviner (the "sangoma"). This often results in a conspiracy of silence; the patients are reluctant to admit such a visit and in most instances deny both the consultation, and subsequent ingestion of prescribed herbal therapy [2]. This handicaps the planning of management, particularly as some toxins have multi-system effects, e.g. acute kidney injury accompanied by hepatitis and colitis, as occurs in dichromate poisoning [3]. While the majority of patients admitted with poisoning have been prescribed by traditional healers, approximately 12% of the patients have obtained their medications from "African" shops (equivalent of a western-style chemist) [1]. It is not always the diviner who is responsible for the prescribing these toxins, but rather the patients who buy medicines without completely understanding their content.

De Smet [4] and others [5] have advocated the need to disseminate knowledge about the risks and benefits of herbal and alternative medicines. Such information would allow 'ingestors' of such medicines the knowledge to decide whether or not to consume herbal concoctions.

The ingestion of alternative medicines for the improvement of well-being is a global problem. This probably reflects, in part, the dissatisfaction many patients express concerning western style medical practice. Larrey [6] points out that the trend in the use of herbal medicines is growing due to a belief that natural products are both good and innocuous when compared with western style medicines. De Smet [4] summarized this global problem using a series of selected case reports. In the summary he described the intake of herbal tea (contained the toxic pyrolizidine alkaloids) leading to hepatotoxicity and death. Another example was the use of azarcon in Mexico (lead tetroxide) causing severe lead poisoning with resultant seizures, encephalopathy and death in a three-year old child. Furthermore, he presented another tragic case of a woman, whom, despite repeated warnings, had continued to eat raw dried rattlesnake meat, contaminated with Salmonella Arizona. She succumbed from sepsis. He concludes that there is a strong placebo effect derived from the ritual of taking herbal medicines and this entices many to try alternative treatments.

Psychosomatic complaints may benefit from this ritual and where health resources are restricted – as in South Africa - may save the State millions of rands in health costs! Chan [7] supports this view and mentions that in many developing countries, traditional methods of treatment (as opposed to the conventional western style prescription methods) are the only affordable and available forms of health care for the majority of the population.

We are all aware of the substantial benefits patients have derived from the use of botanical derivatives to treat medical conditions (digitalis comes to mind immediately). The clinical results with feverfew, which has benefits as an anti-migraine agent, is but one example [4]. However, the acceptability of these plant extracts arose only after safety and efficacy was assured. An example is research conducted by the Chinese on the leaves of Artemisia annua and the discovery of the anti-malarial artemisinin. While the anti-febrile effects of Artemisia annua herb have been recognized in China since the 4th century AD [8], it was only in 1972 that the research into the anti-malarial properties began.

A starting point would be to assemble a catalogue of safe herbal remedies, which the traditional healers could use for their patients. Watt and Breyer-Brandwijk [9] published such a catalogue and listed the local names of numerous medicinal plants. The poisonous ones were also identified in their publication. However, ensuring that this information is easily accessible to the traditional healers is challenging. In addition to the need for a revised, updated and expanded version, the document must be written in the language of the traditional healer and be user friendly.

Bye and Dutton [2] have researched the culture of the Zulu people (concentrated mainly in the KwaZulu/Natal region) and the use of traditional remedies. The Zulu believe that disease is a reflection of disharmony between an afflicted person and his/her ancestors. The sangoma (diviner) diagnoses the problem by consulting with the spirits and thus identifies the source of the disharmony. The inyanga prepares and dispenses the herbal treatment required to dispel the disharmony and in so doing hopes to cure the affliction. Although this work concentrated on the Zulu population [2], there exists this common thread of belief throughout Africa that, during times of illness amongst the blacks, there is a need for ancestral placation. Therefore, the administration of toxic herbal substances (or chemical substances e.g. mixtures of solutions with battery acid and others with dichromates) is intrinsic to the whole African continent.

The lack of good toxicological services in a large part of the African continent is a major contributor to the inability to identify most of the culprit toxins. Another major problem is that the registration of herbalists has not been uniform, which can lead to a situation where ignorant persons are dispensing substances of which they, and anyone else for that matter, know little. When herbal remedies are recommended, there are no checks and balances in the treatment protocols. Unhappily, fatalities as a result of herbal use, are a major problem in infants including the death of healthy babies. Similar to western-type medical practice, charlatans are encountered amongst the sangomas and inyangas. These quacks are usually ignorant of the safer, tried and tested traditional remedies. They may prescribe the hard-core, more toxic substances. An example of such an occurrence is a case of cresol poisoning discussed below.

This chapter will attempt to outline the extent of the problem in South Africa. We have confined our comments to toxins that have a major impact on renal function - although some (if not most!) toxins have secondary effects with consequent kidney failure.

We have also incorporated a description of toxins, which are taken for cosmetic and suicidal purposes, but also by accident and for recreational reasons (and therefore the sangoma and inyanga is definitely innocent in this instance).

Potassium dichromate

The excellent work done by Wood et al [3] in describing the extent of the toxicity of potassium dichromate has been of great educational value. Potassium dichromate is the principal active ingredient in purgative solutions; the indications for its use are broad and may encompass any complaint. The substance is toxic in the hexavalent state but metallic chromium is inert. It is used in the leather industry for tanning, as an industrial cleaning agent and in electroplating. It is a bright yellow crystalline substance in its natural state.

When taken orally or rectally it is irritant to the mucosa and can cause acute tubular necrosis, hepatitis and colitis. The toxic hexavalent chromium becomes rapidly bound to tissue (in the trivalent form). Therefore clinical measures to reduce absorption must be administered immediately in order to have an effect. When inhaled, it causes chronic bronchitis, interstitial pneumonitis and fibrosis. The indications for which dichromates may be prescribed are numerous. Figure 1 is an example of a purgative, the contents of which, on analysis was found to have a mixture of dichromates and faeces. This mixture was given to a patient to relieve mild constipation. The patient initially denied that she had consulted a sangoma but later, after she had undergone dialysis for two weeks followed by complete recovered from her acute tubular necrosis (ATN), brought in the medicine bottle and admitted that she had taken the substance orally on prescription of a healer. This had produced severe diarrhea and dehydration with subsequent ATN. Note (Figure 1) the healer has used western-style prescription methods including standard abbreviations such as t.d.s. and p.o. Furthermore note that the indications for use of the medicine range from "blood" disorders to diarrhea to libido problems!

Wood has presented several cases of known dichromate poisoning [3]. In six of the seven cases, the patients were able to produce the ingested compound for analysis and dichromate proved to be the principal active ingredient. All his patients had blood levels of chromium well in the toxic range. They all required dialysis support and in one tissue was obtained at post-mortem examination. This patient died from sepsis and massive gastrointestinal hemorrhage. It is noteworthy that the liver had the highest chromium content followed by the kidney and this was found 26 days after the initial presentation!

The clinical presentation of these 7 cases was that of a spectrum involving the kidneys with GIT manifestations in all, as well as hepatic failure in two. Sepsis and hemorrhage were secondary manifestation of mucosal damage and in one case, rectal perforation (probably traumatic enema) was an additional finding.

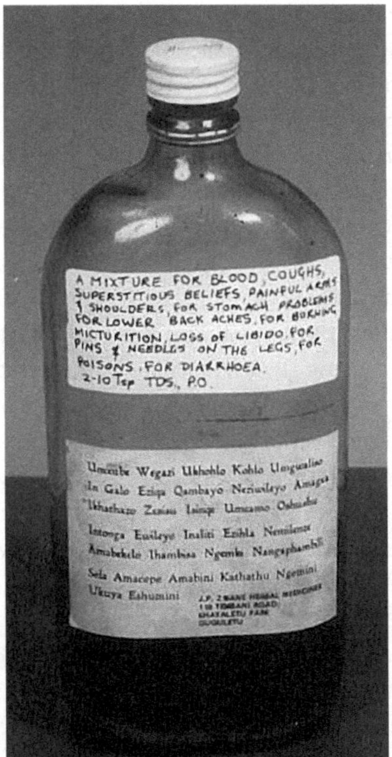

Figure 1. *Medicine bottle containing dichromates. Note indications for use. By courtesy of Prof Wood.*

Treatment consists of early hemodialysis to remove a larger amount of chromium (due to the rapid tissue binding). There is no role for chelating agents. Otherwise, treatment for dichromate poisoning is entirely supportive. Fortunately, the renal failure is reversible. The chromium is taken up by the kidneys and produces a nephrogram on straight abdominal X-ray (Figure 2).

It is intriguing to know that dichromate use is common (personal communication with a sangoma), but the disease is uncommon. Therefore there are unknown mechanisms at play which render the dichromate poison less toxic. It may be related to dose of dichromate, accompanying ingredients in the sangoma preparation or an individual's idiosyncratic metabolism.

Cresols

Transcutaneously absorbed substances may lead to severe toxic systemic effects. Substances, which fall into this category, include the phenols and the closely related compounds, cresols. The commercially available Jeyes fluid is a cresol. Jeyes fluid ingestion and administration by enema are well-documented forms of poisoning in South Africa. Berg et al. (personal communication) are the first in South Africa to describe the development of ATN following the transcutaneous absorption of a cresol. The case was a woman who may have presented to a healer (Berg cannot be sure that it was not a charlatan that was consulted) complaining of nausea. She was "painted" with a solution of Jeyes fluid. Whilst being painted she immediately lost consciousness and was taken to a nearby hospital. In addition to being deeply comatose, superficial chemical burns where noted on admission. Her vital signs were normal including a normal blood pressure. She regained consciousness after approximately 3 hours; her urine was bloody and she became oliguric. It was thought that she had aspirated and she was subsequently treated for pneumonia (confirmed on X-ray and located to the right upper lobe).

Examination of the urine revealed macroscopic blood and granular casts. Her serum biochemistry was abnormal with hyperkalemia and an elevated urea and creatinine. She ultimately required dialysis but recovered sufficient renal function within 3 days to allow cessation of dialysis therapy. In view of the close association between the exposure to the Jeyes fluid and the development of ATN, a renal biopsy was not performed and a causal role was assumed.

It appears that cresols are absorbed across intact skin [10]. Once absorbed, phenols are widely distributed throughout the body and are toxic to various cell types. Green reports on a one-year old child who died 4 hours following the accidental application of a phenol solution to his head. At post-mortem examination, the presence of the phenols in the internal organs was detectable by the typical odor of phenol [10]. ATN was also documented histologically. Bruce et al. document 2 cases of cresol poisoning and their resultant deaths [11].

Cantharidin

Is commonly known as Spanish fly and is derived from blister beetles. Karras speculates that it may be a more common cause of morbidity than is recognized [12]. It is used as a sexual stimulant and is an ingredient in some wart removal remedies [13]. Poisoning is noteworthy for its dramatic effect on the gastrointestinal and urinary tracts, as well as occasionally inducing cardiac abnormalities and seizures [12, 13]. The patient

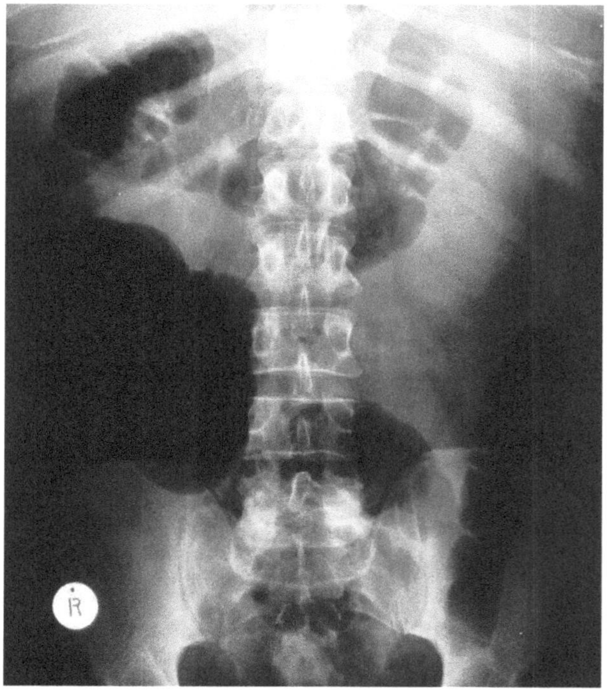

Figure 2. *Straight abdominal XRay illustrating a nephrogram (and dilated colon because of a concurrent colitis).*

may present with massive hematemesis and hematuria. The kidney is often involved with ATN and glomerular damage. Treatment is supportive and includes dialysis when indicated.

Ox-eye daisy or Impila (Callilepsis Laureola)

Seedat, in 1978 [14], concluded that the commonest medical causes of acute kidney injury in the east of South Africa were toxins. The toxins were mainly herbal in nature and the composition of the majority was unknown. However the best studied toxin from this area is the impila [15].

The **impila** (which means health in Zulu) bears a root similar to a sweet potato. It is harvested in winter and stored after drying and crushing. It is boiled in water for 30 min and thereafter administered either rectally or orally [2]. It is a multi-purpose muthi (medicine) and is given for general health, impotence and HIV symptoms. It is also believed that if the root is buried near a person's home, then it will intercept any evil directed towards that household [2].

Impila causes massive centrilobular liver necrosis with hypoglycemia and liver failure. It also causes acute tubular necrosis [16, 17]. Atractyloside is a component in the root of the impila and it is this substance, which has been demonstrated to cause acute tubular necrosis in rats [17].

Watson described 50 black children who had died following the administration of this toxin [16]. Post-mortem examination was conducted in all cases confirming the diagnosis of impila poisoning. No common trend was noted in the clinical presentation of these children. It was concluded that hypoglycemia and evidence of hepatic and renal dysfunction, were strong indicators of impila poisoning.

A substantial experience of toxin induced renal failure has been gained at the Chris Hani Baragwanath Hospital, Soweto. This 3000-bed teaching hospital serves approximately 4 million people from Soweto. Once again patients often visit traditional healers, usually prior to, or instead of consultation with a medical doctor [1, 18]. A study done at the hospital [Katz - personal communication] revealed that 13% of cases of AKI were caused by herbal toxins.

Segal and others reported on ritual-enema-induced colitis [19]. Their report incorporates 11 patients where the clinical hallmarks of the injury were peritonitis and rectal bleeding. The injury in some cases extended to involve the whole colon. Of the enema ingredients, potassium dichromate was prominent. Therefore this is a ubiquitous toxic substance used widely throughout South Africa. Other ingredients were vinegar, caustic soda and dettol. The severe cases were complicated by renal failure. Obviously – with the exception of the dichromates, which we know are directly nephrotoxic - the cause of the renal impairment was multifactorial. Sepsis probably played a major role in the pathogenesis of the acute kidney injury.

Males predominate in the group with herbal induced AKI. This observation is supported by a report from Zimbabwe describing the pattern of poisoning from traditional medicines in that country [20]. Apparently men resort to taking muthi because it is perceived as being manly and also because they have easier access to the sangomas than do women.

There is an interesting report [21], which described a male who presented in AKI after drinking one spoonful of a sangoma prescription. He had visited the sangoma with the complaint of vomiting and abdominal cramps. He required 2 months of dialysis and recovery was incomplete. A sample of the ingested compound was found to contain Cape Aloe. This was a surprise finding, since the aloe is considered to be safe. Therefore one must be cautious in interpreting this as the agent responsible for the AKI, since there may have been other substances present in the concoction, which could not be detected. An unanswered question here is what was the cause of the vomiting and cramps, which led the man to consult the sangoma in the first place? Did that have any deleterious, causal effect on renal function?

Aloes occur throughout the world. The genus Aloe includes herbs, shrubs and trees. The leaves are used for the preparation of medicine or cosmetics [9, 22, 23].

Cape aloe

This is a common species of aloe and is derived from Aloe ferox. It is reported to be the most extensively used plant substance as an herbal remedy in South Africa [9]. The aloe is also identified as one of the most commonly used herbal propriety products [22]. It is not considered toxic. Therefore the case [21] discussed above, must have had other additives that were not measurable or the "dose" may have been too high. Or, as must always be considered, did the original disease for which help was sought from the sangoma, not play a role in causing the AKI [31]?

To support its safety, Van Wyk [23] mentions the medicinal uses of the Cape aloe. The yellow juice from the leaves is dried and a small crystal (the size twice that of a match head) of the dried substance is taken orally as a laxative. Its use as a laxative has also been important from a commercial point of view. The export market has been a valuable source of revenue for SA. It may also be used for arthritis, but at a much smaller dose than that required for a catharsis. Van Wyk mentions that eczema, hypertension and stress have also been included in the list of indications for this product. One is uncertain as to how these indications were arrived at and whether there is any substantive evidence of efficacy, with the use of aloes, in the treatment of these conditions.

The active purgative ingredient in the aloe is called barbaloin. The barbaloin is a prodrug and once in the colon is it converted to the active substance, aloe-emodin anthrone [22, 23]. The conversion to active drug is facilitated by the colonic flora. The laxative action results from the inhibition of colonic Na–K-ATPase with the resultant increase in the water content of the colon.

Senecio

Rose described the toxicity of the senecio plant in 1972 [24]. It is the most common plant species to contain the pyrolizidine alkaloids. Toxicity includes hepatic necrosis and later intrahepatic veno-occlusion. A major secondary component is ATN. There are over 50 species of senecio plants in the south east of South Africa. The plants are used extensively as enemas and purgatives. Rose mentions that, despite the deaths resulting from the use of these plants, the local inhabitants are not aware of the danger these plants pose to their well-being.

Figure 3 is a photograph of a cow horn and segment of hollowed out reed. These objects in the photograph have actually been used in sangoma/inyanga treatment procedures. They were obtained from a sangoma practicing in Cape Town. They are the standard instruments used by the sangomas to administer the various herbal remedies, via the rectum. The Higginson's syringe has also been used [3]. The funnel-shape of the cow horn makes it easy to use this form of treatment – however we must remember the report from Segal [19] in which the complications of rectal perforation and colitis are ascribed to the instruments and methods used to administer treatments rectally. The hollowed out reed is only used in children. Here the prescribed solution is first aspirated into the hollow reed and the blackened tip is inserted into the rectum. The sangoma will then blow through the hollow reed forcing the herbal medicine into the rectum of the child.

Mercury

Barr in 1972, discussed the nephrotic syndrome in adult Africans in Nairobi [25]. In this report he showed that young, English-speaking women, with the nephrotic syndrome, were in the majority. They were able to separate these patients from the rest by the cosmetics that they used. In fact, more specifically, by the habit of applying skin lightning creams. On further analysis, it was found that they had used creams containing amino-mercuric chloride. Analysis of the urine revealed high levels of mercury. After cessation of the mercury containing creams, the urinary mercury levels rapidly fell to normal. This study was of interest in that only 12% of the biopsies obtained were diagnosed as membranous nephropathy. The majority (50%) had minimal change disease.

The mean duration of use of the creams before presentation with leg edema, was 13 months. The remission rate was 50% in those with minimal change

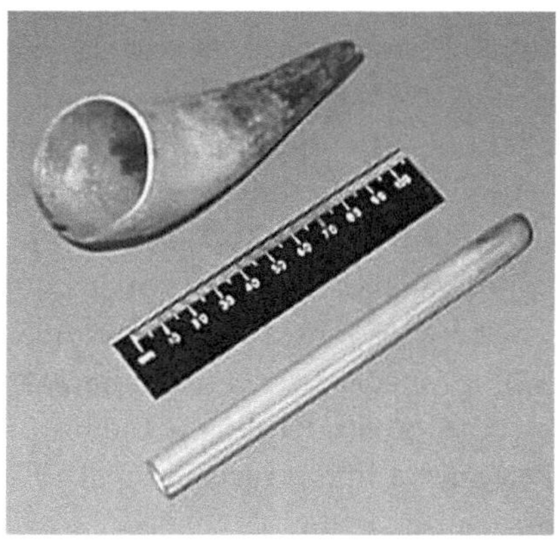

Figure 3. *Cow horn and hollow reid used by the traditional healers for the administration of herbal enemas.*

disease after withdrawal of the creams.

Human exposure is either to mercury vapor or methyl mercury compounds [26]. See also chapter 36. Both of these forms of mercury can lead to kidney involvement with nephrotic range proteinuria. The effect on the kidney is suggested to be on the basis of mercury-stimulated T lymphocytes [26]. These T lymphocytes produce damaging antibodies to the basement membrane with consequent heavy proteinuria. The damage may manifest as membranous nephropathy with the nephrotic syndrome [27, 28] or as minimal change disease [25]. Of importance, there are no case reports of nephrotoxicity resulting from exposure to mercury from amalgam tooth fillings [29].

There is no specific treatment for mercury poisoning of the kidneys but removal of the source of the metal is important. This maneuver may result in spontaneous improvement in 50% of cases [25]. Brown, in a study from Malawi, described the failure to improve in 2 out of 6 patients with membranous nephropathy who were known to have used skin creams [28]. This occurred despite removal from exposure to the mercury as well as the administration of steroids.

Paraphenylene diamine (hair dye)

This dye, paraphenylenediamine, when mixed with henna, blackens the hair in a very short time. The substance is a common cause of ATN in the Sudan [30]. It is also toxic to the heart and liver. It is absorbed through the skin but individuals have ingested the dye in suicide attempts. Within 3-4 hours after ingestion they develop angioneurotic oedema soon followed by renal failure. Renal biopsy shows the typical features of acute tubular necrosis. See chapter 40.

Sodium bromate

This compound is a constituent of hair waving/curling lotions used in the hairdressing salon for perms.

A male patient was admitted to our institution with a history of the intentional ingestion of the "American Look" hair preparation. It contained sodium bromate. He presented 2 days after ingestion with vomiting and deafness. There was no accompanying history of renal impairment, no past history of hypertension and he was not on regular medications. Progressive oliguric renal failure ensued, necessitating hemodialysis. His Hb fell from 7.9 to 2.4 over the course of 5 days and hemolysis was diagnosed. The clinical features in keeping with bromate toxicity were rapid onset of sensorineural deafness and acute kidney injury with progression to anuria [31]. The hemolysis stopped spontaneously and he eventually recovered renal function but remained totally deaf. He did not develop a peripheral neuropathy which is another toxic effect of bromate, as is hemolysis. The mechanisms are unknown.

Bromate is rapidly absorbed from the GIT and within 15 minutes maximum plasma levels are achieved. It is converted to bromide in liver and kidney by glutathione and excreted as bromate and predominantly bromide in urine. The potential toxicity is related to direct renal, cochlea and haematological damage. The exact mechanism of toxicity is unsure but is thought to be due to free radical formation. Ototoxicity, leading to sensorineural deafness may occur within 4 - 16 hrs of exposure [32]. Kidney histology shows epithelial separation in the proximal tubules under light microscopy. Electron microscopy confirms this separation but shows an intact basement membrane, in keeping with tubular necrosis [33]. The glomeruli are unaffected.

There has been a report suggesting that rapid removal of bromates, by hemodialysis, prevents the occurrence of irreversible hearing loss and post ATN renal dysfunction [34].

Copper Sulphate

Copper sulphate is a readily available chemical substance in Africa. It is widely used commercially in painting and the leather industry. The containers in which it is sold, clearly state "poisonous". The bright blue colour makes it attractive for children to want to taste and adults to ingest, either following on from an inyanga preparation or for suicidal purposes. There are reports of a suicide attempt using copper sulphate intravenously [35, 36]. The biggest reported series of poisoning comes from India [37, 38]. In Africa anecdotes are commonly mentioned but not substantiated in published reports.

The toxic effects on the kidneys occur via the induction of acute intravascular hemolysis with the development of acute tubular necrosis. One of the cases mentioned above, who administered the copper sulphate intravenously, had a kidney biopsy 8 weeks following on from presentation and this showed chronic tubulo-interstitial nephritis [36]. Hemodialysis is ineffective in removing copper as it rapidly enters red blood cells (it is also taken up by the liver where it is incorporated into ceruloplasmin). This copper-protein structure circulates until eventually metabolized and is excreted in bile. As for Wilson's disease, chelation treatment is recommended; Oldenquist and Salem (35) successfully used EDTA infusions. Takeda and his group [39] reported the successful use of chelation therapy (dimercaprol and penicillamine) together with hemoperfusion and hemodiafiltration in a patient with cupric sulphate intoxication.

Paraquat

This is a dipyridilium compound and is used as a herbicide. The common methods of paraquat poisoning are either accidental or with suicide intent. Mortality rates are high. The incidence however has decreased in South Africa when compared with the early 1980s (personal observation). It was particularly prevalent in the farming communities. Accidental poisoning resulting from drinking the solution from a softdrink bottle, in which the farmers had stored the poison, was not unusual.

The major toxic effect is on the lungs. The poison causes pulmonary oedema initially, followed by the rapid (within days) development of pulmonary fibrosis, respiratory failure and in most cases by this stage, death [40]. Renal failure usually ensues due to tubular necrosis (direct nephrotoxic effect and from shock and superimposed sepsis). There have been reports of paraquat-induced Fanconi syndrome [41] with severe hypophosphataemia and tubular necrosis on biopsy. The postulated mechanism was an effect of paraquat on the sodium-phosphate transporter in the proximal tubules. The patient made a full recovery after 23 days hospitalization. Intravenous phosphate was administered. An interesting report comes from Bairaktari and others [42]. In this article mention is made of nuclear magnetic resonance spectroscopy of urine from 2 patients who ingested paraquat intentionally. The investigators were able to confirm that the paraquat damage was to the pars recta of the proximal tubule. This may explain the pathogenesis of the development of the Fanconi syndrome [41].

Whilst hemodialysis does remove paraquat, it is far less efficient than charcoal hemoperfusion, which is the treatment of choice. 30% Fuller's earth (a diatomaceous earth) must be administered orally as soon as possible to act as a sorbent of the paraquat in the gut after oral ingestion. Cathartics are administered simultaneously.

The policy at our institution is to start hemoperfusion and administer Fuller's earth as soon as the patient arrives in the hospital and not to wait for the results of paraquat blood levels. This practice followed from the knowledge that prognosis is related to the plasma paraquat level and the duration of such levels [40].

An article from Korea [43], which reported on 147 patients following paraquat ingestion, showed that the mortality rate was high at 44.2%. The authors were able to show that certain laboratory parameters could predict poor outcome. It was suggested that with the aid of these parameters, unhelpful and invasive (hemoperfusion) treatments can be avoided (and by implication, the patients are beyond help). The parameters used as prognosticators were abnormal liver enzymes, renal dysfunction, metabolic acidosis and abnormal urine analysis. They were supported in this observation when Yamaguchi et al found – after examining laboratory data from 160 paraguat poisoning patients – that renal function and acid-base imbalance were useful in judging prognosis [44].

Crystal metamphetamine ("Tik") and methylenedioxymethamphetamine (MDMA, Ecstasy)

These amphetamines are used mostly as a recreational substance in "rave" parties and clubs. Crystal methamphetamine is also known as Ice, Straws, Globes and **Tik** (called tik, because of a clicking sound when heated), is cheap (price ranges from R30-R60) and is easily available in the streets of Cape Town. The crystals are large and are smoked from a heated light bulb from which the base and element have been removed. Crank and Speed are the same substance but are in powder form (smaller granules than Tik). Tik is structurally related to noradrenaline. It has an indirect sympathomimetic effect; it blocks the presynaptic reuptake of dopamine and noradrenaline. The increased catecholamine activity causes intense systemic vasoconstriction and the stimulant effects are longlasting (up to 12 hours). There is an accompanying "rush 'causing a state of high self-esteem and agitation.

A 21 year old male presented to the emergency room complaining of vomiting, diarrhea, headache and visual disturbances. There was a strong history of recreational drug abuse and included mostly Tik, but also ecstasy, cocaine and cannabis. He occasionally used alcohol. His blood pressure was recorded at 220/140 mmHg in both arms. The examination findings of note were on fundoscopy and included retinal infarcts, bleeds and papilloedema. ECG evidence of hypertension was present. Blood biochemistry revealed normal electrolytes but an elevated urea of 59 mmol/L and a creatinine at a high of 2394 umol/L. He had a markedly elevated serum creatinine kinase (in keeping with rhabdomyolysis) HBV, HCV and HIV serology were negative. An ultrasound examination of his kidneys showed them to be equal and normal sized but reported that they were highly echogenic. A renal biopsy confirmed advanced interstitial fibrosis and tubular fall-out. There were areas of tubular necrosis and all glomeruli seen were sclerosed. The vessels showed hypertensive changes. A CT scan of the brain found multiple low densities in both grey and white matter in keeping with hypertensive damage. His blood pressure was very easily controlled on two agents and dialysis. The patient became dialysis dependent. The presentation could have been that of end-stage glomerulonephritis; however there was no preceding history or report of a clinical examination prior to his admission to confirm this. The ease of blood pressure control once the substance abuse was halted, leads one to believe that the hypertension was possibly consequent on Tik abuse. He additionally used ecstasy, which may have played a synergistic role, with Tik inhalation, in the pathogenesis of the hypertension and kidney disease.

Recreational drugs cause a spectrum of glomerular, interstitial and vascular diseases

The effects of amphetamines on the kidney are mainly acute tubular necrosis on the basis of rhabdomyolysis (with myoglobinuria) and a disseminated intravascular coagulopathy. But, malignant hypertension and the resultant effects on the kidneys, must always be a consideration in the differential diagnosis of renal failure [45-50]. These effects are likely to be chronic and irreversible. Bingham et al reported a case of necrotising vasculopathy after the ingestion of both "tik" and "ecstasy" [51]. A renal biopsy confirmed the presence of fibrinoid necrosis involving arterioles and small arteries. The lumina were occluded by intimal thickening. The glomeruli contained necrotising lesions. The hepatitis serology was negative in this patient. The association with Hepatitis B and C and drug abuse (intravenous use with contaminated needles) is well known; Hepatitis C may give rise to a mesangiocapillary glomerulonephritis (MCGN) with cryoglobulinaemia. Methamphetamine-induced acute interstitial nephritis has also been described [52]. Hyperpyrexia and hyponatraemia are other complications encountered in cases of amphetamine abuse [53, 54]. The hyponatraemia results from water intoxication or inappropriate ADH secretion.

Ethylene glycol

Ethylene glycol (EG) is the constituent found in all anti-freeze products. It is commonly used for suicidal intent, or taken by mistake or drank in the belief that it is alcohol. Ethylene glycol is toxic to the kidneys, producing acute tubular necrosis and nephrocalcinosis. The early impressions were that the metabolic product - oxalate - was responsible for the renal impairment. However work on the proximal tubular segments of the mouse kidney, has shown that glycoaldehyde and glyoxylate are responsible for EG nephrotoxicity [55]. This pathogenetic mechanism is via the depletion of ATP. Studies from Prague have reiterated the known fact that concurrent ethanol use with the EG - or the administration of ethanol soon after EG intake - improves the outcome [56-57]. Recovery is expected and supportive dialysis is recommended when necessary. However the lethal blood level of EG is 2 g/L, resulting in multi-organ failure [57].

Steenkamp and Stewart have published an excellent article, providing guidance on the use of analytic methods, to examine the constituents of plants [58]. Some of the constituents so analysed have not been shown to produce toxicity in humans. Clearly they have the potential to produce adverse effects, but as we know with dichromates, administration of the toxin does not always produce adverse effects in humans. Most of what follows is derived from this article [58].

Europe was stunned with the outbreak of Chinese herb nephropathy. There have been no reports from Africa and - because of the superb epidemiological work done to find the culprit and to advertise its toxicity - it may well turn out to be a toxin that does not reach Africa. Aristocholic acid (AA) is a naturally occurring carcinogen and nephrotoxin; it induces a chronic relentlessly progressive tubulo-interstitial nephritis ([59]. The toxic effects caused a number of Belgian women to become dialysis dependent. They took a Chinese herb, contaminated by AA, in the belief that the herb was a safe slimming agent. Steroids slow the progressive nature of the disease [60].

Yams (make up the everyday diet for many in Africa. It is therefore surprising to learn that they contain a toxic substance called dioscorine(, which has convulsive properties and causes hepatic and renal failure [61, 62]. The toxicity is related to the incomplete preparation of the food.

Khat leaf ((Catha Edulis) (chewing is common in East Africa and the Yemen. It produces renal toxicity in rabbits [63]. The leaves contain S-Cathinone (which is metabolised to norephidrine and norpseudoephidrine [64]. No reports of human cases of nephrotoxic adverse effects can be found.

Violet tree

Violet tree ((Wild Wisteria) (has produced poisoning in the Congo. The roots of this plant when taken orally or intravaginally, in search for a cure for dysmenorrhoea, can produce renal ischaemia and death [9] A strychnine-(like substance has been found in the root; additionally a high concentration of methyl salicylate (is found in the oils from the root [9, 58].

Discussion

The study and identification of all the herbal medicines in Africa will be an important contribution to the well-being of the majority of the population. Collaboration with the sangomas is ongoing but limits in the financial capabilities of organizations make it a slow process of accumulating information. The benefits from such collaboration are not limited to defining a therapeutic option, but also will provide education on the culture behind the sangoma/inyanga influence.

The existence of "secret" formulations handed down in families of sangomas/inyangas is still another stumbling block in the analysis of traditional medicines. The belief exists among these traditional healers, that once the "secret" is known, the "medicine" will then lose its power. This must be counteracted by evidence of efficacy.

There is much distrust of traditional healers. This is perhaps justified in some instances; it is particularly relevant when no formal register of traditional healers is in place. Traditional healers are therefore not held accountable.

In turn, Savage and Hutchings [65] point out the failings of the western-style doctors. Many symptoms are unfairly ascribed to the herbal treatment administered. The original disease for which the aid of the sangoma is sought, is often ignored. This situation was described as "an aloof attitude of mild contempt" by Savage and Hutchings [65].

Only once trust is established will the necessary knowledge be made available for the benefit of all those who prescribe medicines. Steenkamp and Stewart provide guidance for analysis of suspected toxins [58]. Unfortunately, the costs of such analyses will not be borne by the South African government and only privately-funded or/and university endeavours will enable any meaningful investigation into the ingredients of presumed toxic concoctions.

Ongoing education against the dangers of substance abuse must continue at school level and in the home. The widespread use of Tik and others has lead to the situation where any individual, admitted to the emergency room, with severe hypertension, must be questioned about the use of amphetamines.

Industrial chemicals must be safeguarded from the general public and information - on the dangers of these substances - advertised in the media for the population to be adequately informed.

Acknowledgements

We are indebted to the contribution made by the co-authors of this chapter in the 2nd Ed of Clinical Nephrotoxins. This edition has built on their contribution and the work has been enlarged and updated.

References

1. Joubert PH. Poisoning admissions of Black South Africans. Clin Toxicology 1990; 28(1): 85-94.
2. Bye SN, Dutton MF. The inappropriate use of traditional medicines in South Africa. J Ethnopharmacol 1991; 34: 253-259.
3. Wood R, Mills PB, Knobel GJ, Hurlow WE, Stokol JM. Acute dichromate poisoning after use of traditional purgatives. A report of seven cases. S Afr Med J 1990; 77: 640-642.
4. De Smet PAGM. Is there any danger in using traditional remedies? J Ethnopharmacol 1991; 32: 43-50.
5. Perharic L, Shaw D, Colbridge M, House I, Leon C, Murray V. Toxicological problems resulting from exposure to traditional remedies and food supplements. Drugs Safety 1994; 11(4): 284-294.
6. Larrey D. Hepatotoxicity of herbal remedies. J of Hepatol 1997; S26: 47-51.
7. Chan TYK. Monitoring the safety of herbal medicines. Drug Safety 1997; 17(4): 209-214.
8. De Smet PAGM. The role of plant-derived drugs and herbal medicines in healthcare. Drugs 1997; 54(6): 801-840.
9. Watt JM, Breyer-Brandwijk MG. The medicinal and poisonous plants of Southern and Eastern Africa. Livingstone, Edinburgh, 1962.
10. Green MA. A household remedy misused – fatal cresol poisoning following cutaneous absorption (a case report). Med Sci Law 1975; 15(1): 65-66.
11. Bruce AM, Smith H, Watson AA. Cresol poisoning. Med Sci Law 1976; 16(3): 171-176.
12. Karras DJ, Farrell SE, Harrigan RA, Henretig FM, Gealt L. poisoning from "Spanish fly" (cantharidin) 1996; 14(5): 478-483.
13. Till JS, Majmudar BN. Canthanridin poisoning. South Med J. 1981; 74(4): 444-447.
14. Seedat YK. Acute renal failure among blacks and Indians in South Africa. S Afr Med J 1978; 54: 427-431.
15. Bhoola KDN. A clinicopathological and biochemical study of the toxicity of Callilepsis laureola (impila). MD thesis. University of Natal 1983.
16. Watson AR, Coovadia HM, Bhoola KD. The clinical syndrome of Impila (Callilepis laureola) poisoning in children. S Afr Med J 1979; 55: 290-293.
17. Wainwright J, Schonland MM, Candy HA. Toxicity of Callilepsis laureola. S Afr Med J 1977; 52: 313-315.
18. Buchanan N, Cane RD. Poisoning associated with witchdoctor attendance. S Afr Med J 1976; 50: 1138-1140.
19. Segal I, Tim LO, Hamilton DG, Lawson HH, Solomon A, Kalk F, Cooke SAR. Ritual –enema-induced colitis. Dis Col Rect 1979; 22(5): 195-199.
20. Kasilo OMJ and Nhachi CFB. The pattern of poisoning from traditional medicines in urban Zimbabwe. S Afr Med J 1992; 82: 187-188.
21. Luyckx VA, Ballantine R, Claeys M, Cuyckens F, Van den Heuvel H, Cimanga RK, Vlietinck AJ, De Broe ME, Katz IJ. Herbal remedy - associated acute renal failure secondary to Cape aloes (Case report). Am J Kidney Dis 2002; 39(3): E13 (www.ajkd.org).
22. Iwu MM. Handbook of African Medicinal Plants. CRC press 1993.
23. Van Wyk B-E, Van Oudtshoorn B, Gericke N. Medicinal plans of South Africa, 1st edition. Briza publications 1997.
24. Rose EF. Senecio species: toxic plants used as food and medicines in the Transkei. S Afr Med J 1972;1039-1043.
25. Barr RD, Rees PH, Cordy PE, Kungu A, Woodger BA, Cameron HM. Nephrotic syndrome in adult Africans in Nairobi. B Med J 1972; 2: 131-134.
26. Clarkson TW. Mercury-an element of mystery. N Engl Med J 1990; 323(16): 1137.
27. Oliviera DBG, Foster G, Savill J, Syme PD, Taylor A. Membranous nephropathy caused by mercury-containing skin lightening cream. Postgr Med J 1987; 63: 303-304.
28. Brown KGE, Abrahams C, Meyers AM. The nephrotic syndrome in Malawian Blacks. S Afr Med J 1977; 55: 275-278.
29. Sandborgh-Englund G, Nygren AT, Ekstrand L, Elinder CG. No evidence of renal toxicity from amalgam fillings. Am J Physiol 1996; 271(4 pt 2): R941-R945.
30. Suleiman SM, Homeida M, Aboud OI. Paraphenylenediamine induced acute tubular necrosis following hair-dye ingestion. Hum Toxicol 1983; 2(4): 633-635.
31. Sashiyama H, Irie Y, Ohtake Y, Nakajima K, Yoshida H, Sakai T, Okuda K. Acute renal failure and hearing loss die to sodium bromate poisoning: a case report and review of the literature. Clin Nephrol 2002; 58(6): 455-457.
32. Campbell KC. Bromate-induced ototoxicity. Toxicology 2006; 221(2-3):205 – 211
33. Watanabe T, Abe T, Satoh M, Oda Y, Takada T, Yanagihara T. Two children with bromate intoxication due to ingestion of the second preparation for permanent hair waving. Acta Paediatr Jpn 1992;34(6):601-605.
34. Uchida HA, Sugiyama H, Kanehisa S, Harada K, Fujiwara K, Ono T, Yamakido M, Makino H. An elderly patient with severe acute renal failure due to sodium bromate intoxication. Intern Med 2006; 45(3):151-154.
35. Oldenquist G and Salem M. Parenteral copper sulphate poisoning causing acute renal failure. Nephrol Dial Transplant 1999;14:441-443

36. Bhowmik D, Mathur R, Bhargava Y, Dinda AK, Agarwal SK, Tiwari SC, Das SC. Chronic interstitial nephritis following parenteral copper sulphate poisoning. Ren Fail 2001;23(5):731-735
37. Chugh KS, Sharma BK, Singhal PC, Das KC, Datta BN. Acute renal failure following copper sulphate intoxication. Postgrad Med J 1977;53(615):18-23.
38. Chugh KS, Singal PC, Sharma BK, Makakur AC, Pal Y, Datta BN, Das KC. Acute renal failure due to intravascular hemolysis in the North Indian patients. Am J Med Sci 1977; 274(2):139-146.
39. Takeda T, Yukioka T, Shimazaki S. Cupric sulphate intoxication with rhabdomyolysis, treated with chelating agents and blood purification. Intern Med 2000;39(3):253-255.
40. Proudfoot AT, Stewart MS, Levitt T, Widdop B. Paraquat poisoning: significance of plasma-paraquat concentrations. Lancet 1979;2:330-332.
41. Gil HW, Yang JO, Lee EY, Hong SY. Case report. Paraquat-induced Fanconi syndrome.Nephrology 2005;10:430-432.
42. Bairaktari E, Katapodis K, Siamopoulos KC, Tsolas O. Paraquat-induced renal injury studied by 1H nuclear magnetic resonance spectroscopy of urine. Clinical Chemistry 1998;44(6):1256-1261.
43. Hong S-Y, Yang D-H, Hwang K-Y. Associations between laboratory parameters and outcome of paraquat poisoning. Toxicology Letters 2000;118:53-59 (www.elsevier.com/locate/toxlet)
44. Yamaguchi H, Shigehito S, Watanabe S, Naito H. Pre-embarkment prognostication for acute paraquat poisoning. Hum Exp Toxicol 1990;9:381-384.
45. Karch SB, Stephens BG, Ho CH. Methamphetamine-related deaths in San Francisco: demographic, pathologic, and toxicologic profiles. J Forensic Sci 1999;44:359–368.
46. Ruttenber AJ, McAnally HB, Wetli CV. Cocaine-associated rhabdomyolysis and excited delirium: different stages of the same syndrome. Am J Forensic Med Pathol 1999;20:120–127.
47. Richards JR. Rhabdomyolysis and drugs of abuse. J Emerg Med 2000;19:51–56.
48. Kendrick WC, Hull AR, Knochel JP. Rhabdomyolysis and shock after intravenous amphetamine administration. Ann Intern Med 1977;86:381–387.
49. Richards JR, Johnson EB, Stark RW, Derlet RW. Meth-amphetamine abuse and rhabdomyolysis in the ED: a 5-year study. Am J Emerg Med 1999;17:681–68
50. Fahal IH, Sallomi DF, Yaqoob M, Bell GM. Acute renal failure after ecstasy. BMJ 1992; 305(6844):29.
51. Bingham C, Beaman M, Nicholls AJ, Anthony PP. Necrotising renal vasculopathy resulting in chronic renal failure after ingestion of methampethamine and 3, 4- methylenedioxymethamphetamine ('ecstasy'). Nephrol Dial Transplant 1998;13:2654-2655.
52. Foley RJ, Kapatkin K, Verani R, Weinman EJ. Amphetamine-induced acute renal failure. South Med J 1984;77:258-259.
53. White SR. Amphetamine toxicity. Semin Respir Crit Care Med 2002;23(1):27-36.
54. Milroy CM, Clark JC, Forrest AR. Pathology of deaths associated with "ecstasy" and "eve" misuse. J Clin Pathol 1996;49(2):149-153.
55. Poldelsky V, Johnson A, Wright S, Rosa VD, Zager RA. Ethylene glycol-mediated tubular injury; identification of critical metabolites in injury pathways. Am J Kidney Dis 2001;38(2):339-348.
56. Krenova M, Pelclova D. Course of intoxications due to concurrent ethylene glycol and ethanolic ingestion. Przegl Lek. 2005;62(6):508-510
57. Krenova M, Pelclova D, Navratil T, Merta M. Experiences of the Czech toxicological information centre with ethylene glycol poisoning. Biomed Pap Med Fac Univ Palacky Olomouc Czech Repub. 2005;149(2):473-475.
58. Steenkamp V and Stewart MJ. Nephrotoxicity associated with exposure to plant toxins, with particular reference to Africa. Ther Drug Monit 2005;27(8):270-277.
59. Vankerweghem JL, Depierreux M, Tielemans C, et al. Rapidly progressive interstitial renal fibrosis in young women; association with slimming regimen including Chinese herbs. Lancet 1993;41:387-391.
60. Vanherweghem JL, Abromowicz D, Tielemans C, Depierreux M. Effects of steroids on the progression of renal failure in chronic interstitial renal fibrosis: a pilot study in Chinese herbs nephropathy. Am J Kidney Dis 1996;27:209-215.
61. Neuwinger HD. African ethnobotany. Poisons and drugs. London:Chapman and Hall 1996.
62. Bevan CWL and Hirst J. A convulsant alkaloid of Discorea Dumetorum. 1958;25:103.
63. Al-Mamary A, Al-Habori M, Al-Aghbari AM. Investigation into the toxicological effects of Catha Edulis: a short term study in animals. Phytother.Res. 2002;16:127-132.
64. Brenneisen R, Geisshuslers S, Schorno X. Metabolism of cathinone to (-) norephedrine and (-) norpseudoephedrine. J Pharm Pharmacol 1986;38:298-300.
65. Savage A, Hutchings A. Poisoned by herbs. Br Med J 1987; 295; 1650-1651.

40

Paraphenylene diamine hair dye poisoning

Mohamed I. HAMDOUK[1], Mohamed B. ABDELRAHEEM[2], Ahbab A. TAHA[1], Mohamed BENGHANEM[3] and Marc E. DE BROE[4]

[1]Bahry Renal Centre, Khartoum, Sudan
[2]Soba University Hospital, University of Khartoum, Sudan
[3]Ibn Rochd University Hospital Center, Casablanca, Morocco
[4]University of Antwerp, Belgium

Introduction

Since 1883, paraphenylene diamine (PPD) has traditionally been used for dyeing (dark color) hair in Europe [1-2] as a fresh preparation mixed with hydrogen peroxide (H_2O_2) [3]. In Sudan PPD is used by women to color their hair and as a body dye when added to henna (*Lawasonia alba*). Henna on it's own need to be applied two or three times for several hours to give the desired color (dark red or black). In contrast this can be achieved with one single application in less than one hour by adding PPD to the henna. The toxicity of PPD, when added to henna occurs through skin absorption. This toxicity can not be attributed to henna, (*L. Alba*) which is a herb used for cosmetic purposes and also used in folk medicine for the treatment of some skin diseases, as an antiinflammatory, antipyretic and analgesic agent [4-5]. In Morocco, Takaout beldia indicates a non-toxic vegetable product extracted from the gallnut of Tamaris Orientalis (Figure 1). This non-toxic substance is highly appreciated by women for its hair dyeing properties. Its rarefaction resulted in the use of paraphenylene diamine as substitute under the name of Takaout Erroumia. If nowadays accidental ingestion is exceptional, its use for suicidal attempt in young women in Morocco and Tunisia is increasing [6].

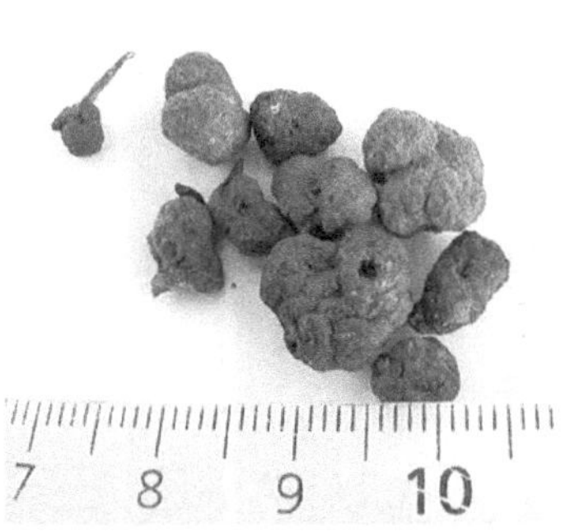

Figure 1. *Natural Takaout beldia (Morocco).*

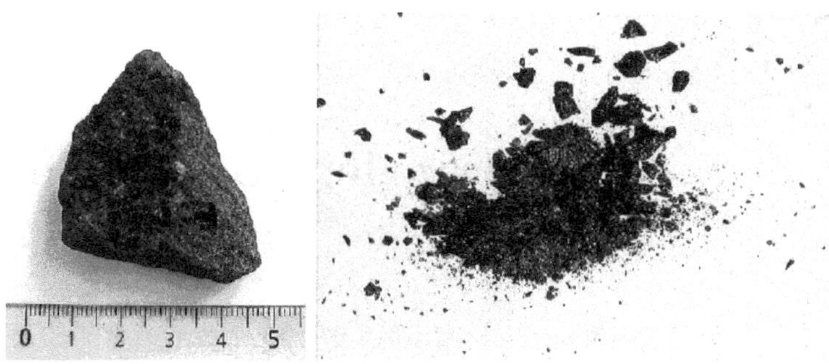

Figure 2. *PPD from the local market.*

For the last seventy-five years the dermatological effects of PPD are well studied and as a result of these studies the European Union restricted the concentration of PPD in hair dye formulations to a maximum of 6% [3]. Systemic intoxication is not well studied although there are many studies of its mutagenicity and carcinogenicity [7-8]. Its ingestion is responsible for a respiratory (cervico-facial edema), muscular (rhabdomyolysis) and a renal syndrome (acute kidney injury due to hypovolemia and myoglobulinuria). The respiratory syndrome mainly determines its prognosis.

Paraphenylene diamine characteristics

Paraphenylene diamine (PPD) [$C_6H_4\,(NH_2)_2$] is an aromatic amine not found in nature. It is a derivative of paranitroanaline and it is available in the form of white crystals when pure and rapidly turns to brown when exposed to air [9]. Paraphenylene diamine has a molecular weight of 108 Dalton; its boiling point is 267°C and melting point 140°C. It is soluble in ethanol, ether, benzene, chloroform, and acetone and with agitation in water [10].

Rinne and Zinke first prepared PPD in 1874 by reducing 1,4 dinitrobenzene with tin and hydrochloric acid. Now it is produced commercially by reducing 1-amino-4-nitrobenzene by (1) iron and hydrochloric acid or (2) iron, ammonium polysulphide and hydrogen or (3) iron and ferrous chloride [2].

PPD is used in a variety of industrial products. Along with its derivatives, it has important antioxidant actions - used in the manufacturing of synthetic and natural rubbers, petroleum products, cellulose ethers and alfalfa meals [2]. PPD also has commercial application as photographic developers and in a variety of antioxidants and is also used in dyeing furs and for printing of cellulosic textile materials. PPD hydrochloride has been used as an analytical reagent in the testing of blood, hydrogen sulphide, amyl alcohol and milk [11].

PPD is used in hair dye formulations and can produce a variety of shades depending on the formulation. The concentration of PPD in hair dye formulation range from 0.20% in golden blond dyes to 3.75% in black hair dyes. Exact concentrations of PPD in different formulations are not known because most hair dye formulations are proprietary.

For safety reasons, different occupational health authorities, in the countries where PPD is produced, have developed standards regarding the degree of air contamination. It has been stated that employees' exposure to PPD should not exceed 0.1 mg/m^2 in the working atmosphere in any eight-hour work shift of forty-hour week. This is the maximum allowable concentration in Germany, Japan and UK [9].

Pharmaco-toxicology

PPD has two modes of reactions by which it has a biological effect:

Oxidation: PPD gives benzoquinone imines as a result of oxidation. The imines react rapidly with the couplers (another chemical material in the formulation) and/or an oxidized PPD to produce indo dyes. The most frequent couplers are 2, 4-diaminoanisole (blue forming coupler), resorcinol (green brown), metaminophenol (magenta/brown) and 1-naphtol (purple blue color). The most commonly used oxidant is hydrogen peroxide. Free ammonia is present to promote the oxidation reaction and the pH of the mixture on the dyed area is about 9.5 [3].

Deamination: Deamination has been suggested as a

mode of action of PPD, which results in the production of aniline, which may contribute in part to the toxic effects of the compound [12].

PPD induces one of the most severe edema both in humans and animal studies. The edema appears to be grossly specific and selectively localized in the head and neck. It was suggested that the toxic effect of the PPD might be produced by the conversion of the PPD on mucus surfaces to its oxidation product quinondimine, which is responsible for intense local irritation [13]. Some authors believed that PPD toxicity is due to some effect either on the blood colloids or on vascular permeability [15]. Also it was believed that the PPD toxicity is due to altered vascular permeability and involvement of the parasympathetic nervous system [13]. Deamination and formation of analine is claimed to be responsible in part for the toxic symptoms [12]. These different views as to the cause of PPD edema appear to be due to the fact that the exact number and nature of the oxidation products is not known [14].

At high concentrations and after a long period of exposure PPD produces cell death. This effect together with lipid peroxidation can be the cause of the production of superoxide and hydrogen peroxide by the autooxidation of PPD [15].

It was proved that at non-toxic doses, PPD induces intercellular adhesion molecule-1 (ICAM-1) expression on the keratinocytes [16]. These results were consistent with the view that oxidative stress may be an essential part of the pre-immunological phase in the induction of the allergic contact dermatitis by PPD [16].

PPD can cause methemoglobinemia by oxidation of the ferrous form (Fe^{2+}) of hemoglobin to the ferric (Fe^{3+}) form. Aniline, nitrobenzene, phenacetin and other nitro and amino organic compounds are powerful methemoglobin formers.

From the studies of the intracutaneous sensitization of guinea pigs using PPD, hydroquinone, quinhydrone and benzoquinone it has been suggested that benzoquinone formation plays an important role in the allergic action of PPD [15].

Studies in rats demonstrate that subcutaneous administration of 3 mg of the PPD hydrochloride induces skeletal muscle lesions in the form of rhabdomyolysis with infiltration of inflammatory cells, necrosis and accumulation of neutral lipids and dilatation of sacroplasmic reticulum [17].

In rats, teratogenicity was studied by testing four commercially available hair dye formulations containing 1, 2, 3 and 4% PPD and several aromatic amine derivatives among their constituents [18]. No abnormal foetal effects were noted, except with the formulation containing 2% PPD, which induced skeletal deformities [18].

Experimental studies in guinea pigs when dermally exposed to PPD revealed that, PPD is absorbed through the skin into the serum and excreted in the urine. There was an increase in malondialdehyde (MDA), which indicates lipid peroxidation, suggesting that increased free radical formation is responsible for the histopathologically tissue damage in the kidney, liver and skin [15]. The increase in histamine level in the blood is a sign of hypersensitive reaction associated with increased permeability of the Mast cells [15]. There were also increased activities of the cytoplasmic enzymes AST and ALT and that of tyrosinase, observed in skin following repeated exposure to PPD. This indicates a metabolic disturbance in amino acid metabolism, which may be responsible for the epidermal thickening and erythematous changes [15].

There are many reports about the dark coloration of urine after topical application of commercial hair dye formulations containing PPD. It was shown that PPD is excreted in urine after topical application [19]. It is believed that the darkening of urine was caused by oxidizing agents and was taken as evidence of the excretion of unchanged PPD [19].

It was found that the LD50 of PPD was 250 mg/kg bw in rabbits and 100 mg/kg/BW in cats. The subcutaneous LD50 was found to be 170 mg/kg bw in rats, 200 mg/kg bw in rabbits and 100 mg/kg bw in dogs. The intraperitoneal LD50 was found to be 37 mg/kg bw in rats [3]. The lethal dose for humans was estimated to be 10 grams of pure PPD [6].

Clinical presentation

Epidemiology

In Sudan, PPD in its pure form (90-99%) is available in the local markets and there are no restrictions for its use or trade (Figure 2).

The major problem of PPD toxicity results from the ingestion of the compound accidentally, in suicidal or homicidal attempts. However, there are some reported cases of severe intoxication after topical application of

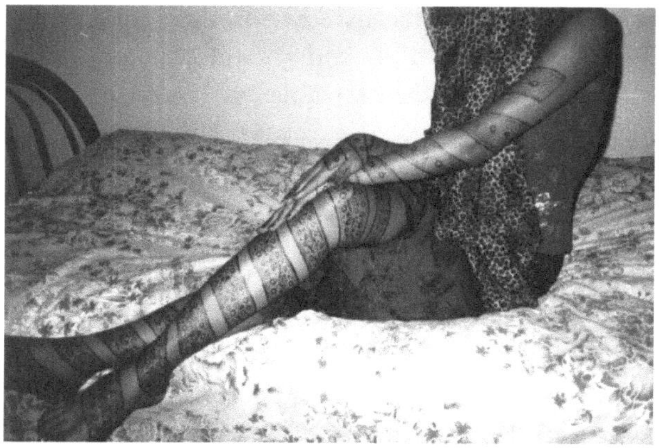

Figure 3. *Intoxication due to massive topical use (Sudan).*

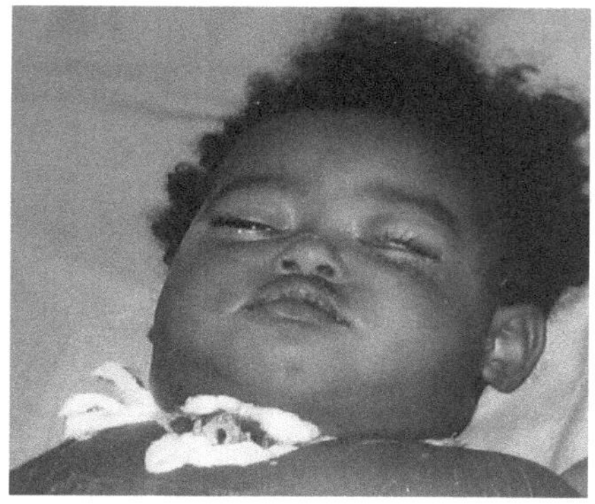

Figure 4. *Accidental PPD intoxication in a child.*

the pure PPD mixed with henna or for dyeing hair [20] (Figure 3). In a recent study, PPD intoxication due to inhalation was seen in 2.7% [21]. Samples of the PPD collected from the local market were found to have a purity of 97% when analyzed [6]. A survey of suicidal attempts in Khartoum, the capital of Sudan, in the period 1987-1990 revealed a number of 264 cases, with an age range between 10 to 30 years. In 35% of these cases PPD was used [22]. In reported series of 24 patients who presented with PPD intoxication and were admitted to Om Durman hospital in Sudan within a period of 12 months, twelve patients took the PPD intentionally and eight of them died [23]. Over a period of 2 years a series of 18 cases were reported in Khartoum North Hospital and there were two babies among them aged eighteen months, 70% were suicidal attempts. The mortality rate in this series was 22% [6]. A number of 150 cases with PPD intoxication had been admitted to the renal unit in Khartoum Teaching Hospital from 1985 to 1995. Sixty percent of them developed ARF requiring dialysis [24].

Recent statistics from the ENT teaching hospital in Khartoum from 1995 to 2005 showed that the total number of patients admitted with PPD intoxication was 3159 patient with an average of 287.1 per year. The common age group affected was 15 - 24 years (52%), this was shown also in other studies [21]. There was a predominance of females 80.7%, and the majority of cases 87% were due to suicidal attempts. The average mortality rate over 10 years was 10.6% peaking up to 27% in 1995 and declining to 5.5% in 2005 which reflects better care.

A 10 year review of acute PPD intoxication during 1989 to 1999 from Wad Medani (Main Gazira State hospital-Sudan), revealed 122 cases. 93.4% was due to suicidal intent and 3.3% was due to accidental and homicidal equally, 90% of the cases were females. The mortality rate was 22.1% [25].

The experience of PPD intoxication in children is even worse. A reported series of 31 Sudanese children between 1984 and 1989, all children presented with acute and severe angioneurotic oedema, 15 required tracheotomy. ARF was reported in 5 children and the mortality rate was 41% and most children died within the first 24 hours. [27]. In another report of Wad Medani teaching hospital 2.6% from their series were children and the common cause of poisoning was accidental [25] (Figure 4). Statistics from the ENT teaching hospital in Khartoum from 1995 to 2005 showed that of 3159 patient admitted with PPD intoxication 568.6 (18%) were children below the age of 14 years. In a report from the poison control centre of Morocco, PPD intoxication was reported in 43 (11.5%) children below the age of 15 years. [21]

In Morocco, intoxication with PPD is a major health problem. A reported series of 171 cases of PPD poisoning admitted to the medical resuscitation service in Ibn Roshd hospital between January 1994 and October 1997. In this series, there were 5 men and 166 women, with a mean age around 26 years. Twenty four percent of the patients developed severe ARF and 55 deaths (38.7%) were observed in this study [26]. In 90% of the cases PPD was ingested in the context of a suicidal attempt. The amount ingested varied between 3 and 15 grams.

Recent evolution of the problem from the Poison

control centre of Morocco (1992 - 2002) reported 374 cases. There were female predominance 77%, the majority of poisoning was intentional 78.1% and the younger population 15-25 years accounted for 54.3%. The mortality rate remained high 21.1% [21]

Cases with PPD poisoning were reported in the UK, France, Israel, Japan and other countries [28-32].

Clinical features and systemic toxicity

Acute systemic toxicity

Cases reported with systemic toxicity of PPD had shown various clinical manifestations as well as biochemical and histological changes, the intoxication represents 30% of the intensive care admittance. It was the second reason for hospitalization in the intensive care unit of the Casablanca University hospital in 1999 and the first reason for admission in the emergency unit (Portes Médicales) of Rabat University hospital in 2003. Acute poisoning by PPD ingestion is ranked amongst the most frequent causes of suicidal poisoning requiring hospitalization in Morocco [21]. Patients with acute poisoning have a characteristic presentation of painless swelling of the face and neck with bulging eyes, a swollen dry hard protruding tongue and chocolate brown colour of the urine (25). The onset of symptoms usually occurs within hours of ingestion or contact with the dye. The frequency of clinical manifestations seen in Sudanese and Moroccan experience is seen in Tables 1 and 2 [25-26].

Nephrotoxicity

The kidneys are particularly vulnerable to effects of noxious agents because of their high perfusion rate. Renal damage induced by chemicals is well known. Renal lesions associated with PPD intoxication received much attention because most of the clinical investigators reported renal failure [6, 34-35]. Experimental studies in mice exposed to PPD showed no histological changes in the kidneys [37]. However, evidence of severe nephrotoxicity has been reported in humans [25-28]. Histological changes typical of acute tubular necrosis have been also reported [39]. A case report of systemic vasculitis and crescentic glomerulonephritis has been published in patients chronically exposed to henna containing PPD [40]. In a prospective study performed in Khartoum Kidney Dialysis Centre and Sheffield Kidney Institute 19 renal biopsies out of a series of 23 patients with severe (39%), moderate (35%) and mild intoxication (26%) were studied under light microscopy. Glomerular injury observed in 94% of the biopsies in the form of hypercellularity, membranous proliferation, glomerular swelling, and capsular drop and accentuated lobular architecture [41]. Tubular lesions were found in 78.9% of the studied samples. Different epithelial necrosis is the most common lesion observed (78.9%) while tubular atrophy had been found in (15.8%) of the studied samples. Interstitial lesions were observed in 16 samples from the studied biopsies (84.2%). Focal inflammation (neutrophils and eosinophils) was the most common injury (47.3%). No vascular injury was observed in all of the studied biopsies [41].

Dermatological manifestations

PPD is a top listed allergen [42-43]. It is well known to cause irritation and dermatitis when conveyed to the skin of susceptible people [12, 30]. Erythematous

Table 1. Frequency of clinical symptoms observed in 171 patients with PPD intoxication in Morocco.

Clinical symptoms	Percentage
Oedema	94%
Acute respiratory insufficiency - Trachial intubations (72%) - Tracheostomy (21%)	56%
Signs of rhabdomyolysis	88%
Gastrointestinal symptoms (abdominal pain)	53%
Oliguric acute renal failure	32%

Table 2. Presenting symptoms and signs in 122 patients with PPD intoxication in Sudan.

Presenting signs and symptoms	No. of Patients	Percentage
Angioneurotic edema and stridor	50	41%
Dark discoloration of urine	122	100%
Flaccid paraplagia	51	42%
Convulsions	5	4%
Cranial nerve palsies (Bulbar)	10	8%
Abdominal pains	20	17%

urticarial papules, plaques and target lesions (erythema multiform like eruptions) were described. These skin manifestations occur as a result of an allergic contact dermatitis, which generally manifest as an eczematous rash [44].

Cardiovascular system

In many reports of PPD toxicity cardiac arrest was the main cause of death. In these cases cardiac arrest is attributed to arrhythmia (Figure 5). Most notably ventricular tachyarrhythmia including ventricular fibrillation has been the major feature of PPD cardiac toxicity [31-32]. Cases of myocardial infarction associated with cardiac rhabdomyolysis have been reported [45].

Respiratory system

On admission the first clinical presentation consists mainly of edema, which is of sudden onset and localized to the cervico-facial region [33]. Dyspnoea, tachypnoea and asphyxia with chest pain following acute PPD poisoning have been reported in a number of studies [6] [12] [28]. PPD was proved to be the cause of asthmatic attacks in the sensitive individuals [46]. A case of Goodpasture's syndrome was reported to be induced by exposure to PPD [47]. Extrinsic allergic alveolitis also has been reported [48].

Ophthalmic effects

In animal study it was reported that 89% of the mice fed PPD developed lenticular changes indicating that PPD has cataractogenous effects, which are related to the duration, amount and individual sensitivity [49]. It was concluded that PPD is potentially toxic to human lens. Exophthalmia and permanent blindness due to optic nerve atrophy following PPD poisoning were reported [6]. Using a patch test to determine PPD phototoxicity, it was proved that PPD could cause a phototoxic reaction and photoallergy [50- 51].

Hepatotoxicity

Subacute toxic hepatitis due to PPD poisoning was early reported with post-mortem small fibrosed liver and fibrous adhesions [33].There was a case report of liver enlargement with progressive neurological symptoms followed by death [52].On other series tender palpable livers were found,lobular inflammation of variable degree,and mild in sinusoids and portal tract inflammation, individual cell necrosis and inflammatory cells around and a granulomatous appearance in sinusoids[41].Radiological examination showed congested liver with prominent hepatic veins and low echogenicity[41].

The histopathological findings of the livers of the sacrificed animals showed signs of focal and early degenerative changes in hepatocytes, along with mild fatty changes. There was a moderate congestion of sinusoids and a focal granulomatous reaction with occasional Langerhans type giant cells [17].. In contrast others reported that there were no hepatic changes seen in their patients [6].

Neuromuscular toxicity

In animal studies it was proved that PPD has a toxic effect on the parasympathetic nerves [14]. In humans, neurotoxicity consist of mental status alterations ranging from drowsiness to coma were reported. Also flaccid paraparesis has been published [6] [25]. Foot drop, palatopharyngeal and laryngeal paralysis were also reported (25). Rhabdomyolysis following intoxication with PPD has been reported [28-30]. Skeletal muscle biopsy of patients showed scattered coagulation necrosis and inflammatory cellular infiltration [30].

Psychiatric

The psychiatric manifestations were studied in 50 patients with PDD poisoning in Wad Medani teaching hospital, 34 (70%) patients showed significant psychiatric manifestations, 24 of them showed depressive disorder while 11 showed conversion disorder. The patients who completed suicide and 62.1% who attempted suicide were from the depressive group (53)

Chronic systemic toxicity

Repeated and prolonged exposure to PPD is believed to increase the risk of non-Hodgkin's lymphomas and multiple myeloma and cancer of the bladder [34–35]. Hair dye formulations containing PPD was incriminated in the increased risk of systemic lupus erythematosus (SLE) and breast cancer; however other studies, showed that there is no significant relationship [36-37]. Aplastic anemia due to PPD exposure also has been reported [38].

Diagnosis

Determination of PPD has a great value in the diag-

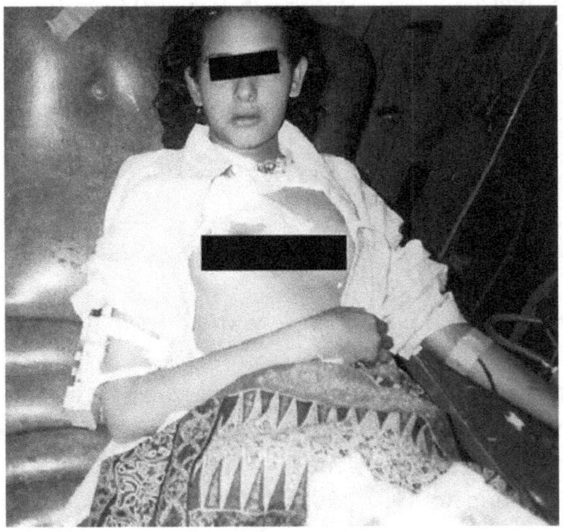

Figure 5. *Complete heart block (Pace Maker) following PPD intoxication.*

nosis; follow up of the treatment and also for medico-legal purposes. PPD was detected first in the urine of experimental animals [19] and in urine of humans by Yagi and colleagues, using thin layer chromatography [6]. Determination of PPD in the serum is not mentioned in the literature.

Treatment

There is no specific antidote for the PPD. The early challenge threatening the patient's life is asphyxia due to edema of the upper respiratory tract and the airways. Tracheostomy is a life saving measurement in this condition [6] (Figure 6). Nasotracheal intubation was proven also to be effective [29].

Vascular refilling is installed promptly in order to prevent as much as possible the development of acute kidney injury.

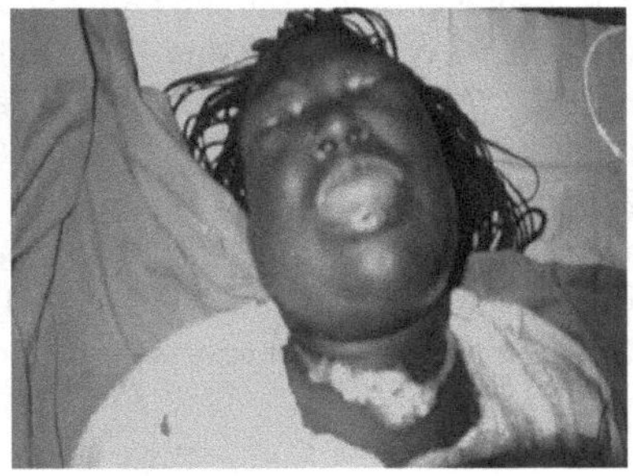

Figure 56. *Severe PPD intoxication in a female showing tongue swelling, neck swelling and tracheostomy.*

Acute kidney injury (ARF) was found to be the second life threatening effect. Hemodialysis had been used as a method of treatment with variable success [27-29]. On the other hand, peritoneal dialysis was used in the treatment of the ARF due to PPD toxicity in other reports [39].

Symptoms related to PPD poisoning seem to be due to histamine release; the use of antihistamines was suggested [54]. Intensive medical treatment by steroids and chlorpheneramine maleate was given to all patients together with prophylactic penicillin in one report [6]. Pethidine was given for relief of muscle pain in another report [30].

Numerous questions concerning PPD remain: physiopathological mechanisms of neurological myocardial and renal damage induced by the toxin, availability of an antidote and the extraction by hemodialysis/hemoperfusion.

References

1. Proger B, Jacobson P, Shmidt P and Stern D. Beilsteins handbouch der organischen chemie. In: IARC monograph on evaluation of the carcinogenic risk of chemical to man. 1977; 16: 127.
2. Thirtle JR. Phenylene diamines and toluen diamines. In: Encyclopedia of chemical technology (2nd edition, volume 15). Kirk RE, Othmer OE (editors). John Wiley and Sons, New York 1968, p. 216-224.
3. Burnett C, Goldenthal EI, Harris SB, Wazeter FX, Strausburg J, Kapp R, Voelker R. Teratology and percutaneous toxicity studies on hair dyes. J Toxicol Environ Health 1976; 1(6):1027-1040.
4. Gupta S, Gupta SS. Anti-inflammatory and antihyaluronidase activity of (Lwasonia alba). Indian Pharmacol 1985; 10: 90-91.
5. Singh S, Modi NT, Saifi AGQ. Anti-inflammatory activity of (Lwasonia inermis). Curr Sci1982; 51: 470-471.
6. Yagi H, El hindi AM, Khalil SI. Acute poisoning from hair dye. East African J 1991; 68: 404-411.
7. Searl CE, Havenden DG, Venih S, Gyde OHB. Carcinogenicity and mutagenicity test of some hair colourents and consituents. Nature 1975; 225: 506-509.

8. Nishioka H. The examination of cancer causing property of pigmented cosmetics through microbiol test. Fourth meeting of Environmental Mutagen Society of Japan, Kyoto 1975, September. 27.
9. IARC Working Group 1987. IARC Monographs on the evaluation of the carcinogenic risk of chemical to man. IARC publication.
10. Grasseli JG (editor). CRC Atlas of Spectral Data and Physical Constants for Organic Compounds. Chemcial Rubger Co., Cleveland, Ohio 1973, p. B-223.
11. Windholz M, Budavaria S. Merck index 1983. Published by Merck and Co. Inc. Rathway J. USA, p. 214-227.
12. Nott HW. Systemic poisoning by hair dye Brit Med J 1924; 1: 421-422.
13. Tainter ML, Hanzlik PJ. The mechanism of edema productionby paraphenylene diamine. J Pharmacol Exp Ther 1924; 24: 179-211.
14. Tainter ML, James M, Vandeventer W. Comparative edemic actions of ortho meta and para-phenylene diamines in different species. Arch int Pharmacodyn 1929; 36: 152-162.
15. Mathur AK, Gupta BN, Muther N, Singh A, Shukla IJ, Ravi Shanker. Biochemical and histopathological changes following dermal exposure to paraphenylene diamine in guinea-pigs. J Applied Toxicology 1990; 10: 383-386.
16. Picardo M, Zompella C, Marchese C, De-Luca C, Faggioni A, Schmidt RJ, Santucci B. Paraphenylene diamine a control allergen, induces oxidative stress and ICAM-1 expression in human keratinocytes. Brit J Dermatol 1992; 126: 450-455.
17. Mascres C, Jasmin G. Alterations de la fibre musculaire induites chez la rat par la p-phenylene diamine. Path Biol (Paris) 1975; 23: 193-199.
18. Burnett C, Loehr R, Corbett J. Dominant lethal mutagenicity study on hair dyes. J Toxicol Envirom Hlth 1977; 2: 657-662.
19. Kiese M, Raucher E. The absorption of P-toluene diamine through human skin hair dye. Toxicol Appl Pharmacol1968; 13: 325-327.
20. D'Arcy PF. Fatalities with the use of a henna dye. Pharmacy international 1982; 3: 217-218.
21. Ayoub Filali, Ilham Semlali, Valeria Ottaviano, Canmelo Fumari, Danillo Corradini, Rachida Soulaymani. A retrospective study of Acute systemic poisoning of paraphenylene Diamine (Occidental Takawt). Afr. J. Trad. CAM (2006) 3 (1): 142 – 149
22. Abdelkarim EE, Ali HM, Harron DWG and Ali KhM. Suicide attempt with Paraphenylene diamine (PPDA) dye in Sudan. Health Services Journal of the Eastern Mediterranean Region. WHO 1992; 6, 2: 44-48.
23. El-Ansary EH, Ahmed MEK, Adam SE. Systemic toxicity of paraphenylene diamine. Lancet 1983; 1: 1341-1342.
24. Salma MS, Mirghani F, Mohamed EN, et al. Poisoning with hair dye containing Paraphenylene diamine: ten years experience. Saudi J Kidney Dis Transplant 1995; 6: 286-289.
25. Othman Mohamed Mustafa. Acute Poisoning with Hair dye Containing Paraphenylene Diamine – The Gazira Experience. Journal of the Arab Board of Specialization 2001: 3 (2)
26. Charra B, Menebhil L, Bensalama A, Mottaoukkil S. Systemic toxicity of paraphenylene diamine. Works of the Sixth Congress of the Arab Society of Nephrology and Renal Transplantation. February 21-24, 2000- Marrakech, Morocco.
27. M. Sir Hashim, Y.O.Hamza, B.Yahia, F.M.Khogali, G.I.Sulieman. Poisoning from henna dye and para-phenylenediamine mixtures in children in Khartoum. Annals of Tropical Paediatrics 1992: 12 3-6
28. Averbukh Z, Modai D, Leonov Y, Weissgarten J, Lewinsohn G, Fucs L, Golik A, Rosenmann E. Rhabdomyolysis and acute renal failure induced by paraphenylenediamine. Hum Toxicol 1989; 8(5): 345-348.
29. Bourquia A, Jabrane AJ, Ramdani B, Zaid D. Systemic toxicity of paraphenylene diamine 4 cases. Press Med 1988; 17: 1798-1800.
30. Saito K, Murai T, Yabe K, Hara M, Watanabe H, Hurkawa T. Rhabdomyolisis due to paraphenylene diamine (hair dye). Report of an autopsy case. Nippon-Hoigaku-Zasshi 1990; 44: 469-474.
31. Lifshits M, Yagoubsky P, Sofer S. Fatal paraphenylene diamine (hair dye) intoxication in child resembling Ludwig's angina. J Toxicol Clin Toxicol 1993; 31: 653-656.
32. Ashraf W, Dawling S, Farrow LJ. Systemic paraphenylene diamine (PPD) poisoning a case report and review. Hum Exp Toxicol 1994; 13: 167-170.
33. Israels MGG, Manch MB, William S. Systemic poisoning by paraphenylene diamine with report of fatal case. Lancet 1934; 1: 505-510.
34. Pearce N, Bethwaite P. Increasing incidence of non-Hodgkin's lymphoma: occupational and environmental factors. Cancer Res 1992; 52: 5496-5500.
35. Brown LM, Evert GD, Burmeister LF, Blair A. Hair dye use and multiple myeloma in white men. Am J Public Health 1992; 82: 1673-1674.
36. Petri M, Allbritton J. Hair product use in systemic lupus erythematosus. A case control study. Arthritis Rheum 1992; 35: 625-629.
37. Koening KL, Pasternack BS, Shore RE, Strax P. Hair dye use and breast cancer: a case control study among screening participants. Am J Epidemiol 1991; 133: 985-995.

38. Hopkins JE, Manoharan A. Severe aplastic anaemia following the use of hair dye: report of two cases and review of literature. Postgrad Med J 1985; 61: 1003-1005.
39. Suliman SM, Homeida M, Aboud OI. Paraphenylene diamine induced acute tubular necrosis following hair dye ingestion. Human Toxicol 1983; 2: 633-635.
40. Brown JH, Conway B, Hill CM. Chronic renal failure associated with topical application of paraphenylene diamine. Brit Med J 1987; 294: 155-156.
41. Hamdouk M. PPD nephrotoxicity. In: Paraphenylene diamine (Hair Dye) Acute Systemic toxicity. Thesis for MMed Sci in Nephrology, Sheffield Kidney Institute, UK. 2001, p. 34-47.
42. Burnett C, Corbett JF. The Chemistry and Toxicology of Hair Dyes. Academic press, New York 1977, p. 203-224.
43. Seidnari S, Di-Nardo A, Motolese A, Pincelli C. Erythema multiforme associated with contact sensitization description of six clinical cases. J Ital Dermato Venerol 1990; 125: 35-40.
44. Nethercott JR, Macpherson M, Choi BC, Nixon B. Contact dermatitis in hairdressers. Contact Dermatitis 1986; 14: 73-79.
45. Ababou A, Ababou K, Mosadik A, Lazreq C, Sbihi A. Myocardial rhabdomyolysis following paraphenylene diamine poisoning. Ann Fr Anesth Reanim 2000; 19: 105-107.
46. Bardana EJ, Andrach RH. Occupotional asthma secondary to low molecular weight agents used in the plastic and resin industries. Eur J Respr Dis 1983; 64: 241-251.
47. Bernis P, Homles J, Quoidbach A, Mahier PH, Bouvy P. Remission of Goodpasture's Syndrome after withdrawal of an unusual toxic. Clinical Nephrol 1985; 23: 312-317.
48. Wang GH, Jiang XF, Luo WC. Report of two cases of extrinsic allergic alveolitis and review of the relevant literature. Chung Hua Chich Chih 1994; 1: 376-8, 384.
49. Jain IS, Jain GC, Kaul RL, Dhir SP. Catractogenous effect of hair dye. A clinical and experimental study. Ann Ophtalmol 1979; 11: 686-687.
50. Kroons S. Standard photopatch testing with waxter, para-aminobenzonic acid, potassium chromate and balsam of Peru. Contact Dermatitis 1983; 9: 5-9.
51. Horio T. Allergic and photoalergic dermatitis from diphenhydramine. Arch Dermatol 1976; 112: 1124-1126.
52. Davison C. Paraphenylene diamine with changes in the central nervous system. Arch Neural psych 1943, 49: 254-56
53. Diaa E. El Gaili, Osman M. Mustafa. Psychiatric Manifestations in Hair Dye poisoning. Journal of the Arab Board of Medical Specializations 2001; 3: 2
54. Gleason MN, Glosselin RE, Hodge HC. Clinical Toxicology of commercial Products. Williams and Wilkins Co., 1963, p. 93.

D

The Renal Failure Patient

41

Trace metal disturbances in end-stage renal failure patients

Patrick C. D'HAESE

Laboratory of Pathophysiology, University of Antwerp, Belgium

Introduction

The association between metal exposure and renal failure can be approached from two points of view. On the one hand environmental/industrial exposure to heavy metals, more particularly, lead, cadmium and mercury and other inorganic substances such as silicon has been linked to a reduced renal function and/or the development of acute or chronic renal failure [1]. This issue has been dealt with in other chapters of this book. On the other hand patients with chronic renal failure, especially those treated by dialysis are at an increased risk for trace element disturbances (Figure 1). Indeed in these subjects the reduced renal function, the presence of proteinuria, metabolic alterations associated with renal insufficiency, the dialysis treatment, medication etc. all may contribute to either accumulation or deficiency of trace metals. With regard to aluminum intensive research on the element's toxic effects has been performed in the past. Recently, new metal-containing medications have been introduced of which the potential toxic effects should be considered and put in a justified context.

Sources and mechanisms of trace element disturbances in uremia

Trace metal disturbances may be due to the *uremia per se*. Indeed, as the urinary excretion route is an important pathway of elimination of many trace elements, i.e. silicon, strontium, aluminum, ... impairment of the kidney will be an important determinant of their accumulation, whilst in the presence of a reabsorptive defect a number of trace elements, especially those that are reabsorbed because of their essential role, be lost resulting in a deficient state. The presence of proteinuria may reasonably result in losses of protein bound elements. It has also been shown also that residual renal function may importantly alter the accumulation and hence toxic effects of aluminum [2]. In uremia translocation of a particular metal from one tissue to another may also occur. As an example, under normal circumstances the kidney is an important target organ for cadmium. In chronic renal failure however, possibly as a consequence of a reduction in binding proteins (e.g. metallothionein), the concentration of cadmium in this tissue decreases to extremely low levels which however, goes along with an increased concentration in other tissues such as the liver because of the failure of the diseased kidney to excrete the element [3]. Since the biosynthesis of the active 1α,25-$(OH)_2$VitaminD_3 compound is significantly reduced in renal failure, the uptake of elements which follow the calcium; i.e. vitamin D mediated pathway for their gastrointestinal absorption such as e.g. strontium [4] or lead [5] may be altered. On the other hand has an increased gastrointestinal absorption of particular elements (e.g. aluminum, lanthanum) in uremia, as compared to health, been attributed to a possible effect of atrophic alterations of the intestinal mucosa; a situation frequently observed in chronic renal failure [6].

In addition may *medication* related to the uremic state lead to important trace element accumulation. In the past this has clearly been established for aluminum resulting from the use of aluminum hydroxide as a phosphate binding agent. As aluminum-based phosphate binders may be contaminated with other elements, e.g. strontium the possibility for a simultaneous accumulation of different elements has been suggested [7]. Strontium is mainly eliminated by the kidney and has been associated with bone mineralization defects when present at high concentrations. In view of this the use of strontium ranelate for the treatment and prevention of osteoporosis should be avoided in patients with a GFR below 30 ml/min [8,9]. Till now, evidence has been presented that in contrast to aluminum hydroxide which is mainly eliminated via the kidney, lanthanum carbonate, which recently has been introduced as an alternative phosphate binding agent, does not pose dialysis patients at an increased risk for accumulation as the element is eliminated via the bile (Figure 2) [10]. Erythropoietin when used to correct the patients' anemia may lead to a relative iron deficiency, or indirectly to iron overload [11]. To which extent and by which mechanism erythropoietin also affects the status of other elements as suggested for silicon, zinc, nickel and manganese [12] needs further confirmation. Various reports in the literature have indicated that solutions for parenteral nutrition and albumin replacement fluids may contain non-negligible amounts of aluminum, chromium and nickel which may accumulate in the body when administered to patients with impaired renal function [13,14]. In various recent papers an association between gadolinium-based contrast agents and the development of nephrogenic systemic fibrosis has been reported in patients with reduced renal function [15].

In patients with uremia, trace element disturbances may also occur by the *dialysis treatment per se*. Indeed,

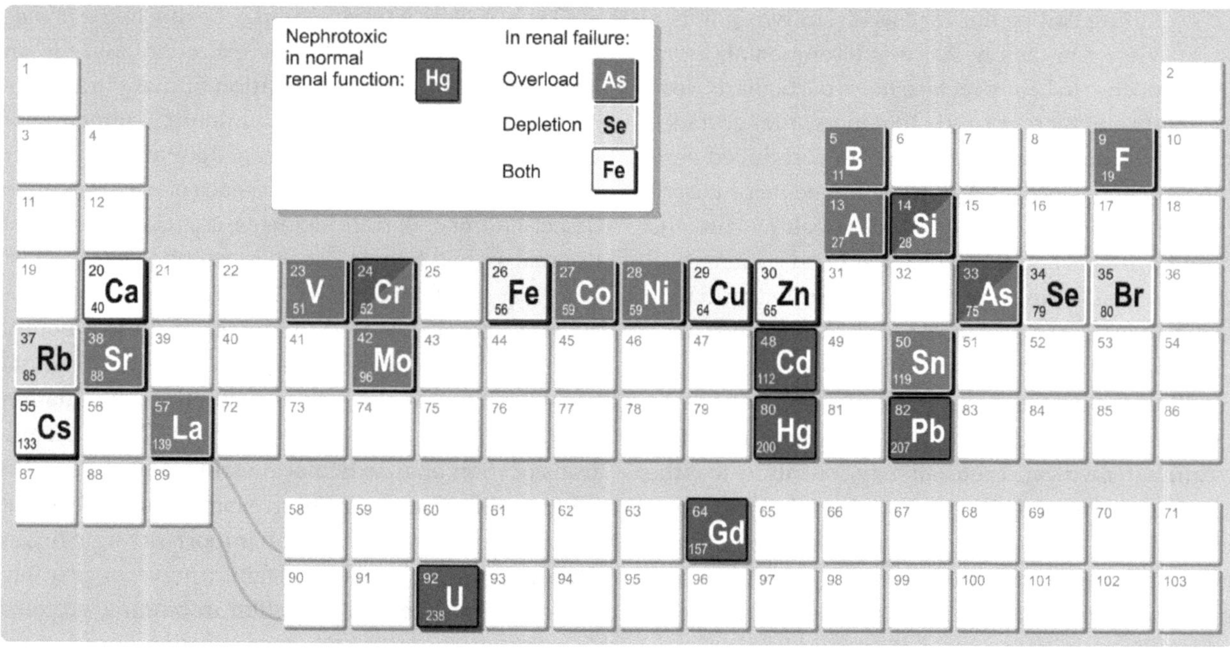

Figure 1: *Overview of trace elements and metals that may either be nephrotoxic after environmental or occupational exposure or of whom the concentration may be disturbed in patients already having chronic renal failure.*

according to the concentration gradient between the ultrafiltrable amount of a particular element in serum and its concentration in the dialysis fluid, some trace elements may be removed whereas others present as contaminants in the dialysis solution will be transferred to the patients. Due to the *hemodialyis* treatment each patient is exposed to 15000-30000 liters of dialysis fluid/year. Hence, the minor dialysate contamination with a given element may already result in its distinct accumulation in those subjects. Serious acute and chronic intoxications as well as metal deficiencies have been reported [16,17].

In *hemodialysis* the dialysis fluids are prepared from the tap water which may contain considerable amounts of trace metals. In the absence of adequate water treatment procedures it must be considered the main source of trace metal dialysate contamination. Some domestic tap water contains aluminum in high concentrations either naturally or as a result of the addition of the element as a flocculant to the water basins, a procedure which is part of the water purification process and has led to an acute, fatal intoxication of a considerable number of patients in a Portuguese dialysis center (see also below) [17,18]. Worth noting is that concentrations of particular elements in tap water may vary seasonally, e.g. silicon, or even on a day-to-day basis, e.g. aluminum. Trace elements can adequately be removed during water treatment, provided that in addition to softening and deionization the water is treated by reverse osmosis (RO). Carrying out these procedures however, does not necessarily imply the total removal of the elements from the final dialysis fluid [17-19]. Aside from the water treatment procedure The use of commercial salts used to prepare the final dialysis fluid may also be a cumbersome issue. Here besides aluminum, identification of other elements that might be responsible for pathological effects in dialysis patients, e.g. strontium, is warranted [20]. In line with this statement, Padovese *et al.* [21] demonstrated that dialysis fluids used for either continuous ambulatory peritoneal dialysis (CAPD), hemodialysis and hemofiltration may contain trace metals in various concentrations depending on the chemical composition of the salts used to prepare the final dialysis fluids. They demonstrated that for a series of trace elements including gold, barium, gallium, thallium, vanadium, nickel, chromium, etc. the weekly exposure via the dialysis fluid appeared to be 50- to 12,000-fold higher than the corresponding estimated amount absorbed via the diet. In this context are the recent findings from multicenter surveys demonstrating the addition of concentrates to result in high silicon or strontium

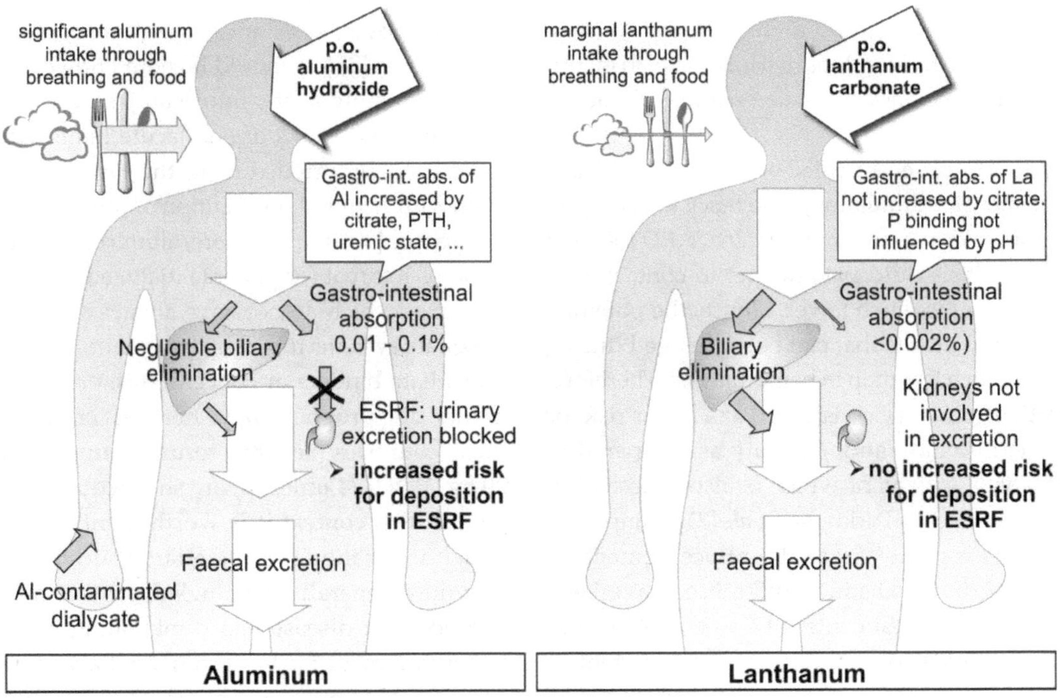

Figure 2: *Comparison of the aluminum and lanthanum metabolism.*

containing dialysates of particular interest [19,20]. Whether the type of the dialysate, i.e. bicarbonate vs. acetate importantly influences the trace metal concentration and subsequent trace metal disturbances is not yet clear. Findings by Schrooten et al. [20] point to a higher risk for strontium accumulation when acetate-based concentrates are used.

It might be anticipated that under certain conditions trace elements used in plasticizers or alloys such as mercury, iron, cadmium, tin and chromium could be introduced into the dialysis fluid also and thus transferred to the patient resulting in either acute or chronic intoxication. The driving force for the transfer of trace elements during dialysis is the gradient between their concentration in the dialysis fluid and the free diffusible fraction in the blood compartment. As a consequence, with highly protein bound elements an even low concentration of these substances in the dialysis fluid may promptly result in a transfer of the element across the dialysis membrane. Hence, in dialysis patients having a serum aluminum level around 20 μg/L (0.74 μmol/L) and of which 80-90% is protein bound, there might already be a transfer to the systemic circulation at aluminum levels in the dialysis fluid as low as 5 μg/L (0.19 μmol/L). In contrast to this, low dialysate levels of a number of elements; e.g. boron [22], fluoride [23], selenium [24], vanadium [25], may result in an adequate intra-dialytic removal of these components from the blood compartment which in turn may result in deficiency of some essential elements, e.g. selenium [24].

Compared to patients treated by hemodialysis, data on trace element accumulation/deficiency in *CAPD* are rather scanty and less documented. In CAPD the total volume of dialysis fluid patients get in contact with during treatment is much lower. Hence, the potential amount of trace metals that can be exchanged during treatment is much less than in hemodialysis. Therefore, CAPD patients must be considered at a lower risk for trace element accumulation/toxicity as compared to hemodialysis; a statement which is also reflected by the data presented of Padovese *et al.* [21] comparing the estimated exposure of forty-four trace elements in both patient groups. Distinct differences have been noted in the trace metal content between CAPD and hemodialysis fluids. Also the trace metal content of CAPD fluids may greatly differ between each other, which has been ascribed to the wide range of trace metal concentration in the salts added to prepare the final dialysis fluid [21,26].

To which extent techniques such as on-line hemodiafiltration and biofiltration or sorbent charcoal-based ultrafiltrate regeneration may alter trace metal levels in chronic renal failure patients is not yet clear and can only be evaluated by long-term longitudinal monitoring.

Trace metal accumulation/toxicity in uremic and dialysis patients

Aluminum

Aluminum is without any doubt the most intensively studied trace metal in dialysis patients and its harmful effects have been well documented during the last decades. So, aluminum overload has been implicated in the pathogenesis of several clinical disorders of the musculoskeletal, central nervous, and hematologic systems [27]. Due to the introduction of adequate water treatment systems and the (partial) withdrawal of aluminum-containing phosphate binders together with the establishment of regular monitoring programs, chronic, caricatural aluminum overload is nowadays rarely seen. At the present day the issue has switched towards more subtle disorders at the level of the parathyroid gland function and bone turnover, resistance to erythropoietin therapy and anemia [28]. It should be noted however, that the risk for, mainly acute, intoxications not be neglected as several outbreaks of (sub)acute fatal intoxications have been reported during the last 2 decades [29] even with criminal prosecution of physicians for gross negligence [30]. Furthermore, aluminum accumulation remains a threat for patients dialyzed in centers from countries which do not have always at their disposal adequate systems for water treatment, aluminum-free phosphate binders or concentrates, or where regular monitoring programs have not been organized yet. In these countries elevated serum aluminum levels (> 20 μg/L, > 0.74 μmol/L) are still frequently observed [29]. In this context it is worth mentioning that the Renal Association (RA) standard states that although it is now generally acknowledged that aluminium-related bone disease is a diminishing problem and water treatment facilities in hemodialysis units have considerably improved, the serum aluminum concentration should be measured every three months in all patients on hemodialysis and all peritoneal dialsysis patients receiving oral aluminium hydroxide, whilst the water aluminum content should be tested on a monthly base. The KDOQI guidelines are slightly less stringent than the RA guidelines, with the recommendation that serum aluminium should be measured at least yearly and every 3 months in patients receiving aluminium-containing medications [31]. Aside from regular monitoring it has been advised recently that products and drugs destinated for chronic renal failure aptients should have their composition re-evaluated in order to contain only components with negligible aluminum contamination [32].

Recent research on the speciation and protein binding characteristics of aluminum has led to a better insight in the mechanisms underlying the element's tissue distribution and toxicity [33, 34]. In this context, the provocative hypothesis linking the widespread use of erythropoietin to the increasing prevalence of adynamic bone disease is of particular interest [35].

Lanthanum

Lanthanum carbonate, together with sevelamer hydrochloride belongs to the new generation of calcium-free phosphate binders that can control hyperphosphatemia without adding to the patients calcium load. Lanthanum is only minimally absorbed (0.00127 ± 0.00080% in healthy humans; being 2 to 3 orders of magnitude lower than the values reported for aluminium) [36] and serum lanthanum levels > 2 µg/L (> 0.014 µmol/L) are only rarely seen during long-term treatment in dialysis patients [37],

Available bone biopsy data in dialysis patients treated for up to 4 years with lanthanum carbonate indicate low-level bone deposition, the highest concentration ever measured in any patient being 9.4 µg/g (0.067 µmol/L). Unlike aluminium, no direct effects of lanthanum on bone have been reported so far in any clinical or experimental setting [37-39]. Ultrastructural localization demonstrated a heterogeneous distribution of lanthanum in the bone of rats and man, which was independent of the underlying type of renal osteodystrophy [40].

The exclusive presence of lanthanum in the bile and in the lysosomes of the liver cell is consistent with excretion of lanthanum by the liver via the transferrin receptor-endosomal-lysosomal-bile canaliculus pathway [41]. Clinical studies of up to 4 years have not disclosed any hepatotoxic effect of the drug in patients treated with this phosphate binder.

Brain lanthanum levels did not exceed 10 ng/g [0.072 nmol/g] in the brain of rats fed orally during 20 weeks or after intravenous administration of high doses of lanthanum over 4 weeks [42]. No neurological effects have been observed during long-term treatment in dialysis patients [43].

Further studies unraveling the speciation of lanthanum in biological fluids will contribute to a further understanding of its metabolism and kinetics. Strictly spoken, there is no risk for dialysis patients to be prone to increased uptake of the element via the use of dialysis fluids or parenteral solutions.

Strontium

Strontium levels are increased in plasma of renal failure patients. In dialysis patients the accumulation of the element has been reported to be strongly centre and country-dependent and values up to 50 times those noted in subjects with normal renal function have been reported within the latter population [20]. In addition to the renal failure, accumulation of the element turned out to be due to the use of strontium-contaminated dialysis fluids secondary to the addition of contaminated acetate-based concentrates. To which other factors such as age, medication, treatment modalities etc ... also contribute to the increased levels is not yet fully understood.

The distribution of the element is similar to that of calcium which means that 99% of the body burden is deposited in bone [44]. Within the dialysis population, bone strontium levels were found to be significantly higher in subjects with osteomalacia as compared to this presenting the other types of renal osteodystrophy [45]. A causal, dose-dependent role of strontium in the development of this bone disease has been established in a chronic renal failure ratmodel [46,47]. Moreover the bone osteomalacic lesions were found to be reversible after withdrawal of strontium [9,48].

Silicon

Serum silicon levels correlate with the degree of renal failure [49] and once enrolled in a dialysis program patients not only accumulate the element via the oral intake of high silicon drinking water but especially by the use of silicon contaminated dialysis fluids [19,50,51]. Contamination of the dialysis fluid was found to be due to either the use of RO membranes that insufficiently retain the element during water treatment or by the addition of concentrates containing high amounts of silicon [19].

The clinical significance of increased silicon levels is not yet understood. Parry *et al.* [52] suggested silicon and aluminum to interact with each other. In their dialysis patients high serum silicon levels were associated with low serum aluminum concentrations inferring either a reduced intestinal absorption -which had been postulated earlier in subjects with normal renal function [53] - or an increased removal of aluminum through dialysis by the formation of the aluminum-silicon complex. To which extent increased silicon levels in the dialysis population may inhibit superoxide dismutase activity [54], favors dextran deposition by linking polysaccharide chains [55, 56] or gives yield to the development of a so-called 'silicon-related syndrome', expressed as by painful, nodular skin eruptions and aberrant hair growth and characterized as perforating folliculitis on skin biopsy [57], is not yet fully understood.

Selenium

Blood selenium levels in dialysis patients are frequently lower than in controls [58]. This is either due to a deficient dietary intake of the element in dialysis patients and/or losses through dialysis membranes [24].

Selenium is known to play a critical role in the glutathione peroxidase activity; an enzyme that protects membrane lipids and other cellular and extracellular components from oxidative damage [58] and an aggravation of oxidative stress during dialysis resulting from low serum serum selenium levels (in combination with decreased serum copper and zinc) has been reported in children with end-stage renal disease as compared to healthy subjects [59]. In view of this oral supplementation of the element to dialysis patients has been recommended and resulted in a significant rise in glutathione peroxidase activity [24, 60]. Selenium supplementation to hemodialysis patients resulted in a progressive increase in T-cell response to phytohemoagglutin and in delayed-type hypersensitivity in the absence of severe side-effects [60].

Chromium

Chromium may enter the body via the dialysis fluid [61]. We (data not published) as well as others [62] noted serum chromium concentrations to be increased up to twenty-fold those observed in subjects with normal renal function. In its hexavalent state, the element may act as a carcinogenic substance. Whether the increased levels in the dialysis population are of clinical significance is not yet clear, nor is it elucidated if the increased serum chromium levels in these patients are accompanied by an increased body burden of the element. In view of the latter, it is worth mentioning that in a previous study of our group, in which we assessed the bone trace element content in end-stage renal failure, bone chromium levels in dialysis patients were significantly increased as compared to those noted in subjects with intact renal function. The accumulation of the element in bone, however, could not be associated with the development of a particular type of renal osteodystrophy [63].

Zinc

Although there are still some discrepancies in the literature regarding zinc levels in dialysis patients, most studies have found decreased levels of the element in serum [64,65] and muscles whereas the levels in bone [63] and other tissues seem to be normal or even increased suggesting translocation of the element in uremia. The dialysis treatment itself seems to have little or no effect on the serum zinc concentrations. Zinc deficiency in uremic patients has been associated with anorexia, disturbances in taste and sexual performance [66] whereas decreased plasma zinc seem to correlate with erythrocyte superoxide dismutase levels [67]. As evaluated by Türk *et al.* [68], zinc supplementation did not have any effect on the restoration of immune parameters or enhancement of the antibody response to multivalent influenza vaccine in hemodialysis patients. On the other hand however, has zinc supplementation been reported an effective means of improving serum levels of zinc and cholesterol in the hemodialysis patient [69].

Copper

Copper levels in serum of CAPD patients tend in general to be lower than those noted in the presence of a normal function. As for zinc however, its deficiency seems not to be due to the dialysis treatment itself. Here, loss of the element as the ceruloplasmin compound into the peritoneum has been suggested

[70]. The effect of copper deficiency is not fully understood. The element is required for lysil oxidase activity which is necessary for cross-linking of collagen. Its deficiency has been associated with growth retardation and anemia. Also has in dialysis patients a correlation been demonstrated between serum copper levels and superoxide dismutase activity.

Iron

Whereas until a decade ago, the development of iron overload secondary due to blood transfusions to correct for the patients' anemia, was one of the major problems in dialysis patients, the issue has now switched towards a relative iron deficiency with the introduction of erythropoietin. It has been demonstrated that relative iron depletion may favor the binding of aluminum to transferrin leading to a preferential uptake of the element in transferrin receptor expressing tissues such as e.g. the parathyroid gland which in turn may lead to a reduced parathyroid secretion and hence the development of adynamic bone disease [33]. On the other hand however, may iron overload, by preventing the binding of aluminum to transferrin, result in an increased deposition of the non-protein bound aluminium at the bone calcification front [71].

Gadolinium

Free gadolinium, a rare earth that is mainly eliminated by the kidney (97%) is toxic to tissues and therefore unsafe in human use. The trivalent gadolinium is very close to the divalent calcium ion as reflected in size, bonding, coordination and donor atom preference [72]. Gadolinium-containing compounds however, are widely used as contrast agents and when used for this application the element is sequestered by binding to a chelate. These stable complexes have long been thought to be safe, even in patients with impaired renal function. Recently however, exposure to gadolinium-containing contrast agents has been associated with the development of 'Nephrogenic Systemic Fibrosis' (NSF). Initially named 'Nephrogenic Fibrosing Dermopathy' (NFD) in 2001, NSF is a recently characterized systemic fibrosing disorder occurring in patients with underlying renal disease. This condition principally leads to skin thickening and hardening and may induce joint immobility and inability to walk and potentially leads to death when several organ systems are involved. Since its recognition in 1997 and the first description in 2000, more than 215 cases have been reported worldwide [73,74]. Clusters of NSF were associated to an exposure to gadolinium containing contrast agents during magnetic resonance imaging [75]. Gadolinium has been detected in skin tissue of patients with NSF [76]. Gadodiamide, a linear gadolinium chelate appears to be particularly at risk as reflected by an odds ratio of 32.5 to acquire NSF when exposed to this particular compound [73,77]. During renal failure, gadodiamide accumulation may explain the development of NSF. Evidence for gadolinium to play an etiological role in the development of the disease is supported by the notion that before the introduction of gadolinium-containing contrast media, NSF has not been known [73]. Regulatory decisions have been taken to contraindicate gadodiamide in patients with severe renal impairment [78]. To date it is uncertain whether other gadolinium-based contrast media are involved in some of the affected patients, but this is a matter of current evaluation [79]. *See also chapter 30.*

Metal-metal interactions

It should be noted that in the majority of the above mentioned studies, metal-induced renal injury was considered as if exposure occurred to only one metal at a time. In reality it is clear that environmental and occupational exposure may involve several metals at the same time and in varying concentrations [34]. It has been shown that with combined exposure various metals may interact with each other and that one metal may alter the potential toxicity of another in either a beneficial or deleterious way. As an example, whilst arsenic has been shown to worsen cadmium-induced nephrotoxicity, data from experimental studies have shown that selenium may protect against the renal effects induced by cadmium [52]. Other studies have shown that the iron status may alter the toxic effects of aluminium at the level of the bone and the parathyroid gland [53,54], whilst in a recent increased lead accumulation was associated with disturbances in the concentration of a number of essential trace elements [55].

References

1. Nuyts GD, Van Vlem E, Thys J, De Leersnijder D, D'Haese PC, Elseviers MM, De Broe ME. Defined and undefined occupational risk factors of chronic renal failure. Lancet 1995; 346: 7-11.
2. Altmann P, Butter KC, Plowman D, Chaput de Saintonge DM, Cunningham J, Marsh FP. Residual renal function in hemodialysis patients may protect against hyperaluminemia. *Kidney Int* 1989; 32: 710-13.
3. Smythe WR, Alfrey AC, Craswell PW, Crouch CA, Ibels LS, Kubo H, Nunnelly LL, Rudolph H. Trace metal abnormalities in chronic uremia. *Ann Intern Med* 1982; 96: 302-310.
4. Blumsohn A, Morris B, Eastell R. Stable strontium absorption as a measure of intestinal calcium absorption: comparison with the double-radiotracer calcium absorption test. *Clin Science* 1994; 87: 363-368.
5. Barton JC, Conrad ME, Harrison L, Nuby S. Effects of calcium on the absorption and retention of lead. *J Lab Clin Med* 1978; 91: 366-376.
6. Ittel TH. Determinants of gastrointestinal absorption and distribution of aluminium in health and uremia. *Nephrol Dial Transplant* 1993; 8 (Suppl 1): 17-24.
7. Canavese C, Pacitti M, Salomone M, Santoro A, Strata P, Mangiarotti G, Talarico S, Sabbioni E, Pietra R, Vercellone A. Strontium overload in uremic patients on regular dialytic treatment. *Trans Am Soc Artif Inter Organs* 1986: 32: 120-122.
8. Lehmann G, Hein G, Wolf G. The osteoporosis patient with renal insufficiency: what has to be taken into account in the selection and administration of antiosteoporosis medication? *Z Rheumatol* 2006; 65: 380-382.
9. Oste L, Bervoets AR, Behets GJ, Dams G, Marijnissen RL, Geryl H, Lamberts LV, Verberckmoes SC, Van Hoof VO, De Broe ME, D'Haese PC. Time-evolution and reversibility of strontium-induced osteomalacia in chronic renal failure rats. *Kidney Int* 2005; 67: 920-930.
10. Damment SJP, Pennick M. Systemic lanthanum is excreted in the bile of rats. *Toxicol Lett.* 2007; 171: 69-77.
11. Singh H, Reed J, Noble S, Cangiano JL, Van Wyck DB. Effect of intravenous iron sucrose in peritoneal dialysis patients who receive erythropoiesis-stimulating agents for anemia: A randomized, controlled trial. *Clin J Am Soc Nephrol* 2006; 1: 475-482.
12. Hosokawa S, Yoshida O 1993 Effects of erythropoietin on trace elements in patients with chronic renal failure undergoing hemodialysis. *Nephron* 1993; 65: 414-417.
13. Gammelgaard B, Sandberg E. Aluminium and nickel in human albumin solutions. *J Trace Elem Electrolytes Health Dis* 1989; 3: 39-42.
14. D'Haese PC, Lamberts LV, Liang L, Boone LP, Van Waeleghem, De Broe ME. Contribution of parenteral and dialysate solutions to the aluminum accumulation in dialysis patients. *Blood Purif* 1990; 8: 359-362.
15. Reilly RF. Risk for nephrogenic systemic fibrosis with gadoteriol (ProHance) in patients who are on long-term hemodialysis. *Clin J Am Soc Nephrol* 2008; 3: 747-751.
16. D'Haese PC, De Broe ME. Adequacy of dialysis: trace elements in dialysis fluids. *Nephrol Dial Transplant* 1996; 11 (Suppl 2): 92-97.
17. Simoes J, Barata JD, D'Haese PC, de Broe ME. Cela n'arrive qu'aux autres. *Nephrol Dial Transplant* 1994; 9: 67-68.
18. Barata JD, D'Haese PC, Pires C, Lamberts LV, Simoes J, De Broe ME. Low-dose (5mg/kg) desferrioxamine treatment in acutely aluminum-intoxicated hemodialysis patients using two drug administration schedules. *Nephrol Dial Transplant* 1996; 11: 125-132.
19. D'Haese PC, Shaheen FA, Huraib SO, Djukanovic L, Polenakovic MH, Spasovski G, Shikole A, Schurgers ML, Daneels RF, Lamberts LV, Van Landeghem GF, De Broe ME. Increased silicon levels in dialysis patients due to the high silicon content in the drinking water, inadequate water treatment procedures, and concentrate contamination: A multicentre study. *Nephrol Dial Transplant* 1995; 10: 1838-1844.
20. Schrooten I, Elseviers MM, Lamberts LV, De Broe ME, D'Haese PC. Increased serum strontium levels in dialysis patients. An epidemiological survey. *Kidney Int* 1999; 56: 1888-1892.
21. Padovese P, Gallieni M, Brancaccio D, Pietra R, Fortaner S, Sabbioni E, Minoia C, Markakis K, Berlin A. Trace elements in dialysis fluids and assessment of the exposure of patients on regular hemodialysis, hemofiltration and continous ambulatory peritoneal dialysis. *Nephron* 1992; 61: 442-448.
22. Mauras Y, KS Ang KS, P Simon P, B Tessier B, F Cartier F, P Allain P. Increase in blood plasma levels of boron and strontium in hemodialyzed patients. *Clin Chim Acta* 1986; 156: 315-320.
23. Chaleil D, Simon P, Tessier B, Cartier F, Allain P. Blood plasma fluoride in haemodialysed patients. *Clin Chim Acta* 1986; 156: 105-108.
24. Saint-Georges MD, DJ Bonnefont DJ, BA Bourely BA, M-CT Jaudon M-CT, P Cereze P, P Chaumeil P, C Gard C, CL D'Auzac CL. Correction of selenium deficiency in hemodialyzed patients. *Kidney Int* 1989; 36 (suppl 27): 274-277.
25. Hosokawa S, Yoshida O. Serum vanadium levels in chronic hemodialysis patients. *Nephron* 1993; 64: 388-394.

26. Wallaeys B, Cornelis R, Mees L, Lameire N. Trace elements in serum, packed cells, and dialysate of CAPD patients. *Kidney Int* 1986; 30: 599-604.
27. De Broe ME, Coburn JW (eds). *Aluminum and renal failure.* Dordrecht: Kluwer Acad Publ, 1989.
28. De Broe ME, Drüeke TB, Ritz E. Consensus Conference: diagnosis and treatment of aluminum overload in end-stage renal failure patients. *Nephrol Dial Transplant* 1993; 8 (Suppl 1): 1-4.
29. D'Haese PC, De Broe ME. Trace elements in dialysis patients. In: Hörl WE, Koch KM, Lindsay RM, Ronco C, Winchester JF (eds). *Replacement of Renal Function by Dialysis.* Dordrecht: Kluwer Acad Publ, 2004 pp 903-925.
30. Berend K, Knoops GJ, De Wolff FA. Prosecution after an outbreak of subacute aluminum intoxication in a hemodialysis center. *Leg Med* 2004; 6: 1-10.
31. Lamb EJ, Hodsman A, van Schalkwyk D, Ansell D, Warwick G. Serum calcium, phosphate, parathyroid hormone, albumin, aluminium and cholesterol achievement on replacement therapy (Chapter 9). *Nephrol Dial Transplant* 2007; 22 (suppl 7): 105-118.
32. Bohrer D, Bertagnolli DC, de Oliveira SMR, do Nascimento PC, de Carvalho LM, Pomblum SG. Drugs as a hidden source of aluminium for chronic renal patients. *Nephrol Dial Transplant* 2007; 22: 605-611.
33. Smans KA, D' Haese PC, Van Landeghem GF, Andries LJ, Lamberts LV, Hendy GN, De Broe ME. Transferrin-mediated uptake of aluminium by human parathyroid cells results in reduced parathyroid hormone secretion. *Nephrol Dial Transplant* 2000; 15: 1328-1336.
34. Van Landeghem GF, De Broe ME, D'Haese PC. Al and Si: Their speciation, distribution, and toxicity - A critical review. *Clin Biochem* 1998; 31: 385-397.
35. Smans KA, Van Landeghem GF, D'Haese PC, Couttenye MM, De Broe ME. Is there a link between erythropietin therapy and adynamic bone disease? *Nephrol Dial Transplant* 1996; 11: 1248-1249.
36. Pennick M, Dennis K, Damment SJ. Absolute bioavailability and disposition of lanthanum in healthy human subjects administered lanthanum carbonate. *J Clin Pharmacol* 2006; 46: 738-746.
37. D'Haese PC, Spasovski GB, Sikole A, Hutchison A, Freemont TJ, Sulkova S, Swanepoel C, Pejanovic S, Djukanovic L, Balducci A, Coen G, Sulowicz W, Ferreira A, Torres A, Curic S, Popovic M, Dimkovic N, De Broe ME. A multicenter study on the effects of lanthanum carbonate (Fosrenol) and calcium carbonate on renal bone disease in dialysis patients. *Kidney Int* 2003; 85 (Suppl): 73-78.
38. Persy VP, Behets GJ, Bervoets AR, De Broe ME, D'Haese PC. Lanthanum: a safe phosphate binder. *Semin Dial* 2006; 19:195-199.
39. Behets GJ, Dams G, Vercauteren SR, Damment SJ, Bouillon R, De Broe ME, D'Haese PC. Does the phosphate binder lanthanum carbonate affect bone in rats with chronic renal failure? *J Am Soc Nephrol* 2004; 15: 2219-2228.
40. Behets GJ, Verberckmoes SC, Oste L, Bervoets AR, Salomé M, Cox AG, Denton J, De Broe ME, D'Haese PC. Localization of lanthanum in bone of chronic renal failure rats after oral dosing with lanthanum carbonate. *Kidney Int* 2005; 67: 1830-1836.
41. Yang Z, Schryvers D, Roels F, D'Haese PC, De Broe ME. Demonstration of lanthanum in liver cells by energy-dispersive X-ray spectroscopy, electron energy loss spectroscopy and high-resolution transmission electron microscopy. *J Microsc* 2006; 223: 133-139.
42. Bervoets ARJ, Yang Z, Schryvers D, Roels F, Behets GJ, Verberckmoes SC, Dauwe S, Blust R, De Broe ME, D'Haese PC. Transhepatocellular transport and increased gastro-intestinal absorption of lanthanum in chronic renal failure. *Kidney Int* (Submitted).
43. Altmann P, Barnett ME, Finn WF; SPD405-307 Lanthanum Carbonate Study Group. Cognitive function in Stage 5 chronic kidney disease patients on hemodialysis: no adverse effects of lanthanum carbonate compared with standard phosphate-binder therapy. *Kidney Int* 2007; 71: 252-259.
44. Cabrera WE, Schrooten I, De Broe ME, D'Haese PC. Strontium and bone. *J Bone Miner Res* 1999; 14: 661-668.
45. D'Haese PC, Schrooten I, Goodman WG, Cabrera WE, Lamberts LV, Elseviers MM, Couttenye M-M, De Broe ME. Increased bone strontium levels in hemodialysis patients with osteomalacia. *Kidney Int* 2000; 57: 1107-1114.
46. Schrooten I, Cabrera W, Dauwe S, Lamberts LV, Marynisen R, Dorriné W, Goodman WG, De Broe ME, D'Haese PC. Strontium causes osteomalacia in chronic renal failure rats. *Kidney Int* 1998; 54: 448-456.
47. Schrooten I, Behets GJ, Cabrera WE, Vercauteren SR, Lamberts LV, Verberckmoes SC, Bervoets AJ, Dams G, Goodman WG, De Broe ME, D'Haese PC. Dose-dependent effects of strontium on bone of chronic renal failure rats. *Kidney Int* 2003; 63: 927-935.
48. Oste L, Verberckmoes SC, Behets GJ, Dams G, Bervoets AR, Van Hoof VO, Bohic S, Drakopoulos M, De Broe ME, D'Haese PC. Strontium incorporates at sites critical for bone mineralization in rats with renal failure. *X-Ray Spectrometry* 2007; 36: 42-44.
49. Gitelman HJ, Alderman F, Perry SJ. Renal handling of silicon in normals and in patients with renal insufficiency. *Kidney Int* 1992; 42: 957-959.
50. Dobbie JW, Smith MJB Urinary and serum silicon in normal and uremic individuals. *Ciba Found Symp* 1986; 121: 194-213.
51. Gitelman HJ, Alderman FR, Perry SJ. Silicon accumulation in dialysis patients. *Am J Kidney Dis* 1992; 19: 140-143.
52. Parry R, Plowman D, Delves HT, Roberts NB, Birchall JD, Bellia JP, Davenport A, Ahmad R, Fahal I, Altmann. Silicon and aluminum interactions in haemodialysis patients. *Nephrol Dial Transplant* 1998; 13: 1759-1762.

53. Edwardson JA, Moore PB, Ferrier IN, Lilley JS, Newton GWA, Barker J, Templar J, Day JP. Effect of silicon on gastrointestinal absorption of aluminium. *Lancet* 1993; 342: 211-212.
54. Shainkin-Kestenbaum R, Adler AJ, Berlyne GM. Inhibition of superoxide dismutase activity by silicon. *J Trace Elem Electrolytes Health Dis* 1990; 4: 97-99.
55. Bergonzi G, Paties C, Vassallo G, Zangrandi A, Poisetti PG, Ballocchi S, Fontana F, Scarpioni L. Dextran deposits in tissues of patients undergoing hemodialysis. Nephrol *Dial Transplant* 1990; 5: 54-58.
56. D'Haese PC, Van Landeghem GF, De Broe ME. Increased silicon levels in dialysis patients due to the high silicon content in the drinking water, inadequate water treatment procedures, and concentrate contamination: A multicentre study. *Nephrol Dial Transplant* 1996; 11: 1188-1189 (Reply Letter to the Editor).
57. Saldanha LF, Gonick HC, Rodriguez HJ, Marmelzat JA, Repique EV, Marcus CL. Silicon related syndrome in dialysis patients. *Nephron* 1997; 77: 48-56.
58. Hsieh Y-Y, Shen W-S, Lee L-Y, Wu T-L, Ning H-C, Sun C-F. Long-term changes in trace elements in patients undergoing chronic hemodialysis. *Biol Trace Elem Res* 2006; 109: 115-121.
59. Zwolińska D, Grzeszczak W, Szczepańska M, Kiliś-Pstrusińska K, Szprynger K. Lipid peroxidation and antioxidant enzymes in children on maintenance dialysis. *Pediatr Nephrol* 2006; 21: 705-710.
60. Bonomini M, Forster S, De Risio F, Rychly J, Nebe B, Manfrini V, Klinkmann H, Albertozzi A. Effects of selenium supplementation on immune parameters in chronic uraemic patients on haemodialysis. *Neprol Dial Transplant* 1995; 10: 1654-1661.
61. Rukgauer M, Schmitt Y, Schneider H, Krusejarres JD. Trace element balance in patients undergoing hemodialysis. *Trace Elem & Electrolytes* 1994; 11: 155-168.
62. Henderson I, Leung A, Halls D, Fell G, Dobbie J, Kennedy AC. Hyperchromiumaemia in chronic dialysis patients. *Proc EDTA-ERA* 1985; 22: 270-275.
63. D'Haese PC, Couttenye M-M, Lamberts LV, Elseviers MM, Goodman WG, Schrooten I, Cabrera W, De Broe ME. Al, Fe, Pb, Cd, Cu, Zn, Cr, Mg, Sr and Ca content in bone of end-stage renal failure patients. *Clin Chem* 1999; 45: 1548-1556.
64. Esfahani ST, Hamidian MR, Madani A, Ataei N, Mohseni P, Roudbari M, Marzieh Haddadi. Serum zinc and copper levels in children with chronic renal failure. *Pediatr Nephrol* 2006; 21: 1153-1156.
65. Navarro-Alarcon M, Reyes-Pérez A, Lopez-Garcia H, Palomares-Bayo M, Olalla-Herrera M, Lopez-Martinez MC. Longitudinal study of serum zinc and copper levels in hemodialysis patients and their relation to biochemical markers. *Biol Trace Elem Res*; 2006; 113: 209-222.
66. Mahajan SK, Bowersox EM, Rye DL, Abu-Hamdam DK, Prasad AS, McDonald FD, Biersack KL . Factors underlying abnormal zinc metabolism in uremia. *Kidney Int* 1989; 36 (Suppl): 269-273.
67. Richard MJ, Arnud J, Jurkovitz C, Hachache T, Meftahi H, Laporte F, Foret M, Favier A, Cordonnier D. Trace element lipid peroxidation abnormalities in patients with chronic renal failure. *Nephron* 1991; 57: 10-15.
68. Türk S, Bozfakioglu S, Ecder ST, Kahraman T, Gürel N, Erkoç R, Aysuna N, Türkmen A, Bekiroglu N, Ark E. Effects of zinc supplementation on the immune system and on antibody response to multivalent influenza vaccine in hemodialysis patients. *Int J Artif Organs* 1998; 21: 274-278.
69. Chevalier CA, Liepa G, Murphy MD, Suneson J, Vanbeber AD, Gorman MA, Cochran C. The effects of zinc supplementation on serum zinc and cholesterol concentrations in hemodialysis patients. *J Ren Nutr* 2002; 12: 183-189.
70. Thomson NP, Stevens BJ, Humphery TJ, Atkins RC. Comparison of trace elements in peritoneal dialysis, hemodialysis and uremia. *Kidney Int* 1983; 23: 9-14.
71. Van Landeghem GF, D'Haese PC, Lamberts LV, Djukanovic L, Pejanovic S, Goodman WG, De Broe ME. Low serum aluminum values in dialysis patients with increased bone aluminum levels. *Clin Nephrol* 1998; 50: 69-76.
72. Evans C (ed). Biochemistry of lanthanides. Plenum Press New York 1990.
73. Rosenkranz AR, Grobner T, Mayer GJ. Conventional or gadolinium containing contrast media: the choice between acute renal failure or nephrogenic systemic fibrosis. *Wien klin Wochenschr* 2007, 119: 271-275.
74. Evenepoel P, Zeegers M, Segaert S, Claes K, Kuypers D, Maes B, Flamen P, Fransis S, Vanrenterghem Y. Nephrogenic fibrosing dermopathy: a novel, disabling disorder in patients with renal failure. Nephrol Dial Transplant 2004, 19: 469-473.
75. Grobner T, Prischl. Gadolinium and nephrogenic systemic fibrosis. Kidney Int 2007; 72: 260-264.
76. Boyd AS, Zic JA, Abraham JL. Gadolinium deposition in nephrogenic fibrosing dermopathy. *J Am Acad Dermatol* 2007; 56: 27-30.
77. Marckmann P, Skov L, Rossen K, Dupont A, Brimnes Damholt M, Goya Heaf J, Thomsen HS. Nephrogenic systemic fibrosis: suspected causative role of gadodiamide used for contrast-enhanced magnetic resonance imaging. *J Am Soc Nephrol* 2006; 17: 2359 - 2362.
78. Andréjak M, Thuillier D, Lok C, Gras-Champel V. Fibrose systémique néphrogénique et produits à base de gadolinium: données disponibles début 2007 Nephrogenic Systemic Fibrosis and Gadolinium-based Contrast Media. *Thérapie* 2007; 62: 169-172.

79. Thomsen HS, (ed) Contrast Media. Safety Issues and ESUR Guidelines. Springer: Berlin, Heidelberg, New York, 2006.
80. Liu J, liu Y, Habeebu SM, Waalkes MP, Klaassen CD. Chronic combined exposure to cadmium and arsenic exacerbates nephrotoxicity, particularly in metallothionein-I/II null mice. *Toxicology* 2000, 147:157-166.
81. El-Sharaky AS, Newairy AA, Badreldeen MM, Eweda SM, Sheweita SA. Protective role of selenium against renal toxicity induced by cadmium in rats. *Toxicology* 2007; 235: 185-93.
82. Van Landeghem GF, D' Haese PC, Lamberts LV, De Broe ME. Competition of iron and aluminium for transferrin: the molecular basis for aluminium deposition in iron-overloaded dialysis patients? *Exp Nephrol* 1997; 5: 239-245.
83. Ahamed M, Singh S, Behari JR, Kumar A, Siddiqui MKJ. Interaction of lead with some essential trace metals in the blood of anemic children from Lucknow, India. *Clin Chim Acta* 2007; 377: 92-97.

42

Smoking and the kidney

Eberhard RITZ

Ruperto-Carola-University, Heidelberg, Germany

Introduction

Smoking, mostly cigarette smoking, is one of the most important modifiable renal risk factor. In contrast to the long known potential of cigarette smoking to promote carcinogenesis, lung disease and cardiovascular events, even in the renal community the renal risk has only recently attracted attention [1], although the renal risk conferred by smoking had been known to diabetologists for more than 2 decades [2].

Acute effects of smoking on the kidney

As early as in 1907 Hesse had described in his doctoral thesis the transient increase of blood pressure and heart rate during cigarette smoking [3]. Nevertheless it had long been claimed that there was no excess hypertension in smokers [4], presumably hypertension is masked because the body weight of smokers is low. Cryer et al [5] documented marked sympathetic activation during cigarette smoking and the release of blood pressure active hormones such as AVP, aldosterone, cortisone and ACTH. The effect of smoking on blood pressure outlasts the period of smoking. In a controlled study Ritz documented higher night time blood pressure on a day when occasional smokers smoked compared to a day when they did not smoke (Figure 1) [6]. She found that this was accompanied by commensurate changes in heart rate. The effects of smoking are complex as illustrated by the findings that smoking also increases arterial stiffness [7] and causes a curious "reversed" office hypertension, i.e. normal office blood pressure in patients with high home blood pressure measurements [8].

The effects of smoking on renal hemodynamics are pronounced. We showed that smoking caused an acute increase in circulating epinephrine, in heart rate and in blood pressure; this is accompanied by a decrease in the filtration fraction with a significant increase of renal vascular resistance [9]. This renal hemodynamic pattern could be reproduced in healthy volunteers by chewing a nicotine containing gum, suggesting that nicotine is the main culprit. Interestingly in patients with IgA glomerulonephritis smoking failed to consistently reduce the filtration fraction; on average filtration fraction remained unchanged and a transient increase

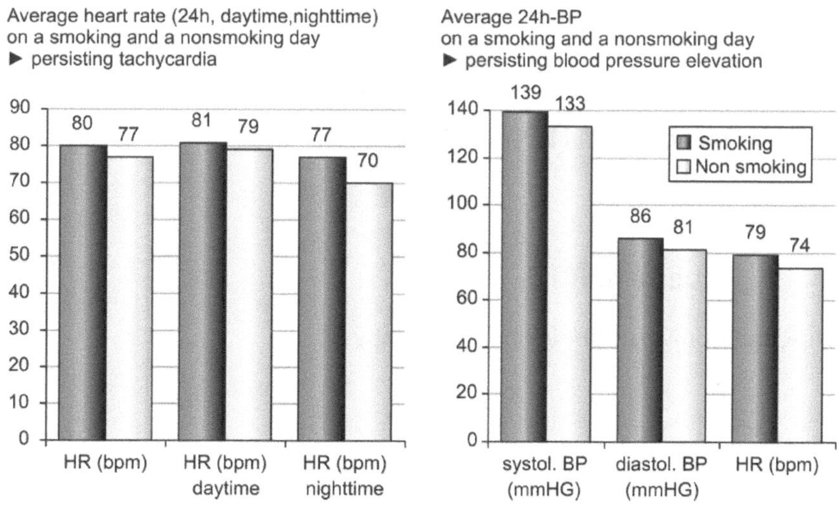

Figure 1. *Systolic and diastolic blood pressure as well as heart rate in healthy occasional smokers – comparison of a smoking day with a non-smoking day [6].*

in urinary albumin excretion was seen, consistent with (but not proof for) acute glomerular hypertension. Plasma renin activity in the circulation did not increase, but even this is inappropriate to the blood pressure increase. Nevertheless the renin-angiotensin system may play a role in the genesis of the acute hemodynamic changes in the kidney, since they were abrogated by ß-1 selective blockers [10].

In animal experiments we produced severe of proteinuria, pronounced glomerulosclerosis and marked interstitial fibrosis when we applied an acetone extract of cigarette smoke to the oral mucosa of subtotally nephrectomized rats [11].

Despite these acute alterations of glomerular function and morphology, in the long run the damage from smoking seems to be mainly mediated by damage to the renal vasculature. Halimi [12] found that acutely cigarette smoking increased the excretion of cGMP in the urine, pointing to compensatory vasodilatation in response to nicotin mediated vasoconstriction. In contrast in long-term observations Gambaro [13] found increased endothelin-1 concentrations in cigarette smokers and this was associated with increased renovascular resistance. The concept of a primary vascular problem in the kidneys of smokers is in line with the observation of Lhotta [14]: he examined renal biopsies of patients with primary renal disease. In smokers he found more severe myointimal hyperplasia and arteriolar hyalinosis. The concept of primarily vascular damage is also in line with our recent observation [15] that diabetic patients with microalbuminuria/proteinuria had a more rapid increase of serum creatinine concentration with time compared to non smokers despite no difference in urinary protein excretion.

Smoking and renal disease

Smoking and microalbuminuria

In early studies on microalbuminuria smoking was identified as a powerful predictor of microalbuminuria [16, 17]. This has recently been confirmed and extended in large population based studies. In the PREVEND study Pinto-Sietsma [18] found that current smokers had an adjusted relative risk of microalbuminuria of 1.65, former smokers a RR of 1.27, but heavy smokers > 20 cigarettes per day a RR of 1.96. This finding was confirmed in the ARIC study where the odds ratio for current smokers was 2.33 and in former smokers 1.58 [19].

In Okinawa Tozawa found in a prospective follow up study that the relative risk to develop proteinuria was 1.32 in a prospective follow up study [20].

Atherosclerotic renal artery stenosis

Many investigators identified smoking as a strong risk factor for atherosclerotic renal artery stenosis; Hadj-Abdelkader [21] found that 70-80% of patients with this diagnosis were smokers and frequently these stenoses are bilateral [22] and frequently the source of cholesterol microembolism [23].

Ischemic nephropathy

A selective decrease of renal plasma flow (RBF) with no decrease in glomerular filtration rate in smokers

[24] is most likely the result of smoking induced endothelial cell dysfunction and possibly also the result of increased production of endothelin 1 [13].

Smoking specific glomerulopathy (including "idiopathic nodular glomerulosclerosis")

Markowitz described "idiopathic nodular glomerulosclerosis", a distinct entity linked to hypertension and smoking [25]. Even in the absence of hypertension a more recent series [26] in nondiabetic heavy smokers showed as smoking specific glomerular damage - apart from nodular glomerulosclerosis - a broader spectrum with segmental or focal glomerulosclerosis, glomerular ischemia, interstitial fibrosis and tubular atrophy as well ad arterial sclerosis and hyalinosis. Electron microscopy showed capillary basement thickening and reduplication.

Diabetic nephropathy

Since the seminal description of Christiansen [2] cigarette smoking had been known to diabetologists as a risk factor for the onset and progression of microangiopathy. Cigarette smoking diabetics have a higher risk to develop microalbuminuria, a greater rate of progression to proteinuria and a greater risk to experience an elevation of serum creatinine. This has been confirmed in numerous studies [27-32]. In diabetic patients with overt diabetic nephropathy and elevated serum creatinine the measured rate of loss of creatinine clearance was twice as high in smokers compared to non-smokers [33]. For obvious reasons there are no controlled prospective studies on whether cessation of smoking attenuates the rate of loss of GFR, but the observation of Sawicki is telling [32]: in type I diabetic patients diabetic nephropathy progressed in 11% of non-smokers, in 33% of ex-smokers and in 53% of current smokers, suggestive of (but not proof for) a beneficial effect of cessation of smoking.

It is of interest that several recent studies confirm that smoking increases not only the risk to develop diabetic nephropathy, but also the risk to develop type 2 diabetes as found in the nurses health study [34] and recently confirmed by other studies [35].

Nondiabetic primary renal disease

There had been some past reports that the risk of progression was higher in patients with lupus nephritis who smoked [36] and in patients with autosomal dominant polycystic kidney disease [37]; but it had remained uncertain, whether smoking affected the immune response and - in view of the two hit hypothesis to explain the generation of renal cysts in ADPKD - whether the higher renal risk of smoking in ADPKD patients is not explained by DNA mutations resulting from smoking.

In a retrospective case control study, however, examining both patients with inflammatory (IgA glomerulonephritis) and non-inflammatory (ADPKD) primary renal disease, Orth et al. [38] found an increased odds ratio of progression to end stage renal disease in patients with 5–15 pack years [odds ratio 3.5 (1.3–9.6)] and in patients with > 15 pack years [5.8 (2.0–17.0; $p < 0.001$)]. Interestingly the increased odds ratio was found only in patients who were not on ACE inhibitors (Table 1).

ACE inhibitors do not provide complete protection, however. In type 2 diabetics Chuahirun found that despite treatment with ACE inhibitors reaching target blood pressure values, serum creatinine had risen to significantly higher values in smokers (1.78 ± 0.2 mg/dl) compared to non-smokers (1.32 ± 0.01) during a 61 months follow up [39].

Chronic kidney disease and end-stage renal disease

The adverse effect of smoking on renal function in patients without primary renal disease has also been well documented. Smoking was the most powerful predictor of progression in patients with severe essential hypertension in the study of Regalado [40] and, as reflected by an increase of serum creatinine > 3 mg/dl, also in the study of Bleyer [41].

In a large prospective population sample, primarily a cancer research project (CLUE study), Haroun [42] noted that smoking accounted for no less than 30% of the "attributable risk" of chronic kidney disease (CKD), defined as serum creatinine > 2 mg/dl, and this was particularly true in the elderly.

Table 1. Smoking – ESRF in men (n=144) with primary renal disease (retrospective case-control study) [27].

Pack-years	Odds ratio (95%-CI)	*p*-value
0-5	1.0	-
5-15	3.5 (1.3-9.6)	0.017
>15	5.8 (2.0-17.0)	0.001

In a nationwide study Ejerblad [43] found a relative risk of major serum creatinine (>3.4 mg/dl) elevation of 1.51 for smokers > 20 cigarettes/day and a risk of 1.52 for smokers with > 30 packyears. A similar magnitude of risk was noted by Ishani [44] in the MRFIT study (RR1.84).

Based on NHANES data 1976–1980 Stengel [45] found in individuals smoking 1–20 cigarettes/day a relative risk of 1.2 and in individuals smoking > 20 cigarettes/day a relative risk of 2.3 for endstage renal disease.

Renal transplants

The adverse effect of cigarette smoking on renal function was not seen only in the kidneys of patients with primary renal disease but also in renal allograft recipients [46]. The hazard ratio of graft loss censored for patient death was 1.48. Sung even found a relative risk of 2.3 for patient s with a history of pretransplant smoking [47].

Conclusion

It emerges from the above that smoking is a major renal risk factor, causing onset and progression of renal disease. The magnitude of the risk is comparable to that conferred by blood pressure elevation and proteinuria. It is a modifiable risk factor [48] but the attention which the medical community devotes to this risk factor is far from what it should be.

References

1. Orth SR, Ritz E, Schrier RW: The renal risks of smoking. *Kidney Int* 51:1669-1677, 1997.
2. Christiansen JS: Cigarette smoking and prevalence of microangiopathy in juvenile-onset insulin-dependent diabetes mellitus. *Diabetes Care* 1:146-149, 1978.
3. Hesse E: Einfluss des Rauchens auf den Kreislauf. *Deutsches Archiv klinische Medizin* 89:565-575, 1907.
4. Green MS, Jucha E, Luz Y: Blood pressure in smokers and nonsmokers: epidemiologic findings. *Am Heart J* 111:932-940, 1986.
5. Cryer PE, Haymond MW, Santiago JV, Shah SD: Norepinephrine and epinephrine release and adrenergic mediation of smoking-associated hemodynamic and metabolic events. *N Engl J Med* 295:573-577, 1976
6. Ritz S: Einfluss des Rauchens auf Blutdruck und Herzfrequenz bei Probanden mit und ohne primäre Nierenerkrankung. *Inauguraldissertation (Medizinische Fakultät der Ruprecht-Karls-Universität Heidelberg)*, 2003.
7. Yasmin, Falzone R, Brown MJ: Determinants of arterial stiffness in offspring of families with essential hypertension. *Am J Hypertens* 17:292-298, 2004.
8. Narkiewicz K, Kjeldsen SE, Hedner T: Is smoking a causative factor of hypertension? *Blood Press* 14:69-71, 2005.
9. Ritz E, Benck U, Franek E, Keller C, Seyfarth M, Clorius J: Effects of smoking on renal hemodynamics in healthy volunteers and in patients with glomerular disease. *J Am Soc Nephrol* 9:1798-1804, 1998.
10. Benck U, Clorius JH, Zuna I, Ritz E: Renal hemodynamic changes during smoking: effects of adrenoreceptor blockade. *Eur J Clin Invest* 29:1010-1018, 1999.
11. Odoni G, Ogata H, Viedt C, Amann K, Ritz E, Orth SR: Cigarette smoke condensate aggravates renal injury in the renal ablation model. *Kidney Int* 61:2090-2098, 2002.
12. Halimi JM, Giraudeau B, Vol S, Caces E, Nivet H, Lebranchu Y, Tichet J: Effects of current smoking and smoking discontinuation on renal function and proteinuria in the general population. *Kidney Int* 58:1285-1292, 2000.
13. Gambaro G, Verlato F, Budakovic A, Casara D, Saladini G, Del Prete D, Bertaglia G, Masiero M, Checchetto S, Baggio B: Renal impairment in chronic cigarette smokers. *J Am Soc Nephrol* 9:562-567, 1998.
14. Lhotta K, Rumpelt HJ, Konig P, Mayer G, Kronenberg F: Cigarette smoking and vascular pathology in renal biopsies. *Kidney Int* 61:648-654, 2002.
15. Orth SR, Schroeder T, Ritz E, Ferrari P: Effects of smoking on renal function in patients with type 1 and type 2 diabetes mellitus. *Nephrol Dial Transplant* 20:2414-2419, 2005.
16. Mimran A, Ribstein J, DuCailar G, Halimi JM: Albuminuria in normals and essential hypertension. *J Diabetes Complications* 8:150-156, 1994.
17. Hörner D, Fliser D, Klimm HP, Ritz E: Albuminuria in normotensive and hypertensive individuals attending offices of general practitioners. *J Hypertens* 14:655-660, 1996.
18. Pinto-Sietsma SJ, Mulder J, Janssen WM, Hillege HL, de Zeeuw D, de Jong PE: Smoking is related to albuminuria and abnormal renal function in nondiabetic persons. *Ann Intern Med* 133:585-591, 2000.

19. Hogan S.H.,Colindres R.E., Cai J., Coresh J.: Association of Smoking with Albuminuria in a cross-sectional Probability Sample of US Adults. *J.Am.Soc.Nephrol.* 12:209a, 2001.
20. Tozawa M, Iseki K, Iseki C, Oshiro S, Ikemiya Y, Takishita S: Influence of smoking and obesity on the development of proteinuria. *Kidney Int* 62:956-962, 2002.
21. Hadj-Abdelkader M, Alphonse JC, Boyer L, Younes H, Deteix P: [Smoking and atheromatous stenosis of the renal arteries]. *Arch Mal Coeur Vaiss* 94:925-927, 2001.
22. Shurrab AE, Mamtora H, O'Donoghue D, Waldek S, Kalra PA: Increasing the diagnostic yield of renal angiography for the diagnosis of atheromatous renovascular disease. *Br J Radiol* 74:213-218, 2001.
23. Scolari F, Tardanico R, Zani R, Pola A, Viola BF, Movilli E, Maiorca R: Cholesterol crystal embolism: A recognizable cause of renal disease. *Am J Kidney Dis* 36:1089-1109, 2000.
24. Baggio B, Budakovic A, Casara D, Gambaro G, Saladini G, Piccoli A, Verlato F: Renal involvement in subjects with peripheral atherosclerosis. *J Nephrol* 14:286-292, 2001.
25. Markowitz GS, Lin J, Valeri AM, Avila C, Nasr SH, D'Agati VD: Idiopathic nodular glomerulosclerosis is a distinct clinicopathologic entity linked to hypertension and smoking. *Hum Pathol* 33:826-835, 2002.
26. Liang KV, Greene EL, Oei LS, Lewin M, Lager D, Sethi S: Nodular glomerulosclerosis: renal lesions in chronic smokers mimic chronic thrombotic microangiopathy and hypertensive lesions. *Am J Kidney Dis* 49:552-559, 2007.
27. Telmer S, Christiansen JS, Andersen AR, Nerup J, Deckert T: Smoking habits and prevalence of clinical diabetic microangiopathy in insulin-dependent diabetics. *Acta Med Scand* 215:63-68, 1984.
28. Rossing P, Hougaard P, Parving HH: Risk factors for development of incipient and overt diabetic nephropathy in type 1 diabetic patients: a 10-year prospective observational study. *Diabetes Care* 25:859-864, 2002.
29. Scott LJ, Warram JH, Hanna LS, Laffel LM, Ryan L, Krolewski AS: A nonlinear effect of hyperglycemia and current cigarette smoking are major determinants of the onset of microalbuminuria in type 1 diabetes. *Diabetes* 50:2842-2849, 2001.
30. Chase HP, Garg SK, Marshall G, Berg CL, Harris S, Jackson WE, Hamman RE: Cigarette smoking increases the risk of albuminuria among subjects with type I diabetes. *Jama* 265:614-617, 1991.
31. Bangstad HJ, Osterby R, Rudberg S, Hartmann A, Brabrand K, Hanssen KF: Kidney function and glomerulopathy over 8 years in young patients with Type I (insulin-dependent) diabetes mellitus and microalbuminuria. *Diabetologia* 45:253-261, 2002.
32. Sawicki PT, Didjurgeit U, Muhlhauser I, Bender R, Heinemann L, Berger M: Smoking is associated with progression of diabetic nephropathy. *Diabetes Care* 17:126-131, 1994.
33. Biesenbach G, Grafinger P, Janko O, Zazgornik J: Influence of cigarette-smoking on the progression of clinical diabetic nephropathy in type 2 diabetic patients. *Clin Nephrol* 48:146-150, 1997.
34. Hu FB, Manson JE, Stampfer MJ, Colditz G, Liu S, Solomon CG, Willett WC: Diet, lifestyle, and the risk of type 2 diabetes mellitus in women. *N Engl J Med* 345:790-797, 2001.
35. Patja K, Jousilahti P, Hu G, Valle T, Qiao Q, Tuomilehto J: Effects of smoking, obesity and physical activity on the risk of type 2 diabetes in middle-aged Finnish men and women. *J Intern Med* 258:356-362, 2005.
36. Ward MM, Studenski S: Clinical prognostic factors in lupus nephritis. The importance of hypertension and smoking. *Arch Intern Med* 152:2082-2088, 1992.
37. Chapman AB, Johnson AM, Gabow PA, Schrier RW: Overt proteinuria and microalbuminuria in autosomal dominant polycystic kidney disease. *J Am Soc Nephrol* 5:1349-1354, 1994.
38. Orth SR, Stockmann A, Conradt C, Ritz E, Ferro M, Kreusser W, Piccoli G, Rambausek M, Roccatello D, Schafer K, Sieberth HG, Wanner C, Watschinger B, Zucchelli P: Smoking as a risk factor for end-stage renal failure in men with primary renal disease. *Kidney Int* 54:926-931, 1998.
39. Chuahirun T, Wesson DE: Cigarette smoking predicts faster progression of type 2 established diabetic nephropathy despite ACE inhibition. *Am J Kidney Dis* 39:376-382, 2002.
40. Regalado M, Yang S, Wesson DE: Cigarette smoking is associated with augmented progression of renal insufficiency in severe essential hypertension. *Am J Kidney Dis* 35:687-694, 2000.
41. Bleyer AJ, Shemanski LR, Burke GL, Hansen KJ, Appel RG: Tobacco, hypertension, and vascular disease: risk factors for renal functional decline in an older population. *Kidney Int* 57:2072-2079, 2000.
42. Haroun MK, Jaar BG, Hoffman SC, Comstock GW, Klag MJ, Coresh J: Risk factors for chronic kidney disease: a prospective study of 23,534 men and women in washington county, Maryland. *J Am Soc Nephrol* 14:2934-2941, 2003.
43. Ejerblad E, Fored CM, Lindblad P, Fryzek J, Dickman PW, Elinder CG, McLaughlin JK, Nyren O: Association between smoking and chronic renal failure in a nationwide population-based case-control study. *J Am Soc Nephrol* 15:2178-2185, 2004.
44. Ishani A, Grandits GA, Grimm RH, Svendsen KH, Collins AJ, Prineas RJ, Neaton JD: Association of single measurements of dipstick proteinuria, estimated glomerular filtration rate, and hematocrit with 25-year incidence of end-stage renal disease in the multiple risk factor intervention trial. *J Am Soc Nephrol* 17:1444-1452, 2006.

45. Stengel B, Tarver-Carr ME, Powe NR, Eberhardt MS, Brancati FL: Lifestyle factors, obesity and the risk of chronic kidney disease. *Epidemiology* 14:479-487, 2003.

46. Woo YM, McLean D, Kavanagh D, Ward L, Aitken S, Miller GJ, Egan P, Hughes K, Clark L, Carswell K, Morris ST, Northridge DB, Rodger RS, Jardine AG: The influence of pre-operative electrocardiographic abnormalities and cardiovascular risk factors on patient and graft survival following renal transplantation. *J Nephrol* 15:380-386, 2002.

47. Sung RS, Althoen M, Howell TA, Ojo AO, Merion RM: Excess risk of renal allograft loss associated with cigarette smoking. *Transplantation* 71:1752-1757, 2001.

48. Remuzzi G, Schieppati A, Ruggenenti P: Clinical practice. Nephropathy in patients with type 2 diabetes. *N Engl J Med* 346:1145-1151, 2002.

43

Star fruit

Miguel M. NETO[1], Ruither O. CAROLINO[2],
Norberto P. LOPES[4] and Norberto GARCIA-CAIRASCO[3]

Departments of [1]Nephrology, [2]Biochemistry and Immunology,
[3]Physiology, Faculty of Medicine, [4]Physics and Chemistry, Faculty of Pharmacy,
University of São Paulo, Ribeirão Preto, SP, Brazil

Introduction

The carambola or star fruit belongs to the *Oxalidaceae* family, species *Averrhoa carambola.* Slices cut in cross-section have the form of a star (Figure 1). It is believed to have originated in Ceylon and the Moluccas but it has been cultivated in southeast Asia and Malaysia for many centuries. It is commonly grown in some provinces in southern China, in Taiwan and India. It is rather popular in the Philippines and Queensland, Australia and moderately so in some of the South Pacific Islands, particularly Tahiti, New Caledonia and Netherlands New Guinea, and in Guam and Hawaii. There are some subspecies in the Caribbean Islands, in Central America and in tropical West Africa. It is also common in Brazil, where it is served as fresh beverage, *in natura,* or as an industrialized juice, as it is also served throughout the world. It was introduced into Southern Florida before 1887 and the fruits are also available in many European countries and Canada. It is widely used in restaurants for decorative purposes. In India, ripe fruit is administered to halt hemorrhages and to relieve bleeding hemorrhoids. In Brazil, star fruit is recommended as a diuretic for kidney and bladder complaints [1, 2].

There are 2 distinct classes of carambola: the smaller, very sour type, richly flavored, with more oxalic acid and the larger, so-called "sweet type", mild flavored, rather bland, with less oxalic acid. The oxalic content of ripe carambolas could reach to an average of 0.5 g per 100 mL of juice, the acid being mostly in the free state. Physicians should be informed of this because there are some individuals who may be adversely affected by ingestion of even small amounts of oxalic acid or oxalates. The acid types of carambola have been used to clean and polish metal, especially brass, as they dissolve tarnish and rust [1].

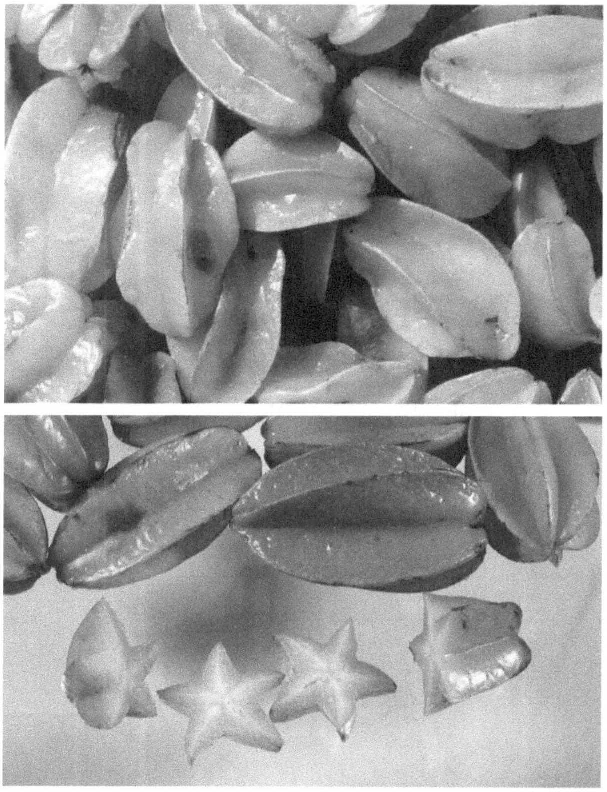

Figure 1. *Averrhoa carambola*

The first description of a patient intoxication outbreak was reported by Martin LC et al in 1993 [3]. They described an outbreak of intractable hiccups in patients on a regular program of hemodialysis. Of the 10 patients, 8 developed intractable hiccups. The other 2 patients who did not present hiccups ingested the fruit immediately before the hemodialysis sessions. Treatment with lidocaine, chlorpromazine, metoclopramide, flunitrazepam was useless. All patients with hiccups improved only after they were submitted to hemodialysis sessions. The authors did not describe any signs of neurological involvement such as behavioral disturbances or mental confusion. The hiccups had been seen as a curiosity and hallmark of star fruit intoxication and not as a threat till 1998. In that year, our group described 6 patients under dialysis that presented hiccups with neurological disturbances after eating star fruit: one patient died with convulsions, others presented mental confusion, psychomotor agitation, insomnia and 5 patients improved after a few hemodialysis sessions [4]. Most of the patients (5 patients) had intractable hiccups as their first symptoms.

Clinical manifestations of neurotoxicity

In 2000 Chang JM et al [5] reported 19 patients with renal failure under dialysis and one also with renal failure but in supportive treatment who after star fruit ingestion developed signs and symptoms of intoxication such as: hiccups, mental confusion, paresis, muscular weakness and convulsions. Eight of those patients died (including the patient in supportive treatment)

After those reports many other reports confirmed these findings and are summarized in Table 1 [3-19].

The most common symptom of star fruit intoxication is persistent and intractable hiccups, observed in almost all 88 patients reported in Table 1. After star fruit ingestion, hiccups start in a variable fashion from 2.5 hours to 14 hours (average 4.6 h) [5] or half to 10 hours (average 2 to 3 hours) [13]. In most of the intoxication cases, attempts to treat hiccups with chlorpromazine and metoclopramide were unsuccessful. The amount of fruit ingested varied in the literature from small pieces to large amounts as 500 mL of juice in 1 to 3 days [13]. Even a small amount of star fruit can cause severe neurological complications and death. According to Chang JM et al [5] presenting symptoms were predominantly neuromuscular. Report of limb numbness were noted in 75%, persistent hiccups in 60%, disturbed consciousness of various degrees in 50%, decreased muscle power in 35%, dyspnea in 25%. Eight of the 10 patients with abnormal consciousness died (80%). According to Neto MM et al [13] persistent hiccups were noted in 93.7%, vomiting in 68.7%, disturbed consciousness of variable degrees (mental confusion that progressed to coma in some cases, psychomotor agitation) in 65.6%, decreased muscle power, limb numbness, paresis, insomnia and paresthesias) in 40.6%, seizures in 21.8% and hemodynamic instability (hypotension and shock) in 9.3%. Seven of the 32 patients who presented seizures and severe consciouness disturbances died.

Star fruit intoxication can be classified into three levels according to signs and symptoms that might provide a useful guideline for institution of proper treatment: mild, moderate and severe (Table 2).

Certain cases of mild intoxication progress to a severe level if patients are not treated and the velocity of progression is extremely variable, depending on the characteristics of each patient. In some cases this progression happens with less than 24 hours after star fruit ingestion [5, 13, 9, 10, 15, 17, 18, 19]. Therefore,

Table 1. Reports of star fruit intoxication.

Reports	Number of cases	Treatment before intoxication	Symptoms described
Martin LC et al, 1993 [3]	08	HD: 7 PD: 1	Hiccups, insomnia
Neto MM et al, 1998 [4]	06	HD: 4 PD: 2	Hiccups, vomiting, insomnia, consciousness disturbance, seizures
Chang JM et al, 2000 [5]	20	HD: 15 PD: 4 Supportive: 1	Hiccups, consciousness disturbance, numbness of limbs, decreased muscle power, skin paresthesia, seizures
Wang JL et al, 2000 [6]	02	Supportive: 2	Hiccups, consciousness disturbance, seizures
Lo KY et al, 2001 [7]	01	PD	Hiccups, insomnia
Ho MP et al 2001[8]	02	Suppportive: 2	Hiccups, vomiting, consciousness disturbance, seizures
Wu CC et al, 2002 [9]	02	Supportive: 2	Hiccups, consciousness disturbance
Yap HJ et al, 2002 [10]	03	HDI: 1 Supportive: 2	Hiccups, insomnia, vomiting, consciousness disturbance, seizures
Chan YL et al, 2002 [11]	01	PD: 1	Hiccups, consciousness disturbances, seizures
Tse KC et al, 2003 [12]	06	PD: 4 HD: 1 Supportive: 1	Hiccups, vomiting, consciousness disturbances, hyperkalemia
Neto MM et al, 2003 [13]	32*	HD: 20 PD: 8 Supportive: 4	Hiccups, vomiting, consciousness disturbances, seizures
Neto MM et al 2004 [14]	04	Supportive: 4	Hiccups, vomiting, diarrhea, consciousness disturbances, seizures
Chang CH et al 2004[15]	01	HD	Vomiting, consciousness disturbances, seizures
Hung SW et al 2004[16]	01	Supportive	Hiccups, vomiting, diarrhea, numbness of the lower limbs, seizures
Tsai MH et al 2005[17]	02	Supportive: 2	Hiccups, nausea, consciousness disturbances, seizures
Chen LL et al 2005 [18]	01	Supportive	Hiccups, consciousness disturbances,
Wu MY et al 2007[19]	02	Supportive: 1 HD: 1	Hiccups, vomiting, consciousness disturbances, seizures
Total	**88**	**HD: 46 PD: 19 Supportive: 23**	

HD: Hemodialysis, PD: peritoneal dialysis, supportive: not yet on a dialysis program

** Included 6 patients of Ref 4.*

Table 2. Clinical levels of star fruit intoxication.

Intoxication level	Signs and symptoms
Mild	• Hiccups • Vomiting • Insomnia
Moderate	• Psychomotor agitation • Numbness, paresthesias and decreased muscle power of the limbs • Mild mental confusion
Severe	• Moderate to severe mental confusion progressing to coma • Seizures progressing to status epilepticus • Hemodynamic instability progressing to hypotension and shock

any patient with renal failure (stages 3 to 5) with a suspected star fruit intoxication should not be discharged and should be observed very closely.

The severe cases may be difficult to diagnose promptly, since the symptoms mimic either strokes (brain stem strokes) or may even resemble "metabolic" or uremic disturbances [9, 13, 15, 16, 19]. Due to suspicion of organic neurologic problems, many patients with severe intoxication had cerebrospinal fluid collected, and were submitted to CT or MRI. No specifical findings were detected in any of this examinations according to review of the literature. A single exception has been the report by Chan YL et al (11) in which the authors claim that star fruit poisoning can induce hyperintense lesions at the thalami and right temporo-occipital cortex revealed by single voxel proton MR spectroscopy.

According to Martin LC et al [3] from 10 patients that ingested the fruit only 8 developed hiccups, the other 2 ate the fruits before their hemodialysis sessions and did not present any symptom.

Although star fruit has enriched potassium content, hyperkalemia has not been suggested as causing of death in reported cases [5, 13].

Most of the patients that were reported in literature were on a regular program of peritoneal dialysis (PD) or hemodialysis (HD). From 88 described patients, 23 patients were without need of regular dialysis or they did not know that they have kidney problems (Table 1). Their creatinine levels ranged from 2.3 mg/dL to 20.5 mg/dL. These patients developed signs and symptoms varying from mild to severe levels of intoxication.

Seizures are present in 30% of patients with star fruit intoxication [17], and most patients have convulsive [6, 8, 10, 11, 13, 14, 17, 18, 19] or non-convulsive [16] *status epilepticus*. The mortality rate of patients with seizures occurring after star fruit intoxication (severe intoxication) is significantly higher than of patients without seizures [13, 17]. Phenytoin, midazolam, diazepam and phenobarbital seem to have little or no effect on the control of persistent seizures provoked by star fruit toxicity. However, significant clinical improvement of seizure was demonstrated in one patient after the use of profofol [20].

Sometimes there is a poor correlation with the degree of underlying renal function and the symptoms, while more severe symptoms may develop in those patients with pre-dialyzed conditions as opposed to those with end stage renal disease [17]. These variations of symptoms among individuals might be explained by individual biological responses, genetic factors, patient age, the amount of toxin content in each fruit, various star fruit subespecies, and the detoxification, excretion, or both, of the toxin from the blood stream [7, 13].

Treatment and outcome: a literature review

According to the revised literature there are 88 patients described, 46 previously on hemodialysis (HD), 19 on peritoneal dialysis (PD) and 23 without previous dialytic treatment (supportive treatment). These patients were described in 16 reports in the medical literature with their symptoms and treatment outcomes [3-19].

In one of the first observations, Martin LC et al [3] reported that hemodialysis eliminated all symptoms, although all of them presented clinical pictures of mild intoxication (hiccups and vomiting). None of those patients had mental confusion or seizures. In another report 6 patients who were described by Neto et al [4], one patient died and PD was offered as the only treatment. The other five received conventional hemodialysis and improved without sequelae (mild and moderate levels of intoxication, and in one case the patient had severe mental confusion without seizures or hemodynamic instability). Unfortunately there is no neurological follow up of any kind in any of the studies in order to look for eventual neurological sequelae in survivors after what we may call the hemodialysis rescue.

Chang et al [5] in a retrospective study of 20 patients described that among 10 patients with abnormal consciousness 8 died despite additional emergent hemodialysis. They did not specify the length of dialysis and the time this emergent dialysis was performed after ingestion. The patients who died had an earlier onset of symptoms (average 4.6 hours after ingestion) than survivors (average 8.8 hours after ingestion).

In their series of 32 patients Neto et al [13] showed that seven patients died after intoxication episodes. The main characteristics of the patients who died were convulsive activities in 6 and severe mental confusion in all 7 patients, while 2 of them presented hemodynamic instability (hypotension and shock). Most of the patients who died were treated by peritoneal dialysis or did not receive any other kind of treatment. The other 25 patients improved without sequelae and they were treated either by conventional hemodialysis, daily hemodialysis (6 to 8 hours duration) or even by continuous methods of dialysis. A few patients were treated by peritoneal dialysis. Complete recovery time in these 25 patients ranged from 1 to 12 days (mean 4.4 days and median 4.0 days).

Tse KC et al [12] presented 6 cases with mild or moderate intoxication. Three patients were treated with intensive hemodialysis and improved, 3 were treated with peritoneal dialysis and also improved. Most patients responded after 2-3 days of treatment.

Neto MM et al [14] presented 4 cases, 3 with mild intoxication and 1 with severe intoxication. Patients with mild intoxication recovered spontaneously and were not dialysed. The patient with severe intoxication and end-stage renal disease was submitted to daily hemodialysis of 6 to 10 hours duration and woke up after 10 days and 80 hours of hemodialysis (extended daily dialysis - EDD). This patient was discharged after 20 days of hospitalization and was enrolled in a program of regular hemodialysis.

Wang JL et al [6] reported 2 cases of patients with severe intoxication who died despite hemodialysis but the time of hemodialysis initiation after ingestion is not known.

Lo KY et al [7] reported one patient with mild intoxication who improved maintaining previous treatment (continuous ambulatory peritoneal dialysis - CAPD).

Ho MP et al [8] described 2 patients, one with moderate and other with severe intoxication who improved after hemodialysis. The patient with moderate intoxication recovered with 2 sessions of HD and the other recovered after 14 days of HD.

Wu CC et al [9] described 2 cases: one with mild intoxication that recovered with only one 6 hour HD session and a severe case who improved with HD after 5 days. Hemodialysis was performed at the same day when the patients were admitted to the hospital.

Yap HJ et al [10] presented 3 cases: one with mild intoxication that improved after HD in 2 days; the second patient presented with mild intoxication that progressed to moderate intoxication after one week without treatment, and improved after 2 days of HD; the third patient who had severe intoxication, was treated with 2 sessions of plasmapheresis without improvement and received HD later. He died after 25 days after admission.

Chan YL et al [11] described one patient with severe intoxication who was submitted to HD 2 days after intoxication and died 7 weeks later with worsening of consciousness disturbances.

Hung SW et al [15] reported a severe case of a patient with intoxication who died. A continuous method of renal replacement therapy was started on the fourth day of intoxication.

Chang CH et al [16] reported one case of severe intoxication that improved with HD in 11 days.

Tsai MH et al [17] reported 2 cases of severe intoxication. Both patients were submitted to hemodialysis, one, 2 days and the other, 3 days after admission, and both died after 23 days and 7 days of treatment respectively.

Chen LL et al [18] reported one severe case of a patient who started hemodialysis 3 days after admission. His state of consciousness did not modify with hemodialysis. Charcoal hemoperfusion was performed during 6 hours and his consciousness improved progressively. About 24 hours after the 6 hours session of hemoperfusion, his consciousness returned to normal without subsequent mental confusion.

Wu MY et al [19] reported 2 severe cases of intoxication. One patient ingested 2 fruits, arriving to the hospital with persistent hiccups, nausea and vomiting. During the next 24 hours, agitation, subsequent drowsy consciousness developed. He was intubated and seizures occurred with a generalized tonic-clonic pattern, evolving to *status epilepticus*. Hemodialysis was performed in the first hospital day. On the second hospital day hemoperfusion was performed due to persistent comatose state after hemodialysis. The condition improved after 20 hours of hemoperfusion. The other patient ingested 1 star fruit in the afternoon and at the same night she presented with hiccups, agitation, bizarre behaviour and mental confusion. Due to deterioration of consciousness and respiratory distress, the trachea was intubated. On the first day the patient underwent a hemodialysis session and remained comatose. A neurologist suspected of a brain stem stroke. Daily dialysis was arranged for 2 days, but she remained comatose. Charcoal hemoperfusion was performed on the third hospital day for 8 hours and consciousness recovered 16 hours after the hemoperfusion session on the fourth hospital day. The patient was weaned off a ventilator on the fifth hospital day.

Treatment and outcome summary

Seven patients who were in supportive treatment (without need for dialysis) at the time of star fruit ingestion had mild intoxication presenting hiccups or diarrhea. Six patients improved without dialysis. Time to improve was up to 24 hours in 4 patients, 5 days in another one, and there is no information in one patient. One patient improved after IPD (intermittent peritoneal dialysis)[13, 14]. Peritoneal dialysis was not an efficient method of treatment although 1 patient with signs and symptoms of moderate intoxication and 2 with mild intoxication changed from CAPD to IPD (intermittent peritoneal dialysis) and improved [13]. Two patients that remained in CAPD also improved [7, 12]. In one case [13] patient presented diplopia that continued for 6 weeks after improvement of the acute intoxication episode. Patients with severe intoxication did not benefit from peritoneal dialysis treatment [13].

Hemodialysis was an efficient method in 30 reported cases especially if initiated early, together with aggressive supportive care including mechanical ventilation in some severe cases [8, 9, 10, 12, 13, 14, 16]. Many patients presented rebound effects after dialysis, with symptoms starting a few hours after the end of the dialytic procedures. These rebound effects included persistence of hiccups or worsening of consciousness disturbances [13]. Interestingly, 2 surviving patients with severe intoxication presenting with seizures and hemodynamic instability, were given continuous replacement therapy as first choice treatment [13]. The recovery time in these 2 cases was 8 and 12 days. Another patient treated with EDD woke up after 10 days of treatment (14). In other 14 reported patients hemodialysis was not effective and patients died despite treatment [5, 6, 10, 11, 15, 17]. In 8 cases reported by Chang JM et al [5] the study was retrospective and we do not know the emergent dialysis starting time and neither the dialysis dose. We also do not have this information in the 2 cases reported by Wang JL et al [6]. Yap HJ et al [10]. describes one severe case of intoxication submitted twice to plasma exchange without improvement. Hemodialysis was started later and the patient died 25 days later due to pneumonia and septic shock without improving consciousness disturbance. In the other 4 reported cases hemodialysis was started within 2 or more days [10, 11, 15, 17]. Early recognition of star fruit intoxication and prompt and properly treatment with hemodialysis seem to be an important factor affecting the survival of patients. In severe cases, prolonged coma duration may be associated with increased morbidity and mortality [10, 11, 13, 14, 17].

Hemoperfusion was used for the first time as an option of treatment in a severe case by Chen LL et al [18] and patient consciousness returned to normal without subsequent mental confusion. Wu MY et al [19] submitted 2 patients with severe intoxication to 20 hours and 8 hours of hemoperfusion and also had good and fast improvement of the intoxication condition. In this 3 cases, 2 hemodialysis sessions in the first described patient, 1 hemodialysis session and 2 daily hemodialysis session in the patients of the second report failed to counterbalance neurotoxicity; however consciousness improved dramatically after hemoperfusion [19]. A dramatic decrease in comatose time and rapid weaning from the ventilator may help reduce morbidity and mortality [19]. Hemoperfusion seems to be a promising kind of treatment to severe cases of star fruit intoxication. However this issue requires further analysis with large trials [19].

Clinical manifestations of nephrotoxicity

Chen CL et al [21] described 2 patients who developed nausea, vomiting, abdominal pain and lumbar pain and presented acute renal failure due to acute interstitial nephritis after the ingestion of great amounts of star fruit juice. Both patients were submitted to hemodialysis, and kidney histology showed typical alterations due to acute oxalate nephropathy such as intraluminal and intraepithelial deposition of colorless oxalate crystals with a pattern of birefringence including all colours of the rainbow under polarized light. These crystals also appear blue in hematoxylin-eosin stain and black in von Kossa´s stain. In both cases renal function recovered in 4 weeks. One of the patients ingested 1600 mL of the juice and the other 3000 mL in a short time interval. The authors determined the oxalate content of sour carambola juice ingested by the patients. The results showed the oxalate contents of star fruit juice ingested in both cases; in one case were 820 mg/dL and in the other case 308 mg/dL. The estimated amounts of ingested oxalate were 13.1 g in one case and 9.2 g for the other case. There are 2 types of star fruit, sour and sweet. The sour type contains more oxalate than the sweet type [1].

Oxalic acid and its soluble salts are poisonous to humans and animals, whereas insoluble salts of calcium and magnesium oxalate are not. Oxalates ingested by humans may be precipitated by calcium as an insoluble complex, which then is excreted in feces [21, 22, 23]. In both cases reported by Chien et al [21], patients ingested sour carambola juice on an empty stomach so that the protective effect of calcium and magnesium in food was not present. The dehydration state may have contributed to the development of carambola- associated acute nephropathy. The authors do not report any concomitant neurological signs or symptoms [21].

Fang HC et al [24] in their report intended to establish a connection between star fruit and acute oxalate nephropathy. They administered star fruit juice, 4 mL/100 g of body weight, in male Sprague-Dawley rats of 180 to 200 g, with an oxalate concentration of 2.4g/dL, approximately 1 g/kg. The authors established a strong relationship between star fruit and acute oxalate nephropathy. This relationship was found only in the experimental group under both fasting and water deprivation conditions.

The acute interstititial nephritis after oxalate overload may be due to calcium oxalate crystals inducing obstructive effect, nephrocalcinosis and also by inducing apoptosis of renal epithelial cells [22, 23, 25].

Recently, Niticharoenpong K et al [26] reported a patient with underlying chronic renal disease, who developed a rapid increase in serum creatinine and oxalate nephropathy after chronic ingestion of star fruit juice without overt neurotoxicity. Urinalysis of this patient revealed numerous crystals, consistent with oxalate crystals. A kidney biopsy was performed and light microscopy showed crystals deposition consistent with oxalate crystals. The patient had been given star fruit by his family for over 3 years. The exact quantity of star fruit juice varied, and could not be ascertained with certainty.

Although there are not many other cases of star fruit oxalate nephrotoxicity described, it seems reasonable to avoid consumption of large amounts of star fruit juice especially on an empty stomach and chronic consumption in patients with underlying chronic renal disease.

Mechanisms of neurotoxicity

Molecular and biochemical aspects

Despite the recent reports of neurotoxicity of star fruit in uremic patients, the first one on star fruit toxicity was described by Muir and Lam [27] in 1980. They related toxic effects of star fruit extract after its intraperitoneal administration in mice. This extract induced seizures and death. In 1993, Martin LC et al. reported the outcome of intractable hiccups in uremic patients associated to star fruit consume [3]. However, the first report of neurotoxicity in human beings was performed by Moyses-Neto M et al (4). Subsequently, many similar case reports were described, but only in 2002 an etiological agent was proposed; oxalic acid would be the star fruit neurotoxin [28].

In fact, oxalic acid (Figure 2), a substance associated to intoxications, is found in other vegetables. The oxalic acid poisoning is well exemplified in the Sorrel poisoning. Sorrel refers to two species of plants belonging to the genus Rumex; *R.acetosa L.* and *R. acetosella L.*, which present high content of oxalate. Sorrel poisoning has been known to occur in man, horse and sheep and is associated to ingestion of these plants . Succinctly, the symptoms of Sorrel poisoning in human is due to the sequestering of serum calcium by the oxalic acid to form insoluble calcium oxalate. This reduction in available calcium leads to violent muscular stimulation with convulsions and collapse, associated to derangement of the blood-clotting mechanism. *Post-mortem*,

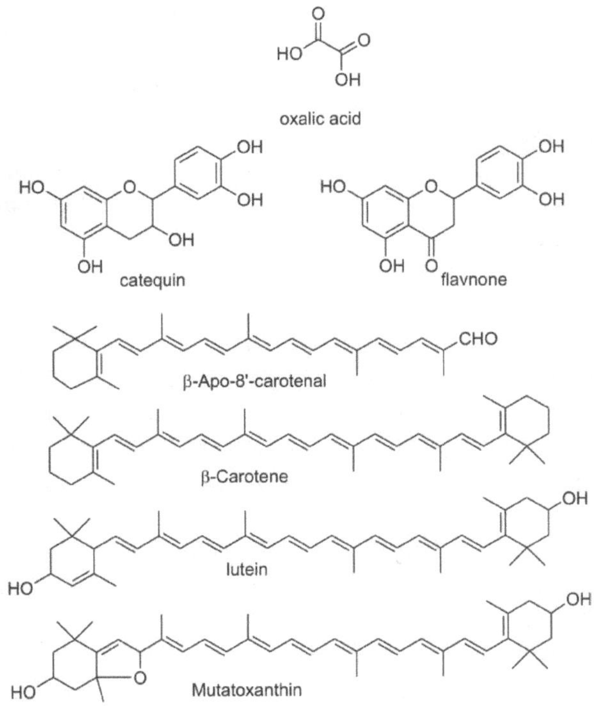

Figure 2. *Examples of chemical constituents presenting on star fruit juice.*

calcium oxalate crystals are found in the renal tubules and in others tissues. The kidney shows cloudy swelling, hyaline-degeneration and tubular sclerosis. The mouth, esophagus and stomach show corrosive effects, and cerebral edema is commonly found [29]. Hence, oxalic acid was considered a logical putative neurotoxin of star fruit.

In fact, this hypothesis was recently supported by a study that described the star fruit juice or oxalate solution administered by gavage could evoke seizures (convulsion associated to electroencephalographic recordings showing generalized spike-waves in parietal and frontal lobes) and death in nephrectomized rats. Furthermore, neither seizure nor death was reported when calcium-treated star fruit juice was administered. These observations are similar to those made after the administration of star fruit juice or oxalate solution administration to sham-operated rats [30]. These data showed the oxalate neurotoxicity in this animal model and gave support for the involvement of oxalate in the intoxication by star fruit in uremic patients.The hipothesis above is not supported by the fact that foods presenting comparable or higher oxalic acid content (i.e. rhubarb and spinach, respectively) [31]; do not induce similar intoxication in uremic patients. Considering this, star fruit may also accumulate secondary natural metabolites that may act as a potent toxin for mammals as occur in other vegetal species (32). Phytochemical investigation of the star fruit juice revealed the occurrence of a large number of volative terpenoids [33] that can not be correlated with the observed neurotoxic effects. In addition to the volatile constituents the star fruit juice has also several carotenoids and flavonoids and some of them are shown in Figure 3. These compounds exhibit potent antioxidant activity [34, 35, 36, 37, 38, 39] and may preserve other unstable structures against the oxidative reaction induced by O_2 during the juice preparation. These facts are well known in current chemistry literature and had encouraged the development of several hyphenated techniques and analytical methodologies for the identification of antioxidant polyenes and vitamins [40, 41, 42, 43].

Some neurotoxic compounds are small molecules and some of them contain functional groups that can react with O_2. Considering this hypothesis the presence of the carotenoids and flavonoids may preserve the toxin chemical structure. Recently, Carolino RO et al isolated and partially characterized a neurotoxic fraction from star fruit applying soft purification steps. This fraction was referred to as AcTx and was able to evoke seizures in mice and rats [44]. Initial insights into the mechanism of action of convulsant activity of AcTx were performed focused on GABA (γ-aminobutyric acid) and glutamate neurotransmitter systems, since it is well-established that an imbalance between these systems may lead to hyperexcitability, provoking seizures [45, 46]. The release and uptake of GABA and glutamate were assayed in synaptosomes. This is a well-recognized model for studying neurotransmitter nerve-terminal-related mechanisms since it retains all machinery for the uptake, storage, release of neurotransmitter, and ionic conductance, while being sufficiently simple and homogeneous for meaningful biochemical studies [47]. In that preparation, AcTx was not able to alter significantly both GABA and glutamate release and re-uptake. The AcTx ability to bind to GABA and glutamate receptors was also evaluated, and we demonstrated it was able to bind only to GABA receptors. Preliminary chemical studies on AcTx content indicated that it was free of oxalic acid and proteinogenic amino acids. In addition, AcTx is a small molecule, with molecular weight less than 500, compatible with renal excretion [44]. These data indicate that star fruit contains at least one other neurotoxin in addition to oxalic acid.

Neurobiological aspects

When behavioral recordings are coupled with electroencephalography, in a digital format, the so-called Video-EEG, allows to prove, in freely moving animals, the behavioral and EEG effects after star fruit ingestion or after local application in specific brain regions of either, the crude or the purified toxin. In the first case the hypothesis that experimentally uremic animals, induced by $HgCl_2$, a known model of renal failure [48], will reproduce the star fruit intoxication effects found in the patients can be tested (see above). In the second case, the hypothesis that the crude or purified toxin *per se* will be able to induce behavioral and EEG activity compatible with brain hyperexcitability, possibly associated to seizures is tested. As a positive effect, the latter experimental protocol (with not relationships with renal alterations) will even validate the potential of this neurotoxin as a new tool in the neuroscience field.

Currently, rats are implanted with electrodes and cannulas in their cortices following known stereotaxic coordinates according to the Atlas of Paxinos and Watson [49]. Control electroencephalograms (EEG) (baseline) are recorded prior to (controls) and after vehicle (0.9% saline solution) injections, for 30 min prior to AcTx application. The Video-EEG recordings are made using specific equipment [50] and only animals that had the electrodes and cannulas in the right position, confirmed by histology, are used (Figure 4C). Control behavior and EEGs were examined in the basal situation that is, in the absence of vehicle or AcTx microinjections. Usually, animals explore the cage and, being awake, display typical desynchronized, high frequency-low amplitude EEG activity. Subsequent microinjections of 1μL of the 0.9% saline vehicle did not modify the EEG, nor induce any behavioral alterations of the animals (Figure 3A; two upper recordings). Animals (n=3) submitted to cortical microinjection of 170 mM AcTx presented strong progression of epileptiform EEG activity from 10 to 240 min (Figure 3) [44] .

The continued phenomenon observed over such a long period of time in both cases is called *status epilepticus*, a mimetic of the clinical situation. This is

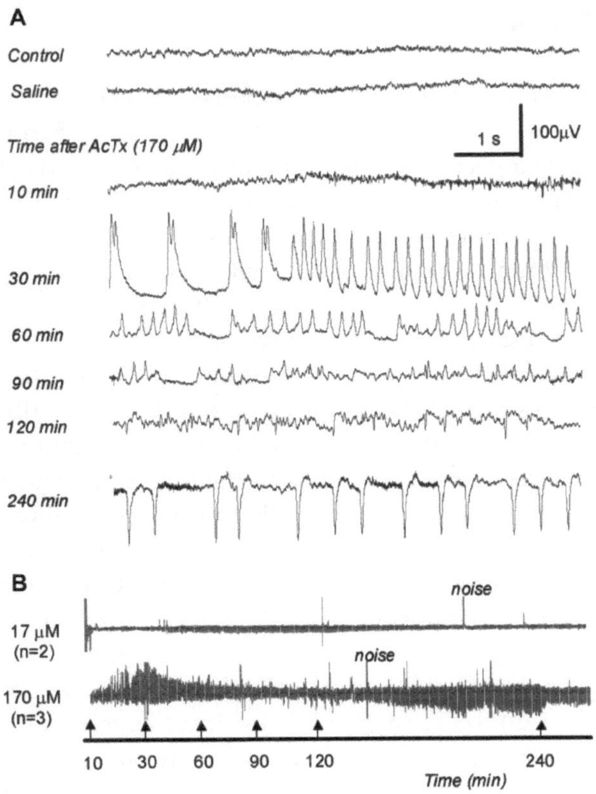

Figure 3. *Evolution of epileptiform activity in rat 02 after cortical microinjection of AcTx (170 μM). **A:** Control and saline recordings express typical desynchronized EEG in the waking state. Ten minutes after AcTx injection, the EEG activity recording indicates subtle baseline alterations with poly-spikes that thereafter, from 20 to 240 min, evolved into a sustained electrographic status epilepticus. Note that at 30 min EEG recording activity was of opposite polarity when compared for example, to the EEG recording at 240 min. **B:** Observe the very weak EEG epileptiform activity following cortical injection of 17 μM/1 μL AcTx, in comparison with the strong EEG epileptiform activity shown after cortical injection of 170 μM/1 μL of the toxin. Notice also, as shown in **A**, that in the second half of the recording period (at around 140 min), there occurred a clear-cut inversion of EEG polarity. Reprinted with permission from Carolino et al [44].*

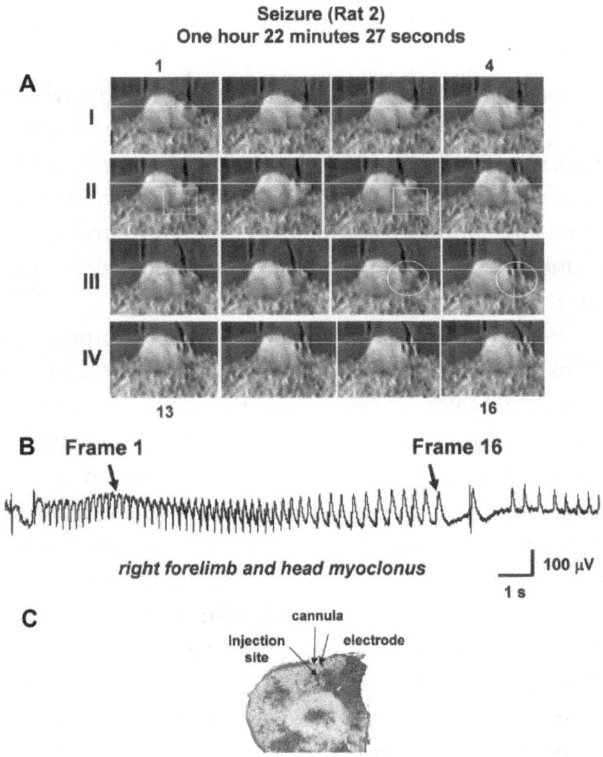

Figure 4. *Behavioral and EEG effects of a cortical AcTx (170 μM/1 μL) microinjection. **A:** Digitalized behavior sequence (16 frames captured in a video-EEG setup). Aligned frames allow the detection of subtle behavioral alterations such as forelimb (white rectangles) and head (white circles) and myoclonic activity. **B:** Observe the EEG window with hypersynchronous epileptiform activity coinciding with video frames ranging from the 1st to the 16th in **A**. **C:** Cellular Nissl staining showing cortical localization of chemitrodes used for AcTx microinjection. Reprinted with permission from Carolino et al [44].*

a protocol interesting for the evaluation of long term effects of the star fruit intoxication, and allows us to look for chronic behavioral, EEG and structural or cellular alterations in these animals. Behavioral and EEG effects of a cortical AcTx (170 μM/1 μL) microinjection are shown in Figure 4.

A preliminary characterization of the video-EEG after crude star fruit juice had been given to animals bearing induced acute renal failure [51]. In addition to that, Video-EEG recordings following cortical administration of AcTx showed behavioral changes, including partial limbic seizures (forelimb and head myoclonus), evolving to a status epilepticus, accompanied by sustained cortical EEG epileptiform activity, particularly after the 170 μM AcTx injection (Figures 3 and 4).

Star fruit juice also induced seizures when applied to cortical areas, showing that convulsant activity is present in crude star fruit extracts. The present data confirm the excitatory profile of AcTx and star fruit extracts. The progressive and sustained EEG epileptiform activity induced by AcTx is a characteristic of known excitatory convulsants, although with potentially different mechanisms of action, such as pilocarpine and kainic acid [52].

In the case of patients, the only report in which the authors claim that star fruit intoxication induce brain lesions (in this case thalamic and cortical) is the one from Chan YL et al [11]. Unfortunately there is no neurological follow up of the eventual neurological sequelae that patients who survive will display in their future lives after the treatment's rescue.

Based on the characteristics of star fruit intoxications and of the isolated neurotoxic fraction (AcTx), we postulated a hypothesis on how the star fruit ingestion would induce intoxication in uremic patients. Initially, the fact that only uremic patients are involved in star fruit intoxications [4, 5, 13] indicate that the neurotoxic substance should be filtered by the kidneys and eliminated in urine, so the star fruit toxin would be hydrosoluble and must have low molecular weight. Actually, AcTx is hydrosoluble and has a low molecular weight (less than 500). Therefore, after star fruit ingestion, the neurotoxin would be absorbed in digestive system, and its plasmatic concentration would increase while its renal excretion would initiate. Conversely, in uremic patients, the renal excretion is impaired or absent, so the plasmatic concentration of star fruit neurotoxin would increase until a serum level which could significantly cross the blood-brain-barrier. In the central nervous system, the star fruit neurotoxin would probably bind to GABAergic receptors inducing excitotoxicity, which would culminate in seizures and, probably, other symptoms of the star fruit intoxication.

It is interesting to notice that the characterization of the cellular and molecular mechanisms of the star fruit intoxication needs to pass through a group of different experimental protocols among them *in vivo* and the *in vitro* bioassays. The correlation between *in vivo* and *in vitro* models is then more complex that we should think it is [53]. Thus, the particular case of synaptosomes and GABA and glutamate release and re-uptake, shows neurochemical dynamics associated to star fruit intoxication mechanisms in a preparation which consists of isolated synaptic terminals (44). However, additional studies are needed with brain slices from control brains treated with the AcTx and even the use of *ex vivo* models (*in vitro* bioassays from tissue after *in vivo* experiments), for example, in our case, brain slices from treated animals.

Conclusions

All observations in our reports and reports from others show that star fruit intoxication may be harmful and even life threatening in patients with renal failure on supportive or dialytic treatment. Hiccups and vomiting, which are common symptoms, could be used as an indication of star fruit intoxication in renal patients presenting with neurological and consciousness disturbances that have no apparent cause.

Hemodialysis, especially on a daily basis is an effective treatment for star fruit intoxication in the majority of cases, if started earlier, according to the literature. In severe cases, continuous methods of replacement may provide a superior initial procedure. In those severe cases that do not respond to these methods, hemoperfusion could be an effective and fast method of treatment. Peritoneal dialysis is useless as a treatment, especially when consciousness disorders ensue.

Although there are not many described cases of star fruit oxalate nephrotoxicity, it seems reasonable to avoid consumption of large amounts of star fruit juice especially on an empty stomach and chronic consumption in patients with underlying chronic renal disease.

The star fruit toxin seems to be a small molecule (molecular weight less than 500), differing from oxalate and common amino acids. It is a potent neurotoxin able to induce seizures and death. Preliminary assays, in synaptosomes, indicated that star fruit neurotoxin binds to GABA receptors.

Acknowledgements

We thank Prof. Dr. Joaquim Coutinho Netto, from the Biochemistry Department, Faculty of Medicine of Ribeirão Preto, University of São Paulo (FMRP-USP), for the investigations of biochemical aspects of the star fruit neurotoxin. To Flavio Del Vecchio for the video-EEG recordings as well as to José Antonio Cortes Oliveira for the behavioral evaluations, both from the Neurophysiology and Experimental Neuroethological Laboratory, Department of Physiology, FMRP-USP. We also thank FAPESP-Brazil (proc. 2003/00873-2), Cinapce-FAPESP (Proc 05/56447-7) and CNPq-Brazil (proc 473448/2003-3) for their financial support to the star fruit projects held at the Neurophysiology and Experimental Neuroethology Laboratory at the FMRP-USP.

References*

1. Morton JF. *Fruits of warm climates*. Flair Books, Miami, FL, 1987:pp125-128.
2. Margen S. *The Wellness Encyclopedia of Food and Nutrition*. Health Letter Assoc. New York, NY; 1992:pp271-272.
3. Martin LC, Caramori JST, Barretti P, Soares VA. Soluço intratável desencadeado por ingestão de carambola (*averrhoa carambola*) em portadores de insuficiência renal crônica. J Bras Nefrol 1993; 15:92-94.
4. Neto MM, Robl F, Netto JC. Intoxication by star fruit (*averrhoa carambola*) in six dialysis patients? (Preliminary report). Nephrol Dial Transpl 1998;13:570-572.
5. Chang JM, Hwang SJ, Kuo HT, Tsai JC, Guh JY, Chen HC, Tsai JH, Lai YH. Fatal outcome after ingestion of star fruit (*averrhoa carambola*) in uremic patients.Am J Kidney Dis 2000; 35:189-193.
6. Wang JL, Cheng CH, Wu MJ, Chen CH, D, Shu KH. (In Chinese) *Status epilepticus* in two patients with chronic renal failure after ingestion of star fruit. Kidney Dialysis 2000; 8:166-169.
7. Lo KL, Tong GMW, Wong PN, Mak SK, Wong AKM. Persistent hiccup in a continuous ambulatory peritoneal dialysis patient following ingestion of star fruit. Hong Kong Journal of Nephrology 2001; 3(1):45-46.
8. Ho MP, Pai MF, Fan CD, Chang KS. Neurological Manifestations Induced by Star fruit (*Averrhoa carambola*) Intoxication in Patients with Chronic Renal Failure: Two Cases Report. J Taiwan Emerg Med 2001; 3:2-7
9. Wu CW, Denq JC, Tsai WS, Lin SH. Star fruit-induced neurotoxicity in two patients with chronic renal failure. J Med Sci 2002; 22(2).
10. Yap HJ, Chen YC, Fang JT, Huang CC. Star fruit: a neglected bu serious fruit intoxicant in chronic renal failure. Dialysis & Transplantation. 2002; 31:564.
11. Chan YL, Leung CB, Yeung DKW. Phosporus and single voxel proton MR spectroscopy and diffusion-weighted imaging in a case of star fruit poisoning. Am J Neuroradiol 2002; 23: 1557-1560.
12. Tse KC, Yip PS, Lam MF, Choy BY, Li FK, Lui SL, Lo WK, Chan TM. Star fruit intoxication in uraemic patients: case series and review of the literature. Internal Medicine Journal 2003; 33:314-316.
13. Neto MM, Costa JAC, Garcia-Cairasco N, Netto JC, Nakagawa B, Dantas M. Intoxication by star fruit (*averrhoa carambola*) in 32 uraemic patients: treatment and outcome. Nephrol Dial Transpl 2003; 18: 120-125.
14. Moyses Neto M, Nardim MEP, Vieira-Neto OM, Vannuchi MTI, Raspanti EO. Intoxicação por carambola (*averrhoa carambola*) em quatro pacientes renais crônicos pré-dialíticos e revisão da literatura. J Bras Nefrol 2003; 26:228-232
15. Hung SW, Lin ACM, Chong CF, Wang TL, Ma HP. Fatal outcome after Star fruit (*Averrhoa carambola*) ingestion in patients with chronic renal insufficiency. Ann Disaster Med 2004; 3:56-59.
16. Chang CH, Yeh JH. Non-convulsive status epilepticus and consciousness disturbance after star fruit (*Averrhoa carambola*) ingestion in a dialysis patient. Nephrology 2004; 9:362-365
17. Tsai MH, Chang WN, Lui CC, Chung KJ, Hsu KT, Huang CR, Lu CH, Chuang YC. Status epilepticus induced by star fruit intoxication in patients with chronic renal disease. Seizure 2005; 14:521-525
18. Chen LL, Fang JT, Lin JL. Chronic renal disease patients with severe star fruit poisoning: hemoperfusion may be an effective alternative therapy. 2005; 43:181-183
19. Wu MY, Wu IW, WuSS, Lin JL. Hemoperfusion as an effective alternative therapy for star fruit intoxication: a report of 2 cases. Am J Kidney Dis 2007; 49:E1-E5
20. Wang YCL, Liu BM, Supernaw RB, Lu YH, Lee PY. Management of star fruit-induced neurotoxicity and seizures in a patient with chronic renal failure. Pharmacotherapy 2006; 26:143-146
21. Chien CL, Fang HC, Chou KJ, Wang JS, Chung HM. Acute oxalate nephropathy after ingestion of star fruit. Am J Kidney Dis 2001; 37:418-422
22. Hruska KA, Seltzer JR, Grieff M: Nephrolithiasis, in Schrier RW, Gottschalk CW(eds): Diseases of the Kidney(ed 6). New York, Little Brown, 1977, pp 739-764.
23. Sanz P. Reig R: Clinical and pathological findings in fatal plant oxalosis: A review. Am J Forensic Med Pathol, 1992; 13: 342-345
24. Fang HC, Chen CL, Wang JS, Chou KJ, Chiou YS, Lee PT, Yeh JH, Yeh MY, Chung HM. Acute oxalate nephropathy induced by star fruit in rats. Am J Kidney Dis 2001; 38:876-880.
25. Fang HC, Lee Po-Tsang, Lu PJ, Chen CL, Chang TY, Hsu CY, Chung HM, Chou KJ. Mechanisms of star fruit-induced acute renal failure. Food Chem Toxicol 2008; 46:1744-1752.
26. Niticharoenpong K, Chalermsanyakorn P, Panvichian R, Kitiyara C. Acute deterioration of renal function induced by star fruit ingestion in a patient with chronic kidney disease. J Nephrol 2006; 19:682-686
27. Muir, CK, Lam, CK. Depressant action of Averrhoa carambola. Med J Malaysia. 1980; XXXIV: 279-80.
28. Chen CL, Chou KJ, Wang JS, Yeh JH, Fang HC, Chung HM. Neurotoxic effects of carambola in rats: the role of oxalate. J Formos Med Assoc. 2002; 101(5): 337-41.

29. Watt JM, Breyer-Brandwijk MG. The medicinal and poisonous plants of Southern and Eastern Africa. 2nd edition, Edinburgh, Livingstone, 1962.
30. Fang HC, Chen CL, Lee PT, Hsu CY, Tseng CJ, Lu PJ, Lai SL, Chung HM, Chou KJ. The role oif oxalate in star fruit neurotoxicity of Five-sixths nephrectomized rats. Food Chem Toxicol 2007; 45:1746-1749.
31. Wilson CW, Shaw PE, Knight-Jr RJ. Analysis of oxalic acid in carambola (Averrhoa carambola L.) and spinach by High-performance liquid chromatography. J. Agric Food Chem 1982; 30(6): 1106-8.
32. Oliveira RB, Godoy SAP, Costa, FB. Plantas tóxicas: conhecimento e prevenção de acidentes. Ribeirão Preto, Holos, 1. ed., 2003. p64
33. Wilson CW Shaw PE, Kinght RJ, Nagy S, Klim M. Volatile constituents of carambola (*Averrhoa carambola L.*). J. Agric. Food Chem.1985; 33:199-201.
34. Artain N, Maárifa Y, Hanafi M. Isolation and identification of active antioxidant compound from star fruit (*Averrhoa carambola*) mistletoe (*Dendrophthoe pentandra (L.) Miq.*) ethanol extract J Appl Science 2006; 8: 1659-1663.
35. Shui G, Leong, Lai P. Residue from star fruit as valuable source for functional food ingredients and antioxidant nutraceutical. Food Chemistry 2006; 97: 277-284
36. Gross JIR., Eckhardt G. Carotenoids of the fruit of *Averrhoa carambola*, Phytochemistry 1983; 22: 1479-1481
37. Gunasegaran R. Flavonoids and anthocyanins of three oxalidaceae, Fitoterapia, 1992, 63: 89-90.
38. Jabbar A, Taleb M, Rashid MA, Hasan CM. 5-Hydroxymethyl-2-furfural from *Averrhoa carambola* Fitoterapia 1995; 66: 377
39. Shui G, Leong LP. Analysis of polyphenolic antioxidants in star fruit using liquid chromatography and mass spectrometry. J Chromatogr A 2004; 1022: 67-75
40. Guaratini T, Vessecchi RL, Lavarda FC, Maia Campos PM, Naal Z, Gates PJ, Lopes NP. New chemical evidence for the ability to generate radical molecular ions of polyenes from ESI and HR-MALDI mass spectrometry. Analyst 2004;129: 1223-1226
41. Guaratini T, Vessecchi R, Pinto E, Colepicolo P, Lopes NP. Balance of xanthophylls molecular and protonated molecular ions in electrospray ionization. J Mass Spectrom 2005; 40: 963-968.
42. Guaratini T, Gates PJ, Cardozo KH, Campos PM, Colepicolo P, Lopes NP. Letter: Radical ion and protonated molecule formation with retinal in electrospray and nanospray. Eur J Mass Spectrom 2006; 12:71-74.
43. Guaratini T, Lopes NP, Pinto E, Colepicolo P, Gates PJ. Mechanism for the elimination of aromatic molecules from polyenes in tandem mass spectrometry. Chem Commun 2006;39: 4110-4112.
44. Carolino RO, Beleboni RO, Pizzo AB, Vecchio FD, Garcia-Cairasco N, Moyses-Neto M, Santos WF, Coutinho-Netto J. Convulsant activity and neurochemical alterations induced by a fraction obtained from fruit Averrhoa carambola (Oxalidaceae: Geraniales). Neurochem Int. 2005; 46: 523-31.
45. Bradford HF. Glutamate, GABA and epilepsy. Prog Neurobiology 1995; 47:477-511.
46. Engelborghs S, D'Hooge R, De Deyn PP. Pathophysiology of epilepsy. Acta Neurol Belgica 2000; 100: 201-13.
47. Gray EG, Whittaker VP. The isolation of nerve ending brain: and electron-microscopic study of cell fragments derived by homogenization and centrifugation. J Anat 1962; 96:79-87
48. Coimbra TM, Cielisnki DA, Humes HD. Epidermal growth factor accelerates renal repair in mercuric chloride nephrotoxicity. Am.J.Physiol 1990; 259: F438-F443.
49. Paxinos, G., Watson, C.H., 1998. The rat brain in stereotaxic coordinates, Academic Press, New York, 256p.
50. Moraes MF, Galvis-Alonso OY, Garcia-Cairasco N. Audiogenic kindling in the Wistar rat: a potential model for recruitment of limbic structures. Epilepsy Research 2000; 39:251-259.
51. Garcia-Cairasco N, Del Vecchio F, Oliveira JAC, Dantas M, Moyses-Neto M. A video-EEG study of the neurotoxic effects of star fruit (*Averrhoa carambola*) juice ingestion in animals with acute renal failure. Proceedings of the 39th European Renal Association and the European Dialysis and Transplantation Meetings, Copenhagen, Denmark. Nephrol Dial Transpl 2000; 17: 89
52. Leite JP, Garcia-Cairasco N, Cavalheiro EA. New insights from the use of pilocarpine and kainate models. Epilepsy Research 2002; 50: 93-103
53. Tiffany-Castiglioni E, Ehrich M, Dees L, Costa LG, Kodavanti PRS, Lasley SM, Oortgiesen M, Durham HD. Bridging the gap between *in vitro* and *in vivo* models for neurotoxicology. Toxicol Sci 1999; 51:178-183.

44

Drug dosage in renal failure

Ali J. OLYAEI[1] and William M. BENNETT[2]

[1]Oregon Health Sciences University, Portland, Oregon, USA
[2]Legacy Good Samaritan Hospital, Portland, Oregon, USA

Introduction

Evolution within the field of dialysis and advances in surgical procedures providing for superior access for shunt placement have made it possible to treat patients with end-stage renal disease with dialysis therapy for more than 50 years. Improved pharmacotherapy of pre- and post- dialysis has also contributed to these remarkable advancements. Drug therapy is also evolving. Health care provider for patients with renal diseases needs to understand the latest drug therapy and ensure appropriateness of therapy in each individual patient [1].

Renal insufficiency and dialysis alter the pharmacokinetics and pharmacodynamics of most commonly used drugs. Of note, an average of eight different classes of drugs per patient are prescribed in patients with renal failure. In comparison to the general population, patients with renal insufficiency experience significantly more adverse drug reactions. Therefore, clinicians caring for these patients must be familiar with the pharmacokinetic behavior of each agent and of the impact of renal failure on the drug elimination process. Understanding the time course of pharmacotherapy is based on knowledge of the relationship between drug concentration and effect. Drugs act by affecting biochemical and physiological processes in the body. Most drugs act at specific receptors but may produce multiple effects because of the location of the receptor in various organs. Knowledge of these properties helps to predict the behavior of a drug in the body and is an important guide in the selection of appropriate doses and dosage intervals.

A particular area of concern is that many patients with renal insufficiency are elderly which in itself may effect drug disposition. Most therapeutic agents or their metabolites are completely or partially eliminated by the kidneys. In patients with renal insufficiency both metabolism and elimination is impaired, therefore, these patients are at a greater risk of adverse drug reactions or drug toxicity. Because of co-morbid conditions, most patients with advanced renal diseases require multiple medications for the treatment of hypertension, hyperlipidemia, hyperuricemia and congestive heart failure. Patients with chronic renal failure are at a greater risk of drug-drug interactions. Finally, depending on various factors such as the size of the drug molecule and degree of protein binding, a significant amount of drug removal may occur during dialysis. Most drug dosages may be adjusted based on plasma therapeutic concentrations (Table 1). To prevent toxicity and optimize efficacy, it is critical that these factors be taken into account and appropriate dosage adjustments made when prescribing drugs for dialysis patients [2-12]. This chapter discusses the pharmacological principles for prescribing drugs in this population and provides specific dosage recommendations (Tables 2-13).

Principles of pharmacokinetics in uremia

Pharmacokinetics is the study of drug behavior (absorption, distribution, metabolism and elimination) in the body. The ability of the body to remove a drug is called clearance. Clearance indicates the intrinsic ability of the body to decrease plasma drug concentration. The three major processes effecting drug clearance are metabolism by the liver, metabolism by the gastrointestinal tract (cytochrome P-450 and P-glycoproteins) or elimination and metabolism by the kidney. At steady state, the overall rate of clearance is equal to rate of drug absorption [1]. The important elements of a drug's pharmacokinetics are shown in Figure 1.

All important pharmacokinetic parameters, such as drug absorption, volume of distribution, protein-protein binding, and drug metabolism must be considered when dose modifications are made in uremic patients. For example, gastroparesis in diabetic patients, slow gastric emptying time and edema of gastrointestinal tract in patients with advanced renal failure may affect drug absorption. Iron preparations and phosphate binders may also alter drug absorption [2].

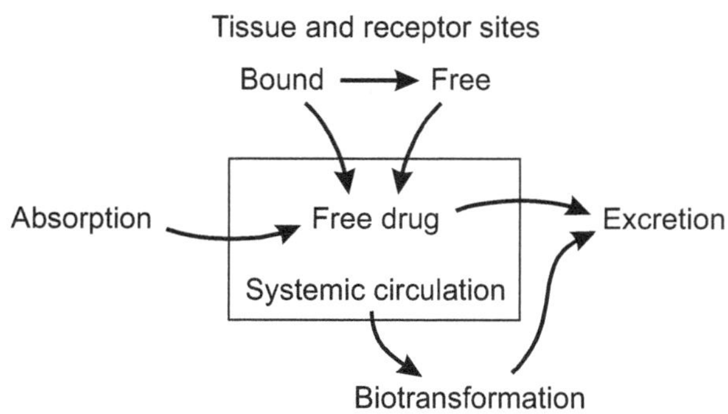

Figure 1. *Interrelationship of absorption, distribution, biotransformation and excretion.*

Absorption

Following oral drug administration, only a certain proportion of the drug is absorbed reaching systemic circulation (F or bioavailability). The percentage of a drug dose that appears in the systemic circulation following oral administration compared with the intravenous route for the same drug defines its bioavailability. In general, drugs given by the intravenous route reach the central compartment directly and usually have a more rapid onset of action. Drugs given by other routes must pass through a series of biologic membranes before entering the systemic circulation. For many drugs, only a fraction of the administered dose may reach the circulation to exert any pharmacodynamic effect [3]. Chronic renal failure may influence drug absorption and bioavailability. The dissolution rate, chemical forms, rout of administration, the gastrointestinal stability and dosage form may alter drug's bioavailability. Bioavailability only indicates the extent of drug absorption not the rate of drug absorption. Drugs can be highly bound to plasma proteins (e.g. aspirin) or unbound (free active moiety). Only the free or unbound concentration of the drug interacts with specific receptors at the site of pharmacologic action. The liver can either metabolize drugs in the 'first pass' as the drug is absorbed into the portal circulation, or later when the drug is delivered to the liver via the systemic blood flow prior to reaching systemic circulation. First pass metabolism can significantly reduce the rate and extent of drug absorption. For renal failure patients, gastric pH is often high due to the use of antacids or anti-ulcer medications that may result in decreased absorption of medications requiring an acid milieu. Aluminum- or calcium-containing antacids may also form non-absorbable chelation products with certain drugs, such as digoxin or tetracycline and impair these agents's absorption [4-6].

Volume of distribution

Following drug absorption, individual drugs distribute throughout the body in a characteristic manner. The apparent volume of distribution (V_d) is the quantity of drug in the body (L/kg body weight) divided by the plasma concentration at steady state. Volume distribution also represents the amount of water that is needed for a drug to dissolve to reach an observed plasma concentration. Therefore, lipophilic agents or drugs with high tissue binding capacity most commonly have a large volume of distribution. In contrast, drugs with high circulating protein binding or water-soluble drugs have a small volume of distribution. Drugs that are largely confined to the intravascular compartment usually have a volume of distribution less then 0.2 L/kg. Uremia, edema and renal failure may alter the volume of distribution of most commonly used agents in patients with renal insufficiency [7-9]. Changes in volume of distribution are usually not clinically significant except for those drugs which have a small volume of distribution under normal circumstances (i.e., >0.7 L/kg).

Protein binding

Unbound or free drugs are pharmacologically active. Therefore, the degree of protein binding is an important issue in adjustment of drug dosing in renal failure. Low plasma albumin or increase in plasma albumin can potentially increase the pharmacodynamic effects of highly bound drugs. Organic acids usually have a single binding site on albumin whereas organic bases tend to have multiple binding sites and their behavior in the presence of increasing renal insufficiency is less predictable. In general, acidic drugs have reduced plasma protein binding in patients with renal failure; this reduction is attributable to a combination of decreased albumin concentration and a reduction in albumin affinity, which is, in turn, influenced by either structural changes in the albumin molecule or accumulation of competing endogenous inhibitors of protein binding. For some agents with high protein binding, the reduced sites or decreased plasma protein can cause potentially important pharmacologic consequences. For example in patients with renal failure, the free plasma concentration of phenytoin increases from 0.1 to 0.35. Therefore, the observed plasma concentration of 4 mg/L is comparable to 10-15 mg/L in patients with normal renal function. Finally only unbound or free drugs are available for drug metabolism or excretion. Uremia decreases binding capacity of most drugs and result in increased metabolism in patients with renal failure. For any given drug therapeutic concentration (bound plus unbound), the proportion of free or active drug is increased. It is more desirable to obtain free drug plasma concentrations in patients with renal failure [10-13].

Eliminations

The presence of progressive renal insufficiency affects most body biochemical processes including drug biotransformation. In addition, some drugs have pharmacologically active metabolites, which, although unimportant in patients with normal renal function, may accumulate in patients with renal insufficiency causing adverse drug reactions [13-17]. Some of these pharmacologically active metabolites may account for the high incidence of adverse drug reactions in patients with renal failure. Some of the best-known examples of this phenomenon are the accumulation of pharmacologically active metabolites of meperidine causing seizures, nitrofurantoin causing peripheral neuropathy and morphine sulfate causing excess respiratory depression. The metabolic biotransformation of drugs to another more water-soluble chemical moiety also may be altered in uremia. In patients with renal failure, chemical reduction, acetylating, ester or peptide hydrolysis may be delayed, whereas metabolism by hepatic microsomal oxidation is usually normal. Drug elimination rate is usually expressed as elimination half-life (t_2). Drug half-life is the time required for the plasma concentration to decrease by 50%. The half-life is dependent upon V_d and clearance (renal, hepatic, or other) as expressed by the formula:

$t_2 = 0.693 \times V_d/\text{clearance}$

For drugs eliminated primarily intact through the kidneys, as the renal clearance decreases, t_2 will increase (assuming that V_d is unchanged). It should be noted that active drug metabolites may also be excreted by the kidney and therefore have a prolonged half-life in renal failure.

Dosing regimens

Most drugs or their metabolites that are normally excreted unchanged by the kidney will require dosage modification in advanced renal failure. The loading dose of a drug will stay the same unless the V_d is significantly altered. The maintenance regimen may be modified by the interval extension method or dosage reduction. The interval extension method utilizes the same dose at greater intervals and is useful for drugs with long half-lives. The dosage reduction method reduces the dosage and leaves the interval between doses unchanged. This method generally leads to more constant serum levels. Therapeutic drug monitoring is a useful method in guiding drug therapy and preventing toxicity. Interpretation of drug levels must be made in light of the amount of drug given; the time elapsed since the last dose, and the route of administration and clinical scenario of the patients [14-18].

Therapeutic drug monitoring

Dosage and interval modifications do not necessarily protect against drug toxicity. Therefore, monitoring drug levels in some specific agents with a narrow therapeutic window is essential in the patient with renal impairment. In order to correctly interpret therapeutic drug monitoring it is important to know the exact time when a dose given, the route of administration, time since the last dose and the particular drug's half-life. Peak drug levels represent the highest drug concentration achieved after initial rapid distribution and in most drugs predict overall drug efficacy. Trough drug levels are obtained immediately before the next dose, represent the lowest serum concentration and predict drug toxicity and accumulations.

Drug level monitoring can be expensive and is not always available. Drug level monitoring does not always reduce the incidence of toxicity. Aminoglycoside antibiotics, for instance, can concentrate in tissues such as the inner ear and renal cortex and toxicity is not always correlated with high blood levels. Ongoing clinical assessment is important even when drug levels are within the established therapeutic range. In the presence of metabolic acidosis or hypokalemia, digoxin toxicity may occur despite acceptable therapeutic levels. Most assays do not distinguish between free and protein-bound drug in the plasma. An increase in unbound drug is common in patients with renal failure. Table 1 summarized the therapeutic drug monitoring in renal insufficiency for drugs which monitoring of drug levels is routinely recommended.

Dialysis and drug clearance

Dialysis and renal replacement therapy (RRTx) are common treatments option for the treatment of acute renal failure in the hospital setting. Many drugs are substantially cleared by dialysis. Therefore, scheduling of drug administration and the possibility of dosage supplementation should be considered in patients receiving dialysis. Scheduled doses should be given upon completion of dialysis therapy. If this is not possible and dialytic treatment increases total body clearance of a given drug by greater than 30%, dosage supplementation may be necessary. Dialyzability is primarily determined by molecular weight (< 500 daltons), water solubility of the drug and extent of protein binding (unbound drugs are more readily cleared). Other factors of a drug which determine dialyzability include Vd, non-renal excretion, ionic charge and erythrocyte partitioning. Some properties of the dialysate and the dialyzer membrane also affect drug clearance and include flow rate, temperature, pH, solute composition, volume (peritoneal dialysis), pore size and surface area.

Creatinine clearance rates of up to 30 to 50 ml/min are currently being achieved with continuous renal replacement therapies (CRRTs) such as continuous venovenous hemofiltration and continuous arteriov-

Table 1. Therapeutic drug monitoring.

Drug name	Therapeutic range	When to draw sample	How often to draw levels
Aminoglycosides (Conventional dosing) Gentamicin, Tobramycin, Amikacin	Gentamicin and Tobramycin: Trough: 0.5–2 mg/L Peak: 5–8 mg/L Amikacin: Peak: 20–30 mg/L Trough: < 10 mg/L	Trough: Immediately prior to dose Peak: 30 min after a 30-45 min infusion	Check peak and trough with 3rd dose For therapy less than 72 h, levels not necessary. Repeat drug levels weekly or if renal function changes
Aminoglycosides (24-h dosing) Gentamicin, Tobramycin, Amikacin	0.5–3 mg/L	Obtain random drug level 12 h after dose	After initial dose. Repeat drug level in 1 week or if renal function changes
Carbamazepine	4–12 mcg/mL	Trough: Immediately prior to dosing	Check 2–4 days after first dose or change in dose
Cyclosporin	150–400 ng/mL	Trough: Immediately prior to dosing	Daily for first week, then weekly.
Digoxin	0.8–2.0 ng/mL	12 h after maintenance dose	5–7 days after first dose for patients with normal renal and hepatic function; 15–20 days in anephric patients
Lidocaine	1–5 mcg/mL	8 h after i.v. infusion started or changed	
Lithium	Acute: 0.8–1.2 mmol/L Chronic: 0.6–0.8 mmol/L	Trough: Before a.m. dose at least 12 h since last dose	
Phenobarbital	15–40 mcg/mL	Trough: Immediately prior to dosing	Check 2 weeks after first dose or change in dose. Follow-up level in 1–2 months.
Phenytoin Free Phenytoin	10–20 mcg/mL 1–2 mcg/mL	Trough: Immediately prior to dosing	5–7 day after first dose or after change in dose
Procainamide NAPA (n-acetyl procainamide) a procainamide metabolite	4–10 mcg/mL Trough: 4 mcg/mL Peak: 8 mcg/mL 10–30 mcg/mL	Trough: Immediately prior to next dose or 12–18 h after starting or changing an infusion Draw with procainamide sample	
Quinidine	1–5 mcg/mL	Trough: Immediately prior to next dose	
Sirolimus	10–20 ng/dL	Trough: Immediately prior to next dose	
Tacrolimus(FK-506)	10–15 ng/mL	Trough: Immediately prior to next dose	Daily for first week, then weekly
Theophylline p.o. or Aminophylline i.v.	15–20 mcg/mL	Trough: Immediately prior to next dose	
Valproic acid (divalproex sodium)	40–100 mcg/mL	Trough: Immediately prior to next dose	Check 2–4 d after first dose or change in dose
Vancomycin	Trough: 5–15 mg/L Peak: 25–40 mg/L	Trough: Immediately prior to dose Peak: 60 min after a 60 min infusion	With 3rd dose (when initially starting therapy, or after each dosage adjustment). For therapy less than 72 h, levels not necessary. Repeat drug levels if renal function changes

enous hemofiltration. CRRTs are enjoying widespread application in both medical and surgical intensive care units. Limited data is available regarding drug removal during CRRT. Dosage adjustments can be determined through close monitoring of drug levels and clinical status of the patient. During CRRT solutes and drugs are removed by convective transport. Drugs also may be substantially removed by membrane-drug binding. Drugs and solutes not bound to plasma proteins and dissolved in the plasma cross the dialysis membrane through plasma water ultrafiltration. The ulltrafiltrate drug concentration is equal to the plasma concentration multiplied by the percentage of unbound drug.

References

1. Winters ME, Basic clinical pharmacokinetics. Winter ME, Applied Therapeutic Inc. Vancouver, WA 1994.
2. Zhang Y. Benet LZ. The gut as a barrier to drug absorption: combined role of cytochrome P450 3A and P-glycoprotein. Clinical Pharmacokinetics. 40(3):159-68, 2001
3. Olyaei AJ, Bennett WM. "The Effect of Renal Failure on Drug Handling". Oxford Textbook of Critical Care, 1996.
4. Benedetti P. de Lalla F. Antibiotic therapy in acute renal failure. Contributions to Nephrology. (132):136-45, 2001.
5. Olyaei AJ, deMattos AM, Bennett WM. "Prescribing Drugs in Renal Failure". Brenner and Rector's, The Kidney, 2000.
6. Olyaei AJ, deMattos AM, Bennett WM. "Drug-drug Interaction and most Commonly Used Drug in Transplant Recipients". Primer on Transplantation, American Society of Transplantation. 2000
7. Olyaei AJ " Drug Dosing in Renal Failure " in Treatment Strategies In Nephrology and Hypertension. By Bennett 1st edition. PocketMedicine.com Inc 2001
8. Olyaei AJ, deMattos AM, Bennett WM "Principle of Drug Usage in Dialysis Patients" Dialysis Therapy, Hanley & Belfus Inc. Medical Publishers. May 2001
9. Olyaei AJ, deMattos, Bennett WM, Drug usage in dialysis patients. In: Nissenson AR, Fine RN, Gentile DE, eds. Clinical dialysis. Norwalk, NJ: Appleton and Lange; 2001.
10. Bennett WM. Guide to drug dosage in renal failure. In: Speight TM, Holford N, eds. Avery's drug treatment, 4th edn. Auckland: ADIS International; 1997:1725–92.
11. Beauchamp D, Labrecque G. Aminoglycoside nephrotoxicity: do time and frequency of administration matter?. Current Opinion in Critical Care 2001:7: 401-408.
12. Livornese LL, Jr., Slavin D, Benz RL, Ingerman MJ, Santoro J. Use of antibacterial agents in renal failure. Infectious Disease Clinics of North America 2001:15: 983-1002.
13. Chertow GM, Lee J, Kuperman GJ et al. Guided medication dosing for inpatients with renal insufficiency. JAMA 2001:286: 2839-2844.
14. Bugge JF. Pharmacokinetics and drug dosing adjustments during continuous venovenous hemofiltration or hemodiafiltration in critically ill patients. Acta Anaesthesiologica Scandinavica 2001:45: 929-934.
15. Izzedine H, Launay-Vacher V, Baumelou A, Deray G. An appraisal of antiretroviral drugs in hemodialysis. [Review] [47 refs]. Kidney International 2001:60: 821-830.
16. Subach RA, Marx MA. Drug dosing in acute renal failure: the role of renal replacement therapy in altering drug pharmacokinetics. Advances in Renal Replacement Therapy 1998:5: 141-147.
17. Joy MS, Matzke GR, Armstrong DK, Marx MA, Zarowitz BJ. A primer on continuous renal replacement therapy for critically ill patients. Annals of Pharmacotherapy 1998:32: 362-375.
18. Joos B, Schmidli M, Keusch G. Pharmacokinetics of antimicrobial agents in anuric patients during continuous venovenous haemofiltration. Nephrology Dialysis Transplantation 1996:11: 1582-1585.

Appendix: **Drug dosing in renal failure**

Abbreviations used:

ACE: angiotensin-converting enzyme
AV: atrioventricular
BUN: blood urea nitrogen
C_{Cr}: Creatinine clearance
CAPD: continuous ambulatory peritoneal dialysis
CHF: congestive heart failure
CMV: cytomegalovirus
CNS: central nervous system
CRRT: continuous renal replacement therapy
CSA/FK: cyclosporine A and tacrolimus
CVD: cardiovascular disease
CVVH: Continuous venovenous hemofiltration
DVT: deep vein thrombosis
ESRD: end-stage renal disease
GI: gastrointestinal
GFR: glomerular filtration rate
HBV: hepatitis B virus
HD: hemodialysis
HDL: high-density lipoprotein
HIT: heparin-induced thrombocytopenia
HSV: herpes simplex virus
INR: international normalized ratio
IV: intravenous
MI: myocardial infarction
MMF: mycophenolate mofetil
NA: not applicable
NC: No data: no change required
NSAIDs: nonsteroidal anti-inflammatory drugs
TB: tuberculosis
TDM: therapeutic drug monitoring
V_D: volume of distribution
VZV: varicella zoster virus.

Table 2. Antibacterial agents

Drug	Normal dosage	% of drug excreted renally	Dosage adjustment for renal failure with GFR (ml/min): >50	10–50	<10	Comments	Method of dosage adjustment: HD	CAPD	CVVH
Aminoglycosides									
Group toxicity: all agents in this group are nephrotoxic and ototoxic; ototoxicity is worse when the patient is hyperbilirubinemic; measure serum levels for efficacy and toxicity; peritoneal absorption increases with presence of inflammation. V_D increases with edema, obesity, and ascites									
Streptomycin	7.5 mg/kg q. 12 hr (1.0 g q. 24 hr for TB)	60%	q. 24 hr	q. 24–72 hr	q. 72–96 hr	May be less nephrotoxic than other members of class	Half **normal** dose after dialysis	20–40 mg/L/day	Dose for GFR 10–50 ml/min; measure levels
Kanamycin	7.5 mg/kg q. 8 hr	50%–90%	60%–90% q. 12 hr; 100% q. 12–24 hr	30%–70% q. 12–18 hr; 100% q. 24–48 hr	20%–30% q. 24–48 hr; 100% q. 48–72 hr	Avoid once-daily dosing in patients with C_{Cr} < 30–40 ml/min or in patients with acute renal failure or an uncertain level of kidney function	Half **full** dose after dialysis	15–20 mg/L/day	Dose for GFR 10–50 ml/min; measure levels
Gentamicin	1.7 mg/kg q. 8 hr	95%	60%–90% q. 8–12 hr; 100% q. 12–24 hr	30%–70% q. 12–18 hr; 100% q. 24-48 hr	20%–30% q. 24–48 hr; 100% q. 48–72 hr	Concurrent penicillin treatment may result in subtherapeutic aminoglycoside levels Peak, 6–8; trough, < 2	Half **full** dose after dialysis	3–4 mg/L/day	Dose for GFR 10–50 ml/min; measure levels
Tobramycin	1.7 mg/kg q. 8 hr	95%	60%–90% q. 8–12 hr; 100% q. 12–24 hr	30–70% q. 12–18 hr; 100% q. 24-48 hr	20–30% q. 24–48 hr; 100% q. 48–72 hr	Concurrent penicillin treatment may result in subtherapeutic aminoglycoside levels Peak, 6–8; trough, < 2	Half **full** dose after dialysis	3–4 mg/L/day	Dose for GFR 10–50 ml/min, measure levels
Netilmicin	2 mg/kg q. 8 hr	95%	50%–90% q. 8–12 hr; 100% q. 12–24 hr	20–60% q 12 hr; 100% q 24–48 hr	10–20% q. 24–48 hr; 100% q 48–72 hr	May be less ototoxic than other members of class Peak, 6–8; trough, < 2	Half **full** dose after dialysis	3–4 mg/L/day	Dose for GFR 10–50 ml/min; measure levels
Amikacin	7.5 mg/kg q. 12 hr	95%	60%–90% q. 12 hr: 100% q. 12–24 hr	30–70% q. 12–18 hr; 100% q. 24–48 hr	20–30% q. 24–48 hr; 100% q. 48–72 hr	Monitor levels Peak, 20–30; trough, <5	Half **full** dose after dialysis	15–20 mg/L/day	Dose for GFR 10–50 ml/min; measure levels
Cephalosporins (oral)									
Group toxicity: Adverse effects: coagulation abnormalities, transitory elevation of BUN, rash, and serum sicknesslike syndrome									
Cefaclor	250–500 mg q. 8 hr	70%	100%	100%	50%	Group toxicity	250 mg after dialysis	250 mg q. 8–12 hr	No data
Cefadroxil	500 mg to 1 g q. 12 hr	80%	100%	100%	50%	Group toxicity	0.5–1.0 g after dialysis	0.5 g/day	No data
Cefixime	200–400 mg q. 12 hr	85%	100%	100%	50%	Group toxicity	300 mg after dialysis	200 mg/day	Not recommended
Cefpodoxime	200 mg q. 12 hr	30%	100%	100%	100%	Group toxicity	200 mg after dialysis	Dose for GFR<10 ml/min	No data
Ceftibuten	400 mg q. 24 hr	70%	100%	100%	50%	Group toxicity	300 mg after dialysis	No data: Dose for GFR <10 ml/min	Dose for GFR 10–50 ml/min
Cefuroxime axetil	250–500 mg q. 8 hr	90%	100%	100%	100%	Malabsorbed in presence of H_2 blockers; absorbed better with food	Dose after dialysis	Dose for GFR<10 ml/min	No data
Cephalexin	250–500 mg q. 8 hr	95%	100%	100%	100%	Rare allergic interstitial nephritis; absorbed well when given intraperitoneally; may cause bleeding from impaired prothrombin biosynthesis	Dose after dialysis	Dose for GFR<10 ml/min	No data

Drug	Normal dosage	% of drug excreted renally	Dosage adjustment for renal failure with GFR (ml/min):			Comments	Method of dosage adjustment		
			>50	10–50	<10		HD	CAPD	CVVH
Cephradine	250–500 mg q. 8 hr	100%	100%	100%	50%	Rare allergic interstitial nephritis; absorbed well when given intraperitoneally; may cause bleeding from impaired prothrombin biosynthesis	Dose after dialysis	Dose for GFR<10 ml/min	No darta
Cephalosporins (IV)									
Group toxicity: may cause coagulation abnormalities, transitory elevation of BUN, rash, and serum sicknesslike syndrome									
Cefamandole	1–2 g IV q. 6–8 hr	100%	q. 6 hr	q. 8 hr	q. 12 hr	Group toxicity	0.5–1.0 g after dialysis	0.5–1.0 g q. 12 hr	Dose for GFR 10–50 ml/min
Cefazolin	1–2 g IV q. 8 hr	80%	q. 8 hr	q. 12 hr	q. 12–24 hr	Group toxicity	0.5–1.0 g after dialysis	0.5 g q. 12 hr	Dose for GFR 10–50 ml/min
Cefepime	1–2 g IV q. 8 hr	85%	q. 8–12 hr	q. 12 hr	q. 24 hr	Group toxicity	1 g after dialysis	Dose for GFR < 10 ml/min	Not recommended
Cefmetazole	1–2 g IV q. 8 hr	85%	q. 8 hr	q. 12 hr	q. 24 hr	Group toxicity	Dose after dialysis	Dose for GFR <10 ml/min	Dose for GFR 10–50 ml/min
Cefoperazone	1–2 g IV q. 12 hr	20%	No renal adjustment required.			Displaced from protein by bilirubin; may prolong prothrombin time; reduce dose by 50% in patients with jaundice	1 g after dialysis	NC	NC
Cefotaxime	1–2 g IV q. 6–8 hr	60%	q. 8 hr	q. 12 hr	q. 12–24 hr	Group toxicity	1 g after dialysis	1 g/day	1 g q. 12 hr
Cefotetan	1–2 g IV q. 12 hr	75%	q. 12 hr	q. 12–24 hr	q. 24 hr	Group toxicity	1 g after dialysis	1 g/day	750 mg q. 12 hr
Cefoxitin	1–2 g IV q. 6 hr	80%	q. 6 hr	q. 8–12 hr	q. 12 hr	May produce false increase in serum creatinine level by interference with assay	1 g after dialysis	1 g/day	Dose for GFR 10–50 ml/min
Ceftazidime	1–2 g IV q. 8 hr	70%	q. 8 hr	q. 12 hr	q. 24 hr	Group toxicity	1 g after dialysis	0.5 g/day	Dose for GFR 10–50 ml/min
Ceftriaxone	1–2 g IV q. 24 hr	50%	No renal adjustment required		Dose after dialysis	750 mg q. 12 hr	Dose for GFR 10–50 ml/min		
Cefuroxime sodium	0.75–1.5 g IV q. 8 hr	90%	q. 8 hr	q. 8–12 hr	q. 12–24 hr	Absorbed well when given intraperitoneally; may cause rare allergic interstitial nephritis; may cause bleeding from impaired prothrombin biosynthesis	Dose after dialysis	Dose for GFR <10	1.0 g q. 12 hr
Clindamycin	150–450 mg q. 8 hr	10%	No renal adjustment required			Increase CSA/FK level	NC	NC	NC
Imipenem-cilastatin	250–500 mg IV q. 6 hr	50%	500 mg q. 8 hr	250–500 q. 8–12 hr	250 mg q. 12 hr	Causes seizures in ESRD; nonrenal clearance in acute renal failure is less than in chronic renal failure; administer with cilastin to prevent nephrotoxicity of renal metabolite	Dose after dialysis	Dose for GFR <10 ml/min	Dose for GFR 10–5 ml/min
Macrolides									
Azithromycin	250–500 mg q. 24 hr	6%	No renal adjustment required			No drug-drug interaction with CSA/KF	NC	NC	NC
Clarithromycin	500 mg q. 12 hr	20%	No renal adjustment required				NC	NC	NC
Dirithromycin	500 mg q. 24 hr		No renal adjustment required			Nonenzymatically hydrolyzed to active compound erythromycylamine.	NC	NC	Dose for GFR 10–50 ml/min

Drug	Normal dosage	% of drug excreted renally	Dosage adjustment for renal failure with GFR (ml/min):			Comments	Method of dosage adjustment		
			>50	10–50	<10		HD	CAPD	CVVH
Erythromycin	250–500 mg q. 8 hr	15%	No renal adjustment required			Increase CSA/FK levels; avoid in transplant patients	NC	NC	NC
Meropenem	1 g IV q. 8 hr	65%	1 g q. 8 hr	0.5–1g q. 12 hr	0.5–1 g q. 24 hr		Dose after dialysis	Dose for GFR<10 ml/min	Dose for GFR 10–50 ml/min
Metronidazole	500 mg IV q. 6 hr	20%	No renal adjustment required			Peripheral neuropathy; disulfiram reaction with alcoholic beverages; increase frequency of liver function tests (1%)	Dose after dialysis	Dose for GFR<10 ml/min	Dose for GFR 10–50 ml/min
Penicillins (oral)						Group toxicity: may cause bleeding abnormalities, hypersensitivity, seizures			
Amoxicillin	500 mg q. 8 hr	60%	100%	100%	50%–75%	Group toxicity	Dose after dialysis	250 mg q. 12 hr	No data
Ampicillin	500 mg q. 6 hr	60%	100%	100%	50%–75%	Group toxicity	Dose after dialysis	250 mg q. 12 hr	Dose for GFR 10–50 ml/min
Dicloxacillin	250–500 mg q. 6 hr	50%	100%	100%	50%–75%	Group toxicity	NC	NC	No data
Penicillin V	250–500 mg q. 6 hr	70%	100%	100%	50%–75%	Group toxicity	Dose after dialysis	Dose for GFR<10 ml/min	No data
Penicillins (IV)									
Ampicillin	1–2 g IV q. 6 hr	60%	q. 6 hr	q. 8 hr	q. 12 hr		Dose after dialysis	250 mg q. 12 hr	Dose for GFR 10–50 ml/min
Nafcillin	1–2 g IV q. 4 hr	35%	No renal adjustment is required				None	None	Dose for GFR 10–50 ml/min
Penicillin G	2–3 million Units IV q. 4 hr	70%	q. 4–6 hr	q. 6 hr	q. 8 hr	Adverse effects: seizures, false positive urine protein reactions; 6 million units/day upper limit dose in ESRD	Dose after dialysis	Dose for GFR<10 ml/min	Dose for GFR 10–50 ml/min
Piperacillin	3–4 g IV q. 4–6 hr		No renal adjustment is required			High sodium, content 1.9 mEq/g	Dose after dialysis	Dose for GFR <10 ml/min	Dose for GFR 10–50 ml/min
Ticarcillin/clavulanate	3.1 g IV q. 4–6 hr	85%	1–2 g q. 4 hr	1–2 g q. 8 hr	1–2 g q. 12 hr	Specific toxicity: sodium, 5.2 mEq/g	3.0 g after dialysis	Dose for GFR <10 ml/min	Dose for GFR 10–50 ml/min
Piperacillin/tazobactam	3.375 g IV q. 6–8 hr	75%–90%	q. 4–6 hr	q. 6–8 hr	q. 8 hr	Specific toxicity: sodium, 1.9 mEq/g	Dose after dialysis	Dose for GFR <10 ml/min	Dose for GFR 10–50 ml/min
Pentamidine	4 mg/kg/day	5%	q. 24 hr	q. 24 hr	q. 48 hr	Inhalation may cause bronchospasm; IV administration may cause hypotension, hypoglycemia, and nephrotoxicity	NC	NC	NC
Quinolones									
Group toxicity: agents in this group are malabsorbed in the presence of magnesium, calcium, aluminum, and iron; photosensitivity, **food**, dairy products, tube feeding, may also impair absorption; theophylline metabolism is impaired; higher oral doses may be needed to treat CAPD peritonitis									
Cinoxacin	500 mg q. 12 hr	55%	100%	50%	Avoid	Group toxicity	Avoid	Avoid	Avoid
Fleroxacin	400 mg q.12 hr	70%	100%	50%–75%	50%	Group toxicity	Dose for GFR<10 ml/min	400 mg/day	NA

Drug	Normal dosage	% of drug excreted renally	Dosage adjustment for renal failure with GFR (ml/min):			Comments	Method of dosage adjustment		
			>50	10–50	<10		HD	CAPD	CVVH
Ciprofloxacin	200–400 mg IV q. 24 hr	60%	q. 12 hr	q. 12–24 hr	q. 24 hr	Poorly absorbed with antacids, sucralfate, and phosphate binders; decreases phenytoin levels; IV dose is one third of oral dose	250 mg q. 12 hr (200 mg if IV)	250 mg q. 8 hr (200 mg if IV)	200 mg IV q. 12 hr
Lomefloxacin	400 mg q. 24 hr	76%	100%	200–400 mg q. 48 hr	50%	Group toxicity	Dose for GFR<10 ml/min	Dose for GFR<10 ml/min	No data
Levofloxacin	500 mg q. 24 hr	70%	q. 12hr	250 q. 12 hr	250 q. 12 hr	L-isomer of ofloxacin: appears to have similar pharmacokinetics and toxicities	Dose for GFR<10 ml/min	Dose for GFR<10 ml/min	Dose for GFR 10–50 ml/min
Moxifloxacin	400 mg q. 24 hr	20%	No renal adjustment is required			Group toxicity	No data	No data	No data
Nalidixic acid	1.0 g q. 6 hr	High	100%	Avoid	Avoid	Group toxicity	Avoid	Avoid	No data
Norfloxacin	400 mg q. 12 hr	30%	q. 12 hr	q. 12–24 hr	q. 24 hr	Group toxicity	Dose for GFR <10 ml/min	Dose for GFR<10 ml/min	No data
Ofloxacin	200–400 mg q. 12 hr	70%	q. 12 hr	q. 12–24 hr	q. 24 hr	Group toxicity	100–200 mg after dialysis	Dose for GFR<10 ml/min	300 mg/day
Pefloxacin	400 mg q. 24 hr	11%	100%	100%	100%	Excellent bidirectional transperitoneal movement	NC	NC	Dose for GFR 10–50 ml/min
Sparfloxacin	400 mg q. 24 hr	10%	100%	50%–75%	50% q. 48 hr	Group toxicity	No data: dose for GFR <10 ml/min	No data	Dose for GFR 10–50 ml/min
Trovafloxacin	200–300 mg q. 12 hr	10%	No renal adjustment is required			Group toxicity	No data	No data	No data
Pentamidine	4 mg/kg/day	5%	q. 24 hr	q. 24 hr	q. 48 hr	Inhalation may cause bronchospasm; IV administration may cause hypotension, hypoglycemia, and nephrotoxicity	NC	NC	NC
Rifampin	300–600 mg	20%	No renal adjustment is required.			Many drug interactions; decrease CSA/FK level	NC	Dose for GFR<10 ml/min	Dose for GFR <10 ml/min
Trimethoprim-sulfamethoxazole	800/160 mg q. 12 hr	70%	q. 12 hr	q. 18 hr	q. 24 hr	May cause hyperkalemia; increase serum creatinine level	Dose after dialysis	q. 24 hr	q. 18 hr
Vancomycin (oral)	125–250 mg q. 8 hr	0%	100%	100%	100%	Oral vancomycin is indicated only for the treatment of *Clostridium difficile* infections	100%	100%	100%
Vancomycin (IV)	1 g IV q. 12 hr	90%	q. 12 hr	q. 24–36 hr	q. 48–72 hr	Nephrotoxic, ototoxic; may prolong the neuromuscular blockade effect of muscle relaxants Peak, 30; trough, 5–10	500 mg q. 12–24 hr	1.0 g q. 24–96 hr	500 mg q. 12 hr
Antifungal Agents									
Amphotericin B	0.5–1.5 mg/kg/day	<1%	No renal adjustment required			Nephrotoxic; may cause infusion-related reactions; give 250 ml normal saline before each dose	q. 24 hr	q. 24 hr	q. 24–36 hr
Amphotec	4–6 mg/kg/day	<1%	No renal adjustment required						
Abelcet	5 mg/kg/day	<1%	No renal adjustment required						
AmBisome	3–5 mg/kg/day	<1%	No renal adjustment required						

Drug	Normal dosage	% of drug excreted renally	Dosage adjustment for renal failure with GFR (ml/min):			Comments	Method of dosage adjustment		
			>50	10–50	<10		HD	CAPD	CVVH
Fluconazole	200–800 mg IV q. 24 hr	70%	100%	100%	50%	Increase CSA/FK level	200 mg after dialysis	Dose for GFR <10 ml/min	Dose for GFR 10–50 ml/min
Flucytosine	37.5 mg/kg	90%	q. 12 hr	q. 16 hr	q. 24 hr	Hepatic dysfunction; marrow suppression more common in azotemic patients: increase CSA/FK level	Dose after dialysis	0.5–1.0 g/day	Dose for GFR 10–50 ml/min
Griseofulvin	125–250 mg q. 6 hr	1%	100%	100%	100%	Increase CSA/FK level	NC	NC	NC
Itraconazole	200 mg q. 12 hr	35%	100%	100%	50%	Poor oral absorption; increase CSA/FK level	100 mg q. 12–24 hr	100 mg q. 12–24 hr	100 mg q. 12–24 hr
Ketoconazole	200–400 mg q. 24 hr	15%	100%	100%	100%	Hepatotoxic; increase CSA/FK level	NC	NC	NC
Miconazole	1,200–3,600 mg/day	1%	100%	100%	100%	Increase CSA/FK level	NC	NC	NC
Terbinafine	250 mg q. 24 hr	>1%	100%	100%	100%	May cause CHF	NC	NC	NC
Antiviral Agents									
Acyclovir	200–800 mg 5x/day	50%	100%	100%	50%	Poor absorption; neurotoxicity in ESRD; IV preparation can cause renal failure if injected rapidly	Dose after dialysis	Dose for GFR<10 ml/min	3.5 mg/kg/day
Amantadine	100–200 mg q. 12 hr	90%	100%	50%	25%		NC	NC	Dose for GFR 10–50 ml/min
Cidofovir	5 mg/kg weekly × 2 (induction); 5 mg/kg every 2 wk	90%	100%	No data: avoid	No data: avoid	Dose-limiting nephrotoxicity with proteinuria, glycosuria, renal insufficiency; nephrotoxicity and renal clearance reduced with coadministration of probenecid	No data: avoid	No data: avoid	No data avoid
Delavirdine	400 mg q. 8 hr	5%	No data: 100%	No data: 100%	No data: 100%		NC	No data	No data: dose for GFR 10–50 ml/min
Didanosine	200 mg q. 12 hr (125 mg if < 60 kg)	40%–69%	q. 12 hr	q. 24 hr	50% q. 24 hr	Adverse effects: pancreatitis	Dose after dialysis	Dose for GFR<10	Dose for GFR < 10 ml/min
Famciclovir	250–500 mg p.o., q. 8–12 hr	60%	q. 8 hr	q. 12 hr	q. 24 hr	For VZV: 500 mg p.o., q. 8 hr; for HSV: 250 p.o. , q. 12 hr; metabolized to active compound penciclovir	Dose after dialysis	No data	No data: dose for GFR 10–50 ml/min
Foscarnet	40–80 mg IV q. 8 hr	85%	40–20 mg q. 8–24 hr, according to C_{Cr}			Nephrotoxic, neurotoxic; adverse effects are hypocalcemia, hypophosphatemia, hypomagnesemia, and hypokalemia	Dose after dialysis	Dose for GFR<10 ml/min	Dose for GFR 10–50 ml/min
Ganciclovir (oral)	1,000 mg q. 8 hr	95%	1,000 mg q. 8 hr	1,000 mg q. 8 hr	1,000 mg q. 24 hr	Oral ganciclovir should be used only for prevention of CMV infection; always use IV ganciclovir for the treatment of CMV infection	No data: dose after dialysis	No data: dose for GFR <10 ml/min	No data
Ganciclovir (oral)	1,000 mg q. 8 hr	95%	1,000 mg q. 8 hr	1,000 mg q. 8 hr	1,000 mg q. 24 hr	Oral ganciclovir should be used only for prevention of CMV infection; always use IV ganciclovir for the treatment of CMV infection	No data: dose after dialysis	No data: dose for GFR <10 ml/min	No data

Drug	Normal dosage	% of drug excreted renally	Dosage adjustment for renal failure with GFR (ml/min):			Comments	Method of dosage adjustment		
			>50	10–50	<10		HD	CAPD	CVVH
Ganciclovir (IV)	5 mg/kg q. 12 hr	95%	q. 12 hr	q. 24 hr	2,5 mg/kg/day	Adverse effects: granulocytopenia and thrombocytopenia	Dose after dialysis	Dose for GFR <10 ml/min	2.5 mg/kg/day
Indinavir	800 mg q. 8 hr	10%	No data: 100%	No data: 100%	No data: 100%	Adverse effects: nephrolithiasis and acute renal failure due to crystalluria or tubulointerstitial nephritis	NC	No data: dose for GFR <10 ml/min	No data
Lamivudine	150 mg b.i.d.	80%	q. 12 hr	q. 24 hr	50 mg q. 24 hr	For HBV infection	Dose after dialysis	No data: dose for GFR <10 ml/min	Dose for GFR 10–50 ml/min
Nelfinavir	750 mg q. 8 hr	No data	No data	No data	No data		No data	No data	No data
Nevirapine	200 mg q. 24 hr for 14 days	< 3	No data: 100%	No data: 100%	No data: 100%	May be partially cleared by hemodialysis and peritoneal dialysis	Dose after dialysis	No data: dose for GFR < 10 ml/min	No data: dose for GFR 10–50 ml/min
Ribavirin	500–600 mg q. 12 hr	30%	100%	100%	50%	Adverse effects: hemolytic uremic syndrome	Dose after dialysis	Dose for GFR<10 ml/min	Dose for GFR 10–50 ml/min
Rifabutin	300 mg q. 24 hr	5–10%	100%	100%	100%		NC	NC	No data: dose for GFR 10–50 ml/min
Rimantadine	100 mg q. 12 hr	25%	100%	100%	50%				
Ritonavir	600 mg q. 12 hr	3.50%	No data: 100%	No data: 100%	No data: 100%	Associated with many adverse drug interactions	NC	No data: dose for GFR < 10 ml/min	No data: dose for GFR 10–50 ml/min
Zalcitabine	0.75 mg q. 8 hr	75%	100%	q. 12 hr	q. 24 hr		No data: dose after dialysis	No data	No data: dose for GFR 10–50 ml/min
Zidovudine	200 mg q. 8 hr or 300 mg q. 12 hr	8%–25%	100%	100%	100 mg q. 8 hr	Enormous interpatient variation; metabolite renally excreted	Dose for GFR <10 ml/min	Dose for GFR <10 ml/min	100 mg q. 8 hr

Table 3. Analgesic agents

Drug	Normal dosage	Route of drug clearance	Dosage adjustment for renal failure with GFR (ml/min):			Comments	Method of dosage adjustment		
			>50	10-50	<10		HD	CAPD	CVVH
Narcotics and narcotic antagonists									
Alfentanil	Anesthetic induction 8-40 g/kg	Hepatic	100%	100%	100%	Titrate the dose regimen	No data	No data	No data
Butorphanol	2 mg q. 3-4 hr	Hepatic	100%	75%	50%		No data	No data	No data
Codeine	30-60 mg q. 4-6 hr	Hepatic	100%	75%	50%		No data	No data	Dose for GFR 10-50 ml/min
Fentanyl	Anesthetic induction (individualized)	Hepatic	100%	75%	50%		No data	No data	No data
Meperidine	50-100 mg q. 3-4 hr	Hepatic	100%	avoid	avoid	Normeperidine, an active metabolite, accumulates in ESRD and may cause seizures; protein binding is reduced in ESRD; 20%-25% of meperidine is excreted unchanged in acidic urine	Avoid	Avoid	Avoid
Methadone	2.5-5 mg q. 6-8 hr	Hepatic	100%	100%	50%-75%		NC	NC	No data
Morphine	20-25 mg q. 4 hr	Hepatic	100%	75%	avoid	Increased sensitivity to drug effect in ESRD	NC	No data	Dose for GFR 10-50 ml/min
Naloxone	2 mg IV	Hepatic	100%	100%	100%		No data	No data	Dose for GFR 10-50 ml/min
Pentazocine	50 mg q. 4 hr	Hepatic	100%	75%	75%		NC	No data	Dose for GFR 10-50 ml/min
Propoxyphene	65 mg q. 6-8 hr	Hepatic	100%	100%	Avoid	Active metabolite norpropoxyphene accumulates in ESRD	Avoid	Avoid	No data
Sufentanil	Anesthetic induction	Hepatic	100%	100%	100%		No data	No data	No data
Nonnarcotics									
Acetaminophen	650 mg q. 4 hr	Hepatic	q. 4 hr	q. 6 hr	q. 8 hr	Overdose may be nephrotoxic; major metabolite of phenacetin.	NC	NC	Dose for GFR 10-50 ml/min
Acetylsalicylic acid	650 mg q. 4 hr	Hepatic (renal)	q. 4 hr	q. 4-6 hr	Avoid	Nephrotoxic in high doses; may decrease GFR when renal blood flow is prostaglandin dependent; may add to uremic GI and hematologic symptoms; protein binding reduced in ESRD	Dose after dialysis	None	Dose for GFR 10-50 ml/min

Table 4. Antihypertensive and cardiovascular agents

Drug	Normal dosage		Percentage of drug excreted renally	Dosage adjustment for renal failure with GFR (ml/min):			Comments	Method of dosage adjustment		
	Starting dose	Maximum dose		>50	10–50	<10		HD	CAPD	CVVH
Adrenergic agonist agents										
Clonidine	0.1 mg b.i.d. or t.i.d.	1.2 mg/day	45%	100%	100%	100%	Adverse effects: sexual dysfunction, dizziness, portal hypotension	NC	NC	Dose for GFR 10–50 ml/min
Dobutamine	2.5 mcg/kg/min	15 mcg/kg/min	10%	100%	100%	100%		No data	No data	Dose for GFR 10–50 ml/min
Angiotensin-converting enzyme (ACE) inhibitors										
Group toxicity: hyperkalemia, acute renal failure, angioedema, rash, cough, anemia, and liver toxicity										
Benazepril	10 mg/day	80 mg/day	20%	100%	75%	25%–50%	Group toxicity	NC	NC	Dose for GFR 10–50 ml/min
Captopril	6.25–25 mg t.i.d.	100 mg t.i.d.	35%	100%	75%	50%	Adverse effects: rare proteinuria, nephrotic syndrome, dysgeusia, granulocytopenia; increases serum digoxin levels	25%–30%	NC	Dose for GFR 10–50 ml/min
Enalapril	5 mg/day	20 mg b.i.d.	45%	100%	75%	50%	Enalaprilat is the active moiety formed in liver	20%–25%	NC	Dose for GFR 10–50 ml/min
Fosinopril	10 mg/day	40 mg b.i.d.	20%	100%	100%	75%	Less likely than other ACE inhibitors to accumulate in renal failure; fosinoprilat is the active moiety formed in liver	NC	NC	Dose for GFR 10–50 ml/min
Lisinopril	2.5 mg/day	20 mg b.i.d.	80%	100%	50%–75%	25%–50%	Lysine analogue of a pharmacologically active enalapril metabolite	20%	NC	Dose for GFR 10–50 ml/min
Pentopril	125 mg q. 24 hr		80%–90%	100%	50%–75%	50%	Group toxicity	No data	No data	Dose for GFR 10–50 ml/min
Perindopril	2 mg q. 24 hr		< 10%	100%	75%	50%	Active metabolite is perindoprilat; clearance of perindopril and its metabolites is almost exclusively renal; approximately 60% of circulating perindopril is bound to plasma proteins, whereas 10% to 20% of perindoprilat is bound	25%–50%	No data	Dose for GFR 10–50 ml/min
Quinapril	10 mg/day	20 mg/day	30%	100%	75%–100%	75%	Active metabolite is quinaprilat; 96 % of quinaprilat is excreted renally	25%	NC	Dose for GFR 10–50 ml/min
Ramipril	2.5 mg/day	10 b.i.d.	15%	100%	50%–75%	25-50%	Active metabolite is ramiprilat; data pertain to ramiprilat	20%	NC	Dose for GFR 10–50 ml/min
Trandolapril	1–2 mg/day	4 mg/day	33%	100%	50%–100%	50%	Group toxicity	NC	NC	Dose for GFR 10–50 ml/min

Drug	Normal dosage		Percentage of drug excreted renally	Dosage adjustment for renal failure with GFR (ml/min):			Comments	Method of dosage adjustment		
	Starting dose	Maximum dose		>50	10–50	<10		HD	CAPD	CVVH
Angiotensin-II-receptors antagonists (ARA)										
Group toxicity: hyperkalemia, angioedema (less common than ACE-inhibitors)										
Candesartan	16 mg/day	32 mg/day	33%	100%	100%	50%	Candesartan cilexetil is rapidly and completely bioactivated by ester hydrolysis during absorption from the GI tract to candesartan	NC	NC	NC
Eprosartan	600 mg/day	400–800 mg/day	25%	100%	100%	100%	Eprosartan pharmacokinetics more variable in ESRD; decreased protein binding in uremia	NC	NC	NC
Irbesartan	150 mg/day	300 mg/day	20%	100%	100%	100%	Group toxicity	NC	NC	NC
Losartan	50 mg/day	100 mg/day	13%	100%	100%	100%	Group toxicity	No data	No data	Dose for GFR 10–50 ml/min
Valsartan	80 mg/day	160 mg b.i.d.	7%	100%	100%	100%	Group toxicity	NC	NC	NC
Telmisartan	20–80 mg/day		<5%	100%	100%	100%	Group toxicity	NC	NC	NC
Beta blockers										
Group toxicity: agents can decrease HDL level and mask symptoms of hypoglycemia; can cause bronchospasm, fatigue, insomnia, depression, and sexual dysfunction										
Acebutolol	400 mg q..24 hr or b.i.d.	600 mg q. 24 hr or b.i.d.	55%	100%	50%	30%–50%	Active metabolites with long half-lives	NC	NC	Dose for GFR 10–50 ml/min
Atenolol	25 mg/day	100 mg/day	90%	100%	75%	50%	Accumulates in ESRD	25–50 mg	NC	Dose for GFR 10–50 ml/min
Betaxolol	20 mg q. 24 hr	80–90%	100%	100%	50%	50%	Group toxicity	NC	Dose for GFR 10–50 ml/min	Dose for GFR 10–50 ml/min
Bopindolol	1 mg q. 24 hr	4 mg q. 24 hr	< 10%	100%	100%	100%	Group toxicity	NC	NC	Dose for GFR 10–50 ml/min
Carteolol	0.5 mg q. 24 hr	10 mg q. 24 hr	< 50%	100%	50%	25%	Group toxicity	No data	No date: no change required	Dose for GFR 10–50 ml/min
Carvedilol	3.125 mg t.i.d.	25 mg t.i.d.	2%	100%	100%	100%	Kinetics are dose dependent; plasma concentrations are reported to be increased in patients with renal impairment	NC	NC	Dose for GFR 10–50 ml/min
Celiprolol	200 mg q. 24 hr		10%	100%	100%	75%	Group toxicity	No data	NC	Dose for GFR 10–50 ml/min
Dilevalol	200 mg b.i.d.	400 mg b.i.d.	< 5%	100%	100%	100%	Group toxicity	NC	NC	No data
Esmolol (IV only)	50 mcg/kg/min	300 mcg/kg/min	10%	100%	100%	100%	Active metabolite retained in renal failure	NC	NC	No data
Labetalol	50 mg p.o., b.i.d.	400 mg b.i.d.	5%	100%	100%	100%	For IV use: 20 mg slow injection over a 2-min period; additional injections of 40 mg or 80 mg can be given at 10-min intervals until a total of 300 mg is administered; alternatively, dose may be administered by continuous infusion of 2 mg/min	NC	NC	Dose for GFR 10–50 ml/min
Metoprolol	50 mg b.i.d.	100 mg b.i.d.	< 5%	100%	100%		See group toxicity	NC	NC	NC

Drug	Normal dosage		Percentage of drug excreted renally	Dosage adjustment for renal failure with GFR (ml/min):			Comments	Method of dosage adjustment		
	Starting dose	Maximum dose		>50	10–50	<10		HD	CAPD	CVVH
Nadolol	80 mg/day	160 mg b.i.d.	90%	100%	50%	25%	Start with prolonged interval and titrate	40 mg	NC	Dose for GFR 10–50 ml/min
Penbutolol	10 mg q. 24 hr	40 mg q 24 hr	< 10	100%	100%	100%		NC	NC	Dose for GFR 10–50 ml/min
Pindolol	10 mg b.i.d.	40 mg b.i.d.	40%	100%	100%	100%		NC	NC	Dose for GFR 10–50 ml/min
Propranolol	40–160 mg t.i.d.	320 mg/day	<5%	100%	100%	100%	In ESRD: bioavailability of propranolol may increase; metabolites may cause increased bilirubin by assay interference; hypoglycemiamay occur	NC	NC	Dose for GFR 10–50 ml/min
Sotalol	80 bid	160 mg b.i.d.	70%	100%	50%	25%–50%	Extreme caution should be exercised in the use of sotalol in patients with renal failure undergoing hemodialysis; to minimize the risk of induced arrhythmia, patients initiated or reinitiated on BETA-PACE should be placed for a minimum of 3 days (on their maintenance dose) in a facility that can provide cardiac resuscitation and continuous electrocardiographic monitoring	80 mg	NC	Dose for GFR 10–50 ml/min
Timolol	10 mg b.i.d.	20 mg b.i.d.	15%	100%	100%	100%		NC	NC	Dose for GFR 10–50 ml/min
Calcium channel blockers Group toxicity: dihydropyridines can cause headache, ankle edema, gingival hyperplasia and flushing; nondihydropyridine can cause bradycardia, constipation, gingival hyperplasia, and AV block										
Amlodipine	2.5/day	10 mg/day	10%	100%	100%	100%	May increase digoxin and cyclosporine levels	NC	NC	Dose for GFR 10–50 ml/min
Bepridil	No data	< 1%	No data	No data	No data	Weak vasodilator and anti-hypertensive	Group toxicity	NC	No data	No data
Diltiazem	30 mg t.i.d.	90 mg t.i.d.	10%	100%	100%	100%	Acute renal dysfunction; may exacerbate hyperkalemia; may increase digoxin and cyclosporine levels	NC	NC	Dose for GFR 10–50 ml/min
Felodipine	5 mg b.i.d.	20 mg/day	1%	100%	100%	100%	May increase digoxin levels	NC	NC	Dose for GFR10–50 ml/min
Isradipine	5 mg b.i.d.	10 mg b.i.d.	<5%	100%	100%	100%	May increase digoxin levels	NC	NC	Dose for GFR 10–50 ml/min
Nicardipine	20 mg t.i.d.	30 mg t.i.d.	<1%	100%	100%	100%		NC	NC	NC
Nifedipine XL	30 mg/day	90 mg b.i.d.	10%	100%	100%	100%	Avoid short-acting nifedipine formulation	NC	NC	NC

Drug	Normal dosage		Percentage of drug excreted renally	Dosage adjustment for renal failure with GFR (ml/min):			Comments	Method of dosage adjustment		
	Starting dose	Maximum dose		>50	10–50	<10		HD	CAPD	CVVH
Nimodipine	30 mg q. 8 hr		10%	100%	100%	100%	May lower blood pressure	NC	NC	Dose for GFR 10–50 ml/min
Nisoldipine	20 mg/day	30 mg b.i.d.	10%	100%	100%	100%	May increase digoxin levels	NC	NC	Dose for GFR 10–50 ml/min
Verapamil	40 mg t.i.d.	240 mg/day	10%	100%	100%	100%	Acute renal dysfunction; active metabolites accumulate particularly with sustained-release forms.	NC	NC	Dose for GFR 10–50 ml/min
Digoxin	0.125 mg q.o.d./q.d. (daily or every other day)	0.25 mg/day	25%	100%	100%	100%	In ESRD: V_D and total body clearance decreased; decrease loading dose by 50%; serum level 12 hr after dose is best guide to clearance; use digoxin-immune antibodies to treat severe toxicity Radioimmunoassay may overestimate serum levels in uremia; clearance decreased by amiodarone, spironolactone, quinidine, and verapamil; hypokalemia and hypomagnesemia enhance toxicity	NC	NC	Dose for GFR 10–50 ml/min
Diuretics										
Group toxicity: agents may cause hypokalemia, hyperkalemia, hyperuricemia, hyperglycemia, and hypomagnesemia; may increase serum cholesterol; use of potassium-sparing agents is recommended										
Acetazolamide	125 mg t.i.d.	500 mg t.i.d.	90%	100%	50%	Avoid	May potentiate acidosis; ineffective as diuretic in ESRD; may cause neurologic side effects in dialysis patients	No data	No data	Avoid
Amiloride	5 mg/day	10 mg/day	50%	100%	100%	Avoid	Hyperkalemia with GFR < 30 ml/min, especially in diabetics; may cause hyperchloremic metabolic acidosis	No data	No data	No data
Bumetanide	1–2 mg/day	2-4 mg/day	35%	100%	100%	100%	Ototoxicity increased in ESRD in combination with aminoglycosides; may cause muscle pain, gynecomastia; high doses effective in ESRD	NC	NC	No data
Chlorthalidone	25 mg q. 24 hr	50%	q. 24 hr	q. 24 hr	Avoid	Ineffective with low GFR	Group toxicity	No data	No data	No data
Ethacrynic acid	50 mg/day	100 mg b.i.d.	20%	100%	100%	100%	Ototoxicity increased in ESRD in combination with aminoglycosides	NC	NC	No data
Furosemide	40–80 mg/day	120 mg t.i.d.	70%	100%	100%	100%	Ototoxicity increased in ESRD, especially in combination with aminoglycosides; high doses effective in ESRD	NC	NC	No data
Indapamide	2.5 mg q. 24 hr	< 5%	100%	100%	Avoid	Ineffective in ESRD	Group toxicity	NC	No data	NC
Metolazone	2.5 mg/day	10 mg b.i.d.	70%	100%	100%		Adverse effects: gynecomastia and impotence; high doses effective in ESRD	NC	NC	No data: no change requrired
Piretanide	6 mg q. 24 hr	12 mg q. 24 hr	40-60%	100%	100%	100%	Ototoxicity; high doses effective in ESRD	NC	NC	No data

Drug	Normal dosage		Percentage of drug excreted renally	Dosage adjustment for renal failure with GFR (ml/min):			Comments	Method of dosage adjustment		
	Starting dose	Maximum dose		>50	10–50	<10		HD	CAPD	CVVH
Spironolactone	100 mg/day	300 mg/day	25%	100%	100%	Avoid	Active metabolites with long half-life; hyperkalemia common when GFR < 30 ml/min, especially in diabetics; may cause gynecomastia and hyperchloremic acidosis; increases serum by immunoassay interference	No data	No data	Avoid
Thiazides	25 mg b.i.d.		50 mg b.i.d.	> 95%	100%	100%	Usually ineffective with GFR < 30 ml/min; effective at low GFR in combination with loop diuretic; hyperuricemia may occur	Avoid	No data	No data
Torasemide	5 mg b.i.d.	20 mg/day	25%	100%	100%	100%	Ototoxicity; high doses effective in ESRD	NC	NC	No data; no change reqiured
Triamterene	25 mg b.i.d.	50 mg b.i.d.	5%–10%	q. 12 hr	q. 12 hr	Avoid	Active metabolite with long half-life in ESRD; hyperkalemia common when GFR < 30 ml/min, especially in diabetics; may cause acute renal failure; acts as folic acid antagonist; may cause urolithiasis or crystalluria in acid urine	Avoid	Avoid	Avoid
Midodrine	No data	No data	75%–80%	5–10 mg q. 8 hr	5–10 mg q. 8 hr	No data	Increases blood pressure	5 mg q. 8 hr	No data	Dose for GFR 10–50 ml/min
Phosphodiesterase enzyme inhibitors										
Amrinone	5 mg/kg/min daily dose <10 mg/kg	10 mg/kg/min daily dose <10 mg/kg	10%–40%	100%	100%	100%	Adverse effects: thrombocytopenia; nausea, vomiting in ESRD	No data	No data	Dose for GFR 10–50 ml/min
Milrinone	0.375 mcg/kg/min	0.75 mcg/kg/min		100%	100%	100%		No data	No data	Dose for GFR 10–50 ml/min
Vasodilators										
Hydralazine	10 mg q.i.d.	100 mg q.i.d.	25%	100%	100%	100%	May cause lupuslike reaction	NC	NC	Dose for GFR 10–50 ml/min
Minoxidil	2.5 mg b.i.d.	10 mg b.i.d.	20%	100%	100%	100%	May cause pericardial effusion, fluid retention, hypertrichosis, and tachycardia	NC	NC	Dose for GFR 10–50 ml/min
Nitroprusside	1 mcg/kg/min	10 mcg/kg/min	<10%	100%	100%	100%	Cyanide is metabolic byproduct; may cause cyanide toxicity	NC	NC	Dose for GFR10–50 ml/min

Table 5. Endocrine and metabolic agents

Drug	Normal dosage		Percentage of drug excreted renally	Dosage adjustment for renal failure with GFR (ml/min):			Comments	Method of dosage adjustment		
	Starting dose	Maximum dose		>50	10–50	<10		HD	CAPD	CVVH
Hypoglycemic agents (oral)										
Group toxicity: avoid all oral hypoglycemic agents on CRRT										
Acarbose	25 mg t.i.d.	100 mg t.i.d.	35%	100%	50%	Avoid	Abdominal pain, nausea, vomiting, and flatulence	Avoid	Avoid	Avoid
Acetohex-amide	250 mg q. 24 hr	1,500 mg q. 24 hr	None	Avoid	Avoid	Avoid	Diuretic effect; may falsely elevate serum creatinine level; active metabolite has a half life of 5–8 hr in healthy persons and is eliminated by the kidney; prolonged hypoglycemia in azotemic patients	Avoid	Avoid	Avoid
Chlorprop-amide	100 mg q. 24 hr	500 mg q24h	47%	50%	Avoid	Avoid	Impairs water excretion; may cause prolonged hy-poglycemia in azotemic patients	Avoid	Avoid	Avoid
Glibornuride	12.5 mg q. 24 hr	100 mg q. 14 hr	No data	No data	No data	No data		Avoid	Avoid	Avoid
Gliclazide	80 mg q. 24 hr	320 mg q. 24 hr	< 20%	50%–100%	Avoid	Avoid		Avoid	Avoid	Avoid
Glipizide	5 mg/day	20 mg b.i.d.	5%	100%	50%	50%		Avoid	Avoid	Avoid
Glyburide	2.5 mg/day	10 mg b.i.d.	50%	100%	50%	Avoid		Avoid	Avoid	Avoid
Gimepiride	1 mg/day	8 mg daily	50%	100%	50%	Avoid		Avoid	Avoid	Avoid
Metformin	500 mg b.i.d.	2,550 mg/day (b.i.d. or t.i.d.)	95%	100%	Avoid	Avoid	Causes lactic acidosis	Avoid	Avoid	Avoid
Repaglinide	0.5–1 mg	4 mg t.i.d.						Avoid	Avoid	Avoid
Tolazamide	100 mg q. 24 hr	250 mg q. 24.hr	7%	100%	100%	100%	Diuretic effects	Avoid	Avoid	Avoid
Tolbutamide	1 g q. 24 hr	2 g q. 24 hr	None	100%	100%	100%	Impairs water excretion	Avoid	Avoid	Avoid
Troglitazone	200 mg/day	600 mg/day	3%	100%	Avoid	Avoid	Hepatotoxic; decrease CSA level	Avoid	Avoid	Avoid
Hypoglycemic agents (parenteral)										
Dosage guided by blood glucose levels										
Insulin	Variable		None	100%	75%	50%	Renal metabolism of insulin decreases with azote-mia	NC	NC	Dose for GFR 10–50
Lispro insulin	Variable		No data	100%	75%	50%	Avoid all oral hypoglycemic agents on CRRT	NC	NC	NC
Hyperlipidemic agents										
Atorvastatin	10 mg/day	80 mg/day	<2%	100%	100%	100%	Liver dysfunction, myalgia, and rhabdomyolysis as-sociated with concurrent CSA/FK treatment	NC	NC	NC
Bezafibrate	200 mg b.i.d. or q.i.d. 400 mg SR q. 24 hr		50%	50%–100%	25%–50%	Avoid		NC	NC	NC
Cholestyr-amine	4 gm b.i.d.	24 gm/day	None	100%	100%	100%	No data	NC	NC	NC
Clofibrate	500 mg b.i.d.	1,000 mg b.i.d.	40%–70%	q. 6–12 hr	q. 12–18 hr	Avoid	No data	NC	NC	NC
Colestipol	5 g b.i.d.	30 g/day	None	100%	100%	100%	No data	NC	NC	NC
Fluvastatin	20 mg/day	80 mg/day	<1%	100%	100%	100%	No data	NC	NC	NC
Gemfibrozil	600 b.i.d.	600 b.i.d.	None	100%	100%	100%	No data	NC	NC	NC
Lovastatin	5 mg/day	20 mg/day	None	100%	100%	100%	No data	NC	NC	NC
Nicotinic acid	1 g t.i.d.	2 g t.i.d.	None	100%	50%	25%	No data	NC	NC	NC

Drug	Normal dosage		Percentage of drug excreted renally	Dosage adjustment for renal failure with GFR (ml/min):			Comments	Method of dosage adjustment		
	Starting dose	Maximum dose		>50	10–50	<10		HD	CAPD	CVVH
Pravastatin	10–40 mg/day	80 mg/day	<10%	100%	100%	100%	No data	NC	NC	NC
Probucol	500 mg b.i.d.		< 2%	100%	100%	100%		NC	NC	NC
Rosuvastatin	5–40 mg/day	40 mg/day	10%	100%	100%	50%	5 mg/day; maintenance, not to exceed 10 mg/day	50%	50%	50%
Simvastatin	5–20 mg/day	20 mg/day	13%	100%	100%	100%	No data	NC	NC	NC
Antithyroid drugs										
Methimazole	5–20 mg t.i.d.		7	100%	100%	100%		NC	NC	NC
Propylthio-uracil	100 mg t.i.d.		< 10	100%	100%	100%		NC	NC	NC

Table 6. Gastrointestinal agents

Drug	Normal dosage		Percentage of drug excreted renally	Dosage adjustment for renal failure with GFR (ml/min):			Comments
	Starting dose	Maximum dose		>50	10–50	<10	
Cimetidine	300 mg t.i.d.	800 mg b.i.d.	60%	100%	75%	25%	Multiple drug-drug interactions (e.g., beta blockers, sulfonylurea, theophylline, warfarin)
Famotidine	20 mg b.i.d.	40 mg b.i..d.	70%	100%	75%	25%	Adverse effects: headache, fatigue, thrombocytopenia, alopecia
Lansoprazole	15 mg/day	30 mg b.i.d.	None	100%	100%	100%	Adverse effects: headache, diarrhea
Nizatidine	150 mg b.i.d.	300 mg b.i.d.	20%	100%	75%	25%	Adverse effects: headache, fatigue, thrombocytopenia, alopecia
Omeprazole	20 mg/day	40 mg b.i.d.	None	100%	100%	100%	Adverse effects: headache, diarrhea
Rabeprazole	20 mg/day	40 mg b.i.d.	None	100%	100%	100%	Adverse effects: headache, diarrhea
Pantoprazole	40 mg/day	80 mg b.i.d.	None	100%	100%	100%	Adverse effects: headache, diarrhea
Ranitidine	150 mg b.i.d.	300 mg b.i.d.	80%	100%	75%	25%	Adverse effects: headache, fatigue, thrombocytopenia, alopecia
Cisapride	10 mg t.i.d.	20 mg q.i.d.	5%	100%	100%	50%–75%	Avoid with azole antifungal agents, macrolide antibiotics, and other P450 3A-4 inhibitors
Metoclo-pramide	10 mg t.i.d.	30 mg q.i.d.	15%	100%	100%	50%–75%	Neurotoxic; increase CSK/FK level
Misoprostol	100 mcg b.i.d.	200 mcg q.i.d.		100%	100%	100%	Adverse effects: diarrhea, nausea, vomiting; abortifacient agent
Sucralfate	1 g q.i.d.	1 g q.i.d.	None	100%	100%	100%	Adverse effects: constipation; decreased absorption of MMF

Table 7. Neurologic and anticonvulsant agents

Drug	Normal dosage		Percentage of drug excreted renally	Dosage adjustment for renal failure with GFR (ml/min):			Comments	Method of dosage adjustment		
	Starting dose	Maximum dose		>50	10–50	<10		HD	CAPD	CVVH
Carbamazepine	2–8 mg/kg/day; adjust for side effect and TDM		2%	100%	100%	100%	Plasma concentration: 4–12 mcg/ml; adverse effects: double vision, fluid retention, myelosuppression	NC	NC	NC
Clonazepam	0.5 mg t.i.d.	2 mg t.i.d.	1%	100%	100%	100%	Although no dose reduction is recommended, the drug has not been studied in patients with renal impairment; recommendations based on known drug characteristics not clinical trials data	NC	NC	NC
Ethosuximide	5 mg/kg/day; adjust for side effect and TDM		20%	100%	100%	100%	Plasma concentration: 40–100 mcg/ml; adverse effects: headache	NC	NC	NC
Felbamate	400 mg t.i.d.	1,200 mg t.i.d.	90%	100%	50%	25%	Adverse effects: anorexia, vomiting, insomnia, nausea	Dose after dialysis	Dose for GFR < 10 ml/min	Dose for GFR 10–50 ml/min
Gabapentin	150 mg t.i.d.	900 mg t.i.d.	77%	100%	50%	25%	Less CNS side effects compared to other agents	300 mg load, then 200–300 mg after hemodialysis	300 mg QID.	Dose for GFR 10–50
Lamotrigine	25–50 mg/day	150 mg/day	1%	100%	100%	100%	Autoinduction, major drug-drug interaction with valproate	No data	No data	Dose for GFR 10–50 ml/min
Levetiracetam	500mg b.i.d.	1,500 mg b.i.d.	66%	100%	50%	50%		250–500 mg after dialysis	Dose for GFR < 10	Dose for GFR 10–50 ml/min
Oxcarbazepine	300 mg b.i.d.	600 mg b.i.d.	1%	100%	100%	100%	Less effect on P450 compared to carbamazapine	NC	NC	NC
Phenobarbital	20 mg/kg/day; adjust for side effect and TDM		1%	100%	100%	100%	Plasma concentration: 15–40 mcg/ml; may cause insomnia	NC	NC	NC
Phenytoin	20 mg/kg/day; adjust for side effect and TDM		1%	Adjust for renal failure and low Albumin			Plasma concentration: 10–20 mcg/ml; may cause nystagmus; check free phenytoin level	NC	NC	NC
Primidone	50 mg	100 mg	1%	100%	100%	100%	Plasma concentration: 5–20 mcg/ml	NC	NC	NC
Sodium valproate	7.5 to 15 mg/kg/day; adjust for side effect and TDM		1%	100%	100%	100%	Plasma concentration: 50–150 mcg/ml; side effects include weight gain, hepatitis; check free valproate level	NC	NC	NC
Tiagabine	4 mg/day; increase 4mg/day, titrate weekly		2%	100%	100%	100%	Total daily dose may be increased by 4 to 8 mg at weekly intervals until clinical response is achieved, or up to 32 mg/day; the total daily dose should be given in divided doses two to four times daily	NC	NC	Dose for GFR 10–50 ml/min
Topiramate	50 mg/day	200 mg b.i.d.	70%	100%	50%	Avoid		Avoid	Avoid	Dose for GFR 10–50 ml/min
Trimethadione	300 mg t.i.d. or q.i.d.	600 mg t.i.d. or q.i.d.	None	q. 8 hr	q. 8– 12 hr	q. 12–24 hr	Active metabolites with long half-life in ESRD; may cause nephrotic syndrome	No data	No data	Dose for GFR 10–50 ml/min

Drug	Normal dosage		Percentage of drug excreted renally	Dosage adjustment for renal failure with GFR (ml/min):			Comments	Method of dosage adjustment		
	Starting dose	Maximum dose		>50	10–50	<10		HD	CAPD	CVVH
Vigabatrin	1 g b.i.d.	2 g b.i.d.	70%	100%	50%	25%	Encephalopathy may arise with drug accumulation	No data	No data	Dose for GFR 10–50 ml/min
Zonisamide	100 mg/day	100–300 mg q.d.–b.i.d.	30%	100%	75%	50%	Manufacturer recommends that zonisamide not be used in patients with renal failure (estimated GFR <50 ml/min); dose recommendations for renal impairment based on clearance ratios: initial dose should be 100 mg/day; after 2 wk, the dose may be increased to 200 mg/day for at least 2 wk; further dosage increases to 300 mg and 400 mg/day can then be made with a minimum of 2 wk between adjustments to achieve steady state at each dosage level; zonisamide doses of 100–600 mg/day appear effective for normal renal function	Dose for GFR < 10 ml/min	Dose for GFR < 10 ml/min	Dose for GFR 10–50 ml/min

Table 8. Rheumatologic agents

Agent	Normal dosage	Percentage of drug excreted renally	Dosage adjustment for renal failure with GFR (ml/min):			Comments	Method of dosage adjustment		
			>50	10–50	<10		HD	CAPD	CVVH
Arthritis and gout agents									
Allopurinol	300 mg q. 24 hr	30%	75%	50%	25%	Adverse effects: interstitial nephritis, exfoliative dermatitis, and rarely, xanthine stones; renal excretion of active metabolite with half life of 25 hr in normal renal function, half life 1 wk in patients with ESRD	Half dose	No data	Dose for GFR 10–50 ml/min
Auranofin	6 mg q24h	50%	50%	Avoid	Avoid	Proteinuria and ephritic syndrome.	NC	NC	NC
Colchicine	Acute: 2 mg then 0.5 mg q. 6 hr Chronic: 0.5–1.0 mg q. 24 hr	5%–175	100%	50-100%	25%	Avoid prolonged use if GFR < 50 ml/min	NC	No data	Dose for GFR 10–50 ml/min
Gold sodium	25–50 mg	60%–90%	50%	Avoid	Avoid	thiomalate proteinuria; ephritic syndrome, membranous nephritis	NC	NC	Avoid
Penicillamine	250–1,000 mg q. 24 hr	40%	100%	Avoid	Avoid	Nephrotic syndrome	One-third dose	No data	Dose for GFR 10–50 ml/min
Probenecid	500 mg bid	< 2%	100%	Avoid	Avoid	Ineffective at decreased GFR	Avoid	No data	Avoid
Nonsteroidal anti-Inflammatory drugs (NSAIDs) Group toxicity: decreases renal function and platelet aggregation; may cause nephrotic syndrome, interstitial nephritis, hyperkalemia , sodium retention; carries increased risk of CVD, MI, and stroke									
Diclofenac	25–75 mg b.i.d.	< 1%	50%–100 %	25%–50%	25%	Group toxicity	NC	NC	Dose for GFR 10–50 ml/min
Diflunisal	250–500 mg b.i.d.	< 3%	100%	50%	50%	Group toxicity	NC	NC	Dose for GFR 10–50 ml/min
Etodolac	200 mg b.i.d.	Negligible	100%	100%	50%	Group toxicity	NC	NC	Dose for GFR 10–50 ml/min
Fenoprofen	300–600 mg q.i.d.	30%	100%	100%	50%	Group toxicity	NC	NC	Dose for GFR 10–50 ml/min
Flurbiprofen	100 mg b.i.d. or t.i.d.	20%	100%	100%	50%	Group toxicity	NC	NC	Dose for GFR 10–50 ml/min
Ibuprofen	800 mg t.i.d.	1%	100%	100%	50%	Group toxicity	NC	NC	Dose for GFR 10–50 ml/min
Indomethacin	25–50 mg t.i.d.	30%	100%	100%	50%	Group toxicity	NC	NC	Dose for GFR 10–50 ml/min
Ketoprofen	25-–5 mg t.i.d.	< 1%	100%	100%		Group toxicity	NC	NC	Dose for GFR 10–50 ml/min
Ketorolac	30–60 mg load then 15–30 mg q. 6 hr	30%–60%	100%	50%	25-50%	May cause acute hearing loss in ESRD	NC	NC	Dose for GFR 10–50 ml/min
Meclofenamic acid	50–100 mg t.i.d. or q.i.d.	2%– 4%	100%	100%	50%	Group toxicity	NC	NC	Dose for GFR 10–50 ml/min
Mefanamic acid	250 mg q.i.d.	< 6%	100%	100%	50%	Group toxicity	NC	NC	Dose for GFR 10–50 ml/min
Nabumetone	1.0-2.0 g q. 24.hr	< 1%	100%	50-100%	50%	Group toxicity	NC	NC	Dose for GFR 10–50 ml/min

Agent	Normal dosage	Percentage of drug excreted renally	Dosage adjustment for renal failure with GFR (ml/min):			Comments	Method of dosage adjustment		
			>50	10–50	<10		HD	CAPD	CVVH
Naproxen	500 mg b.i.d.	< 1%	100%	100%	50%	Group toxicity	NC	NC	Dose for GFR 10–50 ml/min
Oxaproxin	1200 mg q. 24 hr	< 1%	100%	100%	50%	Group toxicity	NC	NC	Dose for GFR 10–50 ml/min
Phenylbutazone	100 mg t.i.d. or q.i.d.	1%	100%	100%	50%	Group toxicity	NC	NC	Dose for GFR 10–50 ml/min
Piroxicam	20 mg q. 24 hr	10%	100%	100%	50%	Group toxicity	NC	NC	Dose for GFR 10–50 ml/min
Sulindac	200 mg b.i.d.	7%	100%	100%	50%	Active sulfide metabolite in ESRD	NC	NC	Dose for GFR 10–50 ml/min
Tolmetin	400 mg t.i.d.	15%	100%	100%	50%	Group toxicity	NC	NC	Dose for GFR 10–50 ml/min
Biologic agents									
		Route of drug clearance							
Etanercept	50 mg S.C. weekly	Hepatic	100%	100%	100%	Increased risk of TB and other infections	100%	100%	100%
Infliximab	3 mg/kg IV at 0, 2, and 6 wk, then q. 8 wk; combine with methotrexate	Hepatic	100%	100%	100%	Increased risk of TB and other infections	100%	100%	100%
Adalimumab	40 mg S.C. every other week	Hepatic	100%	100%	100%	May be continued during therapy; may increase to 40 mg S.C. q. wk in patients not receiving concomitant methotrexate; may cause glomerulonephritis	100%	100%	100%
Anakinra	100 mg/day S.C.	Renal	100%	50%	Avoid	Renal impairment: plasma clearance is reduced up to 75% in patients with severe or end stage renal disease (C_{Cr} less than 30 ml/min); no formal studies have been conducted	100%	50%	Avoid
Rituximab	375 mg/mm every other week	Hepatic	100%	100%	100%	Increased risk of TB and other infections	100%	100%	100%

Table 9. Sedative agents

Drug	Normal dosage	Route of drug clearance	Dosage adjustment for renal failure with GFR (ml/min):			Comments	Method of dosage adjustment		
			>50	10–50	<10		HD	CAPD	CVVH
Barbiturates									
Group toxicity: may cause excessive sedation.; increased osteomalacia in ESRD; charcoal hemoperfusion and hemodialysis more effective than peritoneal dialysis for poisoning									
Pentobarbital	30 mg q. 6–8 hr	Hepatic	100%	100%	100%	Group toxicity	NC	No data	Dose for GFR 10–50 ml/min
Phenobarbital	50–100 mg q. 8–12 hr	Hepatic (renal)	q. 8–12 hr	q. 8–12 hr	q. 12–16 hr	Up to 50% unchanged drug excreted with urine with alkaline diuresis	Dose after dialysis	hale normal dose	Dose for GFR 10–50 ml/min
Secobarbital	30–50 mg q. 6–8 hr	Hepatic	100%	100%	100%	Group toxicity	NC	NC	No data
Thiopental	Anesthesia induction (individualized)	Hepatic	100%	100%	100%	Group toxicity	No data	No data	No data
Benzodiazepines									
Group toxicity: may cause excessive sedation and encephalopathy in ESRD									
Alprazolam	0.25–5.0 mg q. 8 hr	Hepatic	100%	100%	100%	Group toxicity	NC	No data	No data
Clorazepate	15–60 mg q. 24 hr	Hepatic (renal)	100%	100%	100%	Group toxicity	No data	No data	No data
Chlordiazepoxide	15–100 mg q. 24 hr	Hepatic	100%	100%	50%	Group toxicity	NC	No data	Dose for GFR 10–50 ml/min
Clonazepam	1.5 mg q. 24 hr	Hepatic	100%	100%	100%	Although no dose reduction is recommended, the drug has not been studied in patients with renal impairment; recommendations are based on known drug characteristics not clinical trials data	NC	No data	NA
Diazepam	5–40 mg q. 24 hr	Hepatic	100%	100%	100%	Active metabolites desmethyldiazepam and oxazepam may accumulate in renal failure; dose should be reduced if given longer than a few days; protein binding decreases in uremia	NC	No data	NC
Estazolam	1 mg qhs Au: define qhs	Hepatic	100%	100%	100%	Group toxicity	No data	No data	NC
Flurazepam	15–30 mg **qhs**	Hepatic	100%	100%	100%	Group toxicity	NC	No data	No data
Lorazepam	1–2 mg q. 8–12 hr	Hepatic	100%	100%	100%	Group toxicity	NC	No data	Dose for GFR 10–50 ml/min
Midazolam	Individualized	Hepatic	100%	100%	50%	Group toxicity	NA	NA	NA
Oxazepam	30–120 mg q. 24 hr	Hepatic	100%	100%	100%	Group toxicity	NC	No data	Dose for GFR 10–50 ml/min
Quazepam	15 mg **qhs**	Hepatic	No data	No data	No data	Group toxicity	No data	No data	No data
Temazepam	30 mg **qhs**	Hepatic	100%	100%	100%	Group toxicity	NC	NC	No data
Triazolam	0.25–0.50 mg **qhs**	Hepatic	100%	100%	100%	Protein binding correlates with alpha-1 acid glycoprotein concentration	NC	NC	No data
Benzodiazepine antagonists									
Flumazenil	0.2 mg IV over 15 sec	Hepatic	100%	100%	100%	May cause excessive sedation and encephalopathy in ESRD	NC	No data	No data
Miscellaneous sedative agents									
Buspirone	5 mg q.8 hr	Hepatic	100%	100%	100%		No data	No data	No data
Ethchlorvynol	500 mg **qhs**	Hepatic	100%	Avoid	Avoid	Removed by hemoperfusion; may cause excessive sedation	Avoid	Avoid	No data

Drug	Normal dosage	Route of drug clearance	Dosage adjustment for renal failure with GFR (ml/min):			Comments	Method of dosage adjustment		
			>50	10–50	<10		HD	CAPD	CVVH
Haloperidol	1–2 mg q. 8–12 hr	Hepatic	100%	100%	100%	Adverse effects: hypertension, excessive sedation	NC	NC	Dose for GFR 10–50 ml/min
Lithium carbonate	0.9–1.2 g q. 24 hr	Renal	100%	50-75%	25-50%	Nephrotoxic; adverse effects include nephrogenic diabetes insipidus, nephrotic syndrome, renal tubular acidosis, and interstitial fibrosis; acute toxicity when serum levels > 1.2 mEq/L; serum levels should be measured periodically 12 hr after dosing; half life does not reflect extensive tissue accumulation; plasma levels rebound after dialysis; toxicity enhanced by volume depletion, NSAIDs, and diuretics	Dose after dialysis	NC	Dose for GFR 10–50 ml/min
Meprobamate	1.2–1.6 g q. 24 hr	Hepatic (renal)	q. 6 hr	q. 9–12 hr	q. 12–18 hr	Side effects: excessive sedation; excretion enhanced by forced diuresis	NC	No data	No data

Table 10. Anti-Parkinson agents

Drug	Normal dosage	Percentage of drug excreted renally	Dosage adjustment for renal failure with GFR (ml/min):			Comments	Method of dosage adjustment		
			>50	10–50	<10		HD	CAPD	CVVH
Carbidopa	1–2 tablets t.i.d. or q.i.d. (30 mg/day to 200 mg/day)	30	100%	100%	100%	Require careful titration of dose according to clinical response	No data	No data	No data
Levodopa	1–2 tablets t.i.d. or q.i.d. (300 mg/day to 2,000 mg/day)	None	100%	50%–100%	50%–100%	Active and inactive metabolites excreted in urine; active metabolites with long half life in ESRD	No data	No data	Dose for GFR 10–50 ml/min
Rasagiline (MAO-b inhibitor)	1 mg/day	<1%	100%	100%	100%				

Table 11. Antipsychotic agents

Drug	Normal dosage	Percentage of drug excreted renally	Dosage adjustment for renal failure with GFR (ml/min):			Comments	Method of dosage adjustment		
			>50	10–50	<10		HD	CAPD	CVVH
Clozapine	12.5 mg p.o.; 25–50 to 300–450 mg/day by end of 2 weeks; maximum: 900 mg/day	Metabolism nearly complete	100%	100%	100%		No data	No data	Dose for GFR 10–50 ml/min
Haloperidol	1–2 mg q. 8–12 hr	Hepatic	100%	100%	100%	Hypotension, excessive sedation.	No data	No data	Dose for GFR 10–50 ml/min
Loxapine	12.5–50 mg I.M. q. 4–6 hr		100%	100%	100%	Do not administer drug IV	No data	No data	Dose for GFR 10–50 ml/min
Melperone olanzapine	5–10 mg	Hepatic	100%	100%	100%	Potential hypotensive effects	No data	No data	Dose for GFR 10–50 ml/min
Phenothiazines									
Group toxicity: orthostatic hypotension, extrapyramidal symptoms, and confusion									
Chlorpromazine	300–800 mg q. 24 hr	Hepatic	100%	100%	100%	Group toxicity	NC	NC	Dose for GFR 10–50 ml/min
Perphenazine	8 to 16 mg p.o., b.i.d., t.i.d., or q.i.d.; increase to 64 mg/day	Hepatic	100%	100%	100%	Group toxicity	No data	No data	Dose for GFR 10–50 ml/min
Promazine	20–100 mg q. 24 hr	Hepatic	100%	100%	100%	Group toxicity; excessive sedation may occur in ESRD	No data	No data	Dose for GFR 10–50 ml/min
Thioridazine	50–100 mg p.o. , t.i.d.; increase gradually; max dose 800 mg/day	Hepatic	100%	100%	100%	Group toxicity	No data	No data	Dose for GFR 10–50 ml/min
Trifluoperazine	1–2 mg b.i.d.; increase to no more than 6 mg/day	Hepatic	100%	100%	100%	Group toxicity	No data	No data	Dose for GFR 10–50 ml/min
Quetiapine	25 mg p.o., b.i.d.; increase in increments of 25–50 b.i.d or t.i.d. to achieve 300–400 mg/day by day 4	Hepatic	100%	100%	100%		No data	No data	Dose for GFR 10–50 ml/min
Risperidone	1 mg p.o., b.i.d.; increase to 3 mg b.i.d.		100%	100%	100%		No data	No data	Dose for GFR 10–50 ml/min
Thiothixene	2 mg p.o., t.i.d.; increase gradually to 15 mg/day	Hepatic	100%	100%	100%		No data	No data	Dose for GFR 10–50 ml/min
Ziprasideone	20–100 mg q. 12 hr	Hepatic	100%	100%	100%		No data	No data	Dose for GFR 10–50 ml/min

Table 12. Corticosteroid agents

Drug	Normal dosage	Percentage of drug excreted renally	Dosage adjustment for renal failure with GFR (ml/min):			Comments	Method of dosage adjustment		
			>50	10–50	<10		HD	CAPD	CVVH
Group toxicity: may aggravate azotemia; adverse effects: sodium retention, glucose intolerance, hypertension									
Betamethasone	0.5–9.0 mg q. 24 hr	5	100%	100%	100%	Group toxicity	NC	NC	NC
Budesonide	No data	None	100%	100%	100%	Group toxicity	NC	NC	NC
Cortisone	25–500 mg q. 24 hr	None	100%	100%	100%	Group toxicity	NC	NC	NC
Dexamethasone	0.75–9.0 mg q. 24 hr	8	100%	100%	100%	Group toxicity	NC	NC	NC
Hydrocortisone	20–500 mg q. 24 hr	None	100%	100%	100%	Group toxicity	NC	NC	NC
Methylprednisolone	4–48 mg q. 24 hr	< 10	100%	100%	100%	Group toxicity	NC	NC	NC
Prednisolone	5–60 mg q. 24 hr	34	100%	100%	100%	Group toxicity	NC	NC	NC
Prednisone	5–60 mg q. 24 hr	34	100%	100%	100%	Group toxicity	NC	NC	NC
Triamcinolone	4–48 mg q. 24 hr	No data	100%	100%	100%	Group toxicity	NC	NC	NC

Table 13. Anticoagulant agents

Drug	Normal dosage		Percentage of drug excreted renally	Dosage adjustment for renal failure with GFR (ml/min):			Comments	Method of dosage adjustment		
	Starting dose	Maximum dose		>50	10–50	<10		HD	CAPD	CVVH
Alteplase	60 mg over 1 hr then 20 mg/hr for 2 hr		No data	100%	100%	100%	Tissue-type plasminogen activator	No data	No data	Dose for GFR 10–50 ml/min
Anistreplase	30 U over 2–5 min		No data	100%	100%	100%		NC	NC	NC
Aspirin	81 mg/day	325 mg/day	10%	100%	100%	100%	GI irritation and bleeding tendency	NC	NC	NC
Clopidogrel	75 mg/day	75 mg/day	50%	100%	100%	100%		NC	NC	NC
Dalteparin	2,500 units S.C. daily	5,000 units S.C. daily	Unknown	100%	100%	NA	Check anti-factor Xa activity 4 hr after 2nd dose in patients with renal dysfunction	NC	NC	NC
Dipyridamole	50 mg t.i.d.		No data	100%	100%	100%		NC	NC	NC
Enoxaparin	20 mg/day	30 mg b.i.d.	8%	100%	75%–50%	50%	1 mg/kg q. 12 hr for treatment of DVT; check anti-factor Xa activity 4 hr after second dose in patients with renal dysfunction; some evidence of drug accumulation in renal failure	NC	NC	NC
Fondaparinux	2.5mg S.C. daily	10 mg S.C. daily	No data	100%	75%–50%	Avoid	Half life increases with renal failure; should be used for patients with HIT only	NC	NC	NC
Heparin	75 U/kg load then 15 U/kg/hr		None	100%	100%	100%	Half life increases with dose	NC	NC	NC
Iloprost	0.5–2.0 ng/kg/min for 5–12 hr		No data	100%	100%	50%		NC	NC	NC
Indobufen	100 mg b.i.d.	200 mg b.i.d.	< 15%	100%	50%	25%		NC	NC	NC
Streptokinase	250 000 U load, then 100 000 U/hr		None	100%	100%	100%		NC	NC	NC
Sulfinpyrazone	200 mg b.i.d.		25-50%	100%	100%	Avoid	May cause acute renal failure; uricosuric effect at low GFR	NC	NC	NC
Sulotroban	No data		52-62%	50%	30%	10%		NC	NC	NC
Ticlopidine	250 mg b.i.d.	250 mg b.i.d.	2%	100%	100%	100%	Adverse effects: severe neutropenia and thrombocytopenia; decrease CSA level	NC	NC	NC
Tranexamic acid	25 mg/kg t.i.d. or q.i.d.		90%	50%	25%	10%		NC	NC	NC
Urokinase	4400 U/kg load then 4,400 U/kg q. hr		No data	No data	No data	No data		NC	NC	NC
Warfarin	5 mg/day	Adjust per INR	<1%	100%	100%	100%	Monitor INR very closely; start at 5 mg/day; 1 mg vitamin K IV over 30 min or 2.5–5 mg p.o. can be used to achieve INR	NC	NC	NC

Clinical Nephrotoxins

Renal Injury from Drugs and Chemicals

Third Edition

LIST OF ABBREVIATIONS

AA	aristolochic acid
AAN	aristolochic acid nephropathy
AAP	alanine aminopeptidase
AAS	atomic absorption spectrometry
ABC	ATP-binding cassette
ABCD	amphotericin B colloidal dispersion
ABLC	amphotericin B in lipid complex
ACAM	N-cadherin
ACE	angiotensin converting enzyme
ACEI	angiotensin converting enzyme inhibitor
ACGIH	American Conference of Governmental Industrial Hygienists
AcP	acid phosphate
ADH	antidiuretic hormone or alcohol dehydrogenase
ADP	adenosine diphosphate
ADPKD	autosomal dominant polycystic kidney disease
ADR	adverse drug reaction
AE	adverse event
AER	adverse event reaction
AGT	alanine glyoxylate aminotransferase
AH-SOD	hexamethyl-enediamine-conjugated super-oxide dismutase
AHS	allopurinol hypersensitivity syndrome
AIDS	acquired immunodeficiency syndrome
AIN	acute interstitial nephritis
AKI	acute kidney injury
ALB	albumin
α_1-AG	α_1-acid glycoprotein
α_1-m	α_1-microglobulin
α -KG	α –ketoglutarate
ALT	alanine aminotransferase
AmB	amphotericin B
AMI	acute myocardial infarction
AMP	adenosine monophosphate
Amph	amphotericin
ANA	antinuclear antibody
ANCA	anti-neutrophil cytoplasmic antibody
ANDA	abbreviated new drug application
ANF	atrial natriuretic factor
ANT	adenine nucleotide translocator
ANZDATA	Australian and New Zealand Dialysis and Transplant Registry
AP	alkaline phosphatase
APA	aminopeptidase 1 (angiotensinase)
APACHE	Acute Physiology And Chronic Health Evaluation
APC	antigen presenting cell
APhN	acute phosphate nephropathy
APN	aminopeptidase N
AQP	aquaporin
ARBs	angiotensin II receptor antagonists
ARDS	acute respiratory distress syndrome
5-ASA	5-aminosalicylic acid
AST	aspartate aminotransferase
ATHENA	AIDS Therapy Evaluation National Centre
ATG	anti-thymocyte globulin
ATN	acute tubular necrosis
ATP	adenosine triphosphate
AUC	area under the curve
AV	atrioventricular
AVP	arginine vasopressin
AZT	azidothymidine
β_1-m	β_1-microglobulin
BBA	brush border antigen

BBM	brush border membrane
BBMV	brush border membrane vesicle
BC	breast cancer
BCNU	carmustine
bFGF	basic fibroblast growth factor
BEN	Balkan endemic npehropathy
BID	twice daily
BM	basolateral membrane
BMDL	benchmark dose low
BMI	body mass index
BMT	bone marrow transplantation
BN	Brown-Norway
BP	blood pressure
BQ123	cyclo [Trp-Asp-Pro-Val-Leu]
BSA	bovine serum albumin
BSP	bromosulfophthalein
BUN	blood urea nitrogen
BW	body weight
CA	carbonic anhydrase
CABG	coronary artery bypass graft
cADPR	cyclic ADP-ribose
Calc	calcitonin
CAM	cell adhesion molecule
cAMP	cyclic adenosine monophosphate
CAPD	continuous ambulatory peritoneal dialysis
CAPE	caffeic acid phenethyl ester
CaSR	calcium sensing receptor
CC	cytochemistry
CCB	calcium channel blocker
CCD	cortical collecting duct
CCNU	lomustine
Ccr	creatinine clearance
CD	collecting duct
CDC	Center for Disease Control and Prevention
CD-IC	collecting duct intercalated cell
CdMT	cadmium-metallothionein
CD-PC	collecting duct principal cell
CFS	colony-stimulating factor
CG	density gradient centrifugation
CHD	coronary heart disease
CHF	congestive heart failure
CHN	Chinese herb nephropathy
CI	confidence interval
CIN	chronic interstitial nephritis
CKD	chronic kidney disease
CLOD	clodronate
CM	contrast media
CMIN	contrast media induced nephropathy
CMV	cytomegalovirus
CNI	calcineurin inhibitors
CNS	central nervous system
cNOS	constitutive nitric oxide synthase
CNT	connecting tubule
COPD	chronic obstructive pulmonary disease
COX	cyclooxygenase
CPH	cephaloridine
CPK	creatinine phosphokinase
cPLA2	cytosolic phospholipase A2
CPP	calcium phosphorus product
CREB	cAMP response element-binding
CRF	chronic renal failure
CRRT	continuous renal replacement therapy
CsA	cyclosporine A
CSF	colony-stimulating factor
CSFL	cerebrospinal fluid
CT	computer tomography
CTGF	connective tissue growth factor
CTIN	chronic tubulointerstitial nephritis
C_{urea}	urea clearance
CVD	cardiovascular disease
CVVH	continuous venovenous hemofiltration
CVVHD	continuous venous-venous hemodialysis
Cx	clearance of a marker
CYP	cytochrome P450
dA-AAI	7(desoxyadenosin-N^6-yl) aristolactam I
dA-AAII	7(deoxyadenosin-N^6-yl) aristolactam II
DAC	diacylglycerol
DCAA	dichloroacetic acid
DCT	distal convoluted tubule
DCVC	dichlorovinylcysteine
dDAVP	1-desamino-8-D-arginine-vasopressin
DDT	dichlorodiphenyltrichloroethane
DES	diethyl stilbesterol
DEVD-CHO	Asp-Glu-Val-Asp-aldehyde
DFO	desferoxamine
dG-AAI	7(deoxyguanosine-N^2-yl) aristolactam I
DGFR	delayed graft function recovery
DHEA-S	dehydroepiandrosterone-sulfate
DHG	dehydrogenase
DHP	vitamin D binding protein
DIGE	difference in-gel electrophoresis
DISC	death inducing signaling complex
DMARD	disease modifying antirheumatic drugs
DMEM	Dulbecco's modified Eagle medium
DMPC	dimyristoyl phosphatidylcholine
DMPG	dimyristoyl phosphatidylglycerol
DMPS	dimercaptopropane 1 sulphonate
DMSA	dimercaptosuccinic acid
DMSO	dimethylsulfoxide
DMT	divalent metal transporter
DMTU	dimethylthiourea
DNP-SG	S-(dinitropheny1)-glutathione
DOCA	deoxycorticosterone acetate
DPCPX	1,3-dipropyl-8-cyclopentylxanthine (selective adenosine A1 receptor antagonist)
DPP	dipeptidyl peptidase
DTL	descending thin limb
DTPA	diethylenetriaminepentaacetic acid
DVT	deep vein thrombosis
E217 β G	estradiol-17 β -D-glucuronide
EBV	Epstein Barr virus
ecNOS	endothelial nitric oxide synthase

EDD	extended daily dialysis
EDHF	endothelium-derived hyperpolarizing factor
EDRF	endothelium-derived relaxing factor
EDTA	ethylenediamine tetraacetic acid
EDTA	European Dialysis and Transplant Association
EEG	electroencephalogram
EG	ethylene glycol
EGF	epidermal growth factor
EHDP	etidronate
ELISA	enzyme-linked immunosorbent assay
EMA	epithelial membrane antigen
EP	E-prostanoid
eNOS	endothelial nitric oxide synthase
ER	endoplasmic reticulum
ERK	extracellular regulated kinase
ERPF	effective renal plasma flow
ESRD	end-stage renal disease
estrone-S	estrone sulfate
ET	endothelin
ET-1	endothelin-1
ETA	endothelin A
ETB	endothelin B
FACS	fluorescence-activated cell sorting
FAD	flavin adenine dinucleotide
FAK	focal adhesion kinase
FAT	focal adhesion targeting
FCS	fetal calf serum
FDA	Food and Drug Administration
FE	fractional excretion
FENa	fractional excretion of sodium
FE_{urea}	fractional excretion of urea
FF	filtration fraction
FGS	focal glomerulosclerosis
FHH	familial hypercalcemic hypocalciuria
FITC	fluorescein isothiocyanate
FKBP	FK-binding protein
FMN	flavin mononucleotide
FPPS	farnesyl pyrophosphate synthase
FSGS	focal segmental glomerulosclerosis
G6PD	glucose 6 phosphate dehydrogenase
GBM	glomerular basement mmbrane
GC	gas chromatography
GCCA	gadolinium-containing contrast agents
GFR	glomerular filtration rate
GI	gastrointestinal
GLDH	glutamate dehydrogenase
GMP	guanosine monophosphate
GN	glomerulonephritis
GO	glyoxylate oxidase
GP	glycoprotein
GSC	glomerular sieving coefficient
GSH	glutathione
GSSG	glutathione disulfide
GST	glutathione-S-transferase
GT	glutamyl transferase

HA	hyaluronic acid
H&E	hematoxylin and eosin
HCM	hypercalcaemia of malignancy
HCTZ	hydrochlorothiazide
HCV	hepatitis C virus
HD	hemodialysis
HDF	hemodiafiltration
HDL	high-density lipoprotein
HETE	hydroxyeicosatetraenoic acid
HF	hemofiltration
HGF	hepatocyte growth factor
HGPRT	hypoxanthine-guanine phosphoribosyl transferase
HHV	human herpes virus
HIT	heparin-induced thrombocytopenia
HIV	human immunodeficiency virus
HIVAN	HIVassociated nephropathy
HLA	human leukocyte antigen
HMW	high molecular weight
HNL	human neutrophil lipocalin
HO	heme oxygenase
hOAT	human organic anion transporter
HPT	human proximal tubular cells
HPV	human papillomavirus
HR	hazard ratio
HSP	heat shock protein
HSV	herpes simplex virus
hTERT	human telomerase catalytic subunit
HUS	hemolytic uremic syndrome
HUVEC	human umbilical vein endothelial cells
IAKI	ischemic acute kidney injury
IAP	intestinal alkaline phosphatase
IARC	International Agency for Research on Cancer
IBD	inflammatory bowel disease
IBN	ibandronate
IC	information component
ICAD	inhibitor of caspase-activates Dnase
ICAM	intercellular cell adhesion molecule
ICC	immunocytochemistry
ICD	International Classification of Diseases
ICU	intensive care unit
IDDM	insulin-dependent diabetes mellitus
IEG	immediate early gene response
IFN	interferon
Ig	immunoglobulin
IGF	insulin-like growth factor
IL	interleukin
IM	intramuscular
IMCD	inner medullary collecting ducts
iNOS	inducible nitric oxide synthase
INR	international normalized ratio
IPD	intermittent peritoneal dialysis
IP3	inositol 3,4,5 triphosphate
IPRK	isolated perfused rat kidney
ISOM	inner stripe outer medulla

ITAM	immunoreceptor tyrosine activated motive
IV	intravenous
IVIG	intravenous immunoglobulin
IVP	intravenous pyelography
JCAHO	Joint Commission on Accreditation of Healthcare Organizations
JGA	juxtaglomerular apparatus
JNK	c-Jun N-terminal kinase
KAP	kidney androgen-regulated protein
kD or kDa	kilodalton
KDOQI	Kidney Disease Outcomes Quality Initiative
KIM	kidney injury molecule
L-Amph	amphotericin B liposome
LAP	leucine aminopeptidase
LC	lung cancer
LD50	lethal dose for 50%
LDH	lactate dehydrogenase
LDL	low-density lipoprotein
LEHD-CHO	Leu-Glu-His-Asp-aldehyde
LEW	Lewis
LFA	lymphocyte function-associated antigen
LFAB	lipid formulation of amphotericin B
LLC-PK1	renal epithelial cell line from porcine kidney
LMW	low molecular weight
L-NAME	N-nitro-l-arginine methyl ester
LOCM	low osmolar contrast medium
LPS	lipopolysaccharide
LR	likelihood ratio
LRP	LDL-receptor-related protein
LT	leukotriene
LTC4	leukotriene C4
LX	lipoxin
mAb	monoclonal antibody
MAC	minimal alveolar concentration
MACS	magnetic cell separation
magn.	magnification
MAP	mitogen-activated protein or mean arterial pressure
MAPK	mitogen-activated protein kinase
MATE	multidrug and toxin extrusion
MCD	medullary collecting duct
MCP	monocyte chemoattractant protein
MD	macula densa or multiple dose
MDA	malondialdehyde
MDCK	Madin-Darby canine kidney
MDFA	2,2-difluoro-2-methoxyacetic acid
MDMA	methylenedioxymethamphetamine
MDR	multidrug resistance
MDRD	modification of diet in renal disease
MEK	MAP kinase kinase
MHC	major histocompatibility complex
MI	myocardial infarction
MM	multiple myeloma
MMF	mycophenolate mofetil
MMP	matrix metalloproteinases
mPDS	methylprednisolone
MN	membranous nephropathy
MPF+	1-methyl-4-phenylpyridinium
MPGN	membranoproliferative glomerulonephritis
MPO	myeloperoxidase
MPT	mitochondrial permeability transition
MPTP	l-methyl-4-phenyl-l,2,3,6-tetrahydropyridine
MR	magnetic resonance
Mr	molecular weight
MRA	magnetic resonance angiography
MRI	magnetic resonance imaging
MRP	multidrug resistance-associated protein
MRS	magnetic resonance spectroscopy
MRSA	methicillin-resistant Staphylococcus aureus
MS	metabolic syndrome
MT	metallothionein
MTAL	medullary thick ascending limb
MTT	methylthiotetrazole
MTX	methotrexate
NA	not applicable
NAA	neutron activation analysis
NAC	N-acetylcysteine
NADC	Na dependent α-ketoglutarate cotransporter
NADPH	nicotinamide adenine dinucleotide phosphate
NAG	N-acetyl-β-D-glucosaminidase
Na-K-ATPase	sodium-potassium-ATPase
NAME	nitric oxide synthase inhibitor
NAPA	N-acetyl procainamide
NAPAP	N-acetyl-p-aminophenol
NAPQI	N-acetyl-p-benzoquinoneimine
NC	No data: no change required
NCAM	neural cell adhesion molecule
NCX	Na^{+}-Ca^{++} exchanger
NDA	New Drug Application
NDMA	N-methyl-D-aspartate
NEP	neutral endopeptidase
NF-AT-c	nuclear factor of activating T lymphocytes
NGAL	neutrophil gelatinase-associated lipocalin
NHE	Na+/H+ exchanger isoform
NIP	NF-AT interacting protein
NK	natural killer cells
NMN	N-methylnicotinamide
NMTT	N-methyl-tetrazole-thiol
nNOS	neuronal nitric oxide synthase
NO	nitric oxide
NOS	nitric oxide synthase
NPT	sodium-dependent phosphate transporter
NRF	nuclear respiratory factors
NRK52E	normal rat kidney epithelial cells
NRTI	nucleoside analogue reverse transcriptase inhibitor
NSA	neuron specific enolase
NSAID	non-steroidal anti-inflammatory drug
NSF	nephrogenic systemic fibrosis

OA	osteoarthritis
OAT	organic anion transporter
OCT	organic cation transporter
OCTN	organic cation/carnitine transporter
OD	once daily
OFR	oxygen-derived free radicals
OKT3	anti-CD3 monoclonal antibody
OK	opossum kidney
OM	outer medulla
OPN	osteopontin
OR	odds ratio
ORS	oral rehydration solution
OST	other solid tumours
OSHA	Occupational Safety and Health Agency
OSOM	outer stripe outer medulla
OSPS	oral sodium phosphate solution
OTA	ochratoxin
PAA	poly-L-aspartic acid
PAF	platelet activating factor
PAH	para-aminohippurate
PAS	periodic acid Schiff
PAM	periodic acid methenamine
PBMC	peripheral blood mononuclear cells
PC	Pneumocyctis carinii or prostate cancer
PCE	perchloroethylene
PCOP	plasma colloid osmotic pressure
PCP	Pneumocyctis carinii pneumonia or phencyclidine
PCSA	planar cell surface area
PCT	proximal convoluted tubule
PD	peritoneal dialysis
PDB	Paget's disease of bone
PDGF	platelet derived growth factor
PEG	polyethylene glycol
PEEP	positive end-expiratory pressure
PEM	prescription event monitoring
PEPCK	phosphenol pyruvate carboxy-kinase
PEPT	peptide cotransporter
PG	prostaglandin
PGA	poly-L-glutamic acid
PGC	PPAR-gamma-coactivator
PGP	P-glycoprotein
PH1	primary hyperoxaluria type 1
PIDD	primary immune deficiency diseases
PIH	postischemic hydronephrosis
PIP	phosphatidylinositide 4,5 biphosphate
PK	protein kinase
PKB	protein kinase B
PL	phospholipase
PLA	placebo
PMA	phorbol myrastate acetate
PMO	postmenopausal osteoporosis
pmp	per million population
PPAR	peroxisome proliferator-activated receptor
PPD	paraphenylene diamine
PPI	proton pump inhibitor
PRA	plasma renin activity
PR3	proteinase 3
PSS	progressive systemic sclerosis
PST	proximal straight tubule
PT or PTC	proximal tubular cells
PTCA	percutanerous transluminal coronary angioplasty
PTFE	polymeric tetrafluoroethylene
PTH	parathyroid hormone
PTK	protein tyrosine kinase
PTU	propylthiouracil
PTX	polyester
QD	once daily
QTL	quantitative trait locus
RA	rheumatoid arthritis
RAAS	renin-angiotensin-aldosterone system
RANTES	regulated on activation, normal T-cell expressed and secreted
RAP	receptor-associated protein
RAS	renin-angiotensin system
RBF	renal blood flow
RBFV	renal blood flow velocity
RCT	randomized clinical trial
rhIGF	recombinant human insulin growth factor
RIA	radio immunoassay
RIS	risedronate
ROC	receiver-operating characteristic
ROR	reporting odds ratio
ROS	reactive oxygen species
RPF	renal plasma flow
RPGN	rapidly progressive glomerulonephritis
RR	relative risk
RTE	renal tubular epithelial cells
RVR	renal vascular resistance
RXR	retenoic orphan receptor
S-	serum-
SAPK	stress-activated protein kinase
SAT	sulfate-oxalate exchanger
SBP	systolic blood pressure
Scr or SCr	serum creatinine
SDS-PAGE	sodium dodecyl sulphate - polyacrylamide gel electrophoresis
SEM	standard error of the mean
SHAKI	Stuivenberg Hospital Acute Kidney Injury
SHARF	Stuivenberg Hospital Acute Renal Failure
SHR	spontaneously hypertensive rats
SIADH	syndrome of inappropriate antidiuretic hormone
SKF550	(9-fluorenyl)-N-methyl-β-chloroethylamine
SLC	Na^+/Li^+ countertransporter
SLE	systemic lupus erythematosis
SmPC	summary of product characteristics
SMSA	Standard Metropolitan Statistical Area
SMZ	sulfamethoxazole
SNGFR	single nephron glomerular filtration rate

SNS	sympathetic nervous system
SSc	systemic sclerosis
SVV	small vessel vasculitis
t_2	elimination half-life
T3	triiodothyronin
TAC	tacrolimus
TAL	thick ascending limb
T-bet	T-box expressed in T-cells
TB	tuberculosis
TBM	tubular basement membrane
TCA	trichloroacetic acid
TCO2	bicarbonate transport
TCR	T-cell receptor
TDM	therapeutic drug monitoring
TEA	tetraethylammonium
TEER	transepithelial electrical resistance
TER	transepithelial resistance
TFR	transferrin
TGA	Therapeutic Goods Administration
TGF	transforming growth factor or tubuloglomerular feedback
Th	T-helper cell
THP	Tamm-Horsfall protein
TID	trice daily
TLS	tumor lysis syndrome
TLR	toll-like receptors
TLV	threshold limit value
TMA	thrombotic microangiopathic anemia
TMP	trimethoprim
TNAP	tissue non-specific alkaline phosphatase
TNF	tumor necrosis factor
TQ	triple quantum
Treg	regulatory T cells
TRF	transferrin
TRP	tubular reabsorption of phosphorus
TSC	thiazide sensitive Na^+-Cl^- cotransporter
TSH	thyroid-stimulating hormone
TTP	thrombotic thrombocytopenic purpura
TTR	transthryetin
TUNEL	terminal deoxynucleotidyl transferase (Tdt)-mediated dUTP nick end-labeling assay
TxA2	thromboxane A2
TxB2	thromboxane B2
U-	urinary
UP:Ucr	urine protein to creatinine ratio
USRDS	United States Renal Data System
V1aR	vasopressin V1a receptor
V2R	vasopressin V2 receptor
VC	vasoconstriction
VCAM	vascular cell adhesion molecule
Vd	volume of distribution
VD	vasodilatation
VZV	varicella zoster virus
VGEF	vascular endothelial growth factor
VLA	very late antigen
VRE	vancomycin-resistant Enterococci
VSMC	vascular smooth muscle cells
vWF	von Willebrand factor
WHO	World Health Organization
XRF	x-ray fluorescence
ZAG	zinc-α_2-globulin
ZOL	zoledronic acid
ZVAD-fmk	Z-Val-Ala-Asp-fmk

Clinical Nephrotoxins

Renal Injury from Drugs and Chemicals

Third Edition

INDEX

C

D

E

F

G

H

J

K

N

O

Q

S

T

U

Kolibri 360 GmbH
Ferdinand-Jühlke-Straße 7
99095 Erfurt, Deutschland
produktsicherheit@kolibri360.de